PRINCIPLES OF
NEUROLOGY

PRINCIPLES OF NEUROLOGY

Fourth Edition

Raymond D. Adams, M.D.

Bullard Professor of Neuropathology, Emeritus, Harvard Medical School
Senior Neurologist and Formerly Chief of Neurology Service
Massachusetts General Hospital
Director Emeritus, Eunice K. Shriver Center
Boston, Massachusetts

Maurice Victor, M.D.

Professor of Medicine and Neurology, Dartmouth Medical School
Hanover, New Hampshire
Distinguished Physician of the Veterans Administration
White River Junction, Vermont

McGraw-Hill Information Services Company

HEALTH PROFESSIONS DIVISION

New York   St. Louis   San Francisco   Colorado Springs
Auckland   Bogotá   Caracas   Hamburg   Lisbon   London   Madrid
Mexico   Milan   Montreal   New Delhi   Panama   Paris
San Juan   São Paulo   Singapore   Sydney   Tokyo   Toronto

PRINCIPLES OF NEUROLOGY

234567890   HALHAL   892109

ISBN   0-07-000300-9

This book was set in Times Roman by Monotype Composition Company, Inc.
The editors were William Day and Muza Navrozov;
the production supervisor was Robert R. Laffler;
the cover was designed by Edward R. Schultheis;
the index was prepared by Irving Tullar.
Arcata Graphics/Halliday was printer and binder.

Library of Congress Cataloging in Publication Data

Adams, Raymond D. (Raymond Delacy), date
  Principles of neurology.

  Includes bibliographies and index.
  1. Nervous system—Diseases.   2. Neuropsychiatry.
I. Victor, Maurice, date.   II. Title.
[DNLM: 1. Nervous System Diseases.   WL 100 A216p]
RC346.A3   1989   616.8   88-31805
ISBN 0-07-000300-9

CONTENTS

PART V DISEASES OF PERIPHERAL NERVE AND MUSCLE

PART VI PSYCHIATRIC DISORDERS

PREFACE

In the first edition of *Principles of Neurology* we remarked that the preface of a textbook is frequently considered to be a rather useless appendage, doing little more than adding to the book's weight or distracting critics from its content. The value of a book should be judged by its substance and composition. Victor Hugo, in his foreword to *Cromwell,* expressed this sentiment more figuratively by pointing out that one seldom inspects the cellar of a house after visiting its salons or examines the roots of a tree after eating its fruit.

Yet there has to be a place where authors can state the purpose of their work, the manner in which it was conceived, and the reasons for foisting yet another book on a medical public already overburdened with an immense literature. To sustain our analogy, although one seldom derives pleasure from inspecting the cellar of a house, one is not sorry sometimes to have examined its foundations, especially if one is to purchase it.

In the writing of *Principles of Neurology* we have adopted a method of exposition quite unlike that of the standard textbooks of neurology, in which the various diseases of the nervous system are described in endless succession. Instead, we have chosen to introduce the subject with a discussion of the phenomenology, or cardinal manifestations, of neurologic disease—a detailed exposition of the symptoms and signs of disordered nervous function, their anatomic and physiologic bases, and their clinical implications. This is followed by an account of the various syndromes of which these symptoms are a part, and this, in turn, by a consideration of the diseases that express themselves by each syndrome. We believe this to be a logical approach to neurologic disease, for in practice the patient presents with the symptoms of disease, not with a disease already diagnosed. Furthermore, the sequence from symptoms to syndrome to disease recapitulates the rational process by which the neurologist makes a diagnosis. In

teaching students and residents, we have found this method to be eminently successful, and it is to the student and resident that this work is primarily directed. In the strictest sense we believe this work to be an introduction to neurologic medicine.

The compass of our book differs in several other ways from contemporary textbooks of neurology. A significant portion of it has been allotted to psychiatric syndromes and the major psychiatric diseases. This has been done in the belief that all physicians, including neurologists, should be knowledgeable about the diagnosis of the depressive states, neuroses, personality disorders and schizophrenia, and about the biologic facts that pertain to these disorders. The neuropsychiatric effects of alcoholism and drug abuse are also described in detail. Similarly, we have consigned a section of the book to a description of muscle diseases, which more and more are coming under the purview of neurologists. Also, developmental and hereditary metabolic disorders and other aspects of pediatric neurology are emphasized, since these topics are included in all neurology training programs in the United States. Finally, the effects of growth, maturation, and aging on the nervous system are elaborated in detail because all deviations from the normal acquire significance only when viewed against the background of these natural, age-linked changes.

The warm reception accorded the first three editions of *Principles of Neurology* has led us to believe that our plan of exposition has fulfilled a need and has emboldened us to carry this work forward. The preparation of a fourth edition has given us the opportunity to make a deliberate and critical review of the book's contents, with the result that every chapter has been thoroughly revised. The topic of *The Hypothalamus and Neuroendocrine Disorders* has been assigned a chapter of its own. Major new sections have been added on the neurologic manifestations of AIDS and Lyme disease, the use of botulinus toxin in treating torticollis and other restricted dystonias and movement disorders, and the exciting developments in the identification of the abnormal genes in myotonic and Duchenne-Becker muscular dystrophies. Each chapter has been updated to include the important new information that has appeared since the third edition was issued, and this is reflected in the many new references that have been added. Illustrations have been replaced and new ones added. Also, in view of the increasing importance of magnetic resonance imaging, examples of this form of examination have been inserted into appropriate chapters.

We are indebted to numerous colleagues with whom we have repeatedly discussed much of the substantive material of the individual chapters. For many of our concepts of cerebral vascular disease and much of the substance of the chapter on this subject, we are indebted to our colleague of forty years—C. Miller Fisher. Robert Young and Bagwan Shahani, in Boston, and Robert Shields and Asa Wilbourn, in Cleveland, have kept us informed of important developments in clinical neurophysiology. Byron Kakulas, Betty Banker, and Maria Salam-Adams have shared their knowledge of muscle disease, and Arthur Asbury, his knowledge

of peripheral nerve disease. James Corbett critically reviewed the chapter on visual disturbances; David Zee and John Leigh, the chapter on disorders of ocular movement; and Marc Winkelman, the chapter on neoplasms. E. P. Richardson had earlier collaborated with the authors in writing chapters on degenerative diseases, and Robert DeLong, on developmental disorders. Hugo Moser, Edwin Kolodny, and Ira Lott have helped in updating our ideas about hereditary metabolic diseases; Kenneth Johnson and Richard Johnson about demyelinative and viral diseases; David Riley about movement disorders; and Joseph Martin about neuroendocrine disorders. Laurence Cromwell, of the Dartmouth-Hitchcock Medical Center, generously supplied a number of illustrations of magnetic resonance images. Other colleagues too numerous to mention have been sources of constant reference and constructive criticism.

Finally, we would like to express our gratitude to Mrs. Suzanne Chambers, who typed and retyped the material of many chapters, while at the same time attending to her other duties; to Richard Haver and Roger Goldstein, librarians at the Veterans Administration Hospital in White River Junction, Vermont; to Muza Navrozov, for her painstaking editorial efforts, and to William Day and his staff at McGraw-Hill, who have supervised the transcription of a difficult manuscript into the readable chapters of this book.

Raymond D. Adams
Maurice Victor

APPROACH TO THE PATIENT WITH NEUROLOGIC DISEASE

CHAPTER 1

THE CLINICAL METHOD OF NEUROLOGY

Neurology is often regarded as one of the most difficult and exacting specialties of medicine. Students coming to the neurology clinic for the first time are easily discouraged by what they see. Having had brief contact with neuroanatomy, neurophysiology, and neuropathology, they are already somewhat intimidated by the complexity of the nervous system. The ritual they then witness, of putting the patient through a series of maneuvers designed to evoke certain mysterious signs that are difficult to pronounce, is hardly reassuring; in fact the procedure often appears to conceal the very intellectual processes by which neurologic diagnosis is attained. Moreover, the students have had no training in administering the many special tests which are used, such as the lumbar puncture and cerebrospinal fluid examination or the electroencephalographic, electromyographic, arteriographic, and scanning examinations, nor do they know how to interpret the results of such tests. Neurologic textbooks only confirm their fears as they read the myriad details of the many rare diseases of the nervous system.

The authors believe that many of the students' difficulties with neurology can be overcome by adhering to the basic principles of clinical medicine. First and foremost it is necessary to know and acquire facility in use of the *clinical method*. Without a clear comprehension of this method the student is virtually as helpless with a new problem as a botanist or chemist who would attempt to do research without having an understanding of the steps in the scientific method.

The importance of the clinical method stands out more clearly in the study of neurologic diseases than in certain other fields of medicine, but the following remarks have universal application. The solution of any clinical problem is reached by a series of inferences and deductions—each an attempt to explain an item in the history of an illness or a physical finding. Diagnosis is the mental act of integrating all the interpretations and selecting the *one* explanation most compatible with all the facts of clinical observation.

It will be readily perceived that the logical processes involved in diagnosis are not the same in each and every case of neurologic disease and that in some cases the strict adherence to a particular sequence of reasoning is hardly necessary. The clinical picture of Parkinson disease, for example, is usually so characteristic that the nature of the illness is at once apparent. Nevertheless, an analysis of the clinical method will show that in most cases it consists of an orderly series of steps, as follows:

1. The symptoms and signs are secured by history and physical examination.

2. The symptoms and physical signs that are considered relevant to the current problem are interpreted and translated in terms of disordered function of anatomic structures or systems of neurons. Often one recognizes a characteristic clustering of symptoms and signs, constituting a syndrome, and the latter may be particularly helpful in ascertaining the locus and nature of the disease. This step may be called *syndrome diagnosis*.

3. These correlations permit the physician to localize the disease process, i.e., to name the part or parts of the nervous system involved. This step is called the *anatomic diagnosis*.

4. From the anatomic diagnosis and other medical data, particularly the mode of onset, evolution, and course of the illness, the involvement of nonneurologic organ systems, the relevant past and family histories, and the laboratory findings, one deduces the *pathologic diagnosis*; and, when the mechanism and causation of the disease can be determined, the *etiologic diagnosis*.

5. Finally the physician should assess the degree of disability and determine whether it is temporary or permanent. This *functional diagnosis* is important in manage-

3

ment of the patient's illness and judging the potential for restoration of function.

The accurate elicitation of symptoms and signs and their correct interpretation in terms of disordered function of the nervous system are the fundamental steps in diagnosis. When several physicians disagree on the diagnosis, it will often be found that the symptoms of disordered nervous function were incorrectly interpreted in the first place. Thus if a complaint of dizziness is identified as vertigo instead of lightheadedness or if partial continuous epilepsy is mistaken for an extrapyramidal movement disorder such as choreoathetosis, then surely the diagnosis will be erroneous. Repeated examinations may be necessary to establish the fundamental clinical data beyond doubt and, at times, to ascertain the course of the illness. Hence the aphorism that a second examination is the most helpful diagnostic test in a difficult neurologic case.

Different disease processes may cause identical symptoms, which is understandable from the fact that several diseases may involve the same parts of the nervous system. For example, a spastic paraplegia may result from spinal cord tumor, syphilitic meningomyelitis, or multiple sclerosis. Conversely, one disease may cause several different symptoms. However, despite the multitude of possible combinations of symptoms and signs in a particular disease, a few combinations occur with greater frequency than others and can be recognized as the most characteristic clinical features of that disease. The experienced clinician acquires the habit of attempting to categorize every case in terms of one or another syndrome. For example, the symptom complex of right-left confusion and inability to write, calculate, and identify individual fingers constitutes the so-called Gerstmann syndrome. Thus, the anatomic basis of the illness in question is more or less determined, and at the same time the range of possible etiologic factors is narrowed.

The final diagnosis must state the locality of the disease as well as its nature and, to be complete, should express the degree of functional impairment as well. Anatomic diagnosis takes precedence over etiologic diagnosis in neurology. To seek the cause of a disease of the nervous system without first ascertaining the parts or structures that are affected would be analogous in internal medicine to attempting an etiologic diagnosis without knowledge of whether the disease involved the lungs, stomach, or kidneys.

The student must learn the identity and differential diagnosis of the common neurologic syndromes before the details of individual diseases. It should be kept clearly in mind, however, that syndromes are not disease entities but rather abstractions set up by clinicians in order to facilitate the diagnosis of disease. The inherent danger in the method is that it may inculcate a rigidity of thinking and keep one from conceiving of diseases in new relationships.

TAKING THE HISTORY

The following three points about history taking in neurology deserve comment:

1. Special care must be exercised to avoid suggesting to the patient the symptoms that one seeks. The clinical interview is a bipersonal engagement, and the conduct of the examiner has a great influence on the patient. Repetition of this truism may seem tedious, but it is evident that conflicting histories presented on ward rounds can in many cases be traced either to leading questions having suggested symptoms that the examiner expects to find or to an unconscious distortion of the patient's story. Errors and inconsistencies in the recorded history are as often the fault of the physician as of the patient. Here the practice of making bedside notes is particularly to be recommended. The patient given to highly circumstantial and rambling accounts can be kept on the subject of the illness by discreet questions which draw out essential points. Immediate recording of the history assures greater reliability.

2. The mode of onset, evolution, and course of the illness are of paramount importance. Often the nature of the disease process can be decided from these data alone. One must attempt to learn how each symptom began and progressed. If such information cannot be supplied by the patient or his family, it may be necessary to judge the course of the symptoms by what the patient was able to do at different times, (e.g., how far he or she could walk, when it was no longer possible to negotiate stairs, carry on the usual work, etc.) or by changes in the clinical findings between successive examinations, providing the physician has described the findings accurately in his notes and has quantitated them in some way.

3. Since neurologic diseases often derange the mind, it is necessary in every patient with cerebral disease to decide, by an initial assessment of the mental status and the circumstances under which symptoms occurred, whether or not the patient is competent to give a history of the illness. If not, the history must be obtained from a relative, friend, or employer. Certain illnesses, such as those characterized by seizures or other forms of episodic confusion, preclude or impair the patient's knowledge of those parts of the illness. In general, students (and some physicians as well) tend to be careless in estimating the mental capacities of their patients. Attempts are sometimes made to take histories from patients who are feebleminded or so confused

that they have no idea why they are in a doctor's office or a hospital, or from patients who for other reasons could not possibly have been aware of the details of their illnesses.

THE NEUROLOGIC EXAMINATION

The neurologic examination always begins with the history. The manner in which the patient tells the story of his or her illness may betray confusion or incoherence in thinking, impairment of memory or judgment, or difficulty in comprehending or expressing ideas. Observation of such matters is an essential part of the examination and provides information as to the adequacy of cerebral function. The physician should learn how to obtain this type of information without embarrassment to the patient. A common error is to pass lightly over inconsistencies in history and inaccuracies about dates and symptoms, only to discover later that these were the major manifestations of the illness. Asking the patient to give his or her own interpretation of the possible meaning of symptoms may sometimes expose unnatural concern, worry, suspiciousness, or even delusory thinking.

The remainder of the neurologic examination should be performed as the last part of the general physical examination, proceeding from an examination of the cranial nerves, the neck, and the trunk, to the testing of motor, reflex, and sensory functions of the upper and lower extremities, followed by an assessment of sphincteric and autonomic nervous system functions and suppleness of the neck and spine (meningeal irritation). Gait and station should be observed before or after the rest of the examination. The neurologic examination should always be carried out in a sequential and uniform manner, in order to avoid omissions and to facilitate the subsequent analysis of case records.

The thoroughness of the neurologic examination must of necessity be governed by the type of clinical problem presented by the patient. To spend a half hour or more testing cerebral, cerebellar, cranial nerve and motor-sensory function in a patient seeking treatment for a simple compression palsy of an ulnar nerve is pointless and uneconomical. Furthermore, the procedure must be varied according to the condition of the patient. Obviously many parts of the examination cannot be carried out in a comatose patient; infants and small children and psychotic patients need to be examined in special ways. The following comments about the examination procedure apply to these particular clinical circumstances.

THE MEDICAL OR SURGICAL PATIENT WITHOUT NEUROLOGIC SYMPTOMS

In this case, brevity is desirable, but any test that is undertaken should be done carefully and recorded accurately in the patient's chart. With respect to the cranial nerves, the size of the pupils and their reaction to light, ocular movements, visual and auditory acuity (by questioning), and movements of the face, palate, and tongue should be examined. Observing the bare, outstretched arms for atrophy, weakness (drift), tremor, or abnormal movements, inquiring about strength and subjective sensory disturbances, and eliciting the supinator, biceps, and triceps reflexes are usually sufficient for the upper extremities. Inspection of the legs as the feet, toes, and knees are actively flexed and extended, elicitation of the patellar, achilles, and plantar reflexes, and the testing of vibration and position sense in the fingers and toes, complete the essential parts of the neurologic examination. Coordination may be tested by having the patient place a finger on the tip of his nose and run his heel up and down the front of the leg. This entire procedure does not add more than 3 or 4 min to the physical examination. The routine performance of these few simple tests may offer clues to the presence of disease of which the patient is not aware. For example, the finding of Argyll Robertson pupils, absent tendon reflexes, and diminished vibratory and position sense in the legs, alerts the physician to the possibility of tabes when there are no other symptoms of neurosyphilis.

Accurate recording of negative data may be useful in relation to some future illness.

PATIENTS WHO PRESENT SYMPTOMS OF NERVOUS SYSTEM DISEASE

Numerous guides to the examination of the nervous system are available. For a full account of the methods the interested reader is referred to the monographs of Denny-Brown, Ross, DeMyer, Mancall, and the staff members of the Mayo Clinic, each of which approaches the subject from a special point of view. A large number of tests have been devised, and it is not proposed to review all of them here. Some are described in subsequent chapters dealing with disorders of mentation, cranial nerves, and motor, sensory, and autonomic functions. Many tests are of doubtful value and should not be taught to students of neurology. Merely to perform all of them on one patient would require several hours, and probably, in most instances, would not make the examiner any the wiser. The danger with all clinical tests is that the student and physician may regard them as indisputable symbols of disease rather than as ways of uncovering disordered functioning of the nervous system.

The following few tests are relatively simple and provide the most useful information.

TESTING OF HIGHER CORTICAL FUNCTIONS

These functions are tested in detail if the patient's history or behavior during the general examination provide reason to suspect some defect. Questions should then be directed toward determining orientation in time and place and insight into the current medical problem. Attention, speed of response, ability to give relevant answers to simple questions, and the capacity for sustained mental effort, all lend themselves to straightforward observation. Useful bedside tests of attention, memory, and clarity of thought are the immediate repetition of a series of digits in forward and reverse order, serial subtraction of 3s and 7s from 100, recall of three items of information or a short story after an interval of 3 min, and naming the last six presidents or prime ministers. An account of the recent illness, medical consultations, and dates of hospitalizations, and the day-to-day recollection of medical procedures and incidents in the hospital are excellent tests of memory, and a narration of how they were done, of coherence of thinking. Other tests can be devised for the same purpose. Often the examiner can obtain a better idea of the clearness of the patient's sensorium and soundness of intellect by using these few tests and noting the manner in which the patient deals with them than by relying on the score of a formal intelligence test.

If there is any suggestion of aphasia, the nature of the patient's spontaneous speech should be recorded. In addition, the ability to read and write, execute spoken commands, repeat words and phrases of the examiner, name objects and parts of objects and solve simple arithmetical problems should be noted. Bisecting a line, drawing a clock or the floor plan of one's home or a map of one's country and copying figures are useful tests of visual-spatial perception and are indicated in cases of suspected cerebral disease (see Chap. 21).

TESTING THE CRANIAL NERVES

The function of the cranial nerves must be investigated more fully in patients who have neurologic symptoms than in those who do not. Tests of smell are carried out if one suspects a lesion in the anterior fossa, and then it should be determined whether odors can be discriminated in each nostril. The visual fields should be outlined by confrontation testing; if any abnormality is suspected it should be checked on a perimeter and scotomas sought on the Bjerrum screen. Pupil size and reactivity to light and on accommodation and the range of ocular movements should next be observed. Details of these test procedures and their indications are described in Chaps. 11, 12, and 13.

Sensation over the face should be tested with a pin and wisp of cotton, and the presence or absence of the corneal reflexes should be determined. Facial movements should be observed as the patient speaks and smiles, for a slight weakness may be more evident in these circumstances than from movements to command. Audiograms and special tests of auditory and vestibular function are needed if there is any suspicion of disease of the eighth nerve or the labyrinthine end organs (see Chap. 14). The vocal cords should be inspected in cases of suspected medullary disease, especially when there is hoarseness. Corneal and pharyngeal reflexes are of value if there is a difference on the two sides; bilateral absence of these reflexes is seldom significant. Inspection of the protruded tongue is helpful; atrophy, fasciculation, fibrillation, and weakness may be seen. Slight deviation of the protruded tongue as a solitary finding may usually be disregarded. The pronunciation of words should be noted. The jaw jerk and the buccal and sucking reflexes should be sought, particularly if there is a question of dysphagia or dysarthria.

TESTS OF MOTOR FUNCTION

In the assessment of motor function, students must remind themselves that observations of the speed and strength of movements and of muscle bulk, tone, and coordination are usually more informative than the tendon reflexes. It is essential to have the limbs fully exposed and to watch the patient maintain the arms outstretched in the prone and supine positions; perform simple tasks, such as alternately touching his nose and the examiner's finger; make rapid alternating movements that necessitate sudden acceleration and deceleration and changes in direction; and accomplish simple tasks such as buttoning clothes, opening a safety pin, or handling common tools. Estimates of the strength of leg muscles with the patient in bed are often unreliable; there may seem to be little or no weakness even though the patient cannot step up on a chair or arise from a squatting position. Running the heel down the front of the shin, alternately touching the examiner's finger with the toe and then the opposite knee with the heel, and rhythmically tapping the heel on the shin are the only tests of coordination that need be carried out in bed. The maintenance of both arms or both legs against gravity is a useful test; the weak one, tiring first, soon begins to sag. Also, abnormalities of movement and posture and tremors may appear (see Chaps. 4 and 5).

TESTS OF REFLEX FUNCTION

The testing of the biceps, triceps, supinator (radial-periosteal), knee, ankle, and the cutaneous abdominal and plantar reflexes permits an adequate sampling of reflex activity of the spinal cord. The plantar response offers special difficulty because several different reflex responses can be evoked by stimulating the sole of the foot along its outer border from heel to toes. These are (1) the high-level, quick avoidance response, (2) the slower, spinal flexor nocifensor reflex (flexion of knee and hip and dorsiflexion of toes and foot), or Babinski sign, (3) grasp, and (4) support reactions.

TESTING OF SENSORY FUNCTION

This is undoubtedly the most difficult part of the neurologic examination. Usually sensory testing is reserved for the end of the examination, and if the findings are to be reliable, it should not be prolonged for more than a few minutes. Each test should be explained briefly; too much discussion of it with a meticulous, introspective patient may encourage the reporting of useless minor variations of stimulus intensity.

It is not necessary to examine all areas of the skin surface. A quick survey of the face, neck, arms, trunk, and legs with a pin takes only a few seconds. One is of course seeking differences between the two sides of the body (it is preferable to ask whether stimuli on opposite sides of the body feel the same, rather than to ask if they feel different), a level below which sensation is lost, or a zone of relative or absolute anesthesia. Regions of sensory deficit can then be tested more carefully and mapped out. The finding of a zone of hyperesthesia may call attention to a disturbance of superficial sensation. Variations in the sensory findings from one examination to another reflect differences in technique of examination as well as inconsistencies in the responses of the patient.

The details of sensory testing methods are described in Chap. 8.

TESTING OF GAIT AND STANCE

No examination is complete without watching the patient stand and walk. An abnormality of gait may be the only neurologic abnormality, as in certain cases of cerebellar degeneration or frontal lobe disorder. Stance, posture, and lack of highly automatic adaptive movements may provide the most definite clues in an early stage of paralysis agitans (see Chap. 6).

THE COMATOSE PATIENT

Although subject to obvious limitations, examination of the stuporous or comatose patient may yield considerable information concerning the function of the nervous system. The demonstration of signs of focal cerebral or brainstem disease or of meningeal irritation is particularly useful in the differential diagnosis of the diseases that cause stupor and coma. The adaptation of the neurological examination to the comatose patient is considered in Chap. 16.

THE PSYCHIATRIC PATIENT

One is compelled in the examination of psychiatric patients to rely less on the cooperation of the patient and to be unusually critical of his statements and opinions. The depressed patient, for example, may claim to have impaired memory or weakness when actually there is no amnesia or diminution in muscular power; or the sociopath may feign paralysis. The opposite is sometimes true—psychotic patients may make accurate observations of their own symptoms, only to have them ignored because of their mental state.

If the patient will speak and cooperate even to a slight degree, much may be learned about the functional integrity of different parts of the nervous system. Aphasia can, in nearly every instance, be recognized by the manner in which the patient expresses ideas, reads and writes, and responds to spoken or written commands. Often it is possible to determine whether there are hallucinations or delusions, defective memory, or other symptoms of recognizable brain disease merely by watching and listening to the patient. The visual fields can be tested with fair accuracy by observing the patient's response to a moving stimulus or threat in all four quadrants of the fields. The tests of cranial nerve, motor, and reflex functions in the arms and legs, as outlined for the examination of the stuporous or comatose patient (Chap. 16), will yield even more information if minimal cooperation is obtained from the mentally impaired patient. It must be remembered, however, that the neurologic examination is never complete unless the patient will speak and carry out the usual tests. On numerous occasions mute and resistive patients judged to be schizophrenic prove to have some widespread cerebral disease such as hypoxic or hypoglycemic encephalopathy, a brain tumor, a vascular lesion, or extensive demyelinative lesions.

INFANTS OR SMALL CHILDREN

The reader is referred to the methods of examination described by Gesell and Amatruda, Andre-Thomas, Paine and Opfré, and the staff members of the Mayo Clinic, summarized in Chap. 27.

IMPORTANCE OF A WORKING KNOWLEDGE OF NEUROANATOMY AND NEUROPHYSIOLOGY

Once the technique of obtaining reliable clinical data is mastered, students may find themselves handicapped in the interpretation of the findings by a lack of knowledge of neuroanatomy and neurophysiology. For this reason, each of the later chapters dealing with the motor system, sensation, special senses, etc., will be introduced by a review of the anatomic and physiologic facts that are necessary for an understanding of the clinical disorders.

At a minimum, students should know the anatomy of the corticospinal tract, the motor unit (spinal cord, nerve, and muscle), the basal ganglionic and cerebellar motor connections, the sensory pathways, the cranial nerves, the hypothalamus and pituitary connections, the reticular formation of brainstem and thalamus, the limbic system, the areas of cerebral cortex and their major connections, the visual system, the auditory system, the autonomic system, and the cerebrospinal fluid pathways. A working knowledge of neurophysiology should include an understanding of the nerve impulse, neuromuscular transmission, and the contractile process of muscle; spinal reflex activity; central neurotransmission; the processes of neuronal excitation, inhibition, and release; and cortical activation and seizure production.

DIFFERENTIAL (ETIOLOGIC) DIAGNOSIS

The differential diagnosis of the cause of a clinical syndrome requires knowledge of an entirely different order. One must be conversant with the clinical details and the course and natural history of the more common disease entities. Many of these facts are simple and well known and will be presented in later chapters of this textbook.

The findings in the general medical examination are of importance. To illustrate: low-grade fever, anemia, heart murmur, and splenomegaly in a case of unexplained apoplexy point to the diagnosis of subacute bacterial endocarditis with embolic occlusion of a brain artery. Pleocytosis in the cerebrospinal fluid with elevated protein and gamma globulin levels, and a positive serologic reaction establishes a syphilitic etiology in a patient with symptoms of apoplexy, a progressive dementia, or blindness.

The anatomic diagnosis may suggest the cause of a disease. Thus, when a unilateral Horner syndrome, cerebellar ataxia, paralysis of a vocal cord, and analgesia of the face are combined with loss of pain and temperature sensation in the opposite arm, trunk, and leg, an occlusion of the vertebral artery is the most likely cause, because all the involved structures lie in the lateral medulla, within the territory of this artery. In a sense the anatomic diagnosis determines and limits the disease possibilities. If the signs point to disease of the peripheral nerves, it is usually not necessary to consider the causes of disease of the spinal cord. Some signs themselves are almost specific, e.g., Argyll Robertson pupils for neurosyphilis and oculogyric crises for postencephalitic parkinsonism or phenothiazine-induced dyskinesia.

If one adheres faithfully to the clinical method outlined here, neurologic diagnosis becomes relatively simple. In most patients one can reach an anatomic diagnosis. The cause of the disease may prove more elusive. It usually entails the intelligent and selective employment of a number of the laboratory procedures described in the next chapter. Even the most experienced neurologist is unable to ascertain the cause of many neurologic syndromes.

THE PURPOSE OF THE CLINICAL METHOD OF NEUROLOGY

Finally, a few words about the purpose of the clinical method of neurology. Actually, accurate diagnosis accomplishes three main purposes: (1) it enables the physician to determine the proper method of treating the patient; (2) it is also helpful in prognosis, i.e., in predicting the outcome of the illness; and (3) it is the essential initial step in the scientific study of clinical phenomena and disease. The medical profession is primarily concerned with the prevention and cure of illness, and all our knowledge is applied to this well-defined end. A major aim of the neurologist is not to overlook a disease for which there is an effective treatment. Each of the treatable causes of a given syndrome must be carefully considered and excluded by clinical and laboratory methods. For example, in the study of a patient with disease of the spinal cord one must take special care to exclude the presence of a tumor, subacute combined degeneration, spinal syphilis, epidural abscess, prolapsed disc, and cervical spondylosis, for these are treatable spinal cord diseases. Failure to recognize amyotrophic lateral sclerosis is a less serious error as far as the patient is concerned.

Even when no therapy is possible, neurologic diagnosis is more than an intellectual pastime. There is no doubt that the first step in the scientific study of a disease process is its identification in the living patient. Until this is achieved it is impossible to apply adequately the ''master method of controlled experiment.'' The clinical method of neurology thus serves both the physician, in the practical diagnosis and treatment of a patient's condition, and the clinical scientist, in the search for the mechanism and cause of the disease.

LABORATORY DIAGNOSIS

From the foregoing description of the clinical method and its application, it is evident that the use of laboratory aids in the diagnosis of disease of the nervous system is always preceded by rigorous clinical examination. Laboratory study can only be planned intelligently on the basis of clinical information. To reverse this process is wasteful of medical resources. However, in neurology the ultimate goal is the prevention of disease, because the brain changes induced by many neurologic diseases are irreversible. In the prevention of neurologic disease the clinical method is inadequate, and of necessity one resorts to two other methods, viz., the use of genetic information and laboratory screening. Genetic information enables the neurologist to identify patients at risk of developing a disease, and it prompts the search for biologic markers before the advent of symptoms or signs. Biochemical screening tests are applicable to an entire population and permit the identification of neurologic disease in individuals who have yet to show their first symptom; in some of these diseases treatment can be instituted before the nervous system has suffered damage. In preventive neurology, therefore, laboratory methodology may take precedence over clinical methodology.

The laboratory methods that are available for neurologic diagnosis are discussed in the next chapter. The relevant principles of genetic and laboratory screening methods that are presently available for the prediction of disease will be presented in the discussion of the disease(s) to which they are applicable.

REFERENCES

ANDRÉ-THOMAS, CHESNI Y, DARGASSIES ST-ANNE S: *The Neurological Examination of the Infant.* London, National Spastics Society, 1960.

DEMEYER W: *Technique of the Neurological Examination,* 3rd ed. New York, McGraw-Hill, 1980.

DENNY-BROWN D: *Handbook of Neurological Examination and Case Recording,* rev ed. Cambridge, Mass, Harvard, 1957.

GESELL A, AMATRUDA CS: in Knoblock H, Pasamanick B (eds): *Gesell and Amatruda's Developmental Diagnosis,* 3rd ed. Hagerstown, Md, Harper & Row, 1974.

HOLMES G: *Introduction to Clinical Neurology,* 3rd ed. Revised by Bryan Matthews, Baltimore, Williams & Wilkins, 1968.

MANCALL EL: *Alpers and Mancall's Essentials of the Neurologic Examination,* 2nd ed. Philadelphia, Davis, 1981.

MAYO CLINIC AND MAYO FOUNDATION: *Clinical Examinations in Neurology,* 5th ed. Philadelphia, Saunders, 1981.

ROSS RT: *How to Examine the Nervous System,* 2nd ed. New York, Medical Examination Publishing Co., 1985.

CHAPTER 2

SPECIAL TECHNIQUES FOR NEUROLOGIC DIAGNOSIS

The analysis and interpretation of the data elicited by a careful history and examination may prove to be adequate for diagnosis. Special laboratory examinations can then do no more than corroborate the initial impression. However, it happens more often that the conclusion as to the nature of the disease is not reached by simple "case study" alone; the diagnostic possibilities may be reduced to two or three, but the correct one is uncertain. Under these circumstances one resorts to the ancillary examinations outlined below. The aim of the neurologist is to arrive at a final diagnosis by artful analysis of the clinical data, aided by the *least* number of laboratory procedures. Similarly, the strategy of laboratory study of disease should be based purely on therapeutic and prognostic considerations, not on the physician's curiosity or presumed medicolegal exigencies.

A few decades ago the only laboratory procedures available to the neurologist were examination of a sample of cerebrospinal fluid, radiology of the skull and spinal column, radiopaque myelography, pneumoencephalography, and electroencephalography. Now, through formidable advances in scientific technology, the physician's armamentarium has been expanded to include a multitude of laboratory methods. Some of these new methods are so impressive that there is a temptation to substitute them for a careful, detailed history and physical examination; this must be avoided. The neurologist should always keep in mind the primacy of the clinical method and that he or she is the final judge of the relevancy and significance of each laboratory datum. Hence the neurologist must be familiar with all the laboratory procedures and their reliability.

Below is a description of those laboratory procedures that have application to a diversity of neurologic diseases. Procedures that are pertinent to a single disease or category of disease will be presented in the chapter devoted to that disease.

LUMBAR PUNCTURE AND EXAMINATION OF CEREBROSPINAL FLUID

The information yielded by examination of the cerebrospinal fluid (CSF) is often of crucial importance in the diagnosis of neurologic disease.

INDICATIONS FOR LUMBAR PUNCTURE

1. To obtain pressure measurements and to procure a sample of CSF for cellular, chemical, and bacteriologic examination.

2. To aid in therapy by the administration of spinal anesthetics and occasionally antibiotics or antitumor agents.

3. To inject a radiopaque substance (Pantopaque), a water-soluble contrast medium, or air, as in myelography; a radioactive agent, as in scintigraphic cisternography; and rarely air, as in pneumoencephalography.

Lumbar puncture carries a certain risk if the CSF pressure is high (evidenced by headache and papilledema), for it increases the possibility of a fatal cerebellar or tentorial pressure cone. The risk is considerable when papilledema is due to an intracranial mass and much less so in patients with subarachnoid hemorrhage or pseudotumor cerebri, conditions in which repeated lumbar punctures have actually been employed as a therapeutic measure. In patients with a suspected elevation of intracranial pressure, therefore, lumbar puncture should be preceded by a computerized tomography (CT) scan or magnetic resonance (MR) imaging whenever possible. If the latter procedures do not disclose a mass lesion and it is considered essential to have the information yielded by CSF examination, the lumbar puncture should be performed, with certain precautions. A fine-bore (no. 22 or 24) needle should be used, and if the pressure proves to be very high—over 400 mmH$_2$O—one should obtain the necessary sample of fluid and then, according to the suspected disease and patient's condition, administer a unit of urea or mannitol and watch the manometer until the pressure falls. Dexamethasone (Decadron) should then be given in an initial intravenous dose of 10 mg followed by doses of 4 to 6 mg every 6 h.

Cisternal puncture and *cervical subarachnoid puncture,* although safe in the hands of the expert, are too hazardous to entrust to those without experience. The lumbar puncture is to be preferred except in obvious instances of spinal block requiring a sample of cisternal fluid or myelography above the lesion.

Experience teaches the importance of meticulous technique. Lumbar puncture should always be done under sterile conditions. If procaine is injected in and beneath the skin, the procedure should be painless. The puncture is easiest to perform at the L3-L4 interspace or in the space above or below; in infants and young children, in whom the spinal cord may extend to the level of the L3-L4 interspace, lower spaces should be used. Failure to enter the lumbar subarachnoid space after two or three trials can usually be overcome by doing the puncture with the patient in the sitting position and then assisting him to lie on one side for pressure measurements and fluid removal. The "dry tap" is more often due to an improperly placed needle than to an obliteration of the subarachnoid space by a compressive lesion of the spinal cord or chronic adhesive arachnoiditis.

EXAMINATION PROCEDURES

Once the subarachnoid space has been entered, the pressure and "dynamics" of the CSF are determined and a sample of fluid is obtained. The gross appearance of the CSF is noted, after which it is subjected to some or all of the following determinations: (1) number and type of cells and presence of micro-organisms; (2) protein and glucose content; (3) exfoliative cytology, using a Millipore filter or similar apparatus; (4) protein electrophoresis and immunoelectrophoresis for determination of gamma globulin, other protein fractions, and oligoclonal bands, and radioimmunodiffusion procedures for estimating the IgG-albumin index; (5) biochemical tests for pigments, lactate, NH$_3$, pH, CO$_2$, enzymes, etc.; and (6) bacteriologic cultures and virus isolation.

Pressure and Dynamics   When the CSF pressure is measured by a water manometer attached to a needle in either the lumbar subarachnoid space or the cisterna magna with the patient horizontal in the lateral decubitus position,

the opening pressure normally varies from 65 to 195 mmH$_2$O. When measured with the needle in the lumbar region and the patient in a sitting position, the fluid in the manometer rises to the level of the cisterna magna (about 280 mmH$_2$O). It fails to reach the level of the ventricles because the latter are in a closed system under slight negative pressure, whereas the fluid in the manometer is influenced by atmospheric pressure. Normally, with the needle properly placed in the subarachnoid space, the fluid in the manometer oscillates through a few millimeters in response to the pulse and to respiration, and rises promptly with coughing or straining or abdominal compression.

If a spinal subarachnoid block is suspected, jugular compression should be performed. The examiner stands behind the patient and slips a hand around the patient's neck, compressing first one side, then the other, and then both sides simultaneously, exerting enough pressure to compress the veins but not the carotid arteries (Queckenstedt test). In the absence of a subarachnoid block, there should be a rapid rise in pressure of 100 to 200 mmH$_2$O, and the pressure should return to its original level within 10 s after release. A graded degree of jugular compression can be applied by wrapping a narrow (pediatric size) sphygmomanometer cuff around the neck, and observing the pressure responses as the cuff is inflated rapidly to 20 mmHg for 10 s and then released, the procedure being repeated with inflation to 40 and then to 60 mmHg. If there is no rise or only a slow rise and fall in CSF pressure with jugular compression, the effect of abdominal compression is checked to make certain that the needle is still in the subarachnoid space. A failure of the pressure to rise with compression of one jugular vein but not the other (Tobey-Ayer test) may indicate lateral sinus thrombosis. Except for this circumstance, jugular compression should not be performed when intracranial disease is suspected.

Gross Appearance and Pigments   Normally the CSF is clear and colorless, like water. Minor degrees of color change are best detected by comparing tubes of CSF and water against a white background or by looking down the tubes from above. A pleocytosis imparts a hazy or ground glass appearance; at least 200 cells per cubic millimeter (mm^3) must be present to detect this change. The presence of red cells (1000 to 6000 mm^3) imparts a pink to red color, depending on the amount of blood; centrifugation of the fluid or allowing it to stand causes a sedimentation of the red blood cells.

A traumatic tap may seriously confuse the diagnosis if it is incorrectly interpreted to indicate a preexistent subarachnoid hemorrhage. To distinguish between traumatic and nontraumatic types of "bloody tap," three samples of fluid should be taken at the time of the lumbar puncture. Usually, with a traumatic tap, there is a decreasing number of red cells in the second and third tubes. Also, the CSF pressure is usually normal, and if a large amount of blood is mixed with the fluid, it will clot or form fibrinous webs. These are not seen with preexistent hemorrhage because the blood has been greatly diluted with spinal fluid and defibrinated. In subarachnoid hemorrhage the red cells begin to hemolyze after a few hours, giving rise to a yellow discoloration (xanthochromia) in the supernatant fluid. Prompt centrifugation of bloody fluid from a traumatic tap will yield a colorless supernatant; only with large amounts of blood (RBC over 100,000 mm³) will the supernatant fluid be faintly xanthochromic due to contamination with serum bilirubin and lipochromes.

The fluid from a traumatic tap should contain about 1 white blood cell per 700 red cells, assuming that the hemogram is normal, but this ratio varies widely and unpredictably. With subarachnoid hemorrhage, the proportion of white cells rises as red cells hemolyze, sometimes reaching a level of several hundred per cubic millimeter, but the vagaries of this reaction are such that it, too, cannot be relied upon to distinguish traumatic from preexistent bleeding. The same can be said for crenation of red cells, which occurs in both types of bleeding.

The reason that red corpuscles undergo rapid hemolysis in the CSF is not clear. It is surely not due to osmotic differences, for the osmolarity of plasma and CSF are essentially the same. Fishman suggests that the low protein content of CSF disequilibrates the red cell membrane in some way. The reason for the rapid phagocytosis of red cells in the CSF, which takes place within 48 h, is also obscure. Histiocytes engulf the red cells, forming macrophages, and hemosiderin appears in their cytoplasm within 5 to 6 days.

The pigments that discolor the CSF following subarachnoid hemorrhage are oxyhemoglobin, bilirubin, and methemoglobin; in pure form, these pigments are colored red (orange to orange-yellow with dilution), canary yellow, and brown, respectively. Mixtures of these pigments produce combinations of these colors. Oxyhemoglobin appears first, within several hours of the hemorrhage, becomes maximal in about 36 h, and, if no further bleeding occurs, diminishes over a 7- to 9-day period. Bilirubin appears in 2 to 3 days and increases in amount as the oxyhemoglobin decreases. Following a single, brisk bleed, bilirubin persists in the CSF for 2 to 3 weeks, the duration varying with the number of red cells that were present originally. Methemoglobin appears when hemorrhage is loculated in the meninges or in adjacent brain tissue.

If blood is added to spinal fluid in a test tube and allowed to stand for several days, oxyhemoglobin and then methemoglobin will form, but not bilirubin, suggesting that the action of living cells is necessary for the formation of the latter pigment. Barrows and his colleagues have devised three simple biochemical tests that reliably indicate the presence or absence of these pigments—the benzidine reaction (for oxyhemoglobin), a modified Van den Bergh reaction (for bilirubin), and a potassium cyanide test for methemoglobin.

Not all xanthochromia of the CSF is due to hemolysis of red blood cells. With severe jaundice, bilirubin of both the direct and indirect reacting types will diffuse into the CSF. The quantity of bilirubin is from one-tenth to one-hundredth of that in the serum. Elevation of CSF protein from whatever cause results in a faint xanthochromia, more or less in proportion to the albumin-bound fraction of bilirubin. Only at levels of more than 150 mg per 100 mL does the coloration due to protein become visible to the naked eye. Hypercarotenemia and hemoglobinemia (through its breakdown products, particularly oxyhemoglobin) also impart a yellow tint to the CSF. Myoglobin does not enter the CSF, probably because a low renal threshold for this pigment rapidly clears the blood.

Cellularity Normally the CSF contains no cells or at most up to five lymphocytes or other mononuclear cells per cubic millimeter. An elevation of white cells in the CSF always signifies a reactive process to bacteria or other infectious agents, blood, chemical substances, or neoplasm. The white cells can be counted in an ordinary counting chamber, but their identification requires centrifugation of the fluid and a Wright stain of the sediment or the use of a Millipore filter, cell fixation, and staining. One can then recognize and count differentially neutrophilic and eosinophilic leukocytes, lymphocytes, plasma cells, mononuclear cells, arachnoidal lining cells, macrophages, and tumor cells. Bacteria, fungi, fragments of echinococci and cysticerci can also be seen in cell-stained or Gram-stained preparations. An India-ink preparation is useful in distinguishing between lymphocytes and cryptococci or monilia. Dufresne's monograph is an excellent reference on CSF cytology. Special techniques applied to the cells of the CSF, such as immune staining, permit the recognition of glial fibrillary protein and carcinoembryonic and other antigens; and electron microscopy permits the more certain identification of cells and may demonstrate such substances as phagocytosed fragments of myelin (e.g., in multiple sclerosis). These and other special methods for the examination of cells in the CSF will be mentioned in the appropriate chapters.

Proteins In contrast to the protein content of blood, of 5500 to 8000 mg/dL, that of the lumbar spinal fluid is 45 mg/dL or less. The protein content of fluid from the basal cisterns is 10 to 25 mg/dL and that from the ventricles is 5 to 15 mg/dL, reflecting a ventricular-lumbar gradient in the permeability of capillary endothelial cells to protein (blood-CSF barrier) and a lesser degree of circulation in the lumbosacral region. Levels higher than these indicate a pathologic process in or near the ependyma or meninges, though the cause of modest elevations of the CSF protein frequently remains obscure.

As one would expect, bleeding into the ventricles or subarachnoid space results in spillage not only of blood cells but of proteins. If the serum proteins are normal, the CSF protein should increase by 1 mg for every 1000 red cells, providing the same tube of CSF is used in determining the cell count and protein content. Usually the irritating effect of hemolyzed red cells increases the CSF protein to many times this ratio.

The protein content of the CSF in bacterial meningitis, which increases capillary perfusion in choroidal and meningeal vessels, reaches 500 mg/dL, or more. Viral infections induce a less intense and mainly lymphocytic reaction and a lesser elevation of protein—usually 50 to 100 mg but sometimes up to 200 mg/dL; in some instances it is normal. Paraventricular tumors, by reducing the blood-CSF barrier, often raise the total protein to over 100 mg/dL. Protein values as high as 500 mg/dL or even higher are found in exceptional cases of the Guillain-Barre syndrome. Values of 1000 mg/dL, or more, usually indicate loculation of the lumbar CSF (CSF block); the fluid is then deeply yellow and clots readily because of the presence of fibrinogen. This combination of CSF changes is called the *Froin syndrome*. Low CSF protein values sometimes are found in meningismus (a febrile illness with signs of meningeal irritation but normal CSF), in the condition known as meningeal hydrops (see Chap. 30), in hyperthyroidism, or after a recent lumbar puncture. In young children the CSF protein is normally low (less than 20 mg/dL).

The use of precipitation tests (e.g. colloidal gold reaction) has long been replaced by electrophoretic and immunochemical methods. The quantitative partition of CSF proteins by these methods demonstrates the presence of most of the serum proteins with a molecular weight of less than 150,000 to 200,000. The following protein fractions have been identified electrophoretically: prealbumin and albumin, alpha$_1$, alpha$_2$, beta$_1$, beta$_2$, and gamma globulin. Quantitative values of the different fractions are given in Table 2-1. Immunoelectrophoretic methods have also demonstrated the presence of glycoproteins, haptopro-

teins, ceruloplasmin, transferrin and hemopexin. Large molecules, such as fibrinogen, IgM, and lipoproteins, are mostly excluded from the CSF.

There are other notable differences between the protein fractions of CSF and plasma. The CSF always contains a prealbumin fraction, and the plasma does not.

Table 2-1
Average values of constituents of normal CSF and serum

	Cerebrospinal fluid	Serum
Osmolarity	295 mosmol/L	295 mosmol/L
Sodium	138.0 meq/L	138.0 meq/L
Potassium	2.8 meq/L	4.1 meq/L
Calcium	2.4 meq/L	5.2 meq/L
Magnesium	2.7 meq/L	1.9 meq/L
Chloride	124.0 meq/L	101.0 meq/L
Bicarbonate	23.0 meq/L	23.0 meq/L
Carbon dioxide tension	48 mmHg	38 mmHg (arterial)
pH	7.31	7.41 (arterial)
Nonprotein nitrogen	19.0 mg/dL	27.0 mg/dL
Ammonia	30.0 μg/dL	70.0 μg/dL
Uric acid	0.24 mg/dL	4.0 mg/dL
Urea	4.7 mmol/L	5.4 mmol/L
Creatinine	1.1 mg/dL	1.6 mg/dL
Phosphorus	1.6 mg/dL	4.0 mg/dL
Total lipid	1.25 mg/dL	876.0 mg/dL
Total cholesterol	0.4 mg/dL	180.0 mg/dL
Cholesterol esters	0.3 mg/dL	126.0 mg/dL
Glucose	>45.0 mg/dL	90.0 mg/dL
Lactate	1.6 meq/L	1.0 meq/L
Total protein	15–50 mg/dL	6.5–8.4 g/100/dL
Prealbumin	1–7%	Trace
Albumin	49–73%	56%
Alpha$_1$ globulin	3–7%	4%
Alpha$_2$ globulin	6–13%	10%
Beta globulin (beta$_1$ plus tau)	9–19%	12%
Gamma globulin	3–12%	18%

Source: Fishman.

Although derived from plasma, this fraction, for an unknown reason, concentrates in the CSF, and the level is greater in ventricular than in lumbar CSF (perhaps because of its concentration by choroidal cells). The CSF also has a beta$_2$ or tau fraction (transferrin) which is proportionally larger than that in the plasma and again higher in the ventricular than in the spinal fluid. The gamma globulin fraction in CSF is about 70 percent of that in serum.

At present only a few of these proteins are known to be associated with specific diseases of the nervous system. The most important is IgG, which may exceed 12 percent of the total CSF protein in diseases such as multiple sclerosis, neurosyphilis, and subacute sclerosing panencephalitis and other viral meningoencephalitides. The serum IgG is not correspondingly increased, which means that this immune globulin must originate in the nervous system. However, an elevation of serum gamma globulin, as occurs in cirrhosis, sarcoidosis, myxedema, and multiple myeloma, will be accompanied by a rise in the CSF gamma globulins. Therefore, in patients with an elevated CSF gamma globulin, it is necessary to determine the serum protein electrophoretic patterns as well. Certain qualitative changes in the CSF gamma globulin pattern, particularly the demonstration of discrete (oligoclonal) bands, are of special diagnostic importance in multiple sclerosis and subacute sclerosing panencephalitis.

The albumin fraction of the CSF increases in a wide variety of CNS and craniospinal nerve root diseases which increase the permeability of the blood-CSF barrier, but no specific clinical correlations can be drawn.

Glucose   Normally the range of CSF glucose is 45 to 80 mg/dL, i.e., about two-thirds that in the blood. Higher levels parallel the blood glucose, but with marked hyperglycemia the ratio of CSF to blood glucose is less than 0.6. Values below 40 mg/dL are abnormal. After the intravenous injection of glucose, 2 to 4 h is required to reach equilibrium with the CSF; a similar delay follows the lowering of blood glucose. For these reasons, proper evaluation of the CSF glucose requires that blood glucose be measured simultaneously, in the fasting state. Only abnormally low concentrations are of diagnostic significance. Such values in the presence of pleocytosis usually indicate pyogenic, tubercular, or fungal meningitis, although the CSF glucose is sometimes reduced in sarcoidosis, in subarachnoid hemorrhage (most often in the first week), and in widespread neoplastic infiltration of the meninges.

The almost invariable rise of *CSF lactate* in purulent meningitis informs us that some of the glucose is undergoing anaerobic glycolysis by polymorphonuclear leukocytes and cells of the meninges and adjacent brain tissue. For a long time it was assumed that in meningitis the bacteria lowered the CSF glucose by their active metabolism, but the fact that the glucose remains at a subnormal level for 1 to 2 weeks after effective treatment of the meningitis indicates that another mechanism for the hypoglycorrhachia must be operative. Theoretically, at least, an inhibition of the entry of glucose into the CSF, due to an impairment of the membrane transfer system, can be implicated. Interestingly, viral infections of the meninges and brain do not lower the CSF glucose nor raise the lactate levels, though Wilfert has reported low glucose values in a small proportion of patients with mumps meningoencephalitis and rarely in herpes simplex and zoster infections.

Serologic Tests for Syphilis   The nontreponemal antibody tests of the blood—veneral disease research laboratories (VDRL) slide flocculation test and rapid plasma reagin (RPR) agglutination test—can also be performed on the CSF. When positive, they indicate neurosyphilis, but false-positive tests may occur with collagen diseases, malaria, and yaws, or when the CSF is contaminated with seropositive blood. Tests which depend on the use of treponemal antigens, including the *Treponema pallidum* immobilization test and the fluorescent treponemal antibody test, are more specific and assist in the interpretation of false-positive reactions. The value of the CSF in the diagnosis and treatment of neurosyphilis is discussed in Chap. 31.

CHANGES IN SOLUTES AND OTHER COMPONENTS

The average osmolality of the CSF (295 mosmol/L) is identical to that of plasma. As the osmolality of the plasma is increased by the injection of hypertonic intravenous solutions such as mannitol or urea, there is a delay of several hours in the rise of osmolality of the CSF. It is during this period that the hyperosmolality of the blood dehydrates the brain and decreases the volume of CSF.

The CSF and serum levels of sodium, potassium, calcium, and magnesium are listed in Table 2-1. Neurologic disease does not alter the CSF concentrations of these constituents in any characteristic way. The low CSF concentration of chloride that occurs in bacterial meningitis is not specific but a reflection of hypochloremia and elevated CSF protein.

Acid-base balance in the CSF is of considerable interest in relation to metabolic acidosis and alkalosis. Normally the pH of the CSF is about 7.31 and is lower than that of arterial blood, which is 7.41. The P_{CO_2} is higher in the CSF than in arterial blood, 48 to 40 mmHg.

The bicarbonate levels of the two fluids are about the same, 23 meq/L. There is a very precise regulation of CSF pH, and it tends to remain relatively unchanged even in the face of severe systemic acidosis and alkalosis. Studies of acid-base balance in the CSF, while of interest, have only limited clinical value. Acid-base changes in the lumbar CSF do not necessarily reflect the presence of similar changes in the brain, nor are the CSF data as accurate an index of the systemic changes as direct measurements of arterial blood gases.

The *ammonia content* of the CSF is one-third to one-half that of the arterial blood; it rises in hepatic encephalopathy and in the Reye syndrome, and the level correlates with the degree of encephalopathy. The *uric acid* content of CSF is about 5 percent of that in serum and varies with changes in the serum level (e.g., high in uremia and meningitis and low in Wilson disease). The *urea* concentration in the CSF is slightly less than in the serum (see Table 2-1), and in uremia it rises in parallel with that in the blood. An intravenous injection of urea raises the blood level immediately and the CSF level more slowly, during which interval it exerts an osmotic effect. All 24 of the *amino acids* have been isolated from the CSF. The concentration of the total amino acids is about one-third that of plasma. The CSF-to-plasma ratios of the individual amino acids vary from about 1.0 for glutamic acid to 0.1 for glutamate and even less for phenylalanine. Specific transport systems have been delineated for some of the acidic, basic, and neutral amino acids. Elevations of glutamine are found in hepatic coma and the Reye syndrome and of phenylalanine, histidine, valine, leucine, isoleucine, tyrosine, and homocystine in the corresponding aminoacidurias.

Many of the *enzymes* found in serum are known to rise in CSF under conditions of disease, usually in relation to a rise in CSF protein. None of the enzyme changes has proved to be a specific indicator of neurologic disease, with the possible exception of *lactic dehydrogenase,* especially isoenzymes 4 and 5, which are derived from granulocytes and are elevated in bacterial meningitis but not in aseptic or viral meningitis. Lactic dehydrogenase is also elevated in cases of carcinomatous meningitis, as is carcinoembryonic antigen; the latter, however, is not elevated in bacterial or viral or fungal meningitis. As to *lipids* the quantities in CSF are small, and their measurement is difficult. In multiple sclerosis the proportions of the different types of lipid are said to change.

The catabolites of the *catecholamines* are now being measured in the CSF. Homovanillic acid (HVA), the major catabolite of dopamine, and 5-hydroxyindoleacetic acid (5-HIAA), the major catabolite of serotonin, are normally present in the spinal fluid; both are five or six times higher in the ventricular than in the lumbar CSF. The levels of both catabolites are reduced in patients with idiopathic and drug-induced parkinsonism.

Finally, it may be said that with continued development of microchemical techniques for the analysis of the CSF, we can look forward to a better understanding of the metabolic mechanisms of the brain, particularly of the hereditary metabolic diseases. Ultrarefined methods such as gas-liquid chromatography will probably reveal many new catabolic products, the measurement of which will be of value in diagnosis and therapy.

RADIOGRAPHIC EXAMINATION OF SKULL AND SPINE

Although plain films of the cranium and vertebral column have for a long time been considered a "routine" part of the study of the neurologic patient, it has gradually become evident that the yield of useful information from this procedure is relatively small. Even in patients with head injury, where radiography of the skull would seem to be the optimal method of examination, a fracture is found in only 1 out of 16 cases, at a cost of thousands of dollars per fracture and a small but definite risk from radiation exposure.

Sequential refinements of technique such as pneumoencephalography, carotid and vertebral arteriography, and serial autotomography greatly increased the yield of valuable information in special cases, but without question the most important recent advances in neuroradiology, and indeed in neurology, have been computerized tomography (CT) scanning and magnetic resonance (MR) imaging. They have replaced pneumoencephalography entirely, and arteriography to a large extent, and have greatly extended our ability to visualize living pathology. A new field of bioneuropathology has been created.

COMPUTERIZED TOMOGRAPHY (CT SCANNING)

In this procedure the attentuation coefficient of the skull, CSF, cerebral gray and white matter, and blood vessels is measured, with computer assistance, by more than thirty thousand 2- to 4-mm beams of x-ray directed successively at several horizontal levels of the cranium. The differing densities of bone, CSF, blood, and gray and white matter are distinguishable in the resulting picture. One can see hemorrhage, softened and edematous brain, abscess, and tumor tissue and also the precise size and position of the

Figure 2-1

Computerized tomography (CT) scans of cerebrum, orbit, and cervical spine. Scale of densities, ranging from bone (+53) to water (+13) are shown on the left side of each figure. A. Cerebral hemispheres in the horizontal plane, at a level above the lateral ventricles. Note the differences in density between the skull, cerebral cortex, and white matter. Each of the major sulci are seen. B. Plane through the thalami and basal ganglia. The lower parts of the anterior horns are visible as two dark ovals. The lenticular nuclei and caudate nuclei are separated by the anterior limbs of the internal capsules. The thalami are separated from lenticular nuclei by the posterior limbs of the internal capsules. C. The eyeball and the optic nerve are seen in the orbit, as well as the lateral rectus and medial rectus muscles. D. The upper lumbar spine, including vertebral body, laminae, and spinous processes are white; the psoas muscles, on each side of the vertebral body, and the paravertebral muscles are gray. The spinal cord is visible within the spinal canal. (Courtesy of Medical Systems Division, General Electric Company.)

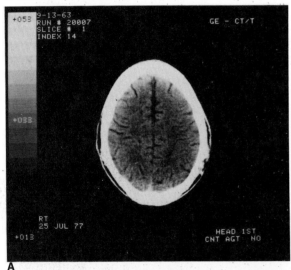

A

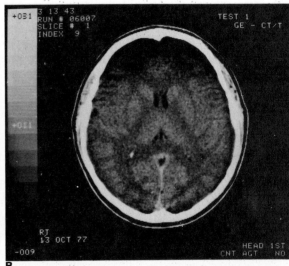

B

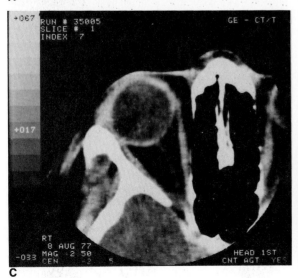

C

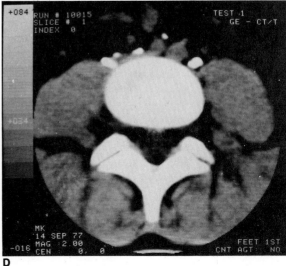

D

ventricles. The radiation exposure is not significantly greater than that from plain skull films.

The results obtained by the first CT scanners were relatively crude, but new machines now afford pictures of brain, spine, and orbit of truly remarkable clarity. As illustrated in Fig. 2-1, in transverse section of the brain one actually sees displayed the caudate and lenticular nuclei and the internal capsules and thalami. The position and width of all the main sulci can be measured, and the optic nerve and medial and lateral rectus muscles stand out clearly in the posterior parts of the orbit. The brainstem, cerebellum, and spinal cord are easily visible in the body scan at appropriate levels.

A novelty less than a decade ago, the CT scan is now an integral part of diagnostic neurology and within reach of virtually every patient who needs it. CT pictures of many of the common lesions of the brain have been inserted in the appropriate chapters.

MAGNETIC RESONANCE IMAGING (MRI)

Magnetic resonance, formerly referred to as nuclear magnetic resonance or NMR, is the newest form of imaging of the brain. Like the CT scan, MR provides ''slice'' images of the brain in any plane, but it has the great advantage of using nonionizing energy.

MRI is accomplished by placing the patient within a powerful magnetic field, which causes the protons of the tissues and CSF to align themselves in the orientation of the magnetic field. Introduction of a specific radio frequency (RF) pulse into the field causes the protons to resonate and to change their axis of alignment. When the RF pulse is removed the protons relax, so to speak, and return to their original alignment. The radio frequency energy which was absorbed and then emitted is subjected to computer analysis, from which an image is constructed (Fig.2-2).

Increasing experience with MR has demonstrated a number of advantages over CT scanning—a higher level of contrast between gray and white matter; a greatly increased capacity for demonstrating lesions in the brainstem, posterior fossa, and deep in the temporal lobe (because of a lack of bone artifact); an increased sensitivity to the presence of white matter lesions, particularly demyelinative lesions; and a lack of known hazard (Bydder et al). Abnormalities of the hindbrain and cervicomedullary junction and syringomyelia are especially well shown by MRI (Fig. 2-2). The recent approval, by the Food and Drug Administration, of gadolinium, a so-called paramagnetic agent that enhances the process of proton relaxation, permits even sharper MR definition of lesions than has been possible heretofore. The degree of cooperation required limits the use of MR in young children and in the mentally retarded. The only

danger in its use is displacement of metal clips on blood vessels and similar devices.

The MR device is costly and requires special housing to contain its powerful magnetic field. Nevertheless, like CT before it, the number of MR devices has proliferated, and MR has become an important adjunct to existing CT techniques for neurologic diagnosis. In particular clinical circumstances, as noted above, it is advantageous to proceed directly to MR.

Other radiologic methods of value to neurology and neurosurgery are angiography, contrast myelography and ventriculography, and, rarely, pneumoencephalography.

ANGIOGRAPHY

This technique has been developed over the last 40 years to the point where it is relatively safe and an extremely valuable method for the diagnosis of aneurysms, vascular malformations, occluded arteries and veins, and sometimes for mass lesions (hemorrhages, tumors, and abscesses). Following local anesthesia, a needle or cannula can be placed percutaneously into the lumen of any of the large arteries of the neck; or, even better, a catheter can be used to cannulate any of the major cervical vessels in a retrograde fashion after being introduced into the brachial or femoral artery. In these ways radiopaque contrast media can be injected to visualize the arch of the aorta, the origins of the carotid and vertebral systems and their extent through the neck into the cranial cavity. Highly experienced arteriographers can visualize the spinal cord arteries, cerebral arteries down to about 0.1 mm in lumen diameter (under optimal conditions), and small veins of comparable size. The procedure is not altogether without risk, and the indications should be clear. Approximately 1 percent of our patients have had a worsening of their condition or even a frank ischemic lesion in the territory of the catheterized artery. High concentrations of the injected media may induce vascular spasm and occlusion, and clots may form on the catheter tip and embolize the artery.

A refinement of angiographic technique—*digital subtraction angiography*—uses digital computer processing to produce an image of the major cervical and intracranial arteries. The great advantage of this radiographic procedure is that the contrast medium can be injected intravenously, and a vessel can be visualized with small amounts of contrast material in it. The resolution achieved by the ''venous angiogram'' does not match that of standard angiography, but the former procedure is considerably safer and more economical and reliably visualizes occlusions and

Figure 2-2

Nuclear magnetic resonance (NMR) images of the brain and spinal cord. Upper illustrations are from a young man with an Arnold-Chiari malformation. The brain and upper part of the cervical cord are visualized in the midsagittal plane. A major portion of the medulla protrudes below the foramen magnum, into the upper cervical canal.

Lower illustrations are from separate patients. Left: *An area of decreased signal is observed in the central portion of the cervical cord and medulla, probably representing a syringomyelia and syringobulbia.* Right: *An area of decreased signal in the upper thoracic cord, representing a cystic tumor. (Courtesy of Technicare Corporation, Cleveland, Ohio.)*

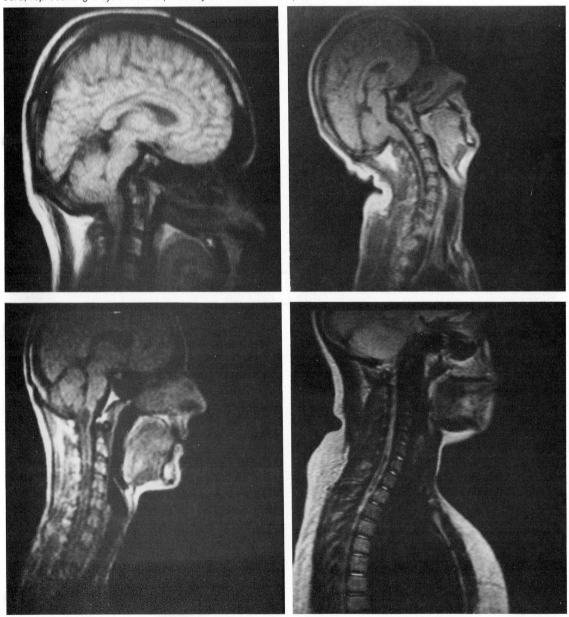

stenoses of the carotid vessels, as well as large ulcerative plaques and aneurysms. The main contraindication is cardiac failure, which may be worsened by the rapid injection of large volumes of fluid. The use of this and other methods for the investigation of carotid artery disease (Doppler flow, ultrasound) are discussed further in the chapter on cerebral vascular disease (page 651). They have the advantage of being safe, inexpensive, and noninvasive.

PNEUMOENCEPHALOGRAPHY (PEG) AND VENTRICULOGRAPHY

The injection of air or oxygen into the lumbar subarachnoid space (PEG) with the patient in the sitting position permits visualization in considerable detail of the size and position of the ventricles, the subarachnoid space (upper spinal and cerebral), and, indirectly, the structures which lie between the ventricles and the meninges. On rare occasions, in cases of greatly elevated intracranial pressure, air is injected directly into the ventricles (ventriculography) through burr holes placed in the skull. Air can also be used in the visualization of the spinal subarachnoid space for the demonstration of such abnormalities as spinal tumors and ruptured intervertebral discs. The advent of CT scanning has virtually precluded the need for air studies.

RADIOPAQUE MYELOGRAPHY (AND VENTRICULOGRAPHY)

By injecting 5 to 25 mL of Pantopaque through a lumbar puncture needle and then tipping the patient on a tilt table, the entire spinal subarachnoid space may be seen. The procedure is almost as harmless as the lumbar puncture, provided that the Pantopaque is afterward removed through the needle. Ruptured lumbar and cervical discs, cervical spondylotic bars and bony spurs encroaching on the spinal cord or roots, and spinal cord tumors can be diagnosed accurately. Occasionally, Pantopaque is injected into the lateral ventricles in order to visualize the third and fourth ventricles and the aqueduct of Sylvius. Some clinics have used air in preference to Pantopaque myelography because of the lesser risk of arachnoiditis (which results occasionally from the failure to remove all of the Pantopaque, particularly if there has been subarachnoid bleeding.) Air myelography, when combined with polytomography, is of special value in visualizing the size and position of the spinal cord and the relation to it of spondylotic bars and spurs. Both air and pantopaque myelography have been superseded by the use of water-soluble, self-absorbing, contrast media, such as metrizamide. The CT body scan also provides excellent images of the spinal canal and intervertebral foramens in three planes. The combination of metrizamide and CT scanning is a particularly useful means of visualizing spinal

and posterior fossa lesions, but this technique also promises to be replaced eventually by MRI.

RADIOACTIVE ISOTOPES

Radioactive isotopes of mercury, technetium, and arsenic have been in regular use for the visualization of tumors, inflammatory masses, subdural hematomas, and some vascular lesions. Since this is a simple, noninvasive procedure, the only limitation in its use is the expense. The more vascular the lesion, the more consistent its demonstration by these methods. *Ultrasound* can also be used to show displacement of central structures of the brain by a mass lesion. Ultrasound also has the advantage of being nonionizing and therefore applicable to the study of the fetal and infant brain.

CRANIAL AND SPINAL BONE SCANS

These procedures are of inestimable value in visualizing tumors and inflammatory processes in cranial and spinal bones. Often the lesions can be visualized when plain films are negative. The bone scan can be combined with the gallium scan for the opacification of soft tissues.

ELECTROENCEPHALOGRAPHY

The electroencephalographic examination is an essential part of the study of the patient suspected of having seizures. It is also used in evaluating the cerebral effects of many medical diseases and the study of sleep. It is described here in some detail, since it cannot suitably be assigned to any other single chapter.

The modern electroencephalograph has 8 to 16 or more separate amplifying units capable of recording from many areas of the scalp at the same time. The amplified brain rhythms are strong enough to move an ink-writing pen, which produces the waveform of brain activity in the frequency range of 0.5 to 30 Hz (cycles per second) on paper moving at a standard speed of 3 cm/s. The resulting electroencephalogram (EEG), or *voltage-versus-time graph*, appears as a number of parallel, wavy lines, as many as there are amplifying units, or "channels." Electrodes, which usually are solder or silver–silver chloride discs 0.5 cm in diameter, are placed on the head by means of adhesive material such as bentonite or collodion, using ECG paste under the electrode to make contact with the scalp. Patients are usually examined with their eyes closed and while relaxed in a comfortable chair or bed. The procedure is entirely painless and takes ¾ to 1¼ h. The ordinary EEG, therefore, represents the electrocerebral activity that is recorded under restricted circumstances, usually during the waking state, from several parts of the cerebral convexities, during an almost infinitesimal segment of the person's life.

In addition to the resting record, a number of so-called activating procedures are usually carried out.

1. The patient is requested to breathe deeply 20 times a minute for 3 min. The resulting alkalosis and cerebral vasoconstriction may activate characteristic seizure patterns or other abnormalities.

2. A powerful light (stroboscope) is placed about 15 in from the patient's eyes and flashed at frequencies from 1 to 20 per second with the patient's eyes opened and closed. The EEG leads may then show waves corresponding to each flash of light (photic driving, Fig. 2-3B) or abnormal discharges (Fig. 2-3C).

3. The EEG is recorded after the patient is allowed to fall asleep naturally or following sedative drugs by mouth or by vein. Sleep is extremely helpful in bringing out abnormalities, especially where temporal lobe epilepsy and certain other seizures are concerned.

4. Special activating procedures, such as the parenteral administration of pentylenetetrazol (Metrazol) or insulin, are hazardous and rarely used now. Their purpose was to produce diagnostically useful abnormalities without actually inducing convulsions.

Through the medium of all-night EEG recordings, many abnormalities associated with sleep can be demonstrated (see Chap. 18). Some of these are important clinically, and the same may be said of EEGs recorded by telemetry from freely moving ambulatory patients.

The EEG consists of 150 to 300 or more pages, each representing 10 s in time. These are obtained by a technician who is primarily responsible for the entire procedure, including notation of movements or other events responsible for artifacts and successive modifications of technique based upon what the record shows. Certain preparations are necessary if electroencephalography is to be most useful. The patient should not be sedated (except as noted above) and should not have been without food for a long time, for both sedative drugs and relative hypoglycemia modify the normal EEG pattern. The same may be said of mental concentration and extreme nervousness or drowsiness, all of which tend to suppress the normal alpha rhythm and increase muscle and other artifacts. When dealing with patients who are suspected of having epilepsy and who are

already being treated for it, most physicians prefer to record the first EEG while the patient continues to receive drugs. If it is normal, and if the referring physician and the electroencephalographer agree, the test can be repeated 24 h after withdrawal of anticonvulsants; it is well known that these drugs reduce the incidence of abnormal interictal records in patients with proved epilepsy. Though it is unusual for seizures to begin during this short interval, it may happen; longer periods without therapy are hazardous. It is helpful to indicate on the request form the suspected site of the lesion or the question to be answered.

TYPES OF NORMAL RECORDINGS

The normal record in adults usually shows somewhat asymmetric 8- to 13-per-second, 50-μV sinusoidal *alpha* waves in both occipital and parietal regions. These waves wax and wane spontaneously and disappear promptly when patients open their eyes or concentrate on something (Fig. 2-3A). Also, waves faster than 13 per second and of lower amplitude (10 to 20 μV), called *beta* waves, are recorded from the frontal regions symmetrically. When the normal subject falls asleep, the rhythm slows symmetrically, and characteristic wave forms (vertex sharp waves and sleep spindles) appear; if sleep is induced by barbiturates, an increase in the fast frequencies occurs and is considered to be normal.

During stroboscopic stimulation, an occipital response to each flash of light may be seen in the normal EEG and is called the *evoked response,* or, at fast rates of stimulation, "photic driving." The visual response arrives in the calcarine cortex 20 to 30 ms after the flash of light. This evoked occipital response from flashes of light or a shifting pattern stimulus (see further on) has increased the scope of electroencephalography in several ways: (1) one can be sure that a person with such a response can at least perceive light, and a patient with such a response who claims to be totally blind is either hysterical or malingering; (2) when this evoked response is absent on one side of the head but present on the other, there is interruption of transmission between the lateral geniculate body and the occipital lobe (geniculocalcarine pathway) on the one side; (3) when there is delay in the evoked response from one eye, there is usually disease in that optic nerve; (4) spread of the occipital response to photic stimulation, with the production of abnormal waves, provides evidence of abnormal excitability (Fig. 2-3B and C). If the activation procedure is continued, seizure patterns may be produced in the EEG, accompanied by gross myoclonic jerks of the face, neck, and limbs, or major convulsions (photomyoclonus and photoconvulsions). This finding is to be differentiated from the purely muscular response, also my-

Figure 2-3

A. *Normal alpha (9 to 10 per second) activity is present posteriorly (bottom channel). The top channel contains a large blink artifact. Note the striking reduction of the alpha rhythm with eye opening. B. Photic driving. During stroboscopic stimulation of a normal subject a visually evoked response is seen posteriorly after each flash of light (signaled on the bottom channel). C. Stroboscopic stimulation at 14 flashes per second (bottom channel) has produced a photoparoxysmal response in this epileptic patient, evidenced by the abnormal spike and slow-wave activity toward the end of the period of stimulation.*

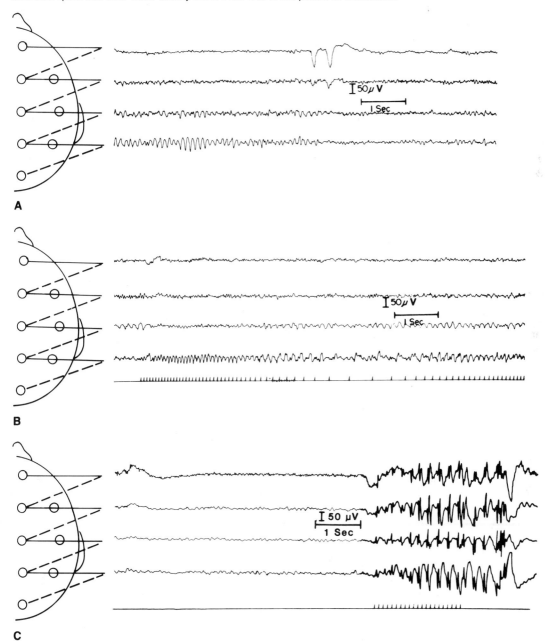

Figure 2-3 *(continued)*

D. *EEG from patient with focal motor seizures of the left side. Note focal spike discharge in right frontal region (channels 1–3). The activity from the left hemisphere (not shown here) was relatively normal.* E. *Petit mal epilepsy, showing generalized 3-per-second spike-and-wave discharge. The abnormal activity ends abruptly and a normal background appears.* F. *Large, slow, irregular delta waves are seen in the right frontal region (channels 1 and 2). In this case a glioblastoma was found in the right cerebral hemisphere, but the EEG picture does not differ basically from that produced by a stroke, abscess, or contusion.*

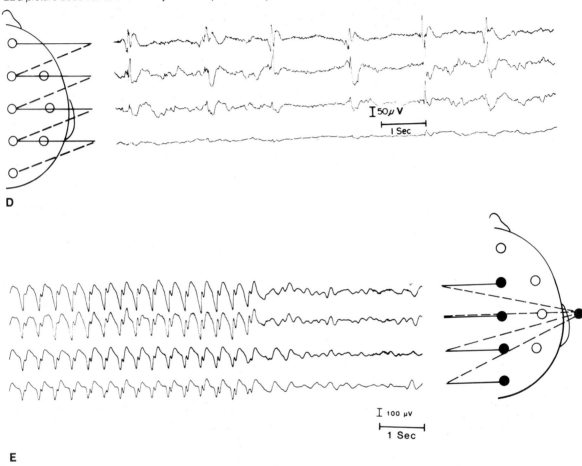

50µ V

1 Sec

D

100 µv

1 Sec

E

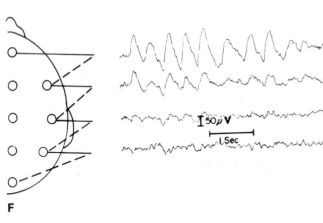

50µ V

1 Sec

F

Figure 2-3 *(continued)*

G. Grossly disorganized background activity interrupted by repetitive discharges consisting of large, sharp waves from all leads about once per second. This pattern is characteristic of Creutzfeldt-Jakob disease. H. Advanced hepatic coma. Slow (about 2 per second) waves have replaced the normal activity in all leads. This record demonstrates the triphasic waves sometimes seen in this disorder (channel 1). I. Deep coma following cardiac arrest, showing electrocerebral silence. With the highest amplification, ECG and other artifacts may be seen, so that the record is not truly "flat" or isoelectric. However, no cerebral rhythms are visible. Note the ECG (channel 5). (Illustrations courtesy of Dr. Susan Chester.)

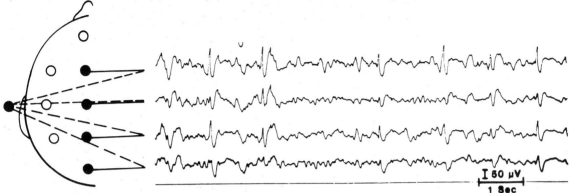

G

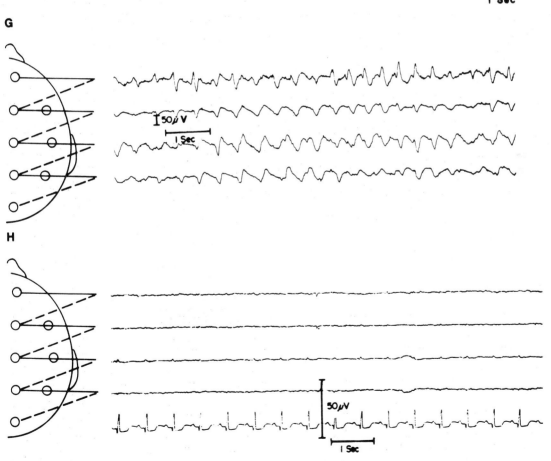

H

I

oclonic, produced normally in contracting scalp muscles and often visible in routine EEGs.

Children and adolescents are more sensitive than adults to all the activating procedures mentioned. It is customary for children to develop slow activity (3 to 4 per second) during the middle and latter parts of a period of overbreathing. This disappears soon after the hyperventilation has stopped. The frequency of the dominant rhythms in infants is normally about 3 per second, and they are very irregular. With maturation, there is a gradual increase in frequency and rhythmicity of these occipital rhythms, and by the age of 12 to 14 years, normal 9- to 10-per-second alpha waves are the dominant pattern (see Chap. 27 for further discussion of maturation of the brain as expressed in the EEG). Children's and infants' records are difficult to interpret because the wide range of normal values at each age makes rigid classification, using frequency criteria, impossible. Nevertheless, asymmetric records, or records with seizure patterns, are clearly abnormal in children of any age.

TYPES OF ABNORMAL RECORDINGS

The most pathologic finding of all is the replacement of the normal EEG pattern by "electrocerebral silence," which means that the electrical activity of the cortical mantle, measured at the scalp, is less than 2 μV or absent. Artifacts of various types are seen as the gains are increased. Acute intoxication with anesthetic levels of drugs, such as barbiturates, can produce this sort of isoelectric EEG (Fig. 2-3I). However, in the absence of nervous system depressants or hypothermia, a record which is "flat" (except for artifacts) over all parts of the head is almost always a result of cerebral hypoxia or ischemia. Such a patient, without EEG activity, reflexes, and spontaneous respiratory or muscular activity of any kind for 6 h or more, is said to be in "irreversible coma." The brain of such patients is largely necrotic, and there is no chance for neurologic recovery.

Localized regions of absent brain waves may rarely be seen when there is a particularly large area of softening or tumor or when an extensive clot lies between the cerebral cortex and the electrodes. With such a finding, the localization of the abnormality is precise, but of course the nature of the lesion is not disclosed. However, most such lesions are too small, relative to the recording arrangement, to be recognized, and the EEG may then record abnormal waves arising from functional though damaged brain at the borders of the lesion.

The abnormal waves are decreased in frequency and of higher amplitude than normal. Waves of fewer than 4

per second with amplitudes from 50 to 350 μV are called *delta* waves (Fig. 2-3G and H); those with a frequency of 4 to 7 per second are called *theta* waves; and the higher-voltage, faster waves are known as *spikes* or *sharp* waves (Fig. 2-3D). These fast and slow waves may be combined, and when a series of them interrupts relatively normal EEG patterns in a paroxysmal fashion, they are highly suggestive of epilepsy. The ones associated with *petit mal* are 3-per-second spike-and-wave complexes that characteristically appear in all leads of the electroencephalogram at the same time and disappear almost as suddenly at the end of the seizure (Fig. 2-3E). This finding led to the theoretic localization of a pacemaker for petit mal discharges in the thalamus or other deep gray structures ("centrencephalon"), but such a center has not been verified anatomically or physiologically.

NEUROLOGIC CONDITIONS WITH ABNORMAL EEG

Epilepsy (see also Chap. 15) All types of generalized epileptic seizures (grand mal and petit mal) are associated with some abnormality in the EEG, provided it is being recorded at the time. Also, the EEG is usually abnormal during the more restricted types of seizure activity (psychomotor, myoclonic, jacksonian). One exception is the seizure state that originates in a deep temporal lobe focus, in which case the discharge fails to reach the scalp in sufficient amplitude to be seen against the normal background activity of the EEG, particularly if there is a strong alpha rhythm. In these cases an anterior temporal electrode, which is the freest of occipital alpha frequencies, or a nasopharyngeal lead may pick up the discharge, especially during sleep. In some such cases, the only way in which this deep activity can be sampled is by inserting an electrode into the substance of the brain, but this procedure is applicable only to the few who are having a craniotomy. Occasionally one may fail to record an EEG abnormality in the course of one of the types of focal seizure (sensory, jacksonian, partial complex, epilepsia partialis continua) or in polymyoclonus. This fact presumably means that the neuronal discharge is too deep, discrete, fast, or asynchronous to be transmitted by volume conduction through the skull and recorded via the EEG electrode, which is some 2 cm from the cortex. Much more frequently, a completely normal EEG during a seizure indicates a "pseudoseizure" or hysteria.

Some of the different types of seizure patterns are shown in Fig. 2-3C, D, and E. The petit mal, myoclonic jerk, and grand mal patterns correlate closely with the clinical seizure type and may be present in the interictal EEG.

A fact of importance is that between seizures as many as 20 percent of patients with petit mal and 40 percent with grand mal epilepsy show a normal pattern. Anticonvulsant therapy also tends to diminish the interictal EEG abnormalities. The records of another 30 to 40 percent of epileptics, though abnormal between seizures, are nonspecifically so, and therefore the diagnosis of epilepsy can be made only by the correct interpretation of clinical data in relation to the EEG abnormality.

Brain Tumor, Abscess, and Subdural Hematoma

Intracranial mass lesions are associated with characteristic abnormalities in the EEG, depending on their type and location, in some 90 percent of patients. In addition to diffuse changes, described below, the classic abnormalities are focal or localized slow wave activity (usually delta, as in Fig. 2-3F) or, occasionally, seizure activity and decreased amplitude and synchronization of normal rhythms. As a rule, the more rapidly expanding lesions (abscess, some metastases, glioblastoma), especially those situated supratentorially, are associated with the greatest frequency of EEG abnormalities. More slowly growing and infratentorial tumors (astrocytomas) particularly those outside the cerebral hemispheres (meningiomas, pituitary tumors) and small deep abscesses often produce no change in the EEG, though they may be very evident clinically. The EEG abnormality is found on the same side as the lesion in as many as 75 to 90 percent of patients with subdural hematomas and supratentorial tumors or abscesses. Therefore, when a patient in whom one of these conditions is suspected has a normal EEG, there are nine chances to one against its presence. Thus the EEG may be helpful in both a negative and positive way, particularly when integrated with the other laboratory and clinical findings. The finding of both a normal EEG and radionuclide scan almost excludes the presence of a supratentorial brain tumor or abscess. These clinical rules are still useful, although presently much more reliance is placed on CT and MR.

Cerebrovascular Disease

The EEG may be useful in the differential diagnosis of vascular hemiplegia. Both the diffuse and the localized EEG changes produced by vascular lesions such as cerebral infarcts and intracranial hemorrhages depend on the location and size of the lesion rather than its type. If the lesion responsible is in the distribution of the internal carotid or other major cerebral artery, an area of excessive slowing is practically always seen acutely in the appropriate region. If the hemiplegia is due to small-vessel disease, i.e., a lacunar infarction deep in the cerebrum or brainstem (see Chap. 34), the EEG is usually normal. Large hemispheral lesions, associated acutely with depressed levels of consciousness, produce widespread, diffuse, slow-wave activity, as is seen with stupor or coma from any cause; a few very large infarctions are manifest initially by ipsilaterally depressed EEG activity. After a few days, as resolution begins and cerebral edema subsides, focal abnormalities may be seen (slow-wave activity or suppression of normal background rhythms). Smaller infarctions may be associated with focal abnormalities initially; they lateralize the lesion well but do not localize it precisely. After 3 to 6 months, roughly 50 percent of patients with cerebrovascular accidents have a normal EEG despite the persistence of clinical abnormalities. Once this occurs, the prognosis for further recovery is poor. Perhaps half these patients will have had normal EEGs even in the week or two following the stroke. Large lesions of the diencephalon or midbrain produce bilaterally synchronous slow waves, but, interestingly, those of pons and medulla, i.e., below the mesencephalon, may be associated with a normal or near-normal EEG pattern, despite catastrophic clinical changes. The EEG may be of lateralizing value in acute subarachnoid hemorrhage, depending upon the extent to which the adjacent cerebrum is affected.

Brain Injury

Cerebral concussion in animals is accompanied by a transitory disturbance in the EEG, but in humans this is usually no longer evident by the time a recording can be made. Cerebral contusion or laceration produces EEG changes similar to those described for cerebrovascular disease. Diffuse changes often give way to focal ones, especially if the lesions are on the lateral or superior surface of the brain, and these in turn usually disappear over a period of weeks or months. Sharp waves or spikes sometimes emerge as the focal slow-wave abnormality resolves and may precede the occurrence of posttraumatic epilepsy. Following head injury, therefore, serial EEGs may be of prognostic value as regards the prospect of epilepsy. They may also aid, as mentioned above, in evaluating patients for subdural hematoma.

Diseases That Cause Coma and States of Impaired Consciousness

The EEG is abnormal in almost all conditions in which there is impairment of consciousness. With hypothyroidism the brain waves are normal in configuration but are usually of decreased frequency. In general, the more profound the change in consciousness, the more abnormal the EEG recording. In these latter situations the slow (delta) waves are bilateral and of high amplitude, and tend to be more conspicuous over the frontal regions (Fig. 2-3H). This pertains to such differing conditions as acute meningitis or encephalitis, severe disorders of blood gases, glucose, electrolyte and water balance, uremia, diabetic coma, and impairment of consciousness accompanying the large cerebral lesions discussed above. In hepatic coma, the degree of abnormality in the EEG corresponds with the degree of confusion, stupor, or coma. Moreover, paroxysms of bilaterally synchronous large, sharp "triphasic waves" are characteristic (Fig. 2-3*H*), though they may also be seen with encephalopathies related to renal or pulmonary failure. Diffuse degenerative diseases (e.g., Alzheimer disease) causing serious affection of the cerebral cortex are accompanied by relatively slight degrees of diffuse, slow-wave abnormality in the theta (4- to 7-Hz) range, occurring relatively late in their course. More rapidly progressive ones, such as subacute sclerosing panencephalitis (SSPE), Creutzfeldt-Jakob disease, and to a lesser extent the cerebral lipidoses often have, in addition, very characteristic, and almost pathognomonic EEG changes, consisting of periodic bursts of high-amplitude, sharp waves, usually bisynchronous and symmetric (Fig. 2-3*G*). Even in situations where the EEG abnormality is not specific or diagnostic, it is useful in emphasizing the presence of physiologic, biochemical, and, sometimes, structural abnormalities of the brain. A normal EEG in a patient who is apathetic, slow, and depressed is a point in favor of the diagnosis of an affective disorder or schizophrenia.

An EEG may also be of help in the diagnosis of coma when the pertinent history is unavailable. It may point to an otherwise unexpected cause such as hepatic encephalopathy, intoxication with barbiturates or other sedative-hypnotic drugs, clinically inapparent continuous epileptic discharges, or diffuse anoxia-ischemia.

Other Diseases of the Cerebrum Many disorders of nervous function cause little or no alteration in the EEG. Multiple sclerosis and other demyelinating diseases are examples, though as many as 50 percent of advanced cases will have an abnormal record of nonspecific type (slow wave frequencies in a focus or over a hemisphere). Delirium tremens and Wernicke-Korsakoff disease, despite the dramatic nature of the clinical picture, cause little or no change in the EEG. Some degree of slowing usually accompanies confusional states which have been designated elsewhere as hypokinetic delirium (see Chap. 19). Interestingly, neuroses and psychoses, such as manic-depressive disorders or schizophrenia, intoxication with hallucinogenic drugs such as LSD, and the majority of cases of mental retardation, are associated either with no modification of the normal record or with minor nonspecific abnormalities.

CLINICAL SIGNIFICANCE OF MINOR EEG ABNORMALITIES

The gross EEG abnormalities discussed above are, by themselves, clearly abnormal and any formulation of the patient's clinical state should attempt to account for them. They include seizure discharge, generalized and extreme slowing, definite slow waves with a clear-cut asymmetry or a focus, and absence of normal rhythms. Certain other findings are of more doubtful significance and represent lesser degrees of abnormality which form a continuum between the undoubtedly abnormal and the completely normal. These records—which comprise such activity as 14- and 6-per-second positive spikes, small sharp waves, scattered 5- or 6-per-second slowing, voltage asymmetries, and moderate "breakdown" with hyperventilation—are termed *borderline* and are most difficult to interpret. The minor EEG abnormalities may be meaningful, but only if correlated with certain clinical phenomena. Whereas borderline deviations in an otherwise entirely normal person have no clinical significance, the same EEG findings, when associated with certain clinical signs and symptoms—even if they, too, are of minimal severity—become important. For example, a patient with tension headaches for 20 years is under neurologic study because of insomnia, weight loss, and an increase in the frequency of headaches. The neurologic examination, CSF, and skull films are all within normal limits. The EEG shows a reduction of voltage in the left occipitoparietal area and less alpha than the same area on the right side. The finding of such an asymmetry in the brain waves has no clinical significance in this case and may be disregarded. On the other hand, the same finding in someone who was rendered unconscious in an accident 9 days before and who shows slight awkwardness in the right hand and a continuous dull headache with a lack of usual alertness has considerable diagnostic meaning. It points to a left hemispheric lesion, perhaps a contusion, or to the presence of a subdural hematoma. The value of a normal or "negative" EEG in certain patients suspected of having a cerebral lesion has been discussed above.

In conclusion, the results of the EEG, like those of the EMG and ECG, are meaningful only in relation to the clinical state of the patient at the time the recordings were made.

SPECIAL APPLICATIONS OF THE EEG

The EEG is useful in the operating room to monitor cerebral activity during the increasingly extensive procedures of modern cardiovascular surgery. EEG apparatus has long been available for indicating the level of anesthesia, and such simple equipment should be used by the anesthetist to monitor both the cardiac and cerebral activity of *all* patients during surgical anesthesia.

In the neurosurgical operating room the EEG can be recorded from the exposed brain (electrocorticogram); seizure patterns can be localized more precisely than from the scalp, so that resection of such physiologically abnormal tissue may be undertaken.

The routine EEG can be of value in the diagnosis of hysterical blindness, as stated above. Similarly, a response evoked by noise during light sleep can be of help in confirming the presence of hearing in a patient who feigns total deafness. These responses may also be helpful in evaluating hearing and vision in infants. However, the visual and auditory evoked responses are usually too small to be visible in the melange of baseline noise and background activity of the routine EEG. Averaging techniques (computerized) may then be used to record them. This interesting branch of electroencephalography is discussed below.

The EEG has become increasingly useful in neonatal and infant neurology. The normal patterns from the seventh month of fetal life through infancy and childhood have been established. Full maturation, viz., the time when the stable adult pattern is achieved, varies considerably, making interpretation difficult. However, certain changes, as described by Werner et al, are clearly indicative of a developmental disorder or disease.

COMPUTERIZED EVOKED POTENTIALS

The stimulation of sense organs or peripheral nerves evokes a response in the appropriate cortical receptive areas and a number of subcortical relay stations as well. However, one cannot place a recording electrode near the relay stations, nor can one detect tiny potentials of only a few microvolts among the much larger background activity in the EEG or EMG. The use of averaging methods, introduced by Dawson, in 1954, and the more recent development of digital computers have provided the means of overcoming these problems. A series of waveforms, modified at each relay station and recorded by distant electrodes (''far-field recording'') can be maximized by the computer to a point where they can be easily measured in terms of their voltage and latency.

For many years it had been known that a light stimulus, flashing on the retina, initiated a discernible waveform over the occipital lobes. In 1969, it was observed by Regan and Heron that a visual evoked response could be produced by the sudden change of a viewed checkerboard pattern. The responses produced in this way were easier to

measure than flash responses and more consistent in waveform from one individual to another. It was found also that this type of stimulus, applied first to one eye and then to the other, could demonstrate conductional delays in the visual pathways of patients who had formerly suffered a disease of the optic nerve—even though there were no residual signs of reduced visual acuity, visual field abnormalities, alterations of the optic nerve head, or changes in pupillary reflexes.

This procedure, which is called *pattern-shift visual evoked responses* (PSVER), has been widely adopted as one of the most delicate tests of lesions in the visual system. Figure 2-4 illustrates the normal PSVER and two types of

Figure 2-4

Pattern-shift visual evoked responses (PSVER). Upper two tracings, from right and left eye, are normal. Latency measured to first major positive peak (b); duration measured from beginning of positive peak (a) to return to baseline (c). Middle tracings: PSVER from the right eye is normal but the latency of the response from the left eye is prolonged and its duration is increased. Lower tracings: PSVER from both eyes show abnormally prolonged latencies, somewhat greater on the left than on the right. Calibration: 50 ms, 2.5 µV. (Redrawn from Shahrokhi et al.)

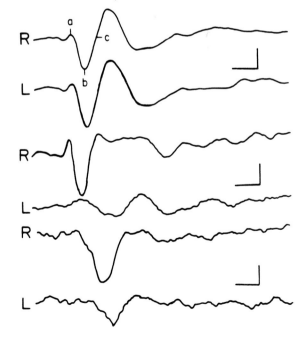

delayed responses. Examinations of large numbers of patients who were known to have had retrobulbar neuritis showed that among 51 such patients only 4 had normal latencies (Shahrokhi et al). These authors found similar abnormalities of the PSVER in about one-third of multiple sclerosis patients who had no history or clinical evidence of optic nerve involvement. Usually, abnormalities of the amplitude and duration of PSVER accompany the abnor-

mally prolonged latencies. A difference between responses from the two eyes signifies involvement of one optic nerve; bilateral prolongation of latencies could be due to lesions in both optic nerves or in the visual pathways posterior to the optic chiasm. A compressive lesion of an optic nerve will have the same effect as a demyelinative one. Glaucoma and other diseases involving structures anterior to the retinal ganglion cells may also produce increased latencies. Impaired visual acuity has little effect on the latency but does correlate well with the amplitude of the PSVER. Many other diseases of the optic nerve, including toxic and nutritional amblyopias, ischemic optic neuropathy, and the Leber type of hereditary optic neuropathy show abnormalities of the PSVER. As indicated above, the test is especially

Figure 2-5

Far-field brainstem auditory evoked responses (BAER). Diagram of the proposed electrophysiologic-anatomic correlations in human subjects.

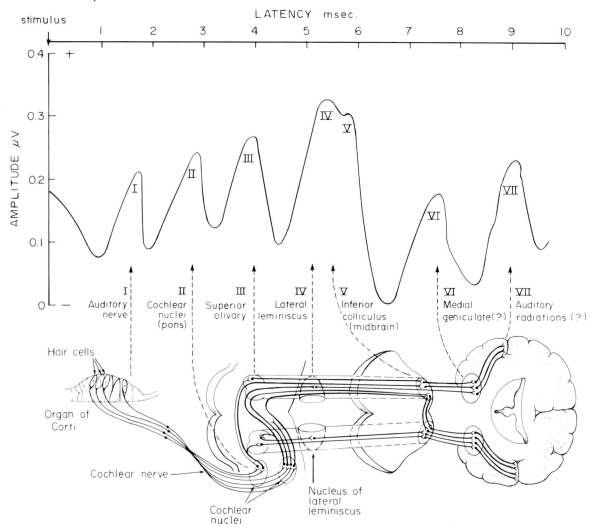

valuable in proving the existence of active or residual disease of an optic nerve. The finding of abnormal PSVER in a patient with a clinically apparent lesion elsewhere in the central nervous system is presumptive evidence of multiple sclerosis.

The cortical effects of auditory stimuli can be studied in the same way as visual ones, by a procedure called *far-field brainstem auditory evoked responses* (BAER). A large number of clicks, delivered first to one ear and then the other, are recorded through scalp electrodes and maximized by computer. A series of seven waves appear at the scalp within 10 ms after each stimulus. On the basis of depth

Figure 2-6

Short-latency somatosensory evoked potentials produced by stimulation of the median nerve at the wrist.

The set of responses shown at left is from a normal subject, and the set at right is from a patient with multiple sclerosis who had no sensory symptoms or signs. In the patient, note the preservation of the brachial-plexus component (EP), the absence of the cervical-cord (N11) and lower-medullary components (N13/P13), and the latency of the thalamo-cortical components (N19 and P22), prolonged markedly above the normal mean +3 SD for the separation from the brachial plexus. Unilateral stimulation occurred at a frequency of 5 per second. Each trace is the averaged response to 1024 stimuli; the superimposed trace represents a repetition to demonstrate waveform consistency. Recording-electrode locations are as follows: FZ denotes midfrontal, EP Erb's point (the shoulder), C2 the middle back of the neck over the C2 cervical vertebra, and Cc the scalp overlying the sensoriparietal cortex contralateral to the stimulated limb.

Relative negativity at the second electrode caused an upward trace deflection. Amplitude calibration marks denote 2 μV. (Reproduced with permission from Chiappa and Ropper, p 1206.)

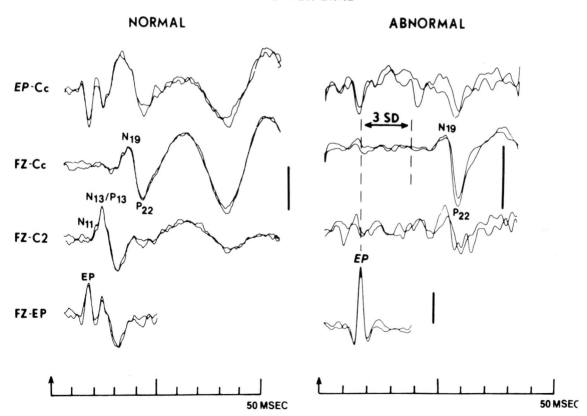

UPPER LIMB

recordings and the study of lesions produced in cats and pathologic studies of the brainstem in humans, it has been determined that each of the first five waves are generated by the brainstem structures indicated in Fig. 2-5. The generators of waves VI and VII are uncertain. A lesion that affects one of the relay stations or its immediate connections is said to be manifested by lower voltage of the wave or a delay in its appearance and an absence or reduction in amplitude of subsequent waves. These effects are more pronounced on the side of the stimulated ear than contralaterally, which is difficult to understand since the majority of the cochlear-superior olivary-lateral lemniscal-medial geniculate fibers cross to the opposite side. It is also surprising that a severe lesion of one relay station would allow impulses to continue their ascent and be recordable in the cerebral cortex.

Short-latency somatosensory evoked potentials (SLSEP) are now being used in most clinical neurophysiology laboratories to confirm lesions in the somatic sensory systems. The technique consists of applying 5 per-second painless electrical stimuli over the median, peroneal, and tibial nerves and recording them (for the upper limb) over Erb's point above the clavicle, over the C_2 spine, and the opposite parietal cortex, and (for the lower limb) over the lumbar and cervical spines and the opposite parietal cortex. The impulses generated in large touch fibers by 500 or more stimuli and averaged by computer can be traced through the peripheral nerves, spinal roots, and posterior columns to the nuclei of Burdach and Goll in the lower medulla, through the medial lemniscus to the contralateral thalamus, and thence to the sensory cortex of the parietal lobes. Delay between the stimulus site and Erb's point or lumbar spine indicates peripheral nerve disease; delay from Erb's point (or lumbar spine) to C_2 implies an abnormality in the appropriate nerve roots or in the posterior columns; the presence of lesions in the medial lemniscus and thalamoparietal pathway can be inferred from delays of subsequent waves recorded from the parietal cortex (Fig. 2-6). The normal wave forms are designated by the symbol P (positive) or N (negative) with a number indicating the interval of time from stimulus to recording, e.g., N 11, N 13, P 13. For purposes of clinical interpretation SLSEPs are assumed to be linked in series, so that interwave abnormalities in latency indicate a conduction defect between the generators of the two peaks involved (Chiappa and Ropper). Recordings with pathologically verified lesions at these levels are to be found in the monograph by Chiappa. This test has been most helpful in establishing the existence of lesions in spinal roots, posterior columns, and brainstem

in such disorders as Guillain-Barre syndrome, multiple sclerosis, and cervical spondylosis, even when the clinical data are uncertain.

MOTOR CORTEX STIMULATION

In intact human beings it is now possible, by using single pulse-high voltage stimulation of the motor cortex and the cervical spine segments, to detect delays or lack of conduction in descending pathways. This technique, introduced by Marsden et al, stimulates only the largest motor neurons (presumably Betz cells) and the fastest conducting axons. Cervical cord stimulation is believed to actuate the anterior roots. The difference in time between the motor cortex and cervical activation of hand or forearm muscles represents the conduction velocity of the cortical-cervical cord motor neurons. Berardelli et al, who have applied the technique to 20 hemiplegic patients with a cerebrovascular lesion, found that in 15 of them there was no descending influence in comparison to the normal side. Although the degree of functional deficit does not correlate with the degree of electrophysiologic change, one expects that refinements of this technique will be useful in evaluating the status of the corticospinal motor system.

ELECTROMYOGRAPHY AND NERVE CONDUCTION STUDIES

These will be discussed in Chap. 44.

PSYCHOMETRY, PERIMETRY, AUDIOMETRY, AND TESTS OF LABYRINTHINE FUNCTION

These methods, drawn largely from the field of physiologic psychology, are used in quantitating and defining the nature of the psychic or sensory deficits produced by disease of the nervous system. The indications for doing these tests are (1) to obtain confirmation of a disorder of function in particular parts of the nervous system and to ascertain its nature or (2) to quantitate the disorder in order to determine, by subsequent examinations, the natural course of the underlying illness. A description of these methods and their clinical use will be found in the chapters dealing with developmental disorders of the cerebrum (Chap. 28), with dementia (Chap. 20), and with disorders of vision (Chap. 12) and of hearing and equilibrium (Chap. 14).

BIOCHEMICAL TESTS

With advances in the biochemistry of metabolic diseases a number of highly specific tests of serum, CSF, and circulating red and white blood cells have become available. These diagnostic procedures and the indications for their use are too numerous and varied to describe here. Each will be presented in relation to the metabolic disease of which it is diagnostic.

BIOPSY OF MUSCLE, NERVE, SKIN, AND CONJUNCTIVUM

The application of light, phase, and electron microscopy to the study of these tissues may be highly informative. The findings will be discussed in Chaps. 45 (muscle), 46 (nerve), and 38 (skin and conjunctivum, in the diagnosis of storage disease).

REFERENCES

BARROWS LJ, HUNTER FT, BANKER BQ: The nature and clinical significance of pigments in the cerebrospinal fluid. *Brain* 78:59, 1955.

BERARDELLI A, INGHILLERI M, MANFREDI M, ET AL: Cortical and cervical stimulation after hemispheric infarctions. *J Neurol Neurosurg Psychiatry* 50:861, 1987.

BRANT-ZAWADZKI M, NORMAN D: *Magnetic Resonance Imaging of The Central Nervous System.* New York, Raven Press, 1987.

BYDDER GM, STEINER RE, YOUNG IR ET AL: Clinical NMR imaging of the brain: 140 cases. *Am J Roentgenol* 139:215, 1982.

CHIAPPA KH: *Evoked Potentials in Clinical Neurology.* New York, Raven Press, 1983.

CHIAPPA KH, ROPPER AH: Evoked potentials in clinical medicine, *N Engl J Med* 306: 1140, 1205, 1982.

DUFRESNE JJ: *Cytopathologie de CSF.* Basel, Ciba Foundation, 1973.

EARNEST F. HOUSER OW, FORBES GS, et al: The accuracy and limitations of intravenous digital subtracation angiography in the evaluation of atherosclerotic cerebrovascular disease: Angiographic and surgical correlation. Mayo Clin Proc 58:735, 1983.

FISHMAN RA: *Cerebrospinal Fluid in Diseases of the Nervous System.* Philadelphia, Saunders, 1980.

HALLIDAY AM (ED): *Evoked Potentials in Clinical Testing.* Edinburgh, Churchill Livingstone, 1982.

HARWOOD-NASH DC, FITZ CR: *Neuroradiology in Infants and Children,* vols 1–3. St Louis, Mosby, 1976.

HUGHES JR: *EEG in Clinical Practice.* Woburn, Mass, Butterworth, 1982.

KILOH LG, McCOMAS AJ, OSSELTON JW, U A: *Clinical Electroencephalography,* 4th ed. London, Butterworth, 1981.

KLASS DW, DALY DD (EDS): *Current Practice of Clinical EEG.* New York, Raven Press, 1979.

KOOI KA, TUCKER RP, MARSHALL RE: *Fundamentals of Electroencephalography,* 2nd ed. Hagerstown, Md, Harper & Row, 1978.

MARSDEN CD, MERTON PA, MORTON HB: Direct electrical stimulation of corticospinal pathways through the intact scalp and in human subjects. *Adv Neurol* 39:387, 1983.

NEWTON TH, POTTS DG (EDS): *Modern Neuroradiology, vol I: Computed Tomography of the Spine and Spinal Cord.* San Anselmo, Calif, Clavadel Press, 1983.

NEWTON TH, POTTS DG: *Modern Neuroradiology, vol II: Advanced Imaging Techniques.* San Anselmo, Calif, Clavadel Press, 1983.

NEWTON TH, HASSO AN, DILLON WP: *Modern Neuroradiology, vol III: Computer Tomography of the Head and Neck.* San Anselmo, Calif, Clavadel Press, 1988..

NIEDERMEYER E, daSILVA FL: *Electroencephalography,* 2nd ed. Baltimore, Urban and Schwarzenberg, 1987.

REGAN D, HERON JR: Clinical investigation of lesions of the visual pathway: A new objective technique. *J Neurol Neurosurg Psychiatry* 32:479, 1969.

SHAHROKHI F, CHIAPPA KH, YOUNG RR: Pattern shift visual evoked responses. *Arch Neurol* 35:65, 1978.

SPEHLMANN R: *EEG Primer.* Amsterdam, Elsevier/North Holland Biomedical Press, 1981.

STARK DD, BRADLEY WG: *Magnetic Resonance Imaging.* St Louis, Mosby, 1988.

WERNER SS, STOCKARD JE, BICKFORD RG: *Atlas of Neonatal Electroencephalography.* New York, Raven Press, 1977.

WESTMORELAND BF, KLASS DW, SHARBROUGH FW, REAGAN TJ: Alpha-coma: Electroencephalographic, clinical, pathological and etiologic correlations. *Arch Neurol* 32:713, 1975.

WILFERT CM: Mumps meningoencephalitis with low cerebrospinal fluid glucose, prolonged pleocytosis and elevation of protein. *N Engl J Med* 280:855, 1969.

WILLIAMS A. HAUGHTON V: *Cranial Computer Tomography: A Comprehensive Test.* St Louis, Mosby, 1985.

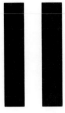

**CARDINAL MANIFESTATIONS
OF NEUROLOGIC DISEASE**

DISORDERS OF MOTILITY

Motor control, to which much of the human nervous system is committed, is accomplished through the integrated action of a vast array of segmental and suprasegmental motor neurons, the latter including the motor and sensory cortices, the supplementary motor cortex, the striatum, pallidum, and other basal ganglionic and thalamic nuclei, the cerebellum, and the vestibular and reticular nuclei of the brainstem. And at each of these levels of the nervous system, all forms of motor activity are guided by sensory feedback. Even injury to certain parts of the brain that are not primarily motor or sensory in function may affect motility since these parts of the human nervous system are concerned with motor behavior and the planning of present and future action.

Although the large repertoire of reflex, postural, emotional-instinctive, and voluntary movements are interrelated, the following parts of the nervous system are known to be engaged primarily in the control of movement, and in the course of disease, to yield a number of characteristic derangements of motor function:

1. The large motor nerve cells in the anterior horns of the spinal cord and the motor nuclei of the brainstem, the axons of which extend into the anterior spinal roots and spinal nerves and into the cranial nerves en route to the skeletal muscles. These constitute the primary, or lower, motor neurons, complete lesions of which result in a loss of all movement—voluntary, automatic, postural, and reflex. The lower motor neurons are the "final common path" by which all nervous impulses are transmitted to muscle.

2. The motor cells in the cerebral cortex near the rolandic fissure and their connections with the spinal motor neurons by a system of fibers known, because of their collective shape in transverse sections through the medulla, as the pyramidal tract. Since the motor fibers that extend from the cerebral cortex to the spinal cord are not confined to the pyramidal tract, they are more accurately designated as the corticospinal tract, or, alternately, as the upper motor neuron, to distinguish them from the lower motor neuron.

3. Several brainstem nuclei that project to the spinal cord, notably pontine and medullary reticular nuclei, vestibular nuclei, and red nuclei. These structures subserve the neural mechanisms of posture and movement, particularly when movement is highly automatic and repetitive. Certain brainstem nuclei are influenced by the motor and/or premotor regions of the cortex, e.g., via corticoreticulospinal relays.

4. Two subcortical systems, the basal ganglia (striatum, pallidum and related structures, including the substantia nigra and subthalamic nucleus) and the cerebellum. These two groups of structures play im-

portant roles in the control of muscle tone, posture, and coordination of movement by virtue of their connections, via the thalamocortical fibers and premotor cortex, with the corticospinal system and other descending pathways from the cortex.

5. Many other parts of the cerebral cortex, particularly the premotor and accessory motor cortex, which are involved in planning and programming of all voluntary movement and assuring that the purposes of the organism are achieved. In addition, those parts of the nervous system concerned with tactile, visual, and auditory sensation are connected by fiber tracts with the motor cortex. These association pathways provide for the sensory regulation of motor function and facilitate the coordination of thought and action.

The impairment of motor function which results from lesions of these various parts of the nervous system may be somewhat arbitrarily divided into (1) paralysis due to affection of lower motor neurons, (2) paralysis due to affection of upper motor (corticospinal) neurons, (3) apraxic or nonparalytic disturbances of purposive movement due to involvement of the association pathways in the cerebrum, (4) involuntary movements and abnormalities of posture due to disease of the basal ganglia, and (5) abnormalities of coordination (ataxia) due to lesions in the cerebellum. The first two types of motor disorder and the apraxic disorders of movement are discussed in Chap. 3; "extrapyramidal" motor abnormalities and disorders of coordination will be considered in Chap. 4. A miscellaneous group of movement disorders—tremor myoclonus, spasms, and tics—and disorders of stance and gait are the subjects of Chaps. 5 and 6. The impairment or loss of motor function which is due to primary disease of striated muscle or to a failure of neuromuscular transmission will be considered further on, in relation to diseases of striated muscle.

CHAPTER 3

MOTOR PARALYSIS

Definitions The term *paralysis* is derived from the Greek words *para,* "beside, off, amiss," and *lysis,* a "loosening" or "breaking up." In medicine it has come to refer to an abolition of function, either sensory or motor. When applied to motor function, *paralysis* means loss of voluntary movement due to interruption of one of the motor pathways at any point from the cerebrum to the muscle fiber. A lesser degree of paralysis is sometimes spoken of as *paresis,* but in everyday medical parlance paralysis may stand for either partial or complete loss of function. The word *plegia* comes from a Greek word meaning "stroke," and the word *palsy,* from an old French word which has the same meaning as *paralysis.* All these words are used interchangeably, though generally one uses *paresis* for slight and *paralysis* or *plegia* for severe loss of motor function.

AFFECTION OF THE LOWER MOTOR NEURON

ANATOMIC AND PHYSIOLOGIC CONSIDERATIONS

Each spinal and cranial motor nerve cell, through the extensive arborization of the terminal part of its efferent fiber, comes into contact with only a few or up to 100 to 200 or more muscle fibers; altogether they constitute "the motor unit." All the variations in force, range, rate, and type of movement are determined by the number and size of motor units called into activity and the frequency with which the muscle fibers are activated. Feeble movements involve only a few small motor units; powerful movements recruit many more units of increasing size. When a motor neuron becomes diseased, as in progressive spinal muscular atrophy, it may manifest increased irritability, and all the muscle fibers that it controls may discharge sporadically, in isolation from other units. The result of contraction of one or several such units is a visible twitch, or *fasciculation,* which can be recognized in the electromyogram as a large

diphasic or multiphasic action potential. If the motor neuron is destroyed, all the muscle fibers which it innervates undergo a profound atrophy, viz., denervation atrophy. Within a few days after motor nerve section the individual denervated muscle fibers become hypersensitive possibly to circulating acetylcholine and contract spontaneously, though they can no longer do so in response to a nerve impulse as a part of the motor unit. This isolated activity of individual muscle fibers, called *fibrillation,* is so fine that it cannot be seen through the intact skin but it can be recorded as a small, repetitive, short-duration spike potential in the electromyogram (Chap. 45).

The motor nerve fibers of each ventral root intermingle with those of neighboring roots to form plexuses, and although the muscles are innervated roughly according to segments of the spinal cord, each large muscle comes to be supplied by two or more roots. In contrast, a single peripheral nerve usually provides the complete motor innervation of a muscle or group of muscles. For this reason the paralysis due to disease of the anterior horn cells or anterior roots has a different pattern than the weakness that follows a lesion of a peripheral nerve.

All motor activity, even the most elementary reflex type, requires the cooperation of many muscles. The analysis of a relatively simple movement, such as clenching the fist, affords some idea of the complexity of the underlying neural arrangements. In this act the primary movement is a contraction of the flexor muscles of the fingers, the flexor digitorum sublimis and profundus, the flexor pollicis longus and brevis, and the abductor pollicis brevis. In the terminology of Beevor, these muscles act as *agonists,* or *prime movers.* In order that flexion of these muscles may be smooth and forceful, the contractibility of the extensor muscles (*antagonists*) must diminish, i.e., they must relax, at the same rate as the flexors contract. The muscles which flex the fingers also flex the wrist; and since it is desired that only the fingers flex, the muscles which extend the wrist must be brought into play to prevent its flexion. The action of the wrist extensors is synergic, and these muscles are called *synergists* in this particular act. Lastly, during this action of the hand, the wrist, elbow, and shoulder need to be stabilized by appropriate flexor and extensor muscles; the muscles which accomplish this serve as *fixators*. The coordination of agonists, antagonists, synergists, and fixators involves reciprocal innervation and is managed entirely by segmental spinal reflexes under the guidance of proprioceptive sensory stimuli. In general, the more delicate the movement, the more precise must be the coordination between agonist and antagonist muscles.

All phasic (ballistic) movements and postures are effected by the activation of motor neurons, large ones supplying large motor units and small ones, small motor units. Small motor units are more efficiently activated by sensory afferents from muscle spindles, are more tonically active, and are more readily recruited in reflex activities and postural maintenance, walking, and running. The large motor units participate mainly in phasic movements which are characterized by an initial burst of activity in the agonist muscles, then a burst in the antagonists, followed by a third burst in the agonists. The strength of the initial agonist burst determines the speed and distance of the movement, but always there is the same triphasic pattern of agonist, antagonist, and agonist (Hallett et al). The basal ganglia and cerebellum set the pattern and the timing of the muscle action in any projected motor performance. This will be discussed further in Chap. 4.

Unlike phasic movements, certain basic motor activities do not involve reciprocal innervation. In the support of the body in an upright posture, when the legs must act as rigid pillars, and in shivering, the agonists and antagonists contract simultaneously. Locomotion requires that the extensor pattern of reflex standing be inhibited, and that an alternating coordinated pattern of stepping movements be substituted; the latter is accomplished by multisegmental spinal and brainstem reflexes, the so-called locomotor centers (Grillner). Suprasegment control of antigravity postural mechanisms is mediated primarily by the reticulospinal and vestibulospinal tracts and independent flexion movements of the extremities by the rubrospinal and corticospinal tracts. These are discussed further on.

The tonus of muscle and the tendon reflexes depend on the status of alpha motor neurons, on muscle spindles and their afferent fibers, and on the small anterior horn cells whose axons terminate on the small (intrafusal) muscle fibers within the spindles. The specialized small motor neurons are called *gamma neurons*, in contrast to the large

alpha neurons which activate all nonspindle muscle fibers. The beta motor neurons effect contraction in both spindle and nonspindle fibers, and, while recognized physiologically, are omitted from most schemes of motor activity. Some of the gamma neurons are tonically active at rest, keeping the intrafusal muscle fibers taut and sensitive to external stretch. A tap on a tendon, by stretching the spindle muscle fibers, activates afferent nerve fibers which synapse with alpha motor neurons in the same and adjacent spinal segments, and they in turn send impulses to the skeletal muscle fibers, resulting in the familiar brief muscle contraction or phasic (myotatic) stretch reflex (Fig. 3-1). The alpha neurons of antagonist muscles are simultaneously inhibited. Thus the setting of the spindle fibers and the state of excitability of the alpha and gamma neurons (influenced by descending fiber systems) determine the level of activity of the tendon reflexes and the responsiveness of muscle to stretch. Other mechanisms, of an inhibitory nature, involve the Golgi tendon organs for which the adequate stimulus is tension produced by active contraction of muscle. These receptors activate afferent fibers that end on internuncial cells, which in turn project to alpha motor neurons, thus forming a disynaptic reflex arc. They have mainly a protective function, preventing excessive muscle contraction, but they also play a role in naturally occurring limb movements, particularly in locomotion.

The segmental and intersegmental mechanisms of the spinal cord are far more complex than this simple sketch might indicate. The alpha neurons of the medial parts of the anterior horn supply trunk or axial muscles and the lateral parts (Rexed lamina IX), the appendicular muscles (see Fig. 7-1B). They receive input from intermediate neurons in laminae V to VIII and from propriospinal neurons in the fasiculi proprii of adjacent spinal segments. All the facilitatory and inhibitory influences supplied by cutaneous and proprioceptive afferent and descending suprasegmental neurons are coordinated at a spinal level in such activities as phasic and tonic reflexes, flexor withdrawal and crossed extension reflexes, postural support, tonic neck and lumbar relexes, and more complex synergies such as rhythmic stepping (e.g., the reflex stepping of neonates). (For details, see Brodal and Baldineta et al.)

Also, there has now accumulated considerable information concerning the pharmacology of motor neurons. The large neurons of the anterior horns of the spinal cord contain high concentrations of choline acetyltransferase, and acetylcholine is their transmitter. Glycine is the neurotransmitter of the interneurons that mediate reciprocal inhibition during relex action. It is also the transmitter for Renshaw inhibitory cells. GABA is the inhibitory neurotransmitter of interneurons in the posterior horn. There are also glutaminergic and aspartergic pathways subserving

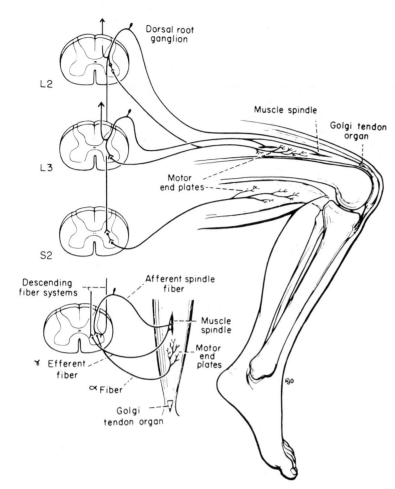

Figure 3-1

Patellar tendon reflex. Sensory fibers of the femoral nerve derived from spinal segments L2 and L3 mediate this myotatic reflex. The principal receptors are the muscle spindles, which respond to a brisk stretching of the muscle effected by tapping the patellar tendon. Afferent fibers from muscle spindles are shown entering only the L3 spinal segment, while afferent fibers from the Golgi tendon organ are shown entering only the L2 spinal segment. In this monosynaptic reflex, afferent fibers entering spinal segments L2 and L3 and efferent fibers issuing from the anterior horn cells of these and lower levels complete the reflex arc. Motor fibers shown leaving the S2 spinal segment and passing to the hamstring muscles demonstrate the disynaptic pathway by which inhibitory influences are exerted upon an antagonistic muscle group during the reflex.

The small diagram below illustrates the gamma loop. Gamma efferent fibers pass to the polar portions of the muscle spindle. Contractions of the intrafusal fibers in the polar parts of the spindle stretch the nuclear bag region and thus cause an afferent impulse to be conducted centrally. The afferent fibers from the spindle synapse with many alpha motor neurons, the peripheral processes of which pass to extrafusal muscle fibers, thus completing the loop. Both alpha and gamma motor neurons are influenced by descending fiber systems from supraspinal levels. (Redrawn from MB Carpenter and J Sutin, Human Neuroanatomy, 8th ed, Baltimore, Williams & Wilkins, 1983.)

excitatory functions in the spinal cord, as well as descending cholinergic, adrenergic, and dopaminergic axons which play a less well defined role in reflex functions.

PARALYSIS DUE TO DISEASE OF THE LOWER MOTOR NEURONS

If all or practically all peripheral motor fibers supplying a muscle are destroyed, all voluntary, postural, and reflex movements are abolished. The muscle becomes lax and soft and does not resist passive stretching, a condition known as *flaccidity*. Muscle tone—the slight resistance that normal relaxed muscle offers to passive movement—is reduced (*hypotonia* or *atonia*). The denervated muscle undergoes extreme atrophy, being reduced to 20 or 30 percent of its original bulk within 3 months. The reaction of the muscle to sudden stretch, as by tapping its tendon, is lost. If only a portion of the motor fibers supplying the muscle is affected, partial paralysis or paresis will ensue and the speed of contraction is also proportionately diminished. The atrophy will be less and the tendon reflex will be reduced instead of lost. The electrodiagnosis of denervation depends upon finding certain abnormalities of nerve conduction and fibrillations, fasciculations, and other abnormalities on needle electrode examination (see Chap. 45).

Lower motor neuron paralysis is the direct result of loss of function or destruction of anterior horn cells or their axons in anterior roots and nerves. The signs and symptoms vary according to the location of the lesion. Probably the most important question for clinical purposes is whether sensory changes coexist. The combination of flaccid, areflexic paralysis and sensory changes usually indicates in-

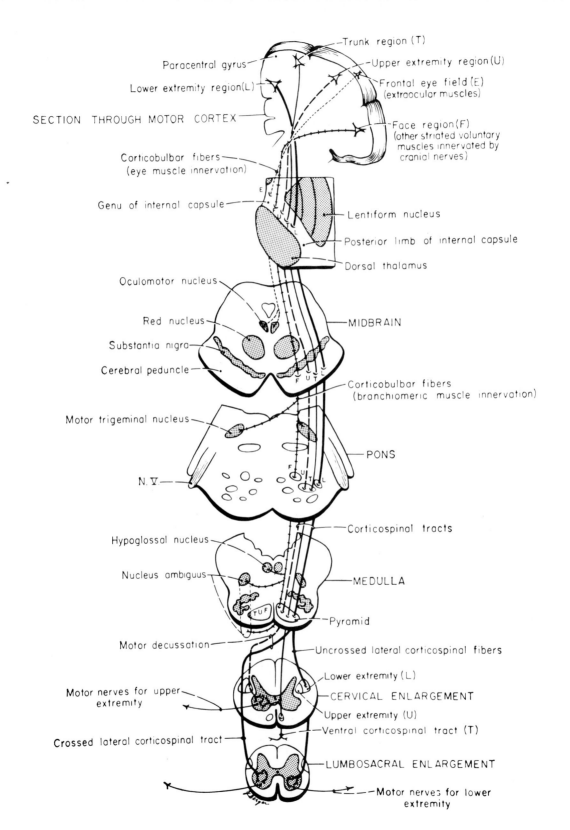

Trunk region (T)

Paracentral gyrus

Upper extremity region (U)

Lower extremity region (L)

Frontal eye field (E)
(extraocular muscles)

SECTION THROUGH MOTOR CORTEX

Face region (F)
(other striated voluntary
muscles innervated by
cranial nerves)

Corticobulbar fibers
(eye muscle innervation)

Genu of internal capsule

Lentiform nucleus

Posterior limb of internal capsule

Dorsal thalamus

Oculomotor nucleus

Red nucleus

MIDBRAIN

Substantia nigra

Cerebral peduncle

Corticobulbar fibers
(branchiomeric muscle innervation)

Motor trigeminal nucleus

PONS

N. V

Corticospinal tracts

Hypoglossal nucleus

Nucleus ambiguus

MEDULLA

Pyramid

Motor decussation

Uncrossed lateral corticospinal fibers

Lower extremity (L)

Motor nerves for upper
extremity

CERVICAL ENLARGEMENT

Upper extremity (U)

Crossed lateral corticospinal tract

Ventral corticospinal tract (T)

LUMBOSACRAL ENLARGEMENT

Motor nerves for lower
extremity

volvement of mixed motor and sensory nerves or affection of both anterior and posterior roots. If sensory changes are absent, the lesion must be situated in the anterior gray matter of the spinal cord, in the anterior roots, in a purely motor branch of a peripheral nerve, or in motor axons alone. At times it may be impossible to distinguish between nuclear (spinal) and anterior root (radicular) lesions. Preserved tendon reflexes and spasticity in muscles weakened by lesions of the corticospinal systems point to the integrity of the spianl segments below the level of the lesion.

AFFECTION OF THE CORTICOSPINAL (PYRAMIDAL), CORTICOBULBAR, AND OTHER UPPER MOTOR NEURONS

ANATOMIC AND PHYSIOLOGIC CONSIDERATIONS

The terms *pyramidal, corticospinal,* and *upper motor neuron* are often used interchangeably, but this is not altogether correct. The pyramidal tract, strictly speaking, refers only to those fibers which course longitudinally in the pyramid of the medulla oblongata. Of all the fiber bundles in the brain, the pyramidal tract has been known for the longest time, the first accurate description having been given by Türck in 1851. It descends from the cerebral cortex, traverses the internal capsule, basis pedunculi, basis pontis and the pyramid of the upper medulla, decussates in the lower medulla, and continues its caudal course in the lateral funiculus of the spinal cord; hence the alternate name, *corticospinal tract.* The corticospinal tract is the only *direct* long-fiber connection between the cerebral cortex and the spinal cord (Fig. 3-2). The other important *indirect* pathways, are the corticorubrospinal, corticoreticulospinal, corticovestibulospinal, and corticotectospinal which do not run in the pyramid and through which the cortex influences the spinal motor neurons. All of these pathways, direct and indirect are currently embraced by the term *upper motor neuron.* All of these descending corticofugal fibers utilize L-glutamate and aspartate as excitatory transmitters.

A major source of confusion about the pyramidal tract stems from the traditional view, formulated at the turn of the century, that it originates entirely from the large motor cells of Betz in the fifth layer of the precentral convolution, or area 4 of Brodmann (Fig. 3-3). However, there are only some 25,000 to 35,000 Betz cells, whereas the medullary pyramid contains about 1 million axons (Lassek). The pyramidal tract, therefore, must contain many fibers that arise from other cortical neurons, particularly those in area 4 and area 6 (the frontal cortex immediately rostral to area 4, including the posterior portion of the superior frontal gyrus, i.e. the supplementary motor area), in the primary somatosensory cortex (Brodmann's areas 3, 1, and 2), and in the superior parietal lobule (areas 5 and 7). The data concerning the origin of the pyramidal tract

Figure 3-3

Lateral (A) and medial (B) surfaces of the human cerebral hemispheres, showing the areas of excitable cortex. (Adapted from Foerster.)

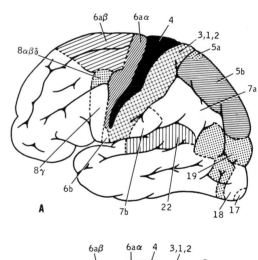

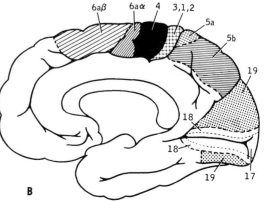

Figure 3-2

◀ *Corticospinal and corticobulbar tracts. The letters on the fiber tracts at various levels correspond to the letters which mark the origin of these fibers in the cortex. (From EC Crosby et al, Correlative Anatomy of the Nervous System, New York, Macmillan, 1962.)*

in humans are scanty, but in the monkey, counting the pyramidal axons that remained after cortical excisions and long survival periods, Russell and DeMyer found that 40 percent of the descending axons arose in the parietal lobe, 31 percent in area 4, and the remaining 29 percent in area 6.

The fibers from areas 4 and 6, the supplementary motor area, and portions of the parietal lobe (areas 1, 3, 5, and 7) converge in the corona radiata and descend through the posterior limb of the internal capsule, crus cerebri, basis pontis, and medulla. As the corticospinal tracts descend in the cerebrum and brainstem, they send collaterals to the striatum, thalamus, red nucleus, cerebellum, and reticular formations. Accompanying the corticospinal tract in the brainstem are the corticobulbar tracts, which are distributed to the motor nuclei of the cranial nerves, ipsilaterally and contralaterally. (Fig. 3-2). Insofar as the corticobulbar and corticospinal fibers have a similar origin and the motor nuclei of the brainstem are the homologues of the motor nuclei of the spinal cord, the term "upper motor neuron" may suitably be applied to both these systems of fibers.

The corticospinal tracts *decussate* at the lower end of the medulla, although some of their fibers may cross above this level. The proportion of crossed and uncrossed fibers varies greatly from one person to another. Most textbooks state that 75 percent of the fibers cross and that the remainder descend ipsilaterally, the latter being more or less equally divided between the lateral and ventral uncrossed corticospinal tracts. In exceptional cases, these tracts cross completely or, very rarely, remain uncrossed. These variations are probably of functional significance in determining the amount of neurologic deficit that results from unilateral lesions such as capsular infarction.

The corticospinal tracts and other upper motor neurons terminate mainly in relation to nerve cells in the intermediate zone of spinal gray matter (internuncial neurons), from which motor impulses are then transmitted to the anterior horn cells. Only 10 to 20 percent of corticospinal fibers (presumably the thick, rapidly conducting axons derived from Betz cells) establish direct synaptic connections with the large motor neurons of the anterior horns.

The *motor area of the cerebral cortex* is defined physiologically as the region of electrically excitable cortex from which isolated movements can be evoked by stimuli of minimal intensity (Fig. 3-3). The muscle groups of the contralateral face, arm, trunk, and leg are represented in the primary motor cortex (area 4), those of the face being in the most inferior part of the precentral gyrus on the lateral surface of the hemisphere and those of the leg in the

paracentral lobule on the medial surface of the cerebral hemisphere. The parts of the body capable of the most delicate movements have, in general, the largest cortical representation.

Area 6, the premotor area, is also electrically excitable, but requires more intense stimuli than area 4 to evoke movements. Stimulation of its caudal aspect (area 6a) produces responses that are similar to those elicited from area 4; these responses probably depend upon transmission of impulses to area 4 (since they cannot be obtained after ablation of this area) and discharge via the corticospinal tract. Stimulation of its rostral portion (area 6aβ) elicits more general movement patterns, which discharge via pathways other than those derived from area 4 ("extrapyramidal"). Very strong stimuli elicit movements from a wide area of premotor frontal and parietal cortex, and the same movements may be obtained from several widely separated points. From this it may be assumed that one of the functions of the motor cortex is to synthesize agonist actions into an infinite variety of finely graded, highly differentiated patterns.

Stimulation of the supplementary motor area (the most anterior portion of area 6 on the medial surface of the cerebral cortex, just anterior, or rostral to the primary motor cortex) may induce relatively gross homolateral or contralateral movements bilateral tonic contractions of the limbs, controversive movements of the head and eyes with tonic contraction of the contralateral arm, and sometimes inhibition of voluntary motor activity and vocal arrest. Presumably, much of the residual motor function following hemispherectomy depends on the ipsilateral innervation contributed by the supplementary motor area of the remaining hemisphere.

How the motor cortex controls movements is still a controversial matter. The traditional view, based on the interpretations of Hughlings Jackson and of Sherrington, is that the motor cortex is organized not in terms of individual muscles but in terms of movements, i.e., the coordinated contraction of groups of muscles. Jackson visualized a widely overlapping representation of muscle groups in the cerebral cortex, based on his observation that a patient could recover the use of the limb following destruction of the limb area as defined by cortical stimulation. This view was supported by Sherrington's observations that stimulation of the cortical surface activated not solitary muscles but a combination of muscles, and always in a reciprocal fashion, i.e., in a manner that maintained the expected relationship between agonists and antagonists. He noted also the inconstancy of stimulatory effects; the stimulation of a given cortical point which initiated flexion of a part at one time might initiate extension at another.

These interpretations must be viewed with circumspection, as must all observations that are based on the electrical stimulation of the surface of the cortex. It has been shown that to stimulate motor cells from the surface, the electric current has to penetrate the cortex to layer V, where the output neurons are located, inevitably activating a large number of cortical neurons. The elegant experiments of Evarts and of Asanuma and their colleagues, who stimulated the depths of the cortex with a microelectrode, have demonstrated the existence of discrete zones of efferent neurons which control the contraction of individual muscles; further stimulation of a given efferent zone often facilitates rather than inhibits the contraction of the antagonists. They have shown also that cells in the efferent zone receive afferent impulses from the particular muscle to which the efferent neurons project. When the effects of many stimulations at various depths were correlated with the exact sites of each penetration, it was found that the cells which projected to a particular pool of spinal motoneurons were arranged in a radially aligned column, about 1 mm in diameter. The columnar arrangement of cells in the motor-sensory cortex has been appreciated for many years and the wealth of radial interconnections between the cells in these columns led Lorente de Nó to suggest that these ''vertical chains'' of cells were the elementary functional units of the cortex. On the sensory side, this notion received strong support from Mountcastle's discovery that the neurons in somatic sensory columns all receive impulses of the same sensory modality from the same part of the body. In regard to the functional organization of the motor columns, it is still not entirely clear whether they contribute to a movement as units or whether individual cells within many columns are selectively activated to produce a movement. The evidence for these disparate views has been summarized by Henneman and by Asanuma.

The role of cerebral-cortical motoneurons in sensory-evoked or planned movement has been elucidated by Evarts and his colleagues. Using single cell recording techniques they showed that the pyramidal cells fire about 60 ms prior to the onset of movement in a sequence determined by the required pattern and force of the movement. But other more complex properties of the pyramidal cells were also noted. Some of them received a somatosensory input transcortically from the parietal lobe (areas 3, 1, and 2), which could be turned on or off or gated according to whether the movement was to be controlled, i.e., guided by sensory input. Many neurons were utilized in a ''set discharge'' that preceded (anticipated) the planned movement. Thus motor neurons were prepared for the oncoming activation, i.e., they were triggered by a number of sensory transcortical inputs from the parietal, prefrontal, premotor and the auditory and visual areas of the cortex. This set signal could occur in the absence of any segmental activity in the spinal cord and muscles. The source of this ''set signal'' was found to be in the supplementary motor cortex which appears to be under the direct influence of the instructing stimuli reaching it from the prefrontal and parietal cortices. The blood flow to each of the cortical motor zones increases with their increase in synaptic activity, and its measurement has been used to follow the neural events (Roland, 1984).

Thus the prefrontal cortex, supplementary motor cortex, premotor cortex, and motor cortex are all responsive to various sensory stimuli and are involved in set discharges prior to and in coordinated fashion during a complex movement. And, as will be remarked later on, the strio-pallidum and cerebellum, which project to these cortical areas, are also activated prior to or concurrently with the discharge of corticospinal neurons.

The termination of the corticospinal and other descending motor tracts has been studied in the monkey by interrupting these pathways in the medulla and more rostral parts of the brainstem and tracing the distribution of the degenerating elements in the spinal gray matter. On the basis of such experiments and a considerable body of physiologic data, Kuypers has suggested that the functional organization of the descending cortical and subcortical pathways is determined more by their patterns of termination and the motor capacities of the internuncial neurons upon which they terminate than by the location of their cells of origin. On the basis of their differential terminal distribution, three groups of motor fibers can be distinguished: (1) A ventromedial pathway, which arises in the tectum, vestibular nuclei, and pontine and medullary reticular cells and terminates principally on the internuncial cells of the ventromedial part of the spinal gray matter. This system is mainly concerned with axial movements—the maintenance of posture, integrated movements of body and limbs, and total-limb movements. (2) A lateral pathway, which is derived mainly from the magnocellular part of the red nucleus and terminates in the dorsal and lateral parts of the internuncial zone. This pathway adds the capacity for independent use of the extremities, especially of the hands. (3) The corticospinal pathway, the major portion of which terminates diffusely throughout the nucleus proprius of the dorsal horn and the intermediate zone and greatly amplifies the control of hand movements. This portion of the corticospinal projection arises from the sensory cortex and appears to function in the control of afferent projection neurons. In addition, a portion of the corticospinal tract synapses directly with the large motor neurons that innervate the distal parts of the extremities, face, and tongue; this system provides the capacity for a high degree of fractionation of movements, as exemplified by independent finger movements.

PARALYSIS DUE TO DISEASE OF THE UPPER MOTOR NEURONS

The corticospinal pathways may be interrupted by lesions at many levels, including the cerebral cortex, subcortical white matter, internal capsule, brainstem, and spinal cord. Practically always, when paralysis is severe and permanent as a consequence of disease, much more is involved than the long, uninterrupted corticospinal pathway. In the cerebral white matter (corona radiata) and internal capsule the corticospinal fibers are intermingled with corticostriate, corticothalamic, corticorubral, corticopontine, cortico-olivary, and corticoreticular fibers. It is noteworthy that thalamocortical fibers, which are a vital link in an ascending fiber system from the basal ganglia and cerebellum, also pass through the internal capsule and cerebral white matter. Thus lesions in these parts simultaneously affect both corticospinal and extrapyramidal systems. The terms *corticospinal* and *pyramidal* as designations for the spastic hemiplegia that results from a capsular lesion are misnomers, therefore. *Upper motor neuron paralysis* is a more suitable term, provided that it is used in a collective sense, indicating involvement of the collaterals of the pyramids and the several other descending fiber systems that influence and modify the lower motor neuron.

In primates, lesions limited to area 4, the motor cortex, cause hypotonia and weakness of the distal limb muscles; there is no spasticity. Lesions of the premotor cortex (area 6) result in spasticity and increased stretch reflexes. Lesions of the supplementary motor cortex, which is believed to have an inhibitory effect on the motor cortex, lead to involuntary grasping. Since it has a major role in motor programming, lesions here may also be responsible for some of the akinesia and mutism seen in striatal disease (major output of basal ganglia is directed to the sensorimotor cortex, via the thalamus). These clinical effects have not been as clearly defined in humans. Removal of cortical areas 4 and 6 for relief of epilepsy causes complete and permanent paralysis and spasticity (Laplane et al).

The one place where corticospinal fibers are isolated as the pyramidal tract is in the medullary pyramids. In humans there are a few documented cases of a lesion more or less confined to this locality (see Ropper et al). The result of such lesions has been a flaccid hemiplegia (with sparing of the face), from which there is considerable recovery. Similarly in monkeys, as shown by Tower in 1940, and more recently by Lawrence and Kuypers, and by Gilman and Marco, interruption of both pyramidal tracts results in a hypotonic paralysis; ultimately these animals recover control over a wide range of movements, though slowness of all movements and loss of individual finger movements remain as permanent deficits. Also, the cerebral peduncle has been sectioned in patients in an effort to abolish involuntary movements (Bucy et al); in some patients a slight degree of weakness or only a Bakinski sign was produced but no spasticity developed. These observations and the ones in monkeys indicate that a pure pyramidal tract lesion does not result in spasticity and that control over a wide range of voluntary movements depends at least in part on nonpyramidal motor pathways. Animal experiments suggest that the corticorubrospinal and corticoreticulospinal pathways are particularly important in this respect, since their fibers are arranged somatotopically and are able to influence stretch reflexes. Further studies of human material are necessary to settle problems related to volitional movement and spasticity. The motor organization of the cat and even of the monkey is so different from that of humans and the range of volitional activity and motor skills so much less that direct comparisons are not justified.

The distribution of the paralysis due to upper motor neuron lesions varies with the locale of the lesion, but certain features are characteristic of all of them. A group of muscles is always involved, never individual muscles, and if any movement is possible, the proper relationships between agonists, antagonists, synergists, and fixators are preserved. The paralysis never involves all the muscles on one side of the body, even in the severest forms of hemiplegia. Movements that are invariably bilateral, such as those of the eyes, jaw, pharynx, larynx, neck, thorax, and abdomen, are little if at all affected. Upper motor neuron paralysis is rarely complete for any long period of time; in this respect it differs from the absolute paralysis due to destruction of anterior horn cells or interruption of their axons.

Upper motor neuron lesions are characterized further by certain peculiarities of residual movement. There is decreased voluntary drive on spinal motor neurons (fewer motor units recruitable and their firing rates are slower). Single motor units are less variable in the intervals between discharges. There is an increased degree of cocontraction of antagonistic muscles reflected in the decreased rate of rapid alternating movements. Another phenomenon is the activation of paralyzed muscles as parts of certain automatisms (synkinesias). The paralyzed arm may suddenly move during yawning and stretching. Attempts by the patient to move the hemiplegic limbs may result in a variety of associated movements. Thus, flexion of the arm may result in involuntary pronation; flexion of the leg may cause the foot to dorsiflex and evert automatically. Also, attempted volitional movements of the normal limb may evoke imitative (mirror) movements in the paretic one or vice versa. In some patients, as they recover from hemiplegia, a variety of movement abnormalities emerge, such as hemitremor, hemiataxia, hemiathetosis, and hemichorea. These are expressions of damage to a number of basal ganglionic and thalamic structures and will be discussed in Chap. 4.

If the upper motor neurons are interrupted above the level of the facial colliculus in the pons, hand and arm muscles suffer most severely and the leg muscles next; of the cranial musculature only the muscles of the tongue and lower part of the face are involved to any significant degree. Broadbent was the first to call attention to this distribution of paralysis, sometimes referred to as ''Broadbent's law.'' At lower levels, such as the cervical cord, acute lesions of the upper motor neuron may cause not only a paralysis of voluntary movement but also abolish temporarily the spinal reflexes subserved by segments below the lesion. This condition is referred to as *spinal shock.* After a few days to weeks the flaccidity and areflexia give way to a state of excessive muscular tonus (hypertonus) and heightened stretch reflexes, a phenomenon known as *spasticity* (see below). This sequence of changes is not sharply defined in cerebral lesions but is typical of spinal ones. With some acute cerebral lesions, spasticity and paralysis develop together; in others the limbs remain flaccid but reflexes are retained.

A predilection for involvement of certain muscle groups, a specific pattern of response to stretch (resistance increases linearly in relation to velocity of stretch), and manifestly exaggerated tendon reflexes are the identifying characteristics of spasticity. The antigravity muscles— flexors of the arms and the extensors of the legs—are predominantly affected. The arm tends to assume a flexed and pronated position and the leg an extended and adducted one, indicating that certain spinal neurons are reflexly more active than others. At rest, with the muscles shortened to midposition, they are flaccid to palpation and electromyographically silent. If the arm is extended or the leg flexed very slowly, there may be little or no change in muscle tone. In contrast, if the muscles are stretched rapidly, the limb moves freely for a very short distance, beyond which there is an abrupt catch and then a rapidly increasing muscular resistance up to a point; thereafter, as the passive extension of the arm or flexion of the leg continues, the resistance melts away. This sequence constitutes the classical ''clasp-knife'' phenomenon. With the limb in the extended or flexed position, a new passive movement may not encounter the same sequence; this whole combination constitutes the lengthening and shortening reaction. Thus the essential feature of spasticity is an increased reactivity to a stretch stimulus.

Until recently it was taught that the heightened phasic and tonic myotatic or stretch reflexes of the spastic state are a ''release'' phenomenon, the result of interruption of descending inhibitory pathways. This appears to be only half the story. Animal experiments have demonstrated that

spasticity (and decerebrate rigidity, see Chap. 16) are due not only to the removal of inhibitory influences. These states are mediated through spindle afferents (increased tonic activity of gamma motoneurons) and, centrally, through reticulospinal and vestibulospinal pathways that act mainly on alpha motoneurons. The clasp-knife phenomenon appears to derive from lesions (or presumably a change in central control) of a specific portion of the reticulospinal system.

Although a clasp-knife relaxation following peak resistance is highly characteristic of cerebral hemiplegia, it is by no means constantly present. In some cases, the arm flexors and leg extensors are spastic, while the antagonist muscles show an even resistance throughout the range of passive movement, i.e., rigidity (Chap. 4); or rigidity may be more prominent than spasticity in all muscles. This plastic resistance, in Denny-Brown's view, is the mild form or precursor of the altered posture or attitude that he called dystonia, a feature that he considered to be characteristic of hemiplegic spasticity. Nor is there a constant relationship between spasticity and weakness. In some cases, severe weakness may be associated with only the mildest signs of spasticity, detectable as a ''catch'' in the pronators on passive supination of the forearm and in the flexors of the hand on extension of the wrist. Contrariwise, the most extreme degrees of spasticity, observed in certain cases of cervical spinal cord disease, may so vastly exceed paresis of voluntary movement as to suggest that these two states depend on separate mechanisms. Indeed, the selective blocking of small gamma neurons is said to abolish spasticity as well as hyperactive segmental tendon jerks, but to leave motor performance unchanged.

The hyperreflexic state that characterizes spasticity often takes the form of *clonus,* a series of rhythmic involuntary muscular contractions, occurring at a frequency of 5 to 7 Hz, in response to an abruptly applied and sustained stretch stimulus. It is usually designated in terms of the part of the limb to which the stimulus is applied (e.g., patella, ankle). The frequency is constant within 1 Hz and is not appreciably modified by altering peripheral or central nervous system activities. Clonus depends for its elicitation on the degree of voluntary relaxation of appropriate muscles, integrity of the spinal stretch reflex mechanisms, sustained hyperexcitability of alpha and gamma motor neurons (suprasegmental effects), and synchronization of the contraction-relaxation cycle of muscle spindles (see Dimitrijevic et al). The cutaneomuscular abdominal and cremasteric reflexes are usually abolished in these circumstances, and a Babinski sign is usually, but not invariably, present.

Irradiation or *spread of reflexes* is regularly associated with the spastic state, although this phenomenon may be observed in normal persons with brisk tendon reflexes. Tapping the radial periosteum, for example, may elicit a reflex contraction not only of the brachioradialis but also of the biceps or triceps and finger flexors. This spreading of reflexes is probably not due to an irradiation of impulses in the spinal cord, as is often taught, but can be accounted for by the propagation of a vibration wave from bone to muscle, stimulating the excitable muscle spindles in its path (Lance). Also reflexes may be "inverted" as in the case of a lesion of the fifth or sixth cervical segments; here the biceps and brachioradialis reflexes are abolished and only the triceps and finger flexors, whose reflex arcs are intact, respond to the radial tap. This mechanism probably explains other manifestations of the hyperreflexic state, such as the Hoffmann sign and the crossed adductor reflex of the thigh muscles.

There have been but few investigations of the biochemical changes in spinal segments which underlie spasticity. Since glutamic acid is the neurotransmitter of the corticospinal tracts, one would expect its action on inhibitory interneurons to be lost. GABA, the inhibitory transmitter of interneurons, has not been measured in the spastic state. Baclofen is thought to act on a specific subtype of GABA receptor, inhibiting glutamate release from supersensitive glutamate receptors, but this notion is still speculative. Actually, baclofen has not been an effective drug in the treatment of spasticity. Glycine, the other inhibitory neurotransmitter in the spinal cord, is measurably reduced in quantity, uptake, and turnover in the spastic animal, and there is some evidence that infusions of glycine reduce spasticity (Davidoff). The changes resulting from interruption of cholinergic, dopaminergic, and noradrenergic fibers and their role in spasticity are unknown.

In addition to hyperactive *phasic myotatic reflexes,* ("tendon jerks"), certain lesions, particularly of the cervical segments of the spinal cord, may result in great enhancement of *tonic myotatic reflexes.* These are stretch reflexes in which a stimulus produces a prolonged asynchronous discharge of motor neurons, causing sustained muscle contraction. In standing or attempting voluntary movement, the entire limb becomes involved in intense muscular spasm that may last for several minutes. During this period the limb is quite useless. Presumably there is both an interruption of bulbar inhibitory influences on the anterior horn cells and a release of the facilitatory effects needed in antigravity support (Henneman).

The *nociceptive spinal flexion reflexes,* of which the Babinski sign is a part, are not an essential component of spasticity. They, too, are exaggerated because of disinhi-

bition or release in cases of paraparesis or paraplegia of spinal origin. Important characteristics of these responses are their capacity to be induced by weak superficial stimuli (such as a series of pinpricks) and their tendency to persist long after the stimulation ceases. In its most complete form a nocifensive flexor synergy involves flexion of the knee and hip (tensor fascia lata) and dorsiflexion of the foot and big toe. It may be fractionated in incomplete suprasegmental lesions. For example the hip and knee may flex but the foot may not dorsiflex, or vice versa.

With bilateral cerebral lesions, exaggerated stretch reflexes can be elicited in cranial as well as in limb and trunk muscles, because of interruption of the corticobulbar pathways. In advanced cases this takes the form of spastic bulbar ("pseudobulbar") paralysis, characterized by dysarthria, dysphonia, dysphagia, and bifacial weakness (see pages 390 and 414).

Table 3-1 summarizes the main attributes of upper motor neuron lesions and contrasts them with those of the lower motor neurons.

APRAXIA AND OTHER NONPARALYTIC DISORDERS OF MOTOR FUNCTION

All that has been said about the cortical and spinal control of the motor system gives one little idea of human motility.

Table 3-1
Differences between upper and lower motor neuron paralysis

Upper motor neuron or supranuclear paralysis	Lower motor neuron or nuclear-infranuclear paralysis
Muscles affected in groups, never individual muscles	Individual muscles may be affected
Atrophy slight and due to disuse	Atrophy pronounced, up to 70 to 80% of total bulk
Spasticity with hyperactivity of the tendon reflexes and extensor plantar reflex (Babinski sign)	Flaccidity and hypotonia of affected muscles with loss of tendon reflexes. Plantar reflex, if present, is of normal flexor type
Fascicular twitches absent	Fascicular twitches may be present
Normal nerve conduction studies; no denervation potentials in EMG	Abnormal nerve conduction studies; denervation potentials (fibrillations, fasciculations, positive sharp waves) in EMG

Viewed objectively, the conscious and sentient human organism is continuously active—fidgeting, adjusting posture and position, sitting, standing, walking, running, speaking, manipulating tools, or performing the intricate sequences of movements involved in athletic or musical activity. Some of these activities are relatively simple, automatic, and stereotyped. Others have been learned and mastered by great conscious effort and through practice have become habitual, i.e., reduced to an automatic level. Still others are complex and voluntary, parts of a carefully formulated plan, and demand continuous attention and thought. What is more remarkable, one can be occupied in several of these variably conscious and habitual activities simultaneously, such as driving through heavy traffic while lighting a cigarette and engaging in animated conversation. Moreover, when an obstacle prevents a sequence of movements from accomplishing its goal, a new sequence can be undertaken automatically for this purpose. These activities represent the third and highest level of motor function in the scheme of Jackson, the activities of the motor cortex and spinal neurons being the second and first levels.

How is all this made possible? Neuropsychologists, studying patients with lesions of different parts of the cerebrum, tell us that the planning of complex activities, conceptualizing their final purpose, and continuous modification of the individual components of a motor sequence until the goal is achieved are under the control of the frontal lobes. Every intended action sets the stage for the movement sequence by first activating "set neurons" in the premotor and motor cortices, caudate and lenticular nuclei, the cerebellum, and brainstem reticular formation. Frontal lesions have the effect of reducing the impulse to think, speak, and act ("cortical tone," to use Luria's expression, is reduced), and a complex activity will not be initiated or sustained long enough to permit its completion. Some have called a defect at this level *ideational apraxia,* a term which the authors consider ambiguous, and incorrect because such disintegrations of complex motor sequences and the substitution of echopraxic and stereotyped patterns parallel many nonmotor deficits of human behavior, as will be explained in several subsequent chapters (Sec. 5).

There is, however, another level of disordered motility for which the term *apraxia* is more appropriate. In this state, a patient with no weakness, no ataxia or other extrapyramidal derangement, and no loss of the primary modes of sensation, loses the ability to execute previously learned skills and gestures. This was the meaning given apraxia by Liepmann, who introduced the term in 1900. It was his view, on the basis of careful case study, that apraxia could be subdivided into three types—ideational, ideomotor, and kinetic. His anatomic data indicated that planned or commanded action is normally developed in the parietal lobe of the dominant hemisphere, where visual, auditory, and kinesthetic information is integrated. Presumably the

formation of engrams of skilled movement depends on the integrity of this part of the brain, and if it is damaged, planned action cannot be formulated. There results an *ideational apraxia*, a view earlier advanced by Pick. From this region there are connections, possibly via the arcuate fasciculus, with the supplementary and premotor cortices of both cerebral hemispheres, wherein the innervatory patterns of movement are initiated. The patient knows and remembers the planned action but because of a disconnection cannot execute it with either hand. This was Liepmann's concept of ideomotor apraxia. *Kinetic limb apraxia*, a condition studied more by Kleist than Liepmann, refers to a clumsiness and maladroitness of a limb in the performance of a skilled act that cannot be accounted for by paresis, ataxia, or other abnormality of movement.

These high-order abnormalities of learned movement patterns have several unique features. Seldom are they evident to the patient himself and therefore are not sources of complaint. For this reason they are often overlooked by the examining physician. Their evocation requires special types of testing which may be interfered with by the condition of the patient. Obviously, if he is confused or aphasic, spoken or written requests to perform an act will not be understood and one must find ways of persuading him to initiate the movements of the examiner. Many of the common tests such as waving good-bye, blowing a kiss, shaking a fist, or saluting are intransitive gestures and are more symbolic than practical. The patient may fail in their execution and yet have no difficulty with habitual actions. In the same vein, requests to demonstrate the imaginary use of common utensils such as "show me how you would brush your teeth, comb your hair, hammer a nail" may result in failure, whereas the patient may later have no difficulty with the real task.

In a practical sense, the lesions responsible for ideomotor apraxia of both arms usually reside in the left parietal region; only a small percentage of right-handed individuals have right parietal lesions. Kertesz et al have provided evidence that separate lesions are responsible for aphasia and apraxia, though the two conditions are not infrequently associated. Surprisingly there are but few cases of ideomotor apraxia with proven premotor lesions. Uncertain still is the exact location of the parietal lesion, whether subcortical or cortical. Geschwind accepted Liepman's proposition that a lesion of a subcortical tract (presumably the arcuate fasciculus) disconnects the parietal from the frontal cortex, accounting for the ideomotor apraxia of the right limbs, and that the left limb apraxia is due to a disconnection of the left and right premotor cortices. In a right-handed person, the lesion that gives rise to a left limb apraxia is usually in the left frontal lobe and includes Broca's area and the left motor cortex. Clinically there is a speech disorder, a right hemiparesis, and apraxia of the nonparalyzed hand, i.e., "sympathetic apraxia," the lesion having separated the language areas from the right motor cortex but not from the left. Such patients can write with the right hand but not with the left. They may write correctly with the right hand and aphasically with the left. That such a syndrome depends upon a disconnection of a pathway that traverses the genu of the corpus callosum, as depicted by Geschwind, is questionable, insofar as it has not been observed in patients subjected to total callosotomy (for the treatment of intractable epilepsy). The disconnection syndromes are discussed further in Chaps. 21 and 22.

Facial apraxia is probably the most common of all apraxias. It may occur with lesions that undercut the left supramarginal gyrus or the left motor association cortex and may be associated with apraxia of the limbs. Such patients are unable to carry out facial movements to command (lick the lips, blow out a match, etc.), although they may do better when asked to imitate the examiner or when holding a lighted match. With lesions that are restricted to the facial area of the left motor cortex, the apraxia will be limited to the facial musculature and may be associated with a so-called verbal apraxia or cortical dysarthria (page 387). So-called apraxia of gait will be considered in Chap.6, "Disorders of Stance and Gait."

Testing for apraxia is carried out in several ways. First, one observes the actions of the patient as he engages in such tasks as dressing, washing, shaving, and using eating utensils. Second, he is asked to wave good-bye, shake his fist as though angry, salute, and blow a kiss—symbolic acts. Third, if he fails, he is asked to imitate the examiner, who performs these acts. Finally he is asked to show how he would hammer a nail, brush his teeth, comb his hair, and so forth, or to execute a complex series of acts, such as lighting and smoking a cigarette or opening and drinking a bottle of beer. The latter are tests of ideational apraxia, the others of ideomotor apraxia, using first auditory and then visual signals. To perform these tasks in the absence of the tool or utensil is always more demanding, because the patient must formulate a plan of action rather than engage in a habitual motor sequence. There may be failure in a commanded or suggested activity (e.g., to take a pipe out of his pocket), yet a few minutes later the patient may perform the same motor sequence automatically.

One may think of such a motor deficit, if it can be singled out, as a kind of amnesia for certain learned patterns of movement, analogous to the amnesia for words in aphasia.

Of course, the physician must always be certain that a failure to follow a spoken or written request is not due to an aphasia that prevents understanding of what is asked, or to an agnosia that prevents recognition of the tool or object to be used. And the presence of mental confusion may obscure an apraxia. Children with cerebral diseases that retard mental development are unable to learn the sequences of movement required in hopping, jumping over a barrier, hitting or kicking a ball, or dancing. They suffer a developmental motor apraxia. Certain tests quantitate failure in these age-linked motor skills (see Chap. 27).

In the authors' opinion, the time-honored division of apraxia into kinetic, ideokinetic or ideomotor, and ideational types is confusing and not useful clinically. It is more helpful to think of the various types in an anatomic sense, as disorders of association between different parts of the cerebral cortex as described above. We have been unable with confidence to separate ideomotor from ideational apraxia. The patient with a severe ideomotor apraxia always has difficulty at the ideational level, shown best in the attempted execution of a complex series of actions. Furthermore, in view of the complexity of the motor system, we are frequently uncertain whether clumsiness of a hand in performing a motor skill represents a kinetic apraxia or some other fault in the intrinsic organization of hand control.

Finally it should be remarked that the complexity of motor activity is almost beyond imagination. Reference was made above to the reciprocal innervation involved in "making a fist." But what is involved in playing a piano concerto? Over a century ago Hughlings Jackson commented that "There are, we shall say over thirty muscles in the hand; these are represented in the nervous centers in thousands of different combinations, that is, as very many movements; it is just as many chords, musical expressions and tunes can be made out of a few notes." The effectuation of these complex movements, many of them learned and habituated, is made possible by the cooperative activities of the basal ganglia, cerebellum, reticular formation of the brainstem, and sensory and motor spinal neurons. All are continuously integrated and controlled by feedback mechanisms. Even the spinal stretch reflex has connections with the motor cortex. These points already touched upon in this chapter will be elaborated in Chaps. 4 and 5.

DIFFERENTIAL DIAGNOSIS OF PARALYSIS

The diagnostic considerations of paralysis may be simplified by the following subdivision, based on the location and distribution of weakness.

1. *Monoplegia* refers to weakness or paralysis of all the muscles of one limb, whether the leg or arm. It should

not be applied to paralysis of isolated muscles or groups of muscles supplied by a single nerve or motor root.

2. *Hemiplegia* is the commonest form of paralysis, involving arm, leg, and sometimes face on one side of the body.

3. *Paraplegia* indicates weakness or paralysis of both legs. It is most commonly the result of spinal cord disease.

4. *Quadriplegia* or *tetraplegia* indicates weakness of all four extremities. It may result from lesions involving the peripheral nerves, the gray matter of the spinal cord, or the upper motor neurons bilaterally in the cervical cord, brainstem, or cerebrum. *Diplegia* is a special form of quadriplegia in which the legs are affected more than the arms.

5. Isolated paralysis of one or more muscle groups.

6. Nonparalytic disorders of movement.

7. Hysterical paralysis.

8. Muscular paralysis without visible changes in nerve and muscle.

MONOPLEGIA

The examination of patients who complain of weakness of one extremity often discloses an asymptomatic weakness of another limb, and the condition is actually a hemiparesis or paraparesis. Or instead of weakness of all the muscles in a limb, only isolated groups are found to be affected. Ataxia, sensory disturbances, or pain in an extremity will often be interpreted by the patient as weakness, as will the rigidity or bradykinesia of parkinsonism or the mechanical limitation resulting from arthritis and bursitis.

In general, the presence or absence of atrophy of muscles in a monoplegic limb is of particular diagnostic help, as indicated below.

Monoplegia without Muscular Atrophy This is due most often to a lesion of the cerebral cortex. Only occasionally does it occur in diseases that interrupt the motor pathways at the level of the internal capsule, brainstem, or spinal cord. A vascular lesion (thrombotic or embolic infarction) is the commonest cause, and of course, a circumscribed tumor or abscess may have the same effect. Multiple sclerosis and spinal cord tumor, early in their course, may cause weakness of one extremity, usually the leg. Weakness due to a lesion of the upper motor neuron is usually accompanied by spasticity, increased reflexes, and an extensor plantar reflex (Babinski sign); exceptionally a lesion of the motor cortex does not result in spasticity. In either event, nerve conduction studies are normal. Also, acute destruction of the motor tracts in the spinal cord may

at first (for several days) reduce tendon reflexes and cause hypotonia (spinal shock). The latter does not occur with partial or slowly evolving lesions and only to a slight degree, if at all, with lesions of the brainstem and cerebrum. In acute diseases of the lower motor neurons the tendon reflexes are always reduced or abolished, but atrophy may not appear for several weeks. Hence, before reaching an anatomic diagnosis one must take into account the mode of onset and the duration of the disease.

Monoplegia with Muscular Atrophy This is more frequent than monoplegia without muscular atrophy. Long-continued disuse of a limb may lead to atrophy, but it is usually of lesser degree than atrophy due to lower motor neuron disease. In disuse atrophy, the tendon reflexes are retained and nerve conduction studies are normal. In diseases that denervate muscles, in addition to paralysis and reduced or abolished tendon reflexes, there may be visible fasciculations. If the limb is partially denervated, the electromyogram shows reduced numbers of motor unit potentials (often of large size), as well as fasciculations and fibrillations. The location of the lesion (whether it is due to nerve, spinal root, or spinal cord involvement) can usually be determined by the pattern of weakness, by the associated neurologic symptoms and signs, and by special tests (cerebrospinal fluid examination, roentgenogram of the spine, electrical studies of nerve and muscle, and myelogram).

Atrophic brachial monoplegia is relatively rare; when present in an infant, it should suggest brachial plexus trauma; in a child, poliomyelitis or other viral infection; and in an adult, poliomyelitis, syringomyelia, amyotrophic lateral sclerosis, or a brachial plexus lesion. Crural monoplegia is more frequent and may be caused by any lesion of the thoracic or lumbar cord, i.e., trauma, tumor, myelitis, multiple sclerosis, etc. Multiple sclerosis rarely causes severe atrophy, and a prolapsed intervertebral disc and the several varieties of mononeuropathy almost never paralyze all or most of the muscles of a limb. A unilateral retroperitoneal tumor may paralyze the leg by implicating the lumbosacral plexus.

HEMIPLEGIA

This is the most frequent form of paralysis in humans. With rare exceptions (a few unusual cases of poliomyelitis or motor system disease), this pattern of paralysis is due to involvement of the corticospinal pathways.

Location of Lesion Producing Hemiplegia The site or level of the lesion, i.e., cerebral cortical, capsular, brainstem, or spinal cord, can usually be deduced from the associated neurologic findings. Diseases localized to the cerebral cortex, cerebral white matter (corona radiata), and internal capsule usually manifest themselves by weakness or paralysis of the face, arm, and leg on the opposite side. The occurrence of convulsive seizures or the presence of a language disorder (aphasia), a loss of discriminative sensation (astereognosis, impairment of tactile localization, etc.), anosognosia, or a homonymous defect in the visual fields suggest a cortical or subcortical location.

Damage to the corticospinal and corticobrainstem tracts in the upper portion of the brainstem (see Fig. 3-2) also causes paralysis of the face, arm, and leg of the opposite side. The lesion in such cases is localized by the presence of a third nerve palsy (Weber syndrome) or other segmental abnormalities on the same side as the lesion. Unilateral lesions of the upper part of the basis pontis have been shown by Fisher to cause a contralateral ataxic hemiplegia, i.e., cerebellar ataxia on the same side as the signs of corticospinal deficit. With low pontine lesions a unilateral abducens or facial palsy is combined with a contralateral weakness or paralysis of the arm and leg (Millard-Gubler syndrome). Lesions in the medulla affect the tongue and sometimes the pharynx and larynx on one side and the arm and leg on the other. These ''crossed paralyses,'' so characteristic of brainstem lesions, are described further in Chap. 46.

Even lower in the medulla, a unilateral infarct in the pyramid causes a flaccid paralysis followed by slight spasticity of the contralateral arm and leg, with sparing of the face and tongue. Some motor function may be retained, as happened in the case of Ropper et al; interestingly, in their patient and in three others previously reported, there was considerable recovery of voluntary power even though the pyramid was almost completely destroyed.

Rarely, a homolateral hemiplegia may be caused by a lesion in the lateral column of the cervical spinal cord. At this level, however, the pathologic process more often induces bilateral signs, with resulting quadriparesis or quadriplegia. Homolateral paralysis, if combined with a loss of vibratory and position sense on the same side and a contralateral loss of pain and temperature, signifies disease of one side of the spinal cord (*Brown-Séquard syndrome*).

As indicated above, the muscle atrophy that follows upper motor neuron lesions never reaches the proportions seen in diseases of the lower motor neuron. The atrophy in the former cases is due to disuse. When the motor cortex and adjacent parts of the parietal lobe are damaged in infancy or childhood, the normal development of the muscles and the skeletal system in the affected limbs is retarded. The limbs and even the trunk are smaller on the one side than on the other. This does not occur if the paralysis occurs after puberty, by which time the greater part of skeletal growth has been attained. In hemiplegia due to spinal cord lesions, muscles at the level of the lesion may atrophy as a result of damage to anterior horn cells or ventral roots.

In the causation of hemiplegia, vascular diseases of the cerebrum and brainstem exceed all others in frequency. Trauma (brain contusion, epidural and subdural hemorrhage) ranks second. Other important causes, in order of frequency, are brain tumor, brain abscess, demyelinative diseases, and complications of meningitis and encephalitis. Most of these diseases can be recognized by their mode of evolution and the conjoined clinical and laboratory findings, which are presented in the chapters on neurologic diseases. Alternating transitory hemiparesis may be due to a special type of migraine (see discussion in Chap. 9).

PARAPLEGIA

Paralysis of both lower extremities may occur with diseases of the spinal cord, spinal roots, or peripheral nerves. If the onset is acute, it may be difficult to distinguish spinal from neuropathic paralysis because the element of spinal shock may result in abolition of reflexes and flaccidity. In acute spinal cord diseases with involvement of corticospinal tracts, the paralysis or weakness affects all muscles below a given level; and often, if the white matter is extensively damaged, sensory loss below a particular level is conjoined (loss of pain and temperature sense due to spinothalamic tract damage, and loss of vibratory and position sense due to posterior column involvement). Also, in bilateral disease of the spinal cord, the bladder and bowel may be paralyzed. Alterations of the CSF (dynamic block, increase in protein or cells) are frequent. In peripheral nerve diseases, motor loss tends to involve the distal muscles of the legs more than the proximal ones (exceptions are certain varieties of acute idiopathic polyneuritis and diabetic neuropathy), and sphincteric function is usually spared or impaired only transiently. Sensory loss, if present, is also more prominent in the distal segments of the limbs. The CSF protein level may be normal or elevated.

For clinical purposes it is helpful to separate the acute paraplegias from the chronic ones and to divide the latter into two groups—those which occur in infancy and those which begin in adult life.

The most common cause of acute paraplegia (or quadriplegia, if the cervical cord is involved) is spinal cord trauma, usually combined with fracture-dislocation of the spine. Spontaneous hematomyelia due to a vascular malformation, thrombosis of the anterior spinal artery, or occlusion of a spinal branch of the aorta (due to dissecting aneurysm or atheroma) with resulting infarction (myelomalacia) are less common causes. Paraplegia or quadriplegia due to postinfectious or postvaccinial myelitis, acute demyelinative or necrotizing myelopathy, and epidural abscess or tumor with spinal cord compression tend to develop somewhat more slowly, over a period of hours or days, or longer. Epidural or subdural hemorrhage from bleeding diseases or warfarin therapy has caused acute paraplegia in a number of our cases; in a few instances the bleeding followed a lumbar puncture. Paralytic poliomyelitis and acute idiopathic polyneuritis—the former a purely motor disorder with mild meningitis, the latter predominantly motor but often with minimal sensory disturbances—must be distinguished from the acute myelopathies and from each other.

In pediatric practice, delay in starting to walk and difficulty in walking are common problems. These conditions may indicate a systemic disease (such as rickets), mental deficiency, or, more commonly, some muscular or neurologic disease. Congenital cerebral disease accounts for a majority of cases of infantile diplegia (weakness predominantly of the legs, with minimal affection of the arms). Present at birth, it becomes manifest in the first months of life and may appear to progress, but actually the disease is stationary and the progression is only apparent, as the motor system develops. Later there may seem to be slow improvement as a result of the normal maturation processes of childhood. Congenital malformation of the spinal cord or birth injury of the spinal cord are other possibilities. Friedreich ataxia and familial paraplegia, progressive muscular dystrophy, and the chronic varieties of polyneuropathy tend to appear later during childhood and adolescence and are slowly progressive. Acute leukomyelopathy with total sensory and motor paralysis below a thoracic level is a rare condition of childhood. Normal CSF and myelography leave one without a tenable etiology, and few cases have been studied pathologically.

In adult life, multiple sclerosis, subacute combined degeneration (vitamin B_{12} deficiency), tumor, protruded cervical disc and cervical spondylosis, syphilitic meningomyelitis, epidural abscess and other infections (tuberculous, fungal, and other granulomatous diseases), motor system disease, syringomyelia, and degenerative disease of the lateral and posterior columns of unknown cause represent the most frequently encountered forms of spinal paraplegia. (See Chap. 36 for discussion of these spinal cord diseases.) Several varieties of polyneuropathy and polymyositis must also be considered in the differential diagnosis of paraplegia or paraparesis.

QUADRIPLEGIA (TETRAPLEGIA)

All that has been said about the spinal causes of paraplegia applies to quadriplegia, the lesion being in the cervical rather than the thoracic or lumbar segments of the spinal cord. If the lesion is situated in the low cervical segments and involves the anterior half of the spinal cord, as in the anterior spinal artery syndrome and certain fracture-dislocations of the cervical spine, the paralysis of the arms may be flaccid and areflexic in type and that of the legs, spastic. Dislocation of the odontoid process with compression of C1 and C2 spinal cord segments may occur with rheumatoid arthritis and Morquio disease; in the latter there may also be pronounced meningeal thickening. Bilateral infarction of the medullary pyramids from occlusion of the vertebral arteries or their anterior spinal branches is a very rare cause of quadriplegia. In infants, aside from developmental abnormalities and anoxia of birth, certain cerebral diseases (Schilder disease, metachromatic and other forms of leukoencephalopathy, lipid storage disease) may be responsible for a quadriparesis or quadriplegia. Congenital forms of muscular dystrophy and infantile muscular atrophy (Werdnig-Hoffmann disease) may be recognized soon after birth.

In adults, repeated cerebral vascular accidents may lead to bilateral hemiplegia, usually accompanied by pseudobulbar palsy.

PARALYSIS OF ISOLATED MUSCLE GROUPS

This condition usually indicates a lesion of one or more peripheral nerves, occasionally of several adjacent spinal roots. The diagnosis of an individual peripheral nerve lesion is made on the basis of weakness or paralysis of a particular muscle or group of muscles and impairment or loss of sensation in the distribution of the nerve in question. Complete or severe interuption of a peripheral nerve is followed by atrophy of the muscles it innervates and by loss of their tendon reflexes. Paralysis of vasomotor and sudomotor functions and trophic changes in the skin, nails, and subcutaneous tissue may also occur.

Knowledge of the motor and sensory functions of the peripheral nerve in question is needed for a satisfactory diagnosis. Since lesions of individual nerves are relatively uncommon in civil life, it is not practical to memorize the precise motor-sensory distribution of each peripheral nerve; special manuals, such as the ones listed in the references, should be consulted. It is, however, of considerable importance to decide whether the lesion is a temporary one of conduction only or whether there has been a pathologic dissolution of continuity, requiring nerve regeneration or corrective surgery for recovery. Electromyography and nerve conduction studies may be of value here.

If there is no evidence of upper or lower motor neuron disease, but certain acts are nonetheless imperfectly performed, one should look for a disorder of position sense or cerebellar coordination, or for rigidity with abnormalities of posture and movement due to disease of the basal ganglia (Chap. 4). In the absence of these disorders, the possibility of an apraxic disorder should be investigated by the methods outlined in the preceding part of this chapter.

HYSTERICAL PARALYSIS

In hysterical paralysis one arm or leg, or both legs, or all one side of the body may be affected. This is usually distinguishable from chronic lower motor neuron disease by absence of areflexia and of severe atrophy. Diagnostic difficulty arises only in certain acute cases of upper motor neuron disease that lack the usual changes in reflexes and muscle tone. The hysterical gait is often diagnostic (Chap. 6). Sometimes there is loss of sensation in the paralyzed parts and loss of sight, hearing, and smell on the paralyzed side—a group of sensory changes that is never seen in organic brain disease. When the hysterical patient is asked to move the affected limbs, the movements tend to be slow and jerky, often with contraction of both agonist and antagonist muscles simultaneously and intermittently. Hoover's sign and the trunk-thigh sign of Babinski are helpful in distinguishing hysterical from organic hemiplegia. To elicit Hoover's sign the examiner places both hands under the heels of the recumbent patient, who is asked to press the heels down forcefully. With organic hemiplegia, pressure will be felt entirely or almost entirely from the nonparalyzed leg. The examiner then places a hand on top of the nonparalyzed foot and asks the patient to raise that leg. In true hemiplegia, no added pressure will be felt by the hand that remained beneath the heel of the paralyzed leg. In hysteria, the heel of the supposedly paralyzed leg will press down on the palm. To carry out Babinski's trunk-thigh test the recumbent patient is asked to sit up while keeping the arms crossed in front of the chest. In the patient with organic hemiplegia there is an involuntary flexion of the paretic limb; in paraplegia, both legs are raised as the trunk is flexed. In hysterical hemiplegia, only the normal leg may be elevated, while in hysterical paraplegia neither leg is raised.

MUSCULAR PARALYSIS AND SPASM UNATTENDED BY VISIBLE CHANGES IN NERVE OR MUSCLE

A discussion of motor paralysis would not be complete without some reference to a group of diseases in which there are no overt structural changes in motor nerve cells, nerve fibers, motor end plates, and muscle fibers. This group is comprised of myasthenia gravis, myotonia congenita (Thomsen disease), familial periodic paralysis, disorders of potassium, sodium, calcium, and magnesium metabolism, tetany, tetanus, botulinus poisoning, black widow spider bite, and the thyroid myopathies. In these diseases, each of which possesses a fairly distinctive clinical picture, the abnormality is purely biochemical, and even if the patient survives for a long time, no light-microscopic changes develop. An understanding of these diseases requires knowledge of the processes involved in nerve excitation, neuromuscular transmission, and in the contraction of muscle. They will be discussed in Chaps. 45, 52, and 53.

REFERENCES

ASANUMA H: Cerebral cortical control of movement. *Physiologist* 16:143, 1973.

ASANUMA H: The pyramidal tract, in Brooks VB (ed): *Handbook of Physiology, Sec 1: The Nervous System, vol 2: Motor Control.* Bethesda, Maryland, American Physiological Society, 1981, chap 15, pp 702–733.

ASANUMA H, SAKATA H: Functional organization of a cortical efferent system examined with focal depth stimulation in cats. *J Neurophysiol* 30:35, 1967.

BALDISSERA F, HULTBORN H, ILLERT M: Integration in spinal neuronal systems, in Brookhart JM, Mountcastle VB (eds): *Handbook of Physiology, sec 1: The Nervous System,* vol 2, part 1. Bethesda, American Physiological Society, 1981, pp 509–595.

BRODAL A: Pathways mediating supraspinal influences on the spinal cord—The basal ganglia, in *Neurological Anatomy in Relation to Clinical Medicine,* 3d ed. New York, Oxford, 1981, chap 4.

BUCY PC, KEPLINGER JE, SIQUEIRA EB: Destruction of the pyramidal tract in man. *J. Neurosurg* 21:385, 1964.

BUCY PC, LADPLI R, EHRLICH A: Destruction of the pyramidal tract in the monkey. *J Neurosurg* 25:1, 1966.

DAVIDOFF RA: Pharmacology of spasticity. *Neurology* 28: part 2 46, 1978.

DENNY-BROWN D: *The Cerebral Control of Movement.* Springfield, Ill, Charles C Thomas, 1966.

DIMITRIJEVIC MR, SHERWOOD AN, NATHAN PW: Clonus, peripheral and central mechanisms, in Desmedt JE (ed): *Physiological Tremor, Pathological Tremors and Clonus.* New York, Karger, 1978, pp 173–182.

EVARTS EV, SHINODA Y, WISE SP: *Neurophysiological Approaches to Higher Brain Functions.* Neurosciences Research Foundation. New York, Wiley, 1984.

FAGLIONI P, BASSO A: Historical perspectives on neuroanatomical correlates of limb apraxia, in Roy EA (ed): *Neuropsychological Studies of Apraxia and Related Disorders.* Amsterdam, North Holland, 1985, pp 3–44.

GESCHWIND N: The apraxias: Neural mechanisms of disorders of learned movement. *Am Sci* 63:188, 1975.

GILMAN S, MARCO LA: Effects of medullary pyramidotomy in the monkey. *Brain* 94: 495, 515, 1971.

GRILLNER S: Locomotion in vertebrates: Central mechanisms and reflex interaction. *Physiol Rev* 55:247, 1975.

HALLET M, SHAHANI BT, YOUNG RR: EMG analysis of patients with cerebellar deficits. *J Neurol Neurosurg Psychiatry* 38:1163, 1975.

HAYMAKER WE, WOODHALL B: *Peripheral Nerve Injuries: Principles of Diagnosis,* 2nd ed. Philadelphia, Saunders, 1953.

HENNEMAN E: Organization of the spinal cord and its reflexes, in Mountcastle VB (ed): *Medical Physiology,* 14th ed, vol 1. St Louis, Mosby, 1980, pp 762–786.

HENNEMAN E: Motor functions of the cerebral cortex, in Mountcastle VB (ed): *Medical Physiology,* 14th ed, vol 1. St. Louis, Mosby, 1980, pp 859–889.

KERTESZ A, FERRO JM, SHEWAN CM: Apraxia and aphasia. The functional anatomical basis for their dissociation. *Neurology* 34:40, 1984.

KLEIST K: KORTICALE (Innervatorische) Apraxie. *Jahrb Psychiatry Neurol* 28:46, 1907.

KUYPERS HGJM: The anatomical organization of the descending pathways and their contributions to motor control especially in primates, in Desmedt JE (ed): *New Developments in EMG and Clinical Neurophysiology.* Basel, Karger, 1973, p 38.

LANCE JW: The control of muscle tone, reflexes and movement: Robert Wartenburg Lecture. *Neurology* 30:1303, 1980.

LANDAU WM: Spasticity and rigidity, in Plum F (ed): *Contemporary Neurology Series,* vol 6: *Recent Advances in Neurology.* Philadelphia, Davis, 1970, chap 1, pp 1–32.

LAPLANE D, TALAIRACH J, MEININGER V ET AL.: Motor consequences of motor area ablations in man. *J Neurol Sci* 31:29, 1977.

LASSEK AM: *The Pyramidal Tract.* Springfield, Ill, Charles C Thomas, 1954.

LAWRENCE DG, KUYPERS HGJM: The functional organization of the motor system in the monkey. *Brain* 91:1, 15, 1968.

LIEPMANN H: Das Krankheitsbild der Apraxie (motorische Asymbolie auf Grund eines falles von einseitiger Apraxie). *Monatsschr Psychiatry Neurol* 8:15, 102, 182, 1900.

LORENTE DE NÓ R: Cerebral cortex: architecture, intracortical connections, motor projections, in Fulton JF (ed): *Physiology of the Nervous System,* 3rd ed. New York, Oxford University Press, 1949, 1, pp 288–330.

LURIA AR: *The Working Brain: An Introduction to Neuropsychology.* New York, Basic Books, 1973.

MEDICAL RESEARCH COUNCIL: *Aids to the Examination of the Peripheral Nervous System,* Memorandum no 45. London, HM Stationery Office, 1976. New edition published 1986 by Bailliere Tindall.

MOUNTCASTLE VB: Modality and topographic properties of single neurons of cat's somatic sensory cortex. *J Neurophysiol* 20:408, 1957.

NYBERG-HANSEN R, RINVIK E: Some comments on the pyramidal tract with special reference to its individual variations in man. *Acta Neurol Scand* 39:1, 1963.

PICK A: *Studien uber motorische Apraxie und ihre nahestehende Erscheinungen: Ihre Bedeutung in der Symptomatologie psychopathologischer Symptomenkomplexe.* Leipzig, Deuticke, 1905.

ROLAND PE: Organization of motor control by the normal human brain. *Hum Neurobiol* 2:205, 1984.,

ROPPER AH, FISHER CM, KLEINMAN GM: Pyramidal infarction in the medulla: A cause of pure motor hemiplegia sparing the face. *Neurology* 29:91, 1979.

RUSSELL JR, DEMYER W: The quantitative cortical origin of pyramidal axons of *Macaca rhesus,* with some remarks on the slow rate of axolysis. *Neurology* 11:96, 1961.

TOWER SS: Pyramidal lesion in the monkey. *Brain* 63:36, 1940.

CHAPTER 4

ABNORMALITIES OF MOVEMENT AND POSTURE DUE TO DISEASE OF THE EXTRAPYRAMIDAL MOTOR SYSTEMS

In this chapter are discussed the disorders of the automatic, static, postural, and other less modifiable motor activities of the human nervous system. They are believed, on good evidence, to be an expression of the older, or "extrapyramidal," motor system, meaning, according to S. A. K. Wilson, who introduced this term, the motor structures in the basal ganglia and certain related brainstem nuclei.

In health, the activities of the basal ganglia and the cerebellum are blended and modulate the corticospinal and cortical-brainstem-spinal systems. The static postural activities of the former are indispensable to the voluntary or willed movements of the latter. The close association of these two systems is also shown by human disease. Lesions that involve the corticospinal tracts predominantly result not only in paralysis of volitional movements of the contralateral half of the body but also in the appearance of a fixed posture or attitude in which the arm is maintained in flexion and the leg in extension (predilection type of Wernicke-Mann or hemiplegic dystonia of Denny-Brown). Interruption of the motor projection pathways by a lesion in the upper pons or midbrain releases another posture in which all four extremities or the arm and leg on one side (ipsilateral to a unilateral lesion) are extended and the cervical and thoracolumbar portions of the spine are dorsiflexed (decerebrate rigidity). In these released motor patterns one has evidence of postural reflexes which are mediated through nonpyramidal bulbospinal and other brainstem systems. Observations such as these and the anatomic data presented in the preceding chapter have blurred the classical distinctions between pyramidal and extrapyramidal motor systems. Nevertheless, this division remains a useful if not an essential concept in clinical work, since it compels us to distinguish between several distinctive motor syndromes—one that is characterized by a loss of volitional movement and spasticity, a second one by akinesia, rigidity, and tremor, without loss of voluntary movement, another by involuntary movements, choreoathetosis, and dystonia, and a fourth by incoordination (ataxia). The clinical differ-

ences between the first two of these, the corticospinal and extrapyramidal disorders, are summarized in Table 4-1.

Much of the criticism of the pyramidal-extrapyramidal concept derives from the terms themselves. The ambiguity related to the use of the term *pyramidal* has been discussed in the preceding chapter, where it was pointed out that pure pyramidal lesions do not cause total paralysis and when the latter exists there is always involvement of other descending corticoreticulospinal pathways. The term *extrapyramidal* is equally imprecise. Strictly interpreted, it refers to all the motor pathways except the pyramidal one, a term so all-embracing as to be practically meaningless. The concept of an extrapyramidal motor system becomes more meaningful if it is subdivided into two parts: (1) the striatopallidonigral and (2) the cerebellar. Disease in either of these parts will result in particular disturbances of movement and posture without significant paralysis. These two major systems and the symptoms that result when they are diseased are described on the following pages.

THE STRIATOPALLIDONIGRAL SYSTEM (BASAL GANGLIA)

ANATOMIC CONSIDERATIONS

As an anatomic entity the basal ganglia have no precise definition. In addition to the caudate and lenticular nuclei, one usually includes the claustrum, the subthalamic nucleus (corpus Luysii), and the substantia nigra. The amygdaloid nuclear complex, because of its largely different connections and functions, is usually excluded. For reasons indicated below, some physiologists have expanded the list of basal ganglionic structures to include the red nucleus and the reticular formation of the brainstem. The latter structures receive direct cortical projections and give rise to rubrospinal and reticulospinal fibers; although these nonpyramidal linkages form indirect connections with the corpus striatum, they appear to be structurally independent of the latter structure.

The anatomic features of the extrapyramidal motor structures and the connections between them and other parts of the brain are too intricate to present in a textbook of neurology (cf. *Brodal, Neurological Anatomy;* also Carpenter and Sutin, *Human Neuroanatomy*). Only a simplified version will be provided here. Knowledge of these anatomic data is essential to an understanding of normal motor function and provides a rational explanation for certain abnormalities of motor function as well, particularly for involuntary movements and tremor.

The main structures composing the basal ganglia are the caudate nucleus and the lentiform nucleus with its two subdivisions, the putamen and globus pallidus (pallidum). Insofar as the caudate and putamen are really a single

structure (separated only incompletely by fibers of the internal capsule), cytologically and functionally distinct from the pallidum; a more meaningful division of these nuclear masses is into the neostriatum (or striatum), comprising the caudate and putamen, and the paleostriatum or pallidum, with its medial (internal) and lateral (external) segments. The putamen and pallidum lie on the lateral aspect of the internal capsule, which separates them from the caudatum, thalamus, subthalamic nucleus, and substantia nigra on its medial side (Figs. 4-1 and 4-2).

The most important connections between these nuclei and with other structures are indicated in Figs. 4-1, 4-2, 4-3, and 4-7. The striatum, which is the receptive part of the basal ganglia, receives topographically organized fibers from all parts of the cerebral cortex (Figs. 4-1, 4-4), particularly the motor-sensory and association areas, as well as from the substantia nigra, parts of the amygdala, and certain thalamic nuclei. The centromedian and parafascicular nuclei project to the putamen; the rostral intralaminar nuclei project mainly to the head of the caudate. In turn, the caudate and putamen project topographically upon the lateral and medial segments of the pallidum and upon the substantia nigra (the efferent part of the basal ganglia), particularly on the portion composed of nonpigmented cells (pars reticulata). Available evidence indicates that striatonigral and nigrostriatal fibers are topographically and reciprocally organized. Projections from the striatum, as they converge in an orderly, radial arrangement in the medial tip of the pallidum, give off collaterals that form dense plexuses of fibers around the long, smooth dendrites of pallidal neurons. The pallidum in turn receives fibers from the substantia nigra.

At one time it was thought that the efferent fibers of the striatum were axons of the large cells that make up 1 to 2 percent of striatal neurons. However, it is now certain that efferent fibers arise from the small and medium-sized neurons as well. The main efferent systems of the basal ganglia originate in the pallidum, particularly its medial segment, and in the pars reticulata of the substantia nigra. The fiber bundles from the pallidum to the thalamus are the ansa and fasciculus lenticularis (Fig. 4-3). The ansa lenticularis sweeps around the internal capsule; the fasciculus lenticularis traverses the internal capsule in a number of small fascicles (Forel's field H_2) and then sweeps medially and caudally to join the ansa in the prerubral field (Forel's field H). Both these fiber bundles then join the *thalamic fasciculus* (Forel's field H_1), which contains not only pallidothalamic projections but also rubrothalamic and dentatothalamic ones. Together they project onto the ventro-

Table 4-1
Clinical differences between corticospinal and extrapyramidal syndromes

	Corticospinal	Extrapyramidal
Character of the alteration of muscle tone	Clasp-knife effect (spasticity)	Plastic, equal throughout passive movement (rigidity), or intermittent (cogwheel rigidity); hypotonia in cerebellar disease
Distribution of hypertonus	Flexors of arms, extensors of legs	Flexors (predominantly) and extensors of all four limbs; flexors of trunk
Shortening and lengthening reaction	Present	Absent
Involuntary movements	Absent	Presence of tremor, chorea, athetosis, dystonia
Tendon reflexes	Increased	Normal or slightly increased
Babinski sign	Present	Absent
Paralysis of voluntary movement	Present	Absent or slight

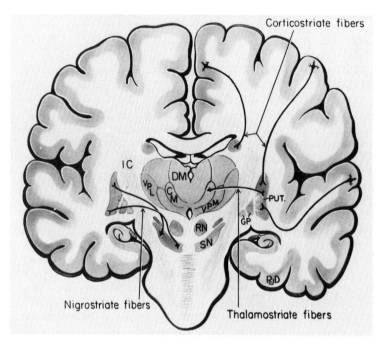

Corticostriate fibers

IC

DM

VPL

CM

VPM

PUT.

GP

RN

SN

R.D

Nigrostriate fibers

Thalamostriate fibers

Figure 4-1

Diagram of the striatal afferent pathways. Corticostriate *fibers from broad cortical areas project to the putamen; fibers from the cortex on the medial surface project largely to the caudate nucleus.* Nigrostriatal *fibers arise from the pars compacta of the substantia nigra.* Thalamostriate *fibers arise from the centromedian-parafascicular complex of the thalamus. CM, centromedian nucleus; DM, dorsomedial nucleus; GP, globus pallidus; IC, internal capsule; PUT., putamen; RN, red nucleus; SN, substantia nigra; VPL, ventral posterolateral nucleus; VPM, ventral posterior medial nucleus. (From MB Carpenter, J Sutin, Human Neuroanatomy, 8th ed, Baltimore, Williams & Wilkins, 1983.)*

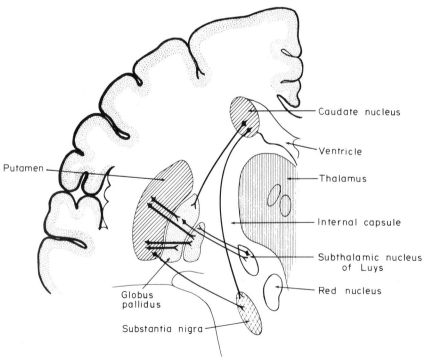

Caudate nucleus

Ventricle

Thalamus

Putamen

Internal capsule

Subthalamic nucleus of Luys

Red nucleus

Globus pallidus

Substantia nigra

Figure 4-2

Diagram of the basal ganglia in the coronal plane, illustrating the main striatal efferent pathways (details in text). The pallidothalamic connections are illustrated in Fig 4-3.

lateral nucleus of the thalamus and to a lesser extent onto the ventral anterior and intralaminar thalamic nuclei. The outer segment of the globus pallidus is connected to and receives fibers from the subthalamic nucleus. The subthalamic nucleus also sends fibers to the substantia nigra. The major projection of the ventrolateral nucleus of the thalamus is to the precentral motor cortex (area 4). The pars reticulata of the substantia nigra projects to the ventromedial thalamic nucleus, pedunculopontine nucleus, and deep layers of the superior colliculus.

The principal anatomic datum to emerge from these observations is the central role of the ventrolateral (and anterior) nucleus of the thalamus. It is a vital link in an ascending fiber system from the basal ganglia and cerebellum to the frontal eye field and supplementary motor area but not (according to Evarts) to the primary motor cortex. Indeed, it would seem that most of the basal ganglionic and cerebellar influence on motor activity is funneled through the ventral tier of thalamic nuclei, which serve to integrate the extrapyramidal impulses and bring them to bear, via the thalamocortical fibers and premotor cortex, on the corticospinal system and on other descending pathways from the cortex. The existence of direct descending pathways from the basal ganglia to the spinal cord has not been established; a small group of fibers projects from the pallidum to the tegmentum of the lower midbrain and probably from there, via polysynaptic pathways through the reticular formation of the pons and medulla, to the

motor neurons of the spinal cord. Another important feature of basal ganglionic physiology, only recently appreciated, is the nonequivalence of all parts of the caudate nucleus and putamen. Zones of cells within these structures appear to have different receptive and executive functions, as described below.

PHYSIOLOGIC CONSIDERATIONS

Although it has been known for a long time that lesions in the basal ganglia are associated with disorders of voluntary movement and posture, physiologists for many years found it difficult to define their functions. Denny-Brown and Yanagisawa, who studied the effects of ablation of individual extrapyramidal structures in monkeys, concluded that the basal ganglia function as a kind of clearinghouse where, during an intended or projected movement, one set of activities is facilitated and all other unnecessary ones are suppressed. Based on the most recent physiologic studies of Evarts, Thach, Alexander, and DeLong, two distinct functional loops have been identified in the basal ganglia. One is a motor loop from the premotor, motor, and supplementary motor areas 5 and 7 to the striatum, pallidum, substantia nigra, thalamus, and back to the supplementary

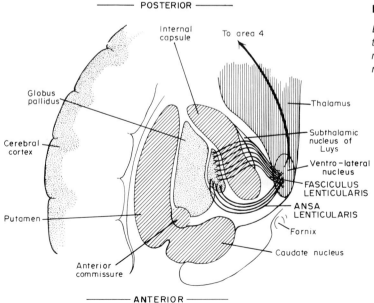

— POSTERIOR —

Internal capsule

To area 4

Globus pallidus

Cerebral cortex

Putamen

Anterior commissure

Thalamus

Subthalamic nucleus of Luys

Ventro-lateral nucleus

FASCICULUS LENTICULARIS

ANSA LENTICULARIS

Fornix

Caudate nucleus

— ANTERIOR —

Figure 4-3

Basal ganglia in the horizontal plane, illustrating the main efferent projections from the medial segment of the pallidum to the ventral nuclei of the thalamus (details in text).

motor areas. The other is a more complex loop, begining in the association areas of the cortex and projecting to the caudate nucleus, and eventually returning to parts of the prefrontal cortex. The subthalamic nucleus and other ganglionic structures (pedunculopontine) also participate in the regulation of the motor circuit.

Thus the prefrontal cortex, where the planning of intended movements is believed to take place, has access through the complex loop to the motor cortex only indirectly, via a circuitous route through the striatum, pallidum, subthalamic nucleus, substantia nigra, and thalamic nuclei.

Figure 4-4

Lateral (A) and medial (B) surfaces of the brain, showing the areas of the cerebral cortex which project to the extrapyramidal motor system. (From EL House et al, A Systematic Approach to Neuroscience, 3rd ed, New York, McGraw-Hill, 1979.)

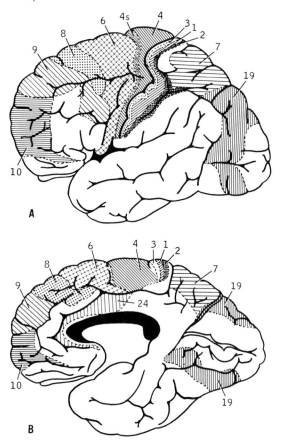

The cognitive (complex) loop is involved more in the selection of the pattern of muscles needed in an act (both rapid ballistic and slow ramp movements). The motor loop seems more important in regulating the amplitude, velocity, and possibly the initiation of the movements. (The cerebellum is mainly responsible for timing the elements in the motor sequence.)

If the striatum is defective, the natural triphasic sequence of agonist-antagonist-agonist contractions during a single ballistic movement (described in Chap. 3), while still properly integrated, does not involve sufficient numbers of motor units to complete the act (Hallett and Khoshbin). A series of such triphasic bursts is then required for a simple movement. This appears to be the basis of hypokinesia. Rigidity and athetosis may be viewed as complete or partial failures of selective activation and suppression and chorea as released fragments of phasic and tonic units. Repeated cycles of triphasic agonist-antagonist-agonist contractions merge with cogwheel rigidity and tremor.

PHARMACOLOGIC CONSIDERATIONS

During the past three decades a series of exciting pharmacologic observations has considerably broadened our understanding of basal ganglionic function and has led to the discovery of a rational treatment of Parkinson disease and other extrapyramidal syndromes. Whereas physiologists had for years failed to discover the functions of the basal ganglia by stimulation and ablation experiments, clinicians became aware that the use of certain drugs, such as reserpine and the phenothiazines, regularly produced extrapyramidal syndromes (parkinsonism, choreoathetosis, dystonia, etc.). These observations greatly stimulated the study of transmitter substances in the central nervous system. These are substances which are synthesized and stored in presynaptic terminals and released, in response to an appropriate stimulus, across the synaptic gap to combine with specific receptor sites on the postsynaptic cell.

The most important neurotransmitter substances from the point of view of basal ganglionic function are glutamate, which activates the corticostriatal excitatory projections, acetylcholine, dopamine, gamma aminobutyric acid (GABA), and serotonin. Norepinephrine is present in relatively low concentrations and its function as a basal ganglionic transmitter is less clearly defined. In addition, the basal ganglia contain other biologically active substances, viz., substance P, enkephalin, cholecystokinin, and somatostatin which may enhance or dimish the effects of the neurotransmitters (hence *neuromodulators*). The neurons utilizing these substances are just now being identified.

Acetylcholine (ACh), long established as the neurotransmitter at the neuromuscular junction as well as in the autonomic ganglia, is also physiologically active in this part of the brain. The highest concentration of ACh as well as of choline acetylase and acetylcholinesterase (the enzymes necessary for the synthesis and degradation of ACh respectively) is in the striatum. ACh is synthesized and released by the small (Golgi type 2) neostriatal neurons, upon which it has an excitatory effect; dopamine has a disinhibitory effect on these neurons. It is likely that the effectiveness of the belladonna alkaloids, which had been used empirically for many years in the treatment of Parkinson disease, also depends on their capacity to antagonize ACh centrally.

Of the catecholamines—dopamine, epinephrine, and norepinephrine—the first has excited the greatest attention. The steps in the pathway for the biosynthesis of the catecholamines and the enzymes involved in each step are tabulated below:

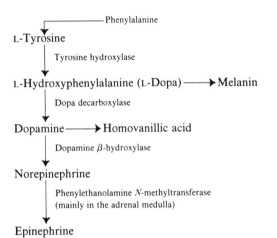

In the brain dopamine is metabolized by the enzymes monoamine oxidase (MAO) and catechol-*o*-methyltransferase (COMT); the end products are homovanillic acid (HVA) and dihydroxyphenylacetic acid (DOPAC). HVA is readily measured in the CSF and both these metabolites can be measured in the plasma.

Dopamine has a specific function in the central nervous system, apart from being a precursor of norepinephrine. The areas richest in dopamine are the substantia nigra, where it is synthesized in the nerve cell bodies of the pars compacta, and the striatum, where it is localized in synaptic endings of nigral fibers. Stimulation of the substantia nigra induces a specific response in the striatum, viz., a release of dopamine, which has an inhibitory effect on neostriatal neurons. Striatonigral fibers in the pars reticulata contain glutamic acid decarboxylase (GAD), the enzyme utilized in the synthesis of GABA, suggesting that these fibers also transport it.

In Parkinson disease (both the idiopathic and postencephalitic varieties), the concentration of dopamine is greatly

decreased in the striatum and substantia nigra, and the content of its major metabolite, HVA, is also decreased in these parts, as well as in the globus pallidus and spinal fluid. The degree of dopamine and HVA deficiency appears to correlate with the degree of cell loss in the substantia nigra, i.e., with the major pathologic change in Parkinson disease.

Certain drugs, namely reserpine, the phenothiazines, and the butyrophenones, notably haloperidol, may induce parkinsonian syndromes in humans. Reserpine acts by depleting the striatum and other parts of the brain of dopamine; haloperidol and the phenothiazines produce parkinsonism by a different mechanism, probably by causing a blockade of dopamine receptors within the striatum.

New insight into the parkinsonian syndrome has come from the discovery that it can be reproduced in humans and primates by the toxin 1-methyl-4-phenyl-1,2,3,6-tetrahydropyridine (MPTP), which destroys the nigral cells and their dopaminergic connections with the striatum (see also page 941). The mesolimbic and mesocortical dopamine pathways that arise from the ventral tegmental area and are affected in Parkinson disease are spared in MPTP intoxication. To Alexander and DeLong this indicates that loss of nigral cells is responsible for the rigidity, akinesia, and tremor. Not excluded, however, is a nigral projection to the thalamus (see further on).

Dopamine as such cannot pass the blood-brain barrier and has no therapeutic effect. However, the immediate dopamine precursor, L-dopa, does cross the barrier and is effective in decreasing the akinesia, rigidity, and the tremor of paralysis agitans (Parkinson disease) and drug-induced parkinsonism. This effect is greatly enhanced by the inhibition of MAO, an important enzyme in the catabolism of dopamine. The addition of an MAO inhibitor to L-dopa results in a marked increase of dopamine concentration in the brain.

Because of the pharmacologic activities of ACh and dopamine, it has been postulated that a functional equilibrium exists in the striatum between the excitatory cholinergic and the inhibitory dopaminergic mechanisms (Hornykiewicz). In Parkinson disease, the decreased release of dopamine within the striatum disinhibits the neurons that synthesize ACh, resulting in a predominance of the cholinergic activity, a notion supported by the observation that parkinsonian symptoms are aggravated by centrally acting cholinergic drugs and improved by anticholinergic drugs. According to this theory, administration of anticholinergic drugs restores the ratio between dopamine and acetylcholine, with the new equilibrium being set at a lower-than-normal level, because of the low striatal dopamine level to begin with. The use of drugs that enhance dopamine synthesis and release (L-dopa) or that directly stimulate dopaminergic receptors (bromocriptine) represents a more physiologic method of treatment of Parkinson disease.

GABA is found in high concentrations in the substantia nigra, striatum, and globus pallidus, where it probably acts as an inhibitory neurotransmitter. Specific neural pathways for this transmitter activity remain to be defined, however. GABA has been implicated in the pathogenesis of Huntington chorea (probably due to a loss of small striatal neurons, which synthesize this transmitter), vitamin B_6–dependent seizures, and many other neurologic disorders, as will be indicated at appropriate points in the text. Other central neurotransmitters such as glutamate, norepinephrine and serotonin will also be considered in relation to the disorders in which they play a part.

The known transmitter substances and pathways of importance in basal ganglionic function are summarized in Fig. 4-5 (adapted from Growdon and Scheife). The release of dopamine at the terminals of the nigrostriatal pathway is well established as is that of GABA at the terminals of a striatonigral pathway, and of serotonin from neurons that originate in the raphe nuclei of the brainstem. However, the chemical transmitter(s) that are involved in other basal ganglionic projection systems—striatopallidal, pallidotha-

lamic, thalamostriate, and luysial-pallidal–have not been established.

A more complete account of this subject than is possible here may be found in the writings of Klawans, of Hornykiewicz, of Growdon and Scheife, and of Young and Penney, referred to at the end of this chapter.

SYMPTOMS OF BASAL GANGLIA DISEASE

In broad terms, all motor disorders may be considered to consist of primary functional deficits (or *negative* symptoms) and secondary effects (*positive* symptoms), the latter being ascribed to the release or disinhibition of the activity of undamaged parts of the motor nervous system. When diseases of the basal ganglia are analyzed along these classic lines, then akinesia and loss of normal postural reflexes stand out as the primary deficits, or negative symptoms, and tremor, rigidity, and involuntary movements (chorea, athetosis, and dystonia) as the positive ones. Disorders of phonation, articulation, and locomotion are more difficult to classify. In some cases they are clearly consequent upon rigidity and postural disorder; in others, where rigidity is slight or negligible, they seem to represent a primary deficiency. Difficulty in the performance of rapid alternating movements probably represents another negative effect in diseases of both the basal ganglia and the cerebellum. In fact, this latter symptom, presenting as clumsiness, may be the only fault manifest in certain maladroit children. Stress and nervous tension characteristically worsen both the motor deficiency and the abnormal movements in all extrapyram-

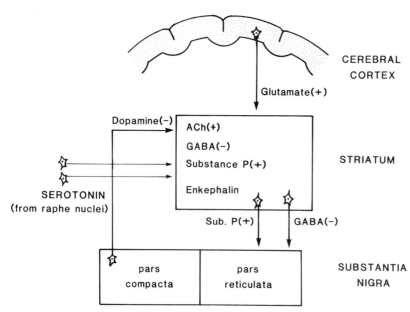

Figure 4-5

Diagram of the chemical transmitters and pathways involved in basal ganglionic function. The symbols (+) and (−) indicate excitatory and inhibitory effects, respectively. The striatal transmitters are synthesized and released by small cells within that structure. Arrows indicate putative transmitter pathways. (Adapted from Growdon and Scheife.)

idal syndromes, just as relaxation helps the motor performance. The involuntary movements are described further on.

HYPOKINESIA AND BRADYKINESIA

Hypokinesia or akinesia refers to the disinclination of the
patient to use an affected part, and to engage it freely in
all the natural actions of the body, as well as slowness in
initiating and executing a movement. In contrast to what
occurs in paralysis (the primary or negative symptom of
corticospinal lesions), strength is not significantly diminished in the part. Also, hypokinesia is unlike apraxia, where
a lesion erases the memory of the pattern of movements
necessary for the intended act. The phenomenon of hypokinesia or akinesia is expressed most clearly as an extreme
underactivity (poverty of movement). The frequent automatic habitual movements observed in the normal state,
such as putting the hand to the face, folding the arms, or
crossing the legs, are absent or greatly reduced in parkinsonian patients. In looking to one side the eyes move, not
the head. In arising from a chair, they fail to make the
usual small adjustments such as pulling the feet back,
putting the hands on the arms of the chair, and so forth.
Blinking is infrequent. Saliva is not swallowed as fast as
it is produced, and sialorrhea results. The face lacks
expressive mobility (hypomimia). An affected arm is neglected.

Bradykinesia, which connotes slowness rather than
lack of movement, is probably another aspect of the same
physiologic difficulty. Not only is the parkinsonian patient
"slow off the mark" (longer interval between a command
and the first contraction of muscles, i.e., increased reaction
time), but the velocity of movement is lower than normal.
Formerly, bradykinesia was attributed to the frequently
associated rigidity, which could reasonably hamper all
movements, but the incorrectness of this explanation became
apparent when it was discovered that an appropriately
placed stereotactic lesion in a patient with paralysis agitans
may abolish rigidity but leave the akinesia unaltered. Thus
it would appear that apart from their contribution to the
maintenance of postures, the basal ganglia provide an
essential element for the performance of the large variety
of voluntary and semiautomatic actions that make up the
full repertoire of natural human motility. As was pointed
out above, Hallett and Khoshbin, in an analysis of ballistic
(rapid) movements in the parkinsonian patient, found that
the normal triphasic sequence of agonist-antagonist-agonist
is intact but lacks the energy (number of activated motor
units) to complete the movement. Several triphasic sequences are then needed, which slows the movement. That
cells in the basal ganglia participate in the initiation of
movement is evident from the fact that the firing rates in
these cells increase before movement is detected clinically.

In terms of pathologic anatomy and physiology,
bradykinesia may be caused by any morbid process or drug
that interrupts the cortico-striato-pallido-thalamic circuit.
Rigidity (discussed further on) is frequently combined.
Examples are reduced dopaminergic input from the substantia nigra to the striatum, as in Parkinson disease;
dopamine receptor blockade by neuroleptic drugs; extensive
degeneration of striatal neurons, as in striatonigral degeneration, multiple system atrophy, and the rigid form of
Huntington chorea; and destruction of the medial pallidum,
as in Wilson and Hallervorden-Spatz disease.

A number of other disorders of voluntary movement
may also be observed in patients with diseases of the basal
ganglia. A persistent contraction of rigid hand muscles, as
in holding a pencil, may not be inhibited in time so that
there is interference with the next willed movement. Attempts to perform a sequence of movements may be blocked
at one point (digital impedance, see page 938) and a tremor
then appears. Voluntary muscles fatigue more readily on
repeated activity. In still other cases, performance of a
simple movement (e.g., touching finger to nose) is rendered
impossible by the simultaneous contraction of antagonist
muscles, not only of the arm and hand but also of the neck,
trunk, and even of the legs ("intention spasm").

DISORDERS OF POSTURAL FIXATION, EQUILIBRIUM, AND RIGHTING

These deficits are also demonstrated most clearly in the
parkinsonian patient. They take the form of an involuntary
flexion of the trunk and limbs and of the head, reminiscent
of a person who falls asleep in an upright position. The
inability of the patient to make appropriate postural adjustments to tilting or falling and to change from the reclining
to the standing position are closely related phenomena.
These postural abnormalities are not the result of weakness,
nor are they related to obvious defects in proprioception or
labyrinthine or visual function, the principal forces that
control the normal posture of the head and trunk. Anticipatory and compensatory righting reflexes are impaired
early in supranuclear ophthalmoplegia and late in Parkinson
disease. These postural abnormalities have been compared
to the flexed postures of the head and neck and disorders
of equilibrium and righting that have been produced in
monkeys by the ablation of the globus pallidus bilaterally
(Richter).

A point of interest is whether akinesia and disorders
of postural fixation are invariable manifestations of all
extrapyramidal diseases and whether without them there

could be any secondary release effects such as dystonia, choreoathetosis, and rigidity. The question has no clear answer. Akinesia and abnormalities of posture are invariable features of Parkinson and Wilson disease; they seem to be present also in Huntington and Sydenham chorea and in double athetosis, but one cannot be sure of their existence in hemiballismus.

ALTERATIONS OF MUSCLE TONE

In the form of hypertonus known as *rigidity* the muscles are continuously or intermittently firm and tense. Although brief periods of electromyographic silence can be obtained in selected muscles by persistent attempts to relax the limb, there is obviously a low threshold for involuntary sustained muscle contraction, and this is present during most of the waking state, even when the patient appears quiet and relaxed. In contrast to spasticity, the increased resistance on passive movement that characterizes rigidity is not preceded by an initial "free interval" and has an even or uniform quality throughout the range of movement of the limb, like that noted in bending a lead pipe or pulling a strand of toffee. When released, the limb does not resume its original position as may happen in spasticity.

Rigidity is present in all muscle groups, both flexor and extensor, but it tends to be more prominent in those which maintain a flexed posture, i.e., the flexor muscles of trunk and limbs. It appears to be somewhat greater in the large muscle groups, but this may be merely a matter of muscle mass. Certainly the small muscles of the face and tongue and even those of the larynx are often affected. The tendon reflexes are not enhanced. Nevertheless, like spasticity, rigidity is said to be abolished by the extradural or subarachnoid injection of local anesthesia, and Foerster demonstrated long ago that it is eradicated by posterior root section, presumably by interrupting the afferent fibers of the gamma loop. Nevertheless, recording from muscle spindles has not confirmed excessive gamma motor neuron drive. In the electromyographic tracing, motor-unit activity is more continuous than in spasticity, persisting even after apparent relaxation.

A special type of rigidity, first noted by Negro in 1901, is the cogwheel phenomenon. When the hypertonic muscle is passively stretched, e.g., when the hand is dorsiflexed, one encounters a rhythmically interrupted, ratchet-like resistance. Wilson postulated that this phenomenon is a minor form of the lengthening-shortening reaction, but it more likely represents an associated static or action tremor that is masked by the rigidity but emerges faintly during manipulation.

Rigidity is a prominent feature of many extrapyramidal diseases such as the advanced forms of paralysis agitans and the postencephalitic variety of Parkinson disease, Wilson disease, striatonigral degeneration, and dystonia musculorum deformans, intoxication, with certain neurolepic drugs, progressive supranuclear palsy, multiple system degenerations, and calcinosis of the basal ganglia. The rigidity is characteristically variable in degree and in some patients, particularly those with choreoathetosis, the limbs are intermittently or persistently hypotonic.

A special type of variable resistance to passive movement is that in which the patient seems unable to relax a group of muscles on command. When the muscles are passively stretched, the patient's inability to cooperate interferes. This is sometimes called *gegenhalten* or *counterholding*. Actually, relaxation requires concentration on the part of the patient. If there is inattentiveness, as happens with diseases of the frontal lobes or senility or confusional states, the question of parkinsonian rigidity may arise. A similar difficulty in relaxing is observed in children.

The pathophysiology of rigidity is not fully understood. Marsden has suggested that overactivity of long-latency and tonic stretch reflexes may contribute to the rigidity of Parkinson disease. Undoubtedly, a more important factor is the greatly excessive supraspinal influence upon alpha motor neurons. Presumably this comes about by disinhibition of cerebral structures that are normally inhibited by the basal ganglia. It is generally agreed that rigidity results from lesions of the nigrostriatal system and can be relieved by dopamine agonists and by stereotactic lesions of the ventral-caudal pallidum or ventrolateral thalamus, which receives the inner pallidal connections.

TREMOR, MYOCLONUS, AND TICS

Of the several types of tremor, only the so-called rest tremor of the Parkinson syndrome can be ascribed to lesions of the basal ganglia, and even this one has an uncertain anatomy. Polymyoclonus is not a manifestation of basal ganglionic diseases and is most often an expression of lesions of the cerebellum, brainstem, and spinal cord. Tics are often ascribed to disordered function of the basal ganglia, but there is no sound pathologic evidence to support this contention. Tremor, tics, and myoclonus are discussed in the next chapter.

INVOLUNTARY MOVEMENTS (CHOREA, BALLISM, ATHETOSIS, DYSTONIA)

In deference to usual practice, these symptoms will be described separately, as though each represents a discrete clinical phenomenon, readily distinguished one from the other. In fact, they usually occur together and have many points of similarity, and there are reasons to believe that they have a common anatomic and physiologic basis. One must be mindful that chorea, athetosis, and dystonia are symptoms and are not to be equated with disease entities which happen to incorporate one of these terms in their names (e.g., Huntington chorea, dystonia musculorum deformans). Here the discussion will be limited to the symptoms. The diseases of which these symptoms are a part are considered in Chap. 43.

Chorea Derived from the Greek word meaning "dance," *chorea* refers to involuntary arrhythmic movements of a forcible, rapid, jerky type. These movements may be simple or quite elaborate and of variable distribution. Although the movements are purposeless, the patient may incorporate them into a deliberate movement, as if to make them less noticeable. When superimposed on voluntary movements, they may assume an exaggerated and grotesque character. Grimacing and peculiar respiratory sounds may be other expressions of the movement disorder. Usually the movements are discrete, but if very numerous, they become confluent and then resemble athetosis. If the involuntary movements can be held in abeyance, normal volitional movements are possible for there is no paralysis, but the latter tend also to be excessively quick and poorly sustained. The limbs are often slack or hypotonic, and because of this, the knee jerks tend to be pendular; with the patient sitting on the edge of the bed and the foot free of the floor, the leg swings back and forth four or five times in response to a tap on the patellar tendon, rather than once or twice, as it does normally. A choreic movement may be superimposed on the reflex movement, checking it in flight, so to speak, and giving rise to the "hung-up" reflex.

The hypotonia in chorea as well as the pendular reflexes contribute to the disorder of movement and may suggest a disturbance of cerebellar function. Lacking, however, are intention tremor and true incoordination or ataxia. Chorea differs from polymyoclonia only with respect to speed of the movements; the myoclonic jerk is much faster and may involve single muscles or part of a muscle as well as groups of muscles. Failure to recognize this difference accounts for inaccurate attribution of chorea to hypernatremia and other metabolic disorders.

Chorea appears in typical form in Sydenham chorea and in the variety of that disease associated with pregnancy (chorea gravidarum). It is a feature also of Huntington chorea (hereditary or chronic chorea), in which the movements tend more typically to be choreoathetotic. Intoxication with phenothiazine drugs or haloperidol, and, rarely, hyperthyroidism, polycythemia vera, or cerebral arteritis may cause chorea.

Chorea may be limited to one side of the body (*hemichorea*), and, when proximal limb muscles are involved, the movements may be unusually violent and flinging in nature, in which case the disorder is referred to

as *hemiballismus*. The lesion in such cases is in or near the opposite subthalamic nucleus of Luys. As the severity of the hemiballismic movements decreases, the patient is left with irregular flexions and extensions of the wrist and fingers, movements that are indistinguishable from chorea and athetosis of mild degree

The anatomic basis of chorea is uncertain. In Huntington chorea there are obvious lesions in the caudate nucleus and putamen. Yet one often observes vascular lesions in these parts, without chorea. The localization of lesions in Sydenham chorea and other choreic diseases is unkown. One suspects that chorea and hemiballismus relate to disorders of the same system of neurons.

Athetosis This term stems from a Greek word meaning "unfixed" or "changeable." The condition is characterized by inability to sustain the fingers and toes, tongue, or any other part of the body in one position. The maintained posture is interrupted by relatively slow, sinuous, purposeless movements which have a tendency to flow into one another. As a rule, the abnormal movements are most pronounced in the digits and hands, face, tongue, and throat, but no group of muscles is spared. One can detect as basic patterns of movement an alternation between extension-pronation and flexion-supination of the arm, and between flexion and extension of the fingers, the flexed and adducted thumb being trapped by the flexed fingers as the hand closes. Other characteristic movements are eversion-inversion of the foot, retraction and pursing of the lips, twisting of the neck and torso, and alternate wrinkling and relaxation of the forehead or opening and closing of the eyelids. The movements appear to be slower than those of chorea, but all gradations between the two are seen, and in some cases it is impossible to distinguish between them, hence the term choreoathetosis. Discrete voluntary movements of the hand are executed more slowly than normal and attempts to perform them may result in a cocontraction of antagonistic muscles and a spread (overflow) of contraction to muscles not normally required in the movement ("intention spasm"). The overflow appears to relate to a failure of the striatum to suppress the activity of unwanted muscle groups. Some of the spasms appear to occur spontaneously, i.e., they are involuntary, and if persistent give rise to fixed dystonic postures (Yanagisawa and Goto).

Athetosis may affect all four limbs or may be unilateral, especially in children who have suffered a hemiplegia at some previous date (posthemiplegic athetosis). Many athetotic patients exhibit variable degrees of motor deficit, due to associated corticospinal tract disease, and variable degrees of rigidity, and these may account for the slower quality of athetosis, in contrast to chorea. In other patients with generalized choreoathetosis, as pointed out above, the limbs may be hypotonic.

The combination of athetosis and chorea of all four limbs is a cardinal feature of Huntington chorea and of a state known as double athetosis, which begins in childhood. Athetosis appearing in the first years of life is usually the result of a congenital or postnatal condition such as hypoxia or kernicterus. Postmortem examinations in some of the cases have disclosed a peculiar pathologic change of probable hypoxic etiology, a *status marmoratus*, in the striatum (Chap. 43); in others, of probable kernicteric etiology, there has been a loss of medullated fibers, a *status dysmyelinatus*, in the same regions. In adults, athetosis may occur as an episodic or persistent disorder in hepatic encephalopathy, as a manifestation of chronic intoxication with phenothiazines or haloperidol, as an effect of excess L-dopa in a parkinsonian patient, and as a feature of certain degenerative diseases, most notably Huntington chorea, but also Wilson disease, Hallervorden-Spatz disease, and Leigh disease (see Chap. 43). Localized forms of athetosis may occasionally follow vascular lesions of the lenticular nucleus or thalamus.

Dystonia, or Torsion Spasm Dystonia is a persistent attitude or posture in one or other of the extremes of athetoid movement. It may take the form of an overextension or overflexion of the hand, inversion of the foot, lateral- or retroflexion of the head, torsion of the spine, with arching and twisting of the back, or forceful closure of the eyes and a fixed grimace (Fig. 4-6). Defined in this way, dystonia is closely allied to athetosis, differing only in the duration or persistence of the postural abnormality and the disproportionate involvement of the larger axial muscles (those of the trunk and limb girdles). The term *dystonia* is generally used in this way, but it has been given other meanings as well. S. A. K. Wilson designated any variability in muscle tone as dystonia. This term has also been applied to fixed abnormalities of posture which may be the end result of certain diseases of the motor system; thus Denny-Brown speaks of "hemiplegic dystonia" and the "flexion dystonia of parkinsonism." If the term is to be used in the latter sense, it would be better to speak of the persistent but reversible athetotic movements of the limbs and trunk as "torsion spasms" or "phasic dystonia," in contrast to "fixed dystonia." The former, like athetosis, may vary considerably in severity and may show remarkable fluctuations in individual patients. Torsion spasm may be limited to the facial, cervical, or trunk muscles or to those of one limb and may cease when the body is in repose. Severe

dystonia results in grotesque movements and distorted positions of the body; sometimes the whole musculature of the body may be thrown into spasm by an effort to move an arm or to speak.

The term *dystonia* was introduced by Oppenheim and Vogt, in 1911, to describe the relatively slow, long-sustained, frequently forceful contorting movements of an uncommon heritable disease, dystonia musculorum deformans. Dystonia, or torsion spasm, is seen in its most pronounced form in this disease, but also occurs as a manifestation of many other diseases ("symptomatic dystonias"). These latter include double athetosis due to hypoxic damage to the brain, kernicterus, Hallervorden-Spatz disease, Huntington chorea, Wilson hepatolenticular degeneration, Parkinson syndrome (both paralysis agitans and the postencephalitic type), lipid storage diseases, striatopallidodentatal calcification, Leigh disease, and acute and chronic phenothiazine and haloperidol poisoning. Dystonia may also be a prominent feature of certain, as yet unnamed, heredodegenerative disorders such as familial striatal necrosis with affection of the optic nerves and other parts of the nervous system (Marsden et al, Novotny et al). Finally, restricted forms of athetosis and dystonia, sometimes called dyskinesias, involve only the orbicularis oculi and face or mandibular muscles (blepharospasm-oromandibular dystonia), the tongue, the cervical muscles (spasmodic torticollis), the hand (writer's cramp), etc. These are described in the next chapter, as well as in Chap. 43.

The most frequent cause of acute dystonic reactions are drugs—phenothiazines, butyrophenones, or metoclopramide—and these respond to intravenous diazepam, given two or three times in 24 to 48 h. All manner of drugs have been used in the treatment of chronic dystonia, with a notable lack of success. However, Fahn has reported beneficial effects (more so in children than in adults) with the anticholinergic agents trihexyphenidyl (Artane) and ethopropazine (Parsidol) given in massive doses—achieved by increasing the dosage very gradually. Stereotactic surgery on the pallidum and ventrolateral thalamus have given rather unpredictable results.

Paroxysmal Choreoathetosis and Dystonia Under the names of "familial paroxysmal choreoathetosis" and "periodic dystonia," among others, there has been described an uncommon familial disorder, characterized by paroxysmal attacks of choreoathetotic movements and/or dystonic spasms of the limbs and trunk. Children and young adults are mainly affected.

There are two main forms of the familial disorder. In the most common form, which has an autosomal dominant or recessive pattern of inheritance, there are numerous, brief (less than 2-s) attacks of choreoathetosis, provoked by startle or sudden movement—hence the title *paroxysmal kinesigenic choreoathetosis.* This disorder responds well to anticonvulsant medication, notably to clonazepam.

In some families, such as those originally described by Mount and Reback and more recently by Lance and by Plant et al, the attacks take the form of a persistent (5-min to 4-h) dystonic spasm and have reportedly been precipitated by the ingestion of alcohol or coffee, by fatigue, and rarely by prolonged exercise (nonkinesigenic). The attacks may be bilateral, predominantly unilateral, or confined to one side and associated with rare bilateral attacks. This form of the disease is inherited as an autosomal dominant trait. A favorable response of this disorder to benzodiazepines

Figure 4-6

A. *Characteristic dystonic deformities of the hands and feet observed in parkinsonism.* B. (Left) *Severe dystonic retrocollis in a young woman.* (Right) *Incapacitating kyphoscoliotic postural deformity in a young man with dystonia.* (A, *from IS Cooper, Parkinsonism: Its Medical and Surgical Therapy, Springfield, Ill, Charles C Thomas, 1961; B, from IS Cooper, Involuntary Movement Disorders, Hagerstown, Md, Harper & Row, 1969.)*

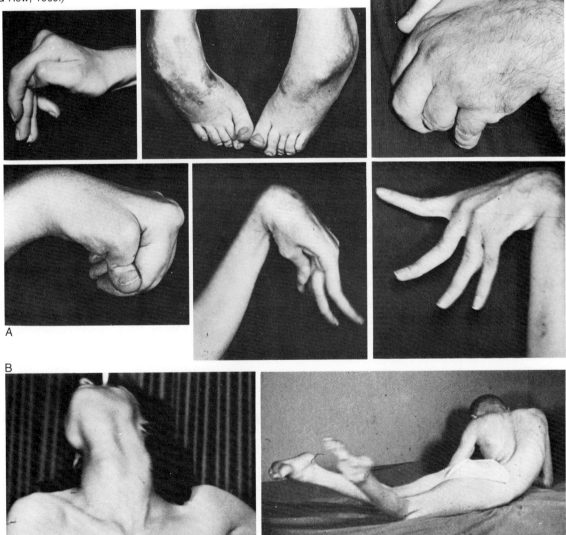

has been reported, particularly if the drug has been given on alternate days (Kurlan and Shoulson).

Because of their paroxysmal nature and the response (of the kinesigenic type) to anticonvulsant drugs, these familial disorders have been thought to represent seizures originating in the basal ganglia. However, consciousness is not lost and the EEG is normal, even when recorded during an attack of choreoathetosis. Also, it should be recalled that oculogyric crises and other spasms occur episodically in basal ganglionic diseases such as postencephalitic parkinsonism and acute and chronic phenothiazine intoxication.

In addition to these familial disorders, sporadic instances of paroxysmal choreoathetosis and dystonia have been described. These latter instances are usually an expression of some serious neurologic or metabolic disease, such as perinatal anoxia, multiple sclerosis, hypoparathyroidism, and thyrotoxicosis.

The Identity of Chorea, Athetosis, and Dystonia
It must be evident, from the foregoing descriptions, that the distinctions between chorea and athetosis are probably not fundamental. Even their most prominent differences—the discreteness and rapidity of choreic movements and the slowness and confluence of athetotic ones—may be more apparent than real. As pointed out by Kinnier Wilson, involuntary movements may follow one another in such rapid succession that they become confluent and therefore appear to be slow. In practice, one finds that the patient with relatively slow, confluent movements also shows discrete, rapid ones, and vice versa, and that many patients with chorea and athetosis also exhibit the persistent disorder of movement and posture that is generally designated as dystonia.

In a similar vein, no meaningful distinction, except one of degree, can be made between choreoathetosis and ballismus. Particularly forceful movements of large amplitude (ballismus) are observed in certain patients with Sydenham and Huntington chorea, who according to traditional teaching, exemplify pure forms of chorea and athetosis, respectively. The intimate relationship between these involuntary movements is illustrated by the patient with hemiballismus, who, at the onset of the illness, exhibits wild flinging movements of the arm and, after a period of partial recovery, shows only choreoathetotic flexion-extension movements that are limited to the fingers. For this reason, the terms *hemiballismus* and *hemichorea* are often used interchangeably.

Finally, it should be pointed out that all disorders of

movement due to lesions of the extrapyramidal system have certain attributes in common. The abnormalities of movement are superimposed on relatively intact praxic and voluntary movements, implying integrity of corticospinal systems; their persistence indicates they are veritable release phenomena; they are abolished by sleep and enhanced by anxiety and excitement; they are caused by a variety of diseases, some of which evoke one type of movement disorder more than another; and they can be altered by certain pharmacologic agents and by stereotaxic lesions in certain parts of the motor systems.

The Anatomic Basis of Choreoathetosis and Dystonia
For many years it had been known that the abrupt onset of violent hemichorea or hemiballismus was associated with a lesion in the contralateral subthalamic nucleus or its immediate connections (Martin). The implications of this relationship were not fully appreciated until relatively recently, however. In 1949, Whittier, Mettler, and Carpenter demonstrated that in monkeys a similar movement disorder, which they termed "choreoid dyskinesia," could be produced consistently in the limbs of one side of the body by a lesion localized to the opposite subthalamic nucleus. They showed also that for such a lesion to provoke dyskinesia, the adjacent pallidum and pallidofugal fibers had to be preserved; furthermore, a secondary lesion, placed in the pallidum, particularly in its medial segment, or in the fasciculus lenticularis, or in the ventrolateral thalamic nuclear group, could abolish the dyskinesia. In a series of sequential studies, Carpenter and his colleagues demonstrated convincingly that this experimental hyperkinesia could be abolished permanently by interruption of the lateral corticospinal tract, but not by interruption of the other motor or sensory pathways in the spinal cord. These observations were interpreted to indicate that the subthalamic nucleus normally exerts an inhibitory or regulating influence on the globus pallidus and ventral thalamus. Removal of this influence, by selective destruction of the subthalamic nucleus, is expressed physiologically by bursts of irregular choreoid activity which arise from the intact pallidum and are conveyed by pallidofugal fibers to the ventrolateral thalamic nuclei, thence by thalamocortical fibers to the premotor cortex, and from there by short association fibers to the motor cortex. Ultimately the abnormal movement expresses itself via the lateral corticospinal tract. In this instance a part of the "extrapyramidal" motor system functions not as an independent motor system but as a facilitatory and inhibitory element in complex motor activities for which the corticospinal tract is the final executive pathway.

Conceivably, the abnormal movements that characterize Huntington chorea or other disorders of the striatum have a similar explanation. Here there is a release of pallidal and thalamic activity by virtue of a loss of striatal neurons, which normally have a modulating effect upon the pallidum. Again, the upper motor neurons must be intact. In post-hemiplegic choreoathetosis the corticospinal tract must have remained relatively intact and recovered function (Dooling and Adams).

Some of these observations and interpretations can be corroborated in humans. It has been appreciated for many years that if patients with involuntary movements suffer a stroke, the movement disorder is abolished on the paralyzed side. Indeed it was this observation that led surgeons to interrupt the corticospinal tract—at its origin in the precentral gyrus, in the cerebral peduncle, or in the dorsolateral funiculus of the spinal cord—in order to obtain the same effect. This operation was given up, however, because of the attendant paresis and spasticity. The most important advance in our understanding of extrapyramidal motor function, credited largely to the pioneering efforts of neurosurgeons (Meyers; Cooper), was the demonstration that tremor, rigidity, and involuntary movements of the limbs could be abolished by a surgical lesion in the medial segment of the globus pallidus or, preferably, in the ventrolateral nucleus of the thalamus (Fig. 4-7), without causing paralysis of voluntary movement. Again the effects are always contralateral. In the treatment of paralysis agitans, the oral administration of L-dopa has largely obviated the need for this surgical procedure, but it is still being used in certain cases of unilateral athetosis, dystonia, and tremor. Apart from these practical considerations, the salutary effects of ventrolateral thalamotomy indicate that the ventrolateral nucleus, probably through its connections with the premotor cortex and the corticospinal pathway, is an essential link in the expression of the extrapyramidal syndromes, both of striatonigral and cerebellar types.

DIAGNOSIS OF DISEASES OF THE BASAL GANGLIA

The fully developed striatonigral syndromes can be recognized without difficulty once the physician has become familiar with their typical modes of clinical presentation. The picture of the Parkinson syndrome, with its slowness of movement, poverty of facial expression, flexed posture, immobility, and static tremor should be fixed in mind; it is the particular combination of these features that stamps the patient unmistakably as parkinsonian. Similarly, the torsion spasms and postural abnormalities of dystonia, whether widespread or involving only a group of neck muscles, as in spasmodic torticollis, once seen, should thereafter be familiar. Choreoathetosis, with its instability of postures and ceaseless movements of fingers, hands, head, and facial muscles, and the shock-like movements of myoclonus that flit over the body, are other standard syndromes. Charac-

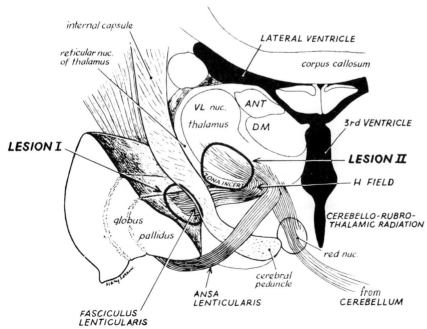

Figure 4-7

Basal ganglia and their connections, illustrating the location of lesions which abolish contralateral parkinsonian tremor. Lesion I involves the medial globus pallidus and fasciculus lenticularis; lesion II involves the ventrolateral nucleus of thalamus. (From TH Lin et al, Electroencephalogr Clin Neurophysiol 13:631, 1961.)

teristic of all is the relatively mild defect in motor power of the affected parts.

Early or mild forms of the basal ganglionic disorders, like all diseases, may offer special difficulties in diagnosis. Cases of paralysis agitans, seen before the appearance of tremor, are often overlooked. The patient may complain of difficulty in performing a particular movement, of trembling, of being nervous and restless or may have experienced an indescribable fatigue, stiffness and aching in certain parts of the body. Because of the absence of weakness and of reflex changes, the condition may be considered psychogenic or arthritic. It is well to remember that the parkinsonian syndrome often has a hemiplegic distribution at its outset, and for this reason the illness may for a time be mistakenly attributed to a mild stroke. A slight masking of the face, the suggestion of a limp, an inability to inhibit blinking when the bridge of the nose is tapped, the failure of an arm to swing naturally in walking, or loss of other automatic movements will help in diagnosis at this time. Every patient presenting with a parkinsonian syndrome or other abnormality of movement and posture in adolescence or early adult life should be investigated for hepatolenticular degeneration by tests of liver function, slit-lamp examination for corneal pigmentation (Kayser-Fleischer ring), and estimations of serum ceruloplasmin and urinary copper excretion. Dystonia in its early stages may be interpreted as an annoying mannerism or hysteria, and only later—in the face of persisting postural abnormality, lack of the usual psychologic picture of hysteria, and the emerging character of the illness—is the correct diagnosis made.

INCOORDINATION OF MOVEMENT (ATAXIA) DUE TO DISEASE OF THE CEREBELLUM

Incoordination of movement may have more than one cause. It may be due to a lesion in the cerebellum or in the sensory pathways that control movement, i.e., cerebellar ataxia and sensory ataxia; there are also forms that are due to neither. This part of the chapter is devoted to cerebellar ataxia. Sensory and other types of ataxia are considered in Chaps. 6, 8, and 14.

The cerebellum is concerned with the *regulation* or *control* of *muscular tone*, with the *coordination of movement*, especially skilled voluntary movement, and with the *control of posture and gait*. The mechanisms by which the cerebellum accomplishes these functions have been the subject of intense investigation in the last few decades. These investigations have yielded a mass of data, testimony

to the complexity of the organization of the cerebellum and its afferent and efferent connections. A coherent picture of cerebellar function is just beginning to emerge, although it is not yet possible, with a few notable exceptions, to relate the symptoms of cerebellar disease to discrete anatomic or functional units of the cerebellum. The following outline of cerebellar structure and function has of necessity been simplified; a full account can be found in the writings of Jansen and Brodal, Gilman and his colleagues, and Thach, listed at the end of this chapter.

ANATOMIC AND PHYSIOLOGIC CONSIDERATIONS

The classic studies of the comparative anatomy and the fiber connections of the cerebellum have led to the subdivision of the cerebellum into three parts (Fig. 4-8*A* and *B*): (1) The *flocculonodular lobe,* which is phylogenetically the oldest portion of the cerebellum (hence *archicerebellum*) and much the same in all animals, is separated from the main mass of the cerebellum, or corpus cerebelli, by the posterolateral fissure. (2) The *anterior lobe,* or *paleocerebellum,* which is the portion of the corpus cerebelli rostral to the primary fissure, constitutes most of the cerebellum in lower animals, but in humans it is relatively small, consisting of the anterior vermis and the contiguous paravermian cortex. (3) The *posterior lobe,* or *neocerebellum,* consists of the middle portions of the vermis and their large lateral extensions; the major portion of the cerebellar hemispheres fall into this subdivision.

This anatomic subdivision corresponds roughly with a functional subdivision of the cerebellum, based on the arrangement of its afferent fiber connections. The flocculonodular lobe receives special proprioceptive impulses from the vestibular nerves and nuclei and is therefore referred to as the "vestibulocerebellum"; it is concerned essentially with equilibrium of the body. The anterior vermis and part of the posterior vermis are referred to as the "spinocerebellum," since the fibers to these parts are derived to a large extent from the proprioceptors of muscles and tendons in the limbs and are conveyed to the cerebellum by the dorsal spinocerebellar tract (from the lower limbs) and the ventral spinocerebellar tract (upper limbs). The main influence of the "spinocerebellum" appears to be on posture and muscle tone. The neocerebellum derives its afferent fibers from the cerebral cortex, via the pontine nuclei and brachium pontis, hence the designation "pontocerebellum"; this portion of the cerebellum is concerned primarily with the coordination of skilled movements that are initiated at a cerebral cortical level.

On the basis of ablation experiments in animals, three rather characteristic clinical syndromes have been delineated, corresponding to these major divisions of the cerebellum. Lesions of the nodulus and flocculus have been found to cause a disturbance of equilibrium of the body and frequently a positional nystagmus as well; individual movements of the limbs are not affected, however. The main effects of anterior lobe ablation in primates are increased shortening and lengthening reactions, somewhat increased tendon reflexes, and an exaggeration of the postural reflexes, particularly the "positive supporting reflex," which consists of an extension of the limb in response to light pressure on the foot pad. Ablation of the cerebellar hemisphere in cats and dogs yields inconsistent results, but in monkeys it causes hypotonia and clumsiness of the ipsilateral limbs; if the dentate nucleus is included in the

hemispheric ablation, these abnormalities are more enduring and the limbs also show an ataxic or "intention" tremor.

It should be emphasized that cerebellar function and structure are hardly as simple or precise as the foregoing outline might suggest. The studies of Chambers and Sprague and of Jansen and Brodal indicate that in respect to both afferent and efferent connections, the cerebellum is organized into longitudinal (sagittal) rather than transverse zones. There are three longitudinal zones—the vermian, paravermian or intermediate, and lateral, and there seems to be considerable overlapping between them. Chambers and Sprague, on the basis of their investigations in cats, concluded that the vermian zone coordinates movements of eyes and the body with respect to gravity and movement

Figure 4-8

Cerebellum, illustrating (A) *major fissures, lobes, and lobules, and* (B) *major divisions, on the basis of phylogenesis and function. (From EL House et al, A Systematic Approach to Neuroscience, 3rd ed, New York, McGraw-Hill, 1979.)*

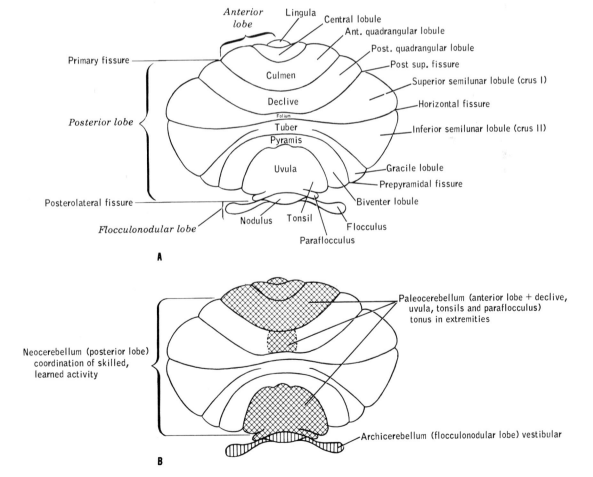

of the head in space. Defects in vestibulocerebellar function disturb the posture, tone, locomotion, and equilibrium of the entire body. The intermediate zone, which receives both peripheral and central input (from cortical area 4), influences postural tone, but also individual movements of the ipsilateral limbs; and the lateral zone is concerned mainly with the coordination of movements of the ipsilateral limbs, but is involved in other functions as well.

The efferent fibers of the cerebellar cortex, which consist essentially of the axons of Purkinje cells, project onto the deep cerebellar nuclei. According to the scheme of Jansen and Brodal, the vermis sends its fibers mainly to the fastigial nucleus; the intermediate zone, to the globose and emboliform nuclei (represented by the interpositus nucleus in animals); and the lateral zone, to the dentate nucleus. The deep cerebellar nuclei, in turn, project to the cerebral cortex and certain brainstem nuclei via two main pathways: (1) Fibers from the dentate, emboliform, and globose nuclei form the superior cerebellar peduncle, enter the upper pontine tegmentum as the brachium conjunctivum, decussate completely at the level of the inferior colliculus, and ascend to the ventrolateral nucleus of the thalamus and, to a lesser extent, to the intralaminar nuclei (Fig. 4-9). Some of the ascending fibers, soon after their decussation, synapse in the red nucleus, but others traverse this nucleus without synapsing. Ventral thalamic nuclear groups that receive projections from the cerebellum project directly to the motor cortex. A small group of fibers of the superior cerebellar peduncle, following their decussation, descend in the ventromedial tegmentum of the brainstem and project to the reticulotegmental and paramedian reticular nuclei. These nuclei in turn project via the inferior cerebellar peduncle to the cerebellum, mainly the anterior lobe, thus completing a cerebelloreticular-cerebellar feedback system (Fig. 4-10). (2) The fastigial nucleus projects onto the vestibular nuclei of both sides, and to a lesser extent onto other nuclei of the reticular formation of the pons and medulla. The inferior olivary nuclei project via the restiform body to the contralateral cerebellar cortex and the corresponding parts of the central nuclei. Thus, although the cerebellum has no direct pathways to the spinal cord comparable to the corticospinal tracts, it influences motor activity through its connections with the motor cortex and brainstem nuclei and their descending motor pathways.

The physiologic studies of Thach et al and Allen and Tsukahara have greatly expanded our knowledge of the role of the dentate and interpositus nuclei. The dentate nucleus receives inhibitory projections from the Purkinje cells of the lateral parts of the cerebellar cortex, and the interpositus

nucleus, from the Purkinje cells of the intermediate zones (between vermis and lateral parts of the hemisphere). Both nuclei also receive excitatory impulses from outside structures, both central (cerebral cortex) and peripheral (peripheral nerve, muscle, cutaneous, and joint receptors of spinal segments). But the two nuclei differ—the interpositus receives a stronger peripheral input than the dentate; the former also receives a stronger input from the sensorimotor cortex than from the premotor and supplementary cortices.

Allen et al and Thach et al have studied the effects of cooling these nuclei during a projected movement in the macaque monkey and conclude that the lateral cerebellum and the dentate nucleus are involved with the premotor cortex in the programming of movements before their initiation, while the intermediate cerebellum and interpositus nucleus are involved in the regulation of movement once it is started, via sensory feedback from the contracting muscles. The latter structures are also activated by collaterals from the corticospinal tract at the same time as the anterior motor neurons. Thach has shown that the dentate neurons actually fire earlier than the interpositus neurons which would affirm the role of the dentate in the planning of movement before the motor cortex discharges.

During projected swift (ballistic) movements in humans, Hallett and Khoshbin have demonstrated the correctness of Holmes' theory that the cerebellum is essential for the proper timing of muscle action in a coordinated act. With cerebellar lesions there is a prolongation of the interval between the command and the triphasic agonist-antagonist-agonist motor sequence referred to above, but also the agonist burst may be too long or too short or continue into the antagonist burst. This could explain the decomposition of movement, the dysmetria, and the slowness of alternating movements. In addition, Thach points out that the nucleus interpositus, and to a lesser extent the dentate nucleus, normally damp physiologic tremor; with lesions of these parts, the tremor increases in amplitude.

NEUROPHARMACOLOGY OF THE CEREBELLUM

The five cell types in the cerebellar cortex (Purkinje, stellate, basket, Golgi, and granule cells) are all inhibitory, except the granule cells. The afferent mossy fibers utilize aspartate, but the neurotransmitter of the climbing fibers is unknown. The transmitter of the afferent fibers from the locus ceruleus is noradrenalin. The granule cell axons that form the parallel fibers elaborate glutamate. All the inhibitory cerebellar cortical neurons appear to utilize GABA. High concentrations of glutamic acid decarboxylate are found in the Purkinje cells. The neurotransmitters of the roof nuclei are unknown.

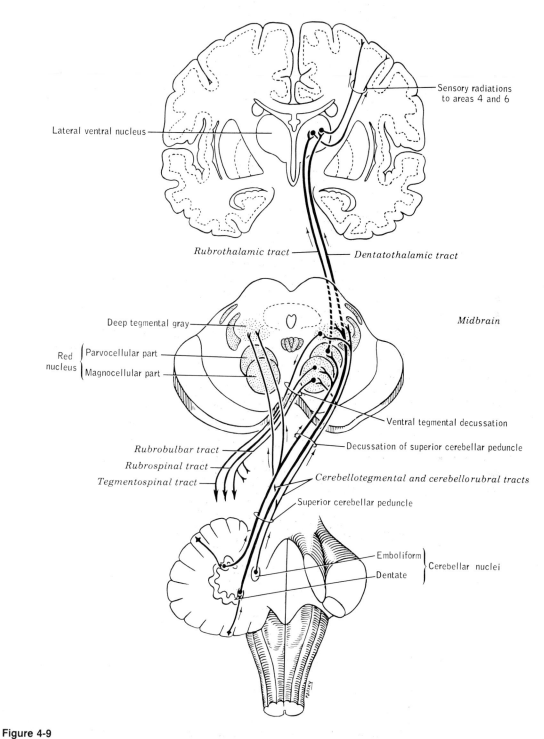

Sensory radiations
to areas 4 and 6

Lateral ventral nucleus

Rubrothalamic tract — *Dentatothalamic tract*

Deep tegmental gray

Midbrain

Red
nucleus { Parvocellular part

Magnocellular part

Ventral tegmental decussation

Decussation of superior cerebellar peduncle

Rubrobulbar tract
Rubrospinal tract
Tegmentospinal tract

Cerebellotegmental and cerebellorubral tracts

Superior cerebellar peduncle

Emboliform } Cerebellar nuclei

Dentate

Figure 4-9

*Cerebellar projections to the red nucleus, thalamus, and cerebral cortex. (Adapted from
EL House et al, A Systematic Approach to Neuroscience, 3rd ed, New York, McGraw-Hill,
1979.)*

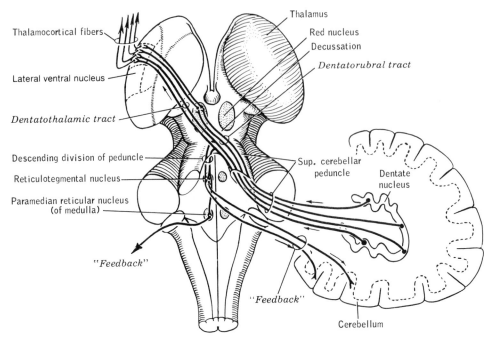

Figure 4-10

Dentatothalamic and dentatorubrothalamic pathways via the superior cerebellar peduncle. The "feedback" circuit via the reticular nuclei and reticulocerebellar fibers is also shown. (From EL House et al, A Systematic Approach to Neuroscience, 3rd ed, New York, McGraw-Hill, 1979.)

CLINICOANATOMIC CORRELATIONS

The symptoms produced in animals by ablation of discrete anatomic or functional zones of the cerebellum bear only an imperfect relationship to the symptoms of cerebellar disease in humans. This is understandable for several reasons. Most of the lesions that occur in humans do not respect the boundaries established by experimental anatomists. However, even when the lesions are confined to discrete functional zones (e.g., flocculonodular lobe, anterior lobe), the clinical syndromes cannot be identified with those produced by the ablation of analogous zones in cats, dogs, and even in monkeys, indicating that the functional organization of these parts varies from species to species.

The evidence that flocculonodular lesions in humans cause a disturbance of equilibrium is quite flimsy. It rests on the observation that with certain tumors of childhood, viz., medulloblastomas, there may be a gross ataxia of stance and gait, but no tremor or incoordination of the limbs when the child is examined in the recumbent position.

Insofar as these tumors are thought to originate from cell rests in the posterior medullary velum, at the base of the nodulus, it has been inferred that the disturbance of equilibrium results from involvement of this portion of the cerebellum. The validity of this deduction remains to be proved, however; by the time such tumors are inspected at operation or autopsy, they have spread beyond the confines of the nodulus, and a strict clinicopathologic correlation is not justified.

Patients in whom accurate clinicoanatomic correlations can be made indicate that the syndrome of ataxia of stance and gait, with normality of movements of the limbs, corresponds more closely with lesions of the anterior vermis than with lesions of the flocculus and nodulus. This conclusion is based on the study of a highly stereotyped form of cerebellar degeneration in alcoholics (see Chap. 39). In such patients the cerebellar disturbance may be limited to one of stance and gait, and in these cases the pathologic changes are restricted to the anterior parts of the superior vermis. In more severely affected patients, there is also incoordination of individual movements of the limbs; in these patients the lesion will be found to extend laterally from the vermis, to involve the anterior portions of the anterior lobes (in patients with ataxia of the legs) and the more posterior portions of the anterior lobes (in patients whose arms are affected). Similar clinicopathologic relationships pertain in patients with familial cerebellar degeneration of the "Holmes type." In either circumstance, despite a serious disturbance of equilibrium, the flocculo-nodular lobe may be spared completely.

These clinicopathologic observations suggest that the cerebellar cortex, and the anterior lobe in particular, is organized somatotopically, a view that has been amply confirmed experimentally (Fig. 4-11). Originally, afferent projections to the cerebellum were thought to be entirely vestibular and proprioceptive, but now it is known that large portions of the hemispheres are involved in tactual, visual, auditory, and even visceral mechanisms. The mapping of evoked potentials from the cerebellar cortex, elicited by a variety of sensory stimuli, and an analysis of the motor effects produced by stimulation of specific parts of the cerebellar cortex, indicate that there is somatotopic localization of function in the cerebellum. The topographic representation of body parts, based on these experimental observations, is illustrated in Fig. 4-11. The similarities between this scheme and the one derived from the study of human disease are at once apparent.

CEREBELLAR SYMPTOMS

Lesions of the cerebellum in humans give rise to the following abnormalities: (1) loss of muscle tone, (2) incoordination (ataxia) of volitional movement, and (3) disorders of equilibrium and gait. Extensive lesions of one cerebellar hemisphere, especially of the anterior lobe, cause hypotonia, postural abnormalities, ataxia, and mild weakness of the ipsilateral arm and leg. Lesions of the cerebellar peduncles have the same effects as extensive hemispheral lesions. If the lesion is limited to portions of the cerebellar cortex and subcortical white matter, there may be surprisingly little disturbance of function, or the abnormality may be greatly attenuated with the passage of time. Lesions

involving the superior cerebellar peduncle or the dentate nucleus cause the most severe and enduring cerebellar symptoms. Disorders of equilibrium and gait depend more upon vermian than upon hemispheral or peduncular involvement.

Hypotonia refers to the decrease in the normal resistance offered by the muscles to palpation or to passive manipulation (usually extension of a limb). It appears to be related to a depression of gamma and alpha motor neuron activity. In experimental animals (cats and monkeys), acute cerebellar lesions and hypotonia are associated with a depression of fusimotor efferent and spindle afferent activity; both static and dynamic afferents are depressed but not the secondary afferents. With the passage of time the fusimotor activity is restored as hypotonia disappears (Gilman, 1970). In the view of Gordon Holmes, hypotonia is the fundamental defect in cerebellar disease, accounting not only for the defects in postural fixation (see below) but also for the ataxia and tremor.

Hypotonia is much more apparent with acute than with chronic lesions and may be demonstrated in a number of ways. There may be undue flabbiness of the muscles on the affected side. Segments of the limbs may be displaced by the examiner through a wider range than normal. With recent, severe cerebellar lesions there may be gross asymmetries of posture, so that the shoulder slumps or the body tilts to the ipsilateral side. After flexing one arm against resistance that is suddenly released, the patient may be unable to check the flexion movement to the point where

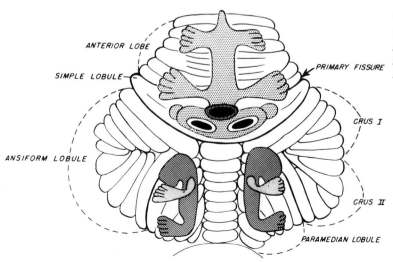

Figure 4-11

Somatotopic localization of motor and sensory function in the cerebellum. See text for explanation. (From M Victor et al, Arch Neurol 1:579, 1959.)

ANTERIOR LOBE

SIMPLE LOBULE

PRIMARY FISSURE

ANSIFORM LOBULE

CRUS I

CRUS II

PARAMEDIAN LOBULE

the arm may strike the face; this is due to a delay in contraction of the triceps muscle, which ordinarily would arrest overflexion of the arm. This response, incorrectly referred to as Holmes' rebound phenomenon, is more appropriately designated as an impairment of the check reflex. Stewart and Holmes, who first described this test, were careful to point out that when the resistance to flexion is suddenly removed, the normal limb moves only a short distance in flexion and then recoils or rebounds in the opposite direction. In this sense, rebound of the limb is actually deficient in cerebellar disease but exaggerated in spastic states.

A preferable method of testing for hypotonia is to tap the wrists of the outstretched arms, in which case the affected limb (or both limbs, in diffuse cerebellar disease) will be displaced through a wider range than normal, because of the failure of toneless muscles to fixate the arm at the shoulder. When an affected limb is shaken, the flapping movements of the hands are of wider excursion than normal. If the patient places his elbows on the table, with the arms flexed and the hands allowed to hang limply, the hand of the hypotonic limb will sag lower than the normal one. Forced flexion of a hypotonic arm at the elbow may obliterate the space between the volar aspect of the wrist and the deltoid. Pendularity of the knee jerk, due to defective tonic contraction of the quadriceps and hamstring muscles, is another manifestation of cerebellar hypotonia. Patients with these abnormalities of tone may show little or no impairment of corticospinal function, indicating that the maintenance of posture involves more than the voluntary contraction of muscles.

The most prominent manifestations of cerebellar disease, namely, the abnormalities of *intended (volitional) movement,* are embraced under the general heading of cerebellar incoordination or ataxia. The terms dyssynergia, dysmetria, and dysdiadochokinesis, among others, refer to particular aspects of ataxia and are commonly used to describe cerebellar abnormalities of movement. Gordon Holmes' characterization of these disturbances, as abnormalities in the rate, range, and force of movement, is at once less confusing and more accurate, as is apparent from an analysis of even a simple movement, e.g., the one elicited by finger-to-nose or by toe-to-finger testing.

The speed of initiating movement is slowed somewhat in cerebellar disease. Motor programs are degraded and the predictive control of movement patterns is lost. Contractions of opposing muscle groups for the maintenance of postures are decomposed and corrective movements are inaccurate. As a result, there is irregularity in both acceleration and

deceleration of movement, these being sometimes slower and sometimes faster than intended. These abnormalities are particularly prominent as the finger or toe approaches its objective. Normally, deceleration of the movement is smooth and accurate, even if sharp changes in direction are demanded by moving the target. With cerebellar disease, the velocity and force of the movement are not checked in the normal manner. The excursion of the limb may be arrested prematurely, and the objective is then attained by a series of jerky movements. Or the limb overshoots the mark (hypermetria); then the error is corrected by a series of secondary movements, in which the finger or toe sways around the target before coming to rest, or moves from side to side a few times on the target itself. This side-to-side movement of the finger as it approaches its target may assume a rhythmic quality and is then referred to as "intention tremor." To some extent, as pointed out by Holmes, this defect is due to hypotonia, i.e., an instability of the arm at the shoulder and elbow (or at the hip and knee, in heel-to-shin testing), the result of defective postural fixation at these joints, and to the voluntary acts of deviation by which the patient attempts to correct the excessive swaying of the limb. Gilman has provided evidence that more than hypotonia is involved in the tremor of cerebellar disease. He found that deafferentation of the forelimb of a monkey resulted in dysmetria and kinetic tremor; subsequent cerebellar ablation significantly increased both the dysmetria and tremor, indicating the presence of a mechanism, as yet unidentified, in addition to depression of the fusimotor efferent-spindle afferent circuit.

All the defects in volitional movement are more noticeable in acts that require alternation of movement, such as pronation-supination of the forearm or the successive touching of each finger to the thumb. The normal rhythm of these movements is interrupted by irregularities of force and speed, a disorder which Babinski named *adiadochokinesis.*

Another notable cerebellar disturbance is "decomposition" of a movement into its constituent parts. Electromyographic analysis has shown that decomposition of movement is due to abnormal duration and timing of bursts of contraction and relaxation of the involved muscles. This abnormality is most evident with compound movements, which involve a change in posture at two or more joints (e.g., in bringing finger to nose or heel to knee), but even a simpler movement may be fragmented, each component being effected with greater or lesser force than is required.

Cerebellar lesions commonly give rise to a disorder of *speech,* which may take one of two forms, either a simple slowing and slurring resembling that which follows interruption of the corticobulbar tracts, or a *scanning dysarthria* with variable intonation, so called because words are broken up into syllables, much as a line of poetry is scanned for meter. The latter disorder is uniquely cerebellar; in addition to its scanning quality, speech is slow, and each syllable, after an involuntary interruption, may be uttered with less force or more force (''explosive speech'') than is natural (Darley et al).

A head tremor of moderate speed (3 to 4 per second) in the anterior-posterior direction often accompanies midline cerebellar lesions. This is called *titubation*. It is much faster than the nodding or bobbing of the head that accompanies lesions of the thalamus.

Ocular movement may be impaired as a result of cerebellar disease. Voluntary gaze is accomplished by a series of jerky movements (saccadic dysmetria). On attempted fixation, the eyes may overshoot the target and then may oscillate through several cycles until precise fixation is attained. It will be recognized that these abnormalities, as well as those of speech, resemble those which characterize volitional movements of the limbs. Smooth pursuit movements are also impaired, being slower than normal and causing the patient to make catch-up saccades in an attempt to keep the moving target near the fovea. Patients with cerebellar lesions are unable to hold eccentric positions of gaze, resulting in the need to make repetitive saccades to look eccentrically, i.e., *gaze-paretic nystagmus* (Zee and others). Downbeat nystagmus, rebound nystagmus, and sustained horizontal nystagmus may also be observed occasionally. The pathogenesis of nystagmus is discussed in Chap. 13. Currently it is believed that nystagmus depends upon lesions of the vestibulocerebellum (Thach and Montgomery). Whether lesions in other parts of the cerebellum cause nystagmus is uncertain; in at least one patient, however, the lesion was confined to the cerebellar territory of the posterior inferior cerebellar artery (Duncan et al). Skew deviation and ocular myoclonus may also be related to cerebellar disease; these abnormalities and other effects of cerebellar lesions on ocular function are discussed in Chap. 13.

A slight *loss of muscular power* and *excessive fatigability* of muscle may occur with acute cerebellar lesions. Also, in unilateral cerebellar disease, the ipsilateral arm may not swing normally in walking. Insofar as these symptoms cannot be explained by a loss of tone or other motor disorder, they must be regarded as primary manifestations of cerebellar disease, but they are never severe or persistent and are of little clinical importance.

Cerebellar disorders of equilibrium and gait are described in Chap. 6.

CLINICOPATHOLOGIC CORRELATIONS OF THE EXTRAPYRAMIDAL MOTOR DISORDERS

The extrapyramidal motor syndrome, as we know it today, was first delineated and so named by S. A. Kinnier Wilson,

in 1912. The most striking abnormality in the nervous system of his patients was a degeneration of the putamens,

Table 4-2
Clinicopathologic correlations of extrapyramidal motor disorders

Symptoms	Principal location of morbid anatomy
Unilateral plastic rigidity with static tremor (Parkinson syndrome)	Contralateral substantia nigra plus (?) other structures
Unilateral hemiballismus and hemichorea	Contralateral subthalamic nucleus of Luys or luysialpallidal connections
Chronic chorea of Huntington type	Caudate nucleus and putamen
Athetosis and dystonia	Contralateral striatum. Pathology of dystonia musculorum deformans (Oppenheim) unknown.
Cerebellar incoordination, intention tremor, and hyptonia	Homolateral cerebellar hemisphere or middle and inferior cerebellar peduncles, brachium conjunctivum (ipsilateral if below decussation, contralateral if above)
Decerebrate rigidity, i.e., extension of arms and legs, opisthotonos	Usually bilateral in tegmentum of upper brainstem, at level of red nucleus or between red and vestibular nuclei
Palatal and facial myoclonus (rhythmic)	Contralateral dentate nucleus or superior cerebellar peduncle or ipsilateral central tegmental tract or inferior olivary nucleus (dentato-olivary pathway)
Diffuse myoclonus	Neuronal degeneration, usually diffuse or predominating in cerebral or cerebellar cortex and dentate nuclei

to the extent of cavitation, and to these lesions Wilson attributed the characteristic symptoms of rigidity and tremor. Shortly thereafter, von Woerkom described a similar clinical syndrome in a patient with acquired liver disease (Wilson's cases were familial); in this case also the most prominent lesions consisted of foci of neuronal degeneration in the striatum. In 1920, Oskar and Cecile Vogt gave a detailed account of the neuropathologic changes in several patients who had been afflicted with choreoathetosis since early infancy; the changes, which they described as a status fibrosus or status dysmyelinatus, were confined to the caudate and lenticular nuclei. The studies of Huntington chorea, beginning with those of Meynert (1871) and followed by those of Jelgersma (1908) and Alzheimer (1911), also related the movement disorder to a loss of nerve cells in the striatum. Tretiakoff (1919) was the first to demonstrate the consistent affection of the substantia nigra in cases of paralysis agitans. A long series of observations, the most recent ones being those of J. Purdon Martin, have related hemiballismus to lesions in the subthalamic nucleus of Luys and its immediate connections.

Unfortunately, many of the classic cases leave much to be desired. We now know that in certain diseases, such as Wilson disease, Huntington chorea, Hallervorden-Spatz disease, and postencephalitic parkinsonism, parts of the brain other than the basal ganglia are involved. Also, lack of quantitative neuropathologic methods has hampered progress in this field. Even now the nature and topography of the pathologic findings in several of these diseases (e.g., dystonia musculorum deformans) have not been determined. The difficulties of clinicoanatomic correlations in cases of cerebellar disease have already been indicated. The lesions responsible for so-called palatal myoclonus have a specific localization in the central tegmental tract, inferior olivary and contralateral dentate nuclei, whereas the anatomic basis of diffuse myoclonus is quite vague (see Chap. 6).

Table 4-2 summarizes the clinicopathologic correlations accepted by most neurologists, but it must be reemphasized that there is still much uncertainty as to finer details.

REFERENCES

ALEXANDER GE, DeLONG ME: Macrostimulation of the primate neostriatum. *J Neurophysiol* 53:1417, 1433, 1985.

ALLEN GI, TSUKAHARA N: Cerebrocerebellar communication systems. *Physiol Rev* 54:957, 1974.

BROOKS VB: *The Neural Basis of Motor Control*. New York, Oxford, 1986.

CARPENTER MB: Brainstem and infratentorial neuraxis in experimental dyskinesia. *Arch Neurol* 5:504, 1961.

CARPENTER MB: Anatomy of the corpus striatum and brainstem integrating systems, in Brooks V (ed): *Handbook of Physiology*, sec 1: *The Nervous System*, vol 2: *Motor Control*. Bethesda, American Physiological Society 1981, chap 19, pp 947–995.

CARPENTER MB, WHITTIER JR, METTLER FA: Analysis of choreoid hyperkinesia in the rhesus monkey: Surgical and pharmacological analysis of hyperkinesia resulting from lesions of the subthalamic nucleus of Luys. *J Comp Neurol* 92:293, 1950.

CARPENTER MB, SUTIN J: The corpus striatum, in *Human Neuroanatomy*, 8th ed. Baltimore, Williams and Wilkins, 1983, chap 17, pp 579–607.

CHAMBERS WW, SPRAGUE JM: Functional localization in the cerebellum. I. Organization in longitudinal cortico-nuclear zones and their contribution to the control of posture, both extrapyramidal and pyramidal. *J Comp Neurol* 103:104, 1955.

CHAMBERS WW, SPRAGUE JM: Functional localization in the cerebellum. II. Somatotopic organization in cortex and nuclei. *Arch Neurol Psychiatry* 74:653, 1955.

COOPER IS: *Involuntary Movement Disorders*. New York, Hoeber-Harper, 1969.

COOPER JR, BLOOM FE, ROTH RH: *The Biochemical Basis of Neuropharmacology*, 4th ed. Oxford, Oxford University Press, 1982.

DARLEY FL, ARONSON AE, BROWN JR: *Motor Speech Disorders*. Philadelphia, Saunders, 1975.

DeLONG MR, ALEXANDER GE: Organization of basal ganglia, in Asbury AK, McKhann GM, McDonald WI (eds): *Diseases of the Nervous System*. Philadelphia, Saunders, 1986, chap 28.

DENNY-BROWN D, YANAGISAWA N: The role of the basal ganglia in the initiation of movement, in Yahr MD (ed): *The Basal Ganglia*. New York, Raven Press, 1976, pp 115–148.

DOOLING EC, ADAMS RD: The pathological anatomy of posthemiplegic athetosis. *Brain* 98:29, 1975.

DUNCAN GW, PARKER SW, FISHER CM: Acute cerebellar infarction in the PICA territory. *Arch Neurol* 32:364, 1975.

EVARTS EV, THACH WT: Motor mechanism of the CNS: Cerebrocerebellar-interrelations. *Ann Rev Physiol* 31:451, 1969.

FAHN S: High-dosage anticholinergic therapy in dystonia. *Neurology* 33:1255, 1983.

GILMAN S: The nature of cerebellar dyssynergia, in Williams D (ed): *Modern Trends in Neurology—5*. London, Butterworth, 1970, chap 4, pp 60–79.

GILMAN S, BLOEDEL J, LECHTENBERG R: *Disorders of the Cerebellum*. Philadelphia, Davis, 1980.

GROWDON JH, SCHEIFE RT: Medical treatment of extrapyramidal diseases, in Isselbacher KJ et al (eds): *Update III, Harrison's Principles of Internal Medicine*. New York, McGraw-Hill, 1982, pp 185–207.

HALLETT M, KHOSHBIN S: A physiological mechanism of bradykinesia. *Brain* 103:301, 1980.

HALLETT M, SHAHANI BT, YOUNG RR: EMG analysis of patients with cerebellar deficits. *J Neurol Neurosurg Psychiatry* 38:1163, 1975.

HASSLER R, REICHERT T, MUNDINGER F, et al: Physiologic observations in stereotaxic operations in extrapyramidal motor disturbances. *Brain* 83:337, 1960.

HOLMES G: The cerebellum of man. Hughlings Jackson Lecture. *Brain* 62:1, 1939.

HORNYKIEWICZ O: Neurochemical pathology and pharmacology of brain dopamine and acetylcholine: Rational basis for the current drug treatment of Parkinsonism, in McDowell FH, Markham CH (eds): *Contemporary Neurology Series,* vol 8: *Recent Advances in Parkinson's Disease.* Philadelphia, Davis, 1971, pp 33–65.

HUDGINS RL, CORBIN KB: An uncommon seizure disorder: Familial paroxysmal choreoathetosis. *Brain* 91:199, 1968.

JANSEN J, BRODAL A: *Aspects of Cerebellar Anatomy.* Oslo, Johan Grundt Tanum Forlag, 1954.

KLAWANS HL JR: *Monographs in Neural Sciences,* vol 2: *The Pharmacology of Extrapyramidal Movement Disorders.* Basel, Karger, 1973.

KURLAN R, SHOULSON I: Familial paroxysmal dystonic choreoathetosis and response to alternate-day oxazepam therapy. *Ann Neurol* 13:456, 1983.

LANCE JW: Familial paroxysmal dystonic choreoathetosis and its differentiation from related syndromes. *Ann Neurol* 2:285, 1977.

MARSDEN CD, LANG AE, QUINN NP, et al: Familial dystonia and visual failure with striatal CT lucencies.. *J Neurol Neurosurg Psychiatry* 49:500, 1986.

MARTIN JP: *Papers on Hemiballismus and the Basal Ganglia.* London, National Hospital Centenary, 1960.

MARTIN JP: *The Basal Ganglia and Posture.* Philadelphia, Lippincott, 1967.

MEYERS R: The surgery of the hyperkinetic disorders, in Vinken PJ, Bruyn GW (eds): *Handbook of Clinical Neurology,* vol 6: *Basal Ganglia.* Amsterdam, North-Holland, 1968, chap 33, pp 844–878.

MOUNT LA, REBACK S: Familial paroxysmal choreoathetosis: Preliminary report on a hitherto undescribed clinical syndrome. *Arch Neurol Psychiatry* 44:841, 1940.

NARABAYASHI H: Tremor mechanisms, in Schaltenbrand G, Walker AE (eds): *Stereotaxy of the Human Brain.* Stuttgart, Thieme, 1982, pp 510–514.

NOVOTNY EJ JR, DORFMAN LN, LOUIS A, et al: A neurodegenerative disorder with generalized dystonia: A new mitochondriopathy? *Neurology* 35(suppl 1): 273, 1985.

PLANT GT, WILLIAMS AC, EARL CJ, MARSDEN CD: Familial paroxysmal dystonia induced by exercise. *J. Neurol Neurosurg Psychiatry* 47:275, 1984.

POIRIER LJ: Experimental and histological study of midbrain dyskinesia. *J Neurophysiol* 23:534, 1960.

RICHTER R: Degeneration of the basal ganglia in monkeys from chronic carbon disulfide poisoning. *J Neuropathol Exp Neurol* 4:324, 1945.

SPRAGUE JM, CHAMBERS WW: Control of posture by reticular formation and cerebellum in the intact, anesthetized and unanesthetized and in the decerebrated cat. *Am J Physiol* 176:52, 1954.

THACH WT JR: The cerebellum, in Mountcastle VB (ed): *Medical Physiology,* 14th ed. St Louis, Mosby, 1980, vol 1, pp 837–858.

THACH WT, MONTGOMERY EB: Motor system, in Pearlman AL, Collins RC (eds): *Neurological Pathophysiology.* New York, Oxford, 1984.

WARD AA JR: The function of the basal ganglia, in Vinken PJ, Bruyn GW (eds): *Handbook of Clinical Neurology,* vol 6: *Basal Ganglia.* Amsterdam, North-Holland, 1968, chap 3, pp 90–115.

WHITTIER JR, METTLER FA: Studies on the subthalamus of the rhesus monkey. *J Comp Neurol* 90:281, 319, 1949.

WILSON SAK: Disorders of motility and of muscle tone, with special reference to the corpus striatum. The Croonian Lectures. *Lancet* 2:1, 53, 169, 215, 1925.

YANAGISAWA N, GOTO A: Dystonia musculatorum deformans. Analysis with electromyography. *J Neurol Sci* 13:39, 1971.

YOUNG AB, PENNEY JB: Pharmacologic aspects of motor dysfunction, in Asbury AK, McKhann GM, McDonald WI (eds): *Diseases of the Nervous System.* Philadelphia, Saunders, 1986, chap 31.

ZEMAN W: Pathology of the torsion dystonias (dystonia musculorum deformans). *Neurology* 20:79, 1970.

CHAPTER 5

TREMOR, MYOCLONUS, SPASMS, AND TICS

The subject of tremor may suitably be considered at this point because of its association with diseases of the basal ganglia and cerebellum. A miscellaneous group of other movement disorders—myoclonus, facial-cervical dyskinesias, occupational spasms, and tics—will also be described in this chapter. The latter disorders are largely involuntary in nature and can be quite disabling, but they have an uncertain pathologic basis and an indefinite relationship to the extrapyramidal motor disorders or to other standard categories of neurologic disease. They are being brought together here mainly for convenience of exposition.

TREMOR

Tremor may be defined as a more or less regular, rhythmic oscillation of a part of the body around a fixed point, usually in one plane. This rhythmic quality distinguishes tremor from other involuntary movements; its biphasic character distinguishes it from clonus. Two general categories are recognized: normal (or physiologic) and abnormal (or pathologic). The former, as the name indicates, is a normal phenomenon; it is present in all muscle groups and persists throughout the waking state and even in certain phases of sleep. The movement is so fine that it can barely be seen by the naked eye and then only if the fingers are firmly outstretched; in most instances special instruments are required for its detection. It ranges in frequency between 8 and 13 Hz, the dominant rate being 10 Hz in adults and somewhat less in childhood and old age. Several hypotheses have been proposed to explain physiologic tremor, the most popular one being that it reflects the ballistocardiogram, i.e., the passive vibration of body tissues produced by mechanical activity of cardiac origin ("BCG tremor"). Assuredly this is not the complete explanation of physiologic tremor. As Marsden points out, it is due to the complex interaction of several additional factors such as spindle input, the unfused grouped firing rates of motor neurons,

and the natural resonating frequencies and inertia of the muscles and other structures. Certain abnormal tremors, namely the metabolic varieties of postural or action tremor and at least one type of familial tremor, are believed by some workers to be variants or exaggerations of physiologic tremor; i.e., "enhanced physiologic tremor" (see further on).

Abnormal or pathologic tremor, which is what one means when the term tremor is used clinically, preferentially affects certain muscle groups—the distal parts of the limbs (especially the fingers and hands), the head, tongue or jaw, and rarely the trunk—and is present only in the waking state. The rate in most forms is from 4 to 7 Hz, i.e., about half that of physiologic tremor. In any one individual the rate is fairly constant in all affected parts, regardless of the size of the muscles or the parts of the body involved. With the advent of EMG and mechanical recording devices, abnormal tremors have been subdivided according to their rate and their relationship to posture of the limbs and volitional movement, the pattern of EMG activity in opposing muscle groups, and their response to certain drugs (Freund et al). The following types of tremor should be familiar to every physician.

PARKINSONIAN (REST) TREMOR

This is a coarse, rhythmic tremor with a frequency of 3 to 5 Hz. Electromyographically, it is characterized by bursts of activity which alternate between opposing muscle groups. The tremor is most often localized in one or both hands and less frequently in the feet, jaw, lips, or tongue. It occurs when the limb is in an *attitude of repose* and is suppressed or diminished by willed movement, at least momentarily, only to reassert itself once the limb assumes a new position. For this reason the parkinsonian tremor is often referred to as a "resting tremor" or "tremor at rest," but these terms need to be qualified. Maintaining the arm in an attitude of repose or keeping it still in other positions requires a certain degree of muscular contraction, albeit slight. If the tremulous hand is fully relaxed, as it is when the arm is fully supported at the wrist and elbow, the tremor usually disappears, but the patient rarely achieves this state. Usually he maintains a state of tonic contraction of the trunk and proximal muscles of the limbs. Under conditions of complete rest, i.e., in all except the lightest phases of sleep, the tremor disappears, as do all abnormal tremors except palatal and ocular myoclonus.

Parkinsonian tremor takes the form of flexion-extension or abduction-adduction of the fingers or the hand; pronation-supination of the hand and forearm is also a common presentation. Flexion-extension of the fingers in combination with adduction-abduction of the thumb yields the classic ''pill-rolling'' tremor. It continues while the patient walks, unlike essential tremor. When the legs are affected, the tremor takes the form of a flexion-extension movement of the foot, and in the jaw and lips an up-and-down and a pursing movement, respectively. The eyelids, if they are closed lightly, tend to flutter rhythmically (blepharoclonus), and the tongue, when protruded, may move in and out of the mouth at about the same tempo as the tremor elsewhere. The rate of the tremor is surprisingly constant over long periods, but the amplitude is variable. Emotional stress, in particular, augments the amplitude, and increasing rigidity of the limbs may reduce it. The tremor interferes surprisingly little with voluntary movement; it is possible, for example, for a tremulous patient to raise a full glass of water to his lips and drain its contents without spilling a drop. Parkinsonian tremor is suppressed to some extent by the phenothiazine derivative ethopropazine (Parsidol), by trihexyphenidil (Artane) and other anticholinergic drugs, and somewhat less consistently by L-dopa. Stereotaxic lesions in the ventrolateral nucleus of the thalamus abolish tremor (and rigidity) contralaterally. A parkinsonian tremor is sometimes associated with tremors of faster frequency (page 938); the latter are of action or postural type and respond better to beta-blocking than to antiparkinson drugs.

Resting tremor is most often a manifestation of the Parkinson syndrome, whether it be the idiopathic variety described by James Parkinson (paralysis agitans) or the postencephalitic or the drug-induced type. In paralysis agitans the tremor is relatively gentle and more or less limited to the distal muscles, whereas the tremor of postencephalitic parkinsonism often has a greater amplitude and involves proximal muscles. In neither disease is there a close correspondence between the degree of tremor and of rigidity or akinesia. A parkinsonian tremor may also be seen in elderly persons without akinesia, rigidity, or masklike facies. In some of these instances it is followed years later by paralysis agitans, but in the majority of cases it is not, the tremor remaining stationary for many years or progressing very slowly. Patients with the familial (wilsonian) or the acquired form of hepatocerebral degeneration may also show a static tremor of parkinsonian type, but usually it is mixed with ataxic tremor and other extrapyramidal motor abnormalities.

INTENTION (ATAXIC) TREMOR

The word *intention* is ambiguous in this context because the tremor itself is not intentional and occurs not when the patient intends to make a movement, but only during the most demanding phases of active movement. In this sense it is a kinetic, or action, tremor, but the latter term has other connotations to neurologists, being used generally as a synonym for postural tremor. The term *ataxic* is a suitable substitute for ''intention'' because this tremor is always combined with and adds to cerebellar ataxia. The salient feature of this tremor is that it requires for its full expression the performance of an exacting, precise, projected movement. The tremor is absent when the limbs are inactive and during the first part of a voluntary movement, but as the action continues and fine adjustments of the movement are demanded (e.g., in touching the tip of the nose or the examiner's finger), an irregular, more or less rhythmic (2 to 3 Hz) interruption of forward progression, with side-to-side oscillation, appears, and may continue for a second or so after the target has been reached. Unlike familial tremor, the oscillations occur in more than one plane (Young). The tremor may seriously interfere with the patient's performance of skilled acts. Sometimes there is a rhythmic oscillation of the head on the trunk (titubation), or of the trunk itself, at approximately the same rate.

This type of tremor invariably indicates disease of the cerebellum or its connections. It may be of such severity that every movement, even lifting the arm slightly from the side, results in a wide-ranging tremor of sufficient violence to throw the patient off balance; in such cases, the lesion is usually in the midbrain, involving the upward projections of the dentatorubrothalamic fibers and the medial part of the ventral tegmental reticular nucleus. Because of the proximity of the lesion to the red nucleus, Gordon Holmes referred to this as a ''rubral tremor.'' However, there is no evidence in animals or in humans that a lesion of the red nucleus per se produces any motor disturbances, other than those attributable to an interruption of the brachium conjunctivum fibers that traverse the nucleus (Carpenter). This type of tremor is seen in multiple sclerosis, and occasionally in Wilson disease and in vascular and other lesions of the tegmentum of the midbrain and subthalamus.

The mechanisms involved in the production of intention or ataxic tremor have been discussed in the preceding chapter (page 69). Beta-adrenergic blocking agents, anticholinergic drugs, and L-dopa have no effect.

POSTURAL OR ACTION TREMOR

These terms refer to a tremor that is present when the limbs and trunk are actively maintained in certain positions (such as holding the arms outstretched) and throughout active movement. More particularly, the tremor is absent when the limbs are relaxed but becomes evident when the muscles are activated; it is accentuated as greater precision of movement is demanded, but it never approaches the degree of augmentation seen in intention tremor. In contrast to static, or parkinsonian, tremor, which is characterized electromyographically by alternate activity in agonist and antagonist muscles, the rhythmicity of most cases of action tremor is accounted for by relatively rhythmic bursts of alpha motor neuron activity that occur almost *synchronously* and simultaneously in the opposing muscle groups. Presumably, inequalities in the strength and timing of contraction of opposing muscle groups account for the tremor.

Action tremors are of several different types, a feature which makes them more difficult to interpret than other tremors. One type seems to be a mere exaggeration of normal or physiologic tremor; it has the same frequency as physiologic tremor but a greater amplitude. Such a tremor, best elicited by holding the arms outstretched with fingers spread apart, is characteristic of intense fright and anxiety, hyperthyroidism, and other toxic states (lithium), and of withdrawal from alcohol and other sedative-hypnotic drugs. Frequently a tremor of the same frequency is observed in certain families (one type of familial tremor). Also it is noteworthy that a transient action tremor of this type can be reproduced by the intravenous injection of epinephrine or beta-adrenergic stimulating agents such as isoproterenol. All these clinical circumstances have in common an increased cardiac output, which may serve to increase the amplitude of physiologic or BCG tremor (see above). However, Young and his colleagues have adduced evidence that the enhancement of physiologic tremor that occurs in these various metabolic and toxic states is due to stimulation of muscular tremorogenic beta-adrenergic receptors by increased levels of circulating catecholamines. Thus it appears that synchronization of motor units in physiologic tremor, though not primarily of neural origin, is nevertheless influenced by central and peripheral nervous activity.

A second type of action tremor is of a slower frequency (4 to 8 Hz) than physiologic tremor. Tremor of this slow-frequency type may occur as the only neurologic abnormality in several members of a family, in which case it is known as *familial tremor.* Such a tremor tends to be inherited as an autosomal dominant trait; it may begin in childhood, but usually comes on later in adult life and persists. If the inherited nature of the tremor is not evident, it is referred to as *essential tremor,* and if it becomes evident only in late adult life, as *senile tremor.* These tremors cannot be distinguished on the basis of their physiologic and pharmacologic properties, and should not therefore be considered as separate entities.

Familial, or *essential, tremor* most often makes its appearance in early adult life, but it may begin in childhood and then persist. It is a relatively common form of tremor, with an estimated prevalence of 415 per 100,000 persons over the age of 40 years (Haerer et al). The usual frequency is 6 to 8 Hz, and it is of variable amplitude. Aging is associated with a decrease in the rate of the tremor, but an increase in amplitude. The tremor may be limited to the upper limbs, or a side-to-side or nodding movement of the head may be added. The tremor of the head may precede the tremor of the hand by several years, but more often it follows the hand tremor. The head tremor is also postural in nature and disappears when the head is supported. In advanced cases there is involvement of the jaw, lips, tongue, and larynx, the latter imparting a quaver to the voice.

The lower limbs are practically always spared. Rare cases, in which the legs are affected disproportionately, have been described under the title of *orthostatic tremor* (Heilman, Thompson et al, Wee et al). This tremor is most prominent during quiet standing, diminishes with walking, and disappears when the patient is seated or reclining. In the latter positions the tremor can be evoked by strong contraction of the leg muscles against resistance. Some of these cases have reportedly responded to the administration of clonazepam.

In distinction to the rapid action tremors, which interfere little with voluntary movements, there are slower (3.5 to 6 Hz), coarser types in which the tremors of hands, head, and voice are much more prominent during active movement than in the maintenance of certain postures (*kinetic tremor*). This type of tremor may increase in severity to a point where handwriting is altered and the patient cannot bring a spoon or glass to the lips without spilling the contents. Eventually all tasks which require manual dexterity are difficult or impossible.

As indicated above, in most patients with essential tremor of fast frequency there is simultaneous activity in agonist and antagonist muscles. In a relatively small proportion of patients, e.g., in the kinetic-predominant tremor, agonist and antagonist muscles are activated alternately.

Some patients with this slow, "alternate beat" form of action tremor may later develop Parkinson disease.

A curious fact about essential or familial tremor is that it can be suppressed by a few drinks of alcohol, but once the effects of the alcohol have worn off the tremor returns and may be even worse. This type of tremor is often suppressed by the beta-adrenergic antagonist propranolol taken orally over a long period of time (between 120 and 240 mg daily), suggesting that the tremor has an autonomic basis. Young et al have shown that neither propranolol nor ethanol, when injected intra-arterially into a limb, decreases the amplitude of essential tremor. These findings suggest that the therapeutic effects of these agents are due less to blockade of the peripheral beta-adrenergic tremorogenic receptors than to their action on structures within the central nervous system. The anticonvulsant drug primidone (50 mg initially, raised slowly to 250 mg daily) has been found to be effective in controlling essential tremor and should be tried in patients who do not respond to or cannot tolerate propranolol. The kinetic-predominant type of essential tremor is said to respond well to clonazepam (Biary and Koller).

An action tremor of varying severity is the most prominent feature of the alcohol withdrawal states. Using surface electrodes on agonist and antagonist muscles of the outstretched limb, Lefebvre-D'Amour and her colleagues have described two somewhat different types of tremor in the alcohol withdrawal state: (1) a tremor of frequency greater than 8 Hz (mean, 8.3 Hz), in which EMG recordings show continuous activity in antagonistic muscles. It resembles physiologic tremor but is of greater amplitude (enhanced physiologic tremor) and is responsive to propranolol (Koller et al); and (2) a tremor of frequency less than 8 Hz (mean, 7.2 Hz), characterized by discrete bursts of EMG activity occurring synchronously in antagonistic muscles, like that observed in one type of familial tremor (see above). Either type may occur in isolated form following relatively short periods of intoxication ("morning shakes"). The mechanisms involved in the genesis of alcohol withdrawal symptoms are discussed in Chap. 41.

Action tremors are seen in a number of neurologic diseases in addition to those already mentioned. A coarse action tremor, sometimes combined with myoclonus, accompanies various types of meningoencephalitis (e.g., general paresis) and certain intoxications (methyl bromide and bismuth). Its anatomy and mechanism are obscure. Also, it is important to note that an action tremor of either the fast-frequency or slower (essential) variety may occur in certain diseases of the basal ganglia, including parkinsonism, in which case both the action and the more typical static tremor may be present. Adams et al have also described a disabling action tremor in patients with steroid-responsive chronic demyelinative polyneuropathy. The EMG pattern in this neuropathic tremor is more irregular than in the essential-familial tremor; it is hypothesized that the tremor is attributable to deafferentation of the muscle spindle. Peroneal muscular atrophy may also be associated with essential-familial tremor.

HYSTERICAL TREMOR

Tremor is a relatively rare manifestation of hysteria, but it may simulate some types of organic tremor, thereby causing difficulty in diagnosis. Hysterical tremors are usually restricted to a single limb and are gross in nature. If the affected limb is restrained by the examiner, the tremor may move to another part of the body. Hysterical tremor is less regular than static tremor. It persists in repose and during movement and is less subject than organic tremors to the modifying influences of posture and willed movement.

TREMORS OF MIXED TYPE

Not all tremors correspond exactly with the ones described above. There is frequently a variation in one or more particulars from the classic pattern, or one type of tremor may show a feature ordinarily considered characteristic of another. In some parkinsonian patients, for example, the tremor is accentuated rather than diminished by active movement; in others the tremor may be very mild or absent "at rest" and only becomes obvious with movement of the limbs. As mentioned above, a patient with classic parkinsonian tremor may also show a fine tremor of the outstretched hands, i.e., a postural or action tremor, and occasionally an element of ataxic tremor as well. In a similar vein, essential or familial tremor may, in its advanced stages, assume the aspects of a cerebellar or intention tremor. Gordon Holmes was careful to note that patients with acute cerebellar lesions sometimes show a parkinsonian tremor in addition to the usual signs of ataxia and ataxic tremor.

The features of one type of tremor may be so mixed with those of another that satisfactory classification is impossible. In certain patients with essential or familial tremor or with cerebellar degeneration, one may observe a rhythmic tremor, characteristically parkinsonian in tempo, which is not apparent in repose but appears with certain sustained postures. It may take the form of an abduction-adduction or flexion-extension of the fingers when the patient's weight is partially supported by the hands, as in the writing position, or it may appear as a tremor of the thigh when the patient is seated or of the arms when they are outstretched.

THE PATHOLOGIC ANATOMY OF TREMOR

The exact anatomic basis of parkinsonian tremor is not known. In paralysis agitans and postencephalitic parkinsonism, the visible lesions predominate in the substantia nigra. In animals, experimental lesions confined to the substantia nigra do not result in tremor, however; neither do lesions in the striatopallidal parts of the basal ganglia. Moreover, not all patients with lesions of the substantia nigra have tremor; in some there are only bradykinesia and rigidity. In a group of eight patients intoxicated with a meperidine analog known as MPTP, which destroys the neurons of the pars compacta of the substantia nigra (page 941), four developed a tremor, and it had more the characteristics of a proximal action or postural tremor than of a rest tremor (Burns et al).

Ward and others have produced a Parkinson-like tremor in monkeys by placing a lesion in the ventromedial tegmentum of the midbrain, just caudal to the red nucleus and dorsal to the substantia nigra. This lesion may also have interrupted ascending fibers from the substantia nigra and descending fibers from the red nucleus. Ward has postulated that interruption of the descending pathway permits a lower brainstem mechanism to oscillate, presumably involving the limb innervation via the reticulospinal pathway. Alternative possibilities are that the lesion in the ventromedial tegmentum interrupts the brachium conjunctivum or a tegmental-thalamic projection or the descending limb of the superior cerebellar peduncle, which functions as a link in a dentate-reticular-cerebellar feedback mechanism (Fig. 4-10).

Tremor has been consistently produced in monkeys by removal of the outflow from deep cerebellar nuclei or section of the superior cerebellar peduncle or brachium conjunctivum, below the decussation. Lesions of the cerebellar nuclei, particularly of the nucleus interpositus, undamp physiologic tremor. The tremor is of the ataxic type, as one might expect, and is associated with other manifestations of cerebellar ataxia. In addition, however, these monkeys show a "simple tremor," which is the term that Carpenter has applied to a "resting" or parkinsonian tremor. The latter tremor is most prominent during the early postoperative period and is less enduring than ataxic tremor, but its presence suggests that ataxic and simple tremors have closely related neural mechanisms. Both forms of tremor can be abolished by ablation of the ventrolateral thalamic nucleus, contralateral to the cerebellar lesion.

In patients with tremor of either the parkinsonian, postural, or intention type, Narabayashi has recorded rhythmic burst discharges of unitary cellular activity in the ventral part of the nucleus intermedius ventralis, synchronous with the beat of the tremor. The neurons which exhibit the synchronous bursts are arranged somatotopically and respond to kinesthetic impulses from the muscles and joints involved in the tremor. Stereotaxic lesions in this area abolish the tremor. The effectiveness of the thalamic lesion may be due to interruption of pallidothalamic and dentatothalamic projections or, what is more likely, to interruption of projections from the ventrolateral thalamus to the premotor cortex, since the impulses responsible for cerebellar tremor, like those for choreoathetosis, are ultimately mediated by the lateral corticospinal tract. This concept explains why a lesion of the subthalamic nucleus causes *contralateral* dyskinesia, whereas a lesion of the brachium conjunctivum, below its decussation, gives rise to *ipsilateral* ataxia and tremor.

In the clinical analysis of tremor in humans the aforementioned types are usually distinguishable on the basis of rhythmicity, amplitude, frequency, relation to movement, postural set, and relaxation. Such testing procedures also differentiate tremors from a large array of nontremorous states, such as fasciculations, lapses of contraction in weak muscles, sensory ataxia, myoclonus, asterixis, epilepsia partialis continua, clonus, and shivering. The anatomical basis of postural and action tremors is unknown.

ASTERIXIS

The movement disorder asterixis, described by Adams and Foley in 1953, consists of arrhythmic lapses of sustained posture. These sudden interruptions in muscular contraction allow gravity or the inherent elasticity of muscles to produce a movement, which the patient then corrects, sometimes with overshoot. The initial movement or lapse in posture is associated with EMG silence for a period of 35 to 200 ms. Therefore asterixis differs physiologically from both tremor and myoclonus with which it was formerly confused; it has incorrectly been referred to as a "flapping tremor" or "negative tremor."

Asterixis is usually evoked by asking the patient to hold his arms outstretched with hands dorsiflexed or to dorsiflex the hands and extend the fingers while resting the forearms on the bed or the arms of a chair. Flexion movements of the hands may then occur once or several times a minute. Usually the lapses in the background EMG activity are generalized and can be provoked by the persistent contraction of any muscle group; sometimes they are confined to one side. If small finger muscles are affected, EMG may be required to separate asterixis from tremor and myoclonus.

This disorder of movement was first observed in patients with hepatic encephalopathy, but was later noted in hypercapnia, uremia, and other metabolic and toxic encephalopathies. However, occasional lapses of this type may appear in the neck and arms during drowsiness in a normal person. They may be evoked by phenytoin and other anticonvulsants. Unilateral asterixis has been noted in an arm and leg on the side opposite an anterior cerebral artery occlusion, and contralateral to a stereotaxic thalamotomy and upper midbrain lesions.

CLONUS, MYOCLONUS, AND POLYMYOCLONUS

The terms *clonus, myoclonus,* and *polymyoclonus* have been used indiscriminately to designate any rhythmic or arrhythmic series of brief muscular contractions attendant upon disease of the central nervous system. In this text, the terms will be used as follows: *Clonus* will refer to a series of *rhythmic, uniphasic or monophasic (i.e., unidirectional) contractions and relaxations* of a group of muscles, thus differing from tremors, which are always diphasic or bidirectional; *myoclonus* will specify the shock-like contraction(s) of a group of muscles, which are irregular in rhythm and amplitude and, with few exceptions, asynchronous and asymmetric in distribution; if such contractions occur singly or are repeated a few times in a restricted group of muscles, such as those of an arm or leg, we shall designate the phenomenon as *segmental myoclonus or myoclonus simplex*. Widespread, lightning-like arrhythmic contractions will be referred to as *polymyoclonus*. This subdivision, as will become evident, is not a matter of mere pedantry. The authors believe that each of the three phenomena has a distinctive pathophysiology and particular clinical implications.

CLONUS

Reference has already been made to the type of clonus that appears in relation to spasticity, in diseases affecting the corticospinal tract (page 45). Here the sustained hyperexcitability of alpha and gamma motor neurons sets the stage for a series of *uniphasic* contractions when the muscles are subjected to sudden and sustained stretch. The condition depends also on the synchronization of the contraction-relaxation cycle of muscle spindles and ceases immediately upon cessation of sustained stretch.

Another type of clonus, called *palatal nystagmus or myoclonus*, depends upon a less well understood central mechanism. It occurs with lesions of any type which interrupt the central tegmental tract(s) in the brainstem, presumably disinhibiting the inferior olivary nucleus and

the olivocerebellar fibers to the contralateral cerebellar cortex and dentate and interpositus nuclei. Lapresle and Ben Hamida have called this circuit (dentate-brachium conjunctivum-central tegmental tract-olivary nuclei-dentate) the triangle of Guillain and Mollaret, after the persons who first carefully studied the condition. Our own pathologic material confirms the central tegmental-olivary lesions but contains no examples of its production by lesions of the cerebellum, or of the dentate and red nuclei. We are impressed with the observations of Matsuo and Ajax who postulate a denervation hypersensitivity of the inferior olivary nucleus and its dentate connections as the basic mechanism. Recently, Kane and Thach have adduced evidence that the critical event in the genesis of palatal myoclonus is denervation not of the olive but of the nucleus ambiguus and the dorsolateral reticular formation adjacent to it. The usual lesions are vascular, neoplastic, or traumatic and lie in the midbrain or pontine tegmentum.

This type of rhythmic clonus occurs at the rate of 60 to 100 times a minute. The uvula and palate elevate, sometimes with an audible click. In some instances the pharynx, facial and extraocular muscles, diaphragm, vocal cords, and even the muscles of the neck, shoulders, and arms partake of the persistent rhythmic movement. Occasionally the movements are unilateral (ipsilateral to the tegmental-olivary lesion). Unlike almost all other involuntary movements they may persist during sleep. It has been suggested that the muscles derived from the branchial clefts are the ones affected in this disorder, and the automatic rhythmicity has been likened to respiration (with which it is not synchronous) and the gill movements of fish.

The use of drugs in treating this movement disorder has met with little success. Serotonin precursors such as 5-hydroxytryptophan (100 mg/day in increasing doses) in conjunction with carbidopa (50 mg tid) is said to be effective in an occasional case (Williams et al). However, the former drug is not commercially available and has not been approved for use in the United States. Tetrabenazine and haloperidol have allegedly been helpful in some cases. Most of our patients have not complained about the movement disorder, and we have had no experience with the aforementioned drug therapy.

Epilepsia partialis continua is yet another type of rhythmic clonus, in which one group of muscles, usually of the face, arm, or leg, is continuously (day and night) involved in a series of rhythmic monophasic contractions. These may continue for weeks, months, or years. In most cases there is a corresponding EEG abnormality. The disorder appears to be cerebral in origin, but its precise anatomic and physiologic basis is unknown (see Chap. 15 for further discussion).

Under the title of *oscillatory myoclonus,* Fahn and Singh have described a clonus-like disorder induced by slow ramp movements made by the patient and by ''stress and anticipation.'' Once started in one part of the body the movements may spread to other parts and then gradually wane. In their three patients there were no other neurologic abnormalities. We are uncertain whether the movement disorder is a tremor (a rhythmic biphasic oscillation around a fixed point) or clonus (a rhythmic monophasic contraction and relaxation of a muscle group).

MYOCLONUS SIMPLEX

One or a few quick contractions of the muscles of a part of the body may occur in epileptic patients. Patients with idiopathic epilepsy may complain of a localized myoclonic jerk or a short burst of myoclonic jerks, occurring particularly on awakening and on the day or two preceding a major generalized seizure, after which they cease. Relatively few of the patients with this type of myoclonus show progressive mental and physical deterioration. One-sided myoclonic jerks are the dominant feature of a particular form of childhood epilepsy—the so-called benign epilepsy with rolandic spikes (page 255). Myoclonus may be associated with atypical petit mal and akinetic seizures in the so-called Lennox-Gastaut syndrome (see page 252). The patient often falls during the brief lapse of postural mechanisms after a single myoclonic contraction. In the West syndrome of infantile spasms, in which the arms and trunk muscles are suddenly flexed or extended in a single myoclonic jerk (''jack-knife'' or ''salaam'' seizures), mental regression occurs in fully 80 to 90 percent of cases, even when the seizures are successfully treated with ACTH.

A special form of arrhythmic, monophasic myoclonus may involve only the legs and regularly disturb sleep at night. Recordings made during sleep have shown the myoclonic jerks to occur about 30 s apart, each lasting 1.5 to 2.5 s. They tend to occur in NREM sleep and according to Coleman et al were observed in 53 of 409 patients being evaluated for sleep disorders. The condition must not be confused with the common hypnic jerk or nocturnal start or with the restless leg syndrome of Ekbom with which it is sometimes associated (see also Chap. 18).

MYOCLONUS MULTIPLEX OR POLYMYOCLONUS

Paramyoclonus Multiplex Under the title *paramyoclonus multiplex,* Friedreich, in 1881, described a sporadic

instance of widespread muscle jerking in adult life. In the course of this description, the term myoclonus was probably used for the first time. All the muscles were involved, particularly those of the lower face and proximal segments of the limbs, and the myoclonus persisted for many years, being absent only during sleep. No other neurologic abnormalities accompanied the movement abnormality. The nature and pathologic basis of this disorder, were never determined and its status as a clinical entity was never secure. Over the years, the term paramyoclonus multiplex has been applied to all varieties of myoclonic disorder (and other motor phenomena as well) to the point where it has nearly lost its specific clinical connotation. The same holds true for many other terms such as electric chorea, fibrillary chorea, and convulsive tremor, which in the past have been identified, on purely speculative grounds, with paramyoclonus multiplex.

Myoclonus multiplex of the type described by Friedreich may occur in pure or ''essential'' form as a benign, often familial, nonprogressive disease or as part of a more complex progressive syndrome which may prove disabling and fatal. Some have specified the first as primary and the latter as secondary forms, but these terms have little to recommend them, serving only to indicate differences in severity and clinical course.

So-called essential myoclonus may begin at any period of life but usually appears first in childhood and is of unknown etiology. An autosomal dominant mode of inheritance is evident in some reports. The myoclonus takes the form of irregular twitches of one or other part of the body, ranging from twitches of groups of muscles to single muscles or even a portion of a muscle. As a result an arm may suddenly flex, the head may jerk backward or forward, or the trunk may curve or straighten. The face, neck, jaw, tongue, and ocular muscles may twitch; also the diaphragm. Some muscle contractions cause no visible displacement of a limb. Even fascicles of the platysma may twitch, according to Wilson. Many of the patients register little complaint, accepting the constant motor activity with stoicism, and lead a relatively normal active life. Seizures, dementia, and other neurologic deficits are notably absent. Occasionally there is hint of a mild cerebellar ataxia and in one family studied by the authors, essential tremor was present as well, both in family members with the polymyoclonia and in those without. The tremor and myoclonus were dramatically suppressed after the ingestion of alcohol. Similar families have been observed by others (Marsden et al). In a Mayo Clinic series, 19 of 94 patients with polymyoclonus were of this type (Aigner and Mulder).

Myoclonic Epilepsy Myoclonic or myoclonus epilepsy constitutes another important syndrome of multiple etiologies. Here the myoclonus is associated with dementia and other signs of progressive neurologic disease (the familial variety of Unverricht and Lundborg) and has as its outstanding feature a remarkable sensitivity of the myoclonus to stimuli of all sorts. If a limb is passively or actively displaced, the resulting myoclonic jerk may lead, through a series of progressively larger and more or less synchronous jerks, to a generalized convulsive seizure. In late childhood this type of myoclonus is usually a manifestation of the juvenile form of lipid storage disease which, in addition to myoclonus, is characterized by seizures, progressive dementia, rigidity, pseudobulbar paralysis, and, in the late stages, by quadriplegia in flexion. Another form of autosomal recessive, stimulus-sensitive (reflex) myoclonus beginning in late childhood or adolescence is caused by the presence of neuronal inclusions (Lafora bodies) in the cerebral and cerebellar cortex and in brainstem nuclei (page 804). In yet another form of familial (probably autosomal recessive) light-sensitive myoclonus, described recently under the title of *Baltic myoclonus* by Eldridge and associates, necropsy has disclosed a loss of Purkinje cells but no inclusion bodies. Unlike Lafora disease, the Baltic variety of myoclonus epilepsy has a favorable prognosis, particularly if the seizures are treated with valproic acid rather than phenytoin.

Under the title of *cherry-red spot–myoclonus syndrome,* Rapin and her associates have drawn attention to a familial (autosomal recessive) form of diffuse incapacitating intention myoclonus associated with visual loss that develops insidiously in adolescence. The earliest sign is a cherry-red spot in the macula which may fade in the chronic stages of the illness. The intellect is relatively unimpaired. The specific enzyme defect appears to be a deficiency of lysosomal α-neuroaminidase (sialidase), resulting in the excretion of large amounts of sialylated oligosaccharides in the urine. Lowden and O'Brien refer to this disorder as *type 1 sialidosis* and distinguish it from a second type in which patients have a short stature (due to chondrodystrophy) and often a deficiency of β-galactosidase in tissues and body fluids. In patients with sialidosis, a mucopolysaccharide-like material is stored in liver cells, but neurons show only a nonspecific accumulation of lipofuscin. A similar clinical syndrome of myoclonic epilepsy is seen in a variant form of neuroaxonal dystrophy and in the late childhood–early adult neuronopathic form of Gaucher disease, where it is associated with supranuclear gaze palsies and cerebellar ataxia (page 810).

In another group of myoclonic disorders, which may be loosely identified as the "myoclonic dementias," the most prominent associated abnormality is a progressive deterioration of intellect. Like the myoclonic epilepsies, the myoclonic dementias may be sporadic or familial and may affect both children and adults. An important childhood type is subacute sclerosing panencephalitis (SSPE), which is a subacute or chronic (occasionally remitting) disease, related in some way to infection with the measles virus

(page 607). Another type, familial in nature and affecting infants and young children, has been described by Ford; it has been called *progressive poliodystrophy.* On a background of normal birth and development over the first few months or years of life, there occurs a progressive psychomotor deterioration, with spastic quadriplegia, seizures, myoclonus, and blindness. The fundamental pathologic alteration is a destruction of nerve cells in the cerebral and cerebellar cortices with replacement gliosis. The transmissible nature of this childhood form has not been established. In adults, there occurs a unique subacute illness characterized by dementia, disturbances of gait and coordination, all manner of mental aberrations, rigidity, and diffuse myoclonus. Originally the jerks are random in character, but late in the disease they may attain a certain rhythmicity and symmetry. In addition there is an exaggerated startle response. This disorder is commonly referred to as *Creutzfeldt-Jakob disease.* In this condition, too, there is a progressive destruction of the nerve cells, mainly but not exclusively of the cerebral and cerebellar cortices, and a striking degree of gliosis. In addition to the parenchymatous destruction, the cortical tissue may show a fine-meshed vacuolation, hence the preferable designation "subacute spongiform encephalopathy." Both the sporadic and rare familial forms of this disease are due to a transmissible agent (see page 609).

Myoclonus in association with signs of cerebellar incoordination, including opsoclonus (rapid, irregular, but predominantly conjugate movements of the eyes in all planes), is another syndrome that has been described both in children and adults under a variety of names. Most cases run a chronic course, waxing and waning in severity. Many of the childhood cases have been associated with occult neuroblastoma, and some have responded to the administration of corticosteroids. In adults a similar syndrome has been described in relation to bronchogenic carcinoma and other tumors, but it also occurs at all ages as a manifestation of a benign postinfectious (possibly viral) illness (Baringer et al). In some cases, myoclonus is associated only with cerebellar ataxia and tremor, opsoclonus being absent, and in others, myoclonus, seizures, retinal degeneration, cerebellar tremor, and ataxia have been combined (dyssynergia cerebellaris myoclonica of Ramsay Hunt).

An acute onset of polymyoclonia with confusion may occur with methyl bromide and lithium intoxication. Once ingestion is discontinued, there is improvement (over days to weeks) and the polymyoclonus is replaced by diffuse action tremors (see above) which themselves later subside.

Finally, it should be noted that myoclonus may occur as a transient or persistent phenomenon in viral encephalitis, suppurative meningitis, general paresis, advanced Alzheimer disease, occasionally in Wilson disease, and with certain intoxications (strychnine, tetanus) and metabolic disorders (uremia, anoxic encephalopathy).

INTENTION OR ACTION MYOCLONUS

Intention or action myoclonus was described by Lance and Adams in 1963 in a group of patients who were recovering from hypoxic encephalopathy. When the patient is relaxed, the limb and other skeletal muscles are quiet (except in the most severe cases). And only seldom does the myoclonus appear during slow, so-called voluntary ramp movements. Fast (ballistic) movements, however, especially when directed to a target, as in touching the examiner's finger, elicit an irregular series of myoclonic jerks that differ in speed and rhythmicity from intention tremor. For this reason it was called *intention myoclonus* or *action myoclonus.* Only the limb that is moving is involved; hence it is a localized, stimulus-evoked myoclonus. It is always associated with cerebellar ataxia. The pathologic anatomy has not been ascertained. Lance and Adams found the irregular discharges to be transmitted via the corticospinal tracts, preceded in some cases by a discharge from the motor cortex. Chadwick et al postulate a reticular loop reflex mechanism. Hallett et al found that a cortical reflex mechanism was operative in some cases, as postulated by Lance and Adams, and a reticular reflex mechanism in others. Whether these are two aspects of one mechanism could not be decided. Some authors have reported 5-hydroxytryptophan, in doses of 100 to 200 mg/day, to be effective in suppressing the disabling myoclonus, but several of our patients could not take the drug because of vomiting, diarrhea, and drowsiness. Mebaral and valproic acid have been helpful in some cases. The benzodiazepam derivative clonazepam (divided doses of 8 to 12 mg daily) is our preference.

SPINAL OR SEGMENTAL MYOCLONUS

The implication that monophasic restricted myoclonus always emanates from the cerebellum or brainstem cannot be sustained for there are forms traceable to a purely spinal lesion. A sharply demarcated segmental myoclonus has been induced in spinal animals by the Newcastle disease virus and examples of myelitis with irregular segmental myoclonic jerks (either rhythmic or arrhythmic) has been reported in humans (page 732).

PATHOPHYSIOLOGY OF MYOCLONUS MULTIPLEX

It seems logical to assume that myoclonus is caused by abnormal discharges of aggregates of motor neurons or interneurons, due to directly enhanced excitability of these cells or to removal of some inhibitory mechanism.

Sensory relations are a prominent attribute of myoclonus multiplex, particularly those related to metabolic disorders, and will eventually shed some light on the mechanism. Flickering light, loud sounds, or abrupt contact with some part of the body initiates a jerk so quickly and consistently that it must utilize a direct sensorimotor pathway or the mechanism involved in the startle reaction. Repeated stimuli may recruit a series of myoclonic jerks that augment to a generalized convulsion, as often happens in the familial myoclonic syndrome of Unverricht-Lundborg. Another type of sensory myoclonus is the audiogenic form, characteristic of Tay-Sachs disease. Each auditory stimulus results in blinking, abrupt elevation of the arms, and other movements. This generalized myoclonic jerk does not fatigue with successive stimuli and is modality specific.

Pathologic examinations have been of little help in determining the essential sites of this unstable neuronal discharge, because in most cases the neuronal disease is so diffuse. The most restricted lesions associated with myoclonus are seemingly located in the cerebellar cortex, dentate nuclei, and pretectal region. A lack of modulating influence of the cerebellum on the thalamocortical system of neurons has been postulated as a likely mechanism, but it is uncertain whether the disinhibited motor activity is then expressed through corticospinal or reticulospinal pathways. Metrazol injections evoke myoclonus in the limbs of animals, and the myoclonus persists after transection of corticospinal and other descending tracts until the lower brainstem (medullary reticular) structures are destroyed. In humans, also, evidence has been adduced that action myoclonus has its basis in reflex hyperactivity of the reticular formation of the medulla. In some such patients, however, the myoclonic jerks have a strict time relationship ("time-locked") to preceding spikes in the contralateral rolandic area, indicating that the cerebral cortex may play an active and perhaps primary role in the elaboration of myoclonus (Marsden et al).

PATHOLOGIC STARTLE SYNDROMES

To some degree, everyone startles or jumps in reaction to a totally unanticipated, potentially frightening stimulus. This is the normal startle reflex. It is probably a protective reaction and its purpose seems to be to prepare the organism for escape. By pathologic startle we refer to a greatly exaggerated startle reflex and to a group of other stimulus-induced disorders of which startle is a predominant part (startle epilepsy, startle disease, or hyperexplexia, "jumping Frenchmen of Maine," and others).

Aside from exaggerated forms of the normal startle reflex, the commonest startle syndrome is so-called startle disease, also referred to as *hyperexplexia* (Suhren et al) or *hyperekplexia* (Gastaut and Villaneuve). The subject has been reviewed most recently by Wilkins and his colleagues.

As an increasing number of cases of startle disease were described, the special attributes of the condition have become more familiar. Any stimulus, most often an auditory one, but also a flash of light, contact with the neck, back, or face, even the presence of someone behind the patient, evinces a stiffening of the body, a flexion of the arms, a jump, and occasionally an involuntary shout and fall to the ground. As pointed out by Suhren et al and by Kurezynski, the condition is transmitted in some families as an autosomal dominant trait. In the proband described by the latter author, affected infants were persistently hypertonic and hyperreflexic and had nocturnal and sometimes diurnal generalized myoclonic jerks, all of which subsided with maturation of the nervous system. At this age the disorder may be mistaken for more common neurologic abnormalities, such as birth injury and spastic quadriplegia. Later in life, excessive startle has to be distinguished from epileptic seizures which may begin with a startle or massive myoclonic jerk (startle epilepsy) and from Gilles de la Tourette syndrome, of which startle may be a prominent manifestation. During the startle, even with a fall, there is no loss of consciousness. The manifestations of tic and other neurologic abnormalities are absent. During the startle, the EEG shows a vertex spike–slow wave complex (? artifactual, due to eye movement and contraction of scalp muscles), followed by a general desynchronization of the cortical rhythms; between startles the EEG is normal.

The mechanism of this startle disorder has been a matter of speculation. Suhren et al and also Fariello et al have postulated a disinhibition of certain brainstem centers. Markand and associates, on the basis of somatosensory-evoked potential testing, have suggested that hyperactive long-loop reflexes constitute the physiologic basis of startle disease. Wilkins et al consider hyperplexia to be an independent phenomenon (different from the normal startle reflex) and to fall within the spectrum of stimulus-sensitive myoclonic disorders. Clonazepam controls the startle disorder to a varying degree. Sedative drugs relieve the rigidity in infants and the startle reaction to a lesser extent.

The relationship of hyperexplexia to the phenomenon displayed by the "jumping Frenchmen of Maine" and other "jumpers" is uncertain. The latter was described originally by James Beard, in 1868, among small pockets of socially backward, French-speaking lumberjacks in northern Maine. The subjects displayed a greatly excessive response to minimal stimuli, to which no adaptation was possible. The reaction consisted of jumping, raising the arms, yelling, hitting, sometimes with echolalia, echopraxia, and a forced obedience to commands, even if this entailed a risk of serious injury. A similar syndrome in Malaysia and Indonesia is known as "latah," and in Siberia as "myriachit." This syndrome has been explained in psychologic terms as operant conditioned behavior (Saint-Hilaire et al) or as culturally determined behavior (Simons). Possibly the complex secondary phenomena can be explained in this way, but the stereotyped onset with an uncontrollable startle and the familial occurrence attest to a biological basis. The primary startle has not been studied sufficiently to identify it with a startle reflex or reflex myoclonus.

SPASMODIC TORTICOLLIS AND OTHER CRANIAL-CERVICAL SPASMS

Spasmodic torticollis and other cranial-cervical spasms are intermittent, arrhythmic, brief or prolonged spasms of contraction of the facial, jaw, lingual, sternomastoid, trapezius, and other neck muscles. The involvement may be restricted to one muscle group: spasms of the orbicularis oculi cause closure of the eyes (blepharospasm); contraction of the muscles of the mouth and jaw may cause forceful opening or closure of the jaw and retraction or pursing of the lips (oromandibular dystonia); the tongue may undergo forceful involuntary protrusion; the throat and neck muscles may be thrown into violent spasm when the patient attempts to speak (spasmodic dysphonia); or the facial muscles may contract in a grimace. When the neck muscles are affected, the spasms may be more pronounced on one side, with rotation and partial extension of the head (torticollis). Occasionally the posterior or anterior neck muscles are involved predominantly, and the head is hyperextended (retrocollic spasm) or inclined forward (antero- or procollic spasm). This movement disorder is involuntary and cannot be inhibited, thereby differing from habit spasm or tic. For many years torticollis was thought to be a type of neurosis, but all neurologists now agree that it is a localized form of dystonia. Typical forms of restricted dystonia may represent tardive dyskinesia (see page 901).

SPASMODIC TORTICOLLIS

This is the most frequent form of limited dystonia, localized to the neck muscles. A condition of unknown cause, it usually begins in early to middle adult life and tends to worsen slowly. Pain in the contracting muscles is a common complaint. The quality of the torticollic movements varies; they may be deliberate and smooth, or jerky. Sometimes an irregular tremor accompanies deviation of the head, possibly representing an effort to overcome the contraction of the neck muscles. The spasms are worse when the patient stands or walks and are characteristically reduced or abolished by a contactual stimulus, such as placing a hand on the chin or neck on the side of the deviation, sometimes on the opposite side, or pressing the occiput against the back of a high chair or pillow. In the majority of cases the spasms cease when the patient lies down. In chronic cases the affected muscles may undergo hypertrophy. Although the most prominently affected muscles are the sternomastoid and trapezius, electromyographic studies also show sustained activity in the posterior cervical muscles on both sides of the neck. Rarely the muscle spasms spread beyond the neck, involving muscles of the shoulder girdle and back, or the limbs. Usually there is no extension to other muscles and the condition persists in unmodified form. No neuropathologic changes were found in the single case that has been studied post mortem (Tarlov).

Spasmodic torticollis is resistant to treatment with L-dopa and other antiparkinsonian agents, including bromocriptine, although occasionally they give slight relief. Psychiatric treatment has been ineffectual. In a few of our patients (four or five of several hundred) the condition disappeared without therapy. In a small proportion of patients (12 percent in the series of Friedman and Fahn) remissions occur—usually in patients with early onset of the disorder, during the first year after onset. Electrical feedback therapy has been proposed but has resulted in sustained improvement in only a few of the milder cases. In severe cases, the sectioning of individual muscles (the sternomastoid) and spinal accessory nerves has helped slightly. A more successful therapy has been a combined sectioning of the spinal accessory nerve (of the more affected sternomastoid) and of the first three cervical motor roots bilaterally—a procedure that reduces spasm without totally paralyzing the muscles. Bilateral thalamotomy has also been tried, but since it is less effective and carries a considerable risk, particularly to speech, it should be reserved for the most severely affected patients with more widespread dystonia.

The use of botulinum toxin for the treatment of torticollis (as for blepharospasm, see further on) is being investigated in several centers. Early reports have been favorable.

BLEPHAROCLONUS AND BLEPHAROSPASM

From time to time, patients in late adult life present with the complaint of inability to keep their eyes open. Any attempt to look at a person or object is associated with a persistent tonic spasm or a series of clonic involuntary contractions of the eyelids. All customary activities are hampered. During conversation the patient struggles to overcome the spasm and is distracted by it. Reading and watching television are impossible at times, but surprisingly easy at others. There is fear even in crossing the street.

One's first inclination is to think of this disorder as photophobia, and indeed the patient may state that bright light is annoying. However, the spasms persist in dim light and even after anesthesia of the corneas. Extraocular movements are quite normal. Blepharospasm may occur as an isolated phenomenon, but just as often it is combined with oromandibular spasms (see below) and sometimes with spasmodic dysphonia, torticollis, and other dystonic fragments. Again it has been postulated that these various focal dystonias have a psychiatric basis, but with the exception of a depressive reaction in some patients, psychiatric symptoms are lacking and treatment of the depression or the use of psychotherapy, acupuncture, aversion therapy, hypnosis, etc., has failed to cure the spasms. No neuropathologic lesion or uniform pharmacologic profile has been established in any of these disorders (Marsden et al).

A variety of antiparkinsonian and tranquilizing medications may be tried, but one should not be sanguine about the chances of success. Sometimes the blepharospasm disappears spontaneously. In extremely persistent and disabling cases, thermolytic destruction of part of the fibers in the branches of the facial nerves which innervate the orbicularis oculi muscles has weakened the spasms and rendered them tolerable.

In recent years blepharospasm (and particularly hemifacial spasm, see page 1081) has been treated successfully by injection of botulinum A toxin into several sites in the orbicularis oculi muscles (2.5 to 5 units of toxin diluted in 0.1 mL saline). Several cycles of treatment are usually required, and benefit lasts for several weeks to months (Dutton and Buckley). There appear to be no adverse systemic effects. It is now the preferred therapy and is being used to treat other focal dystonias, including torticollis and spastic dysphonia.

LINGUAL, FACIAL, AND OROMANDIBULAR SPASMS

These special varieties of involuntary movements also appear in late adult life with a peak age of onset in the sixth decade. Women are affected more frequently than men. The most common type is characterized by forceful opening of the jaw, retraction of the lips, spasm of the platysma, and protrusion of the tongue; or the jaw may be clamped shut and the lips may purse. Common terms for this condition are the *Meige syndrome,* after the French neurologist who gave one of the first clear descriptions of it, and the *Brueghel syndrome,* because of the similarity of the grotesque grimace to that of a subject in a Brueghel painting (''De Gaper''). As indicated above, difficulty in speaking and swallowing (spastic or spasmodic dysphonia) and blepharospasm are frequently conjoined, and occasionally patients with these disorders develop torticollis or dystonia of the trunk and limbs. All these prolonged forceful spasms of facial, tongue, and neck muscles have been provoked by administration of phenothiazine and butyrophenone drugs. More often, however, the disorder induced by neuroleptics is of a different order, consisting of choreoathetotic chewing, lip smacking, and licking movements (orofacial dyskinesia; see page 901).

Only two cases of the Meige syndrome have been studied post mortem. No lesions were found in one, but in the other there were many foci of neuron loss in the striatum (Altrocchi).

A large number of drugs has been used in the treatment of these cranial-cervical spasms, but none has affected a cure. Tetrabenazine, lithium, trihexyphenidyl, and clonazepam have reportedly diminished the spasms in some patients (Jancovic and Ford).

TICS AND HABIT SPASMS

Many persons throughout life are given to habitual movements. They range from simple, highly personalized, idiosyncratic mannerisms (e.g., of the lips and tongue) to repetitive actions such as sniffing, clearing the throat, protruding the chin, or blinking whenever they become tense. Sterotypy and irresistibility are their main identifying features. The patient admits to making the movements and feels compelled to do so in order to relieve tension. For a short time such movements can be suppressed by an effort of will, but they reappear as soon as attention is diverted. In certain cases they become so ingrained that the person is unaware of them and seems unable to control them. An interesting feature of many tics is that they correspond to purposive coordinated acts which normally serve the organism. It is only their incessant repetition when uncalled for that typifies the habit spasm or tic. It varies widely in its expression from a single isolated movement (e.g., blinking, sniffing, throat clearing, or stretching the neck) to a complex of movements.

Children between the ages of 5 and 10 years are especially likely to develop habit spasms. Usually they consist of blinking, hitching up one shoulder, sniffing,

throat clearing, jerking of the head, grimacing, etc. Seldom do they persist for longer than a few weeks if ignored; providing for more rest and a calmer environment are also helpful. In adults, relief of nervous tension by sedative or tranquilizing drugs and psychotherapy may be helpful, but the disposition to tic persists.

Adults often display, when idle, a wide variety of fidgeting types of movement and mannerisms which vary in degree from one person to another. Special types of rocking, head bobbing, and other movements are features of motility unique to the mentally retarded. Apparently they represent a prolongation of some of the rhythmic, repetitive movements (head banging, etc.) of normal infants. If vision is impaired, and in some cases of photic epilepsy, eye rubbing or moving of the fingers rhythmically across the field of vision is observed, especially in mentally retarded children. These ''rhythmias'' have no known pathologic anatomy in the basal ganglia or elsewhere in the brain.

GILLES DE LA TOURETTE SYNDROME

Multiple tics, associated with sniffing, snorting, involuntary vocalization, and troublesome sexual and aggressive impulses, constitute the rarest and most severe tic syndrome. It begins in childhood, usually as a simple tic, and may be precipitated by the administration of CNS stimulants such as methylphenidate and dextroamphetamine, prescribed for the control of hyperactivity. As the condition progresses, new tics are added to the repertoire. Repetitive types of behavior—touching others, repeating the patient's own words (palialia) and the words or movements of others—obsessive-compulsive symptoms, explosive and involuntary cursing, and the compulsive utterance of obscenities (coprolalia) are common manifestations. Feinberg et al have described four patients with arrythmic myoclonus, and vocalization, but it is not clear whether these symptoms represent an unusual variant of Tourette disease or a new syndrome.

In one-third of the cases reported by Shapiro et al, tics have been observed in other members of the family. Several studies have reported a familial clustering of members with Tourette syndrome, but no consistent pattern of inheritance has emerged (Eldridge et al). An ethnic bias (Ashkenazi Jews) has been reported, ranging from 19 to 62 percent in several series, but other series have contained an equally high proportion of northern Europeans of Caucasian stock (Lees et al).

So-called soft neurologic signs are noted in half the patients. Hyperactivity and disorders of attention and perception are frequent. Evidence of "organic" impairment by psychologic tests has been found in 40 to 60 percent of Shapiro's series. However, the intelligence does not deteriorate. Nonspecific abnormalities of the EEG are noted in more than half of the patients.

As to causation, little is known. The disease, if it is such, is unrelated to social class and to psychiatric illness; there is no consistent association with infection, trauma, or other disease. Hyperactive children who have been treated with stimulants appear to be at increased risk of developing or exacerbating tics (Price et al), but a causal relationship has not been established beyond doubt.

No consistent neuropathologic lesion has been established in the only three brains that have been examined. CT, MRI, and PET scanning have shown no abnormalities. In view of the fact that haloperidol (Haldol), the most effective therapy, blocks dopamine (particularly D_2) receptors, the hypothesis has been put forward of dopaminergic overactivity (Chase et al).

The course of the illness is unpredictable. In some adolescents the illness subsides spontaneously and permanently or undergoes long remissions, but in other patients it persists throughout life. This variance emphasizes the difficulty in separating transient habit spasms from the chronic multiple tic syndrome. Haloperidol has proved to be the most useful therapeutic agent. It should be used only in severely affected patients and in small doses (0.25 mg daily) to begin with, gradually increasing the daily dosage to 2 to 10 mg. The addition of benztropine mesylate (0.5 mg daily) at the outset of treatment may help to prevent the adverse effects of haloperidol. Patients who do not respond to haloperidol may do so to the neuroleptic pimozide, which has a more specific antidopaminergic action than haloperidol. Pimozide should be given in small amounts (0.5 mg daily) to begin with, gradually increasing the dosage to 8 to 9 mg daily.

AKATHISIA

The term *akathisia* was coined by Haskovec in 1904 to describe a curious mental state, characterized by an inner restlessness, an inability to sit still, and a compulsion to move about. Later, Sicard recognized a similar state in patients with postencephalitic and idiopathic Parkinson syndrome. When sitting the patient constantly shifts his body and legs, crosses and uncrosses his legs, and swings the uncrossed leg. Walking in place and persistent pacing are also characteristic.

This state is now observed most often in patients receiving neuroleptic drugs (see page 897). It is most prominent in the lower extremities and may not be accompanied, at least in its mildest forms, by perceptible rigidity or other neurologic abnormalities.

WRITER'S CRAMP

This and other so-called craft or occupation cramps or spasms should be mentioned here, if only to indicate their unclassifiable status. The prevailing opinion is that they are restricted or focal dystonias (Sheehy and Marsden). Men and women are equally affected, most often between the ages of 20 and 50 years. The patient observes, upon attempting to write, that all the muscles of thumb and fingers either go into spasm or are inhibited by a feeling of stiffness and pain or in some other inexplicable way. Usually, it is the spasm that interferes, and if prolonged, it may be painful and spread into the forearm or even the shoulder. Sometimes the spasm fragments into a tremor that interferes with the execution of fluid, cursive movements. Immediately upon cessation of writing, the spasm disappears. Although the disturbance in writer's cramp is usually limited to the specific act of writing, it may involve other equally demanding manual tasks. At all other times and in the execution of grosser movements the hand is normal, and there are no other neurologic abnormalities. Many patients learn to write in new ways or to use the other hand, though that, too, may become involved. A few of our younger patients have developed spasmodic torticollis at a later date.

The performance of other highly skilled motor acts, such as piano playing or fingering the violin, may be similarly affected. The "loss of lip" in trombonists and other instrumentalists may represent an analogous phenomenon. In each case a delicate motor skill, perfected by years of practice and performed almost automatically, suddenly comes to require a conscious and labored effort for its execution. Discrete movements are impaired by a spreading innervation of unneeded muscles (intention spasm), a feature common to athetotic states.

The nature of these disorders is quite obscure. They have been classed traditionally as "occupational neuroses," and a psychiatric causation has been suggested repeatedly, but careful clinical analysis does not bear this out. Hypnosis and other forms of psychiatric treatment are usually without effect. Once developed, the disability persists in varying degrees of severity, even after long periods of inactivity of the affected part. It has been claimed that the patient can be helped by a deconditioning procedure that delivers an electric shock whenever the spasm occurs or by biofeedback, but these forms of treatment have not been rigorously tested.

REFERENCES

ADAMS RD, SHAHANI B, YOUNG RR: Tremor in association with polyneuropathy. *Trans Am Neurol Assoc* 34:48, 1972.

AIGNER BR, MULDER DW: Myoclonus. Clinical significance and an approach to classification. *Arch Neurol* 2:600, 1960.

ALTROCCHI PH, FORNO LS: Spontaneous oral-facial dyskinesia: Neuropathology of a case. *Neurology* 33:802, 1983.

BARINGER JR, SWEENEY VP, WINKLER GF: An acute syndrome of ocular oscillations and truncal myoclonus. *Brain* 91:473, 1968.

BIARY N, KOLLER W: Kinetic-predominant essential tremor; successful treatment with clonazepam. *Neurology* 37:471, 1987.

BRUMLIK J: On the nature of normal tremor. *Neurology* 12:159, 1962.

BURNS RS, LEWITT PA, EBERT MH et al: The classical syndrome of striatal dopamine deficiency. Parkinsonism induced by MPTP. *N Engl J Med* 312:1418, 1985.

CARPENTER MB: Functional relationships between the red nucleus and the brachium conjunctivum. Physiologic study of lesions of the red nucleus in monkeys with degenerated superior cerebellar brachia. *Neurology* 7:427, 1957.

CHADWICK D, HALLETT M, HARRIS R et al: Clinical, biochemical, and physiological features distinguishing myoclonus responsive to 5-hydroxytryptophan, tryptophan with a monoamine oxidase inhibitor, and clonazepam. *Brain* 100:455, 1977.

CHASE TN, GEOFFREY V, GILLESPIE M et al: Etudes structurales et functionelles du syndrome de Gilles de la Tourette. *Rev Neurol* 142:851, 1986.

DESMEDT JE (ed): *Progress in Clinical Neurophysiology,* vol 5: *Physiological Tremor, Pathological Tremors and Clonus.* New York, Karger, 1978.

DUTTON JJ, BUCKLEY EG: Botulinum toxin in the management of blepharospasm. *Arch Neurol* 43:380, 1986.

ELDRIDGE R, SWEET R, LAKE CR et al: Gilles de la Tourette's syndrome: Clinical, genetic, psychologic, and biochemical aspects in 21 selected families. *Neurology* 27:115, 1977.

ELDRIDGE R, IIVANAINEN M, STERN R et al: "Baltic" myoclonus epilepsy: Hereditary disorders of childhood made worse by phenytoin. *Lancet* 2:838, 1983.

FAHN S, SINGH N: Segmental tremor versus rhythmic myoclonus: Successful treatment with serotonin precursors. *Neurology* 30:383, 1980.

FAHN S, SINGH N: An oscillating form of myoclonus. *Neurology* 31(4), pt 2:80, 1981.

FARIELLO RG, SCHWARTZMAN RJ, BEALL SS: Hyperekplexia exacerbated by occlusion of the posterior cerebral arteries. *Arch Neurol* 40:244, 1983.

FEINBERG TE, SHAPIRO AK, SHAPIRO E: Paroxysmal myoclonic dystonia with vocalisations: New entity or variant of pre-existing syndromes? *J Neurol Neurosurg Psychiatry* 49:52, 1986.

FORD FR: Degeneration of the cerebral gray matter, in *Diseases of the Nervous System in Infancy, Childhood and Adolescence,* 6th ed. Springfield, Ill, Charles C Thomas, 1973, p 305.

FRIEDMAN A, FAHN S: Spontaneous remissions in spasmodic torticollis. *Neurology* 36:398, 1986.

FREUND HJ, HEFTER H, HOEMBERG V et al: Differential diagnosis of motor disorders by tremor analysis, in Findley LJ, Capildeo R (eds): *Movement Disorders: Tremor.* New York, Oxford University Press, 1984.

GASTAUT R, VILLENEUVE A: A startle disease or hyperekplexia. *J Neurol Sci* 5:523, 1967.

HAERER AF, ANDERSON DW, SCHOENBERG BS: Prevalence of essential tremor. *Arch Neurol* 39:750, 1982.

HALLETT M, CHADWICK P, MARSDEN CD: Ballistic movement overflow myoclonus. A form of essential myoclonus. *Brain* 100:299, 1977.

HALLETT M, CHADWICK D, MARSDEN CD: Cortical reflex myoclonus. *Neurology* 29:1107, 1979.

HALLETT M, CHADWICK D, ADAMS J et al: Reticular reflex myoclonus. A physiological type of human post-hypoxic myoclonus. *J Neurol Neurosurg Psychiatry* 40:253, 1977.

HALLIDAY AM: The neurophysiology of myoclonic jerking—a reappraisal, in Charlton MH (ed): *Myoclonic Seizures,* Roche Medical Monograph Series. Amsterdam, Excerpta Medica, 1975, pp 1–29.

HEILMAN KH: Orthostatic tremor. *Arch Neurol* 41:880, 1984.

HODSKINS MB, YAKOVLEV PI: Anatomico-clinical observations on myoclonus in epileptics and on related symptom complexes. *Am J Psychiatry* 86:827, 1930.

HUNT JR: Dyssynergia cerebellaris myoclonica—primary atrophy of the dentate system: A contribution to the pathology and symptomatology of the cerebellum. *Brain* 44:490, 1921.

JANKOVIC J, FORD J: Blepharospasm and orofacial-cervical dystonia: Clinical and pharmacological findings in 100 patients. *Ann Neurol* 13:402, 1983.

KANE SA, THACH WT JR: Palatal myoclonus and function of the inferior olive: are they related? In Strata P (ed): *Olivocerebellar System in Motor Control.* Published by *Exper Br Res,* Suppl. 11, Berlin, Springer Verlag, 1988.

KOLLER W, O'HARA R, DORUS W, BAUER J: Tremor in chronic alcoholism. *Neurology* 35:1660, 1985.

KUREZYNSKI TW: Hyperekplexia. *Arch Neurol* 40:426, 1983.

LANCE JW, ADAMS RD: The syndrome of intention or action myoclonus as a sequel to hypoxic encephalopathy. *Brain* 87:111, 1963.

LAPRESLE J, BEN HAMIDA M: The dentato-olivary pathway. *Arch Neurol* 22:135, 1970.

LEES AS, ROBERTSON M, TRIMBLE MR, MURRAY HMF: A clinical study of Gilles de la Tourette syndrome in the United Kingdom. *J Neurol Neurosurg Psychiatry* 47:1, 1984.

LEFEBVRE-D'AMOUR M, SHAHANI BT, YOUNG RR: Tremor in alcoholic patients, in Desmedt JE (ed): *Physiological Tremor, Pathological Tremors, and Clonus.* Basel, Karger, 1978, pp 160–164.

LOWDEN JA, O'BRIEN JS: Sialidosis: A review of human neuroaminidase deficiency. *Am J Hum Genetics* 31:1, 1979.

MARKAND ON, GARG BP, WEAVER DD: Familial startle disease (hyperexplexia). *Arch Neurol* 41:71, 1984.

MARSDEN CD: Blepharospasm-oromandibular dystonia syndrome (Brueghel's syndrome). *J Neurol Neurosurg Psychiatry* 39:1204, 1976.

MARSDEN CD: The mechanisms of physiologic tremor and their significance for pathological tremors, in Desmedt JE (ed): *Physiological Tremor, Pathological Tremors and Clonus.* New York, Karger, 1978, pp 1–16.

MARSDEN CD, LANG AE, SHEEHY MP: Pharmacology of cranial dystonia. *Neurology* 33:1100, 1983.

MARSDEN CD, HALLETT M, FAHN S: The nosology and pathophysiology of myoclonus, in Marsden CD, Fahn S (eds): *Movement Disorders.* London, Butterworth, 1982, pp 196–248.

MARSHALL J: Tremor, in Vinken PJ, Bruyn GW (eds): *Handbook of Clinical Neurology,* vol 6: *Basal Ganglia.* Amsterdam, North-Holland, 1968, chap 31, pp 809–825.

MATSU F, AJAX ET: Palatal myoclonus and denervation supersensitivity in the central nervous system. *Ann Neurol* 5:72, 1979.

MOE PG, NELLHAUS G: Infantile polymyoclonia—opsoclonus syndrome and neural crest tumors. *Neurology* 20:7, 1970.

NARABAYASHI H: Surgical approach to tremor, in Marsden CD, Fahn S (eds): *Movement Disorders.* London, Butterworth, 1982, pp 292–299.

PRICE RA, LECKMAN JF, PAULS DL et al: Gilles de la Tourette's syndrome: Tics and central nervous stimulants in twins and nontwins. *Neurology* 36:232, 1986.

RAPIN I, GOLDFISCHER S, KATZMAN R et al: The cherry-red spot–myoclonus syndrome. *Ann Neurol* 3:234, 1978.

SAINT-HILAIRE M-H, SAINT-HILAIRE J-M, GRANGER L: Jumping Frenchmen of Maine. *Neurology* 36:1269, 1986.

SHAHANI BT, YOUNG RR: Action tremors: A clinical neurophysiological review, in Desmedt JE (ed): *Progress in Clinical Neurophysiology,* vol 5. Basel, Karger, 1978, pp 129–137.

SHAPIRO AK, SHAPIRO ES, BRUUN RD et al: Gilles de la Tourette's syndrome: Summary of clinical experience with 250 patients and suggested nomenclature for tic syndromes, in Eldridge R, Fahn S (eds): *Advances in Neurology,* vol 14: *Dystonia.* New York, Raven Press, 1976, pp 277–283.

SHEEHY MP, MARSDEN CD: Writer's cramp—a focal dystonia. *Brain* 105:461, 1982.

SIMONS RC: The resolution of the Latah paradox. *J Nerv Ment Dis* 168: 195, 1980.

SUHREN D, BRUYN GW, TUYMAN JA: Hyperexplexia, a hereditary startle syndrome. *J Neurol Sci* 3:577, 1966.

SUTTON GG, MAYER RF: Focal reflex myoclonus. *J Neurol Neurosurg Psychiatry* 37:207, 1974.

SWANSON PD, LUTTRELL CN, MAGLADERY JW: Myoclonus: A report of 67 cases and review of the literature. *Medicine* 41:339, 1962.

SYMONDS C: Myoclonus. *Med J Australia* 1:765, 1954.

TARLOV E: On the problem of spasmodic torticollis in man. *J Neurol Neurosurg Psychiatry* 33:457, 1970.

THOMPSON PD, ROTHWELL JC, DAY BL et al: The physiology of orthostatic tremor. *Arch Neurol* 43:584, 1986.

VALBO AB, HAGBARTH KE, TOREBJORK HE et al: Somatosensory proprioceptive and sympathetic activity in human peripheral nerves. *Physiol Rev* 59:919, 1979.

WARD AA R: The function of the basal ganglia, in Vinken PJ, Bruyn GW (eds): *Handbook of Clinical Neurology,* vol 6: *Basal Ganglia.* Amsterdam, North-Holland, 1968, chap 3, pp 90–115.

WATSON CW, DENNY-BROWN DE: Myoclonus epilepsy as a symptom of diffuse neuronal disease. *Arch Neurol Psychiatry* 70:151, 1953.

WEE AS, SUBRAMONY SH, CURRIER RD: "Orthostatic tremor" in familial-essential tremor. *Neurology* 36:1241, 1986.

WILKINS DE, HALLETT M, WESS MM: Audiogenic startle reflex of man and its relationship to startle syndromes. *Brain* 109, 561, 1986.

WILLIAMS A, GOODENBERGER D, CALNE DB: Palatal myoclonus following herpes zoster ameliorated by 5-hydroxytryptophan and carbidopa. *Neurology* 28:358, 1978.

WILSON SAK: *Neurology.* London, Edward Arnold & Co., 1940.

YOUNG RR: Tremor, in Asbury AK, McKhann GM, McDonald WI (eds): *Diseases of the Nervous System.* Philadelphia, Saunders, 1986, chap 32.

YOUNG RR, GROWDON JH, SHAHANI BT: Beta-adrenergic mechanisms in action tremor. *N Engl J Med* 293:950, 1975.

YOUNG RR: Pathophysiology and pharmacology of tremors, in Shahani BT (ed): *Electromyography in CNS Disorders: Central EMG.* Stoneham, Mass, Butterworth, 1984. pp 143–159.

CHAPTER 6

DISORDERS OF STANCE AND GAIT

Certain disorders of motor function are manifested most clearly as an impairment of upright stance and locomotion, and their evaluation depends on a knowledge of the neural mechanisms underlying these peculiarly human functions. Analysis of stance and gait is a particularly rewarding medical exercise; with some experience a neurologic diagnosis can sometimes be reached merely by noting the manner in which the patient walks.

NORMAL GAIT

The normal gait seldom attracts attention, but it should be observed with care, if slight deviations from normal are to be appreciated. The body is erect, the head straight, and the arms hang loosely and gracefully at the sides, each moving rhythmically forward with the opposite leg. The feet are slightly everted, and the steps are of moderate length and approximately equal, the internal malleoli almost touching and each foot being placed almost in line with the other. With each step there is coordinated flexion of the hip and knee, dorsiflexion of the foot, and a barely perceptible elevation of the hip so that the foot clears the ground. The heel strikes the ground first, and inspection of the shoes will show that this part is most subject to wear. The muscles of greatest importance in maintaining the erect posture are the erector spinae and the extensors of the hips and knees.

When analyzed in greater detail, the requirements for locomotion in an upright, bipedal position may be reduced to the following elements: (1) antigravity support of the body, (2) stepping, (3) an adequate degree of equilibrium, and (4) a means of propulsion.

The upright support of the body is provided by antigravity reflexes which maintain firm extension of the knees, hips, and back, but are modifiable by position of the head and neck. These reflexes depend on the integrity of the spinal cord and brainstem (transection of the neuraxis

between the red and vestibular nuclei leads to exaggeration of these antigravity reflexes—decerebrate rigidity).

Stepping, the second element, is a basic movement pattern, present at birth and integrated at the midbrain level, as described in Chap. 3. Its appropriate stimuli are contact of the sole with a flat surface and inclination of the body forward and alternately from side to side. The fact that spontaneous walking can be initiated and sustained in decerebrate and in spinal cats is often offered as evidence that this movement pattern depends upon locomotor generators in the subthalamus and midbrain, functioning in conjunction with spinal motor mechanisms (Pierrot-Deseilligny et al). However, their relevance in human locomotion is questionable.

Equilibrium involves the maintenance of balance at right angles to the direction of movement. The center of gravity during the continuously unstable equilibrium that prevails in walking must shift from side to side within narrow limits as the weight is borne first on one foot, then on the other. This is accomplished through the activity of highly sensitive postural and righting reflexes, both peripheral (stretch reflexes) and central (vestibulocerebellar), that are set in motion by each shift in the center of gravity.

Propulsion is provided by leaning forward and slightly to one side and permitting the body to fall a certain distance before being checked by the support of the leg. Here both forward and alternating lateral movements must occur. But in running, where at one moment both feet are off the ground, a forward drive or thrust by the hind leg is also needed. Locomotion may be impaired in the course of neurologic disease when one or more of these mechanical principles is prevented from operating, as we shall see.

There are many variations of gait from one person to another, and it is a commonplace observation that a person may be identified by the sound of his or her footsteps, notably the pace and lightness or heaviness of tread. The manner of walking and the carriage of the body may even provide clues to character, personality, and occupation.

Furthermore, the gaits of men and women differ, a woman's steps being quicker and shorter and movement of the trunk and hips more graceful and delicate. Certain female characteristics of gait, if observed in the male, immediately impart an impression of femininity; or male characteristics in the female, one of masculinity. The changes in stance and gait which accompany aging—the slightly stooped posture and slow, stiff tread—are so familiar that they are not perceived as abnormalities.

ABNORMAL GAIT

Since normal body posture and locomotion require intact labyrinthine function, proprioception, and vision (we see where we are going and pick our steps), the effect of deficits in these senses on normal function is worth noting.

A blind person or a normal one who is blindfolded may walk quite well, moving cautiously with arms slightly forward to avoid collisions, and shortening the step slightly on a smooth surface; with shortening of the step there is less rocking of the body, and the gait seems unnaturally stiff.

A patient without labyrinthine function (as may happen after prolonged administration of streptomycin, kanamycin, or neomycin) shows a slight unsteadiness in walking and an inability to descend stairs without holding onto a banister. Running is more difficult. Such persons have great difficulty in focusing their vision on a fixed target when they are moving or on a moving target when they are stationary. When the body is in motion, objects in the environment appear to jiggle up and down (oscillopsia; see page 219), so that they cannot drive a car or read on a train, and even when walking must stop in order to read a sign. These abnormalities indicate a loss of stabilization of ocular fixation by the vestibular system during body movements. Proof that the gait of such persons is dependent on visual cues comes from their performance blindfolded or in the dark when their unsteadiness and staggering increase to the point of falling.

A loss of proprioception, as occurs with posterior root lesions in tabes dorsalis or with complete interruption of the posterior columns of the spinal cord at a high cervical level, abolishes the capacity for independent locomotion for a long time. After years of training such patients will still have difficulty in starting to walk and in forward propulsion. As Purdon Martin has illustrated, they hold their hands in front of the body, bend the body and head forward, walk with a wide base and irregular uneven steps,

but still rock the body. If they are tilted to one side, they fail to compensate for their abnormal posture. If they fall, they cannot arise without help; they are unable to crawl or to get into an "all-fours" posture. They have difficulty in getting up from a chair. When standing, if blindfolded, they immediately fall. Thus the postural reactions are primarily dependent on proprioceptive rather than on visual or labyrinthine information.

EXAMINATION OF THE PATIENT WITH ABNORMAL GAIT

When confronted with a disorder of gait, the examiner must observe the patient's stance and the attitude and dominant positions of the legs, trunk, and arms. It is good practice to watch patients as they walk into the examining room, when they are apt to walk more naturally than during special tests. They should be asked to stand with feet together, head erect, and with eyes open and then closed. Swaying due to nervousness may be overcome by asking the patient to touch the tip of his nose alternately with the forefinger of one hand and then the other. Next the patient should be asked to walk forward and backward, with eyes open and then closed. A tendency to veer to one side, as in cerebellar disease, can be checked by having the patient walk around a chair. When the affected side is toward the chair, the patient tends to walk into it; and when it is away from the chair, there is a veering outward in ever-widening circles. More delicate tests of gait are walking a straight line heel to toe, and having the patient arise quickly from a chair, walk briskly, stop or turn suddenly, and then sit down again. If all these tests are successfully executed, it may be assumed that any difficulty in locomotion is not due to impairment of proprioceptive or cerebellar mechanisms. Detailed neurologic examination is then necessary in order to determine which of several other disturbances of function is responsible for the patient's disorder of gait.

The following types of abnormal gait are so distinctive that with a little practice they can be recognized at a glance.

Cerebellar Gait The main features of this gait are a wide base (separation of legs), unsteadiness and irregularity of steps, and lateral veering. Steps are uncertain, some are shorter and others longer than intended, and the patient may stagger or lurch to one side or the other. The patient may compensate for these abnormalities by shortening his or her steps and shuffling, i.e., keeping both feet on the ground simultaneously.

The unsteadiness is more prominent on arising quickly from a chair, stopping suddenly while walking, or turning quickly. The irregular swaying of the trunk may be most evident when the patient has to stop walking abruptly and sit down, and it may be necessary for him to grasp the chair for support. Cerebellar ataxia may be so severe that the patient cannot stand without assistance. If less severe, standing with feet together and head erect may be difficult. In its mildest form the ataxia is best demonstrated by having the patient walk a line heel to toe; after a step or two, balance will be lost and it will be necessary to place one foot to the side to avoid falling. The patient with cerebellar ataxia who sways perceptibly when standing with feet together and eyes open will sway somewhat more with eyes closed, as will a normal person. A Romberg sign, i.e., marked swaying or falling with the eyes closed but not with the eyes open, indicates a loss of postural sense, not cerebellar disease (see Chap. 8). Thus the defect in cerebellar gait is not primarily in antigravity support, steppage, or propulsion but in the coordination of proprioceptive, labyrinthine, and visual information in reflex movements, particularly those that are required to make rapid adjustments to changes in posture. Cerebellar abnormalities of stance and gait are usually accompanied by other signs of cerebellar incoordination and intention tremor of the arms and legs, but they need not be. The presence of the latter signs depends on involvement of the cerebellar hemispheres, as distinct from the anterosuperior midline structures. If the lesion of the cerebellum or its peduncles is unilateral, the signs of gait disorder are always on the same side. With thalamic and midbrain lesions (beyond the decussation of the brachium conjunctivum) the ataxic signs are on the opposite side. If the lesion is bilateral, there is often titubation of the head and trunk.

Cerebellar gait is seen most commonly in multiple sclerosis, cerebellar tumors (particularly those which affect the vermis disproportionately—i.e., medulloblastoma), and the cerebellar degenerations. In certain forms of cerebellar degeneration (e.g., the type associated with chronic alcoholism), in which the disease process remains stable for many years, the gait disorder becomes altered as compensations are acquired, and its designation as "drunken" or "reeling" is no longer appropriate. The base is wide and the steps are still short, but more regular; the trunk is inclined slightly forward, the arms are held away from the sides, and the gait assumes a somewhat mechanical, rhythmic quality. In this way the patient can walk for long distances but lacks the capacity to make the necessary postural adjustments in response to sudden changes in position such as occur in walking on uneven ground. Many of these patients show pendularity of the patellar reflexes and other signs of hypotonia of the limbs when they are examined in the sitting and recumbent positions; paradoxically, walking without support brings out a certain stiffness of the legs and firmness of the muscles. Conceivably, the latter abnormality is analogous to the positive supporting reactions, which are observed in cats and dogs following ablation of

the anterior vermis; such animals react to pressure on the foot pad with an extensor thrust of the leg.

Gait of Sensory Ataxia This disorder of gait is due to an impairment of joint-position sense resulting from interruption of afferent nerve fibers in the peripheral nerves, posterior roots, posterior columns of the spinal cords, or medial lemnisci; it may also be produced occasionally by a lesion of both parietal lobes. Whatever the location of the lesion, the effect is to deprive the patient of knowledge of the position of his limbs. The resulting disorder is characterized by varying degrees of difficulty in standing and walking, and in advanced cases there is a complete failure of locomotion, although muscular power is retained. The principal features of the gait disorder are the brusqueness of movement of the legs and the stamp of the feet. The legs are placed far apart to correct the instability, and patients carefully watch the ground and their legs. As they step out, the legs are flung abruptly forward and outward, often being lifted higher than necessary. The steps are of variable length, and many are attended by an audible stamp as the foot is brought down forcibly on the floor (possibly to enhance joint-position sense). The body is held in a slightly flexed position, and some of the weight is supported on the cane that the severely ataxic patient usually carries. Ramsay Hunt characterized this type of gait very well when he said that these patients are recognized by their "stamp and stick." The incoordination is greatly exaggerated when the patient is deprived of visual cues, as in walking in the dark. Such patients, when asked to stand with feet together and eyes closed, show greatly increased swaying or actual falling (Romberg sign). It is said that the shoes are not worn in any one place in cases of sensory ataxia, because the entire sole strikes the ground at once. There is invariably a loss of position sense in the feet and legs and usually a loss of vibratory sense as well.

Formerly, a disordered gait of this type was observed most frequently with tabes dorsalis, hence the term *tabetic gait*, but it is also seen in Friedreich ataxia and related forms of spinocerebellar degeneration, subacute combined degeneration of the cord (vitamin B_{12} deficiency), syphilitic meningomyelitis, chronic sensory polyneuropathy, and those cases of multiple sclerosis or compression of the spinal cord in which posterior column involvement predominates.

Hemiplegic and Paraplegic (Spastic) Gaits In hemiplegia or hemiparesis, the leg is held stiffly and does not flex freely at the hip, knee, and ankle. It tends to rotate outward and to describe a semicircle, first away from and then toward the trunk (circumduction). The foot scrapes the floor, and the toe and outer side of the sole of the shoe are worn. One can recognize a spastic gait by the sound of the slow, rhythmic scuff of the foot along the floor. The arm on the affected side is weak and stiff to a variable degree; it is carried in a flexed position and does not swing naturally. In the hemiparetic child the arm tends to abduct as he steps forward. This type of gait disorder is most often a sequela of cerebral infarction or trauma but may result from a number of other conditions which damage the corticospinal pathway on one side.

The spastic paraplegic or paraparetic gait is in effect a bilateral hemiplegic gait affecting only the lower limbs. Each leg is advanced slowly and stiffly, with restricted motion at the hips and knees. The legs are extended or slightly bent at the knees and may be strongly adducted at the hips, tending almost to cross as the patient walks (scissors gait). The steps are regular and short, and the patient advances only with great effort, as though wading waist-deep in water. An easy way to remember the main features of the hemiplegic and paraplegic gaits is through the letter S, for slow, stiff, and scraping. The defect is in the stepping mechanism and in propulsion, not in support or equilibrium.

The spastic paraparetic gait is a major manifestation of cerebral diplegia, the result of anoxic or other forms of damage to the brain in the perinatal period. This disorder of gait is seen in a variety of chronic spinal cord diseases in which the dorsolateral and ventral funiculi are involved, including multiple sclerosis, syringomyelia, syphilitic meningomyelitis, combined system disease of both the pernicious anemia (PA) and non-PA types, chronic spinal cord compression, and familial forms of spastic paraplegia. Frequently the effects of posterior column disease are added, giving rise to a mixed gait disturbance—a spinal spastic ataxia.

Festinating Gait The term *festinating* is derived from the Latin *festinare*, "to hasten," and appropriately describes the involuntary acceleration or hastening that characterizes the gait of both paralysis agitans and postencephalitic parkinsonism. Rigidity and shuffling, in addition to festination, are the cardinal features of this gait. When they are joined to the typical tremor, unblinking and mask-like facial expression, general attitude of flexion, immobility, and poverty of movement, there can be little doubt as to the diagnosis.

In walking, the trunk is bent forward. The arms are carried slightly flexed and ahead of the body and do not swing. The legs are stiff and bent at the knees and hips. The steps are short, and the feet barely clear the ground as the patient shuffles along. Once forward or backward locomotion has started, the upper part of the body advances ahead of the lower part, as though the patient were chasing his center of gravity. The steps become more and more rapid, and the patient may fall if not assisted. This is festination, and it may occur when the patient is walking forward or backward, taking the form of either propulsion or retropulsion. The defects are in rocking the body from side to side so that the feet may clear the floor and in moving the legs quickly enough to overtake the center of gravity.

Other unusual gaits are sometimes observed in postencephalitic patients. For example, such a patient may be unable to take the first step forward because of an inability to lift one foot, or until he or she takes a few hops or one or two steps backward. Walking may be initiated by a series of short steps or a series of steps of increasing size. Occasionally such a patient may run better than he walks or walk backward better than forward. Walking so preoccupies the patient that simultaneous talking may be impossible.

Choreoathetotic and Dystonic Gaits Diseases that are characterized by involuntary movements and abnormal postures seriously affect gait. In fact, a disturbance of gait may be the initial and dominant manifestation of these diseases, and the testing of gait often brings out abnormalities of movement and posture that are otherwise not conspicuous.

As the patient with congenital athetosis or Huntington chorea stands or walks there is a continuous play of irregular movements affecting the face, neck, hands, and, in the advanced stages, the large proximal joints and trunk. The positions of the upper parts of the body vary with each step. There are jerks of the head, grimacing, squirming and twisting movements of the trunk and limbs, and peculiar respiratory noises. One arm may be thrust aloft and the other one behind the body, with wrist and fingers alternately undergoing flexion and extension, supination and pronation. The head may be inclined in one direction, the lips alternately retract and then purse, and the tongue intermittently protrudes from the mouth. The legs advance slowly and awkwardly, the result of superimposed involuntary movements and postures. Sometimes the foot is plantar-flexed at the ankle, and the weight is carried on the toes; or it may be dorsiflexed or inverted. A superimposed involuntary movement may cause the leg to be suspended in the air momentarily, imparting a lilting or waltzing character to the gait, or it may twist the trunk so violently that the patient may fall.

In dystonia musculorum deformans the first symptom

may be a limp due to inversion or plantar flexion of the foot or a distortion of the pelvis. The patient may stand with one leg rigidly extended or one shoulder elevated, and the trunk may be in a position of exaggerated flexion, lordosis, or scoliosis. Because of the muscle spasms that deform the body in this manner, the patient may have to walk with knees flexed. The gait may seem normal as the first steps are taken, but as the patient walks, the buttocks become prominent, owing to a lumbar lordosis, and one leg or both legs become flexed at the hip, giving rise to the "dromedary gait" of Oppenheim. In the more advanced stages walking becomes impossible, owing to torsion of the trunk or the continuous flexion of the legs.

The general features of choreoathetosis and dystonia have been described more fully in Chap. 4.

Steppage, or Equine, Gait   This is caused by paralysis of the pretibial and peroneal muscles, with resultant inability to dorsiflex and evert the foot. The steps are regular and even, but the advancing foot hangs with the toes pointing toward the ground (foot drop). Walking is accomplished mainly by flexion at the hip, and the leg must be lifted abnormally high in order for the foot to clear the ground. There is a slapping noise as the foot strikes the floor. The anterior and lateral borders of the sole of the shoe become worn. Foot drop may be unilateral or bilateral and occurs in diseases that affect the peripheral nerves of the legs or motor neurons in the spinal cord, such as poliomyelitis, progressive spinal muscular atrophy, and Charcot-Marie-Tooth disease (peroneal muscular atrophy). It may also be observed in certain types of muscular dystrophy in which the distal musculature of the limbs is involved. The most common cause of unilateral foot drop is compression of the common peroneal nerve, where it crosses the head of the fibula.

A particular disorder of gait, also of peripheral origin, may be observed in patients with painful dysesthesias of the soles of the feet. Peripheral neuropathy (most often of the alcoholic-nutritional type), causalgia, and erythromelalgia are the usual causes. Because of the exquisite pain evoked by weight bearing, the patient treads gingerly, as though walking barefoot on hot sand or pavement, with the feet rotated in such a position as to avoid pressure on their most painful portions.

Waddling Gait   This gait is characteristic of progressive muscular dystrophy, but may occur also in chronic forms of spinal muscular atrophy (Wohlfart-Kugelberg-Welander syndrome) and in congenital dislocation of the hips.

In normal walking, as weight is placed alternately on each leg, the hip is fixated by the gluteal muscles, particularly the gluteus medius, allowing for a slight rise of the opposite hip and tilt of the trunk to the weight-bearing side. With weakness of these muscles, there is a failure to stabilize the weight-bearing hip, causing it to bulge outward and the opposite side of the pelvis to drop and the trunk to incline to that side. The alteration in lateral trunk movements results in the roll or waddle.

In progressive muscular dystrophy, an accentuation of the lumbar lordosis is often associated. Also, childhood cases may be complicated by muscular contractures leading to an equinovarus position of the foot, so that the waddle is combined with circumduction of the legs and "walking on the toes."

Staggering, or Drunken, Gait   This is characteristic of alcoholic and barbiturate intoxication. The drunken patient totters, reels, tips forward and then backward, appearing each moment to be about to lose his or her balance and fall. Control over the trunk and legs is greatly impaired. The steps are irregular and uncertain. Such patients appear stupefied and indifferent to the quality of their performance, but under certain circumstances they can momentarily correct the defect.

The adjectives *drunken* and *reeling* are used frequently to describe the gait of cerebellar disease, but the similarities between a drunken and a cerebellar gait are only superficial. The severely intoxicated patient reels or sways in many different directions, and no effort is made to correct the staggering by watching the legs or the ground, as in cerebellar or sensory ataxia. Despite the wide excursions of the body and deviation from the line of march, the drunken patient may walk on a narrow base, and balance may be maintained. In contrast, cerebellar stance and gait are characterized by a wide base, and patients have great difficulty in maintaining their balance if they sway or lurch too far to one side. Milder degrees of the drunken gait more closely resemble the gait disorder that follows loss of labyrinthine function (see above).

Toppling Gait   Toppling, meaning tottering and falling, may occur with brainstem lesions, especially in the older person who has recently had a stroke. It is a feature of the lateral medullary syndrome. In patients with progressive supranuclear palsy (see page 944), where dystonia of the neck is combined with paralysis of vertical gaze and pseudobulbar features, sudden lurches and frequent falls may be an early and prominent feature. The gait, in addition, is uncertain and hesitant, features that are enhanced no doubt by the hazard of falling unpredictably. Toppling is also observed in the more advanced stages of Parkinson disease. The exact cause of the toppling phenomenon is not known; it does not have its basis in weakness, ataxia, or loss of deep sensation. It simply appears to be a disorder of balance that is occasioned momentarily by the wrong placement of a foot and that is due to a failure of the righting reflexes.

Hysterical Gait This may take one of several forms: monoplegic, hemiplegic, or paraplegic. Monoplegic or hemiplegic patients do not lift the foot from the floor while walking; instead, they drag the leg as a useless member or push it ahead of them as though it were on a skate. The characteristic circumduction is absent in hysterical hemiplegia, and the typical hemiplegic posture, hyperactive tendon reflexes, and Babinski sign are missing. The hysterical paraplegic cannot very well drag both legs, and usually depends on canes or crutches or remains helpless in bed or wheelchair; the muscles may be rigid, with contractures, or flaccid. The hysterical gait may take other dramatic forms. Some patients look as though they were walking on stilts, and others lurch wildly in all directions, actually demonstrating by their gyrations a remarkable ability to make rapid and appropriate postural adjustments.

Astasia-abasia, in which patients, though unable either to stand or walk, retain normal use of their legs while in bed, is nearly always a hysterical condition. When such patients are placed on their feet, they may take a few steps and then become unable to advance their legs; they lurch wildly and crumple to the floor if not assisted. On the other hand, one should not assume that a patient who manifests a disorder of gait but no other neurologic abnormality is necessarily suffering from hysteria. Lesions that are restricted to the anterosuperior cerebellar vermis may cause an ataxia that becomes manifest only when the patient attempts to stand and walk; this is true of frontal lobe disease as well (see below).

Gait Disorder in Normal Pressure Hydrocephalus
Progressive difficulty in walking is usually the initial and most prominent symptom of normal-pressure hydrocephalus (NPH), a disorder of CSF circulation that is described in Chap. 30. The gait disturbance in NPH is difficult to characterize. Certainly, it cannot be categorized as an ataxic or spastic gait, or what has been described as an "apraxic" gait (Meyer and Barron, see below).

As with most gait disorders, the natural compensation for the patient with NPH is to shorten the step, widen the base, and spend more of the stride with both feet on the ground, i.e., to shuffle. Sudarsky and Simon, who quantitated these defects by means of high-speed cameras and computer analysis, noted also a diminished cadence (number of steps per minute) and a reduction in the height of step. Walking is perceptibly slower than normal, and the body is held stiffly and moves en bloc, features that are reminiscent of the gait in Parkinson disease. However, the lack of arm swing is more prominent in Parkinson disease than in NPH, and, of course, the other features of Parkinson disease are lacking.

Frontal Lobe Disorder of Gait The capacity to stand and walk may be severely disturbed by diseases that affect the frontal lobes, particularly their medial parts. This disorder of gait is sometimes spoken of as a frontal lobe ataxia or as an apraxia, since the difficulty in walking cannot be accounted for by weakness, loss of sensation, or cerebellar incoordination. Neither designation is entirely accurate, for reasons indicated below. Most likely the disorder represents a loss of integration, at the cortical and basal ganglionic levels, of the essential elements of stance and locomotion which were acquired in infancy and are often lost in senility.

Patients assume a posture of slight flexion, with the feet placed farther apart than normal. They advance slowly, with small, shuffling, hesitant steps. At times they halt, unable to advance without great effort, although they do much better with a little assistance or with exhortation to march in step with the examiner. Turning is accomplished by a series of tiny, uncertain steps that are made with one foot, the other being planted on the floor as a pivot. The initiation of walking becomes progressively more difficult, and in advanced cases patients may be unable to take a step, as though their feet were glued to the floor. Finally they become unable to stand or even to sit, and without support they fall backward or to one side. In patients with untreated NPH, another type of frontal lobe disorder of gait (see above), one observes this progressive deterioration of gait and stance, from an inability to walk, to an inability to stand, sit, and rise from or turn over in bed and the reverse, following treatment.

Some patients are able to make complex movements with their legs, such as drawing imaginary figures, at a time when their gait is seriously impaired. Eventually, however, all movements of the legs become slow and awkward, and the limbs, when passively moved, offer variable resistance (*gegenhalten*). Difficulty in turning over in bed is highly characteristic, and may eventually become complete. These advanced motor disabilities are usually associated with dementia, but the two disorders need not evolve in parallel. Thus, some patients with Alzheimer disease may show a serious degree of dementia for several years before the gait disorder becomes apparent; in other conditions, such as NPH, the opposite pertains. Or both the dementia and gait disorder may evolve together, in a

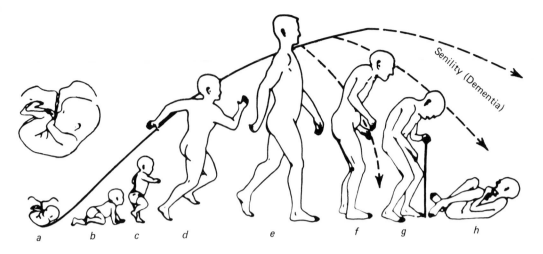

Figure 6-1

The evolution of erect stance and gait and of paraplegia in flexion of cerebral origin according to Yakovlev. The ripening forebrain of the fetus (a) drives the head and body up and moves the individual onward (b through e). When the "driving brain" (frontal lobe, striatum, and pallidum) degenerates, the individual "curls up" again (e through h). (From Yakovlev.)

subacute manner. Grasping, groping, hyperactive tendon reflexes, and Babinski signs may or may not be present. The end result in some cases is a "cerebral paraplegia in flexion" (Yakovlev), in which the patient lies curled up in bed, immobile and mute, the limbs fixed by contractures in an attitude of flexion (Fig. 6-1).

"Senile" Gait　An alteration of gait, unrelated to overt cerebral disease, is an almost universal accompaniment of aging. A slightly flexed posture, slowness and stiffness of walking, and a shortening of the step (marche à petit pas) are its main characteristics. Lost are the speed, balance, and many of the graceful, adaptive movements that one associates with normal gait. A slight misstep, tipping the center of gravity to one side, cannot be corrected. Here also there appears to be a defect in vestibulotruncal righting reflexes. The nature of this gait disorder is not understood. The uncertainty of balance and short-stepped gait in the elderly are often incorrectly attributed to loss of confidence and fear of falling. More likely, they represent a relatively mild degree of the frontal lobe disorder of gait, described above. As noted above, however, a short-stepped, cautious gait lacks specificity, being a general defensive reaction to all forms of defective locomotion. Fisher has remarked upon the similarity of the senile gait to that of NPH and

suggests that this form of hydrocephalus underlies the gait disorder that develops in all mentally competent persons. The changes in gait due to aging are discussed further in Chap. 29.

Gaits of the Mentally Retarded　There are, in addition to the disorders described above, peculiarities of gait that defy analysis. One has only to observe the assortment of gait abnormalities in an institution for the mentally handicapped to appreciate this fact. An ungainly stance with the head too far forward or the neck extended and arms held in odd positions, a wide-based gait with awkward lurches or feet stomping the floor—and each patient with his or her own ungraceful style—these are but a few of the peculiarities that meet the eye. In vain does one try to relate them to a disorder of proprioception, cerebellar deficit, or pyramidal or extrapyramidal disease.

　　The only plausible explanation that comes to mind is that these pathologic variants of gait are based on a retardation of the natural developmental sequences of the spinal mechanisms involved in bipedal locomotion and the supraspinal influences that couple locomotion with posture and righting. The acquisition of the refinements of locomotion, such as running, hopping, jumping, dancing, balancing on one foot, kicking a ball, etc., are age-linked; i.e., each has its average age of acquisition. There are wide individual variations, but the most striking extremes are found in the mentally handicapped, who may be retarded in these ways as well as in scholastic pursuits. Rhythmic rocking movements and hand clapping, odd mannerisms, waving of the arms, tremors, and other stereotyped patterns make their performances even more eccentric. The Lincoln-Oseretsky scale is an attempt to quantitate maturational delays in the locomotory sphere (Chap. 28).

REFERENCES

FISHER CM: Hydrocephalus as a cause of disturbances of gait in the elderly. *Neurology* 32:1358, 1982.

MARTIN JP: The basal ganglia and locomotion. *Ann R Coll Surg Engl* 32:219, 1963.

MEYER JS, BARRON D: Apraxia of gait: A clinico-physiologic study. *Brain* 83:261, 1960.

PIERROT-DESEILLIGNY E, BERGEGO C, MAZIERES L: Reflex control of bipedal gait in man, in Desmedt JE (ed): *Motor Control Mechanisms in Health and Disease*. New York, Raven Press, 1983, pp 699–716.

SUDARSKY L, SIMON S: Gait disorder in late-life hydrocephalus. *Arch Neurol* 44:263, 1987.

YAKOVLEV PI: Paraplegia in flexion of cerebral origin. *J Neuropathol Exp Neurol* 13:267, 1954.

PAIN AND OTHER DISORDERS OF SOMATIC SENSATION, HEADACHE, AND BACKACHE

CHAPTER 7

PAIN

Pain, it has been said, is one of "nature's earliest signs of morbidity," and it stands preeminent among all the sensory experiences by which humans judge the existence of disease within themselves. Only a few maladies do not have painful phases, and in most of them pain is a characteristic without which diagnosis must always be in doubt.

The painful experiences of the sick pose manifold problems for physicians, and students must learn something of these problems in order to prepare themselves for the task ahead. They must be prepared to diagnose disease in patients who have felt only the first rumblings of discomfort, before other symptoms and signs have appeared. Even more problematical are patients who seek treatment for pain that appears to have little or no structural basis, and further inquiry may disclose that fear, worry, and depression have aggrandized some relatively minor ache or that the complaint of pain has become the means of seeking drugs or monetary compensation. They must also cope with the "difficult" pain cases in which no amount of investigation brings to light either medical or psychiatric illness. Finally, the physician must be prepared to manage patients with intractable pain caused by established and incurable disease, who demand relief either by the use of drugs or the "less moderate means of surgery." To deal intelligently with such pain problems requires familiarity with the anatomy of sensory pathways and the sensory supply of body segments, insight into the psychologic factors that influence behavior, and a knowledge of medical and psychiatric diseases.

The dual nature of pain is responsible for some of our difficulty in understanding it. Easier to comprehend is its evocation by particular stimuli and the transmission of pain impulses along certain pathways, i.e., the sensation of pain. Far more abstruse is its quality as a mental state, i.e., the quality of anguish or suffering—"a passion of the soul," in the words of Aristotle—which defies definition and quantification. This duality is of practical importance, for certain drugs or surgical procedures, such as frontal leukotomy, may reduce the patient's reaction to painful stimuli, leaving awareness of the sensation largely intact. By contrast, interruption of certain neural pathways may abolish all sensation in an affected part, but the symptom of pain may persist (viz., denervation dysesthesia or anesthesia dolorosa). Unlike most sensory modalities, which are aroused by a specific (adequate) stimulus such as pressure, heat, or cold, pain may be invoked by each of these stimuli, if it is intense enough.

The authors have noted that even in highly specialized medical centers few, if any, physicians are capable of handling unusual pain problems. In fact, it is to the neurologist that other physicians turn for help with these problems. Although much has been learned recently about the anatomy of pain pathways, their physiologic mechanisms, and which structures to ablate in order to produce analgesia, relatively little is known about which patients should be subjected to these destructive operations or how to manage their pain by medical means. Here is a subspecialty that should challenge every thoughtful physician, for it demands the highest skill in medicine, neurology, and psychiatry.

END ORGANS, AFFERENT PATHWAYS, AND THALAMIC AND CORTICAL TERMINATIONS

PAIN RECEPTORS AND PERIPHERAL AFFERENT PATHWAYS

Traditionally, there have been two major theories of pain sensation. One, known as the *specificity theory* and associated with the name of von Frey, postulated that pain, as well as the modalities of touch, warm and cold, each had a distinctive end organ in the skin, and that each stimulus-specific end organ was connected by its own private pathway to the brain. A second theory, of which Goldscheider was an early protagonist, held that any sensory stimulus, if sufficiently intense, could produce pain. According to the latter theory, there were no distinctive pain receptors and the sensation of pain was the result of the summation of impulses excited by thermal stimuli or pressure applied to the skin. Originally called the *intensivity theory,* it later became known as the "pattern" or "summation" theory. More recent investigations of the anatomy and physiology of pain, as indicated below, have largely reconciled these opposing views.

In terms of peripheral pain mechanisms there is indeed a high degree of specificity, though not an absolute specificity in the von Frey sense. It is now well established that two types of afferent fibers, i.e., the distal axons of primary sensory neurons, respond maximally to noxious stimuli. One type is the very fine, unmyelinated, so-called C fiber (0.4 to 1.1 μm in diameter), and the other is the thinly myelinated A-delta (A-δ) fiber (1.0 to 5.0 μm in diameter). The peripheral terminations of these primary pain afferents, or receptors, are the free profusely branched nerve endings in the skin and other organs; these are covered by Schwann cells and contain little or none of the laminated structure called "myelin." Based on their response characteristics, Yaksh and Hammond found that these small-fiber afferents are of three types: mechanosensitive, thermoreceptive, and polymodal nociceptors. The first two are activated only by intense tissue-damaging pressure or thermal stimulation; their effects are transmitted by both A-δ and C fibers. The polymodal afferents are unmyelinated and respond to both mechanical and thermal stimuli. The A-δ fibers respond to light touch and pressure as well as to pain stimuli and are capable of discharging in proportion to the intensity of the stimulus. The stimulation of single fibers by intraneural electrodes indicates that they can also convey information concerning the nature and location of the stimulus (local sign). These observations on the heterogeneous types of A-δ and C fibers would explain the earlier observations of Weddell and his colleagues that modes of sensation other than pain can be evoked from structures such as the cornea, which is innervated solely by free nerve endings.

The peripheral afferent fibers have their cell bodies in the dorsal root ganglia; central extensions of these nerve cells project, via the dorsal root, to the dorsal horn of the spinal cord (or, in the case of cranial pain afferents, to the nucleus of the trigeminal nerve, i.e., the medullary dorsal horn). The fine myelinated and unmyelinated fibers occupy mainly the lateral part of the root entry zone; and within the spinal cord many of the thinnest fibers form a discrete bundle, the tract of Lissauer (Fig. 7-1A). That Lissauer's tract is predominantly a pain pathway is shown (in animals) by the ipsilateral segmental analgesia that results from its transection, but it contains propriospinal fibers as well. Although it is customary to speak of lateral and medial divisions of the posterior root (the former contain the small pain fibers and the latter the large myelinated fibers), the separation into discrete functional bundles is not complete, and in humans these two groups of fibers cannot be differentially interrupted by selective rhizotomy.

DERMATOMIC DISTRIBUTION OF PAIN FIBERS

Before considering the central terminations of pain fibers, brief reference should be made to their segmental distribution. This subject will be elaborated in the next chapter, which includes maps of the sensory dermatomes, but as a means of quick orientation to the topography of peripheral pain pathways, it should be remembered that the facial structures and anterior cranium lie in the field of the trigeminal nerves; the back of the head, second cervical; the neck, third cervical; the epaulet area, fourth cervical; the deltoid area, fifth cervical; the radial forearm and thumb, sixth cervical; the index and middle fingers, seventh cervical; the little finger and ulnar border of hand and forearm, eighth cervical–first thoracic; the nipple, fifth thoracic; the umbilicus, tenth thoracic; the groin, first lumbar; medial side of knee, third lumbar; the great toe, fifth lumbar; the little toe, first sacral; back of thigh, second sacral; and the genitoanal zones, the third, fourth, and fifth sacral. The distribution of pain fibers from deep structures, though not fully corresponding to those from the skin, also follows a segmental pattern. The first to fourth thoracic nerve roots are the important sensory pathways for the intrathoracic viscera; the sixth to eighth thoracic, for the upper abdominal organs.

THE DORSAL HORN

The afferent pain fibers, after traversing Lissauer's tract, terminate in the posterior gray matter or dorsal horn, predominantly in the marginal zone. Most of the fibers terminate within the segment of their entry into the cord, but some extend rostrally and caudally to one or two adjacent segments ipsilaterally and some, via the anterior commissure, to the contralateral dorsal horn. The cytoarchitectonic studies of Rexed in the cat (the same organization pertains in primates and probably in humans) have shown that neurons in the dorsal horn are arranged in a series of six layers or laminae (Fig. 7-1B). Fine myelinated (A-δ) fibers terminate principally in lamina I of Rexed (marginal cell layer of Waldeyer) and also in the outermost part of

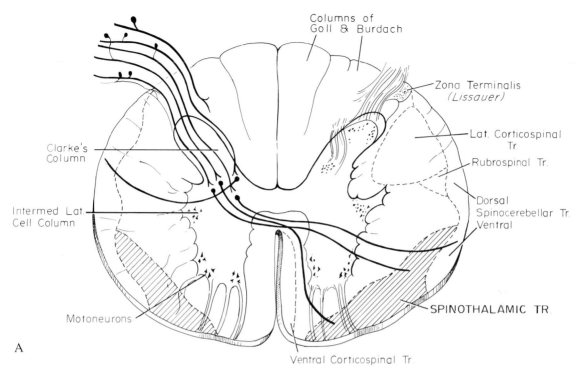

A

Figure 7-1

A. Spinal cord in transverse section, illustrating the course of the afferent fibers and the major ascending pathways. B. Transverse section through the sixth cervical segment of the spinal cord of the cat, illustrating the subdivision of the gray matter into laminae according to Rexed. LM and VM, lateromedial and ventromedial groups of motor neurons. (Adapted from A Brodal, Neurological Anatomy, 3rd ed, New York, Oxford University Press, 1981.)

lamina II; some A-δ pain fibers penetrate the dorsal gray matter and terminate in the lateral part of lamina V. Unmyelinated (C) fibers terminate in lamina II (substantia gelatinosa). From these cells of termination, secondary neurons connect with ventral and lateral horn cells in the same and adjacent spinal segments, and subserve both somatic and autonomic reflexes. Other secondary neurons subserving pain sensation project contralaterally (and to a lesser extent ipsilaterally) to higher levels.

In recent years, several important observations have been made concerning the mode of transmission of pain impulses in the dorsal horn. A-δ pain afferents, when stimulated, release several peptide neurotransmitters, of which the 11-amino acid peptide called *substance P* is present in the greatest concentration and is probably the most important in exciting secondary dorsal horn neurons. The pain-reducing action of opiates supports this view.

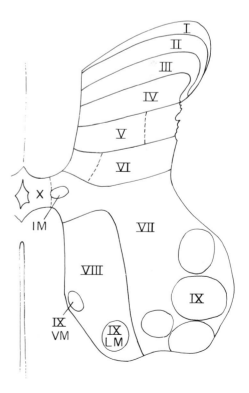

B

Opiates have been noted to decrease substance P; at the same time, flexor spinal reflexes, which are evoked by segmental pain, are reduced. Opiate receptors are found on both presynaptic terminal axons and postsynaptic dendrites. Small neurons in lamina II, capable of releasing enkephalin, are presumably inhibitory in nature. They are believed to modulate nociceptive input in the spinal segments (e.g., flexor reflexes) as well as pain impulses that are transmitted to the brainstem and thalamus. The subject of pain modulation by opiates and endogenous morphine-like substances is elaborated further on.

AFFERENT TRACTS FOR PAIN

As indicated above, axons of secondary neurons that subserve pain sensation decussate in the anterior spinal

Figure 7-2

The main somatosensory pathways. Offsets from the ascending anterolateral fasciculus (spinothalamic tract) to nuclei in the medulla, pons, and mesencephalon, and precise nuclear terminations of the tract are not indicated in the diagram (see text). (Adapted from A Brodal, Neurological Anatomy, 3rd ed, New York, Oxford University Press, 1981.)

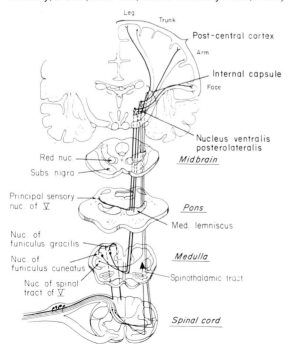

commissure, and ascend in the anterolateral fasciculus to other brainstem and thalamic structures (Fig. 7-2). The axons from each dermatome decussate one to three segments higher than the level of root entry; in this way the dorsal horns and anterior spinal commissure form a continuous pain pathway the full length of the spinal cord. Crossing fibers are added to the inner side of the spinothalamic tract (the principal afferent pathway of the anterolateral fasciculus), so that the longest fibers from the sacral segments come to lie most superficially, and fibers from successively more rostral levels occupy a progressively deeper position (Fig. 7-3). This somatotopic arrangement is of practical importance to the neurosurgeon; the depth to which the funiculus is cut will govern the level of analgesia that is achieved.

In addition to the lateral spinothalamic tract—a fast-conducting pathway that projects directly to the thalamus—the anterolateral fasciculus of the spinal cord contains a more slowly conducting, medially placed system of fibers, which projects via short interneuronal chains to the reticular core of the medulla and midbrain, and then to the medial and intralaminar nuclei of the thalamus. This latter group of fibers is referred to as the *spinoreticulothalamic* or *paleospinothalamic* pathways. It is not clear whether the spinoreticular fibers are collaterals of the spinothalamic tracts, as Cajal originally stated, or whether they represent an independent system, as more recent data suggest. The conduction of diffuse, poorly localized pain arising from deep structures (gut, periosteum) has been ascribed to this paleospinothalamic pathway. Melzack and Casey have proposed that this fiber system (which they refer to as *paramedian*), with its diffuse projection to the limbic and frontal lobes, subserves the *affective-motivational aspects* of pain, i.e., the unpleasant feeling engendered by pain. This is in distinction to the lateral or neospinothalamic pathway, which projects to discrete areas of the sensory cortex and subserves the *sensory-discriminative* aspects of pain, i.e., the processes that underlie the localization and identification, and possibly the intensity, of the noxious stimulus.

There is, in animals at least, a spinal afferent pathway that arises from cells in laminae I, IV, and V of the dorsal horn of the spinal cord and continues *ipsilaterally* in the dorsolateral column as *the spinocervical tract*, terminating in an aggregate of neurons in the cervical cord (C1 to C3 levels)—the *lateral cervical nucleus*. The latter, in turn, projects via the contralateral medial lemniscus to the nucleus ventralis posterolateralis and then to the cortical somatosensory areas I and II (see further on). The exact significance of this tract has yet to be settled. There is no evidence for an analogous tract in humans, even though a lateral cervical nucleus can be identified.

It should be emphasized that the foregoing data,

concerning the cells of termination of cutaneous nociceptive stimuli and the cells of origin of ascending spinal afferent pathways, have all been derived from studies in *animals*. In humans, the cells of origin of the long anterospinal tract fibers have not been fully identified. Information about this pathway in humans has been derived from the study of postmortem material and from the examination of patients subjected to anterolateral chordotomy for intractable pain. Unilateral section of the anterolateral funiculus produces a relatively complete loss of pain and thermal sense on the opposite side of the body, extending to a level three or four segments below the lesion. After a variable period of time, pain sensation usually returns, perhaps because of the presence of pathways that lie outside the anterolateral quadrants of the spinal cord and that gradually assume the capacity to conduct pain impulses. For many years it has been suspected that a longitudinal polysynaptic bundle of small myelinated fibers in the center of the dorsal horn (*the dorsal intracornual tract*) constitutes an ancillary pain conducting pathway.

THALAMIC TERMINUS

The direct spinothalamic fibers, as they approach the thalamus, segregate into two bundles. The lateral division terminates in the ventrobasal and posterior groups of nuclei. The medial contingent terminates mainly in the intralaminar complex of nuclei and in the nucleus submedius. Spinoreticulothalamic fibers (paleospinothalamic tract) project onto the medial intralaminar thalamic nuclei; i.e., they have much the same terminus as the medially projecting, direct spinothalamic pathway. Projections from the dorsal column nuclei, which have a modulating influence on pain transmission, are mainly to the ventrobasal and posterior group of nuclei. Each of the four thalamic nuclear groups that

receives nociceptive projections from the spinal cord has a distinct cortical projection and is thought to play a different role in pain sensation (Fields).

There are also descending fibers from brainstem structures that have an inhibitory effect on pain. One such pathway emanates from nuclei in the periaqueductal region of the midbrain. Presumably it descends in the anterolateral columns of the spinal cord to the posterior horns (laminae I, II, V, VI, and VII). Other stations in the descending pathway are the mesencephalic reticular formation, dorsal raphe nucleus, locus ceruleus, and nucleus reticularis gigantocellularis. The significance of this pain-modulating pathway is discussed further on.

A practical conclusion to be reached from these anatomic and physiologic studies is that at thalamic levels, fibers and cell stations transmitting the sensation of pain are not organized into discrete loci that might provide a feasible site or sites for surgical intervention for relief of pain. In general, neurophysiologic evidence indicates that as one ascends from peripheral nerve to spinal, medullary, mesencephalic, thalamic, and limbic levels, the predictability of neuron responsivity to noxious stimuli diminishes. Thus it comes as no surprise that neurosurgical procedures for interrupting afferent pathways become less and less successful at progressively higher levels of the brainstem and thalamus.

THALAMOCORTICAL PROJECTIONS

The ventrobasal complex, and probably the posterior group of nuclei as well, send their axons to two main cortical

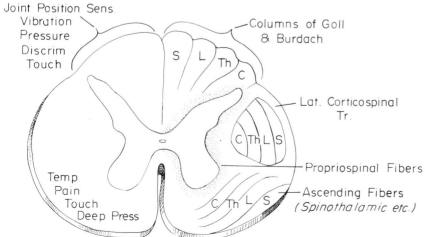

Joint Position Sens.
Vibration
Pressure
Discrim
Touch

Columns of Goll & Burdach

Lat. Corticospinal Tr.

Propriospinal Fibers

Ascending Fibers
(Spinothalamic etc.)

Temp.
Pain
Touch
Deep Press

Figure 7-3

Spinal cord showing the segmental arrangement of nerve fibers within major tracts. On the left side are indicated the "sensory modalities" which appear to be mediated by the two main ascending pathways. Note the broad zone close to the gray matter occupied by propriospinal fibers. C, cervical; L, lumbar; S, sacral; Th, thoracic. (Adapted from A Brodal, Neurological Anatomy, 3rd ed, New York, Oxford University Press, 1981.)

areas: the postcentral cortex (a small number terminate in the precentral cortex) and the upper bank of the sylvian fissure. These cortical areas are described more fully in Chap. 8, but here it can be stated that they are concerned mainly with the reception of tactile and proprioceptive stimuli and with discriminative sensory function, including pain. The extent to which either area is activated by thermal and painful stimuli is uncertain. Certainly, stimulation of these (or any other) cortical areas in a normal, alert human being does not produce pain. Some pain afferents, derived from the mesencephalic offset of the ascending fibers of the anterolateral funiculus, project to subcortical structures, e.g., amygdaloid nuclei, the hypothalamus, and the limbic brain.

PHYSIOLOGY AND PSYCHOLOGY OF PAIN

Stimuli that activate pain receptors vary from one tissue to another. As pointed out above, an adequate stimulus for skin is one that injures tissue, i.e., pricking, cutting, crushing, burning, and freezing. Interestingly these stimuli are ineffective when applied to the stomach and intestine where pain is produced by the local effects of an engorged or inflamed mucosa, distention or spasm of smooth muscle, and traction on the mesenteric attachment. In skeletal muscle, pain is caused by ischemia (the basis of the condition known as intermittent claudication), as well as by injuries of connective tissue sheaths, necrosis, hemorrhage, and the injection of irritating solutions. Prolonged contraction of skeletal muscle evokes an aching type of pain. Ischemia is also the most important cause of pain in cardiac muscle. Joints are insensitive to pricking, cutting, and cautery, but pain is induced in the synovial membrane by inflammation and by exposure to hypertonic saline. Arteries are a source of pain when pierced by a needle or involved in an inflammatory process. Distention and excessive pulsation of arteries are believed to be the basis of migraine; other mechanisms of headache relate to traction on arteries and the meningeal structures by which they are supported (see Chap. 9).

In the painful lesions due to tissue damage, proteolytic enzymes are released which act on gamma globulins to liberate substances that excite peripheral nociceptors. Bradykinins, histamine, prostaglandins, serotonin, and similar polypeptides, as well as potassium ions, which are known to appear in such lesions, elicit pain when injected intra-arterially or applied to the base of a blister. Vascular permeability may also be increased by these substances. Superficial injury to the skin gives rise to vasodilatation,

followed by edema (wheal) and a secondary reddening or flare (the triple response of Lewis).

In addition, direct stimulation of nociceptors releases substances that enhance pain perception. The best studied of these is substance P, which is released from C-fiber terminals in the skin during peripheral nerve stimulation. It causes erythema by dilating cutaneous vessels and edema by release of histamine from mast cells. This reaction, called neurogenic inflammation by White and Helme, is mediated by antidromic action potentials from the small nerve cells in the spinal ganglia (retrograde transport) and is the basis of the axon reflex of Lewis. This reaction is abolished in certain peripheral nerve diseases.

THE GATE-CONTROL THEORY OF PAIN

In 1965, Melzack and Wall propounded a new theory to explain the mechanism of pain. They observed, in decerebrate and spinal cats, that peripheral stimulation of large myelinated fibers produced a negative dorsal root potential and that stimulation of small C (pain) fibers caused a positive dorsal root potential. They postulated that these potentials, which were a reflection of presynaptic inhibition or excitation, modulated the activity of secondary transmitting neurons (T cells) in the dorsal horn, and that this modulation was mediated through an inhibitory interneuron (I cell), as illustrated in Fig. 7-4. In a refinement of this hypothesis, Wall (1980) placed the T cell in lamina V of the dorsal horn and the still unidentified inhibitory cells in laminae II and III. The essence of this theory is that the large diameter fibers excite the I cells, which in turn cause a presynaptic inhibition of the T cells; conversely, the small pain afferents inhibit the I cells, leaving the T cells in an excitatory state. Melzack and Wall emphasized that the transmission of pain impulses from the dorsal horn must also be under the control of a descending system of fibers from the brainstem, thalamus, and limbic lobes. In their view, the descending control mechanism is sensitive to environmental factors and also utilizes information from large primary afferents (Fig. 7-4).

The gate-control mechanism offered a hypothetical explanation of the pain of ruptured disc and of other chronic neuropathies (large fiber outfall). Further, on the basis of this hypothesis, attempts have been made to relieve pain by subjecting the peripheral nerves and dorsal columns (presumably their large myelinated fibers) to sustained, low-intensity, transcutaneous electrical stimulation. Such selective stimulation would theoretically "close" the gate. These procedures have given relief from pain in some clinical situations, although this may not have been due to stimulation of large myelinated fibers alone. Taub and Campbell have presented evidence that analgesia from electrical stimulation may be due to peripheral blockade of the A-δ fibers.

Several other observations are not entirely in keeping with the gate-control hypothesis. In certain forms of peripheral neuropathy, which are characterized by a selective loss of large myelinated fibers (resulting in a pathologic predominance of small C fibers), pain is not a feature; conversely certain neuropathies that are characterized by a predominant loss of small fibers are quite painful. There are experimental difficulties with this theory as well, the most important being that large afferent fibers produce postsynaptic as well as presynaptic inhibition of T cells. These and other aspects of the gate-control theory of pain have been reviewed in detail by P. W. Nathan.

Regardless of the shortcomings of the gate-control theory of pain, it has set neurologists to thinking along new lines. It obviated the necessity of explaining the mechanism of pain by either the specificity theory or the pattern theory. The gate theory acknowledged the physiologic evidence for peripheral specificity and for the central summation of pain impulses, and at the same time emphasized the importance of modulation of afferent impulses at the dorsal horn and control of the dorsal horn mechanisms by descending supraspinal systems. The presence of such pain-modulating mechanisms has now been amply demonstrated (see further on).

PERCEPTION OF PAIN

The *threshold for the perception of pain,* i.e., the lowest intensity of stimulus recognized as pain, is approximately the same in all persons. It is lowered by inflammation and raised by local anesthetics (e.g., procaine), lesions of the nervous system, and certain centrally acting analgesic drugs. Other mechanisms are also important. Distraction and suggestion, by turning attention away from the painful part, reduce the awareness of and response to pain. Strong emotion (fear or rage) suppresses pain, presumably by activation of the descending adrenergic system. Pain is lessened in manic states and enhanced in depression. Neurotic patients in general have the same pain threshold as normal subjects, but their reaction may be excessive or abnormal. The pain thresholds of frontal lobotomized subjects are also unchanged, but they react only briefly or casually, if at all. The degree of emotional reaction and verbalization (complaint) also vary with the personality and character of the patient.

The conscious awareness or perception of pain occurs only when pain impulses reach the thalamocortical level. The precise roles of the thalamus and cortical sensory areas in this mental process are not fully understood, however. Traditionally it has been taught that the recognition of a noxious stimulus as such is a function of the thalamus and that the parietal cortex is necessary for appreciation of the intensity, localization, and other discriminatory aspects of sensation. This seems to be an oversimplification. Probably a close and harmonious relationship between thalamus and cortex must exist in order for a sensory experience to be complete. The traditional separation of sensation (in this instance awareness of pain) and perception (awareness of the nature of the painful stimulus) has been abandoned in favor of the view that sensation, perception, and the various conscious and unconscious responses to a pain stimulus comprise an indivisible process.

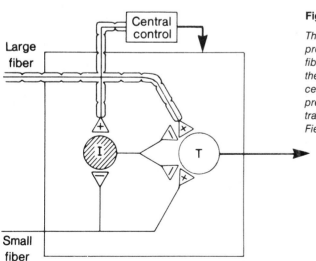

Figure 7-4

The gate control hypothesis of Melzack and Wall: a stimulus presented to the skin activates both large- and small-diameter fibers. If the stimulus is light, large-fiber input predominates, the inhibitory interneuron (I) is excited, and the transmission cell does not fire. If the stimulus is intense, small-fiber input predominates, the inhibitory interneuron is shut off, and the transmission cell (T) is activated, resulting in pain. (From Fields and Levine.)

That the cerebral cortex governs the patient's reaction to pain cannot be doubted, as will be indicated further on. It is also likely that the cortex can suppress or otherwise modify the perception of pain in the same way that corticofugal projections from the sensory cortex modify the rostral transmission of other sensory impulses from thalamic and dorsal column nuclei. It has been shown that central transmission in the spinothalamic tract can be inhibited by stimulation of the sensorimotor areas of the cerebral cortex, and descending fiber systems have been traced to the dorsal horn laminae from which this tract presumably originates.

ENDOGENOUS PAIN CONTROL MECHANISMS

The most important contribution in recent years to our understanding of pain has been the discovery of an endogenous neuronal system for analgesia, which can be activated by the administration of opiates or by naturally occurring brain substances with the pharmacological properties of opiates.

This endogenous analgesia system was first demonstrated by Reynolds (1969), who found that stimulation of the ventrolateral periaqueductal gray matter in the rat produced a profound analgesia without altering behavior or motor activity. Stimulation of other discrete sites, particularly the medial and caudal regions of the diencephalon and rostral bulbar nuclei (notably raphe magnus and paragigantocellularis) were later shown to have the same effect. Under the influence of such electrical stimulation, the animal could be operated upon without anesthesia and move around in an undisturbed manner despite the administration of noxious stimuli. In human subjects, stimulation of the midbrain periaqueductal gray matter through stereotactically implanted electrodes has also been shown to produce a state of analgesia, though not consistently. Further investigation disclosed that stimulation-produced analgesia (SPA) produces its effects by inhibiting the neurons of laminae I and V of the dorsal horn, i.e., the neurons that are activated by noxious stimuli.

As indicated earlier, opiates also act on the neurons of laminae I and V of the dosal horn, suppressing the input from both the A-δ and C fibers. Furthermore, these effects can be reversed by the narcotic antagonist, naloxone. Interestingly, naloxone also reverses SPA. It has already been mentioned that opiates act at several loci in the brainstem, and now it appears that their sites of action correspond with the sites that produce analgesia when stimulated electrically.

The aforementioned observations, summarized here in their briefest form, stimulated the search for opiate binding sites in the central nervous system. High densities of stereospecific binding sites (receptors) for opiates have been found in the spinal cord, in the terminals of primary (A-δ and C) afferents, and in dorsal horn neurons, as well as in the medullary reticular nuclei, medial thalamus, and amygdaloid nuclei. The analgesic effects of opiates are both presynaptic and postsynaptic and their analgesic potency is directly proportional to their affinity for the receptors.

Soon after the discovery of specific opiate receptors in the CNS, several naturally occurring peptides, which proved to have a potent analgesic effect and to bind specifically to opiate receptors, were identified (Hughes et al). These endogenous, morphine-like compounds are generically referred to as *endorphins*, meaning "the morphine within." The most widely studied of these compounds are β-endorphin, a fragment of the pituitary hormone β-lipotropin, and *enkephalin*, and they are found in greatest concentration in relation to opiate receptors in the midbrain. β-Endorphin is not detectable in the dorsal gray matter of the spinal cord; at this level opiate receptors are essentially enkephalin receptors. A theoretical construct of the roles of enkephalin (and substance P) at the point of entry of pain fibers into the spinal cord is illustrated in Fig. 7-5. A subgroup of dorsal horn interneurons also contain enkephalin; they are in contact with spinothalamic tract neurons.

Thus it would appear that the central effects of a painful condition might be determined by the concentration of endorphins in the brain. A deficiency in a particular region would explain persistent or excessive pain. Opiate addiction might be accounted for in this way and also the discomfort that follows withdrawal of the drug. Indeed, it has been shown that β-endorphins not only relieve pain but suppress withdrawal symptoms. In the limbic regions disturbances of formation of endorphin and other neurotransmitters could be the basis of unpleasant and distressing emotional states (e.g., depression). Levine and his colleagues have demonstrated that the narcotic antagonist naloxone not only enhances clinical pain but that it interferes with the pain relief produced by placebos. These observations suggest that the heretofore mysterious beneficial effects of placebos (and perhaps of acupuncture) are due to activation of an endogenous system that shuts off pain through the release of endorphins. Why some patients respond to placebos and others do not is not understood. In general, patients with acute situational anxiety (e.g., soldiers wounded in battle) and severe pain respond better than patients with chronic anxiety and relatively mild pain.

Finally it should be noted that the descending pain control systems probably contain noradrenergic and serotoninergic as well as endorphin-producing links. A descending adrenalin-containing pathway has been traced from the dorsolateral pons to the spinal cord, and its activation blocks spinal nociceptive neurons. The rostroventral medulla contains a large number of serotonergic neurons. Descending fibers from this site inhibit dorsal horn cells concerned with pain transmission, providing a rationale for the use of certain serotonin agonists in patients with chronic pain (see further on).

SOME CLINICAL ASPECTS OF PAIN

As indicated above, the nerve endings in each tissue are activated by different mechanisms, and the pain that results is characterized by its quality, locale, and temporal attributes. *Skin pain* is of two types: a pricking pain, evoked immediately by the penetration of the skin by a needle point, and a stinging or burning pain, which follows in 1 to 2 s. Together they constitute the ''double response'' of Lewis. Ischemia of nerve by the application of a tourniquet to a limb abolishes pricking pain before burning pain. The first pain is thought to be transmitted by the larger (A-δ) fibers and the second (slow) pain, which is somewhat more diffuse and longer lasting, by the thinner, unmyelinated C fibers. Both types of dermal pain are localized with precision, made possible by the overlap of sensory neurons.

Deep pain, from visceral and skeletomuscular structures, is basically aching in quality, but if intense, it may be sharp and penetrating (knife-like). Occasionally there is a burning type of pain, as in the ''heartburn'' of esophageal irritation and rarely in angina pectoris. The pain is felt as being deep to the body surface. The double response is absent, the pain is diffuse and poorly localized, and the margins of the pain are not well delineated, presumably because of the paucity of nerve endings in viscera.

The matter of localization raises a number of problems. Although deep pain has indefinite boundaries, its location always bears a fixed relationship to the skeletal or visceral structure that is involved. It tends to be referred not to the skin overlying the viscera of origin, but to skin innervated by the same spinal segments. This pain, projected to some fixed site at a distance from the source, is called *referred pain.* The fact that primary pain afferents from the skin are far more numerous than visceral afferents and that neurons subserving pain in the dorsal horn are more often activated by skin afferents are the reasons usually given for the projection of visceral pain to the body surface. Since the nerves of any given visceral or skeletal structure may be distributed through several adjacent spinal or brainstem segments, the pain may be fairly widely distributed. For example, cardiac pain arising within the T1 to T4 dermatomes may be projected superficially to the inner side of the arm and the ulnar border of the hand and arm (T1 and T2) and the precordium (T3 and T4), more often to the left, from which side most of the stimuli arise. Once this pool of sensory neurons in the dorsal horns of the spinal

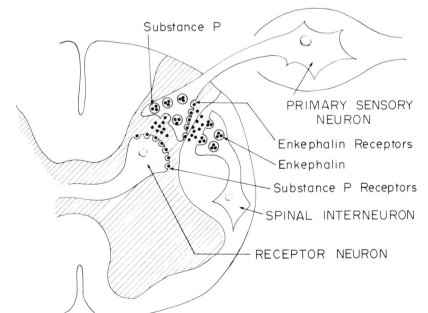

Substance P

PRIMARY SENSORY NEURON

Enkephalin Receptors

Enkephalin

Substance P Receptors

SPINAL INTERNEURON

RECEPTOR NEURON

Figure 7-5

Theoretical mechanism of action of enkephalin (endorphin) and morphine on the transmission of pain impulses from the periphery to the CNS. Spinal interneurons containing enkephalin synapse with the terminals of pain fibers and inhibit the release of the presumptive transmitter, substance P. As a result, the receptor neuron in the dorsal horn receives less excitatory (pain) impulses and transmits fewer pain impulses to the brain. Morphine binds to unoccupied enkephalin receptors, mimicking the pain-suppressing effects of the endogenous opiate enkephalin.

cord is activated, additional noxious stimuli may heighten the activity in the whole sensory field ipsilaterally and, to a lesser extent, contralaterally.

Another peculiarity of localization is *aberrant reference*, explained by an alteration of the physiologic status of the pools of neurons in adjacent segments of the spinal cord. For example, cervical arthritis or gallbladder disease causing low-grade discomfort by constantly activating segmental neurons may induce a shift of cardiac pain cephalad or caudad from its usual locale. Any pain, once it becomes chronic, may spread quite widely in a vertical direction on one side of the body.

The terms *hyperesthesia* and *hyperalgesia* refer to an increased sensitivity and a lowering of the threshold to tactile and painful stimuli. The term *hyperpathia* is used to designate an excessive reaction to pain, but usually with a raised threshold to stimulation. Distinctions between hyperalgesia and hyperpathia are somewhat pedantic. Seldom is it possible in any painful state except inflammation and burns of the skin to demonstrate a distinct hypersensitivity. Instead, in most cases of chronic pain, especially of neuropathic type, there is usually a demonstrable defect in pain perception in the affected part, associated with an increased sensitivity to all stimuli, even those which normally do not evoke pain; and the elicited pain may have unusual features, being diffuse, modifiable by fatigue, emotion, etc., and often mixed with other sensations.

The unmyelinated sprouts of A-δ and C fibers of an injured nerve become capable of spontaneous ectopic excitation and after-discharge and susceptible to ephaptic activation (Rasminsky). They are also sensitive to locally applied or intravenous catecholamines because there are adrenergic receptors on the regenerating fibers. Either this mechanism or ephaptic transmission is thought to be the basis of causalgia or other forms of reflex sympathetic dystrophy, and either mechanism would explain the relief afforded by sympathetic block.

Central structures, e.g., dorsal horns of the spinal cord or thalamus, if chronically bombarded with pain impulses, may become autonomously overactive, i.e., "kindled," and remain so after peripheral pathways are interrupted. Peripheral lesions have been shown to induce enduring changes in the dorsal horn of the spinal cord. Avulsion of nerves or nerve roots may cause chronic pain even in analgesic zones (anesthesia dolorosa or "deafferentation pain"). In experimentally deafferented animals, neurons of lamina V begin to discharge irregularly in the absence of stimulation. Later the abnormal discharge subsides in the spinal cord but can be recorded in the thalamus.

Hence, painful states such as *causalgia, spinal cord pain,* and *phantom pain* are not abolished by simply cutting spinal nerves or spinal tracts.

One of the most remarkable characteristics of pain is the strong feeling tone or affect with which it is endowed, nearly always unpleasant. Furthermore, pain does not appear to be subject to negative adaptation. Other somatic stimuli, if applied continuously, soon cease to be effective, whereas pain may persist as long as the stimulus is operative. Moreover, once a central excitatory state of some kind has been set up, pain may then be evoked by an inappropriate stimulus such as touch or movement, and the sensory experience may outlast the stimulus.

Since pain has this affective element, psychologic conditions assume great importance in all persistent painful states. Furthermore, the patient's tolerance of pain and capacity to experience it without verbalization are also influenced by race, culture, and religion. It is a matter of common knowledge that some individuals, by virtue of training, habit, and phlegmatic temperament, remain stoic in the face of pain and that others react in an opposite fashion. Pain may be the presenting or predominant symptom in a depressive illness (Chap. 56). Then, too, there are rare individuals who seem totally indifferent to pain and others who are incapable of feeling pain, either from a lack of nociceptors and other parts of the primary afferent neuron, or from a congenital deficiency of a neurotransmitter, or from some peculiarity of the central receptive apparatus (see Chap. 8).

Finally, a comment should be made about the devastating effects of chronic pain on a patient's behavior. As Ambroise Paré remarked, "There is nothing that abateth so much the strength as paine." Continuous pain increases irritability and fatigue, disturbs sleep, and impairs appetite. Ordinarily strong persons can be reduced to a whimpering, pitiable state that may arouse the scorn of healthy observers. Persons in pain may seem irrational about their illness and make unreasonable demands on family and physician. Once subjected to the tyranny of chronic pain, the patient requires delicate but firm management (see further on). Depression (possibly reactive?) is a common sequel. The demand for and dependency on narcotics often complicate the clinical problem.

CLINICAL APPROACH TO THE PATIENT WITH PAIN AS THE PREDOMINANT SYMPTOM

One learns quickly in dealing with such patients that not all pain is the consequence of serious disease. Everyday, healthy persons of all ages have pains that must be taken as part of normal sensory experiences. To mention a few, there is the momentary hard pain over an eye, or in the temporal region, occiput, or jaw, which strikes with such alarming suddenness as to raise suspicion of a ruptured intracranial aneurysm; the more persistent ache in the fleshy part of the shoulder, hip, or extremity, relieved spontaneously or by change in position; the fleeting but fluctuant precordial discomfort of gastrointestinal origin, which conjures up fear of cardiac disease; the breath-taking "stitch in the side" due to intercostal or diaphragmatic cramp. These normal pains, as they should be called, tend to be brief and to depart as obscurely as they came. Such pains come to notice only when elicited by an inquiring physician, or when experienced by a patient given to worry and introspection. They must always be distinguished from abnormal pains.

Whenever pain, by its intensity, duration, and the circumstances of its occurrence, appears to be abnormal, or when it constitutes one of the principal symptoms of disease, the physician must attempt to reach a tentative decision as to the mechanism of its production and cause. This is accomplished by a thorough interrogation of the patient, carefully seeking out the main characteristics of the pain in terms of its *location, provoking and relieving factors, quality and time-intensity attributes, mode of onset, duration, severity,* and *time of occurrence.* These diagnostic features are discussed in detail in Harrison's *Principles of Internal Medicine* and are not appropriate for a textbook of neurology. Needless to say, they are put to use everyday in the practice of internal medicine. In conjunction with practical tests designed to reproduce or relieve pain, they enable the physician to identify many diseases.

INTRACTABLE PAIN

Once the pains due to the more common visceral diseases are eliminated, there remains a significant number of chronic pains that fall into one of four categories: intractable pain of inobvious medical disease which may turn out to be carcinomatosis, aneurysm, etc.; pain in association with psychiatric illness; pain with neurologic diseases; and pain of unknown cause.

PAIN DUE TO MEDICAL DISEASES

Carcinomatosis may be presented as the most frequent example. Osseous metastases, peritoneal implants, invasion of retroperitoneal tissues, and implication of nerves of the brachial or lumbosacral plexuses may be extremely painful, and the origin of the pain may be obscure for a long time. Sometimes it is necessary to repeat all diagnostic procedures after an interval of a few months, even though at first they were negative. Once the diagnosis has been established,

therapy must include some type of pain control. Radiation therapy and other medical and surgical measures often fail to relieve the pain. Then comes the delicate decision of whether to administer opiates with the certainty of producing drug addiction, or to resort to one of several neurosurgical procedures for the destruction of pain-sensitive or pain-conducting structures.

One is influenced in reaching this decision by a number of factors, such as the prospect of long survival, attitudes of the patient and the patient's family, location of the pain, and whether the locus is amenable to a surgical procedure. If the patient is ridden with disease and will not live more than a few weeks or months, or is opposed to surgery, or has widespread pain, then surgical measures are out of the question. With pain from widespread osseous metastases, radiation therapy, chemical hypophysectomy by instillation of alcohol into the sella turcica, or radiation hypophysectomy by proton beam bombardment may give relief, even with hormone-insensitive tumors. Pain confined to a restricted area of the jaw or face may be relieved by section or alcohol injection or radio-frequency destruction of nerve, root, or ganglion. Usually section of nerve(s) has not been a satisfactory way of relieving restricted pain of the trunk and limbs, because the overlap of adjacent nerves prevents complete denervation. Section of appropriate sensory roots may be considered in this situation. Bedfast patients with paralysis of the legs and painful flexor spasms have in some cases benefited from crushing of the obturator nerves or intrathecal phenol injections which partially interrupt spinal roots.

Spinothalamic tractotomy, in which the anterior half of the spinal cord on one side is sectioned at an upper thoracic level, effectively relieves pain in the opposite leg and lower trunk. This may be done as an open operation or as a transcutaneous procedure in which a radio-frequency lesion is produced by an electrode. The analgesia and thermoanesthesia may last a year or longer, after which the level of analgesia tends to descend and the pain to return. Bilateral chordotomy is also feasible, but with greater risk of loss of control of sphincters and, at higher levels, of respiratory paralysis. Motor power is nearly always spared because of the position of the corticospinal tract in the posterior part of the lateral funiculus.

Pain in the arm, shoulder, and neck is more difficult to relieve. High cervical transcutaneous chordotomy has been used successfully, with achievement of analgesia up to the chin. Commissural myelotomy by longitudinal incision of the anterior commissure of the spinal cord over many segments has also been performed, with variable success. Lateral medullary tractotomy is another possibility but must be carried almost to the midline to relieve cervical pain. The risks of this latter procedure and also of lateral mesencephalic tractotomy (which may actually produce pain) are so great that neurosurgeons have abandoned these operations.

Stereotactic surgery on the thalamus for one-sided chronic pain is still used in a few clinics, and the results have been instructive. Lesions placed squarely in the nucleus ventralis posterolateralis are said to diminish pain and thermal sensation over the contralateral side of the body, while leaving the patient with all the misery or affect of pain; lesions in the intralaminar or parafascicular-centrum medianum nuclei relieve the painful state without altering sensation (Mark). Thus, at this level there may also be a balance of inhibitory and facilitatory sensory systems, the medial paleospinothalamic and spinoreticulothalamic systems being disinhibited by damage to the neospinothalamic system. Since these procedures have not yielded predictable benefits to the patient, they are now seldom practiced. The same unpredictability pertains to cortical ablations. Patients in whom a severe depression of mood is associated with a chronic pain syndrome have been subjected to bilateral stereotactic cingulotomy or subcaudate tractotomy; the lesions are placed in the white matter above and just lateral to the corpus callosum or in the medial forebrain bundle. A considerable degree of success has been claimed for these operations, but the results are difficult to evaluate. The orbitofrontal leukotomy has been largely discarded because of the personality change which it produces (see Chap. 21).

PAIN IN ASSOCIATION WITH PSYCHIATRIC DISEASES

It is not unusual for patients with endogenous depression to have pain as the predominant symptom. And most patients with chronic pain of all types are depressed. In such cases one is faced with an extremely difficult clinical problem—that of determining whether a depressive state is primary or secondary. In some instances the diagnostic criteria cited in Chap. 56 give the answer, but in others it is impossible to differentiate between the two. Empirical treatment with antidepressant medication or electroconvulsive therapy is one way out of the dilemma. If the pain disappears or recedes to a minor arthritic ache or some similar trivial disorder, one can conclude that depression was the primary problem. If the depression lifts as the pain is brought under medical control, one may assume it was secondary.

Intractable pain may be the leading symptom of both chronic hysteria and compensation neurosis. Every experienced physician is familiar with the "battle-scarred abdomen" of the hysterical woman who has demanded and yielded to one surgical procedure after another, losing appendix, ovaries, fallopian tubes, uterus, gallbladder, etc., in the process. The recognition and management of hysteria are discussed in Chap. 55.

Compensation neurosis is often colored by persistent headaches, neck pain (whiplash injuries), low-back pain, etc. The question of ruptured disc is often raised, and not infrequently laminectomy and spinal fusion are performed on the basis of dubious myelographic and CT findings. Complaints of weakness and fatigue, depression, anxiety, insomnia, nervousness, irritability, palpitations, etc., are woven into the clinical syndrome, attesting to the prominence of psychiatric disorder. Long delay in settlement of litigation, in order allegedly to determine the seriousness of the injury, only enhances the symptoms and prolongs the disability. The medical and legal professions have no certain approach to such problems and are often found to be working at cross-purposes. We have found that a frank objective appraisal of the injury, an assessment of the psychiatric problem, and encouragement to settle the legal claims as quickly as possible, work in the best interest of all concerned. While hypersuggestibility and relief of pain by placebos, etc., may reinforce the physician's belief that there is a prominent factor of hysteria or malingering (see Chap. 55), such data are difficult to interpret and are not acceptable in court.

CHRONIC PAIN WITH NEUROLOGIC DISEASES

Comprising this category are certain chronic mono- and multiple neuropathies, particularly those due to herpes zoster, diabetes, and trauma (including causalgia), and certain polyneuropathies, radiculopathies, spinal arachnoiditis, spinal cord injuries, and the thalamic pain syndrome of Déjerine-Roussy. It is noteworthy that lesions of the cerebral cortex and white matter are not usually associated with pain, but with contralateral hypalgesia; parenthetically it should be mentioned that pain sensation is not entirely abolished by such lesions, even if they include the hemisphere and thalamus on one side.

In most of the pain-producing neurologic diseases or syndromes, the painful phase may not be present at the onset of the illness. For example, the posterolateral thalamic lesion that gives rise to the Déjerine-Roussy syndrome (which may also occur with lesions of white matter of the parietal lobe) is at first characterized by hemianesthesia; as weeks and months pass and sensory function returns to some extent, the pain syndrome develops. Should recovery continue, which it rarely does in thalamic infarcts and hemorrhages, the pain may cease. In other instances, however, pain with little sensory loss is the mode of presentation, and, if confined to the face or arm, is difficult to recognize as neurologic. This sequence of events informs us that persistent pain, like the paresthesias and dysesthesias described in Chap. 8, is based on some mysterious imbalance of afferent sensory impulses, and that it may be abolished if the lesion becomes more extensive or less extensive. The same applies to postherpetic neuralgia and causalgia (Chap. 10) and the painful diabetic neuropathies (Chap. 45). In each of these disorders pain results from the play of natural stimuli on a disequilibrated sensory system.

Uniquely, the patient's description of pain in these several neurologic disorders, particularly in the Déjerine-Roussy syndrome, is more varied and extravagant than in other pain syndromes, probably because the pain is really a dysesthesia combined with sensations of pressure, hotness, coldness, etc. Expressions such as "knife-like, stabbing, crushing, burning (less often, freezing), a constricting band, a storm, a shock, as if the flesh is being torn away, indescribable" are metaphoric attempts to describe a complex of unfamiliar sensory experiences that cause suffering. Another interesting feature of these neurologic pains is the way in which they are affected by various activities and external agencies. Changes in ambient temperature and barometric pressure, increase in static electricity, abrupt contact, certain musical scores and sounds, the use of the painful part or area, a fright or argument, have all been reported to aggravate the condition. Continuously aware of the affected part, the patient may talk about it incessantly in hypochondriacal fashion. The painful part becomes virtually a separate entity, to be watched, shielded, and comforted.

Medical assistance would, in theory, follow several designs: to increase tolerance by altering the perceptual processes in the brain, i.e., the sensitivity and responsivity of the patient (use of tranquilizing and antidepressant medication); to worsen the sensory disorder by reducing the number of functioning elements (interrupting more fibers in the damaged nerve pathway, thus reverting the patient to the original state of anesthesia or analgesia without pain); or to reduce both the sensory input and response by a combination of analgesic and tranquilizing medications. The use of an antidepressant and tranquilizing agent in combination, e.g., amitriptyline or imipramine and thioridazine or fluphenazine, may be more successful as a therapy than neurosurgical procedures which increase the sensory deficit.

Among neurologic disorders that produce intractable pain, the most frequent in our clinical experience, are due to lumbar and cervical disc disease and arachnoiditis. After one or several laminectomies for a ruptured disc and numerous myelograms, there evolves a chronic disabling pain syndrome from which there is no surcease. This is discussed further in Chap. 10.

CHRONIC PAIN OF INDETERMINATE CAUSE

This is the most difficult group of all—pain in the thorax, abdomen, face, or other part which cannot be traced to any visceral abnormality. Supposedly all neurologic sources such as a spinal cord tumor have been excluded by myelography and other tests. The patient's symptoms and behavior are not consonant with any known psychiatric disorder. Yet the patient complains continuously of pain, is disabled, and spends a great deal of effort and money seeking medical aid.

When faced with such a circumstance, sympathetic physicians or surgeons may be persuaded to resort to extreme measures such as exploratory thoracotomy, laparotomy, and laminectomy. Or they may attempt to alleviate the pain and avoid drug addiction by severing roots and spinal tracts, often with the result that the pain moves to an adjacent segment or the other side of the body.

We are inclined to the view that this type of patient should be observed for a time in the hospital and should be seen frequently by the physician. All the medical facts should be reviewed, and the clinical and laboratory examinations repeated, if some time has elapsed since they were last done. Tumors in the hilum of the lung or mediastinum, retropharyngeal, retroperitoneal, and paravertebral spaces, cervix uteri, and prostate are known to offer special difficulty in diagnosis, often not being detected for many months. Neurologic pain is almost invariably accompanied by alterations in cutaneous sensation and other neurologic signs, the finding of which facilitates diagnosis. The possibility of drug addiction as a motivation should be eliminated. It is impossible to assess pain in the addicted individual, for the patient's complaints are woven into the need for medication. Temperament and mood should be evaluated carefully from day to day; the physician must remember that the depressed patient often denies being depressed and may occasionally smile. When no medical, neurologic, or psychiatric disease can be established, we are convinced that it is usually better to let the patient suffer than to prescribe opiates or subject the patient to ablative surgery.

PHARMACOLOGIC MANAGEMENT OF PAIN

The new information about endogenous pain control mechanisms (summarized on pages 110 and 111), in addition to providing an explanation for a number of clinical observations, also provides a theoretical basis for the management of intractable pain by pharmacologic means. In some instances the therapeutic agent may block pain transmission directly by preventing the activation of nociceptors at the periphery; in others, the transmission of pain impulses may be blocked in the central nervous system. In still others, pain may be modulated by the physiologic activation of an intrinsic analgesic system.

Concerning the first of these mechanisms, aspirin and other nonsteroidal anti-inflammatory analgesics are believed to prevent the activation of nociceptors by inhibiting the synthesis of prostaglandins in skin, joints, viscera, etc. Morphine and meperidine given orally, parenterally, or intrathecally presumably produce analgesia by acting as "false" neurotransmitters at receptor sites in the posterior horns of the spinal cord—sites that are normally activated by endogenous opioid peptides (see Fig. 7-5). The separate sites of action of aspirin and opioids provide an explanation for the therapeutic usefulness of combining these drugs. Yet another mechanism consists of the physiologic activation of the intrinsic analgesic system (descending pathways from brain to spinal cord) by electrical stimulation, by administration of placebo, and possibly by acupuncture; short bursts of transcutaneous electrical stimulation may suppress pain in this way ("electroacupuncture"). Not only do opioids act directly on the central pain-conducting sensory systems, but they also exert a powerful action on the affective component of pain. Serotoninergic neurons are also thought to play a role in pain modulation. Tricyclic antidepressants, especially the methylated forms (imipramine, amitriptyline, and doxepin), block serotonin reuptake and thus enhance the action of this neurotransmitter at synapses and facilitate the action of the intrinsic opiate analgesic system.

The actions and use of analgesic and antidepressant drugs in the management of chronic pain are considered in greater detail in Chap. 42.

RARE AND UNUSUAL DISTURBANCES OF PAIN PERCEPTION

Lesions of the parieto-occipital regions of one cerebral hemisphere sometimes have peculiar effects on the patient's capacity to feel and react to pain. One interesting syndrome, discussed by Hécaen and De Ajuriaguerra, goes under the term *pain hemiagnosia*. In the reported cases the left arm and leg have been paralyzed from a right parietal lesion and at the same time rendered hypersensitive to noxious stimuli. When pinched on the affected side, after a delay the patient becomes agitated, moans, and seems distressed but makes no effort to fend off the painful stimulus with the other hand or to withdraw from it. In contrast, if the good side is pinched the patient reacts normally and moves the normal hand at once to the site of the stimulus to remove it. If asked what is being felt when the paralyzed side is hurt, the patient reports unbearable discomfort and cannot identify the source. A hemiagnosia for painful stimuli seems to be present, but the usual autonomic and emotional reactions appear, even in excess. The motor responses are no longer guided by sensory information from one side of the body.

The phenomenon of *asymbolia for pain* is another unusual state, wherein the patient, although capable of distinguishing the different types of pain stimuli from one another and from touch, is said to make none of the usual emotional, motor, or verbal responses to pain. This patient seems totally unaware of the painful or hurtful nature of stimuli delivered to any part of the body, whether on one side or the other. As pointed out by Schilder and Stengel, who first described the condition, not only are the patient's reactions to noxious stimuli judged to be insufficient and incomplete, but the same is true of responses to all signals of danger. In the few reported cases, pain asymboly has been a part of a larger syndrome, including various combinations of sensory aphasia, impairment of body schema and spatial disorientation, right-left confusion, and dyscalculia (i.e., Gerstmann syndrome—see Chap. 21). There is also fluctuation of attention to stimuli and extinction of stimuli on one side of the body, when both sides are simultaneously stimulated, but these abnormalities are thought to be insufficient to explain the asymboly.

The currently accepted interpretation of asymbolia for pain is interruption of transcortical integration. Piéron sees it as a particular type of agnosia (analgagnosia) or apractagnosia (cf. Chap. 21) in which the organism loses its ability to adapt its emotional, motor, and verbal actions to the consciousness of a nociceptive impression. *"Le sujet a perdu la comprehension de la signification de la douleur."* A few verified lesions have involved the supramarginal convolution as well as other parts of the dominant parietal lobe, according to Hécaen and Ajuriaguerra.

REFERENCES

Bonica JJ, (ed): Pain. *Association for Research in Nervous and Mental Disease Publications,* vol 58. New York, Raven Press, 1980.

Dykes RW: Nociception. *Brain Res* 99:229, 1975.

Fields HL: *Pain.* New York, McGraw-Hill, 1987.

Goldscheider A: *Ueber den Schmerz in Physiologischer und Klinischer Hinsicht.* Berlin, Hirschwald, 1884.

Hécaen H, De Ajuriaguerra J: Asymbolie à la douleur, étude anatomoclinique. *Rev Neurol* 83:300, 1950.

HOKFELT T, SKIRBOLL L, LUNDBERG JM, et al: Neuropeptides and pain pathways, in Bonica JJ, Lundblom U, Iggo A (eds): *Advances in Pain Research and Therapy*, vol 5. New York, Raven Press, 1983, pp 227–246.

HUGHES J (ED): Opioid peptides. *Br Med Bull* 39:1–106, 1983.

HUGHES J, SMITH TW, KOSTERLITZ HW, et al: Identification of two related pentapeptides from the brain with potent opiate agonist activity. *Nature* 258:577, 1975.

LELE PP, WEDDELL G: The relationship between neurohistology and corneal sensibility. *Brain* 79:119, 1956.

LEVINE JD, GORDON NC, FIELDS HL: The mechanism of placebo analgesia. *Lancet* 2:654, 1978.

LIGHT AR, PERL ER: Peripheral sensory systems, in Dyck PJ et al (eds): *Peripheral Neuropathy*, 2nd ed. Philadelphia, Saunders, 1984, vol 1, chap 9, pp 210–230.

MARK VH: Stereotactic surgery for the relief of pain, in White JC, Sweet WH (eds): *Pain and the Neurosurgeon*. Springfield, Ill, Charles C Thomas, 1969, chap 18, pp 843–887.

MELZACK R, CASEY KL: Sensory, motivational and central control determinants of pain. A new conceptual model, in Kenshalo D (ed): *The Skin Senses*. Springfield, Ill, Charles C Thomas, 1968, pp 423–439.

MELZACK R, WALL PD: Pain mechanisms: a new theory. *Science* 150:971, 1965.

MOUNTCASTLE VB: Central nervous mechanisms in sensation, in Mountcastle VB (ed): *Medical Physiology*, 14th ed. St Louis, Mosby, 1980, vol 1, part 5, chaps 11–19, pp 327–605.

NATHAN PW: The gate-control theory of pain. A critical review. *Brain* 99:123, 1976.

NICOLL RA, SCHENKER C, LEEMAN SE: Substance P as a transmitter candidate. *Annu Rev Neurosci* 3:227, 1980.

PERL ER: Pain and nociception, in Darian-Smith I (ed): *Handbook of Physiology*, sec 1: *The Nervous System*, vol 3: *Sensory Processes*, part 2. Baltimore, Williams & Wilkins, 1984, chap 20, pp 915–975.

PIERON H: *La Sensation*. Paris, Presses Universitaires de France, 1953.

RASMINSKY M: Ectopic impulse generation in pathologic nerve fibers, in Dyck PJ et al (eds): *Peripheral Neuropathy*, 2nd ed. Philadelphia, Saunders, 1984, vol 1, chap 40, pp 911–918.

REXED B: A cytotectonic atlas of the spinal cord in the cat. *J Comp Neurol* 100:297, 1954.

SCHILDER P, STENGEL E: Asymbolia for pain. *Arch Neurol Psychiatry* 25:598, 1931.

SINCLAIR D: *Mechanisms of Cutaneous Sensation*. Oxford, Oxford University Press, 1981.

SNYDER SH: Opiate receptors in the brain. *N Engl J Med* 296:266, 1977.

TAUB A: The use of psychotropic drugs alone and adjunctively in the treatment of otherwise intractable pain: postherpetic neuralgia; disseminated visceral neoplasm, in Voris HC, Whisler WW (eds): *Treatment of Pain*. Springfield, Ill, Charles C Thomas, 1975, chap 3, pp 32–42.

TAUB A, CAMPBELL JN: Percutaneous local electrical analgesia; peripheral mechanisms, in *Advances in Neurology*, vol 4: *Pain*. New York, Raven Press, 1974, pp 727–732.

WALL PD: The role of substantia gelatinosa as a gate control, in Bonica JJ (ed): *Pain*. New York, Raven Press, 1980, pp 205–231.

WEDDELL G: The multiple innervation of sensory spots in the skin. *J Anat* 75:441, 1941.

WHITE JC, SWEET WH: *Pain and the Neurosurgeon: A Forty Year Experience*. Springfield, Ill, Charles C Thomas, 1969.

WHITE D, HELME RD: Release of substance P from peripheral nerve terminals following electrical stimulation of sciatic nerve. *Brain Res* 336:27, 1985.

WOOLSEY CN, MARSHALL WH, BARD P: Note on the organization of the tactile sensory area of the cerebral cortex of the chimpanzee. *J Neurophysiol* 6:287, 1943.

YAKSH TL, HAMMOND DL: Peripheral and central substrates involved in the rostrad transmission of nociceptive information. *Pain* 13:1, 1982.

ZANDER E, WEDDELL G: Observations on the innervation of the cornea. *J Anat (London)* 85:68, 1951.

CHAPTER 8

OTHER SOMATIC SENSATION

Under normal conditions, sensory and motor functions are interdependent, as was dramatically illustrated by the early animal experiments of Claude Bernard and Sherrington, in which practically all effective movement of a limb was abolished by sectioning only its posterior roots. Interruption of other sensory pathways and destruction of the parietal cortex also have a profound effect upon motility. Sensory and motor neurons are intimately connected at all levels of the nervous system from the spinal cord to the cerebrum. To a large extent, human activity depends upon a constant influx of sensory impulses (most of them not consciously perceived) which are integral to motor adaptations. Truly, in a physiologic sense, "movement is sensation."

However, under conditions of disease, motor and sensory functions may be affected independently. Loss or impairment of sensory function may occur, and these may represent the principal manifestations of neurologic disease. The logic of this is clear enough, since the major anatomic pathways of the sensory system are distinct from those of the motor system and may be selectively disturbed by disease. The analysis of sensory symptoms involves the use of special tests, designed to indicate the nature of the sensory disorder and its locality, and it is from this point of view that disorders of sensory function are considered here.

This chapter will deal with *general somatic sensation,* i.e., afferent impulses which arise from the skin, muscles, or joints. One form of somatic sensation—pain—has already been discussed (Chap. 7) and these two chapters should be read together. The *special* senses—vision, hearing, taste, and smell—are considered in the next section (Chaps. 11 to 14), and visceral (interoceptive) sensation, most of which does not reach consciousness, is considered with the disorders of the autonomic nervous system (Chap. 26).

ANATOMIC AND PHYSIOLOGIC CONSIDERATIONS

An understanding of the sensory disorders depends upon a knowledge of applied anatomy. Ideally, one should be familiar with the sensory receptors in the skin and deeper structures, the distribution of the peripheral nerves and roots, and the pathways by which sensory impulses are conveyed from the periphery and through the spinal cord and brainstem to the thalamus and cortex of the parietal lobe. These aspects of the anatomy of the sensory system and its physiology have already been touched upon in Chap. 7 in relation to the perception of pain, and will be elaborated here to include all forms of somatic sensation. Charts showing the cutaneous distribution of the peripheral nerves (Fig. 8-1) are included in this section, and little more will be said about this aspect of the subject.

Every sensation depends on impulses excited by the adequate stimulation of receptors and is conveyed to the central nervous system by afferent, or sensory, fibers. Sensory receptors are of two general types: those in the skin (exteroceptors) and those in the deeper somatic structures (proprioceptors). The skin receptors are particularly numerous and transduce four types of sensory experience: warmth, cold, touch, and pain; these are conventionally referred to as sensations or senses, e.g., tactile sensation or sense of touch. The proprioceptors inform us of the position of our body in space, of the force, direction, and range of movement of the joints (kinesthetic sense), and of pressure, both painful and painless. Histologically, a wide variety of sensory receptors has been described, varying from simple, free axon terminals to highly branched and encapsulated structures, many of the latter bearing the names of the anatomists who first described them.

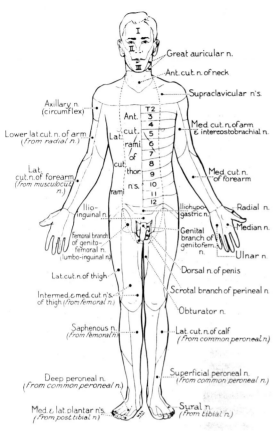

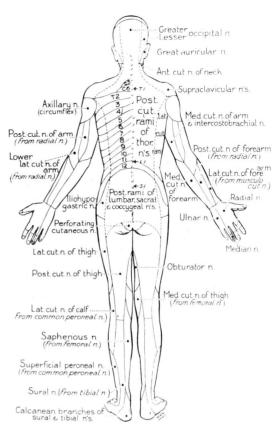

Figure 8-1

The cutaneous fields of peripheral nerves. (From W Haymaker, B Woodhall, Peripheral Nerve Injuries, 2nd ed, Philadelphia, Saunders, 1953.)

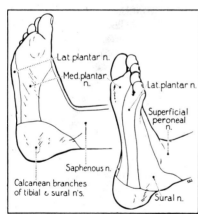

MECHANISMS OF CUTANEOUS SENSATION

As indicated in the preceding chapter, it was common teaching for many years that each of the primary modalities of cutaneous sensation is subserved by a morphologically distinct end organ, each with its separate peripheral nerve

fibers. According to this formulation, traditionally associated with the name of von Frey, each type of end organ responds only to a particular type of stimulus and subserves a specific modality of sensation: Meissner corpuscles—touch; Merkel discs—pressure; Ruffini plumes—heat; Kraus end bulbs—cold; Pacinian corpuscles—vibration and tickle; and freely branching endings—pain.

This specificity theory, as it came to be called, has held up best in respect to the peripheral mechanisms for pain insofar as certain primary afferent fibers, namely the C and A-δ fibers and their free nerve ending type of receptors, respond maximally to noxious stimuli. But even these ''pain fibers'' were shown to convey nonnoxious information, that is to say, their specificity as pain fibers is not absolute (Chap. 7).

Nor has it been possible to ascribe a specific function to each of the many varieties of receptors. Thus, Merkel

119

discs, Meissner corpuscles, nerve plexuses around the hair follicles, and free nerve endings can all be activated by a tactile stimulus. Conversely, a single type of receptor may generate more than one sensory modality. Weddell and his colleagues found that with appropriate stimulation of the cornea each of the four primary modalities of somatic sensibility (touch, warmth, cold, pain) could be recognized, even though the cornea contains only fine, freely ending nerve filaments. In the ear, which is also sensitive to these four modalities, only two types of receptors—freely ending and perifollicular—are present. The lack of organized receptors, e.g., the end bulbs of Krause and Ruffini, in the cornea and ear make it evident that these types of receptors are not essential for the recognition of cold and warmth, respectively, as von Frey and other early anatomists postulated.

Particularly instructive in this regard are the observations of Kibler and Nathan, who studied the responses of warm and cold spots to different stimuli. (Warm and cold spots are those small areas of skin which most consistently respond to thermal stimuli with a sensation of warmth or cold). They found that a cold stimulus applied to a warm spot gave rise to a sensation of cold and vice versa, that a noxious stimulus applied to a warm or cold spot gave rise only to a painful sensation; also they noted that mechanical stimulation of these spots gave rise to a sensation of touch or pressure.

The aforementioned observations such as these indicate that cutaneous receptors are not specific, although each responds preferentially (i.e., has a lower threshold) to one form of stimulation in distinction to another. Such end organs can then be classed as mechanoreceptors, thermoreceptors, or nociceptors, depending on their selective sensitivity to mechanical, thermal, or noxious stimuli, respectively (Sinclair).

More recent physiologic studies have shown that the *quality* of sensation depends on the type of fiber that is stimulated, even though the endings themselves are not specific. Different diseases therefore evoke a variety of sensory deficits determined by which fibers are affected. Microstimulation of single sensory fibers in awake human subjects arouses different sensations depending on which fibers are stimulated and not on the frequency of stimulation. By contrast, the *intensity* of sensation is related to the frequency of stimulation. Afferent impulse frequency *(temporal summation)* is decoded by the brain as expressive of the magnitude of sensation. But in addition, as the intensity of stimulation increases, more sensory units are activated *(spatial summation).*

Localization of a stimulus was formerly believed to be based on the simultaneous activation of overlapping sensory units. Tower defined a peripheral sensory unit as a dorsal root ganglion cell, its central and distal extensions and all the sensory endings in the territory supplied by the distal extension (receptive field). In the very sensitive pulp of the finger, where the error of localization is less than 1.0 mm, there are 240 low-threshold mechanoreceptors per square centimeter, which overlap extensively. Highly refined physiologic techniques, however, have demonstrated that activation of even a single sensory unit is sufficient to localize the point stimulated and that the body map in the parietal lobe is capable of decoding such information.

Although an individual sensory unit may respond to several different types of stimuli, it is most sensitive to one type, which may be termed the adequate stimulus. The stimulus, in order to gain access to the ending, must pass through the skin and the energy of the stimulus must transduce, i.e., depolarize, the nerve ending. Not only does the threshold of stimulation vary but also the nerve impulse that is generated is a graded one, not an all-or-none phenomenon like an action potential. This poorly understood peripheral generator potential determines the *frequency* of impulse in the nerve and to what degree it is sustained or fades out (i.e., adapts to the stimulus or fatigue). The mechanism by which a stimulus is translated into a sensory experience is obscure. It is probably fair to say that each type of specialized ending has a structure that facilitates the transducive process for a particular stimulus. In general the encapsulated endings are of the low threshold type and are connected to large sensory fibers.

PROTOPATHIC AND EPICRITIC SENSIBILITY

Brief reference should be made to this concept of cutaneous sensation, originally formulated by Head and his colleagues on the basis of observations of the sensory changes that followed division of the cutaneous branch of the radial nerve in Head's own forearm. They described an innermost area in which superficial sensation was completely abolished; this was surrounded by a narrower ("intermediate") zone, in which pain sensation was preserved and extreme degrees of temperature were recognized but in which perception of touch, lesser differences of temperature, and two-point discrimination were abolished. Pain in this latter zone was unpleasant and diffuse and could not be localized accurately. To explain these findings, Head postulated the existence of two systems of cutaneous receptors and conducting fibers: (1) a *protopathic* system, subserving pain and extreme differences in temperature and yielding ungraded, diffuse impressions of an all-or-none type, and (2) an *epicritic* system, which mediated touch, two-point discrimination, and lesser differences in temperature. The pain and hyperesthesia that follow damage to a peripheral nerve were attributed to a loss of inhibition that was normally exerted by the epicritic upon the protopathic system.

That an intermediate zone is regularly found between normal and anesthetic areas of denervated skin is generally agreed. However, the nature of the changes in this intermediate zone has been much debated. Trotter and Davies, who repeated Head's experiment, failed to substantiate all of the original observations. They found that the changes in tactile and discriminative sensation in the intermediate zone were not lost but diminished and attributed the changes to hypesthesia of these modalities. The particular structures postulated by Head to underlie each of his functional systems were never established. Actually, the fringe of hypesthetic and altered sensation was later shown by Weddell to be due to collateral regeneration of surrounding nerve fibers, particularly those of pain (collateral regeneration of touch fibers is minimal). Despite these and other criticisms (reviewed in detail by Walshe) the concept of protopathic and epicritic sensibility still has its proponents who use it to explain the alterations in quality of sensation that occur with both peripheral lesions and central ones (e.g., thalamic syndrome). The modulating effects of large primary afferent fibers on small fibers, as postulated in the gate theory of Melzack and Wall (see Chap. 7), has also served to revive interest in Head's hypothesis.

SENSORY PATHWAYS

Fibers that mediate superficial sensation travel in cutaneous sensory or mixed sensory-motor nerves. In cutaneous nerves, unmyelinated pain and autonomic fibers exceed myelinated fibers by a ratio of 3 or 4:1. The myelinated fibers are of two types, small A-δ fibers for pain and temperature and large ones for touch and pressure. The efferent nonmyelinated autonomic fibers are postganglionic and innervate piloerector muscles, sweat glands, and blood vessels. Proprioceptive fibers are carried in deeper, predominantly motor nerves. In addition, these nerves contain afferent and efferent spindle and Golgi tendon organ fibers and thinner pain afferents. The conduction velocities of these fibers are discussed in Chap. 45.

All the sensory neurons have their cell bodies in the dorsal root ganglia; the central projections of these cells enter the spinal cord via the dorsal or posterior roots. Each dorsal root contains all the fibers from skin, muscles, connective tissue, ligaments, tendons, joints, bones, and viscera that lie within the distribution of a single body segment, or somite. This segmental innervation has been amply demonstrated in humans and animals by observing the effects of lesions that involve one or two spinal nerves, such as herpes zoster, which also causes visible vesicles in the corresponding area of skin, or prolapsed intervertebral

Figure 8-2

Distribution of the sensory spinal roots on the surface of the body. (From D Sinclair, Mechanisms of Cutaneous Sensation, Oxford, Oxford University Press, 1981.)

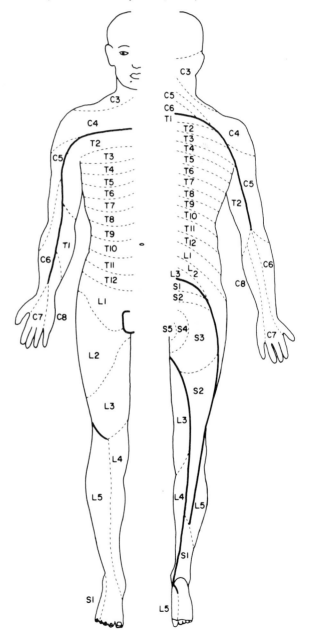

disc, which causes hypalgesia in a single root zone, or surgical section of several roots on each side of an intact root (method of remaining sensibility). Maps of the dermatomes derived from these several types of data are shown in Fig. 8-2. It should be noted that there is considerable overlapping from one segment to the other and that this is more so for touch than for pain (Fig. 8-3). Also the maps differ somewhat according to the methods used in constructing them. In contrast to most dermatomal charts, those of Keegan and Garrett (based on the injection of local anesthetic into single dorsal root ganglia) show bands of hypalgesia to be continuous longitudinally from the periphery to the spine (Fig. 8-4). The segmental distribution of pain fibers from deep structures, though not fully corresponding to that of pain fibers from the skin, also follows a segmental pattern.

In the dorsal roots, the sensory fibers are first rearranged according to function. Large and heavily myelinated fibers enter the cord just medial to the dorsal horn and divide into an ascending and descending branch. The descending fibers and some of the ascending ones enter the gray matter of the dorsal horn within a few segments of their entrance and synapse with nerve cells in the gray matter of posterior and anterior horns, including large

ventral horn cells, subserving segmental reflexes. Some of the ascending fibers run uninterruptedly in the dorsal columns of the same side of the spinal cord, terminating in the gracile and cuneate nuclei. The central axons of the primary sensory neurons are joined in the posterior columns by other secondary neurons whose cell bodies lie in the posterior horns of the spinal cord. The fibers in the fasciculus gracilis are displaced medially as new fibers are added at each successive root. In the posterior column are contained a portion of the fibers for touch and the fibers mediating the senses of pressure, vibration, direction of movement

Figure 8-3

Radicular (A) and peripheral nerve innervation (B) of cutaneous areas showing overlapping of nerve fibers in the dermatomes. (From MB Carpenter and J Sutin, Human Neuroanatomy, 8th ed, Baltimore, Williams & Wilkins, 1983.)

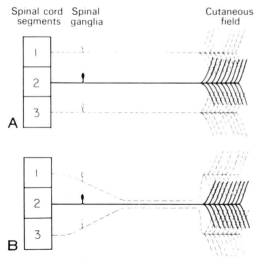

Figure 8-4

Dermatomes of the upper and lower extremities, outlined by the pattern of sensory loss following lesions of single nerve roots. (From Keegan and Garrett.)

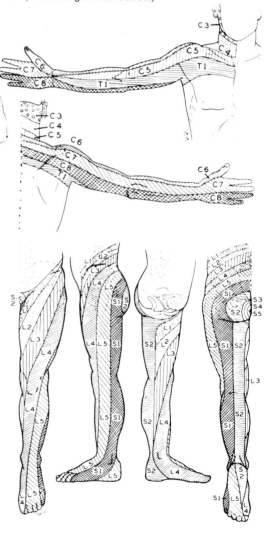

and position of joints and stereognosis (see Fig. 7-3); it is unlikely, however, that the fiber pathways in the posterior columns are the sole mediators of proprioception in the spinal cord (see further on, under "posterior column syndrome"). The nerve cells of the nucleus gracilis and cuneatus give rise to a secondary afferent path, which crosses the midline in the medulla and ascends as the medial lemniscus, to the thalamus (see below).

Thinly myelinated or unmyelinated fibers enter the cord on the lateral aspect of the dorsal horn and synapse with dorsal horn cells, mainly within a segment or two of their point of entry into the cord. The dorsal horn cells in turn give rise to secondary sensory fibers, some of which may ascend ipsilaterally but most of which decussate and ascend in the anterolateral fasciculus of the cord. These anatomic arrangements have already been considered in Chap. 7. Observations based on the surgical interruption of the anterolateral funiculus indicate that fibers mediating pain and temperature occupy the dorsolateral part of the anterolateral funiculus, and those for touch and deep pressure, the ventromedial part.

The pathways mediating cutaneous sensation from the face and head, especially touch, pain, and temperature, are conveyed to the brainstem by the trigeminal nerve; after entering the pons, the pain and temperature fibers run caudally as the descending trigeminal root and terminate in a long vertically oriented nucleus that lies beside it and extends to the second or third cervical segment of the cord, where it becomes continuous with the posterior horn of the spinal gray matter. Axons from the neurons of this nucleus cross the midline and ascend as the trigeminal lemniscus, along the medial side of the spinothalamic tract (Fig. 7-2). Ascending fibers from the reticular nuclei, medial lemniscus, trigeminal lemniscus, and spinothalamic pathways merge in the midbrain and terminate in the posterior complex of thalamic nuclei, particularly in the nucleus ventralis posterolateralis (VPL).

The posterior thalamic complex projects mainly to two somatosensory cortical areas: the first area (S1), corresponds to the postcentral cortex or Brodmann's areas 3, 1, and 2. S1 afferents are derived primarily from VPL and VPM and are distributed somatotopically, with the leg represented uppermost and the face lowermost. Electrical stimulation of this area yields sensations of tingling, numbness, and warmth in specific regions on the *opposite* side of the body. The information transmitted to S1 is tactile and proprioceptive, derived mainly from the dorsal column—medial lemniscus system, and is concerned mainly with sensory discrimination. The second somatosensory area (S2) lies on the upper bank of the sylvian fissure, adjacent to the insula. Localization of function is less discrete in S2 than in S1, but S2 is also organized somatotopically, with the face rostrally and hind leg or leg

caudally. The sensations evoked by electrical stimulation of S2 are much the same as those of S1 but, in distinction to the latter, may be felt bilaterally.

Undoubtedly, the perception of sensory stimuli involves more of the cerebral cortex than the two discrete areas described above. Some sensory fibers probably project to the precentral gyrus and others to the superior parietal lobule. Conversely, S1 and S2 are not purely sensory in function; motor effects can be obtained by stimulating them electrically. It has been shown that sensory neurons in VPL, cuneate and gracile nuclei, and sensory neurons in the dorsal horn of the spinal cord all receive descending cortical projections as well as ascending ones. This reciprocal arrangement probably influences movement and the transmission and interpretation of pain.

Provided that the subcortical structures, especially the thalamus, are intact, certain sensations such as pain, touch, pressure, and extremes of temperature can reach consciousness. Their accurate localization, however, as well as the patient's ability to make fine sensory discriminations, depends to a large extent on the integrity of the sensory cortex. This clinical distinction will be elaborated in the discussion of the sensory syndromes.

EXAMINATION OF SENSATION

Most neurologists would agree that sensory testing is the most difficult part of the neurologic examination. For one thing, test procedures are relatively crude and inadequate, and are unlike natural modes of stimulation with which the patient is familiar. Embarrassingly often, no objective sensory loss can be demonstrated despite symptoms that indicate the presence of such a deficit. Contrariwise, one may discover a sensory deficit when there has been no complaint of sensory symptoms. In the former instance, sensory symptoms, in the nature of paresthesias or dysesthesias, may be generated along axons of nerves not sufficiently diseased to impair or reduce sensory function. In the latter instance, loss of function may have been so gradual as to pass unnoticed. Always there is some difficulty in evaluating the response to sensory stimuli, since it depends on the patient's interpretation of sensory experiences. This in turn will depend on the patient's general awareness and responsiveness, desire to cooperate, as well as intelligence, education, and suggestibility. At times, children and relatively uneducated persons, by virtue of their simple and direct responses, are better witnesses than more sophisticated individuals who are likely to analyze their feelings minutely and report small, inconsequential differences in stimulus intensity.

Before proceeding to sensory testing, the physician should question patients about their symptoms, and this too may pose special problems. Patients are confronted with derangements of sensation that may be unlike anything they have previously experienced, and they have few words in their vocabulary to describe what they feel. They may say that a limb feels ''numb'' and ''dead'' when in fact they mean that it is weak. Observant individuals may occasionally discover a loss of sensation, e.g., a lack of pain on touching an object hot enough to blister the skin or unawareness of articles of clothing and other objects in contact with the skin. But more often disease induces new and unnatural sensory experiences. If nerves, sensory roots, or spinal tracts are damaged or partially interrupted, the patient may complain of tingling or prickling (''like Novocain,'' ''pins and needles'') feelings, cramp-like sensations, burning or cutting pain that occurs either spontaneously or in response to stimulation; presumably some of the remaining touch, pressure, thermal, and pain fibers are hyperexcitable and capable of generating ectopic impulses along their course, spontaneously or after a natural volley of stimulus-evoked impulses (Ochoa and Torebjörk). These abnormal sensations are called *paresthesias* or *dysesthesias,* and their character and distribution inform us of the anatomy of the lesions involving the sensory system. It has been shown that stimulation of touch fibers gives rise to a sensation of tingling and buzzing; of muscle proprioceptors, to pseudocramp; of thermal fibers, to hotness and coldness; and of A-δ fibers, to prickling and pain. Ectopic discharges can be induced by ischemia (postischemic paresthesias), by hypocalcemia, and by diseases of nerves.

Paresthesias should always raise suspicion of a lesion of the sensory pathways in nerves, spinal cord, or higher structures. However, they may, if evanescent, be of no significance. Every person has had the experience of resting on the ulnar, sciatic, or peroneal nerve and having the limb ''fall asleep.'' Anxiety with hyperventilation may cause paresthesias of the lips and hands (sometimes unilateral) from diminution of CO_2 and of ionized calcium. Tetany has the same effects with added carpopedal spasms. Painful paresthesias, including hyperpathia and causalgia (painful burning sensation caused by all stimuli —see Chap. 7) are referred to as dysesthesias. They are probably due to hyperexcitability or disinhibition of neurons in the posterior horns of the spinal cord or trigeminal neurons of the brainstem (Loh and Nathan).

The detail with which sensation is tested in a routine neurologic examination is determined by the clinical situation. If the patient has no sensory complaints, it is sufficient to test vibration and position sense in the fingers and toes and the perception of pinprick over the face, trunk, and extremities, and to determine whether the findings are the same in symmetric parts of the body. A rough survey of this sort may detect sensory defects of which the patient is unaware. On the other hand, more thorough testing is in order if the patient has complaints referable to the sensory system, or if one finds localized atrophy or weakness, ataxia, trophic changes of joints, or painless ulcers.

A few other general principles should be mentioned. One should not press the sensory examination in the presence of fatigue, for an inattentive patient is a poor witness. The examiner must also avoid suggesting symptoms to the patient. After having explained in the simplest terms what is required, the examiner should interpose as few questions and remarks as possible. Consequently, patients must not be asked, ''Do you feel that?'' each time they are touched; they should simply be told to say ''yes'' or ''sharp'' every time they have been touched or feel pain. Patients should not see the part under examination. For short tests it is sufficient that they close the eyes; during more detailed testing it is preferable to screen the eyes from the part being examined. Finally, the findings of the sensory examination should be accurately recorded on a chart.

Somatic sensation is frequently classified as superficial (cutaneous, exteroceptive) and deep (proprioceptive); the former comprises the modalities of light touch, pain, and temperature; the latter includes the sense of position, passive motion, vibration, and deep pressure-pain.

SENSE OF TOUCH

This is usually tested with a wisp of cotton. Patients are first acquainted with the nature of the stimulus by applying it to a normal part of the body. Then they are asked to say ''yes'' each time various other parts are touched. A patient simulating sensory loss may say ''no'' in response to a tactile stimulus. Cornified areas of skin, such as the soles and palms, will require a heavier stimulus than elsewhere, and the hair-clad parts a lighter one, because of the numerous nerve endings around the follicles. The patient is more sensitive to a moving contactual stimulus of any kind than to a stationary one. The deft application of the examiner's or preferably the patient's roving fingertips is a useful method of mapping out an area of tactile loss, as Trotter originally showed.

More precise testing is possible by using a von Frey hair. By this method, a stimulus of constant strength can be applied and the threshold for tactile sensation determined by measuring the force required to bend a hair of known length. Ideally, degrees of tactile perception should be tested by supraliminal stimuli, but this is seldom practical. Special difficulties arise in the testing of tactile perception when, as a consequence of disease in this system, a series of contactual stimuli lead to a dying out of sensation, either through adaptation of the end organ or because the initial sensation outlasts the stimulus and seems to spread. The patient may then fail to report tactile stimuli in an area where they were previously present or he may report contact without being touched. Sudden loss of sensation may create somatic hallucinations: the limb may feel suspended, disconnected from the body, or as though it had assumed an unnatural position (Nathan et al).

SENSE OF PAIN

This is most efficiently estimated by pinprick, although it may be evoked by a great diversity of noxious stimuli. Patients must understand that they are to report the degree of sharpness of the pin, not simply the feeling of contact or pressure of the point. If the pinpricks are applied rapidly in one area, their effect may be summated and excessive pain may result; therefore, they should be delivered about one per second, and not over the same spot.

It is almost impossible, using an ordinary pin, to apply each stimulus with equal intensity. This difficulty can be largely overcome by the use of an algesimeter, which enables one not only to deliver stimuli of constant intensity but also to grade the intensity and determine threshold values. Even with this instrument an isolated stimulus may be reported as being excessively sharp, apparently because of direct contact with a pain spot.

If an area of diminished or absent touch or pain sensation is encountered, its boundaries should be demarcated to determine whether it has a segmental or peripheral nerve distribution or whether sensation is lost below a certain level on the trunk. Such areas are best delineated by proceeding from the region of impaired sensation toward the normal, and the changes may be confirmed by dragging a pin lightly over the parts in question.

DEEP PRESSURE-PAIN

One can estimate this modality simply by firmly pinching or pressing deeply on the tendons and muscles; no special virtue is attached to the traditional and somewhat sadistic use of the testicle or nipple for this test. Pain can often be elicited by heavy pressure even when superficial sensation is diminished; conversely, in some diseases, such as tabetic neurosyphilis, loss of deep pressure-pain may be more prominent than loss of superficial pain.

THERMAL SENSE

The proper evaluation of this modality requires attention to certain details of procedure. One may fail to evoke a sensation of hot or cold if small test objects are used. The

perception of thermal stimuli is relatively delayed, especially if the test objects are applied only lightly and momentarily against the skin. If the temperature of the test object is below 10°C or above 50°C, sensations of cold or heat become confused with pain. As the temperature of the test object approaches that of the skin, the patient's response will be modified by the temperature of the skin itself.

The following procedure for testing thermal sensation is therefore suggested. The areas of skin to be tested should be exposed for some time before the examination. The test objects should be large, preferably two Erlenmeyer flasks containing hot and cold water. Thermometers, which extend into the water through the flask stoppers, indicate the temperature of the water at the moment of testing. At first, extreme degrees of heat and cold (e.g., 10 and 45°C) are employed to delineate roughly an area of thermal sensory disturbance; the patient should be asked to report whether the flask feels ''less hot'' or ''less cold'' over such an area in comparison to a normal part. If an area of impaired sensation is found, the borders can be accurately determined by moving the flask along the skin from the insensitive to the normal region. The qualitative change should then be quantitated as far as possible by estimating the differences in temperature that the patient is able to recognize. The patient is asked to state whether one stimulus feels warmer or colder than another, not whether a given stimulus is warm or cold. The difference in temperature between the two flasks is gradually reduced by mixing their contents. A normal person can detect a difference of 1°C or less when the temperature of the flasks is in the range of 28 to 32°C; in the warm range, differences between 35 and 40°C can be recognized and in the cold range, between 10 and 20°C. In some normal older persons and in others with poor peripheral circulation (especially in cold weather), the responses may not meet these standards.

The perception of heat or cold depends not only on the temperature of the test object but also on the duration of the stimulus and the area over which it is applied. These particulars of testing may be used to detect slight degrees of sensory impairment; the patient may be able to distinguish small differences in temperature when the bottom of the flask is applied for 3 s but be unable to do so if only the side of the flask is applied for 1 s. Throughout the test procedure, especially when small temperature differences are involved, the area of sensory disturbance should be continually checked against perception in normal parts. For greater precision in quantitating thermal sensibility, as might be desired in the investigation of peripheral nerve disease, a number of refined laboratory instruments have been devised (Dyck et al; Bertelsmann et al).

PROPRIOCEPTIVE SENSE

Awareness of the position and movements of our limbs is derived from receptors in the muscles, tendons, and joints. Skin receptors probably facilitate proprioception. The two modalities that comprise proprioception, i.e., sense of movement and position, are usually lost together, although clinical situations do arise in which perception of the position of a limb or digits is lost while that of passive and active movement (kinesthesia) of these parts is retained. The opposite has also been said to occur, but must be very rare.

Abnormalities of position sense may be revealed in several ways. With the arms outstretched and eyes closed, the affected arm will wander from its original position; if the fingers are spread apart, they may undergo a series of changing postures (''piano-playing'' movements, or pseudoathetosis); in attempting to touch the tip of the nose with the index finger, the patient may miss the target repeatedly but not do so with the eyes open.

The lack of position sense in the legs may be demonstrated by displacing the limb from its original position and having the patient, with eyes closed, point to the large toe or put the other foot or leg in the same position. If position sense is defective in both legs, the patient will be unable to maintain balance with feet together and eyes closed (Romberg sign). This sign should be interpreted with caution. Even a normal person in the Romberg position will sway slightly with the eyes closed. A patient with lack of balance due to cerebellar ataxia or other motor disorder will also sway more if visual cues are removed. Only if there is a marked discrepancy between the state of balance with eyes open and with eyes closed can one confidently state that the patient shows a Romberg sign. Mild degrees of unsteadiness in nervous or suggestible patients may be overcome by diverting their attention, e.g., by having them touch the index finger of each hand alternately to the nose while standing with eyes closed.

Perception of passive movement is first tested in the fingers and toes, since the defect, when present, is reflected maximally in these parts. It is important to grasp the digit firmly at the sides opposite the plane of movement; otherwise the pressure applied by the examiner in displacing the digit may allow the patient to identify the direction of movement. This applies also to the testing of the more proximal segments of the limb. The patient should be instructed to report each movement as being ''up'' or ''down'' from the previous position. It is useful to demonstrate the test with a large and easily identified movement, but once the idea is clear to the patient, the smallest detectable changes in position should be determined. The part being tested should be moved rapidly. The range of a quick movement that is normally appreciated in the digits is said to be as little as 1°. In practice, defective perception of passive movement is judged by comparison with a normal limb or, if perception is bilaterally defective, on the basis of what the examiner has learned through experience to be normal. Slight impairment may be disclosed by a slowness of response or, if the digit is displaced very slowly, by an unawareness or uncertainty that movement has occurred; or, after the digit has been displaced in the same direction several times, the patient may misjudge the first movement in the opposite direction; or, after the examiner has moved the toe, the patient may make a number of small voluntary movements of the toe, in an apparent attempt to determine its position or the direction of the movement. Inattentiveness will cause some of these errors.

The sources of information for these several types of proprioception are receptors in the skin, joint or articulatory nerve endings, and receptors in the tendon and muscle (probably Golgi tendon organs according to Roland et al). Moberg believes that cutaneous afferents, activated by movement of the skin, and joint afferents are the most important.

THE SENSE OF VIBRATION

This is a composite sensation comprising touch and rapid alterations of deep-pressure sense. Its conduction depends on both cutaneous and deep afferent fibers which ascend in the dorsal columns of the cord. It is therefore rarely affected by lesions of single nerves but will be disturbed in patients with disease of multiple peripheral nerves, dorsal columns, medial lemniscus, and thalamus. Vibration and position sense are usually lost together, although one of them (most often vibration sense) may be affected disproportionately. With advancing age, vibration sense may be diminished at the toes and ankles.

Vibration sense is tested by placing a tuning fork with a low rate and long duration of vibration (128 dv) over the bony prominences. The examiner must make sure that the patient responds to the vibration, not simply to the pressure of the fork, and that the patient is not trying to listen to it. There are mechanical devices to quantitate vibration sense, but it is sufficient for clinical purposes to compare the point tested with a normal part of the patient or the examiner. Thus, the vibrating fork is allowed to run down until the moment that vibration is no longer perceived, and the fork is then transferred quickly to the corresponding point on the opposite limb; if vibration is then perceived and if this finding is consistent, one can be certain of an impairment of vibration sense. The perception of vibration at the tibial tuberosity after it has disappeared at the ankle, or at the anterior iliac spine after it has disappeared at the tibial tuberosity, is an indication of a peripheral nerve lesion. The level of vibration sense loss due to spinal cord lesions can be estimated by placing the fork over the iliac crests and successive vertebral spines.

DISCRIMINATIVE SENSORY FUNCTIONS

Damage to the sensory cortex or to the thalamocortical projections results in a special type of disturbance that affects mainly the patient's ability to make sensory discriminations. Lesions in these structures usually disturb position sense but leave the so-called primary modalities (touch, pain, temperature, and vibration sense) relatively little affected. In such a situation, or if a cerebral lesion is suspected on other grounds, discriminative function should be tested further by the following tests:

Two-Point Discrimination The ability to distinguish two points from one is tested by using a compass, the points of which should be blunt and applied simultaneously and painlessly. The distance at which such stimuli can be recognized as double varies but is roughly 1 mm at the tip of the tongue, 2 to 3 mm on the lips, 3 to 5 mm at the fingertips, 8 to 15 mm on the palm, 20 to 30 mm on the dorsa of the hands and feet, and 4 to 7 cm on the body surface. It is characteristic of the patient with a lesion of the sensory cortex to mistake two points for one, although occasionally the opposite occurs.

Cutaneous Localization and Figure Writing (*Graphesthesia*) The ability to localize cutaneous tactile or painful stimuli is tested by touching or pricking various parts of the body and asking the patient to point to the part stimulated or to the corresponding part on the examiner's limb. Recognition of numbers or letters (these should be larger than 4 cm) or of the direction of lines drawn on the skin also depends on localization of tactile stimuli. According to Wall and Noordenbos, figure writing and detection of the direction of movement on the skin are the most useful and simplest tests of posterior column function.

Appreciation of Texture, Size, and Shape Appreciation of texture depends mainly on cutaneous impressions, but the recognition of the shape and size of objects is based on impressions from deeper receptors as well. The lack of recognition of shape and form, therefore, though frequently a manifestation of cortical disease, may occur also with lesions of the spinal cord and brainstem because of interruption of tracts transmitting proprioceptive and tactile sensation. The latter type of sensory defect, called *stereoanesthesia*, should be distinguished from *astereognosis*, which connotes an inability to identify an object by palpation, the primary sense data (touch, pain, temperature, and vibration) being intact. In practice, a pure astereognosis is rarely encountered, and the term is employed where the impairment of superficial and vibratory sensation in the hands seems to be of insufficient severity to account for the defect. Defined in this way, astereognosis is either right- or left-sided, and, with the qualifications mentioned below, is the product of a lesion in the opposite hemisphere, involving the postcentral gyrus or the thalamoparietal projections.

The traditional teaching that somatic sensation is represented only in the contralateral parietal lobe is not strictly correct. Beginning with Oppenheim, in 1906, there have been sporadic reports of patients who showed bilateral astereognosis or loss of tactile sensation, as a result of an apparently unilateral cerebral lesion. The validity of these observations was established by Semmes et al, who tested a large series of patients with traumatic lesions involving either the right or left cerebral hemisphere. They found that a substantial number of such patients showed an ipsilateral or bilateral impairment of "cortical" or discriminative sensation (pressure, two-point discrimination, point localization, and passive movement) as a result of unilateral cerebral disease, right or left. These observations, with minor qualifications, have been confirmed by Carmon and also by Corkin et al, who investigated the sensory effects of cortical excisions in patients with focal epilepsy.

Thus it appears that certain somatic sensory functions are mediated not only by the contralateral hemisphere, but also by the ipsilateral one, although the contribution of the former is undoubtedly the more significant.

Finally, astereognosis needs to be distinguished from *tactile agnosia*, in which a one-sided lesion, lying posterior to the postcentral gyrus of the *dominant* parietal lobe, results in an inability to recognize an object by touch in *both* hands. Tactile agnosia is a disorder of conceptualization and perception of symbols akin to the defect in naming parts of the body, or visualizing a plan or a route, or understanding the meaning of the printed or spoken word (visual or auditory verbal agnosia).

Recent observations have called into question the traditional concept of left hemispheric dominance in respect to tactile perception. The findings of Carmon and Benton, that the right hemisphere is particularly important in perceiving the direction of tactile stimuli, and of Corkin, that patients with right-hemisphere lesions show a consistently greater failure of tactile-maze learning than those with left-sided lesions, point to a relative dominance of the right hemisphere in the mediation of tactile performance involving a spatial component. Also, the phenomenon of sensory inattention or extinction is most prominent with lesions of the right parietal lobe (stimuli applied to the left side of the body are neglected or extinguished) and is most informative if the primary and secondary sensory cortical areas are spared. These matters are considered further on in this chapter and in Chap. 21.

A few other terms require definition, since they may be encountered in reading about sensation. Many of them lack precision and others are pedantic. It is recommended that the simplest possible terms be used. *Dysesthesia* refers to any unpleasant or painful sensory experience induced by a stimulus that is ordinarily painless, such as the pressure of bedclothes. *Paresthesias* refer to crawling, burning, tingling, or "pins-and-needles" feelings that arise spontaneously. *Anesthesia* refers to a complete loss of all forms of sensation, and *hypesthesia* to a diminution of sensation. Loss or impairment of specific cutaneous sensations may be indicated by an appropriate prefix or suffix, e.g., thermoanesthesia or thermohypesthesia, analgesia (loss of pain) or hypalgesia, tactile anesthesia and pallanesthesia (loss of vibratory sense). The term *hyperesthesia* refers to an increased sensitivity to various stimuli, and is usually used with respect to cutaneous sensation. The term implies a heightened activity of the sensory apparatus. Under certain conditions (e.g., sunburn) there does appear to be an enhanced sensitivity of cutaneous receptors, but usually the presence of hyperesthesia betrays an underlying sensory defect; careful testing will demonstrate an elevated threshold to tactile, painful, or thermal stimuli, but once the stimulus is perceived it may have a severely painful or unpleasant quality (*hyperpathia*). Some clinicians use the latter term to denote an exaggerated response to a painful stimulus. In *alloesthesia* or *allesthesia*, a tactile or painful stimulus delivered on the side of hemisensory loss is experienced in a corresponding area of the opposite side. This abnormality is observed most frequently with right-sided putaminal lesions (usually hemorrhage) and with anterolateral lesions of the cervical spinal cord. Presumably this phenomenon depends on the existence of an uncrossed ipsilateral spinothalamic pathway (Ray and Wolff).

EFFECT OF AGE ON SENSORY FUNCTION

A matter of general importance in the testing of sensation is the progressive impairment of sensory perception that occurs with advancing age. This finding requires that sensory thresholds, particularly in the feet and legs, always be assessed in relation to age standards. This feature is discerned most readily in relation to vibratory sense, but proprioception, touch, and fast pain are also diminished with age. Sweating and vasomotor reflexes are reduced as well. These changes, which are discussed further in Chap. 29, are probably due to neuronal loss in dorsal root ganglia and are reflected in a progressive depletion of fibers in the posterior columns.

SENSORY SYNDROMES

SENSORY CHANGES DUE TO INTERRUPTION OF A SINGLE PERIPHERAL NERVE

These changes will vary, depending on whether the nerve involved is predominantly muscular, cutaneous, or mixed. Following division of a cutaneous nerve the area of sensory loss is always less than its anatomic distribution because of overlap from adjacent nerves. That the area of tactile anesthesia is greater than the one for pain appears to relate to lack of collateralization (regeneration) from adjacent tactile fibers (in contrast to rapid collateral regeneration of pain fibers). If a large area of skin is involved, the sensory defect characteristically consists of a central portion, in which all forms of cutaneous sensation are lost, surrounded by a zone of partial loss, which becomes less marked as one proceeds from the center to the periphery. The perception of deep pressure and passive movement are intact because these modalities are mediated by nerve fibers from subcutaneous structures and joints. Along the margin of the hypesthetic zone the skin becomes excessively sensitive. A light contact may be felt as smarting and mildly painful. According to Weddell, this is because of collateral regeneration from surrounding healthy pain fibers into the denervated region.

Particular types of lesions have differing effects upon sensory nerve fibers. Compression may ablate the function of large touch and pressure fibers and leave the small pain, thermal, and autonomic fibers intact; procaine and cocaine and ischemia have the opposite effect. The tourniquet test is instructive in this respect. A sphygmomanometer is applied above the elbow, inflated to a point well above the systolic pressure, and maintained there for as long as 30 min. Paresthesias appear within a few minutes, followed by a sensory loss—first of touch and vibration, then of cold, fast pain, heat and slow pain, in that order and spreading centripetally. The condition is not particularly painful if the forearm muscles are not contracted. Recent physiologic studies have confirmed the theory of Lewis et al that a preferential susceptibility to ischemia blocks the function of nerve fibers in order of their size. Release of the cuff results in postischemic paresthesias, which have been shown to arise ectopically along the medullated nerve fibers. Function is recovered in an order inverse to that in which it was lost.

SENSORY CHANGES DUE TO MULTIPLE NERVE INVOLVEMENT (POLYNEUROPATHY)

In most instances of polyneuropathy the sensory changes are accompanied by varying degrees of motor and reflex loss. Usually the sensory impairment is symmetric, with notable exceptions in some instances of diabetic and periarteritic neuropathy. Since the longest and largest fibers tend to be the most affected, the sensory loss is most severe over the feet and legs and over the hands, if the upper limbs are affected. The abdomen, thorax, and face are spared except in the most severe cases. The sensory loss usually involves all the modalities, and although it is manifestly difficult to equate the degree of impairment of pain, touch, temperature, vibration, and position senses, one modality may seemingly be impaired out of proportion to the others. This clinical feature can probably be explained by the fact that disease of the peripheral nerves may damage sensory fibers selectively. For example, selective axonal degeneration or demyelination of the large kinesthetic fibers causes a loss of vibratory sensation and relative sparing of pain, temperature, and tactile perception, and results in severe sensory ataxia. Involuntary movements of digits may also be based on a loss of sense of position and movement. Affection of pain, temperature, and autonomic fibers produces a pseudosyringomyelic syndrome. Prolonged analgesia may lead to trophic ulcers and Charcot joints. These special patterns of loss are discussed in Chaps. 38 and 45. One cannot accurately predict, from the patient's symptoms, which mode of sensation will be disproportionately affected. The term *glove-and-stocking anesthesia*, frequently employed to describe the sensory loss of polyneuropathy, draws attention to the predominantly distal pattern of involvement but fails to indicate that the change from normal to impaired sensation is gradual. In hysteria, by contrast, the border between normal and absent sensation is sharply defined.

SENSORY CHANGES DUE TO INVOLVEMENT OF MULTIPLE SPINAL NERVE ROOTS

Because of considerable overlap from adjacent roots, division of a single sensory root does not produce complete loss of sensation in any area of skin. Compression of a single sensory cervical or lumbar root (e.g., in herniated intervertebral disc) causes varying degrees of impairment of cutaneous sensation in a segmental pattern, however. When two or more roots have been completely divided, a zone of sensory loss can be found, surrounded by a narrow zone of partial loss, in which a raised threshold accompanied by overreaction (hyperpathia) may or may not be demonstrated. For reasons not altogether clear partial sensory loss from root lesions is easier to demonstrate by the use of painful stimuli than by tactile or pressure stimuli. Tendon and cutaneomuscular reflexes may be lost. The presence of muscle weakness and atrophy indicates involvement of ventral roots or plexuses as well.

THE TABETIC SYNDROME (See Fig. 8-5)

This results from damage to the large proprioceptive and other fibers of the posterior lumbosacral (and sometimes the cervical) roots. It is typically caused by neurosyphilis, but also by diabetes mellitus and other diseases that involve the posterior roots. Numbness or paresthesias and lightning or lancinating pains are frequent complaints; areflexia, abnormalities of gait (Chap. 6), and hypotonia without muscle weakness are found on examination. The sensory loss may involve only vibration and position sense in the lower extremities, but in severe cases, loss or impairment of superficial or deep pain sense or of touch may be added. The feet and legs are most affected, much less often the arms and trunk. Atonicity of the bladder with retention of urine is often associated.

COMPLETE SPINAL SENSORY SYNDROME (See Fig. 8-5)

With a complete transverse lesion of the spinal cord, all forms of sensation are abolished below a level that corresponds to the lesion. There may be a narrow zone of hyperesthesia at the upper margin of the anesthetic zone. Loss of pain, temperature, and touch sensation begins one or two segments below the level of the lesion; vibratory and position senses have less discrete levels. It is important to remember that during the evolution of such a lesion there may be a greater discrepancy between the level of the lesion and that of the sensory loss, the latter ascending as the lesion progresses. This can be understood if one conceives of a lesion evolving from the periphery to the center of the cord, affecting first the outermost fibers carrying pain and temperature sensation from the legs. Conversely, a lesion advancing from the center of the cord may affect these modalities in the reverse order.

PARTIAL SPINAL SENSORY SYNDROME (HEMISECTION OF THE SPINAL CORD, BROWN-SÉQUARD SYNDROME)

In rare instances, disease is confined to one side of the spinal cord; pain and thermal sensation are affected on the opposite side of the body, and proprioceptive sensation is affected on the same side as the lesion. The loss of pain and temperature sensation begins one or two segments below the lesion. An associated motor paralysis on the side of the lesion completes the syndrome (Fig. 8-5). Tactile sensation is not affected, since the fibers from one side of the body are distributed in tracts (posterior columns and anterior spinothalamic) on both sides of the cord.

SYRINGOMYELIC SYNDROME (LESION OF THE CENTRAL GRAY MATTER)

Since fibers conducting pain and temperature cross the cord in the anterior commissure, a lesion in this location of considerable vertical extent will characteristically abolish these modalities on one or both sides over several segments (dermatomes) but will spare tactile sensation (Fig. 8-5). The most common cause of such a lesion is syringomyelia; less common causes are intramedullary tumor, trauma, and hemorrhage. This type of *dissociated sensory loss* usually occurs in a segmental distribution, and since the lesion frequently involves other parts of the gray matter, varying degrees of segmental amyotrophy and reflex loss are usually present as well. If the lesion has spread to the white matter, corticospinal, spinothalamic, and posterior column signs will be conjoined.

Figure 8-5

Some of the sites of lesions that produce characteristic spinal cord syndromes (shaded areas indicate lesions).

POSTERIOR COLUMN SYNDROME (See Fig. 8-5)

Loss of vibratory and position sense occurs below the lesion, but the perception of pain and temperature is affected relatively little or not at all. Since posterior column lesions are due to the interruption of central projections of the dorsal root ganglia cells, they may be difficult to distinguish from an affection of large fibers in sensory roots (tabetic syndrome). In some diseases that involve the dorsal columns, vibratory sensation may be involved predominantly, whereas in others position sense is more affected. With complete posterior column lesions, only a few of which have been verified by postmortem examinations (see Nathan et al for a review of the literature), not only is the subject deprived of knowledge of movement and position of parts of the body below the lesion, but all types of sensory discrimination are impaired as well. If the lesion is in the high cervical region, the palpation of objects is clumsy (ataxic) and there is inability to recognize the qualities of objects by touch even though touch-pressure sensation is relatively intact. The stereoanesthesia is expressed also by impaired graphesthesia, tactile localization, and ability to detect the direction of lines drawn on the skin. There may be unusual disturbances of touch and pressure, manifested as lability of threshold, persistence of sensation after removal of the stimulus, and sometimes tactile and postural hallucinations. Nathan et al have confirmed older observations that lesions of the posterior columns cause only slight defects in touch and pressure sensation and that lesions of

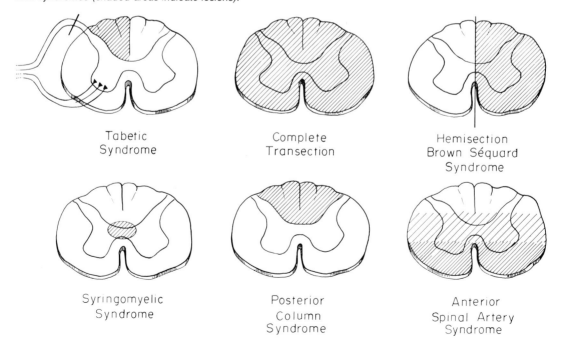

Tabetic
Syndrome

Complete
Transection

Hemisection
Brown Séquard
Syndrome

Syringomyelic
Syndrome

Posterior
Column
Syndrome

Anterior
Spinal Artery
Syndrome

the anterolateral spinothalamic complex cause minimal or no defects in these modalities. However, a combined lesion in both pathways causes a total loss of tactile and pressure sensibility below the lesion.

The loss of sensory functions that follows a posterior column lesion, such as impaired two-point discrimination, figure writing, and the ability to detect the direction and speed of a moving stimulus on the skin, may simulate a parietal "cortical" discriminative lesion, but differs in that vibratory sense is also lost. Paresthesias in the form of tingling and pins-and-needles sensations or girdle- and band-like sensations are common complaints with posterior column disease, and pinprick may produce a diffuse, burning, unpleasant sensation.

In several cases on record, interruption of the posterior columns by surgical incision or other type of injury did not cause a permanent loss of the sensory modalities thought to be subserved by these pathways (Cook and Browder, Wall and Noordenbos). Since postmortem studies of these cases were not carried out, it is possible that some of the posterior column fibers had been spared. Also, it should be realized that not all the proprioceptive fibers ascend to the nuclei of Goll; some proprioceptive fibers leave the posterior columns in the lumbar region and synapse with secondary neurons in the spinal gray matter and ascend in the ipsilateral lateral funiculus. Only cutaneous fibers continue to the nuclei of Goll and Burdach. The proposition of Wall and Noordenbos, which is debatable, is that such patients lose not the modalities conventionally attributed to the posterior columns but the ability to perform tasks that demand simultaneous analysis of spatial and temporal characteristics of the stimulus.

ANTERIOR SPINAL ARTERY SYNDROME (ANTERIOR MYELOPATHY)

With infarction of the spinal cord in the distribution of the anterior spinal artery or other destructive lesions that predominantly affect the ventral portion of the cord, one finds a loss of pain and temperature sensation below the level of the lesion and a relative or absolute sparing of proprioceptive sensation. Since the corticospinal tracts and the ventral gray matter also lie within the area of distribution of the anterior spinal artery, paralysis of motor function forms a prominent part of this syndrome (Fig. 8-5).

DISTURBANCES OF SENSATION DUE TO LESIONS OF THE BRAINSTEM

A characteristic feature of lesions of the medulla is the occurrence, in many instances, of a crossed sensory disturbance, i.e., a loss of pain and temperature sensation on one side of the face and on the opposite side of the body.

This is accounted for by involvement of the trigeminal tract or nucleus and the lateral spinothalamic tract on one side of the brainstem and is nearly always caused by a lateral medullary infarction (Wallenberg syndrome). In the upper medulla, pons, and midbrain, the crossed trigeminothalamic and lateral spinothalamic tracts run together, and a lesion at these levels causes loss of pain and temperature sense on the opposite half of the body and face. In the upper brainstem the spinothalamic tract and the medial lemniscus become confluent, so that an appropriately placed lesion causes a loss of all superficial and deep sensation on the contralateral side. Cranial nerve palsies, cerebellar ataxia, or motor paralysis are often associated, as indicated in Chap. 34.

SENSORY LOSS DUE TO A LESION OF THE THALAMUS (SYNDROME OF DÉJERINE-ROUSSY)

Involvement of the nucleus ventralis posterolateralis of the thalamus, usually due to a vascular lesion, less often to a tumor, causes loss or diminution of all forms of sensation on the opposite side of the body. Position sense is affected more frequently than any other sensory function, and deep sensory loss is usually but not always more profound than cutaneous loss. There may be spontaneous pain or discomfort (*thalamic pain*), sometimes of the most distressing type, on the affected side of the body (see page 115), and any stimulus may then have a diffuse, unpleasant, lingering quality. Emotional disturbance also aggravates the painful state. In spite of this overresponse to pinprick, thermal, or other stimuli, the patient usually shows an elevated pain threshold, i.e., a stronger stimulus than normal is necessary to produce a sensation of pain. The "thalamic" pain syndrome may occasionally accompany lesions of the white matter of the parietal lobe (see page 114) or the medial lemniscus or even the posterior columns of the spinal cord.

SENSORY LOSS DUE TO LESIONS OF THE PARIETAL LOBE

In the best known of the anterior parietal lobe syndromes, that of Verger-Déjerine, there are disturbances mainly of discriminative sensory functions of the opposite face, arm, and leg, without impairment of the primary modalities of sensation (unless the lesion is deep). Loss of position sense, impaired ability to localize touch and pain stimuli (topagnosia), elevation of two-point threshold, astereognosis, and loss of sense of limb position and of movement are the most prominent findings.

Another characteristic manifestation of parietal lobe lesions is sensory inattention or extinction (neglect). In response to bilateral simultaneous testing of symmetric parts, using either tactile or painful stimuli, the patient may acknowledge only the stimulus on the sound side; or, if the face and hand or foot on the affected side is touched, only the stimulus to the face is noticed. Apparently, cranial structures demand more attention than other less richly innervated parts. A similar extinction phenomenon occurs when visual stimuli are simultaneously delivered to both right and left peripheral fields. Yet each stimulus, when applied separately to each side or to each part of the affected side, is properly perceived and localized. This type of sensory extinction, which may also occur occasionally with posterior column and medial lemniscus lesions, may be detected in persons who disclaim any sensory symptoms. This phenomenon and other features of parietal lobe lesions are considered further in Chap. 21.

Yet another parietal lobe syndrome (Déjerine-Mouzon) is featured by a severe impairment of the primary modalities of sensation (pain, thermal, tactile, and vibratory sense) over one-half of the body. It simulates the sensory loss due to a thalamic lesion, hence was called pseudothalamic by Foix et al. Hyperpathia, much like that of the Déjerine-Roussy syndrome (see above), has also been observed in patients with cortical-subcortical parietal lesions. The pseudothalamic syndrome was related by Foix et al to a sylvian infarct; and Bogousslavsky et al traced it to an occlusion of the ascending parietal branch of the middle cerebral artery. In each of the foregoing parietal lobe syndromes, if the dominant hemisphere is involved, there may be an aphasia, a bimanual tactile agnosia, or a Gerstmann syndrome; and in nondominant lesions there may be anosognosia (page 364).

Often with parietal lesions the patient's responses to sensory stimuli are variable. A common mistake is to attribute this abnormality to hysteria, particularly since movements of the affected limbs may be ataxic or seemingly paretic because of loss of proprioception.

A lesion confined to only a part of the parietal cortex (the best examples have been due to glancing bullet wounds of the skull) may result in a circumscribed loss of superficial sensation in an opposite limb, mimicking a root or peripheral nerve lesion.

SENSORY LOSS DUE TO SUGGESTION AND HYSTERIA

The possibility of suggesting sensory loss to a patient is a very real one, as has already been indicated. Hysterical patients rarely complain spontaneously of cutaneous sensory loss, although they may use the term "numbness" to indicate a paralysis of a limb. Examination, on the other hand, may suggest to the patient a complete hemianesthesia, often with reduced hearing, sight, smell, and taste, as well as impaired vibration sense over only half the skull. Anesthesia of one entire limb or a sharply defined sensory loss over part of a limb, not conforming to the distribution of a root or cutaneous nerve, may also be observed. The diagnosis of hysterical hemianesthesia is best made by eliciting the other relevant symptoms of hysteria or, if this is not possible, by noting the discrepancies between this type of sensory loss and that which occurs as part of the usual sensory syndromes. Sometimes in a patient with no other neurologic abnormality or in one with a definite neurologic syndrome, one is dismayed by sensory findings that are completely unexplainable and discordant. In such cases one must try to reason through to the diagnosis by disregarding the sensory findings.

LOCALIZATION OF LESIONS IN SOMATIC SENSORY SYSTEMS BY ELECTRO-PHYSIOLOGIC METHODS

Affirmation of the clinical sensory syndromes is now possible by the application of laboratory tests. Slowing of peripheral nerve conduction is found with lesions of nerve, particularly of demyelinative type. Loss of or slowing of H and M responses corroborates the presence of lesions in proximal parts of nerves, plexuses, and roots. By the use of somatosensory evoked potentials it is possible to demonstrate slowing of conduction in the peripheral nerve (from the stimulus site to Erb's point), in the spinal cord to the lower medulla, in the medial lemniscus to the thalamus, and from the thalamus to the cerebral cortex. These tests require no cooperation of the patient and can be employed in the analysis of sensory systems even in comatose states. (See Chap. 2 for further discussion.)

REFERENCES

BERTELSMANN FW, HEIMANS JJ, WEBER EJM, et al: Thermal discrimination thresholds in normal subjects and in patients with diabetic neuropathy. *J Neurol Neurosurg Psychiatry* 48:686, 1985.

BOGOUSSLAVSKY J, ASSAL G, RAGLI F: Aphasie afférente motrice et hemisyndrome sensitif droite. *Rev Neurol* 138:649, 1982.

BRODAL A: The somatic afferent pathways, in *Neurological Anatomy*, 3rd ed. New York, Oxford University Press, 1981, pp 46–147.

CARMON A: Disturbances of tactile sensitivity in patients with unilateral cerebral lesions. *Cortex* 7:83, 1971.

CARMON A, BENTON AL: Tactile perception of direction and

number in patients with unilateral cerebral disease. *Neurology* 19:525, 1969.

COOK AW, BROWDER ES: Function of posterior columns in man. *Arch Neurol* 12:72, 1965.

CORKIN S, MILNER B, RASMUSSEN T: Tactually guided maze learning in man: Effects of unilateral cortical excision and bilateral hippocampal lesions. *Neuropsychologia* 3:339, 1965.

CORKIN S, MILNER B, RASMUSSEN T: Effects of different cortical excisions on sensory thresholds in man. *Trans Am Neurol Assoc* 89:112, 1964.

DYCK PJ, KARNES J, O'BRIEN PC, ZIMMERMAN IR: Quantitation of cutaneous sensation in man, in Dyck PJ, Thomas PK, Lambert EW, Bunge R (eds): *Peripheral Neuropathy*, 2nd ed. Philadelphia, Saunders, 1984, pp 1103–1138.

FOIX C, CHAVANY JA, LEVY M: Syndrome pseudothalamique d'origine parietale. *Rev Neurol* 35:68, 1965.

HEAD H, RIVERS WHR, SHERREN J: The afferent nervous system from a new aspect. *Brain* 28:99, 1905.

HOLMES GM: *Introduction to Clinical Neurology*, 2nd ed. Baltimore, Williams & Wilkins, 1952, chaps 8, 9.

KEEGAN JJ, GARRETT FD: The segmental distribution of the cutaneous nerves in the limbs of man. *Anat Rec* 102:409, 1948.

KIBLER RF, NATHAN PW: A note on warm and cold spots. *Neurology* 10:874, 1960.

LEWIS T, PICKERING GW, ROTHSCHILD P: Centrifugal paralysis arising out of arrested blood flow to the limb, including notes on a form of tingling. *Heart* 16:1, 1931.

LIGHT AR, PERL ER: Peripheral sensory systems, in Dyck P et al (eds): *Peripheral Neuropathy*, 2nd ed. Philadelphia, Saunders, 1984, vol 1, chap 9, pp 210–230.

LINDBLOM U, OCHOA J: Somatosensory function and dysfunction, in Asbury AK, McKhann GM, McDonald W (eds): *Diseases of the Nervous System*. Philadelphia, Saunders, 1986, pp 283–298.

LOH, L, NATHAN PW: Painful peripheral states and sympathetic blocks. *J Neurol Neurosurg Psychiatry* 41:664, 1978.

MARKEL R: Human cutaneous mechanoreceptors during regeneration: Physiology and interpretation. *Ann Neurol* 18:165, 1985.

MAYO CLINIC: *Clinical Examinations in Neurology*, 5th ed. Philadelphia, Saunders, 1981.

MOBERG E: The role of cutaneous afferents in position sense, kinaesthesia and motor function of the hand. *Brain* 106:1, 1983.

MOUNTCASTLE VG: Central nervous mechanisms in sensation, in Mountcastle VB (ed): *Medical Physiology*, 14th ed. St Louis, Mosby, 1980, vol 1, part 5; chaps 11–19, pp 327–605.

NATHAN PW, SMITH MC, COOK AW: Sensory effects in man of lesions in the posterior columns and of some other afferent pathways. *Brain* 109:1003, 1986.

OCHOA JL, TOREBJÖRK HE: Paraesthesiae from ectopic impulse generation in human sensory nerves. *Brain* 103:835, 1980.

RAY BS, WOLFF HG: Studies on pain: Spread of pain; evidence on site of spread within the neuraxis of effects of painful stimulation. *Arch Neurol Psychiatry* 53:257, 1945.

ROLAND PE, LADEGAARD-PEDERSON H: A quantitative analysis of sensations of tension and of kinaesthesia in man. *Brain* 100:671, 1977.

SEMMES J, WEINSTEIN S, GHENT L, TEUBER H-L: *Somatosensory Changes after Penetrating Brain Wounds in Man*. Cambridge, Mass, Harvard, 1960.

TOREBJÖRK HE, VALLBO AB, OCHOA JL: Intraneural microstimulation in man. Its relation to specificity of tactile sensations. *Brain* 110:1509, 1987.

TOWER SS: Unit for sensory reception in the cornea. *J Neurophysiol* 3:486, 1940.

TROTTER W, DAVIES HM: Experimental studies in the innervation of the skin. *J Physiol* 38:134, 1909.

WALL PD, NOORDENBOS W: Sensory functions which remain in man after complete transection of dorsal columns. *Brain* 100:641, 1977.

WALSHE FMR: The anatomy and physiology of cutaneous sensibility: A critical review. *Brain* 65:48, 1942.

WEDDELL G: The multiple innervaton of sensory spots in the skin. *J Anat* 75:441, 1941.

CHAPTER 9

HEADACHE AND OTHER CRANIOFACIAL PAINS

Of all the painful states that afflict humans, headache is undoubtedly the most frequent. In fact, there are so many vexatious cases of headache in every medical center that it has become necessary to establish special headache clinics where physicians who have extensive experience with this problem may direct diagnostic study and therapy. Insofar as many headaches are due to medical rather than neurologic diseases, the subject is the legitimate concern of the general physician. Yet always there is a question of intracranial disease. Therefore, it is difficult to approach the subject without a knowledge of neurologic medicine.

Why so many pains are centered in the head is a question of some interest. Several explanations come to mind. For one thing the face and scalp are more richly supplied with pain receptors than many other parts of the body, perhaps in order to protect the precious contents of the skull. Then, too, the nasal and oral passages, the eye, and the ear, all delicate and highly sensitive structures, reside here and need to be protected; when afflicted by disease, each is capable of inducing pain in its own way. Finally, for the intelligent person there is greater concern about what happens to the head than to other parts of the body, since the former houses the brain, and headache frequently raises the specter of brain tumor or other cerebral disease. A body without an adequately functioning brain is not of much use.

Semantically, the term *headache* should encompass all aches and pains located in the head, but in practice its application is restricted to discomfort in the region of the cranial vault. Facial, lingual, and pharyngeal pains are put aside as something different, and are discussed separately in the latter part of this chapter.

GENERAL CONSIDERATIONS

In the introductory chapter on pain, reference was made to the necessity, when dealing with any painful state, of determining its quality, severity, location, duration, and time course, and the conditions which produce, exacerbate, or relieve it. When headache is considered in these terms, a certain amount of useful information is obtained, but often less than one might expect. Auscultation of the skull may disclose a bruit (with large arteriovenous malformations or narrowed carotid arteries), and palpation may disclose the tender, hardened arteries of temporal arteritis or sensitive areas overlying a cranial bone metastasis or inflamed sinuses, but apart from such special instances, physical examination of the head itself is seldom useful.

As to the *quality* of cephalic pain, the patient's description is rarely helpful. In fact, persistent questioning on this point may occasion surprise, for the patient often assumes that the word *headache* should have conveyed enough information to the examiner about the nature of the discomfort. Most headaches, regardless of type, tend to be dull, aching, and not sharply localized, as is usually the case with disease of structures deep to the skin. Seldom does the patient describe the pricking or stinging type of pain that is localized to the skin. When asked to compare the pain to some other sensory experience, the patient may allude to tightness, pressure, bursting, sharpness, or stabbing. The most important datum to be obtained is whether the headache throbs with each arterial pulse, indicating a vascular sensitivity. But one must keep in mind that patients often use the word throbbing to refer to a waxing and waning of the headache, without any relation to the pulse.

Similarly, statements about the intensity of the pain must be accepted with caution, since they reflect as much the patient's attitudes and customary ways of experiencing and describing symptoms as their true severity. The bluff, hearty person tends to minimize the discomfort, and the neurotic is more inclined to dramatize it. The degree of incapacity is a better index, especially if the patient is not prone to illness. A severe migraine attack seldom allows performance of the day's work. Another rough index of severity of the headache is its propensity to awaken the patient from sleep or prevent sleep. As a rule the most intense cranial pains are those which accompany meningitis and subarachnoid hemorrhage, which have grave implications, or migraine, cluster headache, or tic douloureux, which do not.

Data regarding *location* of the headache are apt to be more informative. Inflammation of an extracranial artery causes pain localized to the site of the vessel. However, if nerve fibers within the vessel wall are irritated, the pain may be projected toward their source. Lesions of paranasal sinuses, teeth, eyes, and upper cervical vertebrae induce a less sharply localized pain, but one that is still referred to a certain region, usually to the forehead or around the eyes. Intracranial lesions in the posterior fossa cause pain in the occipitonuchal region, homolateral if the lesion is one-sided. Supratentorial lesions induce frontotemporal pain, again homolateral to the lesion. Localization, however, may also be deceiving. Pain in the frontal regions may be due to such diverse lesions and mechanisms as glaucoma, sinusitis, thrombosis of the basilar artery, pressure on the tentorium, or increased intracranial pressure. Similarly, although ear pain may signify disease of the ear itself, more often it is referred from other regions, such as cervical muscles, cervical spine, or structures in the posterior fossa.

The *mode of onset, time-intensity curve,* and *duration* of the headache, with respect both to a single attack and to the natural behavior of the headache over a period of years, are also useful data. The headache of subarachnoid hemorrhage (in the case of a ruptured aneurysm) occurs in a single attack and attains its maximal severity in a matter of minutes; or, in the case of bacterial meningitis, it may come on more gradually, over several hours or days. Brief sharp pain, lasting a few seconds, in the eyeball (ophthalmodynia) or cranium ("icepick" pains) are more common in migraineurs (with or without the characteristic headache) but otherwise are uninterpretable and are significant only for reason of their benignity. Migraine of the classic type has its onset in the early morning hours or daytime, reaches its peak of severity in a half hour or so, and lasts, unless treated, for a period varying from several hours up to 1 to 2 days, often terminated by sleep. More than a single attack of migraine every few weeks is exceptional. A migrainous patient having several attacks per week usually proves to have a combination of migraine and tension headaches. In contrast, the nightly occurrence of unilateral temporo-orbital pain within an hour or two after falling asleep, over a period of several weeks to months, is typical of cluster headache. The pain dissipates in 10 to 30 min. The headache of intracranial tumor may come at any time of the day or night, may interrupt sleep, vary in intensity, and last a few minutes to hours. Tension headaches may persist, with varying intensity, for weeks to months or even longer. In general, headaches that have recurred regularly for many years prove to be vascular or tension in type.

The more or less constant relationship of headache to certain biologic events and also to certain precipitating or aggravating (or relieving) factors must always be noted. Headaches that occur regularly in the premenstrual period in relation to oliguria and edema are usually generalized and mild in degree ("premenstrual tension"), but attacks of migraine may also occur at this time. The headaches of cervical arthritis are most typically intense after a period of inactivity, such as a night's sleep, and the first movements of the neck are stiff and painful. Hypertensive headaches, like those of cerebral tumor, tend to occur early in the morning; as with all vascular headaches, excitement and emotional stress may provoke them. Headache from infection of nasal sinuses may appear, with clocklike regularity, upon awakening or in midmorning, and is characteristically worsened by stooping and changes in atmospheric pressure. Eyestrain headaches naturally follow prolonged use of the eyes, as in reading, peering for a long time against glaring headlights, or exposure for prolonged periods to the glare of video display terminals. In certain individuals, alcohol, intense exercise, stooping, coughing, and sexual intercourse are known to initiate a special type of bursting headache, lasting a few seconds to minutes. If the headache is made worse by sudden movement or by coughing or straining, an intracranial source is suggested. Atmospheric cold may evoke pain in the so-called fibrositic or nodular form of headache or when the underlying condition is arthritic or neuralgic. Anger, excitement, or worry may initiate migraine in certain disposed persons; this is more likely to occur with common migraine than with the classic type. In other patients migraine occurs several hours or a day following a period of intense activity and stress ("weekend migraine"). Easing of the headache by compression of the common carotid artery is characteristic of migraine.

PAIN-SENSITIVE STRUCTURES AND MECHANISMS OF HEADACHE

Understanding of headache has been greatly augmented by observations that have been made during operations on the brain. These observations inform us that the following cranial structures are sensitive to mechanical stimulation: (1) skin, subcutaneous tissue, muscles, extracranial arteries, and periosteum of the skull; (2) delicate structures of the eye, ear, and nasal cavities and sinuses; (3) intracranial venous sinuses and their large tributaries; (4) parts of the dura at the base of the brain and the arteries within the dura and pia-arachnoid, particularly their proximal parts;

and (5) the optic, ocular motor, trigeminal, glossopharyn-geal, vagus, and first three cervical nerves. Interestingly, pain is practically the only sensation produced by stimulation of the aforementioned structures. The bony skull, much of the pia-arachnoid and dura over the convexity of the brain, the parenchyma of the brain, and the ependyma and choroid plexuses lack sensitivity.

The pathways whereby sensory stimuli, whatever their nature, are conveyed to the CNS are the trigeminal nerves, particularly their first divisions, which convey impulses from the forehead, orbit, anterior and middle fossae of the skull, and the upper surface of the tentorium. The ninth and tenth cranial nerves and the first three cervical nerves convey impulses from the inferior surface of the tentorium and all of the posterior fossa. The tentorium demarcates the trigeminal and cervical innervation zones. The central sensory connections through spinal cord and brainstem to thalamus have been described in the preceding chapter.

To summarize, pain from supratentorial structures is referred, by a mechanism already discussed (page 111), to the anterior two-thirds of the head by the trigeminal nerve, and pain from infratentorial structures to the back of the head and neck and forehead by the upper cervical roots. The ninth and tenth cranial nerves refer pain to the ear and throat. There may be local tenderness of the scalp at the site of the referred pain. Dental or temporomandibular joint pain may also have cranial reference. Pain due to disease in other parts of the body is not referred to the head, although it may initiate headache by other means.

By analysis of several types of headache, Wolff and his colleagues have demonstrated that most "spontaneous" cranial pains can be traced to the operation of one or more of the following mechanisms:

1. Traction on and dilatation of the intracranial arteries and distention of extracranial arteries

2. Traction on or displacement of large intracranial veins or the dural envelopes in which they lie

3. Traction on or compression, inflammation or ischemia of sensory cranial and spinal nerves

4. Voluntary or involuntary spasm and possibly interstitial inflammation of cranial and cervical muscles

5. Meningeal irritation and greatly raised or lowered intracranial pressure

More specifically, intracranial mass lesions cause headache only if in a position to deform, displace, or exert traction on vessels and dural structures at the base of the brain, and this may happen long before intracranial pressure rises. In fact the artificial induction of high intraspinal and intracranial pressure by the subarachnoid or intraventricular injection of sterile saline solution does not result in headache. This has been interpreted to mean that raised intracranial pressure does not cause headache, a conclusion that is called into question by the demonstrable relief of headache by lumbar puncture and lowering the CSF pressure in some patients. Actually, most patients with high intracranial pressure complain of bioccipital and bifrontal headache that fluctuates in severity, probably because of traction on vessels or dura. Dilatation of intracranial or extracranial arteries (and possibly sensitization of these vessels), of whatever cause, is likely to produce headache. Headaches that follow seizures, infusion of histamine, and ingestion of alcohol are probably all due to cerebral vasodilatation. Nitrites in cured meats ("hot dog headache") and monosodium glutamate in Chinese food may cause headache by the same mechanism.

The throbbing or steady headache that accompanies febrile illnesses is probably vascular in origin. It may be generalized or predominate in the frontal or occipital regions and is much like histamine headache in being relieved on one side by carotid artery compression and on both sides by jugular vein compression or the subarachnoid injection of saline solution. It is increased by shaking the head. It seems probable that the increased pulsation of meningeal vessels stretches pain-sensitive structures around the base of the brain. In certain cases the pain may be lessened by compression of temporal arteries, and in these cases a component of the headache seems to be derived from the walls of extracranial arteries, as in migraine.

It is likely that a similar mechanism is operative in the severe bilateral throbbing headaches that are associated with extreme rises in blood pressure, as occurs with pheochromocytoma, malignant hypertension, sexual activity, and in patients being treated with monoamine oxidase inhibitors (page 902). So-called cough and exertional headaches may also have their basis in distention of intracranial vessels.

Sensitization of the temporal artery and its branches in the scalp and *basal intracranial arteries* with stretching of surrounding sensitive structures is believed to be the mechanism of most of the pain of migraine, but this statement requires qualification (see below under migraine). Extracranial temporal and occipital arteries, when involved in giant-cell arteritis (cranial or "temporal" arteritis), give rise to severe, persistent headache, at first localized and then more diffuse. Evolving atherosclerotic thrombosis of internal carotid, anterior, and middle cerebral arteries is sometimes accompanied by pain in the forehead or temple; with vertebral artery thrombosis, the pain is postauricular, and basilar artery thrombosis causes pain to be projected to the occiput and sometimes to the forehead.

Infection or *blockage of paranasal sinuses* is accompanied by pain over the affected maxillary or frontal sinuses. Usually it is associated with tenderness of the skin in the same distribution. Pain from the ethmoid and sphenoid sinuses is localized deep in the midline behind the nose, or occasionally in the vertex (especially in disease of the sphenoid sinus) or other part of the cranium. The mechanism in these cases involves changes in pressure and irritation of pain-sensitive sinus walls. Sinus pain may have two remarkable properties: (1) when throbbing, it may be abolished by compressing the carotid artery on the same side, and (2) it recurs and subsides periodically, depending on the drainage from the sinus. With frontal and ethmoidal sinusitis, the pain tends to be worse on awakening and gradually subsides when the person is upright; the opposite pertains with maxillary and sphenoidal sinusitis. These relationships are believed to disclose their mechanism; pain is ascribed to filling of the sinuses and its relief to their emptying, induced by the dependent position of the ostia. Stooping intensifies the pain by causing changes in pressure, as does blowing the nose, if the ostium of the infected sinus is patent; during air flights both earache and sinus headache tend to occur on descent, when the relative pressure in the blocked viscus falls. Sympathomimetic drugs such as phenylephrine hydrochloride, which reduce swelling and congestion, tend to relieve the pain. However, the pain may persist after all purulent secretions have disappeared, probably because of blockage of the orifice by boggy membranes and absorption of air from the blocked sinus (*vacuum sinus headaches*). The condition is relieved when aeration is restored.

Headache of ocular origin, located as a rule in the orbit, forehead, or temple, is of the steady, aching type and tends to follow prolonged use of the eyes in close work. The main faults are hypermetropia and astigmatism (rarely myopia), which result in sustained contraction of extraocular as well as frontal, temporal, and even occipital muscles. Correction of the refractive error abolishes the headache. Traction on the extraocular muscles and on the iris during eye surgery will evoke pain. Another mechanism is involved in iridocyclitis or in *acute glaucoma*, in which raised intraocular pressure causes steady, aching pain in the region of the eye, radiating to the forehead. As for ocular pain in general, it is important that the eyes be refracted, but eyestrain is probably not as frequent a cause as one would expect from the wholesale dispensing of spectacles for its relief.

The headaches accompanying disease of ligaments, muscles, and apophyseal joints in the upper part of the spine, which are referred to the occiput and nape of the neck on the same side and sometimes to the forehead, can be reproduced in part by the injection of hypertonic saline solution into these structures. Such pains are especially frequent in late life, because of rheumatoid and hypertrophic arthritis, and tend also to occur after whiplash injuries or other forms of sudden flexion, extension, or torsion of the head on the neck. If the pain is arthritic in origin, the first movements after being still for some hours are both stiff and painful. The headache of myofibrositis, evidenced by tender nodules near the cranial insertion of cervical and other muscles, is a questionable entity. There are no pathologic data as to the nature of these vaguely palpable lesions, and it is uncertain whether the pain actually arises in them. They may represent only the deep tenderness felt in the region of referred pain or the involuntary secondary protective spasm of muscles. Characteristically, the pain is steady (nonthrobbing) and spreads from one to both sides of the head. Exposure to cold or draft may precipitate it. Though severe at times, it seldom prevents sleep. Massage of muscles, heat, and injection of the tender spots with local anesthetic have unpredictable effects but relieve the pain in some cases. Unilateral occipital headache is often misinterpreted as occipital neuralgia (see below).

The *headache of meningeal irritation* (infection or hemorrhage) is of acute onset, severe, generalized, deep-seated, constant, and associated with stiffness of the neck on forward bending . It has been ascribed by some authorities to increased intracranial pressure. Indeed the withdrawal of CSF may afford some relief. But dilatation and congestion of inflamed meningeal vessels and the chemical irritation of pain receptors in the large vessels and meninges by chemical agents, the most important of which are serotonin and plasma kinins, must also be factors in the production of pain and of spasm of the neck extensors.

Lumbar puncture headache is characterized by a steady occipital-nuchal and frontal pain coming on a few minutes after arising from a recumbent position and relieved within a few minutes by lying down. Its cause is a persistent leakage of CSF into the lumbar tissues through the needle track. The CSF pressure is low (often zero in the lateral decubitus position), and the injection of sterile isotonic saline solution intrathecally relieves the headache. Usually this type of headache is increased by compression of the jugular veins but unaffected by digital obliteration of one carotid artery. It seems probable that in the upright position a low intraspinal and negative intracranial pressure exert traction on dural attachments and dural sinuses by caudal displacement of the brain. Understandably, then, headache following cisternal puncture is rare. As soon as the leakage of CSF stops and CSF pressure is restored (usually from a few days to a week), the headache disappears. "Spontaneous" low-pressure headache may follow a sneeze or strain, presumably because of rupture of the spinal arachnoid along a nerve root (see Chap. 30). Less frequently, lumbar puncture may be complicated by severe stiffness of the neck and pain over the back of the neck and occiput. A second spinal tap discloses pleocytosis but no decrease in glucose—a sterile or chemical meningitis. This benign reaction needs to be distinguished from a suppurative meningitis, the result of introduction of bacteria by the LP needle.

Headaches that are aggravated by lying down occur with chronic subdural hematoma and tumors, especially in the posterior fossa of the skull.

Exertional headaches are usually benign but are sometimes related to pheochromocytoma, arteriovenous malformation, or other intracranial lesions. The same applies to headaches induced by stooping (see further on).

PRINCIPAL VARIETIES OF HEADACHE

There should be little difficulty in recognizing the acute headaches of glaucoma, purulent sinusitis, and bacterial meningitis, and the subacute or more chronic headache of brain tumor, provided these sources of headache are kept in mind. A fuller account of these types of headache will be found where the underlying diseases are described in later sections of the book. When the headache is chronic, recurrent, and unattended by other important signs of disease, the physician faces a more difficult medical problem.

The following types of headaches should then be considered (see Table 9-1).

MIGRAINE

Migraine is a familial disorder characterized by periodic, commonly unilateral, throbbing headaches which begin in childhood, adolescence, or early adult life and recur with diminishing frequency during advancing years.

Two closely related clinical syndromes have been identified. The first is called "classic," or "neurologic," migraine; the second is referred to as "common"; the former occurs in 1 percent of the population, the latter in 5 to 10 percent. In both types, tiredness, yawning, irritability, and lack of concentration may precede an attack. The classic type is ushered in by an evident disturbance of nervous function, most often visual, followed in a few minutes by hemicranial or, occasionally, bilateral headache, nausea, and sometimes vomiting, all of which last for hours

or as long as a day or two. The common migraine syndrome is characterized by an unheralded onset of hemicranial or generalized headache with or without nausea and vomiting but following the same temporal pattern as the typical one. Sensitivity to light and noise attends both types. If severe the patient prefers to lie down in a darkened room and try to sleep. Both headache syndromes usually respond to ergotamine, if administered early in the attack. The genetic nature of classic migraine is evidenced by its occurrence in several members of the family of the same and successive generations in 60 to 80 percent of cases; a family history is less frequently elicited in common migraine, perhaps because diagnosis is less certain, and a group of such cases may include other headache syndromes. Twin and sibling studies have not revealed a consistent mendelian pattern in either form.

Neurologic migraine frequently has its onset soon after awakening, but may occur at any time of day. The patient may have vague premonitory changes in mood and appetite. Then abruptly there is a disturbance of vision consisting usually of unformed flashes of white or multicolored light (photopsia) or formations of dazzling zigzag lines (arranged like the battlements of a castle, hence the term fortification spectra or teichopsia), which move slowly across the visual field for several minutes, leaving scotomatous defects; the latter are usually bilateral and often homonymous (involving corresponding parts of the field of vision of each eye), pointing to their origin in the visual cortex. Retinal and optic nerve migraine have also been observed (see further on). Other focal neurologic symptoms, much less common than visual ones, include: numbness and tingling of the lips, face, hand (on one or both sides), slight confusion of thinking, weakness of an arm or leg, mild aphasia, dizziness and uncertainty of gait, or drowsiness (rarely coma). Only one or a few of these neurologic phenomena are present in any given patient, and they tend to occur in the same combination in each attack. If the weakness or numbness spreads from one part of the body to another or one symptom follows another, it does so relatively *slowly* in a period of minutes (not in seconds, as in a seizure). These symptoms last 5 to 15 min, sometimes longer, and as they begin to recede they are followed by a unilateral throbbing headache (usually on the side of the cerebral disturbance), which slowly increases in intensity. At its peak, in an hour or so, the patient is forced to lie down and to shun light and noise, and nausea and, less often, vomiting may occur. The headache lasts for hours and sometimes for a day or even longer and is always the most unpleasant feature of the illness. The temporal vessels may be tender and the headache may be worsened by strain or jarring of the body.

Much variation occurs. The headache may accompany rather than follow the neurologic abnormalities. Though typically hemicranial (the French word *migraine* is said to be derived from *megrim,* which in turn was derived from the Latin *hemicrania* and its corrupted forms "hemigranea" and "migranea"), the pain may be frontal, temporal, or generalized. Milder forms of migraine, especially if partially controlled by medication, may not force withdrawal from accustomed activities. Any one of the three principal components—neurologic abnormality, headache, and nausea or vomiting—may be absent. With advancing age, there is a tendency for the headache and nausea to become less severe, finally leaving only the neurologic abnormality, which recurs with decreasing frequency. The latter is also subject to variation. Although visual disturbances are by far the most common manifestation, they differ in detail from patient to patient; numbness and tingling of the lips and the fingers of one hand are probably next in frequency, followed by transient aphasia or a thickness of speech and hemiparesis.

A not uncommon variant of the migraine syndrome was first described by Bickerstaff. The patients, usually young women with a family history of migraine, first develop visual phenomena, like those of typical migraine, except that they occupy the whole of both visual fields (temporary blindness may occur). There may be associated vertigo, staggering, incoordination of the limbs, dysarthria, and tingling in both hands and feet and sometimes around both sides of the mouth. Exceptionally there is an alarming period of psychosis, coma, or quadriplegia. These symptoms last 10 to 30 min and are followed by headache, which is usually occipital. Some patients, at the stage when the headache is likely to begin, may faint, and others become confused or stuporous, a state that may persist for several hours or longer. In all respects but their transience, the symptoms closely resemble those due to lesions in the territory of the basilar-posterior cerebral arteries—hence the name *basilar-artery* or *vertebrobasilar migraine.*

Recurrent unilateral headaches associated with extraocular muscle palsies have been called *ophthalmoplegic migraine.* A transient third nerve palsy with ptosis, most often with sparing of the pupil, is the usual picture; rarely, the sixth nerve is affected. The paresis often outlasts the headache by days or weeks and is said to become permanent after many attacks. Retinal and anterior optic nerve ischemia have also been documented. The retinal arterioles are attenuated, sometimes with retinal hemorrhages. In the case reported by Katz and Bamford, there was total blindness in one eye with disc edema and peripapillary hemorrhages. Vision returned only partially after several months. A particularly troublesome migraine variant occurs in a child or adolescent who, after a trivial head injury, may lose sight, suffer severe headache, or be plunged into a state of confusion with belligerent and irrational behavior that lasts for hours or several days before clearing. Another variant

in the child is episodic vertigo and staggering ("paroxysmal disequilibrium") followed by headache (Watson and Steele).

There is also a state known as *hemiplegic migraine,* in which an infant, child, or adult has episodes of unilateral paralysis that may long outlast the headache. Several families have been described in which this condition was inherited as an autosomal dominant trait (familial hemiplegic migraine). Instances of this disorder may account for some of the inexplicable strokes in young women and older adults of both sexes. We have seen several infants and young children who have had attacks of hemiplegia, first on one side then the other, every few weeks. Recovery was complete, and four-vessel arteriography in one child, after more than 70 attacks, was normal. The mode of onset and lack of seizures stamped the illness as vascular, but its relationship to neurologic migraine remains an open question.

The attacks, instead of beginning in childhood and recurring in the usual fashion every few weeks or months with diminishing frequency in middle and late adult years, may have their onset in the latter periods or suddenly increase in frequency during the menopause or in association with hypertension and vascular disease. Some of the transient hemianesthetic or hemiplegic strokes of late life may be of migrainous origin; Fisher has provided some documentation of this hypothesis (see References). In some individuals the migraine, for unaccountable reasons, may increase in frequency for several months. As many as three or four attacks may occur each week, leaving the scalp continuously tender.

A difficult clinical problem is posed by migraine patients who lapse into a condition of daily or virtually continuous migraine (*status migrainosus*). The pain is unilateral, throbbing, and disabling. Relief is sought by increasing the intake of ergot preparations, often to an alarming degree, with only temporary relief. Opioids may have been taken over a period of several weeks, with the threat of addiction. The mechanism of migraine being obscure, one can only surmise that the basic process has been greatly intensified. Always to be considered in diagnosis is the possibility of tension headache combined with an anxious depression (so-called migraine-tension headache syndrome) or a complication of treatment, such as ergot intoxication or narcotic addiction. It has been our practice to admit such patients to the hospital, to discontinue all ergot and narcotic medication, and to administer corticosteroids intravenously. Raskin has found the combination of 0.5 mg of dihydroergotamine and 10 mg of metoclopramide, administered intravenously every 8 h for 2 days,

Table 9-1
Common types of headache

Type	Site	Age and sex	Clinical characteristics	Diurnal pattern	Life profile	Provoking factors	Associated features	Treatment
Common migraine	Frontotemporal Uni- or bilateral	Children, young to middle-aged adults, more common in women	Throbbing; worse behind one eye or ear Becomes dull ache and generalized Sensitive scalp	Upon awakening or later in day Duration: hours to 1–2 days	Irregular intervals, weeks to months Tends to decrease in middle age and during pregnancy	Bright light, noise, tension, alcohol Relieved by darkness and sleep	Nausea and vomiting in some cases	Ergotamine and phenergan at onset Propranolol or amitriptyline for prevention
"Neurologic" migraine	Same as above	Same as above	Same as above Family history frequent	Same as above	Same as above	Same as above	Scintillating lights, blindness, and scotomas Unilateral numbness, weakness, dysphasia, vertigo, confusion—less common	Same as above
Cluster (histamine headache, migrainous neuralgia)	Orbital-temporal Unilateral	Adolescent and adult males (80–90%)	Intense, nonthrobbing pain, uilateral	Usually nocturnal, one or more hours after falling asleep Occasionally diurnal	Nightly or daily for several weeks to months Recurrence after many months or years	Alcohol in some	Lacrimation Stuffed nostril Rhinorrhea Injected conjunctivum	Ergotamine before anticipated attack Amitriptyline Methysergide, corticosteroids, and lithium in recalcitrant cases

	Location	Age/Sex	Quality	Course	Duration	Psychologic factors	Other findings	Treatment
Tension headaches	Generalized	Mainly adults, both sexes, more in women	Pressure (nonthrobbing), tightness, aching	Continuous, variable intensity, for days, weeks, or months	One or more periods of months to years	Fatigue and nervous strain Fear of brain tumor	Depression, worry, anxiety	Antianxiety and antidepressant drugs
Meningeal irritation (meningitis, subarachnoid hemorrhage)	Generalized, or bioccipital or bifrontal	Any age, both sexes	Intense, steady deep pain, may be worse in neck	Rapid evolution—minutes to hours	Single episode	None	Neck stiff on forward bending Kernig and Brudzinski signs	For meningitis or bleeding (see text)
Brain tumor	Unilateral or generalized	Any age, both sexes	Variable intensity May awaken patient Steady pain	Lasts minutes to hours; increasing severity	Once in a lifetime: weeks to months	None Sometimes position	Papilledema Vomiting Impaired mentation Seizures Focal signs	Corticosteroids Mannitol Treatment of tumor
Temporal arteritis	Unilateral or bilateral, usually temporal	Over 50 years, either sex	Throbbing, then persistent aching and burning, arteries thickened and tender	Intermittent, then continuous	Persists for weeks to a few months	None	Loss of vision Polymyalgia rheumatica Fever, weight loss, increased sedimentation rate	Corticosteroids

to be effective in these circumstances. If anxiety and depression emerge as important problems, they are treated along the lines described in Chap. 56.

Rarely, neurologic symptoms, instead of being transitory, may leave a permanent deficit (e.g., a homonymous visual field defect), like an ischemic stroke ("complicated migraine"). Platelet aggregation, edema of the arterial wall, and increased coagulability of the blood have all been implicated in the pathogenesis of arterial occlusion and strokes that complicate migraine (Rascol et al). The reported incidence of this complication has varied. At the Mayo Clinic, in a group of 4874 patients, aged 50 years or younger, who had received a diagnosis of migraine, migraine equivalent, or vascular headache, 20 patients had migraine-associated infarctions (Broderick and Swanson). The use of hormones to prevent pregnancy has increased the frequency and severity of migraine and in several reported instances has resulted in a permanent neurologic deficit. The report by Dorfman et al., in which cerebral infarction was revealed by CT scan in four young adults (16 to 32 years) with migraine, matches our experience and suggests that this complication may be more prevalent than is generally appreciated.

Between attacks the migrainous patient is normal. For a time, when psychosomatic medicine was much in vogue, there was insistence on a migrainous personality, characterized by tenseness, rigidity in thinking, meticulousness, and perfectionism. Further analyses, however, have not established a particular personality type in migrainous patients. Moreover, the fact that the headaches may begin in early childhood, when the personality is relatively amorphous, would argue against this idea. The migrainous attack was said to occur often during the "let-down period," after many days of hard work or stress, but the temporal relations between headache and the day's or week's activities have not proved to be consistent. There is no clear relationship, despite many statements to the contrary, between migraine and neurosis. The relationship to epilepsy is also unclear; the incidence of seizures is slightly higher in migrainous patients and their relatives than in the general population. Lance and Anthony find no mechanism common to migraine and epilepsy.

Migraine is prevalent, found in an estimated 3 to 5 percent of the general population and in a much higher proportion (15 percent) of women during their reproductive years. The incidence in females is about twice that in males, and the headaches tend to occur during periods of premenstrual tension and fluid retention. Estrogen and progesterone levels throughout the menstrual cycle are the same in normal and migrainous women. The onset of migraine in the premenstrual period is thought to be related to the withdrawal of estrogen rather than progesterone (Somerville). The attacks cease during pregnancy in 75 to 80 percent of women, and in others they continue at a reduced frequency; sometimes they first appear during pregnancy, usually in the first trimester. A considerable number of patients link their attacks to certain dietary items, particularly chocolate, cheese, fatty foods, oranges, tomatoes, and onions. Some of these foods are rich in tyramine, which has been incriminated as a cause of migraine. Alcohol, particularly red wine or port, regularly provokes an attack in some persons, and in others headaches are consistently induced by exposure to glare or other strong sensory stimuli, sudden jarring of the head ("footballer's migraine") or by rapid changes in barometric pressure.

So far it has not been possible to educe from the many clinical observations and careful clinical investigations a unifying theory as to the cause and pathogenesis of the common and classic forms of migraine. Tension and other emotional states, which are claimed by some migraineurs to precede their attacks, are so inconsistent as to be no more than aggravating factors. Clearly, the familial occurrence of migraine in the majority of patients implicates an underlying genetic factor, although it is not expressed in a simple mendelian pattern. The puzzle is how this genetic fault is translated periodically into a regional neurologic deficit or unilateral headache, or both. Certainly the throbbing, pulsating quality of the headache and its relief by compression of the carotid artery suggest vascular involvement. Several other facts incriminate blood vessels. The early observations of Graham and Wolff and the later findings by Mathew et al and by Oleson and his colleagues, using the Xenon inhalation method, that the cerebral circulation is reduced in classic migraine, supports this idea. Interestingly, this cerebral oligemia could not be demonstrated in common migraine. The rare but well established migrainous complication of oculomotor or optic nerve ischemic necrosis, recently corroborated by Castaldo et al, Dorfmann et al, and Katz and Bamford, is also in keeping with a vascular hypothesis. The march of the neurologic symptoms, estimated by Lashley to be 3 mm/min, corresponds to the rate of observed spread of hypoperfusion from one occipital lobe anteriorly. This spreading hypoperfusion interferes with the circulation of the cerebral cortex and subcortical white matter (but not with the central ganglionic structures) in the territory of multiple cerebral arteries and is said not to cross major sulci. The linkage of vascular pain and neurologic disorders is believed to relate to the fact that the involved vessels, both intracranial and extracranial, have small unmyelinated fibers in their walls, subserving both pain and autonomic functions. When these fibers are activated via axonal reflexes, substance P was found by Moskowitz to be released into the vessel wall, stimulating pain endings and increasing vascular permeability. In this manner the trigeminovascular complex could cause both the throbbing head pain and neurologic disorder.

These findings leave a number of unanswered questions. Do they mean that classic and common migraine are different diseases or a single disease, involving intracranial arteries in one instance and extracranial in another? Is the neurologic disorder, which seems to have first an excitatory and then an inhibitory phase, the cause or the result of the circulatory change? The resemblance of the slow progression of neurologic migraine to the phenomenon of "spreading cortical depression" first observed by Leao, has invited comparison. The latter investigator demonstrated that a noxious stimulus applied to the rat cortex was followed by slowly spreading waves of inhibition of cortical neurons and release of potassium. These inhibitory waves move at the rate of 3 mm/min; they are initiated by a brief neuronal burst of 5 to 10 s duration and are followed by a depression lasting for many minutes up to an hour. The spreading depression is accompanied by a band of pial hyperperfusion and dilatation (100 percent increase in blood flow) for 1 to 2 min, followed by a decrease in blood flow (25 to 30 percent) for 1 h. The autoregulation of affected vessels in the region of oligemia in migraine was found to respond to blood pressure rises but not to CO_2 inhalation or to volitional activation of the affected cortex during movement. Despite the intriguing similarities of Leao's spreading depression and the hypoperfusion of classic migraine, the Leao phenomenon has not been demonstrated in the human brain and the analogy may not be apt. Moreover, the severity of the reduced blood flow in classic migraine greatly exceeds that found consequent to any metabolic autoregulatory effect observed in the brain. This led Oleson and his colleagues to conclude that the reduction in blood flow was due to a primary vascular disorder. They admit, however, that critical positron emission studies of labeled O_2 and glucose will be necessary to distinguish a primary metabolic suppression of the cerebral cortex from a secondary cortical ischemia.

The neural hypothesis of migraine has not been without its adherents. Living long ago referred to it as a "nerve storm" and Hughlings Jackson as a sensory seizure. Blau as well as Welch also reject the vascular hypothesis in favor of an initial disturbance in the hypothalamus and limbic cortex, thereby activating the intrinsic noradrenergic nervous system and its putative orbitofrontal connections. The possible mechanisms of activation are hypothetically attributable to a reduction in unbound and platelet-bound serotonin (Anthony and Lance).

No final reconciliation of all these conflicting data is possible at this time. The authors continue to favor the unique mechanism of vascular constriction of slow evolution as the best explanation of the neurologic deficit and the headache.

Diagnosis Neurologic migraine should occasion no difficulty in diagnosis if the above facts are kept in mind and a good history is obtained. The difficulties come from a lack of awareness that (1) a progressively unfolding neu-

rologic syndrome may be migrainous in origin, (2) the neurologic disorder may occur without headache, and (3) recurrent headaches, which may be an isolated phenomenon, may take many forms, some of which may prove difficult to distinguish from the other common types of headache. Some of these problems merit elaboration because of their practical importance.

The neurologic part of the migraine syndrome may resemble focal epilepsy, the clinical effects of slow hemorrhage from an arteriovenous malformation or aneurysm, a transient ischemic attack, or a thrombotic or embolic stroke. It is the pace of the neurologic symptoms of migraine, more than their character, that reliably distinguishes the condition from epilepsy. The evolution of an epileptic aura and spread of focal seizure activity are measured in seconds, for they depend on spreading neural excitation, in contrast to the much slower progression of neurologic migraine, which has been attributed by neurophysiologists to "spreading depression"—a phenomenon in which waves of inhibition move across the cerebral cortex at a rate of about 3 mm/min, and which, in migraine, is presumably triggered by vasoconstriction.

Ophthalmoplegic migraine will always suggest a carotid aneurysm, but in very few cases has carotid arteriography revealed such an abnormality. There have been many claims that the habitual occurrence of migraine on the same side of the head increases the likelihood of an underlying vascular malformation, and our studies of numerous cases, both of migraine and of arteriovenous malformations, indicate that among patients with arteriovenous malformations (AVMs) the incidence of classic migraine is more than five times greater than in the general population. Yet there is no close correlation between the size, type, and location of the AVM and headache. Approximately half of the patients with AVM and migraine have a positive family history of migraine. Thus, AVM must be regarded as an acknowledged cause of recurrent headache, and the latter may be frequent and troublesome for years before the malformation is discovered. In more than 900 such patients seen by the authors, many of the headaches, which occur in over 30 percent of cases, do not have the other features of either migraine or cluster headache.

A special problem relates to paroxysms of throbbing headache, not hemicranial in distribution, not preceded by a neurologic aura, and not accounted for by other known cause. Are they examples of common (nonneurologic) migraine or of some other cephalalgia? Unfortunately, since diagnosis depends on the interpretation of the patient's symptoms and since there is as yet no valid confirmatory laboratory test, the controversy as to where migraine begins and ends is of the armchair type. Favoring the diagnosis of migraine are lifelong history, childhood onset, positive family history, and response of the headache to ergotamine.

A variety of episodic attacks have been described as migraine equivalents, especially in children: attacks of abdominal pain with nausea, vomiting, and diarrhea; pain localized in the thorax, pelvis, and extremities; bouts of fever; transient disturbances in mood (psychic equivalents); or episodic vertigo. The only advantage of considering such attacks as migrainous is that this view protects some patients from unnecessary diagnostic procedures and surgical intervention; but by the same token it may delay appropriate investigation and treatment.

CLUSTER HEADACHE

This type of headache has been described under a variety of names, including *paroxysmal nocturnal cephalgia, migrainous neuralgia, (Horton's) histamine cephalgia, red migraine, erythromelalgia of the head*, and many others. It occurs predominantly in young adult men and is characterized by a constant, unilateral orbital localization; it tends to recur nightly or several times during the night and day for a period of 2 to 8 weeks, sometimes much longer, followed by complete freedom for many months or even years (hence the term *cluster*). However, a considerable number of our cases have been chronic over years and overlap the syndrome of chronic paroxysmal hemicrania described below. The pain is felt deep in and around the eye, is intense and nonthrobbing as a rule, and often radiates into the forehead, temple, and cheek. Associated phenomena are a blocked nostril followed by rhinorrhea, injected conjunctivum, and less often by nausea and vomiting, miosis, ptosis, flush and edema of the cheek, all lasting for 10 min to 2 h. The homolateral temporal artery may become prominent and tender during an attack, and the skin over the scalp and face may be hyperalgesic. The pain of a given attack may leave as rapidly as it began or fade away gradually. Almost always the same orbit is involved during a bout of headaches as well as in recurring bouts. A similar type of headache may occasionally occur in the lower face, postauricular, or occipital areas. Ekbom distinguished another lower cluster headache syndrome with infraorbital radiation of the pain, an ipsilateral partial Horner syndrome, and ipsilateral hyperhydrosis. During the period of freedom, alcohol, which commonly precipitates headaches during a cluster, no longer has the capacity to do so.

The picture of cluster headache is usually so characteristic that it cannot be confused with any other disease, though to those unfamiliar with it a diagnosis of migraine,

trigeminal neuralgia, carotid aneurysm, tumors of the sphenoid bone and sinuses, fungus and other granulomatous lesions, or sinusitis may be entertained. Appropriate investigations (CT scan with contrast, carotid arteriography) will always exclude the latter conditions, but are rarely necessary. To be distinguished also are the *Tolosa-Hunt syndrome* of ocular pain and ocular motor paralyses (see further on) and the *paratrigeminal syndrome of Raeder,* which consists of pain, like that of tic douloureux, in the distribution of the ophthalmic and maxillary divisions of the fifth nerve, in association with ocular sympathetic paralysis (ptosis and miosis) but with preservation of sweating; loss of sensation in a trigeminal nerve distribution and weakness of muscles innervated by the fifth nerve are often added. Many of the cases of paroxysmal pain behind the eye or nose or in the upper jaw or temple, associated with blocking of the nostril or lacrimation and described under the titles of sphenopalatine (Sluder), petrosal, vidian, and ciliary (Charlin or Harris) neuralgia, probably represent instances of cluster headache or variants thereof. There is no evidence to support the separation of these neuralgias as distinct entities.

The relationship of the cluster headache to migraine remains conjectural. No doubt certain headaches have some of the characteristics of both migraine and cluster headaches, hence the terms "migrainous neuralgia" and "cluster-migraine" (Kudrow). Lance and others, however, have pointed out differences that seem important to the authors: flushing of the face on the side of a cluster headache and pallor in migraine; increased intraocular pressure in cluster headache, normal in migraine; and increased skin temperature over the forehead, temple, and cheek in cluster headache, decreased in migraine; and notable distinctions in sex distribution, age of onset, rhythmicity, and other clinical features, as described above.

The cause and mechanism of the cluster headache syndrome are unknown. Gardner et al postulated a paroxysmal parasympathetic discharge mediated through the greater superficial petrosal nerve and sphenopalatine ganglion. These authors obtained inconsistent results by cutting the nerve, but others (Kittrelle et al) have reported that local application of cocaine and lidocaine to the region of the sphenopalatine ganglion consistently aborts attacks of cluster headache. Stimulation of the ganglion is said to reproduce the syndrome. Kunkle et al concluded that the pain was arising from the upper branches of the external carotid artery, but Ekbom and Greitz, using arteriography during the attack, could not demonstrate any vascular changes. Sakai and Meyer observed an increase in blood flow during the attack, but it was more on the contralateral side. The cyclical nature of the attacks has been linked to the hypothalamic mechanism that governs the circadian rhythm, on rather speculative grounds. The fact that cluster headache could be reproduced by the intravenous injection of 0.1 mg histamine (an early experimental device for studying the mechanism of headache) led to the notion, popular for many years, that this form of headache was caused by the spontaneous release of histamine, and to a form of treatment which consisted of "desensitizing" the patient by slow intravenous injections of this drug, given daily for several weeks. Experience has shown that this form of treatment accomplishes nothing more than temporization; it can be pointed out that the intravenous injection of histamine induces or worsens many forms of focal or generalized headache (due to fever, trauma, brain tumor) that are dependent upon stretching of pain-sensitive tissue around the vessels derived from the internal carotid artery.

Chronic paroxysmal hemicrania is the name given by Sjaastad and Dale to a unilateral headache syndrome that resembles cluster headache in some respects but has several distinctive features. The headaches are paroxysmal and of short duration (20 to 30 min), invariably affect the temporo-orbital region of one side, and are accompanied by conjunctival hyperemia, rhinorrhea, and in some by a partial Horner syndrome. Unlike cluster headache, however, the paroxysms occur many times each day, recur daily for years on end (the patient of Price and Posner had an average of 16 attacks daily for more than 40 years) and, most importantly, respond dramatically in some instances to the administration of indomethacin.

TENSION HEADACHES

This headache is usually bilateral, often with occipital-nuchal, temporal, or frontal predominance, or with diffuse extension over the top of the cranium. The pain is described as dull and aching, but questioning often uncovers other sensations, such as fullness, tightness, or pressure (as if the head is surrounded by a band or clamped in a vise), on which waves of aching pain are engrafted. The onset of a given attack is more gradual than in migraine, and the headache, once established, may persist with only mild fluctuations for weeks, months, or even years. In fact, this is the only type of headache that exhibits the peculiarity of being absolutely continuous for long periods of time. Although sleep is usually undisturbed, the headache is present when the patient awakens or develops soon afterward, and the common analgesic remedies have no beneficial effect if the pain is intense.

The incidence of tension headache in neurologic practice is probably as great as that of migraine. Like migraine, tension headaches are more common in women than in men. Unlike migraine, they infrequently begin in childhood or adolescence but are more likely to occur in middle age and coincide with anxiety and depression in the trying times of life. In the large series of Lance and Curran, about one-third of patients with tension headaches had

readily recognized symptoms of depression, an experience that coincides with our own. Migraine and traumatic headaches may be complicated by tension headache, which, because of its persistence, often arouses fears of a brain tumor. However, as Patten points out, not more than one or two patients out of every thousand with tension headaches will be found to harbor an intracranial tumor.

For many years it has been taught that tension headaches are due to excessive muscle contraction and an associated constriction of the scalp arteries. However, it is doubtful that either of these mechanisms contributes to the genesis of tension headache, at least in its chronic form. Many persons persistently frown or clench their teeth but do not develop tension headaches. The continuous pressing quality of tension headache, at times when the patient is relaxed, hardly seems attributable to continuous muscle activity. All types of persistent headache may give rise to muscle tension and this has an aching rather than a pressing quality. Moreover, Anderson and Frank found no difference in muscle contraction in migraine and tension headache. In a small group of patients, the headache when severe develops a pulsating quality, to which the term "tension-vascular" headache has been applied (Lance and Curran).

HEADACHE AND OTHER CRANIOFACIAL PAIN WITH PSYCHIATRIC DISEASE

When psychiatric symptoms are sought in patients with headache, it is evident that the majority of those with anxiety neurosis, hysteria, obsessive-compulsive neurosis, and various forms of depressive illness will complain of headache of the tension type. As a corollary, psychologic studies of groups of patients with tension headache have revealed prominent symptoms of anxiety, hypochondriasis, and depression. In our outpatient clinics, the most common cause of generalized intractable headache, both in adolescents and adults, is depression or anxiety in one of its several forms.

The authors have noted that among seriously ill psychiatric patients many have frequent headaches that are not of the tension type. These patients report unilateral or generalized throbbing cephalic pain lasting for hours every day or two. The nature of these headaches, which in some instances resemble common migraine, is unsettled. As the psychiatric symptoms subside, the headaches usually disappear.

Odd cephalic pains, e.g., a sensation of having a nail driven into the head ("clavus hystericus"), may occur in hysteria and raise perplexing problems in diagnosis. The bizarre character of these pains, their persistence in the face of every known therapy, the absence of other signs of disease, and the presence of other manifestations of hysteria provide the basis for correct diagnosis (see Chap. 55).

TRAUMATIC HEADACHE

Severe, chronic, continuous or intermittent headaches appear as the cardinal symptom of several posttraumatic syndromes, separable in each instance from the headache that immediately follows head injury (i.e., that of scalp laceration and cerebral contusion with blood in the CSF and increased intracranial pressure) and that lasts several days or a week or two.

The headache of chronic subdural hematoma is deep-seated, steady, unilateral or generalized, and is accompanied by drowsiness, confusion, stupor, and hemiparesis. The head injury may have been minor and forgotten by the patient and family. Typically the headache and other symptoms increase in frequency and severity over several weeks or months. Diagnosis is usually established by the CT scan or MRI.

Headache is a prominent feature of a complex syndrome comprised of giddiness, fatigability, insomnia, nervousness, trembling, irritability, inability to concentrate, and tearfulness (*posttraumatic nervous instability*). This type of headache and associated symptoms, which resemble the "tension headache syndrome," are described fully in Chap. 35, "Craniocerebral Trauma."

Tenderness and aching pain sharply localized to the scar of the scalp laceration represent in all probability a different problem, raising the question of a *traumatic neuralgia*. With *whiplash injuries* to the neck, unilateral or bilateral retroauricular or occipital pain may occur, due probably to stretching or tearing of ligaments and muscles at the occipitonuchal junction. Much less frequently, cervical intervertebral discs and roots are involved.

Under the heading of *posttraumatic dysautonomic cephalalgia*, Vijayan and Dreyfus have described severe, episodic, throbbing, unilateral headaches, accompanied by ipsilateral mydriasis and excessive sweating of the face. Between bouts of headache, the patients showed partial ptosis and miosis, as well as pharmacologic evidence of partial sympathetic denervation. The condition followed injury to the soft tissues of the neck in the region of the carotid artery sheath. The headaches did not respond to treatment with ergotamine, but prompt relief was obtained in each case with the beta-adrenergic blocking agent propranolol.

HEADACHES OF BRAIN TUMOR

Headache is a significant symptom in about two-thirds of all patients with brain tumor (Rooke). Unfortunately the quality of the pain has no specific features. It tends to be deep-seated, usually nonthrobbing (occasionally throbbing), and is described as aching or bursting. Attacks last a few minutes to an hour or more and occur once or many times during the day. Activity and frequent change in the position of the head may provoke pain, whereas rest diminishes its frequency. Nocturnal awakening because of pain, although typical, is by no means diagnostic. Unexpected forceful (projectile) vomiting may punctuate the illness in its later stages. As the tumor grows, the pain becomes more frequent and severe and eventually continuous, but there are exceptions. Some headaches are mild and tolerable; others are as agonizing as those of bacterial meningitis and subarachnoid hemorrhage. If unilateral, the headache is nearly always on the same side as the tumor. Pain from supratentorial tumors is felt anterior to the interauricular circumference of the skull; from posterior fossa tumors, behind this line. Bifrontal and bioccipital headaches, coming on after unilateral headaches, signify the development of increased intracranial pressure.

CRANIAL ARTERITIS (TEMPORAL ARTERITIS, GIANT-CELL ARTERITIS)

This particular type of inflammatory disease of cranial arteries is an important cause of headache in elderly persons. All of our patients have been over 50 years of age and most of them over 60 years. From a state of normal health they develop an increasingly intense throbbing or nonthrobbing headache, which may be bilateral or unilateral, often localized to the affected arteries, and which persists throughout the day and is particularly severe at night. It lasts for many months if untreated (average duration, 1 year). The superficial temporal and other scalp arteries are frequently thickened and tender and without pulsation. Many of the patients feel generally unwell and have lost weight, and some have a low-grade fever and anemia. The sedimentation rate is frequently but not always elevated, and a few patients have a neutrophilic leukocytosis. As many as 50 percent have generalized aching of muscles, a condition that merges with the syndrome of *polymyalgia rheumatica* (see pages 175 and 674).

The importance of early diagnosis relates to the threat of blindness from thrombosis of the ophthalmic and less often of the posterior ciliary arteries. This may be preceded by several episodes of amaurosis fugax. Ophthalmoplegia may also occur but is less frequent. The intracranial vessels have rarely been affected. Once vision is lost, it is seldom recoverable. For this reason the earliest suspicion of cranial arteritis should lead to hospital admission and biopsy of the appropriate scalp artery; microscopic examination discloses an intense granulomatous or "giant-cell" arteritis. Treatment consists of the administration of prednisone, 45 to 60 mg/day in divided doses over a period of several weeks, with gradual reduction to 10 to 20 mg/day and maintenance at this dosage for several months or for several years if necessary to prevent relapse.

UNUSUAL VARIETIES OF HEADACHE

COUGH AND EXERTIONAL HEADACHE

A patient may complain of transient, severe cranial pain on coughing, sneezing, laughing, heavy lifting, stooping, and straining at stool. Pain is most severe in the front of the head but is also felt in the occipital region and may be unilateral or bilateral. As a rule it follows the initiating action within a few seconds, and lasts a few seconds to a few minutes. Its character is that of a bursting pain and may be of such severity as to cause same patients to cradle their head in their hands.

This syndrome most often occurs as a benign idiopathic state that may last months to a year or two and then may subside. In a report of 103 patients followed for 3 years or longer, Rooke found that additional symptoms of neurologic disease developed in only 10, and Symonds also attested to the usually benign nature of the condition. Its cause and mechanism have not been determined. During the attack the CSF pressure is normal. Bilateral jugular compression may induce an attack, possibly because of traction on the walls of veins and dural sinuses. In a few instances we have observed this type of headache after lumbar puncture or after an angiomatous hemorrhage.

As indicated above, patients with cough or strain headache may occasionally be found to have serious intracranial disease; interestingly, this is most often of the posterior fossa and foramen magnum—arteriovenous malformation, Arnold-Chiari malformation, platybasia, basilar impression, or tumor. It may be necessary, therefore, to supplement the neurologic examination by appropriate skull films, CT scanning, and MRI.

We have tried a variety of medications but can report no consistent therapeutic success with any of them. In some patients, exercise precipitates a typical migraine headache, which can be prevented by ergotamine tartrate or methysergide taken before the activity which habitually causes headache. The cough-strain headache of the Chiari malformation and basilar impression repsonds to the surgical treatment for these conditions, i.e., unroofing the upper cervical cord at the foramen magnum.

HEADACHES RELATED TO SEXUAL ACTIVITY

Lance has described 21 cases of this type of headache, predominantly in males. Two groups were recognized, one in which headache of the tension type developed with sexual excitement, and another in which a severe, throbbing, "explosive" headache occurred at the time of orgasm and persisted for several minutes or hours. The latter headaches were of such abruptness and severity as to suggest a ruptured aneurysm, but the neurologic examination was negative in every instance, as was arteriography in seven patients who were subjected to this procedure. In 18 patients who were followed for a period of 2 to 7 years no other neurologic symptoms developed. Of course, a hypertensive hemorrhage or rupture of an aneurysm or vascular malformation may occur during the exertion and excitement of sexual intercourse.

ERYTHROCYANOTIC HEADACHE

On rare occasions, an intense, generalized, throbbing headache may occur in conjunction with flushing of the face and hands and numbness of the fingers (erythromelalgia or erythermalgia). Episodes tend to be present on awakening from sound sleep. This condition has been reported in a number of unusual settings: (1) in mastocytosis (infiltration of tissues by mast cells which elaborate histamine, heparin, and serotonin), (2) in carcinoid, (3) with serotonin secreting tumors, (4) with some tumors of the pancreatic islets, and (5) with pheochromocytoma. Eighty percent of patients with pheochromocytoma reportedly have vascular-type headaches coincident with paroxysms of hypertension and elaboration of catecholamines (Lance and Hinterberger).

HEADACHE RELATED TO MEDICAL DISEASES

About 50 percent of patients with *hypertension* complain of headache, but the relationship of one to the other is not entirely clear. Minor elevations of blood pressure may be a result rather than the cause of tension headaches. Severe hypertension, with diastolic pressure of more than 120 mmHg, is regularly associated with headache, and measures that reduce the blood pressure relieve the headache. However, it is the moderately severe hypertensive individual with frequent severe headaches who gives the most concern. In many of these patients there is undoubtedly an underlying anxiety or tension state or a common migraine syndrome, but in some the headaches defy explanation. According to Wolff, the mechanism of the hypertensive headache is similar to that of migraine, i.e., increased vascular pulsations. The headaches, however, bear no clear relation to modest peaks in blood pressure. Nevertheless, vasoconstricting drugs such as ergotamine are said to be as effective in some of the common hypertensive headache as in migraine. Curiously, headaches that occur toward the end of renal dialysis or soon after its completion are associated with a fall in blood pressure as well as a decrease in blood sodium levels and osmolality. The mechanism of occipital pain that may awaken the hypertensive patient and wear off during the day is not understood.

The headaches that accompany diseases of the upper cervical spine are well recognized but their mechanism is obscure. Recent writings have focused on the wide range of etiologies such as zygoapophyseal arthropathy, calcified ligamentum flavum, lesions of the posterior longitudinal ligament, and rheumatoid arthritis of the atlanto-axial region. CT scanning has divulged a number of these abnormalities. Their treatment is discussed in Chap. 10.

Experienced physicians are aware of many other conditions in which headache may be a dominant symptom. These include: fevers of any cause, carbon monoxide exposure, chronic lung disease with hypercapnia (headaches often nocturnal), hypothyroidism, Cushing disease, withdrawal from corticosteroid medication, chronic ingestion of ergotamine, chronic exposure to nitrites, occasionally adrenal insufficiency, aldosterone-producing adrenal tumors, use of the "pill," and acute anemia with hemoglobin below 10 g.

TREATMENT

TREATMENT OF MIGRAINE

This topic is logically subdivided into two parts—control of the attack and prevention. The time to initiate treatment of an acute attack is during the neurologic disorder or, if the latter is absent, at the beginning of the headache. If the headaches are mild, the patient may already have learned that 0.6 g acetylsalicylic acid or an equivalent amount of other nonnarcotic analgesics, or small doses of codeine will suffice to control the pain. For more severe attacks ergotamine tartrate is the most effective form of treatment. This drug can be administered subcutaneously or intramuscularly in a dose of 0.25 to 0.5 mg and repeated in 30 min if necessary, but the parenteral route is rarely practical. The use of uncoated 2-mg tablets of ergotamine tartrate, held under the tongue until dissolved and repeated every half hour until the headache is relieved or until a total of 8 mg is taken, is almost as effective. A single dose of promethazine (Phenergan), 50 mg by mouth, given with the ergotamine, relaxes the patient and allays nausea and vomiting. Caffeine, 100 mg, combined with 1 mg of ergotamine (Cafergot) can be taken in tablet form (two at onset of headache and a third in half an hour), but should not be taken late in the day because it prevents sleep, which in itself can relieve an attack of migraine. Patients in whom vomiting prevents oral administration should be given

ergotamine by rectal suppository or inhaler (Medihaler). When ergotamine is administered early in the attack, the headache will be abolished or reduced in severity and duration in some 70 to 75 percent of patients. Once the headache has become intense, ergotamine is of little help, and one must resort to codeine sulfate, 30 mg, or meperidine (Demerol), 50 mg, to control the pain.

Because of the danger of prolonged arterial spasm in patients who have vascular disease or are pregnant, ergotamine must be used cautiously, if at all. Even in healthy individuals, more than 10 to 15 mg of ergotamine per week is risky. Obviously the use of reserpine and "the pill" should be interdicted, because of the propensity of these agents to induce migraine.

In individuals with frequent migrainous attacks, efforts at prevention are worthwhile. Considerable success has been obtained with propranolol (Inderal), beginning with 20 mg thrice daily and raising the dosage gradually to as much as 240 mg daily. In our experience, this regimen reduces the frequency and severity of attacks in 75 percent of patients. Clonidine, 0.05 mg thrice daily, indomethacin 150 to 200 mg daily, Bellergal (a preparation of ergotamine tartrate, 0.3 mg, phenobarbital, 20 mg, and belladonna alkaloids, 0.1 mg) two or three times a day for a few weeks, pizotifen, 1 to 3 mg daily, cyproheptadine (Periactin), 4 to 16 mg/day and correspondingly less in children, or a course of amitriptyline have all reportedly been helpful in some patients. ACTH (40 units/day) or prednisone (45 mg/day for 3 to 4 weeks) has also been helpful in some refractory cases and in terminating migraine status. Methysergide (Sansert), also an ergot preparation, in doses of 2 to 6 mg daily for several weeks or months, is an effective agent in the prevention of migraine. Retroperitoneal fibrosis, which is the most serious complication of methysergide administration, can be avoided by discontinuing the medication for 3 to 4 weeks after every 5-month course of treatment. In patients who cannot tolerate methysergide the monoamine oxidase inhibitor phenelzine (Nardil), 30 to 60 mg daily, may be tried. Evidence suggests that the calcium channel or calcium entry blockers (verapamil, nifedipine) are effective in decreasing the frequency and severity of migraine attacks. Surprisingly, phenytoin has been quite effective in controlling migraine and its variants in children.

Some patients know, or allege to know, that certain items of food induce attacks, and it is obvious enough that they should avoid these foods, if possible. In certain cases it has been claimed that the correction of a refractive error, an elimination diet, or psychotherapy for some personality disorder has relieved migraine. However, this is so exceptional that a cause-and-effect relationship must be doubted, in view of the variability of the disease itself. All experienced physicians appreciate the importance of helping patients rearrange their schedules with a view to controlling tensions and hard-driving ways of living. There is no one way of accomplishing this. In general, long and costly psychotherapy has not been helpful; or at least one can say that there are no substantial data as to its value. Transcendental meditation, acupuncture, progressive relaxation, biofeedback technique all have their advocates, but the results are uninterpretable.

TREATMENT OF CLUSTER HEADACHE

The usual nocturnal attacks of cluster headache should be treated with a single dose of ergotamine at bedtime (3 mg orally or 1 mg by injection). Intranasal lidocaine can be used to abort an attack. In other patients, ergotamine has to be given once or twice during the day, at times when an attack of pain is expected. If ergotamine is not effective or becomes ineffective in subsequent bouts, one should turn to methysergide (3 to 9 mg daily) or preferably prednisone, beginning with 75 mg daily for 3 days, then reducing the dose at 3-day intervals until the headache begins to reappear. If this program of ergotamine, methysergide, and prednisone is not successful, lithium carbonate, in a daily dose of 600 mg (up to 900 mg), should be tried. Ekbom, who introduced this therapy, and Kudrow have found it most effective in chronic cases. The blood level of lithium must be checked frequently and kept between 0.7 and 1.2 meq/L; toxicity is a frequent problem (indicated by nausea, vomiting, blurred vision, fasciculations, and choreoathetosis). Indomethacin has been reported to be efficacious in the chronic form of cluster headache but was ineffective in several of our own cases. We have had greater success with amitriptyline.

TREATMENT OF NONMIGRAINOUS HEADACHES

The most important measures in the treatment of these headaches are those which uncover and remove the underlying disease or functional disturbance.

For common headaches due to fatigue, stuffy atmosphere, or excessive use of alcohol and tobacco, it is simple enough to advise avoidance of the offending activity or agent, and symptomatic therapy in the form of acetylsalicylic acid, 0.6 g (aspirin or Anacin) will suffice. Some patients who invariably have headache when constipated and hypochondriacs who suffer incapacitating headache, fatigue, and depression whenever bowel elimination does not meet their expectations, are not easily helped. Certainly, simple explanation, an anticonstipation regimen, and drugs which counteract depression (see Chap. 56) are preferable to the continuous use of analgesics. Premenstrual headache, if troublesome, can usually be helped by the use of a diuretic compound for the week preceding the menstrual period and mild analgesic and sedative medications (acetylsalicylic acid, 0.6 g, and diazepam, 5 mg).

Hypertensive headaches respond to agents which lower blood pressure and relieve muscle tension. Hydro-chlorthiazide, 50 to 100 mg/day, and methyldopa (Aldomet), 500 to 1500 mg/day, when combined with diazepam, 5 mg bid, have given the best results. Meprobamate, 200 mg tid, or chlordiazepoxide (Librium), 5 mg tid, may be administered in place of diazepam. For the morning occipital ache, a capsule containing sodium nitrite, 30 mg, caffeine sodium benzoate, 0.5 g, and acetophenetidin, 0.6 g, has been useful. A simplified method of treating this kind of headache is to supply the caffeine in a cup of strong black coffee and to give acetylsalicylic acid with it. Blocks under the head of the bed may be helpful.

Muscle contraction and other types of tension headaches respond best to massage, relaxation, and the use of one of several drugs that relieve anxiety (phenobarbital, meprobamate, diazepam, or chlordiazepoxide) or a combination of one of these drugs with amitriptyline or imipramine, when depressive symptoms are present. Simple analgesics such as aspirin are rarely helpful, and with severe tension headaches, stronger analgesic medication (codeine) is usually needed. Psychotherapy is usually not beneficial in this group of patients.

The patient with *posttraumatic nervous instability* requires supportive psychotherapy in the form of reassurance and frequent explanation of the benign and transient nature of the symptoms, a program of increasing physical activity, and the use of drugs that allay anxiety and depression. Tender scars from scalp lacerations may be treated by the repeated subcutaneous injection of 5 mL of 1% procaine. Settlement of litigation as soon as possible works to the patient's advantage.

Heat, massage, salicylates, and indomethacin (Indocin), phenylbutazone (Butazolidin), or one of the newer nonsteroidal anti-inflammatory agents usually effect some improvement in cervical *arthritic diseases* that are associated with cervicocranial pain.

Corticosteroids are highly effective in the treatment of *cranial arteritis*, as has been indicated. The headaches of *cranial tumor* often respond surprisingly well to large doses of prednisone and similar compounds.

In conclusion, it is well to mention the importance of general hygienic measures. Young physicians in particular are apt to seek a specific therapy for each headache syndrome and to give little thought to the general health of the patient. We have observed that most of the recurrent and chronic headaches are likely to be more severe and disabling whenever the patient becomes nervous, sick, and tired. A well-rounded diet, adequate rest, a reasonable amount of physical exercise, and a balanced view of the sources of daily anxieties and how to cope with them should be the goal of all therapeutic programs.

OTHER CRANIOFACIAL PAINS
(See Table 9-2)

TRIGEMINAL NEURALGIA (TIC DOULOUREUX)

This is a disorder of middle age and later life and consists of paroxysms of intense, stabbing pain in the distribution of the mandibular and maxillary divisions (rarely the ophthalmic division) of the fifth cranial nerve. The pain seldom lasts more than a few seconds or a minute or two but may be so intense that the patient winces; hence the term *tic*. The paroxysms recur frequently, both day and night, for several weeks at a time. Another characteristic feature is the initiation of pain by obvious stimuli applied to certain areas of the face, lips, or gums, as in shaving or brushing the teeth, or by movement of these parts in chewing, talking, or yawning—the so-called trigger zones. Sensory or motor loss in the distribution of the fifth nerve cannot be demonstrated in these cases, though there are minor exceptions to this rule. In addition to the paroxysms some of the patients complain of a more or less continuous discomfort and sensitivity of the face, a feature always regarded as atypical even though not infrequent.

In studying the relationship between stimuli applied to the trigger zones and the paroxysms of pain, it is found that the paroxysms are induced by touch and possibly tickle, rather than by a painful or thermal stimulus. Usually a spatial and temporal summation of impulses is necessary to trigger an attack, which is followed by a refractory period of up to 2 or 3 min. This suggests that the mechanism for the paroxysmal pain involves the nucleus of the spinal tract of the fifth nerve.

The diagnosis of tic douloureux must rest upon the strict clinical criteria enumerated above, and the condition needs to be distinguished from other forms of facial and cephalic neuralgia and pain arising from diseases of the jaw, teeth, or sinuses. This form of trigeminal neuralgia is usually without assignable cause (*idiopathic*), in contrast to *symptomatic trigeminal neuralgia,* in which paroxysmal facial pain is a manifestation of other neurologic disease. Thus, tic douloureux is occasionally a manifestation of multiple sclerosis (may be bilateral), an aneurysm of the basilar artery, or a tumor (acoustic or trigeminal neuroma, meningioma, epidermoid) in the cerebellopontine angle. Sometimes it is due to compression of the trigeminal roots by a tortuous blood vessel (usually the posterior cerebellar artery), as originally pointed out by Dandy. The presence of a vascular structure close to the trigeminal nerve is a frequent finding, even in patients without tic douloureux

(Hardy and Rhoton). However, a definite vascular compressive lesion as a cause of such pain is relatively rare (11 percent of the series of Adams et al). Each of these disorders may give rise only to pain in the distribution of the fifth nerve, or they may produce a loss of sensation as well. Other disorders of the fifth nerve, some of which give rise to facial pain, are discussed in Chap. 47, ''Diseases of the Cranial Nerves.''

Antiepileptic drugs such as phenytoin (Dilantin), and particularly carbamazepine (Tegretol) have been found to suppress or shorten the duration of the attacks. Clonazepam and baclofen may be useful in patients who cannot tolerate carbamazepine. Temporizing and using these drugs may permit a spontaneous remission to occur. Most of the patients with severe pain come to surgery. The traditional surgical treatment for tic douloureux has been alcohol or phenol injection of the affected nerve at the foramen ovale and rotundum or section of the root of the trigeminal nerve between the ganglion and the brainstem. These methods have been superseded by stereotactically controlled thermocoagulation of the trigeminal roots using a radio frequency generator (Sweet and Wepsic).

GLOSSOPHARYNGEAL NEURALGIA

This syndrome is much less common than trigeminal neuralgia, but resembles the latter in many respects. The pain is intense and paroxysmal; it originates in the throat, approximately in the tonsillar fossa and is provoked most commonly by swallowing, but also by talking, chewing, yawning, laughing, etc. The pain is localized in the ear or may radiate from the throat to the ear, implicating the auricular branch of the vagus nerve. For this reason White and Sweet have suggested the term *vagoglossopharyngeal neuralgia*. This is the only craniofacial neuralgia which may be accompanied by bradycardia and even by syncope, presumably because of the triggering of cardiovascular regulatory fibers by afferent pain impulses. There is no demonstrable sensory or motor deficit. Rarely, carcinoma or epithelioma of the oropharyngeal-infracranial region or peritonsillar abscess may give rise to pain clinically indistinguishable from glossopharyngeal neuralgia. For idiopathic glossopharyngeal neuralgia, a trial of phenytoin or carbamazepine may be useful, but if these are unsuccessful, the glossopharyngeal nerve and upper rootlets of the vagus near the medulla need to be interrupted surgically.

POSTHERPETIC NEURALGIA

Neuralgia associated with a vesicular eruption, due to infection with the virus of herpes zoster, may affect cranial as well as peripheral nerves. In the region of the cranial nerves, two syndromes are frequent: herpes zoster auric-

Table 9-2
Types of facial pain

Type	Site	Clinical characteristics	Aggravating-relieving factors	Associated diseases	Treatment
Trigeminal neuralgia (tic douloureux)	Second and third divisions of trigeminal nerve, unilateral	Men/women = 1:3 Over 50 years Paroxysms (10–30 s) of stabbing, burning pain; persistent for weeks or longer Trigger points No sensory or motor paralysis	Touching trigger points, chewing, smiling, talking, blowing nose, yawning	Idiopathic If in young adults, multiple sclerosis Vascular anomaly Tumor of fifth cranial nerve	Carbamazepine Phenytoin Alcohol injection, coagulation, or surgical section of nerve
Atypical facial neuralgia	Unilateral or bilateral; cheek or angle of cheek and nose; deep in nose	Predominantly female 30–50 years Continuous intolerable pain Mainly maxillary areas	None	Depressive and anxiety states Hysteria Idiopathic	Antidepressant and antianxiety medication
Postzoster neuralgia	Unilateral Usually ophthalmic division of fifth nerve	History of zoster Aching, burning pain; jabs of pain Paresthesiae, slight sensory loss Dermal scars	Contact, movement	Herpes zoster	Carbamazepine, antidepressants, and sedatives
Costen syndrome	Unilateral, behind or front of ear, temple, face	Severe aching pain, intensified by chewing Tenderness over temporo-mandibular joints Malocclusion, missing molars	Chewing, pressure over temporo-mandibular joints	Loss of teeth, rheumatoid arthritis	Correction of bite Surgery in some
Tolosa-Hunt syndrome	Unilateral, mainly retro-orbital	Intense sharp, aching pain, associated with ophthalmoplegias and sensory loss over forehead; pupil usually spared	None	Lesion of cavernous sinus or superior orbital fissure	Surgery; corticosteroids for granulomatous lesions
Raeder paratrigeminal syndrome	Unilateral, frontotemporal and maxilla	Intense sharp or aching pain, ptosis, miosis, preserved sweating	None	Tumors, granulomatous lesions, injuries in parasellar region	Depends on type of lesion
"Migrainous neuralgia"	Orbitofrontal, temple, upper jaw, angle of nose and cheek	See cluster headache, Table 9-1	Alcohol in some		Ergotamine before anticiapted attack
Carotidynia, lower-half headache, sphenopalatine neuralgia, etc.	Unilateral face, ear, jaws, teeth, upper neck	Both sexes, constant dull ache 2–4 h	Compression of common carotid at or below bifurcation reproduces pain in some	Occasionally with cranial arteritis, carotid tumor, migraine and cluster headache	Ergotamine acutely; methysergide for prevention

ularis and ophthalmicus. Both are exceedingly painful in the acute phase of the infection. In the former, herpes of the external auditory meatus and pinna and sometimes of the palate and occipital region, with or without deafness, tinnitus, and vertigo, is combined with facial paralysis. This syndrome, since its original description by Ramsay Hunt, has been generally known as *geniculate herpes,* despite the lack, to this day, of pathologic proof that it depends upon a herpetic lesion of the geniculate ganglion (see Chap. 47). Pain and herpetic eruption due to herpes zoster infection of the gasserian ganglion and the peripheral and central pathways of the trigeminal nerve are practically always limited to the first division (herpes zoster ophthalmicus). We do not recognize a form of zoster infection with facial or other painful states but no cutaneous eruption. The latter will invariably appear within 4 to 5 days after the onset of the pain.

The acute discomfort associated with the herpetic eruption usually subsides after several weeks, or it may linger on for several months. Treatment with vidarabine and acyclovir, along the lines indicated in Chap. 33, will shorten the period of eruption and pain, but neither drug prevents the occurrence of chronic pain. In the elderly as a rule, the pain becomes chronic and intractable. It is described as a constant burning, with superimposed waves of stabbing pain, and the skin in the territory of the preceding eruption is exquisitely sensitive to the slightest stimuli. This unremitting postherpetic neuralgia of long duration represents one of the most difficult pain problems with which the physician has to deal. Some relief of pain may be provided by massage of the affected areas, infiltration with local anesthesia, and application of a mechanical vibrator or by the administration of phenytoin and carbamazepine. In some patients the pain gradually subsides; others can be managed by the administration of antidepressants and tranquilizing agents (amitriptyline, 75 mg at bedtime, and fluphenazine, 1 mg tid) and strong psychologic support. Recently, capsaicin ointments have been marketed, and it is claimed that they reduce the pain. Extensive trigeminal rhizotomy and nucleotomy or other destructive procedures should be avoided, since these surgical measures are not universally successful and may superimpose a diffuse refractory dysesthetic component upon the radicular neuralgia.

OTALGIA

Pain localized in and around one ear is occasionally a primary complaint. This raises a number of different possible causes and mechanisms. Stimulation of cranial nerves V, VII, IX, and X in awake patients during operations all cause ear pain, yet sections of these nerves usually cause no demonstrable loss of sensation in the ear canal or ear itself. The neurosurgical literature cites examples of otalgia that were relieved by section of the nervus intermedius (sensory part of VII) or nerves IX and X. One is prompted to search for a nasopharyngeal tumor or vertebral artery aneurysm in such cases. But when these are eliminated by appropriate studies, there will always remain examples of primary idiopathic otalgia, lower cluster headache, and glossopharyngeal neuralgia. Some patients with common migraine have pain centered in the ear region and occiput, but we have never observed a trigeminal neuralgia in which the ear was the predominant site of pain.

OCCIPITAL NEURALGIA

Paroxysmal pain may occasionally occur in the distribution of the greater or lesser occipital nerves (suboccipital, occipital, and posterior parietal areas). There may be tenderness where these nerves cross the superior nuchal line, but there is no evidence of an occipital nerve lesion in such cases. Carbamazepine may provide some relief. Sectioning of the nerve or the second cervical dorsal root is rarely successful, and several such patients who had these procedures were later referred to us with disabling anesthesia dolorosa. We have advised repeated injections of local anesthetic agents and the use of steroids, traction, local heat, and analgesic and anti-inflammatory drugs.

CAROTIDYNIA

This term was coined by Temple Fay, in 1927, to designate a special type of cervicofacial pain that could be elicited by pressure on the common carotid arteries of patients with "atypical facial neuralgia," or the so-called lower-half headache of Sluder. Compression of the artery in these patients, or mild faradic stimulation at or near the bifurcation, produced a dull ache which was referred to the ipsilateral face, ear, jaws, and teeth, or down the neck. This type of carotid sensitivity occurs rarely as part of cranial (giant-cell) arteritis and during attacks of migraine or cluster headache, and has also been described with displacement of the carotid artery by tumor and dissecting aneurysm of its wall.

A variant of carotidynia, with a predilection for young adults, has been described by Roseman. This syndrome takes the form of recurrent, self-limited attacks, lasting a week or two. During the attack, aggravation of the pain by head movement, chewing, and swallowing is characteristic. This condition is treated with simple analgesics. Yet another variety of carotidynia appears at any stage of adult life and recurs in attacks lasting minutes to hours, in association with throbbing headaches, indistinguishable from common migraine (Raskin and Prusiner). This form responds favorably to the administration of ergotamine, methysergide, and other drugs that are effective in the treatment of migraine.

COSTEN SYNDROME

This refers to a form of craniofacial pain consequent upon dysfunction of one temporomandibular joint. Malocclusion due to ill-fitting dentures or loss of molar teeth on one side, with loss of the normal masticatory movements, may lead to distortion of and ultimately degenerative changes in the joint and to pain behind or in front of the ear with radiation to the temple and over the face. The diagnosis is supported by the findings of tenderness over the joint, crepitus on opening the mouth, and limitation of jaw opening. Management consists of careful adjustment of the bite by a dental surgeon and should be undertaken only when the patient meets the strict diagnostic criteria of this condition. In our experience, many of the diagnoses of Costen syndrome have been erroneous.

"ATYPICAL" FACIAL PAIN

There remains, after all the aforementioned pain syndromes and all the possible intracranial and local sources of pain from throat, mouth, sinuses, orbit, and carotid vessels have been excluded, a small number of patients with pain in the face for which no cause can be found. These patients are most often young women, who describe the pain as constant and unbearably severe, deep in the face, or at the angle of cheek and nose and unresponsive to all varieties of analgesic medication. Because of the failure to identify an organic basis for the pain, one is tempted to attribute it to psychologic or emotional factors or to abnormal personality traits; these can rarely be defined, however, and only a small proportion of the patients satisfy the diagnostic criteria for hysteria or depression. Always to be differentiated from this group is the condition of trigeminal neuropathy, described in Chap. 47. Facial pain of the "atypical" type, like other chronic pain of indeterminate cause, should be managed by the methods outlined in the preceding chapter, and not by thalamotomy, leukotomy, or other forms of destructive cerebral surgery.

OTHER FACIAL PAINS

A number of other types of facial pain syndromes include ciliary, nasociliary, supraorbital, and Sluder neuralgia. These are vague entities at best, and some are merely different descriptive terms given to pains localized around the eye and nose (see "Cluster Headache" above; also Table 9-2). The Tolosa-Hunt syndrome of pain behind the eye and granulomatous involvement of some combination of cranial nerves III, IV, VI and ophthalmic V, responsive to steroids, is discussed in Chap. 47.

Trigeminal neuritis following dental extractions or oral surgery is another vexing problem. There may be sensory loss in the tongue or lower lip and weakness of the masseter or pterygoid muscle. Eventually the patients recover.

Reflex sympathetic dystrophy of the face is another rare form of persistent facial pain that may follow dental surgery or other forms of penetrating injuries to the face. It is characterized by severe burning pain and hyperpathia in response to all types of stimuli. Sudomotor, vasomotor, and trophic changes are lacking, unlike causalgia that affects the limbs. Nevertheless, this form of facial pain responds to repeated blockade or resection of the stellate ganglion.

Under the title of *neck-tongue* syndrome, Lance and Anthony have described the occurrence of a sharp pain and tingling in the upper neck or occiput on sudden rotation of the neck, associated with numbness of the ipsilateral half of the tongue. They attribute the syndrome to stretching of the C2 ventral ramus, which contains proprioceptive fibers from the tongue; these fibers run from the lingual nerve to the hypoglossal nerve and thence to the second cervical root.

REFERENCES

ADAMS CBT, KAYE AH, TEDDY PJ: The treatment of trigeminal neuralgia by posterior fossa microsurgery. J *Neurol Neurosurg Psychiatry* 45:1020, 1982.

ANDERSON CD, FRANK RD: Migraine and tension headache. Is there a physiological difference? *Headache* 21:63, 1981.

BICKERSTAFF ER: Basilar artery migraine. *Lancet* 1:15, 1961.

BLAU JN: Migraine pathogenesis: The neural hypothesis re-examined. *J. Neurol Neurosurg Psychiatry* 47:437, 1984.

BRODERICK JP, SWANSON JW: Migraine-related strokes. *Arch Neurol* 44:868, 1987.

CASTALDO JE, ANDERSEN M, REEVES AG: Middle cerebral artery occlusion with migraine. *Stroke* 13:308, 1982.

DANDY WE: Concerning the cause of trigeminal neuralgia. *Am J Surg* 24:447, 1934.

DORFMAN LS, MARSHALL WH, ENZMANN DR: Cerebral infarction and migraine: Clinical and radiologic correlations. *Neurology* 29:317, 1979.

DRUMMOND PD, LANCE JW: Extracranial vascular changes and the source of pain in migraine headache. *Ann Neurol* 13:32, 1983.

EKBOM K: cited by Kudrow L. (see below).

EKBOM K, GREITZ T: Carotid angiography in cluster headache. *Acta Radiol [Diagn]* 10:177. 1970.

FISHER CM: Late-life migraine accompaniments—further experience. *Stroke* 17:1033, 1986.

GARDNER WJ, STOWELL A, DUTLINGER R: Resection of the greater superficial petrosal nerve in the treatment of unilateral headache. *J Neurosurg* 4:105, 1947.

GLOVER V, SANDLER M, GRANT E: Transitory decrease in platelet monoamine oxidase activity during migraine attacks. *Lancet* 1:391, 1977.

GURALNICK W, KABAN LB, MERRILL RG: Temporomandibular-joint afflictions. *N Engl J Med* 299:123, 1978.

HARDY DG, RHOTON AL JR: Microsurgical relationships of the superior cerebellar artery and the trigeminal nerve. *J Neurosurg* 49:669, 1978.

HEROLD S, GIBBS JM, JONES AKP et al: Oxygen metabolism in classical migraine. *J Cereb Blood Flow Metab* 5(suppl 5):5445, 1985.

KATZ B, BAMFORD CR: Migrainous ischemic optic neuropathy. *Neurology* 35:112, 1985.

KITTRELLE JP, GROUSE DS, SEYBOLD ME: Cluster headache. *Arch Neurol* 42:496, 1985.

KUDROW L: *Cluster Headache: Mechanisms and Management.* Oxford, Oxford University Press, 1980.

KUNKLE EC, PFEIFFER JB, WILHOIT WM, LAMRICK LW: Recurrent brief headaches in "cluster" pattern *NC Med J* 15:510, 1954.

LANCE JW: Headaches related to sexual activity. *J Neurol Neurosurg Psychiatry* 39:1226, 1976.

LANCE JW: *The Mechanism and Management of Headache,* 4th ed. London, Butterworth, 1982.

LANCE JW, ANTHONY M: Some clinical aspects of migraine: A prospective survey of 500 cases. *Arch Neurol* 15:356, 1966.

LANCE JW, ANTHONY M: Neck-tongue syndrome on sudden turning of the head. *J Neurol Neurosurg Psychiatry* 43:97, 1980.

LANCE JW, CURRAN DA: Treatment of chronic tension headache. *Lancet* I:1236, 1964.

LANCE JW, HINTERBERGER H: Symptoms of phecochromocytoma with particular reference to headache, correlated with catecholamine production. *Arch Neurol* 33:281, 1976.

LASHLEY KS: Pattern of cerebral integration indicated by the scotomas of migraine. *Arch Neurol Psychiatry* 46:331, 1941.

LAURITZEN M, OLESON J: Regional cerebral blood flow during migraine attacks by Xenon 133 inhalation and emission tomography. *Brain* 107:447, 1984.

LEAO AAP: Spreading depression of activity in cerebral cortex. *J Neurophysiol* 7:359, 1944.

MOSKOWITZ MA: The neurobiology of vascular head pain. *Ann Neurol* 16:157, 1984.

OLESON J: The ischemic hypothesis of migraine. *Arch Neurol* 44:321, 1987.

OLSEN TS, FRIBERG L, LASSEN NA: Ischemia may be the primary cause of the neurologic defects in classic migraine. *Arch Neurol* 44:156, 1987.

PATTEN J: *Neurological Differential Diagnosis.* London, Harold Starke, 1977.

PRICE RW, POSNER JB: Chronic paroxysmal hemicrania: A disabling headache syndrome responding to indomethacin. *Ann Neurol* 3:183, 1978.

RASCOL A, CAMBIER J, GUIRAUD B et al: Accidents ischémiques cérébraux au cours de crises migraineuses. *Rev Neurologique* 135:867, 1979.

RASKIN NH: Repetitive intravenous dihydroergotamine as therapy for intractable migraine. *Neurology* 36:995, 1986.

RASKIN NH: Pharmacology of migraine. *Ann Rev Pharmacol Toxicol* 21:463, 1981.

RASKIN NH, PRUSINER S: Carotidynia. *Neurology* 27:43, 1977.

ROOKE ED: Benign exertional headache. *Med Clin North Am* 52:801, 1968.

ROSEMAN DM: Carotidynia. *Arch Otolaryngol* 85:103, 1967.

SACHS H, WOLF A, RUSSELL JAG, CHRISTMAN DR: Effect of reserpine on regional cerebral glucose metabolism in control and migraine subjects. *Arch Neurol* 43:1117, 1986.

SAKAI F, MEYER JS: Abnormal cerebrovascular reactivity in patients with cluster headache and migraine. *Headache* 19:257, 1979.

SIGRID H, GIBBS JM, JONES ADP et al: Oxygen metabolism in migraine. *J Cereb Blood Flow Metab* 5:S445, S446, 1985.

SJAASTAD O, DALE I: A new (?) clinical headache entity "chronic paroxysmal hemicrania." *Acta Neurol Scand* 54:140, 1976.

SOMERVILLE BW: The role of estradiol withdrawal in the etiology of menstrual migraine. *Neurology* 22:355, 1972.

SWEET WH, WEPSIC JG: Controlled thermocoagulation of trigeminal ganglion and rootlets for differential destruction of pain fibers. *J Neurosurg* 40:143, 1974.

SWEET WH: The treatment of trigeminal neuralgia (tic douloureux). *N Engl J Med* 315:174, 1986.

SYMONDS CP: Cough headache. *Brain* 79:557, 1956.

VIJAYAN N, DREYFUS PM: Posttraumatic dysautonomic cephalalgia. *Arch Neurol* 32:649, 1975.

WATSON P, STEELE JC: Paroxysmal dysequilibrium in the migraine syndrome of childhood. *Arch Otolaryngol* 99:177, 1974.

WELCH KMA: Migraine: A behavioral disorder. *Arch Neurol* 44:323, 1987.

WHITE JC, SWEET WH: *Pain and the Neurosurgeon.* Springfield, IL, Charles C. Thomas, 1969, p. 265.

WOLFF HG: in Dalessio DJ (ed): *Headache and Other Head Pain,* 5th ed. New York, Oxford, 1987.

ZIEGLER DK, HURWITZ A, HASSANEIN RS et al: Migraine prophylaxis. A comparison of propranolol and amitriptyline. *Arch Neurol* 44:486, 1987.

CHAPTER 10

PAIN IN THE BACK, NECK, AND EXTREMITIES

The diagnosis of pain in these parts of the body often requires the assistance of a neurologist. The task is to determine whether a disease of the spine, intervertebral discs, or articulations has implicated roots and spinal nerves. Their differentiation, however, demands a knowledge of many diseases outside the specialty of neurology. This is a formidable medical challenge, for approximately one of every five adults has back pain at some time or other. The primary disease often falls within the province of the orthopedist, rheumatologist, or internist, and a proper study of such cases requires a knowledge of diseases outside the specialty of neurology.

The purpose of including a chapter on this subject in a textbook of neurology is to help students appreciate the neurologic implications of back and neck pain and assist them in developing a systematic mode of inquiry and method of examination.

Since pains in the lower part of the spine and legs are caused by rather different types of disease than those in the neck, shoulder, and arms, we shall consider them separately.

PAIN IN THE LOWER BACK AND LIMBS

The lower parts of the spine and pelvis, with their massive muscular attachments, are relatively inaccessible to palpation and inspection. Although some physical signs and radiographs are helpful, it is often necessary to depend on the patient's description of the pain (which may not be altogether accurate) and on the patient's behavior during the execution of certain maneuvers, to assess the nature of the problem. Seasoned clinicians, for these reasons, have come to appreciate the need of a systematic clinical approach, the description of which will be preceded by a brief consideration of the anatomy and physiology of the spine.

ANATOMY AND PHYSIOLOGY OF THE LOWER PART OF THE BACK

The bony spine is a complex structure, roughly divisible into an anterior and a posterior part. The former consists of a series of cylindric vertebral bodies, articulated by the intervertebral discs and held together by the anterior and posterior longitudinal ligaments. The posterior elements are more delicate and extend from the bodies as pedicles and laminas which form, with the posterior aspects of the bodies, the vertebral canal. Stout transverse and spinous processes project laterally and posteriorly, respectively, and serve as the origins and insertions of the muscles which support and protect the spinal column. The bony processes are also held together by sturdy ligaments, the most important being the ligamentum flavum. The vertebrae articulate with one another at the apophyseal joints, each vertebra having a superior and inferior facet. Thus the joint is composed of the inferior facet of the vertebra above and the superior facet of the one below (Figs. 10-1 and 10-2). The apophyseal joints, the compressible intervertebral discs, and the collagenous and elastic ligaments permit flexion, extension, and lateral motion of the spine.

The stability of the spine depends on two types of supporting structures, the ligamentous (passive) and muscular (active). Although the ligamentous structures are quite strong, neither they nor the vertebral body-disc complexes have sufficient integral strength to resist the enormous forces that act on the spinal column, and most of the stability of the lower back is dependent on the voluntary and reflex contractions of the sacrospinalis, abdominal, gluteus maximus, and hamstring muscles.

The vertebral and paravertebral structures derive their innervation from the meningeal branches of the spinal nerves (also known as recurrent meningeal or sinuvertebral nerves). The sinuvertebral nerves spring from the posterior division of the spinal nerves just distal to the dorsal root ganglion, reenter the spinal canal through the intervertebral foramina and supply pain fibers to the intraspinal ligaments, periosteum of bone, outer layers of the annulus fibrosus, and capsule of the articular facets. Each of the sinuvertebral

nerves receives fibers from a neighboring gray ramus or directly from a thoracic sympathetic ganglion; the sympathetic nerves contribute only to the innervation of blood vessels and appear to play no part in voluntary and reflex movement. However, they do contain sensory fibers.

Figure 10-1

The fifth lumbar vertebra viewed from above (A) and from the side (B).

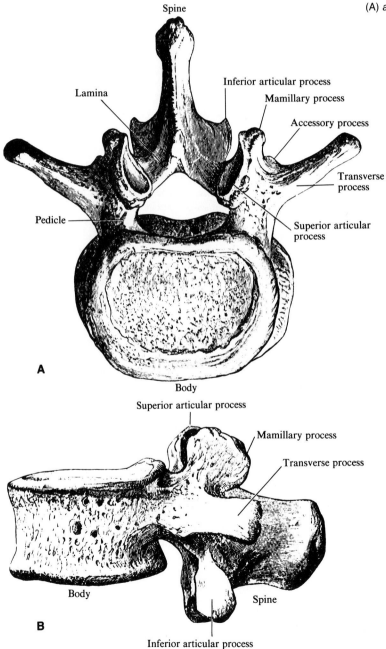

The parts of the back that possess the greatest freedom of movement, and hence are most frequently subject to injury, are the lumbar and cervical. In addition to bending, twisting, and other voluntary movements, many actions of the spine are reflex in nature and are the basis of posture.

Aging Changes in Spinal Structures

Changes in the intervertebral disc tissue and ligaments as a consequence of aging and perhaps minor trauma begin to occur as early as the first part of the third decade. Deposition of collagen and elastin and alterations of glycosaminoglycans combine to decrease the water content of the nucleus pulposus; by measurement, the water content falls from over 90 to 65 percent (Lipson and Muir). The cartilagenous end plate becomes less vascular (Hassler). This dehydrated

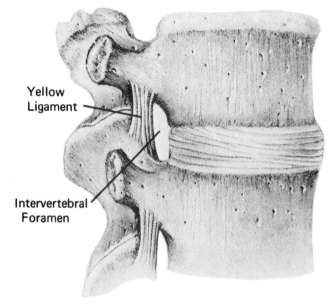

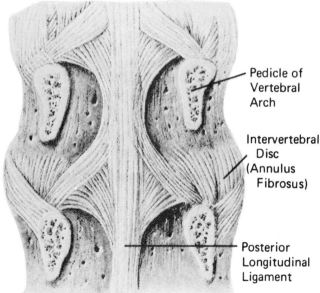

Figure 10-2

The main ligamentous structures of the spine. Buckling of the yellow ligament may compress the nerve roots or the spinal nerve at its origin in the intervertebral foramen, particularly if the foramen is narrowed by osteophytic overgrowth. Fibers of the posterior longitudinal ligament merge with the posteromedial portion of the annulus fibrosus, leaving the posterolateral portion of the annulus relatively unsupported. (From Finneson.)

Yellow Ligament

Intervertebral Foramen

Pedicle of Vertebral Arch

Intervertebral Disc (Annulus Fibrosus)

Posterior Longitudinal Ligament

disc thins out and becomes more fragile. Similar changes occur in the annulus of the disc and ligaments, which fray to an increasing degree in the later decades of adult life, permitting the nucleus pulposus to bulge and, with injury, sometimes to extrude. This process can be followed by MRI, which provides information about the biochemical and structural status of the nucleus. The normal nucleus pulposus has a high signal which is reduced or lost completely as it degenerates. Powell et al examined the lumbar discs in women who had had MR imaging for gynecologic reasons and found an increasing frequency of disc degeneration and bulging, approaching 70 percent by the fiftieth year of life. The shrinking disc changes the alignment of the articular facets and vertebral bodies, leading to hypertrophy of the articular facets and resulting sometimes in facet arthropathy and spur formation. The latter may cause stenosis of the spinal canal and compromise of the lateral recesses and intervertebral canals. Osteoporosis, especially in older women, also increases with age and may result in vertebral flattening or collapse, additionally narrowing the spinal canal.

GENERAL CLINICAL CONSIDERATIONS

Types of Low-Back Pain Of the several symptoms of disease of the spine (pain, stiffness or limitation of movement, and deformity), pain is of foremost importance. Four types of pain may be distinguished: local, referred, radicular, and that arising from secondary (protective) muscular spasm. One identifies these several types of pain by the patient's description; reliance is placed mainly on the character of the pain, its location, and the conditions which modify it.

Local pain is caused by any pathologic process that impinges upon structures containing sensory endings. Involvement of structures that contain no sensory endings is painless. The substance of the vertebral body and intervertebral disc may be destroyed by tumor, for example, without evoking pain, whereas involvement of the periosteum, capsule of apophyseal joints, lumbodorsal fascia, muscles, annulus fibrosus, and ligaments is often exquisitely painful. Swelling of the affected tissues is not apparent if a deep structure of the back is the site of disease. Local pain is often described as steady, and aching, but it may be intermittent and cramp-like. The pain may at times become sharp and, though often diffuse, is always felt in or near the affected part of the spine. Often there is involuntary protective splinting of the corresponding spinal segments by paravertebral muscles, and certain movements or postures that counteract the spasm and alter the position of the injured tissues aggravate or relieve the pain. Firm pressure upon or percussion of superficial structures in the involved region usually evokes tenderness. Muscles that are continually in reflex spasm also become tender and sensitive to deep pressure.

Referred pain is of two types, one that is projected from the spine to viscera and other structures lying within the area of the lumbar and upper sacral dermatomes and another that is projected from pelvic and abdominal viscera to the spine. Pain due to disease of the upper part of the lumbar spine is usually referred to the flank, lumbar region, groin, and anterior thigh. This has been attributed to irritation of the superior cluneal nerves, which are derived from the posterior divisions of the first three lumbar spinal nerves and innervate the superior portions of the buttocks. Pain from the lower part of the lumbar spine is usually referred to the lower buttocks and posterior thighs and is due to irritation of lower spinal nerves, which activate the same pool of intraspinal neurons as the nerves which innervate the posterior thighs. Pain of this type is usually rather diffuse and has a deep, aching quality, but tends at times to be more superficially projected. Kellgren and McCall and his colleagues verified these areas of reference by injecting strong saline solutions into the apophyseal joints. But, as Sinclair et al have pointed out, the sites of reference are inexact and cannot be relied upon for the precise anatomic localization of lesions. In general, the intensity of the referred pain parallels that of the local pain. In other words, maneuvers that alter local pain have a similar effect on referred pain, though not with such precision and immediacy as in "root pain." Usually pain from visceral diseases is felt within the abdomen, flanks, or lumbar region and may be modified by the state of activity of the viscera. Its character and temporal relationships are those of the particular visceral structure involved, and posture and movement of the back have relatively little effect on either the local pain or that referred to the back.

Radicular, or "root" pain, has some of the characteristics of referred pain but differs in its greater intensity, distal radiation, circumscription to the territory of a root, and factors that excite it. The mechanism is stretching, irritation, or compression of a spinal root, within or central to the intervertebral foramen. The pain is sharp, often intense, and usually superimposed on the dull ache of referred pain; it nearly always radiates from a central position near the spine to some part of the lower extremity. Coughing, sneezing, and straining characteristically evoke this sharp radiating pain, although each of them may also jar or move the spine and enhance local pain. In fact, any maneuver that stretches the nerve, e.g., "straight-leg raising," where there is L4, L5, S1 root entrapment, or thigh extension with L3 root entrapment, excites radicular pain;

and jugular vein compression, which raises intraspinal pressure and may cause a shift in position of the root, may have a similar effect. Involvement of L4, L5, and S1 roots, which form the sciatic nerve, causes pain that extends down the posterior aspects of the thigh and the postero- and anterolateral aspects of the leg, into the foot—so-called sciatica. Involvement of the L3 and sometimes L4 root causes pain in the groin and anterior thigh. Paresthesias or superficial sensory loss, soreness of the skin, and tenderness in certain regions along the nerve usually accompany radicular pain. If anterior roots are involved, reflex loss, weakness, atrophy, and fascicular twitching may also occur.

Of importance is the fact that referred pain from the lower back (sometimes called ''pseudoradicular'') does not as a rule project much below the knee and is not accompanied by neurologic change other than a vague numbness without demonstrable sensory impairment. The subcutaneous tissues within the area of referred pain may be tender. Of course, local, referred, and radicular pain may occur together.

Pain resulting from muscular spasm usually occurs in relation to local pain. The spasm is a nocifensive reflexive reaction to protect the diseased parts against injurious motion. Muscle spasm is associated with many disorders of the low back and can distort normal posture. Chronic muscular contraction may give rise to a dull, sometimes cramping ache. One can feel the tautness of the sacrospinalis and gluteal muscles and demonstrate by palpation that the pain is localized to them.

Other pains, often of undetermined origin, are sometimes described by patients with chronic disease of the lower part of the back: drawing and pulling in the legs, cramping sensation (without involuntary muscle spasm), tearing, throbbing, or jabbing pains, and feelings of burning or coldness. These sensations, like paresthesias and numbness, should always suggest the possibility of nerve or root disease.

Since it is often difficult to obtain physical or laboratory confirmation of painful disease of the low back, the importance of an accurate history cannot be overemphasized. In addition to assessing the character and location of the pain, one should determine the factors that aggravate and relieve it, its constancy, and its relationship to activity and rest, posture, and forward bending, and to cough, sneeze, and strain. Frequently the most important lead comes from knowledge of the mode of onset and the circumstances that initiated the pain. Inasmuch as many painful affections of the back are the result of injuries incurred during work or in automobile accidents, the possibility of exaggeration or prolongation of pain for purposes of compensation, or because of hysteria or malingering, must always be kept in mind.

Much information may be gained by *inspection* of the back, buttocks, and lower extremities in various posi-

tions. The normal spine shows a dorsal kyphosis and lumbar lordosis in the sagittal plane, which in some individuals may be somewhat exaggerated (swayback). In the coronal plane, the spine is normally straight or shows a slight curvature, particularly in females. One should observe the spine closely for excessive curvature, list, flattening of the normal lumbar lordosis, presence of a gibbus (a sharp, kyphotic angulation usually indicative of a fracture), pelvic tilt or obliquity, and asymmetry of the paravertebral or gluteal musculature. A sagging gluteal fold suggests an S1 root deficit. In sciatica one may observe a flexed posture of the affected leg, presumably to reduce tension on the irritated nerve.

The next step in the examination is observation of the spine, hips, and legs during certain motions. It is well to remember that no advantage accrues from determining how much pain the patient can tolerate. It is more important to determine when and under what conditions the pain begins. Of considerable value is observation of the patient's natural gait when he is unaware of being watched. One looks for limitation of the natural motions of the patient while standing, sitting, and reclining. When standing, the motion of forward bending normally produces flattening and reversal of the lumbar lordotic curve and exaggeration of the dorsal curve. With lesions of the lumbosacral region that involve the posterior ligaments, articular facets, or sacrospinalis muscles, and with ruptured lumbar discs, protective reflexes prevent stretching of these structures. As a consequence, the sacrospinalis muscles remain taut and prevent motion in the lumbar part of the spine. Forward bending then occurs at the hips and at the thoracolumbar junction; also, the patient bends in such a way as to avoid tensing the hamstring muscles and putting undue leverage on the pelvis. And, in the presence of degenerative disc disease, straightening up from a flexed position is performed with difficulty and only by tucking in and slightly flexing the knees.

Lateral bending is usually less instructive than forward bending. In unilateral ligamentous or muscular strain, bending to the opposite side aggravates the pain by stretching the damaged tissues. With unilateral *sciatica*, the patient lists to one side and strongly resists bending to the opposite side, and, as indicated above, the preferred posture in standing is with the leg slightly flexed at the hip and knee. When the herniated disc lies lateral to the nerve root and displaces it medially, tension on the root is reduced by bending the trunk to the side opposite the lesion; with herniation medial to the root, tension is reduced by inclining the trunk to the side of the lesion.

In the sitting position, flexion of the spine can be performed more easily, even to the point of bringing the knees in contact with the chest. The reason for this is that knee flexion relaxes the often tightened hamstring muscles or relieves stretch of the sciatic nerve. Asking the patient to extend the leg so that the sole of the foot can be inspected is a way of checking for a feigned Lasègue sign (see below).

The study of motions in the reclining position yields much the same information as in the standing and sitting positions. With lumbosacral disc lesions and sciatica, passive lumbar flexion causes little pain and is not limited as long as the hamstrings are relaxed and there is no stretching of the sciatic nerve. With vertebral disease (e.g., arthritis), passive flexion of the hips is free, whereas flexion of the lumbar spine may be impeded and painful. Passive straight-leg raising (possible in normal individuals up to 90° except in those who have unusually tight hamstrings), like forward bending in the standing posture with the legs straight, places the sciatic nerve and its roots under tension, thereby producing pain. It may also cause an anterior rotation of the pelvis around a transverse axis, increasing stress on the lumbosacral joint and thus causing pain if this joint is arthritic or otherwise diseased. Consequently, in diseases of the lumbosacral joints and roots, passive straight-leg raising is limited on the affected side and, to a lesser extent, on the opposite side. Lasègue's sign (pain and limitation of movement during elevation of the leg with knee extended) is a useful indicator of these conditions. Straight raising of the opposite leg may also cause pain on the affected side, believed by some to be an even more reliable sign of prolapsed disc than a Lasègue sign. It is important to remember that the evoked pain is always referred to the diseased side, no matter which leg is elevated. While in the supine position, leg length (anterior-superior iliac spine to medial inalleolus) and the circumference of the thigh and calf should be measured.

Hyperextension may be performed with the patient standing or lying prone. If the condition causing back pain is acute, it may be difficult to extend the spine in the standing position. A patient with lumbosacral strain or disc disease (except in the acute phase) can usually extend or hyperextend the spine without aggravation of pain. If there is an active inflammatory process or fracture of the vertebral body or posterior elements, hyperextension may be markedly limited. In disease of the upper lumbar roots, hyperextension is the motion that is limited and reproduces pain; however, in some cases of lower lumbar disc disease with thickening of the ligamentum flavum, this movement also gives rise to pain. In patients with narrowing of the spinal canal (spondylosis, spondylolisthesis), upright stance and extension may produce neurologic symptoms (see below).

Maneuvers in the lateral decubitus position yield less information as a rule. In cases of sacroiliac joint disease, abduction of the upside leg against resistance reproduces pain in both the sacroiliac region and symphysis pubis; and the pain radiates to the buttock and posterior thigh. Hyperextension of the upside leg with the downside leg flexed is another test for sacroiliac disease. Rotation and abduction of the leg evokes pain in a diseased hip joint. Another helpful maneuver for hip pain is the Patrick test: with the patient supine, the heel of the offending leg is placed on the opposite knee and pain is evoked by depressing the flexed leg.

Gentle palpation and percussion of the spine are the last steps in the examination. It is preferable to first palpate the regions which are the least likely to evoke pain. At all times the examiner should know what structures are being palpated (see Fig. 10-3). Localized tenderness is seldom pronounced in disease of the spine, because the involved structures are so deep. Nevertheless, tenderness of a spinous process (or jarring by gentle percussion) may indicate the presence of inflammation (as in disc space infection), pathologic fracture, or a disc lesion at the site deep to it.

Tenderness over the costovertebral angle often indicates genitourinary disease, adrenal disease, or an injury to the transverse process of the first or second lumbar vertebra [Fig. 10-3, (1)]. Tenderness on palpation of the paraspinal muscles may signify a strain of muscle attachments or injury to the underlying transverse processes of the lumbar vertebrae.

Upon palpation of the spinous processes it is important to note any deviation in the lateral plane (this may be indicative of fracture or arthritis) or in the anteroposterior plane. A "step-off" forward displacement of the spinous process and exaggerated lordosis are important clues to the presence of spondylolisthesis. Tenderness of the interspinous ligaments is indicative of disc lesions [Fig. 10-3, (2)].

Tenderness in the region of the articular facets between the fifth lumbar and first sacral vertebrae is consistent with lumbosacral disc disease [Fig. 10-3, (3)]. Tenderness in this region and in the sacroiliac joints is also a frequent manifestation of ankylosing spondylitis.

Abdominal, rectal, and pelvic examination, in addition to assessment of the integrity of the peripheral vascular systems, are essential elements in the study of the patient with low back symptoms. Neoplastic, inflammatory, or degenerative disorders may produce symptoms referred to the lower part of the spine.

Upon completion of the examination of the back and legs, one turns to a search for motor, reflex, and sensory changes in the lower extremities (see "Protrusion of Lumbar Intervertebral Discs," further on in this chapter).

Laboratory tests often aid in the diagnosis of disorders of the lower spine. Depending on the circumstances, these may include a complete blood count, erythrocyte sedimentation rate (especially helpful in screening for infection or myeloma), measurement of the serum proteins, calcium, phosphorus, uric acid, alkaline phosphatase, acid phosphatase (if one suspects metastatic carcinoma of the prostate), serum protein electrophoresis (myeloma proteins), tuberculin test, agglutination test for *Brucella,* and rheumatoid factor. Radiographs of the lumbar spine should be taken in every case of low-back pain and sciatica, preferably with the patient standing, in the anteroposterior, lateral, and oblique planes. Special spot views or stereoscopic or laminographic films may provide further information in certain cases.

Examination of the spinal canal with a contrast medium (myelogram) may be necessary, especially if a spinal cord tumor is suspected or if a patient thought to have a prolapsed disc fails to improve with conservative measures. This study can be combined with tests of dynamics of the cerebrospinal fluid, and a sample of the fluid should always be removed for cytologic and chemical examination prior to the installation of the contrast medium (preferably metrizamide, which is resorbed). Injection and removal of Pantopaque require special skill and should not be attempted without previous experience with the procedure. If done properly, the procedure has a very low incidence of significant complications.

Increasingly, CT of the spine, with or without metrizamide myelography, and MRI are being utilized. These techniques accurately visualize protruded discs, tumors, etc., and eventually will replace contrast myelography.

The use of epidurography (injection of metrizamide into the epidural space) for the diagnosis of intraspinal lesions not visualized by conventional myelography sometimes reveals a lesion, but the results in our hands have been inconsistent. We have therefore abandoned this method in favor of CT and MRI.

Injection of contrast medium directly into the intervertebral disc (discogram) is a popular procedure in some institutions but is more difficult to interpret than myelography and carries the risk of damage to nerve roots or the introduction of infection. In the authors' opinion, discography is indicated only in special circumstances and should be undertaken only by those who are specialized in its performance. Isotope bone scans are useful in demonstrating tumors and inflammatory processes.

Tests of nerve conduction and EMG are particularly helpful in suspected root and nerve diseases, as will be indicated further on, in the discussion of protruded lumbar discs.

PRINCIPAL CONDITIONS GIVING RISE TO PAIN IN THE LOWER BACK

Congenital Anomalies of the Lumbar Spine Anatomic variations of the spine are frequent, and though rarely of themselves the source of pain and functional derangement, they may predispose an individual to discogenic and spondylotic complications, because of altered mechanics and alignment of the vertebrae or size of the spinal canal.

Figure 10-3

(1) Costovertebral angle. (2) Spinous process and interspinous ligament. (3) Region of articular facet (fifth lumbar to first sacral). (4) Dorsum of sacrum. (5) Region of iliac crest. (6) Iliolumbar angle. (7) Spinous processes of fifth lumbar to first sacral vertebrae (tenderness = faulty posture or occasionally spina bifida occulta). (8) Region between posterior superior and posterior inferior spines. Sacroiliac ligaments (tenderness = sacroiliac sprain, often tender with fifth lumbar to first sacral disc). (9) Sacrococcygeal junction (tenderness = sacrococcygeal injury, i.e., sprain or fracture). (10) Region of sacrosciatic notch (tenderness = fourth to fifth lumbar disc rupture and sacroiliac sprain). (11) Sciatic nerve trunk (tenderness = ruptured lumbar disc or sciatic nerve lesion).

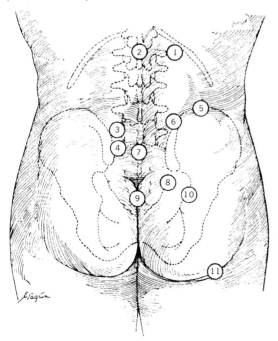

There may be a lack of fusion of the laminae of one or several of the lumbar vertebrae, or of the sacrum (spina bifida). Occasionally, a subcutaneous mass, hypertrichosis, or hyperpigmentation in the sacral area betrays the condition, but in most patients it remains occult until disclosed radiologically. The anomaly may be accompanied by malformation of vertebral joints and usually induces pain only when aggravated by injury. The neurologic aspects of defective fusion of the spine (dysraphism) will be discussed in Chap. 44.

Many congenital anomalies affect the lower lumbar vertebrae: asymmetric facetal joints, abnormalities of the transverse processes, "sacralization" of the fifth lumbar vertebra (in which L5 appears to be fixed to the sacrum), or "lumbarization" of the first sacral vertebra (in which S1 looks like a sixth lumbar vertebra) are seen occasionally in patients with low-back symptoms, but apparently with equal frequency in asymptomatic individuals. Their role in the genesis of low-back derangement is unclear, but in the authors' opinion, they are rarely the cause of specific symptoms.

Spondylolysis consists of a bony defect in the pars interarticularis (a segment near the junction of the pedicle with the lamina) of the lower lumbar vertebrae, probably based on some genetic abnormality. Radiographically, the defect is best visualized on oblique projections. In some individuals it is unilateral; under these circumstances it usually can be traced to single or multiple injuries. In the usual bilateral form, the vertebral body, pedicles, and superior articular facets may move anteriorly, leaving the posterior elements behind. This latter disorder, known as *spondylolisthesis*, is mainly a disease of young people. It may cause little difficulty at first, but eventually becomes symptomatic. The patient complains of pain in the low back, radiating into the thighs, and limitation of motion. Examination discloses tenderness near the segment that has "slipped" (most often L5, occasionally L4), a palpable "step" of the upper spinous processes forward from the segment below, hamstring spasm, and, in severe cases (spondyloptosis), shortening of the trunk and protrusion of the lower abdomen (both of which result from the abnormal forward shift of L5 on S1), and signs of involvement of spinal roots—paresthesias and sensory loss, muscle weakness, and reflex impairment.

Sometimes, the fourth lumbar vertebra may slip forward on the fifth, narrowing the spinal canal, without the presence of a defect in the pars interarticularis. This is spoken of as *intact arch spondylolisthesis* and occurs most often in middle-aged or elderly women. This form of spondylolisthesis is probably due to degenerative disease of the inferior and superior facets. It causes severe low-back pain, made worse by standing or walking and relieved by bed rest. Symptoms of root compression are common. According to Alexander et al, such patients should be treated with laminectomy and medial facetectomy.

Traumatic Disorders of the Low Back Traumatic disorders constitute the most frequent cause of low-back pain; these will be touched upon only briefly, for they are mainly the concern of the orthopedist. In severe acute injuries, the examiner must be careful to avoid further damage. All movements must be kept to a minimum until an approximate diagnosis has been made and adequate measures have been instituted for the proper care of the patient. If the patient complains of pain in the back and cannot move the legs, the spine may have been fractured and the cord compressed or crushed. The neck should not be flexed, and the patient should not be allowed to sit up. (See Chap. 36 for further discussion of spinal cord injury.)

Sprains and strains The terms *lumbosacral strain, sprain,* and *derangement* are used loosely by most physicians, and it is probably not possible to differentiate them. What was formerly referred to as sacroiliac strain or sprain is now known to be due, in many instances, to disc disease. The authors prefer the term "acute low-back or myofascial strain" for minor, self-limited injuries that are usually associated with lifting heavy loads in a mechanically disadvantaged position, a fall, or sudden unexpected motion, as may occur in an auto accident. Sometimes these syndromes are more chronic in nature, being regularly exacerbated by a modicum of bending or lifting and suggesting that postural, muscular, or arthritic factors may play a role.

The discomfort of low-back strain is often severe, and the patient may assume unusual postures related to spasm of the sacrospinalis muscles. The pain is usually confined to the lower part of the back, in the midline or just to one side or another of the spine. The diagnosis of lumbosacral strain depends upon the description of the injury or activity that precipitated the pain, the localization of the pain, the finding of localized tenderness, augmentation by postural changes, e.g., standing up from a sitting position, and alleviation of pain by bed rest, ice massage of the painful area, and nonsteroidal antiflammatory agents. The pain may be relieved by local infiltration of an anesthetic agent, a finding that is also helpful in diagnosis. Sacroiliac strain may seem the most likely diagnosis when there is tenderness over the sacroiliac joint and pain radiating to the buttock and posterior thigh. It is characteristically worsened by abduction of the thigh against resistance and is also felt in the symphysis pubis. It, too, responds to conservative management.

Vertebral fractures Fractures of a lumbar vertebral body are usually the result of flexion injuries. Such trauma may occur in a fall or jump from a height (if the patient lands on the feet, the calcanei may also be fractured) or as a result of auto accidents or other violence. When fractures occur with minimal trauma (or spontaneously), the bone has presumably been weakened by some pathologic process. Most of the time, particularly in older individuals, osteoporosis is the cause of such an event, but there are many other causes, including osteomalacia, hyperparathyroidism, hyperthyroidism, myeloma, metastatic carcinoma, and a number of local conditions. Spasm of the lower lumbar muscles, limitation of movements of the lumbar section of the spine, and the radiographic appearance of the damaged lumbar portion (with or without neurologic abnormalities) are the basis of clinical diagnosis. The pain is usually immediate, though occasionally it may be delayed for days.

Fractured transverse processes, which are almost always associated with tearing of the paravertebral muscles, cause deep tenderness at the site of the injury, local muscle spasm on one side, and limitation of all movements which stretch the lumbar muscles. The radiologic findings confirm the diagnosis. In some circumstances, tears of the paravertebral musculature may be associated with extensive bleeding in the retroperitoneal space and profound shock.

Protrusion of Lumbar Intervertebral Disc This condition is a major cause of severe and chronic or recurrent low-back and leg pain. It is most likely to occur between the fifth lumbar and first sacral vertebrae, and, with lessening frequency, between the fourth and fifth, third and fourth, second and third, and first and second lumbar vertebrae. Rare in the thoracic portion of the spine, disc disease is again frequent at the fifth and sixth and sixth and seventh cervical vertebrae (see further on).

The cause of a protruded lumbar disc is usually a flexion injury, but in a considerable proportion of patients no traumatic episode is recalled. Degeneration of the nucleus pulposus, the posterior longitudinal ligaments, and the annulus fibrosus, which occurs in most adults of middle and advanced years, may have taken place silently or have been manifested by mild, recurrent lumbar ache. A sneeze, lurch, or other trivial movement may then cause the nucleus pulposus to prolapse, pushing the frayed and weakened annulus posteriorly. In more severe cases of disc disease, the nucleus may protrude through the annulus or become extruded and lie as a free fragment in the vertebral canal. Fragments of the nucleus pulposus protrude through rents in the annulus, usually to one side or the other (sometimes centrally), where they impinge upon a root or roots. The latter are compressed against the articular apophysis or adjacent ligament between the articular processes (ligamentum flavum) or, at the lumbar-sacral junction, against the lumbosacral ligament. The protruded material may be resorbed to some extent and become reduced in size, but often it does not, causing chronic irritation of the root or a discarthrosis with posterior osteophyte formation.

The fully developed syndrome of prolapsed intervertebral lumbar disc consists of (1) a stiff, deformed spine, (2) pain radiating into the thigh, calf, and foot, and (3) some combination of paresthesias, weakness, and reflex impairment.

The pain of protruded intervertebral disc is of several types. First there are the spontaneous pains that range from a mild discomfort to the most severe knife-like stabs, radiating the length of the leg and superimposed on a constant intense ache. With the most acute injury the patient must stay in bed, avoiding the slightest movement; a cough, sneeze, or strain is intolerable. The patient is usually most comfortable lying on his or her back with legs flexed at the knees and hips (dorsal decubitus position) and with the shoulders raised on pillows to obliterate the lumbar lordosis. A particular lateral decubitus position may be more comfortable. When the condition is less severe, walking is possible, though fatigue sets in quickly, with a feeling of heaviness and pulling pains. Sitting may be particularly painful. The pain is usually located deep in the buttock, just lateral to and below the sacroiliac joint, and in the posterolateral region of the thigh, with radiation to the calf, heel, and other parts of the foot.

Pain may be characteristically provoked by pressure over the L5 and S1 vertebral spines and along the course of the sciatic nerve at the classic points of Valleix (sciatic notch, retrotrochanteric gutter, posterior surface of thigh, head of fibula). Pressure at one point may cause pain and tingling to radiate down the leg. Elongation of the nerve root by straight-leg raising or by flexing the leg at the hip and extending it at the knee (Lasègue maneuver) is the most consistent of all signs in provoking pain. When the sciatica is severe, straight-leg raising is restricted to 20 to 30°; when less severe, or with improvement, the angle formed by the leg and bed widens, finally to 90° in patients with flexible backs and limbs. The same maneuver with the healthy leg evokes a lesser degree of pain, but always on the side of the spontaneous pain (Fajerstagn sign). The presence of a crossed straight-leg-raising sign is strongly indicative of a ruptured disc as a cause of sciatica (in 56 of 58 cases in the series of Hudgkins). With the patient standing, forward bending of the trunk will cause flexion of the knee on the affected side (Neri sign); the degree of limitation of forward bending approximates that of straight-leg raising. Forced flexion of the head and neck may provoke the sciatica, as does pressure on both jugular veins, a maneuver which increases the intraspinal pressure (Naffziger sign). Marked inconsistencies in response to these tests raise the suspicion of psychologic factors.

In the upright position the posture of the body is altered by the pain. The patient stands with the affected leg slightly flexed at the knee and hip, so that only the ball of the foot rests on the floor. The trunk tends to tilt forward and to one side or the other, depending on the relationship of the protruded disc material to the root (see above). This posture is referred to as "sciatic scoliosis." These antalgic postures are maintained by reflex contraction of the paraspinal muscles which can be both seen and palpated. In walking, the knee is slightly flexed, and weight bearing on the painful leg is brief and cautious, giving a limp. Ascending and descending stairs are particularly painful.

The signs of spinal root involvement are hypotonia, loss or impairment of sensation and tendon reflexes, and muscle weakness. The hypotonia is evident on inspection and palpation of the buttock and calf, and the Achilles tendon tends to be less salient. Paresthesias (rarely hyperesthesia or hypoesthesia) are frequent; they are felt in the foot, usually, sometimes in the leg. Less often there is a diminution of pain perception over the appropriate dermatome(s). Muscle weakness is exceptional. The ankle or knee jerk is usually diminished or lost on the side of the lesion. Bilaterality of symptoms and signs is rare, as is sphincteric paralysis, but they may occur with large central protrusions. The CSF protein is often elevated (50 to 100 mg/dL).

Herniations of the intervertebral lumbar discs most often occur between the fifth lumbar and first sacral vertebrae (compressing the S1 root; see Fig 10-4) and between the fourth and fifth lumbar vertebrae (compressing the L5 root), respectively. It is important therefore to recognize the clinical characteristics of root compression at these two sites. *Lesions of the fifth lumbar root* produce pain in the region of the hip, groin, posterolateral thigh, lateral calf to the external malleolus, dorsal surface of the foot, and the first or second and third toes. Paresthesias may be felt in the entire territory or only in its distal parts. The tenderness is in the lateral gluteal region and near the head of the femur. Weakness, if present, involves the extensors of the big toe and of the foot. The ankle jerk may be lost or diminished (more often it is normal) but hardly ever the knee jerk. Walking on the heels may be more difficult and uncomfortable than walking on the toes, because of weakness of dorsiflexion.

With *lesions of the first sacral root* the pain is felt in the midgluteal region, posterior part of the thigh, posterior region of the calf to the heel, outer plantar surface of the foot and fourth and fifth toes. Tenderness is most pronounced over the midgluteal region (in the region of the sacroiliac joint), posterior thigh areas, and calf. Paresthesias and sensory loss are mainly in the lower part of the leg and outer toes, and weakness, if present, involves the flexor muscles of the foot and toes, abductors of the toes, and hamstring muscles. The Achilles reflex is diminished or absent in the majority of cases. In fact, loss of the Achilles reflex is often the first and only objective sign. Walking on the toes is more difficult and uncomfortable than walking on the heels, because of weakness of the plantar flexors.

The *rarer lesions of the third and fourth lumbar roots* give rise to pain in the anterior part of the thigh and knee and medial part of the leg (fourth lumbar) with corresponding sensory loss. The knee jerk is diminished or abolished.

Rarer still are protrusions of thoracic intervertebral discs (0.5 percent of all surgically verified disc protrusions, according to Love and Schorn). The four lowermost thoracic interspaces are the most frequently involved. Trauma, particularly hard falls on the heels or buttocks, is an important causative factor. Paresthesias below the level of the lesion, loss of sensation, both deep and superficial, and paraparesis or paraplegia are the usual clinical manifestations. Careful myelography is the most important diagnostic maneuver.

Frequently, a herniated disc at one interspace involves more than one root (Fig. 10-4), and it follows that the symptoms will then reflect involvement of two roots. Anomalies of the lumbosacral roots may lead to errors in localization (see descriptions by Postaccini et al). The combined rupture of two or more discs occurs occasionally and further complicates the clinical picture.

Low-back pain may also be caused by degeneration of the intervertebral disc, without frank extrusion of disc tissue. Or the herniation may occur into the adjacent vertebral body, giving rise to a so-called Schmorl nodule. In such cases there are no signs of nerve root involvement, although back pain may be present, sometimes referred to the thigh.

All or part of the above syndromes may be present. Back pain may be present with little or no leg pain; sometimes back pain will disappear and only limb pain and neurologic loss persist; rarely only leg pain will be experienced from the beginning.

When all components of the syndrome are present the diagnosis is easy, but most neurologists prefer to corroborate their clinical impression by CT scans or MR imaging of the L3-S1 spine, with or without contrast myelography. Usually this will demonstrate the protruding disc at the suspected site and also will rule out protrusions at other sites or an unsuspected tumor (Fig. 10-5). Raskin reports CT scanning to be comparable to contrast myelography in visualizing disc tissue and better in distinguishing it from scar tissue. At the lumbosacral junction there may be a wide gap between the posterior margins of the vertebrae and the dural sac, so that a laterally or centrally protruded L5-S1 disc may fail to indent the Pantopaque column. In this situation (and in others where myelography presents technical difficulties) nerve conduction studies and the EMG are useful, as has been indicated above. In fact, we are resorting to electrical studies in the majority of our patients and find, as do Leyshon et al, that they are positive in over 90 percent of cases. Loss or marked asymmetry of the H reflex is a particularly useful sign of S1 radiculopathy. The finding of denervation potentials in the paraspinal muscles (indicating root rather than peripheral nerve lesions) and in other muscles in a root distribution is also helpful, provided that at least 3 weeks has elapsed from the onset of root pain.

Far more difficult is the problem of patients who have had a disc removed but still have back and leg pain (*failed back syndrome*). First one must exclude by myelography and additional studies the possibility of having overlooked a far lateral disc herniation or the extrusion of more disc material at the original site or at another level. Or tomograms may show a foraminal stenosis, or less frequently, a unilateral facet hypertrophy or a congenital or acquired spinal stenosis (see further on), each of which may be surgically correctable. All too often, however, careful study discloses none of these abnormalities, and further exploration reveals only a slight thickening of the arachnoid and adhesions around the roots ("arachnoiditis") or focal epidural scarring with radiculopathy. This subject has been reviewed by Quiles and Marchisello and by Long and has been the subject of a symposium, listed in the references. Freeing the roots from adhesions and fusion of the spine benefits only a minority of such patients, and often both donor and recipient sites of the bone graft become additional sources of pain. Further surgery in patients with no demonstrable disc protrusion should be avoided. It is far better to settle litigation if any is pending, to use nonaddicting pain medication, and to encourage the resumption of activities through a progressive exercise schedule designed to strengthen the abdominal and lumbar

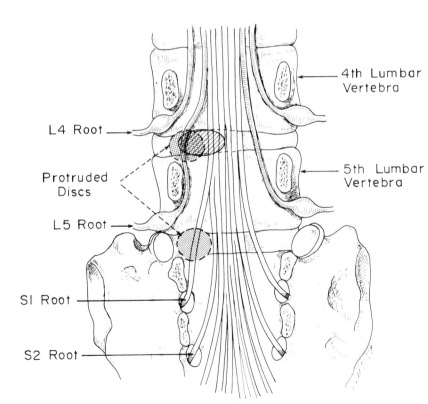

Figure 10-4

Mechanisms of compression of the fifth lumbar and first sacral roots. A lateral disc protrusion at the L4-L5 level usually involves the fifth lumbar root and spares the fourth; a protrusion at L5-S1 involves the first sacral root and spares the fifth lumbar root. Note that a more medially placed disc protrusion at the L4-L5 level may involve the fifth lumbar root as well as the first (or second and third) sacral root.

4th Lumbar Vertebra

5th Lumbar Vertebra

L4 Root

Protruded Discs

L5 Root

S1 Root

S2 Root

muscles. Overweight patients should be urged to lose weight. Tricyclic antidepressants and nonsteroidal anti-inflammatory medications may reduce pain.

OTHER CAUSES OF LOW-BACK PAIN AND SCIATICA

An increasing experience with lumbar back pain, gluteal neuralgia, and sciatica has impressed the authors with the large number of such cases that are unsolvable. Once all these cases were classified as sciatic neuritis or ''sacroiliac strain.'' After Mixter and Barr popularized the concept of ruptured disc, all sciatica and lumbar pain were ascribed to this condition. Operations became widely practiced, not only for frank disc protrusion but also for ''hard discs'' (unruptured) and related pathologies of the spine. The surgical results have become less and less satisfactory, until now in large referral centers, more patients are being seen with postlaminectomy pain than with ruptured discs. To explain these chronic pain cases a number of new pathologic entities, some of uncertain status, have been described. Entrapment of lumbar roots appears not only to be the consequence of disc rupture but also of spondylotic spurs with stenosis of the lateral recess, hypertrophy of apophyseal facets, and arachnoiditis.

Symptoms due to spondylotic spurs and lateral recess stenosis need to be distinguished from those of herniated disc. Disabling pain in one or both legs on standing and walking, relieved by squatting and lying down, with variable motor deficit and reflex and sensory root changes were present in the 35 cases reported by Mikhael et al. Radiologically there was stenosis at one vertebral level. Most often the superior facet of L5 narrowed the lateral recess at the upper border of the pedicle, compressing L5 root and sometimes S1 as well. In polytomograms, the lateral recess was reduced to less than 3 to 4 mm. This condition is more properly designated as a unilateral lumbar spondylosis, or in some instances a spondylolysis. The adjacent articular

Figure 10-5

A. *T1-weighted sagittal MR image showing a large herniated disc at L5-S1. B. FLASH sagittal MR image showing herniated disc (arrow) at C6-C7.*

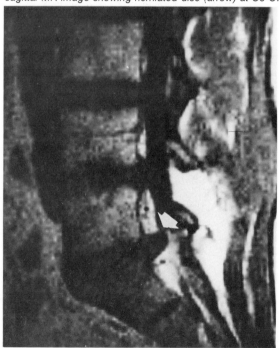

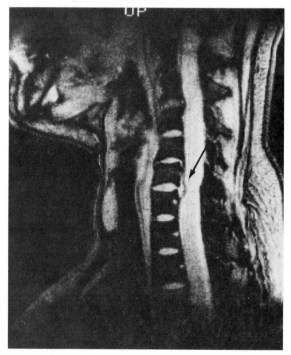

A

B

capsules may suffer injury and add direct and referred pains to a radicular syndrome. Intra-articular lidocaine relieves the pain according to some orthopedists. (See below and Chap. 36 for discussion of the lumbar stenosis syndrome.)

The *unilateral facet syndrome* is closely related to the preceding condition. Reynolds et al observed this in 22 patients in whom there was a lumbar monoradiculopathy indistinguishable from that of a ruptured disc. Sixteen had an L5 radiculopathy, three an S1 radiculopathy, and three an L4 radiculopathy; in 15 there was coexisting back pain. At operation the spinal root was compressed against the floor of the intervertebral canal by an inferior or superior facet. Foraminotomy and facetectomy, after exploration of the root from the dural sac to the pedicle, relieved the pain in 12 of the 15 operated cases. Denervation of lumbar facets by radio frequency electrodes (percutaneous rhizolysis) introduced percutaneously onto nerves supplying the zygoapophyseal joints has been proposed. Collier reported relief in 35 of 122 such patients, but there is considerable doubt as to whether this was due to the rhizolysis or to some other effect.

A surprising finding in myelography is a loculated, cyst-like dilatation of the perineurial sheath, projecting into the intervertebral canal. This may involve multiple lumbar or cervical roots and is sometimes associated with radicular symptoms. There are surgical reports of relief from opening the cyst and freeing the roots.

These are but a few of the large number of spinal abnormalities disclosed by newer radiologic techniques. An atlas of these and others (congenital and developmental stenosis, degenerative disease, Paget disease, zygoapophyseal joint abnormalities, spondylolisthesis) are admirably presented in the symposium on computerized tomography of the lumbar spine (listed in the references under ''Symposium'').

Lumbar adhesive arachnoiditis has also received increasing attention. This is a vague entity in which the arachnoid membrane is thickened and opaque in the vicinity of the cauda equina. The term is also applied to thickening of the sheaths around roots (normally they have no perineurium or epineurium). It can be seen in lumbar myelograms where the contrast material fails to outline the roots and flow freely in the subarachnoid space. According to a British review, lumbar arachnoiditis is rare, being seen in only 80 of 7600 myelograms. Judging by the American literature, it is much more frequent (see under ''Symposium,'' in the References). The usual clinical features are intractable pain and leg pain with combinations of neurologic abnormalities referable to lumbar spinal roots. In our patients, multiple Pantopaque myelograms, uncomplicated disc rupture, operative procedures, infections, and subarachnoid blood have been involved. The syndromes are inseparable from those of discogenic disease. The treatment is unsatisfactory. Operation to lyse adhesions and intrathecal steroids have been of no value.

Finally one must not overlook the possible occurrence of a *lumbosacral plexus neuritis*, a disorder akin to brachial neuritis, and acute or subacute sciatic neuropathy in the diabetic, either of which may produce a syndrome similar to that of ruptured disc (see Chap. 46).

OSTEOARTHRITIS OR OSTEOARTHROPATHY

This, the most frequent type of arthritic disease, usually occurs in later life and may involve all or any part of the spine. It is most prevalent in the cervical and lumbar regions, however, where it is sometimes confused with the discogenic syndromes described above. The pain is centered in the affected part of the spine, is increased by movement, and is associated with stiffness and limitation of motion. There is a notable absence of systemic symptoms such as fatigue, malaise, and fever, and the pain can usually be relieved by rest. A slightly flexed posture is preferred. The sitting position is the most comfortable one. There are no neurologic signs except when associated with disc disease. The severity of the symptoms often bears little relation to the radiologic findings; pain may be present despite minimal radiographic findings, and conversely, marked osteophytic overgrowth with spur formation, ridging, bridging of vertebrae, narrowing of disc spaces, subluxation of posterior joints on flexion, and air in the disc spaces can be seen in both symptomatic and asymptomatic persons.

In the lumbar region, osteoarthritic or spondylotic changes, superimposed on a smaller-than-normal spinal canal, may lead to compression of the caudal roots—so-called *spondylotic caudal radiculopathy* or *lumbar stenosis syndrome*. The roots are actually caught between the posterior surface of the vertebral body and the ligamentum flavum posterolaterally. Upon standing or walking (downhill walking is especially difficult), there is a gradual onset of numbness and weakness of the legs, which forces the patient to sit down. In more severe cases the patient gains relief by lying down with legs flexed at the hips and knees. Usually the numbness begins in one leg, spreads to the other, and ascends as standing or walking continue. Tendon reflexes may disappear, only to return on flexing the spine. Pain in the low back is variable. Disturbances of micturition and impotence are rare. Some patients with lumbar stenosis have neurologic symptoms which persist without relation to body position. The clinical picture, with its intermittency, corresponds to the so-called intermittent claudication of the cauda equina described in 1948, by van Gelderen. It was shown by Verbiest to be due not to ischemia, but to encroachment on the cauda by hypertrophied apophyseal joints, thickened ligaments, and small protrusions of disc material engrafted upon a canal that is developmentally shallow in the anteroposterior diameter. Sometimes a slight subluxation at L3-L4 or at L4-L5 is also present. Later it was shown that the canal in these cases is also narrow from side to side (reduced interpedicular distance radiographically). Decompression of the spinal canal relieves the symptoms in a considerable proportion of the cases.

Spondylotic caudal radiculopathy is the lumbar equivalent of spondylotic cervical myelopathy and radiculopathy. Insofar as the format is a cauda equina syndrome, its differential diagnosis will be discussed in Chap. 36, "Diseases of the Spinal Cord."

Ankylosing Spondylitis This disorder, also called Marie-Strümpell arthritis, affects young males predominantly. The main complaint is pain, usually centered in the low back, at least in the initial stages of the disease. Often it radiates to the back of the thighs and groin. At first the symptoms are vague (tired back, "catches" up and down the back, sore back), and the diagnosis may be overlooked for many years. Although the pain is recurrent, limitation of movement is constant and progressive, and over time dominates the picture. Early in the course, this is experienced as "morning stiffness" or an increase in stiffness after periods of inactivity; these findings may be present long before radiologic changes are manifest. Rarely, a cauda equina syndrome may complicate ankylosing spondylitis, the result apparently of an inflammatory reaction and later a proliferation of connective tissue in the caudal canal (Mathews). Limitation of chest expansion, tenderness over the sternum, and decreased motion and tendency to flexion of the hips may be present early in the course of the disease. The radiologic hallmarks are at first destruction and subsequently obliteration of the sacroiliac joints, followed by bony bridging of the vertebral bodies to produce the characteristic "bamboo spine." When this occurs, the pain usually subsides, but the patient has little motion of the back and neck. Ankylosing spondylitis may also accompany the Reiter syndrome, psoriasis, and inflammatory diseases of the intestine (see also Chap. 36).

Occasionally ankylosing spondylitis is complicated by destructive vertebral lesions. This complication should be suspected whenever the pain returns, after a period of quiescence, or becomes localized. The cause of these lesions is not known, but they may represent a response to nonunion of fractures, taking the form of an excessive production of fibrous inflammatory tissue. Rarely there is collapse of a vertebral segment and compression of the spinal cord. Ankylosing spondylitis, when severe, may involve both hips, greatly accentuating the back deformity and disability.

Rheumatoid arthritis, when it affects the spine, is localized to the cervical region, and is considered further on in this chapter.

Destructive Diseases of the Spine *Infections, neoplastic and metabolic diseases* Metastatic carcinoma (breast, bronchus, prostate, thyroid, kidney, stomach, uterus), multiple myeloma, and reticulum-cell sarcoma are the common malignant tumors that involve the spine. Since the primary lesion may be small and asymptomatic, the presenting complaint caused by these or other tumors may be pain in the back due to metastatic deposits. The pain is described as constant and dull; it is often unrelieved by rest and may be worse at night. At the time of onset of the back pain there may be no radiographic changes, but when they appear they usually take the form of destructive lesions in one or several vertebral bodies with only limited involvement of the disc space, even in the face of a compression fracture. Before such destructive changes become evident, an isotope scan may be helpful in detecting areas of osteoblastic activity due to neoplastic or inflammatory disease.

Infection of the vertebral column is usually the result of pyogenic organisms (staphylococci or coliform bacilli) or tuberculosis. The patient complains of pain in the back, of subacute or chronic nature, which is exacerbated by movement but not materially relieved by rest. Motion becomes limited, and there is tenderness over the spine in the involved segments and pain with jarring of the spine, as occurs with walking on the heels. Usually, these patients are afebrile and do not have a leukocytosis. The erythrocyte sedimentation rate is usually elevated. Radiographs may demonstrate narrowing of a disc space with erosion and destruction of the two adjacent vertebrae. A soft tissue mass may be present, indicating an abscess, which may, in the case of tuberculosis, drain spontaneously, at sites quite remote from the vertebral column.

Special mention should be made of *spinal epidural abscess*, which necessitates urgent surgical treatment. This is usually due to staphylococci, sometimes to *Pseudomonas*, which may be introduced by a contaminated lumbar puncture needle. The main symptom is localized pain, occurring spontaneously and intensified by percussion and pressure upon the vertebral spines; the pain may have a radicular radiation. A rapidly developing flaccid paraplegia appearing in a febrile patient should suggest compression of the spinal cord by epidural abscess. A noninflammatory form of acute epidural compression may be due to hemorrhage (anticoagulant therapy, vascular malformations) and, in the cervical region, to rheumatoid arthritis (see further on).

In so-called *metabolic bone disease* (osteoporosis of

either the postmenopausal or senile type, or osteomalacia), a considerable loss of bone substance may occur without any symptoms whatsoever. Many patients with such conditions do, however, complain of aching in the lumbar or thoracic area and a few have brief paroxysms of pain accompanied by spasms of the muscles of the lower back. This is most likely to occur following an injury, sometimes of trivial degree, which leads to collapse or wedging of a vertebra. Certain movements greatly enhance the pain, and certain positions relieve it. One or more spinal roots may be involved. *Paget disease of the spine* may be associated with aching in the lumbar or thoracic areas; or it may be painless. Occasionally, it may lead to compression of the spinal cord or nerve roots. Patients thought to have neoplastic, infectious, or metabolic disease of the spine need to be thoroughly evaluated by means of radiographs, bone scans, and myelography where indicated, as well as by other laboratory studies.

Referred Pain from Visceral Disease Pain due to disease of the pelvic, abdominal, or thoracic viscera is often referred to the spine. Occasionally back pain may be the first and only symptom. The general rule is that the pain of pelvic disease is referred to the sacral region, lower abdominal disease to the lumbar region (centering around the second to fourth lumbar vertebrae), and upper abdominal disease to the lower thoracic spine (eighth thoracic to the first and second lumbar vertebrae). Characteristically there are no local signs or stiffness of the back, and a full range of motion is possible, without augmentation of the pain. However, some positions, e.g., flexion of the lumbar spine in the lateral recumbent position, may be more comfortable than others.

Low thoracic–upper lumbar back pain in abdominal disease Peptic ulceration and tumor of the stomach and duodenum most typically induce pain in the epigastrium; but if the posterior stomach wall is involved, particularly if there is retroperitoneal extension, the pain may be felt in the dorsal spine, centrally or to one side or in both locations. If very intense, it may seem to encircle the body. The back pain tends to reflect the characteristics of the pain from the affected organ; e.g., if due to peptic ulceration, it appears about 2 h after a meal and is relieved by food and antacids.

Diseases of the pancreas are apt to cause pain in the back, being more to the right of the spine if the head of the pancreas is involved and to the left if the body and tail are implicated.

Retroperitoneal neoplasms, e.g., lymphomas, sarcomas, and carcinomas, may evoke pain in the dorsal or lumbar spine with a tendency to radiate to the lower part of the abdomen, groins, and anterior thighs. A tumor in the iliopsoas region often produces a unilateral lumbar ache with radiation toward the groin and labia or testicle; there

may also be signs of involvement of the upper lumbar spinal roots. An aneurysm of the abdominal aorta may induce pain that is localized to an analogous region of the spine.

The sudden appearance of lumbar pain in a patient receiving anticoagulants should arouse the suspicion of retroperitoneal bleeding.

Inflammatory diseases and neoplasms of the colon cause pain that may be felt in the lower abdomen or in the midlumbar region, or in both places. If very intense, the pain may have a belt-like distribution. Pain from a lesion in the transverse colon or first part of the descending colon may be central or left-sided, and its level of reference is to the second and third lumbar vertebrae. If the sigmoid colon is implicated, the pain is lower, in the upper sacral spine and anteriorly in the midline suprapubic region or left lower quadrant of the abdomen.

Sacral pain in pelvic (urologic and gynecologic) diseases Gynecologic disorders often manifest themselves by back pain, but their diagnosis is seldom difficult. Thorough abdominal palpation, vaginal and rectal examination, supplemented by certain laboratory procedures (sigmoidoscopy, barium enema, pyelography, CT body scan, and culdoscopy), usually disclose the source of pain.

The uterosacral ligaments are the most important pelvic source of chronic back pain. Endometriosis or carcinoma of the uterus (body or cervix) may invade these structures, causing pain that is localized to the sacrum below the lumbosacral joint either centrally or more on one side. In endometriosis the pain begins during the premenstrual phase and often merges with menstrual pain which also may be felt in the sacral region. Malposition of the uterus (retroversion, descensus, and prolapse) characteristically gives rise to sacral pain, especially after the patient has been standing for several hours. Postural adjustments may also evoke pain here when a fibroma of the uterus pulls on the uterosacral ligaments. Low-back pain with radiation into one or both thighs is a common phenomenon during the last weeks of pregnancy.

Pain due to carcinomatous implication of nerve plexuses is continuous and becomes progressively more severe; it tends to be more intense at night. The primary lesion may be inconspicuous, being overlooked on pelvic examination. Papanicolaou smears and an intravenous pyelogram are the most useful diagnostic procedures. Radiation therapy of these tumors may produce sacral pain consequent to swelling and necrosis of tissue, the so-called radiation phlegmon of the pelvis.

Carcinoma of the prostate with metastases to the

lower part of the spine is a common cause of sacral or lumbar pain and may present without urinary symptoms. Spinal nerves may be infiltrated by the tumor, or the spinal cord itself may be compressed if the epidural space is invaded. The diagnosis is established by rectal examination, spine films, and measurement of acid phosphatase (particularly the prostatic phosphatase fraction). Chronic prostatitis, evidenced by prostatic discharge, burning and frequency of urination, and slight reduction in sexual potency, may be attended by a nagging sacral ache; the latter may be mainly on one side, with radiation into one leg if the seminal vesicle is involved on that side. Lesions of the bladder and testes are usually not accompanied by back pain. When the kidney is the site of disease, the pain is ipsilateral, being felt in the flank or lumbar region.

Obscure Types of Low-Back Pain and the Question of Psychiatric Disease A safe rule is to assume that all patients who complain of low-back pain have some type of primary or secondary disease of the spine and its supporting structures or of the abdominal or pelvic viscera. However, even after careful examination there remains a group of patients in whom no pathologic basis can be found for the back pain. Two categories can be recognized: one with postural back pain and another with psychiatric illness, but there are others in whom the diagnosis remains obscure.

Postural back pain Many slender, asthenic individuals and some fat, middle-aged ones have chronic discomfort in the back, and the pain interferes with effective work. The physical examination is negative except for slack musculature and poor posture. The pain is diffuse in the mid or low region of the back; characteristically it is relieved by bed rest and induced by the maintenance of a particular posture over a period of time. Pain in the neck and between the shoulder blades is a common complaint among thin, tense, active women and seems to be related to taut trapezius muscles.

Adolescent girls and boys are subject to an obscure form of epiphyseal disease of the spine (Scheuermann disease) which, over a period of 2 to 3 years, may cause low-back pain with exercise.

Psychiatric illness Low-back pain may be a major symptom in patients with hysteria, malingering, anxiety neurosis, depression, hypochondriasis, and in many nervous persons whose symptoms do not conform to any of these psychiatric illnesses.

Again it is good practice to assume that pain in the back in such patients may signify disease of the spine or adjacent structures, and this should always be carefully sought. However, even when some organic factors are found, the pain may be exaggerated, prolonged, or woven into a pattern of invalidism because of coexistent primary or secondary psychologic factors. This is especially true when there is the possibility of secondary gain (notably compensation). Patients seeking compensation for protracted low-back pain without obvious structural disease tend, after a time, to become suspicious, uncooperative, and hostile toward their physicians or anyone who might question the authenticity of their illness. One notes in them a tendency to describe their pain vaguely and a preference to discuss the degree of their disability and their mistreatment at the hands of the medical profession. The description of the pain may vary considerably from one examination to another. Often, also, the region(s) in which pain is experienced and its radiation are nonphysiologic, and it fails to respond to rest and inactivity. These features and a negative examination of the back should lead one to suspect a psychologic factor. A few patients, usually frank malingerers, adopt the most bizarre gaits and attitudes, such as walking with the trunk flexed at almost a right angle (camptocormia) and being unable to straighten up. Or the patient may be unable to bend forward even 5°, despite the absence of muscle spasm, and he may wince at the slightest pressure, even over the sacrum, which is seldom a site of tenderness, unless there is pelvic disease.

The depressed and anxious patient represents a troublesome problem. A common error is to minimize the importance of anxiety and depression or to ascribe them to worry over the illness and its social effects. In these circumstances common and minor back ailments, e.g., those due to osteoarthritis and postural ache, are enhanced and become intolerable. Such patients are often subjected to surgical procedures, which prove ineffective. The disability seems excessive for the degree of spinal malfunction, and misery, irritability, and despair are the prevailing features of the syndrome. One of the most reliable diagnostic features is the response to drugs that alleviate the depression (see Chap. 56).

PAIN IN THE NECK AND SHOULDER

In this connection, it is useful to distinguish *three major categories of painful disease*—that of the *spine*, *brachial plexus*, and *shoulder*. Although the pain from each of these sources may overlap, the patient usually can indicate its site of origin.

Pain arising from the *cervical part of the spine* is felt in the neck and back of the head (although it may be projected to the shoulder and arm), is evoked or enhanced by certain movements or positions of the neck, and is accompanied by limitation of motions of the neck and tenderness to palpation over the cervical spine.

Pain of brachial plexus origin is experienced in and around the shoulder and in the supraclavicular region, is induced by certain maneuvers and positions of the arm, and is associated with tenderness of structures above the clavicle. There may be a palpable abnormality above the clavicle (aneurysm of the subclavian artery, tumor, cervical rib). The combination of circulatory abnormalities and signs referable to the medial cord of the brachial plexus are characteristic of the *thoracic outlet syndrome,* described further on. These are manifested by diminution or obliteration of the pulse when the patient, seated and with the arm dependent, takes and holds a full breath and tilts the head back and turns it to the affected side (Adson test) or abducts and externally rotates the arm and braces the shoulders (Wright maneuver); by swelling, venous distension and cyanosis of the dependent hand when the subclavian vein is compressed; and blanching and rapid fatigue of muscles being repeatedly contracted with the arm high over the head. A unilateral Raynaud phenomenon, trophic changes in the fingers, and sensory loss over the ulnar side of the hand, with or without interosseous atrophy, complete the clinical picture.

Pain localized to the shoulder region, worsened by motion, and associated with tenderness and limitation of movement (especially internal and external rotation and abduction), points to a tendonitis, subacromial bursitis, or to a tear of the rotator cuff, which is made up of the tendons of the muscles surrounding the shoulder joint. The term *bursitis* is often used loosely to designate these disorders. Shoulder pain, like spine and plexus pain, may radiate into the arm or hand, but sensory, motor, and reflex changes, which always indicate disease of nerve roots, plexus, or nerves, are absent. Shoulder pain of this type is very common in middle and late adult life. It may arise spontaneously or after unusual or vigorous exercise. Local tenderness over the greater tuberosity of the humerus is characteristic. Radiographs of the shoulder may be negative or show a calcium deposit in the supraspinatus tendon or subacromial bursa. In most patients the pain subsides with immobilization and analgesics. If it does not, the injection of 1 mL of hydrocortisone into the bursa is often effective.

Osteoarthritis and osteophytic spur formation of the cervical spine may cause pain which radiates into the back of the head, shoulders, and arms on one or both sides. Coincident compression of nerve roots is manifested by paresthesias, sensory loss, weakness and atrophy, and tendon reflex changes in the arms and hands. Should bony ridges form in the spinal canal (spondylosis), the spinal cord may be compressed, with resulting spastic weakness, ataxia, and loss of vibratory and position sense in the legs.

A cervical myelogram reveals the encroachment on the spinal canal (narrowing to less than 10 to 11 mm in the anteroposterior diameter) and the level at which the spinal cord is affected. There may be great difficulty in distinguishing spondylosis with root and spinal cord compression from a primary neurologic disease (syringomyelia, amyotrophic lateral sclerosis, or tumor) with an unrelated osteoarthritis of the cervical spine, particularly at the C5-C6 and C6-C7 levels, where the disc spaces are often narrowed in the adult. Here the CT scan of the vertebral canal and intervertebral spaces and myelography are of particular importance (see Chap. 36 for differential diagnosis). A combination of osteoarthritis of the cervical spine with injury to ligaments and muscles when the neck has been forcibly extended and flexed (e.g., the acceleration or "whiplash injury" in low-speed rear-end automobile collisions) raises vexatious clinical problems. If the pain is persistent and limited to the neck, the problem will sometimes prove to be due to disruption of a disc, but more often it is associated with tearing of paraspinal muscles and ligaments. Often it is complicated by psychologic and compensation factors (see LaRocca for review of this subject).

Spinal rheumatoid arthritis is localized to the cervical apophyseal joints and atlantoaxial articulation; there is pain, stiffness, and limitation of motion in the neck and pain in the back of the head. In contrast to ankylosing spondylitis, rheumatoid arthritis is rarely confined to the spine. Because of major affection of other joints, the diagnosis is relatively easy to make, but significant involvement of the neck may be overlooked in patients with diffuse disease. In advanced stages of the disease, one or several of the vertebrae may be displaced anteriorly; or a synovitis of the atlantoaxial joint may damage the transverse ligament of the atlas, resulting in forward displacement of the atlas on the axis, i.e., atlantoaxial subluxation. Pain in the neck may project into and cause numbness or burning of one half the tongue (the "tongue-neck syndrome"—see page 1088). In either instance, serious and even life-threatening compression of the spinal cord, gradual or sudden, may occur (see Chap. 36). Cautiously taken lateral roentgenograms in flexion and extension are useful in visualizing atlantoaxial dislocation or subluxation of the lower segments.

CERVICAL DISC PROTRUSION

A common cause of neck, shoulder, and arm pain is disc herniation in the lower cervical region (Fig. 10-6*A* and *B*). It may develop after trauma, which may be major or minor (from sudden hyperextension of the neck, diving, forceful chiropractic manipulations, etc.). The roots most commonly involved in cervical disc protrusion are the seventh (in 70 percent of cases) and the sixth (20 percent); fifth and eighth root involvement make up the remaining 10 percent (Yoss et al).

With a laterally situated disc protrusion between the fifth and sixth cervical vertebrae, the symptoms and signs are referred to the sixth cervical root. The full syndrome is characterized by pain at the trapezius ridge and tip of the shoulder, with radiation into the anterior-upper part of the arm, radial forearm, and often into the thumb; paresthesias and sensory impairment in the same regions; tenderness in the area above the spine of the scapula and in the supra-clavicular and biceps regions; weakness in flexion of the forearm; diminished to absent biceps and supinator reflexes (triceps retained or exaggerated).

When the protruded disc lies between the sixth and seventh vertebrae, there is involvement of the seventh cervical root and the pain is in the region of the shoulder blade, pectoral region and medial axilla, posterolateral upper arm, dorsal forearm and elbow, index and middle fingers, or all the fingers; tenderness is most pronounced over the medial aspect of the shoulder blade opposite the third to fourth thoracic spinous processes, in the supracla-vicular area and triceps region; paresthesias and sensory loss are most evident in the second and third fingers or tips of all the fingers; weakness is found in extension of the forearm and occasionally in the wrist and in the hand grip; the triceps reflex is diminished to absent, and the biceps and supinator reflexes are preserved.

Compression of the eighth cervical root at C7-T1 may mimic an ulnar palsy. The pain is along the medial side of the forearm and the sensory loss is in the distribution of the medial cutaneous nerve of the forearm as well as the ulnar nerve of the hand. The weakness involves the muscles supplied by the ulnar nerve.

These syndromes are usually incomplete in that only one or several of the typical findings are present. The article by Friis et al, listed in the references, describes the distri-bution of pain in 250 cases of herniated disc or spondylo-tic nerve root compression in the cervical region. Virtually every patient, irrespective of the particular root(s) involved, shows a *limitation in the range of motion of the neck and aggravation of pain with movement (particularly hyperexten-sion)*. Coughing, sneezing, and downward pressure on the head in the hyperextended position usually exacerbate the pain, and traction (even manual) tends to relieve it.

In many of the cervical radicular syndromes the onset is acute and there has been no traumatic incident. It is difficult to relate the syndrome to osseous changes that have been present for years. Even more difficult to explain is the tendency to recovery in a few weeks when movement of the neck is limited by traction or a collar. Conservative measures should always be tried before turning to laminec-tomy and foraminotomy.

Unlike lumbar discs, the cervical ones, if large and centrally situated, may result in compression of the spinal cord (central disc, all of the cord; paracentral disc, part of the cord) (Fig. 10-6*B*). The centrally situated disc may be painless, and the cord syndrome may simulate a degenerative disease (amyotrophic lateral sclerosis, combined system disease). A common error is to fail to think of a protruded cervical disc in patients with obscure symptoms in the legs. The diagnosis should be confirmed by CT scan and mye-lography, or MRI if possible (Figure 10-5).

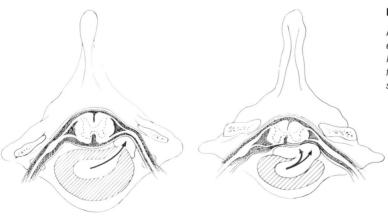

Figure 10-6

A. *Mechanism of root compression in lat-eral herniation of nucleus pulposus.* B. *Mechanism of root and cord compression from central herniation of nucleus pulpo-sus. (Adapted from Kristoff and Odom.)*

A   B

THORACIC OUTLET SYNDROMES

A number of anatomic anomalies occur in the lateral cervical region, which may, under certain circumstances, compress the brachial plexus, the subclavian artery, and the subclavian vein, causing muscle weakness and wasting, pain, and vascular symptoms in the hand and arm. The most frequent of these abnormalities are an incomplete cervical rib, with a sharp fascial band passing from its tip to the first rib; sharp fibrous bands passing from an elongated, down-curving transverse process of C7 to the first rib; less often, a complete cervical rib, which articulates with the first rib; and anomalies of the position and insertion of the anterior and medial scalene muscles. Thus, the sites of potential neurovascular compression extend all the way from the intervertebral foramens and superior mediastimum to the axilla. Depending on the postulated abnormality and mechanism of symptom production, the terms *cervical rib, anterior scalene, costoclavicular,* and *neurovascular compression,* have been applied to this syndrome. The international anatomic term is ''superior thoracic aperture syndrome.''

Variations in regional anatomy could theoretically explain these several postulated mechanisms, but it must be conceded that to this day there is not full agreement about the scalenus anticus and costoclavicular syndromes

(see Gilliatt). An anomalous cervical rib, which arises from the seventh cervical vertebra and extends laterally between the anterior and medial scalene muscles, then under the brachial plexus and subclavian artery to attach to the first rib, obviously disturbs anatomic relationships and may compress these structures (Fig. 10-7). However, since an estimated 1.0 percent of the population has cervical ribs, usually on both sides, and only about 10 percent of these persons have neurologic or vascular symptoms (almost always one-sided), other factors must be operative in most instances. The majority of the patients are women in early or midadult life (male to female ratio 1:5) in whom sagging of the shoulders, large breasts, and poor muscular tone may be of importance. Clavicular abnormalities, both congenital and traumatic, and certain occupational activities may also play a part.

The anterior and middle scalene muscles, the flexors and rotators of the neck, both insert into the first rib, and the subclavian artery and vein and the brachial plexus must pass between them. Hence variations such as abnormalities of insertion of the muscles or their hypertrophy were once

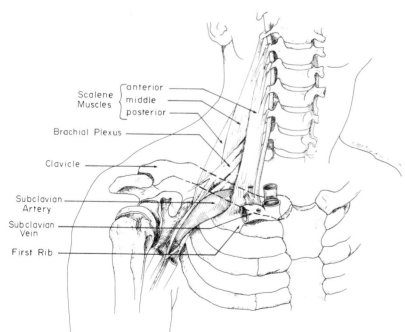

Scalene Muscles
{ anterior
  middle
  posterior

Brachial Plexus

Clavicle

Subclavian Artery

Subclavian Vein

First Rib

Figure 10-7

Course of the brachial plexus and subclavian artery between the anterior scalene and middle scalene muscles. Dilatation of the subclavian artery just distal to the anterior scalene muscle is illustrated. Immediately distal to the anterior and middle scalene muscles is another potential area of constriction, between the clavicle and the first rib. With extension of the neck and turning of the chin to the affected side (Adson maneuver), the tension on the anterior scalene muscle is increased and the subclavian artery compressed, resulting in a supraclavicular bruit and obliteration of the radial pulse.

thought to be the cause of the syndrome. However, section of these muscles (scalenectomy) so rarely altered the symptoms that this mechanism is no longer given credence.

Three neurovascular syndromes have been associated with a rudimentary cervical rib (rarely with a complete cervical rib) and related abnormalities at the thoracic outlet. These syndromes sometimes coexist but more often each occurs in pure form.

1. *Compression of the subclavian vein* causes a dusky discoloration of the arm, venous distention, and edema, and the vein may become thrombosed after prolonged exercise, the so-called effort-thrombotic syndrome of Paget and Schroetter.

2. *Compression of the subclavian artery* may result in ischemia of the limb. It may be complicated by digital gangrene and retrograde embolization. A unilateral Raynaud phenomenon, brittle nails, and ulceration of the finger tips are important diagnostic findings. A supraclavicular bruit, sometimes bilateral, is suggestive but not in itself diagnostic of subclavian compression. The conventional tests for vascular compression—loss of radial pulse during the Adson and Wright maneuvers, described above—are not entirely reliable. Sometimes these maneuvers fail to obliterate the radial pulse in cases of proved compression; contrariwise, these tests may be positive in normal persons. Nevertheless, a positive test on the symptomatic side (with reproduction of the patient's symptoms) but not on the other should always suggest a local lesion.

3. *The neurologic syndrome* is primarily a motor disorder, characterized by slight wasting and weakness of the hypothenar, interosseous, adductor pollicis, and deep flexor muscles of the fourth and fifth fingers, i.e., the muscles innervated by the lower trunk of the brachial plexus and ulnar nerves (pages 1065 and 1068). Weakness of the flexor muscles of the forearms may be present in advanced cases. Tendon reflexes are usually preserved. In addition, most patients complain of an intermittent aching of the arm, particularly of the ulnar side, and about half of them complain also of numbness and tingling along the inner border of the forearm and ulnar distribution of the hand. A loss of superficial sensation in these areas is a variable finding. It may be possible to reproduce these sensory symptoms by firm pressure just above the clavicle or by simple traction on the arm. Interestingly, vascular features are often absent or minimal in patients with the neurologic form of the syndrome.

In all three syndromes, shoulder and arm pain are prominent complaints. The discomfort is of the aching type

and is felt in the posterior hemithorax, pectoral and mammary regions, and upper arm.

Diagnostic measures should include films of the cervical spine, looking for a cervical rib. Typically, nerve conduction studies disclose a reduced amplitude of the ulnar sensory evoked potential. There may be a decrease in the amplitude of the median motor evoked potential, a mild but *uniform* slowing of the median motor conduction velocity, and a prolongation of the F-wave latency. Concentric needle examination of affected hand muscles reveals large amplitude motor units, suggesting collateral innervation. The application of somatosensory evoked potential estimation may prove to be a useful adjunct to the conventional nerve conduction and EMG studies (Yiannikas and Walsh). Digital plethysmography during the Adson, military brace, and abduction maneuvers is more reliable than palpation of the pulse. Brachial artery angiography is usually reserved for patients with a suspected arterial occlusion, an aneurysm, or an obvious cervical rib. The place of venography in the diagnostic work-up is uncertain, for a number of otherwise normal individuals occlude the subclavian vein by fully abducting the arm. We have resorted to this test only if vein thrombosis and extensive collateralization is observed.

In the authors' experience, unambiguous instances of thoracic outlet syndrome are not common. This has also been the experience of Gilliatt, whose review of this subject is recommended. He found only two or three examples annually out of approximately 2000 patients referred to the EMG clinics at the National and Maida Vale Hospitals in London. Neck and arm pain in slender, neurotic women presents particularly difficult problems in diagnosis; often the physician assumes the presence of a thoracic outlet syndrome, only to discover that operation affords little or no lasting relief. One should be skeptical of the diagnosis unless the rigid clinical and EMG criteria, enumerated above, have been met. Common mistakes are to confuse the thoracic outlet syndrome with carpal tunnel syndrome, ulnar neuropathy or entrapment at the elbow, and cervical radiculopathy due to arthritis or disc disease. Myelography and careful nerve conduction and EMG studies may be necessary to rule out these latter disorders.

OTHER CONDITIONS

Metastases to the cervical region of the spine are less common than to other parts of the vertebral column. They are frequently painful and may cause root compression. Extension of the tumor posteriorly or compression fractures may lead to the rapid development of quadriplegia.

The Pancoast tumor, usually a squamous cell carcinoma in the superior sulcus of the lung, may implicate the lower cervical and upper thoracic (T1 and T2) spinal nerves as they exit from the spine. A Horner syndrome, numbness of the inner side of the arm and hand, weakness of all muscles of the hand and of the triceps muscle are combined with pain beneath the upper scapula and in the arm. The neurologic abnormalities may occur long before the tumor becomes visible radiographically.

Shoulder injuries (rotator cuff), subacromial or sub-deltoid bursitis, and "frozen shoulder" (periarthritis or capsulitis), tendonitis, and arthritis may develop in patients who are otherwise well, but these conditions also occur occasionally as a complication of hemiplegia. The pain is often severe and extends toward the neck and down the arm into the hand. The dorsum of the hand may tingle without other signs of nerve involvement. Immobility of an arm following myocardial infarction may be associated with pain in the shoulder and arm and with vasomotor changes and secondary arthropathy of the joints of the hand (shoulder-hand syndrome); after a time, osteoporosis and atrophy of cutaneous and subcutaneous structures occur (Sudeck atrophy or Sudeck-Leriche syndrome). Similar changes may occur in the foot and leg with the painful lesions described in the first part of this chapter. These conditions fall within the province of the orthopedist and will not be discussed in detail. The neurologist, however, must know that they can be prevented by proper exercises and relieved by cooling, exercises, and physiotherapy (see below).

Medial and lateral epicondylitis (tennis elbow) are readily diagnosed by demonstrating tenderness over the affected parts and an aggravation of pain on certain movements of the wrist. We have observed entrapment of the ulnar nerve in some cases of medial epicondylitis.

The pain of the carpal tunnel syndrome (page 1068) often extends into the forearm and sometimes higher, and may be mistaken for disease of the shoulder or neck. Similarly, involvement of the ulnar, radial, or median nerves may be mistaken for brachial plexus or root lesions. EMG and nerve conduction studies are helpful in these circumstances. Tenosynovitis may be associated with the carpal tunnel syndrome or occur separately.

OTHER PAINFUL DISORDERS OF THE UPPER AND LOWER LIMBS

ARTHRITIS OF THE EXTREMITIES

The principal symptom of *osteoarthritis* is pain which is brought on by use and relieved by rest. Stiffness after sitting and immediately upon rising in the morning is common but seldom persists for more than a few minutes. The more common locations are the terminal phalanges, carpal-metacarpal joint of the thumb, knees, hips, and spine.

Rheumatoid arthritis most commonly involves the proximal interphalangeal and metacarpophalangeal joints, toes, wrists, ankle, knee, elbow, hip, and shoulder. Other types of arthritis are numerous—infectious, posttraumatic, and that associated with connective tissue, gastrointestinal, pulmonary, and psoriatic disease. The synovial membranes and periarticular structures are primarily involved in early rheumatoid disease, infectious arthritis, and gout, whereas the cartilage and bone are mainly affected in osteoarthritis and in the later stages of rheumatoid arthritis.

POLYMYALGIA RHEUMATICA

This syndrome is observed in middle-aged and elderly persons and is characterized by severe pain, aching, and stiffness in the proximal muscles of the limbs and a markedly elevated erythrocyte sedimentation rate. Constitutional symptoms (loss of weight, fever, and anemia) and articular swelling are less consistent manifestations. In many patients, polymyalgia rheumatica is associated with giant cell (temporal) arteritis and may be the only symptomatic expression of that disease (pages 146 and 678). This disorder is self-limited, lasting 6 months to 2 years, and responds dramatically to corticosteroid therapy, although the latter may need to be continued for several years.

ARTERIOSCLEROSIS OBLITERANS

Atherosclerosis of large and medium-sized arteries, the most common vascular disease of humans, often leads to symptoms that are induced by exercise (intermittent claudication) but may also occur at rest (ischemic rest pain). The diabetic patient is especially susceptible. The muscle pain that is brought on by exercise and promptly relieved by rest most frequently involves the calf and thigh muscles. If the atherosclerotic narrowing or occlusion involves the aortic and iliac arteries, it may also cause hip and buttock claudication and impotence in the male (Leriche syndrome). Ischemic rest pain, and sometimes attendant ulceration and gangrene, is usually localized to the foot and toes and the consequence of multiple sites of vascular occlusion. Pain at rest is characteristically worse at night and totally or partially relieved by dependency.

The examination of such patients will reveal a loss of one or more peripheral pulses, trophic changes in the skin and nails (in advanced cases), and the presence of bruits over or distal to sites of narrowing. A search (by CT scan) should always be made in such patients for an abdominal aortic aneurysm, since it is prone to rupture and can be corrected by operation. Arteriography is necessary only for confirmation of the location and extent of the vascular narrowing in planning surgical therapy. The upper extremities are rarely involved. Aneurysms of the peripheral arteries do not usually produce pain unless they compress adjacent nerves; they are of importance primarily because they become the source of distal arterial embolization or undergo thrombosis.

PAINFUL CIRCULATORY DISORDERS

In evaluating patients with cold sensitivity it is important to distinguish between Raynaud disease and Raynaud phenomenon. *Raynaud disease* is a benign, symmetric disorder of unknown cause with onset usually in the late teens or early twenties. Females are more commonly affected than males, and cold and emotional stimuli are the factors that trigger the response in the digits. The fingers become white, then blue, and finally red (the triphasic color response). Pain and paresthesias are common during the ischemic phase. Ulcerations are rarely observed.

The *Raynaud phenomenon* is a symptom (sometimes the initial manifestation) of some underlying disease. It may occur at any period of life and may be asymmetric. When severe it is accompanied by tender, painful fingertip ulcers. It is associated most often with one of the collagen-vascular diseases, but also with rheumatoid arthritis, thromboangiitis obliterans, the dysproteinemias, occupational trauma (e.g., working with pneumatic drill, sculling on a cold day), and the thoracic outlet syndrome.

Reflex Sympathetic Dystrophy This is an excessive or abnormal response of the sympathetic nervous system to injury of the shoulder and arm, rarely the leg. It consists of protracted pain in association with cyanosis or pallor, swelling, coldness, pain on passive motion, and osteoporosis. The condition is variously described under such terms as Sudeck atrophy, posttraumatic osteoporosis, and shoulder-hand syndrome. According to Carlson et al, bone scans are positive. Pharmacologic or surgical sympathectomy hastens recovery.

Erythromelalgia This rare disorder of the microvasculature produces a burning pain, usually in the toes and forefoot, in association with changes in ambient temperature. Since it was first described by Weir Mitchell in 1878, many articles have been written about it, but the cause of the primary form is still obscure. Each patient has a temperature threshold above which symptoms appear and the feet become bright red and warm. Those afflicted rarely

wear stockings or regular shoes, since these tend to bring out the symptoms. Patients characteristically relieve the pain by walking on a cold surface or soaking their feet in ice water. The peripheral pulses are intact, and there are no motor, sensory, or reflex changes. There are secondary forms of the disease associated in rare cases with myeloproliferative disorders, particularly polycythemia vera, and occlusive vascular diseases; in some instances it is a manifestation of a painful neuropathy (Chap. 46). According to Abbott and Mitts, aspirin is useful in the treatment of paroxysms of primary erythromelalgia; others recommend methysergide maleate (Pepper).

MANAGEMENT OF BACK AND LIMB PAIN

The pain of muscular and ligamentous strains and minor disc prolapses is usually self-limited, responding to simple measures in a relatively short period of time. The basic principle of therapy in both disorders is rest, in a recumbent position, for several days to weeks. Usually lying on the side with knees and hips flexed is the favored position. With strains of the sacrospinalis muscles and sacroiliac ligaments, the optimal position is hyperextension. This position is best maintained by having the patient lie with a small pillow or blanket under the lumbar portion of the spine or lie face down. Physical measures, such as application of ice in the acute phase (30 min on, 60 min off) and heat after the third or fourth day, diathermy, and massage, are of limited value. Analgesic medication should be given liberally during the first few days [codeine, 30 mg, and aspirin, 0.6 g; acetaminophen, 0.6 g; pentazocine (Talwin), 50 mg; or meperidine (Demerol), 50 mg]. Muscle relaxants are often useful [diazepam (Valium), 10 to 40 mg in divided doses; carisoprodol (Soma), 350 mg twice daily] if only to make bed rest more tolerable. If an inflammatory component is suspected, indomethacin (Indocin), 75 mg/day (in divided doses), or ibuprofen (Motrin), 400 mg three or four times daily, may be helpful. When weight bearing is resumed, discomfort may be diminished by a light lumbosacral support, to be worn until the pain has subsided. Thereafter, corrective exercises are prescribed, designed to strengthen trunk (especially abdominal) muscles, overcome faulty posture, and increase the mobility of the spinal joints.

In the treatment of an *acute or chronic rupture of a lumbar or cervical disc,* complete bed rest is essential, and strong analgesic medication may be required for a few days. The only indication for emergency surgery is an acute compression of the cauda equina by a massive disc protrusion, causing bilateral motor and sensory loss with sphincteric paralysis, or severe unilateral motor loss, such as a foot frop. Traction is of little value in lumbar disc disease, and it is best to permit the patient to find the most comfortable position. In the case of a cervical disc syndrome, traction with a halter may be of considerable benefit. Treatment can be administered with the patient in recumbency, or it can be performed intermittently in the sitting position, using special equipment. During the recumbent phase of treatment of lumbar disc disease, muscle relaxants and anti-inflammatory agents as described above may be of considerable value. After 2 or 3 weeks in bed, the patient can be allowed to resume activities gradually, usually with the protection of a brace or light spinal support (or a soft collar, in the case of cervical disc disease). In lumbar disc disease, exercise programs designed to increase the strength of the abdominal and gluteal muscles should be undertaken at this point. The patient may suffer some minor recurrence of the pain but will be able to continue his or her usual activities and eventually will recover.

If the pain and neurologic findings do not subside on prolonged conservative management or the patient suffers frequent recurrent acute episodes, surgical treatment needs to be considered. This should always be preceded by a CT scan and probably a myelogram to localize the lesion (and rule out the presence of intra- or extradural tumors). The surgical procedure most often indicated is a hemilaminectomy, with excision of the disc involved. In cases with sciatic pain due to L4-L5 or L5-S1 disc ruptures, 85 to 90 percent are relieved. Rerupture occurs in approximately 5 percent (Shannon and Paul). Arthrodesis (spinal fusion) of the involved segments is indicated only in cases in which there is extraordinary instability, usually related to an anatomic abnormality (such as spondylolysis) or, in the cervical region, to an extensive laminectomy that has rendered the spine unstable. A presurgery trial of epidural steroid injection has been recommended by some orthopedists and anesthesiologists, but we have been unable to interpret the results.

Chemonucleolysis has been used for the management of lumbar disc lesions that do not respond to conservative measures. Chymopapain, a polysaccharide-splitting enzyme of plant origin, is introduced into the damaged nucleus pulposus by a laterally placed needle under radiographic control. The enzyme, by its lytic action, causes a decrease in intradiscal pressure. This procedure was used in our hospitals between 1973 and 1975, but the results were not impressive and serious adverse effects were frequent. However, since FDA approval of the drug, its use has been revived. Soon thereafter there appeared a number of reports in which it was claimed that chemonucleolysis successfully relieved sciatic pain, even in patients whose sciatica had been present for many months. However, as experience with this procedure has increased, so have the number of failures, and most neurosurgeons who have used this method at one time or another have now abandoned it. Chemical meningomyelopathy and radiculopathy, with tragic results, may occur if the chymopapain diffuses into the subarachnoid

space. We can only conclude that the treatment is still on trial.

The intradiscal injection of Depomedral has been used as a method of therapy by Wilkinson and Schuman, but their patients had a mixture of radicular and pseudo-radicular pains and were unsuitable for surgical exploration. We find it impossible to evaluate their results.

The choice and performance of such procedures as laminectomy, chemonucleolysis, and spinal arthrodesis should be weighed carefully in the light of the patient's occupation, emotional response, compensation status, etc.

Surely the most difficult patients to manage are those with chronic low-back pain who have already had one or more laminectomies and sometimes a fusion without substantial relief. Our practice has been to repeat the myelogram (usually with metrizamide) and the CT scan. In a small number of the patients it will be found that the disc has reruptured or that there is disc disease at another level. It may happen that the surgeon has not removed all the disc tissue, in which case another operation to remove the rest of it will be successful. EMG and nerve conduction studies, searching for evidence of a radiculopathy, are helpful. If there is evidence of a radiculopathy but no disc material is seen, or only scar tissue, one does not know whether the pain is due to injury from the initial rupture or from the surgery. Various hypothetical explanations are then invoked—radiculitis, lateral recess syndrome, facet syndrome, unstable spine, lumbar arachnoiditis—which for the most part are untestable.

One would suppose that these chronic pain cases could be subdivided into a group with continued radicular pain and another with referred pain from disease of the spine. However, once the pain becomes chronic the separation is not easy. Simple pressure over the spine, buttock, or thigh may cause pain to be projected into the leg. Lidocaine blocks of nerve roots have yielded inconsistent results. Facetectomy and foraminotomy or lysis of arachnoidal adhesions around one or more roots are variably successful. These procedures may be indicated if intra-articular lidocaine injections have a salutary effect on the pain. Lateral lumbar fusions have given unpredictable results. Occupational injuries, in which workman's compensation or litigation are factors, make the patient's report of therapeutic effects almost worthless. Transcutaneous stimulators, posterior column stimulators, and intrathecal morphine have seldom helped for long in our experience. At present the best that can be offered the patient is weight reduction (if the patient is obese), progressive exercise to strenghten abdominal and back muscles, nonsteroidal anti-inflammatory drugs, supportive psychotherapy, and antidepressant drugs in combination with non-habit-forming analgesics.

Spondylosis of the cervical spine, if painful, is helped by bed rest and traction; if signs of spinal cord and root involvement are present, a collar to limit movement may halt the progression and even lead to improvement. Decompressive laminectomy or anterior excision of single spondylotic spurs and fusion is reserved for severe instances of the disease with advancing neurologic symptoms (see Chap. 36).

In the management of the *thoracic outlet syndrome,* a conservative approach is advisable. If the main symptoms are pain and paresthesias, Leffert advises the use of local heat, analgesics, muscle relaxants (see above), and an assiduous program of special exercises to strengthen the shoulder muscles. Twice a day, holding a 1- or 2-lb weight in each hand, the patient intermittently shrugs and relaxes the shoulders forward and upward, then backward and upward, and then upward, each 10 times. In a second exercise, with the weights held at the side, the extended arms are lifted over the head until the backs of the hands meet; again it is done 10 times. In a third exercise the patient faces a corner of a room and places one hand on each wall; with elbows bent, he leans into the wall and at the same time inhales then exhales as he pushes away. A full range of neck motions is then practiced. On such a regime some patients experience a relief of symptoms after two to three weeks.

If severe pain persists, in spite of such a program, surgery is indicated in patients with or without significant motor loss and circulatory compromise. The usual approach is through the supraclavicular space, with cutting of fibrous bands and excision of the rudimentary rib. The procedure favored by some thoracic surgeons is excision of a segment of the first rib, through the axilla. Pain is dramatically relieved but the sensory-motor defects improve only slightly. Atherosclerosis with thrombosis and embolism of the subclavian artery and thrombosis of the vein require decompression and arterioplasty and venous thrombectomy, respectively. Brachial sympathectomy is indicated in exceptional patients with a persistent Raynaud phenomenon. (For further details, see Imparato and Riles.)

As mentioned earlier, vasomotor, sudomotor, and trophic changes in the skin, with atrophy of the soft tissues and decalcification of bone, may follow the prolonged immobilization and disuse of an arm or leg for whatever reason. The patient may be reluctant to move the limb because of pain or, a lack of motivation to get well, or for reasons of monetary gain. Surgery in this group of patients is ill-advised, and the physician's efforts should be directed to mobilization of the affected part through an intensive physical therapy program and settlement of litigation, if this is a factor. If these measures fail, sympathetic blocks and finally sympathectomy are indicated.

PREVENTIVE ASPECTS OF BACK PAIN

Without doubt these are important. There would be many fewer back problems if adults kept their trunk muscles in optimal condition by regular exercise such as swimming, walking briskly, running, and calisthenic programs of the Canadian Air Force type. Morning is the ideal time for exercising, since the back of the older adult tends to be stiffest following a night of inactivity. This happens regardless of whether a bed board or a stiff mattress is used. Sleeping with the back hyperextended and sitting for long periods in an overstuffed chair or a badly designed car seat are particularly likely to aggravate backache. It is estimated that intradiscal pressures are increased 200 percent by changing from a recumbent to a standing position and 400 percent when slumped in an easy chair. Correct sitting posture lessens this pressure. Long trips in a car or plane without change in position put maximal strain on disc and ligamentous structures in the spine. Lifting from a position of flexed trunk, as in removing a heavy suitcase from the trunk of a car, is risky (always lift with the object close to the body). Also, sudden strenuous activity without conditioning and warm-up are likely to injure discs and their ligamentous envelopes. Certain families seem disposed to injury to these structures.

POSTTRAUMATIC PAIN SYNDROMES

Included under this heading are a variety of painful conditions of the extremities caused by trauma or disease of individual peripheral nerves.

Persistent and often incapacitating pain and dysesthesias may follow any type of injury that leads to *neuroma formation or intraneural scarring*—fracture, contusion of the limbs, compression from lying on the arm in a drunken stupor, severing of sensory nerves in the course of surgical operations, or incomplete regeneration after nerve suture. It is stated that the nerves in these cases contain a preponderance of unmyelinated C fibers and a reduced number of A-δ fibers, and this imbalance is presumably related to the genesis of painful dysesthesias. These cases are best managed by complete excision of the neuromas with end-to-end suture of healthy nerve, but not all cases lend themselves to this procedure.

Another special type of neuroma is the one that forms at the end of a nerve severed at amputation (stump neuroma). Pain from this source is occasionally abolished by relatively simple procedures such as resection of the distal neuromas, proximal neurotomy, or resection of the regional sympathetic ganglia. Anterolateral chordotomy with achievement of complete analgesia is the surest way to abolish pain from a stump neuroma (as well as pain from a phantom limb), but is of limited value because of the failure to maintain full analgesia for a protracted time; with some return of sensation (6 months in the case of the lower extremities and earlier in the arms), pain usually returns as well.

NEUROGENIC LIMB PAIN (NONTRAUMATIC)

Many diseases may affect the peripheral nerves and cause pain in the limbs. The nerves may be affected singly (e.g., meralgia paresthetica), or multiple nerves may be affected, in a symmetric or asymmetric fashion. The most painful neuropathies are those associated with alcoholic-nutritional disease (beriberi), polyarteritis, and diabetes mellitus. A transient aching of weakened muscles occurs in about one-half of the patients with idiopathic polyneuritis (Guillain-Barré syndrome). These disorders are considered in Chap. 46.

REFERENCES

ABBOTT KH, MITTS MG: Reflex neurovascular syndromes, in Vinken PJ, Bruyn GW (eds): *Handbook of Clinical Neurology*, vol 8. Amsterdam, North-Holland, 1970, chap 20, pp 321–356.

ALEXANDER E JR, KELLY DL, DAVIS CH JR et al: Intact arch spondylolisthesis. A review of 50 cases and description of surgical treatment. *J Neurosurg* 63:840, 1985.

ARMSTRONG JR: *Lumbar Disc Lesions: Pathogenesis and Treatment of Low Back Pain and Sciatica*, 3rd ed. Baltimore, Williams & Wilkins, 1965.

CARLSON DH, SIMON H, WEGNER W: Bone scanning and the diagnosis of reflex sympathetic dystrophy. *Neurology* 27:791, 1977.

COLLIER B: Treatment for lumbar sciatic pain in posterior articular lumbar joint syndrome. *Anesthesia* 34:202, 1979.

deORIO JK, BIANCO AJ: Lumbar disc excision in children and adolescents. *J Bone Joint Surg* 64:991, 1982.

dePALMA AF, ROTHMAN RH: *The Intervertebral Disc*. Philadelphia, Saunders, 1970.

EVANS BA, STEVENS JC, DYCK PJ: Lumbosacral plexus neuropathy. *Neurology* 31:1327, 1981.

FINNESON BE: *Low Back Pain*, 2nd ed. Philadelphia, Lippincott, 1981.

FRIIS ML, GULLIKSEN GC, RASMUSSEN P: Distribution of pain with nerve root compression. *Acta Neurosurgica* 39:241, 1977.

GILLIATT RW: Thoracic outlet syndromes, in Dyck PJ et al (eds): *Peripheral Neuropathy*, 2nd ed. Philadelphia, Saunders, 1984, pp 1409–1424.

HASSLER O: The human intervertebral disc. A micro-angiographical study on its vascular supply at various ages. *Acta Orthop Scand* 40:765, 1970.

HUDGKINS WR: The crossed straight leg raising sign (of Fajerstagn). *N Engl J Med* 297:1127, 1977.

IMPARATO AM, RILES TS: Peripheral arterial disease, in Schwartz SI et al (eds): *Principles of Surgery*, 5th ed. New York, McGraw-Hill, 1989, pp 933–1010.

KELLGREN JH: On the distribution of pain arising from deep somatic structures with charts of segmental pain areas. *Clin Sci* 4:35, 1939.

KRISTOFF FV, ODOM GL: Ruptured intervertebral disc in the cervical region. *Arch Surg* 54:287, 1947.

KURIHARA K, KATAOKA O: Lumbar disc herniation in children and adolescents and review of 70 cases and their minimum 5-year follow-up studies. *Spine* 5:443, 1980.

laROCCA H: Acceleration injuries of the neck. *Clin Neurosurg* 25:209, 1978.

LASCELLES RG, MOHR PD, NEARY D, BLOOR K: The thoracic outlet syndrome. *Brain* 100:601, 1977.

LEFFERT RD: Thoracic outlet syndrome, in Omer G, Springer M (eds): *Management of Peripheral Nerve Injuries*. Philadelphia, Saunders, 1980.

LEYSHON A, KIRWAN E O'G, PARRY CBW: Electric studies in the diagnosis of compression of the lumbar root. *J Bone Joint Surg* 63–B:71, 1981.

LIPSON SJ, MUIR H: Experimental intervertebral disc degeneration; morphologic and proteoglycan changes over time. *Arthritis Rheum* 24:12, 1981.

LONG DM: Failed back syndrome. In Johnson RT, ed, *Current Therapy in Neurologic Disease - 2*. Toronto, B.C. Decker Inc, 1987, pp 51-53.

LOVE JG, SCHORN VG: Thoracic-disc protrusions. *JAMA* 191:627, 1965.

MATHEWS WB: The neurological complications of ankylosing spondylitis. *J Neurol Sci* 6:561, 1968.

McCALL IW, PARK WM, O'BRIAN JP: Induced pain referral from posterior lumbar elements in normal subjects. *Spine* 4:441, 1979.

McCORMICK CC: Radiology in low back pain and sciatica: An analysis of the relative value of spinal venography, discography, and epidurography in patients with a negative or equivocal myelogram. *Clin Radiol* 29:293, 1978.

MIKHAEL MA, CIRIC I, TARKINGTON JA et al: Neurologic evaluation of lateral recess syndrome. *Radiology* 140:97, 1981.

MIXTER WJ, BARR JS: Rupture of the intervertebral disc with involvement of the spinal canal. *N Engl J Med* 211:210, 1934.

PEPPER H: Primary erythromelalgia: Report of a case treated with methysergide maleate. *JAMA* 203:1066, 1967.

POSTACCINI F, URSO S, FERRO L: Lumbosacral nerve root anomalies. *J Bone Joint Surg* 64-A:721, 1982.

POWELL MC, SZYPRYT P, WILSON M et al: Prevalence of lumbar disc degeneration observed by magnetic resonance in symptomless women. *Lancet* 2:1366, 1986.

QUILES M, MARCHISELLO PJ, TSAIRIS R: Lumbar adhesive arachnoiditis: Etiologic and pathologic aspects. *Spine* 3:45, 1978.

RASKIN SP: Computerized tomographic findings in lumbar disc disease. *Orthopedics* 5:419, 1981.

REYNOLDS AF, WEINSTEIN PR, WACHTER RD: Lumbar mono-radiculopathy due to unilateral facet hypertrophy. *Neurosurg* 10:480, 1982.

SHANNON N, PAUL EA: L4/5, L5/S1 disc protrusions: Analysis of 323 cases operated on over 12 years. *J Neurol Neurosurg Psychiatry* 42:804, 1979.

SHAW MDM, RUSSELL JA, GROSSART KW: The changing pattern of spinal arachnoiditis. *J Neurol Neurosurg Psychiatry* 41:97, 1978.

SINCLAIR DC, FEINDEL WH, WEDDELL G et al: The intervertebral ligaments as a source of segmental pain. *J Bone Joint Surg* 30B:515, 1948.

SYMPOSIUM: Computerized tomography of the lumbar spine. *Spine* 4:281, 1979.

VAN GELDEREN C: Ein orthotisches (lordotisches) Kaydasyndrom. *Acta Psychiatr Neurol Scand* 23:57, 1948.

VERBIEST H: Further experiences on the pathological influence of a developmental narrowness of the bony lumbar vertebral canal. *J Bone Joint Surg* 37B:576, 1955.

WEINSTEIN PR, EHNI G, WILSON CB: *Lumbar Spondylosis. Diagnosis, Management and Surgical Treatment.* Chicago, Year Book, 1977.

WILKINSON HA, SCHUMAN N: Intradiskal corticosteroids in treatment of lumbar and cervical disc problems. *Spine* 5:385, 1980.

YIANNIKAS C, WALSH JC: Somatosensory evoked responses in the diagnosis of the thoracic outlet syndrome. *J Neurol Neurosurg Psychiatry* 46:234, 1983.

YOSS RE, CORBIN KB, MacCARTY CS, LOVE JG: Significance of symptoms and signs in localization of involved root in cervical disc protrusion. *Neurology* 7:673, 1957.

DISORDERS OF THE SPECIAL SENSES

The four chapters in this section are concerned with the highly specialized functions of taste and smell, vision and ocular movement, hearing, and the sense of balance. These special senses and the cranial nerves that subserve them represent the most finely developed parts of the sensory nervous system. The sensory dysfunctions of the eye and ear are, of course, the proprietary interest of the ophthalmologist and otologist, but they are of interest to the clinical neurologist as well. Some of them reflect the presence of serious systemic disease, and others represent the initial or leading manifestation of neurologic disease. It is from both these points of view that they will be considered here. In keeping with the general approach being used in this volume, the disorders of the special senses and of ocular movement will be considered in a particular sequence: first, their cardinal clinical manifestations, along with the certain facts of anatomic and physiologic importance, followed by a consideration of the syndromes of which these manifestations are a part. Because of their specialized nature, some of the diseases which produce these syndromes will be discussed here rather than in other parts of the book.

CHAPTER 11

DISORDERS OF SMELL AND TASTE

The sensations of smell (olfaction) and taste (gustation) are suitably considered together. Physiologically, these modalities share the singular attribute of responding primarily to chemical stimuli, i.e., the end organs that mediate olfaction and gustation are chemoreceptors. Taste and smell are also interdependent clinically. Appreciation of the flavor of food and drink depends to a large extent on their aroma, and an abnormality of one of these senses is frequently misinterpreted as an abnormality of the other. In comparison to sight and hearing, taste and smell play a relatively unimportant role in the life of the individual, and only rarely is the loss of either of these latter modalities a serious handicap. Nevertheless, disorders of taste and smell are persistently unpleasant and sometimes an inability to detect noxious odors (e.g., smoke) or to taste tainted food may have serious results. Also, a loss of taste and smell may serve to identify a number of intracranial and systemic disorders, and they assume clinical importance from this point of view.

OLFACTORY SENSE

ANATOMIC AND PHYSIOLOGIC CONSIDERATIONS

Nerve fibers subserving the sense of smell have their cells of origin in the mucous membrane of the upper and posterior parts of the nasal cavity. The entire olfactory mucosa covers an area of about 2.5 cm and contains three cell types—receptor cells (which number about 6 million in humans), sustenacular or supporting cells, and basal cells, which are the stem cells and the source of both the epithelial and sustenacular cells during regeneration. The *receptor cells* are actually bipolar neurons. Each of these cells has a peripheral process (the olfactory rod), from which project 10 to 30 fine hairs, or cilia. These hair-like processes, which lack motility, are the sites of olfactory receptors. The central processes of these cells, or *olfactory fila*, are very fine (0.2 μm in diameter) unmyelinated fibers that converge to form small fascicles enwrapped by Schwann cells and pass through openings in the cribriform plate of the ethmoid bone into the olfactory bulb (Fig. 11-1). Collectively, the central processes of the olfactory receptor cells constitute the *first cranial*, or *olfactory, nerve*.

In the olfactory bulb, the receptor cell axons synapse with mitral cells (triangular, like a bishop's mitre), the dendrites of which form brush-like terminals or olfactory glomeruli (Fig. 11-1). Smaller, so-called tufted cells in the olfactory bulb also contribute dendrites to the glomerulus. Several thousand olfactory-cell axons converge on a single glomerulus.

The axons of the mitral and tufted cells enter the olfactory tract, which courses along the olfactory groove of the cribriform plate to the cerebrum. Caudal to the olfactory bulbs are scattered groups of cells that constitute the anterior olfactory nucleus (Fig. 11-1). Dendrites of these cells synapse with fibers of the olfactory tract, while their axons project to the olfactory nucleus and bulb of the opposite side; these neurons are thought to function as a reinforcing mechanism for olfactory impulses.

Posteriorly the olfactory tract divides into medial and lateral olfactory striae. The medial stria contains fibers from the anterior olfactory nucleus which pass to the opposite side, via the anterior commissure. Fibers in the lateral stria originate in the olfactory bulb, give off collaterals to the anterior perforated substance, and terminate in the medial and cortical nuclei of the amygdaloid complex and the prepiriform area (also referred to as the lateral olfactory gyrus). The latter represents the *primary olfactory cortex*, which in humans occupies a restricted area on the anterior end of the hippocampal gyrus and uncus (area 34 of Brodmann; see Figs. 21-1 and 21-2). Thus olfactory impulses reach the cerebral cortex without relay through the thalamus; in this respect olfaction is unique among sensory systems. From the prepiriform cortex, fibers project to the neighboring entorhinal cortex (area 28 of Brodmann), the medial dorsal nucleus of the thalamus, and the hypothalamus, but the role of these latter structures in olfaction is not well understood.

Olfactory sense is unlike all others in yet another way. It is common experience that an aroma can restore long-forgotten memories of complex experiences. That olfactory stimuli and emotional stimuli are strongly linked is not surprising, in view of their common roots in the limbic system. Yet the ability to recall an odor is negligible in comparison to one's ability to recall sounds and sights.

Figure 11-1

Diagram illustrating the relationships between the olfactory receptors in the nasal mucosa and neurons in the olfactory bulb and tract. Cells of the anterior olfactory nucleus are found in scattered groups, caudal to the olfactory bulb. Fibers from the anterior olfactory nucleus project centrally (A). A fiber from the contralateral anterior olfactory nucleus is labeled B. Inset. *Diagram of the olfactory structures on the inferior surface of the brain (see text for details).*

As Vladimir Nabokov has remarked: "Memory can restore to life everything except smells."

In quiet breathing, little of the air entering the nostril reaches the olfactory mucosa; sniffing carries the air into the olfactory crypt. To be perceived as an odor, an inhaled substance must be volatile, i.e., spread in the air as very small particles, and soluble in water or lipids. When a jet of scented vapor is directed to the sensory epithelium, a slow negative potential shift called the *electro-olfactogram* (EOG) can be recorded from an electrode placed on the mucosa. The conductance changes that underlie the potential of the receptor are induced by molecules of odorous material dissolved in the mucus overlying the receptor. Intensity of olfactory sensation is determined by a relative frequency of firing of afferent neurons. The quality of the odor is thought to be provided by "cross fiber" activation since the individual receptor cells are responsive to a wide variety of odorants and exhibit different types of responses to stimulants. Evidently excitatory, inhibitory, and on-off responses have been obtained. This olfactory potential can be eliminated by destroying the olfactory receptor surface or the olfactory filaments. The loss of EOG occurs 8 to 16 days after severance of the nerve; the receptor cells disappear, but the sustenacular cells are not altered. Most significant is the fact that the olfactory receptor cells are constantly

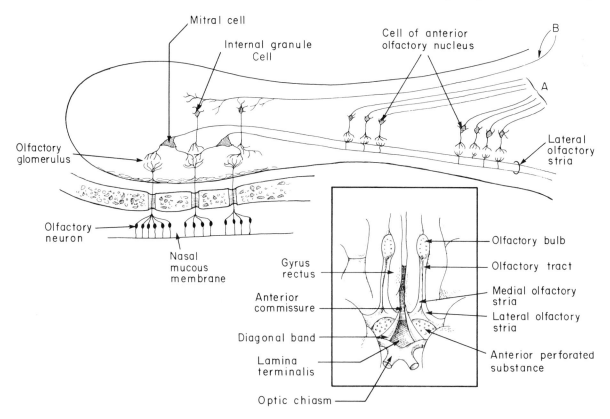

dying and being replaced by new ones, by division of the basal cells of the olfactory epithelium. In this respect the chemoreceptors, both for smell and taste (see below), are unique, constituting the only examples of neuronal regeneration in humans.

CLINICAL MANIFESTATIONS

Disturbances of olfaction may be subdivided into four groups, as follows:

1. Quantitative abnormalities: loss or reduction of the sense of smell (anosmia, hyposmia) or increased olfactory acuity (hyperosmia)

2. Qualitative abnormalities: distortions or illusions of smell (dysosmia or parosmia)

3. Olfactory hallucinations and delusions caused by temporal lobe disorders or psychiatric disease

4. Loss of olfactory discrimination

Anosmia (loss of sense of smell) is the most frequent clinical abnormality and, if unilateral, will not be recognized by the patient. Unilateral anosmia is sometimes demonstrated in the hysterical patient on the side of anesthesia, blindness, and deafness. Bilateral anosmia, on the other hand, is not an uncommon complaint, and the patient is usually convinced that the sense of taste has been lost as well (*ageusia*). This calls attention to the fact that taste depends largely on the volatile particles in foods and beverages, which reach the olfactory receptors through the nasopharynx and that the perception of flavor is a combination of smell and taste. This can be proved by demonstrating that such patients are able to distinguish the elementary taste sensations (sweet, sour, bitter, and salty). The olfactory defect can be verified readily enough by presenting a series of nonirritating olfactory stimuli (vanilla, peanut butter, cigarette, coffee, etc.), first in one nostril, then in the other, and asking the patient to sniff and identify them. If the odors can be detected and described, even if they cannot be identified, it may be assumed that the olfactory nerves are relatively intact (humans can distinguish many more odors than they can identify by name). Ammonia and similar pungent substances should not be used because they test not the sense of smell or taste but the so-called common chemical sense, in which irritants stimulate chemoreceptors (probably the free nerve endings) of the trigeminal nerves.

More elaborate smell identification tests have been developed and standardized by Doty and his colleagues. These tests are reliable and permit the comparison of a patient with age- and sex-matched normal individuals. Doty et al find a pattern of smell loss with age. Air dilution olfactory detection is a useful way of determining thresholds

of sensation and of showing normal olfactory detection in the absence of identification. These special techniques are essentially research tools and are not used in neurologic practice.

Regarding the nasal diseases responsible for bilateral hyposmia or anosmia, the most frequent are those in which hypertrophy and hyperemia of the nasal mucosa prevent olfactory stimuli from reaching the receptor cells. Heavy smoking, it is said, is the most frequent cause of hyposmia. Chronic rhinitis and sinusitis of allergic, vasomotor, or infective types are common causes, though hormonal and metabolic disorders may also cause congestion and swelling of the nasal mucosa. Biopsies of the olfactory mucosa in allergic rhinitis have shown that the sensory epithelial cells are still present, but their cilia are deformed and shortened and are buried under other mucosal cells. Influenza may be followed by hyposmia or anosmia, and this may be permanent, since receptor cells are destroyed by the virus (Douek). These cells may also be affected as a result of atrophic rhinitis (e.g., leprosy) and local radiation therapy, or by a very rare type of tumor ("esthesioneuroepithelioma") that originates in the olfactory epithelium. There is also a group of diseases in which the primary receptor neurons are congenitally absent or hypoplastic and lack cilia. One type is the Kallman syndrome of congenital anosmia and hypogonadotropic hypogonadism. Another type of congenital anosmia occurs in albinos, because of the absence of "olfactory pigment" or some other congenital structural defect.

Head injury causes anosmia by severing the delicate filaments of the receptor cells as they pass through the cribriform plate, especially if the injury is severe enough to cause fracture. The damage may be unilateral or bilateral and is usually permanent. With closed head injury anosmia is less frequent (6 percent of Sumner's series of 584 cases); recovery of olfaction occurs in about one-quarter of such patients. Cranial surgery, subarachnoid hemorrhage, and chronic meningeal inflammation may have a similar effect. Strangely, in some of the traumatic anosmia cases there is also a loss of taste (ageusia). Ferrier, who described one of the first cases of traumatic ageusia, and subsequently Sumner, noted that there was always anosmia as well. Often the ageusia clears within a few weeks. A bilateral lesion near the frontal operculum and paralimbic region, where olfactory and gustatory receptive zones are in close proximity, would best explain this concurrence. Obviously the interruption of olfactory filaments would not explain ageusia.

It has been reported that a large proportion of

unselected patients with multiple sclerosis (Pinching) and Parkinson disease (Quinn et al) show anosmia or hyposmia, for reasons that are quite unclear. Corwin et al have found odor recognition to be reduced in certain dementing diseases, such as Huntington chorea and Alzheimer disease, and it has been known for some time that alcoholics with Korsakoff psychosis have a defect in odor discrimination (see further on). Presumably this is due to degeneration of neurons in the higher order olfactory systems of the medial-temporal and thalamic regions. Hyman et al remark on the early neuronal degeneration near the hippocampus in Alzheimer disease, but there are no studies of the olfactory connections.

Bilateral anosmia is an increasingly common manifestation of malingering, now that it has been recognized as a compensable disability by insurance companies. The fact that the true anosmic will complain inordinately of a loss of taste (but show normal taste sensation) may help to separate them from malingerers.

Meningiomas of the olfactory groove may implicate the olfactory bulbs and tracts and may extend posteriorly to involve the optic nerves sometimes with optic atrophy on one side and papilledema on the other (Foster Kennedy syndrome, page 543). Large aneurysms of the anterior cerebral and anterior communicating arteries may produce a similar syndrome. With tumors confined to one side the anosmia may be strictly unilateral, in which case it will not be reported by the patient but will be found on examination. Children with anterior meningoencephaloceles are usually anosmic and, in addition, may exhibit CSF rhinorrhea when the head is held in certain positions (demonstrated by chemical examination of the fluid, which contains more glucose than mucous secretions, and by watching, under ultraviolet light, fluorescein issue from the nostrils after it has been instilled in the spinal subarachnoid space). Nasal injury and hydrocephalus are other causes of CSF rhinorrhea. These defects in the sense of smell are all attributable to lesions of the receptor cells and their axons or the olfactory bulbs. It is not known whether olfactory symptoms may be produced by lesions of the anterior perforated space or medial and lateral olfactory striae. In some cases of increased intracranial pressure, olfactory sense has been impaired without evidence of lesions in the olfactory bulbs.

Whether a true *hyperosmia* exists is a matter of conjecture. Neurotic individuals may complain of being unduly sensitive to odors, but there is no proof of an actual change in the threshold of perception of odors. During migraine attacks, the patient may be unusually sensitive not only to light and sound but also to odors.

Dysosmia or parosmia (perversion of the sense of smell) may occur with local nasopharyngeal conditions such as empyema of the nasal sinuses and ozena. Partial injuries of the olfactory bulbs may have a similar effect. Parosmia may also be a troublesome symptom in middle-aged and elderly persons who have symptoms of depression. Every article of food is said to have an extremely unpleasant odor (cacosmia). Sensations of disagreeable taste are often associated (cacogeusia). Nothing is known of the basis of this state; there is usually no loss of discriminative sensation.

The treatment of parosmia is difficult. The use of antipsychotic drugs has given unpredictable results. Zinc and vitamins are apparently ineffective. Some reports indicate that repeated anesthetization of the nasal mucosa reduces or abolishes the parosmic disturbance. In many cases the disorder subsides spontaneously. Minor degrees of parosmia are not necessarily abnormal, for unpleasant odors have a way of lingering for several hours and of being reawakened by other olfactory stimuli, as every pathologist knows (phantosmia).

Olfactory hallucinations are always of central origin. The patient claims to smell an odor that no one else can detect. If the patient is convinced of its presence and also gives it personal reference, despite all evidence to the contrary, the symptom assumes the status of a *delusion*. Aside from so-called uncinate seizures, in which the olfactory experience is brief and accompanied by an alteration of consciousness and other epileptic components (see page 253), olfactory hallucinations and delusions usually signify a psychiatric illness. Zilstorff has written informatively on this subject. There is complaint of a large array of odors, most of them foul. In most cases the smell seems to emanate from the patient (intrinsic hallucinations); in others they seem to come from an external source (extrinsic hallucinations). Both types vary in intensity and are remarkable with respect to their persistence. They may be combined with gustatory hallucinations. According to Pryse-Phillips, who took note of the psychiatric illness in a series of 137 patients with olfactory hallucinations, most were associated with endogenous depression and schizophrenia. In schizophrenia the olfactory stimulus is usually interpreted as arising externally and as being induced by someone for the purpose of upsetting the patient. In depression, the stimulus is usually intrinsic and is more overwhelming. All manner of ways are used to get rid of the stench, the usual ones being excessive washing, use of deodorants, and social withdrawal. There is some reason to believe that the amygdaloid group of nuclei is the source of the hallucinations, since stereotactic lesions here have reportedly abolished both the olfactory hallucinations and the psychiatric disorder (Chitanondh).

Olfactory hallucinations and delusions may occur in conjunction with senile dementia, but when this happens one should also consider the possibility of an associated late-life depression. Occasionally olfactory hallucinations occur as part of an alcohol withdrawal syndrome. Peculiar reactions to smell characterize certain sexual psychopathies. Usually the stimuli appear to be extrinsic, but in this regard it should be noted that odors imagined by normal individuals are also perceived as coming from outside the person through inspired air, and unpleasant ones are more clearly represented than pleasant ones.

In interpreting these phenomena, Bromberg and Schilder suggest that smell is an important orienting sense, has value as a "social indicator," and serves to initiate attraction behavior (if pleasant or sexual) or avoidance behavior if disagreeable.

In lower vertebrates, these functions and similar ones (modulation of menstrual and reproductive behavior) have been attributed to the activities of a subset of olfactory receptors in the rostral end of the nasal mucosa. The axons of these cells penetrate the cribriform plate and synapse with secondary neurons in a discrete portion of the olfactory bulb (accessory olfactory bulb). This functionally and anatomically distinct olfactory tissue is referred to as the *vomeronasal system* or *organ* (see the review of Wysocki and Meredith).

Loss of Olfactory Discrimination   Finally one needs to consider a disorder in which the primary perceptual aspects of olfaction (detection of odors, adaptation to odors, and recognition of different intensities of the same odor) are intact but in which the discrimination between odors and their recognition by quality is impaired or lost. To recognize this deficit of olfactory discrimination requires special testing such as matching-to-sample and the identification and naming of a variety of scents. Patients with the alcoholic form of Korsakoff psychosis have been shown to have such an impaired capacity to discriminate between odors; furthermore, this impairment is not attributable to impaired olfactory acuity or to failure of learning and memory (Mair et al). Most likely the olfactory disorder in these patients is due to lesions in the medial dorsal nucleus of the thalamus; several observations in animals indicate that this nucleus and its connections with the orbitofrontal cortex give rise to deficits in odor discrimination (Mair et al; Slotnick and Kaneko). Eichenbaum and his associates demonstrated a similar loss of quality discrimination in a patient who had undergone extensive bilateral medial temporal lobe resection. The operation was believed to have eliminated a substantial portion of the olfactory afferents to the frontal cortex and thalamus, though there was no anatomic verification of this. In patients with sterotactic or surgical amygdalotomies, Andy et al noted a reduction in odor discrimination. Thus it appears that both portions of the higher olfactory pathways (medial temporal lobes and

medial dorsal nuclei) are necessary for the discrimination and identification of odors.

GUSTATORY SENSE

ANATOMIC AND PHYSIOLOGIC CONSIDERATIONS

The sensory receptors for taste (taste buds) are distributed over the surface of the tongue and, in smaller numbers, over the palate, pharynx, and larynx. Mainly they are located in the epithelium along the lateral surfaces of the circumvallate papillae and to a lesser extent in the epithelium of the fungiform papillae. The taste buds are round or oval structures, each composed of up to 200 vertically oriented receptor cells, arranged like the staves of a barrel. The ends of these cells surround a small opening, the taste pore, which opens onto the mucosal surface. The tips of the sensory cells project through the pore as a number of filiform microvilli ("taste hairs"). Fine unmyelinated nerve fibers penetrate the base of the taste bud to innervate the sensory cells. Each receptor is capable of being activated by chemical substances in solution and transmits its activity along the sensory nerves to the brainstem. Any one taste bud is capable of responding to a number of sapid substances, but always it is preferentially sensitive to one type of stimulus. In other words, the receptors are only relatively specific. The sensitivity of these receptors is remarkable: as little as 0.05 mg/dL of quinine sulfate will arouse a bitter taste when applied to the base of the tongue.

As stated above, the four primary taste sensations are salty, sweet, bitter, and sour; more complex flavors are combinations of olfactory and gustatory sensations. All four submodalities are perceived at the tip of the tongue, though this part is more sensitive to sweet and salt. The sides of the tongue are more sensitive to sour and the base to bitter.

If the gustatory impairment is unilateral or topical, taste is tested by withdrawing the tongue with a gauze sponge and using a moistened applicator to place a few crystals of salt or sugar on small discrete parts of the tongue; the tongue is then wiped clean, and the subjects are asked to report what they had sensed. A useful stimulus for sour sensation is a low-voltage direct current, the electrodes of which can be accurately placed on the tongue surface. If the taste loss is bilateral, whole mouth washes with a dilute solution of sucrose, sodium chloride, citric acid, and caffeine may be used. After swishing, the test fluid is spat out and the mouth rinsed with water. The patient indicates whether he or she can taste a substance and is asked to identify it.

Special apparatuses (electrogustometers) have been devised for the measurement of taste intensity and for determining the detection and recognition thresholds of taste and olfactory stimuli (Krarup; Henkin et al), but these are beyond the scope of the usual clinical examination.

The receptor cells of the taste buds have a brief life cycle (about 10 days), being replaced constantly by mitotic division of adjacent basal epithelial cells. The number of taste buds, not large to begin with, diminishes with age. In addition, the perception of taste and smell stimuli diminishes with age (everything begins to taste and smell the same). According to Schiffman, taste thresholds for salt, sweeteners, and amino acids are 2 to 2½ times higher in the elderly than in the young. The reduction in the acuity of taste and smell with aging may contribute to the anorexia, distorted food habits, and weight loss of elderly persons.

From the anterior two-thirds of the tongue, taste fibers first run in the lingual nerve (a major branch of the mandibular nerve). After coursing within the lingual nerve for a short distance the taste fibers diverge to enter the chorda tympani (a branch of the seventh nerve); thence they pass through the pars intermedia and geniculate ganglion of the seventh nerve to the rostral part of the nucleus of the tractus solitarius in the medulla. Fibers from the palatal taste buds pass through the pterygopalatine ganglion and greater superficial petrosal nerve, join the facial nerve at the level of the geniculate ganglion, and proceed to the nucleus of the solitary tract (see Fig. 46-2). Possibly, taste fibers from the tongue may also reach the brainstem via the mandibular division of the trigeminal nerve. The presence of these alternate pathways probably accounts for reported instances of unilateral taste loss that have followed section of the root of the trigeminal nerve and instances in which no loss of taste has occurred with section of the chorda tympani. From the posterior third of the tongue, soft palate, and palatal arches, the sensory taste fibers are conveyed via the glossopharyngeal nerve and ganglion nodosum to the nucleus of the tractus solitarius. Taste fibers from the extreme dorsal part of the tongue and the few that arise from taste buds on the pharynx and larynx run in the vagus nerve. Rostral and lateral parts of the nucleus solitarius, which receive the special afferent (taste) fibers from the facial and glossopharyngeal nerves, constitute the "gustatory nucleus." Probably both sides of the tongue are represented in this nucleus.

The second sensory neuron for taste has been difficult to track. Neurons of the nucleus solitarius project to adjacent nuclei (e.g., dorsal motor nucleus of vagus, ambiguus, salivatorius superior and inferior, trigeminal, and facial) which serve visceovisceral and viscerosomatic reflex functions, but those concerned with the conscious recognition of taste are believed to form an ascending pathway to a pontine parabrachial nucleus. From the latter, two ascending pathways have been traced (in animals). One is the solitariothalamic lemniscus to the ventroposteromedial nucleus. A second passes to the ventral parts of the forebrain, to parts of the hypothalamus (which probably influences autonomic function), and other basal forebrain limbic areas. The ascending fibers lie near the medial lemniscus and are both crossed and uncrossed. Experiments in animals indicate that taste impulses from the thalamus project to the tongue-face area of the postrolandic sensory cortex. This is probably the end station of gustatory projections in humans as well, insofar as gustatory hallucinations have been produced by electrical stimulation of the parietal and/or the rolandic opercula (Hausser-Hauw and Bancaud).

Richter has explored the biologic role of taste in normal nutrition. Animals made deficient in sodium, calcium, certain vitamins, proteins, etc., will automatically select the correct foods, on the basis of their taste, to compensate for their deficiency.

CLINICAL MANIFESTATIONS

Heavy smoking, particularly pipe smoking, is probably the commonest cause of impairment of taste sensation. Extreme drying of the tongue with desquamation and damage to the taste buds may lead to temporary loss or reduction of the sense of taste (*ageusia* or *hypogeusia*). Dryness of the mouth (xerostomia) from inadequate saliva, as occurs in the Sjögren syndrome, irradiation of head and neck, and pandysautonomia, also interferes with taste because taste stimuli, like olfactory ones, are effective only in a fluid medium. If unilateral, ageusia is seldom the source of complaint. Taste is frequently lost over one-half of the tongue (except posteriorly) in cases of Bell's palsy (as indicated on page 1081).

A permanent decrease in acuity of taste and smell (hypogeusia and hyposmia), sometimes associated with perversions of these sensory functions (dysgeusia and dysosmia) may follow influenza-like illnesses. These abnormalities have been associated with pathologic changes in the taste buds, as well as in the nasal mucous membranes. In a group of 143 patients who presented with hypogeusia and hyposmia, 87 were of this postinfluenzal type (Henkin et al); the remainder developed their symptoms in association with scleroderma, acute hepatitis, viral encephalitis, myxedema and adrenal insufficiency, malignancy, deficiency of vitamins B_{12} and A, and the administration of a wide variety of drugs (see below).

Distortions of taste and loss of taste are sources of complaint in patients with a variety of malignant tumors. Oropharyngeal tumors may, of course, abolish taste by invading the chorda tympani or lingual nerves. Malnutrition due to neoplasm or radiation therapy may also cause ageusia, as pointed out by Settle et al. Some patients with certain carcinomas remark on an increase in their threshold for bitter foods, and some breast cancer patients find sour foods intolerable. The loss of taste from radiation of the oropharynx is usually recovered within a few weeks; taste bud turnover, which is reduced by radiation, is only temporary.

An interesting syndrome, called *idiopathic hypogeusia*, in which a decreased taste acuity is associated with dysgeusia, hyposmia, and dysosmia, has been described by Henkin et al. The taste and aroma of food is unpleasant to the point of being revolting (cacogeusia and cacosmia), and the persistence of these symptoms may lead to a loss of weight, anxiety, and depression. Patients with this disorder have been shown to have a decreased concentration of zinc in their parotid saliva, and their symptoms are said to have responded to small oral doses of zinc sulfate.

Persistent misinterpretations and distortions of taste have been reported with a wide variety of drugs (Schiffman), especially with penicillamine, in the course of treatment of Wilson disease and rheumatoid arthritis; with procarbazine, vincristine, and vinblastine, used in the treatment of carcinoma and lymphoma; and with griseofulvin, amitriptyline, antithyroid drugs, chlorambucil, and colestyramine.

Unilateral lesions of the medulla oblongata have not been reported to cause ageusia, perhaps because the nucleus of the tractus solitarius is usually outside the zone of infarction. Unilateral thalamic and parietal lobe lesions have both been associated with contralateral impairment of taste sensation. As indicated above, a gustatory aura occasionally marks the beginning of a seizure originating in the frontoparietal (suprasylvian) cortex. Gustatory hallucinations are much less frequent than olfactory ones. Nevertheless, the former were found in 30 of 718 cases of intractable epilepsy (Hauser-Hauw and Bancaud). During surgery, these investigators produced an aura of disagreeable taste by electrical stimulation of the parietal and frontal opercula and also by stimulation of the hippocampus and amygdala (uncinate seizures). In their view, the low threshold seizure focus for taste in the temporal lobe is secondary to functional disorganization by the seizure state in the opercular gustatory cortex. Gustatory hallucinations were more frequent with right hemisphere lesions, and in half of the cases, the gustatory aura was followed by a convulsion.

REFERENCES

ANDY OJ, JURKO MF, HUGHES JR: The amygdala in relation to olfaction. *Confin Neurol* 37:215, 1975.

BRODAL A: *Neurological Anatomy in Relation to Clinical Medicine*, 3rd ed. Fair Lawn, NJ, Oxford, 1981.

BROMBERG W, SCHILDER P: Olfactory imagination and hallucinations. *Arch Neurol Psychiatry* 32:467, 1934.

CHITANONDH H: Stereotaxic amygdalotomy in the treatment of olfactory seizures and psychiatric disorders with olfactory hallucinations. *Confin Neurol* 27:181, 1966.

CORWIN J, SELBY M, CONRAD P et al: Olfactory recognition deficit in Alzheimer and Parkinsonian dementias. *IRCS Med Sci* 13:260, 1985.

DOTY RL, SHAMAN P, APPLEBAUM SL: Smell identification ability. Changes with age. *Science* 226:1441, 1984.

DOTY RL, SHAMAN P, DANN M: Development of University of Pennsylvania smell indentification test. *Physiol Behav* 32:489, 1984.

DOUEK E: *The Sense of Smell and its Abnormalities*. London, Churchill-Livingstone, 1973.

EICHENBAUM H, MORTON TH, POTTER H, CORKIN S: Selective olfactory deficits in case H.M. *Brain* 106:459, 1983.

HAUSER-HAUW C, BANCAUD J: Gustatory hallucinations in epileptic seizures. *Brain* 110:339, 1987.

HENKIN RI, GILL JR JR, BARTTER FC: Studies on taste thresholds in normal man and in patients with adrenal cortical insufficiency: The effect of adrenocorticosteroids. *J Clin Invest* 42:727, 1963.

HENKIN RI, LARSON AL, POWELL RD: Hypogeusia, dysgeusia, hyposmia and dysosmia following influenza-like infection. *Ann Otol* 84:672, 1975.

HENKIN RI, SCHECHTER PJ, HOYE R, MATTERN CFT: Idiopathic hypogeusia with dysgeusia, hyposmia, and dysosmia. A new syndrome. *JAMA* 217:434, 1971.

HYMAN BT, van HOESEN GW, DAMASIO AR: Alzheimer disease. Cell specific pathology isolates the hippocampal formation. *Science* 225:1168, 1984.

KRARUP B: Electrogustometry: A method for clinical taste examinations. *Acta Otolaryngol* 69:294, 1958.

MAIR R, CAPRA C, McENTEE WJ, ENGEN T: Odor discrimination and memory in Korsakoff's psychosis. *J Exper Psychol: Human Perception and Performance* 6:445, 1980.

PINCHING A: Clinical testing of olfaction reassessed. *Brain* 100:377, 1977.

PRYSE-PHILLIPS W: Disturbances in the sense of smell in psychiatric patients. *Proc Roy Soc Med* 68:26, 1975.

QUINN NP, ROSSOR MN, MARSDEN CD: Olfactory threshold in Parkinson's disease. *J Neurol Neurosurg Psychiatry* 50:88, 1987.

RICHTER CP: Total self-regulatory functions in animals and human beings. *Harvey Lect* 38:63, 1942–1943.

SCHIFFMAN SS: Taste and smell in disease. *N Engl J Med* 308:1275; 1337, 1983.

SETTLE RG, QUINN MR, BREND JG: Gustatory evaluation of cancer patients, in Von Eys J, Nichols BL, Seeling MS (eds): *Nutrition and Cancer*. New York, Spectrum, 1979.

SLOTNICK BM, KANEKO N: Role of mediodorsal thalamic nucleus in olfactory discrimination learning in rats. *Science* 214:91, 1981.

SUMNER D: Post-traumatic ageusia. *Brain* 90:187, 1967.

SUMNER D: Disturbances of the senses of smell and taste after head injuries, in Vinken PJ, Bruyn GW (eds): *Handbook of Clinical Neurology*. Amsterdam, North-Holland, vol 24, 1975, pp 1–25.

WYSOCKI CJ, MEREDITH H: The vomeronasal system, in Finger TE, Silver WL (eds): *Neurobiology of Taste and Smell*. New York, Wiley, 1987, pp 125–150.

ZILSTORFF W: Parosmia. *J Laryngol Otol* 80:1102, 1966.

CHAPTER 12

COMMON DISTURBANCES OF VISION

The faculty of vision is our most important source of information about the world. The largest part of the cerebrum is involved in vision and in the visual control of movement, and in the perception and elaboration of the form and color of objects and words. The optic nerve contains over 1 million fibers, compared to 30,000 in the auditory nerve. The study of the visual system has greatly advanced our knowledge of the nervous system. Indeed we know more about vision than any other sensory system.

In addition, because of its diverse composition of epithelial, vascular, collagenous, neural, and pigmentary tissue, the eye is virtually a medical microcosm, susceptible to manifold diseases. Moreover, its transparency allows direct inspection by the opthalmoscope and affords an opportunity to observe during life many of the specific lesions of medical diseases.

Since the eye is the sole organ of vision, impairment of visual acuity obviously stands as the most frequent and important symptom of eye disease. There are also positive symptoms (phosphenes, visual illusions, and hallucinations), but they are less significant. Irritation, redness, photophobia, pain, diplopia and strabismus, and drooping or closure of the eyelids are the other major symptoms. The impairment of vision may be unilateral or bilateral, sudden or gradual, episodic or enduring. The common causes of failing eyesight vary with age. In late childhood and adolescence, nearsightedness, or *myopia*, is the usual cause, though a pigmentary retinopathy or a retinal, optic nerve, or suprasellar tumor must not be overlooked. In middle age, beginning usually in the fifth decade, farsightedness (presbyopia) is almost invariable. Still later in life, cataracts, glaucoma, retinal hemorrhages and detachments, macular degeneration, and tumor, unilateral or bilateral, are the most frequent causes of visual impairment.

Episodic visual loss in early life, often hemianopic, is due to migraine as a rule; later, transient monocular blindness, or *amaurosis fugax*, is related to stenosis of the carotid artery or less often to embolism of retinal arterioles;

or there may be no discernible cause. Cerebrovascular disease deranges vision with increasing frequency in later life.

A number of terms are commonly used to describe visual loss. *Amaurosis* refers to blindness from any cause, whereas *amblyopia* refers to an impairment or loss of vision which is not due to an error of refraction or to other disease of the eye itself. *Nyctalopia* means poor twilight or night vision and is associated with vitamin A deficiency, retinitis pigmentosa, and, often, color blindness.

APPROACH TO THE PROBLEM OF VISUAL LOSS

In investigating a disturbance of vision one must always inquire as to what the patient means when he or she claims not to see properly, for the disturbance in question may vary from near- or farsightedness to excessive tearing, diplopia, partial syncope, or even giddiness or dizziness. Fortunately the patient's statement can be checked by the measurement of visual acuity, which is the single most important part of the ocular examination. Inspection of the refractive media and the optic fundi, especially the macular region, and the plotting of the visual fields complete the examination.

In the measurement of visual acuity the *Snellen Chart*, which contains rows of letters of diminishing size, is utilized. The height of each letter subtends 5 min of an arc when held at various distances from the eye. The letter at the top of the chart subtends 5 min of an arc at a distance of 200 ft (or roughly 60 m); then follow rows of letters that should be read at lesser distances. Thus if the patient can read only the top letter at 20 rather than 200 ft, the acuity is expressed as 20/200 ($V = 20/200$, or 6/60 if distances are measured in meters rather than feet). If the patient's eyesight is normal, the visual acuity will equal 20/20, or

6/6, using the metric scale. Many persons, especially during youth, can read at 20 ft the line that should be read at 15 ft from the chart ($V = 20/15$). Patients with a corrected refractive error should always wear their glasses for the test. For bedside testing, a ''near card'' can be used. In young children, acuity can be estimated by having them mimic the examiner's finger movements at varying distances or pick up objects of different sizes from varying distances.

If the visual acuity (with glasses) is less than 20/20, either the refractive error has not been properly corrected or there is some other reason for the diminished acuity. The former possibility can be ruled out if the patient can read the 20/20 line at a distance (not on a near card) through a pinhole in a cardboard held in front of the eye; the pinhole permits a narrow shaft of light to fall on the macular fovea (the area of greatest visual acuity) without distortion by the curvature of the lens. Minor degrees of visual impairment may be disclosed by alternately stimulating each eye with a bright white or colored object, enabling the patient to compare the intensity of vision in the two eyes. Objects look less bright and colors less saturated in the faulty eye.

Light entering the eye is focused by the biconvex lens onto the outer layer of the retina. Consequently the cornea, the fluid of the anterior chamber, the lens, the vitreous, and the retina itself must be transparent. The clarity of these media can be determined opthalmoscopically, and this examination requires that the pupil be dilated to at least 6 mm in diameter. This is best accomplished by instilling two drops of 10% phenylephrine (Neo-Synephrine) or cyclopentolate HCl in each eye after the visual acuity has been measured, the pupillary responses recorded, and the intraocular pressure estimated. The mydriatic action of phenylephrine lasts about 4 h. Rarely, an *attack of angle-closure glaucoma* (manifested by diminished vision, ocular pain, nausea, and vomiting) may be precipitated by pupillary dilation; this can be prevented by instilling 2% pilocarpine immediately after the ocular examination. Usually the pupils will have returned to normal size by the time the general physical and neurologic examinations are completed.

By looking through a high-plus lens of the ophthalmoscope, from a distance of 6 to 12 in, the examiner can visualize opacities in the refractive media; by adjusting the lenses from a high-plus to a zero or minus setting, it is possible to ''depth-focus'' from the cornea to the retina. Depending upon the refractive error of the examiner, lenticular opacities are best seen within the $+20$ to $+12$ range. The retina comes into focus with $+1$ to -1 lenses. The pupil appears as a red circular structure (red reflex), the color being provided by blood in the capillaries of the choroid layer. If all the refractile media are clear, reduced vision that is uncorrectable by glasses is due to a defect in the macula, the optic nerve, or the parts of the brain with which they are connected.

NONNEUROLOGIC CAUSES OF REDUCED VISION

It is not feasible to describe all the causes of opacification of the refractive media. Only those with important medical or neurologic implications will be mentioned. In the *cornea*, the most common one is scarring due to trauma and infection. Ulceration and subsequent fibrosis may occur with herpes simplex and herpes zoster infections or may complicate the conjunctivitis and uveitis of certain mucocutaneous-ocular syndromes (Stevens-Johnson, Reiter). Keratitis, meaning inflammation of the cornea, may be a manifestation of congenital syphilis, tuberculosis, and malignant exophthalmos (thyroid ophthalmopathy), or it may be idiopathic, as in ocular pemphigus. More innocent states such as drying and injury of the corneas during coma may result in ulceration and scarring. Hypercalcemia secondary to sarcoid, hyperparathyroidism, and vitamin D intoxication may give rise to precipitates of calcium phosphate and carbonate beneath the corneal epithelium primarily in a plane corresponding to the interpalpebral tissue, so-called band keratopathy. The latter also occurs with multiple myeloma, juvenile rheumatoid arthritis, and faulty lacrimation. Diffuse deposition of calcium in the cornea and conjunctivum is also part of the milk alkali syndrome. Cystine crystals are deposited in the corneas in cystinosis, chloroquine crystals in cases of discoid lupus (treated by this drug), polysaccharides in some of the mucopolysaccharidoses (page 797), and copper in hepatolenticular degeneration (Kayser-Fleischer ring, page 803). Crystal deposits may be observed in multiple myeloma and cryoglobulinemia. The corneas are also diffusely clouded in certain lysosomal storage diseases (page 789). The occurrence of an arcus senilis at an early age is a mark of hypercholesterolemia and may be combined with the yellow periorbital skin deposits of xanthelasma.

In relation to the *anterior chamber* of the eyes, the common problem is one of impediment to the outflow of the aqueous fluid, leading to excavation of the optic disc and visual loss, i.e., *glaucoma*. In more than 90 percent of cases (of the open-angle type) the cause of this syndrome is unknown; a genetic factor is suspected. In about 5 percent the angle between pupil and lateral cornea is narrow and blocked when the pupil is dilated; and in the remaining cases the condition is secondary to some disease process that blocks outflow channels [inflammatory debris of uveitis, red blood cells from hemorrhage in the anterior chamber (hyphema), or new formation of vessels and connective tissue on the surface of the iris (rubeosis iridis), a rare complication of diabetes mellitus and carotid occlusion].

Some degree of increased intraocular pressure is said to occur in 2 percent of all persons over 40 years of age. In most of these cases it is asymptomatic and goes unrecognized for years, but in some it may progress to rapid loss of vision. Pressures above 20 mmHg may damage the optic nerve. The damage is manifest first as a quadrantic defect in the lower nasal field and may lead to blindness. With the ophthalmoscope one can see also that the optic disc is excavated and the margins of the optic cup are broadened.

In the *lens*, cataract formation is the common abnormality. The "sugar cataract" of diabetes mellitus is the result of sustained high levels of blood glucose, which is changed in the lens to sorbitol, the accumulation of which leads to a high osmotic gradient with swelling and disruption of the lens fibers. Galactosemia is a much rarer disease, but the mechanism of cataract formation is similar, i.e., the accumulation of dulcitol in the lens. In hypoparathyroidism, lowering of the concentration of calcium in the aqueous humor is in some way responsible for the opacification of newly forming lens fibers. Prolonged high doses of chlorpromazine and corticosteroids and radiation therapy are believed to induce lenticular opacities. Down syndrome and oculocerebrorenal syndrome (Chap. 44), spinocerebellar ataxia with oligophrenia (Chap. 43), and certain dermatologic syndromes (atopic dermatitis, congenital ichthyosis, incontinentia pigmenti) are also accompanied by lenticular opacities. Myotonic dystrophy (Chap. 50) and, rarely, Wilson disease (Chap. 38) are associated with special types of cataract. Subluxation of the lens, the result of weakening of its zonular ligaments, occurs in syphillis, Marfan syndrome, and homocystinuria.

In the *vitreous humor*, hemorrhage may occur from rupture of a ciliary or retinal vessel. On ophthalmoscopic examination, the hemorrhage appears as a diffuse haziness of part or all of the vitreous or as a sharply defined mass, if the blood is between the retina and the vitreous and displaces the latter rather than mixing with it. The common causes are cranial trauma, rupture of an intracranial aneurysm or AV malformation with high intracranial pressure, rupture of newly formed vessels of proliferative retinopathy in patients with diabetes mellitus, and retinal tears, in which the hemorrhge breaks through the internal limiting membrane. The deep portions of the vitreous humor may also be affected by deposition of calcium soaps, which are seen as small white opacities with the ophthalmoscope; this condition, referred to as *asteroid hyalosis,* is observed in older patients. In systemic amyloidosis there may be amyloid deposits in the vitreous. Occasionally crystals of fatty acids or cholesterol appear as small glistening opacities that fall in a shower when the eyeball is moved (*synchisis scintillans*). The commonest vitreous opacities are the benign "floaters" or "spots before the eyes," which appear as gray dots with changes in the position of the eyes; they may be annoying or even alarming until the person stops looking for them. A sudden increase in floaters associated with a flash of light is characteristic of retinal detachment. Shrinkage of the vitreous humor and retraction from the retina occur with aging and may cause veils or streaks of light (phosphenes), usually in the periphery of the visual field.

NEUROLOGIC CAUSES OF REDUCED VISION

The search begins with an ophthalmoscopic examination of the retina. This thin (100- to 350-μm) sheet of transparent tissue and the nerve head (*optic disc*) into which the visual information is channeled are, properly speaking, parts of the central nervous system and the only parts of this system that can be inspected directly during life. The following anatomic and physiologic facts are requisite for an interpretation of the neurologic lesions that affect vision.

Light entering the eye is focused on the outer (posterior) layer of the retina, which contains two classes of photoreceptor cells, the flask-shaped cones and the slender rods. They rest on a layer of pigmented epithelial cells, which lie behind them. The rods and cones and pigmentary epithelium receive their blood supply from the capillaries of the choroid, not from the retinal arterioles. The rod cells contain rhodopsin, a conjugated protein in which the chromophore group is a carotenoid akin to vitamin A. The rods serve in the perception of visual stimuli in subdued light (twilight or scotopic vision), and the cones are responsible for color discrimination and the perception of stimuli in bright light (photopic vision). Most of the cones are concentrated in the macular and perimacular region and are diminished in number peripherally. Rods and cones transform light rays into electrical impulses, which pass through the bipolar cells of the retina to the superficially (anteriorly) placed neurons, or ganglion cells. The axons of the ganglion cells traverse the optic discs, nerves, and tracts to the lateral geniculate nuclei and superior colliculi (Fig. 12-1).

Three types of cells, referred to as X, Y, and W, have been identified in nonhuman primates on the basis of their functional characteristics and terminations. The X cells are centered in the maculae and project to the striate cortex. The Y cells are distributed throughout the retina and project to both the striate cortex and the superior colliculi. The W cells terminate only in the superior colliculi. Presumably the same neuronal types exist in humans, but in different proportions.

The normal development of these connections requires that the visual system be activated at each of several critical periods of development. The early deprivation of vision in one eye causes a failure of development of the geniculate and cortical receptive fields of that eye. Moreover, the cortical receptive fields of the seeing eye become abnormally large and usurp the monocular dominance columns of the blind eye (Hubel and Wiesel). In children with congenital cataracts, the eye will remain amblyopic if the opacity is removed later, after this critical period of development. A severe strabismus in early life, especially an esotropia, with monocular fixation of the normally positioned eye, will have the same effect.

As they stream across the surface of the retina, the axons of the retinal ganglion cells pursue an arcuate course. Being unmyelinated, they are not visible, although fluorescein retinography shows a tracery of their outlines. The fibers derived from macular cells form a discrete bundle that lies first on the temporal side of the disc and optic nerve and then assumes a more central position within the nerve (papillomacular bundle). They are of smaller caliber than the peripheral optic nerve fibers.

In the optic chiasm the fibers derived from the nasal half of each retina decussate and continue in the optic tract with uncrossed fibers of the other eye (Fig. 12-2). Thus, interruption of the left optic tract causes a right hemianopic defect in each eye (homonymous). In partial tract lesions the visual defects in the two eyes are not exactly congruent, since the tract fibers are not evenly admixed. The optic

Figure 12-1

Diagram of the cellular elements of the retina. Light entering the eye passes through the full thickness of the retina to reach the rods and cones (first system of retinal neurons). Impulses arising in these cells are transmitted by the bipolar cells (second system of retinal neurons) to the ganglion cell layer. The third system of visual neurons consists of the ganglion cells and their axons, which run uninterruptedly through the optic nerve, chiasm, and optic tracts, synapsing with cells in the lateral geniculate body. (Courtesy of Dr EM Chester.)

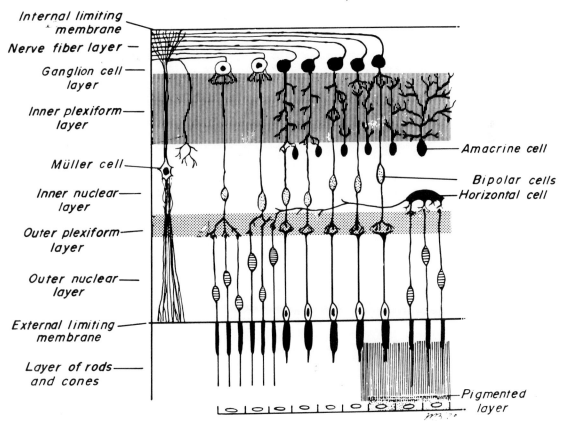

Internal limiting membrane
Nerve fiber layer
Ganglion cell layer
Inner plexiform layer
Müller cell
Inner nuclear layer
Outer plexiform layer
Outer nuclear layer
External limiting membrane
Layer of rods and cones
Amacrine cell
Bipolar cells
Horizontal cell
Pigmented layer

chiasm lies just above the pituitary body and also forms part of the anterior wall of the third ventricle; hence the crossing fibers may be compressed from below by a pituitary tumor, a meningioma of the tuberculum sellae, or an aneurysm, and from above by a dilated third ventricle or craniopharyngioma. The resulting field defect is bitemporal; and if one optic nerve is also implicated, there will be a loss of full-field vision in that eye (Fig. 12-3). Optic tract lesions are relatively rare in comparison to chiasmatic and nerve lesions. Surprisingly, in albinism, there is an abnormality of chiasmatic decussation, in which the majority of the fibers, including many that would not normally cross to the other side, decussate. How this relates to the defect in the pigment epithelium is not known.

Figure 12-2

Diagrammatic representation of the retinal projections, showing the disproportionately large representation of the macula in the lateral geniculate nucleus and visual cortex. (Redrawn from ML Barr and J Kiernan: The Human Nervous System, 4th ed. Philadelphia, Lippincott, 1983.)

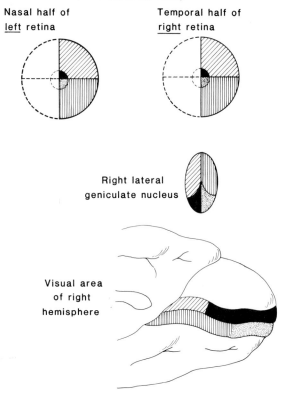

Nasal half of
left retina

Temporal half of
right retina

Right lateral
geniculate nucleus

Visual area
of right
hemisphere

The optic tract terminates mainly in the lateral geniculate nucleus and synapses with the four dorsal laminae of neurons. Two of these laminae receive fibers from the contralateral eye and two from the ipsilateral eye, in an alternating pattern. The geniculate cells project to the visual (striate) cortex, also called area 17. Other optic tract fibers terminate in the superior colliculus and innervate both Edinger-Westphal nuclei, which subserve pupillary constriction. If there is a lesion in one optic nerve, a light stimulus to the ipsilateral eye will have no effect on the pupil of either eye, although the ipsilateral pupil will still constrict consensually, i.e., in response to a light stimulus from the normal eye. This is called the *afferent pupillary defect*. Other tract fibers terminate in the pretectal and suprachiasmatic hypothalamic nuclei. The lateral geniculate body is irrigated by both the posterior choroidal and thalamogeniculate arteries and is rarely infarcted or exclusively involved in any other disease process.

In their course through the temporal lobes the fibers from the lower and upper quadrants of each retina diverge. The lower ones swing out over the temporal horn of the lateral ventricle before turning posteriorly; the upper ones follow a more direct path through the white matter of the uppermost part of the temporal lobe (Fig. 12-4). Both groups of fibers merge more posteriorly at the internal sagittal stratum. Incomplete lesions, for these reasons, cause visual field defects that are partial and not fully congruent.

It is in area 17 (also called V_1) that cortical processing of the retinogeniculate projections occurs. The receptive neurons are arranged in columns, some simple, others complex; some are activated by form and others by moving stimuli, or by color. Some of the afferent fibers terminate in the fourth cortical layer and others just above or below it. The neurons for each eye are grouped together and have concentric center-surround receptive fields.

The deep neurons of area 17 project to the secondary and tertiary visual areas of the occipitotemporal cortex of the same and opposite cerebral hemispheres and also to the multisensory parietal cortices. Several of these extrastriate connections are just now being identified. The classic studies of Hubel and Wiesel have elucidated much of this visual cortical physiology.

The vascular supply of the retina and posterior coats of the eye comes from the ophthalmic branch of the internal carotid artery. This artery gives origin first to the posterior ciliary arteries; the latter give rise to a rich circumferential plexus of vessels (arterial circle of Zinn-Haller) which is located deep to the lamina cribrosa. The arterial circle supplies the optic disc and adjacent part of the optic nerve and the choroid and ciliary body, and anastamoses with the pial arterial plexus that surrounds the optic nerve. The other major branch of the ophthalmic artery is the central retinal artery which issues from the optic disc and divides into four branches, each of which supplies a quadrant of the retina. A short distance from the disc these vessels lose their internal elastic lamina and muscularis and are properly classed as arterioles. The ganglion and bipolar cells receive their blood supply from these arterioles and their capillaries, whereas the deeper photoreceptor elements are nourished by the underlying choroidal vascular bed, by diffusion through the semipermeable Bruch membrane.

ABNORMALITIES OF THE RETINA

As regards the retinal lesions that cause impaired vision, they can usually be seen by ophthalmoscopic examination through a dilated pupil. Common mistakes are a failure to carefully inspect the macular zone (which is located 3 to 4 mm lateral to the optic disc and provides for 95 percent of visual acuity) and to search the periphery of the retina. There are variations in the appearance of the normal macula

and optic disc and these may prove troublesome. A normal macula may be called abnormal because of a slight derangement of the retinal pigment epithelium or a few drusen (see further on).

The normal optic disc varies in color, being paler in infants and in blond individuals; and the prominence of the lamina cribrosa (a sieve-like structure in the central or nasal part of the disc through which run the fascicles of unmyelinated axons of the retinal ganglion cells) differs from one individual to another. The absence of percipient elements in the optic disc or papilla accounts for the normal blind spot. The myelin sheaths of the ganglion-cell axons, which are normally acquired after penetration of the lamina cribrosa, may extend through the disc into the peripapillary

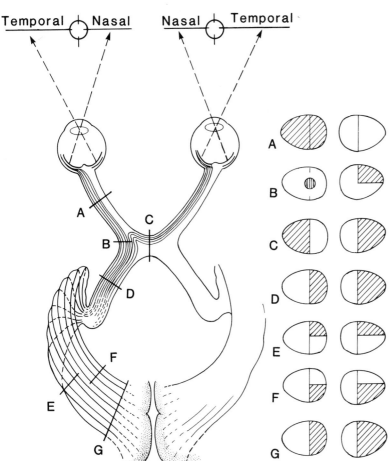

Figure 12-3

Diagram showing the effects on the fields of vision produced by lesions at various points along the optic pathway: A, complete blindness in left eye; B, the usual effect is a left junction scotoma in association with a right upper quadrantanopia. The latter results from interruption of right retinal nasal fibers that project into the base of the left optic nerve (Wilbrand's knee). A left nasal hemianopia could occur from a lesion at this point but is exceedingly rare; C, bitemporal hemianopia; D, right homonymous hemianopia; E and F, right upper and lower quadrant hemianopia; and G, right homonymous hemianopia.

region as another normal variant. They appear as white patches with fine feathered edges, adjacent to the disc, and must not be confused with exudates.

In evaluating *changes in the retinal vessels*, one must remember that these are arterioles and not arteries. Since the walls of the retinal arterioles are transparent, what is seen with the ophthalmoscope is the column of blood within them. The central light streak of many normal arterioles is thought to represent the reflection of light from the ophthalmoscope as it strikes the interface of the column of blood and the concave vascular wall. In *arteriolosclerosis* (usually coexistent with hypertension), the lumina of the vessels appear irregularly narrowed because of fibrous tissue replacement of the media and thickening of the basement membrane. Straightening of arterioles, arteriolar-venular compression, and *segmental narrowing of arterioles* are other signs of hypertension and arteriolosclerosis. It is generally believed that the vein is compressed by the thickened arteriole within the adventitial envelope shared by both vessels at the site of crossing. It is this crossing compression that may lead to occlusions of branches of the retinal veins. Progressive vascular disease, to the point of occlusion of the lumen, results in a narrow, white ("silverwire") vessel with no visible blood column. This change is associated most often with severe hypertension but may follow other types of occlusion of the central retinal artery or its branches. Sheathing of the venules, probably representing focal leakage from the vessels, is observed in some patients with multiple sclerosis, leukemia, malignant hypertension, sarcoid, Behçet disease, or other forms of vasculitis.

In malignant hypertension there are, in addition to the arteriolar changes noted above, a number of extravascular lesions: the so-called soft exudates or cotton-wool patches, sharply marginated, glistening "hard" exudates, retinal hemorrhages, and papilledema; in many patients who show these retinal changes, analogous lesions are to be found in the brain (necrotizing arteriolitis and microinfarcts). This is the picture of hypertensive encephalopathy.

The ophthalmoscopic appearance of retinal hemorrhages is determined by the structural arrangements of the particular tissue in which they occur. In the superficial layer of the retina they are linear or flame-shaped, because of their confinement by the horizontally coursing nerve fibers in that layer. These hemorrhages usually overlie and obscure the retinal vessels. Round or oval ("dot and blot") hemorrhages lie behind the vessels, in the outer plexiform layer (synaptic layer between bipolar cells and nuclei of rods and cones); in this layer, blood accumulates in the form of a cylinder between vertically oriented nerve fibers, and appears round when viewed end-on with the ophthalmoscope. Rupture of arterioles on the inner surface of the retina, such as occurs with ruptured intracranial saccular aneurysms, arteriovenous malformations, and other conditions causing sudden severe elevation of intracranial pressure, permits the accumulation of a sharply outlined lake of blood between the internal limiting membrane of the retina and the coalescing vitreous fibers (hyaloid membrane); this is the subhyaloid or preretinal hemorrhage. Either the small superficial or the deep retinal hemorrhage may show a central or eccentric pale (Roth) spot, which is caused by an accumulation of white blood cells, fibrin, histiocytes, or amorphous material between the vessel and the hemorrhage. This lesion is said to be characteristic of bacterial endocarditis, but we have seen it most often in leukemia and in embolic retinopathy due to carotid disease.

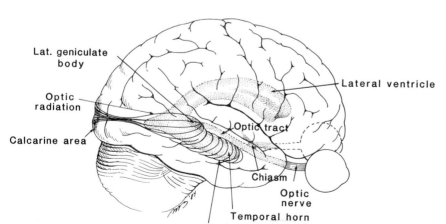

Figure 12-4

The geniculocalcarine projection showing the detour of lower fibers around the temporal horn. Note that practically none of the pathway traverses the parietal lobe.

Lat. geniculate body

Optic radiation

Calcarine area

Lateral ventricle

Optic tract

Chiasm

Optic nerve

Temporal horn

Temporal detour

Cotton-wool patches, like splinter hemorrhages, overlie and tend to obscure the retinal blood vessels. Large patches, or small ones involving the macula, cause serious disturbances of vision. The soft exudates are in reality infarcts of the nerve fiber layer, due to occlusion of arterioles and capillaries; they are composed of clusters of ovoid structures called *cytoid bodies*, representing the terminal swellings of interrupted axons. *Hard exudates* appear as punctate, white or yellow bodies; they lie in the outer plexiform layer, behind the retinal vessels, like the punctate hemorrhages. If present in the macular region, they are arranged in lines radiating toward the fovea (*macular star*). Hard exudates consist of fibrin strands, neutral fat, and fatty acids, and their pathogenesis is not understood. They are observed most often in cases of diabetes mellitus, and accelerated hypertension. *Drusen (colloid bodies)* are difficult to distinguish ophthalmoscopically from hard exudates, except when they occur alone; as a rule, hard exudates are accompanied by other funduscopic abnormalities. The source of drusen is uncertain. Some are probably benign excrescences of Bruch's membrane (which supports the layer of pigment epithelium next to the rods and cones). Others located near the optic disc and simulating papilledema are thought to be mineralized residues of dead axons and can be seen on CT scan in some cases.

Aneurysms of retinal vessels appear as small, discrete red dots and are located, in the largest number, in the paracentral region. They occur with or without other vascular lesions of the retina and are most often a sign of diabetes mellitus, sometimes appearing before the usual clinical manifestations of that disease have become obvious. The use of the red-free (green) light on the ophthalmoscope helps to pick out microaneurysms from the background. Microscopically the aneurysms take the form of small (20- to 90-μm) saccular outpouchings from the walls of capillaries, venules, or arterioles. The vessels of origin of the aneurysms are invariably abnormal, being either acellular branches of occluded vessels or themselves occluded by fat or fibrin.

Finally, the periphery of the retina may harbor a hemangioblastoma, which may appear during adolescence, before the more characteristic cerebellar lesion. A large retinal artery may lead to it and a large vein may be seen draining it. Laser treatment is effective if done early (see page 535). Occasionally, retinal examination discloses the presence of a vascular malformation that may be coextensive with a much larger malformation of the optic nerve and basilar portions of the brain (page 674).

ISCHEMIC LESIONS OF THE RETINA

Occlusion of the internal carotid artery may occasion no disturbance of vision whatsoever, providing there are adequate anastomotic branches from the external carotid artery into the orbit. When ischemic oculopathy does occur, it may be anterior or posterior, or both. Insufficient circulation to the anterior segment is manifested by episcleral vascular congestion, cloudiness of the cornea, anterior chamber flare, rubeosis iridis, and abnormal intraocular pressures. Ischemia of the posterior segment is manifested by circulatory changes in the retina and optic nerve, venous stasis, and low ophthalmodynamometer pressures. Other neurologic signs of carotid disease may be present (page 626).

The central retinal artery or its branches may be occluded by thrombi or emboli. Occlusion of the main artery is attended by sudden loss of sight. The retina becomes cloudy and has a grayish-yellow appearance, and the arterioles are narrowed with segmentation of columns of blood and a cherry-red appearance of the fovea. With branch occlusions by emboli one may be able to see the occluding particles. The most frequent of these are atheromatous particles (glistening, whitish-yellow masses), fibrin-platelet thrombi (red or white masses), and white calcium particles from calcified aortic or mitral valves or atheroma of great vessels. The fibrin-platelet emboli may cause only transient blindness and disappear (amaurosis fugax); they may be difficult to see unless exposed by fluorescein retinography.

Thrombotic ischemic optic neuropathy may occur without visible change in the retinal circulation or at most a slight swelling of the disc. Usually the patient is hypertensive and atherosclerotic. Often the blindness is painless and vision does not return. Later the optic nerve becomes pale.

A transitory ocular ischemia has been reported a few times as a manifestation of migraine; and it has been observed in polycythemia, hyperglobulinemia, sickle-cell anemia, and giant-cell arteritis. In the latter, which assumes importance because of its therapeutic and prophylactic implications, the optic nerve head may undergo infarction, often with permanent blindness. Steroid therapy given for the underlying cranial arteritis or polymyalgia rheumatica is preventative; or if one eye is already affected the other eye may be saved. Massive blood loss may also produce visual loss and ischemic infarction of the retina and optic nerve.

Since the central retinal artery and vein share a common adventitial sheath, atheromatous plaques in the artery are said to be associated in some instances with thrombosis of the retinal vein. There is then a spectacular display of retinal lesions which differs from the picture of central retinal artery occlusion. The veins are engorged and tortuous, and there are diffuse "dot and blot" and streaky linear retinal hemorrhages. This lesion is most frequently observed with diabetes mellitus, hypertension, and leukemia, less frequently with sickle-cell disease, and rarely with multiple myeloma and macroglobulinemia. In retinal vein thrombosis visual loss is more variable and there may be recovery of useful vision.

In summary, sudden painless loss of vision should always raise the question of ischemia of the retina or the optic nerve, due to occlusive disease of the central retinal artery or vein or posterior ciliary arteries. Detachment of the retina and macular or vitreous hemorrhage are somewhat less common causes.

OTHER DISEASES OF THE RETINA

Aside from vascular lesions, other more specific alterations of the retina, namely tears and detachments, may impair vision acutely. The rods and cones may be separated from the pigment layer of the retina; or in cases of proliferative retinopathy secondary to vascular lesions (diabetic retinopathy) the fibrous tissue may contract and pull the entire retina away from the choroid.

Serous retinopathy and chorioretinitis represent another category of retinal disease. In serous retinitis, a condition more frequent in elderly males, the entire perimacular zone is elevated by edema fluid. Vision is usually distorted but acuity is not much impaired. The optic disc remains normal. The retinal change is best revealed by fluorescein angiography. In chorioretinitis there may also be difficulty in diagnosis, and in not a few of our cases the initial diagnosis was retrobulbar neuritis. One cannot depend upon the appearance of a macular star (see above) for diagnosis.

Diseases such as toxoplasmosis, histoplasmosis, syphilis, tuberculosis, sarcoidosis, and the HTLV I virus may affect both the retina and choroid. The ophthalmoscopic picture is characteristic. Destruction of the retina and the pigment epithelium of the choroid produces punched-out lesions, exposing the whitish sclera and deposits of black pigment in various forms. The choroid is also a frequent site of viral and noninfective inflammatory reactions, often in association with recurrent iridocyclitis and lacrimal inflammation.

Degenerations of the retina are an important cause of chronic visual loss. They assume several forms and may be associated with other neurologic abnormalities. The most frequent is a hereditary disease of the outer receptor layer and subjacent pigment epithelium, known as *retinitis pigmentosa*. The retina is thin, and there are fine deposits of

black pigment in the shape of bone corpuscles, more in the periphery. The optic discs later become pale. It may be combined with endocrine or hypothalamic disorders as part of the Laurence-Moon-Biedl syndrome. Another hereditary form with massive central retinal lesions is the Stargardt form of juvenile tapetoretinal degeneration. Like retinitis pigmentosa, it may be accompanied by progressive spastic paraparesis or ataxia. Retinal degeneration is a familiar aspect of a number of other syndromes and diseases, such as Kearns-Sayre syndrome (page 1144), Bassen-Kornzweig disease (page 1059), Refsum disease (page 1058), and Batten-Mayou storage disease (page 809). Drusen arising from Bruch's membrane (see above) are associated with senile macular degeneration, an important cause of visual loss in the elderly. Areas of confluent drusen may give rise to subretinal neovascularization and hemorrhage in patients with pseudoxanthoma elasticum, Paget disease, hyperphosphatemia, sickle-cell anemia, and acromegaly.

Phenothiazine derivatives may conjugate with the melanin of the pigment layer, resulting in degeneration of the outer layers of the retina and a characteristic "bull's eye retinopathy." These drugs should be administered in low dosage, and the patient needs to be tested frequently for defects in visual fields and color vision.

Retinal degeneration may occur also in patients with an oat cell carcinoma of the lung. Antiretinal ganglion cell antibodies, presumably produced by the tumor cells, have been demonstrated in the serum of such patients by Grunwald and Kornguth and their colleagues.

In some of these retinal diseases, minimal changes in the retina or pigment epithelium, enough to reduce visual acuity, may not be readily detected by ophthalmoscopy. In these circumstances it is helpful to estimate the time required for recovery of visual acuity following light stimulation (macular photostress test). This test consists of shining a strong light through the pupil of an affected eye for 10 s and measuring the time necessary for the acuity to return to the pretest level (normally 50 s or less). In macular lesions of the retina it is prolonged. Lesions of the optic nerve do not affect the recovery time. Retinal diseases reduce or abolish the electrical activity generation by the retina and this can be measured in the electroretinogram. Fluorescein retinography is also helpful.

ABNORMALITIES OF THE OPTIC NERVES

These structures, which constitute the axonic projections of the retinal ganglion cells to the lateral geniculate bodies and superior colliculi (the third visual neurons), can only be inspected in the optic nerve head. Observable changes in the optic disc are therefore of particular importance. They may reflect the presence of raised intracranial pressure (papilledema or "choked disc"), congenital defects of the optic nerves (optic pits and colobomas), hypoplasias and atrophy of optic nerves, papillitis, and glaucoma. Illustrations of these and other abnormalities of the disc can be found in the eleventh edition of *Harrison's Principles of Internal Medicine*.

Of the various abnormalities of the optic disc, *papilledema* is of the greatest significance, neurologically speaking, for it provides evidence of increased intracranial pressure. In its mildest form the papilledema may present only as a blurring and slight elevation of the disc, especially of the superior and inferior margins. Since many normal individuals, especially those with hypermetropia, have ill-defined nasal disc margins, this early stage of papilledema may be difficult to detect. Pulsations of retinal veins, best seen where the veins turn to enter the disc, will have disappeared by the time intracranial pressure is raised, but since 10 to 15 percent of normal individuals have no venous pulsations, this criterion is not absolute. On the other hand, the presence of spontaneous venous pulsations is a reliable indicator of an intracranial pressure below 180 to 190 mmH$_2$O and thus usually excludes early papilledema.

The more advanced degrees of papilledema appear as a "mushrooming" of the entire disc and surrounding retina, with edema and obscuration of vessels at the disc margins and peripapillary hemorrhages. When advanced, papilledema is almost always bilateral and may be more pronounced on the side of an intracranial tumor. A purely unilateral edema of the optic disc is usually associated with perioptic meningiomas and other tumors and lesions of the optic nerve, but it can occur at an early stage of increased intracranial pressure. As papilledema becomes chronic, the elevation of the disc margin is less prominent, and pallor of the optic nerve head appears. As the papilledema subsides, once the cause of it is removed, it leaves a secondary optic atrophy. Unlike primary optic atrophy, the disc margins are irregular, often with peripapillary pigment deposits.

Papilledema from increased intracranial pressure must be distinguished from a combined edema of the optic nerve and retina, which typifies both malignant hypertension and posterior uveitis with retinitis. These two conditions are usually divulged by changes in the periphery of the retinas and other data. Papilledema may also occur without raised intracranial pressure in children with cyanotic congenital heart disease and polycythemia. As remarked earlier, visual acuity is usually retained with papilledema, except for enlargement of the blind spots and constriction of the visual fields. The pupillary light reflexes remain normal.

The mechanism of production of papilledema is not fully understood. The essential element is an increase in pressure in the space around the optic nerve, which communicates directly with the subarachnoid space of the brain. This was demonstrated convincingly by Hayreh (1964), who produced bilateral chronic papilledema in monkeys by inflating balloons in the temporal subarachnoid space and then opening the sheath of one optic nerve; the papilledema

promptly subsided on the operated side but not on the opposite side. Many years ago, Paton and Holmes hypothesized that the increased pressure in the perioptic subarachnoid spaces blocks the central retinal vein, leading to congestion in the capillary circulation of the optic nerve head. However, the picture of central retinal vein obstruction, consisting of rapidly evolving retinal edema, peripheral retinal hemorrhages, and marked venous dilatation, is quite different from that of papilledema. Furthermore, the capillaries that become congested in papilledema are derived from the short ciliary arteries (Hayreh). In recent years, the pathogenesis of papilledema has been restudied in terms of orthograde axoplasmic transport (Minckler et al; Tso and Hayreh). These investigators found that with increased intracranial pressure the initial changes consisted of swelling of the nerve fibers due to stasis of anterograde axoplasmic flow, and that these changes were responsible for the swelling of the optic disc and blurring of the disc margins. The vascular changes (hyperemia of the disc, capillary dilatation, and hemorrhages) appeared later and were considered to be secondary to edema of the optic disc.

Fluorescein angiography, red-free fundus photos (which highlight the retinal nerve fibers), and stereoscopic fundus photography may be helpful in detecting early edema of the optic discs.

Congenital cavitary defects due to defective closure of the optic fissure may be a cause of impaired vision because of failure of development of the papillomacular bundle. Usually the optic pit or a larger coloboma is unilateral and unassociated with developmental abnormalities of the brain (optic disc dysplasia and dysplastic coloboma). A hereditary form is known (Brown and Tasman). Children may be born with developmental anomalies of the optic nerves. Their vision may be impaired and the discs are of small diameter (hypoplasia of the optic disc or micropapilla).

SYNDROME OF RETROBULBAR NEUROPATHY

Acute impairment of vision in one eye or both eyes (in the latter case the eyes may be affected either simultaneously or successively) develops in a number of clinical settings. The most frequent is one in which a child, adolescent, or young adult notes a rapid diminution of vision in one eye (as though a veil or haze had covered the eye), sometimes progressing within days or a week or two to complete blindness. The optic disc and retina may appear normal, but if the lesion is near the nerve head, there may be swelling of the disc, i.e., papillitis, and the disc margins are elevated and blurred, and rarely surrounded by hemorrhages. Papillitis is distinguished from the papilledema of increased intracranial pressure by the marked impairment of vision and the scotoma it produces. Pain on movement of the eye, tenderness on pressure of the globe, and a subjective difference in light brightness are other consistent findings. The patient may report an increase in blurring of vision with exertion or following a hot bath. In addition to papillitis, examination may disclose an impairment of color vision and variable haziness of the vitreous. In about 10 percent of cases both eyes are involved, either simultaneously or in rapid succession. In a large proportion of such patients, no cause of the retrobulbar neuropathy can be found, and after several more weeks there is spontaneous recovery. Vision returns to normal in more than two-thirds of all instances; occasionally a scotoma is left; more rarely, the patient is left blind. The optic disc later becomes slightly pale in many of the patients. The CSF may be normal or may contain from 10 to 100 lymphocytes, and the total protein and gamma globulin may be elevated and show oligoclonal bands.

Nearly 75 percent of such patients will develop other symptoms and signs of multiple sclerosis within 15 years, and probably even more will do so if the patients are observed for longer periods. Less is known about children with retrobulbar neuropathy, in whom the disorder is more often bilateral and frequently related to a preceding viral infection. Their prognosis is better than that for adults. Formerly the syndrome was blamed on sinusitis and treated as such, but Cushing long ago proved the error of this assumption. Sinus disease rarely affects vision and should only be considered in the face of other evidence of infection, such as fever, purulent nasal discharge, leukocytosis, etc. Occasionally a sphenoidal or ethmoidal mucocele can compress the optic nerve. Leber hereditary optic atrophy may simulate retrobulbar neuropathy (see page 959). Demyelinative disease is the only common cause of a unilateral retrobulbar neuritis, but the nature of those forms that do not progress to multiple sclerosis remains obscure. Regression of symptoms may occur spontaneously or may be hastened by the administration of ACTH or corticosteroids (see page 766).

TOXIC AND NUTRITIONAL OPTIC NEUROPATHIES

Simultaneous impairment of vision in the two eyes, with central or centrocecal scotomas, usually is caused not by a demyelinative process but by a toxic or nutritional disorder. The latter condition is observed most often in the chronic

alcoholic patient. Impairment of visual acuity evolves over several days or a week or two, and examination discloses bilateral, roughly symmetric central or centrocecal scotomas, the peripheral fields being intact. With appropriate treatment (nutritious diet and B vitamins) instituted soon after the onset of amblyopia, complete recovery is possible; if treatment is delayed, patients are left with varying degrees of permanent defect in central vision and pallor of the temporal portions of the optic discs. This disorder is commonly referred to as "tobacco-alcohol amblyopia," the implication being that it is due to the toxic effects of tobacco or alcohol, or both. In fact the disorder is caused by nutritional deficiency and is properly designated as *nutritional amaurosis* or *nutritional optic neuropathy* (Chap. 39). The same disorder may be seen in nonalcoholic patients, under conditions of severe nutritional deprivation, and in patients with vitamin B_{12} deficiency (pernicious anemia).

Impairment of vision due to *methyl alcohol intoxication* is abrupt in onset and is characterized by large symmetric central scotomas, as well as by symptoms of systemic disease and acidosis. Treatment is directed mainly to correction of the acidosis. The subacute development of central field defects has been attributed to several other toxins and the chronic administration of certain therapeutic agents: halogenated hydroxyquinolines (Enterovioform, Clioquinol), chloramphenicol, ethambutol, isoniazid, streptomycin, chlorpropamide (Diabinese), and ergot. Liebold has catalogued all drugs known to have a toxic effect on the optic nerves.

OTHER OPTIC NEUROPATHIES

A subacute optic neuropathy has been described in Jamaican natives. It is characterized by a bilaterally symmetric central visual loss and is occasionally accompanied by nerve deafness, ataxia, and spasticity. A similar condition has been described in other Caribbean countries. Nothing is known of its cause. A nutritional basis has been suspected but has never been proved.

Congenital and hereditary optic atrophies, including the well-known Leber and related forms, are discussed in Chaps. 38 and 44 (see also Table 14-1).

Chiasmal and optic nerve compression by gliomas, meningiomas, craniopharyngiomas, and metastatic tumors may cause scotomas and optic atrophy (Chap. 31). Thyroid ophthalmopathy is an occasional cause of optic nerve compression. Infiltration of an optic nerve may occur in sarcoidosis and with certain neoplasmas, notably leukemia and lymphoma.

Orbital inflammatory diseases, both acute and subacute types of orbital cellulitis, may affect the optic nerves, but more often they result in pain, proptosis, and ophthalmoplegia. For this reason, they are discussed with the disorders of cranial pain and ocular motility (Chaps. 9 and 13).

Cranial arteritis, systemic lupus erythematosus, diabetes, and AIDS rarely give rise to the syndrome of retrobulbar neuropathy and should only be considered after all other causes of optic nerve compression have been ruled out.

NEUROLOGY OF THE CENTRAL VISUAL PATHWAYS

From the retina there is a point-to-point projection to the lateral geniculate ganglion and from the latter to the calcarine cortex of the occipital lobe. Thus the visual cortex receives a spatial pattern of stimulation that corresponds with the retinal image of the visual field. Visual impairments due to lesions of the central pathways usually involve only a part of the visual fields, and a plotting of the latter provides information as to the site of the lesion.

For purposes of description of the visual fields, each retina and macula are divided into a temporal and nasal half by a vertical line passing through the fovea centralis. A horizontal line represented roughly by the junction of the superior and inferior retinal vascular arcades also passes through the fovea and divides each half of the retina and macula into upper and lower quadrants. The anatomic features of the central projections of the retinas are illustrated in their simplest form in Fig. 12-2.

ABNORMALITIES OF THE VISUAL FIELDS

Visual field defects caused by lesions of the retina, optic nerves, and tracts, lateral geniculate bodies, geniculocalcarine pathway, and striate cortex of the occipital lobe are illustrated in Fig. 12-3. In the alert, cooperative patient, the visual fields can be plotted accurately at the bedside. With one of the patient's eyes covered and the other looking directly into the corresponding eye of the examiner (patient's right eye and examiner's left), a target, such as a moving finger, a cotton pledget, or white disc mounted on a stick, is brought from the outside toward the center of the visual field. With the target at an equal distance between the examiner's and patient's eyes, the patient's fields are compared with those of the examiner. Similarly the patient's blind spot can be aligned with the examiner's, and its size determined by moving the target outward from the blind spot until it is seen. Central and paracentral defects in the field can be outlined the same way. For reasons not known, red-green test objects are more sensitive than white ones in detecting diseases of the optic pathways.

It should be emphasized, however, that movement represents the coarsest stimulus to the retina, so that a perception of motion may be preserved while a stationary target of the same size may not be seen. In other words, moving targets are less useful than static ones in confrontational testing of visual fields. Rapid finger counting, hand comparison, and comparison of color from quadrant to quadrant are simple confrontational tests that will disclose even subtle field defects. Glaser uses a simple and effective method for the detection of hemianopic defects. The examiner's hands are presented simultaneously to either side of the vertical meridian separating the temporal from the nasal hemifield; the hand in the hemianopic depression appears blurred or darker than the other. Similarly, a scotoma may be defined by asking the patient to report changes in color or brightness of a test object as it is moved toward or away from the point of fixation.

A central scotoma is best identified by having the patient fixate on the examiner's nose, on which he places the index finger of one hand or a white-headed pin, and has the patient compare it for brightness, clarity, and color with a finger or pin held in the periphery. Alternately, two test objects can be used, one placed centrally and the other eccentrically, and the patient is asked to describe differences in color intensity. Finally, if any defect is found or suspected by confrontation testing, the fields should be charted on a *perimeter* and scotomas outlined on a *tangent screen*. Computer-assisted perimetry is now available in some centers.

The method of double simultaneous stimulation may elicit visual field defects that are undetected by conventional perimetry. Movement of one finger in all parts of each temporal field may disclose no abnormality, but if movement is simultaneous in analogous parts of both temporal fields, the patient with a parietal lobe lesion, especially on the right, may see only the one in the normal right hemifield. In young children or uncooperative patients the integrity of the fields may be roughly estimated by observing whether the patient is attracted to objects in the peripheral field or blinks in response to sudden threatening gestures in one-half the visual field.

A common abnormality disclosed by visual field examination is *concentric constriction*. This may be due to papilledema, in which case it is usually accompanied by an enlargement of the blind spot. A concentric constriction of the visual field, at first unilateral and later bilateral, associated with pallor of the optic disc (optic atrophy), should suggest chronic syphilitic optic neuritis. Longstanding, untreated glaucoma is another cause of concentric constriction. *Tubular ("gun-barrel," "tunnel") vision*, i.e., constriction of the visual field to the same degree regardless of the distance of the visual test stimulus from the eye, is a sign of hypersuggestibility or hysteria. In organic disease, the constricted visual field naturally enlarges as the distance between the patient and the test object increases.

Visual field defects are always described in terms of the visual field, rather than the retina. The retinal image of an object in the visual field is inverted and reversed from right to left (like the image on the film of a camera). The rules which govern the representation of the visual fields in the geniculae ganglion and cerebral cortex are, therefore, the reverse of those which apply to the retinal representation (see above): (1) The left visual field of each eye is represented in the right geniculate nucleus and the visual cortex of the right occipital lobe. (2) The upper half of the visual field is represented in the lateral part of the geniculate ganglion and below the calcarine fissure in the visual cortex; the opposite holds for the lower half of the visual field.

PRECHIASMAL LESIONS

Lesions of the macula, retina, or optic nerve cause either a scotoma (an island of impaired vision surrounded by normal vision) or a defect which extends to the periphery of one visual field. Scotomas are named according to their position (central, cecocentral) or their shape (ring). A small scotoma in the macular part of the visual field may seriously impair visual acuity. Demyelinative disease (optic neuritis), neuroretinitis, Leber hereditary optic atrophy, toxins (methyl alcohol, quinine, chloroquine, and certain of the phenothiazine tranquilizing drugs), nutritional deficiency (so-called tobacco-alcohol amblyopia), and vascular disease (ischemic optic neuropathy) are the usual causes of scotomas. Orbital or retro-orbital tumors are rare causes. The toxic states are characterized by symmetric bilateral scotomas, and the nutritional disorders by more or less symmetric bilateral central scotomas (involving the fixation point) or centrocecal ones (involving both the fixation point and the blind spot). The centrocecal scotoma, which tends to have an arcuate border, represents a lesion that is predominantly in the distribution of the papillomacular bundle. However, the finding of this visual field abnormality does not establish whether the primary defect is in the cells of the origin of the bundle, i.e., the retinal ganglion cells, or their fibers. Demyelinative disease is characterized by unilateral or asymmetric bilateral scotomas. Vascular lesions which take the form of retinal hemorrhages and infarctions of the nerve-cell layer (cotton-wool patches) give rise to unilateral scotomas; occlusion of the central retinal artery or its branches causes infarction of the retina and gives rise, as

a rule, to altitudinal lesions which respect the horizontal meridian (see further on). As pointed out above, vascular lesions may also occur in the optic nerve (ischemic optic neuropathy), causing sudden blindness or a scotoma with characteristic swelling and pallor of the optic disc and small splinter hemorrhages. Since the optic nerve also contains the afferent fibers for the pupillary light reflex, lesions of the nerve will cause a so-called afferent pupillary defect, which was described briefly above, in the section on anatomy and physiology, and will be considered further, in Chap. 13.

With most diseases of the optic nerve the optic disc will eventually become pale (*optic atrophy*). This usually requires 4 to 6 weeks to develop. If the optic nerve degenerates (e.g., in multiple sclerosis, Leber hereditary optic atrophy, traumatic transection, tumor of nerve, or syphilitic optic atrophy), the disc becomes chalk white, with sharp, clean margins. If the atrophy is secondary (consecutive) to papillitis or papilledema, the disc margins are indistinct and irregular, the disc has a pallid, yellow-gray appearance, like candle tallow, the vessels are partially obscured and may be sheathed, and the adjacent retina is altered.

LESIONS OF THE CHIASM, OPTIC TRACT, AND GENICULOCALCARINE PATHWAY

Hemianopia (hemianopsia) means blindness in one-half the visual field. *Bitemporal hemianopia* indicates a lesion of the decussating fibers of the optic chiasm and is usually caused by tumor of the pituitary gland (disclosed by CT scan). However, it may also be caused by craniopharyngiomas, saccular aneurysms of the circle of Willis, meningiomas of the tuberculum sellae, less often by sarcoidosis, metastatic carcinoma, and ectopic pinealoma or dysgerminoma, and rarely by Hand-Schuller-Christian disease. The lesion is always in the chiasm, involving the decussating nasal fibers from each retina, although in some instances the tumor pushing upward presses the medial parts of the optic nerves against the anterior cerebral arteries. Heteronymous field defects, i.e., scotomas or field defects that differ in the two eyes, are also a sign of involvement of the optic chiasm or the adjoining optic nerves or tracts; they are caused by craniopharyngioma or other suprasellar tumors and rarely by mucoceles, venous angiomas, and opticochiasmic arachnoiditis.

Homonymous hemianopia (a loss of vision in corresponding halves of the visual fields) signifies a lesion of the visual pathway behind the chiasm and, if complete, gives no more information than that. *Incomplete homonymous hemianopia* has more localizing value; as a general rule, if the field defects in the two eyes are identical (congruous), the lesion is likely to be in the calcarine cortex and subcortical white matter of the occipital lobe; if *incongruous*, the visual fibers in the optic tract or in the parietal or temporal lobe are more likely to be implicated. Lesions of the optic tract give the most incongruous defects; these lesions give a congruous defect only when they are complete. Actually, absolute congruity of the field defects is rare, even with occipital lesions.

The lower fibers of the geniculocalcarine pathway (from the inferior retina) swing in a wide arc over the temporal horn of the ventricle into the temporal lobe, before joining the upper fibers of the pathway on their way to the calcarine cortex (Fig. 12-4). This arc of fibers is known as Flechsig's, Meyer's, or Archambault's loop, and a lesion that interrupts these fibers will produce a defect in the upper quadrants of the contralateral visual fields (Fig. 12-3), i.e., an *upper homonymous quadrantanopia*. This clinical effect was first described by Harvey Cushing, so that his name also has been applied to the loop of temporal visual fibers. Parietal lobe lesions are said to affect the lower quadrants of the visual fields more than the upper ones, but this is difficult to document; with a lesion of the right parietal lobe the patient ignores the left half of space, and with a left parietal lesion the patient is usually aphasic.

If the entire optic tract or calcarine cortex on one side is destroyed, the homonymous hemianopia is complete. But often that part of the field subserved by the macula is spared, the reason being that some macular fibers terminate in the ipsilateral striate cortex. With infarction of the occipital lobe due to occlusion of the posterior cerebral artery, the polar region (macular zone) may be spared by virtue of collateral circulation from the anterior cerebral artery. Incomplete lesions of the optic tract and radiation usually spare central (macular) vision. We have nevertheless observed a lesion of the tip of one occipital lobe to produce central homonymous hemianopic scotomata, including the maculae. Lesions of both occipital poles (as in embolization of the posterior cerebral arteries) result in bilateral central scotomas; and if all the calcarine cortex or all the subcortical geniculocalcarine fibers on both sides are completely destroyed, there is ''cortical'' blindness. *Homonymous altitudinal hemianopia* is usually due to lesions of both occipital lobes below or above the calcarine cortex and rarely to a lesion of the optic chiasm or nerves. An altitudinal defect is one that is confined to the upper or lower half of the field but crosses the vertical meridian. The most common cause of an altitudinal homonymous hemianopia is infarction due to occlusion of the posterior cerebral artery. Rarely, the discovery of an altitudinal visual defect, unilateral or bilateral, in an adult denotes an acquired lesion of the retina or optic nerve, and rarely a congenital hypoplasia of the optic nerve. The female offspring of a diabetic mothers are particularly prone to such lesions (Nelson et al).

In some instances of homonymous hemianopia the patient is capable of experiencing some visual sensations in the hemianopic fields, a circumstance that permits the study of the vulnerability of different visual functions. Colored targets may be detected in the hemianopic fields, whereas achromatic ones cannot. But even in complete hemianopic defects, in which the patient admits to being blind, it has been shown that he or she may still react to visual stimuli when forced-choice techniques are used. This type of residual visual function has been called ''blindsight'' by Weiskrantz et al. Blythe et al found that 20 percent of their patients with no pattern discrimination in the hemianopic field could still reach accurately and look at a moving light in the ''blind'' field. These residual visual functions are thought to be subserved by retinocollicular or geniculoprestriate cortical connections.

In distinction to blindness, there is another, less common, category of visual impairment in which patients cannot understand the meaning of what they see, i.e., *visual agnosia*. Primary visual perception is intact, and patients may describe accurately the shape, color, and size of objects that are presented. Despite this, they cannot identify the objects unless they hear, smell, taste, or palpate them. The failure of visual recognition of words alone is called *alexia*. The ability to recognize visually presented objects and words depends upon the integrity not only of the visual pathways and primary visual area of the cerebral cortex (area 17 of Brodmann), but also of those cortical areas which lie just anterior to area 17 (areas 18 and 19 of the occipital lobe and the angular gyrus of the dominant hemisphere). Visual-object agnosia rarely, if ever, occurs as an isolated finding: as a rule it is combined with visual verbal agnosia or homonymous hemianopia, or both. These abnormalities arise from lesions of the dominant occipital cortex and adjacent parietal (angular gyrus) and temporal cortex or from a lesion of the left calcarine cortex combined with one that interrupts the fibers crossing from the right occipital lobe (see page 386). Failure to understand the meaning of an entire picture even though some of its parts are recognized is referred to as *simultagnosia*, and a failure to recognize familiar faces, as *prosopagnosia*. These and other variants of visual agnosia (including visual neglect), and their pathologic bases, are dealt with more fully in Chap. 21.

Other disturbances of vision include various types of distortion in which images seem to recede into the distance (teleopsia), or appear too small (micropsia), or, less frequently, too large (macropsia). If such a disturbance is in one eye only, a local retinal lesion should be suspected. When these phenomena are bilateral, however, they usually signify disease of the temporal lobes, in which case the visual disturbances tend to occur in attacks and are accompanied by other manifestations of temporal lobe seizures (Chap. 15). With parietal lobe lesions, objects may appear to be askew. Lesions of the vestibular nucleus or its immediate connections may also produce the illusion that objects are tilted or that straight lines are curved.

ABNORMALITIES OF COLOR VISION

Normal color vision depends on the integrity of cone cells which are most numerous in the macular region. When activated, they convey information to special columns of cells in the striate cortex. Three different cone pigments with optimal sensitivities to blue, green, and orange-yellow wavelengths are said to characterize these cells; presumably each cone possesses only one of these pigments. Transmission to higher centers for the perception of color is believed to be effected by neurons and axons that encode at least two pairs of complementary colors: red-green in one system and yellow-blue in the other. In the optic nerves and tracts the fibers for color are of small caliber and are preferentially sensitive to noxious agents and pressure. The geniculostriate fibers for color are separate from, but course with, those which convey information about form and brightness; hence there may be a homonymous color hemianopia (hemiachromatopsia). The visual fields for blue-yellow are smaller than those for white light, and the red and green fields are smaller than those for blue-yellow.

Diseases may affect color vision by abolishing it completely (achromatopsia) or partially by quantitatively reducing one or more of the three attributes of color: brightness, hue, and saturation. Or, only one of the complementary pairs of colors may be lost, usually red-green. And the disorder may be congenital and hereditary, or acquired. The commonest form is a male sex-linked inability to see red and green, while retaining normal visual acuity. A genetic abnormality of cone pigments is postulated, but the defect cannot be seen by inspecting the retina. A failure of the cones to develop or a degeneration of cones may cause a loss of color vision, but in the latter condition visual acuity is often diminished, a central scotoma may be present, and, although the macula appears to be normal ophthalmoscopically, fluorescein angiography shows the pigment epithelium to be defective. Congenital color vision defects are usually protan (red) or dentan (green), leaving yellow-blue color vision intact; acquired lesions may affect all colors. Lesions of the optic nerves usually affect red-green more than blue-yellow and the opposite is true of

retinal lesions. An exception is the dominant infantile optic atrophy of Kjer, in which the scotoma mapped by a large blue target is larger than that for red.

Damasio has drawn attention to a group of acquired deficits of color perception, with preservation of form vision, the result of focal damage (usually infarction) of the visual association cortex and subjacent white matter. Color vision may be lost in a quadrant or one-half of the visual field, or in the entire field. The latter, or full-field achromatopsia, is the result of bilateral occipitotemporal lesions, involving the fusiform and lingual gyri, a localization that accounts for its frequent association with visual agnosia (especially prosopagnosia, see page 370) and some degree of visual field defect. A lesion restricted to the inferior part of the right occipitotemporal region, sparing both the optic radiations and striate cortex, causes the purest form of achromatopsia (left hemiachromatopsia). With a similar left-sided lesion, alexia may be associated with the right hemiachromatopsia.

Finally, in addition to the losses of perception of form, movement, and color, lesions of the visual system may also give rise to a variety of positive sensory visual experiences. The simplest of these are called *phosphenes*, i.e., flashes of light and colored spots in the absence of luminous stimuli. Mechanical pressure on the normal eyeball may induce them at the retinal level, as every child discovers. Or they may occur with disease of the visual system at many different sites. Elderly patients commonly complain of flashes of light in the peripheral field of one eye, occurring in the dark; these are related to vitreous tags that rest on the retinal equator. The flashes are quite benign and are known as *Moore's lightning streaks*. In patients with migraine, ischemia of nerve cells in the occipital lobe gives rise to the bright zigzag lines of a fortification spectrum. Stimulation of the cortical terminations of the visual pathways account for the simple or unformed visual hallucinations of epilepsy. *Formed* or complex visual hallucinations (of people, animals, landscapes, etc.) are observed in a variety of conditions, notably in the withdrawal state following chronic intoxication with alcohol and other sedative-hypnotic drugs (Chaps. 41 and 42), in Alzheimer disease (Chap. 43), and in disease of the occipitoparietal or occipitotemporal regions, or the diencephalon (peduncular hallucinosis, see Chap. 21).

Occasionally, patients with an attention hemianopia may displace an image to the nonaffected half of the field of vision (*visual allesthesia*), or a visual image may persist for minutes to hours, or reappear episodically, after the exciting stimulus has been removed (*palinopsia* or *paliopsia*); the latter disorder also occurs in defective, but not blind, homonymous fields of vision. *Polyopia*, the perception of multiple images when a single stimulus is presented, is said to be associated predominantly with right occipital lesions and can be seen with either eye. Usually there is one primary and a number of secondary images and their relationships may be constant or changing. Bender and Krieger, who described several such patients, attributed the polyopia to unstable fixation. *Oscillopsia*, or illusory movement of the environment, occurs mainly with lesions of the labyrinthine-vestibular apparatus, and is described with disorders of ocular movement (see page 219).

Clinical effects and syndromes that result from occipital lobe lesions are discussed further in Chap. 21.

REFERENCES[1]

BENDER MB, KRIEGER HP: Visual function in perimetric blind fields. *Arch Neurol Psychiatry* 65:72, 1951.

BLYTHE IM, KENNARD C, RUDDOCK KH: Residual vision in patients with retrogeniculate lesions of the visual pathways. *Brain* 110:887, 1987.

BROWN GC, TASMAN WS: *Congenital Anomalies of the Optic Disc.* New York, Grune & Stratton, 1983.

CHESTER EM: *The Ocular Fundus in Systemic Disease.* Chicago, Year Book Medical Publishers, 1973.

DAMASIO AR: Disorder of complex visual processing: Agnosia, achromatopsia, Balint's syndrome and related difficulties of orientation and construction, in Mesulam M-M (ed.): *Principles of Behavioral Neurology.* Philadelphia, FA Davis, 1985.

GLASER JS: *Neuro-ophthalmology,* Hagerstown, MD, Harper & Row, 1978.

GRUNWALD GB, KLEIN R, SIMMONDS MA, KORNGUTH SE: Autoimmune basis for visual paraneoplastic syndrome in patients with small cell lung carcinoma. *Lancet* 1:658, 1985.

HAYREH SS: Pathogenesis of oedema of the optic disc (papilloedema). *Br J Ophthalmol* 48:522, 1964.

HAYREH SS: Anterior ischemic optic neuropathy. *Arch Neurol* 38:675, 1981.

HAYREH SS: Blood supply of the optic nerve head and its role in optic atrophy, glaucoma, and oedema of the optic disc. *Br J Ophthalmol* 53:721, 1969.

---

[1]See also references at end of Chap. 13.

HUBEL DH, WIESEL TN: Functional architecture of macaque monkey visual cortex. *Proc R Soc Lond [Biol]* 198:1–59, 1977.

KORNGUTH SE, KLEIN R, APPEN R, CHOATE J: The occurrence of anti-retinal ganglion cell antibodies in patients with small cell carcinoma of the lung. *Cancer* 50:1289, 1982.

LEIBOLD JE: Drugs having a toxic effect on the optic nerve. *Int Ophthalmol Clin,* 11:137, 1971.

LEVIN BE: The clinical significance of spontaneous pulsations of the retinal vein. *Arch Neurol* 35:37, 1978.

McDONALD WI: Diseases of the optic nerve, in Asbury AK, McKhann GM, McDonald WI (eds): *Diseases of the Nervous System.* Philadelphia, Saunders, 1986, Chap. 37.

MINCKLER DS, TSO MOM, ZIMMERMAN LE: A light microscopic autoradiographic study of axoplasmic transport in the optic nerve head during ocular hypotony, increased intraocular pressure, and papilledema. *Am J Ophthalmol* 82:741, 1976.

NELSON M, LESSELL S, SADUN AA: Optic nerve hypoplasia and maternal diabetes mellitus. *Arch Neurol* 43:20, 1986.

PATON L, HOLMES G: The pathology of papilloedema. A histological study of 60 eyes. *Brain* 33:389, 1911.

PEARLMAN AJ: Visual system, in Pearlman AL, Collins RC (eds.): *Neurological Pathophysiology,* 3rd ed. New York, Oxford University Press, 1984, Chap. 7.

RUCKER CW: Sheathing of retinal venus in multiple sclerosis. *Mayo Clin Proc* 47:335, 1972.

SAVINO PJ, PARIS M, SCHATZ NJ et al: Optic tract syndrome. *Arch Ophthalmol* 96:656, 1978.

SMITH JL, HOYT WP, SUSAC JO: Optic fundus in acute Leber's optic atrophy. *Arch Ophthalmol* 90:349, 1973.

TSO MOM, HAYREH SS: Optic disc edema in raised intracranial pressure III: A pathologic study of experimental papilledema. *Arch Ophthalmol* 95:1448, 1977; IV: Axoplasmic transport in experimental papilledema, ibid. 95:1458, 1977.

WEISKRANTZ L, WARRINGTON EK, SANDERS MD: Visual capacity in the hemianoptic field following restricted occipital ablation. *Brain* 97:709, 1974.

YOUNG LHY, APPEN RE: Ischemic oculopathy. *Arch Neurol* 38:358, 1981.

CHAPTER 13

DISORDERS OF OCULAR MOVEMENT AND PUPILLARY FUNCTION

Abnormalities of ocular movement are of two basic types. In one, the disorder of motility can be traced to a lesion of the extraocular muscles themselves or to the cranial nerves that supply them (*nuclear or infranuclear palsy*). In the other, the derangement is in the highly specialized neural mechanisms that enable the eyes to move together (*supranuclear palsy*). Such a distinction, in keeping with the general concept of upper and lower motor neuron paralysis, hardly conveys an idea of the complexity of the neural mechanisms that govern ocular motility; nevertheless it is a useful if not an essential first step in the approach to the patient with defective eye movements. In both cases, it must be recognized, a knowledge of the anatomic basis of normal movement is essential to an understanding of abnormal movement.

SUPRANUCLEAR DISORDERS OF EYE MOVEMENT

ANATOMIC AND PHYSIOLOGIC CONSIDERATIONS

In no aspect of human anatomy and physiology is the sensory guidance of muscle activity more instructively revealed than in the neural control of coordinated ocular movement. To focus the eyes voluntarily in searching the environment, to stabilize objects for scrutiny when the patient is moving, to maintain clear images of moving objects, to bring into sharp focus near and far objects—all require the perfect coordination of six sets of extraocular muscles and three sets of intrinsic muscles (sphincters and dilators of the iris and ciliary muscles). The neural mechanisms that govern these functions reside in the pons, midbrain, cerebellum, basal ganglia, and the frontal and occipital lobes of the brain. Most of the nuclear structures and pathways concerned with ocular movements are now known and much has been learned of their physiology.

Different diseases may elicit particular defects in ocular movement and pupillary function, and these are of diagnostic importance.

Accurate binocular vision is achieved by the associated action of the ocular muscles, which allows a visual stimulus to fall on exactly corresponding parts of the two retinas. The symmetric and synchronous movement of the eyes is termed *conjugate movement* or *gaze* (conjugate = yoked or joined together). The simultaneous movement of the eyes in opposite directions, as in convergence, is termed *disconjugate* or *disjunctive*. These two forms of ocular movement—conjugate and disconjugate—are also referred to as *versional* and *vergence*, respectively. *Vergence movements* are of two types—fusional and accommodative. *Fusional movements* are necessary at all times to prevent visual images from falling on noncorresponding parts of the retinas. *Accommodative vergence movements* are brought into action when one looks at a near object. The eyes turn inward (off their parallel axes) and at the same time the pupils constrict and the ciliary muscles relax to thicken the lens. This synkinesis is called the *near or accommodative triad*.

Area 8 in the frontal lobe is probably the region in which *voluntary* conjugate movements of the eyes to the opposite side are initiated. They can be elicited by instructing the patient to look to the right or left, hence are referred to also as movements on command. These are characteristically rapid (fast eye movements) or *saccadic*. Their purpose is to quickly change ocular fixation, i.e., to bring new images of objects of interest onto the foveas. Saccadic movements (or saccades) may also be elicited *reflexly*, as when a sudden sound or the appearance of an object in the peripheral field of vision triggers an automatic movement of the eyes in the direction of the stimulus. The neuronal firing pattern that produces a saccade has been characterized as "pulse-step" in type. This refers to the sudden increase in neuronal firing (the pulse) that is necessary to overcome the inertia and viscous drag of the eyes and to move them into their new position; this is followed by a return to a new baseline firing level (the step), which maintains the eyes in their new position by the constant tonic contraction of the extraocular muscles. The saccades are so rapid (about 200 ms) that the subject is not aware of any movement and objectively only one swift unbroken conjugate movement is observed.

Saccades are to be distinguished from the slower and smoother, largely involuntary *pursuit, or following, movements*, for which the major stimulus is a moving target upon which the eyes are fixated. The function of pursuit movements is to stabilize the image of a moving object on the foveas as the fixated object is tracked by the eyes (''smooth tracking'') and thus to maintain continuous clear vision of objects moving within the environment. Pursuit movements to each side appear to be generated in the ipsilateral parieto-occipital cortex, but the ipsilateral cerebellum, especially the vestibulocerebellum (flocculus and nodulus) is also involved. Another portion of the cerebellum (posterior vermis) modulates saccadic movements (see further on).

If, when following a moving target, the visual image slips off the foveas, the motor neuron firing rate increases in proportion to the speed of the moving target, so that normally eye velocity matches target velocity. If another visual target enters the field, as when watching a series of stripes on a rotating drum, a quick saccade refocuses the eyes centrally and optokinetic nystagmus results. If the ratio of eye and target velocity is less than unity, i.e., if the eyes fall behind the target, supplementary catch-up saccades are required for refixation. The pursuit movement is then not smooth but jerky (cogwheel). A lesion of one cerebral hemisphere causes pursuit movements to that side to break into saccades. This is often associated with but not dependent upon a homonymous hemanopia. Also, if the parietal lobe is involved optokinetic nystagmus toward the involved hemisphere is lost or impaired.

Vestibular influences are of particular importance in stabilizing images on the retina. By means of the *vestibulo-ocular reflex (VOR)*, a movement of the eyes is produced that is equal and opposite to movement of the head. Mainly the VOR is a response to rapid transient head movements. During sustained rotation of the head, the VOR is supplemented by the *optokinetic system*, which enables one to maintain compensatory eye movements for a prolonged period. If the VOR is lost, as occurs with disease of the vestibular apparatus (e.g., streptomycin intoxication), the slightest movements of the head, even those produced by transmitted cardiac pulsations, cause a movement of images across the retina, large enough to impair vision. If objects are tracked using both eye and head movements, the vestibulo-ocular movements induced by head turning need to be suppressed, otherwise the eyes would remain stabilized

in space; it is likely that the smooth pursuit signals cancel the unwanted vestibular ones (Leigh and Zee).

The corticofugal pathways for conjugate horizontal gaze have been traced in the monkey by Leichnetz. He found that these fibers traverse the anterior limb of the internal capsule and separate at the level of the rostral diencephalon into two bundles: (1) a dorsal ''transthalamic'' one, which is predominantly uncrossed and courses through the internal medullary lamina and paralaminar parts of the thalamus to terminate diffusely in the pretectum, superior colliculus, and periaqueductal gray matter. An offshoot of these fibers (the prefrontal oculomotor bundle) projects to the rostral part of the oculomotor nucleus and to the ipsilateral rostral interstitial nucleus of the medial longitudinal fasciculus (ri MLF) and interstitial nucleus of Cajal (iC), which are involved in vertical eye movements; (2) a more ventral ''capsular-peduncular'' pathway, which descends through the posterior limb of the internal capsule and most medial part of the basis pedunculi. The latter bundle undergoes a partial decussation in the rostral pons, at the level of the trochlear nucleus, and terminates mainly in the paramedian pontine reticular formation (PPRF), which in turn projects to the sixth nerve nucleus (Fig. 13-1).

The cortical pathways for voluntary pursuit movements are less well known. One pathway probably originates in the parietal cortex, mainly area 7, and the adjacent superior temporal and anterior occipital lobes (area MT of the monkey), and descends to the superior colliculus and to the ipsilateral dorsolateral pontine nuclei. The latter, in turn, project to the flocculus and dorsal vermis of the cerebellum.

Ultimately, however, all the pathways mediating impulses for saccadic and pursuit movements, as well as for vestibular and optokinetic movements, converge onto the pontine centers for horizontal gaze. These comprise the PPRF, the sixth nerve nuclei, the vestibular nuclei, and pathways in the pontine and mesencephalic tegmentum connecting the ocular motor nuclei (Fig. 13-1). (Conventionally, the term *ocular motor nuclei* refers to the third, fourth, and sixth cranial nerve nuclei; the term *oculomotor nucleus* refers to the third nerve nucleus alone.) Although the PPRF is essential in generating horizontal and probably vertical saccades, it appears that the neural signals that encode smooth pursuit and vestibular and optokinetic movements project independently to the abducens nuclei (Hanson et al). The abducens nucleus is now known to contain two groups of neurons, each with distinctive morphologic and pharmacologic properties: (1) the abducens motor neurons, which project to the ipsilateral lateral rectus muscle; and

(2) the abducens internuclear neurons, which project via the contralateral MLF to the medial rectus neurons of the oculomotor nucleus. Conjugate lateral gaze is accomplished by the simultaneous innervation of the ipsilateral external rectus and the contralateral internal rectus, the latter through fibers that run in the medial portion of the MLF. It is the interruption of these latter fibers that accounts for the discrete impairment or loss of adduction of the ipsilateral eye, a phenomenon referred to as *unilateral internuclear ophthalmoplegia* (Fig. 13-1). Two other ascending pathways between the pontine centers and the mesencephalic reticular formation have been traced: one traverses the central

Figure 13-1

The supranuclear pathways subserving conjugate horizontal gaze to the left. Pathway originates in the right frontal cortex, descends in the internal capsule, decussates at the level of the rostral pons and descends to synapse in the left pontine paramedian reticular formation (PPRF). Further connections with the ipsilateral sixth nerve nucleus and contralateral medial longitudinal fasciculus are also indicated. Cranial nerve nuclei III and IV are labeled on left; nucleus of VI and vestibular nuclei (VN) are labeled on right. LR, lateral rectus; MR, medial rectus; MLF, medial longitudinal fasciculus.

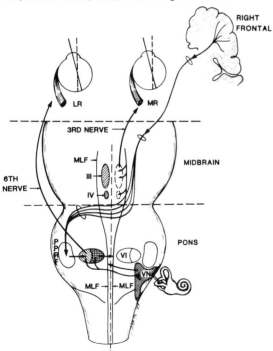

tegmental tract and terminates in the pretectum, in the nucleus of the posterior commissure; the other is a bundle separate from the MLF that passes around the nuclei of Cajal and Darkschewitz to the rostral interstitial nucleus of the MLF. In addition, each vestibular nucleus projects onto the MLF and abducens nucleus of the opposite side (Fig. 13-1).

Although projections from the frontal eye fields to the ocular motor nuclei, as described above, undoubtedly exist, indirect projections are probably more important in the voluntary control of conjugate eye movements. According to Leigh and Zee, a more accurate conceptualization of these voluntary influences is one of a hierarchy of cell stations and parallel pathways that do not project directly to ocular motor nuclei but to adjacent *"premotor"* or *"burst neurons,"* which discharge at high frequencies immediately preceding the saccade. The premotor or burst neurons for horizontal saccades lie within the PPRF and those for vertical saccades in the ri MLF (see below). Yet a third class of neurons is involved in saccadic movement. These cells lie in the midline of the pons and are tonically active except during a saccade (hence *pause cells*). These cells inhibit unwanted discharges of saccadic neurons.

The arrangements of nerve cells and fibers for *vertical upward and downward gaze* are situated in the pretectal areas of the midbrain tegmentum and involve the fibers and nuclei in the region of the posterior commissure. Büttner-Ennever and her colleagues have adduced evidence that the critical lesion for the production of vertical gaze palsies involves the group of cells lying interstitially within the medial longitudinal fasciculus, rostral to the oculomotor nucleus, at the junction of the midbrain and thalamus (ri MLF) and that this nucleus functions as the "premotor" nucleus or "burst cells" for the production of fast (saccadic) vertical eye movements.

In several patients who showed an isolated palsy of downward gaze, autopsy has disclosed bilateral lesions (infarction) of the rostral midbrain, situated in the ventral portion of the pretectal tegmentum, on either side of the aqueduct, just medial and dorsal to the red nuclei. In monkeys, a defect in downward gaze has been produced by the placement of bilateral lesions 1.7 mm in diameter, centered in these regions (Kömpf et al). A unique case, recently described by Bogousslavsky and his colleagues, suggests that a paralysis of vertical gaze may follow a strictly unilateral infarction of the posterior commissure, the ri MLF and the iC.

Finally, there are important vestibulocerebellar influences on both smooth pursuit tracking and saccadic movements (see also Chap. 4). The flocculus and posterior vermis of the cerebellum receive abundant sensory projections from the proprioceptors of the cervical musculature (head velocity), retinas (target velocity), proprioceptors of eye muscles (eye position and eye velocity), from auditory and tactile receptors, and from the superior colliculi and PPRF. Cerebellar efferents concerned with ocular movement project onto the vestibular nuclei. The latter, in turn, influence gaze mechanisms through several projection systems: one, for horizontal movements, consists of direct projections from the vestibular nuclei to the contralateral sixth nerve nucleus; another, for vertical movements, projects, via the contralateral MLF, to third and fourth nerve nuclei (Figs. 13-1 and 14-2).

Lesions of the flocculus and posterior vermis are consistently associated with deficits in smooth pursuit and with an inability of the patient to suppress the vestibulo-ocular reflex with fixation (Baloh et al). Also, as indicated in Chap. 4, patients with cerebellar (floccular) lesions are unable to hold eccentric positions of gaze and need to make repeated saccades to look eccentrically. This phenomenon, referred to as *gaze-paretic nystagmus*, is explained by the fact that with acute, one-sided lesions of the vestibulocerebellum, the inhibitory discharges of the Purkinje cells onto the ipsilateral medial vestibular nucleus is removed and the eyes deviate away from the lesion. When gaze to the side of the lesion is attempted, the eyes drift back to the midline and can only be corrected by a saccadic jerk. There is no attendant vertigo, nausea, or vomiting. The head and neck may also turn away from the lesion (the occiput toward the lesion, and the face away). In addition, the vestibular ocular reflexes, which coordinate eye movements with head movements, are improperly adjusted (Thach and Montgomery).

THE TESTING OF OCULAR MOVEMENTS

It is apparent from the foregoing remarks that there is considerable information to be obtained about ocular movements by the simple expedient of asking the patient to look quickly to each side and up and down, to follow a moving target (a light, the examiner's or the patient's finger, or an optokinetic drum), and of passively turning the head and irrigating the ears in patients with stupor and coma.

With a little practice most individuals make accurate saccades. The persistent impairment of saccadic movements, particularly overshooting of the eyes (*hypermetria*), is characteristic of a midline cerebellar lesion. Such an abnormality may also be observed in patients with Huntington disease, although the most striking abnormality in the latter disorder is a *slowness of saccadic movements*, sometimes extreme in degree. Slow saccades may also be seen in Wilson disease, ataxia-telangiectasia, progressive supranuclear palsy, and certain lipid storage diseases. Lesions involving the PPRF, may be accompanied by slow saccadic movements. Hypometric, slow saccades, occurring only in

the adducting eye on quick lateral gaze, indicate an internuclear ophthalmoparesis from a lesion of the MLF. When slow saccades are first observed to occur in the vertical plane, the likeliest diagnoses are progressive supranuclear palsy or Huntington disease. Yet another saccadic disorder takes the form of an inability to initiate voluntary movement, either vertically or horizontally. This abnormality may be congenital in nature, as in the ocular apraxia of childhood (Cogan syndrome, see below) and ataxia-telangiectasia; as an acquired abnormality, difficulty of initiation of saccadic movements may be seen in Huntington disease and in cases of bilateral cerebral infarction.

Fragmentation of smooth pursuit movement is a frequent neuro-ophthalmologic finding. Drug intoxication—with phenytoin, barbiturates, diazepam and other sedative drugs—is probably the most common cause. As a manifestation of structural disease, it indicates a disorder of the vestibulocerebellum. In extrapyramidal diseases, such as Parkinson disease, Huntington disease, and progressive supranuclear palsy, there is often an impairment of smooth pursuit movements in association with slow, hypometric saccades. Asymmetric impairment of smooth pursuit movements is indicative of a parietal lobe lesion; a right parietal lesion causes an impairment of smooth tracking to the patient's right and a decrease in nystagmus on rotating the optokinetic drum in that direction.

Zee has described a simple means of evaluating the vestibulo-ocular reflex (VOR). In a dimly lit room, the patient is instructed to fixate on a distant target with one eye while the examiner observes the optic nerve head of the other eye with an ophthalmoscope. The subject is then instructed to rotate his head back and forth at a rate of one to two cycles per second. In a normal subject, the optic nerve head remains stationary; if the vestibulo-ocular reflex is impaired, the optic nerve head appears to oscillate. Normally, movement of the head at this rate does not cause blurring of vision, because of the rapidity with which the VOR accomplishes compensatory eye movements. However, with head fixated, to-and-fro movement of the environment will cause blurring of vision, because normal tracking movements are too slow to fixate the object in space. As a rule, the patient with impairment of smooth pursuit movements will have a commensurate inability to suppress the VOR that is part of normal combined head-eye tracking.

Combined fusional-accommodative movements (tested by asking the patient to look at his or her thumbnail as it is brought toward the eyes) are frequently impaired in the elderly and in confused or inattentive patients. In others, the absence or impairment of these movements should suggest the presence of basal ganglionic disease, more particularly progressive supranuclear palsy or Parkinson disease. Convergence spasms may accompany paralysis of vertical gaze and retraction nystagmus. Such spasms, occurring alone, are characteristic of hysteria; a cycloplegic (5% homatropine eyedrops) then abolishes them.

PARALYSIS OF CONJUGATE MOVEMENT (GAZE)

An acute lesion, such as an infarct in one frontal lobe, usually causes paralysis of contralateral gaze, and the eyes will turn toward the side of the cerebral lesion. This rule is not absolute; occasionally a deep cerebral lesion, particularly a thalamic hemorrhage extending into the midbrain, will cause the eyes to deviate conjugately to the side opposite the lesion.

In the case of cerebral infarction, the gaze palsy is temporary, lasting only for a day or two, rarely longer. Almost invariably, it is accompanied by hemiparesis. In this circumstance, forced closure of the eyelids frequently causes the eyes to move conjugately to the side of the hemiparesis, rather than upward. During sleep the eyes deviate conjugately from the side of the lesion to the side of the paralysis. Also, as indicated above, slow pursuit movements to the side of the lesion tend to break up into saccades. With bilateral frontal lesions the patient may be unable to turn the eyes voluntarily in any direction, but retains fixation and following movements, which are believed to be initiated in the parieto-occipital cortex. Gaze paralysis of central origin is not attended by strabismus or diplopia. The usual causes are vascular occlusion with infarction, hemorrhage, and abscess or tumor of the frontal lobe.

Midbrain lesions affecting the pretectum on both sides of the midline (perhaps on one side, as indicated above) and lesions in the region of the posterior commissure interfere with conjugate movements in the vertical plane. Paralysis of gaze in the vertical plane is frequently referred to as the *Parinaud syndrome* or the *syndrome of the sylvian aqueduct*. Upward gaze is affected far more frequently than downward gaze and is often associated with mydriasis, loss of convergence movements and of pupillary light reflexes; occasionally convergence or retractory nystagmus (see page 219), blepharospasm, or rhythmic retraction of the upper eyelids are present as well. Vestibular or optokinetic nystagmus in the vertical plane is usually lost in association with these abnormalities. The range of upward gaze is frequently restricted by a number of extraneous factors, such as aging, drowsiness, and increased intracranial pressure. In patients who cannot elevate their eyes voluntarily, reflex upward deviation of the eyes in response to forced flexion of the head (doll's-head maneuver) or to forced closure of the eyelids (*Bell's phenomenon*) indicates that the nuclear and infranuclear mechanisms for upward gaze are intact and that the defect is supranuclear. It must be remembered, however, that about 15 percent of normal adults do not show a Bell's phenomenon. In the disorder known as progressive supranuclear palsy there may be an early selective paralysis of downward gaze, combined with nuchal dystonia (Chap. 43).

A lesion in the rostral midbrain tegmentum, by interrupting the cerebral pathways for conjugate gaze before their decussation, will cause a palsy of horizontal gaze to the opposite side. A lesion in the pontine horizontal gaze complex, involving the abducens nucleus, causes *ipsilateral* gaze palsy, with the eyes deviating to the opposite side. As a rule, the horizontal gaze palsies of cerebral and pontine origin are readily distinguished. The former are usually accompanied by hemiparesis, and the paralysis of gaze is on the same side as the hemiparesis. Palsies of pontine origin are associated with other signs of pontine disease, particularly peripheral facial and external rectus palsies on the same side as the paralysis of gaze, and the hemiparesis, if present, is on the side opposite to the gaze palsy. Gaze palsies due to cerebral lesions tend not to be as long-lasting as those due to pontine lesions. Also, in the case of a cerebral lesion (but not a pontine lesion), the eyes can be turned to the paralyzed side if a target is fixated and the head is rotated passively to the opposite side.

Skew deviation is a poorly understood disorder of gaze in which there is a maintained vertical deviation of one eye above the other. The deviation may be the same (comitant) in all fields of gaze, or it may be variable for different directions of gaze. The patient complains of vertical diplopia. Skew deviation does not have precise localizing value, but occurs with a variety of lesions of the brainstem and cerebellum. With skew deviation due to brainstem disease, the eye on the side of the lesion is lower than the other eye, in distinction to unilateral internuclear ophthalmoplegia, in which the eye is usually higher on the side of the lesion.

Another unusual disturbance of gaze is the *oculogyric crisis or spasm,* which consists of conjugate spasmodic movements of the eyes, usually upward and less frequently laterally or downward. Recurrent attacks, sometimes associated with spasms of the neck, mouth, and tongue muscles and lasting from a few seconds to an hour or two, are pathognomonic of postencephalitic parkinsonism (pages 604 and 939). This phenomenon is now more commonly observed as an acute reaction in patients being given phenothiazine drugs (page 901). The pathogenesis of these ocular spasms is not known.

Congenital ocular motor apraxia (Cogan syndrome) is a disorder characterized by abnormal eye and head movements during attempts to change the position of the eyes. The patient is unable to make normal voluntary horizontal saccades when the head is stationary. If the head is free to move and the patient is asked to look at an object to either side, the head is turned with a thrusting movement and the eyes turn in the opposite direction. The head overshoots the target and the eyes, as they return to the central position, fixate on the target. Both voluntary saccades and the quick phase of vestibular nystagmus are defective. The pathologic anatomy has never been studied. This phenomenon is also seen in ataxia-telangiectasia (page 794) and in association with agenesis of the corpus callosum.

NUCLEAR AND INFRANUCLEAR DISORDERS OF EYE MOVEMENT

ANATOMIC CONSIDERATIONS

The third (oculomotor), fourth (trochlear), and sixth (abducens) cranial nerves innervate the extrinsic musculature of the eye. Since their actions are closely integrated and many diseases involve all of them at once, they are suitably considered together.

The oculomotor (third nerve) nuclei consist of several paired groups of nerve cells, adjacent to the midline and ventral to the aqueduct of Sylvius, at the level of the superior colliculi. A centrally located group of nerve cells that innervate the pupillary sphincters and ciliary bodies (muscles of accommodation) is situated dorsally in the so-called Edinger-Westphal nucleus; this is the parasympathetic portion of the oculomotor nucleus. Ventral to this nuclear group are the cells which mediate the actions of the levator of the lid, superior and inferior recti, inferior oblique, and medial rectus, in this dorsal-ventral order. This functional arrangement has been determined in cats and monkeys by extirpating individual extrinsic ocular muscles and observing the retrograde cellular changes (Warwick). More recent studies, utilizing radioactive tracer techniques (Büttner-Ennever and Akert), have shown that the medial rectus neurons occupy three disparate locations within the oculomotor nucleus, rather than being confined to its ventral tip. These experiments have also indicated that the medial and inferior recti and the inferior oblique have a strictly homolateral representation in the oculomotor nuclei; the superior rectus receives only crossed fibers; and the levator palpebrae superioris has a bilateral innervation. Vergence movements are under the control of medial rectus neurons and not an

unpaired medial group of cells ("nucleus of Perlia"), as was once supposed.

It is important to note that the efferent fibers of the oculomotor and abducens nuclei have a considerable intramedullary extent (Fig. 13-2*A* and *B*). The fibers of the third nerve nucleus course ventrally in the brainstem, traversing the medial longitudinal fasciculus, the red nucleus, substantia nigra, and the medial part of the cerebral peduncle, and may therefore be interrupted by lesions involving these latter structures. The sixth nerve arises at a considerably lower level, from a paired group of cells in the floor of the fourth ventricle, adjacent to the midline, at the level of the lower pons. The intrapontine portion of the facial nerve loops around the sixth nerve nucleus before it turns anterolaterally to make its exit; a lesion in this locality, therefore, may cause a homolateral paralysis of the lateral rectus and facial muscles. The cells of origin of the trochlear nerves are just caudal to those of the oculomotor nerves. Unlike the third and sixth nerves, the fourth nerve decussates a short distance from its origin, before emerging from the dorsal surface of the brainstem, just caudal to the inferior colliculi.

The oculomotor nerve, soon after it emerges from the brainstem, comes into close relationship with the posterior cerebral artery. Both these structures may be compressed at this point by herniation of the uncus through the tentorium. More anteriorly, the oculomotor nerve crosses the internal carotid artery at its junction with the posterior communicating artery. An aneurysm at the latter site frequently damages the third nerve, and this serves to localize the site of compression or bleeding. The sixth cranial nerve sweeps upward, after leaving the brainstem, and joins the third and fourth cranial nerves; together, the ocular motor nerves course anteriorly, pierce the dura, and run in the lateral wall of the cavernous sinus, where they are closely applied to the various divisions of the fifth nerve. In the posterior part of the cavernous sinus, compressive lesions, notably infraclinoid extradural aneurysms and tumors, tend to involve all three trigeminal divisions, together with the nerves to the extraocular muscles; in the middle portion of the sinus, the ocular nerves and first and second trigeminal divisions are involved; and in the anterior portion, only the ophthalmic division. Together with the latter division, the third, fourth, and sixth nerves enter the orbit through the superior orbital fissure. The oculomotor nerve, as it enters the orbit, divides into superior and inferior branches. The superior branch supplies the superior rectus and the voluntary part of the levator palpebrae (the involuntary part is under the control of sympathetic fibers); the inferior branch supplies the pupillary and ciliary muscles and all the other extrinsic ocular muscles except two—the superior oblique and the external rectus—which are inner-

Figure 13-2

A. Brainstem in horizontal section, at level of third nerve nucleus, indicating structures involved by lesions at different loci in the midbrain. Lesions at 1 result in homolateral third nerve paralysis and homolateral anesthesia of the cornea. Lesions at 2 result in homolateral third nerve paralysis and contralateral tremor (Benedikt syndrome). Lesions at 3 result in homolateral third nerve paralysis and crossed corticospinal tract signs (Weber syndrome). B. Brainstem at the level of the sixth nerve nuclei, indicating structures involved by lesions at different loci. Lesions at 1 result in homolateral sixth and seventh nerve paralyses with varying degrees of nystagmus and weakness of conjugate gaze to the homolateral side. Lesions at 2 result in homolateral sixth nerve paralysis and crossed hemiplegia (Millard-Gubler syndrome). (From DG Cogan, Neurology of the Ocular Muscles, 2nd ed, Springfield, IL, Charles C Thomas, 1956.)

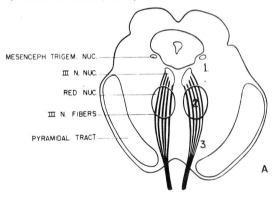

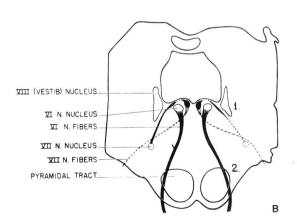

vated by the trochlear and abducens nerves, respectively. Superior branch lesions caused by aneurysm and viral infection have been observed from time to time.

Although all the extraocular muscles probably participate in every movement of the eyes, a movement in a specific direction should clinically be thought of as requiring the action of one particular muscle; e.g., outward rotation of the eye requires the action of the lateral rectus, inward rotation, the medial rectus. The action of the superior and inferior recti and the oblique muscles varies according to the position of the eye. When the eye is turned outward, the elevator is the superior rectus, and the depressor is the inferior rectus. When the eye is turned inward, the elevator and depressor are the inferior and superior oblique muscles, respectively. The actions of the ocular muscles in different positions of gaze are illustrated in Fig. 13-3.

STRABISMUS

Strabismus (*squint*) refers to a muscle imbalance that results in improper alignment of the visual axes of the two eyes. It may be caused by weakness of an individual eye muscle (*paralytic strabismus*) or by an imbalance of muscular tone presumably due to a faulty "central" mechanism that normally maintains a proper angle between the two visual axes (*nonparalytic strabismus*). Almost everyone has a slight tendency to the latter, i.e., to misalign the visual axes (*phoria*), but normally this tendency is overcome by the fusion mechanisms. In persons with strabismus the misalignment becomes manifest and can no longer be overcome (*tropia*). Paralytic strabismus is primarily a neurologic problem; nonparalytic strabismus (referred to as *concomitant strabismus* if the angle between the visual axes is the same in all fields of gaze) is more strictly an ophthalmologic problem.

Once binocular fusion is established, usually by 6 months of age, any type of ocular muscle imbalance will cause diplopia, since images then fall on disparate or noncorresponding parts of the two functionally active retinas. After a time, however, the child learns to eliminate the diplopia by suppressing the image in one eye. After a variable period the suppression becomes permanent, and the individual grows up with a diminished visual acuity in that eye, the result of prolonged disuse (*amblyopia ex anopsia*). With proper early treatment, the amblyopia can be reversed, but if it persists beyond the age of 5 or 6 years, recovery of vision rarely occurs. Occasionally, when the eyes are used alternately for fixation (*alternating strabismus*), visual acuity remains good in each eye.

Nonparalytic strabismus may pose a problem for neurologists. It has a way of appearing in early childhood for unclear reasons and conjures up possibilities of serious neurologic disease. Sometimes it is first noticed after a head injury or an infection, and may be exposed by some other neurologic disorder or drug intoxication that impairs sensory fusional mechanisms (vergence). In a cooperative patient, nonparalytic strabismus may be demonstrated by showing that each eye can be moved fully when the other eye is covered. Also the "cover test" will reveal a misalignment of the eye when first one, then the other is covered, requiring the stimulated eye to focus on a test object. The uncovered eye will be forced to change its position (movement of redress) when alternating from binocular to monocular focusing.

PTOSIS AND RETRACTION OF EYELIDS

In the normal individual, the eyelids on each side are at the same level with respect to the iris, and there is a variable prominence of the eyes depending upon the width of the palpebral aperture. Blinking occurs irregularly, at a rate of 12 to 20 times per minute. A reduced frequency of blinking (<10/min) is a manifestation of Parkinson disease or progressive supranuclear palsy. Orbital tumors and thyroid disease are the commonest causes of unilateral and bilateral exophthalmos. Other causes of staring with retraction of the upper lids are progressive supranuclear palsy and hydrocephalus, in which there is paralysis of upward gaze and downturning of the eyes ("sunset sign"). Retraction of the eyelids (Collier's sign), when part of a dorsal midbrain

Figure 13-3

Muscles chiefly responsible for vertical movements of the eyes in different positions of gaze. (From DG Cogan, Neurology of the Ocular Muscles, 2nd ed, Charles C Thomas, Springfield, IL, 1956.)

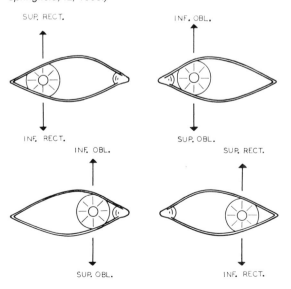

SUP. RECT.   INF. OBL.

INF. RECT.   SUP. OBL.

INF. OBL.   SUP. RECT.

SUP. OBL.   INF. RECT.

syndrome, is accompanied by a light-near pupillary dissociation; unlike lid retraction in dysthyroid orbitopathy, there is no lid lag (Graefe's sign) on downward gaze. Lid retraction has been observed in patients with hepatic cirrhosis, Cushing disease, chronic steroid myopathy, and hyperkalemic periodic paralysis; in these conditions also, lagophthalmos is absent.

Lid retraction on the side of a Bell's palsy is due to the unopposed action of the levator muscle; there is also brow ptosis and laxity of the upper eyelid skin. A unilateral ptosis may be accompanied by overaction of the contralateral levator and frontalis muscles; this combination of abnormalities may be observed with myasthenia gravis, Horner syndrome, and anatomic ptosis (compensatory ptosis in diplopic states). Aberrant regeneration of the third nerve may cause a pseudo-Graefe sign, i.e., retraction of the lid on attempted lateral or downward gaze.

Unilateral retraction of the upper lid occurs with a variety of lesions that stimulate or irritate its homolateral sympathetic fibers (see further on in this chapter). In myotonic dystrophy and other less common myotonic disorders, forceful closure of the eyelids may induce a strong after-contraction. In extrapyramidal disease, gentle closure elicits blepharoclonus.

Ptosis is a characteristic feature of muscular dystrophies, myasthenia gravis, and third nerve lesions (see below).

PARALYSIS OF INDIVIDUAL OCULAR MUSCLES

Characteristic clinical disturbances result from lesions of the third, fourth, and sixth cranial nerves. A complete third nerve lesion causes ptosis or drooping of the upper eyelid (since the levator palpebrae is supplied mainly by the third nerve) and an inability to rotate the eye upward, downward, or inward. When the lid is passively elevated, the eye is found to be deviated outward and slightly downward because of the unopposed intact actions of the lateral rectus and superior oblique muscles; in addition, one finds a dilated nonreactive pupil (iridoplegia) and paralysis of accommodation (cycloplegia), due to interruption of the parasympathetic fibers in the third nerve. However, the extrinsic and intrinsic eye muscles may be differentially affected. Infarction of the central portion of the oculomotor nerve, as occurs in diabetic ophthalmoplegia, may spare the pupil, since the preganglionic fibers lie near the surface. Compressive lesions of the nerve dilate the pupil. After injury, regeneration of the third nerve fibers may be aberrant. Some of the fibers that originally moved the eye now reach the iris; the pupil, which in unreactive to light, may constrict when the eye turns up and in.

Fourth nerve lesions result in extorsion and weakness of downward movement of the affected eye, most marked when the eye is turned inward, so that the patient commonly complains of special difficulty in reading or going downstairs. This defect may be overlooked in the presence of a third nerve palsy if the examiner fails to note the absence of intorsion as the patient tries to move the paretic eye downward. Head tilting to the opposite shoulder (Bielschowsky sign) is especially characteristic of fourth nerve lesions; this maneuver causes a compensatory intorsion of the unaffected eye, and ameliorates the double vision.

Lesions of the *sixth nerve* result in a paralysis of lateral or outward movement and a crossing of the visual axes. With incomplete sixth nerve palsies, turning the head toward the side of the paretic muscle may overcome diplopia.

Diplopia and the Red-Glass Test The foregoing signs of ocular motor palsy may occur with various degrees of completeness. When the ocular paresis is slight, there may be no obvious squint or defect in ocular movement; yet the patient experiences diplopia. Study of the relative positions of the images of the two eyes then becomes a useful way

of determining which muscle might be involved. The image seen by the affected eye is usually less distinct, but a more reliable way of distinguishing the weak muscle is by the *red-glass test*. A red glass is placed in front of the patient's right eye (the choice of the right eye is arbitrary, but if the test is always done in the same way, interpretation is simplified). The patient is then asked to look at a flashlight (held at a distance of 1 m), to turn both eyes to various points in the visual fields, and to state or indicate with the two index fingers the position of the red and white images and the relative distances between them. The positions of the two images are plotted as indicated in Fig. 13-4.

Three rules aid in the analysis of ocular movements by the red-glass test. (1) The direction in which the distance between the images is at a maximum is the direction of

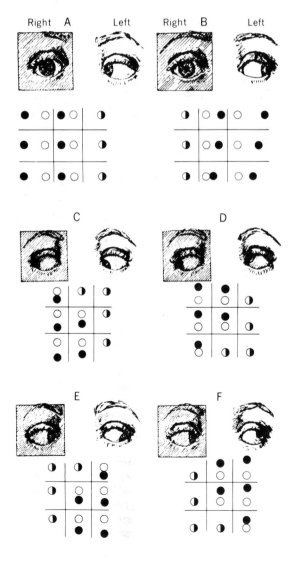

Figure 13-4

Diplopia fields with individual muscle paralysis. The dark glass is in front of the right eye, and the fields are projected as the patient sees the images. A. Paralysis of right external rectus. Characteristic: right eye does not move to the right. Field: horizontal homonymous diplopia increasing on looking to the right. B. Paralysis of right internal rectus. Characteristic: right eye does not move to the left. Field: horizontal crossed diplopia increasing on looking to the left. C. Paralysis of right inferior rectus. Characteristic: right eye does not move downward when eyes are turned to the right. Field: vertical diplopia (image of right eye lowermost) increasing on looking to the right and down. D. Paralysis of right superior rectus. Characteristic: right eye does not move upward when eyes are turned to the right. Field: vertical diplopia (image of right eye uppermost) increasing on looking to the right and up. E. Paralysis of right superior oblique. Characteristic: right eye does not move downward when eyes are turned to the left. Field: vertical diplopia (image of right eye lowermost) increasing on looking to left and down. F. Paralysis of right inferior oblique. Characteristic: right eye does not move upward when eyes are turned to the left. Field: vertical diplopia (image of right eye uppermost) increasing on looking to left and up. (From DG Cogan, Neurology of the Ocular Muscles, 2nd ed, Springfield, IL, Charles C Thomas, 1956.)

action of the paretic muscle. For example, if the greatest horizontal separation is in looking to the right, either the right abductor or the left adductor muscle is weak. (2) If the separation is mainly horizontal, the paresis will be found in one of the horizontally acting recti (a small vertical disparity should be disregarded); if the separation is mainly vertical, the paresis will be found in the vertically acting muscles, and a small horizontal deviation should be disregarded. (3) The image projected farther from the center belongs to the paretic eye. If the patient looks to the right and the red image is farther to the right, then the right lateral rectus muscle is weak. If the white image is to the right of the red, then the left internal rectus muscle is weak. In testing vertical movements, again the image seen with the eye with the paretic muscle is the one projected most peripherally in the visual field. It must be remembered that the red-glass test distinguishes *one* of *two* muscles responsible for the movement in the direction of maximal separation of images. For example, if the maximum vertical separation of images occurs on looking downward and to the *left*, and the white image is projected farther down than the red, the paretic muscle is the left inferior rectus; if the red image is lower than the white, the paretic muscle is the right superior oblique. Separation of images on looking up and to the right or left will similarly distinguish paresis of the inferior oblique and superior rectus muscles.

Monocular diplopia occurs most commonly in relation to diseases of the cornea and lens, rather than the retina; usually the images are overlapping or superimposed rather than discrete. Monocular diplopia has been reported in association with cerebral disease (Safran et al), but this must be a very rare occurrence. In most cases, no disease can be found to explain monocular diplopia. Occasionally patients with homonymous scotomas due to a lesion of the occipital lobe will see multiple images (polyopsia) in the defective field of vision, particularly when the target is moving.

Rarely, the acute onset of convergence paralysis may give rise to diplopia and blurred vision at all near points; most cases are due to head injury, some to encephalitis or multiple sclerosis. Many cases of convergence paralysis do not have an organic basis. The acute onset of divergence paralysis causes diplopia at a distance because of crossing of the visual axes; in patients with divergent paralysis, images fuse at near distance. This disorder, the pathologic basis of which is unknown, is difficult to distinguish from mild bilateral sixth nerve palsies and from convergence spasm, which is common in malingerers and hysterics.

The Causes of Third, Fourth, and Sixth Nerve Palsies
Ocular palsies may be central, i.e., due to a lesion of the nucleus or of the intramedullary portion of the cranial nerve, or they may be peripheral. Weakness of ocular muscles due to a lesion in the brainstem is usually accompanied by involvement of other cranial nerves or long tracts. Peripheral lesions, which may or may not be solitary, have a great variety of causes. Rucker (1958, 1966), who analyzed 2000 cases of paralysis of the ocular motor nerves, found that the most common causes were tumors at the base of the brain (primary, metastatic, meningeal carcinomatosis), trauma to the head, ischemic infarction of a nerve, and aneurysms of the circle of Willis, in that order. In a more recently reported series of 1000 unselected cases (Rush and Younge), trauma was a more frequent cause than neoplasm and the frequency of aneurysm-related cases had declined; otherwise the findings were little changed from the earlier studies. Much less common causes of paralysis of the ocular motor nerves include herpes zoster, subdural hematoma, giant-cell arteritis, ophthalmoplegic migraine, sarcoid, and tuberculous, syphilitic, and other chronic forms of meningitis. Myasthenia gravis must always be considered in cases of acute ocular muscle palsy. Actually, in the single largest group of patients (20 to 30 percent) no cause could be assigned. Fortunately, in most of the cases of undetermined cause, the palsy disappears in a few weeks to months.

The acute development of a sixth, third, or fourth nerve palsy on one side is a relatively common occurrence in the adult. In Rucker's series, the sixth nerve was affected in about one-half the cases; third nerve palsies were about one-half as common as those of the sixth nerve; and the fourth nerve was involved in less than 10 percent of cases.

An isolated sixth nerve palsy frequently proves to be caused by neoplasm. In children, the most common tumor that involves the sixth nerve is a pontine glioma; in adults, it is a metastatic tumor from the nasopharynx. Thus it is essential that the nasopharynx be examined carefully in every case of unexplained sixth nerve palsy, particularly if it is accompanied by sensory symptoms on the side of the face. As the abducens nerve passes near the apex of the petrous bone, it is in close relation to the trigeminal nerve. Both may be implicated by petrositis, manifested by facial pain and diplopia (Gradenigo syndrome). Fractures at the base of the skull may have a similar effect. Infarction and intraorbital cellulitis are less common causes of sixth nerve palsy.

The fourth nerve is particularly vulnerable to head trauma and is practically never involved by aneurysm. The sixth nerve also is rarely damaged by aneurysm. This reflects the relative infrequency of carotid artery aneurysms in the infraclinoid portion of the cavernous sinus, where they can impinge on the sixth nerve. In contrast, supraclinoid aneurysms commonly involve the third nerve. Herpes zoster ophthalmicus may affect any of the ocular motor nerves but particularly the trochlear, which shares a common sheath with the ophthalmic division of the trigeminal nerve.

In third nerve lesions due to compression by aneurysm, tumor, or temporal lobe herniation, enlargement of the pupil is an early sign, because of the peripheral location in the nerve of the pupilloconstrictor fibers. In cases of infarction of the third nerve, as occurs in patients with diabetes, the pupil is usually spared, since the infarction characteristically involves the central portion of the nerve. The oculomotor palsy that occurs with diabetes is of acute onset, developing over a few hours, and is accompanied by pain around the eye and forehead. The prognosis for recovery in cases of diabetic third nerve palsy (as in other nonprogressive lesions of the ocular motor nerves) is usually good, because of the potentiality of nerve regeneration. Infarction of the third nerve probably occurs in nondiabetics as well as in diabetics. In chronic compressive lesions of the third nerve (aneurysm, cholesteatoma, etc.) there may be aberrant regeneration, manifested by pupillary constriction on adduction of the eye or by retraction of the upper lid on downward gaze or adduction.

Rarely, children or young adults may have one or more attacks of ocular palsy in conjunction with an otherwise typical migraine (ophthalmoplegic migraine). The muscles (both extrinsic and intrinsic) innervated by the oculomotor or, very rarely, the abducens nerve are affected. Presumably, intense spasm of the vessels supplying these nerves causes a transitory ischemic paralysis. Arteriograms done after the onset of the palsy usually disclose no abnormality. The patient with oculomotor palsy tends to recover, but after repeated attacks there may be some permanent residual paresis.

The *slow* development of a *unilateral ophthalmoplegia* is most often traced to an aneurysm, a tumor, or an inflammatory process in the anterior portion of the cavernous sinus or at the superior orbital fissure (syndrome of Tolosa-Hunt; see Table 47-1). The various intramedullary and extramedullary syndromes involving the ocular motor and other cranial nerves are summarized in Tables 47-1 and 47-2. See also the diagrams of the angioanatomic syndromes in Chap. 34.

Acute, bilateral ophthalmoplegia, evolving within a day or several days, raises a number of diagnostic considerations. Keane, who analyzed 60 such cases, found the cause to be within the brainstem in 18 (usually Wernicke disease or pretectal infarction), in the cranial nerves in 26 (Guillain-Barré syndrome or tuberculous meningitis), within

the cavernous sinus in 8 (tumors or infection), and at the myoneural junction in 8 (myasthenia gravis or botulism). The *chronic development of bilateral ophthalmoplegia* is most often due to an ocular myopathy (progressive external ophthalmoplegia, see Chap. 50).

Several causes of *pseudoparalysis of ocular muscles* need to be distinguished. In thyroid disease a tight inferior or superior rectus muscle may limit upward and downward gaze; less frequently a tight medial rectus muscle limits abduction (each is demonstrable by forced ductions). In most instances of thyroid ophthalmopathy, diagnosis is not difficult. In a significant number of cases, however (10 to 25 percent, according to Spector and Carlisle), there are no systemic or laboratory signs of thyrotoxicosis, and the signs of infiltrative ophthalmopathy may be limited ("minimal euthyroid Graves disease"). The muscle enlargement can be demonstrated by CT scans and ultrasonography and the inelasticity by duction tests. This disorder is discussed further in Chap. 51.

The Duane retraction syndrome, due to congenital fibrosis of the lateral rectus, causes retraction of the globe on adduction and limitation of abduction. As mentioned above, convergence spasm, in which both eyes converge on attempted fixation straight ahead or to the side, is usually hysterical and can be arrested by the use of a cycloplegic. An old squint or tropia with secondary fibrosis of an ocular muscle should also be considered.

MIXED GAZE AND OCULAR MUSCLE PARALYSIS

We have already considered two types of paralysis of the extraocular muscles: paralysis of conjugate movements (gaze) and neural paralysis of individual ocular muscles. Now we must consider a third, viz., mixed gaze and ocular muscle paralysis. The latter is always a sign of an intrapontine or mesencephalic lesion, due usually to vascular, demyelinative, inflammatory, or neoplastic disease.

A lesion of the lower pons in or near the sixth nerve nucleus causes a homolateral paralysis of the lateral rectus muscle and a failure of adduction of the opposite eye, i.e., a combined paralysis of the sixth nerve and of conjugate lateral gaze. As already indicated, the pontine center accomplishes horizontal conjugate gaze by simultaneously innervating the ipsilateral lateral rectus (via the abducens neurons) and the contralateral medial rectus via fibers that originate in the internuclear neurons of the abducens nucleus and run in the medial longitudinal fasciculus (MLF). With a lesion of the left MLF, the left eye fails to adduct when the patient looks to the right; this condition is referred to as *left internuclear ophthalmoplegia*. With a lesion of the right MLF, the right eye fails to adduct when the patient looks to the left (*right internuclear ophthalmoplegia*). Nystagmus is more prominent in or limited to the abducting eye. Since the MLF also contains axons that originate in the vestibular nuclei and govern vertical eye and head position, a lesion of the MLF causes vertical nystagmus and impairment of vertical fixation and pursuit. Since the two medial longitudinal fasciculi lie close together, each being situated adjacent to the midline, they are frequently affected together, yielding a bilateral internuclear ophthalmoplegia; this condition should always be suspected when only adduction of the eyes is affected. Lesions involving the medial longitudinal fasciculi in the high midbrain may result in a loss of convergence in conjunction with paralysis of the medial recti on attempted lateral gaze ("anterior" internuclear ophthalmoplegia); if the MLF is involved by a lesion in the pons, convergence is spared, but some degree of horizontal gaze or sixth nerve palsy may be associated ("posterior" internuclear ophthalmoplegia, Fig. 13-1). Since lesions of the MLF often spare convergence, the pathways that govern this movement must project to the oculomotor nucleus directly and not via the pathway from abducens internuclear neurons, which mediate adducting versional eye movements.

Another mixed pontine disorder of ocular movement combines an internuclear ophthalmoplegia in one direction and a horizontal gaze palsy in the other direction. One eye lies fixed in the midline for all horizontal movements; the other eye can make only abducting movements, with horizontal nystagmus in the direction of abduction ("one-and-a-half syndrome" of Fisher). The lesion in such cases involves the pontine eye turning center plus the internuclear fibers of the ipsilateral MLF and is usually due to vascular or demyelinative disease. Caplan has described a number of other mixed ocular motor defects with thrombotic lesions of the upper part of the basilar artery ("top of the basilar" syndromes). These include vertical gaze palsy, pseudoabducens paresis, and pupillary abnormalities in combination with visual field defects and behavioral changes.

NYSTAGMUS AND OTHER SPONTANEOUS OCULAR MOVEMENTS

Nystagmus refers to involuntary rhythmic movements of the eyes and is of two general types. In so-called *jerk nystagmus*, the movements alternate between a slow component and a fast corrective component, or jerk, in the opposite direction. In *pendular nystagmus*, the oscillations are roughly equal in rate for the two directions, although on lateral gaze the pendular type may be converted to the jerk type, with the fast component to the side of gaze.

In testing for nystagmus, the eyes should be examined first in the central position and then during upward, downward, and lateral movements. Nystagmus of labyrinthine origin, e.g., the type induced by irrigation of the external auditory canal with hot or cold water, is best brought out

by fitting the patient with Frenzel spectacles, which prevent visual fixation and also magnify the eyes. On the other hand, nystagmus of brainstem and cerebellar origin is brought out best by having the patient fixate upon and follow a moving target. Labyrinthine nystagmus may vary with the position of the head. In particular, the postural nystagmus of Barany is evoked by hyperextension and rotation of the neck, with the patient in the supine position. The head must be below the horizontal plane of the bed and turned to the side. Nystagmus of vertical-torsional type and vertigo develop in 10 to 15 s and persist for another 10 to 15 s. On sitting up quickly, the nystagmus reappears in the opposite direction. Optokinetic nystagmus, the type of nystagmus induced in normal persons by looking at a moving object, should be tested by asking the patient to look at a striped rotating cylinder or at a striped cloth that is moved across the field of vision. Newer methods of recording eye movements have greatly facilitated the definition of different forms of nystagmus.

In some normal individuals a few irregular jerks are observed as they turn their eyes to one side ("nystagmoid" jerks), but no sustained rhythmic movements occur once fixation is attained. Occasionally a fine rhythmic nystagmus may occur in extreme lateral gaze, beyond the range of binocular vision, but if it is bilateral and disappears as the eyes move a few degrees toward the midline it usually has no clinical significance. These movements are probably analogous to the tremulousness of skeletal muscles that are contracted maximally.

Pendular nystagmus is found in a variety of conditions in which central vision is lost early in life, such as albinism and various other diseases of the retina and refractive media (congenital ocular nystagmus). Occasionally it is observed as a congenital abnormality, even without poor vision. The defect is postulated to be an instability of smooth pursuit or gaze-holding mechanisms. Examples are occasionally seen in multiple sclerosis. The nystagmus is always binocular and in one plane; i.e., it will remain horizontal even during vertical movement. It is purely pendular (sinusoidal) except in extremes of gaze, when it may convert to jerk nystagmus. Head oscillation may accompany the nystagmus and is probably compensatory. The syndrome of miner's nystagmus, formerly a common cause of industrial disability, occurs in patients who have worked for many years in comparative darkness. The oscillations of the eyes are usually very rapid, increase on upward gaze, and may be associated with compensatory oscillations of the head and intolerance of light. *Spasmus nutans*, a specific type of pendular nystagmus of infancy, is accompanied by head nodding and occasionally by wry positions of the neck. It begins between the fourth and twelfth months of life, never after the third year. The nystagmus may be horizontal, vertical, or rotatory, is usually more pronounced in one eye than the other (or limited to one eye) and can be intensified by immobilizing or straightening the head. The prognosis is good, and most infants recover within a few months or years.

Jerk nystagmus is the more common type. It may be horizontal or vertical, particularly on ocular movement in these planes, or it may be rotatory and rarely retractory or vergent. By custom, in the English-speaking world, the direction of the nystagmus is named according to the direction of the fast component. There are several varieties of jerk nystagmus. Some occur spontaneously, others are readily induced in normal persons by drugs, or by labyrinthine or visual stimulation. Deviations from the patterns of normally induced nystagmus may provide important clues to the locus of disease.

When one is watching a moving object (e.g., the passing landscape from a train window, or a rotating drum with vertical stripes), a rhythmic jerk nystagmus, *optokinetic nystagmus (OKN)*, normally appears. The usual explanation of this phenomenon is that the slow component of the nystagmus represents an involuntary pursuit movement to the limit of comfortable conjugate gaze; the eyes then make a quick saccadic movement in the opposite direction and fixate a new target coming into the visual field. With unilateral cerebral lesions, specifically of the parietal region (and transiently with acute frontal lobe lesions), OKN may be lost or diminished when a moving stimulus, e.g., the striped OKN drum is rotated *toward* the side of the lesion, whereas rotation of the drum to the opposite side elicits a normal response. It should be noted that patients with hemianopia may show a normal optokinetic response. On the other hand, patients with a parietal lobe lesion, with or without hemianopia, frequently have an abnormal optokinetic response. These observations suggest that an abnormal response does not depend upon a lesion of the geniculocalcarine tract. Presumably it is due to interruption of the efferent pathways from the parietal region to the lower centers for conjugate gaze. Frontal lobe lesions allow the eyes to deviate tonically in the direction of the target, with little or no fast phase correction.

Perhaps the most important fact about OKN is that its demonstration proves that the patient is not blind. Thus it is of particular value in the examination of hysterical patients and malingerers who claim that they cannot see and of neonates and infants (OKN is established within minutes or hours after birth).

Labyrinthine stimulation, e.g., irrigation of the external auditory canal with hot or cold water, produces nystagmus; in addition, cold water induces a slow tonic deviation of the eyes in a direction opposite to that of the nystagmus. The slow component reflects the effect of impulses originating in the semicircular canals, and the fast component is a corrective movement. Smooth pursuit movements remain intact, indicating that the labyrinthine vestibular nystagmus is suppressed during fixation. The production of nystagmus by labyrinthine stimulation and other features of vestibular nystagmus are discussed further in Chap. 14.

Drug intoxication is the most frequent cause of induced nystagmus. Alcohol, barbiturates and other sedative-hypnotic drugs, and phenytoin are the common offenders. This form of nystagmus is most prominent on deviation of the eyes in the horizontal plane, but occasionally it may appear in the vertical plane as well, and rarely in the vertical plane alone, suggesting then a tegmental brainstem lesion. It may be asymmetric in the two eyes, for unknown reasons.

Nystagmus occurring spontaneously in patients may signify the presence of labyrinthine-vestibular, brainstem, or cerebellar disease. Vestibular-labyrinthine nystagmus may be horizontal, vertical, or oblique and that of labyrinthine origin characteristically has a torsional component. Tinnitus and hearing loss are associated with disease of the peripheral labyrinthine mechanism; vertigo, nausea, vomiting, and staggering may accompany disease of any part of the labyrinthine-vestibular apparatus (see Chap. 14).

Brainstem lesions often cause a coarse, unidirectional, gaze-dependent nystagmus, which may be horizontal or vertical; the latter is brought out usually on upward gaze, less often on downward gaze. The presence of vertical nystagmus usually indicates disease in the pontomedullary or pontomesencephalic tegmentum. Vertigo is uncommon, but signs of disease of other nuclear structures and tracts in the brainstem are frequent. Vertical nystagmus of upbeat type is observed frequently in patients with demyelinative or vascular disease, tumors, and Wernicke disease. There is still uncertainty about the precise anatomy of coarse upbeat nystagmus. According to some authors, it has been associated with lesions of the anterior vermis, but we have not observed such an association. Kato et al cite cases with a lesion at the pontomedullary junction, involving the nucleus prepositus hypoglossi, which receives vestibular connections and projects to all brainstem and cerebellar regions concerned with oculomotor functions.

Vertical nystagmus in a downward direction may also be observed in Wernicke disease and is characteristic of syringobulbia, Chiari malformation, basilar invagination, and other lesions in the medullary-cervical region. Halmagyi et al, who studied 62 patients with downbeat nystagmus, found that one-half of them were associated with Chiari malformation and various forms of cerebellar degeneration; in most of the remainder no cause could be found. Downbeat nystagmus, in association with oscillopsia, has been observed in patients with profound magnesium depletion (Saul and Selhorst). Cerebellopontine-angle tumors may cause a coarse bilateral horizontal nystagmus, coarser to the side of the lesion. Nystagmus of several types, including gaze-evoked nystagmus, downbeat nystagmus, and "rebound nystagmus" (gaze-evoked nystagmus which changes direction with fatigue or refixation to the primary position), occurs with cerebellar disease (more specifically with lesions of the vestibulocerebellum) or with brainstem lesions that involve the nucleus prepositus hypoglossi and medial vestibular nucleus (see above, in relation to upbeat nystagmus). Characteristic also of cerebellar disease are the closely related disorders of saccadic movement (opsoclonus, flutter, dysmetria) described below. The nystagmus that occurs only in the abducting eye (dissociated nystagmus) and is a common sign of multiple sclerosis probably represents an incompletely developed form of internuclear ophthalmoplegia; on attempted lateral gaze, the adducting eye (which does not show nystagmus) will lag behind the abducting one.

Convergence nystagmus is a rhythmic oscillation in which a slow abduction of the eyes in respect to each other is followed by a quick movement of adduction. It is usually accompanied by quick rhythmic retraction movements of the eyes *(nystagmus retractorius)* and by one or more features of the Parinaud syndrome. There may also be rhythmic movements of the eyelids, or a maintained spasm of convergence, best brought out on attempted elevation of the eyes to command or downward rotation of an OKN drum. These unusual phenomena all point to a lesion of the upper midbrain tegmentum and are usually manifestations of vascular disease or of tumor, notably pinealoma. *Seesaw nystagmus* is a torsional-vertical oscillation in which the intorting eye moves up and the opposite (extorting) eye moves down, and then both move in the reverse direction. It is occasionally observed in conjunction with bitemporal hemianopia due to sellar or parasellar masses. Rhythmic "palatal nystagmus," due to a lesion of the central tegmental tract, may be accompanied by ocular myoclonus, a pendular nystagmus, or a convergence-retraction nystagmus that has the same beat as the palatal and pharyngeal muscles.

Oscillopsia refers to illusory movement of the environment in which stationary objects seem to move back and forth—either up or down or from side to side. It may be associated with ocular flutter or with coarse nystagmus of any type due to lesions of the brainstem, involving the vestibular nuclei on one or both sides. With lesions of the labyrinths (as in streptomycin toxicity), oscillopsia is characteristically provoked by motion, e.g., riding in an automobile, and indicates a loss of stabilization of ocular fixation by the vestibular system during body movement. In these latter circumstances cursory examination of the eyes may disclose no abnormalities; however, if the patient's head is rapidly oscillated while attempting to fixate a target, one may bring out an impairment of smooth eye movements and substitution with saccades. If briefly episodic and involving only one eye, oscillopsia may be due to myokymia of an ocular muscle.

Similar subjective phenomena may be produced by parietal-occipital lesions. These take the form of visual distortions or illusions in the contralateral homonymous fields. It may seem to the patient, for example, that a venetian blind is continually being opened and closed, or that objects are moving or waving or shimmering in that field.

Ocular bobbing is a term coined by C. M. Fisher to describe a distinctive spontaneous fast jerk of the eyes in a downward direction, followed by a slow drift to the midposition. It occurs usually in comatose patients in whom horizontal eye movements are absent and has been associated most often with large destructive lesions of the pons, less often of the cerebellum. The phenomenon itself and the clinical setting in which it occurs are variable, however (Susac et al, Mehler). There may be a slow conjugate downward movement, followed by a rapid return to the midposition. Or the eyes may initially jerk upward quickly and return slowly, or move slowly upward and return quickly to the midposition. The pathophysiology of these ocular movements is obscure. Also, in some cases of coma, Fisher has noted a slow, side-to-side pendular oscillation of the eyes. This phenomenon has been associated with bilateral hemispheric lesions that have presumably released a brainstem pacemaker.

Opsoclonus is the term applied to rapid, conjugate oscillations of the eyes in a horizontal, rotatory, and vertical direction, made worse by voluntary movement or the need to fixate the eyes. These movements may be continuous and chaotic, as in the "dancing eyes" of children with viral encephalitis or the Kinsbourne syndrome. Often, as indicated in Chap. 5, they are associated with widespread myoclonus (with parainfectious disease and with paraneoplastic syndromes). Similar movements have been produced in monkeys by creating bilateral lesions in the pretectum. Parenthetically, a fine oscillation of the eyes can be produced voluntarily in some otherwise normal persons. *Ocular dysmetria* consists of an overshoot of the eyes on attempted fixation, followed by several cycles of oscillations of diminishing amplitude until precise fixation is attained. The overshoot may occur on eccentric fixation or on refixation in the primary position of gaze. This abnormality probably reflects dysfunction of the anterior-superior vermis and underlying deep cerebellar nuclei. *Ocular flutter* refers to occasional bursts of very rapid, to-and-fro flutter-like horizontal oscillations around the point of fixation; this abnormality is also associated with cerebellar disease. Opsoclonus, ocular dysmetria, and flutter-like oscillations may occur together or a patient may show only one or two of these ocular abnormalities, either simultaneously or in sequence. Although all of these ocular dyskinesias represent abnormal saccadic movements and often occur together, it appears that saccadic dysmetria is mechanistically quite different from opsoclonus and flutter-like oscillations (Zee and Robinson). One hypothesis relates opsoclonus and ocular flutter to a disorder of the saccadic "pause neurons" (see above). Their exact anatomic basis has not been elucidated.

THE PUPILS

The testing of pupillary size and reactivity, which can be accomplished by the use of a flashlight, yields important, often vital, clinical information. Essential, of course, is the proper interpretation of the pupillary reactions, and this requires some knowledge of their underlying neural mechanisms.

The diameter of the pupil is determined by the balance of innervation between the autonomically innervated sphincter and radially arranged dilator muscles of the iris, the sphincter muscle playing the major role. *The pupilloconstrictor (parasympathetic)* fibers arise in the Edinger-Westphal nucleus in the high midbrain, join the third cranial (oculomotor) nerve, and synapse in the ciliary ganglion with the postganglionic neurons, 3 percent of which innervate the sphincter pupillae and 97 percent, the ciliary body. The sphincter of the pupil comprises 50 motor units, according to Corbett and Thompson. *The pupillodilator (sympathetic)* fibers arise in the posterolateral part of the hypothalamus and descend uncrossed, in the lateral tegmentum of the midbrain, pons, medulla, and cervical spinal cord to the eighth cervical and first and second thoracic segments, where they synapse with the lateral horn cells. These cells give rise to preganglionic fibers, most of which leave the cord by the second ventral thoracic root and proceed through the stellate ganglion to synapse in the superior cervical ganglion; the postganglionic fibers course along the internal carotid artery and traverse the cavernous sinus, where they join the first division of the trigeminal nerve, finally reaching the eye as the long ciliary nerve. Some of them also innervate the sweat glands and arterioles of the face and Müller's muscle in the eyelid.

The Pupillary Light Reflex The commonest stimulus for pupillary constriction is exposure of the retina to light. Reflex pupillary constriction is also part of the act of convergence and accommodation for near objects (near synkinesis).

The pathway for the pupillary light reflex consists of three parts (Fig. 13-5): (1) An afferent limb, which has its origin in the retinal receptor cell, passes through the bipolar cell, and synapses with the retinal ganglion cell, the axon of which runs in the optic nerve and tract. The light reflex fibers leave the optic tract just rostral to the lateral geniculate body and enter the high midbrain, where they synapse in the pretectal nucleus. (2) Intercalated neurons, by which the pupillomotor fibers pass ventrally to the ipsilateral Edinger-Westphal nucleus, and, via fibers that cross in the posterior commissure, to the contralateral Edinger-Westphal nucleus. (3) An efferent two-neuron pathway from the Edinger-Westphal nucleus by which all motor impulses reach the pupillary sphincter, as described above.

Alterations of the Pupils The pupils tend to be large in children and small in the aged, sometimes even miotic, but still reactive (senile miosis). Asymmetry of the pupils, of 0.3 to 0.5 mm, is found in an estimated 20 to 25 percent of normal individuals. A disease that destroys only a small number of nerve cells in the Edinger-Westphal or ciliary ganglions will cause paralysis of a sector or sectors of the iris and deform the pupil.

Normally the pupil constricts under a bright light (direct reflex) and the other unexposed pupil also constricts (consensual reflex). With complete or nearly complete interruption of the optic nerve the pupil will fail to react to direct light stimulation; however, the pupil of the blind eye will show a consensual reflex, i.e., it will constrict when light is shone in the healthy eye. The lack of a direct reflex in the blind eye together with a lack of a consensual reflex in the sound one means that the afferent limb of the reflex arc (optic nerve) is the site of the lesion. A lack of direct light reflex with retention of the consensual reflex places the lesion in the efferent limb of the reflex arc, i.e., in the homolateral oculomotor nerve or its nucleus. It is evident that a lesion of the afferent limb of the light reflex pathway will not affect the near responses of the pupil and that lesions of the visual pathway caudal to the point where the light reflex fibers leave the optic tract will not alter the pupillary light reflex (Fig. 13-5).

Following initial constriction, the pupil may dilate slightly in spite of a light shining steadily in one or both eyes. Slowness of response along with failure to sustain pupillary constriction, or "pupillary escape," is sometimes referred to as the Gunn pupil sign; a mild degree of it may be observed in normal persons, but it is far more prominent in cases of damage to the retina or optic nerve. A variant of this abnormal pupillary response may be used to expose mild degrees of retrobulbar neuropathy. If a light is shifted quickly from the normal to the impaired eye, the direct light stimulus is no longer sufficient to maintain the previously evoked consensual pupillary constriction, and both pupils dilate. These abnormal pupillary responses form the basis of ''the swinging-flashlight test,'' in which each pupil is alternately exposed to light at 3-s intervals.

The Gunn pupil sign is not to be confused with the Marcus Gunn or ''jaw-winking'' phenomenon, a congenital and sometimes hereditary anomaly, in which a ptotic eyelid retracts momentarily when the mouth is opened or the jaw is moved to one side. In other cases, inhibition of the levator muscle and ptosis occurs with opening of the mouth (''inverse Marcus Gunn phenomenon''). These associated movements of lid and jaw have been referred to as a trigemino-oculomotor synkinesis and attributed to abnormal connections between the central mechanisms innervating the pterygoid and levator muscles.

Interruption of the sympathetic fibers either centrally, between the hypothalamus and their point of exit from the spinal cord (C8 to T4, mainly T2), or peripherally (cervical sympathetic chain, superior cervical ganglion, or along the carotid artery) results in miosis and ptosis (because of paralysis of the pupillary dilator muscle and of Müller's muscle, respectively), loss of sweating on the same side of the face, and redness of the conjunctiva. The pattern of sweating may be helpful in localizing the lesion (Morris et al). With lesions of the common carotid artery, loss of sweating involves the entire side of the face. With lesions distal to the bifurcation, loss of sweating is confined to the medial aspect of the forehead and side of the nose. Retraction of the eyeball (enophthalmos) probably does not occur but is an illusion created by narrowing of the palpebral fissure. The entire complex is called the *Bernard-Horner,* or *Horner syndrome.* Stimulation or irritation of the sympathetic fibers has the opposite effect, i.e., lid retraction, dilatation of the pupil, and apparent proptosis. The ciliospinal pupillary reflex, evoked by pinching the neck (afferent, C2, C3), is effected through these efferent sympathetic fibers, but we have not found it to be a reliable test. Extreme constriction of the pupils (miosis) is commonly observed with pontine lesions, presumably because of bilateral interruption of the pupillodilator fibers. Interruption of the parasympathetic fibers yields an abnormal dilatation of the pupils (mydriasis),

Figure 13-5

Diagram of the pupillary light reflex. (Redrawn from FB Walsh, WF Hoyt, Clinical Neuro-Ophthalmology, 3rd ed, Baltimore, Williams & Wilkins, 1969.)

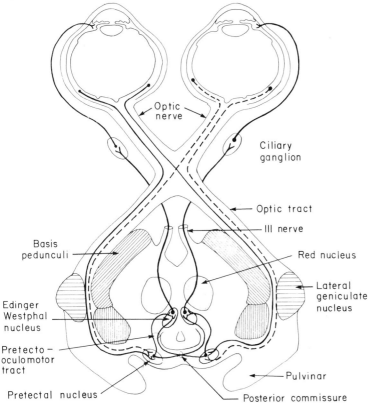

often with loss of pupillary light reflexes; this is frequently the result of midbrain lesions and is a common finding in cases of deep coma.

    The functional integrity of the sympathetic and parasympathetic nerve endings in the iris may also be determined by the use of certain drugs. (See Figs. 13-6 and 13-7.) Atropine and homatropine dilate the pupils by paralyzing the parasympathetic nerve endings; physostigmine and pilocarpine constrict the pupils, the former by inhibiting cholinesterase activity at the neuromuscular junction, and the latter by direct stimulation of the sphincter muscle of the iris. Epinephrine and phenylephrine dilate

the pupils by direct stimulation of the dilator muscle. Cocaine dilates the pupils by preventing the reabsorption of norepinephrine into the nerve endings. Morphine acts centrally to constrict the pupils. *Oculosympathetic palsy* is a frequent neurologic finding (see page 435).

    In diabetes mellitus, where nerves are often invoved, the pupils are affected in the majority of cases. They are smaller than would be expected for age due to involvement of pupillodilator sympathetic fibers, and mydriasis is excessive upon instillation of sympathomimetic drugs (alpha antagonists). The light reflex, mediated by parasympathetic fibers (which are also damaged), is reduced, usually to a greater degree than constriction on accommodation (Smith and Smith). Some of these abnormalities require special methods of pupillometry for their demonstration.

    In chronic syphilitic meningitis and other forms of

Figure 13-6

Pupillary responses to various drugs and stellate block. (Reprinted, with permission, from RH Johnson, JMK Spalding, Disorders of the Autonomic Nervous System, Philadelphia, Davis, 1974.)

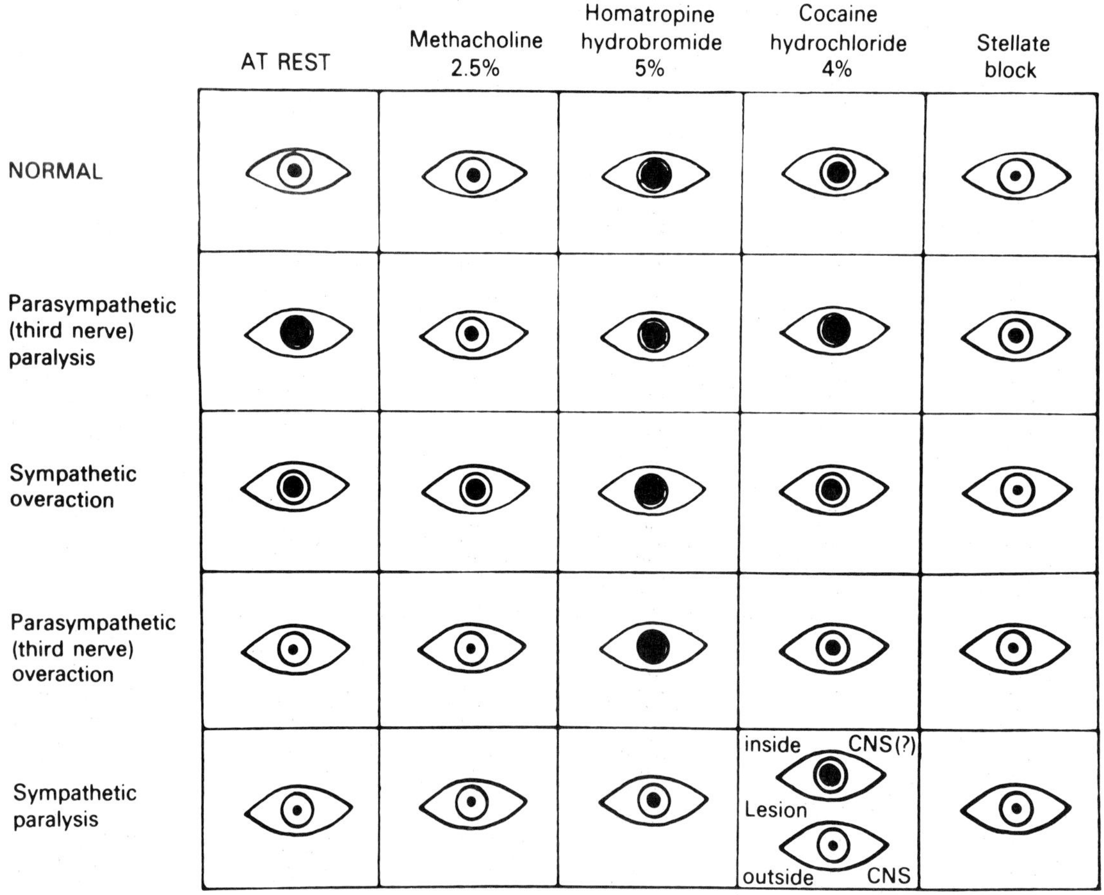

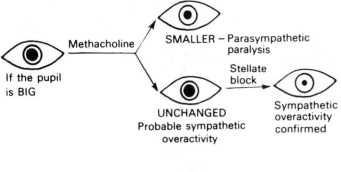

If the pupil is BIG

Methacholine

SMALLER – Parasympathetic paralysis

UNCHANGED
Probable sympathetic overactivity

Stellate block

Sympathetic overactivity confirmed

Figure 13-7

A simplified procedure for the pharmacologic investigation of a pupillary abnormality. (Reprinted, with permission, from RH Johnson, JMK Spalding: Disorders of the Autonomic Nervous System. Philadelphia, Davis, 1974.)

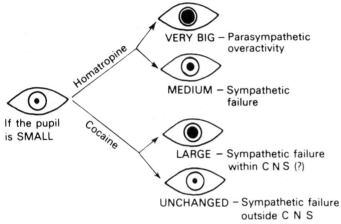

If the pupil is SMALL

Homatropine

VERY BIG – Parasympathetic overactivity

MEDIUM – Sympathetic failure

Cocaine

LARGE – Sympathetic failure within C N S (?)

UNCHANGED – Sympathetic failure outside C N S

late syphilis, particularly tabes dorsalis, the pupils are usually small, irregular, and unequal; they do not dilate properly in response to mydriatic drugs and fail to react to light, although they do constrict on accommodation. In some cases atrophy of the iris is also associated. This is known as the *Argyll Robertson pupil.* The exact locality of the lesion is not certain; it is generally believed to be in the tectum of the midbrain proximal to the oculomotor nuclei, where the descending pupillodilator fibers are in close proximity to the light reflex fibers (Fig. 13-5). The possibility of a partial third nerve lesion or a lesion of the ciliary ganglion seems more plausible to the authors. A similar pupillary abnormality has also been observed in the meningoradiculitis of Lyme disease (also referred to as the Bannworth syndrome). A dissociation of the light reflex from the accommodation-convergence reaction is sometimes observed with other midbrain lesions, e.g., pinealoma, multiple sclerosis, and occasionally in patients with diabetes mellitus; in these diseases, miosis, irregularity of pupils, and failure to respond to a mydriatic are not constantly present. S. A. K. Wilson referred to this condition as the Argyll Robertson pupillary phenomenon, in contrast to the Argyll Robertson pupil.

Another interesting pupillary abnormality is the tonic reaction sometimes referred to as the *Adie pupil.* This syndrome is due to a degeneration of the ciliary ganglia and the postganglionic parasympathetic fibers which normally constrict the pupil and effect accommodation. The patient may complain of blurring of vision or may have suddenly noticed that one pupil is larger than the other. The reaction to light and sometimes to accommodation are absent if tested in the customary manner, although the size of the pupil will change slowly on prolonged maximal stimulation. Once dilated, the pupil remains in this state for many seconds, up to a minute or longer. The loss of accommodation is due to affection of the ciliary muscle. On contraction, paralysis of a segment or segments of the pupil is also characteristic of the Adie syndrome. The affected pupil reacts promptly to the common mydriatic and miotic drugs and is unusually sensitive to a 0.125% solution of pilocarpine, or a 2.5% solution of methacholine, strengths that have only a minimal effect on a normal pupil. The tonic pupil usually appears during the third or fourth decade of life and is much more common in women than in men; it may be associated with the absence of knee or ankle jerks and hence be mistaken for tabes dorsalis. From all available data it represents a mild polyneuropathy.

Finally, mention should be made of a rare pupillary

phenomenon, characterized by transient or periodic mydriasis, for which no cause can be found. The episodes of mydriasis last for minutes to days and may recur at random intervals. Ocular motor palsies and ptosis are notably lacking, but sometimes the pupil is distorted during the attack. Some patients complain of blurred vision and head pain on the side of the mydriasis, suggesting a form of ophthalmoplegic migraine. In children, following a minor or major seizure, one pupil may remain dilated for a protracted period of time.

Ocular movement, pupillary reaction, and visual acuity may be affected by diseases which alter the contents of the orbit. Usually this is accompanied by bilateral exophthalmos, as in thyroid or pituitary disease, or unilateral exophthalmos with thyroid disease, orbital tumors (dermoids, hemangiomas, adenoma of lacrimal gland, optic nerve glioma, neurofibroma, metastatic carcinoma, meningioma), granuloma, orbital cellulitis or abscess, or cavernous sinus thrombosis. Progressive paralysis of the eyelids, which may obstruct vision, occurs separately or as part of an external ophthalmoplegia, as in the ocular myopathy of Kiloh and Nevin or in oculopharyngeal dystrophy.

REFERENCES

BALOH RW, YEE RD, HONRUBIA V: Late cortical cerebellar atrophy. *Brain* 109:159, 1986.

BOGOUSSLAVSKY J, MIKLOSSY J, DERUAZ JP et al: Unilateral left paramedian infarction of thalamus and midbrain: A clinicopathological study. *J Neurol Neurosurg Psychiatry* 49:686, 1986.

BÜTTNER-ENNEVER JA, AKERT K: Medial rectus subgroups of the oculomotor nucleus and their abducens internuclear input in the monkey. *J Comp Neurol* 197:17, 1981.

BÜTTNER-ENNEVER JA, BÜTTNER U, COHEN B, BAUMGARTNER G: Vertical gaze paralysis and the rostral interstitial nucleus of the medial longitudinal fasciculus. *Brain* 105:125, 1982.

CAPLAN LR: "Top of the basilar" syndrome. *Neurology* 30:72, 1980.

COGAN DG: A type of congenital ocular motor apraxia presenting jerky head movements. *Am J Ophthalmol* 36:433, 1953.

COGAN DG: *Neurology of the Ocular Muscles,* 2nd ed. Springfield, IL, Charles C Thomas, 1956.

COGAN DG: *Neurology of the Visual System.* Springfield, IL, Charles C Thomas, 1966.

CORBETT JJ, THOMPSON HS: Pupillary function and dysfunction, in Asbury AK, McKhann GM, McDonald WI (eds): *Disease of the Nervous System.* Philadelphia, Saunders, 1986, Chap 46, pp 606–617.

CORIN MS, ELIZAN TS, BENDER MB: Oculomotor dysfunction in patients with Parkinson's disease. *J Neurol Sci* 15:251, 1972.

DAROFF RB: Ocular oscillations. *Ann Otol Rhinol Laryngol* 86:102, 1977.

FISHER CM: Some neurophthalmological observations. *J Neurol Neurosurg Psychiatry* 30:383, 1967.

GLASER JS: *Neuro-ophthalmology.* Hagerstown, MD, Harper & Row, 1978.

GOLDBERG ME, BUSHNELL MC: Behavioral enhancement of visual responses in monkey cerebral cortex. II. Modulation in frontal eye fields specifically related to saccades. *J Neurophysiol* 46:773, 1981.

HALMAGYI GM, RUDGE P, GRESTY M, SANDERS MD: Downbeating nystagmus. *Arch Neurol* 40:777, 1983.

HANSON MR, HAMID MA, TOMSAK RL et al: Selective saccadic palsy caused by pontine lesions: Clinical, physiological and pathological correlations. *Ann Neurol* 20:209, 1986.

HOTSON R: Cerebellar control of fixation eye movements. *Neurology* 32:31, 1982.

JACOBS L, ANDERSON PJ, BENDER MG: The lesions producing paralysis of downward but not upward gaze. *Arch Neurol* 28:319, 1973.

KATO I, NAKAMURA T, WATANABE J et al: Primary posterior upbeat nystagmus: Localizing value. *Arch Neurol* 42:819, 1985.

KEANE JR: Acute bilateral ophthalmoplegia: 60 cases. *Neurology* 36:279, 1986.

KÖMPF D, PASIK T, PASIK P, BENDER MB: Downward gaze in monkeys. Stimulation and lesion studies. *Brain* 102:527, 1979.

LEICHNETZ GR: The prefontal cortico-oculomotor trajectories in the monkey. *J Neurol Sci* 49:387, 1981.

LEIGH RJ, ZEE DS: *The Neurology of Eye Movements.* Philadelphia, Davis, 1983.

MEHLER MF: The clinical spectrum of ocular bobbing and ocular dipping. *J Neurol Neurosurg Psychiatry* 51:725, 1988.

MORRIS JGL, LEE J, LIM CL: Facial sweating in Horner's syndrome. *Brain* 107:751, 1984.

PIERROT-DESEILLIGNY CH, CHAIN F, SERDARU M et al: The one-and-a-half syndrome. *Brain* 104:665, 1981.

RUCKER CW: Paralysis of the third, fourth, and sixth cranial nerves. *Am J Ophthalmol* 46:787, 1958.

RUCKER CW: The causes of paralysis of the third, fourth and sixth cranial nerves. *Am J Ophthalmol* 61:1293, 1966.

RUSH JA, YOUNGE BR: Paralysis of cranial nerves III, IV, and VI. Cause and prognosis in 1000 cases. *Arch Ophthalmol* 99:76, 1981.

SAFRAN AB, KLINE LB, GLASSER JS, DAROFF RB: Television-induced formed visual hallucinations and cerebral diplopia. *Br J Ophthalmol* 65:707, 1981.

SAUL RF, SELHORST JB: Downbeat nystagmus with magnesium depletion. *Arch Neurol* 38:650, 1981.

SMITH AS, SMITH SC: Assessment of pupillary function in diabetic neuropathy, in Dyck PJ, Thomas PK, Asbury AK et al (eds): *Diabetic Neuropathy.* Philadelphia, Saunders, 1987, Chap 13.

SPECTOR RW, TROOST BT: The ocular motor system. *Ann Neurol* 9:517, 1981.

SPECTOR RH, CARLISLE JA: Minimal thyroid ophthalmopathy. *Neurology* 37:1803, 1987.

SUSAC JO, HOYT WF, DAROFF RB, LAWRENCE W: Clinical

spectrum of ocular bobbing. *J Neurol Neurosurg Psychiatry* 33:771, 1970.

THACH WT, MONTGOMERY EB: Motor system, in Pearlman AL, Collins RC (eds): *Neurological Pathophysiology,* 3rd ed. New York, Oxford University Press, 1984, Chap 9, pp 151–178.

WALL M, WRAY SH: The one and a half syndrome—a unilateral disorder of the pontine tegmentum: A study of 20 cases and review of the literature. *Neurology* 33:971, 1983.

WARWICK R: Representation of the extraocular muscles in the oculomotor nuclei of the monkey. *J Comp Neurol* 98:449, 1953.

WARWICK R: The so-called nucleus of convergence. *Brain* 78:92, 1955.

WHITE OB, ST CYR JA, SHARPE JA: Ocular motor deficits in Parkinson's disease. *Brain* 106:555, 571, 1983.

ZEE DS: Ophthalmoscopy in examination of patients with vestibular disorders. *Ann Neurol* 3:373, 1978.

ZEE DS, YEE RD, COGAN DG et al: Ocular motor abnormalities in hereditary cerebellar ataxia. *Brain* 99:207, 1976.

ZEE DS, ROBINSON DA: A hypothetical explanation of saccadic oscillations. *Ann Neurol* 5:405, 1979.

CHAPTER 14

DEAFNESS, DIZZINESS, AND DISORDERS OF EQUILIBRIUM

ANATOMIC CONSIDERATIONS

The vestibulocochlear or eighth cranial nerve has two components: the cochlear nerve, which subserves hearing or acoustic function, and the vestibular nerve, which is concerned with equilibrium and orientation of the body in space.

The acoustic division has its cell bodies in the spiral ganglion of the cochlea. This ganglion is composed of bipolar cells, the peripheral processes of which convey auditory impulses from the specialized neuroepithelium of the inner ear, the spiral organ of Corti. This is the end organ of hearing, wherein sound is transduced into nerve impulses. It consists of numerous hair cells, aligned in rows along the entire 2½ turns of the cochlea. Each afferent auditory fiber and the hair cell with which it is connected has a minimum threshold at one frequency (''characteristic'' or ''best'' frequency). The basilar membrane, upon which the hair cells rest, vibrates at different frequencies throughout its length, according to the frequency of the sound stimulus. In this way the fibers of the cochlear nerve respond to the full range of audible sound and can differentiate and resolve complexes of sounds.

There are about 30,000 afferent cochlear neurons, the central processes of which constitute the cochlear division of the eighth cranial nerve. In addition, the nerve contains approximately 500 efferent fibers, which arise from the superior olivary nuclei (80 percent from the contralateral nucleus and 20 percent from the ipsilateral one) and synapse with the afferent neurons from the hair cells (Rasmussen). The function of this efferent pathway is not clear. Possibly it plays some part in the auditory activity that is generated in the ear itself; it is thought to enhance the sharpness of sound perception by some feedback mechanism (Kemp). The eighth nerve also contains adrenergic postgaglionic fibers that are derived from the cervical autonomic chain and innervate the cochlea.

The vestibular division arises from cells in the vestibular or Scarpa's ganglion, which is situated in the internal auditory meatus. This ganglion also is composed of bipolar cells, the peripheral processes of which terminate in hair cells of the specialized sensory epithelium of the labyrinth (semicircular canals, saccule, and utricle). The sensory epithelium is located on hillocks (cristae) in the dilated openings or ampullae of the semicircular canals, where they are called the *cristae ampullaris,* and in the utricle and saccule, where they are called *maculae acusticae.* The hair cells of the maculae are covered by the *otolithic membrane* or *otolith,* which is composed of calcium carbonate crystals embedded in a gelatinous matrix. The sensory cells of the cristae are covered by a sail-shaped gelatinous mass called a *cupula.*

The central fibers from the spiral and vestibular ganglia are united in a common trunk, which enters the cranial cavity through the internal auditory meatus (accompanied by the facial and intermediate nerves), traverses the cerebellopontine angle, and enters the brainstem at the junction of the pons and medulla. Here the cochlear and vestibular fibers become separated. The cochlear fibers bifurcate and terminate almost at once in the dorsal and ventral cochlear nuclei. Secondary acoustic fibers project via the trapezoid body and lateral lemniscus to the inferior colliculi and medial geniculate bodies, which in turn project via the auditory radiations (situated in the most posterior part of the internal capsule) to the primary receptive areas for hearing in the transverse temporal gyri of Heschl (Fig. 14-1). Other cortical areas are also excited by auditory stimuli. In humans these comprise at least the superior temporal gyrus and the upper bank of the sylvian fissure, including frontal and parietal operculi (Celesia). In animals there are four representations of the cochlea in the sylvian regions and three polysensory areas which can be activated by auditory, visual, and somatic stimulation. The detailed physiology and anatomy of these ''centers'' and the medial geniculate bodies and other thalamic nuclei are not known.

The vestibular fibers of the eighth nerve terminate in the four vestibular nuclei: superior (Bechterew), lateral (Deiters), medial (triangular or Schwalbe), and inferior (spinal or descending). In addition, some of the fibers from the semicircular canals project directly to the cerebellum, via the juxtarestiform body, to terminate in the flocculonodular lobe and adjacent vermian cortex ("vestibulocerebellum"). Efferent fibers from this portion of the cerebellar cortex project ipsilaterally to the vestibular nuclei and to the fastigial nucleus; fibers from the fastigial nucleus project in turn to the contralateral vestibular nuclei, again via the juxtarestiform body. Thus the cerebellum of each side exerts an influence on the vestibular nuclei of both sides (Fig. 14-2; see also Chap. 4).

Figure 14-1

The ascending auditory pathways. The lower part of the diagram is a horizontal section through the upper medulla. (From CR Noback, The Human Nervous System, 3rd ed, New York, McGraw-Hill, 1981.)

The lateral and medial vestibular nuclei also have important connections with the spinal cord, mainly via the uncrossed lateral vestibulospinal and the crossed and uncrossed medial vestibulospinal tracts (Fig. 14-3). Presumably, vestibular effects on posture are mediated via these pathways—the axial muscles mainly by the medial vestibulospinal tract and the limb muscles by the lateral tract. The nuclei of the third, fourth, and sixth cranial nerves come under the influence of the vestibular nuclei, mainly the superior and medial nuclei, through the projection pathways described in Chap. 13. In addition, all the vestibular nuclei have afferent and efferent connections with the pontine reticular formation (Fig. 14-3). Finally, there are projections from the vestibular nuclei to the cerebral cortex, although the exact anatomic pathways are not known. In the monkey the projections are almost

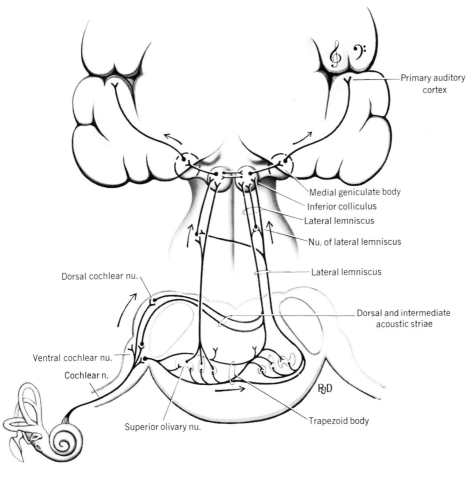

Primary auditory cortex

Medial geniculate body
Inferior colliculus
Lateral lemniscus
Nu. of lateral lemniscus

Lateral lemniscus

Dorsal cochlear nu.

Dorsal and intermediate acoustic striae

Ventral cochlear nu.
Cochlear n.

Superior olivary nu.

Trapezoid body

exclusively contralateral, terminating near the "face area" of the first somatosensory cortex (area 2 of Brodmann).

These brief remarks convey some notion of the complexity of the anatomic and functional organization of the vestibular system (for a full discussion, see the monographs of Brodal and of Baloh, Honrubia, and Jacobson). It is apparent that acoustic and vestibular function (as well as other cranial nerve function) may be affected together in the course of disease, or that each may be affected separately.

DEAFNESS, TINNITUS, AND OTHER DISORDERS OF AUDITORY PERCEPTION

DEAFNESS

This is a problem of immense proportions. In 1969, Konigsmark estimated that there were in the United States at least 6 million persons with hearing loss of sufficient severity to impair the understanding of speech; there were probably three times this many with some impairment of hearing. He estimated that in about one-half the affected children and about one-third the affected adults, the deafness was on a hereditary basis.

Deafness is of three general types: (1) *conductive*

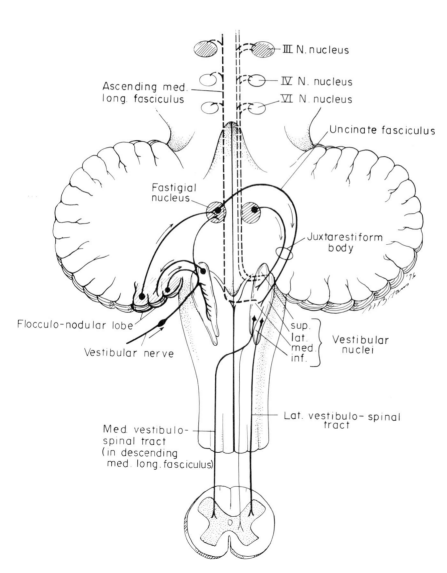

Figure 14-2

A simplified diagram of the vestibulocerebellar and vestibulo-spinal pathways and connections between vestibular and ocular motor nuclei. (See text and also Fig. 13-1.)

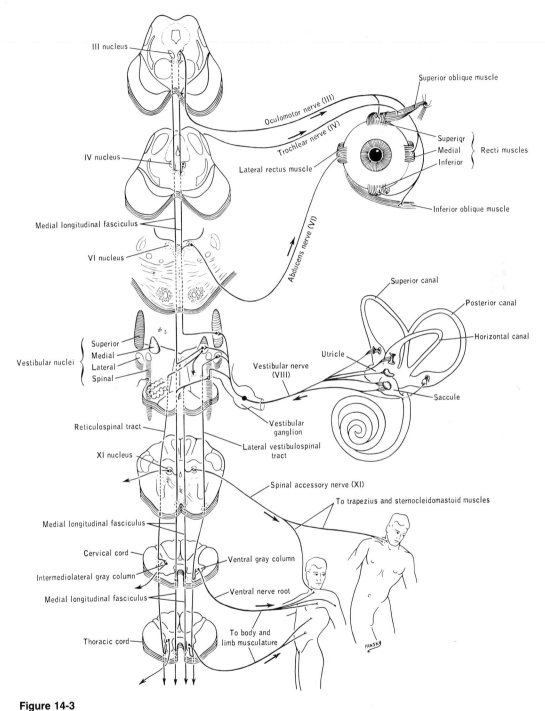

Figure 14-3

The vestibular reflex pathways. (From EL House et al, A Systematic Approach to Neuroscience, New York, McGraw-Hill, 1979.)

deafness, which is a ~~defect in the mechanism by which~~ sound is transformed (amplified) and conducted to the cochlea and is due to disorders of the external or middle ear, such as otosclerosis, chronic otitis, cholesteatoma, or occlusion of the external auditory canal or eustachian tube; (2) *sensorineural deafness* (also called *nerve deafness*), which is due to disease of the cochlea or of the cochlear division of the eighth cranial nerve; and (3) central deafness, due to lesions of the cochlear nuclei and their connections with the primary receptive areas for hearing in the temporal lobes.

Since the cochlear nucleus is connected with the cortex of both temporal lobes, hearing is unaffected by unilateral cerebral lesions. Deafness due to brainstem lesions is observed only rarely, since a massive lesion is required to interrupt both the crossed and uncrossed projections from the cochlear nucleus—so massive as a rule that other neurologic abnormalities make the testing of hearing impossible. The two peripheral forms of deafness need to be distinguished, since important remedial measures are available for conductive deafness.

In differentiating conductive from nerve deafness, the tuning-fork tests are often of value. When a vibrating fork, preferably of 512-Hz frequency, is held about an inch from the ear (the test for air conduction), sound waves can be appreciated only as they are transmitted through the middle ear and will be reduced with disease in this location. When the vibrating fork is applied to the skull (test for bone conduction), the sound waves are conveyed directly to the cochlea, without the intervention of the sound-transmission apparatus of the middle ear, and will therefore not be reduced or lost. Normally air conduction is better than bone conduction. These principles form the basis for several simple tests of auditory function.

In the *Weber test,* the vibrating fork is applied to the forehead in the midline. A normal person hears the sound equally in both ears. In nerve deafness, the sound is localized in the normal ear; in conductive deafness the sound is localized in the affected ear. In the *Rinne test* the fork is applied to the mastoid process. At the moment the sound ceases the fork is held at the auditory meatus. In middle ear deafness the sound cannot be heard by air conduction after bone conduction has ceased (abnormal or negative Rinne test). In nerve deafness the reverse is true (normal or positive Rinne test), although both air and bone conduction may be quantitatively decreased. The *Schwabach test* consists of comparing the patient's bone conduction with the bone conduction of a normal observer.

In general, sensorineural deafness is characterized by a partial loss of perception of high-pitched sounds and conductive deafness by a partial loss of perception of low-pitched sounds. This can be ascertained with the use of tuning forks of different frequencies, but the most accurate results are obtained by the use of an electric audiometer and the construction of an audiogram that reveals the entire range of hearing at a glance. The audiogram represents the nucleus of any diagnostic evaluation of loss of hearing and the point of departure for subsequent diagnostic evaluation.

TINNITUS

This is the other major manifestation of cochlear and auditory disease. *Tinnitus aurium* literally means "ringing of the ears" (Latin *tinnire,* "to ring or jingle") and is a common symptom in adults. Although the term always refers to sounds originating in the ear, they need not be ringing in character. Buzzing, humming, whistling, roaring, hissing, clicking, or pulse-like sounds are also reported. Some otologists use the term *tinnitus cerebri* to distinguish other head noises from those that arise in the ear, but most often the term *tinnitus* is used without qualification and refers to *tinnitus aurium.*

Tinnitus may be defined generally as any sensation of sound for which there is no source outside the individual. It may be divided into two basic types, *tonal* and *nontonal* (nonvibratory and vibratory, in the terminology of Fowler). The tonal type is by far the more common and is also called *subjective tinnitus,* because it can be heard only by the patient. The nontonal form is sometimes *objective,* in the sense that under certain conditions, the tinnitus can be heard by the examiner as well as by the patient. In either case, whether tinnitus is produced in the inner ear or in some other part of the head and neck, sensory auditory neurons must be stimulated, for only the auditory neural pathways can transmit an impulse that will be perceived as sound.

Nontonal (vibratory) head noises are mechanical in origin and conducted to the inner ear through the various hard or soft, fluid or gaseous media of the body. They are not due to a primary dysfunction of the auditory neural mechanism but have their origin in the contraction of muscles of the eustachian tube, middle ear (stapedius, tensor tympani), the palate (palatal myoclonus), or the muscles of deglutition. One type of nontonal tinnitus is caused by opening and closing of the eustachian tubes. The most common form of objective tinnitus is a vascular bruit from the large vessels of the neck or arteriovenous malformations of the brain. In these latter cases, the tinnitus corresponds to the pulse (pulsatile tinnitus), and the examiner may hear a bruit over the mastoid process. One must be cautious in interpreting this symptom because normal persons can hear their pulse when lying with one ear on a pillow, and introspective individuals may worry about it.

Tonal tinnitus arises in the middle or inner ear. Under ideal acoustical circumstances (in a soundproof room, having an ambient noise level of 18 dB or less), it is present in 80 to 90 percent of adults (''physiologic tinnitus''). The ambient noise level in ordinary living conditions usually exceeds 35 dB and is of sufficient intensity to mask physiologic tinnitus, which remains inaudible. However, tinnitus due to disease of the middle ear and auditory neural mechanism may also be masked by environmental noise and hence becomes troublesome only in quiet surroundings—at night, in the country, etc.

Most often, tinnitus signifies a disorder of the inner ear, ossicles of the middle ear, tympanic membrane, or eighth nerve. The large majority of patients who complain of persistent tinnitus have some degree of deafness as well. Tinnitus that is localized to one ear and is described as having a tonal character (such as a ringing or bell-like or high, steady musical tone) is usually associated with an impairment of cochlear or neural function. Tinnitus due to middle ear disease (e.g., otosclerosis) tends to be more constant than the tinnitus of sensorineural disorders, and is of variable intensity and lower pitch. All clicks, pops, rushing sounds, etc., are believed to be due to middle ear disease.

As was remarked, the pitch of tinnitus associated with a conductive hearing loss is of low-frequency (median frequency of 490 Hz, with a range of 90 to 1450 Hz). That which accompanies sensorineural loss is higher (median frequency of 3900 Hz, with a range of 545 to 7500 Hz). This rule does not apply to Ménière disease, in which the tinnitus usually has a low-pitched buzzing or roaring sound (median frequency of 320 Hz, with a range of 90 to 900 Hz), thus resembling the tinnitus that accompanies a conductive rather than a sensorineural hearing loss (Nodar and Graham).

There are many theories as to the mechanism of tonal tinnitus. One postulates an overactivity or disinhibition of hair cells, adjacent to a part of the cochlea that has been injured. Another theory, proposed by Möller, is based on the finding of an abnormal discharge pattern of afferent neurons; the latter is attributed to ephaptic transmission between nerve fibers that have been damaged by vascular compression. Relief of tinnitus has reportedly been achieved by decompression of the eighth nerve (Jannetta).

For most forms of tinnitus there is little effective treatment. Patients reconcile themselves to its presence as a rule, once the nature of the disorder is explained to them. If tinnitus is the basis of repeated complaints, one usually discovers that the patient is anxious or depressed, and a careful medical history will reveal the other symptoms of the psychiatric illness. Treatment then needs to be directed to the psychiatric symptoms.

OTHER DISORDERS OF AUDITORY PERCEPTION

Pontine lesions may be accompanied by *complex auditory illusions* with some of the qualities of a hallucination

(*pontine auditory hallucinosis*). These consist of alternating musical tones, like an organ, or a jumble of sound (like a symphony orchestra tuning up), or siren-like or buzzing sounds, like a swarm of bees. These auditory sense disturbances are more complex than neurosensory tinnitus but less formed than temporal lobe hallucinations. They are usually associated with impairment of hearing in one or both ears and other neurologic signs related to the pontine lesion. Brainstem evoked potentials reveal intact cochlear, auditory nerve, and cochlear nuclear responses. As in the case of peduncular visual hallucinosis, the patient realizes the sounds are unreal, i.e., they have insight into their illusory nature (Cascino and Adams).

Another recognized but inexplicable type of auditory hallucinosis occurs in aged patients with longstanding neurosensory deafness. They hear songs, symphonies, choral music, or unfamiliar melodies all day long, interrupted only by voices in conversation or other ambient noise, or by sleep. Our cases, like those reported by Hammeke et al, were neither depressed nor demented, and anticonvulsant and antipsychotic drugs have had no effect.

Complex auditory hallucinations may occur as part of temporal-lobe epilepsy and with other temporal-lobe lesions. Contrariwise, seizures may be induced by musical sounds, as well as by other auditory stimuli. These topics are discussed in Chaps. 15 and 21.

SPECIAL AUDIOLOGIC PROCEDURES

The differentiation of cochlear from acoustic nerve lesions poses special problems. In general, there is a correlation between the severity of hair cell loss and nerve degeneration; i.e., complete end organ destruction will result in the loss of all afferent fibers (efferent and autonomic neurons are unaltered). If, however, the supporting elements of the organ of Corti are preserved, the hair cells may disappear long before there is secondary degeneration of sensory fibers (Hinojosa and Lindsay). Many noxious agents (trauma, persistent loud noise, drugs, hypoxia) may damage the hair cells before nerve fiber loss occurs. Primary neuronal degeneration as a cause of deafness is less frequent, but does occur, as in advanced age (Suga and Lindsay).

A number of special tests have proved to be helpful, indeed essential, in distinguishing cochlear from retrocochlear (nerve) lesions. Although an absolute distinction cannot be made on the basis of any one test, the results of the tests when taken together make it possible to predict the site of the lesion with considerable accuracy. These tests, usually carried out by an otologist or audiologist, include the following:

1. *Loudness recruitment*. This phenomenon is thought to depend upon selective destruction of low-intensity elements subserved by the external hair cells of the organ of Corti. The high-intensity elements are preserved, so that loudness is appreciated at high intensities. In testing for loudness recruitment, the difference in hearing between the two ears is estimated, and the loudness of the pure tone stimulus of a given frequency delivered to each ear is then increased by regular increments. In nonrecruiting deafness (characteristic of a nerve trunk lesion), the original difference in hearing persists in all comparisons of loudness above threshold, since both high- and low-intensity fibers are affected. In recruiting deafness (which occurs with a lesion in the organ of Corti, e.g., Ménière disease), the more affected ear gains in loudness and may finally be equal to the better one. In bilateral disease, recruitment is assesed by the intensity of stimulus that causes discomfort. In the normal person the threshold of discomfort is about 100 dB.

2. *Speech discrimination*. This consists of presenting the patient with a list of 50 phonetically balanced monosyllabic words (e.g., thin, sin) at suprathreshold levels. Speech-discrimination score is the percentage of the 50 words correctly repeated by the patient. Marked reduction (less than 30 percent) in the speech-discrimination test scores with respect to threshold sensitivity is characteristic of eighth nerve lesions.

3. *Short-increment sensitivity index (SiSi)*. The patient is asked to respond to a series of twenty 1-dB increments in amplitude superimposed on a steady tone of the same frequency presented at a sensation level of 20 dB. In normal persons and in those with retrocochlear lesions, most of these small 1-dB pips of sound are not heard; with cochlear lesions most of them are heard.

4. *Threshold "tone decay" (abnormal auditory adaptation)*. This test requires only a conventional pure-tone audiometer. With lesions of the cochlear nerve, e.g., acoustic neuroma, a continuous tone presented at or above threshold intensity gradually seems to decrease in loudness, in contrast to what happens with cochlear lesions.

5. *Békésy audiometry*. Continuous and interrupted tones are presented at various frequencies. Tracings are made which measure the increments by which the patient must increase the volume in order to continue to hear the continuous and interrupted tones just above threshold. Analysis of many tracings has shown that there are four basic configurations, referred to as types I to IV Békésy audiograms. Types III or IV usually indicate the presence of a retrocochlear lesion, the type II response points to a lesion of the cochlea itself, and type I is considered normal.

6. *Computerized auditory evoked potentials (page 28)*. This is the newest method and provides information as to the integrity of primary and secondary neural pathways from the cochlea to the temporal lobe cortex. This method can be used in uncooperative and even comatose patients. It is also of value in the study of brain death where all waves except the cochlear response are abolished.

Of these special tests, threshold tone decay and auditory recruitment are the most helpful in distinguishing sensorineural hearing loss of cochlear origin from that of primary acoustic nerve affection.

MIDDLE EAR DEAFNESS

The common causes are otosclerosis, otitis media, and trauma. Of the various types of progressive conductive deafness, otosclerosis is the most frequent, being the cause of about half the cases of deafness that have their onset in early adult life (usually in the second or third decade). It is transmitted as an autosomal dominant trait with variable penetrance. Pathologically this disorder is characterized by an overgrowth of labyrinthine capsular bone around the oval window, leading to progressive fixation of the stapes. The remarkable advances in micro-otologic surgery, designed to mobilize or replace the stapes, have greatly altered the prognosis in this disease; significant improvement in hearing can now be achieved in the majority of such patients.

The use of antibiotic drugs has greatly reduced the incidence of suppurative otitis media, both the acute and chronic forms, which in former years were common causes of conductive hearing loss. Chronic serous otitis media is still an important cause of this type of deafness.

Fractures of the temporal bone, particularly those in the long axis of the petrous pyramid, may damage middle ear structures, and frequently there is bleeding into the middle ear as well, from a ruptured tympanic membrane. Transverse fractures through the petrous pyramid are more likely to damage the cochlear-labyrinthine structures and the facial nerve.

SENSORINEURAL DEAFNESS

This has many causes. The cochlea may be damaged by rubella in the pregnant mother. Mumps, acute purulent meningitis, or chronic infection spreading from the middle to the inner ear may cause nerve deafness in childhood. Measles vaccination, mycoplasma pneumonii infection, and scarlet fever are in rare instances associated with acute deafness, with or without vestibular symptoms. It is uncertain whether the deafness in these cases is due to direct infection or represents an autoimmune reaction of the inner ear.

Little is known about the syndrome of sudden unilateral deafness without vertigo. Presumably it is of cochlear origin. A vascular causation has been postulated, on uncertain grounds. A few cases have complicated herpes zoster and mumps parotitis, but there is no proven relationship with the usual viral respiratory infections. In a prospective study of 88 such cases, Mattox and Simmons found that two-thirds of them recovered their hearing completely within a few days or a week or two, and that none of the currently popular treatments, such as histamine and steroids, had any effect on the outcome. In the remaining patients, recovery was much slower and often incomplete; in this latter group, the hearing loss was predominantly for high tones and was associated with varying degrees of vertigo and hypoactive caloric responses. Episodic deafness in one ear, without vertigo, proves in most instances to be Ménière disease (see further on).

Explosions or intense, sustained noise in certain industrial settings or from gun blasts or even rock music may result in a high-tone sensorineural hearing loss. Certain antimicrobial drugs (viz., streptomycin, kanamycin, neomycin, and gentamicin) may damage cochlear hair cells. Quinine and acetylsalicylic acid may impair sensorineural function transiently. The most common type of hearing loss in the aged (presbycusis) is a high-frequency sensorineural type, which is probably due to neuronal degeneration, i.e., progressive loss of spiral ganglion neurons (Suga and Lindsay). Otologists have described a progressive sensorineural type of hearing loss as a late manifestation of congenital syphilis, allegedly occurring despite prior treatment of the latter disorder with adequate doses of penicillin. It has been claimed that the long-term administration of steroids may be useful in these circumstances. The pathologic basis of the hearing loss in such cases has not been determined, and the causal relationship to congenital syphilis remains to be established.

The *auditory nerve* may be involved by tumors of the cerebellopontine angle or by syphilitic or other types of chronic meningitis. Deafness may also result from a demyelinative plaque, infarction, or tumor involving the cochlear nerve fibers or nuclei in the *brainstem*. Rarely, deafness is the result of bilateral lesions of the temporal lobes. (Chap. 21). Pure word deafness is also due to temporal lobe disease. Here, despite normal pure tone perception and audiometry and normal brainstem auditory evoked potentials, spoken words cannot be understood. This condition is discussed in Chap. 22.

A large series of *genetically determined syndromes* which feature a neural or conductive type of deafness, some congenital and others having their onset in childhood or early adult life, have come to light (see articles by Konigsmark and by Proctor and Proctor). Most of them are inherited as an autosomal dominant trait, but others are characterized by a recessive or sex-linked transmission. There are few complete histopathologic studies of congenital and hereditary deafness. Two groups can be recognized— aplasias and degenerations. Four types of inner ear aplasia have been described: (1) *Michel defect,* a complete absence of the otic capsule and eighth nerve; (2) *Mondini defect,* an incomplete development of the bony and membranous labyrinths and the spiral ganglion; (3) *Scheibe defect,* a membranous cochleosaccular dysplasia with atrophy of the vestibular and cochlear nerves; and (4) rare chromosomal aberrations (trisomies) characterized by abnormality of the end organ and absence of the spiral ganglion.

In addition to these more or less pure aplasias of the auditory system, cochleovestibular atrophies and degenerations occur as part of many other developmental and heredodegenerative syndromes. Konigsmark has classified these forms of hereditary deafness on the basis of associated defects caused by the same gene: malformations of the external ear; integumentary abnormalities such as hyperkeratosis, hyperplasia or scantiness of eyebrows, albinism, large hyperpigmented or hypopigmented areas, brittle twisted hairs, and coniform and missing teeth; ocular abnormalities such as hypertelorism, severe myopia, optic atrophy, congenital and juvenile cataracts, and retinitis pigmentosa; neurologic abnormalities such as polyneuropathy and sensory ataxia (Refsum syndrome), progressive ophthalmoplegia and cerebellar ataxia, bilateral acoustic neuromas, photomyoclonic seizures, and mental deficiency; skeletal abnormalities; and renal, thyroid, or cardiac abnormalities. These hereditary syndromes are summarized in Table 14-1. The associations of neurosensory deafness with degenerative neurologic diseases are discussed further in Chap. 43.

HYSTERICAL DEAFNESS

It is possible to distinguish hysterical deafness from organic disease in several ways. In the case of bilateral deafness, the distinction can be made by observing a blink (cochleo-orbicular reflex) or an alteration in skin sweating (psychogalvanic skin reflex) in response to loud sound. Unilateral hysterical deafness may be detected by an audiometer, with both ears connected, or by whispering into the bell of a stethoscope attached to the patient's ears, closing first one and then the other tube without the patient's knowledge. The elicitation of brainstem auditory evoked potentials provides indisputable evidence that the patient can hear. It

Table 14-1
Hereditary cochleovestibular atrophies
Type I: Progressive hearing loss with involvement of kidneys, skin, or bones

Mode of inheritance	Age of onset	Type of hearing loss	Associated abnormalities	Eponymic disease or syndrome
Autosomal dominant	Childhood	Onset with loss of low, mid, or high frequencies, variably progressive	None	
Recessive	Congenital	Neural, rapidly progressive with failure of speech development	None	
Sex-linked recessive	Early childhood	Neural, rapidly progressive with speech impairment	None	
Autosomal dominant or recessive	Early adulthood	Neural, with tinnitus; progressive with unilateral or bilateral vestibular paresis	Episodic paroxysmal vertigo (''hereditary Ménière'')	
Autosomal dominant	Congenital or first decade	Sensorineural; variable severity and progression	Progressive nephritis with uremia	Alport
Autosomal recessive	Childhood	Neural; progressive	Renal tubular acidosis	
Autosomal dominant	Childhood or adolescence	Sensorineural; slowly progressive	Nephrotic syndrome with amyloidosis; recurrent urticaria and fever	Muckle-Wells
Autosomal dominant (probable)	Childhood	Neural; progressive	Ichthyosis of extremities; prolinuria; glomerulosclerosis and uremia in some cases	Goyer
Autosomal dominant	Early adulthood	Neural; progressive	Congenital anhidrosis with absence of sweat and sebacious glands	Helweg-Larsen
Autosomal dominant	Middle age	Conductive loss at onset, then sensorineural; progressive	Osteitis deformans	Paget
Dominant	Childhood	Conductive or neural or mixed; usually progressive	Craniometaphyseal dysplasia with sclerosis of base of skull and narrowing of foramina; sometimes optic atrophy and facial palsy	Pyle
Recessive	Childhood or adolescence	Neural or mixed; progressive	Osteosclerosis of skull and mandible with narrowing of foramina; facial paresis	Van Buchem
Autosomal dominant	Second or third decade	Conductive; sometimes neural or mixed	Osteogenesis imperfecta tarda	Ekman-Lobstein or Van der Hoeve

Table 14-1 *(continued)*
Hereditary cochleovestibular atrophies
Type II: Hereditary hearing loss with retinal disease

Mode of inheritance	Age of onset	Type of hearing loss	Associated abnormalities	Eponymic disease or syndrome
Recessive	Congenital	Sensorineural, with vestibular hypofunction	Progressive retinitis pigmentosa and ataxia beginning in late childhood or adolescence. Sometimes mental defect, cataracts and glaucoma	Usher
Recessive	Early in second decade	Sensorineural; progressive	Retinitis pigmentosa, polyneuropathy, ataxia, mental deterioration	Refsum
Recessive	Infancy	Sensorineural; progressive	Retinal pigmentary degeneration, cataracts, diabetes mellitus	Alström
Recessive	Childhood	Sensorineural; variable progression	Dwarfism, senile appearance, variable mental retardation	Cockayne
Autosomal dominant	Childhood	Neural; variably progressive	Optic atrophy, ataxia, muscle wasting of shoulder girdle and hands, mental dullness, degeneration of optic nerves, posterior columns, spinocerebellar and corticospinal tracts	Sylvester
Recessive	Infancy	Neural; progressive with failure of speech development	Optic atrophy, polyneuropathy	Rosenberg-Chutorian
Autosomal recessive	First decade	Neural; progressive	Optic atrophy, juvenile diabetes mellitus	Turnbridge-Paley
Autosomal recessive	Infancy	Neural; progressive	Opticocochleodentate degeneration, progressive quadriparesis and mental deterioration	Nyssen-Van Bogaert
Sex-linked recessive	Congenital (ocular signs)	Onset of neural deafness in second and third decade; progressive	Retinal vascular and glial proliferation, progressive microphthalmia and mental retardation	Norrie
Recessive	Congenital	Neural	Tortuosity of retinal vessels and exudative retinitis, muscle wasting, immobile facies	Small

Table 14-1 (continued)
Hereditary cochleovestibular atrophies
Type III: Hereditary hearing loss with nervous system disease

Mode of inheritance	Age of onset	Type of hearing loss	Associated abnormalities	Eponymic disease or syndrome
Dominant	Third decade	Neural, progressive	Nephropathy, photomyoclonic seizures, mental deterioration, diabetes mellitus. Diffuse cerebral and cerebellar cortical neuronal loss	Hermann
Dominant	Childhood	Neural, slowly progressive	Myoclonus, progressive ataxia and dysarthria	May-White
Recessive	Congenital	Neural, with failure of speech development	Mild chronic myoclonic epilepsy	Latham-Munro
Dominant	Congenital	Neural, varying severity	Piebald trait and variable absence of pigmentation of skin; ataxia and mental retardation frequent	Telfer
Dominant	Second or third decade	Sensorineural	Hyperuricemia, decreased renal function, progressive ataxia and dysarthria, proximal muscle weakness and wasting	Rosenberg-Bergstrom
Recessive	Childhood	Progressive, severe	Progressive ataxia, hypotonia and dysarthria, mild mental retardation	Lichtenstein-Knorr
Autosomal recessive	Infancy or early childhood	Neural, slowly progressive	Progressive ataxia of gait, hypogonadism, mental deficiency, wasting and weakness of distal limb muscles	Richards-Rundle
Recessive	Childhood	Neural, rapidly progressive	Progressive cerebellar ataxia, mental deficiency, extensor plantar signs, pigmented spots on face and limbs; heart block	Jeune-Tommasi
Autosomal dominant	Second or third decade	Neural; progressive with tinnitus and loss of vestibular function	Bilateral acoustic neuromas	Gardner
Dominant	Childhood	Neural deafness, not in all cases	Progressive sensory radicular neuropathy	Denny-Brown
Dominant	First or second decade	Neural; progressive	Myopia, cataracts and retinitis pigmentosa; sensorimotor peripheral neuropathy; skin atrophy with ulceration; dental caries; kyphoscoliosis, cystic bone changes	Flynn-Aird

Table 14-1 *(continued)*
Hereditary cochleovestibular atrophies
Type III: Hereditary hearing loss with nervous system disease

Mode of inheritance	Age of onset	Type of hearing loss	Associated abnormalities	Eponymic disease or syndrome
Autosomal recessive	Childhood	Neural, progressive	Proteinuria, progressive distal muscle wasting and weakness with claw hand and foot	Lemieux-Neemeh
? Dominant with incomplete penetrance	Congenital	Auditory imperception with failure of speech development	Indifference to pain	Osuntokun
Autosomal recessive	Childhood or adolescence	Progressive; neural with loss of vestibular function	Slowly progressive bulbar palsy	

Source: Konigsmark, 1975.

should be kept in mind that brief episodes of deafness with fully preserved consciousness may be caused by a seizure in one temporal lobe (epileptic suppression of hearing).

DIZZINESS AND VERTIGO

Dizziness and other sensations of imbalance are among the commonest symptoms confronting the neurologist. The significance of these complaints varies greatly. For the most part they are benign, but always there is the possibility that they signal the presence of an important neurologic disorder. Diagnosis of the underlying disease demands that the complaint of dizziness be analyzed correctly—the nature of the disturbance of function being determined first, and then its anatomic localization. This classic approach to neurologic diagnosis is nowhere more valuable than in the patient whose main complaint is dizziness.

The term *dizziness* is applied by the patient to a number of different sensory experiences—a feeling of rotation or whirling, as well as nonrotatory swaying, weakness, faintness, light-headedness, or unsteadiness. Blurring of vision, feelings of unreality, syncope, and even petit mal or other seizure phenomena may be called "dizzy spells." Hence a close questioning as to how the patient is using the term becomes a necessary first step in clinical study. Essentially, the physician must determine whether the symptoms have the specific quality of vertigo—which in this chapter will refer to all subjective and objective illusions of motion or position—or whether they are more properly categorized as nonrotatory giddiness or pseudo-vertigo. The distinction between these two groups of symptoms will be elaborated presently, following a brief discussion of the factors that are involved in the maintenance of equilibrium.

PHYSIOLOGIC CONSIDERATIONS

Several mechanisms are responsible for the maintenance of a balanced posture and for the awareness of the position of the body in relation to its surroundings.

Continuous afferent impulses from the eyes, labyrinths, muscles, and joints inform us of the position of different parts of the body. In response to these impulses the adaptive movements necessary to maintain equilibrium are carried out. Normally we are unaware of these many fine adjustments, since they operate for the most part at a reflex level. The most important of the afferent impulses are:

1. Visual impulses from the retina of both eyes and possibly impulses derived from proprioceptors of the ocular muscles, which enable us to judge the distance of objects from the body. These impulses are coordinated with impulses from the labyrinths and neck (see below) to stabilize gaze during movements of the head and body.

2. Impulses from the labyrinths, which function as highly specialized spatial proprioceptors and register changes in the velocity of motion (either acceleration or deceleration) and position of the body. The cristae of the three semicircular canals respond primarily to angular acceleration of the head, and the saccular and utricular maculae respond to acceleration. In each of these locations displacement of the sensory hair cells is the effective stimulus. In the semicircular canals this is accomplished by movement of the endolymphatic fluid, which in turn is induced by rotation of the head. In the utricle and saccule the hairs are displaced in response to the force of gravity on the otoliths. In either event the movement generates an electrical charge in the hair cells, causing depolarization of the nerve terminals and initiating impulses in the vestibular nerve. Reflexes subserved by the maculae compensate for changes induced by and in the

direction of gravity, whereas reflexes that govern posture, tone, equilibrium, and ocular stability during movement are initiated both by the maculae and cristae.

3. Impulses from the proprioceptors of the joints and muscles, which are essential to all reflex, postural, and volitional movements. Those from the neck are of special importance in relating the position of the head to the rest of the body.

These sense organs are connected with the cerebellum and certain ganglionic centers and pathways in the brainstem, particularly the ocular motor, red, and vestibular nuclei and the medial longitudinal fasciculi. These are the important coordinators of the sensory data and provide for postural adjustments and the maintenance of equilibrium. They are the basis of what is called the "space constancy mechanisms," whereby our perceptions of ourselves and the external environment are matched. Conversely, any disease that disrupts these neural mechanisms may give rise to vertigo and disequilibrium.

Important psychophysiologic mechanisms are involved in the maintenance of equilibrium and the orientation of our bodies to the external world. Early in life we come to coordinate parts of our body in relation to one another and to perceive that portion of space occupied by our bodies. We construct from these integrated sensory data a general concept that has been designated by Russell Brain as the *body schema*. The space around our body is represented by another set of data, the *environmental schema*. These two schemata are neither static nor independent; they are constantly being modified and adapted to one another; their interdependence is ascribed to the fact that the various sense organs which supply the information on which the two schemata are based are usually activated simultaneously by any body movement. Through a process of learning we come to see objects as stationary while we are moving, and moving objects as having motion when we are either moving or stationary. Motion of an individual in space is always relative. At times, especially when our own sensory information is incomplete, we mistake movement of our surroundings for movements of our own body. A well-known example of this is the feeling of movement that one experiences in a stationary train, when actually a neighboring train is moving. Hence, in this frame of reference, orientation of the body in space is made possible only by the maintenance of an orderly relationship between the bodily schema and the schema of the external world; as a corollary, disorientation in space, or disequilibrium, occurs when this relationship is upset.

Yet another factor that influences equilibrium is the effect of aging. Many old people lose their balance on extending their neck, and the postural protective mechanisms are impaired, making falls more frequent. A destructive lesion of one or both labyrinths may leave an elderly person permanently unbalanced, while a younger person compensates for the loss.

CLINICAL CHARACTERISTICS OF VERTIGO AND GIDDINESS

A careful history and physical examination usually afford the basis for separating true vertigo from the dizziness of the anxious patient and from the other types of pseudovertigo. The recognition of vertigo is not difficult when the patient states that objects in the environment spun around or moved in one direction or that there was a sensation of the head and body whirling. (A distinction is sometimes drawn between subjective vertigo, meaning a sense of turning of one's body, and objective vertigo, an illusion of movement of the environment, but its validity is doubtful.) Often, however, the patient is not so explicit. The feeling may be described as a to-and-fro or up-and-down movement of the body, usually of the head. Or the floor or walls may seem to tilt or to sink or rise up. In walking, the patient may have felt unsteady and veered to one side. Or there may have been a sensation of leaning or being pulled to the ground or to one side or another, as though being drawn by a strong magnet. This feeling of impulsion is particularly characteristic of vertigo.

Some patients may be able to identify their symptoms only when they are asked to compare them with the feeling of movement experienced when coming to a halt after rapid rotation. If the patient is unobservant or imprecise in his or her descriptions, a helpful tactic is to provoke a number of dissimilar sensations by rotating the patient rapidly, irrigating the ears with warm and cold water, asking the patient to stoop for a minute and straighten up, to stand relaxed for 3 min and check blood pressure for orthostatic effect, and to hyperventilate for 3 min. Should the patient be unable to distinguish among these several types of induced dizziness or to ascertain the similarity of one of the types to his or her own condition, the history is probably too inaccurate for purposes of diagnosis.

When the patient's symptoms are mild or poorly described, small items of the patient's history—a disinclination to stoop or walk during an attack, a tendency to list to one side, an aggravation of symptoms by turning over in bed, closing the eyes, or riding in a vehicle, and a preference for one position—help to identify them as vertigo.

In some patients an attack of vertigo is so abrupt and violent that they are virtually flung to the ground, sometimes injuring themselves. This attack has been given the quaint term ''otolithic catastrophe of Tumarkin'' and attributed, with little evidence, to involvement of the utricle or saccule. The diagnosis is usually substantiated by the presence of vertigo, nausea, and vomiting while the patient is on the ground, distinguishing it from a seizure or faint. Probably it differs from other forms of labyrinthine vertigo only in its severity.

All but the mildest forms of vertigo are accompanied by varying degrees of nausea, vomiting, pallor, and perspiration. As a rule, patients have some difficulty with walking, and cannot walk at all if the vertigo is intense. Forced to lie down, they realize that one position, usually on one side with eyes closed, reduces the vertigo and nausea and that the slightest motion of the head aggravates them. One form of vertigo, the benign positional vertigo of Bárány (see further on), occurs only for a few seconds after lying down, sitting up, or turning. If the vertigo is less severe, the patient can walk unsteadily but may veer to one side. The source of the ataxia that is associated with vertigo (vertiginous ataxia) is recognized as being ''in the head,'' not as being related to control of the legs and trunk. It is noteworthy that in these circumstances the coordination of the individual movements of the limbs is not impaired—a point of difference from most instances of cerebellar disease. There may be headache, generalized or in the region of the offending ear. Loss of consciousness as part of a vertiginous attack nearly always signifies another type of disorder (seizure or faint).

Giddiness and other types of pseudovertigo are usually described as a feeling of swaying or light-headedness, or a swimming sensation, or, more rarely, as a feeling of uncertainty or walking on air, or being ''queer in the head'' or about to fall or ''pass out.'' These sensory experiences are particularly common in illnesses featured by anxiety attacks, viz., anxiety neurosis, hysteria, and depression. They are in part reproduced by hyperventilation; and then it is appreciated that varying degrees of apprehensiveness, panic, palpitation, breathlessness, trembling, and sweating are concurrent.

Other pseudovertiginous symptoms are less definite. In severe anemic states, weakness and languor may be attended by a light-headedness related to postural change and exertion, the basis of which must be a mild hypoxia. In the emphysematous patient, physical effort may be associated with weakness and peculiar cephalic sensations, and coughing may lead to giddiness and even fainting (tussive syncope) because of impaired return of venous blood to the heart. The dizziness that so often accompanies hypertension is difficult to evaluate; sometimes it is an expression of anxiety, or it may conceivably be due to an unstable adjustment of cerebral blood flow. Postural dizziness is another example of unstable vasomotor reflexes preventing a constancy of cerebral circulation; it is notably frequent in persons with primary orthostatic hypotension and polyneuropathy, in those recently bedfast, in the weak and ill, and possibly in the elderly. Rising abruptly from a recumbent or sitting position may be followed immediately by a swaying type of dizziness, dimming of vision, and spots before the eyes, which last for several seconds. The patient is forced to stand still and steady himself by holding onto a nearby object. Occasionally, a syncopal attack may occur at this time (see page 293).

In practice it is usually not difficult to separate these types of pseudovertigo from true vertigo, for there is none of the feeling of impulsion or rotation or other disturbance of motion so characteristic of the latter. Lacking also are the ancillary symptoms of true vertigo, viz., nausea, vomiting, tinnitus and deafness, staggering, and the relief obtained by sitting or lying still.

THE NEUROLOGIC AND OTOLOGIC CAUSES OF VERTIGO

The fact that vertigo may constitute the aura of an epileptic seizure, the origin of which is in the temporal cortex, supports the view that a cerebral cortical lesion can produce vertigo. Electrical stimulation of the cerebral cortex, either of the posterolateral aspects of the temporal lobe or the inferior parietal lobule, near the sylvian fissure may evoke intense vertigo (page 256). The occurrence of vertigo as the initial symptom in a seizure is infrequent. In such a case, a sensation of movement—either of the body away from the side of the lesion or of the environment in the opposite direction—lasts for a few seconds before being submerged in other seizure activity. Vertiginous epilepsy of this type should be differentiated from vestibulogenic seizures, in which an excessive vestibular discharge serves as the stimulus for a seizure. In this latter form of reflex epilepsy, tests that induce vertigo may provoke the seizure.

Ocular motor disorders, such as recent ophthalmoplegia with diplopia, are a source of spatial disorientation, and may give rise to brief sensations of vertigo, accompanied by mild nausea and staggering. This is maximal when the patient looks in the direction of action of the paralyzed muscle; it is attributable to the receipt of two conflicting visual images. In fact some normal people may experience dizziness for brief periods when adjusting to bifocal glasses or when looking down from a height.

Whether lesions of the cerebellum produce vertigo seems to depend on which part of the cerebellum is involved. Large destructive processes in the cerebellar hemispheres and vermis may cause no vertigo. However, lesions involving the cerebellum in the territory of the posterior inferior cerebellar artery (distal to the branches to the medulla oblongata) may cause an intense vertigo, indistinguishable from that due to labyrinthine disorder (Duncan et al). In two such cases that were studied pathologically, the lesion (ischemic infarction) extended to the midline and involved the flocculonodular lobe. Falling, in these cases, was to the side of the lesion; nystagmus was present on gaze to each side but was more prominent on gaze to the side of the infarct. Labyrinthine disease, on the other hand, usually causes unidirectional nystagmus to the side opposite the lesion and swaying or falling toward the side of the lesion—i.e., the direction of the nystagmus is opposite to that of the falling and past pointing.

The observations of Biemond and DeJong document a kind of nystagmus and vertigo induced by disturbances of the upper cervical roots and the muscles and ligaments that they innervate (so-called cervical vertigo). Spasm of the cervical muscles, trauma to the neck, and irritation of the upper cervical sensory roots are said to produce asymmetric spinovestibular stimulation and thus evoke nystagmus and prolonged vertigo and disequilibrium. Another possible explanation of cervical vertigo might relate to circulatory insufficiency in the vertebral-basilar territory. Toole and Tucker demonstrated a reduced flow through these vessels (in cadavers) when the head was rotated or hyperextended. The existence of this type of vertigo and nystagmus, or at least these interpretations of it, is still open to question.

Although lesions of the cerebral cortex, eyes, cerebellum, and perhaps the cervical muscles may give rise to vertigo, they are not common sources of vertigo, and vertigo is not the dominant manifestation of disease in these parts. For all practical purposes, vertigo indicates a disorder of the vestibular end organs, the vestibular division of the eighth nerve, or the vestibular nuclei in the brainstem and their immediate connections, and the clinical problem resolves itself into deciding which portion of the labyrinthine-vestibular apparatus is primarily involved. Usually this decision can be made on the basis of the form of the vertiginous attack and, particularly, the associated symptoms. The common labyrinthine-vestibular syndromes are described below.

LABYRINTHINE VERTIGO AND MÉNIÈRE DISEASE

Labyrinthine disease is the most common cause of true vertigo. The classic variety, Ménière disease, is characterized by recurrent attacks of vertigo associated with fluc-

tuating tinnitus and deafness. One or the other of the latter symptoms—rarely both—may be absent during the initial attacks of vertigo, but they invariably assert themselves as the disease progresses and increase in severity during an acute attack.

The attacks of vertigo are characteristically abrupt and last for several minutes to an hour or longer. The vertigo is unmistakably whirling or rotational in type and usually so severe that the patient cannot stand or walk. Varying degrees of nausea and vomiting, tinnitus, a feeling of fullness in the ear, and a diminution in hearing are practically always associated. Nystagmus is present during the acute attack. It is horizontal in type, usually with a rotary component; the slow phase of the nystagmus as well as past pointing and falling are to the side of the affected ear. The patient preferentially lies with the faulty ear uppermost and is disinclined to look toward the normal side because of exaggeration of the nystagmus and dizziness.

The attacks vary considerably in frequency and severity. They may recur several times weekly for many weeks on end, or there may be remissions of several years' duration. Frequently recurring attacks may give rise to mild chronic states of disequilibrium and a reluctance to move the head or to turn quickly. With milder forms of the disease the patient may complain more of head discomfort and of difficulty in concentration than of vertigo and may be considered neurotic. Symptoms of anxiety are common in patients with Ménière disease, particularly in those who suffer frequent, severe attacks.

Irrigation of the ear canal with cold and warm water (caloric testing) usually discloses an impairment or loss of thermally induced nystagmus on the involved side. In caloric testing, the patient's head is tilted forward 30° from the horizontal (bringing the horizontal semicircular canal into a vertical plane, which is the position of maximal sensitivity of this canal to thermal stimuli). The external auditory meati are irrigated in turn for 30 s with water at 30°C and 44°C (7°C below and above body temperature), with a pause of at least 5 min between each irrigation. In normal persons, cold water induces a slight tonic deviation of the eyes to the side being irrigated, followed, after a latent period of about 20 s, by nystagmus to the opposite side (direction of the fast phase). Warm water induces nystagmus to the irrigated side. In normal subjects, the nystagmus usually persists for 90 to 120 s, but the range of values is much larger.

Simultaneous irrigation of both canals with cold water causes a tonic downward deviation of the eyes, with nystagmus (quick component) upward. Bilateral irrigation with warm water yields movement and nystagmus in the opposite direction.

Bithermal caloric testing will reliably answer whether or not the vestibular end organs react, and comparison of the responses from the two ears will indicate which one is paretic. The presence of ''directional preponderance'' can be determined (if the two stimuli that induce nystagmus to one side provoke a stronger reaction than the two stimuli that provoke nystagmus to the other side), and is a means of quantifying the caloric responses.

Vestibular (labyrinthine) stimulation can also be produced by rotating the patient in a Bárány chair or any type of swivel chair. The patient's eyes should be kept closed or blindfolded during rotation to avoid the effects of optokinetic nystagmus. Electronystagmography represents a more refined method of detecting disordered labyrinthine function, since it obviates completely the effects of visual fixation (which may suppress nystagmus even in patients wearing Frenzel glasses).

The hearing loss in Ménière disease usually begins before the first attack of vertigo, but may appear later. Episodic deafness without vertigo has been called cochlear Ménière syndrome. Frequently there is a decrement in hearing with each attack; this may improve after a few hours but later it becomes irreversible, i.e., there is a saltatory progressive unilateral hearing loss (in only 10 percent of cases are both ears involved). Early in the disease, deafness affects mainly the low tones and fluctuates in severity. Without the fluctuations in pure tone audiometric thresholds the diagnosis is uncertain. Later the fluctuations cease and high tones are affected. Speech discrimination is relatively preserved. The attacks of vertigo usually cease when the hearing loss is complete. Audiometry reveals a sensorineural type of deafness, with air and bone conduction equally depressed. Provided that deafness is not complete, loudness recruitment can be demonstrated in the involved ear (see above). In general, the association of vertigo and deafness signifies a disease process of the end organ or eighth nerve. The precise locus of the disease is determined by tests of labyrinthine and auditory function and by finding neurologic and radiologic signs of affection of structures adjacent to the eighth cranial nerve.

Ménière disease affects the sexes about equally and has its onset most frequently in the fifth decade of life, although it may occur in younger adults and the elderly. Cases of Ménière disease are usually sporadic, but rare hereditary forms (both autosomal dominant and recessive) have been described (see reviews by Konigsmark). The pathologic changes consist of distention of the endolymphatic system (endolymphatic hydrops), which leads to degeneration of the delicate cochlear hair cells. It has been speculated that the paroxysmal attacks of vertigo are related to ruptures of the membranous labyrinth, leading to disruption of sensory receptors and a dumping of potassium-containing endolymph into the perilymph, which has a paralyzing effect on vestibular nerve fibers (Friedmann).

During an acute attack of Ménière disease, rest in bed is the most effective treatment, since the patient can usually find a position in which vertigo is minimal. The antihistaminic agents dimenhydrinate (Dramamine), cyclizine (Marezine), or meclizine (Bonine, Antivert), and promethazine hydrochloride (Phenergan) in doses of 25 to 50 mg every 4 h are useful in the more protracted cases. Betahistine HCl (Vasomotal), 8 mg tid, has also been recommended. For many years a low-salt diet, ammonium chloride, and diuretics have been used in the treatment of Ménière disease, but their value has never been established. The same is true of dehydrating agents such as oral glycerol. Mild sedative drugs may help the anxious patient between attacks. Trimethobenzamine (Tigan) in 200 mg suppositories every 6 h helps to control the nausea and vomiting. If the attacks are continuous and disabling, permanent relief can be obtained by surgical means. Destruction of the labyrinth is the measure employed in patients with strictly unilateral disease and complete or nearly complete loss of hearing. In patients with bilateral disease or significant retention of hearing, the vestibular portion of the eighth nerve can be sectioned or decompressed (by separating the nerve from an aberrant vessel). An endolymphatic-subarachnoid shunt is the operation favored by some surgeons, and selective destruction of the vestibule by a cryogenic probe is favored by others. The introduction of any surgical procedure must be tempered by the fact that the majority of the patients, who are middle-aged, recover spontaneously in a few years.

BENIGN POSITIONAL VERTIGO

This disorder of labyrinthine function is more frequent than Ménière disease. It is characterized by the occurrence of paroxysmal vertigo and nystagmus with the assumption of certain critical positions of the head, particularly lying down or turning over in bed, bending over and straightening up, and tilting the head backward. First described by Bárány, Dix and Hallpike were responsible for emphasizing its benign nature in most instances. Individual episodes last for less than a minute, and symptoms my recur periodically for several days or for many months, and rarely for years. As a rule, examination discloses no abnormalities of hearing or other identifiable lesions in the ear or elsewhere. However, if patients are subjected to careful bithermal caloric testing, a considerable number will show mild abnormalities of vestibular function (Baloh et al). This is the positional vertigo of Bárány, of the so-called benign paroxysmal type.

The *diagnosis* of this disorder is settled at the bedside by moving the patient from the sitting position to recumbency with the head tilted 30° over the end of the table and

30° to one side (Hallpike maneuver). After a latency of a few seconds, this maneuver produces a paroxysm of vertigo, and the patient may become frightened and grasp the examiner or the table or struggle to sit up. The vertigo is accompanied by nystagmus that is predominantly torsional in type, with the upper pole of the eye beating toward the floor. Electronystagmography discloses a vertical and horizontal nystagmus as well, with the rapid components in the direction of the forehead and away from the floor, respectively (Baloh et al). The vertigo and nystagmus last no more than 30 to 40 s and usually for less than 15 s. Changing from a recumbent to a sitting position reverses the direction of vertigo and nystagmus. With repetition of the maneuver, the vertigo and nystagmus become less apparent, and after three or four trials, can no longer be elicited; they can be reproduced in their original severity only after a protracted period of rest.

There are, in addition, variants of benign positional vertigo in which turning suddenly will induce vertigo for a few seconds. Such attacks of vertigo may come and go for years, particularly in the elderly, and require no treatment. At the other end of the scale is the rare patient with positional vertigo of such persistence and severity as to require surgical intervention.

In their study of 240 patients with benign positional nystagmus, Baloh and his colleagues found that 17 percent had their onset within several days or weeks after cerebral trauma and 15 percent after presumed viral neurolabyrinthitis. The significance of these findings is unclear, insofar as they did not appear to influence the clinical symptoms or course of the otologic disorder. It should be pointed out that sudden changes in position may induce vertigo and nystagmus or cause a worsening of these symptoms in patients with all types of vestibular-labyrinthine disease, including those associated with Ménière disease, vertebral-basilar artherosclerosis, trauma, and posterior fossa tumors. However, only if the paroxysm has the special characteristics noted above, viz., latency of onset, brevity, reversal of direction of nystagmus on lying down and sitting, fatigability with repetition of the test, and the presence of distressing subjective symptoms of vertigo or its persistence for months or years without other symptoms, can it be regarded as "benign positional" in type.

Benign positional vertigo is presumably due to cuprolithiasis of the posterior semicircular canal, meaning dislocation of the otoliths, which move freely with a change in position of the head (Shuknecht and Kitamura). Brandt and Daroff advocate mechanical therapy, consisting of lying first on one side, initiating vertigo and nystagmus, then on the other, each for 30 s in a sequence of five trials and repeated several times a day. This is believed to cause a loosening and dispersion of the otoliths. The condition has been relieved in a few patients with an incapacitating form of the disorder by section of the nerve to the ampulla of the posterior semicircular canal (Gacek), but the operation is difficult and may result in deafness.

VESTIBULAR NEURONITIS (NEUROPATHY)

This is the term applied originally by Dix and Hallpike to a distinctive disturbance of vestibular function, characterized clinically by a paroxysmal and usually a single attack of vertigo and by a conspicuous absence of tinnitus and deafness.

This disorder occurs mainly in young to middle-aged adults (children and older individuals may be affected), without preference for either sex. The patient frequently gives a history of an antecedent upper respiratory infection of nonspecific viral type. Usually the onset of vertigo is abrupt, although some patients describe a prodromal period of several hours or days in which they felt "topheavy" or "off balance." The vertigo is severe as a rule, and is associated with nausea, vomiting, and the need to remain immobile. Examination discloses vestibular paresis on one side (hyporesponsivity or absent response to caloric stimulation). Nystagmus (quick component) and sense of body motion are to the opposite side, whereas falling and past-pointing are to the side of the lesion. Auditory function is normal. In some patients the caloric responses are abnormal bilaterally, and in some the vertigo may recur.

Vestibular neuronitis is a benign disorder. The severe vertigo and associated symptoms subside in a matter of several days, but lesser degrees of these symptoms, made worse by rapid movements of the head, may persist for several weeks. The caloric responses are gradually restored to normal as well.

The portion of the vestibular pathway that is primarily affected in this disease and the nature of the affection are not known; hence the general designation vestibular neuronitis. Dix and Hallpike reasoned that the lesion was located central to the labyrinth, since hearing is spared and vestibular function usually returns to normal. Shuknecht and Kitamura have reported a degeneration of peripheral nerve, possibly of viral origin. For want of specific etiologic data, many neurologists prefer the term *vestibular neuropathy*. It is likely that many of the conditions described under the terms epidemic vertigo, epidemic labyrinthitis, and acute labyrinthitis are examples of the same syndrome.

During the acute stage antihistamine drugs and scopolamine are helpful. The latter may be administered transdermally (Transdermscop).

The term *labyrinthine apoplexy* has been applied to a clinical syndrome consisting of a single abrupt attack of severe vertigo, nausea, and vomiting, without tinnitus or hearing loss, but with permanent ablation of labyrinthine function on one side. It has been suggested that this syndrome is due to occlusion of the labyrinthine division of the internal auditory artery, but so far anatomic confirmation of this idea has not been obtained.

A particular form of paroxysmal vertigo occurs in childhood. The attacks occur in a setting of good health and are of sudden onset and brief duration. Pallor, sweating, and immobility are prominent manifestations, and occasionally vomiting and nystagmus occur. No relation to posture or movement has been observed. The attacks are recurrent but tend to cease spontaneously after a period of several months or years. The outstanding abnormality is demonstrated by caloric testing, which shows impairment or loss of vestibular function, bilateral or unilateral, frequently persisting after the attacks have ceased. Cochlear function is unimpaired. The pathologic basis of this disorder has not been determined.

Cogan has described a not infrequent syndrome in young adults, in which a *nonsyphilitic interstitial keratitis* is associated with vertigo, tinnitus, nystagmus, and rapidly progressive deafness. The prognosis for vision is good, but the deafness and loss of vestibular function are usually permanent. The cause and pathogenesis of this syndrome are unknown, although approximately half of the patients later develop aortic insufficiency or a systemic vasculitis that resembles polyarteritis nodosa. These vascular complications proved fatal in 7 of 78 cases reviewed by Vollertsen and his colleagues.

There are many other causes of aural vertigo, such as purulent labyrinthitis complicating meningitis, serous labyrinthitis due to infection of the middle ear, "toxic labyrinthitis" due to intoxication with alcohol, quinine, or salicylates, motion sickness, and hemorrhage into the internal ear. In these instances the attack of vertigo tends to last longer than in the recurrent form, but in other respects the symptoms are similar. Vertigo with varying degrees of spontaneous or positional nystagmus and reduced vestibular responses is a frequent complication of head trauma, both of the type called "whiplash" injury and of concussion. The vertigo, though sometimes long-lasting, invariably improves in these circumstances and rarely is it accompanied by impairment of hearing, in distinction to the vertigo that follows fractures of the temporal bones (as described earlier in this chapter under deafness). Streptomycin and gentamicin may damage the fine hair cells of the vestibular end organs and cause a permanent disorder of equilibrium (as well as of hearing).

VERTIGO OF VESTIBULAR NERVE ORIGIN

This may occur with diseases that involve the nerve in the petrous bone or the cerebellopontine angle. Except that it is less severe and is less frequently paroxysmal, it has many of the characteristics of labyrinthine vertigo. The adjacent auditory division of the eighth cranial nerve may also be affected, which explains the frequent coincidence of tinnitus and deafness. The function of the seventh and fifth cranial nerves may be disturbed by tumors of the lateral recess (especially acoustic neuroma), as well as by meningeal inflammation in this region, or, rarely, by compression from an abnormal vessel.

The most common cause of vertigo of eighth nerve origin is an acoustic neuroma. Vertigo is rarely observed as the initial symptom; the usual sequence is deafness affecting the high-frequency tones initially, followed some months or years later by chronic vertigo and impaired caloric responses, then additional cranial nerve palsies (involving the seventh, fifth, and tenth nerves), ipsilateral ataxia of limbs, and headache (see page 538). Variations of this sequence of development of symptoms are frequent, however. In the diagnosis of acoustic neuroma, MRI and CT scanning with contrast medium are the most important ancillary examinations. Others include the special audiologic tests which serve to separate lesions of the eighth nerve from those of the cochlea (absence of loudness recruitment, low SiSi scores, poor speech discrimination, pronounced tone decay, and type III or IV Békésy audiograms); examination of the spinal fluid, which shows an elevation of protein content in most cases; roentgenograms of the skull, including polytomography of the temporal bones, and metrizamide cisternography, which is particularly useful in the detection of tumors confined to the internal auditory canal.

VERTIGO OF BRAINSTEM ORIGIN

In these cases, vestibular nuclei and their connections are implicated. Auditory function is nearly always spared, since the vestibular and cochlear fibers diverge upon entering the brainstem, at the junction of the medulla and pons. As a general rule, the vertigo and the accompanying nausea, vomiting, nystagmus, and disequilibrium are more protracted with brainstem than with labyrinthine lesions. Nevertheless one often observes marked nystagmus without the slightest degree of vertigo—which does not happen with labyrinthine disease. The nystagmus which accompanies such central lesions tends also to be more persistent than that from peripheral lesions. The nystagmus may be uni- or bidirectional, purely horizontal, vertical or rotary, and is characteristically worsened by attempted visual fixation. In contrast, nystagmus of labyrinthine origin is unidirectional, and the direction of past pointing and falling is in the direction of the slow phase; a purely vertical nystagmus does not occur, and a purely horizontal nystagmus without a rotary component is unusual. Furthermore, labyrinthine nystagmus is inhibited by visual fixation.

Central localization is confirmed by finding the attendant signs of involvement of other structures within the brainstem (cranial nerves, sensory and motor tracts, etc.). Mode of onset, duration, and other features of the clinical picture depend upon the nature of the causative disease, which is usually vascular, demyelinative, or neoplastic.

Vertigo is a prominent symptom of ischemic attacks and brainstem infarction occurring in the territory of the vertebral-basilar arteries. On the other hand, vertigo as the sole manifestation of disease of the brainstem is rare, and the rule we have found trustworthy is that unless other symptoms and signs of brainstem disorder appear within 1 or 2 weeks, one can postulate an aural origin and nearly always exclude vascular disease of the brainstem. The same is true of multiple sclerosis, which may be the explanation of a persistent vertigo in some adolescents or young adults.

Attacks of vertigo followed by an intense unilateral and often suboccipital headache and vomiting have been described under the title of *basilar artery migraine* (see page 139). Test results of cochlear and vestibular function in these patients are normal, and the visual symptoms of classic migraine are usually absent, although they are said to be present frequently among family members of such patients. The relationship of this "migraine equivalent" to disease of the vertebral and basilar arteries is obscure.

The features of the various vertiginous syndromes are summarized in Table 14-2.

REFERENCES

BALOH RW: *Dizziness, Hearing Loss, and Tinnitus: The Essentials of Neurotology.* Philadelphia, Davis, 1984.

BALOH RW, HONRUBIA V, JACOBSON K: Benign positional vertigo: Clinical and oculographic features in 240 cases. *Neurology* 37:371, 1987.

BÁRÁNY R: Diagnose von Krankheitserscheinungen im Bereiche des Otolithenapparatus. *Acta Otolaryngol* 2:234, 1921.

BIEMOND A, deJONG JMBV: On cervical nystagmus and related disorders. *Brain* 92:437, 1969.

BRANDT TL, DAROFF RB: Physical therapy for benign paroxysmal positional vertigo. *Arch Otolaryngol,* 106:484, 1980.

BRODAL A: The cranial nerves, in *Neurological Anatomy,* 3rd ed. New York, Oxford, 1981, pp 448–577.

CASCINO G, ADAMS RD: Brainstem auditory hallucinosis. *Neurology* 36:1042, 1986.

CELESIA GG: Organization of auditory cortical areas in man. *Brain* 99:403, 1976.

COATES AC: Vestibular neuronitis. *Acta Otolaryngol,* suppl 251, 1969.

COGAN DG: Syndrome of nonsyphilitic interstitial keratitis and vestibuloauditory symptoms. *Arch Ophthalmol* 34:144, 1945.

DIX MR: Modern tests of vestibular function, with special reference to their value in clinical practice. *Br Med J* 3:317, 1969.

DIX M, HALLPIKE C: The pathology, symptomatology and diagnosis of certain common disorders of the vestibular system. *Ann Otol Rhinol Laryngol* 61:987, 1952.

DUNCAN GW, PARKER SW, FISHER CM: Acute cerebellar infarction in the PICA territory. *Arch Neurol* 32:364, 1975.

FOWLER EP: Head noises in normal and in disordered ears. *Arch Otolaryngol* 39:498, 1944.

FRIEDMANN I: Ultrastructure of ear in normal and diseased states, in Hinchcliffe R, Harrison D (eds): *Scientific Foundations of Otolaryngology.* London, Heinemann, 1976, pp 202–211.

GACEK RR: Transection of the posterior ampullary nerve for the relief of benign paroxysmal positional vertigo. *Ann Otol Rhinol Laryngol* 83:596, 1974.

GRAHAM JT: Tinnitus aurium. *Acta Otolaryngol,* suppl 202, 1965.

GRAHAM JT, NEWBY HA: Acoustical characteristics of tinnitus. *Arch Otolaryngol* 75:162, 1962.

HAMMEKE TA, McQUILLEN MP, COHEN BA: Musical hallucinations associated with acquired deafness. *J Neurol Neurosurg Psychiatry* 46:570, 1983.

HELLER MF, BERGMAN M: Tinnitus aurium in normally hearing persons. *Ann Otol Rhinol Laryngol* 62:73, 1953.

HINOJOSO R, LINDSAY JR: Profound deafness. Associated sensory and neural degeneration. *Arch Otolaryngol* 106:193, 1980.

JANNETTA PJ: Neurovascular decompression in cranial nerve and systemic disease. *Am J Surg* 192:518, 1980.

KEMP DT: Stimulated acoustic emissions from within the auditory system. *J Acoust Soc Am,* 64:1386, 1978.

KONIGSMARK BW: Hereditary deafness in man. *N Engl J Med* 281:713, 774, 827, 1969.

KONIGSMARK BW: Hereditary progressive cochleovestibular atrophies, in Vinken PJ, Bruyn GW (eds): *Handbook of Clinical Neurology,* vol 22. Amsterdam, North-Holland, 1975, chap 22, pp 481–497.

KONIGSMARK BW: Hereditary diseases of the nervous system with hearing loss, in Vinken PJ, Bruyn GW (eds): *Handbook of Clinical Neurology,* vol 22. Amsterdam, North-Holland, 1975, chap 23, pp 499–526.

LEIGH RJ, ZEE DS: *The Neurology of Eye Movements.* Philadelphia, Davis, 1983.

MATTOX DE, SIMMONS FB: Natural history of sudden sensorineural hearing loss. *Ann Otol* 86:463, 1977.

MÖLLER AR: Pathophysiology of tinnitus. *Ann Otol Rhinol Laryngol* 93:39, 1984.

NODAR RH, GRAHAM JT: An investigation of frequency charac-

Table 14-2
Vertiginous syndromes with lesions of different parts of the vestibular system

	Findings on ear exam	Other neurologic findings	Disorders of equilibrium	Type of nystagmus*	Hearing	Laboratory exam
Labyrinths (postural vertigo, trauma, Ménière disease, aminoglycoside toxicity, labyrinthitis)	Usually negative	None	Ipsilateral past pointing and lateral propulsion to side of lesion	Horizontal or rotary to side opposite lesion, paroxysmal, positional	Normal or conduction or neurosensory deafness with recruitment	Vestibular paresis by caloric testing, directional preponderance
Vestibular nerve and ganglia (vestibular neuropathy, herpes zoster)	Zoster vesicles in external auditory canal and palate	Auditory eighth, seventh, and sometimes other cranial nerve abnormalities	Ipsilateral past pointing and lateral propulsion to side of lesion	Vestibular, positional	Usually sensorineural deafness, without recruitment Speech discrimination diminished	Radiography and CT may be normal or abnormal Vestibular paresis on caloric testing Directional preponderance
Cerebellopontine angle (acoustic neuroma, glomus and other tumors)	Negative	Ipsilateral fifth, seventh, ninth, tenth cranial nerves, cerebellar ataxia Increased intracranial pressure (late)	Ataxia and falling ipsilaterally	Gaze-paretic, positional, coarser to side of lesion	Sensorineural deafness without recruitment	CT and MRI abnormal Vestibular paresis on caloric testing Directional preponderance Increased CSF protein
Brainstem and cerebellum (infarcts, tumors, viral infections)	Negative	Multiple cranial nerves, brainstem tract signs, cerebellar ataxia	Ataxia present with eyes open	Coarse horizontal and vertical, gaze-paretic	Usually normal	Hyperactive labyrinths or directional preponderance on caloric testing CT and MRI abnormal in some cases
Higher (cerebral) connections	Negative	Aphasia, visual field, hemimotor, hemisensory, and other cerebral abnormalities, seizures	No change	Usually absent	Normal	No change in caloric responses CT and EEG may be abnormal

*See Chap. 13 for description of types of nystagmus.

245

teristics of tinnitus associated with Ménière's disease. *Arch Otolaryngol* 82:28, 1965.

PAGE J: Audiologic tests in the differential diagnosis of vertigo. *Otolaryngol Clin North Am* 6(1):53, 1973.

PROCTOR CA, PROCTOR B: Understanding hereditary nerve deafness. *Arch Otolaryngol* 85:23, 1967.

RASMUSSEN GI: An efferent cochlear bundle. *Anat Rec* 82:441, 1942.

RUDGE P: *Clinical Neuro-otology*. Edinburgh, Churchill-Livingstone, 1983.

SHUKNECHT HF, KITAMURA K: Vestibular neuronitis. *Ann Otol Rhinol Laryngol* 90:1, 1981.

SUGA S, LINDSAY JR: Histopathological observations of presbycusis. *Ann Otol Rhinol Laryngol* 85:169, 1976.

TILLMAN TW: Special hearing tests in otoneurologic diagnosis. *Arch Otolaryngol* 89:51, 1968.

TOOLE JF, TUCKER H: Influence of head position upon cerebral circulation. *Arch Neurol*, 2:616, 1960.

VOLLERTSEN RS, McDONALD TJ, YOUNGE BR, et al: Cogan's syndrome. 18 cases and a review of the literature. *Mayo Clin Proc* 61:344, 1986.

EPILEPSY AND DISORDERS OF CONSCIOUSNESS

CHAPTER 15

EPILEPSY AND OTHER SEIZURE DISORDERS

In contemporary society the frequency and importance of epilepsy can hardly be overstated. From the statistical studies of Hauser and Kurland, who determined the prevalence in a small urban community, it can be estimated conservatively that more than 1 million individuals in the United States are subject to recurrent seizures, or epilepsy, exclusive of those in whom convulsions complicate intercurrent illnesses or injuries. The chronicity of many seizure states adds to their statistical importance. Indeed epilepsy is the second most common neurologic disorder, exceeded only by apoplexy. Therefore it is desirable for every physician, if he or she is to achieve some degree of competency in the diagnosis and treatment of seizure states, to know something of the nature of these disorders.

Epilepsy may be described basically as an intermittent derangement of the nervous system presumably due to a sudden, excessive, disorderly discharge of cerebral neurons. This was the postulate of Hughlings Jackson, the eminent British neurologist of the nineteenth century, and modern electrophysiology offers no evidence to the contrary. The discharge results in an almost instantaneous disturbance of sensation, loss of consciousness, impairment of psychic function, convulsive movements, or some combination thereof. A terminologic difficulty arises from the diversity of the clinical manifestations. The term *convulsion* seems inappropriate for a disorder that consists only of an alteration of sensation or consciousness. *Seizure* is preferable as a generic term, and also for the reason that it lends itself to qualification. The term *motor* or *convulsive seizure* is therefore not tautologic, and one may likewise speak of a *sensory seizure* or *psychic seizure*. The word *epilepsy* is derived from Greek words meaning ''to seize upon'' or a ''taking hold of.'' Our forebears referred to it as the *falling sickness* or the *falling evil*. Although a useful medical term to denote recurrent seizures, the word *epilepsy* still has unpleasant connotations and is probably best avoided in

dealing with patients, until such time as the general public becomes more enlightened.

Viewed in its many clinical contexts, the first solitary seizure or brief outburst of seizures may occur during the course of many medical illnesses. It indicates always that the nervous system has been affected by disease, either primarily or secondarily. By their very nature, if repeated every few minutes as in status epilepticus, seizures may threaten life. Equally important, a seizure or a series of them may be the manifestation of an ongoing neurologic disease that demands the full employment of special diagnostic and therapeutic measures, as in the case of a brain tumor.

A more common and less grave circumstance is for a seizure to be but one in an extensive series occurring over a long period of time, with most of the attacks being more or less similar in type. In this instance they may be the result of a burned-out lesion that originated in the past and remains as a scar. The original disease may have passed unnoticed; or perhaps it occurred in utero, at birth, or in infancy in parts of the brain too immature to manifest signs. Again, it may have affected a silent area in a mature brain. Patients with such old lesions probably make up the majority of those with recurrent seizures, but are necessarily classified as having ''idiopathic epilepsy,'' because it is impossible to ascertain the nature of the original disease; and the seizures may be the only sign of brain abnormality. In this sense, all epilepsy is ''symptomatic,'' or ''secondary,'' although the latter terms generally indicate that the seizures have an identifiable and usually acquired structural cause.

There are other types of epilepsy for which no pathologic basis is established and for which there is no apparent underlying cause, except perhaps a genetic one. These seizures have been referred to as *primary, essential,* or *centrencephalic*. Included in this category are hereditary types, such as certain types of grand mal and petit mal.

Some authors (Lennox and Lennox, Forster) apply the term idiopathic only to seizures of this latter type.

CLASSIFICATION OF SEIZURES

Seizures have been classified in many ways: according to their supposed etiology and site of origin, on the basis of their clinical form (generalized or focal), frequency (isolated, cyclic, prolonged, or repetitive), or physiologic (EEG) correlates, and even in terms of their response to therapy.

The following classification is abstracted from Gastaut (1970), with the addition of certain revisions, proposed by the Commission on Classification and Terminology of the International League Against Epilepsy (1981). This classification, based mainly on the clinical form of the seizure and its electroencephalographic features, has been adopted worldwide and is generally referred to as the International Classification.

A CLASSIFICATION OF SEIZURES

I. Generalized seizures (bilaterally symmetrical and without local onset)
   A. Tonic or clonic or tonic-clonic (grand mal) seizures
   B. Absence (petit mal)
      1. Simple—loss of consciousness only
      2. Complex—with brief tonic, clonic, or automatic movements
   C. Lennox-Gastaut syndrome
   D. Juvenile myoclonic epilepsy
   E. Infantile spasms (West syndrome)
   F. Atonic (astatic, akinetic) seizures (sometimes with myoclonic jerks)
II. Partial (focal) seizures beginning locally
   A. Simple or elementary (usually *without* loss of consciousness)
      1. Motor (including Jacksonian)
      2. Sensory or somatosensory (visual, auditory, olfactory, gustatory, vertiginous)
      3. Autonomic
      4. Psychic
   B. Complex (usually *with* impaired consciousness; may begin as simple partial seizure). Includes cognitive, affective, psychosensory and psychomotor symptomatology—i.e., "temporal lobe" or "psychomotor seizures"
   C. Partial seizures (simple or complex) with secondary generalization
III. Unilateral or predominantly unilateral seizures (tonic, clonic, or tonic-clonic, with or without impaired consciousness)
IV. Unclassifiable (because of inadequate data)

GENERALIZED SEIZURES

THE GENERALIZED CONVULSIVE SEIZURE (GRAND MAL)

The term *convulsion* is most applicable to this form of seizure. The patient may sense its approach by any one of several subjective phenomena (the prodrome). For some hours the patient may feel apathetic, depressed, irritable, or, very rarely, the opposite—ecstatic. One or more myoclonic jerks of the trunk or limbs, on awakening, may herald the occurrence of a seizure later in the day. Abdominal pains or cramps, pallor or redness of the face, throbbing headache, constipation or diarrhea have also been given prodromal status, but we have not found them frequent enough to be helpful. In more than half the cases there is some type of movement (usually turning of the head and eyes or whole body), palpitation, a sinking, rising, or gripping feeling in the epigastrium, or an unnatural sensation in another part of the body, a few seconds before consciousness is lost. Such a remembered experience is called the *aura,* which the patient regards as a sign of an impending seizure, but which is, in reality, a simple partial seizure. The aura may constitute the entire seizure, or it may progress, leading to unconsciousness and a generalized seizure of the complex partial or tonic-clonic type. The aura is important, for it may provide a clue as to the location of the "discharging focus" or lesion.

Less often, the seizure strikes "out of the blue," i.e., without warning, beginning with a sudden loss of consciousness and fall to the ground. The initial motor signs are an opening of the mouth and eyes associated with extension of the legs and abduction of the arms, flexion at the elbows and pronation of the hands ("hands-up" position). These are followed by snapping shut of the jaws, often with biting of the tongue, and there may be a piercing cry as the whole musculature is seized in a spasm and air is forcibly emitted through the closed vocal cords. Since the respiratory muscles are caught in the tonic spasm, breathing is impossible, and after some seconds the skin and mucous membranes become cyanotic. The bladder may empty at this stage or later, during the postictal stupor. The pupils are dilated and unreactive to light. This is the so-called *tonic phase* of the seizure, and lasts for 10 to 20 s.

There then occurs a transition from the tonic to the *clonic phase* of the convulsion. At first there is a mild generalized tremor, which is in effect a repetitive relaxation of the tonic contraction. The tremor becomes coarser and rapidly gives way to violent muscular contractions that come in rhythmic salvos and agitate the entire body. The eyes roll, the face becomes violaceous and contorted by a series of grimaces. The pulse is rapid. There is a bloody froth on the lips from the bitten tongue and excessive salivation; rarely, periorbital hemorrhages appear. Sweating is now abundant. The clonic jerks decrease in amplitude and frequency over a period of about 30 s, the entire clonic phase lasting for a minute or less, as a rule. The patient remains apneic until the end of the clonic phase, which is marked by a deep inspiration.

In the terminal phase of the seizure all movements have ended and the patient lies still and limp in a deep coma. The pupils, equal or unequal, now begin to contract to light. Breathing is quiet, and the skeletal muscles are relaxed. This state persists for about 5 min, after which the patient opens the eyes, begins to look about, and is obviously disoriented and confused. The patient may speak and later not remember anything that was said. If undisturbed, the patient often falls into an exhausted sleep for several hours and may awaken with a pulsatile headache. When fully recovered, such a patient has no memory of any part of the spell except the aura, but knows that something has happened because of the strange surroundings (in ambulance or hospital), the obvious concern of others, and a sore, bitten tongue and aching muscles from the violent contractions. The contractions may even have crushed or fractured a vertebral body, or a serious injury (fracture, subdural hematoma, or burn) may have been sustained in the fall.

Convulsions of this type ordinarily come singly or in groups of two or three and may occur when the patient is awake and active or during sleep. About 5 to 8 percent of such patients will at some time have a series of grand mal seizures without completely regaining consciousness between them. This is called *status epilepticus* and demands urgent treatment. Conversely, instead of the whole dramatic sequence described above, only a part of the seizure may occur. For example, there may be only the aura without loss of consciousness, or only a brief tonic spasm followed by a few moments of confusion, the so-called *tonic seizure*. The latter type of seizure is not followed by a clonic phase and is shorter than the tonic-clonic one. Seizures may be abbreviated by anticonvulsive medications, and the partial motor activity may then point to the site of the discharging lesion.

"ABSENCE" (MINOR EPILEPSY, PETIT MAL)

In contrast to major generalized seizures, absence or petit mal seizures (formerly referred to as *pyknoepilepsy*) are notable for their brevity and the paucity of motor activity. Indeed, they are so brief that sometimes the patients themselves are not aware of them, and to an onlooker they resemble a moment of absentmindedness.

The attack, coming without warning, consists of a sudden interruption of consciousness. The patient stares and stops talking briefly or ceases to respond. Only a few such patients (about 10 percent) are completely motionless

during the attack. Often one observes clonic movements of the eyelids, facial muscles, or fingers or synchronous movements of both arms occurring at a rate of 3 per second, a rate that also characterizes the EEG abnormality. Automatisms, in the form of lip smacking, chewing, and fumbling movements of the fingers, are common during an absence attack. Lip smacking is especially prominent in seizures induced by hyperventilation. Postural tone may be slightly decreased or increased, and occasionally there is a mild vasomotor disorder. As a rule such patients do not fall, and they may even continue such complex acts as walking or riding a bicycle. After 2 to 10 s, occasionally longer, the patient re-establishes full contact with the environment and resumes all preseizure activity. Only a loss of the thread of conversation or the place in reading betrays the occurrence of a momentary "blank" period (an absence). Voluntary hyperventilation for 2 to 3 min is an effective way of inducing these petit mal attacks.

Typical petit mal or absence is the most characteristic epilepsy of childhood; rarely do these seizures begin before 4 years of age or following puberty. Another attribute is their great frequency. As many as several hundred may occur in a single day, sometimes in bursts at certain times of the day. Most often they relate to periods of inattention and occur in the classroom when the child is sitting quietly rather than participating actively in his lessons. If frequent, they may disturb attention and thinking so that the child does poorly in school. Such attacks may last for hours with no interval of normal mental activity between them—so-called *petit mal* or *absence status*. Most cases of the latter type have been described in adults. An attack of petit mal status may be provoked by a burst of grand mal seizures or by the abrupt withdrawal of anticonvulsant drugs—in which case the persistent EEG abnormality need not be of the petit mal type. Hence the term "nonconvulsive generalized status" is preferred.

Petit mal may be the only type of seizure during childhood. The attacks tend to diminish in frequency in adolescence, but rarely do they disappear. Usually grand mal attacks become superimposed upon petit mal.

Petit Mal Variants To be distinguished from typical absence are varieties in which the loss of consciousness is less complete or in which myoclonus is prominent, and others in which the EEG abnormalities are less regularly of a 3-per-second spike-and-wave type (they may be 2 to 2.5 per second, or take the form of 4- to 6-Hz multispike and wave complexes, or there may be no EEG abnormalities).

About 30 percent of children with absence attacks will, in addition, display symmetric or asymmetric myoclonic jerks, without loss of consciousness. About 50 percent of such patients will also at some time have major generalized (tonic-clonic) convulsions. A special variety of benign myoclonic seizures occurs in late childhood and adolescence (*juvenile myoclonic epilepsy*). This form of epilepsy is characterized by myoclonic jerks affecting mainly the flexor muscles of the neck and shoulders, a tendency to clonic-tonic-clonic seizures shortly after awakening, relatively infrequent absence attacks, and a 4- to 6-Hz multispike and wave EEG pattern. Intelligence is not impaired, and the response to treatment, particularly to valproate, is excellent. The same is generally true of the other forms of epilepsy (including ''rolandic epilepsy''; see further on) that have their onset in late childhood and adolescence.

In sharp contrast to the aforementioned epilepsies is a form that has its onset in infancy and early childhood (between 2 and 6 years) and is characterized by the occurrence of atonic (astatic) seizures, often succeeded by various combinations of minor motor tonic-clonic and partial seizures and intellectual impairment, in association with a distinctive, slow (1- to 2½-Hz) spike-and-wave EEG pattern. This is the so-called *Lennox-Gastaut syndrome*. Often it is preceded by infantile spasms, a characteristic EEG picture (''hypsarrhythmia''), and an arrest in development, a triad sometimes referred to as the *West syndrome* (see further on). The notion that absences, myoclonic seizures, and akinetic seizures constitute a petit mal triad, as originally proposed by Lennox, should be abandoned. Akinesia (motionlessness) is not unique to any seizure type. The typical absence, with or without myoclonic jerks, rarely causes the patient to fall and should be considered a separate entity, because of its benignity. The early onset of atonic seizures with abrupt falls and injuries and associated abnormalities always has grave implications, namely, the presence of serious neurologic disease. Also, in contrast to the classical absence, the Lennox-Gastaut syndrome may persist into adult life and is the most difficult to treat of all forms of epilepsy.

FOCAL SEIZURES

All forms of seizures, possibly even the primary generalized types for which no cause is apparent, are believed to originate in a discharging focus or lesion in some part of the cerebrum, and in this sense all epilepsy is focal in nature. But in the generalized seizure without aura and in the petit mal absence, as will be pointed out further on, the location of the focus of origin is unknown, and there is no reason to think—if it exists at all—that it resides in the cerebral cortex. By contrast, what we are referring to here as a focal seizure is clearly the product of a lesion in some part of the cerebral cortex. The specific type and pattern of the seizure vary with the locale of the lesion. So-called psychomotor seizures usually have their focus in the temporal lobe on one side or the other; seizures characterized by auditory and vertiginous sensations emanate from the superior temporal cortex, etc. The seizure types and patterns that are listed in Table 15-1 are so helpful in the localization of the offending lesion that their relationships should be memorized by every student of medicine.

COMPLEX PARTIAL SEIZURES (PSYCHOMOTOR EPILEPSY, TEMPORAL LOBE EPILEPSY)

These differ from the major generalized and petit mal seizures discussed above in that (1) the aura (i.e., the initial event in the seizure) is often a complex hallucination or perceptual illusion, indicating a temporal lobe origin, and (2) instead of a complete loss of control of thought and action, there is a period of altered behavior and consciousness, for which the patient is later found to be amnesic.

Though it is difficult to enumerate all the psychic experiences which may occur during complex partial seizures, they may be categorized into a somewhat arbitrary hierarchy of illusions, hallucinations, dyscognitive states, and affective experiences. Illusions, or distortions of ongoing perceptions, are the most common. Objects or persons in the environment may shrink or recede into the distance, or, less frequently, they may enlarge. Hallucinations are most often visual or auditory (consisting of formed or unformed visual images, sounds, and voices), less frequently olfactory (usually unpleasant, unidentifiable sensations of smell), gustatory, or vertiginous. The dyscognitive states involve feelings of increased reality or familiarity (déjà vu) or of strangeness or unfamiliarity (jamais vu) or depersonalization. A certain old memory or scene may insert itself into the patient's mind and recur with striking clarity, or there may be an abrupt interruption of memory. Epigastric and abdominal sensations are frequent; usually they are difficult to describe but are recognized as not being part of normal experience. Fear and anxiety are the most common affective experiences. Relatively rarely does the patient describe feelings of rage or intense anger as part of a psychomotor seizure.

These subjective experiences may constitute the entire seizure (simple partial seizure), or they may be followed by a *period of unresponsiveness*. The motor components of the psychomotor seizure (automatisms) occur during this latter phase. These include lip smacking, chewing or swallowing movements, fumbling of the hands, or shuffling of the feet. The patient may walk around in a daze or perform acts that are inappropriate (undressing in public, speaking incoherently, etc.). Certain complex acts that were initiated before the loss of consciousness, such as walking, chewing food, turning the pages of a book, or even driving, may continue. However, if asked a specific question or given a command, it becomes evident that the patient is out of contact. There may be no response at all, or the patient may look toward the examiner in a confused way or utter a few stereotyped phrases. Usually such a patient can be led gently but may resist or push the examiner. The violence and aggression that are said to characterize patients with temporal lobe seizures usually take this form of nondirected resistance in response to restraint, during the period of *automatic behavior* (so called because the patient presumably acts like an automaton). Unprovoked assault or outbursts of intense rage or blind fury are unusual. Currie et al found such outbursts in only 16 of 666 patients (2.4 percent) with temporal lobe epilepsy. Rarely, laughter or running may be the most striking feature of an automatism (*gelastic epilepsy* and *epilepsia procursiva*, respectively). Or the patient may walk repetitively in small circles (*volvular*

epilepsy) or simply wander aimlessly, either as an ictal or postictal phenomenon (*poriomania*).

Seizures of this type may proceed to tonic spasms or other forms of secondarily generalized seizures. This tendency to generalization is true of all forms of simple partial or focal epilepsy.

The patient with complex partial seizures may exhibit only one of the foregoing types of seizure activity or various combinations of them. In a series of 414 patients studied by Lennox, 43 percent displayed some of the motor changes; 32 percent, automatic behavior; and 25 percent, the alterations in psychic function. Because of the frequent concurrence of these three symptom complexes, he referred to them as the *psychomotor triad*. Probably the clinical pattern varies with the precise locality of the lesion and the direction and extent of spread of the electrical discharge. Because of their focal origin and complex symptomatology, all these types of seizures are subsumed under the title of *complex partial seizures*. This term is preferable to *temporal lobe*

Table 15-1
Common seizure patterns

Clinical type	Localization
Somatic motor	
Jacksonian (focal motor)	Prerolandic gyrus
Masticatory	Amygdaloid nuclei
Simple contraversive	Frontal
Head and eye turning associated with arm movement	Supplementary motor cortex
Somatic and special sensory (auras)	
Somatosensory	Contralateral postrolandic
Unformed images, lights, patterns	Occipital
Auditory	Heschl's gyri
Vertiginous	Superior temporal
Olfactory	Mesial temporal
Gustatory	Insula
Visceral: autonomic	Insular-orbital-frontal cortex
Complex partial seizures	
Formed hallucinations	Temporal neocortex or amygdaloid-hippocampal complex
Illusions	
Dyscognitive experiences (déjà vu, dreamy states, depersonalization)	
Affective states (fear, depression, or elation)	Temporal
Automatism (ictal and postictal)	Temporal and frontal
Absence	Frontal cortex, amygdaloid-hippocampal complex, reticular-cortical system
Bilateral epileptic myoclonus	Reticulocortical

Source: Modified from Penfield and Jasper.

seizures, since typical *psychomotor* seizures can apparently arise from a focus in the frontal lobe, and the seizure discharge in such cases can be limited to the frontal lobe.

Complex partial seizures are not peculiar to any period of life but show an increased incidence in adolescence and adult years. In the series of Ounsted et al, about one-third of the cases of temporal lobe epilepsy could be traced to the occurrence of severe febrile convulsions in early life (see further on). As a corollary, about 5 percent of their patients with febrile seizures continued to have seizures during adolescence and adult life, and in the latter group there were many in whom the seizures were of temporal lobe type. Also, in Falconer's series of temporal lobectomies for intractable epilepsy, there were many patients who had had this special type of febrile epilepsy. Neonatal convulsions, cerebral palsy, and head trauma are other factors that place a child at risk of developing complex partial seizures (Rocea et al). Two-thirds of patients with psychomotor seizures also have generalized grand mal seizures or have had them at some earlier time, in which case the generalized seizures may have led to secondary damage to the temporal lobes.

Psychomotor seizures are notably variable in duration. Behavioral automatisms rarely last longer than a minute or two, although postictal confusion and amnesia may persist for a considerably longer time. Some psychomotor seizures consist only of a momentary change in facial expression and a blank spell, resembling an absence seizure. Almost always, however, psychomotor seizures of this type are characterized by distinct ictal and postictal phases, whereas patients with absence attacks have an instantaneous return of consciousness following their seizures. EEG recording during natural sleep or following hyperventilation, especially if carried out for more than 3 min, is useful in disclosing the temporal lobe focus.

FOCAL AND JACKSONIAN MOTOR SEIZURES

Focal, or partial, motor seizures are attributable to a discharging lesion of the opposite frontal lobe. Their most common manifestation is a turning movement of the head and eyes to the side opposite the irritative focus, often associated with a tonic contraction of the trunk and extremities on that side. These movements may constitute the entire seizure or may be followed by generalized clonic movements; generalization of the seizure may occur just before or simultaneously with loss of consciousness. On the other hand, a lesion in one or other frontal lobe may give rise to a major generalized convulsion without an introductory turning of the head and eyes. It has been postulated that in both types of seizure, the one with and the one without versive movements, there is an immediate spread of the discharge from the frontal lobe to an integrating center in the thalamic or high midbrain reticular formation, accounting for the loss of consciousness.

Versive or *adversive* are the terms applied to seizures that begin with forceful, sustained deviation of the head and eyes, and sometimes of the entire body. *Contraversive* would be a more correct designation, since the turning movements are almost invariably to the side opposite the irritative focus. Nonforceful, unsustained, or seemingly involuntary lateral head movements do not have localizing value, the ictal movement being either to the side of the focus or away from it. The same is true for the head and eye turning that occurs at the end of the generalized tonic-clonic phase of versive seizures (Wyllie et al). Contraversive deviation of the head and eyes can be induced most consistently by electrical stimulation of the superolateral frontal region (area 8), just anterior to area 6 (Fig. 21-2). However, the same movements can be obtained by stimulation of the more anterior portions of the frontal cortex, the posterior part of the superior frontal gyrus (the supplementary motor area), and the temporal or occipital cortex—presumably through propagation of the ictal discharge to the frontal contraversive area. In seizures of temporal lobe origin, contraversive movements, if they occur, are preceded by quiet staring and automatisms.

Gastaut and his colleagues have drawn attention to the association of versive movements (conjugate deviation of the eyes and head and one to three complete turns of the body) with bilaterally synchronous 3-cps spike-and-wave discharges. Having its onset in late childhood, this combination of events has been referred to as *benign versive* or *circling epilepsy* and may represent a variety of primary generalized epilepsy. In more than half the patients the versive movements are succeeded by generalized seizures, which are usually mild and short-lasting and respond well to treatment with valproate or phenobarbital.

Do most cases of generalized motor seizure (grand mal) of the idiopathic type have a frontal lobe focus? This question cannot be answered unequivocally. Actually an epileptogenic frontal lobe focus, determined by EEG recording or pathologic examination, has been found in only a small number of such cases, and these may not be representative of the whole group.

The *jacksonian motor seizure* begins with a tonic contraction of the fingers of one hand, the face on one side, or one foot. This transforms into clonic movements in these parts, in a fashion analogous to that in a generalized tonic-clonic convulsion. The disorder then spreads ("marches") from the part first affected to other muscles on the same side of the body. In the "classic" form, which is a clinical rarity, the seizure spreads from the hand, up the arm, to the face, and down the leg; or if the first movement is in the foot, the seizure marches up the leg, down the arm, and to the face, usually in a matter of 20 to 30 s. Consciousness is not lost if the motor-sensory symptoms are confined to one side (a small proportion of cases of focal motor epilepsy are associated with sensory symptoms). Rarely, the first muscular contraction may be in the abdomen, thorax, or neck. In some cases the one-sided motor signs are followed by turning of the head and eyes to the convulsing side, occasionally the opposite, and by a generalized seizure with loss of consciousness.

The high incidence of onset of focal motor epilepsy in the lips, fingers, and toes is probably related to the disproportionate cortical representation of these parts of the body. The disease process or focus of excitation is usually in the rolandic cortex, i.e., area 4 (Fig. 3-3); in a few cases it has been found in the postrolandic convolution. Lesions confined to the premotor cortex (area 6) are said to induce tonic contractions of the contralateral arm, face, neck, or all of one side of the body. The occasional occurrence of perspiration and piloerection, in parts of the body involved in a focal motor seizure, suggests that these autonomic functions have a cortical representation in the rolandic area. Some neurologists distinguish *focal motor* and *jacksonian motor seizures* by the absence of a characteristic march in the former, but both have essentially the same localizing significance.

Seizure discharges arising from the cortical language areas may give rise to a brief aphasic disturbance (*ictal aphasia*) or, more frequently, to vocal arrest. Ictal aphasia is usually succeeded by other focal or generalized seizure activity but may occur in isolation, without loss of consciousness, and can be described later by the patient. Postictal aphasia is more common and has much the same localizing value. Vocalization at the outset of a seizure has no such significance. These disturbances should be distinguished from the stereotyped repetition of words or phrases or garbled speech that characterizes the postictal confusional state.

ACQUIRED APHASIA WITH CONVULSIVE DISORDER

This unusual epileptic syndrome of childhood was first described by Landau and Kleffner, in 1957. It is characterized by an acquired disorder of language function, coupled with epileptic discharges in the EEG; convulsive seizures are usually but not always added. More than 100 such cases have now been reported. The language disorder takes the form of a verbal auditory agnosia, progressing to mutism. The abnormal EEG discharges resemble those of rolandic epilepsy (see below) except that they are usually temporal in origin and bilateral. The epileptic activity is responsive to anticonvulsant medication, but the aphasic disorder has persisted to a variable degree in some children. The nature of the Landau-Kleffner syndrome is quite obscure. It is generally considered to be acquired, but some authors have included developmental language disorders under this rubric. The few pathologic studies of surgically removed cerebral cortex have shown no abnormalities; in particular they have not disclosed any evidence of encephalitis (Cole et al).

ROLANDIC EPILEPSY (BENIGN EPILEPSY WITH ROLANDIC SPIKES)

This type of focal motor epilepsy is unique among the partial epilepsies of childhood in that it is a self-limited disorder and is apparently transmitted as an autosomal dominant trait. The convulsive disorder begins between 5 and 9 years of age. It usually announces itself by a nocturnal tonic-clonic seizure with focal onset. Thereafter the seizures take the form of clonic contractions of one side of the face, less often of one arm or leg, and the interictal EEG shows high voltage spikes in the lower rolandic or centrotemporal area. The seizures are readily controlled by a single drug and gradually disappear during adolescence.

EPILEPSIA PARTIALIS CONTINUA

This is another special type of focal motor epilepsy, characterized by clonic twitching of one group of muscles, usually of the face, arm, or leg, which is repeated at fairly regular intervals of a few seconds and persists for hours, days, or months without spreading to other parts of the body. Thus epilepsia partialis continua is in effect a focal motor status epilepticus. The distal muscles of the leg and arm, especially the flexors of the hand and fingers, are affected more frequently than the proximal ones. In the face, seizures involve either the corner of the mouth or one eyelid, or both. Occasionally, isolated muscles of the neck or trunk are affected on one side. The clonic spasms may be accentuated by active or passive movement of the involved muscles and may be reduced in severity, but not abolished, during sleep.

First described by Kozhevnikov, in patients with Russian spring and summer encephalitis, these partial seizures may be induced by a variety of acute or chronic cerebral lesions. In some cases the underlying disease is not apparent, and the twitchings are mistaken for some type of tremor or extrapyramidal movement disorder. Most patients with epilepsia partialis continua show focal EEG abnormalities, either slow-wave abnormalities or sharp waves or spikes over the central areas of the contralateral hemisphere. And in some cases, the spike activity can be related precisely in location and time to the motor activity (Thomas et al). As a rule, this type of seizure activity responds poorly or not at all to anticonvulsant medications.

Whether cortical mechanisms or subcortical ones are responsible for epilepsia partialis continua is an unresolved question. The electrophysiologic evidence adduced by Thomas and his colleagues favors a cortical origin. The pathologic evidence is less definite. In each of eight cases in which the brain was examined post mortem, they found some degree of involvement of the motor cortex or adjacent cortical area, contralateral to the affected limbs. However, all but one of these patients also had some involvement of deeper structures on the same side as the cortical lesion or on the opposite side, or on both sides.

SOMATOSENSORY, VISUAL, AND OTHER TYPES OF SENSORY SEIZURES

Somatic-sensory seizures, either focal or "marching" to other parts of the body on one side, are nearly always indicative of a focus in or near the postrolandic convolution of the opposite cerebral hemisphere. In patients with such seizures, Penfield and Kristiansen found the seizure focus in the postcentral or precentral convolution in 49 out of 55 cases. The sensory disorder is usually described as numbness, tingling, or a "pins-and-needles" feeling, occasionally as a sensation of crawling (formication), electricity, or movement of the part. Pain and thermal sensations may occur but are infrequent. The onset is in the lips, fingers, and toes in the majority of cases, and the spread to adjacent parts of the body follows a pattern determined by sensory arrangements in the postcentral (postrolandic) convolution of the parietal lobe. If the sensory symptoms are localized to the head, the focus is in or adjacent to the lowest part of the convolution, near the sylvian fissure; if the symptoms are in the leg or foot, the upper part of the convolution, near the superior sagittal sinus or on the medial surface of the hemisphere, is involved.

Visual seizures are also of localizing significance. Lesions in or near the striate cortex of the occipital lobe usually produce elemental visual sensations of darkness or of spots or lights, which may be stationary or moving and colorless or colored. According to Gowers, red is the most frequent color, followed by blue, green, and yellow. These images may be referred to the visual field on the side opposite the lesion, or may appear straight ahead of the patient. If they occur on one side of the visual field, patients often report that only one eye is affected, the one opposite the lesion, probably because the average person is aware of only the temporal half of a homonymous field defect. It is curious that a lesion arising in one occipital lobe may cause momentary blindness in both eyes. It has been noted that lesions on the lateral surface of the occipital lobes (Brodmann areas 18 and 19) are likely to cause a sensation of twinkling or pulsating lights. Complex or formed visual hallucinations are usually due to a focus in the posterior part of the temporal lobe, near its junction with the occipital lobe, and may be associated with auditory hallucinations. Often, visual images, either hallucinatory or nonhallucinatory ones, are distorted, being too small (micropsia) or too large (macropsia) or unnaturally arranged.

Auditory hallucinations are infrequent as an initial manifestation of a seizure. Occasionally a patient with a focus in one superior temporal convolution will report a buzzing or a roaring in the ears. A human voice, sometimes repeating unrecognizable words, has been noted a few times with lesions in the more posterior part of one temporal lobe.

Vertiginous sensations of a type suggesting vestibular stimulation may be the first symptom of a seizure. The lesion is usually localized in the superior-posterior temporal region or at the junction between parietal and temporal lobes. In one of the cases reported by Penfield and Jasper, a sensation of vertigo was evoked by stimulating the cortex at the junction of the parietal and occipital lobes. Occasionally, with a temporal focus, the vertigo is followed by an auditory sensation. Giddiness, or lightheadedness, is also a frequent prelude to a seizure, but this has so many different meanings that it is of little diagnostic import.

Olfactory hallucinations are often associated with disease of the inferior and medial parts of the temporal lobe, usually in the region of the hippocampal convolution or the uncus (hence Jackson's term *uncinate seizures*). Usually the perceived odor is exteriorized, i.e., projected to some place in the environment, and is described as disagreeable or foul, though otherwise unidentifiable. Gustatory hallucinations have also been recorded in proven cases of temporal lobe disease (see Chap. 11); salivation and a sensation of thirst may be associated. Electrical stimulation in the depths of the sylvian fissure, extending into the insular region, has reproduced peculiar sensations of taste.

Vague and often indefinable visceral sensations arising in the thorax, epigastrium, and abdomen are among the most frequent of auras, as already indicated. In several such cases the seizure discharge has been localized to the upper bank of the sylvian fissure, but in a few cases the focus was located in the upper or middle frontal gyrus, or in the medial frontal area near the cingulate gyrus. Palpitation and acceleration of the pulse at the beginning of the attack have also been related to a temporal lobe focus.

MYOCLONUS AND OTHER MOTOR SEIZURES

The phenomenon of myoclonus has already been discussed in Chap. 5, where the relationship to seizures was indicated. Characterized by a brusque, brief, muscular contraction, some myoclonic jerks are so small as to involve only one muscle or part of a muscle, and others so large as to implicate a limb on one or both sides of the body or the entire trunk musculature. They may occur intermittently and unpredictably or present as a single jerk or a brief salvo.

As indicated above, single myoclonic jerks occur with varying frequency in patients with absence seizures and in patients with generalized clonic-tonic-clonic or tonic-clonic seizures. As a rule, these types of myoclonic epilepsy are quite benign and respond well to medication. In contrast, disseminated myoclonus, having its onset in childhood, raises the suspicion of an acute viral encephalitis or, if lasting a few weeks, of a progressive subacute sclerosing encephalitis, juvenile lipidosis, Lafora type of familial myoclonic epilepsy, or other chronic familial degenerative diseases of undefined type (paramyoclonus multiplex of Friedreich, dyssynergia cerebellaris myoclonica of Ramsay Hunt). In middle and late adult years, disseminated myoclonus, when joined with dementia, usually indicates the presence of so-called Creutzfeldt-Jakob disease (page 609). At any age, diffuse myoclonus may be a sequel of hypoxic injury to the brain. An interesting feature of all forms of disseminated myoclonus is the tendency for sensory stimulation or movement to elicit the myoclonus. When numerous and generalized, notably in the familial types, the myoclonic jerks may be recruited under certain stimulus conditions into a generalized seizure with loss of consciousness. In a sense, such random, arrhythmic myoclonus might be designated as *epilepsia partialis discontinua* and *disseminata*. The causative diseases are discussed in Chaps. 33, 38, and 40.

Massive myoclonus (West syndrome) is the term applied to a particular form of epilepsy of infancy and early childhood. West described the condition in his own son in the middle of the nineteenth century. The seizure disorder, which in most cases appears during the first year of life, is characterized by recurrent, gross flexion and less frequently by extension movements of the trunk and limbs (hence the alternative terms, *infantile, salaam,* or *jackknife spasms*). Most but not all patients with this disorder show severe EEG abnormalities, consisting of continuous multifocal spikes and slow waves of large amplitude; this pattern, referred to as *hypsarrhythmia* ("mountainous" dysrhyth-

mia) by Gibbs and Gibbs, is not specific for infantile spasms, however. These seizures are frequently associated with developmental or acquired abnormalities of the brain. As the child matures the seizures diminish and usually disappear by the fourth to fifth year. Both seizures and EEG abnormalities may respond dramatically to treatment with ACTH, adrenal corticosteroids, or the benzodiazepine, nitrazepam (the latter drug is probably the safest). However, most patients, even those who were apparently normal when the seizures appeared, are left mentally impaired. Myoclonus may also be part of the Lennox-Gastaut syndrome, a seizure disorder of early childhood of grave prognosis (see above).

Paroxysmal attacks of *choreoathetotic and dystonic movements,* usually without loss of consciousness, are thought by some to be epileptic in nature, perhaps originating in the basal ganglia. We are skeptical of this interpretation (see page 65). Occasionally the movements are in the form of pronounced trembling, torsion movements of the trunk, or ballistic or ataxic movements of the limbs. Paroxysmal cerebellar ataxia is less common but probably of similar nature. It may be suppressed by Diamox. The extrapyramidal paroxysmal disorders are discussed further in Chap. 4 (page 64).

REFLEX EPILEPSY

For a long time it has been known that seizures could be evoked in certain epileptic individuals by a discrete physiologic or psychologic stimulus. Forster has classified the evoking stimuli into five types: (1) *visual*—flashing light (by far the commonest type of seizure-inducing stimulus), visual patterns, closure of the eyes in bright light, and specific colors (especially red); (2) *auditory*—sudden unexpected noise, specific sounds and musical themes, and certain voices; (3) *somatosensory*—either a brisk unexpected tap or sudden movement after sitting or lying still, or a prolonged tactile stimulus to a certain part of the body; (4) *reading* of words or numbers; and (5) *eating.*

The evoked seizure may be focal (beginning often in the part of the body that was stimulated) or generalized, and may take the form of one or a series of myoclonic jerks, or of a petit mal or grand mal seizure. Seizures induced by music, voice, reading, and eating are usually of the temporal lobe type. In a few instances such reflex epilepsy, as it is called, has been due to a focal cerebral disease, such as tumor, but far more often its cause cannot be ascertained.

Anticonvulsant medication is generally ineffective in

controlling reflex epilepsy. Some patients learn to avert the seizure by undertaking a mental task, e.g., thinking about some distracting subject, counting, etc., or by initiating some type of physical activity. [Similarly, spontaneously occurring focal motor seizures, e.g., those beginning in the toes or fingers, may be arrested (inhibited) by applying a ligature above the affected part or, in the case of focal sensory seizures, by applying a vigorous sensory stimulus ahead of the advancing sensory aura.] Forster has demonstrated that in certain types of reflex epilepsy the repeated and carefully controlled presentation of the noxious stimulus may eventually render the stimulus innocuous. This technique requires a great deal of time and assiduous reinforcement, which limits its therapeutic value.

HYSTERICAL SEIZURES

These are also referred to as "psychogenic" seizures and "pseudoseizures" (sham seizures). As these qualifying adjectives indicate, they are nonepileptic in nature; i.e., they are not caused by abnormal neuronal discharge, but they are mentioned here because they are sometimes mistaken for epileptic seizures and treated with anticonvulsant drugs, to which they are characteristically unresponsive. A pseudoseizure may be an isolated hysterical symptom ("conversion reaction") or a manifestation of hysteria in the female (Briquet disease) or of compensation neurosis and malingering in males or females. Usually, the motor display in the course of a pseudoseizure is sufficient to distinguish it from a genuine seizure (see Chap. 55). Where doubt remains, a recording of the ictal or postictal EEG or the combined video and EEG recording of an attack will settle the issue. This subject is discussed further in Chap. 55.

THE NATURE OF THE DISCHARGING LESION

Physiologically, the epileptic seizure has been defined as a sudden alteration of central nervous system function, resulting from a paroxysmal high-frequency or synchronous low-frequency, high-voltage electrical discharge (Schmidt and Wilder). This discharge may arise from an assemblage of neurons in any part of the cerebrum, cortical or subcortical, and perhaps in the brainstem and spinal cord as well, but it is the visible focal lesion in the cerebral cortex that has been the most thoroughly investigated. There need not be a visible lesion, for under the proper circumstances, a seizure discharge can be initiated in an entirely normal cerebral cortex, as when the cortex is activated by a drug or stimulated repeatedly by subconvulsive electrical stimuli ("kindling phenomenon").

Just why the neurons in or near a focal lesion discharge abnormally is not fully understood. Some of the electrical properties of a cortical epileptogenic focus suggest that its neurons have been deafferented. Such neurons are known to be hypersensitive, and they may remain so chronically, in a state of partial depolarization, able to fire irregularly at rates of 700 to 1000 per second. The cytoplasmic membranes of such cells appear to have an increased permeability, which renders them susceptible to activation by hyperthermia, hypoxia, hypoglycemia, hypocalcemia, and hyponatremia, as well as by repeated sensory (e.g., photic) stimulation and during certain phases of sleep (where hypersynchrony of neurons is known to occur).

Experimentally produced epileptic foci in the animal cortex are characterized by the occurrence, from time to time, of spontaneous interictal discharges, during which all the neurons of the discharging focus exhibit a paroxysmal depolarizing shift (DS), reflected as a negative surface wave in the EEG. Following the DS, the cells within the focus show a hyperpolarizing potential, probably due to an increase in chloride conductance across the cell membrane. The surrounding neurons are hyperpolarized from the beginning and inhibit those within the epileptic focus. Seizure spread probably depends on any factor or agent that activates neurons in the focus or inhibits those which surround it. The precise mechanisms which govern the transition from the circumscribed interictal discharge to the widespread seizure state are not understood.

Biochemical studies of the clone of neurons from a seizure focus have not clarified the problem. Epileptic foci are known to be sensitive to acetylcholine and to be slower in binding and removing it than normal cerebral cortex. A deficiency of the inhibitory neurotransmitter, γ-aminobutyric acid (GABA), a disturbance of cytochrome oxidase with decrease in ATP production, a reduction in the Krebs cycle function with a shift to a GABA-succinate shunt, or a disturbance in local regulation of extracellular K, Na, Ca, or Mg are other plausible hypotheses that have been proposed to explain the heightened excitability of epileptogenic neurons. Calcium is of particular interest in this regard, for it is known to stabilize cell membranes and to be essential for transmitter release at presynaptic terminals. Heinemann et al recorded a decrease in Ca in experimental epileptic foci preceding both the onset of ictal activity and the associated increase in K. (See Pedley for a review of the subject.)

Concurrent EEG recordings from an epileptogenic cortical focus and subcortical, thalamic, and brainstem centers have enabled investigators to construct a sequence of electrical and clinical events that characterize an evolving focal seizure. Firing of the involved neurons in the cortical focus is reflected in the EEG as a series of periodic spike discharges, which increase progressively in amplitude and frequency. Once the intensity of the seizure discharge exceeds a certain point, it overcomes the inhibitory influence of surrounding neurons and spreads to neighboring cortical and subcortical regions, via short corticocortical synaptic connections. Probably, if the abnormal discharge remains confined to the cortical focus and the immediate surrounding cortex, there are no clinical symptoms or signs of seizure. If an analogy may be drawn from experimental epileptic foci, the EEG abnormality that persists during the interseizure period reflects this type of confined abnormal cortical activity.

If unchecked, cortical excitation spreads to the contralateral cortex via interhemispheric pathways and anatomically and functionally related pathways to subcortical nuclei (particularly the basal ganglionic, thalamic, and brainstem reticular nuclei). Then it is that the first clinical manifestations of the convulsion begin, the particular signs and symptoms depending upon the portion of the brain from which the seizure originates. The excitatory activity from the subcortical nuclei is fed back to the original focus and to the other parts of the forebrain, a mechanism which serves to amplify the excitatory activity and gives rise to the characteristic high-voltage polyspike discharge in the EEG. There is propagation downward to spinal neurons as well, via corticospinal and reticulospinal pathways.

The spread of excitation to the subcortical, thalamic, and brainstem centers corresponds with the tonic phase of the seizure and loss of consciousness, as well as with the signs of autonomic nervous system overactivity (salivation, mydriasis, tachycardia, increase in blood pressure). Vital functions may be arrested but usually for only a few seconds. In rare instances, however, death may occur owing to a cessation of respiration, derangement of cardiac action, or some unknown cause.

Soon after the spread of excitation, a diencephalocortical inhibition begins and intermittently interrupts the seizure discharge, changing it from the persistent discharge of the tonic phase to the intermittent bursts of the clonic phase. Electrically, a transition occurs from a continuous polyspike to a spike-and-wave pattern. The intermittent clonic bursts become less and less frequent and finally cease altogether, leaving in their wake an "exhaustion" of the neurons of the epileptogenic focus. The latter is thought to be the basis of *Todd's postepileptic paralysis* (and of postictal aphasia and hemianopia) and the diffuse slow waves in the EEG. Plum and his associates have observed a two- to threefold increase in glucose utilization during seizure discharges, and the paralysis that follows might be due to depletion of glucose or some other substrate. However, inhibition of epileptogenic neurons may occur in the absence of neuronal exhaustion and the exact roles

played by each of these factors in postictal paralysis of function is not settled.

The development of unconsciousness and the generalized tonic contraction of muscles is reflected in the EEG by a high-voltage discharge which appears simultaneously over the entire cortex. The generalization of the clinical and electrical manifestations depends upon activation of a deep, centrally located physiologic mechanism which, for reasons outlined in Chap. 16, includes the midbrain reticular formation and its diencephalic extension, the intralaminar and nonspecific thalamic projection systems (originally referred to by Penfield as the centrencephalon, now as the reticulocortical activating system). Apparently, the same central mechanism is operative whether the generalized seizure is triggered by spread from a cortical focus or whether it originates in the "centrencephalon."

The characteristic 3-per-second high-voltage spike-and-wave discharge and seizures resembling absence attacks have been produced in animals by the topical application of epileptogenic substances in both prefrontal regions. The EEG discharges persist after thalamectomy, but are interrupted by callosal section. The spike-and-wave complex, which represents brief excitation followed by slow-wave inhibition, is the type of EEG pattern which characterizes the clonic (inhibitory) phase of the focal motor or grand mal seizure. In contrast to what occurs in grand mal seizures, this strong element of inhibition is present from the beginning of a petit mal attack, a feature perhaps that accounts for the failure of excitation to spread to lower brainstem and spinal structures (tonic-clonic movements do not occur).

Temporal lobe seizures are known to arise in foci in the medial temporal lobe, amygdaloid nuclei, and hippocampus. They may arise also in the convexity of the temporal lobe and propagate to the amygdaloid nuclei and hippocampus. Electrical stimulation in these areas reproduces feelings of depersonalization, emotionality, and automatic behavior. The latter, so characteristic of psychomotor epilepsy, sometimes take the form of a psychosis which appears to be a direct effect of the temporal lobe discharge in some instances and a postexcitatory, inhibitory, or paralytic effect in others. Loss of memory for the events of the episode may be due to the paralytic effect of the discharge on neurons of the amygdaloid nuclei and hippocampus.

A discovery of theoretical importance is that a seizure focus, if active for a time, may establish, via commissural connections, a persistent secondary focus in the corresponding area of cortex in the opposite hemisphere (mirror focus). The nature of this development is not fully understood. It may be similar to the "kindling" phenomenon, mentioned above. No morphologic change is visible in the mirror focus by light microscopy. Possibly Golgi studies, like those performed by the Scheibels on the epileptic temporal lobe, would show the same irregularity and tortuosity of dendrites and loss of dendritic spines which they consider significant (see below). The mirror focus may be a source of confusion in trying to identify electrographically the side of the primary lesion by EEG, but there is little evidence that it can produce chronic seizures in humans. Similarly, there are no data supporting a role for kindling in the diagnosis and management of patients with epilepsy (Goldensohn).

Severe seizures may be accompanied by a systemic lactic acidosis with a fall in arterial pH, reduction in arterial oxygen saturation, and rise in Pco_2. These effects are secondary to the respiratory spasm and excessive muscular activity. In paralyzed and artificially ventilated subjects receiving electroconvulsive therapy, these changes are less marked and the oxygen tension in cerebral venous blood may actually rise. Heart rate, blood pressure, and particularly CSF pressure rise briskly during the seizure. According to Plum and his associates, the rise in blood pressure evoked by the seizure causes a sufficient increase in cerebral blood flow to meet the increased metabolic needs of the brain.

THE ELECTROENCEPHALOGRAM IN EPILEPSY

The electroencephalogram (EEG) provides a delicate confirmation of Hughlings Jackson's theory of epilepsy—that it represents a recurrent, sudden, excessive disorderly discharge of cortical neurons. The EEG is undoubtedly the most sensitive, indeed an indispensable, tool for the diagnosis of epilepsy, but like other laboratory tests it must be used in conjunction with clinical data. Many epileptic patients have a perfectly normal interictal EEG; occasionally, using standard methods of scalp recording, the EEG may even be normal during a simple or complex partial seizure. Conversely, a small number of healthy persons show paroxysmal EEG abnormalities; some of them have a family history of epilepsy and may themselves later develop seizures.

The EEG abnormalities that characterize an evolving epileptogenic focus and generalization of seizure activity, both the grand mal and petit mal types, have been described in the preceding section. At first there was thought to be a characteristic EEG picture for psychomotor epilepsy, but further studies have not confirmed this. The postseizure state, or *postconvulsive paralysis of cerebral function,* also has its EEG correlate, taking the form of random generalized

slow waves. With recovery of normal mentation, the EEG returns to normal or to the preseizure state. The EEG tracing obtained during the interval between seizures is abnormal to some degree in approximately 40 percent of fully conscious and 75 percent of sleeping patients.

A higher yield of abnormalities and a more precise definition of seizure types can be obtained by the use of telemetry systems, in which patients are attached to the EEG machine by cable or radio transmitter, without unduly limiting their freedom of movement. Even greater freedom of movement is possible through the use of a small cassette recorder that is attached to a miniature EEG machine worn by the patient. In some medical centers, the telemetry system is joined to a time-lapse video-audio system, making it possible to record seizure phenomena (even at night, with dim infrared light) and to synchronize them with the EEG abnormalities. The role of intensive neurodiagnostic monitoring in the investigation and treatment of seizures has been reviewed recently by Gumnit.

The EEG changes in epilepsy are discussed further in Chap. 2.

PATHOLOGY OF THE SEIZURE STATE

In some cases of idiopathic (primary) epilepsy of the grand mal and petit mal types the brain has been grossly and microscopically normal, though it is unlikely that the entire brain was subjected to serial sectioning in any single case. The same is true for the convulsive states attending drug withdrawal, intoxication, and hypoglycemia, which must represent derangements at the subcellular level.

Many of the so-called secondary epilepsies have definable pathologies. These include zones of neuronal loss and gliosis (scars), hamartomas, vascular malformations, and tumors. The latter are rare in early life. The frequency of these lesions is not fully known. Certainly the focal epilepsies have the highest incidence of a structural substratum, although in certain cases no morphologic change is visible. In several series of cases of temporal lobe excisions, such as that of Falconer, incisural sclerosis (neuronal loss with gliosis) in the hippocampal and amygdaloid regions were found in the majority of cases; vascular malformations, hamartomas, and astrocytomas were less frequent, and in a small number no abnormalities could be found.

The widespread use of CT scanning and MRI offers another approach to the pathologic study of epilepsy. Gastaut and Gastaut have reported that in primary grand mal and petit mal epilepsies, a CT abnormality was found in approximately 10 percent of cases, whereas in the Lennox-Gastaut syndrome, the West syndrome, and partial complex epilepsies it was found in 52, 77, and 63 percent, respectively. Atrophy, calcification, and malformations were the most frequent abnormalities. MRI is a particularly sensitive means of detecting epileptogenic lesions of the medial-basal portions of the temporal lobes. We have observed several patients in whom MRI disclosed a surgically treatable lesion of the temporal lobe, after CT scanning had failed to do so.

With reference to the focal epilepsies it has not been possible to determine which component of the lesion is responsible for the seizures. In other words, one cannot say from the microscopic examination of focal cerebral lesions whether any given one of them was epileptogenic. Gliosis, fibrosis, vascularization, and meningocerebral cicatrix have all been incriminated, but they are found in nonepileptic foci as well. The Scheibels' Golgi studies of neurons from epileptic foci in the temporal lobe showed distortions of dendrites, loss of dendritic spines, and disorientation of neurons near the scars, but these findings were not compared with similar nonepileptic lesions. Moreover, changes such as these have proved to be nonspecific, and the same changes in Golgi preparations can be seen as a result of poor fixation (Williams et al). Partial disconnection of groups of cortical neurons from those of the neighboring cortex and from those of the other cerebral hemisphere and thalamus seems likely to have occurred, and certain systems of inhibiting neurons may have been destroyed. In the highly epileptogenic experimental lesions produced by application of aluminum cream and penicillin to the cortex, some neurons are surely destroyed, especially in the superficial layers, and the synaptic connections of the remaining ones are reduced in number. Probably a disorganization of these cortical interneuronal relationships is more important than the nature of the lesion since diseases as different as hemorrhage, infarction, and neoplastic invasion, for example, are all epileptogenic at times. Once a gliotic focus of whatever cause, bordered by groups of discharging neurons, becomes epileptogenic, it may remain so throughout the lifetime of the patient.

Another aspect of the pathology of the epileptic brain relates to effects (traumatic, hypoxic) secondary to the seizures themselves—an epileptic encephalopathy, so to speak. Cortical contusions are seen in some cases in which the original seizure disorder did not have a traumatic basis. Norman and his colleagues have called attention to recent lesions in the cerebellum and hippocampus of hypoxic-hypotensive origin in long-standing severe epileptics. According to Salcman et al degeneration of Purkinje cells may occur in chronic epileptics who had never experienced a generalized convulsion; the pathogenesis of these latter neuropathologic changes is unclear but is probably not hypoxic.

A particularly common finding in the brains of epileptics is a bilateral loss of neurons in the CA1 segment (Sommer sector) of the pyramidal cell layer of the hippo-

campus, sometimes extending into the underlying dentate gyrus. Often it cannot be determined whether these lesions were incurred at birth and gave rise to seizures, or happened later, as a result of anoxia in the course of major generalized seizures.

ROLE OF HEREDITY

In the genesis of the epilepsies, heredity plays an important though variable role. The hereditary element is most clearly discerned in classical petit mal (absence attacks with 3-per-second spike-and-wave discharges), which is transmitted as an incompletely penetrant autosomal dominant trait (Metrakos and Metrakos). This is also true for other primary generalized ("centrencephalic") epilepsies that begin in childhood, including the benign astatic type and the myoclonic epilepsy of late childhood and adolescence. In grand mal epilepsy, familial coincidence occurs in 5 to 10 percent of patients (Browne and Feldman). The importance of genetic factors in these epilepsies is emphasized by the findings in twin studies; in six major studies the overall concordance rate was 60 percent for monozygotic twins and 13 percent for dizygotic pairs (Tsuboi).

In the partial or focal epilepsies (which is the form that seizures take in two-thirds of adults and almost half the children with epilepsy) the role of heredity is not nearly so clear. With the exception of the so-called rolandic type, a mendelian pattern of inheritance has not been demonstrated. However, numerous studies have shown a greater-than-expected incidence of seizures or EEG abnormalities or both among first-degree relatives of patients with partial epilepsy. The genetics of epilepsy has been reviewed in detail by Anderson and Hauser.

CLINICAL APPROACH TO THE EPILEPSIES

MEDICAL DISEASES IN WHICH SEIZURES ARE A PROMINENT CLINICAL MANIFESTATION

Among medical diseases that may be complicated by a seizure or a burst of seizures, the following are the most frequent.

1. Generalized convulsions of the "tonic-clonic" type appear prominently during the *abstinence or withdrawal period in patients addicted to alcohol, barbiturates, or other sedative-hypnotic drugs.* Suspicion of this mechanism is raised by the telltale marks of alcohol abuse or the history of prolonged nervousness requiring sedation. Also, disturbances of sleep, tremulousness, disorientation, illusions, and

hallucinations are often associated with the convulsive phase of the illness. Seizures in this setting may occur singly but more often in brief flurries, the entire convulsive period lasting for several hours, rarely for a day or longer, during which time the patient is unduly sensitive to photic stimulation (see Chap. 41).

2. Seizures are a prominent feature of all varieties of *bacterial meningitis*, more so in children than in adults. Fever and stiff neck usually provide the clue, and lumbar puncture yields the salient diagnostic data. Seizure(s) may be the initial manifestation of syphilitic meningitis.

3. *Uremia* is another condition with a strong convulsive tendency. Of interest is the relation of seizures to the development of complete anuria. The latter state is tolerated for 2 or 3 days without neurologic signs, and then there is an abrupt onset of twitching, trembling, myoclonic jerks, and generalized motor seizures. Tetany may be added. The motor display, one of the most dramatic in medicine, lasts several days until the patient sinks into terminal coma or recovers, depending on the outcome of the renal disease. When this twitch-convulsive syndrome accompanies lupus erythematosus, idiopathic epilepsy, or generalized neoplasia, one can nearly always be sure that it has its basis in renal failure.

4. Other acute metabolic illnesses and electrolytic disorders complicated by generalized and multifocal motor seizures are hyponatremia and water intoxication, thyrotoxic storm, porphyria, hypoglycemia, hyperglycemia, hypomagnesemia, pyridoxine deficiency, argininosuccinic aciduria, and phenylketonuria. Lead (in children) and mercury (in children and adults) are the most frequent convulsive metallic intoxicants.

Generalized seizures, with or without twitching, may occur in the terminal phase of many other illnesses, such as gram-negative septicemia with shock, liver coma, and intractable congestive heart failure.

5. Cardiac arrest, suffocation or respiratory failure, NO_2 anesthesia, CO poisoning—the common causes of *hypoxic encephalopathy*—induce a diffuse myoclonic jerking of all the musculature and generalized seizures as soon as cardiac function is resumed. The convulsive phase of this condition may last only a few days, in association with coma, stupor, and confusion; or it may persist indefinitely as an intention myoclonus-convulsive state.

6. Several primary diseases of the brain may be announced by an acute convulsive state. Myoclonic jerking and seizures appear early in acute herpes simplex enceph-

alitis and other forms of viral, treponemal, and parasitic encephalitides, in subacute sclerosing panencephalitis, as well as in lipid storage diseases, subacute spongiform encephalopathy (Creutzfeldt-Jakob disease), and diffuse gliomatosis of the brain.

Convulsive seizures are a relatively uncommon occurrence in the evolving phases of a stroke. Only exceptionally will an acute cerebral embolus cause a focal fit, though old embolic infarcts become epileptogenic in about 25 percent of cases. Similarly, thrombotic infarcts are almost never convulsive at their onset, but may later become so if they involve the cortex. The rupture of an aneurysm is occasionally marked by one or two generalized convulsions. Subcortical hypertensive hemorrhages occasionally become sources of recurrent focal epilepsy. Cortical phlebothrombosis or thrombophlebitis with cortical ischemia and infarction is highly epileptogenic, but fortunately is rare; the same is true for hypertensive encephalopathy.

FEBRILE AND OTHER SEIZURES OF INFANCY AND CHILDHOOD

The well-known *febrile seizure,* peculiar to infants and children between 6 months and 5 years of age (peak incidence 9 to 20 months) and tending to be familial, is generally regarded as a benign condition. Usually it takes the form of a single, generalized motor seizure, occurring as the temperature rises or reaches its peak. Seldom does the seizure last longer than a few minutes, and by the time an EEG can be obtained there is usually no abnormality. Recovery is complete, and the risk of developing epilepsy in later life is little or no greater than that of the general population.

This benign type of febrile seizure should not be confused with a second and more serious type of illness in which an acute encephalitic or encephalopathic state presents as a febrile illness with focal or prolonged seizures, generalized or focal EEG abnormalities, and repeated episodes of febrile convulsions with the same or different illnesses. The seizure disorder may present as status epilepticus and the illness may end fatally; or the child may survive and be left with mental impairment, hemiparesis, or other neurologic abnormalities. The seizures may recur, not only with infections, but at other times. Lennox and others have failed to separate these two types of febrile convulsions and a third one in which an antecedent birth injury of the brain or other disease is exposed by an episode of fever with convulsions. When cases of all three types are lumped together under the rubric of febrile convulsions, it is not surprising that a high percentage are complicated by atypical petit mal and atonic and astatic spells followed by tonic seizures, mental retardation, and psychomotor epilepsy (Lennox-Gastaut syndrome). Falconer, who has studied psychomotor seizures in adult life, notes retrospectively a high incidence of "febrile seizures" during infancy and childhood. The authors believe that he is referring to the second and third types described above, which we prefer not to label as febrile convulsions.

Recent epidemiologic studies have substantiated this clinical point of view. Annegers and his colleagues followed a cohort of 687 children for an average of 18 years after their initial febrile convulsion. Overall, these children had a fivefold excess of unprovoked seizures in later life. Among the children with simple febrile convulsions, the risk was only 2.4 percent. By contrast, children with complex febrile convulsions (focal, prolonged, or repeated episodes of febrile seizures) had a greatly increased risk— 8, 17, or 49 percent, depending on the association of one, two, or three of the complex features. The subsequent occurrence of generalized-onset seizures appeared to be associated with the number of febrile convulsions and a family history of seizures, whereas partial seizures were associated with all three of the complex features.

Other types of epilepsy are also notable with reference to certain diseases of childhood and certain stages in the development of the nervous system. In the young child, a focal vascular or encephalitic lesion may cause hemiparesis or other focal or lateralizing signs. Unilateral seizures follow, and some of these are of the inhibitory type with a sudden hemiplegia representing the seizure; or the seizure may be followed by a Todd's paralysis lasting several hours to days. Some of these patients improve within a few years and have no further seizures. Tumor is rarely the cause of unilateral seizures in the child. An inherited, unilateral form of epilepsy in childhood, characterized by sensory and motor seizure activity (especially of the face), associated with anarthria and a lower rolandic or midtemporal spike focus, has been described above ("Rolandic Epilepsy"). Both the EEG seizure focus and the seizures disappear within a few years.

Infantile spasms ("idiopathic") are of primary and secondary types. The former is probably of metabolic origin, but the specific abnormality is unknown. The latter may be caused by a wide variety of diseases: tuberous sclerosis, phenylketonuria or other amino acid abnormality, Sturge-Weber disease, birth injury, or developmental anomaly of the brain (see Chap. 44).

Neonatal seizures are of special type. They differ sharply, both in their nature and causation, from seizures in children and in adults. Mainly they are caused by perinatal asphyxia and cerebral hemorrhage, and to a lesser extent by certain infectious and inherited diseases, hypoglycemia, and hypocalcemia. Volpe recognized the following seizure patterns, in order of decreasing frequency: *subtle seizures*, consisting of horizontal eye movements and blinking,

"pedaling" movements, and oral automatisms; *tonic seizures*, resembling decorticate or decerebrate posturing in association with eye signs, apnea, or clonic jerks; *multifocal clonic jerks; focal clonic seizures*; bilateral *massive myoclonic jerks* (some of these patients later develop typical infantile spasms).

RECURRENT GENERALIZED AND FOCAL SEIZURES BEGINNING IN ADULT LIFE

The usual causes are traumatic scars, cerebral tumors, old cerebrovascular foci such as small subcortical hemorrhages and embolic or thrombotic infarcts that involve the cortex, suppurative diseases, especially thrombophlebitis and abscesses, and neurosyphilis. Each of these categories of disease will be discussed in its appropriate chapter. Obviously their clinical analysis must be supplemented by the most refined diagnostic procedures available to neurologists, such as localizing EEG, cytology and chemical tests of CSF, arteriography, and CT scans and MRI.

RECURRENT SEIZURES OF UNKNOWN CAUSE (IDIOPATHIC EPILEPSY)

As pointed out in the introduction to this chapter, seizures have a way of appearing long after the inception of a disease that has left in its wake a discharging focus. The latter may attract attention only when it happens to evoke a seizure. Even if tardive epilepsy were fatal—which it rarely is— pathologic study is usually so remote from the active phase of the causative disease that one is left with only an uninterpretable neuronal loss and glial scarring or with a lesion that cannot be discerned even after microscopic study of the brain.

The clinical approach to recurrent seizures in childhood and adolescence is much influenced by these facts. Rarely can the cause be determined. Usually one must conclude that the underlying disease is burned out and further pursuit of the cause will be unsuccessful or that the epilepsy is of primary (hereditary) type for which a morphologic basis has never been determined. In either instance the reality of the seizure problem is equally serious and equally challenging to control. If one surveys the entire population of epileptic patients, the majority will fall into this "idiopathic" category, not into the group with acute medical disease or with an advancing focal lesion.

When analyzed in greater detail, patients with idiopathic epilepsy tend to fall into three groups: (1) those whose seizures begin in infancy and early childhood and who are abnormal in other ways (some neurologists would exclude these cases from the category of idiopathic epilepsy because of the signs of cerebral disease, even though the cause is unknown); (2) those who are thought to be normal or only slightly abnormal until the first seizure at the age of 5 to 10 years; and (3) those who appear entirely normal until about puberty or adolescence, when they have their first generalized convulsion. The first two groups are much larger than the third, because with every passing year after the occurrence of a brain lesion the chances of its becoming an epileptic focus lessen. In the mature brain the usual interval between the brain injury and first seizure is 9 to 15 months, but it may be as brief as a few months or as long as several years. In the immature brain the interval may be longer, but in either instance, once the epilepsy begins there is a tendency for it to lessen in frequency with each passing year, as the static lesion becomes more remote. Children are said to outgrow their epilepsy, but the same trend has been noted in soldiers whose brain injury and subsequent epilepsy were acquired in adult life.

The medical histories of patients whose seizures begin in infancy and early childhood disclose a disproportionately high incidence of parturitional difficulties. Developmental anomalies of the cerebral cortex are also frequent. Seizures may have occurred in the neonatal period, and of this group approximately half turn out to be developmentally retarded. The infantile twitches and brief tonic spasms tend to be replaced after a few months by infantile myoclonic flexor spasms (salaam spasms), which may persist for 4 to 5 years, in diminishing severity, before giving way to atypical petit mal and generalized seizures. The specific seizure pattern is a function, then, not only of the topography of the discharging focus but of the level of maturation of the nervous system. Also, as pointed out earlier, a change in the pattern of seizures may be consequent upon the occurrence of a series of convulsions. Thus, anoxic damage to the hippocampi during seizures may cause an increasing incidence of psychomotor seizures.

The clinical investigation of seizures beginning early in life involves the differentiation of many diseases. The most frequent ones are developmental defects of many types, hypoxic-hypotensive failures of perfusion of the brain, intrauterine and infantile infections, metabolic diseases, and tuberous sclerosis. In this group the control of seizures is only one of many problems including difficulties with training, discipline, and schooling, and the need to correct specific disabilities.

Seizures beginning in the 4- to 8-year period may be typical petit mal, with grand mal appearing some time later, or the initial seizure may be grand mal in type. The neurologic history may disclose no antecedent illness or other disturbance of nervous function. Films of the skull, CSF examination, and CT scans may disclose no abnormalities, or at most some minor one such as a slight enlargement of the temporal horn of a ventricle. If the seizures are infrequent and responsive to anticonvulsant medication, the child's scholastic progress and emotional and social adjustment are unimpaired. Fully 80 percent of cases fall into this favorable group. If the seizures are frequent and not easily suppressed by medication and if they are unusual in other ways (atypical petit mal, psychomotor, or one-sided seizures), the child's life may be seriously deranged. Such a child may fail in school, spend much time in hospitals, and be derailed from the normal developmental track. Poor motivation, parental dependence, immature reactions, difficulty in learning, muddled thinking, bizarre ideation, and religiosity sometimes pose problems as difficult as the seizures themselves. In adult life the seizures may continue to interfere with work, marriage, etc. The most disabled members of this group usually have associated cerebral deficits.

Some patients with temporal lobe seizures, during the interictal period, may exhibit a number of behavioral abnormalities. Often they are slow and rigid in their thinking, subject to outbursts of bad temper and aggressiveness, and tend to be circumstantial and tedious in conversation and preoccupied with rather naive religious and philosophical ideas. Obsessionalism, humorless sobriety, emotionality (mood swings, sadness, and anger) and a tendency to paranoia are other frequently described traits. Diminished sexual interest or potency in men and menstrual problems in women are common among patients with partial seizures of temporal lobe origin. Moreover, in a considerable proportion of such patients, both men and women, reproductive endocrine disorders, not readily attributable to anticonvulsant drugs, can be demonstrated (Herzog et al).

Bear and Fedio have suggested that certain of these traits (obsessionalism, elation, sadness, and emotionality) are more common with *right* temporal lesions and that anger, paranoia, and cosmologic or religious conceptualizing are more characteristic of *left* temporal lesions. However, that such behavioral changes distinguish patients with temporal lobe epilepsy from other groups of epileptics has not been established. Rodin and Schmaltz, who administered the Bear-Fedio inventory to patients with both primary generalized and temporal lobe epilepsy, found no significant differences between the two groups. Moreover, they found no features that would distinguish patients with right-sided temporal foci from those with left-sided foci. The problem of personality disturbances in epilepsy remains to be settled (see review of Trimble).

Despite the widespread belief that temporal lobe epileptics are more prone to develop interictal psychosis than patients with other forms of epilepsy, this question also has not been settled with finality (see reviews of Stevens and of Pincus and Tucker). The data of Rodin et al are noteworthy in this regard. They found that complex partial seizures do not lead to psychiatric disturbances if this is the *only* seizure type from which the patient suffers. However, patients with *both* partial complex and major generalized seizures are significantly more likely to develop psychiatric disorders than those with two or more seizure types of non-temporal lobe origin. Also, it appears that epileptics, particularly those with temporal lobe seizures, are more prone to depression than nonepileptics, and that depression in epileptics is more than a nonspecific reaction to a chronic disability (Mendez et al).

The group with the best outlook are adolescents or young adults who have their first generalized seizure while performing adequately in high school or college. All laboratory tests, including the interictal EEG, may be normal. In the authors' experience, such patients, if treated intelligently, have no more trouble in continuing their education and in social adjustment than they would have if the seizures had never occurred.

The common causes of recurrent seizures according to the age of onset are summarized in Table 15-2.

OTHER PROBLEMS IN DIFFERENTIAL DIAGNOSIS

The clinical differences between a seizure and a syncopal attack are considered in detail in Chap. 17. It must be emphasized that there is no single criterion that will distinguish them unequivocally. The authors have erred in calling akinetic seizures simple faints and in mistaking cardiac or carotid sinus faints for seizures. Petit mal may be difficult to identify because of the brevity of attacks. Helpful maneuvers are to have the patient hyperventilate or to count aloud for 5 to 10 min. Patients who have frequent petit mal attacks will pause in counting or skip one or two numbers. Psychomotor seizures are the most difficult of all to diagnose. These attacks are so variable in character and so likely to induce minor disturbances in conduct—rather than obvious interruptions of consciousness—that they may be misdiagnosed as temper tantrums, hysteria, sociopathic behavior, or acute psychosis. Careful questioning of witnesses of an attack is essential. Verbalizations that cannot be remembered or walking aimlessly from one room into another are characteristic. In all these obscure forms of epilepsy, prolonged EEG monitoring may prove diagnostic (see page 260). Mild psychomotor seizures, characterized by a brief loss of consciousness and lip smacking, may be mistaken for petit mal, unless it is kept in mind that the

former (but not the latter) is almost invariably followed by a period of confusion.

Epilepsy complicated by states of mental dullness and confusion poses a special problem in diagnosis. Most epileptic patients seen in hospital and office practice show no mental deterioration, regardless of the type of seizure. Undoubtedly, seizures are more common in the mentally retarded, but recurrent seizures in themselves do not cause intellectual deterioration (Ellenberg et al). Therefore, the appearance of dementia, persistent confusion, or some other derangement of mental function should suggest the possibility of frequently recurrent subclinical seizures not con-

Table 15-2
Causes of recurrent seizures in different age groups

Age of onset	Probable cause
Neonatal	Congenital maldevelopment, birth injury, anoxia, metabolic disorders (hypocalcemia, hypoglycemia, vitamin B_6 deficiency, phenylketonuria, and others)
Infancy (1–6 months)	As above Infantile spasms
Early childhood (6 months–3 years)	Infantile spasms, febrile convulsions, birth injury and anoxia, infections, trauma
Childhood (3–10 years)	Perinatal anoxia, injury at birth or later, infections, thrombosis of cerebral arteries or veins, or indeterminate cause ("idiopathic" epilepsy)
Adolescence (10–18 years)	Idiopathic epilepsy, including genetically transmitted types, trauma
Early adulthood (18–25 years)	Idiopathic epilepsy, trauma, neoplasm, withdrawal from alcohol or other sedative-hypnotic drugs
Middle age (35–60 years)	Trauma, neoplasm, vascular disease, alcohol or other drug withdrawal
Late life (over 60 years)	Vascular disease, tumor, degenerative disease, trauma

Note: Meningitis and its complications may be a cause of seizures at any age. In tropical and subtropical countries, parasitic infection of the CNS is a common cause.

trolled by medication, drug intoxication, postseizure psychosis, or a brain disease that has caused both dementia and seizures.

TREATMENT

The treatment of epilepsy of all types can be divided into four parts: the removal of causative and precipitating factors, the regulation of physical and mental hygiene, the use of antiepileptic drugs, and the surgical excision of epileptic foci.

REMOVAL OF CAUSATIVE AND PRECIPITATING FACTORS

Central nervous system infections, such as the meningitides and syphilis, which may give rise to convulsive seizures, should be treated by appropriate measures. The same may be said of hyponatremia, hypocalcemia, and similar conditions. Disturbances of the endocrine system resulting from islet-cell adenomas or hypoparathyroidism require surgery and appropriate replacement therapy, respectively. The logic of this approach is self-evident and does not need to be elaborated.

When convulsive seizures are associated with cerebral tumor or abscess, surgical management is usually indicated. It must be remembered, however, that the surgical removal of a meningioma of the brain will relieve seizures in only about 50 percent of cases and that in cases of glioma or abscess of the brain, the percentage is much smaller. In such cases, further treatment with drugs is necessary.

Surgery has also been advocated for the removal of cortical scars secondary to cerebral trauma and birth injuries, on the assumption that such scars are surrounded by irritable foci which trigger the seizures. The neurosurgical treatment of epilepsy is discussed further on.

PHYSICAL AND MENTAL HYGIENE

The most important factors in seizure breakthrough, next to the abandonment of medication, are loss of sleep and alcoholic excess. The need for moderation in the use of alcohol must be stressed, as well as the need to maintain regular hours of sleep.

The epileptic patient should have a wholesome, regular diet consisting of simple foods with an abundance of vegetables and fresh fruits. Constipation can be a troublesome symptom and should be avoided by the establishment of regular bowel habits, proper diet, and the use of mild laxatives when necessary.

A moderate amount of physical exercise is desirable. With proper safeguards, even the more dangerous sports, such as swimming, may be permitted. However, a person with incompletely controlled epilepsy should not be allowed to drive an automobile, operate unguarded machinery, climb ladders, or take tub baths behind locked doors; such a person should swim only in the company of a good swimmer and wear a life preserver when boating.

Simple psychotherapy will frequently prevent or help overcome the feelings of inferiority and self-consciousness of many epileptic patients. Patients and their families will benefit from such therapy, and proper family attitudes should be cultivated. Oversolicitude and overprotection should be discouraged. It is important to emphasize that the patient should be allowed to live as normal a life as possible. Every effort should be made to keep children in school, and adults should be encouraged to work. Once seizures are under medical control for a period varying from 6 months to a year, the driving of an automobile is allowed in most western countries. Many communities have vocational rehabilitation centers and special social agencies for epileptics, and advantage should be taken of such facilities. Patients should be encouraged to participate in available recreational activities as well.

THE USE OF ANTIEPILEPTIC DRUGS— GENERAL PRINCIPLES

Approximately 75 percent of patients with convulsive seizures can have their attacks controlled completely or reduced in frequency and severity by the use of antiepileptic drugs. Although these drugs are not a cure for epilepsy, their use is the most important facet of treatment of convulsive disorders. The most commonly used drugs are listed in Table 15-3, along with their dosages, effective blood levels, and serum half-life. It should be noted that because of the long half-life of phenytoin, phenobarbital, and ethosuximide, these drugs need be taken only once daily, preferably at bedtime. Valproate and carbamazepine have short half-lives and their administration should be spaced during the day.

Certain drugs are more effective in one type of seizure than in another, and it is necessary to use the proper drugs in the optimum dosages for the different types of seizures. If satisfactory results are not obtained with one drug, then another should be tried, but frequent shifting of drugs is not advisable. Each should be given an adequate trial before another is substituted. In some patients a combination of two drugs will produce better results than one alone. Rarely are more than two drugs necessary, and the physician should make an effort to succeed with no more than two drugs, given in adequate dosage.

Initially, only one drug should be used and the dosage increased until therapeutic levels have been assured. If seizures are still not controlled, a second drug can then be added. Changes in medication should be made only if such a program is inadequate. In changing medication, the dosage of the new drug should be gradually increased to an optimum level at the same time that the dosage of the old drug is gradually decreased. The sudden withdrawal of a drug may lead to status epilepticus, even though a new drug is substituted. Once an anticonvulsant or a combination of anticonvulsants is found to be effective, its use should be maintained for a period of years.

The therapeutic dose for any patient must be determined, to some extent, by trial and error. Not uncommonly a drug is discarded as being ineffective, whereas a slightly increased dosage would have led to a disappearance of the attacks. It is, however, a common error to administer a drug to the point where the patient is so dull and stupefied that the toxic effects of the drug are more incapacitating than the seizures. It is highly doubtful whether the prolonged

administration of anticonvulsant medication is a factor in the development of the mental deterioration that occurs in a small percentage of the patients with convulsive seizures. In fact, improvement in mental faculties sometimes occurs following control of the seizures by the use of anticonvulsant drugs.

The management of seizures with drugs is greatly facilitated by having the patient chart daily medication and the number, time, and circumstances of seizures. Ideally such a baseline should be established before medication is begun, since each patient tends to have an individual pattern of seizures, but this is impractical. Some patients find it helpful to use a dispenser that would be filled on Sunday, for example, for the week. This indicates to the patient whether a dose was missed and whether the supply of medications is running low.

The efficacy of anticonvulsant drugs is increased also by frequent measurements of their *serum levels*. The levels

Table 15-3
Common antiepileptic drugs

Generic name	Trade name	Usual daily dosage		Principal therapeutic indications	Serum half-life, hours	Effective blood level, µg/ml
		Children	Adults, mg			
Phenobarbital	Luminal	3–5 mg/kg (8 mg/kg infants)	60–200	Tonic-clonic seizures; simple and complex partial seizures; absence	96 ± 12	10–40
Phenytoin	Dilantin	4–7 mg/kg	300–400	Tonic-clonic seizures; simple and complex partial seizures	24 ± 12	10–20
Carbamazepine	Tegretol	20–30 mg/kg	600–1200	Tonic-clonic seizures; complex partial seizures	12 ± 3	4–10
Primidone	Mysoline	10–25 mg/kg	750–1500	Tonic-clonic seizures; simple and complex partial seizures	12 ± 6	5–15
Ethosuximide	Zarontin	20–40 mg/kg	750–2000	Absence	40 ± 6	50–100
Methsuximide	Celontin	10–20 mg/kg	500–1000	Absence	40 ± 6	40–100
Diazepam	Valium	0.15–2 mg/kg (intravenously)	10–150	Status epilepticus		
ACTH		40–60 units/day		Infantile spasms		
Valproic acid	Depakene	30–60 mg/kg	1000–3000	Absence and myoclonic seizures; as an adjunctive drug in tonic clonic and complex partial seizures	8 ± 2	50–100
Clonazepam	Clonopin	0.01–0.2 mg/kg	1.5–20	Absence; myoclonus	18–50	0.01–0.07

of phenytoin, barbiturate, primidone, ethosuximide, and carbamazepine can all be measured on a single specimen by gas-liquid chromatography. These measurements are helpful in regulating dosage, revealing irregular drug intake, identifying the responsible agent in intoxicated patients who are taking more than one drug, and assuring compliance on the part of the patient. Blood for serum levels should be drawn in the morning, before breakfast (''trough levels''), a procedure that introduces consistency in the measurement of drug concentrations.

The effective serum levels (''therapeutic range'') for each of the commonly used anticonvulsant drugs is indicated in Table 15-3. The upper and lower levels of this range are not to be regarded as immutable confines into which the serum values of a given patient must fit. In some patients, seizures are controlled at serum levels below the therapeutic range and in others the seizures continue despite serum values within the therapeutic range. In the latter patients seizures are often controlled by raising dosage(s) above the therapeutic range but not to the point of producing clinical toxicity. In general, higher serum concentrations of drugs are necessary for the control of simple or complex partial seizures than for the control of tonic-clonic seizures alone (Schmidt et al). It is to be noted that the blood level is not an infallible index of the amount of drug entering the brain. A variable amount is bound to albumin and does not penetrate nervous tissue.

Always to be considered in the use of antiepileptic drugs are their possible adverse interactions with other drugs. Many such interactions have been demonstrated but only a few are of clinical significance, requiring adjustment of drug dosages (Kutt). Chloramphenicol may cause the accumulation of phenytoin and phenobarbital, and erythromycin may cause the accumulation of carbamazepine. Antacids may reduce phenytoin concentration whereas cimetidine does the opposite. Salicylates may lead to decline in plasma levels of anticonvulsant drugs. Among anticonvulsant drugs, valproate often causes accumulation of phenobarbital.

Once an effective anticonvulsant regimen has been established, it must usually be continued for many years. Because of the long-term toxic effects of such a regimen, the occurrence of a single generalized seizure in an otherwise normal child or adult (with a normal CT scan and EEG) does not call for the institution of anticonvulsant therapy. Moreover, withdrawal of anticonvulsant drugs should be undertaken in patients who have been free of seizures for a prolonged period. There are few firm rules to guide the physician in this decision. A recent prospective study has shown that in patients who had been seizure free during two years of treatment with a single drug, one-third relapsed after discontinuation of the drug, and this relapse rate was much the same in adults and children (Callaghan et al). In this group, the relapse rate was less in patients with petit mal and generalized-onset seizures and greater in those with complex partial seizures with secondary generalization. Other authors have suggested that a longer seizure-free period is associated with lesser rate of relapse (see review of Todt). This subject has recently been discussed by Pedley.

THE USE OF SPECIFIC DRUGS IN TREATMENT OF SEIZURES

Tonic-Clonic Seizures (Grand Mal)   Phenytoin and carbamazepine are equally effective (see Table 15-3 for dosages). Since the latter has fewer side effects if properly administered, it is usually preferred. In many cases, phenytoin or carbamazepine alone will control the seizures. If not, the combined use of these two drugs may be effective; therapeutic serum levels of each can be achieved without side effects. An alternative procedure is to add phenobarbital (60 to 200 mg daily) in carefully graded increments; when either phenytoin or carbamazepine is used in combination with phenobarbital, a full therapeutic dose of each drug must be given. Where such a regimen fails to control the seizures, a combination of primidone and phenytoin or primidone and carbamazepine may be successful. Primidone should be *added* to full therapeutic doses of phenytoin or carbamazepine in increments of 50 mg every few days, to a maximum of 750 to 1500 mg daily. In some patients, the addition of valproate to carbamazepine may prove effective. Valproate should not be used with phenobarbital and probably not with phenytoin.

The *toxic effects of phenobarbital,* which are drowsiness and mental dullness, nystagmus, and staggering, should be used as indications of excessive dosage. The adverse effects of primidone are much the same. Rash, fever, lymphadenopathy, eosinophilia and other blood dyscrasias, and polyarteritis are manifestations of *phenytoin hypersensitivity,* and their occurrence calls for discontinuation of the medication. Overdose with phenytoin causes ataxia, diplopia, and stupor. The prolonged use of phenytoin often leads to hirsutism (mainly in young girls), hypertrophy of gums, and coarsening of facial features. Because of this we consider carbamazepine the drug of first choice. Chronic phenytoin intoxication may rarely be associated with peripheral neuropathy, and probably with cerebellar degeneration (see Lindvall and Nilsson). An antifolate effect on blood and interference with vitamin K metabolism have also been reported. The pregnant woman taking Dilantin should be given vitamin K before delivery and the newborn infant should receive vitamin K as well, to prevent bleeding. Phenytoin should not be used together with disulfiram (Antabuse), chloramphenicol, sulfamethizole, and phenylbutazone, and neither phenobarbital nor phenytoin should be used in patients receiving dicumarol. *Carbamazepine* causes many of the same side effects as phenytoin, but to a much lesser degree. Leucopenia and diplopia are the most common side effects, and pancytopenia occurs occasionally. A complete blood count should be made before treatment is instituted, and the white cell count should be checked regularly in patients taking this drug. The major shortcoming of valproate is the occasional production of hepatotoxicity.

Several studies in the past decade have documented a slight but definite increase in the incidence of congenital malformations in the offspring of epileptic women, as compared with nonepileptic ones (Janz). Phenytoin, phenobarbital, and primidone are about equally teratogenic and produce the same types of malformation (Andermann). Also, the chronic administration of valproate during pregnancy is associated with an increased evidence of fetal distress and fetal anomalies (Jager-Roman et al). Trimethadione administration is complicated by a high rate of congenital heart disease and should not be used during pregnancy. Nevertheless, pregnant epileptics need to be maintained on anticonvulsant drugs, because the potential teratogenic effects are outweighed by the danger of seizures (particularly status). There is some evidence that the blood levels of anticonvulsants should be modified for pregnancy, keeping them at the lower limits of the ''therapeutic range'' (Dansky et al).

Complex Partial Seizures   Drugs effective in the treatment of grand mal seizures are also effective in the treatment of complex partial seizures. Phenytoin, 300 to 400 mg/day, and carbamazepine, 0.6 to 1.2 g/day, have given the best results in adults. Most neurologists now use carbamazepine initially in preference to phenytoin. On the whole, the results of anticonvulsant treatment are not as good as in tonic-clonic seizures.

Petit Mal Attacks   Drugs effective in the treatment of grand mal and psychomotor seizures are relatively ineffective in the treatment of patients with petit mal attacks. In the latter, ethosuximide (Zarontin), 750 to 1500 mg/day, has been the most successful and has replaced trimethadione (Tridione) and paramethadione (Paradione). It is good practice to begin with a single dose of 250 mg of ethosuximide per day and increase it every week until the optimum therapeutic effect is achieved. Valproate and to a lesser extent methsuximide (Celontin) are useful in individual cases where ethosuximide has failed. In patients with benign absence attacks that are associated with photosensitive epilepsy, myoclonus, and clonic-tonic-clonic seizures (ju-

venile myoclonic epilepsy), valproate is the drug of choice. Valproate is particularly useful in children with both petit mal and grand mal, since the use of this drug alone often permits the control of both types of seizure.

Minor Seizures and Focal Attacks   The drugs that are effective in the treatment of grand mal and psychomotor seizures are also effective against focal attacks and minor seizures. The latter, which appear in patients whose grand mal attacks have been controlled, can occasionally be checked by simply increasing the dose of the drug(s) that the patient is already taking, making certain that they fall below toxic levels. If the minor attacks are very infrequent and not incapacitating, no great effort need be made to treat them.

Atypical Petit Mal plus Other Types   In patients who are subject to petit mal as well as grand mal or psychomotor seizures, valproic acid should be given as the first drug. Should this drug be ineffective, ethosuximide plus phenytoin, carbamazepine, phenobarbital, or primidone should be tried. The treatment of the special types of convulsions in the neonatal period and in infancy and childhood is discussed by Fenichel and by Volpe.

Probably the form of epilepsy that is most difficult to treat is the atypical petit mal syndrome of *Lennox-Gastaut* (see above). Some of these patients have as many as 50 or more seizures per day, and every combination of anticonvulsant medications has no effect. Recently valproic acid (900 to 2400 mg/day) has been tried, and in approximately half the cases the frequency of spells has been reduced. Clonazepam also has had limited success.

Myoclonus   Seizure states in which myoclonus is a major element (petit mal, juvenile myoclonic, and certain cases of tonic-clonic epilepsy) respond particularly well to valproate. Even the myoclonus of certain progressive diseases, such as the Unverricht-Lundborg syndrome, may be suppressed by this drug.

In the treatment of massive myoclonus in infants, ACTH or adrenal corticosteroids have been the most effective. Postanoxic intention myoclonus (see page 86) can be suppressed by clonazepam (8 to 12 mg/day) and by 5-hydroxytryptophan (1 to 1.5 g/day) combined with carbidopa (150 to 400 mg/day).

Status Epilepticus   Recurrent generalized convulsions at a frequency which does not allow consciousness to be regained in the interval between seizures (grand mal status) probably constitute the most serious therapeutic problem. Most patients who die of epilepsy do so because of uncontrolled seizures of this type (mortality of about 10 percent) or an injury sustained as a result of seizure. Rising temperature, circulatory collapse, and lower-nephron nephrosis is a sequence of events which may be encountered in fatal cases of status epilepticus. Prolonged convulsive status (>90 min) also carries a risk of serious neurologic sequelae.

It must be conceded that at present no known drug will safely control all recurrent convulsions. This is not surprising, for there are many causes of convulsions, and not all cases are alike. Clinical experience teaches that in some patients the convulsive tendency is so overwhelming that no amount of anticonvulsant medication, even anesthetic agents, will prevent recurrence of seizures. In others the liability to recurrent convulsions lasts only a few hours or at most a few days, regardless of whether anticonvulsant medication is given. The real hazard in treating resistant recurrent convulsions is that consciousness and vital functions may be suppressed to a degree incompatible with life. The risk of deep coma without convulsions may be greater than semicoma or stupor with an occasional convulsion.

The many regimens that have been proposed for the treatment of status attest to the fact that no one of them is altogether satisfactory. The authors have had the most success with the following program. When the patient is first seen, diazepam (Valium) is administered intravenously at a rate of about 2 mg/min until the seizures stop or a total of 20 mg has been given. Immediately thereafter a loading dose (13 mg/kg) of phenytoin is administered by vein at a rate of 25 mg/min or by nasogastric tube. Phenytoin should not be given intramuscularly. If seizures continue, an endotracheal tube should be inserted and O_2 administered, and either diazepam *or* sodium phenobarbital should be given: diazepam is given intravenously in doses of 5 to 10 mg and can be repeated every 30 min, to a maximum of 100 to 150 mg per 24 h. Alternatively, phenobarbital is infused at a rate of 100 mg/min until the seizures stop or to a total dose of 20 mg/kg. Cardiac and respiratory function should be monitored throughout the administration of these drugs. If none of these measures controls the seizures, all medication except phenytoin should be discontinued and some form of anesthesia should be administered—ether, pentothal (up to 0.5 g intravenously), or halothane, with neuromuscular blockade. If an anesthetist is not available, an infusion of 4% paraldehyde in normal saline or 50 to 100 mg of lidocaine may be given intravenously. Should the seizures continue despite all these medications, one is justified in the assumption that the convulsive tendency is so strong that it cannot be checked by reasonable quantities of anticonvulsants. One then depends entirely on phenytoin, 0.5 g, and sodium phenobarbital, 0.4 g/day (smaller doses in infants and children, as shown in Table 15-3), and on safeguarding the patient's vital functions. It is estimated that the combination of diazepam and phenytoin will terminate tonic-clonic status epilepticus in 65 percent of cases and an intravenous drip of diazepam in another 20 percent. Lorazepam is five times more potent than diazepam in arresting seizures in animals, and early clinical trials indicate that it may be effective in humans.

Petit mal status should be managed by intravenous diazepam followed by ethosuximide or valproic acid, or both.

SURGICAL TREATMENT OF EPILEPSY

The surgical excision of epileptic foci in simple and complex partial epilepsies that have not responded to intensive and prolonged medical therapy has been used effectively in several neurologic centers. The best known of these in North America are the Montreal Neurological Institute (Penfield, Rasmussen) and the National Institutes of Health in Bethesda (Van Buren et al). It has been estimated, at these centers, that approximately 40 percent of all cases of partial epilepsy are candidates for surgical therapy. To locate the discharging focus requires a careful analysis of clinical and EEG findings, sometimes including those obtained by telemetry and the use of stereotactic or subdural strip electrodes. Approximately one-third of the patients of the Montreal group became seizure free (15 percent after some earlier attacks), and in another third there was a marked reduction in attacks three or more years after surgery. These data are based on a study of 1145 patients over a period of 2 to 45 years. The mortality rate in the Montreal group was 0.2 percent.

Other surgical procedures as yet of unproven value are stereotactic ablations and section of the corpus callosum. Cooper et al implanted a cerebellar stimulator, taking advantage of the inhibitory effects of Purkinje cells on motor activity. They reported some success, but we have not confirmed this in several cases under our care. This has been the experience of others as well (Wright et al). These procedures are best carried out in a few medical centers with a special interest in their study and evaluation.

REFERENCES

Andermann E: Teratogenic effects of anticonvulsant medication, in Robb P (ed): *Epilepsy Updated: Causes and Treatment.* Chicago, Year Book Medical Publishers, 1980, pp 275–277.

ANDERSON VE, HAUSER WA: The genetics of epilepsy, in Bearn AG et al (eds): *Progress in Medical Genetics, vol. VI: Genetics of Neurological Disorders.* New York, Praeger, 1985, pp. 10–52.

ANNEGERS JF, HAUSER WA, SHIRTS SB, KURLAND LT: Factors prognostic of unprovoked seizures after febrile convulsions. *N Engl J Med* 316:493, 1987.

BEAR DM, FEDIO P: Quantitative analysis of interictal behavior in temporal lobe epilepsy. *Arch Neurol* 34:454, 1977.

BROWNE TR, FELDMAN RG: *Epilepsy.* Boston, Little, Brown, 1983.

CALLAGHAN N, GARRETT A, GOGGIN T: Withdrawal of anticonvulsant drugs in patients free of seizures for two years. *N Engl J Med* 318:942, 1988.

COLE AJ, ANDERMANN F, TAYLOR L et al: The Landau-Kleffner syndrome of acquired epileptic aphasia: unusual clinical outcome, surgical experiences, and absence of encephalitis. *Neurology* 38:31, 1988.

COMMISSION ON CLASSIFICATION AND TERMINOLOGY OF THE INTERNATIONAL LEAGUE AGAINST EPILEPSY. Proposal for revised clinical and electroencephalographic classification of epileptic seizures. *Epilepsia* 22:489, 1981.

COOPER IS, AMIN I, GILMAN S: The effect of chronic cerebellar stimulation upon epilepsy in man. *Trans Am Neurol Assoc* 98:192, 1973.

CURRIE S, HEATHFIELD KWG, HENSON RA, SCOTT DF: Clinical course and prognosis of temporal lobe epilepsy. *Brain* 94:173, 1970.

DANSKY L, ANDERMANN E, SHERWIN AL et al: Maternal epilepsy and birth defects: Correlation with anticonvulsant levels during pregnancy. *Can J Neurol Sci* 6:377, 1979.

EADIE MJ, TYRER JH: *Anticonvulsant Therapy: Pharmacological Basis and Practice,* 2nd ed. London, Churchill Livingstone, 1980.

ELLENBERG JG, HIRTZ DG, NELSON KB: Do seizures in children cause intellectual deterioration? *N Engl J Med* 314:1085, 1986.

FALCONER MA: Genetic and related aetiological factors in temporal lobe epilepsy: A review. *Epilepsia* 12:13, 1971–1972.

FENICHEL GM: *Neonatal Neurology,* 2nd ed. New York, Churchill Livingstone, 1985.

FORSTER FM: *Reflex Epilepsy, Behavioral Therapy and Conditional Reflexes.* Springfield, Ill, Charles C Thomas, 1977.

GASTAUT H: Clinical and electroencephalographical classifications of epileptic seizures. *Epilepsia* 11:102, 1970.

GASTAUT H, AGUGLIA U, TINUPER P: Benign versive or circling epilepsy with bilateral 3-cps spike and wave discharges in late childhood. *Ann Neurol* 19:301, 1986.

GASTAUT H, GASTAUT JL: Computerized transverse axial tomography in epilepsy. *Epilepsia* 17(3):325, 1976.

GIBBS FA, GIBBS EL: *Atlas of Electroencephalography.* Vol. 2: *Epilepsy.* Reading, MA, Addison-Wesley, 1952.

GOLDENSOHN E: The relevance of secondary epileptogenesis to the treatment of epilepsy: Kindling and the mirror focus. *Epilepsia* 25(suppl 2):156, 1984.

GOWERS WR: *Epilepsy and Other Chronic Convulsive Diseases: Their Causes, Symptoms and Treatment.* New York, Dover, 1964. (Originally published in 1885; reprinted as Am Acad Neurol Reprint Series, vol 1.)

GUMNIT RJ: Intensive neurodiagnostic monitoring: role in the treatment of seizures. *Neurology* 36:1340, 1986.

HAUSER WA, KURLAND LT: The epidemiology of epilepsy in Rochester, Minnesota. *Epilepsia* 16:1, 1975.

HEINEMANN U, LUX HD, GUTNICK MJ: Extracellular free calcium and potassium during paroxysmal activity in the cerebral cortex of the cat. *Exp Brain Res* 27:237, 1977.

HERZOG AG, SEIBEL MM, SCHOMER OL et al: Reproductive endocrine disorders in men with partial seizures of temporal lobe origin. *Arch Neurol* 43:347, 1986.

JAGER-ROMAN E, DEICHL A, JAKOB S et al: Fetal growth, major malformations, and minor anomalies in infants born to women receiving valproic acid. *J Pediatrics* 108:997, 1986.

JANZ D: Antiepileptic drugs and pregnancy-altered utilization patterns and teratogenesis. *Epilepsia* 23(suppl 1):553, 1982.

KUTT H: Interactions between anticonvulsants and other commonly prescribed drugs. *Epilepsia* 25(suppl 2):188, 1984.

LANDAU WM, KLEFFNER FR: Syndrome of acquired aphasia with convulsive disorder in children. *Neurology* 7:523, 1957.

LENNOX MA: Febrile convulsions in childhood. *Am J Dis Child* 78:868, 1949.

LENNOX W, LENNOX MA: *Epilepsy and Related Disorders.* Boston, Little, Brown, 1960.

LINDVALL O, NILSSON B: Cerebellar atrophy following phenytoin intoxication. *Ann Neurol* 16:258, 1984.

MENDEZ MF, CUMMINGS JL, BENSON DF: Depression in epilepsy. Significance and phenomenology. *Arch Neurol* 43:766, 1986.

METRAKOS K, METRAKOS JD: Genetics of convulsive disorders. II. Genetic and electroencephalographic studies in centrencephalic epilepsy. *Neurology* 11:474, 1961.

NIEDERMEYER E: *Epilepsy Guide.* Baltimore, Urban and Schwarzenberg, 1983.

NORMAN RN, SANDRY S, CORSELLIS JAN: The nature and origin of patho-anatomical change in the epileptic brain, in Vinken PJ, Bruyn GW (eds): *Handbook of Clinical Neurology.* Amsterdam, North-Holland, 1974, vol 15, pp 611–620.

OUNSTED C, LINDSAY J, NORMAN RA: *Biological Factors in Temporal Lobe Epilepsy, Clinics in Developmental Medicine,* vol 22. London, Heineman/Spastic Society, 1966.

PEDLEY TA: The pathophysiology of focal epilepsy: Neurophysiological considerations. *Ann Neurol* 3:2, 1978.

PEDLEY TA: Discontinuing antiepileptic drugs. *N Engl J Med* 318:982, 1988.

PENFIELD W: Ablation of abnormal cortex in cerebral palsy. *J Neurol Neurosurg Psychiatry* 15:73, 1952.

PENFIELD W, JASPER HH: *Epilepsy and Functional Anatomy of the Human Brain.* Boston, Little, Brown, 1954.

PENFIELD W, KRISTIANSEN K: *Epileptic Seizure Patterns.* Springfield, Ill, Charles C Thomas, 1951.

PENRY JK, DALY DD (eds): *Complex Partial Seizures and Their Treatment.* New York, Raven Press, 1975.

PENRY JK, PORTER RV, DREIFUSS FE: Simultaneous recording of absence seizures with video tape and electroencephalography. *Brain* 98:427, 1975.

PINCUS JH, TUCKER GJ: *Behavioral Neurology.* 3rd ed. London, Oxford University Press, 1985.

PLUM F, HOWSE DC, DUFFY TE: Metabolic effects of seizures. *Res Publ Assoc Res Nerv Ment Dis* 53:141, 1974.

PORTER RJ: *Epilepsy. 100 Elementary Principles.* Philadelphia, WB Saunders, 1984.

RASMUSSEN T: Cortical resection in the treatment of focal epilepsy, in Purpura DT et al (eds): *Neurosurgical Management of the Epilepsies: Advances in Neurology,* vol 8. New York, Raven Press, 1975, p 139.

RODIN E, KATZ M, LENNOX C: Differences between patients with temporal lobe seizures and those with other forms of epileptic attacks. *Epilepsia* 17:313, 1976.

RODIN E, SCHMALTZ S: The Bear-Fedio personality inventory and temporal lobe epilepsy. *Neurology* 34:591, 1984.

ROCCA WA, SHARBROUGH FW, HAUSER A et al: Risk factors for complex partial seizures: A population-based case-control study. *Ann Neurol* 21:22, 1987.

SALCMAN M, DEFENDINI R, CORRELL J, GILMAN S: Neuropathological changes in cerebellar biopsies in epileptic patients. *Ann Neurol* 3:10, 1978.

SCHEIBEL ME, SCHEIBEL AB: Hippocampal pathology in temporal lobe epilepsy: A Golgi survey, in Brazier MAB (ed): *Epilepsy: Its Phenomena in Man.* New York, Academic Press, 1973, pp 315–357.

SCHMIDT D, EINICKE I, HAENEL F: The influence of seizure type on the efficacy of plasma concentrations of phenytoin, phenobarbital, and carbamazepine. *Arch Neurol* 43:262, 1986.

SCHMIDT RP, WILDER BJ: *Epilepsy.* Philadelphia, Davis, 1968.

SCHOMER DL: Partial epilepsy. *N Engl J Med* 309:536, 1983.

STEVENS JR: Psychiatric implications of psychomotor epilepsy. *Arch Gen Psychiatry* 14:461, 1966.

SUTHERLAND JM, EADIE MJ: *The Epilepsies.* London, Churchill Livingstone, 1980.

THOMAS JE, REGAN TJ, KLASS DW: Epilepsia partialis continua: A review of 32 cases. *Arch Neurol* 34:266, 1977.

TODT H: The late prognosis of epilepsy in childhood: results of a prospective follow-up study. *Epilepsia* 25:137, 1984.

TRIMBLE MR: Personality disturbances in epilepsy. *Neurology* 33:1332, 1983.

TSUBOI T: Genetic aspects of epilepsy. *Folia Psychiatr Neurol Jpn* 34:215, 1980.

VAN BUREN JM, AJMONE-MARSAN C, MATSUGA N, SADOWSKY D: Surgery of temporal lobe epilepsy, in Purpura DT et al (eds): *Neurosurgical Management of the Epilepsies: Advances in Neurology,* vol 8. New York, Raven Press, 1975, p 155.

VOLPE JJ: *Neurology of the Newborn,* 2nd ed. Philadelphia, WB Saunders, 1986.

WILLIAMS RS, FERRANTI RJ, CAVINESS VS JR: The Golgi rapid method in clinical neuropathology: The morphologic consequences of suboptimal fixation. *J Neuropath Exper Neurol* 37:13, 1978.

WOODBURY DM, PENRY JK, PIPPENGER CE (eds): *Antiepileptic Drugs,* 2nd ed. New York, Raven Press, 1982.

WRIGHT GDS, McLELLAN DL, BRICE JG: A double-blind trial of chronic cerebellar stimulation in twelve patients with severe epilepsy. *J Neurol Neurosurg Psychiatry* 47:769, 1984.

WYLLIE E, LUDES H, MORRIS HH et al: The lateralizing significance of versive head and eye movements during epileptic seizures. *Neurology* 36:606, 1212, 1986.

CHAPTER 16

COMA AND RELATED DISORDERS OF CONSCIOUSNESS

In hospital neurology the clinical analysis of unresponsive and comatose patients becomes a practical necessity. There is always an urgency about such medical problems—a need to determine the underlying disease process and the direction in which it is evolving and to protect the brain against more serious or irreversible damage. When called upon, the attending physician must therefore be fully prepared to implement a systematic investigation of the comatose patient; the need for prompt therapeutic and diagnostic action allows no time for deliberate, scholarly investigation.

Some idea of the dimensions of this category of neurologic disease can be obtained from published statistics. In two large municipal hospitals it was estimated that as many as 3 percent of total admissions to an emergency ward were due to diseases that had caused coma (Table 16-1). Although these statistics were gathered many years ago, they serve to emphasize the frequency and gravity of these diseases.

The terms *consciousness, confusion, stupor, unconsciousness,* and *coma* have been endowed with so many different meanings that it is almost impossible to avoid ambiguity in their usage. They are not strictly medical terms, but literary, philosophic, and psychologic ones as well. The word *consciousness* is the most difficult of all. William James once remarked that everyone knows what consciousness is until he attempts to define it. To the psychologist, consciousness denotes a state of awareness of one's self and one's environment. Knowledge of one's self includes all "feelings, attitudes and emotions, impulses, volitions, and the active or striving aspects of conduct" (English)—in short, an awareness of all one's own mental functioning, particularly of the cognitive processes. These can be judged only by the patients' verbal accounts of their introspections and, indirectly, by their actions. Physicians, being practical people for the most part, have learned to place greater confidence in their observations of the patient's behavior and reactions to overt stimuli than in what the patient says. For this reason they usually give the term

consciousness its commonest and simplest meaning, viz., the state of the patient's awareness of self and environment. This narrow definition has another advantage in that the word *unconsciousness* is the exact opposite—a state of *unawareness of self and environment* or a suspension of those mental activities by which people are made aware of themselves and their environment. To add to the ambiguity, psychoanalysts have given the word *unconscious* a still different meaning; for them it is a repository of impulses and memories of previous experiences that cannot immediately be recalled to the conscious mind.

Much more could be said about the history of our ideas concerning consciousness, and the theoretic problems with regard to its definition, but this would serve no practical purpose. The interested reader is referred to the discussion of consciousness by Frederiks, in the *Handbook of Clinical Neurology* (see References).

DESCRIPTION OF STATES OF NORMAL AND IMPAIRED CONSCIOUSNESS

The following definitions, though probably not acceptable to all psychologists, are of service to clinical medicine, and they will provide the student with a convenient terminology for describing the state of awareness and responsiveness of his patients.

Normal Consciousness This is the condition of the normal person when awake. In this state the individual is fully responsive to stimuli and indicates by behavior and speech the same awareness of self and environment as the examiner. This normal state may fluctuate during the course of the day from keen alertness or deep concentration with a marked constriction of the field of attention, to mild general inattentiveness and drowsiness.

Inattention, Confusion, and Clouding of Consciousness In these conditions the patient does not take into account all elements of the immediate environment. These states always imply, as does delirium, an element of sensorial clouding or imperceptiveness and distractibility. The term *confusion* lacks precision, but in a general way it denotes an inability to think with customary speed and clarity. Here the difficulty is to define *thinking*, a term that refers variably to problem solving or to coherence of ideas about a subject. The patient may fail in either way for several different reasons, viz., inattentiveness, disorder of language, forgetfulness, apathy or abulia (see Chap. 19).

Severely confused and inattentive persons are usually unable to do more than carry out the simplest commands. Few if any thought processes are in operation. Their speech may be limited to a few words or phrases, or they may be voluble. They are unaware of much that goes on around them, do not grasp their immediate situation, and are usually incontinent. Moderately confused persons can carry on a simple conversation for short periods of time, but their thinking is slow and incoherent, and they are unable to stay on one topic and to inhibit inappropriate responses. Usually they are disoriented in time and place. They are distractible and at the mercy of every stimulus. Occasionally, hallucinatory-delusional experiences impart a psychotic cast to the clinical picture, obscuring the deficit in attention. Periods of irritability and excitability may alternate with drowsiness and impaired vigilance. Tremor, asterixis, and myoclonus often mar motor performance. Sequences of movement also betray impersistence. In mild degrees of confusion the disorder may be so slight that it can be overlooked unless the examiner searches for alterations in the patient's behavior and conversation. The patient may even be roughly oriented as to time and place, with only occasional irrelevant remarks betraying an incoherence of thinking.

Patients with mild or moderately severe confusion can be subjected to psychologic testing. The degree of confusion often varies from one time of day to another. It tends to be least pronounced in the morning and most pronounced in the evening or night, when environmental cues are less clear-cut and the patient is fatigued. Many events that happen to the confused patient leave no trace in memory; in fact, the capacity to recall events that had occurred in any given period is one of the most delicate tests of mental clarity. However, careful analysis will show the defect to be one of inadequate perception or registration of information, rather than a fault in retentive memory.

In some medical writings the terms *delirium* and *confusion* are used interchangeably, the former connoting nothing more than a confusional state in which hyperactivity is prominent. However, the vivid hallucinations that characterize delirious states, the inaccessibility of patients to events other than those to which they are reacting at any one moment, their extreme agitation, their tendency to tremble, startle easily, and convulse, and the signs of overactivity of the autonomic nervous system suggest a cerebral disorder of distinctive type. The clearest evidence of the relationship of inattention, confusion, stupor, and coma is that patients may pass through each of these states as they become comatose or emerge from coma. The authors have not observed such a relationship between coma and delirium, with the possible exception of hepatic stupor and coma, which may be *preceded* by a brief period of delirium. No doubt, in certain acute mental syndromes the distinction between delirium and other confusional states is difficult to make, since some of the attributes of delirium may be lacking. These problems are elaborated in Chap. 19.

At times a patient with certain types of aphasia, especially jargon aphasia, may create the impression of

Table 16-1
Relative incidence of diseases which cause coma

Disease	Boston City Hospital series (clinical cases)*			Cook County series+ (autopsied cases)	
	No.	Percent	Mortality, percent	No.	Percent
Alcoholism	690	59.1	2.0	16	4.6
Trauma	152	13.0	31.5	94	27.5
Cerebral vascular disease	118	10.0	77.0	120	35.0
Poisoning	33	3.0	9.0		
Epilepsy	28	2.4	0		
Diabetes	20	1.7	55.0	8	2.3
Bacterial meningitis	20	1.7	100.0	29	8.5
Pneumonia	20	1.7	90.0	18	5.4
Cardiac decompensation	17	1.4	70.0		
Neurosyphilis	7	0.6	0	4	1.2
Uremia	7	0.6	100.0	37	10.9
Eclampsia	7	0.6	68.4		
Miscellaneous	48	1.1	75.0	16	4.6
Total	1167	100.0		342	100.0

*Reported by P Solomon, CD Aring, *Am J Med Sci* 188:805, 1934.
+ Reported by B Holcomb, *JAMA* 77:2112, 1921.
Note: These figures were collected in 1933 before the introduction of most of the sulfonamide drugs or antibiotics.

being confused, but close observation will reveal that the disorder is confined to the sphere of language and that behavior is otherwise natural and appropriate to the situation.

Stupor In this state mental and physical activity are reduced to a minimum. Patients can be roused only by vigorous and repeated stimuli, at which time they open their eyes, look at the examiner, and do not appear to be unconscious; response to spoken commands is either absent or slow and inadequate. Tremulousness of movement, coarse twitching of muscles, restless or stereotyped motor activity, and grasping and sucking reflexes are observed frequently in such patients, and tendon and plantar reflexes may or may not be altered, depending on the way in which the underlying disease has affected the nervous system. In psychiatry, *stupor* refers also to a state in which the perception of sensory stimuli is presumably normal; impressions of the external world are normally received but activity is suspended or marked by negativism, e.g., catatonic schizophrenia.

Coma The patient who appears to be asleep and is at the same time incapable of sensing or responding to external stimuli and inner needs is in a state of coma. Coma may vary in degree, and in its deepest stages no reaction of any kind is obtainable; corneal, pupillary, pharyngeal, tendon, and plantar reflexes are all absent. With lesser degrees of coma, pupillary reactions, reflex ocular movements, and other brainstem reflexes are preserved, and there may or may not be extensor rigidity of the limbs and opisthotonos—signs which, as Sherrington showed, indicate decerebration. Respirations are often slow or rapid, periodic, or deranged in other ways (see further on). In still lighter stages, referred to as *semicoma,* most of the above reflexes can be elicited, and the plantar reflexes may be either flexor or extensor (Babinski sign). Moreover, vigorous stimulation of the patient or distention of the bladder may cause a stirring or moaning and a quickening of respirations.

These physical signs vary somewhat, depending on the cause of coma. For example, patients with alcoholic intoxication may be unresponsive to noxious stimuli and areflexic, even when respirations and other vital signs are not threatened. Drug overdose rarely produces decerebrate rigidity, no matter what the degree of coma. The signs of depth of coma and stupor, when compared in serial examinations, are most useful in assessing the direction in which the disease is evolving.

Thus, in terms of wakefulness and arousal, states of normal alertness, drowsiness, confusion and inattentiveness, stupor and coma represent a continuum. Some clinicians declare that distinctions between these states are of little semiologic significance. The authors disagree. If one employs the terms in conformity with the above definitions,

they provide clues to the underlying disease process and to prognosis. Coma is always a potentially dangerous condition, often with a fatal outcome.

RELATIONSHIP OF SLEEP TO COMA

Persons in sleep give little evidence of being aware of themselves or their environment; in this respect they are unconscious. Sleep shares a number of other features with the pathologic states of drowsiness, stupor, and coma. These include yawning, closure of the eyelids, cessation of blinking and swallowing, upward deviation or divergence or roving movements of the eyes, loss of muscular tone, decrease or loss of tendon reflexes and even the presence of Babinski signs, irregular respirations, sometimes Cheyne-Stokes in type, and occasionally incontinence of urine. Upon being awakened from a deep sleep a person may be confused for a few minutes, as every physician knows. Nevertheless, sleeping persons may still respond to unaccustomed stimuli and at times are capable of some mental activity in the form of dreams that leave their traces in memory, thus differing from persons in stupor or coma. The most important difference, of course, is that persons in sleep, when stimulated, can be roused to normal consciousness. There are important physiologic differences as well. Cerebral oxygen uptake does not decrease during sleep as it often does in coma, and the EEG, which may be similar in sleep and in coma, is much more often different, as will be indicated later in this chapter and in Chap. 18. The anatomic basis for these differences is not clear.

THE PERSISTENT VEGETATIVE STATE, PSEUDOCOMA, AND AKINETIC MUTISM

With increasing refinements in the treatment of severe cerebral injury, more and more patients who formerly would have died have survived for indefinite periods, without regaining any meaningful mental function. For the first week or two after the cerebral injury these patients are in a state of deep coma. Then they begin to open their eyes, at first in response to painful stimuli and later spontaneously and for increasingly prolonged periods. The patient may blink in response to threat. Intermittently the eyes move from side to side, seemingly following objects or fixating momentarily on the physician or a family member, and giving the erroneous impression of cognition. However, the patient remains inattentive, does not speak, and shows no signs of awareness of the environment or inner need;

responsiveness is limited to primitive postural and reflex movements of the limbs. In brief, there is arousal or wakefulness, without awareness or responsiveness. The EEG, which originally may have been isoelectric, approaches normality, even showing alpha rhythm and sleep patterns. If lasting, this syndrome is most appropriately referred to as the *persistent vegetative state* (Jennett and Plum).

The states of coma described above and the persistent vegetative state must be clearly distinguished from a clinical state in which there is little or no disturbance of awareness (consciousness), but only an inability of the patient to respond adequately. The latter state is referred to variously as the *locked-in* syndrome, *coma vigile*, or the *deefferented* state. We prefer the term *pseudocoma*. It is due most often to a lesion of the basis pontis. Such a lesion spares both the somatosensory pathways and the ascending neuronal system responsible for arousal and wakefulness, but interrupts the corticobulbar and corticospinal pathways, depriving the patient of speech and the capacity to respond in any other way. Severe degrees of motor neuropathy (e.g., Guillain-Barré syndrome) or periodic paralysis may have a similar effect. One could logically refer to this state as *akinetic mutism* insofar as the patient is akinetic (motionless) and mute, but this term was originally used by Cairns in a somewhat different sense—to describe a patient who appeared to be awake but was unresponsive (actually Cairns' patient was able to answer in whispered monosyllables). Following repeated evacuation of a third ventricular cyst, the patient would regain consciousness but was unable to remember any of the events that had occurred when she was in the akinetic-mute state. Unfortunately this term has been applied to yet another group of patients who are silent and inert as a result of bilateral frontal lobe lesions, despite the integrity of motor and sensory pathways; lacking to an extreme degree in these latter patients is the psychic drive or impulse to action (abulia). Unlike Cairns' patient, they register most of what is happening about them and form memories.

It is apparent from these remarks that the various states of impaired consciousness shade into one another and are rapidly changeable. Hence there may be considerable imprecision surrounding their use. The student would be better advised to supplement arbitrary designations such as *coma* and *akinetic mutism* with simple descriptive language, indicating whether the patient appears awake or asleep or drowsy or alert, and noting the degree of his patient's awareness of his surroundings and the nature of the responses to a variety of designated stimuli.

BRAIN DEATH

In the late 1950s European neurologists called attention to a state of coma in which the brain was irreversibly damaged and had ceased to function but in which pulmonary and cardiac function could still be maintained by artificial means. Mollaret and Goulon referred to this condition as *coma dépassé* (a state beyond coma). It has also been called *irreversible coma, brain death,* and *cerebral death,* terms that are now used interchangeably. The concept that a person is dead if the brain is dead and that death of the brain may precede the cessation of cardiac function posed a number of important ethical, legal, and social problems as well as medical ones. The various aspects of brain death have been the subject of close study by several professional committees, which have provided rather clear and generally accepted guidelines for determining that the brain is dead.

The central considerations in the diagnosis of brain death are (1) the absence of cerebral functions, (2) the absence of brainstem functions, including spontaneous respiration, and (3) the irreversibility of the state. To this is usually added evidence of catastrophic brain disease (trauma, cardiac arrest, apoplexy, etc.).

The absence of cerebral function is judged by the total lack of spontaneous movement and motor and vocal response to all visual, auditory, and cutaneous stimulation. Spinal reflexes may persist in some cases.

The absence of brainstem function is judged by absence of spontaneous eye movements; midposition of the eyes; lack of response to oculocephalic and caloric testing; dilated, fixed pupils; paralysis of bulbar musculature (no facial movement or gag, corneal, or sucking reflexes); no decerebrate reponses to noxious stimuli; and absence of respiratory movements. For practical purposes, absolute apnea is present if the patient makes no effort to override the respirator for at least 15 min. As a final test, the patient can be disconnected from the respirator long enough (a few minutes) to ensure that arterial P_{CO_2} rises above the threshold for stimulation of respiration.

The EEG is a valuable indicator of cerebral death and most institutions require proof of electrocerebral silence (flat or isoelectric EEG), which is considered to be present if there is no change in electrical potentials of more than 2 μV during two 30-min recordings taken 6 h apart. It needs to be emphasized that cerebral unresponsivity and a flat EEG do not always signify brain death but that both may occur, and be completely reversible, in states of profound hypothermia and intoxication with sedative-hypnotic drugs.

When examination has disclosed that all brain functions are absent, it should be repeated in 6 h, to confirm that the state is irreversible. If an adequate history of cerebral disease is lacking and comprehensive screening procedures for drugs are not available, an observation period of 72 h may be required to assess reversibility. Although they are rarely practical, cerebral perfusion studies, demonstrating complete cessation of intracranial circulation, provide absolute evidence of brain death.

A task force for the determination of brain death in children has recommended the adoption of the same criteria as for adults. Because of the great difficulty in evaluating the status of nervous function in relation to perinatal insults, the task force suggests that a diagnosis of brain death not be made before the seventh postnatal day and that the period of observation be extended to 48 h. As with adults, the main problem is one of eliminating the possibility of reversible brain dysfunction from toxins, drugs, hypothermia, and hypotension.

THE ELECTROENCEPHALOGRAM AND DISTURBANCES OF CONSCIOUSNESS

One of the most delicate confirmations of the fact that the states of impaired consciousness are expressions of neurophysiologic changes is the altered electroencephalogram (EEG). With sleep the EEG shows a number of characteristic changes, which are described and illustrated in Chap. 18. Similarly, some alteration in brain waves occurs in all disturbances of consciousness except the milder degrees of confusion. This alteration usually consists of a disorganization of the EEG pattern, which shows random, slow waves of high voltage in certain stages of confusion; more regular, slow, 2- to 3-per-second waves of high voltage in stupor and semicoma; and slow waves or even suppression of all organized electrical activity (brain death) in the deep coma of hypoxia and ischemia—the so-called brain death syndrome. The EEGs of deep sleep and of light coma resemble each other. In some deeply comatose patients the EEG may show diffuse 8- to 12-Hz activity which may be mistaken for physiologic alpha rhythm. However, the former pattern (so-called alpha coma) is not limited to the posterior cerebral regions and displays no reactivity to sensory stimuli. This alpha-like activity during coma has no localizing significance and does not necessarily have a grave prognosis, as was originally proposed (Iragui and McCutchen).

It should be emphasized that not all diseases that cause confusion, stupor, and coma have the same effect on the EEG. Some, such as barbiturate intoxication, may cause an increase in frequency and amplitude of the brain waves. In epilepsy the disturbance of consciousness is usually attended by paroxysms of sharp waves or "spikes" (fast waves of high amplitude) or by the characteristic alternating slow waves and spikes of petit mal. Other diseases, such as hepatic coma, characteristically cause a decrease in frequency and an increase in amplitude of brain waves and the appearance of bilaterally synchronous triphasic waves. Whether all metabolic diseases of the brain induce similar changes in the EEG has not been determined. Probably

there are differences among them, some of which may be significant (see Chap. 2).

MORBID ANATOMY AND PHYSIOLOGY OF COMA

In recent times there has been some clarification and amplification of earlier neuropathologic observations that the smallest lesions associated with protracted coma are always to be found in the thalamus and upper part of the midbrain. The essence of more recent neurophysiologic studies is that an ascending series of destructive lesions of the spinal cord, medulla, cerebellum, and lower pons has no effect on the state of consciousness, until the level of the upper pons is reached. Destruction of the high brainstem reticular formation invariably induces states of prolonged unresponsiveness, accompanied by a slow, synchronized EEG, whereas stimulation by an electrode placed in the reticular formation causes a drowsy or sleeping animal to become suddenly alert and its EEG to change correspondingly (desynchronization). Furthermore, the state of unresponsiveness induced by destruction of the reticular formation cannot be reversed by strong sensory stimulation, even if the primary sensory pathways from the periphery via the thalamus to the cerebral cortex are preserved. Similarly, as anesthetic agents abolish consciousness, they are found to suppress the activity of the reticular activating system, without interfering, at least at certain stages, with the transmission of somatosensory impulses to the cerebral cortex.

The anatomic boundaries of the reticular activating system of the upper brainstem are indistinct. It is interspersed throughout the paramedian regions of the upper pontine and midbrain tegmentum, the septal region, and the hypothalamus, and includes the functionally related medial, intralaminar, and reticular nuclei of the thalamus. In the brainstem, nuclei of the reticular formation receive collaterals from the direct spinothalamic pathways and project not just to the sensory cortex of the parietal lobe, as do the thalamic relay nuclei for somatic sensation, but to the whole of the cerebral cortex. Sensory stimulation, it would seem, then, has the double effect of conveying to the brain information about the outside world and also of activating those parts of the nervous system on which consciousness depends. The cerebral cortex not only receives impulses from the ascending reticular activating system but also modulates this incoming information via corticofugal connections to the reticular formation.

These new data are in line with the older ideas of Herbert Spencer and Hughlings Jackson—that the diencephalon and cerebral cortex always function together, as a unit, and represent the highest level of integrative nervous activity, called *centrencephalic* by Penfield. Though the anatomic details of the reticular activating system have yet to be worked out and the physiology is more complicated than this simple formulation would suggest, it nevertheless, as a working idea, makes some of the following neuropathologic observations more comprehensible.

The study of a large number of human cases in which coma preceded death by several days has disclosed two major types of lesion. (1) In one group, a readily discernible lesion such as a tumor, abscess, intracerebral, subarachnoid, subdural, or epidural hemorrhage, massive infarct, or meningitis was demonstrable. Usually the lesion involved only a portion of the cortex and white matter, leaving much of the cerebrum intact. Rarely, it was located in the thalamus or midbrain, which would make the coma understandable, but in the other instances the coma was related to a temporal lobe-tentorial herniation with compression, ischemia, and secondary hemorrhage in the midbrain and subthalamic region, or with distortion or displacement of these parts (see Chap. 31). A detailed clinical record will show the coma to have coincided with these herniations and displacements. Exceptionally, widespread bilateral damage to the cortex and subcortical white matter was found—the result of bilateral infarcts or hemorrhages, viral encephalitis, hypoxia, or ischemia—without visible thalamic or midbrain lesions. Presumably, the coma in these cases was the result of complete interruption of the corticofugal impulses that normally sustain diencephalic and midbrain reticular activity. Only if the cerebral lesions were massive was conciousness markedly impaired. (2) In the second group (larger than the first) no lesion was visible to the naked eye. In some instances the grossly normal brain revealed a characteristic microscopic change, which may be hepatic coma. Usually the microscopic lesions were too diffuse for clinicoanatomic correlation. Often no abnormality was divulged by any technique of pathology; the lesion, caused by a metabolic or toxic state, was presumably subcellular or molecular.

Thus pathologic changes are compatible with physiologic deductions—that the state of prolonged coma correlates with lesions of all parts of the cortical-diencephalic system of neurons, but it is only in the upper brainstem that the coma-producing lesions may be small and discrete.

MECHANISMS WHEREBY CONSCIOUSNESS IS DISTURBED IN DISEASE

It is not possible to identify all the different mechanisms by which consciousness is disturbed. Already several ways

in which the mesencephalic-diencephalic-cortical systems are deranged have been identified; there are many others.

In a number of disease processes there is direct interference with the metabolic activities of the nerve cells in the cerebral cortex and the central nuclear masses of the brain. Hypoxia, hypoglycemia, hyper- and hypo-osmolar states, acidosis, alkalosis, hypokalemia, hyperammonemia, and deficiencies of thiamine, nicotinic acid, vitamin B_{12}, pantothenic acid, and pyridoxine are well-known examples (see Chap. 40 and Table 40-1). The relevant point for our discussion is that cerebral metabolism is reduced in all metabolic disorders leading to coma, whereas cerebral blood flow is changed little or not at all. Oxygen values below 2 mL/min per 100 g brain tissue are incompatible with an alert state. In hypoglycemia the cerebral blood flow is normal or above normal, whereas the cerebral metabolic rate is diminished, owing to deficiency of substrate. In thiamine and vitamin B_{12} deficiency the cerebral blood flow is normal or slightly diminished, and the cerebral metabolic rate is diminished, presumably because of insufficiency of coenzymes. Extremes of body temperature (above 41°C or below 30°C) probably induce coma through a nonspecific effect on the metabolic activity of neurons. Diabetic acidosis, uremia, hepatic coma, and the coma of systemic infections are examples of endogenous intoxications. The identity of the toxin(s) responsible for coma is not entirely known. In diabetes, acetone bodies (acetoacetic acid, β-hydroxybutyric acid, and acetone) are present in high concentration, and in uremia there is probably accumulation of dialyzable toxins, perhaps phenolic derivatives of the aromatic amino acids. In both conditions "dehydration" and serum acidosis may also play an important role. In many cases of hepatic coma, elevation of blood NH_3 to levels five to six times normal has been found. Lactic acidosis may affect the brain by lowering arterial blood pH to less than 7.0. The impairment of consciousness that accompanies pulmonary insufficiency is related to both hypoxia and hypercapnia, the elevated carbon dioxide tension probably being the main factor (see Table 39-1). In hyponatremia (≤120 meq/L) from whatever cause, neuronal dysfunction is due to the intracellular movement of water, leading to neuronal swelling and loss of potassium chloride from the cells. The mode of action of bacterial toxins is unknown.

Drugs such as alcohol, barbiturates, bromides, phenytoin, alcohol, glutethimide, and phenothiazines induce coma by their direct effects on neuronal membranes in the cerebrum and diencephalon. Others such as methyl alcohol, ethylene glycol, and paralydehyde act by producing a metabolic acidosis. Many additional pharmacologic agents have no direct action on the nervous system but lead to coma through the mechanism of circulatory collapse and inadequate cerebral blood flow. Although the coma of toxic and metabolic diseases usually evolves through a state of drowsiness, confusion, and stupor (and the reverse sequence occurs during emergence from coma), each disease imparts its own characteristic clinical features. Probably this means that each disease has a distinctive mechanism and that the topography is somewhat different from one disease to another.

A critical decline in blood pressure, usually to a systolic level below 70 mmHg, affects neural structures by causing a decrease in cerebral blood flow and, secondarily, in cerebral metabolic rate. If the decline in blood pressure is abrupt, the corresponding clinical picture is one of syncope, i.e., physical weakness preceding and following the loss of consciousness, the whole process being promptly reversible (Chap. 17).

The sudden, violent, and excessive neuronal discharge that characterizes *epilepsy* is a common coma-producing mechanism. Usually focal seizure activity has little effect on consciousness until it spreads from one side of the brain (and body) to the other. Coma then ensues, presumably because the spread of the seizure discharge to central neuronal structures paralyzes their function. Other types of seizure in which consciousness is interrupted from the very beginning are believed by some neurologists to originate in the diencephalon.

Concussion exemplifies still another special pathophysiologic mechanism of coma. In "blunt" head injury it has been shown that there is an enormous increase in intracranial pressure, on the order of 200 to 700 lb/in^2, lasting a few thousandths of a second. Either the vibration set up in the skull and transmitted to the brain or the sudden marked increase in intracranial pressure was for many years thought to be the basis of the abrupt paralysis of nervous function that follows head injury. That the increased pressure may be the main factor was suggested by the experimental observation that raising the intraventricular pressure to a level approaching diastolic blood pressure abolishes all vital functions. As pointed out in Chap. 34, a blow to the head imparts a swirling motion of the brain with torque of the upper brainstem; this is the mechanism favored by most neurologists.

As was pointed out above, large destructive and space-consuming lesions of the cerebrum, such as hemorrhage, tumor, abscess, or infarction impair consciousness in two ways. One is by direct extension of the lesion into the diencephalon and midbrain. The other, far more frequent, is by lateral and downward displacement of the upper brainstem, with or without herniation of the medial part of the temporal lobe (uncus, hippocampus) through the opening in the tentorium and crushing of the upper midbrain against the opposite free edge of the tentorium or causing ischemia at this level of the neuraxis (see Chap. 30). Plum and Posner subdivide the brainstem displacements by supratentorial masses into two groups: one, a central syndrome

with downward displacement and bilateral compression, and the other, a unilateral displacement with uncal herniation. In their view, the central syndrome takes the form of a rostral-caudal deterioration of function, from diencephalon to medulla, reflected clinically by a sequence of disordered consciousness and respiratory, ocular, and motor signs. More specifically there is first confusion, apathy, and drowsiness, and often Cheyne-Stokes respiration; then the pupils become small and react very little to light; doll's-head eye movements are elicitable as are deviations of the eyes in response to cold water caloric testing. The fast component of the response is impaired or absent, however; bilateral Babinski signs can be detected early, and later grasp reflexes and decorticate postures appear. These signs give way to a downward gradient of brainstem signs—coma, central hyperventilation, medium-sized fixed pupils, bilateral decerebrate postures, loss of oculovestibular responses, slow irregular breathing and death—which are much the same as the late effects of uncal herniation. The uncal syndrome differs mainly, they believe, in that drowsiness in the early stages is accompanied by unilateral pupillary dilatation.

Our own experience does not fully substantiate this distinction between the two syndromes, and seldom have we been able to follow such an orderly sequence of neural dysfunction from the diencephalic to medullary level. With lateral shift and uncal herniation one sometimes observes smallness of the pupils as drowsiness develops, rather than ipsilateral pupillary dilatation. Or the contralateral pupil dilates before the ipsilateral one. And it has not been at all clear that the dilatation of one pupil is always due to trapping or compression of the oculomotor nerve by the herniated uncus. Involvement of the third nerve nucleus or its fibers of exit appears to be responsible in some cases. Ropper and Shafran who studied 12 patients with brain edema and lateral diencephalic-mesencephalic shifts due to hemispheral infarcts found that four of their patients did not have ipsilateral pupillary enlargement; in one the pupillary enlargement was contralateral; and in three the pupils were symmetric. Cheyne-Stokes breathing was frequent and early. In one patient, the first motor sign was an ipsilateral decerebrate rigidity rather than decorticate posturing; most of the patients had bilateral Babinski signs. These signs often progressed to deep coma and decerebration within hours, and they fluctuated widely, worsening with waves of high intracranial pressure (Lundberg waves). Brain death supervened in seven of these 12 patients within 11 days, but severe alterations of brain tissue in these cases made clinicopathologic correlations difficult.

We favor the notion of a single mechanism of lateral displacement, often but not necessarily with temporal lobe herniation, causing a derangement of subthalamic, mesencephalic, and upper pontine tegmental function, probably due to ischemia. This view has been supported by the recent observations of Ropper, who has used CT scanning (and subsequently MRI) to study the structural displacements in patients with acute hemispheral mass lesions. He found that early disturbances of consciousness (drowsiness and stupor) could be related to the degree of lateral displacement of high brainstem structures (judged by distortions of the basal cisterns and shifts in the position of the pineal body and, occasionally, the septum pellucidum), in the apparent absence of transtentorial herniation. This hypothesis will be carefully studied by modern imaging techniques.

CLINICAL APPROACH TO THE COMATOSE PATIENT

It is important to repeat that coma is not a disease per se but is always a symptomatic expression of an underlying disease. Sometimes the underlying disease is perfectly obvious, as with severe cranial trauma. All too often, however, the patient is brought to the hospital in a state of coma, and little or no information is immediately available. The clinical problem must then be scrutinized from many angles. To do this efficiently, the physician must have a broad knowledge of disease and a methodical approach that leaves none of the common and treatable causes of coma unexplored.

When the comatose patient is seen for the first time, one must quickly make sure that the patient's airway is clear. It is equally important to ascertain that the patient is not in shock (circulatory collapse) and, if trauma has occurred, that there is no bleeding from a wound or ruptured organ (e.g., spleen or liver). If shock or bleeding has supervened, certain therapeutic measures (insertion of an endotracheal tube, administration of pressor agents, oxygen, blood, or glucose solutions, *after* drawing blood for glucose determinations) take precedence over diagnostic procedures. In the patient who has suffered a head injury there may be a fracture of the cervical vertebrae, in which case one must be cautious about moving the head and neck lest the spinal cord be inadvertently crushed. There must be an immediate inquiry as to the previous health of the patient, whether there had been a head injury or a convulsion, and the circumstances in which the person was found. The persons who accompany the comatose patient to the hospital should not be permitted to leave until they have been questioned.

From an initial survey many of the common types of disease causing coma, such as severe head injuries, alcoholic or other forms of drug intoxication, and hypertensive brain hemorrhage, are readily recognized. As can be seen in Table 16-1, which summarizes data from the Boston City and the Cook County Hospitals, the aforementioned disorders comprised about two-thirds of all cases of coma admitted to the emergency wards of those hospitals. In large university hospitals, which tend to attract the more obscure and difficult cases, the statistics are quite different. For example, in the series of Plum and Posner (Table 16-2), which resembles more that of the Massachusetts and Cleveland Metropolitan General Hospitals, only 113 of 500

Table 16-2
Final diagnosis in 500 patients admitted to hospital with "coma of unknown etiology"

Supratentorial mass lesions	101
Intracerebral hematoma	44
Subdural hematoma	26
Epidural hematoma	4
Cerebral infarct	9
Thalamic infarct	2
Brain tumor	7
Pituitary apoplexy	2
Brain abscess	6
Closed-head injury	1
Subtentorial lesions	65
Brainstem infarct	40
Pontine hemorrhage	11
Brainstem demyelination	1
Cerebellar hemorrhage	5
Cerebellar tumor	3
Cerebellar infarct	2
Cerebellar abscess	1
Posterior fossa subdural hemorrhage	1
Basilar migraine	1
Metabolic and other diffuse disorders	326
Anoxia or ischemia	87
Hepatic encephalopathy	17
Uremic encephalopathy	8
Pulmonary disease	3
Endocrine disorders (including diabetes)	12
Acid-base disorders	12
Temperature regulation	9
Nutritional	1
Nonspecific metabolic coma	1
Encephalomyelitis and encephalitis	14
Subarachnoid hemorrhage	13
Drug poisoning	149
Psychiatric disorders	8

Note: Listed here are only those patients in whom the initial diagnosis was uncertain and a final diagnosis was established. Thus, obvious poisonings and closed-head injuries are underrepresented.

Source: Plum and Posner.

patients proved to have cerebrovascular disease (60 of the 113 were cerebral, brainstem, and cerebellar hemorrhage), and only in 31 was coma the consequence of trauma (contusions, epidural and subdural hemorrhages). Indeed, all ''mass lesions,'' such as tumors, abscesses, hemorrhages, and infarcts, made up less than one-third of the coma-producing diseases. The majority were the result of exogenous and endogenous intoxications and hypoxia. Subarachnoid hemorrhage, meningitis, and encephalitis made up another 5 percent of the total. Thus the order is reversed, but still intoxication, stroke, and cranial trauma stand as the ''big three'' of coma-producing conditions.

DIAGNOSIS

Alterations in vital signs—temperature, pulse, respiratory rate, and blood pressure—are important aids in diagnosis. *Fever* is most often due to a systemic infection such as pneumonia, or to bacterial meningitis, and only rarely to a brain lesion that has disturbed the temperature-regulating centers. An excessively high body temperature (42 or 43°C) associated with dry skin should arouse the suspicion of heat stroke. *Hypothermia,* on the other hand, is frequently observed in patients with alcoholic or barbiturate intoxication, extracellular fluid deficit, peripheral circulatory failure, and myxedema.

Slow breathing points to morphine or barbiturate intoxication, and occasionally to hypothyroidism, whereas deep, rapid breathing suggests pneumonia, diabetic or uremic acidosis (Kussmaul respiration), pulmonary edema, or, rarely, to intracranial diseases that cause central neurogenic hyperventilation. The *rapid breathing* of pneumonia is often accompanied by an expiratory grunt, cyanosis, and fever. Diseases that elevate intracranial pressure or damage the brain often cause slow, irregular, or periodic (*Cheyne-Stokes*) breathing; the various disordered patterns of breathing and their clinical significance are described below with the neurologic examination of the stuporous or comatose patient.

The *pulse rate,* if exceptionally slow, should suggest heart block, or if combined with periodic breathing and hypertension, an increase in intracranial pressure. A rate of 140 per minute or more calls attention to the possibility of an ectopic cardiac rhythm with insufficiency of cerebral circulation. Marked hypertension is observed in patients with cerebral hemorrhage and hypertensive encephalopathy and, at times, in those with greatly increased intracranial pressure. Hypotension is the usual finding in the states of depressed consciousness that are due to diabetes, alcohol or barbiturate intoxication, internal hemorrhage, myocardial infarction, dissecting aortic aneurysm, gram-negative bacillary septicemia, and Addison disease.

Inspection of the skin may yield valuable information. Cyanosis of the lips and nail beds means inadequate

oxygenation. Cherry-red coloration indicates carbon monoxide poisoning. Multiple bruises, and in particular a bruise or boggy area in the scalp, bleeding or CSF leakage from an ear or the nose, or periorbital hemorrhage always raise the possibility of cranial fracture and intracranial trauma. Telangiectases and hyperemia of the face and conjunctivae are the usual stigmata of alcoholism; myxedema imparts a characteristic puffiness of the face. Marked pallor suggests internal hemorrhage. In pituitary hypoadrenalism the skin is sallow. A maculohemorrhagic rash indicates the possibility of meningococcal infection, staphylococcal endocarditis, typhus, or Rocky Mountain spotted fever. Pellagra may be recognized by the typical skin lesions of the face, arms, and legs. Excessive sweating suggests hypoglycemia or shock, and dry skin suggests diabetic acidosis or uremia. Skin turgor is reduced in dehydration. Blisters, sometimes hemorrhagic, may form over pressure points if the patient has been motionless for a time; such blisters are particularly characteristic of acute barbiturate poisoning.

The *odor of the breath* may provide a clue to the etiology of coma. The odor of alcohol is easily recognized (except for vodka, which is odorless). The spoiled-fruit odor of diabetic coma, the uriniferous odor of uremia, and the musty fetor of hepatic coma are distinctive enough to be identified by physicians who possess a keen sense of smell.

Neurologic examination of the stuporous or comatose patient, although limited in many ways, is of crucial importance. Simply watching the patient for a few minutes may yield considerable information about the functions of different parts of the nervous system. The predominant postures of the body, the presence or absence of spontaneous movements, the position of the head and eyes, and the rate, depth, and rhythm of respiration, should be noted. The state of responsiveness should then be estimated by noting the patient's reaction to calling his or her name, to simple commands, or to painful stimuli such as supraorbital or sternal pressure or pressure on knuckles or pinching the side of the neck or inner parts of the arms or thighs. By grading these stimuli, one may evaluate both the degree of unresponsiveness and changes from hour to hour in the course of the illness. Vocalization may persist in stupor and light coma and is the first response to be lost as coma deepens. Grimacing and deft avoidance movements of parts stimulated are preserved in light coma; their presence substantiates the integrity of corticobulbar and corticospinal tracts. The *Glasgow coma scale,* constructed originally as a quick and simple means of quantitating the responsiveness of patients with severe cerebral trauma, is equally useful in other acute coma-producing diseases (see Chap. 35).

It is usually possible to determine whether coma is accompanied by meningeal irritation or focal disease in the cerebrum or brainstem. In all but the deepest stages of coma, meningeal irritation, from either bacterial meningitis or subarachnoid hemorrhage, will cause resistance to passive flexion of the neck but not to extension, turning, or tipping the head. (It should be noted that in some patients the signs of meningeal irritation do not develop for 12 to 24 h after the occurrence of subarachnoid hemorrhage, during which time the CT scan and lumbar puncture are the most reliable diagnostic measures.) Resistance to movement of the neck in all directions may be part of a generalized muscular rigidity or may indicate disease of the cervical spine. In the infant, bulging of the anterior fontanel is at times a more reliable sign of meningitis than stiff neck. A temporal lobe or cerebellar pressure cone or decerebrate rigidity may also limit passive flexion of the neck and may be confused with meningeal irritation.

As indicated above, a lesion in a cerebral hemisphere, or in the diencephalon or brainstem, can usually be detected even though the patient is comatose, by careful observation of the patient's spontaneous movements, responses to stimulation, prevailing postures of the body, rhythm and frequency of respiration, and by examination of the cranial nerves. This is of more than passing importance, because severe and persistent derangements of these functions are observed frequently with mass lesions of the brain but not with metabolic disorders (except in the terminal stages). A hemiplegia is revealed by a lack of restless movements of an arm and leg and of avoidance or protective movements in response to painful stimuli. The paralyzed limbs are slack; if placed in uncomfortable positions, they tend to remain there, and if lifted from the bed, they "fall flail." The hemiplegic leg lies in a position of external rotation (this may also be due to a fractured femur), and the thigh may appear wider and flatter than the nonhemiplegic one. The cheek puffs out in expiration on the paralyzed side, and with hemispheric lesions the eyes are often turned away from the paralysis (toward the lesion); the opposite may occur with brainstem lesions. In most cases a hemiplegia reflects a contralateral hemispheral lesion, but with temporal lobe herniation and compression of the cerebral peduncle against the opposite tentorium, the hemiparetic signs may be ipsilateral to the lesion (false localizing sign).

A moan or grimace may be provoked by painful stimuli on one side but not on the other, reflecting the presence of a hemianesthesia. A stuporous patient may fail to be attracted to visual stimuli presented on one side and not the other, or fail to blink in reaction to a threatening movement on one side, findings that suggest the presence of a homonymous hemianopia. or occipitofrontal disconnection.

Of the various indicators of brainstem function, the most useful are the pattern of breathing, pupillary size and reactivity, ocular movement, and oculovestibular reflexes. These functions, like consciousness itself, are to a large extent dependent upon the integrity of structures in the midbrain and subthalamus.

A massive supratentorial lesion, bilateral deep-seated cerebral lesions, or metabolic disturbances of the brain give rise to a characteristic pattern of breathing, in which a period of waxing-and-waning hyperpnea regularly alternates with a shorter period of apnea (*Cheyne-Stokes respiration,* or *CSR*). This phenomenon has been attributed to isolation of the brainstem respiratory centers from the cerebrum, rendering them more sensitive than usual to CO_2 (hyperventilation drive). As a result of overbreathing, the blood CO_2 drops below the level where it stimulates the centers, and breathing stops. CO_2 then reaccumulates until it exceeds the respiratory threshold, and the cycle repeats itself. Alternatively, CSR has been attributed to the stimulating effect of a low arterial Po_2 on the depressed respiratory center. In congestive heart failure (and in experimental animals), the occurence of CSR has been related to a prolonged circulation time from lung to brain.

Clinically, the presence of CSR signifies bilateral dysfunction of cerebral structures, usually those deep in the hemispheres or diencephalon. In itself, CSR is not a grave sign. Only when it gives way to other abnormal respiratory patterns, which implicate the brainstem more directly, is the patient in imminent danger. Lesions of the lower midbrain-upper pontine tegmentum, either primary or secondary to a tentorial herniation, may give rise to *central neurogenic hyperventilation* (CNH). This disorder is characterized by an increase in the rate and depth of respiration, to the extent that respiratory alkalosis may result. This disorder is thought to represent a release of the reflex mechanisms for respiratory control in the lower brainstem. The threshold of respiratory activation is low and the respiratory drive continues despite low arterial CO_2 tensions and elevated pH. The administration of oxygen does not modify the pattern (unlike its effect in certain cases of pneumonia and pulmonary congestion, in which hypoxia provides the drive to hyperventilation). The neurologic basis of this state is also uncertain. It has been observed with tumors of the medulla and lower pons as well as midbrain tumors. However, North and Jennett, in a study of the respiration of neurosurgical patients, found no consistent correlation between tachypnea and lesion site. Plum later suggested that the tachypnea was caused by pulmonary edema, and in the tumor cases of Goulon et al, by lactate production by the tumor cells per se.

Low pontine lesions, usually due to basilar artery occlusion, sometimes cause *apneustic breathing* (a pause of 2 to 3 s after full inspiration) or so-called *short-cycle Cheyne-Stokes respiration*, in which the breathing and apneic cycles are very short—there may be three or four rapid, deep breaths, the waxing and waning phases of which consist of only one or two breaths; or seven to ten breaths may alternate with periods of apnea without waxing and waning; or occasional small breaths are interposed between full breaths. In yet other cases a few breaths are omitted from time to time (*respiration alternans*). With lesions of the dorsomedial part of the medulla the rhythm of breathing is chaotic, being irregularly interrupted, each breath varying in rate and depth (Biot breathing). This has also been called "ataxia of breathing," not an appropriate term. The latter progresses to infrequent, prolonged inspiratory gasps and finally to apnea, a sequence that may also be observed with CSR or CNH; in fact, respiratory arrest is the mode of death of most patients with serious central nervous system disease. As has been pointed out by Fisher and by Plum and Posner, when certain supratentorial lesions progress to the point of temporal lobe and cerebellar herniation, one may observe a succession of respiratory patterns (CSR–CNH–Biot breathing), indicating extension of the functional disorder from upper to lower brainstem. Rapidly evolving lesions of the posterior fossa may cause acute respiratory failure, without intervention of any of the aforementioned abnormalities of breathing. Also it should be noted that in patients with acute head injuries and other forms of diffuse brain damage, the patterns of abnormal breathing may overlap and it is difficult to relate particular breathing patterns with discrete sites of brain damage.

With massive midbrain lesions *the pupils* dilate to 4 or 5 mm and become unreactive to light; thus, the preservation of pupillary light reflexes indicates integrity of the pupillary dilatation and constriction mechanisms in the midbrain (see Fig. 13-6). Pontine tegmental lesions cause miotic pupils with only a slight reaction to strong light; this is characteristic of the early phase of pontine hemorrhage. Ciliospinal pupillary dilatation is also lost in brainstem lesions (see page 221). A Horner syndrome (miosis, ptosis, apparent enophthalmos, and reduced sweating) may be observed homolateral to a lesion of one side of the brainstem, thalamus, or hypothalamus or to a dissecting aneurysm of the internal carotid artery. A unilateral dilated pupil (>5.0 mm) may be caused by an ipsilateral mesencephalic lesion or by compression of the midbrain and third nerve by a temporal lobe herniation.

The pupillary reactions are of great importance. Normal pupils indicate integrity of midbrain structures, which is usually the case in drug intoxications and metabolic disorders that cause coma. Exceptions are glutethimide (Doriden) intoxication and deep ether anesthesia, which cause the pupils to be of medium size or slightly enlarged and unreactive for several hours; opiates (heroin and morphine), which cause pinpoint pupils with so slight a constriction to light that it can be seen only with a magnifying glass; and atropine poisoning, in which the pupils are widely dilated and fixed.

Ocular movements are altered in a variety of ways. In light coma of metabolic origin the eyes rove from side to side in random fashion. These movements disappear as brainstem function becomes depressed. Oculocephalic reflexes (doll's-eye movements), elicited by briskly turning or tilting the head, with eyes moving conjugately in the opposite direction, are not present in the normal alert person. Elicitation of these reflexes in comatose patients provides evidence of intactness of the tegmental structures of the midbrain and pons, which integrate ocular movements, and of the third, fourth, and sixth cranial nerve nuclei and nerves. But now cerebral control is impaired. Irrigation of each ear with 30 to 100 mL ice water (or just cold water if the patient is not comatose) will normally cause nystagmus (fast component) away from the stimulated side (see page 240). In comatose patients in whom the fast "corrective" phase of nystagmus is lost, the eyes are deflected to the side irrigated with cold water or away from the side irrigated with hot water. The position is held for 2 to 3 min. These vestibulo-ocular reflexes are also lost with brainstem lesions. If, while one is eliciting lateral conjugate movements, only one eye abducts and the other fails to adduct, one can conclude that the medial longitudinal fasciculus has been interrupted (on the side of adductor paralysis). Irrigating both ears simultaneously with ice water with the head flexed 30° from horizontal will normally induce vertical conjugate movements. An abducens (sixth nerve) palsy is indicated by medial deviation of the eye because of unopposed action of the medial rectus muscle; oculomotor (third nerve) palsy results in an outward and slight downward position of the eye, the result of unopposed action of the lateral rectus and superior oblique muscles. There may be a persistent conjugate deviation of the eyes to one side—away from the side of the paralysis with large cerebral lesions (looking toward the lesion) and toward the side of the paralysis with unilateral pontine lesions (looking away from the lesion). "Wrong-way" conjugate deviation may sometimes occur with thalamic and brainstem lesions (see page 210). And during a one-sided seizure the eyes turn toward the convulsing side (opposite to the irritative focus). The eyes may be turned down and inward (looking at the nose) in thalamic and upper midbrain lesions (Parinaud syndrome; see page 210). Retraction and convergence nystagmus and "ocular bobbing" occur with lesions in the tegmentum of the midbrain and lower pons, respectively (page 219). The coma-producing structural lesions of the brainstem, including those due to temporal lobe herniation, abolish most if not all conjugate ocular movements, whereas metabolic disorders do not. Poisoning with barbiturates and phenytoin (Dilantin) are the only common drugs that abolish ocular movements, but pupillary reactions remain intact.

Restless movements of the arms and legs and grasping and picking movements signify that the corticospinal tracts are more or less intact. Variable resistance to passive movement (paratonic rigidity), complex avoidance movements and discrete protective movements have the same meaning, and if they are bilateral, the coma usually is not profound. Also, the occurrence of focal motor epilepsy usually indicates intactness of the corticospinal pathway. With massive destruction of a cerebral hemisphere, such as occurs in hypertensive hemorrhage or carotid–middle cerebral artery occlusion, focal seizures are seldom seen on the paralyzed side; seizure activity may occur in the ipsilateral limbs alone, with the paralysis probably preventing the contralateral limbs from participating. Often, elaborate forms of semivoluntary movement are present on the "good side" in patients with extensive disease in one hemisphere; they probably represent some type of disequilibrium (or diaschisis) of cortical and subcortical movement patterns. Definite choreic, athetotic, or hemiballistic movements indicate disorder of the basal ganglionic and subthalamic structures, just as they do in the alert patient.

Postural changes are often informative in the comatose patient. One of these is *decerebrate rigidity,* which in its fully developed form consists of opisthotonus, clenched jaws, and stiffly extended limbs, with internal rotation of the arms and plantar flexion of the feet. This postural pattern was first described by Sherrington, who produced it in cats and monkeys by transecting the brainstem at the intercollicular level. Such a precise correlation is rarely possible in patients who develop this stereotyped extensor posturing in a variety of clinical settings—with midbrain compression due to temporal lobe herniation or to cerebellar or other posterior fossa lesions; with certain metabolic disorders such as anoxia and hypoglycemia; and rarely with hepatic coma and profound intoxication. Sometimes the basis of this postural abnormality is unclear, as with certain subacute inflammatory, demyelinative, and infarctive cerebral lesions. In some patients the lesions are clearly in the cerebral white matter or basal ganglia; presumably, in these cases, there is a functional derangement of structures in the midbrain and upper pons due to brain swelling, distortion, and so forth.

Decerebrate posturing, either in experimental preparations or in humans, is usually not a persistent steady state but an intermittent and transient one. Hence the term *decerebrate state* is preferable to decerebrate rigidity, which implies a fixed, tonic extensor attitude (Feldman). The extensor postures, which may be unilateral or bilateral, may seemingly occur spontaneously, but characteristically they are evoked by passive manipulation of the limbs and all variety of noxious stimuli. Also characteristically, the extensor postures can be altered by active or passive movements of the head, i.e., by reflex influences arising in the labyrinths and in the proprioceptors of the neck. Hyperextension of the neck, for example, intensifies the rigid extensor posture of all four limbs. Turning the head to one side may cause an exaggeration of extensor postures on the chin side and a flexion and abduction of the opposite arm. These reactions are analogous to the tonic reflexes described by Magnus in decerebrate animals.

Decorticate rigidity, with arm or arms in flexion and adduction and leg(s) extended, signifies lesions at a higher level—in cerebral white matter, internal capsules, or thalamus. Bilateral decorticate rigidity is essentially bilateral spastic hemiplegia. *Diagonal postures,* e.g., flexion of one arm and extension of the opposite arm and leg, probably indicate a supratentorial lesion. Forceful extensor postures of the arms and weak flexor responses of the legs are probably due to lesions at about the level of the vestibular nuclei. Lesions below this level lead to flaccidity and abolition of all postures and movements. The coma is usually profound.

Lower brainstem reflexes are seldom helpful in the analysis of coma. Only in the most profound forms of intoxication and metabolic coma, as might occur in hypoxic necrosis of the entire brain, are coughing, swallowing, hiccoughing, and spontaneous respirations all abolished. Further, the tendon and plantar reflexes may give little indication of what is happening. Tendon reflexes are sometimes preserved until the late stages of coma due to metabolic disturbances and intoxications. In coma due to a large cerebral infarction or hemorrhage, the tendon reflexes may be normal or only slightly reduced on the hemiplegic side, and the plantar reflexes may be absent or extensor.

A history of headache before the onset of coma, recurrent vomiting, and papilledema are the best clues to increased intracranial pressure. Papilledema may develop within 12 to 24 h in brain trauma and brain hemorrhage, but, if pronounced, it usually signifies brain tumor or abscess, i.e., a lesion of longer duration. Multiple retinal or large subhyaloid hemorrhages are usually associated with ruptured saccular aneurysm or hemorrhage from an arteriovenous malformation. Papilledema, with widespread retinal exudates, hemorrhages, and arteriolar changes, is an almost invariable accompaniment of malignant hypertension. In patients with evidence of increased intracranial pressure a

CT scan should be obtained as a primary procedure. Lumbar puncture, although carrying a certain risk of promoting further herniation, is nevertheless necessary in some instances (to rule out suppurative meningitis, encephalitis, and a primary subarachnoid hemorrhage), not visible by CT scan, as discussed in Chap. 2.

LABORATORY PROCEDURES

Unless the diagnosis is established at once by history and physical examination, it is necessary to carry out a number of laboratory procedures. If poisoning is suspected, aspiration and analysis of the gastric contents is sometimes helpful, but greater reliance should be placed on chemical anaylsis of the blood. Accurate means are available for measuring the blood levels of phenytoin, barbiturates, and a wide range of other toxic substances. A specimen of urine is obtained by catheter for determination of specific gravity, and glucose, acetone, and albumin content. Urine of low specific gravity and high protein content is found in uremia, but proteinuria may also occur for 2 or 3 days after a subarachnoid hemorrhage or with fever. Urine of high specific gravity, glycosuria, and acetonuria are found almost invariably in diabetic coma; but glycosuria and hyperglycemia may result from a massive cerebral lesion. Blood counts are made, and in malarial districts a blood smear is examined for malarial parasites. Neutrophilic leukocytosis occurs in bacterial infections and also with brain hemorrhage and softening. Venous blood should be examined for glucose, nonprotein nitrogen, carbon monoxide, bicarbonate, pH, ammonium, sodium, potassium, chlorides, calcium, phosphorus, and SGOT (serum glutamic oxaloacetic transaminase).

The CSF should be examined, with the qualifications noted above and in Chap. 2. As has been repeatedly indicated, a CT scan should precede lumbar puncture in patients with suspected increase in intracranial pressure. In others, a CT scan should be obtained as soon as possible after these procedures, preferably between the emergency ward and the hospital room.

CLASSIFICATION OF COMA AND DIFFERENTIAL DIAGNOSIS

The demonstration of focal brain disease or of meningeal irritation with abnormalities of the CSF is of particular help in the differential diagnosis of coma, and serves to divide the diseases that cause coma into three classes, as follows:

I. Diseases that cause no focal or lateralizing neurologic signs or alteration of the cellular content of the CSF. Usually brainstem functions and CT are normal.
   A. *Intoxications:* alcohol, barbiturates, opiates, etc. (Chaps. 41 and 42)
   B. *Metabolic disturbances:* anoxia, diabetic acidosis, uremia, hepatic coma, hypoglycemia, Addisonian crisis (Chap. 40)
   C. *Severe systemic infections:* pneumonia, typhoid fever, malaria, septicemia, Waterhouse-Friderichsen syndrome
   D. *Circulatory collapse (shock)* from any cause, and cardiac decompensation in the aged
   E. Epilepsy (Chap. 15)
   F. Hypertensive encephalopathy and eclampsia (Chap. 34)
   G. Hyperthermia or hypothermia
   H. Concussion (Chap. 35)

II. Diseases that cause meningeal irritation with blood or an excess of white cells in the CSF, usually without focal or lateralizing cerebral or brainstem signs. The CT scan may be normal or abnormal.
   A. Subarachnoid hemorrhage from ruptured aneurysm, AV malformation, occasionally trauma (Chaps. 34 and 35)
   B. Acute bacterial meningitis (Chap. 32)
   C. Some forms of viral encephalitis (Chap. 33)

III. Diseases that cause focal brainstem or lateralizing cerebral signs, with or without changes in the CSF. CT scan is usually abnormal.
   A. Brain hemorrhage (Chap. 34)
   B. Cerebral infarction due to thrombosis or embolism (Chap. 34)
   C. Brain abscess, subdural empyema (Chap. 32)
   D. Epidural and subdural hemorrhage and brain contusion (Chap. 35)
   E. Brain tumor (Chap. 31)
   F. Miscellaneous: e.g., thrombophlebitis, some forms of viral encephalitis, focal embolic encephalomalacia due to bacterial endocarditis, acute hemorrhagic leukoencephalitis, disseminated (postinfectious) encephalomyelitis

Using the clinical criteria outlined above, one can usually ascertain whether a given case of coma falls into one of these three categories. Concerning the group without focal or lateralizing or meningeal signs [which includes most of the acquired metabolic diseases of the brain, intoxications (both exogenous and endogenous), concussion, and postseizure states], it should be pointed out that residua from previous neurologic disease may confuse the clinical picture. Thus, an earlier hemiparesis, from vascular disease or trauma, may reassert itself in the course of uremic or hepatic coma, or with hypotension, hypoglycemia, diabetic acidosis, or following a seizure. In hypertensive encephalopathy, focal signs may also be present. Occasionally, for no understandable reason, one leg may seem to move less, or one plantar reflex may be extensor, or seizures may be predominantly or entirely unilateral in a metabolic coma. The diagnosis of concussion or of postepileptic coma depends on observation of the precipitating event or indirect evidence thereof. Usually the diagnosis in the latter case is not long obscure, for another seizure or burst of seizures may occur, and recovery of consciousness, once the seizures cease, is usually prompt. The final determination of the exact toxic or metabolic disorder requires the synthesis of a variety of clinical and laboratory data (see Table 16-3).

With respect to the second group in the above outline, the signs of meningeal irritation (head retraction, stiffness of neck on forward bending, Kernig and Brudzinski legflexion signs) can usually be elicited in both bacterial meningitis and subarachnoid hemorrhage. However, in infants, and in adults, if the coma is profound, stiff neck may be absent. In such cases the spinal fluid has to be examined in order to establish the diagnosis. In bacterial meningitis, unless it is associated with brain swelling and cerebellar herniation, the CSF pressure is not exceptionally high (usually less than 400 mmH$_2$O); if it is, the pupils become fixed and dilated and there are signs of compression of the medulla, with fall in arterial blood pressure and arrest of respiration. Patients in coma from ruptured aneurysms also have high CSF pressure and often a massive hemispheral and ventricular extension of the hemorrhage. The blood is usually visible in the CT scan.

In the third group of patients, it is the focality of sensorimotor signs, the aforementioned changes in respiratory pattern, and the abnormal pupillary and ocular reflexes and postural states that provide the clues to serious structural lesions in the cerebral hemispheres and their effects upon segmental brainstem functions. As the latter become prominent, they may obscure earlier signs of cerebral disease. It is noteworthy that the coma due to bilateral cerebral infarction, traumatic necrosis of the cerebral hemispheres, or massive cerebral hemorrhage may resemble the coma of metabolic and toxic diseases, since brainstem mechanisms may be preserved, at least for a time; contrariwise, hepatic, hypoglycemic, and hypoxic coma will sometimes resemble coma due to brainstem lesions, by causing decerebrate postures. In massive cerebral hemorrhage, the CT scan is diagnostic and makes lumbar puncture unnecessary. Unilateral infarction due to anterior, middle, or posterior cerebral artery occlusion seldom produces more than stupor or light coma; however, with massive unilateral infarction due to carotid artery occlusion or with bilateral infarction, coma may be profound. Evidence of temporal lobe herniation and brainstem displacement is manifested by altered respiration (CSR, CNH), bilateral Babinski signs, dilated pupil and ptosis most often on the side of the lesion, decerebrate postures, and later by dilated pupils and loss of full ocular movements. The coma itself gives no clue as to the nature of the underlying mass lesion. A terminal pattern of descending gradient of diencephalic, mesencephalic, and pontomedullary paralysis of nervous function is identical in all. Differential diagnosis must depend on the clinical and ancillary data.

Finally, it should be stated that diagnosis has as its prime purpose the direction of therapy, and it matters little to the patient whether we diagnose a disease for which there is no treatment. The treatable causes of coma are drug intoxications, shock due to infection or exsanguination, epidural and subdural hematoma, brain abscess, bacterial and fungal meningitis, diabetic acidosis, hypoglycemia, and hypertensive encephalopathy.

CARE OF THE COMATOSE PATIENT

Seriously impaired states of consciousness, regardless of their cause, are often fatal not only because they represent an advanced stage of many diseases but also because they add their own particular burdens to the primary disease. The physician's main objective, of course, is to find the cause of the coma, according to the procedures already outlined, and to treat it appropriately. It often happens, however, that the disease process is one for which there is no specific therapy; or, as in hypoxia or hypoglycemia, the disease process may already have expended itself, before the patient comes to the attention of the physician. Again, the problem may be infinitely complex, for the disturbance may be attributable not to a single cause but to several factors acting in unison, no one of which could account for the total clinical picture. In lieu of direct therapy, supportive measures must be used, and, indeed, the patient's chances of surviving the original disease often depend on the effectiveness of these measures.

The successful management of the insensate patient requires the services of a well-coordinated team of nurses under the constant guidance of a physician. Necessary treatment must be instituted immediately, even if all the diagnostic steps have not been completed; diagnosis and treatment have to proceed concurrently, not seriatim. The following is a brief outline of the principles involved in the treatment of such patients. The details of management of shock, fluid and electrolyte imbalance, and other complications that threaten the comatose patient (pneumonia, urinary tract infections, phlebothrombosis, etc.) are found in *Harrison's Principles of Internal Medicine*.

Table 16-3
Important points in the differential diagnosis of the common causes of coma

General group	Specific disorder	Important clinical findings	Important laboratory findings	Remarks
Coma *with* focal or lateralizing signs of brain disease	Brain tumor	Stertorous breathing, neurologic signs dependent on location, papilledema	CT scan +; CSF pressure elevated; protein often > 100 mg percent	Steady progression of signs and symptoms
	Cerebral hemorrhage	Stertorous breathing, hypertension, flushed skin, hemiplegia	CT scan +; CSF grossly bloody and under increased pressure	Sudden onset, elderly patients
	Cerebral thrombosis	Unilateral and bilateral paralysis of abrupt onset	CT scan + after several days; CSF normal or protein modestly elevated	Stupor or coma
	Cerebral embolism	Sudden onset of paralysis	Same as above; occasionally up to 5000 RBC/mm³ in CSF	Evidence of heart disease
	Fracture or concussion	Signs of skin trauma	CT scan ± skull fracture by x-ray; CSF bloody and under increased pressure	Bleeding from nose or ears; history of trauma
	Subdural hematoma	Slow respiration, rising blood pressure, hemiparesis, dilated pupil	CT scan +; normal or increased CSF pressure; xanthochromia with relatively low protein	History of trauma; progressively severe headache, drowsiness, and confusion
	Brain abscess	Neurolgic signs depending on location; symptoms and signs of increased intracranial pressure	CT scan +; fever, leukocytosis; increased pressure, protein and white cells, but normal glucose in CSF	Subacute evolution of headache and neurologic signs on background of sinus, ear, or lung infection or septicemia
	Hypertensive encephalopathy	Headache, severe hypertension, andretinopathy, convulsions	CT scan ±; CSF pressure normal or increased; protein 50–200 mg	Confusion, stupor or coma evolving over several days
Coma *without* focal or lateralizing signs, *with* meningeal irritation	Meningitis	Stiff neck, positive Kernig sign, fever, headache	CT scan ±; pleseytosis, increased protein, low glucose in CSF	Subacute or acute onset
	Subarachnoid hemorrhage	Stertorous breathing, hypertension, stiff neck, positive Kernig sign	CT scan may show blood and aneurysm; bloody or xanthochromic CSF under increased pressure	Sudden onset with headache
Coma *without* focal neurologic signs or meningeal irritation. CT scan normal	Alcohol intoxication	Hypothermia, hypotension, flushed skin, alcohol breath	Elevated blood alcohol	

General group	Specific disorder	Important clinical findings	Important laboratory findings	Remarks
	Barbiturate intoxication	Hypothermia, hypotension	Barbiturate in urine; EEG often shows fast activity	History of intake of intoxicating substance
	Opium intoxication	Slow respiration, cyanosis, constricted pupils		Administration of naloxone causes withdrawal signs
Coma *without* focal neurologic signs or meningeal irritation. CT scan normal	Carbon monoxide intoxication	Cherry-red skin	Carboxyhemoglobin	
	Anoxia	Rigidity, decerebrate postures, fever, seizures, involuntary movements	CSF normal; EEG may be isoelectric, or show high voltage delta	Abrupt onset following cardiopulmonary failure; damage permanent if anoxia exceeds 3–5 min
	Hypoglycemia	Same as above	Low blood glucose; coeliac angiography may disclose insulinoma	Characteristic slow evolution through stages of nervousness, hunger, sweating, flushed face; then pallor, shallow respirations and seizures
	Diabetic coma	Signs of extracellular fluid deficit, hyperventilation with Kussmaul respiration, "fruity" breath	Glycosuria, hyperglycemia, acidosis; reduced serum bicarbonate; ketonemia and ketonuria	History of polyuria, polydipsia, weight loss, or diabetes
	Uremia	Hypertension; sallow, dry skin, uriniferous breath, twitch-convulsive syndrome	Protein and casts in urine; elevated BUN and serum creatinine; anemia, acidosis, hypocalcemia, etc.	Progressive apathy, confusion, and asterixis precede coma
	Hepatic coma	Jaundice, ascites, and other signs of portal hypertension	Elevated blood NH_3 levels CSF yellow with normal protein	Onset over a few days or after hemorrhage from varices or paracentesis; confusion, stupor, asterixis, and characteristic EEG changes precede coma
	Hypercapnia	Papilledema, diffuse myoclonus, asterixis	Increased CSF pressure; Pco_2 may exceed 75 mmHg; EEG theta and delta activity	Advanced pulmonary disease; profound coma and brain damage uncommon

General group	Specific disorder	Important clinical findings	Important laboratory findings	Remarks
	Severe infections; heat stroke	Extreme hyperthermia, rapid respiration	Vary according to cause	Evidence of a specific infection or exposure to extreme heat
	Idiopathic epilepsy	Episodic disturbance of behavior or convulsive movements	Characteristic EEG changes	History of previous attacks

1. The management of shock, if it is present, takes precedence over all other diagnostic and therapeutic measures.

2. Shallow and irregular respirations, stertorous breathing (indicating obstruction to inspiration), and cyanosis require the establishment of a clear airway and delivery of oxygen. The patient should be placed in a lateral position so that secretions and vomitus do not enter the tracheobronchial tree. Usually the pharyngeal reflexes are suppressed so that an endotracheal tube can be inserted without difficulty. Secretions should be removed by suctioning as soon as they accumulate; otherwise they will lead to atelectasis and bronchopneumonia. Oxygen can be administered by mask in a 100% concentration for 6 to 12 h, alternating with 50% concentration for 5 h. The depth of respiration can be increased by the use of 5 to 10% carbon dioxide for periods of 3 to 5 min every hour. Atropine should not be given; edema of the lungs and fluid in the tracheobronchial passages are not glandular secretions. Furthermore, atropine thickens this fluid and may also disturb temperature regulation. Aminophylline is helpful in controlling Cheyne-Stokes breathing. Respiratory paralysis dictates the use of endotracheal intubation and a positive-pressure respirator, but in the authors' experience neither has been effective in comatose states in which there is disorganization of the respiratory centers.

3. Concomitantly, an intravenous line is established and blood samples drawn for the measurement of the blood elements, glucose, toxins, and electrolytes and for tests of liver and kidney function. Arterial blood gases should also be measured. Naloxone, 0.5 mg, should be given intravenously if a narcotic overdose is a diagnostic possibility.

4. With massive cerebral lesions it is now common practice to put a pressure-measuring device in the skull. This provides constant monitoring of intracranial pressure. When the pressure is elevated, mannitol, 50 g in a 20% solution, should be given intravenously over 10 to 20 min. Corticosteroids help to maintain the reduction in intracranial pressure. Repeated CT scans allow the physician to follow the size of the lesion, and degree of localized edema, and to detect herniations of cerebral tissue.

5. A lumbar puncture should be performed if meningitis or subarachnoid hemorrhage is suspected, keeping in mind the risks of this procedure and the means of dealing with them (page 10). A CT scan may have disclosed a subarachnoid hemorrhage in which case no lumbar puncture is necessary.

6. Convulsions should be controlled by measures outlined in Chap. 15.

7. As indicated above, gastric aspiration and lavage with normal saline may be useful in some instances of coma due to drug ingestion. Salicylates, opiates, and anticholinergic drugs (tricyclic antidepressants, phenothiazines, scopolamine), all of which induce gastric atony, may be recovered many hours after ingestion. Caustic materials should not be lavaged because of the danger of perforation. Lavage of strychnine and other analeptic drugs carries the danger of precipitating seizures and cardiac arrhythmias. Induction of emesis induced by ipecac or apomorphine should be reserved for alert patients.

8. The temperature-regulating mechanisms may be disturbed, and extreme hypothermia, hyperthermia, or poikilothermia may occur. In hyperthermia, the use of alcohol sponges and a cooling mattress are indicated.

9. The bladder should not be permitted to become distended; if the patient does not void, he or she should be fitted with an external drainage apparatus or a retention catheter. If the bladder is found to be greatly distended, decompression should be carried out slowly, over a period of hours. Urine excretion should be kept between 500 and 1000 mL/day. The patient should not be permitted to lie in a wet or soiled bed.

10. Diseases of the central nervous system may upset the control of water, glucose, and salt. The unconscious patient can no longer adjust the intake of food and fluids

by hunger and thirst. Both salt-losing and salt-retaining syndromes have been described with brain disease. Water intoxication and severe hyponatremia may of themselves prove fatal. If coma is prolonged, the insertion of a stomach tube will ease the problems of feeding the patient and maintaining fluid and electrolyte balance.

11. Aspiration pneumonia is avoided by prevention of vomiting (stomach tube), proper positioning of the patient, and restriction of oral fluids. Should it occur, corticosteroid therapy is beneficial. The legs should be examined each day for signs of phlebothrombosis and if found treated by anticoagulants or surgical measures. Deep vein thrombosis, which is a common occurrence in comatose and hemiplegic patients, often does not manifest itself by clinical signs. It can be prevented by the administration of low doses of warfarin (Coumadin) (maintaining a prothrombin time of 15 s) or by the use of inflatable boots or stockings.

12. If the patient is capable of moving, suitable restraints should be used to prevent falling out of bed.

PROGNOSIS OF COMA

Patients whose clinical state indicates that brain death has occurred will usually not survive for more than a few days, so that the decision as to "shutting off the respirator" or "pulling the plug" can be delayed. In patients with preserved brainstem functions, so-called cerebral death, the prediction of outcome is more difficult. If there are no pupillary responses or eye movements within 6 h of the onset of coma, the fatality rate is 95 percent. Other unfavorable prognostic signs are absence of corneal reflexes and eye opening responses and atonia of the limbs at 1 and 3 days after the onset of coma and absence of visual, auditory, and somatosensory evoked responses. It is the unfortunate survivor, from this latter group, who may remain in a persistent vegetative state for months or years, breathing without aid and with preserved hypothalamopituitary functions. Society has yet to reach a consensus as to whether the removal of a feeding tube and other simple support measures is justifiable.

REFERENCES

Bennett DR, Hughes JR, Korein J: *Atlas of Electroencephalography in Coma and Cerebral Death.* New York, Raven Press, 1976.

Caronna JJ, Simon RP: The comatose patient: A diagnostic approach and treatment. *Int Anesthesiol Clin* 17(2/3):3, 1979.

Feldman MH: The decerebrate state in the primate. I: Studies in monkeys. *Arch Neurol* 25:501, 1971.

Feldman MH, Sahrmann S: The decerebrate state in the primate. II: Studies in man. *Arch Neurol* 25:517, 1971.

Fisher CM: The neurological examination of the comatose patient. *Acta Neurol Scand Suppl* 36, 1969.

Frederiks JAM: Consciousness, in Vinken PJ, Bruyn GW (eds): *Disorders of Higher Nervous Function, Handbook of Clinical Neurology,* vol 4. Amsterdam, North-Holland, 1969, chap 4, p 48.

Goulon M, Escourolle R, Augustin S et al: Hyperventilation primitive par glioma bulbo-protuberantiel. *Rev Neurol,* 121:636, 1969.

Guidelines for the detection of brain death in children. *Ann Neurol* 21:616, 1987.

Iragui VJ, McCutchen CB: Physiologic and prognostic significance of "alpha coma." *J Neurol Neurosurg Psychiatry* 46:632, 1983.

Jennett B, Plum F: Persistent vegetative state after brain damage. *Lancet* 1:734, 1972.

Magnus R: Some results of studies in the physiology of posture. *Lancet* 2:531; 585, 1926.

Mollaret P, Goulon M: Le coma dépassé. *Rev Neurol* 101:3, 1959.

North JB, Jennett S: Abnormal breathing patterns associated with acute brain damage. *Arch Neurol* 32:338, 1974.

Plum F: Hyperpnea, hyperventilation, and brain dysfunction. *Ann Int Med* 76:328, 1972.

Plum F: Mechanisms of central hyperventilation. *Ann Neurol* 11:636, 1982.

Plum F, Posner JB: *Diagnosis of Stupor and Coma,* 3rd ed. Philadelphia, Davis, 1980.

Posner JB: The comatose patient. *JAMA* 232:1313, 1975.

Ropper AH: Lateral displacement of the brain and level of consciousness in patients with an acute hemispheral mass. *N Engl J Med* 314:953, 1986.

Ropper AH, Shafran B: Brain edema after stroke: Clinical syndrome and intracranial pressure. *Arch Neurol* 41:26, 1984.

Sherrington CS: Decerebrate rigidity and reflex coordination of movements. *J Physiol* 22:319, 1898.

CHAPTER 17

FAINTNESS AND SYNCOPE

The term *syncope* (Greek, *synkope*) literally means a "cessation," a "cutting short," or "pause." Medically, it refers to an episodic interruption of consciousness due to a diminished flow of blood to the brain, and is synonymous in everyday language with *faint*. The terms *faint* and *faintness* are also commonly used to describe the sudden loss of strength and other symptoms that characterize the impending or incomplete fainting spell. This latter state is referred to as *presyncope,* whereas syncope designates the more advanced or complete state with generalized loss of postural tone, inability to stand, and loss of consciousness. Relatively abrupt onset, brief duration, spontaneous and complete recovery not requiring specific resuscitative measures are other distinguishing features.

Faintness and syncope are among the most common nervous symptoms. Practically every adult has experienced some presyncopal symptoms, if not a fully developed syncopal attack, or has observed such an attack in others. Description of these symptoms, as with other predominantly subjective states, is often ambiguous. The patient, usually untrained in introspection, may refer to them as light-headedness, giddiness, dizziness, "drunk feeling," weak spells, or if consciousness was lost, as "blackouts." Careful questioning may be necessary to ascertain that these words refer to sudden weakness and an impaired alertness. In many instances the condition is clarified by the fact that these symptoms have proceeded to a sensation of faintness and then a momentary loss of consciousness, which is easily recognized as a faint, or syncope. This sequence also informs us that under certain conditions any difference between faintness and syncope is only quantitative. These symptoms must be clearly set apart from certain types of epilepsy, the other major cause of episodic unconsciousness, and from disorders such as cataplexy, transient ischemic attacks, "drop attacks," or vertigo, which are also characterized by episodic attacks of generalized weakness or inability to stand upright, without loss of consciousness.

CLINICAL FEATURES OF SYNCOPE

Faints may vary somewhat, according to their mechanisms, but all of them conform roughly to the following pattern.

Though the syncopal attack may develop rapidly, it is doubtful if consciousness is ever abolished as abruptly as with a seizure. Even with an arrest of cardiac function, i.e., cardiac syncope, the onset requires several seconds. With few exceptions, e.g., the Stokes-Adams syndrome, the patient is usually in the upright position at the beginning of the attack, either sitting or standing. A number of subjective symptoms, known as the prodrome, mark the onset of the faint. The person feels uneasy and queasy, is assailed by a sense of giddiness and swaying, apprehension, and a severe headache. What is most noticeable, even at the beginning of the attack, is a pallor or ashen-gray color of the face, and often the face and body become bathed in a cold perspiration. Salivation, nausea, and sometimes vomiting accompany these symptoms; patients try to protect themselves by yawning, sighing, or breathing deeply. Vision may dim and the ears ring, and it may be impossible to think clearly ("gray-out"). If the person can lie down promptly, the attack may be averted or aborted, short of complete loss of consciousness; otherwise, consciousness is lost and the patient falls to the ground. The deliberate onset of most types of syncope enables patients to lie down or at least to protect themselves as they slump. A hurtful fall is exceptional.

The depth and duration of unconsciousness vary. Sometimes the person is not completely oblivious of the surroundings. It may still be possible to hear voices or see the blurred outlines of people or there may be a complete lack of awareness and responsiveness. The patient may remain in this state for seconds to minutes, rarely longer, unless for some reason he or she is kept in the upright position.

If unconsciousness persists for 15 to 20 s, convulsive

movements may occur (convulsive syncope). These usually take the form of tonic extension of the trunk and clenching of the jaw, or brief, mild, clonic jerks of the limbs and trunk and twitchings of the face. Occasionally the extensor rigidity and jerking flexor movements are more severe, lasting for 2 to 3 min. Very rarely is there a generalized tonic-clonic convulsion. Usually the person who has fainted lies motionless, with skeletal muscles fully relaxed. Sphincteric control is maintained in nearly all cases. The pulse is thin and slow or cannot be felt; the systolic blood pressure is reduced (to 60 mmHg or less, as a rule), and breathing is almost imperceptible. The depressed vital functions, striking facial pallor, and unconsciousness simulate death.

Once the patient is horizontal from having fallen or deliberately lain down, the flow of blood to the brain is no longer hindered. The strength of the pulse soon improves, and color begins to return to the face. Breathing becomes quicker and deeper. Then the eyelids flutter, and consciousness is quickly regained. There is from this moment onward a correct perception of the environment. Confusion, headache, and drowsiness, the common sequelae of a convulsive seizure, do not follow a syncopal attack. The patient is nevertheless keenly aware of physical weakness, and by arising too soon, may precipitate another faint.

CAUSES OF EPISODIC FAINTNESS AND SYNCOPE

The following classification is based on established or assumed physiologic mechanisms.

I. Circulatory (deficient quantity of blood to the brain and extracranial structures)
  A. Inadequate vasoconstrictor mechanisms
    1. Vasodepressor (vasovagal)
    2. Postural hypotension
    3. Primary autonomic insufficiency
    4. Sympathectomy (surgical or pharmacologic, i.e., due to antihypertensive medications)
    5. Peripheral and central nervous system diseases
    6. Carotid sinus irritability (see also bradyrhythmias, below)
  B. Hypovolemia
    1. Blood loss
    2. Addison disease
  C. Mechanical reduction in venous return to heart
    1. Valsalva maneuver
    2. Cough
    3. Micturition
    4. Atrial myxoma (ball-valve thrombus)

  D. Reduced cardiac output
    1. Obstruction to left ventricular outflow: aortic stenosis, hypertrophic subaortic stenosis
    2. Obstruction to pulmonary flow: pulmonic stenosis, tetralogy of Fallot, primary pulmonary hypertension, pulmonary embolism
    3. Myocardial: massive myocardial infarction with "pump" failure
    4. Pericardial: cardiac tamponade
  E. Cardiac arrhythmias
    1. Bradyrhythmias
      a. Atrioventricular (AV) block (second- and third-degree) with Stokes-Adams attacks
      b. Ventricular asystole
      c. Sinus bradycardia, sinoatrial block, sinus arrest, sick-sinus syndrome
      d. Carotid sinus syncope (see also "Inadequate vasoconstrictor mechanism")
      e. Vagoglossopharyngeal neuralgia (and other painful states)
    2. Tachyrhythmias
      a. Episodic ventricular fibrillation with or without associated bradyrhythmias
      b. Ventricular tachycardia
      c. Supraventricular tachycardia without AV block
II. Other causes of episodic faintness and syncope
  A. Altered state of blood to the brain
    1. Hypoxia
    2. Anemia
    3. Diminished CO_2 due to hyperventilation (faintness common, syncope rare)
    4. Hypoglycemia (faintness frequent, syncope rare)
  B. Emotional disturbances
    1. Hysterical fainting
    2. Anxiety attacks (presyncope common, syncope rare)

This list of conditions that cause faintness and syncope is deceptively long and involved. It will be recognized that the usual types are reducible to a few well-established mechanisms resulting in a temporary reduction in the flow of blood to the brain (which in turn is due to a decrease in peripheral resistance, as in vasovagal syncope, or to a diminished cardiac output, as in the Stokes-Adams attack), or an altered state of the blood itself, so that an essential component, such as oxygen or glucose, is not delivered to the brain in adequate amount. In order not to obscure the central problem of fainting by too many details, only the varieties of fainting commonly encountered in clinical practice will be discussed below.

COMMON TYPES OF SYNCOPE

Vasodepressor (Vasovagal) Syncope This is the common faint, seen mainly in young individuals. It always occurs when the patient is in the erect position, and may be averted or relieved by lying down. There is a short premonitory phase of pallor, nausea, salivation, epigastric distress, perspiration, yawning, anxiety, tachypnea, and weakness, with pupillary dilatation and bradycardia. The period of unconsciousness lasts only a few seconds or a minute or two. Jaw clenching, extensor rigidity or clonic movements may occur 15 to 20 s after the loss of consciousness.

Sudden vasodilatation, particularly of intramuscular arterioles, caused by strong emotion, physical injury, or other factors (see below) is thought to be the initial event. Peripheral vascular resistance decreases due to active vasodilatation of "resistance vessels" and blood pressure falls. Cardiac output fails to exhibit the compensatory rise that normally occurs in hypotension. Vagal stimulation may then occur (hence the term *vasovagal*), causing bradycardia, and possibly leading to a further drop in blood pressure and to perspiration, increased peristaltic activity, nausea, and salivation. The loss of consciousness and pallor are caused by inadequate flow of blood to the brain and extracranial structures.

Although bradycardia does appear in the course of the common fainting spell, it probably contributes little to the loss of consciousness. The term vasovagal, used originally by Thomas Lewis to designate this type of faint, is therefore not entirely apt and should be avoided as a synonym for vasodepressor syncope. Atropine is said to reverse the bradycardia without increasing the blood pressure, indicating the presence of reduced peripheral vascular resistance. The initial reduction in cardiac output is at first partially compensated by an increase in heart rate and in peripheral vasoconstriction, but these mechanisms fail just before the loss of consciousness. In the genesis of this type of syncope, the dilatation of intramuscular vessels is more important than splanchnic vesels. Skin vessels are constricted.

The common, or vasodepressor, faint occurs (1) in normal health under the influence of strong emotion (sight of blood or an accident) or in conditions that favor peripheral vasodilatation, e.g., hot, humid, crowded rooms ("heat syncope"), especially if the person is hungry or tired or has had a few drinks, or (2) during a painful illness or after bodily injury as a consequence of fright, pain, and other factors. Where pain is involved, the vasovagal element is more prominent in the genesis of the faint.

Postural (Orthostatic) Hypotension with Syncope

This type affects persons whose vasomotor reflexes are variably unstable or defective. Although the character of the faint differs little from the vasodepressor type, the effect of posture in its initiation is its most typical attribute. Sudden arising from a recumbent position or prolonged periods of standing still are the two circumstances under which it is most likely to happen.

Postural syncope tends to occur under the following conditions: (1) in otherwise normal individuals who for an unknown reason have defective pressor-receptor reflexes (pressor-receptors are pressure-sensitive receptors in the large blood vessels); (2) as part of a syndrome known as chronic orthostatic hypotension or primary autonomic insufficiency (see further on); (3) after prolonged illness with recumbency, especially in elderly individuals with poor muscle tone; (4) in association with diseases of the peripheral nerves, including autonomic nerves (diabetic neuropathy, tabes dorsalis, amyloid and other polyneuropathies), which interrupt vasomotor reflexes and also cause the muscles to be weak and flabby; (5) after sympathectomy; (6) in persons with large varicose veins of the legs, which facilitate the pooling of blood; (7) in patients receiving L-dopa, antihypertensive drugs (particularly ganglionic blocking agents such as guanethidine), and certain sedative and antidepressant drugs; and (8) in patients who are hypovolemic from diuretics, excessive sweating, acute hemorrhage (as occurs with a bleeding peptic ulcer) or Addison disease.

These conditions are easily understood if one keeps in mind that the pooling of blood in the lower parts of the body, on assuming the erect posture, is normally prevented by (1) reflex arteriolar and arterial constriction, (2) reflex acceleration of the heart by means of aortic and carotid reflexes, and (3) muscular activity, which improves venous return. Lipsitz has pointed out that aging is associated with a progressive impairment of these compensatory mechanisms, thus rendering the older person especially vulnerable to syncope. However, even in some younger persons, after the blood pressure has fallen slightly and stabilized at a lower level, the compensatory reflexes may fail suddenly, with a precipitant drop in pressure. A strong autonomic reaction then occurs, with pallor, sweating, nausea, etc., and sometimes a brief faint.

Micturition Syncope This condition is usually seen in men, in young adults as well as in the elderly, who arise from bed at night to urinate. The syncope occurs at the end of micturition or soon thereafter, and the loss of consciousness is abrupt, with rapid and complete recovery. The mechanism is not fully understood. A full bladder causes reflex vasoconstriction; as the bladder empties this gives way to vasodilatation which, in the erect posture, might be sufficient to cause fainting in some individuals. Vagally mediated bradycardia may also be a factor, and alcohol ingestion, hunger, fatigue, and upper respiratory infection are common predisposing factors. In some instances, especially in the elderly, the nocturnal collapse has caused serious head injury.

Syncope may occur occasionally in the course of prostatic examination, but only if the patient is standing (*prostatic syncope*). The Valsalva maneuver and reflex vagal stimulation may be contributing factors.

Hyperbradykininism This is the term applied to a syndrome of orthostatic hypotension, characterized by postural faintness and syncope, a rise in heart rate, facial erythema, and purple discoloration of the legs after standing. Most of the patients have been young females. The syndrome is familial and associated with abnormally high plasma concentrations of the polypeptide bradykinin, which presumably causes dilatation of cutaneous venules and capillaries in the legs and reduction in venous return. Improvement has attended the use of propranolol, fludrocortisone and cyproheptadine.

Primary Autonomic Insufficiency (Idiopathic Orthostatic Hypotension) When the autonomic nervous system is defective for any reason, the patient, on assuming an upright position, shows a steady fall in blood pressure to a level at which the cerebral circulation cannot be supported. Compensatory tachycardia does not occur, however, and contrary to what occurs in vasopressor syncope, there are no autonomic responses such as pallor, sweating, or nausea, and there is no release of norepinephrine. Clouding of the sensorium with staggering or falling may precede unconsciousness or be the only evidence of cerebral disorder.

Primary autonomic insufficiency, also called *idiopathic orthostatic hypotension*, presents in two forms. In one, there is probably a selective degeneration of neurons in the sympathetic ganglia with denervation of smooth muscle and glands (pathology not fully delineated); in the other, there is a degeneration of preganglionic neurons in the lateral columns of gray matter in the spinal cord, leaving postganglionic neurons isolated from spinal control. The latter lesion is often associated with degeneration of other systems of neurons in the central nervous system (Shy and Drager). Three such system degenerations have been identified, occurring singly or in combination: (1) degeneration of the substantia nigra and locus ceruleus, (2) striatonigral degeneration, and (3) olivopontocerebellar degenerations. In the first two syndromes orthostatic hypotension is combined with a parkinsonian syndrome; in the third, with cerebellar ataxia.

All these forms of degenerative disease have their onset in adult life, and the associated hypotension and syncope are usually part of a more widespread paralysis of autonomic function that includes a fixed cardiac rate, a loss of sweating in the lower parts of the body, atonicity of the bladder, constipation, and impotence in the male. These conditions are discussed more fully in Chap. 26.

Syncope of Cardiac Origin This is due to a sudden reduction in cardiac output, usually because of a dysrhythmia. Normally, a pulse as low as 35 to 40 beats per minute or as high as 150 beats per minute is well tolerated, especially if the patient is recumbent. Changes in pulse rate beyond these extremes impair cerebral circulation and lead to syncope. Upright posture, anemia, and coronary, myocardial, and valvular disease all render the individual more susceptible to these alterations. The various valvular, myocardial, and rhythm abnormalities that may compromise cardiac output and lead to syncope have been discussed by Lipsitz.

Syncope of cardiac origin occurs most frequently in patients with complete atrioventricular block and a pulse rate of 40 or less per minute (Adams-Stokes-Morgagni syndrome). The causation of heart block need not concern us here. The block may be persistent or intermittent; it is often preceded by disturbed conduction in two or three fascicles of the conduction system or by a second-degree heart block. When the block is complete and the pacemaker below the block fails to function, ventricular contraction ceases altogether. Ventricular arrest of 4 to 8 s, if the patient is upright, is enough to cause coma; when the patient is supine the asystole must last 12 to 15 s. At 12 s, according to Engel, the patient turns pale and is momentarily weak or may lose consciousness without warning. This may occur at any time of the day or night and regardless of the position of the body. If the duration of cerebral ischemia exceeds 15 to 20 s there may be a few tonic spasms or clonic jerks, and if it persists up to 5 min, the ashen-gray pallor gives way to cyanosis, stertorous breathing, incontinence, fixed pupils, and bilateral Babinski signs. As heart action is resumed, the face and neck become flushed. In cases of prolonged asystole there may be cerebral injury, caused by a combination of hypoxia and ischemia. Coma may persist or may be replaced by confusion and other neurologic signs, and focal ischemic changes, often irreversible, may then be traced to the fields of occluded atherosclerotic cerebral arteries or the border zones between the areas of supply of major arteries. Cardiac faints of the Stokes-Adams type may recur several times a day. Occasionally the heart block is transitory, and between attacks the electrocardiogram (ECG) may show only evidence of myocardial disease. A continuous taped electrocardiogram or monitor is then needed to demonstrate the intermittent AV block.

Less often, faintness and syncope are due to dysfunction of the sinus node (manifested by marked sinus bradycardia, sinoatrial block, or sinus arrest). This is the "sick-sinus syndrome." It has characteristic ECG changes. The nodal block results in prolonged (≥ 3 s) atrial asystole. Initially there may be a failure of sinus rate to accelerate with exercise or fever. The lesion in the node is usually due to ischemia, inflammatory disease (myocarditis), or cardiodepressant drugs (quinidine), but it may immediately follow tachycardia. A bout of ventricular fibrillation or some other tachyrhythmia such as atrial flutter and paroxysmal atrial and ventricular tachycardia with normal AV conduction may also reduce cardiac output to a degree sufficient to cause syncope.

Cardiac syncope may also result from massive myocardial infarction, particularly when associated with cardiogenic shock; fright, pain, or arrhythmias may also assume importance. Aortic stenosis often sets the stage for exertional syncope, because cardiac output cannot keep pace with the demands of exercise. This may result in myocardial and cerebral ischemia and arrhythmias. Idiopathic hypertrophic subaortic stenosis may also lead to exertional syncope, by the same mechanism. In primary pulmonary hypertension, bouts of right-sided heart failure may be associated with syncope. However, vagal overactivity may be responsible for the syncope in this condition, as well as for the syncope that accompanies pulmonary embolism. Ball-valve thrombus in the left atrium, left atrial myxoma, malfunction of a prosthetic valve, or cardiac tamponade from rupture of a dissecting aortic aneurysm may produce sudden mechanical obstruction of the circulation and syncope. Tetralogy of Fallot is the congenital cardiac malformation that most often leads to syncope. Here systemic vasodilatation, possibly associated with infundibular spasm, greatly increases right-left cardiac shunting, thereby producing hypoxia.

In other types of cardioinhibitory syncope, the cardiac slowing is purely reflexive, because of irritation of the vagus nerves (from esophageal diverticula, mediastinal tumors, gallbladder stones, carotid sinus disease, vagoglossopharyngeal neuralgia, bronchoscopy and needling of body cavities). Here the reflex bradycardia is more often of sinoatrial than atrioventricular type. Weiss and Ferris called such faints "vagovagal." Gastaut and Fischer-Williams, who used the oculocardiac inhibitory reflex (pressure on the eyeball) to study syncope, found that the heightened vagal discharge caused momentary cardiac arrest.

Carotid Sinus Syncope   The carotid sinus is normally sensitive to stretch and gives rise to sensory impulses, which are carried via the nerve of Hering, a branch of the glossopharyngeal nerve, to the medulla oblongata. Massage of one of the carotid sinuses or of both of them alternately, particularly in elderly persons, causes (1) a reflex cardiac slowing (sinus bradycardia, sinus arrest, or even atrioventricular block), the so-called vagal type of response, or (2)

a fall of arterial pressure without cardiac slowing, the *depressor type* of response, or (3) possibly an interference with the circulation of the ipsilateral cerebral hemisphere, the so-called *central type.*

Faintness or syncope due to carotid sinus sensitivity has reportedly been initiated by turning of the head to one side while wearing a tight collar, or even by shaving over the region of the sinus. But the absence of a history of such an event is of no aid in diagnosis, since spontaneous attacks may occur. The attack nearly always begins when the patient is upright, usually standing. The onset is sudden, often with falling. Convulsive movements occur quite frequently in the vagal and depressor types of carotid sinus syncope. The "central type" was described by Weiss et al, but the authors have had difficulty in distinguishing it from the effects of carotid stenosis due to atherosclerosis. The latter condition is characterized by homolateral blindness or contralateral sensory or motor deficits, usually without loss of consciousness. The period of unconsciousness in carotid sinus syncope seldom lasts longer than a few minutes, and the sensorium is immediately clear when consciousness is regained. The majority of the reported cases have been in males.

In a patient displaying faintness on massage of one carotid sinus, it is important to distinguish between the benign disorder (hypersensitivity of the carotid sinus) and a much more serious condition—atheromatous narrowing of the opposite carotid or of the basilar artery (see Chap. 34). In testing for carotid sinus sensitivity in the latter circumstances, it is important to avoid compression of the carotid artery, which may represent the major vascular supply to both hemispheres.

Vagoglossopharyngeal Neuralgia   This is known occasionally to induce a reflex type of fainting. The sequence is always pain, then bradycardia and syncope; in this instance the pain is localized to the base of the tongue, pharynx or larynx, tonsillar areas, and an ear. It may be triggered by pressure at these sites or simply by chewing or swallowing. Presumably, the pain activates afferent impulses in the ninth nerve, which in turn activates the vasomotor centers (dorsal motor nuclei of the vagus) via collateral fibers from the nucleus of the tractus solitarius. Wallin et al have provided evidence that, in addition to bradycardia, there is inhibition of peripheral sympathetic activity. Section of the appropriate branches of the ninth and tenth cranial nerve relieves the condition (page 150).

The same mechanism is probably operative in so-called swallow syncope, in which consciousness is lost during or immediately after a forceful swallow. The administration of anticholinergic drugs (propantheline 15 mg tid) has abolished these attacks (Levin and Posner).

Other examples of fainting due to reflex vagal stimulation have been mentioned above, in the discussion of cardiac syncope.

Tussive Syncope ("Laryngeal Vertigo") This is a rare condition that results from a severe paroxysm of coughing, first described by Charcot, in 1876. Patients with this type of syncope are usually heavy-set males who smoke and have chronic bronchitis. Occasionally it occurs in children, particularly following the paroxysmal coughing spells of pertussis and laryngitis. After hard coughing, the patient suddenly becomes weak and may lose consciousness momentarily. This is attributable to the greatly elevated intrathoracic pressure, which interferes with the venous return to the heart. The Valsalva maneuver of trying to exhale against a closed glottis produces the same effect. The unconsciousness that results from *breath holding spells* in infants is probably based on this mechanism as well, although the so-called pallid attacks in infants probably represent reflex vasodepression. The loss of consciousness that occurs during competitive weight lifting ("weight-lifters' blackout") is also due to the Valsalva maneuver, compounded by the effects of vascular dilatation, produced by squatting and hyperventilation. Lesser degrees of this phenomenon (faintness and light-headedness) not infrequently follow other kinds of strenuous activity such as laughing, straining at stool, or heavy lifting.

Syncope Associated with Cerebrovascular Disease This is infrequent and has usually been caused by partial or complete occlusion of the large arteries in the neck. The best examples are found in patients with the "aortic-arch syndrome" (pulseless disease), in which the brachiocephalic and common carotid and vertebral arteries have become narrowed. Physical activity may then critically reduce blood flow to the upper part of the brainstem, causing abrupt loss of consciousness; stenosis or occlusion of vertebral arteries and the "vertebral steal syndrome" are other examples (see Chap. 33). Fainting is said also to occur occasionally in patients with congenital anomalies of the upper cervical part of the spine (Klippel-Feil syndrome) or cervical spondylosis, in which the vertebral circulation is compromised. Head turning may then cause vertigo, nausea and vomiting, visual scotomas, and finally unconsciousness.

Hysterical Fainting Hysterical fainting is rather frequent and usually occurs under dramatic circumstances (Chap. 55). The attack is unattended by any outward display of anxiety. The evident lack of change in pulse and blood pressure or color of the skin distinguishes it from the vasodepressor faint. The diagnosis is based on these negative findings in a person who exhibits the general personality and behavioral characteristics of hysteria. Several interesting instances of mass faintness and syncope of hysterical type have been described in school marching bands (Levine).

Syncope of Unknown Cause Finally, it should be pointed out that after careful evaluation of patients with syncope and the exclusion of the many forms of the condition described above, there remains a significant proportion of patients in which a cause for the syncope cannot be ascertained. Kapoor and his colleagues, who prospectively evaluated 204 patients with syncope, established a cardiovascular cause in 53, and a noncardiovascular cause in 54; no cause could be determined in 97 patients. As one might expect the mortality rate and incidence of sudden death was highest, by far, in the patients with cardiovascular syncope. It is virtually nil in the vasodepressor faints of young people.

PATHOPHYSIOLOGY OF SYNCOPE

In the final analysis, the loss of consciousness in these different types of syncope must be caused by a change in the neural elements in those parts of the brain subserving consciousness (high brainstem reticular activating system). In this respect syncope and primary generalized (so-called centrencephalic) epilepsy have a common ground; yet there is an important difference. In epilepsy, whether major or minor, the arrest in mental function is almost instantaneous, and, as revealed by the EEG, is accompanied by a paroxysm of activity occurring simultaneously in all of the cerebral cortex. Syncope is not so sudden. The difference relates to the essential pathophysiology—a sudden spread of an electric discharge in epilepsy, and a more gradual failure of the cerebral circulation in syncope.

During syncopal attacks, there are demonstrable reductions in cerebral blood flow, cerebral oxygen utilization, and cerebral vascular resistance. A systolic blood pressure of 50 mm Hg, lasting more than a few seconds, is nearly always attended by a loss of conciousness. This reduces the level of blood flow necessary to maintain consciousness, which is about 30 mL per 100 g brain per minute (normal 50 to 55 mL). If the ischemia lasts only a few minutes, there are no lasting effects on the brain. If it persists for a longer time, it may result in necrosis of the border zones between the fields of supply of the major cerebral or cerebellar arteries.

The maintenance of blood pressure during various levels of activity and postural changes depends on baroreceptors in the aorta, carotids, and elsewhere. These receptors send afferent impulses to the brainstem. The vasomotor centers in the brainstem control cardiac rate and vasoconstriction in the skeletal musculature, skin, and splanchnic bed, via vagal and sympathetic fibers. Assuming the upright posture diminishes venous return to the heart and stroke volume, which provokes an immediate compensatory increase in heart rate and peripheral vasoconstriction. Only when these compensations fail does the cardiac output fall. Factors that diminish venous return or reduce cardiac output underlie many types of faint, some of which have already been described: valsalva maneuver (as in heavy lifting, a paroxysm of coughing, singing a long note), squatting, pulmonary hypertension, lying supine during pregnancy, and partial blockage of cardiac output (as in aortic stenosis during exercise). Notably, congestive heart failure is not a cause of syncope. Diseases that denervate autonomic ganglia and structures innervated by the vagus nerves are of crucial importance (Sharpey-Schafer).

The EEG changes during syncope have been investigated by Gastaut and Fischer-Williams. As mentioned above, attacks of cardiac arrest and syncope were produced by compression of the eyeballs (oculovagal reflex) in 20 of 100 patients who had a history of syncopal attacks—mainly of the vasopressor type. These investigators found that after a 7- to 13-s period of cardiac arrest there was a loss of consciousness, pallor, and muscle relaxation. Toward the end of this period, runs of bilaterally synchronous theta and delta waves appeared, predominantly in the frontal lobes, and in some patients one or more myoclonic jerks occurred in time with the slow waves. If the cardiac arrest persisted beyond 14 or 15 s, the EEG became flat. This period of electrical silence lasted for 10 to 20 s and was sometimes accompanied by a generalized tonic spasm with incontinence. Following the spasm, heartbeats and large-amplitude delta waves reappeared, and after another 20 to 30 s the EEG reverted to normal. It is noteworthy that rhythmic clonic seizures or epileptiform EEG activity were not observed at any time during the periods of cardiac arrest, syncope, and tonic spasm.

DIFFERENTIAL DIAGNOSIS

OF CONDITIONS ASSOCIATED WITH EPISODIC WEAKNESS AND FAINTNESS BUT RARELY WITH SYNCOPE

Anxiety Attacks and the Hyperventilation Syndrome These are discussed in detail in Chaps. 24 and 55. The giddiness of anxiety and hyperventilation is frequently described as a feeling of faintness, but a loss of consciousness does not follow. Such symptoms are not accompanied by facial pallor or relieved by recumbency. The diagnosis is made on the basis of the associated symptoms, and part of the attack can be reproduced by having the patient hyperventilate. Two of the mechanisms known to be involved in the attacks are reduction in arterial Pco_2 as the result of hyperventilation, and the release of epinephrine. Hyperventilation results in hypocapnia, alkalosis, increased cerebrovascular resistance, and decreased cerebral blood flow. When anxiety attacks are combined with a Valsalva maneuver or prolonged standing, fainting may occur.

Hypoglycemia Another cause of obscure episodic weakness is hypoglycemia. When severe, hypoglycemia is usually traceable to a serious disease, such as a tumor of the islets of Langerhans or advanced adrenal, pituitary, or hepatic disease. With progressive lowering of blood glucose, the clinical picture is one of hunger, trembling, flushed facies, sweating, confusion, and finally, after many minutes, seizures and coma. When mild, hypoglycemia is usually of the reactive type, occurring 2 to 5 h after eating, and is not associated with a disturbance of consciousness. The diagnosis depends largely upon the history, the documentation of reduced blood glucose during an attack, and the reproduction of the patient's spontaneous attacks by an injection of insulin or an oral dose of tolbutamide (or ingestion of a high-carbohydrate meal, in the case of reactive hypoglycemia)

Acute Hemorrhage Acute blood loss, usually within the gastrointestinal tract, is a cause of weakness, faintness, or even unconsciousness. In the absence of pain and hematemesis, the cause (peptic ulcer is the most common) may remain obscure until the passage of a black stool.

Transient Cerebral Ischemic Attacks These occur in some patients with arteriosclerotic narrowing or occlusion of the cartoid or vertebral-basilar arteries. The main symptoms, varying from patient to patient, include dim vision, hemiparesis, numbness of one side of the body, dizziness, and thick speech; rarely an impairment of consciousness is added. In any one patient the attacks are usually of one type and indicate a temporary deficit of function in a certain region of the brain due to inadequate circulation. The mechanism of the deficit has not been fully elucidated; recurrent embolism is the probable explanation in some cases (see Chap. 34).

The term *drop attack* is generally applied to a falling spell that occurs without warning and without loss of consciousness or postictal symptoms. The patient, usually elderly and more often female, suddenly falls down while walking or standing, rarely while stooping. The knees inexplicably buckle. There is no dizziness or impairment of consciousness, and the fall is usually forward, with scuffing of the knees and sometimes the nose. The patient is able to right herself and to rise immediately, unless obese, and goes her way, quite embarrassed. There may be several attacks during a period of a few weeks and none thereafter. EEGs are normal. Drop attacks also occur in hydrocephalics, and the patient, though conscious, may not be able to arise for several hours. Drop attacks, as defined above, are usually without identifiable mechanism and quite benign, requiring no treatment. They are often attributed to brainstem ischemia, but the evidence is not convincing. In only about one-quarter such cases, according to Meissner et al, can an association be made with cardiovascular or cerebrovascular disease, to which treatment should be directed.

OF SEIZURE AND SYNCOPE

Fully developed syncope must be distinguished from other cerebral disturbances causing loss of consciousness, the most frequent of which are atonic seizures or some other form of epilepsy (see Chap. 15). The epileptic attack may occur day or night, regardless of the position of the patient; syncope rarely appears when the patient is recumbent, the only common exception being the Stokes-Adams attack. The patient's color does not usually change at the very onset of an epileptic attack; pallor is an early and invariable finding in all types of syncope, except chronic orthostatic hypotension and hysteria, and it precedes unconsciousness. Epilepsy is more sudden in onset; if an aura is present, it rarely lasts longer than a few seconds before consciousness is abolished. The onset of syncope is usually more deliberate, and the prodromal symptoms are quite distinctive and different from those of seizures. Injury from falling is frequent in epilepsy and rare in syncope, for the reason that only in the former are protective reflexes instantaneously abolished. Tonic spasm of muscles with upturning of the eyes is a prominent and often an initial feature of epilepsy but occurs only rarely and late in the course of a faint; however, twitching and a few clonic contractions of the limbs may occur several seconds after the patient has fainted (see above). Urinary incontinence is frequent in epilepsy and rare in syncope, but it may not occur during an epileptic attack, in which case it cannot be used as a means of excluding the latter disorder. The return of consciousness is slow in epilepsy, prompt in syncope; mental confusion, headache, and drowsiness are common sequelae of the former state, and physical weakness with clear sensorium of the latter. Repeated spells of unconsciousness in a young person at a rate of several per day or month are much more suggestive of epilepsy than of syncope. No one of these points will absolutely differentiate epilepsy from syncope, but taken as a group and supplemented by electroencephalograms, they usually enable one to distinguish the two conditions.

OF DIFFERENT TYPES OF SYNCOPE

When faintness is related to reduced cerebral blood flow resulting directly from a disorder of cardiac function, there may be a combination of pallor and cyanosis, with pronounced dyspnea, and often the jugular veins are distended. When, on the other hand, the peripheral circulation is at fault, pallor is not accompanied by cyanosis or respiratory disturbances, and the veins are collapsed. During the attack a heart rate faster than 150 beats per minute indicates an ectopic cardiac rhythm, while a rate of less than 40 suggests complete heart block. In a patient with faintness or syncope attended by bradycardia, one has to distinguish between the neurogenic reflex type and the cardiogenic (Stokes-Adams) type. The electrocardiogram is decisive, but even without it, Stokes-Adams attacks can be recognized clinically by their longer duration, the greater constancy of the slow heart rate, the presence of audible sounds synchronous with atrial contraction, and the marked variation in the intensity of the first sound, despite the regular rhythm. The clinical diagnosis may at times be difficult or impossible, however.

The color of the skin, character of the breathing, appearance of the veins, and rate of the heart are therefore valuable data in diagnosis if the patient is seen during the attack. Unfortunately, the physician rarely has the opportunity to witness the syncopal attack and must obtain the proper clues from someone who did. It is essential that the physician be familiar with the circumstances and the precipitating and alleviating factors in a given episode of weakness or fainting. The following points are also helpful in the differential diagnosis of presyncope and syncope.

Type of Onset When the attack begins with relative suddenness, i.e., over the period of a few seconds, carotid sinus syncope, postural hypotension, sudden atrioventricular block or other cardiac arrhythmia is likely. When the symptoms develop gradually during a period of several minutes, hyperventilation (usually without faint) or hypoglycemia should be considered. Onset of syncope during or immediately after exertion is seen occasionally in persons with aortic stenosis or aortic insufficiency and with severe occlusive disease of the basilar artery.

Position at Onset of Attack   Attacks due to hypoglycemia, hyperventilation, or heart block are not dependent upon posture. Faintness associated with a decline in blood pressure (including carotid sinus attacks) and with ectopic tachycardia usually occurs only in the sitting or standing position, whereas the faintness of orthostatic hypotension occurs in response to a change from the recumbent to the standing position.

Associated Symptoms   The associated symptoms during an attack are important; palpitation is likely to be present when the attack is due to anxiety or hyperventilation, to ectopic tachycardia, or to hypoglycemia. Numbness and tingling in the hands and face are frequent accompaniments of hyperventilation. Irregular jerking movements and generalized spasms without loss of consciousness or change in the EEG are typical of the hysterical faint.

Duration and Frequency of Attacks   When the duration is very brief, i.e., a few seconds to a few minutes, carotid sinus syncope or one of the several forms of vasodepressor syncope or postural hypotension is most likely. A duration of more than a few minutes but less than an hour suggests hypoglycemia or hyperventilation. Although the latter types of attack are causes of episodic symptoms that simulate presyncope, they are usually not a cause of syncope.

When an otherwise healthy adult has many fainting attacks over a period of days one must consider myocardial disease with dysrhythmia, action of antihypertensive and psychotropic drugs, and hysteria.

SPECIAL METHODS OF EXAMINATION

In patients who complain of recurrent weakness or syncope but do not have a spontaneous attack while under observation of the physician, an attempt to reproduce attacks may prove to be of great assistance in diagnosis. Here it is important to recall that normal persons can faint if made to squat and overbreathe and then to stand erect and hold their breath (Valsalva maneuver). Prolonged standing at attention in the heat often causes even well-conditioned soldiers to faint, as does compression of the chest and abdomen while holding one's breath, as in the parlor trick of adolescents (fainting lark).

When hyperventilation is accompanied by faintness, the pattern of symptoms can be reproduced readily by having the subject breathe rapidly and deeply for 2 to 3 min. This test may also be of therapeutic value because the underlying anxiety tends to be lessened when the patient learns that symptoms can be produced and alleviated at will simply by controlling breathing.

Other conditions in which the diagnosis is clarified by reproducing the attacks are carotid sinus hypersensitivity (massage of one or the other carotid sinus) and orthostatic hypotension (observations of pulse rate, blood pressure, and symptoms in the recumbent and standing positions or even better, with the patient on a tilt table). Most patients with tussive syncope cannot reproduce an attack by the Valsalva maneuver, but can sometimes do so by voluntary coughing, if severe enough. Another useful procedure is to have the patient perform the Valsalva maneuver for more than 10 s (thus trapping blood behind closed valves in the veins) while measuring the pulse and blood pressure (see tests of autonomic function, page 429). In each of these instances the crucial point is not whether symptoms are produced, but whether they reproduce the exact pattern of symptoms that occurs in the spontaneous attacks. Careful continuous monitoring of the ECG in the hospital or by using a portable tape recorder may identify an arhythmia responsible for the syncopal episode. Monitoring may show that the syncopal attack corresponds with an episode of cardiac standstill, extreme bradycardia, or severe tachyrhythmia.

The EEG may be helpful in differentiating syncope from epilepsy. In the interval between epileptic seizures the EEG with sleep activation shows some degree of abnormality in 75 percent of cases, whereas it should be normal between syncopal attacks.

TREATMENT

Patients seen during the preliminary stages of fainting or after they have lost consciousness should be placed in a position which permits maximal cerebral blood flow, i.e., with head lowered between the knees, if sitting, or in the supine position with legs elevated. All tight clothing and other constrictions should be loosened and the head turned so that the tongue does not fall back into the throat, blocking the airway. Peripheral stimulation, such as sprinkling cold water on the face and neck or the application of cold towels or the cautious inhalation of ammonia is helpful. If the temperature is subnormal, the body should be covered with a warm blanket. Since emesis is frequent, one should be prepared for a possible aspiration of vomitus. Nothing should be given by mouth until the patient has regained consciousness. The patient should not be permitted to rise until the sense of physical weakness has passed, and should be watched carefully for a few minutes after rising.

As a rule, the physician sees the patient after recovery from the faint, and is asked to explain why it happened and how it can be prevented in the future. One should think first of those causes of fainting that constitute a therapeutic emergency. Among them are massive internal hemorrhage and myocardial infarction, which may be painless, and cardiac arhythmias. In an elderly person a sudden faint, without obvious cause, should arouse the suspicion of complete heart block, even though all findings are negative when the physician sees the patient.

The prevention of fainting depends on the mechanisms involved. In the usual vasodepressor faint of adolescents, which tends to occur in circumstances favoring vasodilatation and periods of emotional excitement, fatigue, hunger, etc., it is enough to advise the patient to avoid such circumstances. In postural hypotension, patients should be cautioned against arising suddenly from bed. Instead, they should first exercise the legs for a few seconds, then sit on the edge of the bed and make sure they are not light-headed or dizzy before starting to walk. They should sleep with the headposts of the bed elevated on 8- to 12-in high wooden blocks. A snug elastic abdominal binder and elastic stockings are often helpful. Drugs of the ephedrine group (ephedrine sulfate, 40 to 50 mg) may be useful if they do not cause insomnia.

In the syndrome of chronic orthostatic hypotension, special corticosteroid preparations [flurocortisone acetate (Florinef), 0.01 to 0.02 mg/day in divided doses] and increased salt intake to expand blood volume are helpful. Binding of the legs (i.e., wearing a G suit) and sleeping with head and shoulders elevated are other useful measures. Tyramine and monoamine oxidase inhibitors have given relief in some cases of Shy-Drager syndrome.

The treatment of carotid sinus syncope involves first of all instructing the patient in measures that minimize the hazards of a fall (see below). Loose collars should be worn, and the patient should learn to turn the whole body, rather than the head alone, when looking to one side. Atropine or one of the ephedrine group of drugs should be used, respectively, in patients with pronounced bradycardia or hypotension during attacks. If atropine is not successful and the syncopal attacks are incapacitating, the insertion of a demand pacemaker into the right ventricle should be considered. Radiation or surgical denervation of the carotid sinus has apparently yielded favorable results in some patients, but it is rarely necessary. Once it has been concluded that the attacks are due to a narrowing of major cerebral arteries, some of the surgical measures discussed in Chap. 34 must be considered. Vagovagal attacks usually respond well to anticholinergic drugs (propantheline, 15 mg tid).

Treatment of the hyperventilation syndrome and of hysteria are considered in Chap. 55. For a discussion of the treatment of the various cardiac arhythmias that may induce syncope and of hypoglycemia, the reader is referred to *Harrison's Principles of Internal Medicine*.

In the elderly person a faint carries the additional hazard of a fracture or other trauma due to the fall. Therefore, patients subject to recurrent syncope should cover the bathroom floor and bathtub with rubber mats, and should have as much of their home carpeted as is feasible. Especially important is the floor space between the bed and the bathroom, because this is the route along which faints are most common in elderly persons. Outdoor walking should be on soft ground rather than hard surfaces, and the patient should avoid standing still for prolonged periods, which is more likely to induce an attack than walking.

REFERENCES

COMPTON D, HILL PM, SINCLAIR JD: Weight-lifters' blackout. *Lancet* 2:1234, 1973.

ENGEL GL: *Fainting,* 2nd ed. Springfield, Ill, Charles C Thomas, 1962.

FREIDBERG CK: Syncope: Pathological physiology: Differential diagnosis and treatment. *Mod Concepts Cardiovasc Dis* 40:55, 1971.

GASTAUT H, FISCHER-WILLIAMS M: Electro-encephalographic study of syncope: Its differentiation from epilepsy. *Lancet* 2:1018, 1957.

JOHNSON RH, SPALDING JMK: *Disorders of the Autonomic Nervous System.* Philadelphia, Davis, 1974.

KAPOOR WN, KARPF M, MAHER Y et al: Syncope of unknown origin. *JAMA* 247:2687, 1982.

KAPOOR WN, KARPF M, WIEAND S et al: A prospective evaluation and follow-up of patients with syncope. *N Engl J Med* 309:197, 1983.

KONTOS HA, RICHARDSON DW, NORVELL JE: Norepinephrine depletion in idiopathic orthostatic hypotension. *Ann Intern Med* 82:336, 1975.

LEVINE B, POSNER JB: Swallow syncope: Report of a case and review of the literature. *Neurology* 22:1086, 1972.

LEVINE RJ: Epidemic faintness and syncope in a school marching band. *JAMA* 238:2373, 1977.

LIPSITZ LA: Syncope in the elderly. *Ann Intern Med* 99:92, 1983.

MEISSNER L, WIEBERS DO, SWANSON JW, O'FALLON WM: The natural history of drop attacks. *Neurology* 36:1029, 1986.

SHARPEY-SCHAFER EP: Syncope. *Br Med J* 860, 1953.

SCHOENBERG BS, KUGLITSCH JF, KARNES WE: Micturition syncope—not a single entity. *JAMA* 229:1631, 1974.

SHY GM, DRAGER GA: A neurological syndrome associated with orthostatic hypotension: A clinical-pathologic study. *Arch Neurol* 2:511, 1960.

SILVERSTEIN MD, SINGER DE, MULLEY AG et al: Patients with syncope admitted to intensive care units. *JAMA* 248:1185, 1982.

STREETEN DHP, KERR LP, KERR CB, et al: Hyperbradykininism: A new orthostatic syndrome. *Lancet* 2:1048, 1972.

WALLIN BG, WESTERBERG C-E, SUNDLÖF G: Syncope induced by glossopharyngeal neuralgia: Sympathetic outflow to muscle. *Neurology* 34:522, 1984.

WEISS S, CAPPS RB, FERRIS EB JR, MUNRO D: Syncope and convulsions due to a hyperactive carotid sinus reflex: Diagnosis and treatment. *Arch Intern Med* 58:407, 1936.

WEISS S, FERRIS EB JR: Adams-Stokes syndrome with transient complete heart block of vagovagal reflex origin: Mechanism and treatment. *Arch Intern Med* 54:931, 1934.

WRIGHT KE JR, MCINTOSH MD: Syncope: Review of pathophysiological mechanisms. *Prog Cardiovasc Dis* 13:580, 1971.

ZIEGLER DK, LIN J, BAYER WL: Convulsive syncope: Relationship to cerebral ischemia. *Trans Am Neurol Assoc* 103:150, 1978.

ZIEGLER MG, LAKE CR, KOPIN IJ: The sympathetic nervous system defect in primary orthostatic hypotension. *N Engl J Med* 296:293, 1977.

CHAPTER 18

SLEEP AND ITS ABNORMALITIES

Sleep, that familiar yet inexplicable condition of repose in which consciousness is in abeyance, is obviously not abnormal, yet it is not illogical to consider it in connection with abnormal phenomena. There are no doubt irregularities of sleep, some of which approach serious extremes, just as there are unnatural forms of waking consciousness.

Everyone has had a great deal of personal experience with sleep, or lack of it, and has observed people in sleep, so it requires no special knowledge of neurology to know something about this condition or to appreciate its importance to health and well-being. The psychologic and physiologic benefits of sleep have seldom been so eloquently expressed as in the words of Tristram Shandy:

> 'Tis the refuge of the unfortunate—the enfranchisement of the prisoner, the downy lap of the hopeless, the weary, the broken-hearted; of all the soft delicious functions of nature this is the chiefest; what a happiness it is to man, when the anxieties and passions of the day are over.

Physicians are often consulted by patients who suffer some derangement of sleep. Most often the problem is one of sleeplessness, but sometimes it concerns excessive sleep or other peculiar phenomena occurring in connection with sleep. Certain points concerning the physiology of normal sleep and the sleep-waking mechanisms will first be reviewed, since familiarity with these concepts is necessary for an understanding of sleep disorders and their treatment.

NORMAL SLEEP

Sleep, as everyone knows, is an elemental phenomenon of life and an indispensable phase of human existence. It represents one of the basic 24-h (circadian) rhythms, traceable through all mammalian, avian, and reptilian species. The neural control of circadian rhythms is thought to reside in the ventral-anterior region of the hypothalamus, more specifically in the suprachiasmatic nuclei. Lesions in these nuclei result in a complete disorganization of the sleep-wakefulness cycles, as well as of the rest-activity, temperature, and feeding rhythms.

Observations of the human sleep-wake cycle show it to be age-linked. The newborn baby sleeps from 16 to 20 h a day and the child, 10 to 12 h. Total sleep time drops to 9 to 10 h at age 10, and to about 7 to 7.5 h during adolescence. A gradual decline to about 6.5 h develops in late adult life. However, wide individual differences in the length and depth of sleep are to be noted, due apparently to genetic factors, early-life conditioning, and particular physical and psychologic states.

The pattern of sleeping, which in terrestrial life is adjusted to the 24-h day, also varies in the different epochs of life. A nocturnal predominance begins to appear only after the first few weeks of postnatal life of the full-term infant; as the child matures, the morning nap is omitted, then the afternoon nap, and by the fourth or fifth year the night's sleep becomes consolidated into a single long period. Actually, half of the world's population, or more, continues to have an afternoon nap (siesta) as a lifelong sleep-wake pattern. This alternating pattern of sleeping and waking persists throughout adolescence and adult years, unless altered by emotional or physical disease, and not until old age does fragmentation of the sleep pattern occur. Night awakenings then increase in frequency, and the daytime waking period becomes interrupted frequently by paroxysmal bursts of sleep lasting seconds to minutes (microsleep), as well as by longer naps. From about 35 years of age onward, women tend to sleep slightly more than men.

Seminal contributions to our understanding of the physiology of sleep were made by Loomis and his associates, by Aserinsky, and by Dement and Kleitman, through electroencephalographic (EEG) and polygraphic analysis. Five stages of sleep, representative of two alternating physiologic mechanisms, were defined. Relaxed wakefulness is accompanied by sinusoidal alpha waves of 9 to 11 Hz (cycles per second) and low-voltage fast activity of mixed frequency in the EEG; there are the usual artifacts due to blinking and movements of the eyes and limbs. The electromyogram is silent when the patient is sitting or lying quietly in bed, except for the facial (mimetic) muscles. As a person falls asleep and the muscles relax, the eyelids droop and the EEG pattern changes to one of progressively lower voltage and mixed frequency, with loss of alpha waves; this is associated with slow rolling eye movements and is called *stage 1 sleep*. As sleep changes into stage 2, $\frac{1}{2}$- to 2-s bursts of 12- to 16-Hz waves (sleep spindles) and high-amplitude, sharp slow-wave (K) complexes appear. The deep sleep of stages 3 and 4, also referred to as *slow-wave sleep*, is composed of an increasing proportion of high-amplitude (>100 μV), slow-wave (1 to 2 Hz) activity in the EEG. In the next stage of sleep, muscle tone is reduced further, except in the muscles of the eyes, which undergo bursts of rapid movements (REMs) behind the closed eyelids. Concomitantly, the EEG becomes desynchronized, i.e., it has a lower-voltage and higher-frequency discharge pattern, but 10-Hz alpha bursts are rare. The first four stages of sleep are called *nonrapid eye movement (NREM)* sleep or *quiet* or *synchronized sleep;* the last stage is variously designated as *rapid eye movement (REM), fast-wave, nonsynchronized* or *desynchronized* sleep (Fig. 18-1).

In the first portion of a typical night's sleep the normal young and middle-aged adult passes successively through stages 1, 2, 3, and 4 of NREM sleep. After about 70 to 100 min, a large proportion of which consists of stages 3 and 4 sleep, the first REM period occurs, usually heralded by a transient increase in body movements and a shift in the EEG pattern from stage 4 to 2. This NREM-REM cycle (activity-rest cycle of Kleitman) is repeated at about the same interval four to six times during the night, depending on the length of sleep. The first REM period may be brief, and the later cycles have much less stage 4 NREM sleep (in most cases, actually none). In the latter portion of a night's sleep, the cycles consist essentially of two alternating stages—REM sleep and stage 2 (spindle-K-complex) sleep. Newborn full-term infants spend about 50 percent of sleep in the REM stage (although they have different EEG and eye movement characteristics than adults). The newborn sleep cycle lasts about 60 min (50 percent REM, 50 percent NREM, generally alternating through a 3- to 4-h interfeeding period), but with age the sleep cycle lengthens to 90 to 100 min. About 20 to 25 percent of total sleep time in young adults is spent in REM sleep, 3 to 5 percent in stage 1, 50 to 60 percent in stage 2, and 10 to 20 percent in stages 3 and 4 combined. The amount of sleep in stages 3 and 4 decreases with age, and the elderly (over 70 years) have virtually no stage 4 sleep and only

small amounts of stage 3 sleep (Fig. 18-2). The 90- to 100-min cycle is fairly stable in any one person and is believed to continue to operate in a less perceptible degree during wakefulness in relation to cyclic gastric motility, hunger, degrees of alertness, and capacity for cognitive activity.

PHYSIOLOGIC CHANGES IN SLEEP

A comparison of the physiologic changes in NREM and REM sleep is instructive. The change in the EEG pattern has already been indicated. Cortical neurons tend to discharge in synchronized bursts during NREM sleep and in nonsynchronized bursts in the wakeful states; in REM sleep the unit activity rate is quite high and generally asynchronous. Most complex visual dreaming occurs in the REM period and is recalled most consistently if the subject is awakened at this time. Similar mental activity occurs in non-REM sleep, though to a much lesser extent. Subjects are easily aroused from REM sleep, but arousing a person during stages 3 or 4 of NREM sleep is more difficult and full arousal may take 5 min or more, during which the subject may be disoriented and confused (physicians called at night should not make medical decisions during this period).

As mentioned above, tonic muscle activity is minimal during REM sleep, although small twitching, trembling movements in facial and distal extremity (hand and foot) muscles can still be detected. Gross body movements occur every 15 min or so in all stages of sleep, but are maximal in the transition between REM and NREM sleep, when the sleeping person changes position, usually from side to side (most people sleep on the side). Eye movements of REM sleep are conjugate and occur in all directions (horizontal more than vertical). On closer study, REM sleep has been found to have phasic and tonic components. During the phasic period, in addition to the rapid eye movements, the pupils alternately dilate and constrict and the blood pressure, pulse, and respiration increase and become more irregular. The phasic activities are related to bursts of neuronal activity in the vestibular nuclei and are mediated through the medial longitudinal fasciculi and ocular motor nuclei, the median raphe nuclei, and the corticospinal tracts. In the nonphasic periods of REM sleep, alpha and gamma spinal neurons are inhibited, the H responses diminish, and the tendon (myotatic) and postural and flexor reflexes diminish or are abolished. This flaccidity or atonia, which is prominent in the abdominal, upper airway, and intercostal muscles, may compromise breathing during REM sleep and pose a threat to life in infants with excessive respiratory difficulty and in

Figure 18-1

EEG recordings from a 29-year-old woman in the awake state and various stages of sleep.
Awake state *(uppermost tracing).*
1. Stage 1 sleep: *EEG decreases in amplitude and increases in frequency, giving a "flat" appearance.*
2. Stage 2 sleep: *bursts of 13- to 16-Hz waves (sleep spindles) as well as high-amplitude, single-complex (K) waves appear against a background of low frequency.*
3. Stage 3 sleep: *appearance of high-voltage slow waves (delta activity) with some spindling.*

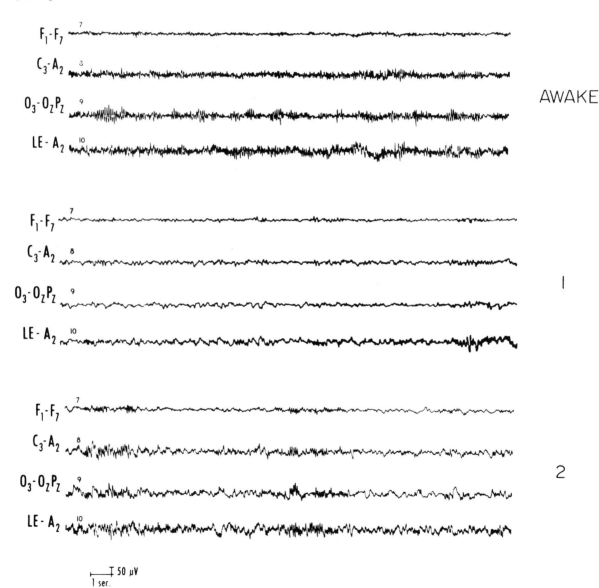

4. Stage 4 sleep: predominant delta slow-wave activity.

REM sleep: concomitant appearance of relatively low-voltage mixed-frequency EEG (stage 1) and REM (rapid-eye-movement) episodes.

Technical note: Four recording sites from the same montage are illustrated in each tracing: $F_1 - F_7$, left frontal; $C_1 - A_2$, left central to right ear; $O_3 - O_z$, P_z (between O_z and P_z), left parietooccipital; LE-A_2, left eye to right ear. Recordings were made at conventional sleep-laboratory speed of 15 mm/s (i.e., half the paper speed of standard clinical EEG recordings). (Adapted from Williams et al.)

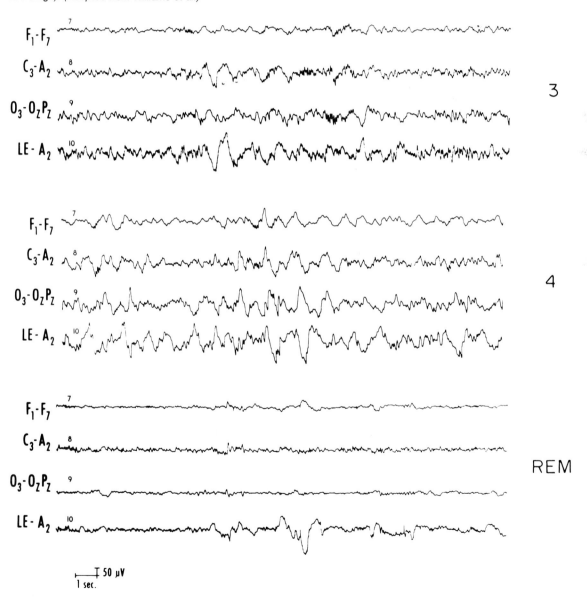

patients with kyphoscoliosis, muscular dystrophy, and paralytic poliomyelitis (Guilleminault and Dement).

It has long been known that the body temperature falls during sleep; however, if sleep does not occur, there still is a drop in body temperature, as part of the circadian (24-h) temperature curve. This fall is also independent of the 24-h recumbency-ambulatory cycle. During sleep, the fall in temperature occurs mainly during the NREM period, and the same is true of the heart beat and respiration, both of which become slow and more regular in this period. Oxygen consumption in muscle diminishes during NREM sleep and increases markedly in the brain during REM sleep. Urine excretion decreases during sleep, and the absolute quantity of sodium and potassium that is eliminated also decreases; however, the specific gravity and osmolality increase, presumably because of increased, antidiuretic hormone excretion and reabsorption of water. Autonomic nervous functions tend to be activated in REM sleep. Breathing is more irregular; heart rate and blood pressure fluctuate, and cerebral blood flow and metabolic rate increase. Penile erections appear about every 90 min, usually in REM periods.

A number of hormonal changes have a regular relationship to the sleep-wake cycle. During the first 2 h of sleep there is a surge of growth hormone secretion, mainly during sleep stages 3 and 4. Three or four episodic bursts of cortisol and ACTH secretion occur in the latter half of night sleep, producing the high concentrations that are characteristically found on awakening. Prolactin secretion increases during the night in both men and women, the highest plasma concentrations being found soon after the onset of sleep. Also, an increased sleep-associated secretion of luteinizing hormone occurs in pubertal boys and girls.

Evidence derived from studies in animals shows that the physiologic mechanisms governing NREM and REM sleep lie in the pontine reticular formation and are influenced by acetylcholine and by the two biogenic amines, 5-hydroxytryptamine (serotonin) and norepinephrine. Serotoninergic neurons are located in and near the midline or raphe regions of the pons; the lower groups of cells project to the medulla and spinal cord; the more rostral raphe nuclei project to the medial temporal (limbic) cortex, and the dorsal raphe nuclei project to the neostriatum, cerebral and cerebellar cortices, and thalamus. Norepinephrine-rich neurons are concentrated in the locus ceruleus and related nuclei in the central tegmentum of the caudal mesencephalon as well as in other lateral-ventral tegmental regions. These neurons project downward to the lateral horn cells of the spinal cord and upward via centrally located tegmental tracts to specific thalamic and subthalamic nuclei and all of the cerebral cortex, and via the superior cerebellar peduncle to the cerebellar cortex. Acetylcholine also appears to function as a neurotransmitter in the brainstem reticular activating system, judging by the activity of the cholinergic giant cells of the gigantocellular tegmental field during sleep. The projection system of this neurotransmitter has not been defined, however.

Hobson has proposed that the basic oscillation of the sleep cycle is the result of the reciprocal interaction of excitatory and inhibitory neurotransmitters. Single cell recordings from the pontine reticular formation suggest that there are two interconnected neuronal populations whose levels of activity fluctuate periodically and reciprocally. During the periods of wakefulness, according to this theory, the activity of aminergic (inhibitory) neurons is high, and, because of this aminergic inhibition, the activity of the

Figure 18-2

Normal sleep cycles. REM sleep (darkened areas) occurs cyclically throughout the night at intervals of approximately 90 min in all age groups. REM sleep shows little variation in the different age groups, whereas stage 4 sleep decreases with age. (From Kales and Kales.)

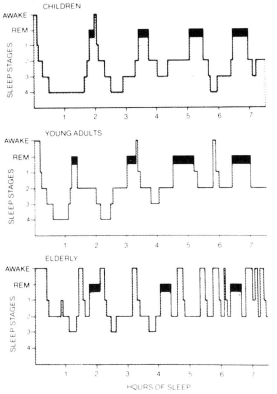

cholinergic neurons is low. During NREM sleep, aminergic inhibition gradually declines and cholinergic excitation increases; REM sleep occurs when the shift is complete. Support for this notion has been provided by the finding that the microinjection of either cholinergic agonists or aminergic antagonists into the pontine brainstem converts an animal from a state of wakefulness to one of REM sleep.

This theory provides a logical explanation for the sleep disorders and their treatment. Thus, excessive wakefulness, i.e., insomnia, as might occur with anxiety, is related to aminergic overactivity (or cholinergic underactivity) and can be countered by aminergic antagonists (e.g., diazepam). Reciprocally, hypersomnia is related to aminergic underactivity (or cholinergic overactivity) and can be countered by aminergic agonists (e.g., amphetamine). Timing errors between the sleep cycle "oscillator" and other neuronal systems are thought to account for parasomnic states such as sleep paralysis and sleep walking.

There is also evidence that certain peptides may play a role in sleep regulation. The plasma of drowsy or sleeping rabbits has been shown by Monnier and Hosli to contain a nonapeptide substance that induces somnolence and delta sleep in alert animals. Pappenheimer and his associates have isolated a different peptide ("S factor") from the brains of goats deprived of sleep; when injected into rats and rabbits it induces slow-wave (delta) sleep lasting several hours. Subsequently, other possible sleep factors, including muramyl peptides and interleukin I, both of which increase slow-wave sleep, have been identified. The precise origin and nature of these substances are as yet unknown.

THE FUNCTION OF SLEEP

This has been pondered by physiologists and psychiatrists. Parkes has reviewed the main theories—body restitution, facilitation of motor function, consolidation of learning and memory—and tends to agree with Popper and Eccles, who are quoted as saying "Sleep is a natural repeated unconsciousness that we do not even know the reason for." There is no convincing proof that we stabilize learned material while asleep. The authors, on the basis of plausibility and reason, favor the simple notion that sleep restores strength and physical and mental energy.

THE EFFECTS OF TOTAL AND PARTIAL SLEEP LOSS

Deprived of sleep, experimental animals will die within a few days to weeks, no matter how well they are fed, watered, and housed (Rechtschaffen et al), but whether insomnia leads to death in humans is unknown (Parkes). Humans deprived of sleep do, nevertheless, suffer a variety of unpleasant symptoms that must be separated from the usual types of insomnia.

Despite many studies of the deleterious emotional and cognitive effects of sleeplessness, we still know too little about them. If deprived of sleep (NREM and REM) for periods of 60 to 200 h, human beings experience increasing fatigue and irritability and find it difficult to concentrate, to perceive accurately, and to maintain their orientation. Feelings of persecution may be experienced, but psychotic behavior is rare (2 to 3 percent of 350 sleep-deprived patients studied by Tyler). Illusions and hallucinations, mainly visual and tactile ones, intrude into consciousness and become more intense as the period of sleeplessness is prolonged. Performance of skilled motor activities deteriorates. If the tasks are of short duration and of slow pace, the subject can manage them but if speed and perseverance are demanded, he cannot. Incentive to work weakens, and sustained thought and action are interrupted by lapses of attention. Neurologic signs to be noted include a mild and fleeting nystagmus, impairment of saccadic eye movements, loss of accommodation with exophoria, a slight tremor of the hands, ptosis of eyelids, expressionless face, and thickness of speech, with mispronunciation and incorrect choice of words. A decrement of alpha waves appears in the EEG, and closing of the eyes no longer generates alpha activity. The concentration of 17-hydroxycorticosteroids increases in the blood, and catecholamine output rises.

Rarely, and probably only in predisposed persons, loss of sleep provokes psychotic episodes; the subject may go berserk, screaming and sobbing, and incoherently muttering about seeing things. Fragmentary delusions and paranoid thoughts are more frequent.

During recovery from prolonged sleep deprivation, the amount of sleep obtained is never equal to the amount lost. This is probably due to the intrusive nature of sleep in the waking period (it is virtually impossible to deprive a human being or animal totally of sleep) and the occurrence of microsleep periods, which represent a sizable amount of time, if summated. When falling asleep after a long period of deprivation, the subject rapidly enters stage 4 of NREM sleep, which continues for several hours at the expense of stage 2 and REM sleep. But by the second recovery night, REM sleep rebounds and exceeds that of the predeprivation period. Stage 4 NREM sleep seems to be the most important sleep stage in restoring the altered functions that result from prolonged sleep deprivation.

Partial and differential sleep deprivation produce somewhat different effects than total or near total deprivation. Subjects in whom REM sleep is prevented night after night show an increasing tendency to hyperactivity, emotional lability, and a diminished ability to control their impulses, a state that corresponds to the heightened activity, excessive appetite, and oversexuality of REM sleep-deprived animals. Differential deprivation of NREM sleep (stages 3 and 4) leads, instead, to hyporesponsiveness and excessive sleepiness.

Since the need for sleep varies considerably from person to person, it is difficult to decide what is partial sleep deprivation. Certain rare individuals apparently function well on 4 h or even less of sleep per 24-h period, and others, who sleep long hours, claim not to obtain the maximum benefit from it.

SLEEP DISORDERS

INSOMNIA

This word signifies a chronic inability to sleep at times when sleep is normally expected to occur, and is used popularly to indicate any impairment in its duration, depth, or restorative properties. Insomnia may consist of difficulty in falling asleep or in remaining asleep, or a too early final awakening; or there may be a combination of these abnormalities. Precision as to what constitutes insomnia is impossible at the present time because of our uncertainty as to the exact amounts of sleep that are required and its role in the economy of the human body. All that can be said is that it is a frequent complaint (15 to 30 percent of the population) and more prominent in the elderly, particularly in thin old ladies who smoke and use alcohol.

Two general classes of insomnious disturbance may be defined—one in which there appears to be a primary abnormality of the normal sleep mechanism, another in which sleep impairment is secondary to a medical or psychologic disorder. Polygraphic studies have defined yet another subgroup of insomniacs—"pseudoinsomniacs"—who actually sleep enough but who perceive their sleep time to be shortened.

The term *primary insomnia* should be reserved for the condition in which nocturnal sleep is disturbed for prolonged periods and in which none of the symptoms of neurosis, depression, or other psychiatric or medical diseases can be elicited to explain the sleep disturbance. In some of the patients, like those of Hauri and Olmstead, the disorder is lifelong. Unlike the rare individuals who seem to be satisfied with 3 to 4 h of sleep a night, insomniacs suffer the effects of partial sleep deprivation and resort to all manner of drugs and various techniques to induce or maintain

sleep. Their life comes to revolve around sleep to such an extent that they have been called "sleep pedants" or "sleep hypochondriacs." Although statements of insomniacs are often not to be trusted, Rechtschaffen and Monroe have confirmed that most of them do indeed sleep poorly. They sleep for shorter periods, move and awaken more often, spend less time in stage 4 sleep than normal persons, and show a heightened physiologic arousal. Personality inventories have disclosed a high incidence of psychologic disturbances in this group of patients, but whether these are a cause or effect is not clear. Although victims of insomnia, regardless of the cause, tend to exaggerate the amount of sleep lost, primary insomnia should be recognized as an entity and not passed off as a quirk of the neurotic.

Secondary insomnia, also called *situational insomnia,* can often be ascribed to pain or some other recognizable bodily disorder, to drug abuse, or to anxiety, worry, or depression. This type of insomnia is usually transient. Of the medical disorders conducive to abnormal wakefulness, pain in the spine with or without nerve root involvement stands out, and also abdominal discomfort from peptic ulcer and carcinoma.

An obscure state known as the "restless legs syndrome" (anxietas tibiarum) may regularly delay the onset of sleep. The patient complains of an unpleasant aching sensation of the legs, often associated with creeping or crawling feelings —symptoms that are temporarily relieved by movement. The syndrome is usually benign but may occasionally be a prelude to a peripheral neuropathy, particularly uremic polyneuropathy. Excessive fatigue may give rise to abnormal muscular sensations of similar nature.

Another syndrome, *nocturnal myoclonus,* has been shown to be a cause of insomnia. This condition, also referred to as *periodic leg movements during sleep,* is to be distinguished from the gross jerks that occur occasionally in normal persons on falling asleep. The former is characterized by prolonged periods of repetitive movements of the legs, occurring every 20 to 40 s; mainly the anterior tibialis is involved, with extension of the big toe, sometimes followed by flexion of the hip, knee, and ankle. These movements produce frequent microarousals or, if severe, periodic full arousals. The patient, usually unaware of these sleep-related movements, is often told of them by a bedmate. This type of periodic movement may be associated with "restless legs" (see above) as well as with narcolepsy, sleep apnea, and other sleep disorders—indicating that it is probably secondary to a chronic sleep-wake disturbance and not a primary sleep-related disorder. Baclofen (20 to 40 mg at bedtime) may reduce the fragmentation of sleep caused by the muscle twitches, but not the twitches themselves (Guilleminault and Flagg).

While nocturnal myoclonus and sleep apnea (see further on) are recognized causes of insomnia and daytime sleepiness, they appear to be infrequent. Kales et al, in a study of 200 insomniacs in a sleep laboratory, encountered no patients with sleep apnea and only about 5 percent with nocturnal leg jerks.

Acroparesthesias, a predominantly nocturnal tingling and numbness of the fingers and palms due to tight carpal ligaments (carpal-tunnel syndrome), may awaken the patient at night. *Cluster headaches* characteristically awaken the patient within 1 to 2 h after falling asleep. In a few patients the headaches were found to occur during or immediately after the REM period.

More frequently, insomnia is secondary to some type of psychologic disturbance. Domestic or business worries may keep the patient's mind in a turmoil (situational insomnia). Also, vigorous mental activity late at night, or excitement, which leaves the muscles tense, may counteract drowsiness and sleep. A strange bed or surroundings may do likewise. Under these circumstances there is mainly a difficulty in falling asleep, with a tendency to sleep late in the morning. These facts emphasize that a certain degree of conditioning and environmental factors (social and learned) are normally involved in readying the mind and body for sleep. Parkes refers to these as "zeitgebers."

Illnesses in which anxiety and fear are prominent symptoms also result in difficulty in falling asleep and in light, fitful, or intermittent sleep. Also, disturbing dreams are frequent and may awaken the patient. Some patients even try to stay awake in order to avoid them, but this is the exception. In contrast, the depressive illnesses characteristically produce early-morning waking and inability to return to sleep; the quantity of sleep is reduced, and nocturnal motility is increased; REM sleep, although not always reduced, comes earlier in the night—this is termed the "increased pressure of REM sleep." If anxiety is combined with depression there is a tendency for both the above patterns to be observed. Yet another pattern of disturbed sleep can be discerned in individuals who are under great tension and worry or are overworked and exhausted. These people sink into bed and sleep through sheer exhaustion, but around 4 or 5 A.M they awaken with their worries and are unable to get back to sleep.

In states of mania and acute agitation, sleep diminishes and REM sleep may be abolished. Chronic intoxication with alcohol, barbiturates, and certain nonbarbiturate sedative-hypnotic drugs markedly reduces REM sleep, as well as stages 3 and 4 of NREM sleep. Following withdrawal of these drugs there is a rapid and marked increase of REM sleep and of dreaming. The patient has difficulty in falling asleep, and once asleep, arousals are frequent. Thus insomnia may be produced by the drugs that were intended to cure the disorder ("drug-withdrawal insomnia"; see Kales et al). Furthermore, a form of drug-withdrawal insomnia ("rebound insomnia") may actually occur during the night

in which the drug is administered. The drug produces its hypnotic effect in the first half of the night and a worsening of sleep during the latter half of the night, as the effects of the drug wear off; the patient and the physician may be misled into thinking that these latter symptoms require more of the hypnotic drug or a different one. Alcohol taken in the evening acts in the same way. It facilitates falling asleep, but after a few hours there is difficulty maintaining sleep.

A wide variety of other pharmacologic agents may give rise to sporadic or persistent disturbances of sleep. Caffeine-containing beverages, steroids, bronchodilators, central adrenergic blockers, amphetamines, and cigarettes are the most common offenders.

The sleep rhythm may be totally deranged in acute confusional states and delirium, and the patient may doze for only short periods, both day and night, the total amount and depth of sleep in a 24-h period being reduced. Frightening hallucinations may prevent sleep. The senile patient tends to catnap during the day and to remain alert for progressively longer periods during the night, until sleep is obtained in a series of short naps throughout the 24 h; the total amount of sleep may be increased or decreased.

Neurologic diseases may derange the total amount and patterns of sleep. This has been reported in pontine infarction with involvement of the tegmental raphe nuclei (Markand and Dyken). The abnormality took the form of a decrease in NREM sleep and a near abolition of REM sleep, lasting for weeks and months. A similar pattern has been described in patients with Huntington chorea, dyssynergia cerebellaris myoclonica of Ramsay Hunt, olivopontocerebellar degeneration, and progressive supranuclear palsy (Parkes). Dreaming is absent in some of these conditions. Following major head injury, abnormalities of sleep may persist for months or years, with a decrease in stages 1 and 2 of NREM sleep and less than the expected amounts of REM sleep and dreaming.

Disturbed and decreased total sleep also occurs when the normal circadian rhythm of the sleep-wake cycle is altered, as in shift workers who periodically change their work schedule from day to night. Sleep loss and disturbed sleep as a result of transmeridional jet flights (jet lag) is now a familiar problem. East-bound travelers fall asleep late and face an early sunrise. The consequent fatigue is a product of both sleep deprivation and a phase change required by changing time zones. The best antidote is to stay awake all day until the usual evening hour for sleep and to take a short-acting sedative (triazolam) at bedtime. These measures facilitate the resetting of the circadian rhythm. West-bound travelers face a late sunset and a long night's sleep, and adjust more readily to the resetting of the circadian rhythm.

Treatment of Insomnia   In general, sedative-hypnotic drugs for the management of insomnia should be prescribed only as a short-term adjuvant during illness or some unusual circumstance. For patients who have difficulty in falling asleep or staying asleep, or both, a quick-acting, fairly rapidly destroyed hypnotic is useful. The ones most commonly used at present are flurazepam (Dalmane), 15 to 30 mg, and triazolam (Halcion), 0.25 to 0.5 mg; much less used are secobarbital (Seconal), 0.1 g given 15 to 20 min before going to bed; chloral hydrate (Noctec), 1 to 2 g; or glutethimide (Doriden), 0.5 g. These drugs are more or less equally effective in inducing and maintaining sleep; however, they affect sleep stages differently. Flurazepam reduces stage 4 but not REM sleep, whereas the barbiturates and glutethimide reduce both stage 4 and REM sleep. If these drugs have to be given for longer than a week or two, all of them, with the possible exception of flurazepam, begin to lose their effectiveness, and larger doses are required to regain the initial effect. Patients who awaken too early in the morning may be given a longer-acting barbiturate, such as barbital, 0.3 g at bedtime. Chloral hydrate may be substituted if barbital is undesirable. Amitriptyline (50 mg at bedtime) appears to be a sleep-enhancing drug even in those who are not anxious or depressed. It is believed to block noradrenaline action.

When pain is a factor in insomnia, the sedative may be combined with acetylsalicylic acid, 0.3 to 0.6 g, or an equivalent dose of acetaminophen (Tylenol), or with codeine phosphate, 30 mg, or a stronger narcotic, when the pain is severe. For cardiac patients with orthopnea or Cheyne-Stokes respiration, an aminophylline suppository, 0.5 g at bedtime, will frequently relieve the respiratory distress. "Restless legs" are often helped by the use of a benzodiazepine (diazepam, clonazepam) or the α-adrenergic blocker tolazoline (Priscoline), 25 mg qid, and nocturnal myoclonus by baclofen, as mentioned above. The use of drugs in patients with delirium and manic-depressive disease is discussed in Chaps. 41 and 56.

The danger of administering fast-acting barbiturates on a nightly basis has been mentioned above. The repeated use of these drugs in an effort to achieve sleep carries a real danger of addiction, which, once developed, is pernicious in character. Withdrawal, unless accomplished skillfully, may cause serious mental disturbance or precipitate convulsions (see Chap. 42). In this respect, flurazepam and other benzodiazepines are less hazardous, but the risk of addiction still exists. Also, the nightly use of these drugs may have a cumulative effect, leading to daytime drowsiness and ataxia. Sedative-hypnotic drugs of all types are a common source of constipation, lead to fatigue and loss of strength, and have slight but definite teratogenic effects.

The chronic insomniac who has no other symptoms should not be permitted to use sedative drugs as a crutch on which to limp through life. The solution of this problem is rarely to be found in medication. One should search out and correct, if possible, any underlying situational or psychologic difficulty, using medication only as a temporary measure. Patients should be encouraged to regularize their daily schedules, including their bedtime, and to be physically active during the day, but to avoid strenuous physical and mental activity before bedtime. Dietary excesses need to be corrected and all nonessential medications interdicted. A helpful approach is to lessen the patient's concern about sleeplessness by pointing out that the human organism will always get as much sleep as needed, and that there is pleasure to be derived from staying awake and reading a good book.

PARASOMNIC DISTURBANCES (SOMNOLESCENT STARTS, SENSORY PAROXYSMS, AND SLEEP PARALYSIS)

A number of characteristic disorders occur in the transitional period between waking and sleep.

As sleep comes on, certain motor centers may be excited to a burst of insubordinate activity. The result is a sudden "start" or bodily jerk of large amplitude that rouses the incipient sleeper. It may involve one or both legs or the trunk (less often, the arms) and be associated with a frightening dream or sensory experience. If the "start" occurs repeatedly during the process of falling asleep and is a nightly event, it may become a matter of great concern to the patient. The "starts" are more apt to occur in individuals in whom the sleep process develops slowly, and are especially frequent under conditions of tension and anxiety. Polygraphic recordings have shown that these bodily jerks occur only during light sleep. Sometimes they appear as part of an arousal response to a faint external stimulus. It is probable that some relationship exists between these brusque nocturnal jerks and the sudden isolated jerk of a leg, or arm and leg, that occurs occasionally in a healthy, fully conscious person.

The recurrent bodily jerks that appear at the moment of falling asleep are not a variant of epilepsy. Oswald, who first studied this phenomenon by means of polygraph recordings, considers the jerks to be physiologic events, exaggerations of the common "somnolescent starts." EEG recordings in relation to the jerks do not disclose any epileptic discharges, and association with other manifestations of epilepsy is exceptional. Nor should these "starts" be referred to as *nocturnal myoclonus,* a term now used to designate the relatively mild, repetitive twitches that occur *during* sleep, mainly in stages 3 and 4 (see above, under "Insomnia").

Sensory centers may be disturbed in a similar way, either as an isolated phenomenon or in association with motor phenomena. The patient, dropping off to sleep, may be roused by a sensation that darts through the body, a sudden clang or crashing sound, or a sudden flash of light. Sometimes there is a sensation of being turned or lifted and dashed to the earth; conceivably these are sensory paroxysms involving the labyrinthine-vestibular mechanism.

A small proportion of otherwise healthy infants exhibits rhythmic jerking of the hands, arms, and legs, both at the onset and in the later stages of sleep. Coulter and Allen differentiate this state from myoclonic epilepsy and neonatal seizures by the absence of EEG changes and its occurrence only during sleep. It disappears by 1 or 2 years of age.

Curious paralytic phenomena, referred to as *pre- and postdormital paralyses,* may occur in the transition from the sleeping to the waking state. Sometimes in the morning, less frequently when falling asleep, otherwise healthy persons, though awake, conscious, and fully oriented, are unable to innervate their muscles (respiratory and diaphragmatic function and eye movements are usually not affected, however). They lie as though still asleep, with eyes closed, and may become quite frightened while engaged in a struggle for movement. They have the impression that if they could move one muscle, the paralysis would be dispelled instantly and they would regain full power. It has been stated that the slightest cutaneous stimulus, such as the touch of a hand, or calling the patient's name, will abolish the paralysis. Such attacks are observed in patients with narcolepsy (discussed later in this chapter) or with the hypersomnia of the pickwickian syndrome and other forms of sleep apnea. Some cases are familial. The weakness or paralysis is thought to be a dissociated form of the atonia of REM sleep. Usually the attacks are brief (minutes) and transient, and if they occur in isolation and only on rare occasions, are of no special significance. If frequent, as in narcolepsy, imipramine, desipramine, or clonipramine can be used to prevent them.

NIGHT TERRORS AND NIGHTMARES

The night terror (*pavor nocturnus*) is mainly a problem of childhood. It usually occurs soon after falling asleep, often within 30 min, during stage 3 or 4 sleep. The child awakens abruptly in a state of intense fright, screaming or moaning, with marked tachycardia (150 to 170 beats per minute) and deep, rapid respirations. Children with night terrors are often sleepwalkers as well, and both kinds of attack may occur simultaneously. The entire episode lasts only a minute or two, and in the morning the child recalls nothing of it or only a vague unpleasant dream. It has been suggested that night terrors, somnambulism, and confusion represent impaired or partial arousal from deep sleep, since EEGs taken during such episodes show a waking type of mixed frequency and alpha pattern. Children with night terrors and somnambulism do not show an increased incidence of psychologic abnormalities and tend to outgrow these disorders. Their persistence into adult life, however, is said to be associated with significant psychopathology (Kales et al). There is evidence that diazepam, which reduces the duration of stages 3 and 4 sleep, will prevent night terrors; this drug can be tried in persistent cases but should not be used for protracted periods.

Frightening dreams or nightmares are far more frequent than night terrors and affect children and adults alike. They occur during periods of normal REM sleep and are particularly prominent during periods of increased REM sleep (REM rebound), following the withdrawal of alcohol or other sedative-hypnotic drugs that had suppressed REM sleep chronically. Autonomic changes are slight or absent, and the content of the dreams can usually be recalled in considerable detail. Some of these dreams (e.g., the ones occurring in the alcohol-withdrawal period) are so vivid that the patient may later have difficulty in separating them from reality.

Nightmares are of little significance as isolated events. Fevers dispose to them, as do conditions such as indigestion, or the reading of bloodcurdling stories, or exposure to terrifying movies or television programs before bedtime. Persistent nightmares may be a pressing medical complaint, and are said to be accompanied frequently by other behavioral disturbances or neuroses. In adults they should always arouse the suspicion of chronic alcohol or barbiturate intoxication and withdrawal.

SOMNAMBULISM AND SLEEP AUTOMATISM

Examples of sleepwalking come to the attention of the practicing physician not infrequently. This condition likewise occurs more often in children (average age, 4 to 6 years) than in adults, and is often associated with nocturnal enuresis and night terrors, as has been indicated. The estimated frequency of sleepwalking in children is 15 percent, and one in five sleepwalkers has a family history. The motor performance and responsiveness during the sleepwalking incident vary considerably. The most common behavioral abnormality is for patients to sit up in bed or on the edge of the bed without actually walking. When walking about the house, they may turn on a light or perform some other familiar act. There may be no outward signs of emotion, or the patient may be frightened (night terror). Usually the eyes are open, and such sleepwalkers are guided by vision, thus avoiding familiar objects; the sight of an unfamiliar object may awaken them. Sometimes these patients make no attempt to avoid obstacles and may injure themselves. If spoken to, they make no response; if told to return to bed, they may do so but more often must be led back to it. Sometimes they repeatedly mutter strange phrases or sentences or perform certain repetitive acts such as pushing against a wall or turning a doorknob back and forth. The episode lasts for only a few minutes, and the following morning they usually have no memory of it.

Half-waking somnambulism, or sleep automatism, is a closely related disorder. This is a state in which an adult, half-roused from sleep, goes through a fairly complex routine such as going to a window, opening it, and looking out, but afterward recalls only a part of the episode.

A popular belief is that the sleepwalker is acting out a dream. Sleep-laboratory observations are at variance with this view, since somnambulism has been found to occur almost exclusively during stages 3 and 4 of NREM sleep, when dreaming is least likely to occur. And the entire nocturnal sleep pattern of such individuals does not differ from normal. Similarly, there is no evidence that somnambulism is a form of epilepsy. It is probably allied to talking in one's sleep, although the two conditions seldom occur together.

Some psychiatrists hold that somnambulism represents a dissociated mental state, similar to the hysterical trance of fugue, except that it begins during sleep. To them sleepwalking is evidence of a psychoneurotic disorder. This interpretation is probably incorrect, at least in children and adolescents, since they usually do not show any other signs of psychopathology. The onset of sleepwalking or night terrors in adult life is most unusual and should suggest the presence of major psychiatric disease. It must be distinguished from fugue states (page 1195) and ambulatory automatisms of complex partial seizures (page 253). Claims have been made that crimes can be committed during sleepwalking, but the evidence is impossible to evaluate. Usually such a patient has been an intoxicated sociopath.

The major consideration in the treatment of somnambulism is to guard patients against injury by locking doors and windows, removing dangerous objects from their usual routes of march, having them sleep on the ground floor,

etc. Children usually outgrow this disorder, and parents should be reassured on this score and disabused of the notion that somnambulism is a sign of psychiatric disease.

NOCTURNAL EPILEPSY

It has long been known that convulsive seizures often occur during sleep, especially in children. This is such a frequent occurrence that the practice of inducing sleep in order to obtain confirmation of epilepsy has been adopted as an activating procedure in most EEG laboratories. Seizures may occur soon after the onset of sleep or at any time during the night, but mainly in stage 4 of NREM sleep or in REM sleep. They are also common during the first hour after awakening. On the other hand, deprivation of sleep may be conducive to a seizure.

Sleeping epileptic patients attract attention to their seizures by a cry, violent motor activity, or labored breathing. As in diurnal seizures, after the tonic-clonic phase, they become quiet and fall into a state resembling sleep but from which they cannot be roused. Their appearance depends on the phase of the seizure they happen to be in when first observed. If the nocturnal seizure is unobserved, the only indication of it may be disheveled bedclothes, a few drops of blood on the pillow, wet bed linen from urinary incontinence, a bitten tongue, or sore muscles. In some, the occurrence of a seizure is betrayed only by confusion or headache, the common aftermaths of a seizure disorder. Rarely, a patient may die in an epileptic seizure during sleep, presumably from smothering in the bedclothes or aspirating vomitus, or for some obscure reason (possibly cardiac dysrhythmia). These accidents, and similar ones in awake epileptics, account for the higher mortality rate in epileptics than in nonepileptics.

Rarely, epilepsy may occur in conjunction with night terrors and somnambulism, and the question then arises whether the latter disorders are in the nature of postepileptic automatisms. Usually no such relationship is established. EEG studies during a nocturnal period of sleep are most helpful in such cases.

EXCESSIVE SLEEP (HYPERSOMNIA) AND REVERSAL OF SLEEP-WAKING RHYTHM

Encephalitis lethargica, or "epidemic encephalitis," the remarkable illness that appeared on the medical horizon as a pandemic following World War I, provided some of the most dramatic instances of pathologic somnolence. In fact, protracted sleep lasting for days to weeks was such a prominent symptom of this disease that it was called *sleeping sickness*. The patient appeared to be in a state of continuous sleep, or *somnosis*, and could be kept awake only by constant stimulation. Although the infective agent was never isolated, the pathologic anatomy was fully divulged by many excellent studies, all of which demonstrated a destruction of neurons in the midbrain, subthalamus, and hypothalamus. Patients who survived the acute phase of the illness often had difficulty in reestablishing their normal sleep-waking rhythm. As the somnolence disappeared, some patients exhibited a reversal of the sleep-wake rhythm, tending to sleep by day and stay awake at night; many of them also developed a Parkinson syndrome, months or years later. Possibly the hypersomnia was related to destruction of epinephrine-rich neurons in the substantia nigra, resulting in overactivity of the raphe (serotoninergic) neurons.

Hypersomnia also occurs in trypanosomiasis, the common cause of "sleeping sickness" in Africa, and with a variety of diseases localized to the mesencephalon and the floor and walls of the third ventricle. Small tumors in this area have been associated with arterial hypotension, diabetes insipidus, hypo- or hyperthermia and protracted somnolence lasting many weeks. Such patients can be aroused, but if left alone, they immediately fall asleep. Traumatic and vascular lesions and other diseases affecting the mesencephalon and diencephalon produce a similar clinical picture. Severe myxedema causes hypersomnia, as does hypercapnia, the latter with nocturnal headache and confusion.

Periodic hypersomnia is a manifestation of the *Kleine-Levin syndrome*. Three or four times a year, for periods lasting a few days to several weeks, these patients (most often adolescent boys) may have daily attacks of prolonged diurnal sleep lasting many hours, or the duration of nocturnal sleep may be greatly prolonged, or they may sleep for days on end. Nevertheless the organization of components of the sleep cycle is normal. The food intake during the period of hypersomnia may exceed three times the normal (bulimia), and to a variable extent there are other behavioral changes such as social withdrawal, negativism, slowness of thinking, incoherence, inattentiveness, and disturbances of memory. The basis of this condition has never been elucidated. A psychogenic mechanism has been proposed but is without foundation. The condition usually disappears during adulthood (see also page 453).

Finally it should be mentioned that sleep laboratories now recognize a form of *idiopathic hypersomnia*, in which there are repeated episodes of drowsiness throughout the day. This condition is discussed more fully following the section on narcolepsy, with which it is most often confused. The chronic use of alcohol or drugs and certain metabolic diseases also cause daytime drowsiness.

SLEEP APNEA AND DAYTIME HYPERSOMNOLENCE

As mentioned above, REM sleep is characterized by irregular breathing, and this may include several brief periods of apnea, up to 10 s in duration. Such apneas, occurring during REM sleep or at the onset of sleep, are not considered to be pathologic. During the past decade it has come to be recognized that in some individuals sleep-induced apneic periods are particularly frequent and prolonged (greater than 10 s) and that such a condition may be responsible for a variety of clinical disturbances in children and adults. This pathologic form of sleep apnea may be due to a cessation of respiratory drive (so-called central apnea) or to an obstruction of the upper airway, or to a combination of these two mechanisms.

The *central form of sleep apnea* has been observed in patients with bulbar poliomyelitis, lower brainstem infarction, spinal (high cervical) surgery, syringobulbia, encephalitis, striatonigral degeneration, Creutzfeldt-Jakob disease, olivopontocerebellar degeneration, and with a disorder referred to as the *primary, or idiopathic, hypoventilation syndrome*. The lesions in these neurologic diseases are localized to the medulla by the presence of ninth and tenth cranial nerve palsies, dysphagia, dysphonia, hiccough, and crossed sensory defects. In some cases, breathing ceases with sleep (so-called Ondine's curse). In the few autopsied cases of central alveolar hyperventilation, Liu et al found the external arcuate nuclei of the medulla to be absent and the neuron population in the medullary respiratory areas to be depleted.

Apnea of the obstructive type is often associated with obesity and adenotonsillar hypertrophy, and less frequently with acromegaly, myxedema, micrognathia, and myotonic dystrophy. This form of sleep apnea is characterized by noisy snoring of a special type. After a period of regular, albeit noisy, breathing, there occurs a waning of breathing efforts; then, despite repeated inspiratory efforts, with contractions of the diaphragms, airflow ceases. After a prolonged period of apnea (10 to 30 s or even longer) the patient makes a series of progressively greater breathing efforts until breathing resumes, accompanied by very loud snorting sounds and a brief arousal.

Obstructive sleep apnea occurs during REM sleep, for the reason that the upper respiratory muscles (genioglossus, geniohyoid, tensor veli palatini, and medial pterygoid) normally contract just before the diaphram contracts, protruding the tongue and helping to keep the oropharynx open. If the airway is obstructed or the muscles are weakened and then go slack during REM sleep, the negative intrathoracic pressure causes collapse of these passages. Kyphoscoliosis, weakened muscles, and lung disease add to the problem.

The occurrence of a prolonged period of sleep apnea, from whatever cause, is accompanied by progressive hypercapnia and hypoxia, a transient increase in systemic and pulmonary arterial pressures, and sinus bradycardia or other arrhythmias. The blood gas changes, or perhaps other stimuli, induce an arousal response, either a lightening of sleep or a very brief awakening, which is followed by an immediate resumption of breathing. The patient quickly falls asleep again and the sequence is repeated, several hundred times a night in severe cases. Paradoxically these patients are very difficult to rouse at all times during the night.

Sleep apnea syndromes occur in persons of all ages. In adults, obstructive sleep apnea is predominantly a disorder of overweight, middle-aged men, and usually presents as *excessive daytime sleepiness,* a complaint that is often mistaken for narcolepsy (see below). Other patients, usually those with the central form of apnea, complain mainly of a disturbance of sleep at night, or insomnia, which may be incorrectly attributed to anxiety or depression. Morning headache, inattentiveness, and decline in school or work performance are other symptoms attributable to sleep apnea. Ultimately, systemic and pulmonary arterial hypertension, cor pulmonale, polycythemia, and heart failure may develop. These symptoms, if combined with obesity, are frequently referred to as the pickwickian syndrome, so named by Burwell et al (1956), who identified this clinical syndrome with that of the extraordinarily sleepy, red-faced fat boy described by Dickens, in *The Pickwick Papers*. The term is no longer apt, since it fails to indicate the fundamental role of sleep apnea in the genesis of the syndrome. Furthermore, obesity is found in only a minority of patients with sleep apnea; conversely, apnea occurs in only a small proportion of obese persons. Severe and life-threatening sleep apnea may occur with lateral medullary infarction and other lower brainstem lesions.

In infants with delayed maturation of the respiratory centers, sleep apnea is not infrequent and not without danger, accounting for a certain number of crib deaths. In approximately half of the observed infants with this latter condition, the apnea represents a respiratory arrest during a seizure. This can be demonstrated by EEG.

The full-blown syndrome of sleep apnea is readily recognized. In patients who complain only of excessive daytime sleepiness or insomnia, the diagnosis may be elusive and require special tests of respiratory function in addition to all-night polygraphic sleep monitoring. Treatment is governed by the severity of symptoms and the predominant type of apnea, central or obstructive. In central apnea, medroxyprogesterone and protriptyline, a nonsedating tricyclic antidepressant, are the drugs most often used. The

latter drug has also been found to be effective in reducing daytime somnolence in patients with mild obstructive sleep apnea (Brownell et al). In the latter patients, weight loss and surgical correction of an anatomic defect are helpful as well. Patients with severe hypersomnia and life-threatening cardiopulmonary signs require tracheostomy and respirator care. (See Parkes for a full account of therapeutic measures.)

NARCOLEPSY AND CATAPLEXY

This clinical entity has long been known to the medical profession. Gelineau gave it the name *narcolepsy* in 1880, although several authors had described the recurring attacks of irresistible sleep even before that time (see historical review by Passouant). Loewenfeld (1902) was probably the first to recognize the common association between the sleep attacks and the temporary paralysis of the somatic musculature during bouts of laughter, anger, and other emotional states; this was referred to as *cataplectic inhibition* by Henneberg (1916) and later as *cataplexy* by Adie (1926). The term *sleep paralysis,* to designate the brief, episodic loss of voluntary movement that occurs during the period of falling asleep (hypnagogic or predormital) or less often, when awakening (hypnopompic or postdormital), was introduced by Kinnier Wilson in 1928. Actually, Weir Mitchell had described this disorder in 1876, under the title of *night palsy*. Sometimes sleep paralysis is accompanied or just preceded by vivid and terrifying hallucinations (*hypnagogic hallucinations*). The hallucinations may be visual, auditory, vestibular (a sense of motion), or somatic (a feeling that a limb or finger or other part of the body is enlarged or otherwise transformed). These four conditions constitute a clinical tetrad. The association of hypnagogic hallucinations with narcolepsy was first noted by Lhermitte and Tournay, in 1927.

Clinical Features   This syndrome is not infrequent, as shown by the fact that Daly and Yoss recorded the occurrence of about 100 new cases a year at the Mayo Clinic. The estimated prevalence rate is 40 per 100,000 population. Males are affected more often than females. Family studies have disclosed an increased incidence of excessive sleep disturbances among the parents, siblings, and children of probands with narcolepsy, but a recessive or dominant pattern of transmission has not been identified (Kessler et al). Nevertheless, tissue typing of narcoleptics defined by strict clinical and laboratory criteria has disclosed an almost universal association with HLA-DR2 antigen, suggesting at least a genetically determined susceptibility to the disease (Neely et al).

As a rule, narcolepsy begins in late childhood, adolescence, or early adult life; in fully 90 percent of narcoleptics the condition is established by the 25th year. Narcolepsy is usually the first symptom, less often cataplexy, and rarely sleep paralysis. The essential disorder is one of irresistible attacks of sleepiness. Several times a day, usually after meals, or while sitting in class or being in other states of physical inactivity, the affected person is assailed by an uncontrollable desire to sleep. The eyes close, the muscles relax, breathing deepens slightly, and by all appearances the individual is dozing. A noise, a touch, or even the cessation of the lecturer's voice is enough to awaken the patient. The periods of sleep rarely last longer than 15 min, unless the patient is reclining, when they may continue for an hour or longer. At the conclusion of a nap the patient feels somewhat refreshed. What distinguishes the narcoleptic sleep attacks from the commonplace postprandial drowsiness is the frequent occurrence of the former (two to six attacks every day, as a rule), their irresistability, and their occurrence in unusual situations, as while standing, eating, or carrying on a conversation. Blurring of vision, diplopia, and ptosis may attend drowsiness and may bring the patient to an ophthalmologist.

It is not generally appreciated that in addition to episodes of outright sleep, narcoleptics frequently experience episodic lapses in consciousness, characterized by automatic behavior and amnesia. These latter phenomena may last for a few seconds or as long as an hour or more. Like true sleep attacks, these lapses of consciousness occur more often in the afternoon and evening than in the morning, usually when the patient is alone and performing some monotonous task, such as driving. Initially the patient feels drowsy and may recall attempts to fight off the drowsiness, but gradually he or she loses track of what is going on. The patient may continue to perform routine tasks correctly but does not respond appropriately to a new demand or answer complex questions. Often there is a sudden burst of words, without meaning or relevance to what was just said. Such an outburst may terminate the attack, for which there is complete or nearly complete amnesia. In many respects the attacks resemble episodes of nocturnal sleepwalking. Such attacks of automatic behavior and amnesia are common, occurring in more than half of a large series of patients with narcolepsy-cataplexy (Guilleminault and Dement). Driving accidents are frequent in these patients, occurring more often than in the epileptic population.

Nocturnal sleep is often troubled and reduced in amount. The number of hours in a 24-h day spent in sleep by the narcoleptic is not much greater than that of a normal individual. Narcoleptics have an increased incidence of sleep apnea and nocturnal myoclonus, but not of somnambulism.

Approximately 70 percent of narcoleptics, if questioned carefully, will admit having some form of cataplexy, and if the narcoleptic attacks can be shown by polygraph

recordings to represent episodes of REM sleep (see below), then almost all such patients will give a history of cataplectic attacks. Cataplexy refers to a sudden loss of muscle tone brought on by strong emotion; circumstances in which hearty laughter, more rarely excitement, surprise, or anger will cause the patient's head to fall forward, the jaw to drop, the knees to buckle, even with falling to the ground, all with perfect preservation of consciousness. In perhaps 5 percent of cases, the cataplectic attacks are unprovoked. The attacks last only a few seconds or a minute or two, and are of variable frequency. In most of our cases they appear at intervals of a few days or weeks. Exceptionally there are many attacks daily and even status cataplexicus, in which the atonia lasts for hours. This is more likely to happen at the beginning of the illness or upon discontinuing tricyclic medication.

Some attacks of cataplexy are partial (e.g., only a dropping of the jaw). Wilson found that the tendon reflexes were abolished during the attack. Pupillary reflexes are absent in some cases and preserved in others. H responses are lost.

Rarely, cataplexy precedes the onset of sleep attacks, but usually it follows them, sometimes by many years. Sleep paralysis and hypnagogic hallucinations (see above) occur in about one-quarter of the patients, and the full tetrad occurs in about 10 percent. Although cataplexy is pathognomonic of narcolepsy, hypnagogic paralysis and hallucinations may occur occasionally in normal persons. Also it should be noted that normal children, especially when tickled, may laugh to the point of cataplexy. About 10 percent of narcoleptics have none of the associated phenomena ("independent narcolepsy"), and in these cases REM periods are not found consistently at the onset of sleep.

Once the condition begins, it usually continues for the remainder of the patient's life, perhaps becoming less severe with age. No other abnormality is associated with it, and none develops later.

Cause and Pathogenesis The cause of narcolepsy is unknown. It bears no relation to epilepsy or migraine. A psychogenesis has been proposed, but the relevance of the psychologic observations remains open to question. Furthermore, narcolepsy and cataplexy, as well as unambiguous sleep-onset REM periods, have been described in animals (dogs and horses)—a finding that certainly challenges the psychiatric view of this condition. No autopsies in which the brain was thoroughly examined have been reported.

Rarely, the narcolepsy-cataplexy syndrome follows

cerebral trauma or accompanies multiple sclerosis, cranio-pharyngioma or other tumors of the third ventricle or brainstem, or diabetes insipidus (*secondary or symptomatic narcolepsy*).

The most important development in our understanding of narcolepsy has been the demonstration, by Dement and his group, that this disorder is associated with an inversion of the two states of sleep, with REM rather than NREM sleep occurring at the onset of the sleep attacks. Not all the diurnal sleep episodes of the narcoleptic begin with REM sleep, but almost always such an onset can be identified in narcoleptic-cataplectic patients in the course of a polygraphic sleep study. The hypnagogic hallucinations (which in this formulation are viewed as dream phenomena), cataplexy, and sleep-onset paralysis (inhibition of anterior horn cells) are all identified as events that characterize the REM period. These investigators have also shown that the night sleep pattern of patients with narcolepsy-cataplexy characteristically begins with a REM period. This, too, almost never occurs in normal subjects or in patients with other types of hypersomnia. Furthermore, the nocturnal sleep pattern is altered in narcoleptics, with frequent body movements and transient awakenings and decrease in sleep stages 3 and 4 and in total sleep. In addition, Passouant and his colleagues, on the basis of continuous 24-h polygraphic monitoring, have presented evidence that in some patients there is a 90- to 120-min periodicity of the narcolepsy-REM sleep attacks all during the day. Also evidence has been presented that *sleep latency* (the time between the point when an individual tries to sleep and the point of onset of EEG sleep patterns), measured repeatedly in diurnal nap situations, is greatly reduced in narcoleptics (Richardson). Thus narcolepsy is not simply a matter of excessive diurnal sleepiness (essential daytime drowsiness) or even a disorder of REM sleep, but a generalized disorganization of sleep-waking functions.

Diagnosis The greatest difficulty in the diagnosis of narcolepsy relates to the problem of separating it from the sleep pattern of certain sedentary, obese adults who, if unoccupied, doze readily after meals, or during a game of bridge, or in the theater. However, characteristic of narcolepsy is the imperative need for sleep, even under unusual circumstances (such as standing up) and the tendency of the sleep attacks to recur many times a day. When cataplexy is conjoined, diagnosis becomes certain. The brief attacks of automatic behavior and amnesia of the narcoleptic need to be distinguished from hysterical fugues and complex partial seizures. Excessive somnolence, easily mistaken for idiopathic narcolepsy, may attend sleep apnea syndromes

(the most frequent cause), obesity, heart failure, hypothyroidism, excessive use of barbiturates and other anticonvulsants, alcohol, cerebral trauma, and certain brain tumors (e.g., craniopharyngioma). Where polygraphic sleep recording facilities are available, the finding of *short latency* (less than 5 min) *REM sleep* during normal waking hours or just after nocturnal sleep begins will confirm the diagnosis of narcolepsy. Cataplexy must be distinguished from drop attacks (Chap. 17) and atonic seizures, in which consciousness is temporarily abolished.

Treatment No single therapy will control all the symptoms. The narcolepsy responds best to (1) strategically placed 15-min naps (during lunch hour, before or after dinner, etc.) and (2) the use of analeptic drugs [dextroamphetamine sulfate (Dexedrine) or methylphenidate hydrochloride (Ritalin)] or tricyclic antidepressants (imipramine or clomipramine). Monoamine oxidase inhibitors (phenelzine, pargyline) are also effective in controlling narcoleptic symptoms, but their severe side effects make them impractical for long-time use. All these drugs presumably produce their effects by inhibiting REM sleep.

The timing and frequency of the scheduled naps has to be determined for each individual according to the usual temporal distribution of the spontaneous attacks. Similarly the time of medication should be adjusted to the study or work habits of the patient. Methylphenidate is the drug of first choice because of its prompt action and relative lack of side effects. It is given in doses of 10 to 20 mg thrice daily, on an empty stomach. The usual dose of amphetamine is 5 to 10 mg given three to five times a day. This is ordinarily well tolerated and does not cause wakefulness at night. These drugs have rather little effect on cataplexy but are partially effective in the Kleine-Levin syndrome. Imipramine (Tofranil), in doses of 25 mg three to four times a day, and clomipramine, in a dose of 10 mg daily, are effective in preventing cataplexy. If these drugs fail, protryptamine may be helpful. Since methylphenidate and amphetamines are particularly effective in reducing the sleep attacks and imipramine or clomipramine in reducing cataplexy and sleep paralysis, the combined use of these drugs is often indicated. A problem with the stimulant drugs is the development of tolerance over a 6- to 12-month period, which requires the switching of drugs and periods of drug cessation. Both the stimulant drug and the tricyclic antidepressants increase catecholamine levels and their chronic administration may produce hypertension. Excessive amounts of amphetamines may induce a schizophreniform psychosis (Chap. 42).

Narcoleptics must be warned of the danger of sleep attacks and analogous lapses of consciousness while driving or during engagement in other activities that require constant alertness. The earliest feeling of drowsiness should prompt the patient to pull off the road and take a nap. Long distance driving should probably be avoided completely.

DAYTIME DROWSINESS (ESSENTIAL HYPERSOMNOLENCE)

As indicated, this may be the presenting symptom in a number of diseases other than narcolepsy and cataplexy. It merges at one extreme with the daytime drowsiness of the normal person, and at the other with a distressing pattern of daytime hypersomnolence that interferes with schooling and work. Some of these patients will eventually be recognized as narcoleptics, others as victims of sleep apnea. In populations of such patients under study in a sleep laboratory, Guilleminault and Dement recorded that a cause could be established in over 90 percent of patients. When chronic daytime drowsiness occurs repeatedly and persistently without known cause, it is classified as essential hypersomnolence. Roth distinguished the state from narcolepsy on the basis of longer daytime sleep periods, deep and undisturbed night sleep, sleep drunkenness, difficult morning awakening, and absence of REM-onset sleep and cataplexy. Admittedly, this condition proves difficult to distinguish from pure narcolepsy and sleep paralysis unless laboratory studies are made. The treatment is the same as that for narcolepsy.

PATHOLOGIC WAKEFULNESS

This state has been induced in animals by lesions in the tegmentum (median raphe nuclei) of the pons. Comparable states are known to occur in humans, but must be rare. The commonest causes of asomnia in hospital practice are delirium tremens and other drug-withdrawal psychoses. Drug-induced psychoses and hypomania may also cause hyposomnia.

SLEEP PALSIES AND ACROPARESTHESIAS

Several types of paresthetic disturbance, sometimes distressing in nature, may develop during sleep. Everyone is familiar with the phenomenon of an arm or leg "falling asleep." The immobility of the limbs and the maintenance of uncomfortable postures without being aware of them permits undue pressure to be applied to exposed nerves. The ulnar, radial, and peroneal nerves are quite superficial in places, and pressure of the nerve against the underlying bone may interfere with intraneural circulation of blood in the compressed segment. If such pressure is continued for half an hour or longer, a sensory and motor paralysis—sometimes referred to as *sleep* or *pressure palsy*—may develop. This condition usually lasts only a few hours or

days, but if the compression is prolonged, the nerve may be severely damaged so that functional recovery awaits regeneration. Unusually deep sleep or stupor, as in alcoholic intoxication or anesthesia, renders patients especially liable to pressure palsies, merely because they do not heed the discomfort of a sustained unnatural posture. A form of familial pressure palsies, in which there is a disposition to involvement of one nerve after another under conditions not usually conducive to the condition, is also known (page 1067).

Acroparesthesias are frequent in adult women and are not unknown to men. The patient, after being asleep for a few hours, is awakened by a numbness, tingling, prickling, "pins and needles" feeling in the fingers and hands. There are also aching, burning pains or tightness and other unpleasant sensations. At first there is a suspicion of having slept on an arm, but the frequent bilaterality of the symptoms and their occurrence regardless of the position of the arms, dispels this notion. Usually the paresthesias are in the distribution of the median nerves. With vigorous rubbing or shaking of the hands the paresthesias subside within a few minutes, only to return later, upon first awakening in the morning. The condition tends not to occur during the daytime unless the patient is lying down or sitting with the arms and hands in one position. In severe cases, the hands at all times feel swollen, stiff, clumsy, slightly numb, and sometimes distressingly painful. Examination may disclose little or no objective sensory loss, though in some cases touch and pain sensation are diminished in parts supplied by the median nerves. Atrophy and weakness of the abductor pollicis brevis and opponens pollicis muscles have also been noted, and in a few cases have been marked in degree (carpal tunnel syndrome; see also pages 175 and 1068). The use of the hands for heavy work during the day seems to aggravate the condition, and a holiday or a period of hospitalization may relieve it. It often occurs in young housewives with a new baby or in factory workers who perform a routine task. The disorder is particularly common in rheumatoid arthritis, myxedema, acromegaly, primary amyloidosis, mucopolysaccharidoses, and multiple myeloma (due to amyloid deposits); common to all of these is a thickening of the transverse carpal ligaments or the synovia of the flexor tendons, with compression of the median nerve. The injection of 50 mg hydrocortisone beneath the carpal ligaments and the use of chlorothiazide (Diuril) or one of its analogues has given relief in a respectable number of cases, particularly those with a tenosynovitis. The section of the transverse carpal ligament and palmar aponeurosis nearly always cures recalcitrant cases.

BRUXISM

Nocturnal grinding of the teeth, sometimes diurnal as well, occurs at all ages and may be as distressing to the bystander as it is to the patient. It may also cause serious dental problems unless the teeth are protected in some way. There are many hypothetical explanations, all without proof. Stress is most often blamed, and claimants point to EMG studies that show the masseter and temporalis muscles to be excessively contracted in states of nervous tension. We are more inclined to regard it as a tic or automatism.

NOCTURNAL ENURESIS

Nocturnal bedwetting with daytime continence is a frequent disorder during childhood, but it may persist into adult life. Approximately one of ten children 4 to 14 years of age is affected, boys more frequently than girls, and even among adults (military recruits) the incidence is 1 to 3 percent. Though the condition was formerly thought to be functional, i.e., psychogenic, the studies of Gastaut and Broughton have revealed a peculiarity of bladder physiology. The intravesicular pressure periodically rises to much higher levels in the enuretic patient than in normal persons, and the arousal time under such conditions is delayed. Also, the bladder of the enuretic patient tends to be smaller. This suggests a maturational failure of certain modulating nervous influences. The urinary incontinence has been found to occur usually during the first third of the night, especially during stage 4 of NREM sleep, and is preceded by a burst of rhythmic delta waves associated with a general body movement. If the patient is awakened at this point, he does not report any dreams. Imipramine (Tofranil) has proved to be an effective agent in reducing the frequency of enuresis. Diseases of the urinary tract, diabetes mellitus or diabetes insipidus, epilepsy, sickle-cell anemia, and spinal cord or cauda equina disease must be differentiated as causes of symptomatic enuresis.

RELATION OF SLEEP TO OTHER MEDICAL ILLNESSES

Patients with duodenal ulcer secrete more HCl during sleep (peaks coincide with REM sleep) than normal subjects. Patients with coronary arteriosclerosis show ECG changes during REM sleep, and nocturnal angina has been recorded at this time. Asthmatics frequently have their attacks at night, but not concomitantly with any specific stage of sleep; they do have a decreased amount of stage 4 NREM sleep and frequent awakenings, however. Patients with hypothyroidism have shown a decrease of stages 3 and 4 NREM sleep, and a return to a normal pattern when they become euthyroid.

The senile dement exhibits reduced amounts of REM sleep and stage 4 NREM sleep, as do patients with Down syndrome, phenylketonurics, and brain-damaged children. A correlation has been demonstrated between the level of intelligence and the amount of REM sleep in all these conditions, and in normal persons as well. Alcohol, barbiturates, and other sedative-hypnotic drugs, which suppress REM sleep, permit extraordinary excesses of it to appear during withdrawal periods, which may in part account for the hyperactivity and confusion seen in these states.

REFERENCES

ASERINSKY E and KLEITMAN N: A motility cycle in sleeping infants as manifested by ocular and gross bodily activity. *J Appl Physiol* 8:11, 1955.

BROWNELL LG, WEST P, SWEATMAN P et al: Protriptyline in obstructive sleep apnea. *N Engl J Med* 307:1037, 1982.

BURWELL CS, ROBIN ED, WHALEY RD, BICKELMANN AG: Extreme obesity associated with alveolar hypoventilation: A Pickwickian syndrome. *Am J Med* 21:811, 1956.

COULTER DL, ALLEN RJ: Benign neonatal sleep myoclonus. *Arch Neurol* 39:192, 1982.

DALY D, YOSS R: Narcolepsy, in Vinken PJ, Bruyn GW (eds): *Handbook of Clinical Neurology,* vol 15: *The Epilepsies.* Amsterdam, North-Holland, 1974, chap 43, pp 836–852.

DEMENT WC, KLEITMAN N: Cyclic variations in EEG during sleep and their relation to eye movements, bodily motility and dreaming. *EEG Clin Neurophysiol* 9:673, 1957.

GUILLEMINAULT C, DEMENT WC: 235 cases of excessive daytime sleepiness: Diagnosis and tentative classification. *J Neurol Sci* 31:13, 1977.

GUILLEMINAULT C, DEMENT WC: *Sleep Apnea Syndromes.* New York, Alan R Liss, 1978.

GUILLEMINAULT C, DEMENT WC, PASSOUANT P (eds): *Narcolepsy, Advances in Sleep Research,* vol 3. New York, Spectrum, 1976.

GUILLEMINAULT C, FLAGG W: Effect of baclofen on sleep-related periodic leg movements. *Ann Neurol* 15:234, 1984.

HAURI P: *The Sleep Disorders,* 2nd ed. Kalamazoo, Michigan, Upjohn, 1982.

HAURI P, OLMSTEAD E: Childhood onset insomnia. *Sleep* 3:59, 1980.

HOBSON JA, BRAZIER MAB (eds): *The Reticular Formation Revisited.* New York, Raven Press, 1980.

KALES A: Chronic hypnotic use: Ineffectiveness, drug withdrawal insomnia and hypnotic drug dependence. *JAMA* 27:513, 1974.

KALE A, CADIEUX RJ, SOLDATOS CR et al: Narcolepsy-cataplexy. I: Clinical and electrophysiologic characteristics. *Arch Neurol* 39:164, 1982.

KALES A, KALES JD: Sleep disorders: Recent findings in the diagnosis and treatment of disturbed sleep. *N Engl J Med* 290:487, 1974.

KALES A, KALES JD, SOLDATOS CR: Insomnia and other sleep disorders. *Med Clin North Am* 66:971, 1982.

KESSLER S, GUILLEMINAULT C, DEMENT W: A family study of 50 REM narcoleptics. *Acta Neurol Scand* 50:503, 1974.

KRAMER RE, DINNER DS, BRAUN WE et al: HLA-DR2 and narcolepsy. *Arch Neurol* 44:853, 1987.

LIU HM, LOEW JM, HUNT CE: Congenital central hypoventilation syndrome; a pathologic study of the neuromuscular system. *Neurology* 28:1013, 1978.

LOOMIS AL, HARVEY EN, HOBART G: Cerebral states during sleep as studied by human brain potentials. *J Exp Psychol* 21:127, 1937.

MARKAND ON, DYKEN ML: Sleep abnormalities in patients with brainstem lesions. *Neurology* 26:769, 1976.

MITLER MM: Toward an animal model of narcolepsy-cataplexy, in Guilleminault C, Dement WC, Passouant P (eds): *Narcolepsy.* New York, Spectrum, 1976, pp 387–409.

MONNIER M, HOSLI L: Humoral regulation of sleep and wakefulness by hypnogenic and activating dialysable factors. *Prog Brain Res* 18:118, 1965.

NEELY SE, ROSENBERG RS, SPIRE JP et al: HLA antigens in narcolepsy. *Neurology* 36(suppl 1):299, 1986.

OSWALD I: Sudden bodily jerks on falling asleep. *Brain* 82:92, 1959.

PAPPENHEIMER JR, MILLER TB, GOODRICH CA: Sleep-promoting effects of cerebrospinal fluid from sleep-deprived goats. *Proc Natl Acad Sci USA* 58:513, 1967.

PARKES JD: *Sleep and Its Disorders*, Philadelphia, Saunders, 1985.

PASSOUANT P: The history of narcolepsy, in Guilleminault C, Dement WC, Passouant P (eds): *Narcolepsy.* New York, Spectrum, 1976, pp 3–13.

POPPER KR, ECCLES JC: *The Self and the Brain.* Berlin, Springer Verlag, 1977.

RECHTSCHAFFEN A, GILLILAND MA, BERGMAN BM et al: Physiological correlates of prolonged sleep deprivation in rats. *Science* 221:182, 1983.

RECHTSCHAFFEN A, KALES A (eds): *A Manual of Standardized Terminology, Techniques, and Scoring System for Sleep Stages of Human Subjects.* Washington, Public Health Service, 1968.

RECHTSCHAFFEN A, MONROE LJ: Laboratory studies of insomnia, in Kales A (ed): *Sleep: Physiology and Pathology, A Symposium.* Philadelphia, Lippincott, 1969, p 158.

RICHARDSON GS: Excessive daytime sleepiness in man: Multiple sleep latency measurement in narcoleptic and control subjects. *EEG Clin Neurophysiol* 45:621, 1978.

ROTH B: *Narcolepsy and Hypersomnia.* Basel, Springer Verlag, 1980.

SOLOMON F, WHITE CC, PARRON DL, MENDELSON WB: Sleeping pills, insomnia and medical practice. *N Engl J Med* 300:803, 1979.

TYLER DB: Psychological change during experimental sleep deprivation. *Dis Nerv Sys* 16:239, 1955.

WEITZMAN ED, BOYAR RM, KAPEN S, HELLMAN L: The relationship of sleep and sleep stages to neuroendocrine secretion and biological rhythms in man. *Recent Prog Horm Res* 31:399, 1975.

WILLIAMS RL, KARACAN I, HURSCH CJ: *Electroencephalography (EEG) of Human Sleep: Clinical Applications.* New York, Wiley, 1974.

WILSON SAK: *Neurology.* London, Arnold, 1940,

ZARCONE V: Narcolepsy. *N Engl J Med* 288:1156, 1973.

DERANGEMENTS OF INTELLECT, BEHAVIOR, AND LANGUAGE DUE TO DIFFUSE AND FOCAL CEREBRAL DISEASE

Physicians sooner or later discover through clinical experience the need for special competence in assessing the mental faculties of their patients. They must be able to observe with detachment and complete objectivity the patient's intelligence, memory, judgment, mood, character, and other attributes of personality, in much the same fashion as they observe the nutritional state and the color of the mucous membranes. The systematic examination of these affective and intellectual functions permits the physician to reach certain conclusions regarding mental status, and to understand the patient and his or her illness. Without such data, errors will be made in evaluating the reliability of the history in the diagnosis of the patient's neurologic or psychiatric disease and in conducting an appropriate therapeutic program.

Perhaps the content of this section will be more clearly understood if we anticipate a few of the introductory remarks to the section on psychiatric diseases. The main thesis of the neurologist is that mental and physical functions of the nervous system are simply two aspects of the same neural process. Mind and behavior both have their roots in the self-regulating, goal-seeking activities of the organism, the same ones that provide impulse to all forms of mammalian life. The prodigious complexity of the human brain permits, to an extraordinary degree, the solving of difficult problems, the capacity for remembering past experiences and phrasing them in a symbolic language that can be written and read, and the planning of events that have not taken place. Somehow there emerges in the course of these complex cerebral functions a more complete and continuous awareness of one's self and of the operation of one's own psychic processes than is found in any other species. It is this continuous inner consciousness of past experiences and ongoing cognitive activities that is called mind. Any separation of the mental from the observable behavioral aspects of nervous system function is illusory. Biologists and psychologists have reached the modern monistic view by placing all protoplasmic activities of the nervous system (growth, development, behavior, and mental function) in a continuum and noting the inherent purposiveness and creativity common to all of them. The physician is persuaded of the truth of this view through daily clinical experience, in which every known aberration of behavior and intellect appears as an expression of cerebral disease. Further, in many brain diseases the physician witnesses parallel disorders of the patient's behavior and introspective awareness of functional capacities.

Chapters 19 and 20 will be concerned with common disturbances of the sensorium and of intellection which have not been discussed previously and which stand as cardinal manifestations of certain cerebral diseases. The most frequent of these are the acute confusional states, delirium, and disorders of learning, memory, and other intellectual functions. A consideration of these abnormalities, indicative as a rule of a diffuse disturbance of cerebral function, leads naturally to an examination of the symptoms consequent upon focal cerebral lesions (Chap. 21), and of language mechanisms (Chap. 22), which fall between the readily localizable functions of the cerebrum and those which cannot be localized.

CHAPTER 19

DELIRIUM AND OTHER ACUTE CONFUSIONAL STATES

The singular event in which a patient with previously intact mentality becomes acutely psychotic is observed almost daily on the medical and surgical wards of a general hospital. Occurring as it often does during an infective fever or in the course of a toxic or metabolic disorder (such as renal or hepatic failure or as an effect of medication or abuse of alcohol), it never fails to create grave problems for the physician, nursing personnel, and family. The physician has to cope with the problem of diagnosis often without the advantage of a lucid history, and any program of therapy to be initiated is constantly threatened by the patient's agitation, sleeplessness, and inability to cooperate. The nursing personnel is burdened with the need of providing satisfactory care for the patient and, at the same time, maintaining a tranquil atmosphere for other patients. The family must be supported as it faces the appalling spectre of insanity and all it signifies.

These difficulties are greatly magnified when the patient arrives in the emergency ward, having behaved in some irrational way, and the physician must begin the clinical analysis without knowledge of the patient's background and underlying medical illnesses. Under such circumstances it is tempting to rid oneself of the clinical problem by transferring the patient to a psychiatric hospital. This is unwise in the authors' opinion, for there may not be adequate facilities for the investigation and management of the great variety of medical diseases with which the psychosis may be associated. It is far better to study such clinical problems initially on a general medical or neurologic ward and to transfer the patient to a psychiatric service only if the behavioral disorder proves impossible to manage in a general hospital, or, if warranted, when the underlying medical problems have been identified and a program of treatment started.

DEFINITION OF TERMS

The definition of normal and abnormal states of mind is difficult, because the terms used to describe these states have been given so many different meanings in both medical and nonmedical writings. Compounding the difficulty is the fact that the pathophysiology of the confusional states, delirium, and dementia is not fully understood, and the definitions depend on their clinical relationships, with all the imprecision that this entails. The following nomenclature, though tentative, has proved useful to us and will be employed in this and subsequent chapters throughout this textbook.

Confusion is a general term denoting an incapacity of the patient to think with customary speed, clarity, and coherence. Disorientation, impaired attention and concentration, an inability to properly register immediate events and to recall them later, and a general diminution of all mental activity are its most conspicuous attributes. Thinking, speech, and the performance of goal-directed actions may be impersistent or abruptly arrested by intrusions of irrelevant thoughts. Reduced perceptiveness with visual and auditory illusions, and even hallucinations and paranoid delusions (a veritable psychosis) are other variable features.

These several psychologic disturbances may appear in many contexts. A confusional state may be an essential element in delirium, in which case it depends mainly on a disorder of perception and is associated with agitation and tremor. A confusional state may appear at a certain stage in the evolution and devolution of a number of diseases that lead to drowsiness, stupor, and coma, as was pointed out in Chap. 16, in which instance it must be aligned with disorders of consciousness. Also, confusion is a characteristic feature of the chronic syndrome of dementia, where already there has been a failure of memory, language facility, and other intellectual functions. Intense emotional disturbances, either hypomania or a retarded depression, may interfere with attentiveness and coherence of thinking. Finally, there are clinical instances of confusion in association with focal cerebral lesions, particularly of the right parietal, frontal, or temporal lobe association areas. Then, instead of tremor, asterixis, and myoclonia—the generalized motor abnormalities that characterize confusional states of toxic-metabolic origin—there may be unilateral neglect of self and environment and motor-sensory defects.

The many mental and behavioral aberrations to be seen in confused patients, and their occurrence in various combinations and clinical contexts, make it unlikely that they all derive from a single psychologic abnormality, such as a disturbance of attention. Phenomena as diverse as drowsiness and stupor, hallucinations and delusions, disorders of perception and registration, impersistence and perseveration, and so forth, cannot logically be reduced to a disorder of one psychologic or physiologic mechanism. More likely, a number of separable disorders of function are involved, all acute and usually reversible. We refer to all of them as the confusional states, for want of a better term.

We shall use the term *delirium* to denote a special type of confusional state. In addition to many of the negative elements mentioned above, delirium is marked by a prominent disorder of perception, terrifying hallucinations and vivid dreams, a kaleidoscopic array of strange and absurd fantasies and delusions, inability to sleep, tendency to convulse, and intense emotional disturbances. All these positive aspects of disordered consciousness, after the classic studies of the French authors, are designated by the term *oneirism* or *oneiric consciousness* (from the Greek *oneiros*, "dream"). The *twilight states* are closely related disorders, but the clinical descriptions have been so divergent that the term now has little useful meaning. We would add that delirium is distinguished also by heightened alertness, i.e., an increased readiness to respond to stimuli, and by marked overactivity of psychomotor and autonomic nervous system functions. Implicit in the term *delirium* are its nonmedical connotations—intense agitation, frenzied excitement, and trembling.

It should be noted that this distinction between delirium and other acute confusional states is not universally accepted. Some authors attach no particular significance to the autonomic and psychomotor overactivity and oneiric or dreamlike features of delirium, or to the underactivity and somnolence that characterize certain other confusional states.

All such states are lumped together under the heading of toxic psychosis, infective-exhaustive psychosis, febrile delirium, exogenous reaction type of psychosis, acute organic reaction, or symptomatic psychosis, with the implication that they are all induced by toxic or metabolic disturbances of the brain. We believe that delirium should be set apart from other confusional states, for the reason that the two conditions are descriptively different and tend to occur in different clinical contexts, as will be indicated further on. Nevertheless, implicit in both is the idea of an acute, transient, completely reversible disorder.

Amnesia is said to be another feature of these conditions. Actually it should refer to both a loss of past memories and an inability to form new ones, despite an alert state of mind. It presupposes an ability to grasp the problem, to use language normally, and to maintain adequate motivation to learn and to recall. The failure is mainly one of retention, recall, and reproduction, and it should be distinguished from states of drowsiness, acute confusion, and delirium, in which information and events seem never to have been adequately perceived and registered in the first place. The amnesic state may be partial or selective, e.g., for words, visual images of faces, patterns, objects, colors, or motor skills. Then it is usually classed as a form of *aphasia, agnosia,* or *apraxia* (see Chap. 22).

Dementia literally means an undoing of the mind and more particularly, a deterioration of all intellectual or cognitive functions, with little or no disturbance of consciousness or perception. Implied by the word is the idea of a gradual enfeeblement of mental powers in a person who formerly possessed a normal mind. *Amentia,* by contrast, indicates a congenital feeblemindedness. Dementia and amnesia are defined further in the next chapter.

OBSERVABLE ASPECTS OF BEHAVIOR AND THEIR RELATION TO CONFUSION, DELIRIUM, AMNESIA, AND DEMENTIA

The intellectual, emotional, volitional, and behavioral activities of the human organism are so complex and varied that one may question the feasibility of using derangements of them as reliable indicators of cerebral disease. Certainly they have not the same reliability and ease of anatomic and physiologic interpretation as sensory and motor paralysis or aphasia. Yet one observes particular disturbances of higher cerebral functions recurring with such regularity in certain diseases as to be useful in clinical medicine; and some of them gain in specificity because they are often combined in certain ways to form syndromes, which are essentially what states of confusion, delirium, amnesia, and dementia are.

The components of mentation and behavior that lend themselves to bedside examination are (1) the processes of sensation and perception; (2) the capacity to memorize; (3) the ability to think and reason; (4) temperament, mood, and emotion; (5) initiative, impulse, and drive; and (6) insight. Of these (1) is sensorial, (2) and (3) are cognitive, (4) is affective, and (5) is conative or volitional. Insight refers to the introspective observations made by patients concerning their own normal or disordered functioning. Each component of behavior and intellection has its objective side, expressed in the behavioral responses that are produced by certain stimuli and its subjective side, expressed in the thinking and feeling described by the patient in relation to the stimuli.

DISTURBANCES OF PERCEPTION

Perception, i.e., the process of acquiring through the senses a knowledge of the ''world about'' or of one's self (apperception in classic psychology), involves much more than the simple sensory process of being aware of the attributes of a stimulus. New stimuli, visual for example, activate the visual striate cortex and association areas wherein lie the storage mechanisms for coded representations of these stimuli. The effects must be lasting if the stimuli are to be remembered. Recognition involves the reactivation of this system by the same stimuli at a later time. Included in the process are the maintenance of attention, the selective focusing on a stimulus, elimination of all extraneous stimuli, and identification of the stimulus by recognizing its relationship to personal remembered experiences.

The perception of stimuli undergoes predictable types of derangement in disease. Most often there is a reduction in the number of perceptions in a given unit of time and a failure to synthesize them properly and relate them to the ongoing activities of the mind. Or there may be apparent inattentiveness or fluctuations of attention, distractibility (pertinent and irrelevant stimuli now having equal value), and inability to persist in an assigned task. Qualitative changes also appear, mainly in the form of sensory distortions, causing misinterpretations and misidentifications of objects and persons (illusions); and these, at least in part, form the basis of hallucinatory experience in which the patient reports and reacts to stimuli not present in the environment. There is an inability to perceive simultaneously all elements of a large complex of stimuli, a defect that is sometimes explained as a ''failure of subjective organization.'' These major disturbances in the perceptual sphere, often referred to as ''clouding of the sensorium,'' are characteristic of deliria and other acute confusional states, but a quantitative deficiency may also become evident in the advanced stages of amentia and dementia.

DISTURBANCES OF MEMORY

Memory, i.e., the retention of learned information and experiences, is involved in all mental activities. It may be arbitrarily subdivided into several parts, viz., (1) registration (also called encoding), which includes all that was mentioned under perception; (2) fixation, mnemonic integration, and retention; (3) recognition and recall; and (4) reproduction. As stated above, there may be a complete failure of learning and memory in patients with impaired perception and attention, for the reason that the material to be learned was never registered and assimilated. In the Korsakoff amnesic syndrome (Korsakoff psychosis), newly presented material appears to be temporarily registered but cannot be retained for more than a few minutes (anterograde amnesia or failure of learning). There is always an associated defect in the recall and reproduction of memories that had been formed several days, or weeks, or even years before the onset of the illness (retrograde amnesia). The fabrication of stories, called *confabulation*, constitutes a third feature of the syndrome, but not a specific or invariable one. Sound retention with failure of recall is at times a normal state; when it is severe and extends to all events of past life it is usually due to hysteria or malingering. Proof that the processes of registration and recall are intact under these circumstances comes from hypnosis and suggestion, by means of which the lost items are fully recalled and reproduced. Patients with the Korsakoff syndrome fail on all tests of learning and recent memory, and their behavior accords with their deficiencies of information. Hypnosis does not facilitate recall. Since memory is involved to some extent in all mental processes, it becomes the most testable component of mentation and behavior.

DISTURBANCES OF THINKING

Thinking, the highest order of intellectual activity, remains one of the most elusive of all mental operations. If by thinking we mean the selective ordering of symbols for learning and organizing information, for problem solving, and the capacity to reason and form sound judgments (the usual definition), then the working units of this type of mental activity are words and numbers. The substitution of words and numbers for the objects for which they stand (symbolization) is a fundamental part of the process. These symbols are formed into ideas or concepts, and the arrangement of new and remembered ideas into certain orders or relationships, according to the rules of logic, constitutes another intricate part of thought, presently beyond the scope of analysis. On page 357, reference is made to Luria's analysis of the steps involved in problem solving in connection with frontal lobe function, but actually, as he points out, the whole cerebrum is implicated. In a general way one may examine thinking for speed and efficiency, ideational content, coherence and logical relationships of ideas, quantity and quality of associations to a given idea, and the propriety of the feeling and behavior engendered by an idea.

Information concerning the thought processes and associative functions is best obtained by analyzing the patient's spontaneous verbal productions and by engaging him or her in conversation. If the patient is taciturn or mute, one may have to depend on responses to direct questions or upon written material, i.e., letters, etc. One notes the prevailing trends of the patient's thoughts; whether the ideas are reasonable, precise, and coherent or vague, circumstantial, tangential, and irrelevant; and whether the thought processes are shallow and fragmented.

Disorders of thinking are prominent in deliria and other confusional states, in mania and hypomania, in dementia, and in schizophrenia. The organization of thought may be disrupted, with fragmentation, repetition, and perseveration. This is spoken of as an "incoherence of thinking" and marks confusional states of all types. The patient may be excessively critical, rationalizing, and hair-splitting; this disturbance of thinking is often seen in depressive psychoses. Derangements of thinking may also take the form of a flight of ideas; patients move nimbly from one idea to another, and their associations are numerous and loosely linked. This is a common feature of hypomanic and manic states. The opposite condition, poverty of ideas, is characteristic both of depression, where it is combined with gloomy thoughts, and of dementing diseases, where it is part of a reduction of all intellectual activity. Thinking may be distorted in such a way that ideas are not checked against reality. When a false belief is maintained in spite of normally convincing contradictory evidence, the patient is said to have a delusion. Delusions are common to many illnesses, particularly manic depressive and schizophrenic states. Some patients believe that ideas have been implanted in their minds by some outside agency, such as radio, television, or atomic energy; these are the "passivity feelings" characteristic of schizophrenia. Other distortions of logical thought, such as gaps in sequential thinking, intrusion of irrelevant ideas, and condensation of associations, are typical of schizophrenia, of which they constitute diagnostic features.

DISTURBANCES OF EMOTION, MOOD, AND AFFECT

The emotional life of the patient is expressed in a variety of ways. In the first place, rather marked individual differences in basic temperament are to be observed in the normal population; some persons are throughout their lives cheerful, gregarious, optimistic, and free from worry, whereas others are just the opposite. The usually volatile, cyclothymic person is said to be liable to manic-depressive psychosis, and the suspicious, withdrawn, introverted person to schizophrenia and paranoia, but there are frequent exceptions to this statement. Strong, persistent emotional states, such as fear and anxiety, may occur as reactions to life situations and may be accompanied by derangements of visceral function. If excessive and disproportionate to the stimulus, they are usually manifestations of an anxiety neurosis or depression. Variations in the degree of responsiveness to emotional stimuli are also frequent, and when extreme and persistent, assume importance. In depression, all stimuli tend to enhance the somber mood of unhappiness. Emotional responses that are excessively labile and poorly controlled or uninhibited are a common manifestation of many cerebral diseases, particularly those involving the corticopontine and corticobulbar pathways. This disorder constitutes part of the syndrome of spastic bulbar (pseudobulbar) palsy. All emotional expression may be lacking, as in apathetic states or severe depressions, or the patient may be vulnerable to every trivial problem in daily life, i.e., unable to control worry. Finally, the emotional response may be inappropriate to the stimulus, e.g., a depressing or morbid thought may seem amusing and be attended by a smile, as in schizophrenia.

Temperament, mood, and other emotional experiences described above are evaluated by observing the patient's appearance and questioning him about his feelings. For these purposes it is convenient to divide emotionality into mood and affect (or feeling). By *mood* is meant the prevailing emotional state of an individual without reference to the stimuli immediately impinging upon him or her. It may be pleasant and cheerful or melancholic. Language (e.g., the adjectives used) and facial expression, attitude, posture, and speed of movement most reliably reflect the patient's mood. By contrast, *affect* (or *feeling*) refers to the emotional reactions evoked by environmental stimuli. According to some psychiatrists, *feeling* is the subjective component, and *affect*, the overt manifestation. Others use either term to describe the subjective state. The difference between mood as a prevailing emotional state and feeling, or affect, as an emotional reaction to stimuli may seem rather tenuous, but these distinctions are considered valuable by psychiatrists. The significance of various types of emotional disturbance is discussed more fully in Chap. 25.

Reference was made, in Chaps. 3 and 4, to motor weakness, akinesia, and bradykinesia as cardinal manifestations of corticospinal and extrapyramidal disease. In these settings, a defect in the motor system interferes with voluntary or automatic movements, much to the distress of the patient. But motility and activity can be impaired for other reasons, one of which is a lack of *conation* or *impulse*. These terms designate that basic biologic urge, driving force, or purpose by which every organism is motivated to achieve its objectives. Indeed motor activity is a necessary and satisfying objective in itself, for few individuals can remain still for long (fidgets, doodling) and even idiots obtain a certain gratification from rocking, etc.

It is the authors' impression that a quantitative reduction in the amount of spontaneous activity per unit of time is one of the most important manifestations of cerebral disease. And an important characteristic of this state, which we call *abulia* or *hypobulia,* is the concomitant reduction in speech, ideation, and emotional reaction (apathy). Individuals are known to vary in strength of impulse, drive, and energy. Some are born low in impulse, with a lifelong tendency to inactivity, a constitutional inadequacy that Kahn has called *asthenic psychopathy;* others are excessively active from early life. But with certain cerebral diseases idleness of body and mind may reach an extreme degree, to a point where a wide-awake person, perceptive of the environment, does not speak of move for weeks on end (akinetic mutism, see page 276). Such patients seem indifferent to what is happening around them and unconcerned about the consequences of their inactivity.

Abulia is clinically distinguishable from two allied states, *catatonia* and the *psychomotor retardation* of depression. Kahlbaum, who first used the term catatonia in 1874, described it as a condition in which the patient sits or lies silent and motionless, with a staring countenance, completely without volition and without reaction to sensory impressions. Sometimes there is resistance to the examiner's efforts to move the patient (negativism) or certain movements or phrases are repeated hour after hour. If the limbs are moved they may retain their new position for a prolonged period (flexibilitas cerea) but usually there is no rigidity except that of voluntary resistance. In the psychomotor retardation of depression, the profundity of the depressed mood may be so great that the patients make no attempt to help themselves in any way. Their speech expresses their sadness and desire to die.

In both catatonia and depression, the mind is usually sufficiently alert to record events and later to remember them, in which respect these states differ from *stupor.* But this distinction is not always valid for we have seen catatonic schizophrenics and retarded depressives who occasionally could not recall what had happened during the period of catatonia or depression. Moreover, Stauder has described a form of lethal catatonia in which the completely immobilized patient develops a fever, collapses, and dies. Recently a similar state has come to be recognized as the consequence of intoxication with neuroleptic drugs, the so-called *neuroleptic malignant syndrome* (see page 901). Probably there is a close relationship, if not identity between catatonia and akinetic mutism.

Pathologic degrees of restlessness and hyperactivity represent the opposite extreme of abulia. *Akathisia* refers to the constant restless movements and inability to sit still that complicate the administration of phenothiazines and buterophenones (see pages 90 and 901). On page 483 is described the hyperactivity-inattention syndrome of children, mostly boys. In the manic form of manic depressive disease (and to a lesser extent in hypomania) continuous activity and relative insomnia are added to the flight of ideas and the euphoric though somewhat irritable mood. Following certain cerebral diseases, as occurred in von Economo encephalitis, the patient may remain in a state of constant movement, destroying uncontrollably whatever could be reached. Kahn referred to this state as "organic drivenness."

LOSS OF INSIGHT

Insight, the state of being fully aware of the nature and degree of one's deficits, becomes manifestly impaired or abolished in relation to all types of cerebral disease that cause complex disorders of behavior. Rarely do patients with any of these diseases seek advice or help for their illness. Instead, the family usually brings the patient to the physician. Thus, diseases that produce the aforementioned abnormalities of mentation not only evoke observable changes in behavior but also alter or reduce the capacity of the patient to make accurate introspections concerning his or her own psychic function. This fact stands as proof that the brain is the organ both of behavior and of all inner psychic experiences; i.e., mind and behavior are but two inseparable aspects of the function of the nervous system.

COMMON SYNDROMES

To summarize, the entire group of acute confusional and delirious states is characterized principally by an alteration of consciousness with prominent disorders of attention and perception that interfere with the speed, clarity, and coherence of thinking, the formation of memories, and the capacity for performance of directed activities. Three major clinical syndromes can be recognized. One is a *confusional state* in which there is manifest reduction in alertness and psychomotor activity. The second syndrome, here called *delirium*, is characterized by overactivity, sleeplessness, tremulousness, and hallucinations, with convulsions often preceding or associated with the delirium. A third syndrome consists of a confusional state occurring in persons with some other cerebral disease. The latter may also dispose the patient to an acute psychosis, which we have chosen to designate as a *beclouded dementia*. These illnesses tend to develop acutely, to have multiple causes, and, except for certain cerebral diseases, to terminate within a relatively short period of time (days to weeks), leaving the patient without residual damage or with whatever defects were present before their onset.

ACUTE CONFUSIONAL STATES ASSOCIATED WITH REDUCED ALERTNESS AND PSYCHOMOTOR ACTIVITY

Clinical Features   Some features of this syndrome have already been described in Chap. 16, "Coma and Related Disorders of Consciousness." In the most typical examples, all mental functions are reduced to some degree; but alertness, attentiveness, and the ability to concentrate and to grasp all elements of the immediate situation suffer most. In its mildest form, the patient appears alert and may pass for normal, and only the failure to recollect and reproduce happenings of the past few hours or days reveals the subtle inadequacy of mental function. The more obviously confused patients spend much of their time in idleness, and what they do may be inappropriate and annoying to others. Only the more automatic acts and verbal responses are performed properly, but these may permit the examiner to obtain from the patient a number of relevant and accurate replies to questions about age, occupation, and residence. Reactions are slow and indecisive. Such patients may repeat every question that is put to them, before answering, and their responses tend to be brief and mechanical. It is difficult or impossible for them to sustain a conversation. Their attention wanders and they have constantly to be brought back to the subject at hand. They may even fall asleep during the interview, and, if left alone, they are observed to sleep more hours each day than is natural, or to sleep the usual number of hours at irregular intervals. Frequently there are perceptual disturbances in which voices, common

objects, and the actions of other persons are misinterpreted. Frank hallucinations may occur but often one cannot discern whether these patients hear voices and see things that do not exist, i.e., whether they are hallucinating, or are merely misinterpreting stimuli in the environment. Inadequate perception and forgetfulness result in a constant state of bewilderment. Some patients are irritable and others are extremely suspicious; in fact, a paranoid trend may be the most pronounced and troublesome feature of the illness, which then takes the form of an acute psychosis. There may also be mild degrees of anomia and dysphasia and a labile affect.

As the confusion deepens, conversation becomes more difficult, and at a certain stage these patients no longer notice or respond to much of what is going on around them. Replies to questions may be a single word or a short phrase spoken in a soft tremulous voice or whisper. The patient may be mute. In its most advanced stages confusion gives way to stupor and finally to coma. As these patients improve, they may pass again through the stage of stupor and confusion in the reverse order. All this informs us that at least one category of confusion is but a manifestation of the same disease processes that in their severest form cause coma.

Typical confusional states, in which impairment of alertness and attention dominate, are readily distinguished from delirium; in others, with more than the usual degree of irritability and restlessness, one cannot fail to notice their resemblance to one another. Further, when a delirium is complicated by an illness that superimposes stupor (e.g., delirium tremens with pneumonia, meningitis, or hepatic encephalopathy), it may be difficult to distinguish from other acute confusional states. Difficulty in distinguishing these two states explains why some psychiatrists (Engel and Romano, Lipowski) insist that there is only one disorder, which they call *delirium*. The present writers disagree, for reasons that were stated earlier in this chapter and are elaborated below.

Etiology   The many causes of this type of confusional state are listed in Table 19-1. The most frequent are drug intoxications and metabolic disorders—electrolyte imbalance, disorders of acid-base and water metabolism, renal and hepatic failure, hyper- and hypoglycemia, and chronic cardiac and pulmonary insufficiency. Concussion and seizures and certain focal cerebral lesions may also be followed by a period of confusion.

Morbid Anatomy and Pathophysiology   All that has been said on this subject in Chap. 16, "Coma and Related Disorders of Consciousness," is applicable to at least one subgroup of the confusional states. In the majority of cases no consistent pathologic change has been found. The EEG

Table 19-1
Classification of delirium and acute confusional states

I. Delirium
   A. In a medical or surgical illness (no focal or lateralizing neurologic signs; CSF usually clear)
     1. Typhoid fever
     2. Pneumonia
     3. Septicemia, particularly erysipelas and other streptococcal infections
     4. Rheumatic fever
     5. Thyrotoxicosis and ACTH intoxication (rare)
     6. Postoperative and postconcussive states
   B. In neurologic disease that causes focal or lateralizing signs or changes in the CSF
     1. Vascular, neoplastic, or other diseases, particularly those involving the temporal and parietal lobes and upper part of the brainstem
     2. Cerebral contusion and laceration (traumatic delirium)
     3. Acute purulent and tuberculous meningitis
     4. Subarachnoid hemorrhage
     5. Encephalitis due to viral causes (e.g., herpes simplex, infectious mononucleosis) and to unknown causes
   C. The abstinence states, exogenous intoxications, and postconvulsive states; signs of other medical, surgical, and neurologic illnesses absent or coincidental
     1. Withdrawal of alcohol (delirium tremens), barbiturates, and nonbarbiturate sedative drugs, following chronic intoxication (Chaps. 41 and 42)
     2. Drug intoxications: scopolamine, atropine, amphetamine, etc.
     3. Postconvulsive delirium
II. Acute confusional states associated with psychomotor underactivity
   A. Associated with a medical or surgical disease (no focal or lateralizing neurologic signs; CSF clear)
     1. Metabolic disorders; hepatic stupor, uremia, hypoxia, hypercapnea, hypoglycemia, porphyria
     2. Infective fevers, especially typhoid
     3. Congestive heart failure
     4. Postoperative, posttraumatic, and puerperal psychoses
   B. Associated with drug intoxication (no focal or lateralizing signs; CSF clear): opiates, barbiturates and other sedatives, Artane, etc.
III. Associated with diseases of the nervous system (with focal or lateralizing neurologic signs and/or CSF changes)
   A. Cerebral vascular disease, tumor, abscess (especially of the *right* parietal, inferofrontal, and temporal lobes)
   B. Subdural hematoma
   C. Meningitis
   D. Encephalitis
IV. Beclouded dementia, i.e., senile or other brain disease in combination with infective fevers, drug reactions, heart failure, or other medical or surgical diseases

is of interest, because it is almost invariably abnormal in more severe forms of this syndrome, in contrast to delirium, where the changes are relatively minor. High-voltage slow waves in the 2- to 4-per-second (delta) range or the 5- to 7-per-second (theta) range are the usual findings.

DELIRIUM

Clinical Features These are most perfectly depicted in the alcoholic patient. The symptoms usually develop over a period of 2 or 3 days. The first indications of the approaching attack are difficulty in concentration, restless irritability, tremulousness, insomnia, and poor appetite. One or several generalized convulsions precede or initiate the delirium in almost 30 percent of the cases. The patient's rest is troubled by unpleasant or terrifying dreams. There may be momentary disorientation, an occasional inappropriate remark, or transient illusions or hallucinations.

These initial symptoms rapidly give way to a clinical picture that, in severe cases, is one of the most colorful in medicine. The ''sensorium is clouded'' in that the patients are inattentive and unable to perceive all elements of their situation. They may talk incessantly and incoherently and look distressed and perplexed; their expression is in keeping with their vague notions of being annoyed or threatened by someone who seeks to injure them. From their manner and the content of their speech it is evident that they misinterpret the meaning of ordinary objects and sounds, misidentify the people around them, and have vivid visual, auditory, and tactile hallucinations, often of a most unpleasant type. At first they can be brought into touch with reality and may in fact identify the examiner and answer other questions correctly; but almost at once they relapse into their preoccupied, confused state, giving wrong answers and being unable to think coherently. Before long they are unable to shake off their hallucinations even for a second and do not recognize their physician or even their family. They are unable to make meaningful responses to the simplest questions and are profoundly disoriented, as a rule.

Tremor and jerky restless movements are usually present and may be violent. Sleep is impossible or occurs only in brief naps. The countenance is flushed, the pupils are dilated, and the conjunctivas are injected; the pulse is rapid and soft, and the temperature may be raised. There is much sweating, and the urine is scanty and of high specific gravity. The signs of overactivity of the autonomic nervous system, more than any other, distinguish delirium from all other confusional states.

The symptoms abate, either suddenly or gradually,

after 2 or 3 days, although in exceptional cases they may persist for several weeks. The most certain indication of the end of the attack is the occurrence of sound sleep and of lucid intervals of increasing length. Recovery is usually complete.

Delirium is subject to all degrees of variability, not only from patient to patient but in the same patient from day to day and even hour to hour. The entire syndrome may be observed in one patient, and only one or two symptoms in another. In its mildest form, as so often occurs in febrile diseases, it consists of an occasional wandering of the mind and incoherence of verbal expression. This form, lacking motor and autonomic overactivity, is sometimes referred to as a *quiet delirium* (or *hypokinetic delirium*) and cannot be distinguished from the confusional states described above. The more severe form of delirium, best exemplified by delirium tremens, ends fatally in 5 to 15 percent of patients depending often on the gravity of associated diseases or injuries (see Chap. 41).

Morbid Anatomy and Pathophysiology The brains of patients who have died in delirium tremens usually show no pathologic changes of significance. Delirium may also occur in association with a number of recognizable pathologic states such as viral encephalitis or meningoencephalitis, Wernicke disease, trauma, or focal embolic encephalomalacia due to subacute bacterial endocarditis or to cardiac surgery. The topography of these lesions is of particular interest. They tend to be localized in the midbrain and subthalamus and in the temporal lobes, where they involve the reticular activating and limbic systems.

Electrical stimulation studies of the human cerebral cortex during surgical exploration have clearly indicated the importance of the temporal lobe in the genesis of complex visual, auditory, and olfactory hallucinations. With subthalamic and midbrain lesions, visual hallucinations may occur that are not unpleasant and may be accompanied by good insight (the ''peduncular hallucinosis'' of Lhermitte). With pontine lesions there may be unformed auditory hallucinations.

The EEG in delirium may show nonfocal slow activity in the 5- to 7-per-second range, a state that rapidly returns to normal as the delirium clears. However, in other cases only activity in the fast beta frequency range is seen, and in milder degrees of delirium there is usually no abnormality at all.

An analysis of the several conditions conducive to delirium suggests at least three different physiologic mechanisms. The withdrawal of alcohol, barbiturates, or other sedative-hypnotic drugs, following a period of chronic intoxication, is the most common one (see Chaps. 41 and 42). These drugs are known to have a strong depressant effect on certain areas of the central nervous system; presumably, the disinhibition and overactivity of these parts, after withdrawal of the drug, are the basis of delirium. In this respect it is interesting to note that the symptoms of delirium tremens are the antithesis of those of alcoholic intoxication. In the case of bacterial infections and poisoning by certain drugs, such as atropine and scopolamine, the delirious state probably results from the direct action of the toxin or chemical agent on these same parts of the brain. Thirdly, destructive lesions, such as those of the under surfaces of the temporal lobes in herpes simplex encephalitis or severe concussive injury, may cause delirium by disturbing the function of these particular areas.

Psychophysiologic mechanisms have also been postulated. It has long been suggested that some persons are much more liable to delirium than others. There is much reason to doubt this hypothesis, for it has been shown that all of a group of randomly selected persons develop delirium if the causative mechanisms are strongly operative (Wolff and Curran). This is not surprising, for any healthy person under certain circumstances may experience phenomena akin to those of delirium. After repeated auditory and visual stimulation, the same impressions may continue to be perceived even though the stimuli are no longer present. A soldier, for example, may continue to hear the whine of artillery shells long after the bombardment has ceased. Also, a healthy person can be induced to hallucinate by being placed for several days in an environment as free as possible of sensory stimulation. A relation between delirium and dream states has been postulated because both are characterized by a loss of appreciation of time, a richness of visual imagery, indifference to inconsistencies, and ''defective reality testing.'' Moreover, patients may refer to some of these delirious symptoms as a ''bad dream,'' and normal persons may experience so-called hypnagogic hallucinations in the period between waking and sleeping. In general, however, formulations in the field of dynamic psychology seem more reasonably to account for the topical content of delirium than to explain its occurrence. Wolff and Curran, having observed the same content in repeated attacks of delirium due to different causes, concluded that the content depends more on age, sex, intellectual endowment, occupation, personality traits, and past experiences of the patient than on the cause or mechanism of the delirium.

The main difficulty in understanding delirium arises from the fact that it has not been possible to ascertain which of the many symptoms have physiologic significance. What is the basis of this altered consciousness, this sensorial disturbance, this lack of harmony between actual sensory impressions of the present and memory of those in the past? Obviously, something has been removed from the perceptive process, something that leaves the patient at the mercy of certain sensory stimuli and unable to attend to others, and at the same time incapable of discriminating between sense impression and fantasy. The lack of inhibition of sensory processes may also be the basis of the sleep disturbance (insomnia).

VASCULAR, SENILE, AND OTHER DEMENTING BRAIN DISEASES COMPLICATED BY MEDICAL OR SURGICAL ILLNESS: BECLOUDED DEMENTIA

A variety of cerebral diseases may be associated with confusional states. Among these are meningitis, encephalitis, disseminated vascular coagulation, tumors, and cerebral trauma. Of particular interest are focal lesions (usually infarcts) of the right cerebral hemisphere. The occurrence of an acute confusional state with infarctions in the territory of the right middle cerebral artery has been described by several authors (Mesulam et al; Caplan et al; Mori and Yamadori); mainly the infarcts involved the posterior parietal lobe or inferior frontal-striatal regions. An acute agitated delirium has been described repeatedly with lesions of the right temporal lobe—either of the fusiform and calcarine regions (Horenstein et al) or of the hippocampal, fusiform, and lingual gyri (Medina et al) or the middle temporal gyrus (Mori and Yamadori). Of course, there may be elements of confusion with stroke in almost any cerebral territory, but in the aforementioned reports the confusional state was frequently unattended by other paralytic motor and sensory disorders.

Apart from such focal lesions, many elderly patients who enter the hospital with a medical or surgical illness are mentally confused. Presumably the liability to this state is determined by preexisting brain disease, most often senile dementia, which may or may not have been obvious to the family before the onset of the complicating illness. Other cerebral diseases (vascular, neoplastic, demyelinative) may have the same effect.

All the clinical features that one observes in the acute confusional states may be present. The severity may vary greatly. The confusion may be reflected only in the patient's inability to relate sequentially the history of the illness, or it may be so severe that the patient is virtually non compos mentis.

Although almost any complicating illness may bring out the confusion in such a person, the most common are infectious diseases, especially in those cases which resist the effects of antibiotic medication; posttraumatic states, notably concussive brain injuries; operations, particularly cardiotomy, prostatectomy, and the removal of cataracts (in which case the confusion is probably related to temporary deprivation of vision); and with congestive heart failure, chronic respiratory disease, and severe anemia, especially pernicious anemia. Often it is difficult to determine which of several possible factors is responsible for the confusion, and there may be more than one. In a cardiac patient with a confusional psychosis for example, there may be fever, a marginally reduced cerebral blood flow, intoxication with one or more drugs, and electrolyte imbalance. The same may be true of a patient in a postoperative confusional state, in which a number of factors such as fever, infection, dehydration, and drug intoxication may be incriminated. Alcoholism may further complicate the problem.

When such patients recover from the medical or surgical illness, they usually return to their premorbid state, though their shortcomings, now drawn to the attention of the family and physician, may be more obvious than before.

COINCIDENTAL DEVELOPMENT OF SCHIZOPHRENIC OR MANIC-DEPRESSIVE PSYCHOSIS DURING A MEDICAL OR SURGICAL ILLNESS

A certain proportion of psychoses of the schizophrenic or manic-depressive type first become manifest during an acute medical illness or following an operation or parturition and need to be distinguished from an acute confusional state. A causal relationship between the psychosis and medical illness is sought but cannot be established. The psychosis may have preceded the medical illness but was not recognized, or it may have emerged during the convalescent period. The diagnostic studies of the psychiatric illness must proceed along the lines suggested in Chaps. 56 and 57. Close observation will usually reveal a clear sensorium and relatively intact memory, which permits differentiation from the acute confusional states.

CLASSIFICATION AND DIAGNOSIS OF DELIRIUM AND OTHER ACUTE CONFUSIONAL STATES

The syndromes themselves and their main clinical relationships are the only satisfactory basis for classification until such time as the actual cause and pathophysiology are discovered (Table 19-1). The practice of classifying the syndromes according to their most prominent symptom or degree of severity, e.g., "picking delirium," "microptic delirium," "acute delirious mania," and "muttering delirium," has no fundamental value.

The first step in *diagnosis* is to recognize that the patient is confused. This is obvious in most cases, but, as pointed out above, the mildest forms of confusion, particularly when some other acute alteration of personality is prominent, may be overlooked. In these mild forms a careful analysis of the patient's thought processes as the history of the illness and the details of personal life are given will usually reveal an incoherence. Digit span and serial subtraction of 3s and 7s from 100 are useful bedside tests of the patient's capacity for sustained mental activity. The task of crossing out all of certain letters on a printed page over a period of a few minutes is a useful measure of attention. Memory of recent events is one of the most delicate tests of adequate mental function and may be accomplished by having the patient relate all the details of entry to the hospital, ancillary examinations, etc., as outlined in Chap. 20.

Once it is established that the patient is confused, the differential diagnosis must be made between delirium, an acute confusional state associated with psychomotor underactivity, a beclouded dementia, and a confusional state that complicates focal cerebral disease. This is done by taking into account the degree of the patient's alertness, wakefulness, psychomotor and hallucinatory activity, disturbances of memory and impulse, and the presence or absence of signs of autonomic nervous system overactivity and of focal cerebral disease.

At times a left hemispheral lesion, causing a mild Wernicke aphasia, resembles a confusional state, in that the stream of thought, as judged by verbal output, is incoherent. The prominence of paraphasias and neologisms in spontaneous speech, difficulties in auditory comprehension, and normal nonverbal behavior, mark the disorder as aphasic in nature.

The distinction between an acute confusional state and dementia may be difficult at times. The patient with acute confusional psychosis is said to have a "clouded sensorium" (a somewhat ambiguous term, usually referring to a symptom complex of inattention, perhaps drowsiness, and an inclination to inaccurate perceptions and sometimes to hallucinations and delusions), whereas the patient with dementia usually has a clear sensorium. However, some demented patients are as beclouded as those with confusional psychosis, and the two conditions are at times indistinguishable, except for a difference in their mode of onset and clinical course. All this suggests that the parts of the nervous system affected may be the same in both conditions. When the physician is faced with this problem, the history of the onset is of prime importance. The confusional psychosis

usually develops abruptly and is reversible, whereas dementia has an insidious onset and chronic course and is more or less irreversible, as will be elaborated in the following chapter. As indicated above, schizophrenia and manic-depressive psychosis can usually be separated from the confusional states by the presence of a clear sensorium and relatively good memory.

Once a case has been appropriately classified, it is important to determine its clinical associations (Table 19-1). A thorough medical and neurologic examination, lumbar puncture, and CT scan should be performed. The medical and neurologic findings determine the underlying disease and its treatment, and they also give information concerning prognosis. In the neurologic examination, particular attention should be given to language functions, visual fields and visual-spatial discriminations, cortical sensory functions, calculation, and other test performances that require normal functioning of the high-order, heteromodal sensory cortices of the temporal, parietal, and occipital lobes.

CARE OF THE DELIRIOUS AND CONFUSED PATIENT

The primary therapeutic effort is directed to the control of the underlying medical disease. Other important objectives are to quiet the patients and protect them against injury. A nurse, an attendant, or a member of the family should be with such patients at all times if this can be arranged. Depending on how active and vigorous they are, a locked room, screened windows that cannot be opened by the patient, and a low bed should be arranged. It is often better to let such patients walk about the room than to tie them into bed, which may excite or frighten them and cause them to struggle to the point of exhaustion and collapse. If they are less active, they can usually be kept in bed by side rails, wrist restraints, or a restraining sheet or net. The patient should be permitted to sit up or walk about the room part of the day, unless this is contraindicated by the primary disease.

All drugs that could possibly be responsible for the acute confusional state or delirium should be discontinued (unless, perhaps, the withdrawal effects are believed to underlie the illness). In these circumstances, chlordiazepoxide (Librium) is the drug favored by most physicians, but paraldehyde, chloral hydrate, chlorpromazine, and diazepam are trustworthy and equally effective sedatives, if given in full doses. Whichever drug is used should be continued until natural sleep is restored. One must be cautious in attempting to suppress agitation completely. To accomplish this may require very large doses of drugs, and vital functions may then be dangerously impaired. The purpose of sedation is to assure rest and sleep so that patients do not exhaust themselves, and to facilitate nursing care. Continuous warm baths are also effective in quieting the delirious patient, but very few general hospitals have proper facilities for this valuable method of treatment.

A fluid intake and output chart should be kept, and any fluid and electrolyte deficit should be corrected. The pulse and blood pressure should be recorded at frequent intervals in anticipation of circulatory collapse. Transfusions of whole blood and the administration of vasopressor drugs may be lifesaving.

Finally, the physician should be aware of the many small therapeutic measures that allay fear and suspicion and reduce the tendency to hallucinations. The room should be kept dimly lighted at night, and if possible, the patient should not be moved from one room to another. Every procedure should be explained in detail, even such simple ones as the taking of blood pressure or temperature. The presence of a member of the family may enable the patient to maintain contact with reality.

It may be some consolation and also a source of professional satisfaction to remember that most delirious patients recover if they receive competent medical and nursing care. The family should be reassured on this point. They must also understand that the patient's abnormal behavior is not willful but rather symptomatic of a brain disease.

See also Chaps. 40 and 41 for specific aspects of management of delirium due to withdrawal of alcohol, barbiturates, and other sedative-hypnotic drugs.

REFERENCES

CAPLAN LR, KELLY M, KASE CS et al: Mirror image of Wernicke's aphasia. *Neurology* 36:1015, 1986.

ENGEL GL, ROMANO, J: Delirium: A syndrome of cerebral insufficiency. *J Chronic Dis* 9:260, 1959.

EY H: Disorders of consciousness in psychiatry, in Vinken PJ, Bruyn GW (eds): *Handbook of Clinical Neurology*. Vol. 3: *Disorders of Higher Nervous Activity*. Amsterdam, North-Holland, 1969, chap 7, pp 112–136.

HORENSTEIN S, CHAMBERLIN W, CONOMY T: Infarction of the fusiform and calcarine regions. Agitated delirium and hemianopia. *Trans Am Neurol Assoc* 92:85, 1967.

KAHN E: *Psychopathic Personalities*. New Haven, Yale University Press, 1931.

LIPOWSKI ZJ: *Delirium: Acute Brain Failure in Man*. Springfield, Ill, Charles C Thomas, 1980.

LISHMAN WA: *Organic Psychiatry. The Psychological Consequences of Cerebral Disorder*. Oxford, Blackwell, 1978.

MEDINA JL, RUBINO FA, ROSS A: Agitated delirium caused by infarction of the hippocampal formation, fusiform and lingual gyri. *Neurology* 24:1181, 1974.

MESULAM MM, WAXMAN SG, GESCHWIND N et al: Acute confusional states with right middle cerebral infarctions. *J Neurol Neurosurg Psychiatry* 39:84, 1976.

MESULAM M-M: Attention, confusional states, and neglect, in Mesulam M-M (ed), *Principles of Behavioral Neurology*. Philadelphia, Davis, 1985, chap 3.

MORI E, YAMADORI A: Acute confusional state and acute agitated delirium. *Arch Neurol* 44:1139, 1987.

STAUDER HK: Die tödliche Katatonie. *Arch Psychiatr Nervenkr* 102:614, 1934.

WOLFF HG, CURRAN D: Nature of delirium and allied states. *Arch Neurol Psychiatry* 33:1175, 1935.

CHAPTER 20

DEMENTIA AND THE AMNESIC (KORSAKOFF) SYNDROME

Increasingly, as the number of elderly in our population rises, the neurologist is consulted because an otherwise healthy person begins to lose his or her capacity to function effectively as a worker or head of a family. This may indicate the beginning of a brain tumor, the formation of a chronic subdural hematoma, or the development of chronic drug intoxication, chronic meningoencephalitis (syphilis), degenerative cerebral disease, normal-pressure hydrocephalus, or a depressive illness. In former times, when there was little that could be done about these clinical states, no great premium was attached to diagnosis. But modern medicine offers the means of treating several of these conditions and in some instances of restoring the patient to normal health and effectiveness. Moreover, a number of modern diagnostic technologies now allow earlier recognition of the underlying pathologic process, improving the chances of recovery.

DEFINITIONS

In current neurologic parlance the term *dementia* usually denotes a clinical syndrome composed of failing memory and loss of other intellectual functions due to chronic progressive degenerative disease of the brain. Such a definition is too narrow. Actually the term covers a number of closely related syndromes that are characterized not only by intellectual deterioration but also by certain behavioral abnormalities and changes in personality. Moreover it is illogical to set apart any one constellation of cerebral symptoms on the basis of their speed of onset, rate of evolution, severity or duration. Alternatively, we would propose that there are several states of dementia of multiple causation and mechanism and that a diffuse degeneration of neurons (usually chronic) is only one of the many causes. Therefore it is more correct to speak of *the dementias* or the dementing diseases.

To understand the phenomenon of intellectual deterioration, it is helpful to have some idea of how intellectual activity is normally organized and sustained by the brain, and the manner in which deficits in intelligence relate to diffuse and focal cerebral disease.

THE NEUROLOGY OF INTELLIGENCE

Intelligence or *intelligent behavior* is "the aggregate or global capacity of the individual to act purposefully, to think rationally, and to deal effectively with his environment" (Wechsler). It is global because it characterizes an individual's behavior as a whole; it is an aggregate in the sense that it is composed of a number of independent and qualitatively distinguishable abilities.

As every educated person knows, intelligence has something to do with normal cerebral function. Further, the level of intelligence obviously differs widely from one person to another, and members of certain families are exceptionally bright and intellectually accomplished while others are just the opposite. Intelligent children, if properly motivated, excel in school and score high on intelligence tests, which are themselves predictive of scholastic success. Indeed the first intelligence tests devised by Binet and Simon in 1905 were for this purpose. The term *intelligence quotient*, or *IQ*, was introduced by Terman in 1916; it denotes a figure that is obtained by dividing mental age (as determined by the Binet-Simon scale) by chronologic age (up to the fourteenth year) and multiplying the result by 100. The IQ correlates with achievement in school and eventual success in professional work. The IQ calls attention to other qualities of intelligence—that it increases with age up to the fourteenth to sixteenth year and that at any given age a large sample of normal children attain test scores that are distributed in conformity with the normal, or Gaussian, curve. The wide application of the Wechsler-Bellevue and later the Wechsler Adult Intelligence Scale (WAIS) has revealed another characteristic—a falling off of intelligence test performance after the age of 35 years.

The original studies of pedigrees of highly intelligent and mentally inferior families, which revealed a striking concordance between parent and child, lent support to the idea that intelligence is mainly inherited. However, it soon became evident that the tests being used depended to a large extent on skill with words and verbal relationships and specific cultural experiences that educated parents provided for their children, and were less reliable in selecting children who were talented but never had similar educational opportunities. In recent times this has led to the widespread belief that intelligence tests are only achievement tests and that environmental factors that foster high performance are the only important ones in determining intelligence. Neither of these two views is entirely correct. The studies of monozygotic and dizygotic twins raised in the same or different families has put the matter in a clearer light. Identical twins reared together or apart are more alike in intelligence than nonidentical twins brought up in the same home (see reviews of Willerman, of Shields, and of Slater and Cowie). There can be no doubt, therefore, that genetic endowment is the more important factor; Piercy has estimated the ratio of the hereditary and environmental components of intelligence to be from 6:4 to 8:2. However, such estimates can only be approximations. There is convincing evidence that early learning may modify the level of ability that is finally obtained. The latter should not be looked upon as the sum of genetic and environmental factors, but as the product of the two. Moreover, all psychometrists have come to appreciate that achievement or success is governed also by factors other than purely intellectual ones—such as a readiness to learn, interest, persistence, and motivation. Wechsler termed these x and z factors; they are variable and unmeasurable in tests of intelligence.

As to psychologic theories of intelligence, three have held sway. One is known as the two-factor theory of Spearman, who noted that all the separate tests of cognitive abilities correlated positively, suggesting that a general (g) factor enters into all performance. Since none of the correlations approached unity, he postulated that every test measures not only this general ability (commonly identified with intelligence), but also a number of subsidiary factors, specific to the individual tests. The latter he designated the s factors. The second theory, the multifactorial theory of Thurstone, proposes that intelligence consists of a number of primary mental abilities, such as memory, verbal facility, numerical ability, visual-spatial perception, and capacity for problem solving, all of them more or less equivalent. These primary abilities, although correlated, are not subordinate to a more general ability. A third theory, that of Alexander, supports Spearman's notion of a g factor but holds that this factor alone is insufficient to explain total correlational variance between tests.

Concerning the way in which adult intelligence develops, the most widely known theory is that of Piaget, who proposed that a child learns by discrete stages related to age—sensorimotor, from 0 to 2 years; preconceptual thought, from 2 to 4 years; intuitive thought, from 4 to 7 years; concrete ''operations'' (conceptualization), from 7 to 11 years; and finally the period of ''formal operations'' (logical or abstract thought), from 11 years on. This concept implies that the capacity for logical thought, developing as it does according to an orderly timetable, is coded in the genes. Surely one can perceive these states of intellectual development in the child, but Piaget's theory has been criticized as being too anecdotal and lacking the quantitative validation that could be derived only from studies of a large normal population. Further, it does not take into account the individual's special abilities, which do not develop and reach their maximum at the same time as the more general intellectual capacities.

Another theory of intelligence is that of Hebb, based on his observations that cerebral injury caused a more diffuse disturbance of intellect in children than in adults. The latter tended to suffer more focal impairment, or else showed little intellectual change, even with large frontal lesions. On the basis of these observations Hebb postulated two forms of intelligence: one, an innate capacity to form concepts (intelligence A), which determines the speed and level of intellectual development and which is delayed or impaired in a nonspecific way by lesions of many parts of the brain. The second, intelligence B, is the level of intellectual efficiency actually attained, which, once developed, is relatively little affected by cerebral lesions. According to Hebb, the cognitive abilities that are seriously impaired by cerebral lesions require an unimpaired brain for their optimal performance, i.e., they involve intelligence A. This subject is discussed further in Chap. 28.

One would suppose that in neurology, where we are confronted with so many diseases affecting the cerebrum, it might be possible to verify one of these several theories of intelligence and to determine its anatomy. Diffuse lesions might be expected to impair the g factor of intelligence in proportion to the mass of brain involved (''mass-action'' principle of Lashley). According to Chapman and Wolff there is a correlation between the volume of tissue lost and a general deficit of cerebral function. Others have disagreed, claiming that no universal psychologic deficit can be recognized with lesions affecting various parts of the cerebrum. Probably the truth lies between these two divergent points of view. With lesions above a certain size (50 mL of tissue, according to Tomlinson et al) there is some general reduction in performance, especially in speed, and an impaired capacity to reason. It is noted also that levels of *g* do not decline consistently with age. On the other hand, in a closely reasoned analysis of specific intellectual deficits, Piercy has found positive correlations between losses of particular functions (Spearman's and Thurstone's *s* factors, so to speak) and lesions of particular parts of the left and right hemispheres. These are discussed in Chap. 21. Thus, the evidence provided by neurologic studies is more consistent with a concept of intelligence as a gestalt of multiple primary abilities, each with a certain degree of anatomic localization, than as a strictly unitary function. However, they do not eliminate the possibility of a *g* factor—perhaps one that is equivalent to thinking or abstract reasoning ability and that is only operative if the connections of the frontal lobes with other parts of the brain are intact. Attention, drive, and motivation have a separate and as yet unidentified anatomy.

THE NEUROLOGY OF DEMENTIA

The study of dementia also shows it to consist of a loss of several relatively separable but overlapping abilities, presenting in a number of different combinations. These varied constellations of intellectual deficits constitute the preeminent clinical abnormalities in several cerebral diseases, and, sometimes, the only abnormalities. The most common types of dementing diseases and their relative frequency are listed in Table 20-1. These figures, which are in accord with our experience, have been compiled by Wells, and are based on the findings in three neurologic centers as well as his own.

What is noteworthy about these figures is the apparently high level of accuracy of diagnosis. In the series of Wade et al, the clinical diagnosis was verified by postmortem examination in 87 percent of 65 cases; we have had a similar degree of success in diagnosis. This is somewhat misleading, however. In the "cerebral atrophy" (Alzheimer disease) group, for example, there is always an incalculable number of cases of Pick disease and other degenerative diseases that cannot be differentiated clinically, although they probably do not make up more than 5 or 10 percent of the entire group. Also, these data do not indicate the frequency of combined types, particularly of Alzheimer and vascular disease(s). Impressive also is the fact that approximately 1 in 20 patients seen in a neurologic center with a question of dementia proves to have a potentially reversible psychiatric illness simulating dementia (pseudodementia).

In the following pages we shall consider the prototype syndromes. The special features of individual diseases of which dementia is a part will be presented in Chap. 43 (degenerative diseases) and other appropriate chapters.

DEMENTIA DUE TO DEGENERATIVE DISEASES

The earliest signs of dementia due to degenerative disease may be so subtle as to escape the notice of the most discerning physician. Often an observant relative of the patient or an employer is the first to become aware of a certain lack of initiative, a lack of interest in work, a neglect of routine tasks, or an abandonment of pleasurable pursuits. Initially, these changes may be attributed to fatigue or boredom. The gradual development of forgetfulness is another prominent early symptom. Proper names are no longer remembered, the purpose of an errand is forgotten, appointments are not kept, a recent conversation or social event has been forgotten. The patient may ask the same question repeatedly, the answers that were previously given not being retained. Sometimes the mental failure is brought to light more dramatically by a severe confusional state that attends a febrile illness, a concussive head injury, or the taking of some new medicine. Later it becomes evident that the patient is easily distracted by every passing incident. No longer is it possible to think about or discuss a problem

Table 20-1

The common types of dementing diseases and their relative frequency

Dementing disease	Relative frequency, %
Cerebral atrophy, mainly Alzheimer-senile dementia	50
Multi-infarct dementia	10
Alcoholic dementia*	5-10
Intracranial tumors	5
Normal-pressure hydrocephalus	6
Huntington chorea	3
Chronic drug intoxications	3
Miscellaneous diseases (hepatic failure; pernicious anemia; hypo- or hyperthyroidism; dementias with Parkinson disease, amyotrophic lateral sclerosis, cerebellar atrophy; neurosyphilis; Cushing syndrome, Creutzfeld-Jakob disease; multiple sclerosis; epilepsy)	7-10
Undiagnosed types	3
Pseudodementias (depression, hypomania, schizophrenia, hysteria, undiagnosed)	7

*Frequency varies with incidence of alcoholism in the population studied.

Source: Wells.

with the usual clarity, and there is a failure to comprehend all aspects of complex situations. One feature of a situation or some relatively unimportant event may become a source of unreasonable concern or worry. Tasks that require several steps cannot be accomplished, and all but the simplest directions cannot be followed. The patient may get lost, even along habitual routes of travel. Day-to-day events are not recalled, and perseveration in speech, action, and thought is noted. In yet other instances, the first abnormality may be in the nature of emotional instability, taking the form of outbursts of anger, tears, or aggressiveness. Frequently a change in mood becomes apparent, deviating more toward depression than elation. Apathy is common. Some patients are grumpy, irascible, and bad-tempered. A few are cheerful and facetious. The direction of the mood change is said to depend on the previous personality of the patient, rather than on the character of the disease, but one can think of glaring exceptions to this dictum. Excessive lability of mood may also be observed, i.e., easy fluctuation from laughter to tears on slight provocation. Loss of social graces and indifference to social customs occur but usually later in the course of illness. Judgment becomes impaired, early in some, late in others. At certain phases of the illness, suspiciousness or frank paranoia may develop. Visual and auditory hallucinations, sometimes quite vivid in nature, may be added. As a rule these patients have little or no realization of such changes within themselves; they lack insight.

As the condition progresses, all intellectual faculties are impaired, but memory most of all. Patients may fail to recognize their relatives or to recall their names. Apractagnosias may be prominent, and the defects may alter the performance of the simplest tasks, such as preparing a meal or setting the table, or even using the telephone or a knife and fork, or dressing, or walking. A disorder of gait may occur in the early stages of some dementing diseases and in the late stages of others (see Chap. 6).

Language functions tend to suffer almost from the beginning. The capacity to understand the nuances of language is lost early as are the suppleness and spontaneity of verbal expression. Vocabulary becomes restricted and conversation, rambling and repetitious. Patients grope for proper names and common nouns and no longer formulate ideas with well-constructed phrases or sentences. There is a tendency to resort instead to clichés, stereotyped phrases, and exclamations, which may hide the underlying defect during conversation. More severe degrees of aphasia, dysarthria, palilalia, and echolalia may be added to the clinical picture, but only in the later stages. As pointed out by Chapman and Wolff, there is loss also of the capacity to express feelings and impulses, to tolerate frustration and restrictions, and to modulate defense reactions. Disagreeable behavior—petulance, agitation, shouting and whining if restrained—may occur.

There is also a physical deterioration. Food intake, which may be increased in the beginning of the illness, is in the end reduced, with resulting emaciation. Any febrile illness, drug intoxication, or metabolic upset is poorly tolerated, leading to severe confusion, stupor, or coma, an indication of the precarious state of cerebral compensation (see ''Beclouded Dementia,'' Chap. 19). Finally, these patients remain in bed most of the time, oblivious of their surroundings, and succumb to pneumonia or to some other intercurrent infection. Should they not succumb in this way, some patients become virtually decorticate—totally unaware of their environment, unresponsive, mute, and incontinent. They lie with eyes open but do not look about. Food and drink are no longer requested but are swallowed if placed in the mouth. Grasping and sucking reflexes are easily elicited. The limbs may exhibit a combination of spasticity and rigidity, the tendon reflexes are hyperactive, and occasionally diffuse choreoathetotic movements or random myoclonic jerking can be observed. Pain or an uncomfortable posture goes unheeded. The course of the disease extends over 5 to 10 years or more.

It would be an error to think that the abnormalities in the atrophic-degenerative dementing diseases are confined to the intellectual sphere. The appearance of the patient and the physical examination alone yield highly informative data. The first impression is helpful; patients may be unkempt, slovenly, and unbathed. They may look bewildered, as though lost, or their expression is vacant, and they do not maintain a lively interest or participate in the interview. There is a kind of psychic inertia. Deference to other members of the family when unable to answer the examiner's questions is characteristic. The posture appears to be stiff and inflexible. All movements are slow, sometimes suggesting an oncoming Parkinson syndrome. Sooner or later the gait becomes altered in a characteristic manner (Chap. 6). Attempts to move the limbs passively encounter a fluctuating resistance (gegenhalten). Grasp and sucking reflexes, mouthing movements, uninhibited blink on tapping the glabella, snout reflex (protrusion of the lips in response to perioral tapping), biting or jaw clamping (bulldog) reflex, corneomandibular reflex (jaw clenching when cornea is touched), and palmomental reflex (retraction of one side of the mouth and chin when the thenar eminence of the palm is stroked), all occur with increasing frequency in the advanced stages of the dementia. Many of these abnormalities will be recognized as mild motor disinhibitions that appear when the premotor areas of the brain are involved.

Naturally every case does not follow the exact sequence outlined above. Not infrequently a patient is brought to a physician because of a loss of facility in language. In other patients impairment of retentive memory with relatively intact reasoning power may be the dominant clinical feature in the first months or even years of the disease; or low impulsivity (apathy and abulia) may be the most conspicuous feature, resulting in an obscuration of the more specialized higher cerebral functions. Gait disorder, though usually a late development, may occur early, particularly in patients in whom the dementia is superimposed on Parkinson disease, cerebellar ataxia, or amyotrophic lateral sclerosis, which sometimes happens. Insofar as the several types of degenerative disease do not affect indentical parts of the brain, it is not surprising that their symptomatology varies. These variations and others will be described in Chap. 43.

In general, one may say that the aforementioned alterations of intellect and behavior are the direct consequence of neuronal loss in the cerebrum. Expressed in another way, the symptoms are the primary manifestations of neurologic disease. However, some symptoms are secondary, i.e., they are the patient's reactions to the catastrophe of losing his or her mind. For example, demented persons may seek solitude to hide their affliction and may thus only appear to be asocial or apathetic. Again, excessive orderliness may be an attempt to compensate for failing memory; apprehension, gloom, and irritability may reflect a general dissatisfaction with a necessarily restricted life. According to Kurt Goldstein, who has written about these "catastrophic reactions," as he called them, even patients in a state of fairly advanced deterioration are still capable of reacting to their illness and to persons who care for them.

Special psychologic tests aid in the quantitation of some of these abnormalities. The Wechsler Adult Intelligence Scale (WAIS) reveals scores well below the patient's norm, with a disproportionate reduction of the nonverbal parts of the test. The Wechsler Memory Scale is highly sensitive to the amnesic feature of the illness. The Reitan battery, popular in certain circles, permits wide testing of many functions, including topographic memory, visual perception, and personality traits, and it includes parts of the above tests.

Arteriosclerotic dementia represents a special problem and merits a few words. Often the term *arteriosclerotic* is applied incorrectly to the dementia of Alzheimer disease or other degenerative diseases. Undoubtedly, the compounded effect of recurrent strokes impairs intellect; usually, but not always, the stroke-by-stroke advance of the disease is apparent in such patients. Moreover, having senile dementia does not indemnify the patient against cerebro-vascular disease; in fact, this combination is very frequent, in which case the clinical picture may be a composite of the two diseases. Certain cerebrovascular lesions may cause highly characteristic syndromes—e.g., pseudobulbar palsy or pathologic emotionality, due to bilateral small lacunar infarcts in the corticobulbar motor pathways; the combination of Korsakoff psychosis with visual field alterations and visual agnosias, caused by bilateral posterior cerebral artery occlusion; and the frontal lobe–sympathetic apraxia syndrome, with anterior cerebral artery occlusion (see Chap. 21, under "Disconnection Syndromes").

The dementia of *normal-pressure hydrocephalus* often simulates that of the degenerative diseases, although the former tends to evolve more rapidly. Normal-pressure hydrocephalus, usually distinguished by the triad of gait disorder, psychomotor slowing, and sphincter incontinence, is discussed further in Chap. 30. Since it is correctible by ventriculoperitoneal shunting, one must now look closely at the whole population of dementing patients and subject them to appropriate clinical and diagnostic tests.

Cerebral tumors, particularly those involving the corpus callosum, right temporal, and frontal lobes, may alter mental function for some time before headaches, seizures, and focal signs of cerebral disease appear, and the latter may be inconspicuous. The same is true of *chronic subdural hematoma.*

MORBID ANATOMY AND PATHOPHYSIOLOGY OF DEMENTIA

Attempts to relate the impairment of particular intellectual functions to lesions in certain parts of the brain have been eminently unsuccessful. Two types of difficulty have obstructed progress in this field. (1) There is the problem of defining, analyzing, and determining the nature of the so-called intellectual functions. (2) The morbid anatomy of the dementing diseases is often so diffuse and complex that it cannot be fully localized and quantitated. The memory impairment, which is a constant feature, may occur with extensive disease in several different parts of the cerebrum. Yet it is important to note that the functions of certain parts of the diencephalon and temporal lobes are more fundamental to retentive memory than the rest of the brain, as will be pointed out further on. Failure in tests of verbal function (the most advanced degree of which is aphasia) is closely associated with disease of the dominant cerebral hemisphere, particularly the perisylvian parts of the frontal, temporal, and parietal lobes. Loss of capacity for reading and calculation is related to lesions in the posterior part of the left (dominant) cerebral hemisphere. Impairment in drawing or constructing simple and complex figures with blocks, sticks, picture arrangements, etc., is observed most often in right (nondominant) parietal lobe lesions. Thus, the clinical picture resulting from cerebral disease depends in part on the extent of the lesion, i.e., the amount of cerebral tissue destroyed, and on the specific locality of the lesion.

Dementia is related usually to obvious structural diseases of the cerebrum, the diencephalon, and possibly the basal ganglia. In some, such as Alzheimer disease and Pick lobar atrophy, the main process appears to be a degeneration and loss of nerve cells in the cortical association areas, with secondary changes in the cerebral white matter. In Pick disease the syndrome is often mainly frontal or temporal, or both. In others, such as Huntington chorea, a similar degeneration of neurons predominates in the caudate nuclei, putamens, and other parts of the basal ganglia. Finally, purely thalamic degenerations may be the basis of a dementia, because of the integral relationship of the thalamus to the cerebral cortex.

Arteriosclerotic vascular disease, which pursues a different course than the degenerative diseases, results in multiple foci of infarction throughout the thalami, basal ganglia, brainstem, and cerebrum and, in the latter, in the motor, sensory, or visual projection areas as well as in the association areas. The aftermath of severe trauma, if it results in a type of dementia, may be found in the cerebral convolutions (mainly frontal and temporal), corpus callosum, and mesencephalon; rarely there is widespread degeneration of the white matter (page 697) and hydrocephalus. Most diseases that produce dementia are quite extensive.

Mechanisms other than the destruction of brain tissue may operate in some cases. *Chronic increased intracranial pressure* or *chronic hydrocephalus* (with large ventricles the pressure may not exceed 180 mmHg), regardless of cause, is often associated with a general impairment of mental function. Compression of cerebral white matter is the main factor. The compression of one or both of the cerebral hemispheres by chronic subdural hematomas may have the same effect. *A diffuse inflammatory process* is at least in part the basis of dementia in syphilis, cryptococcosis, and virus infections such as herpes simplex and subacute sclerosing panencephalitis; presumably there is a loss of some neurons and also an inflammatory derangement of the function of other neurons or the predominant lesions are in the white matter, as in progressive multifocal leukoencephalitis. Lastly, several of the *metabolic* and *toxic* disorders discussed in Chaps. 38 and 42 may interfere with nervous function over a period of time and create a clinical picture similar to, if not identical with, that of dementia. One must suppose that the altered biochemical environment has affected neuronal function.

"SUBCORTICAL" DEMENTIA

This term has been used in a number of different contexts and has little to recommend it. McHugh and Folstein, who introduced the concept, proposed that the dementias of certain predominantly basal ganglionic diseases, such as

Huntington chorea, progressive supranuclear palsy, and Wilson disease, are characterized by slow, dysarthric speech, forgetfulness, slowed thought processes, apathy, and depression; by contrast, the "cortical dementias" (prototype, Alzheimer disease), were distinguished by their severe disturbances of language and memory, apraxia, agnosia, and impaired capacity for abstract thought. This does not appear to be a fundamental distinction, either on clinical or pathologic grounds. It will be recognized that the symptoms allegedly typical of "subcortical dementia" are also characteristic of "cortical dementias," and that any differences between them are probably attributable to differences in severity of the dementing processes—an argument that has been made convincingly by Mayeux and Stern and their colleagues and by Tierney et al. In general, differences in the severity of symptoms are an insecure basis for distinguishing between diseases or categories of disease.

Anatomically, no form of dementia is strictly cortical or subcortical. In practically all dementing diseases, lesions are found in both structures, as Whitehouse has recently emphasized. The attribution of dementia to subcortical gliosis, for example, has always proved to be incorrect; invariably, there are cortical changes as well. In a similar vein, the changes of Alzheimer disease extend far beyond the confines of the cerebral cortex, involving the striatum, the thalamus, and even the cerebellum.

Far more useful than this contrived division into cortical and subcortical would be a careful analysis of the main attributes of any given constellation of dementing symptoms and their correlation with the disease and its cerebral-basal-ganglionic-thalamic localization.

BEDSIDE CLASSIFICATION OF DEMENTING DISEASES OF THE BRAIN

The conventional classification of dementing diseases of the brain is usually according to cause, if known, or to the pathologic changes. Another more practical approach, which follows logically from the method by which the whole subject has been presented in this book, is to subdivide the diseases into three categories on the basis of the neurologic signs and associated clinical and laboratory signs of medical disease. Once it has been determined that the patient suffers from a dementing illness, it must then be decided, from the medical, neurologic, and ancillary data, into which category the case fits. This classification may at first seem somewhat artificial. However, it is likely to be more useful to the student or physician not conversant with the many diseases that cause dementia than a classification based on pathology.

I. Diseases in which dementia is associated with clinical and laboratory signs of other medical disease
   A. Hypothyroidism
   B. Cushing syndrome
   C. Nutritional deficiency states such as pellagra, the Wernicke-Korsakoff syndrome, and subacute combined degeneration of spinal cord and brain (vitamin B_{12} deficiency)
   D. Chronic meningoencephalitis: general paresis, meningovascular syphilis, cryptococcosis
   E. Hepatolenticular degeneration, familial and acquired
   F. Chronic drug intoxications
II. Diseases in which dementia is associated with other neurologic signs but not with other obvious medical disease
   A. Invariably associated with other neurologic signs
      1. Huntington chorea (choreoathetosis)
      2. Schilder disease and related demyelinative diseases (spastic weakness, pseudobulbar palsy, blindness)
      3. Amaurotic familial idiocy and other lipid-storage diseases (myoclonic seizures, blindness, spasticity, cerebellar ataxia)
      4. Myoclonic epilepsy (diffuse myoclonus, generalized seizures, cerebellar ataxia)
      5. Subacute spongiform encephalopathy (one type of Creutzfeldt-Jakob disease) (myoclonic dementia)
      6. Cerebrocerebellar degeneration (cerebellar ataxia)
      7. Cerebral-basal ganglionic degenerations (apraxia-rigidity)
      8. Dementia with spastic paraplegia
      9. Progressive supranuclear palsy
      10. Certain hereditary metabolic diseases (Chap. 38)
   B. Often associated with other neurologic signs
      1. Thrombotic or embolic cerebral infarction
      2. Brain tumor (primary or metastatic) or abscess
      3. Brain trauma, such as cerebral contusion, midbrain hemorrhage, chronic subdural hematoma
      4. Marchiafava-Bignami disease (often with apraxia and other frontal lobe signs)
      5. Communicating (normal-pressure) or obstructive hydrocephalus (usually with ataxia of gait)
      6. Progressive multifocal leukoencephalitis
III. Diseases in which dementia is usually the only evidence of neurologic or medical disease
   A. Alzheimer disease
   B. Pick disease
   C. AIDS dementia
   D. Alcoholic dementia
   E. Degenerative disease of unspecified type

The special clinical features and morbid anatomy of these many dementing diseases are discussed in appropriate chapters throughout this book.

DIFFERENTIAL DIAGNOSIS

Although confusion or dementia per se does not indicate a particular disease, certain combinations of symptoms and neurologic signs are more or less characteristic and may aid in diagnosis. The mode of onset, the clinical course and time span, the associated neurologic signs, and the accessory laboratory data constitute the basis of differential diagnosis. It must be admitted, however, that some of the rarer types of "degenerative" brain disease are at present recognized only by pathologic examination. The correct diagnosis of treatable forms of dementia—neurosyphilis, cryptococcosis, subdural hematoma, brain tumor, chronic drug intoxication, normal-pressure hydrocephalus, pellagra and other deficiency states, hypothyroidism and other metabolic and endocrine disorders—is of course of greater practical importance than the diagnosis of the untreatable ones.

The first task in dealing with this class of patients is to verify the presence of intellectual deterioration and personality change. It may be necessary to examine the patient several times before one is confident of the clinical findings.

There is always a tendency to assume that mental function is normal if a patient complains only of nervousness, fatigue, insomnia, or vague somatic symptoms, and to label the patient psychoneurotic. *This will be avoided if one keeps in mind that psychoneurosis rarely begins in middle or late adult life.* A practical rule is to assume that all mental illnesses beginning during this period are due either to structural disease of the brain or to depression.

A mild dysphasia must not be mistaken for dementia. Aphasic patients appear uncertain of themselves, and their speech may be incoherent. Furthermore, they may be anxious and depressed over their ineptitude. Careful attention to the patient's language performance will lead to the correct diagnosis in most instances. Further observation will disclose that the patient's behavior, except that which is related to the language disorder, is not abnormal.

Depressed patients present another type of problem. They may complain that their mental function is poor or that they are forgetful and cannot concentrate. Scrutiny of their complaints will show, however, that they usually can remember the details of their illness and that no qualitative change in other intellectual functions has taken place. Their difficulty is either a lack of energy and interest or preoccupation with personal worries and anxiety, which prevent the focusing of attention on anything except their own problems. Even during mental tests their performance may be impaired by their emotional state, in much the same way as that of the worried student during examinations. This condition of emotional blocking is called *experiential confusion*. When such patients are calmed by reassurance and encouraged to try harder, their mental function improves, indicating that intellectual deterioration has not occurred. Hypomanic patients fail in tests of intellectual function because of their restlessness, inability to persevere, and distractibility. It is helpful to remember that demented patients rarely have sufficient insight to complain of mental deterioration, and if they admit to poor memory, they do so without conviction or full appreciation of the degree of their disability. The physician must never rely on the patient's statements as to the efficiency of mental function and must always evaluate a poor performance on tests in the light of the emotional state and motivation at the time the test is given. Yet another problem is that of the impulsive, cantankerous, and quarrelsome patient who is a constant source of distress to employer and family. Such changes in personality and behavior, verging at times on psychosis, may precede or mask early intellectual deterioration, as often happens in Huntington disease.

The neuropsychiatric symptoms associated with metabolic, endocrine, or toxic disorders (i.e., ACTH or corticosteroid therapy, hypothyroidism, Cushing syndrome, hypercalcemia, Addison disease, hepatic encephalopathy, hypoglycemia, uremia, chronic barbiturate or other drug intoxication) may present difficulties in diagnosis because of the wide variety of clinical pictures by which they manifest themselves. Some patients appear to be suffering from a dementia, others from an acute confusional psychosis; or, if there are mood changes, negativism, hallucinations, and delusions, a manic-depressive psychosis or schizophrenia is suggested. In the toxic-metabolic disorders, some degree of clouding of the sensorium and impairment of intellectual function can usually be recognized, and these findings, along with the brevity of the illness, should be enough to exclude schizophrenia and manic-depressive psychosis. It is well to remember that the abrupt onset of mental symptoms always points to a confusional psychosis or delirium; inattention, clouding of the sensorium, perceptual disturbances, and often drowsiness are conjoined (Chap. 19). Inasmuch as these latter conditions are practically always reversible, it is important that they be distinguished from dementia.

Once it is decided that the patient suffers from a dementing disease, the next step is to determine by careful physical examination whether there are other neurologic signs or indications of a particular medical disease. This enables the physician to place the case in one of the three categories in the bedside classification (see above). Ancillary examinations, such as CT scanning or MRI, EEG, and lumbar puncture should be carried out in most cases. Usually these procedures necessitate admission to a hospital. The final step is to determine, from the total clinical picture, the particular disease within any one category.

THE AMNESIC SYNDROME (Korsakoff Psychosis; Amnesic- or Amnestic-Confabulatory Syndrome)

These terms are used interchangeably to designate a unique but common disorder of cognitive function, in which memory is deranged out of proportion to all other components of mentation and behavior. It possesses two salient features that may vary in severity but are always conjoined: (1) an impaired ability to recall events and other information that had been well established before the onset of the illness (*retrograde amnesia*) and (2) an impaired ability to acquire certain types of new information, i.e., to learn or to form new memories (*anterograde amnesia*). Other cognitive functions (particularly the capacity for concentration, spatial organization, visual and verbal abstraction), which depend little or not at all on memory, are impaired to a lesser degree. The patient is usually lacking in initiative and spontaneity.

The definition of Korsakoff psychosis is predicated also upon the integrity of certain aspects of behavior and mental function. The patient must be awake and attentive, responsive, and capable of understanding the written and spoken word, of making appropriate deductions from given premises, and of solving such problems as can be concluded within his or her forward memory span. Immediate memory (e.g., digit repetition) is intact and remote memory (early life events) is relatively unaffected. These "negative" features are of particular importance, because they help to distinguish Korsakoff psychosis from a number of other disorders in which the basic defect is not in retentive memory, but in some other psychologic mechanism, e.g., in attention and perception (as in the delirious, confused, or stuporous patient), in recall (as in the hysterical patient), or in volition, i.e., the will to learn (as in the apathetic or abulic patient with frontal lobe disease or depression).

Confabulation, i.e., falsification of memory in an alert, responsive individual, is often included in the definition of Korsakoff psychosis, but it occurs only in certain patients with this syndrome. Most often it can be provoked by questions as to the patient's recent activities; the replies may be recognized as partially remembered events and personal experiences that are related with no regard to their proper temporal sequence. Far less frequent but more dramatic is a spontaneous recital of personal experiences, many of which are fantasies. These two forms of confabulation have been referred to as "momentary" and "fantastic" and it has been claimed, on uncertain grounds, that the latter form reflects an associated lesion in the frontal lobes (Berlyne). In our patients with alcoholic Korsakoff syndrome, so-called fantastic confabulation was observed mainly in the initial phase of the illness, in which it could be related to a state of profound general confusion; "momentary confabulation" came later, in the convalescent stage. In the chronic, stable stage of the illness, confabulation was rarely elicitable, irrespective of how broadly this symptom was defined.

The anatomic structures of particular importance in memory function are the diencephalon (specifically the medial portions of the dorsomedial and adjacent midline nuclei of the thalamus) and the hippocampal formations (gyrus dentatus, hippocampus, parahippocampal gyrus), and amygdaloid nuclei. Bilaterally placed lesions in these regions derange memory and learning out of all proportion to other cognitive functions, and a unilateral lesion in these regions of the dominant hemisphere can probably produce a lesser degree of the same effect. A severe and enduring (5-year) defect in retentive memory has also been observed with bilateral infarction of the septal gray matter, nucleus accumbens, diagonal band of Broca, and paraventricular hypothalomic gray matter (Phillips et al). It is noteworthy that these septal nuclei have connections with the hippocampus through the precommissural fornix and with the amygdala through the diagonal band.

Experimental studies in subhuman primates have confirmed the importance of the diencephalic-hippocampal structures in memory function. (The review of these many studies by Squire and Zola-Morgan is recommended.) The difficulty of evaluating memory function in animals has been largely overcome by the development of a new type of delayed nonmatching-to-sample task, which has proved to be impaired both in patients with the amnesic syndrome and in monkeys with lesions of the medial dorsal nuclei and inferomedial temporal regions (Mishkin and Delacour). Using this method of testing recognition memory, Mishkin and his colleagues found that slight impairment followed ablation of either the hippocampus or the amygdala bilaterally, but that severe impairment could be produced only by the bilateral destruction of both amygdala and hippocampus. Again it should be noted that the hippocampus projects to the anterior nuclei of the thalamus and amygdala to the medial dorsal nucleus. Horel's claim, that the critical structure in the inferomedial temporal lobe is not the hippocampus but the underlying white matter (the so-called temporal stem or albal stalk), has been refuted. The latter structure, which connects the inferior and middle temporal gyri with the pulvinar and medial dorsal nucleus, is essential for visual pattern discrimination, but not for recognition memory (Zola-Morgan et al).

All of these observations suggest that the medial temporal lobe and medial thalamic regions together form a circuit essential for memory function.

The importance assigned to the hippocampal formations and medial thalamic nuclei in memory function does not mean that the mechanisms governing this function are confined to these structures or that these parts of the brain form a "memory center." It means only that these are the sites where the smallest lesions have the most devastating effects on memory and learning. Normal memory function involves many parts of the brain in addition to the diencephalic-hippocampal structures. Integrity of the reticular formation of the upper brainstem is of obvious importance, since a state of alertness and attentiveness is a requisite for any learning. Also, it is known that extensive lesions of the neocortex may cause impairment of retentive memory and learning and that this effect is probably more dependent upon the size of the lesion than upon its locus. Of particular importance are the circumscribed areas of the cerebral cortex that are related to special forms of learning and memory, a subject that is considered in detail in the next chapter. Thus, a lesion of the dominant temporal lobe impairs the ability to remember words, and a lesion of the inferior parietal lobule, to recognize written words and to relearn them; the dominant parietal lobe is related to recollection of geometric figures and numbers; the nondominant parietal lobe, to visual-spatial relations, and so forth.

Any hypothesis concerning the anatomic substratum of learning and retentive memory must include, therefore, not only the diencephalic-hippocampal structures, but also special parts of the neocortex and the midbrain reticular formation. We would propose that the diencephalic-hippocampal structures are involved in all active phases of learning and integration of new information, regardless of the sense avenue through which this information reaches the organism in order to be assimilated or of the final pathway of its expression; and it seems to make little difference whether the acquired experience involves functions that are classed as purely cognitive or emotional. This general aspect of memory function might be designated as the "universal" or "U" factor of memory. Restricted regions of the temporal, parietal, and occipital cortex, which have particular relationships to the several "special memories," may be designated as the "S" factors of memory.

It is a remarkable feature of the Korsakoff amnesic state that no matter how severe the defect in retentive memory, old special memories remain intact. Also noteworthy is the fact that long-standing social habits, automatic motor skills, and memory for words (language) and visual impressions (visual or pictorial attributes of persons, objects, and places) are unimpaired. Long periods of repetition and usage have made these functions virtually automatic; they no longer require the participation of the diencephalic-hippocampal structures that were necessary to learn them originally. All of this suggests that these special memories, or coded forms of them, through a process of relearning and habituation, come to be "stored" or "filed" in other regions of the brain; i.e., they acquire a separate and independent anatomy.

Several fundmental questions concerning the amnesic syndrome remain unanswered. How does a disease process, acting over a brief period of time, not only impair all future learning but also wipe out a vast reservoir of past memories that had been firmly established for many years before the onset of the illness? What are the anatomic and physiologic mechanisms that govern immediate memory, which remains intact in even the most severely damaged patients with the Korsakoff amnesic syndrome? What are the anatomic arrangements that enable the patient with virtually no capacity to retain any newly presented factual information still learn some simple perceptual-motor and cognitive skills? Detailed discussions of these and other aspects of memory function will be found in the references at the end of this chapter.

CLASSIFICATION OF DISEASES CHARACTERIZED BY AN AMNESIC SYNDROME

The amnesic (Korsakoff) syndrome, as defined above, may be a manifestation of several neurologic disorders that are identified by their mode of onset and clinical course, the associated neurologic signs, and ancillary findings.

I. Amnesic syndrome of sudden onset—usually with gradual but incomplete recovery
  A. Bilateral hippocampal infarction due to atherosclerotic-thrombotic or embolic occlusion of the posterior cerebral arteries or their inferior temporal branches
  B. Infarction of the basal forebrain due to occlusion of anterior cerebral-anterior communicating arteries
  C. Trauma to the diencephalic, inferomedial temporal, or orbitofrontal regions
  D. Spontaneous subarachnoid hemorrhage (mechanism of amnesia not understood)
  E. Carbon monoxide poisoning and other hypoxic states (rare)
II. Amnesia of sudden onset and short duration
  A. Temporal lobe seizures
  B. Postconcussive states
  C. "Transient global amnesia"
III. Amnesic syndrome of subacute onset with varying degrees of recovery, usually leaving permanent residua
  A. Wernicke-Korsakoff syndrome
  B. Herpes simplex encephalitis
  C. Tuberculous and other forms of meningitis characterized by a granulomatous exudate at the base of the brain
IV. Slowly progressive amnesic states
  A. Tumors involving the floor and walls of the third ventricle and limbic cortical structures
  B. Alzheimer disease (early stage) and other degenerative disorders with disproportionate affection of the temporal lobes

The foregoing amnesic states, and the disorders of which they are a part, are discussed in the appropriate chapters. The only exception is so-called *transient global amnesia,* the nature of which is not entirely certain. It cannot with assurance be included with the epilepsies, or with the cerebrovascular diseases, or with any other category of disease and is therefore being considered here.

"TRANSIENT GLOBAL AMNESIA"

This is the name applied by Fisher and Adams to a particular type of memory disorder that occurs not infrequently in middle-aged and elderly persons and that is characterized by an episode of confusion and bewilderment lasting for several hours. The patient's symptoms have their basis in a defect in memory for events of the present and the recent past. During the attack there is no impairment in the state of consciousness and no overt sign of seizure activity, and personal identification is intact, as are motor, sensory, and reflex functions. Unlike psychomotor epilepsy the patient is alert, in contact with his surroundings, and capable of high-level intellectual activity and language function during the attack. As soon as the attack has ended, no abnormality of mental function can be detected.

Recurrence of such attacks is relatively uncommon, being noted in only 6 of 33 patients who were followed for periods of 1 to 17 years (Shuping et al) and in 16 of 74 patients followed for 7 to 210 months (Hinge et al). The latter authors estimated the mean annual recurrence rate to be so low (4.7 percent) that most elderly patients are likely to exierience only one attack. In one of the authors' cases there were more than 50 attacks, but in all the rest (more than 100 cases) 5 was the maximum. Most attacks occur spontaneously, but a possible precipitating factor, such as a highly emotional experience, pain, sexual intercourse, and mild head truma, has been reported in some of them (Haas and Ross). Two patients in the series of Shuping et al had multiple attacks of transient global amnesia, which ceased after treatment of an associated medical condition (polycythemia vera in one and myxomatous degeneration of the mitral valve in the other). Shuttleworth and Wise also described the occurrence of transient global amnesia consequent upon embolism; of course, embolic or thrombotic infarction in the posterior artery territories is known to cause strokes with permanent loss of memory (see Chap. 34). One of the difficulties in reading the many published reports of global amnesia is whether the patient, during the attack, was in contact with the environment and capable of high-level mental performance. Most if not all patients with temporal lobe seizures and concussion are not.

The pathogenesis of transient global amnesia has not been settled. It has been suggested that it represents an unusual form of temporal lobe epilepsy, but this seems unlikely. EEG recordings during an attack or shortly thereafter do not show epileptic activity (Miller et al). Moreover, amnesic episodes due to seizures are usually much briefer than those of transient global amnesia. More likely, the latter represent transient ischemic attacks; rarely does this disorder progress to stroke, however. In the series of Hinge et al, the observed rates of death and stroke were similar to the expected rates in the Danish population matched for age and sex. Using EEG and nasopharyngeal leads, Rowan and Protass found independent mesial temporal spike discharges in five of seven patients. They attributed the discharges to ischemic lesions. In some reported cases such spike discharges disappeared after a few months, an unlikely happening if the attacks were due to hippocampal epilepsy.

The benignity and infrequency of episodic global amnesia in most patients is noteworthy. No treatment is required, other than an explanation of the nature of the attack and reassurance.

THE CLINICAL APPROACH TO THE PROBLEM OF DEMENTIA AND THE AMNESIC STATE

The physician presented with a patient suffering from dementia and amnesia must adopt an examination technique designed to expose fully the intellectual defect. Abnormalities of posture, movement, sensation, and reflexes cannot be relied upon to disclose the disease process, since the association areas of the brain may be severely damaged without demonstrable neurologic signs of these types. Suspicion of a dementing disease is aroused when the patient presents multiple complaints that seem totally unrelated to one another and to any known syndrome, when irritability, nervousness, and anxiety are vaguely described by a patient and the symptoms do not fit exactly into one of the major psychiatric syndromes, and when the patient is incoherent in describing the illness and the reasons for consulting a physician.

Three categories of data are required for the recognition and differential diagnosis of dementing brain disease:

1. A reliable history of the illness

2. Findings on mental examination, i.e., the so-called "mental status," as well as on the rest of the neurologic examination

3. Ancillary examinations: CT scanning, MRI, and sometimes lumbar puncture, EEG, and appropriate laboratory procedures to rule out luetic, toxic, metabolic, and endocrine disorders.

The history should always be supplemented by information obtained from a person other than the patient, because, through lack of insight, patients are often unaware of their illness; indeed, they may be ignorant even of their chief complaint. Special inquiry should be made about the patient's general behavior, capacity for work, personality changes, language, mood, special preoccupations and concerns, delusional ideas, hallucinatory experiences, personal habits, and such faculties as memory and judgment.

The examination of the mental status must be systematic. At a minimum it should include the following:

1. *Insight* (patient's replies to questions about the chief symptoms): What is your difficulty? Are you ill? When did your illness begin?

2. *Orientation* (knowledge of personal identity and present situation): What is your name, your address, current location (building, city, state)? What is your occupation? Are you married?

Place: What is the name of the place where you are now (building, city, state)? How did you get here? What floor is it on? Where is the bathroom?

Time: What is the date today (day of week, of month, month, year)? What time of the day is it? What meals have you had? When was the last holiday?

3. *Memory.*

Remote: Tell me the names of your children and their birth dates. When were you married? What was your mother's maiden name? What was the name of your first school teacher? What jobs have you held?

Recent past: Tell me about your recent illness (compare with previous statements). What did you have for breakfast today? What is my name (or the nurse's name)? When did you see me for the first time? What tests were done yesterday? What were the headlines of the newspaper today? Give the patient a simple story, oral or written, and ask him to retell it after 3 to 5 min.

Immediate recall ("short-term memory"): Repeat these numbers after me (give series of 3, 4, 5, 6, 7, 8 digits at speed of one per second). Now when I give a series of numbers, repeat them in reverse order.

Memorization (learning): The patient is given four simple data (examiner's name, date, time of day, and a fruit, structure, or trait, such as honesty) and is asked to repeat them until he or she can do so without prompting. The capacity to reproduce them at intervals after committing them to memory is a test of *retentive memory span*. Another useful test is to ask the patient to give the names of 12 flowers, 12 vegetables, and 12 trees.

Visual span: Show the patient a picture of several objects; then ask him or her to name the objects and note any inaccuracies.

4. *General information:* Ask about names of the current president, first president, and recent presidents, well-known historic dates, the names of large rivers, of large cities, number of weeks in a year, definition of an island, etc.

5. *Capacity for sustained mental activity:* Crossing out all the a's on a printed page; counting forward and backward; saying the months of the year forward and backward.

Calculation: Test ability to add, subtract, multiply, and divide. Subtraction of serial 7s from 100 is a good test of calculation as well as of concentration.

Constructions: Draw a clock and place hands at 7:45; map of U.S.A.; floor plan of your house; copy a cube.

Abstract thinking: See if the patient can detect similarities and differences between classes of objects (orange and apple, horse and dog, desk and bookcase), or explain a proverb or a fable.

6. *General behavior:* Attitudes, general bearing, stream of thought, attentiveness, mood, manner of dress, etc.

7. *Special tests of localized cerebral functions:* Grasping, sucking, aphasia battery, praxis with both hands, and cortical sensory function.

In order to enlist the full cooperation of patients, the physician must prepare them for questions of this type. Otherwise, the first reaction will be one of embarrassment or anger because of the implication of unsound mind. It should be pointed out to the patient that some individuals are rather forgetful or have difficulty in concentrating, or that it is necessary to ask specific questions in order to form some impression about their degree of nervousness when being examined. Reassurance that these are not tests of intelligence or of sanity is helpful. If the patient is extremely agitated, suspicious, or belligerent, intellectual functions must be inferred from his or her remarks and from information supplied by the family.

This type of mental status survey can be accomplished in about 10 min. In our experience, high performance on all tests eliminates the possibility of dementia in 95 percent of cases. It may fail to identify a dementing disease in an uncooperative patient and in a highly intelligent individual in the earliest stages of disease.

The question of whether to resort to formal psychologic tests is certain to arise. Such tests yield quantitative data of comparative value but cannot of themselves be used for diagnostic purposes. Pfeiffer's test and Roth's dementia index rely essentially on the points mentioned above and a report of the patient's performance of the activities of daily living, which are lost in the later stages of disease. All the clinical and psychologic tests measure the same aspects of behavior and intellectual function. Probably the Wechsler Adult Intelligence Scale (WAIS) is the most widely used. The Wechsler Memory Scale is useful in estimating the degree of memory failure and in distinguishing the amnesic state from a more general dementia (discrepancy of more than 25 points between the WAIS and the memory scale). Using the WAIS, the discrepancy between the vocabulary, picture-completion, and object-assembly tests as a group (these correlate well with premorbid intelligence and are relatively insensitive to dementing brain disease) and arithmetic, block-design, digit-span, and digit-symbol tests provide an index of deterioration. The Mini-Mental Status of Folstein et al is a useful bedside method of scoring cognitive impairment and following its progress.

MANAGEMENT OF THE DEMENTED PATIENT

Dementia is a clinical state of the most serious nature, and usually it is worthwhile to admit patients to the hospital for a period of observation. The physician then has an opportunity to see them on different occasions in a new and fairly constant hospital environment, where the laboratory procedures mentioned above can be carried out (blood counts, vitamin B_{12} and drug levels, evaluation of thyroid, adrenal, renal, and liver function and cardiac and vascular status, examination of CSF for syphilis, and the special tests of CNS function such as EEG, CT scan, MRI, etc.). The management of demented patients in the hospital may be relatively simple if they are quiet and cooperative. If the disorder of mental function is severe, it is helpful if a nurse, attendant, or member of the family can stay with the patient at all times. Provision must be made for adequate food and fluid intake and control of infection, using the same measures outlined for the delirious patient.

The primary responsibility of the physician is to diagnose the treatable forms of dementia and to institute appropriate methods of therapy. Once it is established that the patient has an untreatable dementing brain disease, a responsible member of the family should be informed of the medical facts and prognosis, if the diagnosis is sufficiently certain for this to be done. Patients themselves need only be told that they have a nervous condition for which they are to be given rest and treatment. Nothing is accomplished by telling them more. If the dementia is slight and circumstances are suitable, patients should remain at home, continuing activities of which they are capable. They should be spared responsibility and guarded against injury that might result from imprudent action. If they are still at work, plans for occupational retirement should be carried out. In more advanced stages of the disease, when mental and physical enfeeblement become pronounced, nursing home or institutional care should be arranged. Seizures should be treated symptomatically. Nerve tonics, vitamins, vasodilators, and hormones are of no value in checking the course of the illness or in regenerating atrophic tissue. They may, however, offer some support to the patient and family. Sometimes stimulants in the form of dextroamphetamine, caffeine, and nicotinic acid cause transitory improvement in mental function. Undesirable restlessness, nocturnal wandering, belligerency, or anxiety may be reduced by administration of one of the antianxiety drugs (see Chap. 42), and emotional lability and paranoid tendencies, by imipramine and chlorpromazine.

REFERENCES

ALEXANDER WP: Intelligence, concrete and abstract. *Br J Psychol* 1:1, 1935.

BERLYNE N: Confabulation. *Br J Psychiatry* 120:31, 1972.

BRUN A, ENGLUND E: A white matter disorder in dementia of Alzheimer type: A pathoanatomical study. *Ann Neurol* 19:253, 1986.

CHAPMAN LF, WOLFF HF: The cerebral hemispheres and the highest integrative functions. *Arch Neurol* 1:357, 1959.

FISHER CM, ADAMS RD: Transient global amnesia. *Acta Neurol Scand*, vol 40, suppl 9, 1964.

FOLSTEIN M, FOLSTEIN S, McHUGH PR: ''Mini-mental status.'' A practical method for grading the cognitive state of patients for the clinician. *J Psychiatr Res* 12:189, 1975.

GOLDSTEIN K: *The Organism. A Holistic Approach to Biology.* New York, American Book Company, 1939, pp 35–61.

HAAS DC, ROSS GS: Transient global amnesia triggered by mild head trauma. *Brain* 109:251, 1986.

HEBB DO: Intelligence, brain function and the theory of mind. *Brain* 82:260, 1959.

HINGE H-H, JENSEN TS, KJAER M et al: The prognosis of transient global amnesia. *Arch Neurol* 43:673, 1986.

HOREL JA: The neuroanatomy of amnesia: A critique of the hippocampal memory hypothesis. *Brain* 101:403, 1978.

LASHLEY KS: *Brain Mechanisms and Intelligence.* University of Chicago, 1929.

MAYEUX R, STERN Y: Subcortical dementia. *Arch Neurol* 44:129, 1987.

MILLER JW, YANAGIHARA T, PETERSON RC, KLASS DW: Transient global amnesia and epilepsy. *Arch Neurol* 44:629, 1987.

MISHKIN M: A memory system in the monkey. *Phil Trans R Soc Lond* B298:85, 1982.

MISHKIN M, DELACOUR J: An analysis of short term visual memory in the monkey. *J Exp Psych Anim Behav Proc* 1:326, 1975.

MISHKIN M, SPIEGLER BJ, SAUNDERS RC, MALAMUT BL: An animal model of global amnesia, in Corkin S et al (eds): *Alzheimer's Disease: A Report of Progress in Research* (Aging, vol 19), New York, Raven Press, 1982, pp 235–237.

NAUTA WJH: Fiber degeneration following lesions of the amygdaloid complex in the monkey. *J Anat* 95:515, 1961.

NEWMANN M, COHN R: Progressive subcortical gliosis: A rare form of presenile dementia. *Brain* 90:405, 1967.

PHILLIPS S, SANGELANG V, STERNS G: Basal forebrain infarction. *Arch Neurol* 44:1134, 1987.

PIAGET J: *The Psychology of Intelligence.* London, Routledge and Kegan Paul, 1950.

PIERCY M: Neurological aspects of intelligence, in Vinken PJ, Bruyn GW (eds): *Handbook of Clinical Neurology,* vol 3: *Disorders of Higher Nervous Activity.* Amsterdam, North-Holland, 1969, chap 18, pp 296–315.

ROWAN AJ, PROTASS LM: Transient global amnesia: Clinical and electroencephalographic findings in 10 cases. *Neurology* 29:869, 1979.

SHIELDS J: *Monozygotic Twins Brought Up Apart and Brought Up Together: An Investigation into the Genetic and Environmental Causes of Variation in Personality.* London, Oxford University Press, 1962.

SHIELDS J: Heredity and psychological abnormality, in Eysenck HJ (ed): *Handbook of Abnormal Psychology,* 2nd ed. London, Pitman, 1973.

SHUPING JR, ROLLINSON RD, TOOLE JF: Transient global amnesia. *Ann Neurol* 6:159, 1979.

SHUTTLEWORTH EC, WISE GR: Transient global amnesia due to arterial embolism. *Arch Neurol* 29:340, 1973.

SLATER E, COWIE V: *The Genetics of Mental Disorders.* London, Oxford University Press, 1971, pp 196–200.

SPEARMAN CE: *The Abilities of Man.* London, Macmillan, 1927.

SQUIRE LR, ZOLA-MORGAN S: The neurology of memory, in Deutsch JA (ed): *The Physiological Basis of Memory,* 2nd ed. New York, Academic, 1983, pp. 199–268.

TIERNEY MC, SNOW WG, REID DW et al: Psychometric differentiation of dementia. *Arch Neurol* 44:720, 1987.

THURSTONE LL: *The Vectors of the Mind.* Chicago, University of Chicago Press, 1953.

TOMLINSON BE, BLESSED G, ROTH M: Observations on the brains of demented old people. *J Neurol Sci* 11:205, 1970.

VICTOR M, ADAMS RD, COLLINS GH: *The Wernicke-Korsakoff Syndrome,* 2nd ed. Philadelphia, Davis, 1989.

WADE JPH, MIRSEN TR, HACHINSKI VC et al: The clinical diagnosis of Alzheimer disease. *Arch Neurol* 44:24, 1987.

WECHSLER D: *The Measurement of Adult Intelligence,* 3rd ed. Baltimore, Williams and Wilkins, 1944.

WELLS C (ed): *Dementia.* Philadelphia, Davis, 1977, p 250.

WHITEHOUSE PJ: The concept of subcortical and cortical dementia: Another look. *Ann Neurol* 19:1, 1986.

WILLERMAN L: *The Psychology of Individual and Group Differences.* San Francisco, Freeman, 1978, pp 106–129.

ZOLA-MORGAN S, SQUIRE LR, MISHKIN M: The neuroanatomy of amnesia: Amygdala-hippocampus versus temporal stem. *Science* 218:1337, 1982.

CHAPTER 21

NEUROLOGIC DISORDERS CAUSED BY LESIONS IN PARTICULAR PARTS OF THE CEREBRUM

The age-old controversy about cerebral functions—whether they are diffusely represented in the cerebrum, with all parts roughly equivalent, or localized to certain lobes or regions—was resolved long ago. Clinicians and physiologists have demonstrated beyond doubt that particular cortical regions are related to certain functions. For example, the pre- and postrolandic zones are motor and sensory, the striate-parastriate occipital zones are visual, the superior temporal and transverse gyri of Heschl are auditory. Yet there is no doubt that many complex behavioral and mental operations depend upon interrelated networks of neurons, widely distributed in the cerebrum.

One may suitably ask just what is meant by cerebral localization. Does it refer to the physiologic function of a circumscribed aggregate of neurons in the cerebral cortex, indicated clinically by a loss of that function (negative symptom) when the neurons in question are paralyzed or destroyed? From what we know of the rich connectivity of all parts of the cortex one must assume that this is not the case, but only that lesions in the particular part, or in the fiber systems with which it is connected, are most consistently involved in that function. To be distinguished also are the disinhibited functions (positive symptoms) of closely related intact parts of the cerebrum.

Morphologic data support this conceptualization of cerebral cortical localization. Along strictly histologic lines Brodmann was able to distinguish 47 different areas of cerebral cortex (Figs. 21-1 and 21-2), and von Economo identified more than twice this number. Although this parcellation was criticized by Bailey and von Bonin, it is still used by physiologists and clinicians today. Also, the cortex has been shown to differ in its various parts by virture of its myelination pattern (Fig. 28-3) and particular connections with other areas of the cortex in the same and opposite cerebral hemispheres and with the thalamus and other lower centers. Hence, one must regard the cortex as a heterogeneous array of many anatomic systems, each

with rather complex intercortical and central (thalamic) arrangements.

Some general aspects of cerebral cortical anatomy are noteworthy. The sheer size of the cortex is remarkable. Unfolded, it has a surface extent of about 4000 cm^2—about the size of a full sheet of newsprint (right and left pages). Contained in the cortex are an estimated 50 billion neurons and more than five times this number of glial cells (Angevine and Cotman).

Most of the human cerebral cortex is phylogenetically recent, hence *neocortex* or *neopallium*. It is also referred to as *isocortex* (Vogt) and homogenetic cortex (Brodmann) because of its uniform embryogenesis and morphology. These latter features distinguish the neocortex from the older and less uniform cortex, which is comprised mainly of hippocampus and olfactory cortex and is referred to as the *archipallium* or *allocortex* (''other cortex'').

Concerning the detailed histology of the neocortex, six layers can be distinguished, from the pial surface to the underlying white matter (molecular or plexiform; external granular; external pyramidal; internal granular; ganglionic or internal pyramidal; multiform or fusiform). These are illustrated in Figs. 21-3 and 21-4. Two cell types—relatively large pyramidal cells and smaller, more numerous stellate cells—predominate, and variations in the lamination of the neocortex are largely determined by variations in the size and density of these neuronal types. Despite the many variations in lamination described by the cortical map makers, two main types of neocortex are recognized: (1) *the homotypical cortex,* in which the six-layered arrangement is readily discerned. The association cortex—the large areas of cortex (75 percent of the surface) that are not obviously committed to primary motor or sensory functions—is generally of this type; (2) *the heterotypical cortex,* in which the layers are less distinct than those of the homotypical cortex. The heterotypical cortex is characterized by a granular or agranular specialization. The precentral

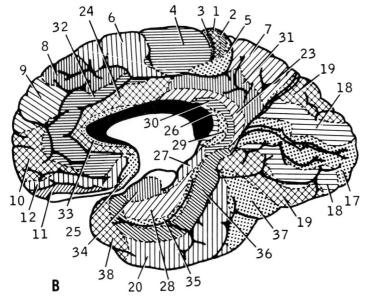

Figure 21-1

Cytoarchitectural zones of the human cerebral cortex. A. *Lateral surface.* B. *Medial surface.*

Figure 21-2 ▶

Cytoarchitectural zones of the cerebral cortex, basal surface, adapted from Brodmann.

cortex (areas 4 and 6) is dominated by pyramidal rather than granular cells, especially in layer IV; hence the term *agranular* (Fig. 21-3). In contrast, primary sensory cortex [postcentral gyrus (areas 3, 1, 2), banks of the calcarine sulcus (area 17), and the transverse gyri of Heschl] where layers II and IV are strongly developed for the receipt of afferent impulses, has been termed *granular cortex* or *koniocortex* (Greek *konio,* ''dust''), because of the marked predominance of granular cells (Fig. 21-3).

The intrinsic organization of the isocortex follows the pattern elucidated by Lorente de Nó. He described vertical chains of neurons that are arranged in cylindrical modules or columns, each containing 100 to 300 neurons, which are heavily interconnected up and down between cortical layers and to a lesser extent horizontally. Figure 21-5 illustrates the fundamental vertical (columnar) organization of these neuronal systems. Afferent fibers activated by various sensory stimuli terminate in layers IV, III, and II. These impulses are then transmitted by internuncial neurons to adjacent superficial and deep layers and then to appropriate efferent neurons in layer V. Neuronal connections are mainly through axonal-dendritic synapses. In the macaque brain, each pyramidal neuron in layer V has about 60,000 synapses, and one afferent axon may encompass an area that contains up to 5000 neurons; these figures convey some idea of the wealth of cortical connections. These columnar ensembles of neurons, on both the sensory and motor sides, function as the elementary working units of the cortex, in a manner that has been indicated in Chap. 3.

Whereas certain regions of the cerebrum are committed to special perceptual, motor, mnemonic, and other activities, the intricacy of the anatomy and psychophysical mechanisms in each region are just beginning to be envisioned. The lateral geniculate-occipital organization in relation to color vision and recognition of form, stemming from the work of Hubel and Wiesel, may be taken as an example. In area 17 there are specialized groups of neurons activated in lamina 4C by spots of light or lines projected onto each retina and transmitted by particular cells in the lateral geniculate bodies. And other groups of cortical neurons are essential for the perception of color. Preparedness for all types of visual stimulation, recognition of objects, faces, and verbal and mathematical symbols also involve these areas but are integrated in others beyond areas 17 and 18.

Cortical-subcortical integrations are reflected in praxis. The simplest willed or commanded movement of the hand requires the activation of premotor cortex (also called accessory motor cortex) which projects to the striatum and cerebellum and back to the motor cortex in a complex circuitry, before direct and indirect corticospinal pathways can activate certain combinations of spinal motor neurons.

Interregional connections of the cerebrum are required not only for certain natural functions, but, if de-

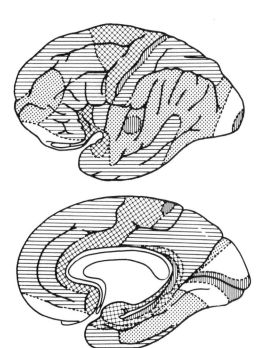

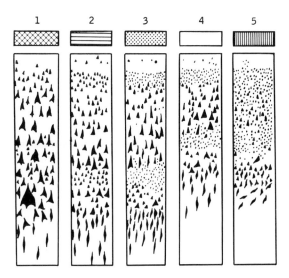

Figure 21-3

The five fundamental types of cerebral cortex, according to von Economo: 1, agranular; 2, frontal; 3, parietal; 4, polar; and 5, granulous.

stroyed, they disinhibit or release other areas. Denny-Brown has referred to these as cortical tropisms. Destruction of the premotor areas, leaving precentral and parietal lobes intact, results in the release of the sensory-motor mechanisms of groping, grasping, and sucking reflexes. Parietal lesions result in complex avoidance movements to contactual stimuli. Temporal lesions lead to a visually activated reaction to every observed object and its oral exploration.

Some of the aforementioned disorders and others known as *disconnection syndromes* depend not merely on involvement of cortical regions but on the interruption of interhemispheral and intrahemispheral fiber tracts. Some of these disconnections are indicated in Figs. 21-6 and 21-7;

the involved fiber systems include the corpus callosum, anterior commissure, uncinate temporal-frontal fasciculus, occipito- and temporo-parietal tracts, etc. Extensive lesions in white matter may virtually isolate certain cortical zones. An example is the isolation of the Wernicke and Broca areas from the rest of the cortex as in the case of hypoxic encephalopathy described by Geschwind and his colleagues.

These aspects of cerebral localization, brought out so clearly in the writings of Wernicke, Déjerine, Liepmann, and Geschwind have been elaborated by the Soviet school of physiologists and psychologists. They do not view function as the direct property of a particular, highly specialized group of cells in one region of the cerebrum, but as the product of complex reflex activity by which sensory stimuli are analyzed and integrated at various levels of the nervous system and are united, through a system of temporary connections, into a working mosaic, adapted to

Figure 21-4

The basic cytoarchitecture of the cerebral cortex, adapted from Brodmann.

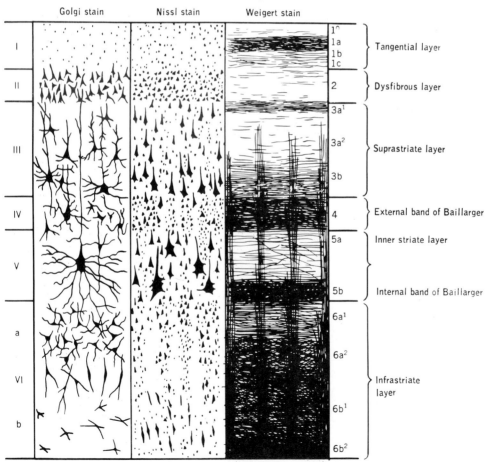

accomplish a particular task. Within such a functional system, the initial and final links (the task and the effect) remain unchanged but the intermediate links (the means of performance of a given task) may be modified within wide limits, and will never be exactly the same on two consecutive occasions. Thus, when a certain act is called for by a spoken command, the dominant temporal lobe must receive the message and transmit it to the premotor areas; or it may be initiated by the intention of the patient in which case the first measurable cerebral activity (a negative readiness potential) occurs anterior to or in the premotor cortex. The motor cortex is always under the dynamic control of the proprioceptive, visual, and vestibular systems. These are some of the recognizable elements in the motor performance, and the symptom, which is a loss of the skilled act, may be caused by a lesion which affects any one of several elements in the act, either the motor centers or their connections with the other elements. All parts comprise a

recognizable functional system, and the purpose of neuropsychology is to localize defects in particular parts of the system.

This conception of cerebral function and localization, which applies to all mental activities, differs from that which postulates the functional equivalence of all cerebral regions and also from that which assumes strict localization of any given activity within one part of the brain. It is open to neuropsychologic analysis, which has been the approach of A. R. Luria and others of the Soviet school.

Another theoretical scheme of cerebral anatomy and function systematizes cortices of similar overall structure and divides the cerebral mantle into three longitudinally oriented zones. The central or medial zone (allocortex and

Figure 21-5

The organization of neuronal systems in the granular cortex, following the plan of Lorente de Nó. The black spheres represent points of synapse. A. Connections of efferent cortical neurons. B. Connections of intracortical neurons. C. Connections of afferent (thalamocortical) neurons. D. Mode of termination of afferent cortical fibers. P, pyramidal cell; M, Martinotti cell; S, spindle cell; 1, projection efferent; 2, association efferent; 3, specific afferent; 4, association afferent.

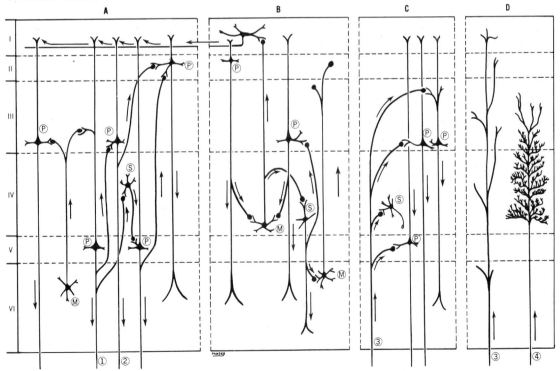

hypothalamus) provides the mechanisms for all internal functions—the milieu interne of Bernard and Cannon. The outer zone, comprising the sensory-motor and association cortices and their projections, provides the mechanisms for perceiving the external world and interacting with it. The region between (limbic-paralimbic cortices) provides the bridges that permit the adaptation of organismal needs to the external environment. This mode of conceptualizing brain activity, first proposed by Broca, was elaborated by Yakovlev and has more recently been adopted by Mesulam. And it incorporates the parcellation schemes of von Economo and Brodmann.

From these remarks it follows that subdivision of the cerebrum into frontal, temporal, parietal, and occipital lobes has only a limited functional validity. It was made long before our first glimmer of knowledge about the function of the cerebrum. Even when the neurohistologists began parcellating the neocortex, they found that their areas did not fall within zones bounded by sulci and fissures. Therefore, when the words *frontal, parietal, temporal,* and *occipital* are used in the text below, it is mainly to provide the reader with a familiar anatomic reference.

SYNDROMES CAUSED BY LESIONS OF THE FRONTAL LOBES

ANATOMIC AND PHYSIOLOGIC CONSIDERATIONS

The frontal lobes lie anterior to the central, or rolandic, sulcus and superior to the sylvian fissure (Fig. 21-8). They are larger in humans (30 percent of the cerebrum) than in any other primate (9 percent in the macaque) (Fig. 21-9). Several different systems of neurons are located here, and they subserve different functions. Areas 4, 6, and 8 relate specifically to motor activities. The primary motor cortex, i.e., area 4, is directly connected with somatic sensory neurons of the anterior part of the postcentral gyrus (Chap. 3), as well as with other parietal areas, thalamic nuclei, and reticular formation of the upper brainstem. As was pointed out in earlier chapters, all motor activity needs sensory guidance, and this comes from the somesthetic, visual, and auditory cortices and from the cerebellum via the ventral tier of thalamic nuclei.

Area 8 is concerned with turning the eyes and head contralaterally. Area 44 of the dominant hemisphere (Broca's area) and the contiguous part of area 4 are "centers" of motor speech and related functions of the lips, tongue, larynx, and pharynx, and bilateral lesions in these areas cause paralysis of articulation, phonation, and deglutition.

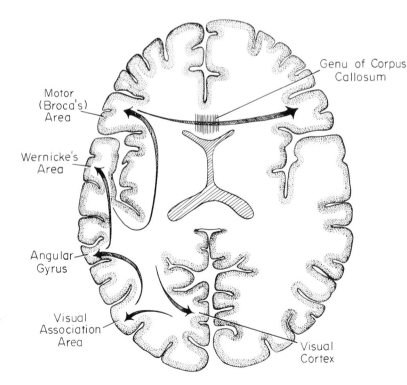

Figure 21-6

Intrahemispheric connections involved in naming a seen object, according to Wernicke's model. The visual pattern is transferred from the visual cortex and association areas to the angular gyrus, which contains the memories for arousing the auditory pattern in Wernicke's (auditory association) area. The auditory form, in turn, is transmitted, via the arcuate fasciculus, to the motor (Broca's) association area. There the articulatory form is aroused and transferred to the face area of the motor cortex, and the word is spoken. (Redrawn, with permission, from N Geschwind, Sci Am 226:76, 1972.)

Genu of Corpus Callosum

Motor (Broca's) Area

Wernicke's Area

Angular Gyrus

Visual Association Area

Visual Cortex

The cingulate and medial-orbital gyri, which are the frontal components of the limbic system, take part in the control of respiration, blood pressure, peristalsis, and other autonomic functions. The most anterior parts of the frontal lobes (areas 9 to 12 and 45 to 47), sometimes referred to as the *prefrontal areas,* are particularly well developed in human beings but have no clearly assigned functions. These parts do not belong to the motor areas, in the sense that electrical stimulation evokes no direct movement; the prefrontal cortex is said to be inexcitable. Yet they are involved in the initiation of planned action.

The frontal agranular cortex (areas 4 and 6) and,

more specifically, the pyramidal cells of layer V of the pre- and postcentral convolutions provide most of the cerebral efferent system known as the pyramidal, or corticospinal, tract (see Figs. 3-2 and 3-3). Another massive projection is the frontopontocerebellar tract. In addition there are other fiber systems which pass from frontal cortex to caudatum, putamen, subthalamic nucleus, red nucleus, brainstem reticular formation, substanta nigra, inferior olive, as well as

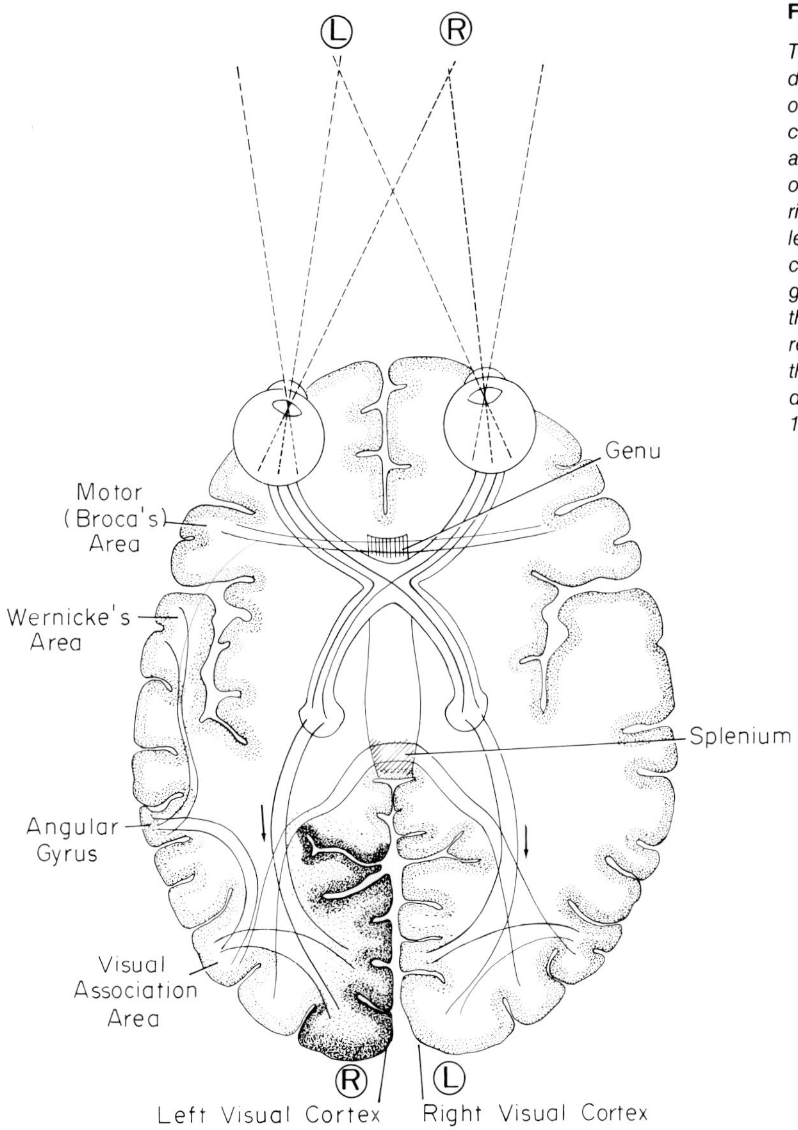

Figure 21-7

The visual part of the disconnection syndrome, based on the classic case study of J. J. Déjerine (1892). The left visual cortex and splenium were destroyed as a result of a left posterior cerebral artery occlusion. The patient was blind in his right visual field (R), and words from the left (L), perceived in the right visual cortex, could not cross over to the language areas because of destruction of the splenium. The patient was unable to read, despite normal visual acuity and the capacity to copy written words. (Redrawn from N Geschwind, Sci Am 226:76, 1972.)

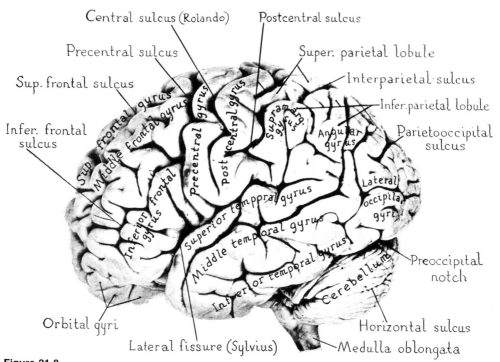

Figure 21-8

Photograph of lateral surface of the human brain. (From MB Carpenter and J Sutin, Human Neuroanatomy, 8th ed, Baltimore, Williams & Wilkins, 1982.)

to the ventrolateral, medial dorsal, and dorsolateral nuclei of the thalamus. Areas 8 and 6 are connected with the oculomotor, abducens, and other brainstem motor nuclei, and with identical areas of the other cerebral hemisphere through the corpus callosum. Area 44 also has transcortical connections. A massive bundle connects the frontal with the occipital lobes. An uncinate bundle connects the orbital part of the frontal lobe with the temporal lobe.

The granular frontal cortex has a rich system of connections both with lower levels of the brain (medial and ventral nuclei and pulvinar of the thalamus) and with virtually all other parts of the cerebral cortex including its limbic and paralimbic parts (Fig. 21-10).

In respect to its limbic connections, the frontal lobe is unique among cerebral cortical areas. The orbital-frontal cortex and cingulate gyrus, when electrically stimulated, induce manifest effects on respiratory, circulatory, and other vegetative functions. These parts of the frontal cortex also receive major sensory projections from all parts of the limbic system, presumably to mediate the emotional coloring of sensory experiences, and are connected to other parts of the limbic and paralimbic cortices (hippocampus, parahippocampus, anterior pole of the temporal lobe, amygdala,

and midbrain reticular formation). The frontal limbic connections are described in greater detail in Chap. 25.

Figure 21-9

Diagram to show the progressive enlargement of the frontal granular cortex in the phylogenetic scale: cat (A), dog (B), rhesus monkey (C) and man (D). The brains are not drawn to scale.

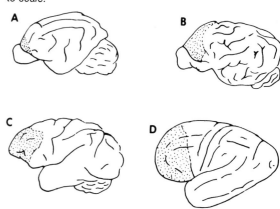

The clinical effects of lesions in the frontal lobes can be grouped under the following headings:

1. Motor abnormalities

2. Impairment of cognitive function

3. Lack of initiative and spontaneity (apathy and abulia)

4. Other changes in personality, particularly disinhibition of behavior

Motor Abnormalities Of the various effects of frontal lobe lesions, most is known about the motor abnormalities. Lesions in its posterior part, involving the frontoparietal cortex and subcortical white matter, cause spastic paralysis of the contralateral face, arm, and leg. Involved are the corticospinal tract and other indirect tracts that descend from the motor, premotor, and anterior parietal cortex via red nuclei and pontomedullary reticular nuclei in the brainstem to the spinal cord, as was pointed out above and in Chap. 3. Lesions of the more anterior parts of the motor cortex (area 6 and supplementary motor area of 8—*the premotor cortex*) result in less paralysis and more spasticity as well as a release of sucking, groping, and grasping

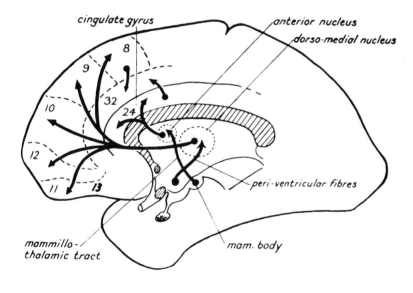

Figure 21-10

Diagram of the major connections of the frontal lobe. Above: Major afferent projections to the premotor frontal areas and cingulate gyrus. Shown also are the projections from the mammillary body to the anterior nucleus of the thalamus and from the hypothalamus, via periventricular fibers, to the dorsomedial nucleus. Below: Major efferent projections from the premotor frontal areas to the thalamus, hypothalamus and brainstem. The numbers in both diagrams refer to Brodmann's cytoarchitectonic areas (see Figs. 21-1 and 21-2). (Redrawn from LeGros Clark, Lancet 1:353, 1948.)

reflexes, the mechanisms of which reside in the parietal lobe and which, according to Denny-Brown, are normally inhibited by the frontal cortex. Mutism, unilateral neglect, and impairment of bibrachial coordination was found by Laplane et al to follow ablation of the supplementary motor areas.

Electrical stimulation of the motor cortex elicits contraction of the corresponding muscle groups, and focal seizure activity has a similar effect. Temporary paralysis of contralateral eye turning, and sometimes head turning, follows a destructive lesion in the lateral (convexity) part of area 8. Seizure activity in this area causes a tonic deviation of the head and eyes to the opposite side. Destruction of Broca's and adjacent insular and motor cortex results in a motor speech disorder, agraphia, and apraxia of the face, lips, and tongue (see Chap. 22).

When the lesions of the motor parts of the frontal lobe are bilateral, there is a quadriplegia or quadriparesis, in which the weakness is not only more severe but more extensive, affecting cranial muscles (pseudobulbar palsy) as well as spinal ones.

Damage to the cortices anterior to areas 6 and 8, i.e., to areas 9, 10, 45, and 46—the *prefrontal cortex*, have less easily defined effects on motor behavior. The prefrontal cortex is heteromodal and has strong reciprocal connections with the visual, auditory, and somatosensory cortices. It is involved in the planning and initiation of sequences of movement, as indicated in Chap. 4. In the monkey, for example, when a visual signal evokes movement, some of the prefrontal neurons become active immediately preceding the response; other prefrontal neurons are activated if the response is to be delayed. Blood flow and glucose utilization increase at the same time. With prefrontal lesions on one side or the other, slight grasping and sucking, imitation of the examiner's gestures and compulsive manipulation of objects that are in front of the patient (imitation and utilization behavior of Lhermitte), reduced motor activity, motor perseveration, paratonic rigidity on passive manipulation of the limbs (gegenhalten or counterholding), can be elicited in various combinations by appropriate tests.

A contralateral ataxia has been described with prefrontal lesions but has not been verified anatomically; in our cases of contralateral ataxia after a cerebral lesion the parietal lobe has always been involved. There may also occur a characteristic disturbance of stance and gait with bilateral frontal (and probably basal ganglionic) lesions. Steps shorten to a shuffle, balance is precarious, and with further deterioration the patient can no longer walk or even stand (so-called Bruns' apraxia of gait). *Cerebral paraplegia in flexion* is the end stage; the affected individual lies curled up in bed, unable even to turn over (see Chap. 6).

Frontal lobe incontinence is another manifestation of frontal lobe disease. Right- or left-sided lesions involving the posterior part of the superior frontal and anterior cingulate gyri and intervening white matter result in a loss of control of micturition and defecation (Andrew and Nathan). There is no warning of fullness of the bladder and imminence of urination or bowel evacuation, and the patient is surprised and embarrassed at suddenly being wet or soiled. Less complete forms of the syndrome are associated with frequency and urgency of urination during waking hours. An element of indifference to being incontinent is added when the more anterior (nonmotor) parts of the frontal lobes are the site of disease.

In the spheres of speech and language, a number of abnormalities, other than Broca's aphasia, appear in conjunction with disease of the frontal lobes—laconic speech, lack of spontaneity of speech, telegraphic speech, loss of fluency, perseveration of speech, whispering, and dysarthria. These are more prominent with left-sided lesions, and are fully described in Chap. 22.

Cognitive and Intellectual Changes In general, when one speaks of the frontal lobes, reference is made to the more anterior (prefrontal), nonmotor, nonlinguistic parts. Here one faces a paradox. These most recently developed parts of the human brain, sometimes called the "organ of civilization," have the most elusive functions.

The effects of lesions of the frontal lobes was first divulged by the famous case of Harlow, published in 1868. His patient, Phineas Gage, was a capable, God-fearing foreman, who became irreverent, dissipated, irresponsible, and vacillating and confabulated freely following an injury in which a crowbar was driven by a dynamite explosion through his frontal lobes. In Harlow's words, "he was no longer Gage." Another similarly dramatic example was Dandy's patient (the subject of a monograph by Brickner) who underwent a bilateral frontal lobotomy during the removal of a meningioma. In chimpanzees, Jacobsen and his collaborators observed that the removal of the premotor parts of the frontal lobes led to social indifference, tameness, placidity, forgetfulness, and difficulty in problem solving—findings that led Egaz Moniz to perform prefrontal lobotomies on psychotic patients. This operation provided the opportunity to study the effects of a wide range of frontal lobe lesions.

The findings in patients subjected to frontal leukotomy have been the subject of endless controversy. Some workers such as Hebb and Penfield claimed that there were no discernible effects, even with bilateral lesions. Others, such as Goldstein, Rylander, Chapman and Wolff, Halstead and

Reitan, and Hécaen, insisted that if the proper tests were used, there could be demonstrated a series of predictable and diagnostic changes in cognition and behavior. The arguments, pro and con, and the inadequacies of many of the studies, both in method of testing and in anatomic verification of the lesions, have been well summarized by Walsh.

Admittedly, in patients who underwent bilateral frontal lobotomy, there was little if any impairment in performance on intelligence tests and certainly no loss of alertness and orientation. There is less consensus regarding memory. Hécaen stated that in 20 percent of his series of 131 frontal tumors there was an element of forgetfulness. But the memory loss was different from the characteristic Korsakoff amnesic syndrome of diencephalic-temporal lobe origin. The frontal lobe memory defect appeared to be part of a more general disturbance in thinking. The patient could recall the details of a problem and his or her errors in trying to solve it and could discuss them as an intellectual exercise, but could not put them to use in the correction of further performances. Tissot et al view this as a failure to assimilate new material and integrate it with actual experience. Benton probably refers to the same phenomenon when he describes a generally impaired integration of behavior over a period of time. In dealing with problems the patient may be unable to think of all the options and to select the appropriate one, which is what Goldstein means by inability to think abstractly. The patient fails to conceptualize all the demands of the situation, but thinks ''concretely,'' i.e., he thinks and reacts directly to the stimulus situation. Lesions in the basal forebrain region differ strikingly from anterolateral ones in that they cause a Korsakoff amnesic syndrome, indistinguishable from that of diencephalic-hippocampal disorder, as well as apathy and loss of volition (Phillips et al).

Luria has offered an interesting conception of the role of the frontal lobes in intellectual activity. His general premise is that meaningful correlations of disturbed behavior and brain lesions must be preceded by a qualitative analysis of the patient's behavior. He postulates that problem solving of whatever type (perceptual, contructive, arithmetic, psycholinguistic or logical—definable also as goal-related behavior) proceeds in four steps: (a) the specification of a problem and the conditions in which it has arisen (in other words, a goal is perceived and the conditions associated with it are set); (b) a plan of action or strategy for the solution of the problem is formulated, which requires that certain linguistic activities be simultaneously initiated in orderly sequence; (c) the execution, including implementation and control of the plan; (d) checking or comparison of the results against the original plan to see if it was adequate. Obviously such a complex psychologic activity must implicate many parts of the cerebrum and will suffer as a result of a lesion in any of the parts that contribute to the functional system. Luria finds that when the frontal lobes are injured by disease, there is not only a general psychomotor slowing but an erroneous analysis of the conditions of the problem. ''The plan of action that is selected quickly loses its regulating influence on behavior as a whole and is replaced by a perseveration of one particular link of the motor act or by the influence of some connection established during the patient's past experience.'' Furthermore, there is a failure to distinguish the essential links in the analysis and to compare the final solution with the original conception of the problem. Expressed otherwise, failure to initiate and sustain mental activity results in a kind of incoherence of the reasoning process, with easy distraction by irrelevant data and perseveration.

Plausible as this scheme appears, like Goldstein's ''loss of the abstract attitude,'' such psychophysiologic analyses of the mental processes are highly theoretical, and the factors to which they refer are not easily measured.

Impairment or Lack of Initiative and Spontaneity These are the most common effects of frontal lobe disease and much easier to observe in the clinic than to quantitate. With relatively mild forms of this disorder, patients exhibit an idleness of thought, speech, and action, and lapse into this state without complaint. They are tolerant of any condition in which they are placed, though if irritated by circumstances they may act unreasonably, not seeming to be able to think through the consequences of their remonstrances. They let members of the family answer questions and ''do the talking,'' and interject a remark only rarely. Questions directed to the patient may evoke only a brief, unqualified answer. Placidity is a notable feature of the behavior. Worry, anxiety, self-concern, hypochondriasis, chronic pain, and depression are all reduced by the frontal lobe disease, as they are by frontal lobotomy.

Extensive bilateral disease is accompanied by a quantitative reduction in all psychomotor activity. The number of movements, of spoken words, and thoughts per unit of time diminish. Lesser degrees of this are called *abulia;* the most severe form is *akinetic mutism* (page 276), wherein a nonparalyzed patient, alert and capable of movement and speech, lies totally motionless and silent for days or weeks on end. This condition has been attributed to bilateral lesions in the anterior frontal regions or frontal-diencephalic connections (see Fig. 21-10). The opposite state, in a sense, is the hyperactivity syndrome or ''organic drivenness,'' described by von Economo and by Kahn.

When this syndrome has occurred in our patients, it has been associated with frontal and temporal lobe lesions, usually encephalitic, although exact clinicopathologic correlations could not be determined. The hyperactivity of small boys and the mania or hypomania of manic-depressive disease are also equally lacking a known anatomic basis.

Other Changes in Personality In addition to the disorders of initiative and spontaneity, frontal lobe lesions result in a number of other changes in personality, best appreciated by the patient's family. It has been difficult to find a term for all these personality changes. Some have referred to them as a loss of ego strength, a lessening of the integrative and constructive forces within the personality. Some patients, particularly those with low frontal lesions, have a tendency to make silly jokes that are inappropriate to the situation—so-called Witzelsücht, or ''moria''; they are socially uninhibited. The patient is no longer the sensitive, compassionate, effective human being he or she once was. These changes, observed characteristically in lobotomized patients, came to be recognized as too great a price to pay for loss of neurotic traits, pain, depression, and ''tortured self-concern,'' for which reasons lobotomies, even limited ones, were done; hence the procedure became obsolete.

The question of the effect of unilateral prefrontal lesions continues to vex all clinicians. If small they are completely undetectable; even with large lesions, as in extensive frontal lobe glioma, the impairments may be so subtle as to escape detection unless the patient is studied at home or in the workplace. Rylander, by careful psychologic testing, has shown that patients with lesions of either frontal lobe manifest a slight elevation of mood with increased talkativeness and tendency to joke, lack of tact, inability to adapt to a new situation, instability of mood, and loss of initiative—changes that are more readily recognized in patients with bilateral frontal lobe lesions.

Our experience with patients with frontal lobe lesions affirms most of the statements above. Most apparent is the abulic-hypokinetic disorder which seems to slow the mental processes involved in all forms of cerebral performance. Inattentiveness, impersistence in all assigned tasks, and sometimes drowsiness, are the major features of this disorder. Luria refers to this as an impairment in ''cortical tone,'' a failure of the frontal lobes to prepare and to regulate the ''activation processes lying at the basis of voluntary attention.'' Such a state cannot be specifically ascribed to the prefrontal regions since it may be a reflection of a more general impairment of the thalamolimbic or reticular activating thalamocortical system. In general we agree that the greatest cognitive-intellectual deficits relate to lesions in the dorsolateral parts of the prefrontal lobes and the personality and behavioral changes to lesions of the medial-orbital parts. The diagnosis of lesions in these latter parts is facilitated by the finding of unilateral anosmia or optic atrophy, such as occurs with a meningioma of the olfactory groove.

Finally it should be emphasized that the function of the frontal lobes or other discrete part of the brain cannot be determined simply by the study of patients who have suffered injury or disease of that part. *Symptoms from lesions of a part of the nervous system are not to be equated with the function of that part.* The symptoms of frontal lobe deficit are the product of both a loss of certain functions and the functional activity (sometimes overactivity) of the portions of the nervous system that remain intact. Although frontal lobe function is the subject of a vast literature and endless speculation (see reviews of Stuss and Benson and of Damasio), it is obvious that a unified concept of this function has not emerged—mainly, perhaps, because the frontal lobes include several heterogeneous systems. There is no doubt that the mind is changed by disease of the prefrontal parts of the frontal lobes, but it is difficult to say exactly how it is changed. Perhaps at present it is best to regard the frontal lobes as the part of the brain that quickly and effectively orients and drives the individual, with all the percepts and concepts formed from past life experiences, toward action that is projected into the future.

Effects of frontal lobe diseases may be summarized as follows:

I. Effects of unilateral frontal disease, either left or right
   A. Contralateral spastic hemiplegia
   B. Slight elevation of mood, increased talkativeness, tendency to joke, lack of tact, difficulty in adaptation, loss of initiative
   C. If entirely prefrontal, no hemiplegia; grasp and suck reflexes may be released
   D. Anosmia with involvement of orbital parts
II. Effects of right frontal disease
   A. Left hemiplegia
   B. Changes as in IB, C, and D.
III. Effects of left frontal disease
   A. Right hemiplegia
   B. Motor speech disorder with agraphia, with or without apraxia of the lips and tongue (see Chap. 22)
   C. Loss of verbal associative fluency
   D. Sympathetic apraxia of left hand
   E. Changes as in IB, C, and D
IV. Effects of bifrontal disease
   A. Bilateral hemiplegia
   B. Spastic bulbar (pseudobulbar) palsy

C. If prefrontal, abulia or akinetic mutism, lack of ability to sustain attention and solve complex problems, rigidity of thinking, bland affect and labile mood, and varying combinations of grasping, sucking, decomposition of gait, and sphincteric incontinence

SYNDROMES CAUSED BY LESIONS OF THE TEMPORAL LOBES

ANATOMIC AND PHYSIOLOGIC CONSIDERATIONS

The boundaries of the temporal lobes are indicated in Fig. 21-8. The sylvian fissure separates the superior surface of each temporal lobe from the frontal lobe and anterior parts of the parietal lobe. There is no definite anatomic boundary between the temporal lobe and the occipital or posterior part of the parietal lobe. The temporal lobe includes the superior, middle, and inferior temporal, lateral occipitotemporal, lingual, parahippocampal, and hippocampal convolutions and the transverse gyri of Heschl; the last constitute the primary auditory receptive area and are located within the sylvian fissure. This area has a tonotopic arrangement; fibers carrying high tones terminate in the medial portion of the gyrus and those carrying low tones, in the lateral and more rostral portions (Merzenich and Brugge). There are rich reciprocal connections between the medial geniculate bodies and Heschl's gyri. The latter project to the unimodal association cortex of the superior temporal gyrus, which in turn project to the paralimbic and limbic regions of the temporal lobe and to temporal and frontal heteromodal association cortices and inferior parietal lobe. The cortical receptive zone for labyrinthine impulses is not so well demarcated as that for hearing but probably is situated on the banks of the sylvian fissure, just posterior to the auditory receptive area.

The superior part of the dominant temporal lobe is concerned with the acoustic aspects of language (page 378) and the middle and inferior convolutions with visual discriminations. The latter convolutions receive fiber systems from the striate and peristriate cortex and in turn project to the contralateral visual association cortex, to the prefrontal heteromodal cortex, to the superior temporal cortex, and to the limbic and paralimbic cortex. Presumably these systems subserve visual discriminative functions such as spatial orientation, depth and distance estimation, stereoscopy, and hue perception. Similarly, the unimodal auditory cortex is closely connected with a series of auditory association areas in the superior temporal convolution, and the latter are connected with prefrontal and temporal-parietal heteromodal areas and the limbic areas (Mesulam). Most of these auditory systems have been worked out in the macaque, but they are probably involved in complex verbal and nonverbal auditory discriminations in humans.

The hippocampal convolution was formerly thought to be related to the olfactory system, but now it is known that lesions here do not alter the sense of smell. In addition, along with the orbitofrontal cortex, a major part of the paralimbic formations lie in the medial temporal lobes, as pointed out in the section on the frontal lobes.

Most of the temporal lobe cortex, including Heschl's gyri, has fairly equally developed pyramidal and granular layers. In this respect it resembles more the granular cortex of the frontal and prefrontal regions and inferior parts of the parietal lobes (see Fig. 21-4). Unlike the six-layered neocortex, the hippocampus and gyrus dentatus are typical of the three-layered allocortex, the phylogenetically older portion of the cerebral cortex (archipallium).

A massive fiber system connects the striate and parastriate zones of the occipital lobes to the inferior and medial parts of the temporal lobes. The temporal lobes are connected to one another through the anterior commissure and middle part of the corpus callosum, and the inferior, or uncinate, fasciculus passes between the anterior temporal and orbital frontal regions. The arcuate fasciculus connects the posterosuperior temporal lobe to the motor cortex and Broca's area (see page 378).

CLINICAL EFFECTS AND SYNDROMES

Visual Field Defects Lesions of the temporal lobe characteristically produce a contralateral upper homonymous quadrantanopia, due to involvement of the lower arching fibers of the geniculocalcarine pathway (as described on page 203). Lesions that interrupt the peristriate temporal projections interfere with visual memory, recognition of written language (alexia), visual naming (anomia), pattern discrimination, and possibly the recognition of colors (achromatopsia) and objects. The latter phenomena are discussed further on, with the manifestations of parieto-occipital lesions.

Cortical Deafness Bilateral lesions of the transverse gyri of Heschl are known to cause deafness. Henschen, in his famous review of 1337 cases of aphasia that had been reported up to 1922, found nine in which these parts were destroyed by restricted vascular lesions, with resulting deafness. There are now some 20 cases of this type in the medical literature; lesions in other parts of the temporal lobes have no effect on hearing. These observations are the basis for the concept that the primary auditory receptive area is located in the cortex of the transverse gyri (chiefly the first), in the posterior part of the superior temporal convolution (primary auditory koniocortex—areas 41 and 42). Subcortical lesions which interrupt the fibers from both medial geniculate bodies to the transverse gyri have the same effect. With superior temporal lesions there is usually an aphasia as well because of the proximity of the transverse gyri to the left superior temporal association cortex. Hécaen has remarked that cortically deaf persons may seem to be unaware of their deafness, a state similar to blind persons who act as though they can see (Anton syndrome; see further on, under "Visual Anosognosia").

Unlike the marked visual and somatic sensory defects with unilateral cerebral lesions, unilateral lesions of Heschl's gyri were for a long time believed to have no effect on hearing; but it has been found that if very brief auditory stimuli are delivered, the threshold of sensation is elevated in the ear opposite the lesion. Also, while unilateral lesions do not diminish the perception of pure tones or clearly spoken words, the ear contralateral to a temporal lesion is less efficient if the conditions of hearing are rendered more difficult (binaural test). For example, if words are slightly distorted (electronically filtered to alter consonants), they are heard less well in that ear; also the patient has more difficulty in equalizing sounds that are presented to both ears and in perceiving rapidly spoken numbers or different words presented to the two ears (dichotic listening).

Auditory Agnosias Lesions of the secondary (unimodal association) zones of the auditory cortex—area 22 and part of area 21 of Brodmann—have no effect on the perception of sounds and pure tones. However, the perception of complex combinations of sounds is severely impaired. This impairment, or auditory agnosia, takes several forms— inability to recognize sounds, music (amusia), and words— and presumably each has a slightly different anatomic basis.

In agnosia for sounds, all noises are indistinguishable. Such varied sounds as the tinkling of a bell, the rustling of paper, running water, or a siren all sound alike. The condition is usually associated with auditory verbal agnosia or with amusia. Hécaen states that an agnosia for sounds alone has been reported in only two cases; one patient could identify only half of 26 familiar sounds, and the other could recognize no sound other than the ticking of a watch. Yet in both patients the audiogram was normal, and neither had trouble understanding spoken words. In both, the lesion

involved the right temporal lobe, and the corpus callosum was intact.

Amusia proves to be more complicated, for the appreciation of music has several aspects: the recognition of a familiar melody and the ability to name it, the perception of pitch and timbre, and the ability to produce, read, and write music. There are many reports of musicians who became word-deaf with lesions of the dominant temporal lobe and retained their recognition of music and their skill in producing it. Others became agnosic for music but not for words, and still others were agnosic for both words and music. According to Segarra and Quadfasel, impaired recognition of music depends on lesions in the middle temporal gyrus and not on lesions at the pole of the temporal lobe, as had been postulated by Henschen.

That the appreciation of music is impaired by lesions of the nondominant temporal lobe finds support in Milner's studies of patients who had undergone temporal lobectomy. She found a statistically significant lowering of the patient's appreciation of the duration of notes, timbre, intensity of sounds, and memory of melodies following right temporal lobectomy; these abilities were preserved in patients with left temporal lobectomies, regardless of whether Heschl's gyri were included. Similar observations were made by Shankweiler, but in addition he found that patients had difficulty in the denomination of a note or the naming of a melody following left temporal lobectomies.

These data suggest that the nondominant hemisphere is important for the perception of musical notes and melodies but that the naming of musical scores and all the semantic (writing and reading) aspects of music require the integrity of the dominant temporal lobe.

The effects of electrical stimulation of the temporal lobe cortex in conscious humans are described on page 253 (Table 15-1).

Word Deafness (Auditory Verbal Agnosia) This is the essential element in Wernicke's aphasia and is discussed in Chap. 22. While often combined with agnosia for sounds and music, there is no doubt that it can occur separately. In essence, the left temporal lobe fails in its function of decoding the acoustic signals of speech and converting them to appropriate motor expressions. Not infrequently patients with Wernicke aphasia have uncontrollable emotional outbursts.

Auditory Illusions Temporal lobe lesions that leave hearing intact may cause paracusia; i.e., sounds may be heard more loudly or less loudly than normally. There may also be modifications of timbre or tonality. Sounds or words may seem strange or disagreeable, or they may seem to be repeated, a kind of sensory perseveration. If auditory hallucinations are also present, they may undergo similar alterations. Such paracusias may last indefinitely and alter musical appreciation as well.

Auditory Hallucinations These may be elementary (murmurs, blowing, sound of running water or motors, whistles, clangs, sirens, etc.), or they may be complex (musical themes, choruses, voices). Usually sounds and musical themes are heard more clearly than voices. Patients may recognize the illusions and hallucinations for what they are (i.e., abnormalities of hearing), or they may be convinced that the voices are real and respond to them with intense emotion. Hearing may fade before or during the hallucination.

In temporal lobe epilepsy the auditory hallucinations may occur alone or in combination with visual or gustatory hallucinations, visual distortions, dizziness, and aphasia. There may be hallucinations based on remembered experiences (experiential hallucinations, in the terminology of Penfield and Rasmussen).

The anatomy of the lesions underlying auditory illusions and hallucinations has been incompletely studied. In some instances these sensory phenomena have been combined with auditory verbal (or nonverbal) agnosia; the superior and posterior parts of the dominant or both temporal lobes were then involved. Clinicoanatomic correlation is difficult in cases of tumors that distort the brain without completely destroying it and also cause edema of the surrounding tissue. Moreover, it is often uncertain whether some of the symptoms have been produced by destruction of cerebral tissue or by excitation, i.e., by way of seizure discharges, which act in a fashion similar to electrical stimulation of the audiopsychic zones during surgical operations. Elementary hallucinations and dreamy states have been reported with lesions of either temporal lobe, whereas the more complex auditory hallucinations and particularly polymodal ones (visual plus auditory) occur more often with left-sided lesions. Also it should be noted that elementary (unformed) auditory hallucinations (e.g., the sound of an orchestra tuning up) occur with lesions that appear to be restricted to the pons (''pontine auditory hallucinosis'').

It is tempting to relate complex auditory hallucinations to disorders in the auditory association areas surrounding Heschl's gyri, but the data do not fully justify such an assumption. The most one can say is that the superolateral part of the temporal lobe is usually affected, and if the hallucinations are polymodal, the lesions lie more posteriorly, usually in the dominant hemisphere.

Vestibular Disturbances In the superior and posterior part of the temporal lobe (posterior to the auditory cortex, in the first and second temporal convolutions) there is an area which responds to vestibular stimulation. If it is destroyed on one side, the only clinical effect is a change

in the pattern of eye movements on optokinetic stimulation. Epileptic activation of this area may occur inducing vertigo or a sense of disequilibrium. As was pointed out on page 239, pure vertiginous epilepsy is a rarity, and if vertigo does precede a seizure, it is usually momentary and is quickly submerged in the other components of the seizure.

Disturbances of Time Perception These may occur with lesions of either temporal lobe. In a temporal lobe seizure, time may seem to stand still or to pass with great speed. On recovery from such a seizure the patient, having lost all sense of time, may repeatedly look at the clock. Serious cerebral diseases (amentias and dementias) may prevent or abolish the capacity to reckon personal events in terms of a time scale. The patient with Korsakoff psychosis is unable to correlate experiences in their proper time relationships, presumably because of failure of retentive memory. Other than these clinical instances the authors have not been impressed with derangements of the sense of time as having any importance in clinical neurology.

Other (Nonauditory) Syndromes Between the hippocampal formation (on the inferomedial surface of the temporal lobe) and the primary and secondary auditory areas (Heschl's transverse gyri and superior temporal convolution, respectively) there is a large inferolateral expanse of temporal lobe that has only vaguely assignable functions. With lesions in these parts of the dominant temporal lobe, a defect in the retrieval of words (amnesic dysnomia) has been a frequently observed abnormality.

Careful psychologic studies have disclosed a difference between the effects of dominant and nondominant temporal lobectomy. With the former there is impairment in the learning of material presented through the auditory sense; with the latter there is failure in the learning of visually presented material. In addition, about 20 percent of patients who had undergone temporal lobectomy, left or right, showed a syndrome similar to that which results from lesions of the prefrontal regions. Perhaps a more significant observation is that the remainder of the cases showed little or no defect in personality or behavior. The study of cases of uncinate epilepsy, with the characteristic dreamy state, olfactory or gustatory hallucinations, and masticatory movements, suggests that all these functions are organized through the limbic parts of the temporal lobes. Similarly, stimulation of the posterior parts of the first and second temporal convolutions of fully conscious epileptic patients can arouse complex memories and visual and auditory images, some with strong emotional content. Penfield and Roberts, who reported these observations, call this part of the temporal lobe the "interpretive cortex."

Stimulation of the amygdaloid complex of nuclei has evoked olfactory sensations. Complex emotional experiences from the past may be recalled. There are also notable autonomic effects: blood pressure rises, pulse rate increases, and the patient looks frightened. Sexual aberrations (excessive arousal, overactivity, reduced capacity) have also been reported in some patients, and MacLean has reproduced some of these and other visceral effects in monkeys by stimulation of the medial periamygdaloid regions, i.e., the part that he has labeled the "visceral brain" (see also page 409). Some seizures arising from foci in this region are manifested as a complex of disordered thought, hallucinations, and strange, detached, and at times violent, uncontrollable behavior. This complex of symptoms resembles schizophrenia and hypomania. Aggressive behavior in some sociopaths has been associated with discharging foci in one or both temporal lobes. There are cases on record in which ablation of the amygdaloid nuclei has eliminated uncontrollable rage reactions in psychotic patients. Temporal lobe epileptics with psychosis, on the other hand, while improved with respect to seizures, tend to persist in their psychotic behavior. Hippocampal and adjacent convolutions have been excised bilaterally, for a distance of 7 cm from the temporal pole, with a disastrous loss of ability to learn or to establish new memories (Korsakoff psychosis). Patients with lesions of the right posterior-inferior temporal lobe may exhibit an acute confusional psychosis, as was pointed out in Chap. 20. All this indicates an important role of the temporal lobes in auditory and visual perception and imagery, in learning and memory, and in the emotional life of the individual.

Bilateral removal of the temporal lobes in the macaque monkey produces a behavioral state in which the animal reacts to every visual stimulus without seeming to recognize it (psychic blindness, or visual agnosia). The animal sees small objects, but in order to recognize them must examine them by oral and manual contact. Placidity, i.e., lack of the usual emotional response to stimuli, and increase in sexual activity are other prominent features. This is the Klüver-Bucy syndrome, and the precise form, as produced in monkeys, has so far not been observed in humans (Marlowe et al). In a person with a stable personality, unilateral temporal lobectomy has had little recognizable effect on emotion and temperament. However, if the lesions are bilateral, a syndrome resembling that of Klüver and Bucy has been described, though always, in humans, there is an associated amnesic defect, aphasia, bulimia, or

dementia (Lilly et al). A contrasting syndrome, resembling the sham rage of animals, may also be observed in patients with bilateral lesions of the inferomedial and anterior parts of the temporal lobes. In this disorder, which is usually the result of trauma or herpes simplex encephalitis, the patient reacts to every stimulus with extreme belligerence, screaming, cursing, biting, and spitting (see also Chap. 25).

To summarize, human temporal lobe syndromes include the following:

 I. Effects of unilateral disease of the dominant temporal lobe
   A. Homonymous upper quadrantanopia
   B. Wernicke's aphasia
   C. Amusia (some types)
   D. Impairment in tests of verbal material presented through the auditory sense
   E. Dysnomia or amnesic aphasia
 II. Effects of unilateral disease of nondominant temporal lobe
   A. Homonymous upper quadrantanopia
   B. Inability to judge spatial relationships in some cases
   C. Impairment in tests of visually presented nonverbal material
   D. Agnosia for sounds and some qualities of music
III. Effects of disease of either hemisphere
   A. Auditory illusions and hallucinations
   B. Psychotic behavior (aggressivity)
 IV. Effects of bilateral disease
   A. Korsakoff amnesic defect (hippocampal formations)
   B. Apathy and placidity ⎫ Klüver-Bucy
   C. Increased sexual activity ⎬ syndrome
   D. "Sham rage"

SYNDROMES CAUSED BY LESIONS OF THE PARIETAL LOBES

ANATOMIC AND PHYSIOLOGIC CONSIDERATIONS

This part of the cerebrum is the least well demarcated from the rest (Fig. 21-8). Lying behind the central sulcus and above the sylvian fissure, it has no sharp boundaries inferiorly and posteriorly, where it merges with the temporal and occipital lobes respectively. On its medial side the parieto-occipital sulcus marks the posterior border which is completed by extending the line of the sulcus downward to the preoccipital notch on the inferior border of the hemisphere. Within the parietal lobe there are two important sulci: the postcentral sulcus, which forms the posterior boundary of the somesthetic cortex, and the interparietal sulcus, which runs anteroposteriorly from the middle of the posterior central sulcus and separates the mass of the parietal lobe into superior and inferior parietal lobules (Fig. 21-3). The posterior extremity of the sylvian fissure curves upward to terminate in the inferior parietal lobule where it is surrounded by the supramarginal gyrus (Brodmann's area

40). The superior temporal sulcus also turns up, into the more posterior part of the inferior parietal lobule, and is surrounded by the angular gyrus (area 39). The supramarginal and angular gyri are sometimes referred to as Ecker's inferior parietal lobule. These two gyri and the posterior third of the first temporal gyrus make up what continental neuroanatomists call Wernicke's speech area.

The architecture of the postcentral convolution is typical of all primary receptive areas (koniocortex or homotypical granular cortex). The rest of the parietal lobe resembles the associational cortex, both unimodal and heteromodal, of the frontal and temporal lobes. The superior and inferior parietal lobules and adjacent parts of the temporal and occipital lobes are much larger in humans than in any of the other primates and are relatively slow in development, not being fully functional until the seventh year of age. This area of heteromodal cortex has large fiber connections with the frontal, occipital, and temporal lobes of the same hemisphere and, through the middle part of the corpus callosum, with corresponding parts of the opposite hemisphere.

The postcentral gyrus or primary somatosensory cortex receives its main input from the ventroposterior thalamic nucleus, which is the terminus of the ascending somatosensory pathways. The contralateral half of the body is represented somatotopically on the posterior bank of the rolandic sulcus. It has been shown in the macaque that spindle afferents project to area 3a, cutaneous afferents to areas 3b and 1, and joint afferents to area 2 (Kaas). The homotypic sensory cortex projects to the superior parietal lobule (area 5) which is the somatosensory association cortex. Some parts of areas 1, 3, and 5 (except the hand and foot representations) probably connect, via the corpus callosum, with the opposite somatosensory cortex. There is some uncertainty as to whether area 7 (which lies posterior to area 5) is unimodal somatosensory or heteromodal visual and somatosensory; certainly it receives a large contingent of fibers from the occipital lobe.

In humans, electrical stimulation of the cortex of the superior and inferior parietal lobules evokes no specific motor or sensory effects. Overlapping here, however, are the tertiary zones for vision, hearing, and somatic sensation, the supramodal integration of which is essential to our awareness of space and person and certain aspects of language and calculation, as will be described below.

THE FUNCTIONS OF THE PARIETAL LOBES

Within the brain no other territory surpasses the parietal lobes in the rich variety of clinical phenomena that are exposed under conditions of disease. Our current understanding of the effects of parietal lobe disease contrasts sharply with that of the late nineteenth century, when these lobes, in the classic textbooks of Oppenheim and Gowers, were considered to be "silent areas." However, the clinical manifestations may be subtle, requiring special techniques for their elicitation; and even more difficult is the interpretation of these abnormalities of function in terms of a coherent and plausible physiology.

Despite Critchley's pessimistic prediction that to establish a formula of normal parietal function will prove to be a "vain and meaningless pursuit," our concepts of the activities of this part of the brain are beginning to assume some degree of order. There is now little reason to doubt that the anterior parietal cortex contains the mechanisms for tactile percepts. Discriminative tactile functions are organized in the more posterior, secondary sensory areas. But the greater part of the parietal lobe functions as a center for integrating somatic sensory with visual and auditory information, for the purpose of constructing an awareness of the body (body schema) and of its relation to extrapersonal space. Frontal connections provide the necessary proprioceptive and visual information for movement of the body and manipulation of objects and for certain constructional activities, and impairment of these functions implicates the parietal lobes, more clearly the right. The understanding of the grammatical and syntactical aspects of language is a function of the dominant parietal lobe, as will be elaborated in Chap. 22. The recognition and utilization of numbers, arithmetic principles and calculation, which have important spatial attributes, are other functions integrated principally through the dominant parietal lobe.

CLINICAL EFFECTS AND SYNDROMES

Cortical Sensory Syndromes   The effects of a parietal lobe lesion on somatic sensation were first described by Verger and then more completely by Déjerine, in his monograph *L'agnosie corticale,* and by Head and Holmes. In the French medical literature these effects are sometimes referred to as the Verger-Déjerine syndrome. As was pointed out in Chap. 8 the defect is essentially one of sensory discrimination, i.e., an impairment or loss of the sense of position and passive movement and of the ability to localize tactile, thermal, and noxious stimuli applied to the body surface, to distinguish objects by their size, shape, and texture (astereognosis), to recognize figures written on the skin, and to distinguish between single and double contacts (two-point discrimination). In contrast, the perception of pain, touch, pressure, vibratory, and thermal stimuli is relatively intact. This type of sensory defect is sometimes referred to as "cortical," although these effects can be produced just as well by lesions of the subcortical connections. Clinicoanatomic studies implicate the contralateral postcentral gyrus, particularly the hand area; parietal-cortical lesions that spare the postcentral gyrus produce only transient somatosensory changes or none at all (Corkin et al; Carmon and Benton).

The question of unilateral versus bilateral sensory deficits with lesions in only one postcentral convolution was raised by the studies of Semmes et al and Corkin et al. In tests of pressure sensitivity, two-point discrimination, point localization, position sense, and tactual object recognition, they found bilateral disturbances in nearly half of their patients with unilateral lesions, but the deficits were always most severe contralaterally and mainly in the hand. These disturbances of discriminative sensation and the subject of tactile agnosia are discussed more fully in Chap. 8.

Déjerine and Mouzon have described another sensory syndrome in which touch, pressure, pain, thermal, vibratory, and position sense are lost on one side of the body or in a limb. This syndrome usually occurs with large, acute lesions (infarcts, hemorrhages) in the central and subcortical white matter of the contralateral parietal lobe and recedes in time, leaving more subtle defects in sensory discrimination. As indicated in Chap. 8, smaller lesions, particularly ones that result from a glancing blow to the parietal region, or a small infarct or hemorrhage, may cause a defect in cutaneous-kinesthetic perception in a discrete part of a limb, e.g., the ulnar or radial half of the hand and forearm; these cerebral lesions may mimic a peripheral nerve or root lesion.

Head and Holmes drew attention to a number of interesting points about patients with parietal sensory defects—the easy fatigability of their sensory perceptions, the inconsistency of responses to painful and tactile stimuli, the difficulty in distinguishing more than one contact at a time, the tendency of superficial pain sensations to outlast the stimulus and to be hyperpathic, and the occurrence of hallucinations of touch.

The Asomatognosias   The idea that visual and tactile sensory information is synthesized during development into a body schema or image (perception of one's body and of the relations of bodily parts to one another) was first clearly formulated by Pick and extensively elaborated by Brain. Long before their time, however, it was suggested that such information was the basis of our emerging awareness of ourselves as persons, and philosophers had assumed that this comes about by a constant interplay between percepts of ourselves and those of the surrounding world.

The formation of the body schema is believed to be based on the constant influx of sensations from our bodies as we move about; hence, motor activity is important in its development. Always, however, a sense of extrapersonal space is involved as well, and this depends upon visual and labyrinthine impulses. The mechanisms upon which these perceptions depend are best appreciated by studying their derangements in the course of neurologic disease.

Unilateral asomatognosia (Anton-Babinski syndrome)   The observation that a patient with a dense left hemiplegia may be indifferent to, or unaware of, the paralysis was first made by Anton. Babinski named this disorder *anosognosia*. It may express itself in several ways: The patient may act as if nothing were the matter. If asked to raise the paralyzed arm, the patient may raise the intact one or do nothing at all. If asked whether the paralyzed arm has been moved, the patient may say "yes." If the failure to do so is pointed out, the patient may admit that the arm is slightly weak. If told it is paralyzed, the patient may deny that this is so or offer an excuse: "My shoulder hurts." If asked why the paralysis went unnoticed, the response may be, "I'm not a doctor." Some patients report that they feel as though their left side has disappeared, and when shown their paralyzed arm, they may deny it is theirs and assert that it belongs to someone else, or even take hold of it and fling it aside. This mental derangement, which Hughlings Jackson referred to as a kind of "imbecility," obviously includes a somatic sensory defect as well as a conceptual negation of paralysis, and even a disturbed visual perception and neglect of half of the body.

Anosognosia is usually associated with other abnormalities. Often in this state there is a blunted emotionality. The patient looks dull, is inattentive and apathetic, and shows varying degrees of general confusion. There may be an indifference to failure, a feeling of something missing, visual and tactile illusions when sensing the paralyzed part, hallucinations of movement, and allocheiria (one-sided stimuli are felt on the other side).

A particularly common group of parietal symptoms consists of neglect of one side of the body in dressing and grooming ("dressing apraxia"), recognition only on the intact side of bilaterally and simultaneously presented stimuli ("sensory extinction"), deviation of head and eyes to the side of the lesion and torsion of the body in the same direction (failure of directed attention to the body and to extrapersonal space on the side opposite the lesion). The patient may fail to shave one side of the face, or to apply lipstick or to comb the hair on one side, or find it impossible to put on eyeglasses or insert dentures or put on a dressing gown, one sleeve of which has been turned inside out. Unilateral spatial neglect is brought out by having the patient bisect a line or draw a daisy or a clock, or name all the objects in the room. Homonymous hemianopia, visual inattention, and varying degrees of hemiparesis may or may not be present, and there may be grasping and groping with the nonparalyzed hand.

Disturbances of the perception of space, other than language-related ones, are most evident in patients with lesions of the right, nondominant parietal lobe. These include disorders of topographic (extrapersonal) orientation and topographic and geographic memory, with resulting difficulties in route finding, and an inability to reproduce geometric figures ("constructional apraxia"). A number of tests have been designed to elicit these disturbances, such as indicating the time by placement of the hands of a clock, drawing a map, spontaneous (free) drawing, copying a complex figure, reproducing stick-pattern constructions and block designs, three-dimensional constructions, and reconstruction of puzzles. In the majority of cases, as remarked above, the lesions responsible for these deficits prove to be in the right hemisphere, though the dominance is not as striking as that of language and language-associated functions.

According to Denny-Brown et al, the basic disturbance in such cases is an inability to summate a series of "spatial impressions"—tactile, kinesthetic, visual, or auditory—a defect they refer to as *amorphosynthesis*. In their view, imperception or neglect of one side of the body and of extrapersonal space represents the full extent of the disturbance, which in lesser degree consists only of tactile and visual extinction. They make the additional points that the disorder of spatial summation is strictly contralateral to the damaged parietal lobe, right or left, and has to be distinguished from a true agnosia, which is a conceptual disorder and involves both sides of space as a result of damage to one (the dominant) hemisphere. More recent observations indicate that patients with right parietal lesions show elements of ipsilateral neglect in addition to the striking degree of contralateral neglect, suggesting that in respect to spatial attention the right parietal lobe is truly dominant (Weintraub and Mesulam).

The lesion responsible for the various forms of unilateral asomatognosia lies in the cortex and white matter of the superior parietal lobule but may extend variably into the postcentral gyrus, frontal motor areas, and temporal and occipital lobes, which accounts for some of the associated abnormalities. Rarely, a deep lesion of the ventrolateral thalamus and juxtaposed white matter of the parietal lobe will produce contralateral neglect. Unilateral asomatognosia is seven times as frequent with right (nondominant) parietal lesions as with left-sided ones, according to Hécaen's statistics. The apparent infrequency of right-sided symptoms is attributable in part to their obscuration by an associated aphasia.

Bilateral asomatognosia (Gerstmann syndrome)

The symptoms that make up this syndrome provide the most striking examples of bilateral asomatognosia and are due to a left, or dominant, parietal lesion. The characteristic features are: confusion of the right and left sides of the body; inability to designate or name the different fingers of the two hands; and inability to calculate and to write. One or more of these manifestations may be associated with word blindness, in which case the lesion can be placed in the angular gyrus or subjacent white matter ("angular gyrus syndrome"). There has been a dispute as to whether the four main elements of the Gerstmann syndrome have a common basis or only a chance association. Benton states that they occur together in a parietal lesion no more often than do constructional apraxia, alexia, and loss of visual memory and that every combination of these symptoms and those of the Gerstmann syndrome occurs with equal frequency in parietal lobe disease. Others disagree and believe that right-left confusion, digital agnosia, agraphia, and acalculia have special significance, being linked through a unitary defect in spatial orientation. The authors favor the latter interpretation. Lesions of the superior parietal lobule may interfere with voluntary movement of the opposite limbs, particularly the arm. In reaching for a visually presented target in the contralateral visual field, and to a lesser extent in the ipsilateral field, the movement is misdirected and dysmetric (the distance to the target is misjudged). This disorder of movement, sometimes referred to as optic ataxia, resembles cerebellar ataxia. This is explained by the fact that cortical areas 7 and 5 receive visual projections from the peristriate areas and proprioceptive ones from the cerebellum, both of which are integrated in multimodal parietal neurons. Areas 5 and 7 in turn project to frontal areas 6, 8 and 9, where ocular scanning and reaching are coordinated.

From the above descriptions it is evident that the left and right parietal lobes function differently. The most obvious difference, of course, is that language and arithmetic functions are centered in the left hemisphere. It is hardly surprising therefore that verbally mediated or verbally associated spatial functions are more affected with left-sided than right-sided lesions. It must also be realized that speech involves cross-modal connections and is central to all cognitive functions. Hence cross-modal matching tasks (auditory-visual, visual-auditory, visual-tactile, tactile-visual, auditory-tactile, etc.) are most clearly impaired with dominant hemisphere lesions. Indeed this is what Butters and Brody have found. Similarly, faults in what Luria has called logicogrammatical and syntactic aspects of language (which he considers to be quasispatial) occur with left parietal lesions. Such patients can read and understand spoken words but cannot grasp the meaning of a sentence if it contains elements of relationship (e.g., the mother's daughter versus the daughter's mother; the father's brother's son; Jane's complexion is lighter than Marjorie's but darker than her sister's). In calculation there are similar effects; the patient may be able to read numbers and describe the rules of a required computation but not be able to carry it out with pencil and paper. It should be noted that addition, subtraction, multiplication, and division all require the placing of numbers in specific spatial relationships. The recognition and naming of parts of the body and the distinction of right from left and up from down are other learned, verbally mediated spatial concepts which are disturbed by lesions in the dominant parietal lobe.

Ideomotor and ideational apraxia As was pointed out in Chap. 3, patients with dominant parietal lesions who exhibit no defects in motor or sensory function lose the ability to perform learned motor skills on command or by imitation. Common implements and tools can no longer be used, either in relation to the patient's body (e.g., comb or brush) or to objects in the environment. It is as though the patient has forgotten the learned sequences of movement. The effects are bilateral. It is of interest that in both agraphia and acalculia, the motor defect appears to be marred by agnosic defects, hence the common term *apractagnosia*.

Consciousness of Self and Depersonalization
There are many circumstances in which the patient's appreciation of self in relation to the environment is disturbed in a more general sense. Some of these, such as diplopia and labyrinthine vertigo (see Chaps. 13 and 14), are readily understandable, since in these disorders conflicting data about the external world, e.g., double images or unnaturally moving images are presented to the sensorium. In other clinical conditions, however, there is no evidence of sensory deficit. Rather, some disorder occurs in the state of continuous self-consciousness, which depends on the influx of sensations and their association with past memories, the stream of life experiences, and feelings that keep us continuously aware of ourselves as entities. Patients with depression of mood may say that they do not feel natural as they move about; it is as though they were frozen in their reactions, as though something has altered their way of feeling and experiencing. The schizophrenic may feel unreal, or *depersonalized*. Extreme degrees of this are observed in the delusions of negativism (*délire de negativisme*), in which such patients deny their own existence. In a manic attack every experience may be more vivid, enjoyable, and personalized than ever before. Also, delusions of transformation, of being someone else (a royal figure, God, or Jesus) occur in schizophrenia, manic states, and general paresis (delusions of grandeur). It is tempting to view all these elusive clinical phenomena as manifestations of more general disturbances of the body-environmental schemata, but the evidence is inconclusive.

The effects of disease of the parietal lobes may be summarized as follows:

I. Effects of unilateral disease of the parietal lobe, right or left
    A. Cortical sensory syndrome and sensory extinction (or total hemianesthesia with large acute lesions of white matter)
    B. Mild hemiparesis, unilateral muscular atrophy in children
    C. Homonymous hemianopia (incongruent) or visual inattention, and sometimes anosognosia, neglect of one-half of the body and of extrapersonal space (observed more frequently with right than with left parietal lesions)
    D. Abolition of optokinetic nystagmus to one side
II. Effects of unilateral disease of the dominant parietal lobe (left hemisphere in right-handed patients); additional phenomena include:
    A. Disorders of language (especially alexia)
    B. Gerstmann syndrome
    C. Tactile agnosia (bimanual astereognosis; see page 127)
    D. Bilateral ideomotor and ideational apraxia
III. Effects of unilateral disease of the nondominant (right) parietal lobe
    A. Topographic memory loss
    B. Anosognosia and dressing apraxia. These disorders may occur with lesions of either hemisphere but have been observed more frequently with lesions of the nondominant one.

In all these lesions, if the disease is sufficiently extensive, there may be a reduction in the capacity to think clearly, inattentiveness, and impaired memory.

It is still not possible to present an all-embracing formula of parietal lobe function. It does seem reasonably certain that in addition to the perception of somatosensory impulses (postcentral gyrus) the parietal lobe participates in the integration of all sensory data, especially those which provide consciousness of one's surroundings, of the relation of objects in the environment to one another, and of the position of the body in space. In this respect, the parietal lobe may be regarded as a special, high-order sensory organ, the locus of transmodal (intersensory) integrations, particularly tactile and visual ones, which are the basis of our concepts of spatial relations.

SYNDROMES CAUSED BY LESIONS OF THE OCCIPITAL LOBES

ANATOMIC AND PHYSIOLOGIC CONSIDERATIONS

The occipital lobes are the terminus of the geniculocalcarine pathways and are essential for visual perception and recognition. This part of the brain has a large medial surface and somewhat smaller lateral and inferior surfaces. The parieto-occipital fissure is its obvious medial boundary with the parietal lobe, but laterally it merges with the parietal and the temporal lobes. The large calcarine fissure courses in an anteroposterior direction from the pole of the occipital lobe to the splenium of the corpus callosum, and area 17, the primary idiotypic visual receptive cortex, lies on its banks (Fig. 21-1). It is typical koniocortex but is unique in that its fourth layer is divided into two granular cell layers by a greatly thickened band of myelinated fibers, the external band of Baillarger. This stripe in area 17, also called the *line* or *band of Gennari,* is grossly visible and has given the name of *striate cortex* to this area. The largest part of area 17 is the terminus of the macular fibers (see Fig. 12-1). The parastriate cortex (areas 18 and 19) lacks the line of Gennari and resembles the granular unimodal association cortex of the rest of the cerebrum. Area 17 contains cells that are activated by the homolateral geniculocalcarine pathway and that send fibers to other cells in area 17 as well as to cells in areas 18 and 19. The latter are connected with one another and with the angular gyri, lateral and medial temporal and parietal gyri, frontal motor areas, limbic and paralimbic areas, and with corresponding areas of the opposite hemisphere through the posterior third (splenium) of the corpus callosum.

The connections among these several areas in the occipital lobe are complicated, and the old idea that area 17 is activated by the lateral geniculate neurons and that their activity is then transferred and elaborated in areas 18 and 19 is surely not the complete story. Actually there are four or five occipital receptive fields, activated by the lateral geniculate neurons, and as Hubel and Wiesel have shown, the response patterns of neurons in both occipital lobes to edges and moving visual stimuli, to on-and-off effects of light, and to colors are much different than was originally supposed. The monographs of Polyak and of Walsh and Hoyt contain detailed information about the anatomy and physiology of this part of the brain.

CLINICAL EFFECTS AND SYNDROMES

Visual Field Defects The most familiar clinical disorder resulting from a lesion of *one* occipital lobe, homonymous hemianopia, has already been discussed in Chap. 12. Extensive destruction abolishes all vision in the corresponding half of each visual field. With a neoplastic lesion that eventually involves the entire striate region, the field defect may extend from the periphery toward the center, and loss of color vision (hemiachromatopsia) precedes loss of black and white. Lesions that destroy only part of the striate cortex on one side yield characteristic field defects that accurately indicate the loci of the lesions. A lesion confined

to the pole of the occipital lobe results in a central hemianopic defect which splits the maculas and leaves the peripheral fields intact. This observation indicates that half of each macula is unilaterally represented and settles once and for all the old debate as to whether they may be spared in hemianopia. Bilateral lesions of the occipital poles, as in embolism of the posterior cerebral arteries, result in bilateral central hemianopias. Quadrant defects and altitudinal field defects due to striate lesions indicate that the cortex on one side of the calcarine fissure is damaged. The cortex below the fissure is the terminus of fibers from the lower half of the retina, and the resulting field defect is in the upper quadrant, and vice versa. Most bilateral altitudinal defects are traceable to incomplete occipital lesions (cortex or terminal parts of geniculocalcarine pathways). Head and Holmes described several such cases due to gunshot wounds; embolic or thrombotic infarction has been the usual cause in our material.

As indicated in Chap. 12, the homonymous hemianopia that results form ablation of one occipital lobe is not absolute. In monkeys, visuospatial orientation and the capacity to reach for moving objects in the defective field are preserved (Denny-Brown and Chambers). In humans also, flashing light and moving objects can sometimes be seen in the blind field. Weiskrantz et al have referred to these preserved functions as "blindisms."

Cortical Blindness With bilateral lesions of the occipital lobes (destruction of area 17 of both hemispheres), there is a loss of sight. The degree of blindness may be equivalent to that which follows enucleation of the eyes or severance of the optic nerves. The pupillary light reflexes are preserved, since they depend upon visual fibers that terminate in the midbrain, short of the geniculate bodies (see Fig. 13-6). Usually no changes are detectable in the retinas, though van Buren has described slight optic atrophy in monkeys long after occipital ablations. The eyes are still able to move through a full range, but optokinetic nystagmus cannot be elicited. Visual imagination and visual imagery in dreams are preserved. With very rare exceptions (Chap. 2), no cortical potentials can be evoked in occipital lobes by light flashes, and the alpha rhythm is lost in the EEG.

Less complete lesions leave the patient with varying degrees of visual perception. There may also be visual hallucinations of either elementary or complex types, as described on page 204. The mode of recovery from cortical blindness has been studied carefully by Gloning and his colleagues, who describe a regular progression from cortical blindness, through visual agnosia and partially impaired perceptual function to recovery. Even with recovery the patient may complain of visual fatigue (asthenopia) and difficulties in fixation and fusion.

The usual cause of cortical blindness is occlusion of the posterior cerebral arteries (embolic or thrombotic). The infarct may also involve the medial temporal regions and thalami with resulting Korsakoff psychosis and a variety of other neurologic deficits referable to the high midbrain and diencephalon (see page 342). Hypoxic encephalopathy, Schilder disease and other leukodystrophies, and bilateral gliomas are other causes of cortical blindness. A transitory form of cortical blindness may occur with head injury.

Visual Anosognosia (Anton's Syndrome)   The main characteristic is denial of blindness in patients who obviously cannot see. The patients act as though they can see, and when attempting to walk, they collide with objects, even to the point of injury. Excuses may be offered for their difficulties: "I lost my glasses," "The light is dim," etc., or there may be only an indifference to the loss of sight. The lesions in cases of negation of blindness extend beyond the striate cortex to involve the visual association areas.

Rarely, the opposite condition may arise: a patient can see small objects, but claims to be blind. This individual walks about avoiding obstacles, picks up crumbs or pills from the table, and catches a small ball thrown from a distance. Damasio suggests that this might be a type of visual disorientation but with sufficient residual visual information to guide the hand, and that the lesion will be in the visual association areas superior to the calcarine cortex.

Visual Illusions and Hallucinations   While these may occur in relation to lesions in any part of the visual system, they are particularly frequent with occipital lobe lesions. Electrical stimulation of the occipital cortex elicits visual phenomena of this type, and it seems likely, therefore, that seizures reproduce them by activating the visual system directly. In these instances the hallucinations are *positive phenomena*. Certain lesions disturb the equilibrium of the visual system in other ways, possibly by disinhibiting other parts, thereby liberating the hallucinations (*negative* phenomena). Difficulties in distinguishing between positive and negative hallucinatory phenomena also arise in the interpretation of the effects of drugs and withdrawal from drugs. Although illusions and hallucinations are considered separately here, they may be difficult to separate, especially in epilepsy and delirium.

Visual Illusions (Metamorphopsias)   These may present as distortions of form, size, movement, or color; also visual

images may fail to arouse visual memories and their associated affect, resulting in a sense of strangeness or inexplicable familiarity, as occurs in the "dreamy state" of temporal lobe epilepsy. Some of these have already been mentioned in Chaps. 12 and 15.

Visual illusions take the form of objects seeming too small (micropsia) and distant or too large (megalopsia or macropsia) and moving toward the patient. In other cases, objects may appear elongated, swollen, or run together, or the vertical and horizontal orientation of the image may shift. Inverted vision, irradiation of contour, disappearance of color (achromatopsia), illusional coloring (erythropsia), polyopia (one object appearing as two or more objects) or monocular diplopia (vertical, concentric, especially triplopia), illusions of movement of stationary objects, too rapid displacement of moving objects, or imperception of movement are other forms of illusory visual experience. Also, there may be a loss of stereoscopic vision, perseveration or periodic reappearance of visual images long after the cessation of the visual stimulus (palinopsia or paliopsia), or a false orientation of objects in space (optic allesthesia). In a group of 83 patients with visual perceptual abnormalities Hécaen found that 71 fell under one of four headings: deformation of the image, change in size, illusion of movement, or a combination of all three.

Illusions of these types have been reported with lesions of the occipital, occipitoparietal, or occipitotemporal regions, and the right hemisphere appears to be involved more often than the left. Illusions of movement occur more frequently with posterior temporal lesions, polyopsia more frequently with occipital lesions, and palinopsia with both parietal and occipital lesions. Visual field defects are present in many of the cases.

Hoff and Pötzl have insisted that an element of vestibular disorder underlies the metamorphopsias of parieto-occipital lesions (the vestibular system is represented in the parietal as well as in the temporal lobe; see pages 239 and 256). *Polyopia* (the perception of several images of the same object), ascribed to faulty ocular fixation, has usually proved to be a manifestation of occipital lesions, although it may occur in hysteria.

Pharmacologic agents may also alter vision, and one may surmise that occipital or temporo-occipital regions are involved. Atropine, lysergic acid, and mescaline cause many of these illusory phenomena. Faulty integration of sensory information due to parietal lesions may explain some of the failures to synthesize ocular movement and vestibular function.

Visual Hallucinations   These phenomena may be elementary or complex, and both have sensory as well as cognitive aspects. Elementary (or unformed) hallucinations include flashes of light, colors, luminous points, stars, multiple lights (like candles), and geometric forms (circles, squares, and hexagons). They may be stationary or moving (zigzag, oscillations, vibrations, or pulsations). Complex, or formed, hallucinations include objects, persons, or animals. They may be of natural size, lilliputian, or grossly enlarged. With hemianopia they may appear in the defective field or move from the intact field toward the hemianopic one. The patient may realize that the hallucinations are false experiences or may be convinced of their reality. Since the patient's response is usually in accord with the nature of the hallucination, he or she may react with fear to a threatening vision, or with amusement if its content is benign.

The clinical setting for the occurrence of visual hallucinations varies. Often they are associated with a homonymous hemianopia, as indicated above. Frequently the background is one of confusion and clouding of consciousness, as in the syndrome of delirium (Chap. 19). In the "peduncular hallucinosis" of Lhermitte, the hallucinations are purely visual, appear natural in form and color, move about as in an animated cartoon, and are usually considered to be unreal, abnormal phenomena (preserved insight). Similar phenomena may occur as part of hypnagogic hallucinations in the narcolepsy-cataplexy syndrome (see page 314).

A special syndrome of ophthalmopathic hallucinations occurs in the blind or partially blind person (syndrome of Bonnet). The visual images may be of elementary or complex type, usually of people or animals and are polychromic (vivid colors). The hallucinations appear in the blind field. They may occupy all of the visual field (in the totally blind person) or the field of one eye, or corresponding blind fields in the patient with homonymous hemianopia. Moving the eyes or closing the affected eye has variable effects, sometimes abolishing the hallucinations.

In patients with visual hallucinations, the lesions, if they can be identified, are usually situated in the occipital lobe or posterior part of the temporal lobe. According to Penfield and Rasmussen, elementary hallucinations have their origin in lesions of the occipital cortex, and complex ones, in the temporal cortex.

In our material, so-called peduncular hallucinosis has been associated mainly with diencephalic lesions and not strictly with mesencephalic ones. As indicated above, the hallucinations in this disorder are purely visual; if hallucinations are polymodal, the lesion is always in the cerebrum.

The hallucinatory phenomena of delirium are nonlocalizable, as was pointed out in Chap. 19, but sometimes the evidence points to an origin in the temporal lobe. In ophthalmopathic hallucinations there is visual loss from ocular, optic nerve or tract, or occipital lobe lesions, and also a slight impairment of mental function.

The Visual Agnosias *Object agnosia* This rare condition consists of a failure to name and indicate the use

of a seen object by spoken or written word or by gesture. The patient cannot even tell the generic class of the seen object. Vision is intact, the mind is clear, and the patient is not aphasic—conditions requisite for the diagnosis of agnosia. If the object is palpated, it is recognized at once, and it can also be identified by smell or sound if it has an odor or makes a noise. Movement of the object or placing it in its customary surroundings facilitates recognition. In most reported instances of object agnosia, first described by Lissauer in 1890, the patient retains normal visual acuity but cannot identify, match, or name objects presented in any part of the visual fields. Lissauer conceived of visual object recognition as consisting of two distinct processes— the construction of a perceptual representation from vision (apperception) and the mapping of this perceptual representation onto stored percepts of the object's functions and associations. Lissauer proposed that impairment of either of these processes could give rise to a defect in visual object recognition.

As indicated in Chap. 12, visual object agnosia is a rare phenomenon, and is usually associated with visual verbal agnosia (alexia) and homonymous hemianopia. Prosopagnosia (see below) is also present in most cases. The underlying lesions are usually bilateral, involving the inferolateral parts of the occipital lobes, although McCarthy and Warrington have related an instance of visual object agnosia to a restricted lesion of the left occipitotemporal region (by MR imaging).

Simultanagnosia Wolpert originally described a patient in which there was a "spelling dyslexia" (an inability to read all but the shortest words, spelled out letter by letter) and a failure to perceive simultaneously all the elements of a scene and to properly interpret the scene. In the framework of Gestalt psychology the patient could see the parts but not the whole. A cognitive defect of synthesis of the visual impressions was thought to be the basis of this condition, which Wolpert called *simultanagnosia*. Some of the patients with this disorder have a right homonymous hemianopia; in others the visual fields are "full." This is part of the Balint syndrome (see below), the other components of which are faulty visual scanning (ocular apraxia) and visual reaching (optic ataxia), suggesting that a fault in ocular scanning might underlie all the defects. Through tachistoscopic testing, Kinsbourne and Warrington have noted that, by reducing the time of stimulus exposure, single objects are perceived in an instant, but not two objects. Levine and Calvanio, whose review of this subject is recommended, find the basis of simultanagnosia to be a quantitative defect in "the capacity for perceptual analysis and form synthesis, resulting in a decrease in the span of visual form apprehension.'' Nielsen has attributed this disorder to a lesion of the inferolateral part of the dominant occipital lobe (area 18). Also Kinsbourne and Warrington reported the case history of a patient who presented with an isolated ''spelling dyslexia'' and simultanagnosia; there was a localized lesion within the inferior part of the left occipital lobe.

Prosopagnosia (Greek *prosopon*, ''face'') This is the name that has been given to a particular form of visual defect or agnosia in which the patient cannot identify a familiar face, either by looking at the person or a picture, even though he knows that a face is a face and can point out the features. Such patients cannot learn to recognize new faces. They may also be unable to interpret the meaning of facial expressions or to judge the ages or distinguish the genders of faces. In identifying persons, the patient depends on other data, such as the presence and type of spectacles or moustache, the type of gait, or sound of the voice. Similarly, species of animals and birds cannot be distinguished from one another, but generic recognition is preserved. As a rule, other agnosias are present in such cases (color agnosia, simultanagnosia), and there may be topographical disorientation, disturbances of body schema, and constructional or dressing apraxia. Visual field defects are nearly always present, a left upper quadrantanopia being the most frequent. Some neurologists have interpreted this condition as a simultanagnosia involving facial features. Another interpretation is that the face, though satisfactorily perceived, cannot be matched to a memory store of faces. Levine has found a deficit in perception, characterized by insufficient feature analysis of visual stimuli. The small number of cases that have been studied anatomically and by CT scan indicate that prosopagnosia is associated with bilateral lesions of the ventromesial occipitotemporal regions (Damasio et al).

Closely allied, and often associated, with prosopagnosia is the syndrome of *loss of environmental familiarity*, in which the patient is unable to recognize familiar places. The patient may be able to describe a familiar environment from memory and locate it on a map, but he experiences no sense of familiarity when faced with the actual landscape. In essence, this is an environmental agnosia. This syndrome is associated with right-sided, medial temporal-occipital lesions, although in some patients, as in those with prosopagnosia, the lesions are bilateral (Landis et al).

Visual agnosia for words See Chap. 22 and below in the present chapter, under ''Corpus Callosum and the Disconnection Syndromes.''

Visual disorientation and disorders of spatial (topographic) localization Spatial orientation, which depends upon visual, tactile, and kinesthetic perceptions, has already been discussed under ''Parietal Lobes.'' There are instances, however, where the defect in visual perception predominates. Patients cannot draw the floor plan of their house or a map of their town or the United States and cannot describe a familiar route, say from their home to their place of work, or find their way in familiar surroundings. In brief, they have lost topographic memory. Furthermore, they may have difficulty visualizing and describing the shapes of common objects and also in localizing objects seen in their own visual field. Yet, there is no agnosia for the objects themselves or of the word symbols that represent them. Most of such patients described by Holmes had bilateral occipitoparietal lesions.

Color agnosia Here one must distinguish several different aspects of the identification of colors such as the correct perception of color (the loss of which is called *color blindness*) or the naming of a color. The common form of color blindness is congenital, and is readily tested by the use of Ishihara plates. Acquired color blindness with retention of form vision, due to a cerebral lesion, is referred to as central *achromatopsia*. Here the disturbance is one of hue discrimination; the patient cannot sort a series of colored wools according to hue (Holmgren test), and may complain that colors have lost their brightness or that everything looks gray. Achromatopsia is frequently associated with visual field defects and with prosopagnosia. Most often the field defects are bilateral and affect the upper quadrants. However, full field achromatopsia may exist with retention of visual acuity and form vision. There may also be a hemi- or quadrantachromatopsia, without other abnormalities. These features, together with the associated prosopagnosia, point to involvement of the inferomesial occipital and temporal lobe(s) and the lower part of the striate cortex or optic radiation (Meadows 1974a; Damasio et al). These clinical findings are explained by the animal studies of Hubel, which unequivocally identified sets of cells in areas 17 and 18 that are activated only by color stimuli.

A second group of patients with color agnosia have no difficulty with color perception (i.e., they can match seen colors), but they cannot reliably name seen colors or point out colors in response to their names. They have a *color anomia*, of which there are at least two varieties. One is typically associated with pure word blindness, i.e., alexia without agraphia, and is best explained by a disconnection of the primary visual areas from the language areas (see further on). In the second variety, the patient fails not only in tasks that require the matching of a seen color with its spoken name, but in purely verbal tasks pertaining to color naming, such as naming the colors of common objects (e.g., grass, banana). This latter disorder is probably best regarded as a form of anomic aphasia, in which the aphasia is more or less restricted to the naming of colors (Meadows, 1974b). According to Damasio, the lesion has invariably involved the mesial part of the left hemisphere at the junction of occipital and temporal lobes, just below the splenium of the corpus callosum. All the patients also had a right homonymous hemianopia, because of destruction of the left lateral geniculate body, optic radiation, or calcarine cortex.

Balint Syndrome This consists of (1) an inability to look voluntarily into and to scan the peripheral field, despite the fact that eye movements are full (psychic paralysis of fixation of gaze); (2) a failure to precisely grasp or touch an object under visual guidance, as though hand and eye were not coordinated (optic ataxia); and (3) visual inattention (disorientation) affecting mainly the periphery of the visual field, attention to other sensory stimuli being intact. Balint, a Hungarian neurologist, was the first to recognize this constellation of findings.

The psychic paralysis of gaze is apparent when the patient attempts to turn his or her eyes to fixate an object in the right or left visual field and to follow a moving object into all four quadrants of the field once the eyes are fixated on it. Optic ataxia is detected when the patient reaches for an object, either spontaneously or in response to verbal command. To reach the object, the patient engages in tactile search with the palm and fingers, presumably using somatosensory cues to compensate for a lack of visual information. This may give the erroneous impression that the patient is blind. In contrast, movements which do not require visual guidance, such as those directed to the body, or movements of the body itself, are performed naturally. This disorder may involve one or both hands. The presence of visual inattention is tested by asking the patient to carry out tasks such as looking at a series of objects or connecting a series of dots by lines; often only one of a series of objects can be found even though the visual fields seem to be full.

The essential feature in the Balint syndrome appears to be a failure to properly direct oculomotor function in the exploration of space. Thus it is closely related, if not identical, to simultanagnosia and to a disorder of spatial summation (amorphosynthesis). In all the reported cases of the Balint syndrome the lesions have been bilateral, often in the border zones (areas 19 and 7) of the parieto-occipital regions, although instances of optic ataxia alone have been described within a single visual field, contralateral to a right or left parieto-occipital lesion.

The effects of disease of the occipital lobes may be summarized as follows:

I. Effects of unilateral disease, either right or left
   A. Contralateral (congruent) homonymous hemianopia, which

may be central (splitting the macula) or peripheral; also homonymous hemiachromatopsia
   B. Irritative lesions—elementary (unformed) hallucinations
II. Effects of left occipital disease
   A. Right homonymous hemianopia
   B. If deep white matter or splenium of corpus callosum is involved, alexia and color-naming defect
   C. Object agnosia
III. Effects of right occipital disease
   A. Left homonymous hemianopia
   B. With more extensive lesions, visual illusions (metamorphopsias) and hallucinations; more frequent with right-sided than left-sided lesions
   C. Loss of topographic memory and visual orientation
IV. Bilateral occipital disease
   A. Cortical blindness (pupils reactive)
   B. Loss of perception of color
   C. Prosopagnosia, simultanagnosia
   D. Balint syndrome

THE THEORETICAL PROBLEM OF VISUAL AND OTHER AGNOSIAS

From the foregoing discussion it is apparent that the term *visual agnosia* applies to a series of visual perceptive disorders which include, in varying combinations, faults of discrimination, identification, and recognition of faces, objects, pictures, colors, spatial arrangements, and words. The diagnosis of these states is predicated on the assumption that the failure in perception occurs in spite of intact visual acuity and adequate mental function, and an essentially normal language mechanism. When examined carefully, agnosic patients usually do not satisfy all these criteria and instead have a number of derangements that may at least in part explain their perceptual incompetence. Often there is a unisensory or polysensory disturbance, or an inadequacy of memory or of naming, or an impairment of visuo-oculomotor control. Anatomic studies have established that disturbances of recognition of complex forms, human faces, and spatial arrangements accompany right (nondominant) parieto-occipital lesions more often than left-sided ones. Disturbances of perception of graphic symbols of objects, of color discrimination and naming—in short all of the lexical aspects of recognition—are virtually always associated with left parieto-occipital lesions. Variations in the clinical effects of such lesions are dependent to a large extent on the tests used to elicit them and whether they involve learning, recognition, and recall.

There have been many critics of the concept of agnosia as a higher-order perceptual disturbance that can be clearly separated from loss of elementary sensation. Such a division is said to perpetuate an archaic view of sensory reception in the brain as consisting of two separable functional attributes, elementary sensation and perception. Bay, for example, claims that careful testing of patients with visual agnosia always brings to light some degree of diminished vision, in combination with general defects such as confusion and mental deterioration. Others (Geschwind; Sperry, Gazzaniga, and Bogen) emphasize that the visual agnosias depend upon disconnections of the visual receptive zones of the brain and the language areas of the left hemisphere, the learning and memory zones of the temporal lobes, the suprasensory zones of the parietal lobes, and the motor regions. Hécaen and Gassel and McCarthy and Warrington have presented the evidence for and against these points of view.

The reported cases of visual agnosia emphasize the complexity of the perceptive process and the inadequacy of our knowledge of the physiology of the several receptive zones of the occipital lobes. The fact that in some cases there are impairments of primary sensation that can be elicited by careful testing of visual function—using visual adaptation, perception of pattern, flicker-fusion, etc., as Bay recommends—cannot be disputed. However, even when present, such abnormalities would not fully explain the loss of discrimination and the inability to visualize or imagine the form and color of objects, their spatial arrangements, and their names. Failure of a sensation to activate these visual memories must involve a higher-order disturbance of cerebral function in the heteromodal association areas. Here sensory and motor functions are always integrated, the latter being used by the scanning and exploring sense organs. To reduce the agnosias to a series of disconnections between the striate and parastriate cortex and other parts of the brain, although an interesting approach, leads to an overly simplified mechanistic view of cerebral activity which probably will not be sustained as more knowledge of cerebral physiology is acquired. There is still a great need of cases in which sensation and perception have been tested in detail and in which the anatomy of the lesion, in its stable end stage, has been studied by serial microscopic sections of the whole brain.

SPECIAL PSYCHOLOGIC TESTS

In the study of focal cerebral disease there are two approaches—the clinical-neurologic and the psychometric. The first consists of the observation and recording of qualitative changes in behavior and performance and the identification of syndromes from which there may be deductions as to the locus and nature of certain diseases.

The second consists of recording a patient's level of performance on a variety of psychologic tests that have been standardized in a large population of age-matched normal individuals. These tests provide data that can be graded and treated statistically. An example is the *deterioration index* deduced from the difference in performance on subtest items of the Wechsler Adult Intelligence Scale which hold up well in cerebral diseases (vocabulary, information, picture completion, and object assembly) and those which undergo impairment (digit span, similarities, digit symbol, and block design). The main criticism of this and other scatter patterns, such as the Halstead-Reitan impairment index, is the implicit assumption that cerebral activity is a unitary function, the defects of which are quantitative and related to the volume of the lesion rather than its location. The neurologic arguments against this notion were given in the introduction to this chapter.

Nonetheless it cannot be denied that there are certain psychometric scales which reveal disease in certain parts of the cerebrum more than in others and provide data that allow comparison of the patient's deficits from one point in the course of an illness to another. Walsh has listed those that he finds most valuable in his text on neuropsychology. In addition to the Wechsler Adult Intelligence Scale, Wechsler Memory Scale, and an aphasia screening test he recommends the following for quantitation of:

I. *Frontal lobe disorders*
  A. Milan sorting test, Halstead category test, and Wisconsin card-sorting test, as tests of ability to abstract
  B. The Porteus Maze Test, Reitan Trail Making Test, the recognition of figures in the Figure of Rey as tests of planning, regulating, and checking programs of action
  C. Benton's Verbal Fluency Test for estimating verbal skill and verbal regulation of behavior

II. *Temporal lobe disorders*
  A. Figure of Rey, Benton Visual Retention Test, Illinois Nonverbal Sequential Memory Test, Recurring Nonsense Figures of Kimura, and Facial Recognition Test as modality specific memory tests
  B. Milner's Maze Learning Task and Lhermitte-Signoret amnesic syndrome tests for general retentive memory
  C. Seashore Rhythm Test, Speech-Sound Perception Test from the Halstead-Reitan battery, Environmental Sounds Test, and Austin Meaningless Sounds Test, as measures of auditory perception

III. *Parietal lobe disorders*
  A. Figure of Rey, Wechsler Block Design and Object Assembly, Benton Figure Copying Test, Halstead-Reitan Tactual Performance Test, and Fairfield Block Substitution Test as tests of constructional praxis
  B. Several mathematical and logicogrammatical tests as tests of spatial synthesis
  C. Cross-modal association tests as tests of suprasensory integration

D. Benson-Barton Stick Test, Cattell's Pool Reflection Test, and Money's Road Map Test, as tests of spatial perception and memory

IV. *Occipital lobe disorders*

A. Color naming, color form association, visual irreminiscence, as tests of visual perception; recognition of faces of prominent people, map drawing

It is the authors' opinion that the data obtained from the above tests should supplement clinical observations. Taken alone, they cannot be depended upon for the localization of cerebral lesions.

DISTURBANCES OF THE NONDOMINANT CEREBRAL HEMISPHERE

Surgical sectioning of the corpus callosum (see below) has stimulated interest in the functions of the right cerebral hemisphere, when isolated from the left. It is in the sphere of visual-spatial perception that right hemispheric dominance is most convincing. Lesions of the right posterior cerebral region result in an inability to utilize information about spatial relationships in making perceptual judgments and in responding to objects in a spatial framework. This is manifest in constructing figures (constructional apraxia), in the spatial orientation of the patient (topographic agnosia), in identifying faces (prosopagnosia), and in relating to one another a scattering of visual stimuli (simultanagnosia). Also there are claims that the right hemisphere is more important than the left in visual imagery, in attention, in emotion (both in feeling and the perception of emotion in others), but the evidence is less firm. The idea of its importance in attention derives from the neglect of left visual space and of somatic sensation in the anosognosic syndrome, and also the apparent apathy of such patients.

DISCONNECTION SYNDROMES

Several clinical syndromes, the result of interruption of the connections between the two cerebral hemispheres in the corpus callosum or adjacent white matter (commissural syndromes) or between different parts of one hemisphere (intrahemispheric disconnection syndromes), have been delineated. Some of these are illustrated in Figs. 21-6 and 21-7.

When the entire corpus callosum has been destroyed by tumor or surgical section, the language and perception areas of the left hemisphere are isolated from the right hemisphere. These patients, if blindfolded, are unable to match an object held in one hand with that in the other. Objects placed in the right hand are named correctly, but not those in the left. Furthermore, if rapid presentation is used to avoid bilateral visual scanning, they cannot match an object seen in the right half of the visual field with one

in the left half and they cannot read words projected to the left visual field. They are alexic in the left visual fields since the verbal symbols that are seen there have no access to the language areas of the left hemisphere. If given a verbal command, they execute it correctly with the right hand, but not with the left. For example, if asked to write from dictation with the left hand, they produce only an illegible scrawl.

In most lesions confined to the posterior fifth of the corpus callosum (splenium), only the visual part of the disconnection syndrome occurs. Occlusion of the left posterior cerebral artery provides the best examples of the latter. Since infarction of the left occipital lobe causes a right homonymous hemianopia, all visual information needed for activating the speech areas of the left hemisphere must thereafter come from the right occipital lobe. Patients with a lesion of the splenium of the corpus callosum or the adjacent white matter cannot read or name colors because the visual information cannot reach the left angular gyrus. There is no difficulty in copying words; presumably the visual information for activating the left motor area crosses the corpus callosum more anteriorly. Spontaneous writing and writing to dictation are also intact because the language areas, including the angular gyrus, Wernicke's and Broca's areas, and the left motor cortex are intact and connected. The patients are unable to read what they have written unless it is memorized.

A lesion that is limited to the anterior third of the corpus callosum (or a surgical section of this part, as in patients with intractable epilepsy) does not result in an apraxia of the left hand, i.e., a failure of only the left hand to obey spoken commands, the right one performing normally. A section of the entire corpus callosum does result in such an apraxia, indicating that the fiber systems that connect the left to the right motor areas cross in the corpus callosum posterior to the genu (but anterior to the splenium). Object naming and matching of colors without naming them are done without error.

Of interest to the authors is the fact that one often encounters patients with a lesion in all or some part of the corpus callosum without being able to demonstrate the aforementioned disconnection syndromes. Is the lesion incomplete? Probably not in every case. Notable is the observation that in some patients with a congenital absence of the corpus callosum (a not uncommon developmental abnormality) none of the interhemispheral disconnection syndromes can be found. One can only suppose that in such patients information is transferred by another route—perhaps the anterior or posterior commissure.

Of intrahemispheric disconnections, the following have received the most attention. They are mentioned here only briefly and are considered in detail in the following chapter.

1. *Conduction* (also called "central") *aphasia.* The patient has fluent, but paraphasic, speech and writing, impaired repetition, and relatively intact comprehension of spoken and written language. Wernicke's area in the temporal lobe is separated from Broca's area, probably by a lesion in the arcuate fasciculus.

2. *Sympathetic apraxia in Broca's aphasia.* By destroying the origin of the fibers that connect the left and right motor association cortices, a lesion in the subcortical white matter underlying Broca's area and contiguous cortex or anterior corpus callosum causes an apraxia of command movements of the left hand.

3. *Pure word deafness.* Although the patient is able to hear and to identify nonverbal sounds, there is loss of ability to comprehend spoken language. The patient's speech remains normal. This defect has been attributed to a subcortical lesion of the left temporal lobe, spanning Wernicke's area, interrupting also those fibers that cross from one Wernicke's area to another in the corpus callosum, and preventing them from activating the left auditory region. Bilateral temporal lesions have the same effect.

OTHER BEHAVIORAL DISORDERS ASSOCIATED WITH CEREBRAL DISEASE

When one attempts to categorize all the patients with relatively acute or subacute disorders of mentation and behavior discussed above, there remains a considerable number that defy classification. These patients present an almost infinite variety of syndromes in which the following abnormalities of function may occur: reduced or increased levels of speech, thought, and action; disorientation as to time and place; idleness and lack of interest; loss of sense of humor, or inappropriate jocularity; resistiveness and negativism; lack of observance of social custom, use of abusive and vulgar language; inexplicable euphoria and lack of proper concern; complaint of excess sensitivity to sounds; distortions of smell and taste; inability to follow a conversation or to think coherently; sexual indiscretion, lack of modesty, and other signs of disinhibition; and disturbances of sleep. Obviously not all these many symptoms have the same basic significance, and the majority possess only relative localizing value. They may be associated with definite hemiparesis, hemihypesthesia, aphasia, or hom-

onymous hemianopia; but even without these lateralizing signs they point to the existence of cerebral disease.

Syndromes comprising these elements may be observed in subacute inclusion body encephalitis, Behçet meningoencephalitis, adult toxoplasmosis, infectious mononucleosis, acute or subacute demyelinative diseases (acute or subacute recurrent multiple sclerosis), granulomatous and other forms of angiitis, gliomatosis cerebri, carcinomatous meningitis, endothelial angiomatosis, multiple tumor metastases, acute and subacute bacterial endocarditis, widespread atheromatous or myxomatous embolization, Whipple disease, and thrombopenia with small vessel thrombosis. A fuller account of some of these cerebral symptoms will be found in the chapters dealing with these diseases.

REFERENCES

ANDREW J, NATHAN PW: Lesions of the anterior frontal lobes and disturbances of micturition and defaecation. *Brain* 87:233, 1964.

ANGEVINE JB JR, COTMAN CW: *Principles of Neuroanatomy.* New York, Oxford University Press, 1981.

BAY E: Disturbances of visual perception and their examination. *Brain* 76:515, 1953.

BAILEY P, VON BONIN G: *The Isocortex in Man.* Urbana, IL, University of Illinois Press, 1951.

BALINT R: Seelenlahmung des "Schauens" optische Ataxie, raumliche Storung der Aufmerksamkeit. *Monatsschr Psychiat Neurol* 25:51, 1909.

BENTON AL: The fiction of Gerstmann's syndrome. *J Neurol Neurosurg Psychiatry* 24:176, 1961.

BODAMER J: Die Prosop Agnosie. *Arch Psychiatr Nervenkr* 179:6, 1947.

BRAIN R: Visual disorientation with special reference to lesions of the right hemisphere. *Brain* 64:244, 1941.

BRICKNER RM: *The Intellectual Functions of the Frontal Lobes.* New York, Macmillan, 1936.

BUTTERS N, BRODY BA: The role of the left parietal lobe in the mediation of intra- and cross-modal associations. *Cortex* 4:328, 1968.

CARMON A: Sequenced motor performance in patients with unilateral cerebral lesions. *Neuropsychologia* 9:445, 1971.

CARMON A. BENTON AL: Tactile perception of direction and number in patients with unilateral cerebral disease. *Neurology* 19:525, 1969.

CHAPMAN LF, WOLFF HF: The cerebral hemispheres and the highest integrative functions of man. *Arch Neurol* 1:357, 1959.

CLARK WE LEG: The connexions of the frontal lobes of the brain. *Lancet* 1:353, 1948.

CORKIN S, MILNER B, RASMUSSEN T: Effects of different cortical excisions on sensory thresholds in man. *Trans Am Neurol Assoc* 89:112, 1964.

CRITCHLEY M: *The Parietal Lobes.* London, Arnold, 1953.

DAMASIO AR: The frontal lobes, in Heilman KM, Valenstein E (eds): *Clinical Neuropsychology,* 2nd ed. New York, Oxford University Press, 1985, pp 339–375.

DAMASIO AR, BENTON AL: Impairment of hand movements under visual guidance. *Neurology* 29:170, 1979.

DAMASIO AR, DAMASIO H, VAN HOESEN GW: Prosopagnosia: Anatomic basis and behavioral mechanisms. *Neurology* 32:331, 1982.

DAMASIO AR, VAN HOESEN GW: Emotional disturbances associated with focal lesions of the limbic frontal lobe, in Heilman KM, Satz P (eds): *Neuropsychology of Human Emotion,* New York, Guilford Press, 1983, pp 85–110.

DAMASIO A, YAMADA T, DAMASIO H et al: Central achromatopsia: Behavioral, anatomic, and physiologic aspects. *Neurology* 30:1064, 1980.

DÉJERINE J, MOUZON J: Un nouveau type de syndrome sensitif corticale observe dans un cas de monoplégie corticale dissociée. *Rev Neurol* 28:1265, 1914–1915.

DENNY-BROWN D: The frontal lobes and their functions, in Feiling A (ed): *Modern Trends in Neurology.* New York, Hoeber-Harper, 1951, pp 13–89.

DENNY-BROWN D, BANKER B: Amorphosynthesis from left parietal lesion. *Arch Neurol Psychiatry* 71:302, 1954.

DENNY-BROWN D, CHAMBERS RA: Physiologic aspects of visual perception. 1. Functional aspects of visual cortex. *Arch Neurol* 33:219, 1976.

DENNY-BROWN D, MEYER JS, HORENSTEIN S: Significance of perceptual rivalry resulting from parietal lesions. *Brain* 75:433, 1952.

FISHER CM: Anger associated with dysphasia. *Trans Am Neurol Assoc* 95:240, 1970.

GASSEL MM: Occipital lobe syndromes (excluding hemianopia), in Vinken PJ, Bruyn GW (eds): *Handbook of Clinical Neurology,* vol 2. New York, American Elsevier, 1969, chap 19, pp 640–679.

GESCHWIND N: The clinical syndromes of cortical disconnections, in Williams D (ed): *Modern Trends in Neurology,* vol 5. London, Butterworth, 1970, p 29.

GESCHWIND N, QUADFASEL FA, SEGARRA J: Isolation of the speech area. *Neuropsychologia* 6:327, 1968.

GLONING I, GLONING K, HAFF H: *Neuropsychological Symptoms and Syndromes in Lesions of the Occipital Lobes and Adjacent Areas.* Paris, Gauthier-Villars, 1968.

GOLDSTEIN K: The significance of the frontal lobes for mental performance. *J Neurol Psychopathol* 17:27, 1936.

GUARD O, DELPY C, RICHARD D et al: Une cause malconnue de confusion mentale: le ramollissement temporal droit. *Rev Med* 40:2115, 1979.

HARLOW JM: Quoted in Denny-Brown D: The frontal lobes and their functions, in Feiling A (ed): *Modern Trends in Neurology.* New York, Hoeber, 1951, p 65.

HEAD H, HOLMES G: Sensory disturbances from cerebral lesions. *Brain* 34:102, 1911.

HEBB DO, PENFIELD W: Human behavior after extensive bilateral removal of the frontal lobes. *Arch Neurol Psychiatry* 44:421, 1940.

HÉCAEN H: Clinical symptomatology in right and left hemispheric lesions, in Mountcastle VB (ed): *Interhemispheric Relations and Cerebral Dominance.* Baltimore, Johns Hopkins, 1962, chap 10, pp 215–263.

HEILMAN KA, VALENSTEIN E: *Clinical Neuropsychology.* New York, Oxford University Press, 1979.

HENSCHEN SE: *Klinische und Anatomische Beiträge zur Pathologie des Gehirns,* vols 5–7. Stockholm, Nordiska Bokhandel n, 1920–1922.

HOFF H, PÖTZL O: Zur diagnostischen Bedeutung der Polyopie bei Tumoren des Occipitalhirnes. *Z Gesamte Neurol Psychiatr* 152:433, 1935.

HOLMES G: Disturbances of spatial orientation and visual attention with loss of stereoscopic vision. *Arch Neurol Psychiatry* 1:385, 1919.

HUBEL D: Exploration of the primary visual cortex. *Nature* 299:515, 1982.

HUBEL DH, WIESEL TN: Receptive fields, binocular interaction and functional architecture in the cat's visual cortex. *J Physiol* 160:106, 1962.

JACOBSEN CF: Functions of frontal association in primates. *Arch Neurol Psychiatry* 33:558, 1935.

JOYNT RJ, GOLDSTEIN MN: Minor cerebral hemisphere, in Friedlander WJ (ed): *Advances in Neurology,* vol 7. New York, Raven Press, 1975, pp 147–183.

KAAS JH: What if anything is S_1? Organization of the first somatosensory area of cortex. *Physiol Rev* 63:206, 1983.

KINSBOURNE M, WARRINGTON EK: A disorder of simultaneous form perception. *Brain* 85:461, 1962.

KINSBOURNE M, WARRINGTON EK: The localizing significance of limited simultaneous visual form perception. *Brain* 86:697, 1963.

KLÜVER H, BUCY PC: An analysis of certain effects of bilateral temporal lobectomy in the rhesus monkey with special reference to psychic blindness. *J Psychol* 5:33, 1938.

LANDIS T, CUMMINGS JL, BENSON F, PALMER EP: Loss of topographic familiarity. An envrionmental agnosia. *Arch Neurol* 43:132, 1986.

LAPLANE D, TALAIRACH J, MEININGER V et al: A motor consequence of motor area ablations in man. *J Neurol Sci* 31:29, 1977a.

LAPLANE D, TALAIRACH J, MEININGER V et al: Clinical consequence of corticectomies involving supplementary motor area in man. *J Neurol Sci* 34:301, 1977b.

LEVINE D: Prosopagnosia and visual object agnosia. *Brain Lang* 5:341, 1978.

LEVINE DN, CALVANIO R: A study of the visual defect in verbal alexia–simultanagnosia. *Brain* 101:65, 1978.

LHERMITTE F: Human autonomy and the frontal lobes. II. Patient behavior in complex and social situations. The "environmental dependency syndrome." *Ann Neurol* 19:335, 1986.

LHERMITTE F: Utilization behavior and its relation to lesions of the frontal lobes. *Brain* 106:237, 1983.

LILLY R, CUMMINGS SL, BENSON F, FRANKEL M: The human Klüver-Bucy syndrome. *Neurology* 33:1141, 1983.

LURIA AR: *Higher Cortical Functions in Man.* New York, Basic Books, 1966.

LURIA AR: Frontal lobe syndromes, in Vinken PJ, Bruyn GW (eds): *Handbook of Clinical Neurology,* vol 2. Amsterdam, North-Holland, 1969, chap 23, pp 725–759.

LURIA, AR: *The Working Brain.* London, Allen Lane, 1973.

MacLean PD: Chemical and electrical stimulation of hippocampus in unrestrained animals. II. Behavioral findings. *Arch Neurol Psychiatry* 78:128, 1957.

McCarthy RA, Warrington EK: Visual associative agnosia: A clinico-anatomical study of a single case. *J Neurol Neurosurg Psychiatry* 49:1233, 1986.

Marlowe WB, Mancall EL, Thomas JJ: Complete Kluver-Bucy syndrome in man. *Cortex* 11:53, 1975.

Meadows JC: The anatomical basis of prosopagnosia. *J Neurol Neurosurg Psychiatry* 37:489, 1974a.

Meadows JC: Disturbed perception of colors associated with localized cerebral lesions. *Brain* 97:615, 1974b.

Merzenich MM, Brugge JF: Representation of the cochlear partition on the superior temporal plane of the macaque monkey. *Brain Res* 50:275, 1973.

Milner B: Interhemispheric differences in the localization of psychological processes in man. *Br Med Bull* 27:272, 1971.

Nielsen JM: *Agnosia, Apraxia, Aphasia: Their Value in Cerebral Localization,* 2nd ed, New York, Hoeber, 1946.

Obrador S: Temporal lobotomy. *J Neuropathol Exp Neurol* 6:185, 1947.

Penfield W, Rasmussen P: *The Cerebral Cortex of Man.* New York, Macmillan, 1950.

Penfield D, Roberts L: *Speech and Brain Mechanisms.* Princeton, New Jersey, Princeton University Press, 1956.

Phillips S, Sangalang V, Sterns G: Basal forebrain infarction. A clinicopathologic correlation. *Arch Neurol* 44:1134, 1987.

Polyak SL: *The Vertebrate Visual System.* University of Chicago Press, 1957.

Reitan RW: Psychological deficits resulting from cerebral deficits in man, in Warren JM, Akert K (eds): *The Frontal Granular Cortex and Behavior.* New York, McGraw-Hill, 1964, chap 14.

Rylander G: Personality changes after operations on the frontal lobes. *Acta Psychiatr Scand Suppl* 20: 1939.

Segarra JM, Quadfasel FA: Destroyed temporal lobe tips: Preserved ability to sing. *Proc VII Internat Cong Neurol* 2:377, 1961.

Semmes J, Weinstein S, Ghent L, Teuber HL: *Somatosensory Changes After Penetrating Brain Wounds in Man.* Cambridge, Massachusetts, Harvard University Press, 1960.

Shankweiler DP: Performance of brain-damaged patients on two tests of sound localization. *J Comp Physiol Psychol* 54:375, 1961.

Sperry RW, Gazzaniga MS, Bogen JE: The neocortical commissures: Syndrome of hemisphere disconnection, in Vinken PJ, Bruyn GW (eds): *Handbook of Clinical Neurology,* vol 4. Amsterdam, North-Holland, 1969, chap 14, pp 273–290.

Stuss DT, Benson DF: *The Frontal Lobes.* New York, Raven Press, 1986.

Tissot R, Constantinidis J, Richard J: *La Maladie de Pick,* Paris, Masson et Cie, 1975.

van Buren JM: Trans-synaptic retrograde degeneration in the visual system of primates. *J Neurol Neurosurg Psychiatry* 26:402, 1963.

Walsh FB, Hoyt WF: The visual sensory system: Anatomy, physiology and topographic diagnosis, in Vinken PJ, Bruyn GW (eds): *Handbook of Clinical Neurology,* vol 2. Amsterdam, North-Holland, 1969, chap 18, pp 506–639.

Walsh KW: *Neuropsychology: A Clinical Approach.* Edinburgh, Churchill Livingstone, 1978.

Weintraub S, Mesulam M-M: Right cerebral dominance in spatial attention. *Arch Neurol* 44:621, 1987.

Weiskrantz L, Warrington EK, Saunders MD et al: Visual capacity in the blind field following a restricted occipital ablation. *Brain* 97:709, 1974.

Wolpert I: Die Simultanagnosie-Störung der Gesamtauffassung. *Z Gesamte Neurol Psychiatr* 93:397, 1924.

CHAPTER 22

AFFECTIONS OF SPEECH AND LANGUAGE

Speech and language functions are of fundamental human significance, both in social intercourse and in private intellectual life. When they are disturbed as a consequence of brain disease, the resultant functional loss exceeds all others in gravity—even blindness, deafness, and paralysis.

The neurologist is concerned with all derangements of speech and language, including those of reading and writing, because they are the source of great disability and are almost invariably manifestations of disease of the brain. In a narrower context, language is the means whereby patients communicate their complaints and problems to the physician and at the same time the medium for all the delicate interpersonal transactions between physician and patient. Therefore any disease process that interferes with speech or the understanding of spoken words touches the very core of the physician-patient relationship. Finally, the clinical study of language disorders serves to illuminate the abstruse relation between psychologic functions and the anatomy and physiology of the brain. Language mechanisms fall somewhere between the well-localized sensorimotor functions and the more complex mental operations such as imagination and thinking, which cannot be localized.

GENERAL CONSIDERATIONS

It has been remarked that as human beings our commanding position in the animal world rests on the possession of two faculties: (1) the ability to develop and employ verbal symbols as a background for our own ideation and as a means of transmitting thoughts, by spoken and written word, to others of our kind; and (2) the remarkable facility in the use of our hands. One curious and provocative fact is that the evolution of both language and manual dexterity occurs in relation to particular aggregates of neurons and pathways in one (the dominant) cerebral hemisphere. This is a departure from most other localized neurophysiologic activities, which are organized according to a contralateral or bilateral and symmetrical plan. The dominance of one

hemisphere, usually the left, emerges with speech and the preference for the right hand, especially for writing; and a lack of development or loss of cerebral dominance as a result of disease entails a disturbance of both these traits.

There is abundant evidence that higher animals are able to communicate with one another by vocalization and gestures. However, the content of their communication is their feeling tone of the moment. This emotional language, as it is called, was studied by Charles Darwin, who noted that it undergoes increasing differentiation in the animal kingdom. Only in the chimpanzee are the first semblances of propositional speech recognizable.

Similar instinctive patterns of emotional expression are observed in human beings. They are the earliest modes of expression to appear (in infancy) and may have been the first forms of speech in primitive human beings. Moreover, the language we use to express joy, anger, and fear is retained even after destruction of all the language areas in the dominant cerebral hemisphere. The neural arrangements for this paralinguistic form of communication (by means of intonation, facial expression, eye movements, body gestures), which subserves emotional expression, are bilateral and symmetrical and do not depend solely on the cerebrum. The experiments of Cannon and Bard amply demonstrated that emotional expression is possible in animals after removal of both cerebral hemispheres, provided the diencephalon and particularly the hypothalamic part of it remains intact. In the human infant, emotional expression is well developed at a time when much of the cerebrum is still immature.

Propositional or symbolic language differs from emotional language in several ways. Instead of communicating feeling it is the means of transferring ideas from one person to another, and it requires in its development the substitution of a series of sounds or marks for objects, persons, and concepts. This is the essence of language. As was stated, propositional or symbolic speech is not found in animals or in the human infant. It is not instinctive but learned and is therefore subject to all the modifying influences of social environment and culture. However, the learning process becomes possible only after the nervous system has reached a certain degree of development. Facility in symbolic language, which is acquired over a period of 15 to 20 years, depends then both on the maturation of the nervous system and on education.

Although speech and language are closely interwoven functions, they are not strictly synonymous. A derangement of language function is always a reflection of an abnormality of the brain and, more specifically, of the dominant cerebral hemisphere. A disorder of speech may have a similar origin, but not necessarily; it may be due to abnormalities in different parts of the brain, or to extracerebral mechanisms. Language function involves the comprehension, formulation, and transmission of ideas and feelings by the use of conventionalized signs, marks, sounds, and gestures and their sequential ordering according to accepted rules of grammar. Speech, on the other hand, refers more to the articulatory and phonetic aspects of verbal expression.

The profound importance of language in contemporary society may be overlooked unless one reflects on the proportion of our time devoted to purely verbal pursuits. *External speech,* or *exophasy,* by which is meant the expression of thought by spoken or written words and the comprehension of the spoken or written words of others, is an almost continuous activity when human beings are gathered together; *inner speech,* or *endophasy,* i.e., the silent processes of thought and the formulation in our minds of unuttered words on which thought depends, is ''the coin of mental commerce.'' The latter is almost incessant during our preoccupations, since we think always with words. Thought and language are inseparable. In learning to think, the child talks aloud to itself and only later learns to suppress the vocalization. Even adults may mutter subconsciously when pondering a difficult proposition. As Gardiner remarks, any abstract thought can only be held in mind by the word or mathematical symbol denoting it. It is entirely impossible to comprehend what is meant by ''religion'' without the controlling and limiting consciousness of the word itself. Words have thus become part of the mechanism of our thinking and remain for ourselves and for others the guardians of our thought (quoted by Brain). This is the reasoning that persuaded Head, Wilson, Goldstein, and others that any theory of language must include explanations not only in terms of cerebral anatomy and physiology, but also of physical processes, no one of which is superimposable on the other.

ANATOMY OF THE LANGUAGE FUNCTIONS

The conventional teaching is that there are three main language areas, situated, in most persons, in the left cerebral hemisphere (Fig. 22-1). Two are receptive and one is executive. The two receptive areas are closely related and embrace what may be referred to as the central language zone. One, subserving the perception of spoken language, occupies a crescentic zone in the posterior one-third of the first temporal convolution (areas 41 and 42, or Wernicke's area), just lateral to the primary auditory receptive area in Heschl's gyri; another, subserving the perception of written language, occupies the angular convolution (area 39) in the inferior parietal lobule, anterior to the visual receptive areas. The supramarginal gyrus, which lies between these auditory and visual language ''centers,'' and the inferior temporal region (area 37), just anterior to the visual association cortex, are probably part of this central language zone as well. Here are located the integrative centers for crossmodal visual and auditory functions. The third area situated at the posterior end of the inferior frontal convolution is referred to as Broca's area or Brodmann's area 44 and is concerned with motor aspects of speech. The entire language zone is perisylvian, i.e., it borders the sylvian fissure.

These sensory and motor areas are intricately connected by nerve fibers, one large bundle of which, the arcuate fasciculus, passes through the isthmus of the temporal lobe and around the posterior end of the sylvian fissure; other connections may traverse the external capsule of the lenticular nucleus (subcortical white matter of the

Figure 22-1

Diagram of the brain showing the classic language areas, numbered according to the scheme of Brodmann. The elaboration of speech and language probably depends on a much larger area of cerebrum, indicated roughly by the entire shaded zone (see text).

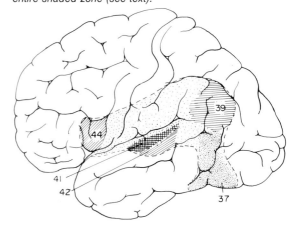

insula). There are also many corticocortical connections and other fiber systems leading into these perisylvian zones and projecting from them to other parts of the brain. The visual receptive and somatosensory cortices connect via the parietal lobe, and the auditory receptive zones, via the temporal lobe. Short association fibers join Broca's area with the lower rolandic cortex, which in turn innervates the speech apparatus, i.e., the muscles of the lips, tongue, pharynx, and larynx. These language areas are also connected with the striatum and thalamus and to corresponding areas in the minor cerebral hemisphere through the corpus callosum and anterior commissure (Figs. 21-6 and 21-7).

There has been much difference of opinion concerning these cortical areas, and objection has been made to calling them centers, for they do not represent histologically circumscribed structures of constant function. Actually there is relatively little information concerning their anatomy and physiology. A competent neuroanatomist could not distinguish these cortical language areas microscopically from the cerebral cortex that surrounds them. Some of the receptor zones are polymodal, i.e., are activated by auditory, visual, and tactile stimuli. Presumably their function is integrative. Electrical stimulation of the anterior cortical language areas while the patient is alert and talking (during craniotomy under local anesthesia) may induce a simple vocalization, usually a single-vowel monotone, but otherwise causes only an arrest of speech. Electrical stimulation of Wernicke's area causes errors of speech, such as stumbling over a word or saying the wrong word.

Knowledge of the location of language functions has come almost exclusively from the postmortem study of humans with focal brain diseases. Two major theories have emerged. One, enunciated by Lichtheim, subdivides the language zone into separate afferent and efferent channels and auditory and visual perceptive parts, connected by identifiable tracts to the executive centers. Depending on the exact anatomy of the lesions, a number of special syndromes are elicited. The other theory, advanced by Marie, and favored by Head, Wilson, Brain, and Goldstein, favors a single central language mechanism, whose physiology is even more complicated than that underlying voluntary movement of the hand in skilled acts. In recent years, Geschwind has popularized the first theory, resurrecting the original postulations of Wernicke and Déjerine. From the available evidence, the authors are unable to accept the idea that the language structure and mechanism are divisible into discrete parts, each specifiable language function depending on a certain fixed group of neurons. Instead, language must be regarded as an integrated sensorimotor process, roughly localized in the opercular, or perisylvian, region of the dominant cerebral hemisphere. Undeniably there is, within the language area, a kind of afferent and

efferent localization, as discussed below, but there is also a presently undifferentiable central mass action, in which the degree of deficit is to a considerable extent influenced by the size of the lesion.

Carl Wernicke, of Breslau, more than any other person, must be credited with the anatomic-psychologic scheme upon which many contemporary ideas of aphasia rest. Earlier, Paul Broca (1865), and even before him, Dax (1836), had made the fundamental observations that a lesion of the insula and the overlying operculum deprived a person of speech, and that such lesions were always in the left hemisphere. Wernicke's thesis was that there were two major anatomic loci for language: (1) an anterior locus, in the posterior part of the inferior frontal lobe (Broca's area), in which were contained the "memory images" of speech movements, and (2) the insular region and adjoining parts of the posterior perisylvian cortex, which was the center for the images of sounds (Meynert had already shown that aphasia could occur with lesions in the temporal lobe, Broca's area being intact). Wernicke believed that the fibers between these regions ran in the insula and mediated the psychic reflex arc between the heard and spoken word. Later, Wernicke came to accept von Monakow's view that the connecting fibers ran around the posterior end of the sylvian fissure, in the arcuate fasciculus.

Wernicke gave a comprehensive description of the receptive or sensory aphasia that now bears his name. The four main features, he pointed out, were a disturbance of comprehension of spoken and written language (alexia), agraphia, and fluent paraphasic speech. In Broca's aphasia, by contrast, comprehension was intact, but the patient was mute or employed only a few simple words. Wernicke theorized that a lesion interrupting the connecting fibers between the two cortical speech areas would give rise to a disturbance in which the patient's comprehension would be undisturbed, but the intact sound images would be unable to exert an influence on the choice of words. Wernicke proposed that this variety of aphasia be called *Leitungsaphasie*, or conduction aphasia; later it was given the name "central aphasia" by Kurt Goldstein.

This anatomic scheme was the basis of Wernicke's classification of aphasia, and although it was much criticized by Pierre Marie, Henry Head, von Monakow, Arnold Pick, and Goldstein, the anatomic plans which they proposed coincided roughly with that of Wernicke. Careful case analyses since the time of Broca and Wernicke have repeatedly documented an association between the receptive (Wernicke) type of aphasia and lesions in the posterior perisylvian region and between a predominantly (Broca) motor aphasia and lesions in the posterior part of the inferior frontal convolution and the adjacent motor, insular, and opercular regions of the cortex. The concept of a conduction aphasia, based upon an interruption of pathways between Wernicke's and Broca's zones, has been the most difficult to accept, because it presupposes a neat separation of sensory and motor functions, which is not in line with contemporary views of sensorimotor physiology of the rest of the nervous system. Nevertheless, there are in the medical literature a few descriptions of cases that conform to the Wernicke model of conduction aphasia; the lesion in these cases most often lies in the parietal operculum, involving the white matter deep to the supramarginal gyrus, where it presumably interrupts the arcuate fasciculus or insular subcortex.

Thus it appears that human language function depends upon the integrity of an anatomic region situated between the primary receptive areas of the temporal and occipital lobes (and their association areas in the parietal and temporal lobes) and the motor areas in the inferior frontal lobe of the dominant hemisphere. This places the language area in close connection with the cortical sensory association and cross-modal elaboration areas of the superior temporal and inferior parietal lobes, with the corresponding parts of the opposite cerebral hemisphere through the corpus callosum, and with the medial parts of the temporal lobes and diencephalon (learning-memory mechanism). But just how these regions of the brain are organized, and how they can be activated (controlled) by a variety of visual and auditory stimuli and bifrontal motivational mechanisms, resulting in the complex behavior of which we make casual daily use in interpersonal communication, remain to a large extent unknown.

Although localization of the lesion that produces aphasia is in most instances roughly predictable from the clinical deficit, there are wide variations in the degree of deficit that follows focal brain disease. Inconsistency of anatomic findings in certain types of aphasia has been explained in several ways. The most popular explanation has been that the net effect of any lesion depends not only on the locus and extent of the lesion but also on the degree of cerebral dominance, i.e., on the degree to which the minor hemisphere assumes language function after damage to the major one. According to this view, a left-sided lesion has less effect on language function if cerebral dominance is poorly established than if dominance is strong. Another explanation invokes the poorly understood concept that individuals differ in the way they acquire language as

children. This is believed to play a role in making available alternative means for accomplishing language tasks when the method initially learned has been impaired through brain disease. The extent to which improvement of aphasia represents ''recovery'' of function or generation of new response methods has not been settled to the present day.

CEREBRAL DOMINANCE AND ITS RELATION TO SPEECH AND HANDEDNESS

The functional supremacy of one cerebral hemisphere is crucial to language function. There are five ways of determining that the left side of the brain is dominant: (1) the loss of speech when disease occurs in certain parts of the left hemisphere and its preservation with lesions involving corresponding parts of the right hemisphere; (2) preference for and greater facility in the use of the right hand, foot, and eye; (3) the arrest of speech immediately after stimulation of the anterior language are during a surgical procedure (see above) or after the injection of sodium amytal (165 mg over a period of 3 to 5 s) into the left internal carotid artery (Wada test). The latter produces mutism for a minute or two, followed by misnaming (including perseveration and substitution), misreading, and paraphasic speech—these effects lasting 8 to 9 mins altogether; and (4) Kimura test of dichotic hearing (the right ear hears words when different ones are delivered to each ear simultaneously; and (5) increased blood flow in the left inferior frontal region when talking, and in the left superior temporal region when listening (Lassen et al).

Approximately 90 to 95 percent of the general population is right-handed; i.e., they choose the right hand for intricate, complex acts and are more skillful with it. The preference is more complete in some persons than in others. Most individuals are neither completely right-handed nor completely left-handed but favor one hand for more complicated tasks.

The reason for hand preference is still controversial. There is strong evidence of a hereditary factor, but the mode of inheritance is uncertain. Yakovlev and Rakic observed in infant brains that the corticospinal tract coming from the left cerebral hemisphere contains more fibers and decussates higher than the tract from the right hemisphere. Learning is also a factor; many children are shifted at an early age from left to right (shifted sinistrals), because it is a handicap to be left-handed in a right-handed world. Many right-handed persons sight with the right eye, and it has been said that eye preference determines hand preference. Even if true, this still does not account for eye dominance. It is noteworthy that handedness develops simultaneously with language, and the most that can be said at present is that localization of language and preference for one eye, hand, and foot are all manifestations of some fundamental, inherited tendency not yet defined. There are slight but definite anatomic differences between the dominant and the nondominant cerebral hemispheres. The *planum temporale*, the region on the superior surface of the temporal lobe between Heschl's gyri and Wernicke's language zone, has been found to be slightly larger on the left in 65 percent of brains and larger on the right in only 11 percent (Geschwind and Levitsky). In angiograms, LeMay and Culebras noted that the left sylvian fissure is longer and more horizontal than the right and that there is a greater mass of cerebral tissue in the area of the left temporoparietal junction. CT scans have shown the right occipital horn to be smaller than the left, possibly indicative of a greater right-sided development of visual-spatial connections. Also, subtle cytoarchitectonic asymmetries of the auditory cortex and posterior thalamus have been described; these and other biologic aspects of cerebral dominance are reviewed by Geschwind and Galaburda.

Left-handedness may result from disease of the left cerebral hemisphere in early life, and this probably accounts for its higher incidence among the feebleminded and brain-injured. Presumably the neural mechanisms for language then become centered in the right cerebral hemisphere. Handedness and cerebral dominance may fail to develop in some individuals, and this is particularly true in certain families. Developmental defects in speech and reading, stuttering, mirror writing, and general clumsiness are much more frequent in these individuals.

In right-handed individuals, aphasia is almost invariably related to a left cerebral lesion; aphasia in such individuals as a result of purely right cerebral lesions (''crossed aphasia'') is very rare, occurring in only 1 percent of cases (see review by Joanette). Cerebral dominance in ambidextrous and left-handed persons is not nearly so uniform. In a large series of left-handed patients with aphasia, 60 percent had lesions confined to the left cerebral hemisphere (Goodglass and Quadfasel). Further, in the relatively rare case of an aphasia due to a right cerebral lesion, the patient is nearly always left-handed; moreover, the language disorder in some such patients is less severe and enduring than in right-handed patients with comparable lesions (Gloning, Subirana). These latter findings suggest a bilateral, albeit unequal, representation of language functions in nonright-handed patients. Using the technique of intracarotid injection of sodium amytal (Wada test, see above) Milner et al found evidence of bilateral speech representation in about 15 percent of 212 consecutively studied nonright-handed patients.

The language capacities of the minor hemisphere have not been documented by careful anatomic studies. As mentioned above, there is always some uncertainty as to whether any residual function after lesions of the major hemisphere can be traced to recovery of parts of its language

zones or to activity of the minor hemisphere. The observations of Levine and Mohr suggest that the nondominant hemisphere has only a limited capacity to produce oral speech after extensive damage of the dominant hemisphere; their patient recovered the ability to sing, recite, curse and utter one or two-word phrases, all of which were abolished by a subsequent minor hemisphere infarction. The fact that varying amounts of language function may remain after dominant hemispherectomy in adults with glioma also suggests a definite though limited capacity of the minor hemisphere for language production. Kinsbourne's observations of the effect of intra-arterial amytal on the right hemisphere of patients aphasic from left-sided lesions makes the same point. Congenital absence (or surgical section) of the corpus callosum, permitting the testing of each hemisphere, has shown virtually no language functions of the right hemisphere.

SPEECH AND LANGUAGE DISORDERS DUE TO DISEASE

These may be divided into four categories:

1. A cerebral disturbance in which there is a loss more or less exclusively of the production or of comprehension of spoken or written language, or both. This condition is called *aphasia* or *dysphasia*.

2. Disturbances of speech and language with diseases that affect the higher nervous integrations, i.e., with diseases causing delirium and dementia. Speech is seldom lost in these conditions but is deranged as part of a general impairment of perceptual and intellectual functions. In Alzheimer disease, a gradual impairment of all elements of language constitutes an important part of the clinical picture (Chap. 20).

Palilalia is a special disorder of speech in which the patient compulsively repeats a phrase or word with decreasing volume and increasing rapidity, finally making only silent articulatory movements of the lips (aphonic palilalia). This abnormality is observed mainly in patients with progressive supranuclear palsy, postencephalitic parkinsonism, and pseudobulbar palsy, but also in other diseases with bilateral upper brainstem lesions. *Echolalia* is a somewhat different disorder, in which the patient repeats, parrot-like, words and phrases that he or she hears. Its most striking occurrence is in patients with transcortical aphasia, in whom there is a marked impairment of auditory comprehension (see further on).

3. A defect in articulation, with intact mental functions and normal comprehension and memory of words. This is a pure motor disorder of the muscles of articulation and may be due to flaccid or spastic paralysis, rigidity, repetitive spasms (stuttering), or ataxia. The terms *dysarthria* and *anarthria* have been applied to some of these conditions.

4. Loss of voice due to a disorder of the larynx or its innervation—*aphonia* or *dysphonia*. Articulation and language are unaffected.

CLINICAL VARIETIES OF APHASIA

Systematic examination will usually enable one to decide whether a patient has a predominantly *motor*, or *Broca's*, *aphasia*, sometimes called "expressive," "anterior," or "nonfluent" aphasia; a *sensory*, or *Wernicke's*, *aphasia*, referred to also as *receptive*, posterior, or fluent aphasia; a *total*, or *global*, *aphasia*, with loss of all or nearly all speech and language functions; or one of the *dissociative language syndromes*, such as conduction aphasia, word deafness (auditory verbal agnosia), word blindness (visual verbal agnosia or alexia), and several types of mutism. Anomia (nominal or amnesic aphasia) and the impaired ability to communicate by writing (agraphia) are found to some degree in practically all types of aphasia. Only rarely does agraphia exist alone. When viewed in relation to the patient's capacity to carry on a conversation, i.e., to speak spontaneously, the fluent and nonfluent forms of language disorder represent extremes on a continuum, in which fluency is affected in all gradations of severity.

MOTOR, OR BROCA'S, APHASIA

Although the precise nature of Broca's aphasia remains somewhat in doubt, we have chosen to apply the term, as have others, to a primary deficit in language output or speech production. In our experience there is a wide range of variation in the motor deficit from the mildest type of so-called cortical dysarthria with intact comprehension and ability to write, to a complete loss of all means of communication through lingual, phonetic, and manual action. Since the muscles that can no longer be used in speaking may still function in other learned acts, i.e., they are not paralyzed, the term *apraxia* seems applicable to certain elements of the deficit.

In the most advanced form of the syndrome patients will have lost all power of speaking aloud. Not a word can

be uttered in conversation, in attempting to read aloud, or to repeat words that are heard. One might suspect that the lingual and phonatory apparatus are paralyzed, until patients are observed to have no difficulty chewing, swallowing, clearing the throat, and even vocalizing without words. Occasionally, the words *yes* and *no* can be uttered, usually in the correct context. Or patients may repeat a few stereotyped utterances over and over again, as if compelled to do so, a disorder referred to as *monophasia* (Critchley), *recurring utterance* (Hughlings Jackson), or *verbal stereotypy* or *automatism*. If speech is possible at all, certain habitual expressions, such as "Hi," "Fine, thank you," or "Good morning," seem to be the easiest, and the words of well-known songs may be sung. When angered or excited, patients may utter an expletive, thus emphasizing the fundamental distinction between propositional and emotional speech (see above). Patients recognize their ineptitudes and mistakes. Repeated failures in speech may cause exasperation or despair.

Often the lower part of the face and arm are weak on the opposite (right) side, and occasionally the leg as well. The tongue may deviate away from the lesion, i.e., to the right, and be slow and awkward in rapid movements. For a time, despite the relative preservation of auditory comprehension and ability to read, commands to purse, smack, or lick the lips, or to blow and whistle and make other purposeful movements are poorly executed, which means that an apraxia has extended to certain other learned oropharyngeal acts. In these circumstances, imitation of the examiner's actions is better performed than execution of acts on command. Self-initiated actions, by contrast, may be normal.

In the milder form of Broca's aphasia and in the recovery phase of the severe form, patients are able to speak aloud to some degree. Words are uttered slowly and laboriously. Enunciation (articulation) and the melody of language (prosody) are disordered. This dysfluency takes the form of improper accent or stress on certain syllables and incorrect intonation and phrasing of words in a series and pacing of word utterances. Speech is sparse (10 to 15 words per minute compared to the normal 100 to 115 words per minute) and consists mainly of nouns, transitive verbs, or important adjectives; phrase length is abbreviated and many of the small words (articles, prepositions, conjunctions) are omitted, giving the speech a telegraphic character (so-called agrammatism). The substantive content allows the patient to communicate ideas to some extent, despite the gross expressive difficulties. Repetition of spoken language is always abnormal. If a patient with nonfluent aphasia has no difficulty in repetition, the condition is one of transcortical aphasia (see further on).

Most patients with Broca's aphasia have a correspondingly severe impairment in writing. Should the right hand be paralyzed, the patient cannot print with the left one, and if the right hand is spared, the patient fails as miserably in writing requests or replies to questions as in speaking them. Letters are malformed and words are misspelled. While writing to dictation is impossible, letters and words can still be copied.

The comprehension of spoken and written language, though normal under many conditions of testing, is usually defective in Broca's aphasia and will break down under stringent testing, especially when novel or complicated material is introduced. Confrontation naming is usually faulty. These are the most variable and controversial aspects of Broca's aphasia. In some patients with a loss of motor speech and agraphia as a result of cerebral infarction, the understanding of spoken and written language may be virtually normal. Mohr has pointed out that in such patients the initial mutism is usually replaced by a rapidly improving dyspraxic and effortful articulation, leading later to complete recovery; the lesion in these cases is restricted to a zone in and immediately around the posterior part of the inferior frontal convolution (Broca's area). Mohr has stressed the distinction between this relatively mild and restricted aphemic type of motor speech disorder and the more complex syndrome that is traditionally referred to as Broca's aphasia. The latter is characterized by greater difficulty in understanding spoken and written language and by protracted mutism; verbal stereotypes, agrammatism, and dysprosody are prominent during the recovery phase. The lesion in this latter disorder involves the inferior frontal gyrus and deep subcortical tissue, the anterior insula and frontal-parietal operculum, and adjacent cerebrum. In other words, the lesion in this form of Broca's aphasia extends well beyond the so-called Broca's area.

It is noteworthy that in one of Broca's original patients, whose expressive language had been limited to a few verbal stereotypes for 10 years before his death, inspection of the surface of the brain (the brain was never cut, although CT scans have since been made) disclosed an extensive lesion, encompassing the left insula, the frontal, central, and parietal operculum, and even part of the inferior parietal lobe, posterior to the sylvian fissure. The Wernicke area was spared, refuting the prediction of Marie. Curiously, Broca attributed the aphasic disorder to the lesion of the frontal operculum alone. (The term *operculum* refers to the cortex around the sylvian fissure, which covers or forms a lid over the insula, or island, of Reil.) Broca ignored the rest of the lesion, which he considered to be a later spreading effect of the stroke. Perhaps Broca was influenced by the prevailing opinion of that time (1861) that articulation was a function of the inferior parts of the frontal lobes. The fact that Broca's name later became attached to a discrete part of the inferior frontal cortex (Brodmann's area 44) helped to entrench the idea that Broca's aphasia equated with a

lesion in Broca's area. However, as pointed out above, a lesion confined to Broca's area gives rise to a relatively modest and transient motor speech disorder (Mohr et al) or to no disorder of speech at all (Goldstein).

Motor speech disorders, both severe Broca's aphasia and the more restricted and transient types, are most often due to a vascular lesion. Embolic infarction in the territory of the upper main (rolandic) division of the middle cerebral artery is probably the most frequent type of vascular lesion and results in the most abrupt onset and sometimes the most rapid regression (occurring in hours or days), depending on whether the ischemic paralysis proceeds to tissue necrosis. Even with the latter, however, transient ischemia around the zone of infarction causes a more extensive syndrome than that of the infarct alone. In other words, the physiologic impairment exceeds the pathologic. Because of the distribution of this artery, there are frequently an associated *right*-sided faciobrachial paresis and a *left*-sided brachial apraxia (due probably to interruption of the fibers that connect the left and right motor cortices). Atherosclerotic thrombosis, tumor, subcortical hypertensive hemorrhage, traumatic hemorrhage, etc., should they involve the appropriate parts of the motor cortex, may also declare themselves by a Broca's aphasia.

A closely related syndrome, *pure word mutism*, also causes the patient to be wordless but leaves inner speech intact and writing undisturbed. Anatomically, this is believed to be in the nature of a disconnection of the motor cortex for speech from lower centers and will be described with the dissociative speech syndromes further on in this chapter.

WERNICKE'S APHASIA

This syndrome comprises two main elements: (1) an impairment in the comprehension of speech—basically an inability to differentiate word elements or phonemes, both spoken and written—which reflects involvement of auditory association areas or their separation from the angular gyrus and the primary auditory cortex (Heschl's transverse gyri); and (2) a fluently articulated but paraphasic speech, which reveals the major role of the auditory region in the regulation of language. The defect in auditory language functions is manifest further by a varying inability to repeat spoken words. The defect in visual language functions is reflected in an inability to read (alexia).

The patient talks volubly, gestures freely, and appears strangely unaware of the deficit. Speech is produced without effort; the phrases and sentences appear to be of normal length and are properly intonated and articulated. Despite the fluency and normal prosody, the patient's speech is remarkably devoid of meaning. In contrast to Broca's aphasia, the patient with Wernicke's aphasia produces words that are nonsubstantive. Also, the words themselves are often malformed or inappropriate, a disorder referred to as *paraphasia*. A phoneme (the minimum unit of sound that permits the differentiation of the meaning of a word) or a syllable may be substituted within a word (e.g., "The grass is greel"); this is called *literal paraphasia*. The substitution of one word for another ("The grass is blue") is called *verbal paraphasia* or *semantic substitution*. Neologisms, i.e., phonemes, syllables, or words that are not part of the language, may also appear ("The grass is grumps"). Fluent paraphasic speech may be entirely incomprehensible (*gibberish* or *jargon aphasia*). Fluency is not an invariable feature of Wernicke's aphasia. Speech may be hesitant, in which case the block tends to occur in that part of a phrase which contains the central communicative (predicative) item, such as a key noun, verb, or descriptive phrase. The patient with such a disorder conveys the impression of constantly searching for the correct word and of having difficulty in finding it.

Although the motor apparatus required for the expression of language may be quite intact, patients with Wernicke's aphasia are unable to function as social organisms because they are deprived of all means of communication. They cannot understand what is said to them; a few simple commands may still be executed, but there is failure to carry out complex ones. They cannot read aloud or silently with comprehension, tell others what they want or think, or write spontaneously. Written letters are often combined into meaningless words, but there may be a scattering of correct words. When trying to designate an object that they see or feel, they cannot find the name, even though they may be able to repeat it from dictation; nor can they write from dictation the very words that they can copy. The copying performance is notably slow and laborious and conforms to the contours of the model, including the examiner's handwriting style. All these defects, of course, may be present in varying degrees of severity. In general, the defects in reading, writing, naming, and repetition parallel in severity the defect in comprehension. There are, however, exceptions in which either reading or the understanding of spoken language is more affected. Some aphasiologists thus speak of two Wernicke syndromes.

In terms of the Wernicke schema, the motor language area is no longer under control of the auditory and referent areas. The latter term designates the cortical areas in the posterior perisylvian region, where visual, tactile, and auditory memories are integrated. The referent centers are also connected with the motor language area, allowing the expression of self-generated verbal thoughts. The language disturbance caused by lesions in the referent centers was called "central aphasia" by Brain and Goldstein. The disconnection of the motor speech area from the auditory and referent centers accounts for the impairment of repetition as well as the ability to read aloud. Reading may remain fluent but with the same paraphasic errors that mar conversational language. The explanation of dyslexia (visual perception of letters and words) in lesions that are centered in the temporal lobe is that most individuals learn to read by transforming the printed word into the auditory form before it can gain access to the referent centers. Only in the congenitally deaf is there a direct pathway between the visual and referent centers.

Wernicke's aphasia that is due to stroke usually improves in time, sometimes to the point where the deficits can be detected only by asking the patient to repeat unfamiliar words from dictation, to name unusual objects or parts of objects, to spell difficult words, or to write complex self-generated sentences. A more favorable prognosis attends those forms of Wernicke's aphasia in which some of the elements, e.g., reading, are only slightly impaired.

As a rule, the lesion lies in the posterior perisylvian region (comprising posterosuperior temporal, opercular supramarginal, angular, and posterior insular gyri) and usually it is due to embolic (less often thrombotic) occlusion of the lower division of the left middle cerebral artery. A "slit hemorrhage" in the subcortex of the temporoparietal region or involvement of this area by tumor, abscess, or extension of a small putaminal or thalamic hemorrhage may have similar effects but a different prognosis. A lesion that involves structures deep to the posterior temporal cortex will cause an associated homonymous hemianopia. Sometimes there are no associated neurologic signs, and the aphasic patient may be misdiagnosed as psychotic.

The posterior perisylvian region appears to encompass a variety of language functions, and seemingly minor changes in size and locale of the lesion are associated with important variations in the elements of Wernicke's aphasia or lead to *conduction aphasia* or to *pure word deafness* (see below). The interesting theoretical problem is whether all the deficits observed are indicative of a unitary language function that resides in the posterior perisylvian region or, instead, of a series of separate sensorimotor activities whose anatomic pathways happen to be crowded together in a small region of the brain. In view of the multiple ways in which language is learned and deteriorates in disease, the latter hypothesis seems more likely.

TOTAL, OR GLOBAL, APHASIA

This syndrome is due to a lesion that destroys a large part of the language area of the major cerebral hemisphere. The lesion is usually due to occlusion of the left internal carotid or middle cerebral artery, but it may be caused by hemorrhage, tumor, or other lesions, and it may occur as a postictal effect. The middle cerebral artery nourishes all of the language area, and nearly all the aphasic disorders due to vascular occlusion are caused by involvement of this artery or its branches.

All aspects of speech and language are affected in global aphasia, as the term implies. At the most, the patients can say only a few words, usually some cliché or habitual phrase. They may understand a few words and phrases, but they characteristically fail to carry out a series of simple commands or to name a series of objects because of rapid fatigue and verbal and motor perseveration (the obligate repetitive evocation of a word or motor act just after it has been employed in another context). They cannot read or write or repeat what is said to them. The patient may participate in common gestures of greeting, show modesty and avoidance reactions, and engage in self-help activities. With the passage of time some degree of comprehension of language may return, and what then is most likely to emerge is the clinical picture of a severe Broca's aphasia.

Varying degrees of right hemiplegia, hemianesthesia, and homonymous hemianopia almost invariably accompany global aphasia of vascular origin. In such patients, language function rarely recovers to a significant degree. On the other hand, improvement frequently occurs when the main cause is cerebral edema, postconvulsive paralysis, or a transient metabolic derangement such as hypoglycemia, hyponatremia, etc., which may worsen an old lesion that had involved language areas. Although speech loss from a disintegrating embolus of the left middle cerebral artery may be transient, some part of the deficit may persist, being easily demonstrated by presenting the patient with complex words or sentences.

DISSOCIATIVE SYNDROMES

This term refers to certain disorders of language that result *not* from lesions of the cortical language areas themselves, but from an alleged interruption of association pathways joining the primary receptive areas to the language areas. Included also in this category are aphasias due to lesions that separate the more strictly receptive parts of the language mechanism from the purely motor ones ("conduction aphasia") and to lesions that isolate the perisylvian speech areas from the other parts of the cerebral cortex ("transcortical aphasias").

The anatomic basis for most of these so-called disconnection syndromes is poorly defined. The concept,

however, is an interesting one and emphasizes the importance of afferent, intercortical, and efferent connections of the language mechanisms. The weakness of the concept is that it may lead to premature acceptance of anatomic and physiologic arrangements that are overly simplistic.

Conduction Aphasia As indicated earlier, Wernicke theorized that certain clinical symptoms would follow a lesion that effectively separated the auditory and motor speech centers, without damaging either of them. Since then, many cases have been described that conform to Wernicke's proposed model of conduction aphasia, which is the name he gave to it.

In many respects the features of conduction aphasia resemble those of Wernicke's aphasia. There is a similar fluency and paraphasia in self-initiated speech, in repeating what is heard, and in reading aloud, and writing is invariably impaired. Dysarthria and dysprosody are lacking or may be present, to a slight degree, in some patients. Speech output may be normal or somewhat reduced. In contrast to Wernicke's aphasia, *patients have little or no difficulty in understanding words that are heard or seen, and are aware of their deficit.* Comprehension is preserved because the connections between the auditory and referent centers are unaffected, according to Levine and Calvanio. Characteristically, *repetition is severely affected*, and the contrast between defective repetition and relatively normal comprehension is said to be an essential feature of the syndrome. One of the best ways of eliciting the defect is to have the patient repeat nonsense syllables. The mistakes are then of the literal paraphasic type, i.e., substitution of a closely but detectably different letter or syllable.

The lesion in autopsied cases has been located in the cortex and subcortical white matter in the upper bank of the sylvian fissure, involving the supramarginal gyrus of the inferior parietal lobule and occasionally the most posterior part of the superior temporal region. It has been said that the critical structure involved is the arcuate fasciculus. This is a fiber tract that streams out of the temporal lobe, proceeding somewhat posteriorly, around the posterior end of the sylvian fissure; there it joins the superior longitudinal fasciculus, deep in the anteroinferior parietal region, and proceeds forward through the suprasylvian opercular region to the motor association cortex, including Broca's area (Figs. 21-6 and 21-7). However, in most of the reported cases, such as those of the Damasios, the external capsule, claustrum, capsula externa and putamen were also involved. Mohr has questioned the purity of conduction aphasia as an aphasic syndrome. In his survey, he found the separation of the conduction from the Wernicke syndrome to be ambiguous and the lesions to be much the same.

The usual cause of conduction aphasia is an embolic occlusion of the ascending parietal or posterior temporal branch of the middle cerebral artery, but other forms of vascular disease, neoplasm, or trauma in this region may produce the same syndrome.

"Pure" Word Deafness (Auditory Verbal Agnosia)

This uncommon disorder originally described by Lichtheim, in 1885, is characterized by an impairment of auditory comprehension, repetition, and ability to write to dictation. The impaired repetition distinguishes word deafness from transcortical aphasia, and the preservation of reading, writing, and spontaneous speech distinguishes it from Wernicke aphasia. In patients with word deafness self-initiated utterances are correctly phrased and the patient's writing and ability to comprehend written language are normal. Such patients may declare that they cannot hear, but shouting does not help, sometimes to their surprise. By audiometric testing no hearing defect is found and nonverbal sounds, such as a doorbell, can be distinguished. The patient is forced to depend heavily on visual cues and frequently uses them well enough to understand most of what is said. However, tests that prevent the use of visual cues readily uncover the deficit. If able to describe the auditory experience, the patient says that words sound like a jumble of noises. As with visual verbal agnosia, the syndrome of "pure" auditory verbal agnosia is not pure, particularly at its onset, and paraphasic and other elements of Wernicke aphasia may be detected (Buchman et al).

In most recorded autopsy studies the lesion has been bilateral, in the middle third of the superior temporal gyri, in a position to interrupt the connections between the primary auditory cortex in the transverse gyri of Heschl and the association areas of the superoposterior cortex of the temporal lobe. The few unilateral lesions have been localized in this part of the dominant temporal lobe. Requirements of small size and superficiality of the lesion in the cortex and subcortical white matter are best fulfilled by an embolic occlusion of a small branch of the lower division of the middle cerebral artery.

"Pure" Word Blindness (Alexia without Agraphia, Visual Verbal Agnosia)

This also is a rare syndrome, in which a literate person loses the ability to read aloud and to understand written script and, often, to name colors, i.e., to match a seen color to its spoken name—*visual verbal color anomia*. Such a person can no longer name or point on command to letters or words although often able to read numbers. Understanding spoken language, repetition of what is heard, writing spontaneously and to dictation, and conversation are all intact. The ability to copy words is better preserved than reading, and the patient may even be able to spell a word or to identify a word that is spelled to him or her. The most striking feature of this syndrome is the retained capacity to write fluently, after which the patient cannot read what has been written (*alexia without agraphia*). Often no complaint about the difficulty is registered; it is discovered almost by accident. In lesser degrees of the affection, the patient manages to read single letters but not to join them together (asyllabia). In this respect the disorder resembles simultanagnosia (see page 369). And when the patient with alexia or dyslexia also has difficulty in auditory comprehension and in repeating spoken words, the syndrome corresponds to Wernicke aphasia.

Autopsies of such cases have usually demonstrated a lesion that destroys the left visual cortex and underlying white matter, particularly the geniculocalcarine tract, as well as the connections of the right visual cortex with the intact language areas of the dominant hemisphere. In the case originally described by Déjerine (1892), this disconnection occurred in the posterior part (splenium) of the corpus callosum, wherein lie the connections between the visual association areas of the two hemispheres (Fig. 21-7). More often the callosal pathways are interrupted in the forceps major or in the paraventricular region (Damasio and Damasio). In either event, the patient is blind in the right half of each visual field by virtue of the left occipital lesion, and visual information reaches only the right occipital lobe; however, this information cannot be transferred, via the callosal pathways, to the angular gyrus of the left (dominant) hemisphere.

A rare variant of this syndrome takes the form of *alexia without agraphia and without hemianopia*. A lesion, deep in the white matter of the left occipital lobe, at its junction with the parietal lobe, interrupts the projections from the intact visual cortex to the angular gyrus but spares the geniculocalcarine pathway (Greenblatt). This lesion, coupled with one in the splenium, prevents all visual information from reaching the angular gyrus.

In yet other cases, the lesion is confined to the angular gyrus and/or the subjacent white matter. In such cases, a right homonymous hemianopia will also be absent but the *alexia may be combined with agraphia,* with anomic aphasia (see below) and other elements of the Gerstmann syndrome, i.e., right-left confusion, acalculia, and finger agnosia (page 365). The entire constellation of symptoms is sometimes referred to as the *syndrome of the angular gyrus.*

"Pure" Word Mutism (Subcortical Motor Aphasia of Wernicke, Anarthria of Marie, Pure Motor Aphasia of Déjerine, Aphemia of Bastian, "Cortical Dysarthria," "Verbal Apraxia") Occasionally, as a result of a vascular lesion or other type of localized injury of the dominant frontal lobe, the patient loses all capacity to speak, while retaining perfectly the ability to write, to understand spoken words, and to read silently with comprehension. Faciobrachial palsy may be associated. From the time speech becomes audible, language may be syntactically complete, showing neither loss of vocabulary nor agrammatism; or there may be varying degrees of dysarthria (hence "cortical dysarthria"), anomia and paraphasic substitutions, especially for consonants. The essential point is that this type of speech disorder is nearly always transitory. Within a few weeks or months language is restored to normal. Bastian and more recently other authors have called this syndrome "aphemia," a term that was used originally by Broca in another context—to describe the severe motor aphasia that now carries his name. Probably the syndrome is closely allied to what Mohr has called "small Broca's aphasia."

The anatomic basis of pure word mutism has not been determined precisely, although reference is made in a few postmortem cases to a lesion in Broca's area. Bastian speculated that there was a separation of Broca's convolution from subcortical motor centers; hence the complete escape of intellectual function, even in the stage of mutism. A particularly well-studied case has been reported by Roch-LeCours and Lhermitte. Their patient uttered only a few sounds for 4 weeks, after which he recovered rapidly and completely. From the onset of the stroke the patient showed no disturbance of comprehension of language or of writing. Autopsy, 10 years later, disclosed an infarct that was confined to the cortex and subjacent white matter of the lowermost part of the precentral gyrus. Broca's area, one gyrus forward, was completely spared.

Anomic (Amnesic, Nominal) Aphasia Some degree of word-finding difficulty is probably the most frequent type of aphasic disturbance. In fact, without some degree of anomia, a diagnosis of aphasia is usually incorrect. Only when this feature is the most notable aspect of language difficulty is the term anomic aphasia employed. In this latter, relatively uncommon form of aphasia, the patient loses only the ability to name objects. There are typical pauses in speech, groping for words, circumlocution, and substitution of another word or phrase that conveys the meaning. Less frequently used words give more trouble. When shown a series of common objects, the patient may tell of their use instead of giving their names. The difficulty applies not only to objects seen but to the names of things

heard or felt (Geschwind), but this is more difficult to demonstrate. Beauvois et al have described a form of bilateral tactile aphasia in which objects seen and verbally mentioned could be named but not those felt with either hand. Recall of the names for letters, digits, and other printed verbal material is almost invariably preserved, and immediate repetition of a spoken name is intact. That the deficit is principally one of naming is shown by the patient's correct use of the object and, usually, by an ability to point to the correct object on hearing or seeing the name. The understanding of what is heard or read is normal. There is a tendency for patients to attribute their failure to forgetfulness or to give some other lame excuse for the disability, suggesting that they are not completely aware of the nature of their difficulty.

Of course, there are patients who not only fail to name objects, but also will not recognize the correct word when it is given to them. In such patients, the understanding of what is heard or read is not normal, i.e., the naming difficulty is but one symptom of another type of aphasic disorder.

Anomic aphasia has been associated with lesions in different parts of the language area. In some cases the lesion has been deep in the basal portion of the posterior temporal lobe, in position probably to interrupt connections between sensory language areas and the hippocampal regions concerned with learning and memory. Mass lesions, such as a tumor or an otogenic abscess, are the most frequent causes, and as they enlarge a contralateral upper quadrantic visual field defect or a Wernicke's aphasia is added. Occasionally, anomia appears with lesions due to occlusion of the temporal branches of the posterior cerebral artery. Anomia may be a prominent manifestation of transcortical motor aphasia and may be associated with the Gerstmann syndrome, in which case the lesions are found in the frontal lobe and angular gyrus respectively. In Beauvois' case of tactile aphasia there had been a hemorrhage from a vascular malformation in the left parieto-occipital region. A diffuse disease such as Alzheimer disease may begin with an anomic type of aphasia and minor degrees of it are common in old age. This deficit may also be discovered in testing patients with a confusional state caused by metabolic or infectious disease, but then it has no localizing value. By the time the patient's difficulty is fully recognized, other disorders of speech and indifference, apathy, and abulia are conjoined. Finally, anomic aphasia may be the only residual abnormality after partial recovery from Wernicke's, conduction, transcortical sensory, or (rarely) Broca's aphasia (Benson).

Isolation of the Speech Areas (Transcortical Aphasias) Destruction of the border zones between anterior, middle, and posterior cerebral arteries, usually as a result of prolonged hypotension, carbon monoxide poisoning, or other forms of anoxia, may effectively isolate the intact motor and sensory language areas from the rest of the cortex of the same hemisphere. In the case of Assal et al, multiple infarcts had isolated all of the language area. In *transcortical sensory aphasia,* so named by Lichtheim and later defined by Goldstein, the patient suffers a deficit of auditory and visual word comprehension, and writing and reading are impossible. Presumably information from the nonlanguage areas of the cerebrum cannot be transferred to Wernicke's area for conversion into verbal form. Speech remains fluent, with marked paraphasia, anomia, and empty circumlocutions; *repetition, however, is remarkably preserved,* unlike the deficit in Wernicke's and conduction aphasia, in which ability to repeat the spoken word is lost or severely impaired. Facility in repetition, in extreme degree, takes the form of echoing, parrot-like, word phrases and songs that are heard (echolalia). In a series of 15 such patients, CT and isotope scans have uniformly disclosed a lesion in the posterior parietal-occipital region (Kertesz et al). This locale explains the frequent concurrence of transient visual agnosia and hemianopia. This disorder has a good prognosis, in general.

In terms of the Wernicke schema, the lesion disconnects the auditory language area from the referent centers. The paraphasia is thought to result from the weakened control of the motor speech center by the auditory center, though the direct connection between them (presumably the arcuate fasciculus, see above) is preserved. Preservation of this direct connection accounts for the ability to repeat. Reading and auditory comprehension suffer because the sensory information does not reach the referent centers.

In *transcortical motor aphasia* ("anterior isolation syndrome," "dynamic aphasia" of Luria) the patient is unable to initiate conversational speech, producing only a few grunts or syllables. Comprehension is relatively preserved but again repetition is strikingly intact. This type of aphasia occurs in two clinical contexts: (1) in a mild, partially recovered Broca's aphasia in which repetition remains superior to conversational speech (repeating and reading aloud are generally easier than self-generated speech); and (2) in states of abulia and akinetic mutism with frontal lobe damage, for the same reason.

These syndromes are of great theoretical interest and are more common than is currently appreciated.

THE AGRAPHIAS

Writing is of course an integral part of language function but a less essential and universal component, for a considerable segment of the world's population speaks but does not read or write.

It might be supposed that all the rules of language derived from the study of motor aphasia would be applicable to agraphia. In part this is true. One must be able to formulate ideas into words and phrases in order to have something to write as well as to say; hence disorders of writing like disorders of speaking reflect all the basic defects of language. But there is an obvious difference between these two expressive modes. In speech only one final motor pathway coordinating the movements of lips, tongue, larynx, and respiratory muscles is available, whereas if the right hand is paralyzed, one can still write with the left one, or with a foot, and even with the mouth by holding a pencil between the teeth.

The writing of a word can be performed either by the direct lexical method of recalling its spelling or by sounding out its phonemes and transforming them into learned graphemes (motor images), i.e., the phonologic method. Some authors state that in agraphia there is a specific difficulty in transforming phonologic information, acquired through the auditory sense, into orthographic forms; others see it as a block between the visual form of phonemes and the cursive movements of the hand (see Basso et al). In support of the latter idea is the fact that reading and writing usually develop together and are long preceded by the development of auditory-articular mechanisms.

Pure agraphia as the initial and sole disturbance of language function must be a great rarity, but such cases have been described (see review of Rosati and de Bastiani). Pathologically verified cases are virtually nonexistent, but CT examination of the case of Rosati and de Bastiani disclosed a lesion of the posterior perisylvian area. This is in keeping with the observation that a lesion in or near the angular gyrus will occasionally cause a disproportionate disorder of writing as part of the Gerstmann syndrome (page 365). The notion of a specific center for writing in the posterior part of the second frontal convolution ("Exner's writing area") has been abandoned (Leischner). Stimulation of different parts of the inferior frontal cortex always deranges both speech and writing.

Quite apart from the *aphasic agraphias* in which spelling and grammatical errors abound, there are special forms of agraphia caused by abnormalities of spatial perception and praxis. Disturbances in the perception of spatial relationships appear to underlie *constructional agraphia.* In this circumstance letters and words are formed clearly enough but wrongly arranged on the page. Words may be superimposed, written diagonally, in haphazard arrangement, from right to left, or reversed, and with right parietal lesions only the right half of the page is used. Usually other constructional difficulties such as inability to copy geometric figures or to make drawings of clocks, flowers, and maps, etc., will be found as well.

A third group may be called the *apraxic agraphias.* Here language formulation is correct and the spatial arrangements of words respected, but the hand has lost its skill in forming letters and words. Handwriting becomes a scrawl, losing all personal character. There may be an uncertainty as to how the pen should be held and applied to paper. As a rule, other learned manual skills are simultaneously disordered. Speculations as to the basic fault here are similar to those discussed in Chap. 3, under ''Nonparalytic (Apraxic) Motor Disorders,'' and in Chap. 21, in relation to functions of the frontal and parietal lobes.

OTHER CEREBRAL DISORDERS OF LANGUAGE

It would be incorrect to conclude that the syndromes described above, all related to perisylvian lesions of the dominant cerebral hemisphere, represent all the ways in which cerebral lesions disturb language. The effects on speech and language of diffuse cerebral disorders, such as delirium tremens and Alzheimer disease, have already been mentioned (see page 381). Pathologic changes in parts of the cerebrum other than the perisylvian regions may secondarily affect language function. The lesions that occur in the border zones between major cerebral arteries and effectively isolate perisylvian areas from other parts of the cerebrum fall into this category (transcortical aphasias, see above). Another example is the lesion in the medial and orbital parts of the frontal lobes, which impairs all motor activity, to the point of abulia or akinetic mutism (see page 276). The mute patient, in contrast to the aphasic one, emits no sounds. If less severely hypokinetic, the patient's speech tends to be laconic with long pauses and an inability to sustain a monologue. Not only do extensive occipital lesions impair reading but they also reduce the utilization of all visual and lexical stimuli. Deep cerebral lesions, by causing fluctuating states of inattention and disorientation, induce fragmentation of words and phrases and sometimes protracted uncontrollable talking (logorrhea). Strong stimulation, which momentarily stabilizes behavior and speech, proves the essential integrity of language mechanisms.

Severe mental retardation often results in failure to acquire even spoken language, as pointed out in Chaps. 28 and 44. If there is any language skill it consists only of the understanding of a few simple commands.

A lesion of the dominant *thalamus,* usually vascular and involving the posterior nuclei, may cause an aphasia, the clinical features of which are not entirely uniform. Usually there is mutism to begin with and comprehension

is impaired. With partial recovery, spontaneous speech is reduced; less often it is fluent and paraphasic, to the point of jargon. Reading and writing may or may not be affected. Anomia has been described with a ventrolateral lesion (Ojemann). Characteristically the patient's ability to repeat dictated words and phrases are unimpaired. Complete recovery, in a matter of weeks, is the rule, often with persistence of the thalamic lesion. This suggests that in some cases the aphasic disturbance is secondary to local pressure on, or edema of, the language areas.

Aphasia has also been described with dominant *striatal-capsular lesions,* particularly if they extend laterally into the subcortical white matter of the temporal lobe and into the insula. The head of the caudate, anterior limb of the internal capsule, and the anterior-superior aspect of the putamen appear to be the critically involved structures. The aphasia is characterized by nonfluent, dysarthric, paraphasic speech, and varying degrees of difficulty with comprehension of language, naming, and repetition. The lesion is vascular as a rule and a right hemiparesis is usually associated. In general, striatal-capsular aphasia recovers more slowly and less completely than thalamic aphasia.

These two subcortical aphasias—thalamic and striatal-capsular—resemble, but are not identical to, the Broca and Wernicke types of aphasia. For further discussion of the subcortical aphasias the reader is directed to the articles of Naesser and Alexander, and their colleagues.

DISORDERS OF ARTICULATION AND PHONATION

The act of speaking is a highly coordinated sequence of contractions of the respiratory musculature, larynx, pharynx, palate, tongue, and lips. These structures are innervated by the vagal, hypoglossal, facial, and phrenic nerves. The nuclei of these nerves are controlled by both motor cortices through the corticobulbar tracts. As with all movements, there are also extrapyramidal influences from the cerebellum and basal ganglia. For speaking, air has to be expired in regulated bursts, and each expiration must be maintained long enough (by pressure mainly from the intercostal muscles) to permit the utterance of phrases and sentences. The current of expired air is then finely regulated by the activity of the various muscles engaged in speech.

Phonation, or the production of vocal sounds, is a function of the larynx, more particularly the vocal cords. The pitch of the speaking or singing voice depends upon the length and mass of the membranous parts of the vocal cords and can be varied by changes in tension of the vocal cords, which is adjusted by means of the intrinsic laryngeal muscles before any audible sound emerges. The controlled intratracheal pressure forces air past the glottis and separates the margins of the cords, setting up a series of vibrations and recoils. Sounds thus formed are modified as they pass through the nasopharynx and mouth, which act as resonators. *Articulation* consists of contractions of the pharynx, palate, tongue, and lips, which interrupt or alter the vocal sounds. Vowels are of laryngeal origin, as are some consonants, but the latter are formed for the most part during articulation; the consonants *m*, *b*, and *p* are labial, *l* and *t* are lingual, and *nk* and *ng* are guttural (throat and soft palate).

Defective articulation and phonation are recognized at once by listening to the patient speak during ordinary conversation or read aloud from a newspaper or a book. Test phrases or attempts at rapid repetition of lingual, labial, and guttural consonants (e.g., *la-la-la-la*, *me-me-me-me*, or *k-k-k-k*) bring out the particular abnormality. Disorders of phonation call for a precise analysis of the voice and its apparatus during speech and singing. The movements of the vocal cords should be inspected with a laryngoscope, and those of the tongue, palate, and pharynx by direct observation.

DYSARTHRIA AND ANARTHRIA

In pure dysarthria or anarthria there is no abnormality of the cortical language mechanisms. The dysarthric patient is able to understand perfectly what is heard, and, if literate, has no difficulty in reading and writing, although unable to utter a single intelligible word. This is the strict meaning of being inarticulate.

Defects in articulation may be subdivided into several types: lower motor neuron dysarthria, spastic and rigid dysarthria, ataxic dysarthria, and hypo- and hyperkinetic dysarthrias.

Lower Motor Neuron Dysarthria, Atrophic Bulbar Paralysis This is due to weakness or paralysis of the articulatory muscles, the result of disease of the motor nuclei of the medulla and lower pons or their intramedullary or peripheral extensions, the cranial nerves (*lower motor neuron paralysis*). In advanced forms of this disorder, the shriveled tongue lies inert and fasciculating on the floor of the mouth, and the lips are lax and tremulous. Saliva constantly collects in the mouth because of dysphagia, and drooling is troublesome. The voice is altered to a rasping monotone because of vocal cord paralysis. As the condition

develops, speech becomes slurred and progressively less distinct. There is special difficulty in the enunciation of vibratives, such as *r*, and as the paralysis becomes more complete, lingual and labial consonants are finally not pronounced at all. Bilateral paralysis of the palate, causing nasality of speech, may occur with diphtheria and poliomyelitis, and most often with progressive bulbar palsy, a form of motor neuron disease (page 954). Bilateral paralysis of the lips, as in the facial diplegia of Guillain-Barré disease, interferes with enunciation of labial consonants; *p* and *b* are slurred and sound more like *f* and *v*. Degrees of these abnormalities are also observed in myasthenia gravis.

Spastic and Rigid Dysarthrias These are more frequent than the lower motor neuron variety. Diseases that involve the corticobulbar tracts, usually vascular disease or motor system disease, result in the syndrome of spastic bulbar (pseudobulbar) palsy. The patient may have had a clinically inevident vascular lesion at some time in the past, affecting the corticobulbar fibers on one side. Since the bulbar muscles are probably innervated by both motor cortices, there may be no impairment in speech or swallowing from a unilateral lesion. Should another stroke then occur, involving the other corticobulbar tract at the pontine, midbrain, or capsular level, the patient immediately becomes dysphagic, dysphonic, and anarthric or dysarthric, often with paresis of the tongue and facial muscles. This condition, unlike bulbar paralysis due to lower motor neuron involvement, entails no atrophy or fasciculations of the paralyzed muscles; the jaw jerk and other facial reflexes soon become exaggerated, the palatal reflexes are retained or increased, emotional control is impaired (spasmodic crying and laughing), and sometimes breathing becomes periodic (Cheyne-Stokes).

When the dominant frontal operculum alone is involved, speech may be dysarthric usually without the impairment in emotional control. In the beginning, with vascular lesions, the patient is usually mute but with recovery or in mild degrees of the same condition, speech is notably slow, thick, and indistinct, much like that of partial bulbar paralysis. The terms *cortical dysarthria* and *anarthria*, among many other terms, have been applied to this disorder, which is more closely related to mild forms of Broca's aphasia than to the dysarthrias being considered in this section (see discussion of "Pure Word Mutism," under "The Aphasias," above). Also, in many cases of partially recovered Broca's aphasia the patient is left with a dysarthria that may be difficult to distinguish from a pure articulatory defect. Careful testing of other language functions, especially writing, will in this instance reveal the aphasic nature of the defect.

In paralysis agitans, and in the postencephalitic Parkinson syndrome, one observes an extrapyramidal disturbance of articulation, characterized by slurring of words and syllables and trailing off the end of sentences. The voice is low-pitched, monotonous, and lacks both volume and inflection. The words are uttered hastily and run together in a pattern different from spastic dysarthria. In advanced cases speech is almost unintelligible; only whispering is possible. It may happen that the patient finds it impossible to talk while walking but can speak better if standing still, sitting, or lying down. The term *hypokinetic* aptly describes one aspect of parkinsonian speech.

With chorea and myoclonus, speech may also be affected in a highly characteristic way. The speech is loud, harsh, variably stressed and poorly coordinated with breathing (*hyperkinetic dysarthria*). Unlike the defect of pseudobulbar palsy or paralysis agitans, chorea and myoclonus cause abrupt interruptions of the words by superimposition of abnormal movements. The latter abnormality is best described as "hiccup speech," in that the breaks are unexpected, as in singultus. Grimacing and other characteristic motor signs must be depended upon for diagnosis.

Corticobulbar and extrapyramidal disturbances of speech may be combined in double athetosis (page 993) and Hallervorden-Spatz disease (page 800). The speech is loud, slow, and labored. And in diffuse cerebral diseases such as general paresis, slurred speech is one of the cardinal signs.

Ataxic Dysarthria This is characteristic of acute and chronic cerebellar lesions. It may be observed in multiple sclerosis, in various degenerative disorders involving the cerebellum, as a sequel of anoxic encephalopathy, and in heatstroke. The principal abnormality is slowness of speech; slurring, monotony, and unnatural separation of the syllables of words (scanning) are other features. Again, coordination of speech and of respiration is disordered. There may not be enough breath to utter certain words or syllables, and others are uttered with greater force than intended (explosive speech). *Scanning dysarthria* (see page 74) is distinctive and is due most often to mesencephalic lesions involving the brachium conjunctivum. However, in some cases of cerebellar disease, especially if there is an element of spastic weakness of the tongue from corticobulbar tract involvement, there may be only a slurring dysarthria, and it is not possible to predict the anatomy of disease from analysis of speech alone. Myoclonic jerks involving the speech musculature may be superimposed on cerebellar ataxia in a number of diseases.

Acquired Stuttering This abnormality, characterized by interruptions of the normal rhythm of speech by involuntary repetition, and prolongation or arrest of uttered letters or syllables, is a common developmental disorder, to be discussed in Chap. 44. But as pointed out by Rosenbek

and by Helm and their colleagues, it may appear in patients who are recovering from aphasic disorders and who had never stuttered in childhood. Acquired stuttering differs from the developmental type in that the repetitions, prolongations, and blocks are restricted to the initial syllables and there is no adaptation; it involves grammatical as well as substantive words and is unaccompanied by grimacing and associated movements. In many instances, acquired stuttering is transitory, but if permanent, according to Helm et al, bilateral cerebral lesions are present. Nevertheless we have observed some cases in which only a left-sided, predominantly motor aphasia provided the background for stuttering and others in which stuttering was an early sign of cerebral glioma that originated in the parietal region. Benson also sites patients in whom stuttering accompanied fluent aphasia.

APHONIA AND DYSPHONIA

Finally, a few points should be made concerning the fourth group of speech disorders, i.e., those due to disturbances of voice. In adolescence there may be a persistence of the unstable "change of voice" normally seen in boys during puberty. As though by habit, the patient speaks part of the time in falsetto, and the condition may persist into adult life. Its basis is unknown. Probably the larynx is not masculanized, i.e., there is a failure in the spurt of growth (length) of the vocal cords that ordinarily occurs in pubertal boys. Voice training has been helpful in the majority of patients.

Paresis of respiratory movements, as in poliomyelitis and acute idiopathic polyneuritis, may affect the voice because insufficient air is provided for phonation. Also, disturbances in the rhythm of respiration may interfere with the fluency of speech. This is particularly noticeable in so-called extrapyramidal diseases, where one may observe that the patient tries to talk during part of inspiration. In the latter conditions, another common feature is reduced volume of the voice (hypophonia) due to limited excursion of the breathing muscles; the patient is unable to shout or to speak above a whisper. Whispering speech is also a feature of stupor and occasionally of concussive brain injury, but strong stimulation may make the voice audible.

With paresis of both vocal cords, the patient can speak only in whispers. Since the vocal cords normally separate during inspiration, their failure to do so when paralyzed may result in an inspiratory stridor. If one vocal cord is paralyzed, as a result of involvement of the tenth cranial nerve by tumor, for example, the voice becomes hoarse, low-pitched, rasping, and somewhat nasal in quality, like cleft palate speech, because the posterior nares do not close during phonation. The pronunciation of certain consonants such as *b, p, n,* and *k* is followed by an escape of air into the nasal passages. The abnormality is sometimes less pronounced in recumbency and increased when the head is thrown forward.

Another curious condition about which little is known is *spastic dysphonia*. Spasmodic dysphonia would be a better term; the adjective *spastic* suggests corticospinal involvement, whereas the disorder is probably of extrapyramidal origin. The authors have seen many patients, middle-aged or elderly men and women, otherwise healthy, who gradually lost the ability to speak quietly and fluently. Any attempt to speak results in contraction of all the speech musculature so that the patient's voice is strained and speaking is a great effort. The patient sounds as though he or she were trying to speak while being strangled. Shouting is easier than quiet speech, and whispering is unaltered. Other actions utilizing approximately the same muscles (swallowing and singing) are usually unimpeded.

Spastic dysphonia is usually nonprogressive and occurs as an isolated phenomenon, but we have observed exceptions in which it occurs in various combinations with blepharoclonus, spasmodic torticollis, writer's cramp, or some other type of segmental dystonia.

The nature of spastic dysphonia is unclear. As a neurologic disorder it is apparently akin to writer's cramp, i.e., a restricted dystonia (see page 90). Speech therapists watching such a patient strain to achieve vocalization often assume that relief can be obtained by making the patient relax; and psychotherapists believe at first that a search of the patient's personal life around the time when the dysphonia began will enable the patient to understand the problem and regain a normal mode of speaking. But both these methods have failed without exception. Drugs useful in extrapyramidal diseases such as paralysis agitans have only exceptionally proved beneficial. Crushing of one recurrent laryngeal nerve is said to be beneficial (Dedo). Injections of botulinus toxin in one vocal cord provide relief for several months. An anatomic abnormality has not been demonstrated, but careful neuropathologic studies have not been made.

Glottis spasm, as in tetanus and tetany, results in crowing, stridulous phonation. Hoarseness and raspiness of the voice may also be due to structural changes in the vocal cords, the result of cigarette smoking, acute or chronic laryngitis, polyps, etc.

CLINICAL APPROACH TO THE PATIENT WITH SPEECH AND LANGUAGE DISORDERS

APHASIA

In the investigation of aphasia it is first necessary to inquire into the patient's native language, handedness, and previous level of literacy and education. For many years it has been taught that following the onset of aphasia, individuals who had been fluent in more than one language (polyglots) improved more quickly in their native tongue than in a subsequently acquired language (Ribot's law). This rule seems to hold if the patient is not truly fluent in, or has not used, the acquired language for a long time. More often, the language most used before the onset of the aphasia will recover first (Pitres' law). Usually, if adequate testing is possible, more or less the same aphasic abnormalities are found in both the first and the more recently acquired language. Many naturally left-handed children are trained to use the right hand for writing; therefore, in determining handedness we must ask which hand is used for throwing a ball, threading a needle, sewing, or using a spoon or common tools such as a hammer, saw, or bread knife. It is important before the beginning of the examination to determine whether the patient is alert and can be made to participate reliably in testing, as accurate assessment of language depends on these factors.

One should quickly ascertain whether the patient has other signs of a gross cerebral lesion such as hemiplegia, facial weakness, homonymous hemianopia, or cortical sensory loss. When such a constellation of major neurologic signs is present, the aphasic disorder is usually of the total (global) type. Dyspraxia of limbs and speech musculature, in response to spoken commands or to visual mimicry, is generally associated with Broca's aphasia and sometimes with Wernicke's aphasia. Bilateral or unilateral homonymous hemianopia without motor weakness tends often to be linked to pure word blindness, to alexia with or without agraphia, and to anomic aphasia.

The special types of aphasia—Broca's, Wernicke's, conduction, pure word deafness or blindness—are sometimes associated with evidence of embolism to the nondominant cerebral hemisphere or to other organs.

Conversational testing permits quick assessment of the motor aspects of speech (praxis and prosody), fluency, language formulation, and auditory comprehension. If the disability consists mainly of sparse, laborious speech, it suggests, of course, Broca's aphasia, and this possibility can be pursued further by tests of repeating from dictation and by special tests of praxis of the oropharyngeal muscles. Fluent, empty, paraphasic speech with impaired comprehension is indicative of Wernicke's aphasia. Impaired comprehension but perfectly normal formulated speech and intact ability to read suggest the rare syndrome of pure word deafness. Disorders confined to naming, generally without paraphasias, when other language functions (reading, writing, spelling, etc.) are found adequate, are diagnostic of amnesic or anomic aphasia.

When conversation discloses virtually no abnormalities, other tests may still be revealing. The most important of these are reading, writing, repetition, and naming. Reading aloud single letters, words, and text may reveal the dissociative syndrome of pure word blindness. Except for this syndrome and for Bastian's aphemia (''Pure Word Mutism,'' see above), writing is disturbed in all forms of aphasia. Literal and verbal paraphasic errors may appear in milder cases of Wernicke's aphasia as the patient reads aloud from a text or from words in the examiner's handwriting. Similar errors appear even more frequently when the patient is asked to explain the text, read aloud, or give an explanation in writing.

Testing the patient's ability to repeat spoken language is a simple and important maneuver in the evaluation of aphasic disorders. As with other tests of aphasia, it may be necessary to increase the complexity of the test, from digits and simple words to complex words, phrases, and sentences, in order to disclose the full disability. Defective repetition occurs in all forms of aphasia (Broca's, Wernicke's, and global) due to lesions in the perisylvian language areas. The patient may be unable to repeat despite adequate comprehension—the hallmark of conduction aphasia. Contrariwise, normal repetition in an aphasic patient indicates that the perisylvian area is intact. Thus the capacity for repetition may be preserved despite grossly disordered visual and auditory comprehension, as in transcortical sensory aphasia. In fact, in the latter circumstance, the tendency to repeat may be excessive (echolalia). Preserved repetition is also characteristic of transcortical motor aphasia, anomic aphasia, and of the aphasia that occurs occasionally with subcortical lesions.

These deficits can be quantitated by the use of any one of several examination procedures. Those of Goodglass and Kaplan and of Kertesz are the most widely used in the United States. Careful examination of aphasic patients will enable one to predict the type and localization of the lesion in approximately two-thirds of the patients. Broca, Wernicke, conduction, global, and anomic types accounted for 392 of 444 cases studied by Benson and his group. He concedes that localization of aphasia-producing lesions is still inexact and that there are increasing opportunities for clinicopathologic correlation, especially with MRI.

ARTICULATION-PHONATION DISORDERS

Disturbances of articulation point to involvement of a different set of neural structures, such as the motor cortices, the corticobulbar pathways, the fifth, seventh, ninth, tenth, and twelfth cranial nerve nuclei or their peripheral extensions, and extrapyramidal nuclei and tracts. Often it is necessary to use neurologic findings other than those related to speech and language to decide which of these structures are implicated. The fundamental distinction between the atrophic bulbar (nuclear or infranuclear) and the spastic bulbar (pseudobulbar or supranuclear) palsies is grasped only with difficulty by most students. The information obtained by localizing these two major types of dysarthria is essential in differential diagnosis.

Dysphonia should lead to an investigation of laryngeal disease, either primary or secondary to an abnormality of innervation. Inspection of the vocal cords is a necessary step in the clinical study.

TREATMENT

The sudden onset of aphasia would be expected to cause great apprehension, but except for cases of pure or almost pure motor disorders of speech, most patients show remarkably little concern. It appears that the very lesion that deprives them of speech also causes at least a partial loss of insight into their own disability. This reaches almost a ludicrous extreme in some cases of Wernicke's aphasia, in which patients become indignant when others cannot understand their jargon. Nonetheless, as improvement occurs, many patients do become discouraged. Reassurance and a positive program of speech rehabilitation are the best ways of helping the patient at this stage.

Whether contemporary methods of speech therapy accomplish more than can be accounted for by spontaneous recovery is still uncertain. Most aphasic disorders are due to vascular disease and trauma and nearly always they are accompanied by some degree of spontaneous improvement in the days, weeks, and months that follow the stroke or accident. The results obtained in clinical trials on groups of patients by heterogeneous methods have been equivocal. Nevertheless, Howard et al have shown increased efficacy of word retrieval in a group of chronic stable aphasics by two different techniques. More studies of this type, which control the effects of interest and motivation, are needed.

PROGNOSIS AND RECOVERY PATTERNS

In general, recovery from aphasia due to cerebral trauma is faster and more complete than from aphasia due to stroke. The type of aphasia and particularly its initial severity (extent of the lesion) clearly influence recovery: global aphasia usually improves very little and the same is true of severe Broca and Wernicke aphasia (Kertesz and McCabe). The various dissociative speech syndromes and pure word mutism tend to improve rapidly and often completely. Also, in general, the outlook for recovery of any particular aphasia is more favorable in a left-handed person than in a right-handed one. Characteristically, in the course of recovery, one type of aphasia evolves into another type (global into severe Broca's; Wernicke's, transcortical, and conduction into anomic)—patterns that may mistakenly be attributed to the effects of therapy. Because so many factors may influence the mode of recovery of aphasia, the effectiveness of formal speech therapy has never been fully evaluated.

One must decide for each patient whether speech training is needed and when it should be started. As a rule, therapy is not advisable in the first few days of an aphasic illness, because one does not know how lasting it will be. Also, if the patient suffers a severe global aphasia and can neither speak nor understand spoken and written words, the speech therapist is helpless. Under such circumstances, one does well to wait a few weeks until one of the language functions has begun to return. Then the physician may begin to encourage and help the patient to use the function to a maximum degree. In milder aphasic disorders the patient may be sent to the speech therapist as soon as the illness has stabilized.

The methods of speech training are specialized, and it is advisable to call in a person who has been trained in this field. However, inasmuch as the benefit is largely psychologic, an interested member of the family or a schoolteacher can be of help if a speech therapist is not available in the community.

Frustration, depression, and paranoia, which may complicate some aphasias, require psychiatric evaluation and treatment. The language problems of children pose special problems and demand skillful diagnosis and treatment. These are considered fully in Chap. 28.

REFERENCES

ALEXANDER MP, NAESER MA, PALUMBO CL: Correlation of subcortical CT lesion sites and aphasia profiles. *Brain* 110:961, 1987.

ASSAL G, REGLI F, THUILLARD A et al: Syndrome de l'isolement de la zone du language. *Revue Neurol* 139:417, 1983.

BASSO A, TABORELLI A, VIGNOLO LA: Dissociated disorders of reading and writing in aphasia. *J Neurol Neurosurg Psychiatry* 41:556, 1978.

BEAUVOIS MF, SAILLANT B, MEININGER V, LHERMITTE F: Bilateral tactile aphasia: A tacto-verbal dysfunction. *Brain* 101:381, 1978.

BENSON DF: *Aphasia, Alexia and Agraphia*. New York, Churchill Livingstone, 1979.

BRAIN R: *Speech Disorders,* 2nd ed. Washington, DC, Butterworth, 1965.

BROCA P: Portée de la parole. Ramollissement chronique et destruction partielle du lobe anterieur gauche du cerveau. *Paris Bull Soc Anthrop* 2:219, 1861.

BUCHMAN AS, GARRON DC, TROST-CARDOMONE JE et al: Word deafness: One hundred years later. *J Neurol Neurosurg Psychiatry* 49:489, 1986.

CRITCHLEY M: Aphasiological nomenclature and definitions. *Cortex* 3:3, 1967.

DAMASIO AR, DAMASIO H: The anatomic basis of pure alexia. *Neurology* 33:1573, 1983.

DAMASIO H, DAMASIO AR: The anatomical basis of conduction aphasia. *Brain* 103:337, 1980.

DEDO HH: Recurrent laryngeal nerve section for spastic dysphonia. *Ann Otol* 85:451, 1976.

DÉJERINE J: Contribution a l'étude anatomo-pathologique et clinique des differentes varietés de cécité verbale. *Memoires Societé Biologique* 4:61, 1892.

GARDINER AH: *The Theory of Speech and Language*. Westport, CT, Greenwood Press, 1979.

GESCHWIND N: Disconnection syndromes in animals and man. *Brain* 88:237, 585, 1965.

GESCHWIND N: Wernicke's contribution to the study of aphasia. *Cortex* 3:449, 1967a.

GESCHWIND N: The varieties of naming errors. *Cortex* 3:97, 1967b.

GESCHWIND N, GALABURDA AM: *Cerebral Dominance. Biological Foundations*. Cambridge, MA, Harvard University Press, 1984.

GESCHWIND N, LEVITSKY W: Human brain: Left-right asymmetries in temporal speech region. *Science* 161:186, 1968.

GLONING K: Handedness and aphasia. *Neuropsychologia* 15:355, 1977.

GOLDSTEIN K: *Language and Language Disturbances*. New York, Grune & Stratton, 1948, pp 190–216.

GOODGLASS H, KAPLAN E: *The Assessment of Aphasia and Related Disorders*. Philadelphia, Lea & Febiger, 1972.

GOODGLASS H, QUADFASEL FA: Language laterality in left-handed aphasics. *Brain* 77:521, 1954.

GREENBLATT SH: Alexia without agraphia or hemianopsia. *Brain* 96:307, 1973.

HEAD H: *Aphasia and Kindred Disorders*. London, Cambridge University Press, 1926.

HELM NA, BUTLER RB, BENSON DF: Acquired stuttering. *Neurology* 28:1159, 1978.

HOWARD D, PATTERSON K, FRANKLIN S: Treatment of word retrieval deficits in aphasia. A comparison of two therapy methods. *Brain* 108:817, 1985.

JOANETTE Y, PUEL JL, NESPOULOSIS A et al: Aphasie croisée chez les droities. *Revue Neurol* 138:375, 1982.

KERTESZ A: *Aphasia and Associated Disorders*. New York, Grune & Stratton, 1979.

KERTESZ A, MCCABE P: Recovery patterns and prognosis in aphasia. *Brain* 100:1, 1977.

KERTESZ A, SHEPPARD A, MACKENZIE R: Localization in transcortical sensory aphasia. *Arch Neurol* 39:475, 1982.

KINSBOURNE M: *Hemispheric Disconnection and Cerebral Function.* Springfield, IL, Charles C Thomas, 1974.

LASSEN NA, INGVAR NH, SKINHOF E: Brain function and blood flow. *Sci Am* 239:62, 1978.

LEISCHNER A: The agraphias, in Vinken PJ, Bruyn GW (eds): *Handbook of Clinical Neurology,* vol 4: *Disorders of Speech, Perception and Symbolic Behavior.* Amsterdam, North-Holland, 1969, pp 141–180.

LeMAY M, CULEBRAS A: Human brain morphologic differences in the hemispheres demonstrable by carotid angiography. *N Engl J Med* 287:168, 1972.

LESSER RP, LUEDERS H, DINNER DS et al: The location of speech and writing functions in the frontal language area. *Brain* 107:275, 1984.

LEVINE DN, CALVANIO R: Conduction aphasia, in Kirshner HS, Freeman FR (eds): *The Neurology of Aphasia.* Lisse, Swets and Zeitlinger, 1982.

LEVINE DN, MOHR JP: Language after bilateral cerebral infarctions: Role of the minor hemisphere in speech. *Neurology* 29:927, 1979.

LICHTHEIM L: On aphasia. *Brain* 7:433, 1885.

MARIE P: Revision de la question de l'aphasie. *Sem Med* 26:241, 1906.

MILNER B, BRANCH C, RASMUSSEN T: Evidence for bilateral speech representation in some non-right-handers. *Trans Am Neurol Assoc* 91:306, 1966.

MOHR JP: Broca's area and Broca's aphasia, in Whitaker H, Whitaker H (eds): *Studies in Neurolinguistics,* vol 1. New York, Academic, 1976, pp 201–235.

MOHR JP: The vascular basis of Wernicke aphasia. *Trans Am Neurol Assoc* 105:133, 1980.

MOHR JP, PESSIN MS, FINKELSTEIN S et al: Broca aphasia: Pathologic and clinical. *Neurology* 28:311, 1978.

NAESSER MA, ALEXANDER MP, HELM-ESTABROOK N et al: Aphasia with predominantly subcortical lesion sites. *Arch Neurol* 39:2, 1982.

NIELSEN JM: *Agnosia, Apraxia, Aphasia: Their Value in Cerebral Localization,* 2nd ed. New York, Hafner, 1962.

OJEMANN G: Subcortical language mechanisms, in Whitaker H, Whitaker H (eds): *Studies in Neurolinguistics,* vol 1. New York, Academic, 1976, pp 103–138.

ROSENBEK J, MESSERT B, COLLINS M et al: Stuttering following brain damage. *Brain Lang* 6:82, 1975.

ROCH-LeCOURS H, LHERMITTE F: The pure form of the phonetic disintegration syndrome (pure anarthria). *Brain Lang* 3:88, 1976.

ROSATI G, DE BASTIANI P: Pure agraphia: A discrete form of aphasia. *J Neurol Neurosurg Psychiatry* 42:266, 1979.

SUBIRANA A: Handedness and cerebral dominance, in Vinken PJ, Bruyn GW (eds): *Handbook of Clinical Neurology,* vol 4: *Disorders of Speech, Perception and Symbolic Behavior.* Amsterdam, North-Holland, 1969, pp 284–292.

SYMONDS C: Aphasia. *J Neurol Neurosurg Psychiatry* 16:1, 1953.

WERNICKE K: *Der Aphasische Symptomkomplex.* Breslau, Kohn & Weigert, 1874. English translation by Eggert GH: *Wernicke's Works on Aphasia. A Source Book and Review.* The Hague, Moulon, 1977.

WILSON SAK: *Aphasia.* London, Kegan Paul, 1926.

YAKOVLEV PI, RAKIC P: Patterns of decussation of bulbar pyramids and distribution of pyramidal tracts on the two sides of the spinal cord. *Trans Am Neurol Assoc* 91:366, 1966.

ANXIETY AND DISORDERS OF ENERGY, MOOD, EMOTION, AND AUTONOMIC FUNCTIONS

CHAPTER 23

LASSITUDE AND FATIGUE

In this chapter and the next we will consider the clinical phenomena of lassitude, fatigue, anxiety, and depression. These cardinal manifestations of disease, though more abstruse than paralysis, sensory loss, seizures, or aphasia, are no less important, if for no other reason than their frequency. They may provide clear indication of the existence of a psychiatric illness, as will be pointed out later. Often, however, they are only slight aberrations of normal reactions to all manner of medical and neurologic diseases, in which case it may be difficult to separate their effects from those of the underlying diseases.

The terms *weakness* and *tiredness*, among many others, are used by patients to describe a variety of symptoms which vary in their diagnostic and prognostic import. The complaints can usually be fitted into one of the following categories:

I. *Lassitude, fatigue, lack of energy, listlessness, and languor.* (These terms, though not synonymous, shade into one another; all refer to a weariness and a loss of the sense of well-being that is typical of persons who are healthy in mind and body.)
II. *Weakness, loss of strength, paresis, paralysis.* These may be persistent or episodic.
  A. *Persistent weakness.* This may be (1) restricted to certain muscles or groups of muscles (see Chap. 3), or (2) more or less generalized, i.e., involving the entire musculature (see Chap. 48).
  B. *Episodic.* Attacks of weakness may occur in myasthenia and the periodic paralyses. Many patients confuse "attacks of weakness" with a diminished sense of alertness, light-headedness, or feeling of faintness. These usually turn out to be episodes of vertigo, seizures, or presyncope (Chaps. 14, 15, and 17, respectively) or of anxiety (Chap. 24).

Of all the symptoms in this group lassitude and fatigue are the most frequent and often the most vague. More than half of all patients entering a general hospital register a direct complaint of fatigability or admit to it when questioned. During the Second World War, fatigue was such a prominent symptom in combat personnel as to be given a separate place in medical nosology, viz., "combat fatigue," which referred to all acute psychiatric illnesses that happened on the battlefield. The common clinical antecedents and accompaniments of fatigue, its significance, and its physiologic and psychologic bases should, therefore, be matters of interest to all physicians.

Patients who complain of lassitude and fatigue have a more or less characteristic way of describing their symptoms. They say that they are "all in," "tired all the time," "weary," "exhausted," "turned off," "fed up," or "pooped out" or that they have "no pep," "no ambition," or "no interest." They manifest their condition by showing an indifference to the tasks at hand, by talking much about how hard they are working; they are inclined to sit around or lie down, or occupy themselves with trivial tasks. On closer analysis one observes that they have a difficulty in initiating activity and also in sustaining it.

This condition is the familiar aftermath of sleeplessness, prolonged labor or great physical exertion, and under such circumstances it is accepted as a normal, physiologic reaction. When, however, the same symptoms or similar ones appear without relation to such antecedents, they are suspected of being the manifestations of disease.

The physician's task begins, then, with an attempt to determine whether the patient is merely suffering from the physical and mental effects of overwork without realizing it. Overworked, overwrought people are everywhere observable in our society. Their actions are both instructive and pathetic. Some personal inadequacy seems to prevent them from deriving pleasure from any activity except their work, in which they indulge themselves as a kind of defense mechanism. Their behavior is said to be irrational in that they will not listen to reason; they seem to be impelled by certain notions of duty and refuse to think of themselves.

They work with great intensity and persistence, which reveals a high degre of emotional involvement. Such persons frequently show other symptoms, such as irritability, restlessness, and sleeplessness. Their symptoms and behavior may be better understood by considering certain psychologic studies of the effects of fatigue on the normal individual.

EFFECTS OF FATIGUE ON THE NORMAL PERSON

According to several authoritative sources, fatigue has both explicit and implicit effects, grouped under (1) a series of biochemical and physiologic changes in many organs of the body, (2) an overt disorder in behavior taking the form of a reduced output of work (*work decrement*), and (3) an expressed dissatisfaction and a subjective feeling of tiredness.

As to the biochemical and physiologic changes, continuous muscular work leads to depletion of muscle glycogen and an accumulation of lactic acid and other metabolites, which in themselves reduce the power of muscular contraction and delay the recovery of muscle strength. Even in normal persons, extreme degrees of muscular effort, in which activity exceeds provision of substrate, may result in a necrosis of fibers and rise in serum concentrations of creatine kinase and aldolase (this effect is much more evident in individuals with one of the hereditary metabolic diseases of muscle described in Chap. 51). The muscles are slightly swollen and sore for several days. It is said that the injection of blood from a fatigued animal into a rested one will produce overt manifestations of fatigue in the latter, but the authors are skeptical of such reports. With repeated contraction of muscles, their actions become tremulous, movements are less adept, and the coordination of agonist, antagonist, and synergist muscles is less precise. Other well-known changes induced by exercise include an increase in the rate of breathing, a quickening of the pulse, a rise in blood pressure, a widening of the pulse pressure, and an increase in the white blood cell count and metabolic rate. These alterations bear out the hypothesis that fatigue is in part a manifestation of altered metabolism.

The decreased productivity and capacity for work, which is a direct consequence of fatigue, has been investigated by industrial psychologists. Their findings show clearly the importance of the motivational factor on work output, whether it be in manual or mental tasks. Also, individual differences in energy potential appear to be important, as are differences in physique, intelligence, and temperament.

True muscle weakness is not found in the majority of persons complaining of fatigue. This may be difficult to prove, for many such individuals are disinclined to exert full effort in tests of peak-power contractions or endurance. In general, we agree with Rowland et al that physiologic fatigue is a normal process and that weakness and exercise intolerance are symptoms of muscle disease.

The subjective aspects of fatigue have been carefully recorded. Aside from feeling weary and tired, the fatigued person is unable to deal effectively with complex problems and tends to be unreasonable, often about trivialities. The number and quality of his associations in psychologic tests are reduced. The ability to deliberate and to make sound judgments is impaired; decisions made late at night may appear unsound the next day. The worker, after a long, hard day, is unable to perform adequately the demanding duties of head of the household; the tired business executive who becomes the tyrant of the family is proverbial. A disinclination to try and the appearance of ideas of inferiority are other characteristics of the fatigued mind.

Instances of fatigue and lassitude resulting from overwork are not difficult to recognize. A description of the patient's daily routine and a talk with family members and associates will usually suffice. Moreover, if the person can be persuaded to live at a more reasonable pace and allow time for outside pleasurable activities, the symptoms will subside. A common error in diagnosis, however, is the ascription of fatigue to overwork when actually it is a manifestation of a neurosis or depression.

FATIGUE AS A MANIFESTATION OF PSYCHIATRIC DISORDER

The great majority of patients who enter a hospital because of unexplained chronic fatigue and lassitude are found to have some type of psychiatric illness. Formerly this state was called "neurasthenia," but since fatigue rarely exists as an isolated phenomenon, the current practice is to label such cases according to the total clinical picture. The usual associated symptoms are nervousness, irritability, anxiety, depression, insomnia, headaches, difficulty in concentrating, reduced sexual impulse, and loss of appetite. In one series, 75 percent of persons admitted to a general hospital because of a chief complaint of chronic fatigue were diagnosed, finally, as having *anxiety neurosis* and *tension states*. Depression accounted for another 10 percent, and the remainder of the patients had a miscellany of medical and psychiatric illnesses.

Several features are common to the psychiatric group. The fatigue may be worse in the morning. There is an inclination to lie down and rest, but sleep does not come. The fatigue is worsened by mild exertion and relates more to some activities than to others. Inquiry may disclose that the fatigue was first experienced in temporal relation to a grief reaction, a surgical operation, a medical illness, or some other unpleasant event. The feeling of fatigue interferes with mental as well as physical activities; the patient is easily worried, is mentally inactive, and finds it difficult to concentrate in attempting to solve a problem or in carrying on a complicated conversation.

Depression, as will be elaborated in the following chapter, has a characteristic effect on impulse and energy. Also, sleep is disturbed, with a tendency to early-morning waking, so that such persons are at their worst in the morning, both in spirit and in energy output. Their tendency is to improve as the day wears on, and they may even feel fairly normal by evening. It is difficult to decide whether the fatigue is a primary manifestation of the disease or is secondary to a lack of interest.

Not all chronically fatigued individuals deviate enough from normal to justify the diagnosis of neurosis or depression. Many people in society, because of circumstances beyond their control, have little or no purpose in life and much idle time. They are bored with the monotony of their routine. Such circumstances are conducive to fatigue, just as the opposite, a strong emotion or a new enterprise that excites optimism and enthusiasm, will dispel fatigue. Other persons seem normal until some adversity is encountered, arousing worry or fear, and then it becomes apparent that their adjustment was marginal. Such reactions are understandable to anyone who has ever had stage fright and who remembers the sense of physical weakness, the utter incapacity to act, the intellectual chaos that overwhelms the previously well-ordered mind, and the exhaustion that follows.

PSYCHOLOGIC THEORIES

The enervating effect of certain emotional states, such as anxiety, is well known, and one might suppose that the simple prolongation of the emotional experience would explain the chronic fatigue of anxiety neurosis. However, this explanation would not account for the occurrence of fatigue at a time when no emotional disorder is apparent.

One psychoanalytic theory postulates that chronic fatigue, in the broadest sense, is like the anxiety from which it derives; it is a danger signal that something is wrong—that some attitude or activity has been too intense or too persistent. Fatigue is then a means of self-preservation, serving not merely to protect the person against physical injury but also to protect his self-esteem and self-confidence. As to mechanism, it is claimed that the fatigue is the result of exhaustion of the store of psychic energy required to maintain the repression of unacceptable ideas. Another psychoanalytic theory holds that fatigue is not a negative symptom, i.e., a lack or depletion of energy, but an unconscious desire for inactivity. A reciprocal relation is said to exist between fatigue and anxiety. Both are protective, but anxiety is the more imperative. It calls for taking some positive action to get out of a predicament, whereas fatigue calls for inactivity. Both operate blindly, however, for the person cannot perceive what it is that must be done or stopped. All this allegedly happens at the subconscious level.

Another psychologic theory holds that some persons are low in impulse and energy throughout life. They are born "tired," being more so at times of stress. Some psychiatrists believe that such persons have a constitutional inadequacy. Janet described them as having a low psychological tension. Kahn classified them as "psychopaths weak in impulse"; in his description he pointed out their inability, from infancy and throughout life, to play games vigorously, to compete successfully, to work hard without exhaustion, to withstand or recover quickly from illness, or to assume a dominant role in a social group.

It is obvious that these several psychologic hypotheses could not all be correct, nor could they be applicable to all situations in which chronic fatigue is the complaint. Undoubtedly there are persons who, because of genetic or constitutional factors, are underactive and lacking in stamina and the capacity to sustain physical or mental activity. It is equally clear that psychic and physical energy are closely linked to mood. The more chronic varieties of acquired fatigue, without associated medical disease, have psychiatric significance in nearly all instances.

LASSITUDE AND FATIGUE WITH MEDICAL DISEASE

Acute or chronic infection is an important cause of fatigue. Everyone, of course, has at some time or other sensed the abrupt onset of exhaustion, a tired ache in the muscles or an inexplicable listlessness, only to discover later that he or she was "coming down with the flu." More chronic infections such as hepatitis, tuberculosis, brucellosis, infectious mononucleosis, and Lyme disease may not be evident immediately but should always be suspected when the fatigue is a new symptom and out of proportion to other symptoms such as mood change, nervousness, and anxiety. More often the fatigue begins with an obvious infection but persists for several weeks after the overt manifestations of infection have subsided, and it may then be difficult to decide whether there is still a lingering infection (as in hepatitis or Epstein-Barr viral infections), or the infection has been complicated by psychologic symptoms during convalescence.

An even more difficult problem is that of the patient who remains severely fatigued for many months or even a year or longer after a bout of infectious mononucleosis or some other viral illness. Some such patients were found to have extrordinarily high antibody titers to the Epstein-Barr virus (EBV), which suggested a causal relationship and gave rise to terms such as the chronic infectious mononucleosis or EBV syndrome (Straus et al). However, subsequent studies have made it clear that the vast majority of patients with complaints of chronic fatigue have neither a clear-cut history of infectious mononucleosis—or serologic evidence of such an infection (Strauss; Holmes et al), and that in these patients the etiology of the chronic fatigue remains obscure. It is difficult to dispel the notion that the symptoms are psychoneurotic; it seems that in the diseases mentioned above and in other systemic viral infections, long-standing neurotic symptoms have been uncovered. Nevertheless, the possibility of some obscure secondary metabolic or immunologic derangement, consequent to the infection, cannot be dismissed (Swartz).

Metabolic and endocrine diseases (Chaps. 27 and 40) of various types may cause inordinate degrees of lassitude and fatigue. Sometimes there is in addition a true muscular weakness. In Addison disease and Simmonds disease, fatigue may dominate the clinical picture. Aldosterone deficiency is another established cause of chronic fatigue. In persons with hypothyroidism, with or without frank myxedema, lassitude and sluggishness are frequent complaints, and also muscle aching and joint pains. Fatigue may also be present in patients with hyperthyroidism but is usually less troublesome than nervousness. Uncontrolled diabetes mellitus may be accompanied by excessive fatigability, as are hyperparathyroidism, hypogonadism, and Cushing disease.

Anemia, when moderate or severe, should be considered as a possible cause of unexplained lassitude. Mild grades of anemia are usually asymptomatic; lassitude is far too often ascribed to it. An occult malignant tumor may also announce itself by inordinate fatigue.

Any type of nutritional deficiency may, when severe, cause lassitude, and in its earlier stages this may be the chief complaint. Weight loss and a history of alcoholism and dietary inadequacy may provide the only other clues to the nature of the illness.

For several weeks or months following myocardial infarction, most patients complain of fatigue out of all proportion to effort. In many of these patients there is an accompanying anxiety or depression. Much more difficult to understand is the complaint of fatigue that may precede myocardial infarction.

Among neurologic diseases in which fatigability is a prominent symptom one should mention the syndrome of posttraumatic nervous instability (page 710), Parkinson disease, and multiple sclerosis. The fatigue of the parkinsonian patient may precede the recognition of neurologic signs by months or even years. It is probably a reaction to the subjective awareness of increasing disability resulting from the akinesia. The fatigue that accompanies multiple sclerosis may be greatly worsened by exposure to high temperatures, e.g., a hot bath. The majority of patients who recover from a stroke complain of being weak and tired.

DIFFERENTIAL DIAGNOSIS

If one looks critically at the patients who enter a hospital because of incapacitating exhaustion, lassitude, and fatigability (sometimes incorrectly called "weakness"), it is evident that the most commonly overlooked diagnoses are anxiety neurosis and depression. The correct conclusion can usually be reached by keeping these illnesses in mind as one elicits the history from patient and family. Difficulty arises when symptoms of the psychiatric illness are so inconspicuous as not to be appreciated; one comes then to suspect the diagnosis only by having eliminated the common medical causes. Observation in the hospital may bear out the existence of an anxiety state or gloomy mood, as the patient resists rehabilitation. Strong reassurance in combination with a therapeutic trial of antianxiety or antidepression drugs may suppress symptoms of which the patient was barely aware, thus clarifying the diagnosis. The so-called asthenic psychopath described above is recognized by the characteristic lifelong behavioral pattern revealed in his or her biography.

Tuberculosis, brucellosis, Lyme disease, anicteric hepatitis, subacute bacterial endocarditis, Mycoplasma pneumonia, Epstein-Barr, Coxsackie B and other viral infections, malaria, hookworm, giardiasis, and other parasitic infections should always be included in the differential diagnosis and a search made for their characteristic symptoms and signs and laboratory findings. There should be a search for occult tumor. An endocrine survey is also in order in all obscure cases. The measurement of thyroid hormones, cortisol, and electrolytes in the serum may help to identify an endocrine cause of a fatigue syndrome.

It should be remembered that chronic intoxication with alcohol, barbiturates, or other sedative drugs, some of which are given to suppress nervousness or insomnia, may contribute to fatigability. Finally, the rapid and recent onset of fatigue should always suggest the presence of an infection, a disturbance in fluid balance, or rapidly developing circulatory failure of either peripheral or cardiac origin.

GENERALIZED WEAKNESS

As was emphasized in the foregoing remarks, weakness must be distinguished from lassitude and fatigue. The demonstration of reduced muscular power sets the case analysis along different lines, bringing up for particular consideration diseases of the peripheral nervous system or of the musculature. It must be kept in mind that weakness may be so slight as to be detectable only after sustained exercise.

True neural or myopathic weakness is probably never caused by psychologic factors, though the hysteric or malingerer may claim weakness. Usually this can be detected by the criteria outlined in Chap. 55. In anemia, chronic infection, malignancy, and nutritional depletion (except when polyneuropathy is present), the thin muscles are always stronger during tests of peak contraction than one would expect, though strength may fall short of that of a healthy individual (see Chap. 44 for description of tests of peak power and endurance of muscles).

The presence of muscular weakness is ascertained by (1) obtaining a history of reduced strength and (2) demonstrating a failure to contract the muscles with normal force. By testing each of the major groups of muscles from head to foot, one may ascertain whether all or certain groups fall below standard. Quantitative and qualitative changes (myasthenia, inverse myasthenia, myotonia, paramyotonia, pathologic cramping) may also be detected by the methods outlined in Chaps. 52 and 53. The topography of weakness and associated neurologic findings permit distinction between the various types of spinal, peripheral nerve, and myopathic pareses. Rare diseases, difficult to diagnose, that cause inexplicable muscle weakness and exercise intolerance are masked hyperthyroidism, hyperparathyroidism, ossifying hemangiomas with hypophosphatemia, some of the kalemic periodic paralyses, hyperinsulinism, disorders of carbohydrate and lipid metabolism, the mitochondrial myopathies, and possibly adenylate deaminase deficiency.

REFERENCES

ADAMS RD: Thayer lectures: I. Principles of myopathology. II. Principles of clinical myology. *Johns Hopkins Med J* 131:24, 1972.

HOLMES GP, KAPLAN JE, GLANTZ NM et al: Chronic fatigue syndrome. A working case definition. *Ann Intern Med* 108:387, 1988.

JANET P: *Les Neuroses.* Paris, Flammarion, 1895.

KAHN E: *Psychopathic Personalities.* New Haven, Yale University Press, 1931.

MAYER-GROSS W: *Clinical Psychiatry,* 3rd ed., Slater E, Roth M (eds), Baltimore, Williams & Wilkins, 1969.

ROWLAND LP, LAYZER RB, DiMAURO S: Pathophysiology of metabolic muscle disorders, in Asbury AK, McKhann GM, McDonald WI (eds): *Diseases of the Nervous System.* Philadelphia, Saunders, 1986, Chap 16.

STRAUSS SE: The chronic mononucleosis syndrome. *J Infect Dis* 157:405, 1988.

STRAUSS SE, DALE JK, TOBI M et al: Acyclovir treatment of the chronic fatigue syndrome. *N Engl J Med* 319: 1692, 1988.

SWARTZ MN: The chronic fatigue syndrome—one entity or many? *N Engl J Med* 319:1726, 1988.

CHAPTER 24

NERVOUSNESS, IRRITABILITY, ANXIETY, AND DEPRESSION

The world is full of nervous, tense, apprehensive, and worried people. The stresses of contemporary society are often blamed for their plight. The poet W. H. Auden referred to our time as "the age of anxiety." But history informs us that our own age is not unique in this respect. Medical historians have identified comparable periods of anxiety dating back to the time of Marcus Aurelius and Constantine, when societies were undergoing rapid and profound changes and individuals were assailed by an overwhelming sense of insecurity, personal insignificance, and fear of the future (Rosen).

Like lassitude and fatigue, nervousness, irritability, anxiety and depression are among the most frequent symptoms encountered in office and hospital practice. A British survey (Lader) found that more than 40 percent of the population, at some time or other, experienced symptoms of anxiety, and about 5 percent suffered from lifelong anxiety states. The vast amounts of antianxiety drugs and alcohol that are consumed in our society would tend to corroborate these figures. Of course, some degree of anxiety is experienced by everyone facing a challenging event or threatening task, for which one may feel inadequate. In such cases, anxiety is not abnormal, and the alertness and attentiveness that accompany this state may actually improve performance. In a similar vein, if worry or depression stands in clear relation to economic reverses or loss of a loved one, the symptom is usually accepted as normal. Only when excessively intense, uncontrollable, or prolonged, or when the visceral derangements that accompany these symptoms are prominent, do anxiety and depression become matters of medical concern. Admittedly, the line that separates normal emotional reactions and pathologic (neurotic) ones is not a sharp one. These matters are dealt with more fully in Chap. 55.

In this chapter we will be concerned with nervousness, anxiety, irritability and depression as symptoms, together with currently accepted views of their origins and biologic significance. The diseases of which these symptoms may be a part are discussed in Chaps. 55 and 56.

NERVOUSNESS

By this vague term the lay person usually refers to a state of restlessness, tension, uneasy apprehension, irritability, or hyperexcitability, but it may connote other states, such as thoughts of suicide, fear of killing one's child or spouse, a distressing hallucination, a paranoid idea, a frankly hysterical outburst, or even tics or tremulousness. Careful inquiry as to what the patient means when complaining of nervousness is always a necessary first step.

Most often nervousness represents no more than a psychic and behavioral state in which the person is maximally challenged or threatened by difficult personal problems. This is more likely to happen at certain times in life than at others. For example, adolescence rarely passes without its period of turmoil, as the young attempt to emancipate themselves from parental dominance or to adjust to scholastic demands, a work situation, or to the opposite sex. The menses are regularly accompanied by increased tension and moodiness, referred to, in its most severe form, as the premenstrual tension syndrome. In the postpartum period it is exceptional for the new mother not to experience transient anxiety and depression, i.e., the "postpartum blues," associated possibly with hyperprolactinemia. Some persons, because of early patterning or character formation, claim to have been nervous in all their social relationships throughout life; one should then suspect a neurosis, depression, or schizophrenia, even though performance within the family unit, at school, and at work were adequate. Others complain of a recent development of nervousness, and one must consider such possibilities as an upheaval in personal affairs, the first attack or exacerbation of a neurosis, an endogenous depression, an endocrine disease (hyperthyroidism, adrenal cortical disease, or corticosteroid therapy), or withdrawal from alcohol or other sedative drugs. Some patients complain of a nervousness that attends the onset of a medical or neurologic disease; it would then appear to be secondary, occasioned by fear of disability, dependency, or death.

Nervousness, even in its simplest form, is reflected in a number of behavioral changes. There are often a mild somberness of mood, an increased tendency to tears and anger (irritability), fatigue that bears no proper relation to activity and rest, and disturbed sleep, eating, and drinking habits. Headaches may increase in number and intensity. There is a tendency to sweat, tremble, be aware of heart action, feel a bit ''queer in the head'' or giddy, have an upset stomach, and urinate more often, though these autonomic accompaniments are seldom as conspicuous as in anxiety neurosis.

Thus, it would appear that what is being described here as nervousness and anxiety constitute a graded series of reactions and that the latter in many instances is only a more intense and protracted form of the former.

THE ANXIETY STATE

There is no unanimity among psychiatrists as to whether anxiety is a single emotional reaction, varying only in its severity or duration, or a group of discrete reactions, each with distinctive clinical features (Hoehn-Saric). In some writings anxiety is classified as a form of subacute or chronic *fear*. However, there is reason to question this assumption. Anxious patients, when frightened under experimental conditions, state that a fear reaction differs in being more overwhelming. The frightened patient is ''frozen,'' unable to act or to think clearly, and his responses are automatic and sometimes irrational. The fear reaction is characterized by overactivity of both the sympathetic and parasympathetic nervous systems, and the parasympathetic effects (bradycardia, sphincteric relaxation) may predominate, unlike other forms of anxiety, in which sympathetic effects are the more prominent. Long ago, Cicero distinguished between an acute and transient attack of fear provoked by a specific stimulus (angor) and a protracted state of fearfulness (anxietas). This distinction was elaborated by Freud, who regarded fear as an appropriate response to a sudden, unexpected external threat and anxiety as a neurotic maladjustment (see below).

The authors take no position in this dispute and would only make the point that in this chapter anxiety will be defined as an intermittent or sustained emotional state characterized by a subjective feeling of fear and uneasy anticipation (apprehension), usually with a definite topical content and associated with the physiologic accompaniments of strong emotion, i.e., breathlessness, tightness in the chest, choking sensation, palpitation, restlessness, increased muscular tension, giddiness, trembling, sweating, and flushing. By topical content is meant the idea, person, or object about which the person is anxious. The several vasomotor and visceral alterations that underlie the symptoms are mediated through the autonomic nervous system, particularly its sympathetic part, and involve also the thyroid and adrenal glands.

FORMS OF ANXIETY

Anxiety is manifested in acute episodes, each lasting several minutes, or as a protracted state that may last for weeks, months, or years. In the *acute attacks,* or *panics,* as they are called, patients are plunged into an inexplicable mental state in which they fear they will die, lose their reason or self-control, become insane, or commit some horrible crime. Breathlessness, a feeling of suffocation, sweating, trembling, palpitation and gastric distress are the physical accompaniments. As a persistent protracted state the patient experiences fluctuating degrees of nervousness, restlessness, irritability, fatigue, insomnia, intolerance of physical exertion, and tension headaches. Discrete anxiety attacks and persistent states of anxiety merge with one another.

Episodic or sustained anxiety without a disorder of mood (i.e., without depression) is classified as *anxiety neurosis.* The chronic form with prominent exercise intolerance is called *neurocirculatory asthenia,* among many other terms. Anxiety may, however, be combined with other somatic symptoms in hysteria and is the most prominent feature of *phobic neurosis.* Persistent anxiety with insomnia, lassitude, and fatigue, regardless of mood, should always raise the suspicion of a *depressive* illness, especially when it begins in middle adult life or beyond. Also panic attacks may occur at the beginning of a schizophrenic illness. Both anxiety and depression are prominent features of the syndrome of posttraumatic nervous instability (see page 710).

Thus, the differential diagnosis of an anxiety state includes all the major syndromes in psychiatry. Often it is but one component of a far more serious condition, one which may result in suicide or some other antisocial act. Also, when visceral symptoms predominate or the psychic counterparts of fear and apprehension are absent, the presence of thyrotoxicosis, corticosteroid overdosage, pheochromocytoma, hypoglycemia, and menopause should be suspected.

PHYSIOLOGIC AND PSYCHOLOGIC BASIS

The cause, mechanism, and biologic meaning of anxiety have been the subjects of much speculation, and completely satisfactory explanations are not available. The psychologist regards anxiety as anticipatory behavior, i.e., a state of uneasiness about something that may happen in the future. William McDougall spoke of it as "an emotional state arising when a continuing strong desire seems likely to miss its goal." The primary emotion, somewhat muted perhaps, is that of fear, and its arousal under conditions not overtly threatening may be explained as a conditioned response to some recondite component of a formerly threatening stimulus.

Freud originally attributed anxiety to a repression of sexual urges and later to a situation which in some manner deprived the individual of a "love object." The topical content or cause of potential danger lies in the "subconscious." The postulated danger is internal rather than external; a primitive drive has been aroused that is not compatible with current social practices, and it can be satisfied only at the risk of harming the person. This and other psychoanalytic theories are reviewed by Hoehn-Saric and by Nemiah.

Physicians have searched for evidence of impairments of visceral function without success. The patient with neurocirculatory asthenia is in poor physical condition and has an increased blood lactate concentration in the resting state and after exercise, and infusions of lactic acid are said to make the symptoms worse. The patient will not tolerate the work or exercise needed to build up his stamina. The urinary excretion of epinephrine has been found elevated in some patients; in others, there is an increased urinary excretion of norepinephrine and its metabolites. Aldosterone excretion is raised to two or three times the normal level during intense anxiety. Medical students experiencing fear and anxiety while preparing for an examination also excrete increased amounts of aldosterone. The meaning of these effects, i.e., whether they are primary or secondary, is not certain, but it is becoming increasingly evident that prolonged and diffuse anxiety is a pattern of behavior related to certain biochemical abnormalities of blood, and probably of the brain.

Animal studies have related acute anxiety to the locus ceruleus and the septal and hippocampal areas—the principal norepinephrine-containing nuclei. It is noteworthy that the locus ceruleus is involved in REM sleep and that drugs such as the tricyclic antidepressants and monoamine oxidase inhibitors, which suppress REM sleep, also decrease anx-

iety. But surely these are not the only parts involved; bifrontal orbital leukotomy also diminishes anxiety, possibly by interrupting the medial forebrain connections with the limbic parts of the brain.

Anxiety, being so ubiquitous, is probably not without biologic significance. It strengthens social bonds at certain moments in life, as when there is a threat of separation of child and mother (separation anxiety); even in the adult period, marriage, companionship, and work are stabilized by the threat of anxiety. Also intense intellectual activity is facilitated by anxiety. Barratt and White found that mildly anxious medical students performed better on examinations than those lacking in anxiety. As anxiety increases, so does the standard of performance, but only to a point, after which increasing anxiety causes a rapid decline in performance (Yerkes-Dodson law).

IRRITABILITY, IRRITABLE MOOD, AND AGGRESSIVE BEHAVIOR

The phenomenon of irritability, or an irritable mood, must be familiar to almost everyone, exposed as we are to all of the noise and niggling inconveniences and annoyances of daily life. It is, nevertheless, a difficult symptom to interpret in the context of psychopathology.

Freud used the term ("Reisbarkeit") in a restricted sense—to denote an undue sensitivity to noise, and considered it a manifestation of anxiety, but obviously this symptom has a much broader connotation and significance. For one thing, some people are by nature irritable, throughout life. Also, irritability is an almost expected reaction in overworked, overwrought individuals, who become irritable by force of circumstances. An irritable mood or feeling may be present without observed manifestations (inward irritability), or there may be an overt loss of control of temper, with irascible verbal and behavioral outbursts, provoked by trivial but frustrating events.

Irritability, in the foregoing circumstances, can hardly be considered a departure from normal. However, when it appears in a person of normally placid temperament, it assumes significance, for it may then signify an ongoing anxiety state or depression. Irritability is also a common symptom of obsessional neurosis. Here the irritability tends to be directed inwardly, indicating perhaps that there is a greater sense of frustration with personal disability (Snaith and Taylor). Depressed patients are frequently irritable; as a corollary, this symptom should always be sought in patients suspected of being depressed, since it is so readily recognized, both by patients and their families. The postnatal mood disorder, referred to earlier in this chapter, is characterized by high levels of outwardly directed irritability. The most extreme degrees of irritability, exemplified by repeated quarrelsome and assaultive behavior (irritable aggression)—rarely observed in anxiety neurosis and endogenous depression—are the mark of sociopathy and ''organic'' neurologic conditions.

DEPRESSION

There are few persons who do not experience periods of discouragement and despair. As with nervousness, irritability, and anxiety, depression of mood that is appropriate to a given situation in life is a natural reaction and seldom is the basis of medical concern. Patients in these situations tend to seek help only when their grief or unhappiness are persistent and beyond control, but there are numerous instances in which these symptoms assert themselves for reasons that are not apparent. Often the symptoms are interpreted as a medical illness, bringing the patient first to the internist. Sometimes another disease is found (such as chronic hepatitis or other infection, or postinfluenzal asthenia) in which chronic fatigue is confused with depression, but often the opposite pertains, i.e., an endogenous depression is the essential problem even when there has been evidence earlier of a viral or bacterial infection. Since the risk of suicide is not inconsiderable in depression, an error in diagnosis may be life-threatening.

Information about depression, like that of all psychiatric syndromes, is gained from three sources: the history obtained from the patient, the history obtained from the family or a close friend, and the findings on examination.

From the patient and the family it is learned that the patient has been ''feeling unwell,'' ''low in spirits,'' ''blue,'' ''glum,'' ''unhappy,'' or ''morbid.'' There has been a change in emotional reactions of which the patient may not be fully aware. Activities that were formerly pleasurable are no longer so. Often, however, change in mood is less conspicuous than reduction in psychic and physical energy, and it is this type of case that is so often misdiagnosed by internists and neurologists. A complaint of fatigue is almost invariable; not uncommonly, it is worse in the morning after a night of restless sleep. The words ''loss of pep,'' ''weak,'' ''tired,'' ''no energy,'' ''my job seems more difficult'' appear in the language of the patient. The outlook is pessimistic. The patient is irritable and preoccupied with uncontrollable worry over trivialities. With excessive worry the ability to think with accustomed efficiency is reduced; there are complaints of the mind not functioning properly, and of being forgetful and unable to concentrate. If the patient is naturally of suspicious nature, paranoid tendencies may assert themselves.

Particularly troublesome in medical diagnosis is the patient's tendency to hypochondriasis. Indeed, most cases formerly diagnosed as hypochondriasis are now regarded

as depression. Pain from whatever cause—a stiff joint, a toothache, fleeting abdominal pains, or other disturbances such as constipation, frequency of urination, insomnia, pruritus, burning tongue, weight loss—may become an obsessive focus of complaint. The patient passes from doctor to doctor seeking relief from symptoms that would not trouble the normal person, and no amount of reassurance relieves his or her state of mind. The anxiety and depressed mood of these persons may be obscured by their preoccupation with visceral functions.

When examined, the patient's facial expression is often plaintive, troubled, pained, or anguished. The attitude and manner of the patient betray a prevailing mood of depression, discouragement, and despondency. In other words, the affect, which is the outward expression of feeling, is consistent with the depressed mood. During the interview the patient may be tearful. Occasionally, such patients cry openly. In some there is a kind of immobility of the face that mimics parkinsonism, though others are restless and agitated (pacing, wringing their hands, etc.). Occasionally the patient will smile, but the smile impresses one as more a social gesture than an expression of feeling.

The stream of speech, from which the ideational content is determined, is slow. At times the patient is mute and speaks neither spontaneously nor in response to questions. There may be a long pause between questions and answers. The latter are brief and may be monosyllabic. There is a paucity of ideas. The retardation extends to all topics of conversation and affects movement of the limbs as well. The most extreme forms of decreased motor activity, rarely seen in the medical clinic, border on stupor.

The content of speech is found to be abnormal if examined carefully. Conversation is replete with pessimistic thoughts, fears, expressions of unworthiness, inadequacy, inferiority, hopelessness and sometimes guilt. In severe depressions, bizarre ideas, delusions about the body (''blood drying up,'' ''bowels are blocked with cement,'' ''I am half dead'') may be expressed.

CAUSATION AND DIAGNOSIS

Three theories have emerged concerning the cause of the pathologic depressive state: (1) the endogenous form is hereditary; (2) a biochemical abnormality results in a periodic depletion in the brain of serotonin and norepinephrine; (3) a basic fault in character development exists. These theories will be elaborated in Chap. 56.

Apart from the masked depression, in which a somatic complaint directs medical thinking along other lines, the problem for the physician is to distinguish the mild moodiness of some individuals from a serious endogenous depression. Of importance is the enduring quality of the latter. Symptoms of anxiety may be the main feature and obscure the depressive symptoms, only to have the patient commit suicide while receiving an inappropriate tranquilizer. In elderly persons, depressive symptoms may be misinterpreted as those of an early dementia.

It is the authors' belief that depression is one of the most commonly overlooked diagnoses in clinical medicine. Part of the trouble is with the word itself, which implies being unhappy about something. The persistent or recurrent endogenous depression should be suspected in all chronic states of ill health, hypochondriasis, disability that exceeds manifest signs of a medical disease, neurasthenia, chronic pain syndromes, and suicide attempts. Inasmuch as recovery is the rule, suicide is a tragedy for which the medical profession must often share responsibility.

REFERENCES

BARRATT ES, WHITE R: Impulsiveness and anxiety related to medical students' performance and attitudes. *J Med Educ* 44:604, 1969.

CASSIDY WL, FLANAGAN NB, SPELLMAN M, COHEN ME: Clinical observations in manic depressive disease. *JAMA* 164:1535, 1953.

FREUD S: On the grounds for detaching a particular syndrome from neurasthenia under the description "anxiety neurosis," in *Standard Edition of the Complete Psychological Works of Sigmund Freud,* vol. 3. London, Hogarth Press, 1962, p 90.

HOEHN-SARIC R: Anxiety: Normal and abnormal. *Psychiatric Ann* 9:11, 1979.

LADER M: The nature of clinical anxiety in modern society, in Spielberger CD, Sarason IG (eds): *Stress and Anxiety,* vol 1. New York, Halsted, 1975, pp 3–26.

LEHMANN HE: Affective disorders: Clinical features, in Kaplan HI, Sadock BJ (eds): *Comprehensive Textbook of Psychiatry,* 4th ed. Baltimore, Williams & Wilkins, 1985, chap 18.5, pp 786–811.

NEMIAH JC: Neurotic disorders, in Kaplan HI, Sadock BJ (eds): *Comprehensive Textbook of Psychiatry,* 4th ed. Baltimore, Williams & Wilkins, 1985, chap 20, pp 883–957.

ROSEN G: Emotions and sensibility in ages of anxiety: A comparative historical review. *Am J Psychiatry,* 124:771, 1967.

SNAITH RP, TAYLOR CM: Irritability: Definition, assessment, and associated factors. *Br J Psychiatry* 147:127, 1985.

WHEELER EO, WHITE PD, REED EW, COHEN ME: Neurocirculatory asthenia (anxiety neurosis, effort syndrome, neurasthenia). *JAMA* 142:878, 1950.

CHAPTER 25

THE LIMBIC LOBES AND THE NEUROLOGY OF EMOTION

The medical literature is replete with references to illnesses believed to be based on emotional disorders. Careful examination of clinical records reveals that a diversity of phenomena are being so classified: anxiety states, cycles of depression and mania, reactions to distressing life situations, so-called psychosomatic diseases, and illnesses of obscure nature. Obviously great license is being taken with the term *emotional,* the result no doubt of its indiscriminate nonmedical usage. Such ambiguity discourages neurologic analysis. Nevertheless, in certain clinical states patients appear to be inappropriately apathetic or excessively emotional under conditions that normally are not conducive to emotionality. It is to these disturbances that the following remarks pertain. First, however, one must be clear as to what is meant by emotion.

According to the *Dictionary of Psychology* (Drever) emotion is a complex state of the organism involving certain types of bodily changes (mainly visceral and under the control of the autonomic nervous system) in association with a mental state of excitement or perturbation, and leading usually to an impulse to action or to a certain type of behavior. If the emotion is intense, there may ensue a disturbance of intellectual functions, viz., a measure of disorganization of normal sequences of ideas and actions, and a tendency toward a more automatic behavior of ungraded, stereotyped character.

In its most easily recognized human form, emotion is initiated by a stimulus (real or imagined), the perception of which involves recognition, memory, and specific associations. The emotional state that is engendered is mirrored in a psychic experience, i.e., a feeling, or affect, which is purely subjective and known to others only through the patient's verbal expressions or by judgment of his or her behavior. The latter, which is in part hormonal-visceral and in part motor, may show itself in the patient's facial expression, bodily attitude, vocalizations, or directed voluntary activity. Subdivided, the components of emotion appear to consist of (1) the stimulus, (2) the affect or

feeling, (3) the autonomic-visceral changes, and (4) the impulse to a certain type of activity. In many cases of neurologic disease, however, it is not possible to separate these components from one another, and to emphasize one of them does no more than indicate the particular bias of the examiner.

ANATOMIC RELATIONSHIPS

The occurrence of deviant emotional reactions in the course of disease has been more regularly attended by lesions in certain parts of the nervous system than in others. These have been grouped under the term *limbic* and are among the most complex and least understood parts of the nervous system. The Latin word *limbus* means a border or margin. Credit for introducing the term limbic to neurology is usually given to Broca (of aphasia fame) who used it to describe the ring of gray matter (formed primarily by the cingulate and parahippocampal gyri) that encircles the corpus callosum and underlying upper brainstem. Actually Thomas Willis had pictured this region of the brain and referred to it as the limbus in 1664. Broca preferred his term *le grand lobe limbique* to *rhinencephalon,* which refers more specifically to structures having an olfactory function. Neuroanatomists of more recent times have affirmed his position and have extended the boundaries of the *limbic lobe* to include not only the cingulate and parahippocampal gyri, but also the underlying hippocampal formation (hippocampus, dentate gyrus, and subiculum, i.e., the portion of the parahippocampal gyrus in direct continuity with the hippocampus), subcallosal gyrus, amygdala, and the parolfactory area. The terms ''visceral brain'' and ''limbic system,'' introduced by Paul MacLean, have an even wider designation; in addition to all parts of the limbic lobe, they include a number of associated subcortical nuclei, such as those of the amygdaloid complex, septal region, preoptic area, hypothalamus, anterior thalamus, habenula, and central midbrain tegmentum, including the raphe nuclei and interpeduncular nucleus. The major structures comprising the limbic system and their relationships are illustrated in Figs. 25-1 and 25-2.

The cytoarchitectonic arrangements of the limbic cortex clearly distinguish it from the surrounding neocortex (isocortex). The latter, as stated in Chap. 21, differentiates into a characteristic six-layered structure. In contrast, the inner part of the limbic cortex (hippocampus) is composed of irregularly arranged aggregates of nerve cells that tend to be trilaminate (archi- or allocortex). The cortex of the cingulate gyrus, which forms the outer ring of the limbic lobe, is transitional between neocortex and allocortex—hence mesocortex or juxtallocortex. The hippocampal formation has a highly specialized architecture, consisting of

two interlocking convolutions, the dentate gyrus and hippocampus proper; the latter extends via the subiculum (gateway) to the parahippocampal gyrus. The main component of the hippocampal formation is a band of pyramidal neurons, one segment of which (Sommer sector, or CA1) is known to be especially susceptible to hypoxia. The amygdaloid complex, a subcortical nuclear component of the limbic lobe, also has a unique composition, consisting of several separable nuclei each with special connections to other limbic structures.

The connections between the orbital-frontal neocortex and limbic lobes, between the individual components of the limbic lobes, and between the limbic lobes and the hypothalamus and midbrain reveal some of the potential functional relationships. At the core of this system lies the medial forebrain bundle, a complex set of ascending and descending fibers that connect the orbital-frontal cortex, the septal nuclei, the hypothalamus, and caudally, certain nuclei

Figure 25-1

Sagittal schematic of the limbic system. The location of the major limbic structures and of the thalamus, hypothalamus, and midbrain tegmentum are shown. (From Angevine and Cotman.)

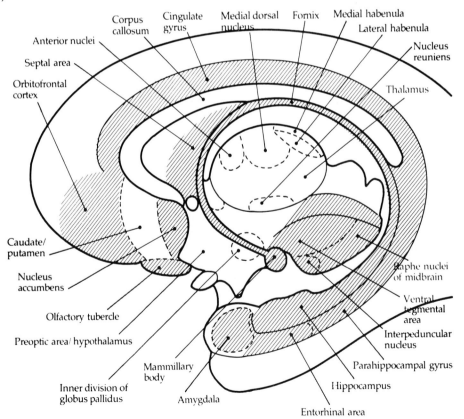

in the midbrain and pons. The major *afferent projections* to this system are from the amygdala and hippocampus rostrally, and from the spinal cord and lower brainstem caudally. The *major efferent projections* are to the thalamus, visceral-motor system, and hypophyseal complex. This system, of which the hypothalamus is the central part, has been designated by Nauta as the *septohypothalamomesencephalic continuum*, and represents the principal connecting pathway between the limbic forebrain (limbic lobe, orbitofrontal cortex, hippocampus, amygdala) and limbic midbrain areas.

Another connection between the limbic forebrain and midbrain structures is via the striamedullaris-fasciculus retroflexus route. This is a two-stage connection that runs over the thalamus to the habenula (a midline diencephalic nucleus located medial to the pulvinar) and then descends to the paramedian midbrain tegmentum.

There are many other interrelationships between various parts of the limbic system, only a few of which can be indicated here. The best known of these is the so-called Papez circuit. It leads from the hippocampus, via the fornix, to the mammillary body and septal and preoptic regions. The bundle of Vicq d'Azyr connects these latter parts with the anterior nuclei of the thalamus, which in turn project to the cingulate gyrus, and then, via the cingulum, to the hippocampus. The cingulum runs concentric to the curvature of the corpus callosum; it connects various parts of the limbic lobe to one another and projects also to the striatum and to certain brainstem nuclei. Also, the cingulum receives fibers from the inferior parietal lobule, which is a multimodal suprasensory center for the integration of visual, auditory, and tactile perceptions. According to Baleydier and Mauguiere, the posterior cingulate gyrus (area 23) is specifically connected with the associative temporal cortex, the medial temporal and orbitofrontal cortices, and the medial pulvinar (a thalamic nucleus which receives multisensory projections) and sends fibers to the parietal lobe. The anterior cingulate gyrus (area 24) projects to the amygdala, nucleus accumbens septi, and the medial dorsal, intralaminar, and anterior thalamic nuclei. Finally, the

Figure 25-2

Diagrams of the medial surface of the brain, illustrating: A. The topography of the mesocortex and allocortex, which constitute the cortical parts of the limbic system, or limbic lobe. B. Two major pathways that interconnect various parts of the limbic lobe. C. Topography of allocortical subicular projections to the limbic lobe. D. Topography of amygdaloid projections to the limbic lobe. (Reprinted, with permission, from Damasio and Van Hoesen.)

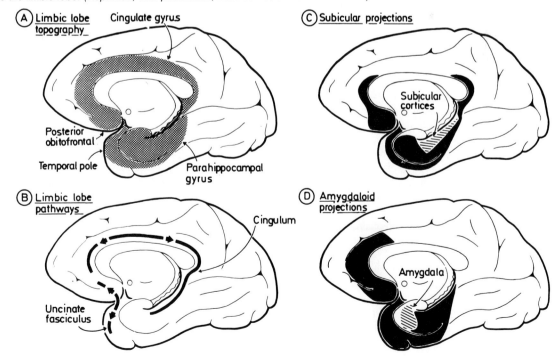

cingulate convolutions are connected with one another through the corpus callosum.

PHYSIOLOGY OF THE LIMBIC SYSTEM

The functional properties of the limbic structures first became known during the third and fourth decades of this century. From ablation and stimulation studies, Cannon, Bard, and others established the fact that the hypothalamus contained the suprasegmental integrations of the autonomic nervous system, both the sympathetic and parasympathetic parts (see Chap. 26). Soon after, anatomists found efferent pathways from the hypothalamus to the neural structures subserving the segmental parasympathetic and sympathetic reflexes. Bard localized the central regulatory apparatus for emotional reactions as well as that for respiration, wakefulness, and sexual activity in the hypothalamus. As described in Chap. 27, the hypothalamus was also found to contain neurosecretory cells, which control the secretion of the pituitary hormones; within it also are special sensory receptors for the regulation of hunger, thirst, body temperature, and levels of circulating electrolytes. Gradually there emerged the idea of a hypothalamic-pituitary-autonomic system that is essential to both the basic homeostatic and emergency reactions of the organism.

The impressions of the great psychologists of the nineteenth century that autonomic reactions were an essential motor part of instinctual emotions were corroborated. In fact, for a time, it was proposed that emotional experience was merely the awareness of these visceral activities (the James-Lange theory of emotion). The fallacy of this theory became evident when it was demonstrated by Sherrington that the capacity to manifest emotional changes remained after all visceral afferent fibers had been interrupted.

Although emotion involves the same neortical perceptive-cognitive activities as does any nonemotional sensorimotor experience, it was realized that the important difference relates to its prominent visceral effects, and the particular behavioral reactions that are evoked. Clearly, specific parts of the nervous system must be utilized.

As mentioned above, Bard, in 1928, first produced "sham rage" in cats by removal of the cerebral hemispheres, leaving the hypothalamus and brainstem intact. This is a state in which the animal reacts to all stimuli with an expression of intense anger and the signs of autonomic overactivity. In subsequent studies, Bard and Mountcastle found that only if the ablations included the amygdaloid nuclei on both sides would sham rage be produced; removal of all the neocortex, but sparing the limbic lobe, resulted in a placid animal. Interestingly, in the macaque monkey, a normally aggressive and recalcitrant animal, removal of the amygdaloid nuclei bilaterally greatly reduced the reactions of fear and anger.

On the basis of the physiologic observations of Cannon and Bard and his knowledge of neuroanatomy, Papez postulated that the limbic parts of the brain "elaborate the functions of central emotion as well as participate in emotional expression." Their intermediate position enables them to transmit neocortical effects, from their outer side, to the hypothalamus and midbrain, on their inner side.

The discovery that the hippocampus and underlying white matter is important in memory and learning emerged more recently through the observations of Scoville and Milner and others who observed the effects of medial temporal lobectomies, infarction, and anoxic lesions of these parts (page 342). The role of the cingulate gyrus in behavior of animals and humans has been the subject of much discussion. Stimulation is said to produce autonomic effects similar to the vegetative correlates of emotion (increase in heart rate and blood pressure, dilatation of pupils, piloerection, respiratory arrest, breath-holding). More complex responses such as fear, anxiety, or pleasure have been reported by neurosurgeons, although the results are inconstant. Bilateral cingulectomies have been performed, mainly in psychotic and neurotic patients (Meyer et al, Ballantine et al) with a diminution of emotional reactions. Some investigators believe that the cingulate gyri are involved in memory processing (functioning presumably in connection with the medial dorsal thalamic nuclei and medial temporal lobes) and in exploratory behavior and attention toward visual stimuli. In humans this system appears to be more efficient in the nondominant hemisphere, according to Bear. Baleydier and Mauguiere emphasize the dual function of the cingulate gyrus in alert and cognitive as well as emotional mentation.

Another aspect of limbic function has come to light as information is being acquired about neurotransmitters. The level of norepinephrine is highest in the hypothalamus and next in the medial parts of the limbic system, and at least 70 percent of it is concentrated in axon terminals of neurons that lie in the medulla and in the locus ceruleus in the pons (see Chap. 18). The axons of other ascending fibers, especially those coming from the reticular formation of the midbrain and terminating in the amygdala and septal nuclei as well as in lateral parts of the limbic lobe, are rich in serotonin. The axons of neurons in the ventral tegmental parts of the midbrain, which ascend in the medial forebrain bundle and the nigrostriatal pathway, contain much of the brain dopamine. Also notable is the fact that the zinc content of the limbic system is the highest of any part of the nervous system.

EMOTIONAL DISTURBANCES DUE TO DISEASES INVOLVING THE LIMBIC SYSTEM

Many of the foregoing ideas about the role of the limbic system have come from experimentation in laboratory animals. Only in relatively recent years have neurologists, primed with the knowledge of these studies, begun to observe emotional disturbances in patients with disease of limbic structures. These clinical observations, summarized in the following pages, are beginning to form an interesting chapter in neurology. The authors have listed the most readily recognized derangements of emotion in Table 25-1. The list is tentative, since our understanding of many of these states is incomplete. Whether these derangements can be used as pathognomonic indicators of lesions and diseases in particular parts of the human brain is not certain. Panksepp thinks of disturbances of emotional experiences and their expression as reflective only of "spheres of influence" of certain brain mechanisms. The authors believe that taken in context they are useful diagnostically. And, as knowledge of emotional disorders increases, it will undoubtedly bring together large segments of psychiatry and neurology.

EMOTIONAL DISTURBANCES IN HALLUCINATING AND DELUDED PATIENTS

These are best portrayed by the patient with a florid delirium. Threatened by imaginary figures and hearing their admonitions, which seem real and inescapable, the patient trembles, cowers, asks for protection, and displays the full picture of terror. The patient's affect, emotional reaction, and visceral and somatic motor responses are altogether appropriate to the content of the hallucinations, which are real to the patient. We have seen a patient slash his wrists and another try to drown himself in response to hallucinatory

Table 25-1
Neurology of emotional disturbances

I. Disturbances of emotionality due to:
   A. Perceptual abnormalities (illusions and hallucinations)
   B. Cognitive derangements (delusions)
II. Disinhibition of emotional expression
   A. Emotional lability
   B. Pathologic laughing and crying
III. Rage reactions and aggressivity
IV. Apathy and placidity
   A. Klüver-Bucy syndrome
   B. Other syndromes
V. Altered sexuality
VI. "Diencephalic" epilepsy
VII. Endogenous fear, anxiety, depression, and euphoria

voices that admonished them for their worthlessness and the shame they had brought upon their families. The abnormality under these circumstances is one of disordered perception and thinking, and we have no reason to believe that there is a derangement of the mechanism for emotional expression.

An emotional outburst, seemingly inappropriate or excessive, is a common occurrence in a psychotic person. Here the patient's emotional experience and impulse to action are a response to a delusion. Believing that somebody is threatening him, the patient may in a state of fury injure or kill the imagined tormentor. Again the emotional state becomes comprehensible once the content of the delusion has been divulged.

However, many psychotic patients whose hallucinations and delusions persist for months or years appear to become inured to them. No longer do the natural emotional reaction and impulse follow. The patient either denies having hallucinations or appears to disregard them. Perhaps we observe here the emergence of the bland affect and inappropriate emotional reaction of the schizophrenic. We have had occasion, in patients with alcoholic auditory hallucinosis, to trace this state from the early terrifying hallucinosis with appropriate emotional response to a state indistinguishable from paranoid schizophrenia with inappropriate reaction (see Chap. 41). Tolerance has developed to the morbid ideation, and the blunting of affect and emotional expression is secondary.

In these aforementioned conditions the clinician appreciates that although the emotional outburst is the overt manifestation of abnormal nervous functioning, the basic abnormality is in the sphere of perception and cognition. The emotional state is secondary.

DISINHIBITION OF EMOTIONAL EXPRESSION

Emotional Lability It is commonplace clinical experience that cerebral disease of many types, seemingly without respect to location, weakens the mechanism of control of emotional expression—a mechanism that has been acquired over years of maturation. To be grown up implies an ability to inhibit one's emotions; not that one has less feeling with maturation, but rather that it can be hidden from others. The degree to which this pertains varies with sex and ethnicity. In certain cultures, women are permitted to cry in public, but men are not. Men and women of Mediterranean races exhibit their feelings more openly than Anglo-Saxons.

A patient whose cerebrum has been damaged by one or more vascular lesions may suffer the humiliation of crying in public upon meeting an old friend or hearing the national anthem. Less often a mildly amusing remark or an attempt to tell a funny story may cause excessively prolonged and loud laughter. There may also be easy vacillation from one state to another; this is called *emotional lability* and has for more than a century been accepted as a sign of "organic brain disease." In this type of emotional disturbance, the response is appropriate to the stimulus and the affect is congruent with the visceral and motor components of the expression. The anatomic substrate is recondite. Perhaps lesions of the frontal lobes more than those of other parts of the brain are conducive to this state, but the authors are unaware of a critical clinicoanatomic study that substantiates this impression. It is certainly a frequent accompaniment of diffuse cerebral diseases such as Alzheimer disease, but of course these diseases also involve the limbic cortex.

Pathologic (Forced, Spasmodic) Laughing and Crying

This form of disordered emotional expression, characterized by outbursts of involuntary, uncontrollable laughing or crying, has been well recognized since the late nineteenth century. Numerous references to these conditions (the *Zwangslachen* and *Zwangsweinen* of German neurologists and the *rire et pleurer spasmodiques* of the French) are to be found in the writings of Oppenheim, von Monakow, and Wilson. Not included under this heading are the depression of spirits with tearfulness and irritability that so often accompanies chronic diseases of the nervous system; the facile moods and outbursts of the neurotic; or the euphoria and witzelsucht (silly behavior and shallow facetiousness) of frontal lobe disease.

Forced laughing and crying always signify a pathologic substratum in the brain, either diffuse or focal; hence it stands as a syndrome of multiple causes. It may occur with degenerative and vascular diseases of the brain and no doubt is the direct result of them, but often their diffuse nature precludes useful topographic analysis and clinicoanatomic correlation. More instructive in this regard are those cases in which a vascular, degenerative, or demyelinative process is discretely localized, but unfortunately few well-documented clinical cases of these types have been studied by proper anatomic methods.

The best examples of pathologic laughing and crying are provided by lacunar vascular disease and less often by amyotrophic lateral sclerosis and multiple sclerosis. They may also be part of the residue of the more widespread lesions of hypoxic-hypotensive encephalopathy, cerebral trauma, or encephalitis. Most often by far, a sudden hemiplegia or double hemiplegia sets the stage for the pathologic emotionality that emerges as part of the syndrome of *pseudobulbar palsy* (page 46). In the latter there is a striking incongruity between the loss of voluntary movements of muscles innervated by the motor nuclei of the lower pons and medulla (inability to forcefully close the eyes, elevate and retract the corners of the mouth, open and close the mouth, chew, swallow, phonate, articulate, and move the tongue) and the preservation of movement of the same muscles in yawning, coughing, throat clearing, and spasmodic laughing or crying (i.e., in reflexive pontomedullary activities). In some such cases, on the slightest provocation and sometimes for no apparent reason, the patient is thrown into hilarious laughter that may last for many minutes to the point of exhaustion. Or, far more often, the opposite happens—the mere mention of the patient's family or the sight of the doctor provokes an uncontrollable spasm that resembles crying. The severity of the emotional incontinence or the ease with which it is provoked does not always correspond with the severity of the faciobulbar paralysis. In some patients with forced crying and laughing there is little or no detectable weakness of facial and bulbar muscles; in others, forced laughing and crying is lacking, despite severe weakness. Therefore the pathologic emotional state cannot be equated with pseudobulbar palsy even though the two usually occur together.

Is this pathologic state, whether one of involuntary laughing or crying, activated by an appropriate stimulus? Does the emotional response accurately reflect the patient's affect, or feeling? There are no simple answers to these questions. One problem, of course, is to determine what constitutes an appropriate stimulus for the patient in question. Virtually always the emotional response is set off by some stimulus or thought, but in most cases it is trifling, or at least it appears so to the physician; merely addressing the patient or making some casual remark in his or her presence may suffice. Certainly in such cases the emotional response is out of all proportion to the stimulus. As to the affect, Oppenheim and others stated that these patients need not feel sad when crying or mirthful when laughing, and at least in some cases this is in agreement with our experience. Other patients, however, report a congruence of affect and expression.

Noteworthy also are the invariability of the initial motor response and the relatively undifferentiated nature of the emotional reaction. Laughter and crying, as they proceed, may merge with one another. Poeck puts great emphasis on the latter point, but it does not seem surprising when one considers the closeness of these two forms of emotional expression. Moreover, some normal persons cry when happy and smile when sad. More impressive to us is the fact that in some patients with pseudobulbar palsy, laughing and crying are the only available forms of emotional expression; intermediate phenomena, such as smiling and frowning, are lost. Impressive also are the patients with complete loss of voluntary bulbar motor function, in whom spasmodic laughing or crying, or a caricature thereof, is the only available form of expression, emotional or voluntary.

Wilson, in his discussion of the anatomic basis and mechanism of this state, pointed out that laughing and crying involve the same facial, vocal, and respiratory musculature and have similar visceral accompaniments (dilatation of facial vessels, secretion of tears, etc.). Two major supranuclear pathways control the pontomedullary mechanisms of facial and other movements required in laughing and crying. One is the familiar corticobulbar pathway, from motor cortex through the posterior limb of the internal capsule, for the control of volitional movements; the other is a more anterior frontothalamopontomedullary connection, for emotional expression. The latter is believed to descend just rostral to the knee of the internal capsule and to contain facilitatory and inhibitory fibers, but it has not been traced to the lower pons. Unilateral involvement of this anterior pathway leaves the opposite side of the face under volitional control but paretic during laughing, smiling, and crying (emotional facial paralysis); the opposite is observed with a unilateral corticobulbar lesion. Wilson's argument, based to some extent on clinicopathologic evidence, was that in pseudobulbar palsy the descending motor pathways, which naturally inhibit the expression of the emotions, are interrupted, but he could not decide where. Almost 40 years later, Poeck, after reviewing all the published pathologic anatomy in 30 verified cases, was able to do no more than conclude that supranuclear motor pathways are always involved with loss of a control mechanism somewhere in the brainstem, between thalamus and medulla. However, this clinical state is observed in amyotrophic lateral sclerosis where the corticobulbar tracts may be involved at a cortical and subcortical level. The lesions are bilateral in practically all instances (see references under Poeck).

A rare but probably related syndrome is *le fou rire prodromique* (prodromal laughing madness) of Féré, in which uncontrollable laughter begins abruptly and is followed after several hours by hemiplegia. Martin cites examples where patients laughed themselves to death. Again the pathologic anatomy is unsettled. Laughing and (less often) crying may occur also as a manifestation of epileptic seizures, usually of psychomotor type. Ictal laughter is usually without affect. Daly and Mulder have referred to these as "gelastic" seizures. The concurrence of gelastic seizures and precocious puberty should suggest an underlying hamartoma of the hypothalamus (see Chap. 27)

AGGRESSIVITY, VIOLENCE, ANGER AND RAGE

Aggressivity is an integral part of social behavior. During early life the emergence of aggressive action enables the individual to secure a position in the family and later in an ever-widening social circle. Individual differences, probably inherited, are noteworthy from infancy on, and males are generally more aggressive than females.

The degree to which excessively aggressive behavior is tolerated varies in different cultures. In most civilized societies, tantrum behavior, rage reactions, violence, and destructiveness are not condoned, and one of the principal objectives of training and education is the suppression and sublimation of such behavior. The rate at which this developmental process proceeds varies from one individual to another. In some, especially males, it is not complete until 25 to 30 years of age, and until that time the deviant behavior is called sociopathy (see Chap. 28).

That groundless outbreaks of unbridled rage may present as the main manifestation of disease is an idea not fully appreciated by the medical profession. Such patients may, with little provocation, change from an entirely reasonable state to one of the wildest rage, with a blindly furious impulse to violence and destruction. They charge at those around them, strike, kick, bite, and throttle whomever they can reach; they smash every object which they can lay hands on, tear their clothes, shout, and curse; their eyes flash and roll; their faces are suffused with blood, and their hearts beat violently. Every incoming sensation excites them to the point of frenzy. On attempting to subdue the patient, one finds that he has the strength of five people. In such states the patient appears out of contact with reality and is impervious to all argument or pleading. As well as one can tell, this pattern of behavior is associated with a feeling of anger. What is so obviously abnormal is the provocation of the attack by some trifling event and a degree of violence that is out of all proportion to the stimulus. There are examples also of dissociation of affect and behavior, in which the patient may spit, cry out, attack, or bite without seeming to be angry. This is especially true of the mentally retarded.

Rage reactions of the intensity described above may be encountered in the following medical settings: (1) as part of a psychomotor seizure (temporal lobe epilepsy); (2) as an episodic reaction without recognizable seizures or other neurologic abnormality, as in certain sociopaths; or (3) in the course of some recognizable acute or chronic neurologic disease. Each of these is considered below.

Rage in Psychomotor Seizures According to Gastaut et al a directed attack of uncontrollable rage may occur both as part of a seizure and as an interictal phenomenon. Some patients describe a gradual heightening of excitability for 2 to 3 days, either before or after a seizure, before bursting into a rage. Certainly such attacks have been observed, but they are not common, according to the survey of Gloor and Feindel. Aggressive behavior as part of a temporal lobe seizure is usually part of the ictal or postictal behavioral automatism and tends to be brief in duration and poorly directed (see page 253). Usually the lesion is in the temporal lobe of the dominant hemisphere. Similarly, a feeling of rage or severe anger is rare as an ictal emotion—much less common than feelings of fear, sadness, or pleasure (only 17 cases of anger among 165 patients with ictal emotion were reported by Williams). Geschwind has emphasized the frequency of a profound deepening of the patient's emotional experiences in temporal lobe epilepsy.

Rage Attacks without Visible Seizure In some instances of this type the patient has always been hot-headed, intolerant of frustration, and impulsive, exhibiting behavior that would be classed as sociopathic (Chap. 56). There are others, however, who, at certain periods of life, usually adolescence or early adulthood, begin to have episodes of wild, aggressive behavior. A small amount of alcohol or some other drug may set them off. One suspects epilepsy but there is no history of recognizable seizure and no interruption of consciousness so typical of complex partial epilepsy. The EEG is either normal or nonspecifically abnormal. In a few such patients, where aggression has caused serious injury to others (or homicide), depth electrodes have been placed in the amygdaloid nuclear complex and seizure discharges recorded. Attacks of excitement and various autonomic accompaniments have been aroused by stimulation of the same regions, and the abnormal behavior has in some instances been relieved by electrocoagulation of the abnormally discharging structures. Mark and Ervin have documented a number of impressive examples of this "dyscontrol syndrome."

Violent Behavior in Acute or Chronic Neurologic Disease From time to time one encounters patients in whom intense excitement, rage, and aggressivity begin abruptly in association with an acute neurologic disease. One of our patients, who was brought to the hospital in coma and with bloody cerebrospinal fluid after an occipital injury, became exceedingly violent as he regained consciousness and could only be controlled by the use of restraints and heavy sedation. When he died several days later, the medial portions of the orbital and temporal lobes were found to be reduced to a hemorrhagic pulp. Hemorrhagic leukoencephalitis, herpes simplex encephalitis, and traumatic necrosis of these regions may have the same effect. Fisher has noted the occurrence of intense rage reactions in association with a Wernicke type aphasia. Akert and Hess and Poeck and Pillieri have described cases of this type with a ruptured aneurysm of the circle of Willis and a hypophyseal adenoma (see Poeck and Pillieri for references).

Of interest also in this connection are the effects of slow-growing tumors of the temporal lobe. Of 18 such patients with mental disorder reported by Malamud, several had fits of rage; all the latter were cases of temporal lobe glioma. Other patients harboring such tumors had no rage reactions but exhibited a clinical picture resembling schizophrenia. It is noteworthy that eight of his nine patients with temporal lobe glioma also had seizures. Zeman and King, Cushing, Dott, Alpers, MacLean, and Bingley have reported other examples (see Poeck for references). The anteromedial part of the left temporal lobe has been the site of the tumor in the majority of cases. Falconer and Serafetinides have described patients with rage reactions in which there was a hamartoma or sclerotic focus in this region. However, the precise anatomy has not been demarcated.

Although the functional anatomy of these states of anger, rage, and aggressivity has not been fully established, all the human and animal data point to lesions in the temporal lobes. Stimulation of the corticomedial amygdaloid nuclei, through depth electrodes, evokes a display of anger, whereas stimulation of the basal-lateral nuclei does not. Destruction of the amygdaloid complex bilaterally reportedly reduces aggressivity in humans (Kiloh, Narabayashi et al). Presumably the amygdala activates the hypothalamus in the rage reaction either through the stria terminalis or the ventral amygdalofugal pathway, or both; Burzaco reduced the rage reaction by making lesions in the stria terminalis. Lesions in the medial dorsl nuclei, which receive projections from the amygdaloid nuclei, render humans more placid and docile. Sex hormones influence the activity of these temporal-lobe circuits. Testosterone promotes aggressivity and estradiol suppresses it, suggesting an explanation for sex differences in the disposition to anger.

PLACIDITY AND APATHY

The healthy organism normally displays highly energized, exploratory acitivity of its environment. Some of this is motivated by the drive for sexual satisfaction and procurement of food, and in humans it may be a matter of curiosity. According to Panksepp, these activities are governed by "expectancy circuits," involving nuclear groups in meso-limbic and mesocortical dopaminergic circuits, connected with the diencephalon and mesencephalon via forebrain bundles; lesions that interrupt these connections abolish the expectancy reactions.

In our experience, a quantitative reduction in all activity is the most frequent of all psychobehavioral alterations in patients with cerebral disease. There are fewer thoughts, fewer words uttered, fewer movements per unit of time. That this is not a purely motor phenomenon is disclosed in conversation with the patient, who seems to perceive and think more slowly, to make fewer associations with a given idea, and to exhibit less inquisitiveness and interest. This reduction in psychomotor activity is recognized as a personality change by the family.

Depending upon how this state is viewed, it may be interpreted as a heightened threshold to stimulation, inattentiveness or inability to maintain an attentive attitude, impaired thinking, apathy, or lack of impulse (abulia). All are correct in a sense, for each represents a different aspect of the reduced mental activity. Clinicoanatomic correlates are inexact, but bilateral interruption of the inferomedial frontal connections are sometimes observed to result in a striking lack of impulse, spontaneity, and conation, i.e., akinetic mutism. The patient is fully concious, wide awake, and looks around. In this respect abulia differs from stupor and hypersomnolence. Insofar as there is no paralysis, it differs from *pseudocoma* or *locked-in syndrome*. In abulia we assume the apathy and placidity to be secondary to reduced impulse.

Patients who exhibit abulia are difficult to test because they respond slowly or not at all to every type of test. Yet on rare occasions when intensely stimulated they may speak and act normally. It is as though some central diencephalic-cortical energizing mechanism, different from the reticular activating system of the upper brainstem, is impaired.

Quite apart from this abulic syndrome, which has already been discussed in relation to extensive lesions of the frontal lobes (Chap. 21), there are lesser degrees of it where a lively, sometimes volatile, person has been rendered placid by a disease of the nervous system. The patient is hypobulic. The most consistent changes of this type were observed to follow bilateral medial-orbital frontal leukotomy. If the lesions interrupted the anteromedial frontothalamic connections, anxiety, depression, and agitation were eliminated, but always at the expense of certain personality alterations such as indifference, lack of concern, and superficiality of thinking. These effects, too, have been discussed in relation to the frontal lobes. Barris and Schuman and many others have documented states of extreme placidity with lesions of the anterior cingulate gyri. Unlike retarded

depression (Chap. 56), the mood is neutral; the patient is apathetic rather than depressed.

The alteration in emotional behavior described above was also found by Klüver and Bucy to be part of a syndrome resulting from total bilateral temporal lobectomy in adult rhesus monkeys. In addition, their animals lost the ability to recognize objects visually (they could not distinguish edible from inedible objects), had a striking tendency to examine everything orally, were unusually alert and responsive to visual stimuli (they touched or mouthed every object in their visual fields), became hypersexual, and increased their food intake.

This constellation of behavioral changes has been sought in human beings, but the complete syndrome has been described only infrequently (Marlowe et al). Pillieri and Poeck have collected some of the cases that come closest to reproducing the syndrome (Fig. 25-3A and B). Unfortunately many human examples have occurred in conjunction with diffuse diseases (Alzheimer and Pick cerebral atrophies, meningoencephalitis of toxoplasmic or herpes simplex type) and hence are of little use for anatomic analysis. With bitemporal surgical ablations placidity and enhanced oral behavior were the most frequent consequences and altered sexual behavior and visual agnosia less so. In all patients who showed placidity and an amnesic state the hippocampi had been destroyed, but not the amygdaloid nuclei. It is also of interest that the cingulate gyri, where lesions have sometimes been made to reduce anxiety and depression, were involved in only one of five cases with placidity.

Perhaps the most consistent type of reduced emotionality in humans is the one associated with acute lesions (usually infarcts or hemorrhages) in the right or nondominant parietal lobe. Not only is the patient indifferent to the paralysis but, as Bear points out, is unconcerned about other diseases and personal and family problems, is less able to interpret the emotional facial expressions of others, and is inattentive in general. Dimond et al interpret this to mean that the right hemisphere is more involved in affective-emotional experience than the left, which is committed to language. This has been confirmed in the split-brain preparation. Bear speculates that in the right hemisphere there are two pathways subserving visual exploration for affective relevant stimuli—one that passes to the inferior parietal lobe, cingulate gyrus, and frontal lobe for attentive surveillance, the other to the medial temporal, amygdaloid, and inferior frontal cortex for the effectuation of the corresponding emotional response.

The full range of placidity reactions in neurology has

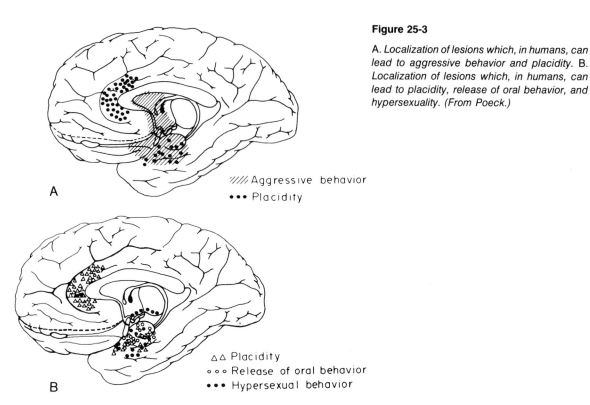

Figure 25-3

A. *Localization of lesions which, in humans, can lead to aggressive behavior and placidity.* B. *Localization of lesions which, in humans, can lead to placidity, release of oral behavior, and hypersexuality. (From Poeck.)*

A

///// Aggressive behavior
••• Placidity

B

△△ Placidity
ooo Release of oral behavior
••• Hypersexual behavior

not been cataloged. Unfortunately neurologists and psychiatrists have tended to neglect this aspect of behavior.

ALTERED SEXUALITY

The normal pattern of sexual behavior in both male and female may be altered by cerebral disease quite apart from impairment due to obvious physical disability or to diseases that destroy or isolate the segmental reflex mechanisms (see Chap. 26).

Hypersexuality in either sex is a rare but well-documented complication of neurologic disease. Kleist pointed out that lesions of the orbital parts of the frontal lobes remove moral-ethical restraints and may lead to indiscriminate sexual behavior, and that superior frontal lesions may be associated with a general loss of initiative which reduces all impulsivity, including sexual. In rare cases, extreme hypersexuality marks the onset of encephalitis or develops gradually with tumors of the temporal region. Persistence of this behavior suggests disinhibition rather than stimulation as the mechanism. Presumably the limbic parts of the brain are affected, the ones from which MacLean and Ploog could evoke penile erection and orgasm by electrical stimulation (medial dorsal thalamus, medial

forebrain bundle, and septal preoptic region). In humans, Heath has observed that stimulation of the ventral-septal area (through depth electrodes) evokes feelings of pleasure and lust. However, we know of no case in which a stable lesion that caused abnormal sexual behavior has been studied carefully by serial sections of the whole brain.

In our clinical work we find that *hyposexuality*, meaning loss of libido, is most often due to a depressive illness. Certain drugs, notably antihypertensive agents, anticonvulsants, and neuroleptics, may cause a loss of libido. A variety of cerebral diseases may also have this effect. Lesions that involve the tuberoinfundibular region of the hypothalamus are known to cause disturbances in sexual function. If acquired early in life, pubertal changes are prevented from occurring; hamartomas of the hypothalamus, as in von Recklinghausen neurofibromatosis and tuberous sclerosis, may cause sexual precocity. Panautonomic neuropathy and lesions involving the sacral parts of the parasympathetic system also abolish normal sexual performance.

Blumer and Walker have reviewed the literature on the association of epilepsy and abnormal sexual behavior. They note that sexual arousal is apt to occur only in relation to temporal lobe seizures, particularly when the discharging focus is in the medial temporal region. These have been called *sexual seizures*. They also cite the high incidence of the global hyposexuality in patients with temporal lobe epilepsy. Temporal lobectomy in such patients has sometimes been followed by a period of hypersexuality.

"DIENCEPHALIC" AUTONOMIC EPILEPSY

Penfield, in 1929, recorded a clinical illness characterized by episodes of flushing of the face, lacrimation, salivation, shivering, hiccups, an initial increase and then decrease in respiratory rate, tachycardia, hypertension, sweating, and dilatation or contraction of the pupils. Consciousness was altered so that it was impossible to ascertain the patient's emotional state. Such attacks occurred several times a day and lasted for 4 to 10 min. The cause was a tumor wedged into the foramina of Monro and compressing the dorsal (or anterior) nuclei of the thalamus on either side.

Most neurologists have found it impossible to evaluate this case. The nature of the lesion and its location leave open the possibility of intermittent hydrocephalus. Although certain autonomic changes commonly appear in the course of seizures (dilatation of one or both pupils, sweating, hyperpnea, etc.; see page 250), we have never observed a seizure of precisely the type described by Penfield nor have any convincing examples been reported by others. However, attacks of autonomic overactivity without loss of consciousness may occur with basal ganglionic disease and with pheochromocytomas (see Chap. 26).

ANXIETY, FEAR, AND DEPRESSION

The phenomenon of acute fear and anxiety occurring as a prelude to, or part of, a seizure is familiar to every physician. Williams' study, already alluded to, is of particular interest; in a series of about 2000 epileptics, he was able to cull 100 patients in whom an emotional experience was part of the seizure. Of these latter cases, 61 experienced feelings of fear and anxiety and 21 experienced depression. Daly has made similar observations. These clinical data call to mind the effects of stimulating the upper, anterior, and inferior parts of the temporal lobe and cingulate gyrus during surgical procedures (Penfield and Jasper); frequently the patient described feelings of strangeness, uneasiness, and fear. Consciousness was variably impaired at the same time in most instances, and some patients had hallucinatory experiences as well.

Neuronal circuits subserving fear are coextensive with those of anger; both are thought to lie in the medial part of the temporal lobe. Both in animals and in humans, electrical stimulation in this region can arouse each emotion, but the circuitry subserving fear is located lateral to that of anger and rage. Destruction of the central part of the amygdaloid nuclear complex abolishes fear reactions. These nuclei are connected to the lateral hypothalamus and midbrain tegmentum, from which Monroe and Heath and Nashold et al have been able to evoke feelings of fear and anxiety by electrical stimulation.

Depression is less frequent as an ictal emotion, although this state may occur as an interictal phenomenon. Of interest is the observation that lesions of the dominant hemisphere are more likely to be attended by a pervasive depression of mood than lesions of the nondominant one. We have observed this tendency and Robinson and Szetela have more fully documented this relationship. They found that approximately two-thirds of their patients with left hemispheric infarcts (shown by CT scans) had significant depressions. It appeared that the nearer the lesion was to the frontal lobe, the greater the likelihood of depression.

Odd mixtures of depression and anxiety are often associated with temporal lobe tumors, and less often with tumors of the hypothalamus and third ventricle (see review by Alpers).

Elation and euphoria are less well documented as limbic phenomena, nor has the elevation in mood in some patients with multiple sclerosis ever been adequately explained. Feelings of pleasure, satisfaction, and "stirring sensations" are unusual but well-described emotional experiences in patients with temporal lobe seizures, and this type of affective response, like that of fear, has been elicited by Penfield and Jasper by stimulating several different parts of the temporal lobe. In hypomania and mania every experience may be colored by feelings of delight and pleasure and a sense of power, and these experiences may be remembered after the patient has recovered.

DIFFERENTIAL DIAGNOSIS

Aside from clinical observation there are no reliable means of evaluating the above-described emotional disorders. While neurologic medicine has done little more than describe and classify some of the clinical states dominated by emotional derangements, an activity considered by some to be the lowest level of science, knowledge of this type is nonetheless of both theoretical and practical importance. In theory it prepares one for the next step, of passing from a superficial to a deeper order of inquiry, where questions of pathogenesis can be broached. Practically, it provides certain clues that are useful in the differential diagnosis of disease, as the following clinical problems indicate.

Uninhibited Laughter and Crying and Emotional Lability As indicated earlier, one may confidently assume that the syndrome of forced or spasmodic laughing and crying signifies cerebral disease and more specifically bilateral disease of the corticobulbar tracts. Usually the motor and reflex changes of pseudobulbar palsy are associated, especially heightened facial and mandibular reflexes, and often corticospinal tract signs are present as well. Extreme emotional lability also indicates bilateral cerebral disease, although here, too, only the signs of unilateral disease may be apparent clinically. The most common pathologic states are lacunar infarction or other cerebrovascular lesions, diffuse hypoxic-hypotensive encephalopathy, amyotrophic lateral sclerosis, and multiple sclerosis. Abrupt onset, of course, points to vascular disease.

Placidity and Apathy　These may be the earliest and most important signs of cerebral disease. Clinically, placidity and apathy must be distinguished from the retardation of Parkinson disease and depressive illness. Alzheimer disease, normal-pressure hydrocephalus, and frontal–corpus callosum tumors are the usual pathologic bases of apathy and placidity, but these disturbances may occur in conjunction with a variety of other frontal and temporal lesions (see also the remarks on stupor, pseudocoma or locked-in syndrome, and retarded depression on pages 275, 276, and 407).

An Outburst of Violent Anger and Aggressive Action　Most often such an outburst is but another episode in a lifelong sequence of sociopathic behavior (see Chap. 56). More significance attaches to its abrupt appearance as a sudden departure from normal character. If there are seizures, and if rage accompanies the seizures, the outburst of rage should be viewed as the consequence of the seizure activity on temporal lobe function. The usual causes are birth injury, cranial trauma, encephalitis, and earlier seizures. Amygdaloid seizures as a cause of blind rage are suggested by (1) abruptness of onset, (2) easy provocation, (3) evocation by alcohol or small amounts of other drugs, (4) other signs (clinical or EEG) of temporal lobe disease. Rarely, rage and aggressivity are expressive of an acute neurologic disease of the medial temporal and orbital-frontal regions. We have several times observed such states transiently in a stable individual as an expression of an obscure encephalopathy.

　Rage reactions with continuous violent activity must be distinguished from *mania*, in which there is flight of ideation to the point of incoherence, euphoric or irritable mood, and incessant activity; *organic driveness*, in which continuous activity is accompanied by no clear ideation;

and extreme instances of *akathisia,* where incessant restless movements and pacing may occur in conjunction with extrapyramidal symptoms (see Chaps. 56, 21, and 42, respectively).

An Acute Panic Attack, Extreme Fright and Agitation　Here the central problem must be clarified by determining whether the patient is delirious (clouding of consciousness, psychomotor overactivity, and hallucinations), deluded (schizophrenia), in an anxiety attack (anxiety neurosis, anxious depression), or hypomanic (overactive, flight of ideas). Rarely does panic prove to be an expression of temporal lobe epilepsy.

Depression, Anxiety, Bizarre Ideation Developing over Weeks, Months, or a Few Years　While these symptoms are usually due to a psychosis (schizophrenia or manic-depressive disease), one should consider a tumor or other lesion of the temporal lobe when there are psychomotor seizures, aphasic difficulty, rotatory vertigo (rare), and quadrantic visual field defect. Such states have been described in hypothalamic disease, suggested by somnolence, diabetes insipidus, visual field defects, and hydrocephalus.

REFERENCES

ANGEVINE JB JR, COTMAN CW: *Principles of Neuroanatomy.* New York, Oxford University Press, 1981, pp 253–283.

AKERT K, HESS WR: Über die neurobiologischen Grundlagen akuter affektiver Erregungszustände. *Schweiz Med Wochenschr* 92:1524, 1962.

ALPERS BJ: Personality and emotional disorders associated with hypothalamic lesions. *Res Publ Assoc Nerv Ment Dis* 20:725, 1939.

BALEYDIER C, MAUGUIERE F: The duality of the cingulate gyrus in monkey. *Brain* 103:525, 1980.

BALLANTINE HT, CASSIDY WL, FLANAGAN NB et al: Stereotaxic anterior cingulotomy for neuropsychiatric illness and chronic pain. *J Neurosurg* 26:488, 1967.

BARD P: A diencephalic mechanism for the expression of rage with special reference to the sympathetic nervous system. *Am J Physiol* 84:490, 1928.

BARD P, MOUNTCASTLE VB: Some forebrain mechanisms involved in the expression of rage with special reference to suppression of angry behavior. *Assoc Res Nerv Ment Dis Proc* 27:362, 1947.

BARRIS RW, SCHUMAN HR: Bilateral anterior cingulate gyrus lesions: Syndrome of the anterior cingulate gyri. *Neurology* 3:44, 1953.

BEAR DM: Hemispheric specialization and the neurology of emotion. *Arch Neurol* 40:195, 1983.

BINGLEY T: Mental symptoms in temporal lobe epilepsy and temporal lobe gliomas. *Acta Psychiatr Scand* 33(suppl 120):1958.

BLUMER D, WALKER AE: The neural basis of sexual behavior, in Benson F, Blumer D (eds): *Psychiatric Aspects of Neurologic*

Disease. New York, Grune & Stratton, 1975, chap 11, pp 199–217.

BURZACO JA: Fundus stria terminalis, an optional target in sedative sterotaxic surgery, in Laitinen LV, Livingston KE (eds): *Surgical Approaches in Psychiatry.* Baltimore, University Park Press, 1973, pp 135–137.

CANNON WB: *Bodily Changes in Pain, Hunger and Fear,* 2nd ed. New York, Appleton-Century, 1929.

CUSHING H: *Pituitary Body, Hypothalamus and Parasympathetic Nervous System.* Springfield, IL, Charles C Thomas, 1932.

DALY DD: Ictal affect. *Am J Psychiatry* 115:97, 1958.

DALY DD, MULDER DW: Gelastic epilepsy. *Neurology* 7:189, 1957.

DAMASIO AR, VAN HOESEN GW: The limbic system and the localization of herpes simplex encephalitis. *J Neurol Neurosurg Psychiatry* 48:297, 1985.

DIMOND SJ, FARRINGTON L, JOHNSON P: Differing emotional responses from right and left hemisphere. *Nature* 261:690, 1976.

DOTT NM: Surgical aspects of the hypothalamus, in Clark WE et al (eds): *The Hypothalamus: Morphological, Functional, Clinical and Surgical Aspects.* Edinburgh, Oliver & Boyd, 1938.

FALCONER MA, SERAFETINIDES EA: A follow-up study of surgery in temporal lobe epilepsy. *J Neurol Neurosurg Psychiatry* 26:154, 1963.

FÉRÉ MC: Le fou rire prodromique. *Rev Neurol* 11:353, 1903.

FISHER CM: Anger associated with dysphasia. *Trans Am Neurol Assoc* 95:240, 1970.

GASTAUT H, MORIN G, LEFEVRE N: Etude de comportement des epileptiques psychomoteurs dans l'intervalle de leurs crises. *Ann Med Psychol* 1:1, 1955.

GESCHWIND N: The clinical setting of aggression in temporal lobe epilepsy, in Field WS, Sweet WH (eds): *The Neurobiology of Violence.* St Louis, Warren H Green, 1975.

GLOOR P, FEINDEL W: Affective behavior and the temporal lobe, in *Physiologie und Pathophysiologie des Vegetativen Nervensystems,* vol 2: *Pathophysiologie.* Stuttgart, Hippokrates-Verlag, 1963, pp 685–716.

HEATH RG: Pleasure and brain activity in man. *J Nerv Ment Dis* 154:3, 1972.

ISAACSON RL: *The Limbic System.* New York, Plenum, 1974.

KILOH LG: The treatment of anger and aggression and the modification of sex deviaiton, in Smith JS, Kiloh LG (eds): *Psychosurgery and Psychiatry.* Oxford, Pergamon Press, 1977, pp 37–54.

KLEIST K: Gehirnpathologie und lokalisatorische Ergebnisse; die Störungen der Ichleistungen und ihre Lokalisation im Orbital-, Innen- und Zwischenhirn. *Monatsschr Psychiatr Neurol* 79:338, 1931.

KLÜVER H, BUCY PC: An analysis of certain effects of bilateral temporal lobectomy in the rhesus monkey with special reference to psychic blindness. *J Psychol* 5:33, 1938.

MACLEAN PD: Contrasting functions of limbic and neocortical systems of the brain and their relevance to psychophysiological aspects of medicine. *Am J Med* 25:611, 1958.

MACLEAN PD, PLOOG DW: Cerebral representation of penile erection. *J Neurophysiol* 25:29, 1962.

MALAMUD N: Psychiatric disorder with intracranial tumors of limbic system. *Arch Neurol* 17:113, 1967.

MARK VH, ERVIN FR: *Violence and the Brain.* New York, Harper & Row, 1970.

MARLOWE WB, MANCALL EL, THOMAS JJ: Complete Klüver-Bucy syndrome in man. *Cortex* 11:53, 1975.

MARTIN JP: Fits of laughter (sham mirth) in organic cerebral disease. *Brain* 70:453, 1950.

MEYER G, MACELHANEY M, MARTIN W et al: Stereotaxic cingulotomy with results of acute stimulation and serial psychological testing, in Laitinen LV, Livingston KE (eds): *Surgical Approaches in Psychiatry.* Lancaster, Medical and Technical Publishers, 1973, pp 38–58.

MONROE RR, HEATH RC: Psychiatric observations on the patient group, in Heath RC (ed): *Studies in Schizophrenia.* Cambridge, MA, Harvard University Press, 1983, pp 345–383.

NARABAYASHI H, NACAO Y, YOSHIDA M, NAGAHATA M: Stereotaxic amygdalectomy for behavior disorders. *Arch Neurol* 9:1, 1963.

NASHOLD BS, WILSON WP, SLAUGHTER DE: Sensations evoked by stimulation in the midbrain of man. *J Neurosurg* 30:14, 1969.

NAUTA WJH: The central visceromotor system: A general survey, in Hockman CH (ed): *Limbic System Mechanisms and Autonomic Function.* Springfield, IL, Charles C Thomas, 1972, chap 2, pp 21–33.

PANKSEPP J: Mood changes, in Vinken PJ, Bruyn GW, Klawans HL (eds): *Handbook of Clinical Neurology,* vol 45. Amsterdam, North-Holland, 1985, chap 21.

PAPEZ JW: A proposed mechanism of emotion. *Arch Neurol Psychiatry* 38:725, 1937.

PENFIELD W, JASPER H: *Epilepsy and the Functional Anatomy of the Human Brain.* Boston, Little, Brown, 1954, pp 413–416.

PILLIERI G: The Klüver-Bucy syndrome in man. *Psychiatr Neurol* 152:65, 1967.

POECK K: Pathophysiology of emotional disorders associated with brain damage, in Vinken PJ, Bruyn GW (eds): *Handbook of Clinical Neurology,* vol 3: *Disorders of Higher Nervous Activity.* Amsterdam, North-Holland, 1969, chap 20, pp 343–367.

POECK K: Pathological laughter and crying, in Vinken PJ, Bruyn GW, Klawans HV (eds): *Handbook of Clinical Neurology,* vol 45. Amsterdam, North-Holland, 1985, chap 16.

ROBINSON RG, SZETELA B: Mood change following left hemisphere injury. *Ann Neurol* 9:447, 1981.

SCOVILLE WB, MILNER B: Loss of recent memory after bilateral hippocampal lesions. *J Neurol Neurosurg Psychiatry* 20:11, 1957.

WILLIAMS D: The structure of emotions reflected in epileptic experiences. *Brain* 79:29, 1956.

WILSON SAK: Some problems in neurology: II. Pathological laughing and crying. *J Neurol Psychopathol* 16:299, 1924.

ZEMAN W, KING FA: Tumors of the septum pellucidum and adjacent structures with abnormal affective behavior: An anterior or midline structure syndrome. *J Nerv Ment Dis* 127:490, 1958.

CHAPTER 26

DISORDERS OF THE AUTONOMIC NERVOUS SYSTEM

The human internal environment is regulated in large measure by the autonomic nervous system and endocrine glands and by the integrated activity of these two systems. The visceral and homeostatic functions, essential to life and the survival of our species, are involuntary. Why nature has divorced them from volition is an interesting question. One would like to think that the mind, being preoccupied with discriminative, moral, and esthetic matters, should not have to be troubled with such mundane activities as breathing, regulation of heart rate, lactating, hunger, and sleep. Claude Bernard expressed this idea in more sardonic terms when he wrote that "nature thought it prudent to remove these important phenomena from the caprice of an ignorant will."

Diseases that exert their morbid effects exclusively on the neuroendocrine axis, i.e., are primary, are not numerous and would deserve only passing notice in a textbook on neurology. On the other hand, there are many medical diseases whose symptoms are to some extent expressed by a derangement of autonomic and neuroendocrine function (e.g., hypertension, syncope, asthma). Also a wide variety of pharmacologic agents influence these functions, making them the concern of every physician. What is more, autonomic parts of the neuraxis and parts of the endocrine system represent the effector apparatus utilized in all emotional and affective experience.

For purposes of exposition, the disorders of the autonomic nervous system and neuroendocrine system are accorded separate chapters—this chapter dealing with the autonomic nervous system and the following one with the hypothalamus and neuroendocrine disorders. The following discussion of anatomy and physiology serves as a necessary introduction to both chapters.

ANATOMIC AND PHYSIOLOGIC CONSIDERATIONS

Probably the most remarkable feature of the autonomic nervous system (also called the visceral or vegetative nervous system) is the location of a major part of it outside the cerebrospinal axis, in proximity to the structures that it innervates. This position alone seems to symbolize its relative independence from the cerebrospinal system. Also, in distinction to the somatic neuromuscular system, where a single motor neuron bridges the gap between the central nervous system and the effector organ, in the autonomic nervous system there are always two motor neurons (Fig. 26-1).

From a strictly anatomic viewpoint the autonomic nervous system is divided into thoracolumbar (sympathetic) and craniosacral (parasympathetic) divisions (Figs. 26-2 and 26-3). The *parasympathetic division* consists of the special visceral nuclei in the brainstem, viz., the antero-median and dorsal visceral cell columns of the oculomotor nucleus, the superior and inferior salivatory nuclei, and the dorsal motor nucleus of the vagus. The axons (preganglionic fibers) of the anteromedian nucleus and dorsal visceral cell columns (only the latter constitute the Edinger-Westphal nucleus) course in the oculomotor nerve and synapse in the ciliary ganglion in the orbit; axons of the ciliary ganglion cells innervate the ciliary muscle and sphincter pupillae (Fig. 13-6). The preganglionic fibers of the superior salivatory nucleus enter the facial nerve, and at a point near the geniculate ganglion they form the greater superficial petrosal nerve, through which they reach the sphenopalatine ganglion; the cells of this ganglion innervate the lacrimal gland (see also Fig. 46-1). Other fibers of the facial nerve traverse the tympanic cavity as the chorda tympani and eventually join the submandibular ganglion; the cells of this ganglion innervate the submandibular and sublingual glands. Axons of the inferior salivatory nerve cells enter the glossopharyngeal nerve and reach the otic ganglion through the tympanic plexus and lesser superficial petrosal nerve; cells of the otic ganglion send fibers to the parotid gland. Preganglionic fibers, derived from the dorsal motor nucleus, enter the vagus nerve and terminate in ganglia situated in the walls of the many thoracic and abdominal viscera; their postganglionic fibers activate smooth muscle and glands of the pharynx, esophagus, and the gastrointestinal tract (to midcolon), as well as the heart, pancreas, liver, gallbladder, kidney, and ureter.

The *sacral part of the parasympathetic system* is made up largely of preganglionic neurons originating in the lateral horns of the second, third, and fourth sacral segments. Axons of these sacral neurons traverse the sacral nerves and synapse in ganglia that lie within the walls of the distal colon, bladder, and other pelvic organs. These sacral autonomic neurons, like the cranial ones, have long preganglionic and short postganglionic fibers, which would be expected from the peripheral location of the ganglion cells.

The separation of autonomic and motor neurons at the sacral level has been difficult, because some neurons activate the external sphincter (voluntary muscle) and others supply the smooth muscle of the bladder. At the turn of the century, Onufrowicz, calling himself Onuf, described a discrete, compact group of relatively small cells in the

anterior horns of the sacral segments. These neurons were originally thought to be autonomic in function, mainly because of their anatomic features. There is now compelling evidence that they are somatomotor, innervating the skeletal muscle of the external urethral and anal sphincters (Holstege and Tan). Neurons in the intermediolateral cell column (probably parasympathetic motor) innervate the detrusor of the bladder wall. In passing, it is worth noting that in motor system disease, in which bladder and bowel functions are usually preserved, the neurons in Onuf's nucleus (in contrast to other somatomotor neurons in the sacral cord) remain intact (Mannen et al).

The *preganglionic neurons of the sympathetic division* originate in the intermediolateral cell column of the spinal

Figure 26-1

Sympathetic outflow from the spinal cord and the course and distribution of sympathetic fibers. The preganglionic fibers are in heavy lines; postganglionic fibers are in thin lines. (From Pick.)

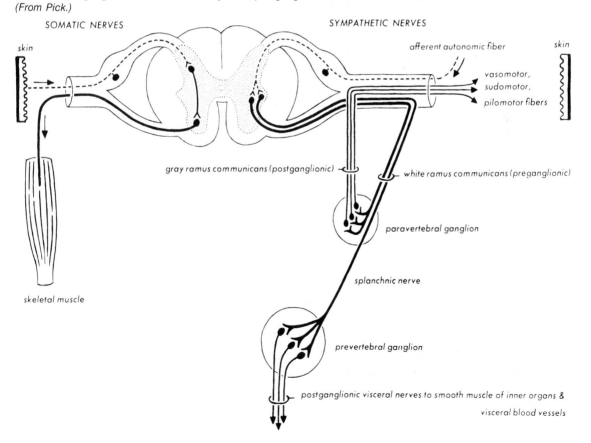

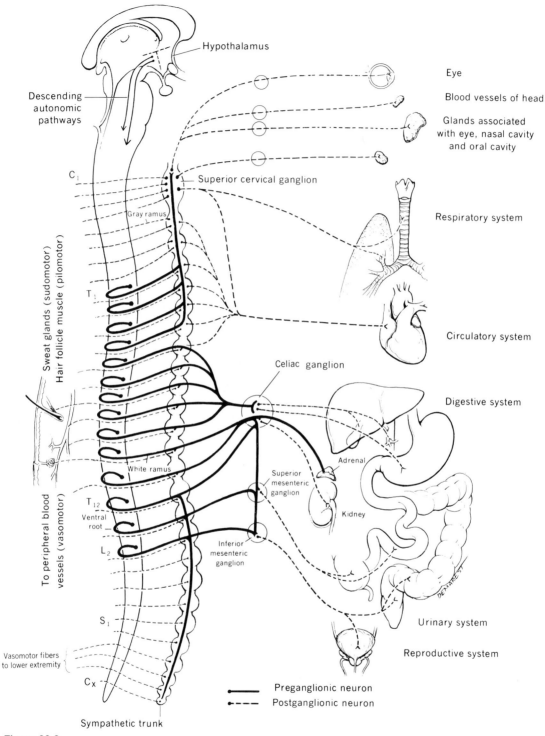

Figure 26-2

The sympathetic (thoracolumbar) division of the autonomic nervous system. Preganglionic fibers extend from the intermediolateral nucleus of the spinal cord to the peripheral autonomic ganglia, and postganglionic fibers extend from the peripheral ganglia to the effector organs, according to the scheme in Fig. 26-1. (From CL Noback, R Demarest, The Human Nervous System, 3rd ed, New York, McGraw-Hill, 1981.)

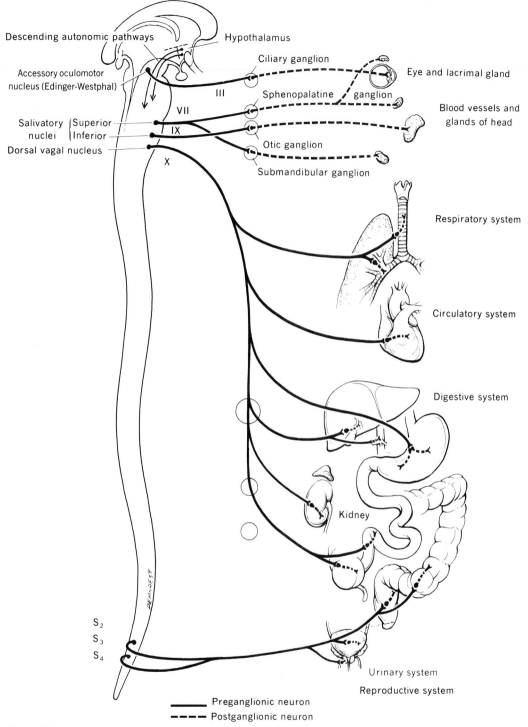

Figure 26-3

The parasympathetic (craniosacral) division of the autonomic nervous system. Preganglionic fibers extend from nuclei of the brainstem and sacral segments of the spinal cord to peripheral ganglia. Short postganglionic fibers extend from the ganglia to the effector organs. The lateral-posterior hypothalamus is part of the supranuclear mechanism for the regulation of parasympathetic activities. The frontal and limbic parts of the supranuclear regulatory apparatus are not indicated in the diagram (see text). (From CL Noback, R Demarest, The Human Nervous System, 3rd ed, New York, McGraw-Hill, 1981.)

gray matter, from the eighth cervical to the second lumbar segments. Low and Dyck have estimated that each cord segment contains 5000 lateral horn cells and that in late adult life there is an attrition of 5 to 7 percent per decade. The postganglionic neurons consist of aggregates of motor neurons whose cell bodies are collected into two large ganglionated chains or cords, one on each side of the vertebral column (paravertebral ganglia) and several single prevertebral ganglia.

The axons of the preganglionic neurons traverse the anterior roots and enter the sympathetic ganglia via the white (medullated) communicating rami. A preganglionic sympathetic fiber may pass through several ganglia before it finally synapses with a postganglionic neuron (see Figs. 26-1 and 26-4), and its terminals make contact with 20 or more postganglionic neurons. In addition, one ganglion cell is supplied by several preganglionic fibers; thus a diffuse discharge of the sympathetic system is possible. Some preganglionic fibers pass through the paravertebral ganglia as splanchnic nerves to synapse in prevertebral ganglia (celiac, superior, and inferior mesenteric ganglia, see Fig. 26-4).

The axons of the sympathetic ganglion cells are unmyelinated or thinly myelinated. Those that pass via the gray communicating rami to spinal nerves supply the blood vessels, sweat glands, and hair follicles, and also form plexuses which supply the heart, bronchi, kidneys, intestines, pancreas, bladder, and sex organs. The postganglionic fibers of the prevertebral ganglia form the hypogastric, splanchnic, and mesenteric plexuses, which innervate the glands, smooth muscle, and blood vessels of the abdominal and pelvic viscera (Figs. 26-1 and 26-2).

The sympathetic innervation of the adrenal medulla is peculiar in that its secretory cells receive preganglionic fibers directly from the splanchnic nerves. This is an exception to the rule that organs innervated by the autonomic nervous system receive only postganglionic nerves. This unique arrangement can be explained by the fact that the cells of the adrenal medulla are the morphologic homologues of the postganglionic sympathetic neurons, and they secrete epinephrine and norepinephrine, the postganglionic transmitters, directly into the bloodstream.

There are three cervical (superior, middle, and inferior, or stellate), eleven thoracic, and four to six lumbar ganglia. The head receives its sympathetic supply from the eighth cervical and first two thoracic cord segments, the fibers of which pass through the inferior and middle cervical ganglia and synapse with the nerve cells of the superior cervical ganglia. Postganglionic fibers from the latter cells follow the internal and external carotid arteries and innervate the blood vessels, smooth muscle, and the sweat, lacrimal, and salivary glands of the head. Included among these postganglionic fibers are the pupillodilator fibers and those innervating Müller's muscle of the upper eyelid. The arm receives its postganglionic innervation from the upper thoracic segments via the stellate ganglion. The cardiac plexus and other thoracic sympathetic nerves are derived from the upper thoracic segments and the abdominal visceral plexuses, from the fifth to the ninth or tenth thoracic segments. The lower three lumbar and first sacral ganglia, however, have no visceral connections; they supply only the legs.

The nerve terminals, and the neuromuscular and neuroglandular junctions of the autonomic nervous system have been more difficult to visualize and study than the motor end plates of striated muscle. As the postganglionic axons enter an organ, usually via the vasculature, they ramify into many smaller branches and pass, without a Schwann cell covering, among the smooth muscle fibers,

Figure 26-4

The principle of the preganglionic innervation of paravertebral ganglia which are placed beyond the limits of the preganglionic sympathetic outflow from the spinal cord. Preganglionic fibers (heavy lines) emerging from a spinal segment do not synapse exclusively in the corresponding paravertebral ganglion. Some pass as splanchnic nerves to prevertebral ganglia; some fibers enter the sympathetic trunk, in which they pass up or down for a variable number of segments. (From Pick.)

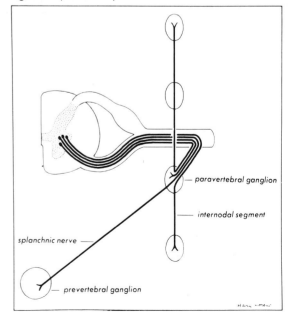

the glands, and, in largest number, to small arteries, arterioles, and precapillary sphincters (Burnstock). Some of these terminals penetrate the smooth muscle of the arterioles; others remain in the adventitia. At the ends of the postganglionic fibers and in part along their course there are swellings that lie in close proximity to the sarcolemma or gland cell membrane; often the muscle fiber is grooved to accommodate these swellings. The axonal swellings contain synaptic vesicles, some clear and others with a dense granular core. The former contain acetylcholine and those with a dense core, catecholamines, particularly nor-adrenalin (Falck, Richardson). This is well illustrated by the iris, where the nerves to the dilator muscle (sympathetic) contain dense-core vesicles and those to the constrictor (parasympathetic), clear vesicles. A single nerve fiber innervates multiple smooth muscle and gland cells.

Somewhat arbitrarily, anatomists have declared the autonomic nervous system to be purely efferent motor and secretory in function. However, most autonomic nerves are mixed and contain afferent fibers that convey sensory impulses from the viscera and blood vessels. The cell bodies of these sensory neurons lie in the posterior root ganglia; some of their central axons synapse with the lateral horn cells of the spinal cord, subserving visceral reflexes, and others synapse in the dorsal horn; secondary afferents carry sensory impulses to certain brainstem nuclei and the thalamus via the lateral spinothalamic as well as via a polysynaptic sensory pathway (page 106).

The central control mechanisms of the autonomic nervous system are considered further on in this chapter, and the modes of interaction between this system and the endocrine glands are considered in the next chapter.

PHYSIOLOGIC AND PHARMACOLOGIC CONSIDERATIONS

The function of the autonomic nervous system is to regulate the activities of a group of organs, mainly visceral ones, which possess a high degree of independence. When the autonomic nerves are interrupted, these organs continue to function (the organism survives), but their activities cannot be effectively organized in maintaining homeostasis and adapting to the demands of changing emotional conditions and stress.

It was learned long ago that most viscera have a double nerve supply, sympathetic and parasympathetic, and that these two parts of the autonomic nervous system exert opposite effects. For example, the heart is excited by the sympathetic nervous system and inhibited by the parasympathetic. Some structures, however, such as the sweat glands, somatic blood vessels, and hair follicles, receive only sympathetic postganglionic fibers, and the adrenal gland, as indicated above, has only a preganglionic sym-

pathetic innervation. Also, some parasympathetic neurons have been identified in sympathetic ganglia.

All autonomic functions are mediated through the release of chemical transmitters, the most important of which are acetylcholine (ACh) and norepinephrine (NE). ACh is synthesized at the terminals of axons and stored in presynaptic vesicles until released by the arrival of nerve impulses. It is released at the ends of all preganglionic fibers (both in the sympathetic and parasympathetic ganglia) as well as at the ends of all postganglionic parasympathetic and some postganglionic sympathetic fibers. ACh is also the chemical transmitter of nerve impulses to the skeletal muscle fiber. The arrival of nerve impulses releases ACh which traverses the synaptic cleft and attaches to receptor sites on the next neuron, smooth or striated muscle cell, or glandular cell. There are two distinct types of ACh receptors. Those in ganglia and muscle respond to the nicotinic effects of ACh. The postganglionic parasympathetic receptors are muscarinic. Removal of ACh is accomplished by diffusion into the blood stream and by destruction locally, through the action of anticholinesterases.

As a general rule, postganglionic sympathetic fibers release NE at their terminals, but there are exceptions. The sweat glands, for example, are innervated by postganglionic sympathetic fibers, but their terminals release ACh. The NE that is discharged into the synaptic space activates specific receptor sites (*adrenergic receptors*) on the postsynaptic membrane of target cells.

The adrenal medulla, as has been remarked, represents a special case. Stimulation of the splanchnic nerve (equivalent to a preganglionic sympathetic nerve) releases ACh from its terminals, which in turn depolarizes the chromaffin cells and releases large amounts of epinephrine directly into the blood stream. In this way the sympathetic nervous system and the adrenal medulla act in unison to produce diffuse effects—as one would expect from their role in emergency reactions. The parasympathetic responses (as in the pupil and urinary bladder) tend to be more discrete.

The effects of sympathetic nervous system activation are diverse. The cardiovascular responses consist of arteriolar constriction, tachycardia, enhanced cardiac contractility and renin release, all of which maintain or raise the blood pressure. Other effects are mydriasis, ejaculation, sweating, and bronchodilatation. The metabolic effects include lipolysis, glycogenolysis, and release of antidiuretic hormone. The effects of parasympathetic activation are to slow the sinoatrial rate and atrial-ventricular conduction, stimulate bronchial, salivary, and gastric glands, constrict the pupil, activate smooth muscle cells in the bronchi and intestine, sustain penile erection, and influence micturition and defecation (see further on).

There are two types of adrenergic receptor, classified by Ahlquist as *alpha* and *beta*. In general, the effects of catecholamines on alpha receptors are excitatory, and the effects on beta receptors are inhibitory. This distinction is not absolute, however. The contractility of heart muscle, for example, is increased when its beta receptors are activated; and the inhibitory effects of catecholamines on the gut are mediated by both alpha and beta receptors. The beta-adrenergic receptor sites can be subdivided on the basis of the relative selectivity of effects of excitatory drugs and antagonists. Beta$_1$ receptors are for all practical purposes limited to the heart and increase the heart rate and contractility. Beta$_2$ receptors relax the smooth muscle of the bronchi.

The two divisions of the autonomic nervous system, acting in conjunction with the endocrine glands, with which they are closely related, maintain the homeostasis of the organism. The integration of these two systems is achieved primarily in the hypothalamus. In addition, the endocrine glands are influenced by circulating catecholamines, and some of them are innervated by adrenergic fibers, which terminate not only on blood vessels but in some cases directly on secretory cells. These autonomic-endocrine relations are elaborated in the following chapter.

THE CENTRAL REGULATION OF VISCERAL FUNCTION

Among the most important recent advances in neuroanatomy has been the discovery of autonomic regulating mechanisms in the brain. Small, insignificant-appearing nuclei in the walls of the third ventricle beneath the thalami (hypothalamus) and in buried parts of the cerebral (limbic) cortex, formerly judged to have purely olfactory functions, are now known to have rich to-and-fro connections. In fact, the hypothalamus serves as the integrating mechanism of the autonomic nervous system and limbic system, as has been indicated in Chap. 25. The regulatory activity of the hypothalamus is accomplished in two ways—through direct descending pathways in the spinal cord, and through the pituitary and thence other endocrine glands. The latter neuroendocrine relationships are the subject of Chap. 27.

This supranuclear regulatory apparatus of the autonomic nervous system consists of three main groups of structures: (1) the frontal lobe cortex; (2) the limbic lobe and amygdaloid nuclei; and (3) the hypothalamus.

The *frontal lobe cortex*—the least understood and most uniquely human arrangement—appears to be the highest level of integration of autonomic function. Stimulation of one frontal lobe may evoke changes in temperature and sweating in the contralateral arm and leg, and massive lesions here, which usually cause a hemiplegia, may modify these functions in the direction of either inhibition or facilitation. Lesions involving the posterior part of the superior frontal and anterior part of the cingulate gyri (usually bilateral, occasionally unilateral) result in loss of voluntary control of the bladder and bowel (see page 356). Most likely a large contingent of these fibers terminates in the transitional mesocortex (cingulate gyrus) and archicortex (hippocampus) and in the hypothalamus, which in turn send fibers to the brainstem and spinal cord. The descending spinal pathways are believed to lie ventromedial to the corticospinal fibers.

The archicortex and transitional mesocortex and their associated subcortical structures (substantia innominata, amygdaloid, septal, piriform, habenular, and midbrain tegmental nuclei) have been identified as important parts of the so-called cerebral autonomic centers. Together they have been called the *visceral brain:* the anatomy and the effects of stimulation and ablation of these structures or parts of them have been illustrated and discussed in Chap. 25. Of central importance in the autonomic regulatory apparatus is the amygdaloid group of nuclei. Electrical stimulation in or near these nuclei in the unanesthetized cat yields a variety of motor and vegetative responses. One of these has been referred to as the *fear,* or *flight,* response, in which the animal appears frightened and runs away and hides; another is the *anger,* or *defense,* reaction, characterized by growling, hissing, and piloerection. However, not only the amygdaloid nuclei are concerned in these reactions. Lesions in the ventromedial nuclei of the hypothalamus (which receives an abundant projection of fibers from the amygdaloid nuclei via the stria medullaris) have also been shown to cause aggressive behavior, and bilateral ablation of neocortical area 24 (rostral cingulate gyrus) has produced the opposite state—tameness and reduced aggressiveness, at least in some species.

In addition to these central relationships, interaction between the autonomic nervous system and the endocrine glands also occurs at a peripheral level. The best-known example of this interaction is in the adrenal medulla, as indicated above. A similar relationship holds for the pineal gland; release of norepinephrine from postganglionic fibers which end on pineal cells has been shown to stimulate several of the enzymes which are involved in the biosynthesis of melatonin. Similarly, the juxtaglomerular apparatus of the kidney and the islets of Langerhans of the pancreas may be considered to function as neuroendocrine transducers, since they convert a neural stimulus (in these cases adrenergic) to an endocrine secretion (renin and glucagon and insulin, respectively).

Finally, the central role of the hypothalamus in the initiation and regulation of autonomic activity is now generally recognized. Sympathetic responses are most readily obtained by stimulation of the posterior and lateral regions of the hypothalamus, and parasympathetic responses from the anterior regions. The descending sympathetic fibers are largely or totally uncrossed, but their exact course is not clear. As indicated in Chap. 25, the fibers from the lateral hypothalamic area at first run in the prerubral field, dorsal and slightly rostral to the red nucleus; they then traverse the lateral tegmentum of the midbrain and pons and descend to the intermediolateral cell column of the spinal cord via the lateral part of the medullary reticular formation. Luhan and Pollock demonstrated that a small infarct in the territory of supply of the superior cerebellar artery, involving an area just posterior to the medial lemniscus and extending laterally to the periphery of the rostral pons, causes an ipsilateral ptosis, miosis, and anhidrosis (Horner syndrome). In the medulla, the descending pathway is located in the posterolateral retro-olivary area, and in the cervical cord the fibers run in the posterior angle of the anterior horn (Nathan and Smith). According to the latter authors, some of the fibers supplying sudomotor neurons run outside this area, but remain ipsilateral.

EMERGENCY AND ALARM REACTIONS

Inasmuch as the autonomic nervous system and the adrenal glands have been accepted for many years as the neural and humoral basis of all instinctive and emotional behavior, it is remarkable how little sound information has been acquired about their role in disease. In chronic anxiety and acute panic reactions, in depressive psychosis, mania, and schizophrenia, all of which are characterized by an altered emotionality, no consistent autonomic or endocrine dysfunction has been demonstrated. This has been disappointing, since Cannon, with his emergency theory of sympathoadrenal action, had given us such a promising concept of the neurophysiology of acute emotion and Selye had extended this theory so plausibly to explain all the reactions to stress in animals and humans. According to these theories, strong emotion, such as anger or fear, excites the sympathetic nervous system and the adrenal glands, which are under direct neural as well as endocrine (CRF and ACTH) control. These sympathoadrenal reactions are brief and sustain the animal in "flight or fight." Prolonged stress and production of ACTH activates all the adrenal hormones referred to collectively as *steroids* (glucocorticoids, mineralocorticoids, and androcorticoids). According to Selye, the more prolonged defensive and adaptive reactions develop in three stages: (1) the alarm reaction, i.e., the initial

arousal of the body's defensive forces; (2) the stage of resistance, which develops if the stress is not too strong and if the adaptation is effective; and (3) the final stage of exhaustion and death.

Animals deprived of adrenal cortex or human beings with Addison disease cannot tolerate stress, because they are incapable of mobilizing both the adrenal medulla and adrenal cortex. In animals, exercise, cold, oxygen lack, and surgical injury all are said to evoke the same sympathoadrenal reactions as anger or fear. Some of these reactions are accompanied by adrenal enlargement, thymic and lymphatic hyperplasia, and gastric ulceration and other irreversible tissue changes. Selye's extension of Cannon's theory, although attractive, has received little support. Critics have pointed out that the conditions to which his experimental animals had been subjected are so different from human disease that conclusions as to the unity of the two cannot be drawn. More critical studies of the anatomy and physiology of the hypothalamus, hypophysis, adrenal glands, and autonomic nervous system are needed to fully test these hypotheses.

TESTS FOR ABNORMALITIES OF THE AUTONOMIC NERVOUS SYSTEM

With few exceptions, such as testing pupillary reactions and examination of the skin for abnormalities of color and sweating, the neurologist tends not to be precise in evaluating the function of the autonomic nervous system. Nonetheless, several simple tests can be used to confirm clinical impressions. Some of the more important ones are described below and are summarized in Table 26-1. Pupillary responses to pharmacologic agents and stellate block are illustrated in Fig. 13-6 and 13-7.

RESPONSE OF BLOOD PRESSURE AND HEART RATE TO CHANGES IN POSTURE

This is one of the simplest and most important tests of autonomic function. McLeod and Tuck state that in changing from the recumbent to the standing position, a fall of more than 30 mmHg systolic and 15 mmHg diastolic is abnormal; others give figures of 20 and 10 mmHg. They caution that the arm of which the cuff is placed be held horizontally when standing, so that the fall in arm pressure will not be obscured by hydrostatic pressure. In response to the drop in blood pressure, the pulse rate (under vagal control) normally increases by 11 to 29 beats per minute, then slows

Table 26-1
Clinical tests of autonomic function

Test	Normal response	Part of reflex arc tested
Noninvasive bedside tests		
Blood-pressure response to standing or vertical tilt	Fall in BP ≤ 30/15 mmHg	Afferent and efferent limbs
Heart rate response to standing	Increase 11–29 beats/min; 30:15 ratio ≥ 1.04	Afferent and efferent limbs
Isometric exercise	Increase in diastolic BP, 15 mmHg	Sympathetic efferent limb
Heart rate variation with respiration	Maximum-minimum heart rate ≥ 15 beats/min; E:I ratio ≥ 1.2*	Vagal afferent and efferent limbs
Valsalva ratio	≥ 1.4*	Afferent and efferent limbs
Sweat tests	Sweating over all body and limbs	Sympathetic efferent limb
Axon reflex	Local piloerection, sweating	Postganglionic sympathetic efferent fibers
Plasma noradrenaline level	Rises on tilting from horizontal to vertical	Sympathetic efferent limb
Plasma vasopressin level	Rise with induced hypotension	Afferent limb
Invasive tests		
Valsalva maneuver	Phase I: Rise in BP Phase II: Gradual reduction of BP to plateau; tachy-cardia Phase III: Fall in BP Phase IV: Overshoot of BP, bradycardia*	Afferent and efferent limbs
Baroreflex sensitivity	(1) Slowing of heart rate with induced rise of BP* (2) Steady-state responses to induced rise and fall of BP	(1) Parasympathetic afferent and efferent limbs (2) Afferent and efferent limbs
Infusion of pressor drugs	(1) Rise in BP (2) Slowing of heart rate	(1) Adrenergic receptors (2) Afferent and efferent parasympathetic limbs
Other tests of vasomotor control		
Radiant heating of trunk	Increased hand blood flow	Sympathetic efferent limb
Immersion of hand in hot water	Increased blood flow of opposite hand	Sympathetic efferent limb
Cold pressor test	Reduced blood flow	Sympathetic efferent limb
Emotional stress	Increase BP	Sympathetic efferent limb
Tests of pupiliary innervation		
4% Cocaine	Pupil dilates	Sympathetic innervation
0.1% Adrenaline	No response	Postganglionic sympathetic innervation
1% Hydroxyamphetamine hydrobromide	Pupil dilates	Postganglionic sympathetic innervation
2.5% Methacholine, 0.125% pilocarpine	No response	Parasympathetic innervation

* Age-dependent response.   BP = blood pressure; E:I = expiration:inspiration.   *Source:* McLeod and Tuck.

after 15 beats to a stable state by the thirtieth beat. The ratio of RR (ECG) intervals corresponding to the thirtieth and fifteenth beats (the 30:15 ratio) is a measure of integrity of vagal inhibition. A ratio in young adults of less than 1.04 is abnormal.

Another simple but reliable means of testing autonomic function is to quantitate the *variation in heart rate* during quiet breathing. The ECG is recorded while the patient breathes at a regular rate of six per minute. Normally, the heart rate varies by 15 beats per minute or more; differences of less than 10 beats per minute are considered abnormal. The ratio of the longest RR interval during expiration to the shortest RR interval during inspiration constitutes the expiration-inspiration (E:I) ratio. Up to age 40, ratios less than 1.2 are abnormal; the ratio decreases with age.

TESTS OF VASOMOTOR REACTIONS

Measurement of the skin temperature is a useful index of vasomotor function. Vasomotor paralysis results in vasodilatation of skin vessels and a rise in temperature; vasoconstriction lowers the temperature. With a skin thermometer one may compare affected and normal areas under standard conditions. The normal skin temperature is 31 to 33°C when the room temperature is 26 to 27°C. Vasoconstrictor tone may also be tested by measuring the temperature of the area in question before and after immersing the hands in cold water.

The integrity of the sympathetic reflex arc, which includes baroreceptors in the aorta and carotid sinus and their afferent pathways, vasomotor centers, and the sympathetic and parasympathetic outflow, can be tested in a general way by combining the cold pressor test, Valsalva maneuver, and mental arithmetic test.

Vasoconstriction induces an elevation of the blood pressure and bradycardia. This is the basis of the *cold pressor test*. In normal persons, immersing the hands in ice water for 60 s raises the systolic pressure by 15 to 20 mmHg and the diastolic pressure by 10 to 15 mmHg.

In the *Valsalva maneuver*, the patient exhales into a manometer or against a closed glottis for 10 to 15 s, creating a markedly positive intrathoracic pressure. Normally, this causes a sharp reduction in venous return and cardiac output, so that the blood pressure falls; the effect on the baroreceptors is to cause a reflex tachycardia and peripheral vasoconstriction. With release of intrathoracic pressure, the venous return, stroke volume, and blood pressure return to higher than normal levels; parasympathetic influence then predominates and results in bradycardia.

The stress involved in doing *mental arithmetic* in noisy and distracting surroundings will normally stimulate a mild but measurable increase in pulse rate and blood pressure. This response does not depend upon the afferent limb of the sympathetic reflex arc.

Failure of the heart rate to increase during the positive intrathoracic pressure phase of the Valsalva maneuver points to sympathetic dysfunction, and failure of the rate to slow during the period of blood pressure overshoot points to a parasympathetic disturbance. If the response to the Valsalva maneuver is abnormal and the response to the cold pressor test is normal, the lesion is probably in the baroreceptors or their afferent nerves; such a defect has been found in diabetic and tabetic patients. A failure of the pulse rate and blood pressure to rise during mental arithmetic, coupled with an abnormal Valsalva maneuver, suggests a defect in the central or peripheral efferent sympathetic pathways.

The sustained isometric contraction of a group of muscles (e.g., forearm) for 5 min normally increases the heart rate and the systolic and diastolic pressures by 15 mmHg or more. The response is reduced or absent with lesions of the sympathetic reflex arc, particularly of the efferent limb.

TESTS OF SUDOMOTOR FUNCTION

The integrity of sympathetic efferent pathways can be assessed further by *tests of sudomotor activity*. There are several of these. Sweat can be weighed after it is absorbed by small squares of filter paper. Powdered charcoal dusted on the skin will cling to moist areas and not to dry ones. The galvanic skin-resistance test is an easy but not entirely reliable way of measuring sweating. A string galvanometer indicates the resistance offered by the skin to the passage of a weak galvanic current through the skin. Increase in sweating lowers the resistance; anhidrosis raises it. This method can be used to outline the area of a peripheral nerve lesion which reduces sweating. The starch test or a color indicator such as quinizarin (gray when dry, purple when wet) may be used. If the amount of sweat is not sufficient to show by these tests, the patient should be warmed with blankets or a heating cradle and given a diaphoretic such as hot tea or a dose of pilocarpine. Failure to sweat in response to these tests indicates an impairment of the efferent sympathetic pathway, somewhere between the hypothalamus and the skin.

LACRIMAL FUNCTION

Tearing can be estimated in a rough manner by the Schirmer test, in which one end of a 5-mm-wide and 25-mm-long strip of thin filter paper is inserted into the lower conjunctival sac while the other end hangs over the edge of the lower lid. The moisture of the tears wets the strip of filter paper, producing a moisture front. In normal patients, after 5 min, the moistened area extends over a length of approximately 15 mm. Values below 10 mm are suggestive of hypolacrimia.

TESTS OF BLADDER AND GASTROINTESTINAL FUNCTION

Bladder function is best assessed by the cystometrogram, i.e., by measuring intravesicular pressure as a function of the volume of sterile saline solution permitted to flow by gravity into the bladder. Relatively simple apparatus is available for this purpose. The rise of pressure as 500 mL of fluid is allowed to flow gradually into the bladder and the emptying contractions of the detrusor can be recorded by a manometer. (A detailed account of cystometric techniques can be found in the monograph of Krane and Siroky.) A quick and simple way of determining bladder atony (prostatic obstruction and overdistention having been excluded) is to measure the residual urine (by catheterization of the bladder) immediately after voluntary voiding or by estimating its volume by intravenous pyelography.

Disorders of gastrointestinal motility are readily demonstrated by radiologic examination. In dysautonomic states a barium swallow may disclose a number of abnormalities, including atonic dilatation of the esophagus, gastric atony and distention, delayed gastric emptying time, and a characteristic small-bowel pattern consisting of an increase in frequency and amplitude of peristaltic waves and rapid intestinal transit. A barium enema may demonstrate colonic distention and a decrease in propulsive activity. Sophisticated manometric techniques are now available for the measurement of gastrointestinal motility (see Low et al).

PHARMACOLOGIC TESTS OF AUTONOMIC FUNCTION

The topical application of pharmacologic agents is useful in evaluating *pupillary denervation*. Part of the rationale behind these special tests is "Cannon's law," or the phenomenon of denervation hypersensitivity, in which an effector organ, 2 to 3 weeks after denervation, becomes hypersensitive to its particular neurotransmitter substance and to related drugs.

The instillation of a 1:1000 solution of epinephrine into the conjunctival sac has no effect on the normal pupil but will cause the sympathetically denervated pupil to dilate (3 drops instilled 3 times at 1-min intervals). The pupillary size is checked after 15, 30, and 45 min. As a rule,

hypersensitivity to epinephrine is greater with lesions of postganglionic fibers than of preganglionic fibers. In lesions which involve central sympathetic pathways, the pupil rarely reacts. If denervation is incomplete, the hypersensitivity phenomenon may not be demonstrable.

The topical application of a 4% cocaine solution as a test for sympathetic denervation may be more reliable. The test should be carried out as described above. Cocaine potentiates the effect of the adrenergic transmitter since it probably prevents the reuptake of epinephrine into nerve endings. A normal response to cocaine consists of pupillary dilatation. In sympathetic denervation caused by lesions of the post- or preganglionic fibers, no change in pupillary size occurs, since no transmitter substance is available. In cases of central sympathetic lesions, slight mydriasis occurs.

A freshly prepared solution of 2.5% methacholine (Mecholyl) can be used in a similar fashion to demonstrate parasympathetic denervation. The normal pupil will not respond to this concentration of methacholine whereas the denervated pupil will constrict.

These and other pharmacologic methods of evaluating pupillary disturbances are illustrated in Figs. 13-6 and 13-7.

The intracutaneous injection of 0.05 mL of histamine phosphate in a dilution of 1:1000 normally causes a 1-cm wheal after 5 to 10 min. This is surrounded by a narrow red areola, and this in turn by an erythematous flare which extends 1 to 3 cm from the border of the wheal. A similar triple response follows the release of histamine into the tissue as the result of a scratch. The wheal and the deeply colored red areola are caused by direct action of histamine on blood vessels, while the flare depends upon the integrity of the axon reflex mediated along sensory fibers by antidromic transmission. In familial dysautonomia the flare response is absent. It may also be absent in peripheral neuropathies that involve sympathetic nerves (e.g., diabetes, alcoholic-nutritional disease, Guillain-Barré syndrome, amyloidosis, porphyria, etc.).

Finally, *the systemic administration of pharmacologic agents* may provide information about the autonomic innervation of the heart. These include the infusion of methacholine at a steady rate. In dysautonomic states this will produce a drop in blood pressure without an increase in heart rate, at a lower infusion rate than in normal subjects. In cases of familial dysautonomia, methacholine restores temporarily the sense of taste, deep tendon reflexes, and the flare response to histamine. The mechanism by which this occurs is unknown.

The infusion of norepinephrine causes a rise in blood pressure which is usually more pronounced in dysautonomic states than with normal subjects for a given infusion rate. In patients with familial dysautonomia, the infusion of norepinephrine also produces erythematous blotching of the skin, like that which occurs under emotional stress. Thus, bouts of hypertension and blotching of the skin in dysautonomic children are believed to be due to an exaggerated response to endogenous norepinephrine.

The infusion of angiotensin II into patients with idiopathic orthostatic hypotension also causes an exaggerated blood pressure response. The response to methacholine and norepinephrine has been interpreted as a denervation hypersensitivity to neurotransmitter or related substances. Since angiotensin II is not one of those substances, a different mechanism needs to be invoked, perhaps defective baroreceptor function. Thus, hypertension induced by angiotensin II, methacholine, or norepinephrine would not lead to compensatory peripheral reflex vasodilatation and bradycardia.

The integrity of autonomic innervation of the heart can be evaluated by the intramuscular injection of atropine, ephedrine, and neostigmine while the heart rate is monitored. Normally, the intramuscular injection of 0.8 mg of atropine causes a parasympathetic block and an increase in heart rate because of unopposed sympathetic activity. No such change occurs in cases of sympathetic denervation of the heart. Similarly, 25 mg of ephedrine administered intramuscularly results in increased heart rate under normal conditions; in cases of sympathetic denervation, this response is absent. Conversely, 1 mg of neostigmine given intramuscularly results in bradycardia, provided the parasympathetic innervation of the heart is intact.

Micromethods are now available for the measurement of noradrenalin and dopamine β-hydroxylase in the serum. Normally, when a person changes from a recumbent to a standing position, the levels rise (see below).

In summary, the noninvasive tests listed in Table 26-1 and described above are quite adequate for the clinical testing of autonomic function. According to McLeod and Tuck, abnormal findings in these tests correlate well with the results of tests using intra-arterial catheterization and infusion of pressor drugs. Abnormalities in any two of the bedside tests are indicative of autonomic dysfunction.

CLINICAL DISORDERS OF THE AUTONOMIC NERVOUS SYSTEM

COMPLETE AUTONOMIC PARALYSIS (DYSAUTONOMIC POLYNEUROPATHY)

This condition has now been reported in many adults and children. Over a period of a week or a few weeks the patient develops anhidrosis, orthostatic hypotension, paralysis of pupillary reflexes, loss of lacrimation and salivation, impotence, impaired bladder and bowel function, reduced gastric acidity (ulcer symptoms may disappear), and loss of certain pilomotor and vasomotor responses in the skin.

The CSF protein may be normal or increased. Although no autopsy studies have been done, it is assumed that both the sympathetic and parasympathetic parts of the autonomic nervous system are affected, mainly at the postganglionic level. In some patients the abnormalities are more pronounced in the cholinergic autonomic system. Somatic sensory and motor nerve fibers appear to be spared. However, in one of the patients described by Low and his colleagues, there was morphologic and physiologic evidence of loss of small myelinated and unmyelinated somatic fibers. The patient originally reported by Young et al, and most of the other patients with pure dysautonomia, recovered within a few months. However, in some of the children with this disease, called cholinergic dysautonomia (Kirby et al), there has been no postural hypotension and the course was more chronic. It seems likely that this is an autoimmune autonomic polyneuropathy, similar to that of acute idiopathic polyneuritis (Guillain-Barré syndrome).

BOTULISM

Here the clostridial toxin interferes with the release of acetylcholine at the neuromuscular junctions, more specifically at the presynaptic terminals, causing an acute paralysis. Surprisingly, autonomic effects, both parasympathetic and sympathetic, are slight. Dry eyes, dry mouth, and gastrointestinal ileus may occur but are lost in the welter of paralytic effects. The pupils are usually spared (see page 909).

ORTHOSTATIC HYPOTENSION (See Also Chap. 17)

This condition results from a disturbance of the circulation upon assuming the upright posture. Normally, standing up results in the pooling of blood in dependent parts of the body, due to the effects of gravity. Some 500 to 700 mL of blood collects in the distensible (capacitance) veins in the legs and splanchnic area and is temporarily removed from the effective circulation. The venous return to the heart is reduced and the cardiac output falls by about 10 percent; the stroke volume diminishes and there is a transient, slight reduction in blood pressure.

The decrease in blood pressure and cardiac stroke volume are sensed by stretch receptors (baroreceptors) in the aortic arch, carotid sinus, atria and ventricles. Afferent fibers project from the baroreceptors mainly in the nerves of Hering (ninth cranial nerve) and vagus nerves to medullary vasomotor centers and provoke an almost instantaneous reflex increase in sympathetic vasomotor outflow. This causes constriction of the capacitance venous system, thus facilitating venous return to the heart, and arteriolar constriction, which raises total peripheral resistance and increases the diastolic blood pressure. Simultaneously there occurs a reflex tachycardia, mediated either by decrease in vagal tone or by an increase in sympathetic stimulation; also, plasma catecholamine and renin levels are increased because of increased sympathetic stimulation and other factors. Increased blood pressure acting on baroreceptors has the opposite effects, i.e., it inhibits the medullary vasomotor centers and causes bradycardia.

The combination of these several reflex mechanisms assures the maintenance of blood pressure at steady levels. In general, cardiac output is lower in the erect posture, with lower systolic pressure (10 mmHg) and higher diastolic pressure (10 mmHg) and more rapid heart beat (5 to 10 per min).

Idiopathic Orthostatic Hypotension (*Progressive Autonomic Failure*)

This clinical state is now known to be caused by at least two conditions. In one, a degenerative disease of middle and late adult life first described by Bradbury and Eggleston in 1925, the lesions are said to involve mainly the postganglionic sympathetic neurons (Petito and Black), the parasympathetic system being relatively spared and the central nervous system being uninvolved. In the second disorder, described by Shy and Drager, the preganglionic lateral horn neurons of the thoracic spinal segments degenerate; cerebellar and basal ganglionic signs are added to the clinical picture. In both conditions, anhidrosis, orthostatic hypotension, impotence, and atonicity of the bladder may develop.

The differentiation of these two types of orthostatic hypotension—the chronic peripheral postganglionic and the central preganglionic—is based on pharmacologic evidence. In the former type, plasma levels of norepinephrine, while the patient is recumbent, are subnormal because of failure of the damaged nerve terminals to synthesize or release catecholamines. When the patient stands up, the norepinephrine levels do not rise as they do in a normal person. In this type there is also (denervation) hypersensitivity to injected norepinephrine. In the central type, the resting norepinephrine levels in the plasma are normal but on standing, again, there is no rise. However, sensitivity to exogenously administered norepinephrine is normal. Cohen et al, who studied the postganglionic sudomotor and vasomotor functions of 62 patients with idiopathic orthostatic hypotension, found that postganglionic denervation was uncommon in patients

with multiple system atrophy, i.e., the central type—a finding that distinguished it from the first (postganglionic) type. In both types the plasma levels of dopamine β-hydroxylase, the enzyme that converts dopamine to norepinephrine, are subnormal (Ziegler et al).

Unfortunately, pathologic studies have not established the existence of a uniform central type. Oppenheimer, who has collected all reported cases with complete autopsies, finds that the central cases fall into two groups—one in which autonomic failure is associated with the Parkinson syndrome and Lewy bodies, the other with involvement of the striatum, cerebellum, pons, and medulla (olivopontocerebellar degeneration and striatonigral degeneration) but without Lewy bodies. The latter condition is now being loosely referred to as multiple system atrophy. In both groups the autonomic failure appears to be related to degeneration of lateral horn cells. In multiple system atrophy, nerve cells of the vagal nuclei, of the nuclei of the tractus solitarius and locus ceruleus, and of the sacral autonomic nuclei are also degenerated, accounting for laryngeal abductor weakness (laryngeal stridor), incontinence, and impotence. Noradrenalin and dopamine are depleted in the hypothalamus (Spokes et al). The sympathetic ganglia have been normal except for the case of Rajput and Rozdilsky in which most of the ganglion cells had degenerated.

Lewis has described a family in which orthostatic hypotension was associated with muscular atrophy, ataxia, rigidity, tremor, and sphincteric incontinence. The disease develops and progresses slowly during midadult life and is inherited as an autosomal dominant trait.

Peripheral Neuropathy with Secondary Orthostatic Hypotension

Impairment of autonomic function, of which orthostatic hypotension is the most serious feature, may occur as part of the more common peripheral neuropathies (Guillain-Barré, chronic inflammatory neuropathy, infectious mononucleosis, porphyric, diabetic, and alcoholic-nutritional). Disease of the peripheral nervous system may affect the circulation in two ways: baroreceptors may be affected, interrupting normal homeostatic reflexes on the afferent side, or postganglionic sympathetic fibers may be affected in the spinal nerves. The severity of the autonomic failure need not parallel the degree of motor weakness. In some patients with acute polyneuropathy (notably the Guillain-Barré and porphyric types), transient hypertension may occur, possibly due to overactivity of the sympathetic nervous system.

Of particular importance is the autonomic disorder of the diabetic, due presumably to a special type of neuropathy. It presents as impotence, nocturnal diarrhea, hypotonia of the bladder, and orthostatic hypotension, in some combination. Its pathologic basis has been difficult to assess because of the frequency of artifact in the sympathetic ganglia in autopsy material. Duchen has attributed the autonomic disorder to vacuolization of sympathetic ganglionic neurons, cell necrosis and inflammation, loss of myelinated fibers in the vagi and white rami communicantes, and loss of lateral horn cells in the spinal cord. He believes the spinal cord changes to be secondary.

A particular polyneuropathy with an unusually prominent dysautonomia is that due to amyloidosis (Andrade disease). Extensive analgesia and thermohypesthesia and, to a lesser degree, impairment of other forms of sensation may also be present. Motor function is much less affected. Sympathetic function is more impaired than parasympathetic. Iridoplegia (pupillary paralysis) and other glandular and smooth muscle functions are variably disturbed.

Poisoning with organophosphate insecticides (e.g., Parathion), which are anticholinesterase drugs, causes a combination of parasympathetic overactivity and motor paralysis (see page 914). The most severe degree of autonomic disturbance, involving postganglionic sympathetic and parasympathetic function, is produced by ingestion of the rodenticide *N*-3-pyridylmethyl-*N'*-*p*-nitrophenylurea (PNU, Vacor). The drugs guanethidine and guanacline selectively destroy sympathetic ganglion cells in the monkey (Palmatier et al).

Both the primary and secondary types of orthostatic hypotension are also discussed in connection with syncope, in Chap. 17.

AUTONOMIC NEUROPATHY IN INFANTS AND CHILDREN (RILEY-DAY SYNDROME)

In this familial disease, with an autosomal recessive pattern of inheritance, the main symptoms are postural hypotension and lability of blood pressure, faulty regulation of temperature, diminished hearing, hyperhidrosis, blotchiness of the skin, insensitivity to pain, emotional lability, and vomiting. There is denervation sensitivity of the pupils and other structures. A deficiency of neurons has been described in the superior cervical ganglia and in the lateral horns of the spinal cord. Also a decreased number of unmyelinated nerve fibers in the sural nerve has been reported by Aguayo and by Dyck and their colleagues (see also page 1060).

AUTONOMIC FAILURE IN THE ELDERLY

Orthostatic hypotension is prevalent in the elderly. Caird et al reported that in individuals over 65 years living at home, 24 percent had a fall of systolic blood pressure on standing of 20 mmHg, 9 percent had a fall of 30 mmHG, and 5 percent, a fall of 40 mmHg. An increased frequency of thermoregulatory impairment has also been documented. Goldman et al, in a survey of hospital admissions for elderly

patients, found 3.6 percent to have a temperature of 35°C or below. The elderly are also more liable to hyperthermia when exposed to high ambient temperature. Loss of sweating of the lower parts of the body and increased sweating of the head and arms probably reflect a senile neuropathy. Impotence and incontinence increase with age. Brocklehurst noted a surprisingly high incidence of incontinence in persons over 65 years of age (two or more times a month in 7.6 percent of men and 12.5 percent of women). The anatomic and physiologic basis of these changes have not been ascertained (see reference to Collins for review and bibliography).

PARTIAL OR RESTRICTED AUTONOMIC SYNDROMES

Bernard-Horner and Stellate Ganglion Syndromes

Interruption of the sympathetic fibers at any point along the internal carotid arteries (postganglionic fibers), or the removal of the superior cervical ganglion results in miosis, drooping of the eyelid, apparent enophthalmos, and abolition of sweating over one side of the face (see also page 221). The same syndrome may be caused by interruption of the preganglionic fibers from their origin in the intermediolateral cell column of the eighth cervical and first through third thoracic spinal segments, or by interruption of the descending, uncrossed hypothalamospinal pathway in the tegmentum of the brainstem or cervical cord. The common causes of the syndrome are tumorous or inflammatory involvement of cervical lymph nodes, surgical and other types of trauma to cervical structures, neoplastic invasion of the proximal part of the brachial plexus, basilar skull fractures, tumor, syringomyelia, or traumatic lesions of the first and second thoracic spinal segments, and infarcts or other lesions of the lateral part of the medulla (Wallenberg syndrome). There is also an idiopathic variety which may at times be hereditary. If a Horner syndrome develops early in life, the iris on the side of the lesion fails to become pigmented and remains blue or mottled gray-brown and blue. A lesion of the stellate ganglion, e.g., compression by a tumor arising from the superior sulcus of the lung, produces the interesting combination of a Horner syndrome and paralysis of sympathetic reflexes in the arm (hand and arm are dry and warm).

Keane has provided data as to the relative frequency of the lesions causing oculosympathetic paralysis. In 100 successive cases, 63 were of central type due to brainstem strokes, 21 were preganglionic due to trauma or tumors of the neck, 13 were postganglionic due to miscellaneous causes, and in 3 cases the localization was indeterminate (see Chap. 13 for further discussion).

Other Pupillary and Salivatory Disturbances A disorder of the oculomotor nerve, in addition to paralyzing four of the extraocular muscles and the levator muscle of the eyelid, causes a dilatation of the pupil, with an abolition of the constriction which normally occurs as a reaction to light and on accommodation; also there may be an associated loss of near vision and accommodation, owing to paralysis of the ciliary muscle. The Holmes-Adie pupil and other parasympathetic and sympathetic abnormalities of pupillary function are considered further in Chap. 13 (Figs. 13-6 and 13-7).

Diseases which involve the facial, glossopharyngeal, and vagus nerves seldom induce recognizable parasympathetic changes. However, Bell's palsy, or less commonly, head injury, operations on the ear, or surgical resection of the greater superficial petrosal nerve may be followed by imperfect regeneration and misdirection of nerve fibers. For example, fibers which should innervate the salivary glands may reach either the lacrimal or the sweat glands in the preauricular and temporal regions. Eating (or even thinking of good food), with its attendant reflex salivation, then provokes lacrimation (syndrome of crocodile tears) or temporal sweating (auriculotemporal syndrome).

Sympathetic and Parasympathetic Paralysis in Tetraplegia and Paraplegia Lesions of the C4 or C5 segments of the spinal cord, if complete, will sever all suprasegmental control of the sympathetic and sacral parasympathetic nervous systems. The same effects are observed with lesions of the upper thoracic cord (above T6). Lower thoracic lesions leave much of the descending sympathetic outflow intact, with only sacral parasympathetic control being interrupted. Traumatic necrosis of the spinal cord is the usual cause of these states, but it may happen with infarct necrosis, certain forms of myelitis, and tumors.

The initial effect of a cervical cord transection of acute type is abolition of all autonomic as well as sensory-motor functions of the isolated spinal cord. There is hypotension, loss of sweating and pilo-erection, paralytic ileus, and paralysis of the bladder. Plasma adrenalin and noradrenalin are reduced. This state lasts for several weeks. The basic mechanisms accounting for spinal shock are not known. Interest is focused on neurotransmitters (catechol-amines, endorphins, substance P, and 5-hydroxytrypt-amine).

After spinal shock dissipates, the sympathetic and parasympathetic functions return (since the afferent and efferent autonomic connections with the isolated segments of the spinal cord are intact) but are no longer under the control of higher centers. With cervical cord lesions, there are no longer any sympathetically mediated cardiovascular changes in response to stimuli reaching the medulla. However, cutaneous stimuli (pinprick or cold) in segments of the body below the transection will raise the blood pressure. A fall in blood pressure is not compensated by sympathetic vasoconstriction. Hence tetraplegics are prone to orthostatic hypotension. Pinching the skin below the lesion causes gooseflesh in adjacent segments. Heating the body results in flushing and sweating over the face and neck, but not the trunk and legs. Bladder and bowel, including their sphincters, which were at first flaccid, become automatic as spinal reflex control returns. There may be reflex penile erection or priapism and even ejaculation, and the female may become pregnant even though voluntary control of sexual activity has been abolished.

After a time the tetraplegic may develop a "mass reflex"—with leg flexion and micturition, there may be a rise in blood pressure in association with bradycardia, and sweating and pilomotor reactions in parts below the cervical segments ("autonomic dysreflexia"). These reactions may also be evoked by pinprick, passive movement, contact with limbs and abdomen, and pressure on the bladder. An exaggerated vasopressor reaction also occurs when norepinephrine is injected. In such attacks the patient complains of paresthesias of the neck, shoulders, and arms; tightness in the chest and dyspnea; pupillary dilatation; pallor followed by flushing of the face; fullness in the head and ears; and a throbbing headache. Plasma noradrenaline and dopamine rise slowly during the autonomic discharge. When prolonged, myocardial infarction, seizures, and visual defects have been observed. Clonidine has been useful in preventing the hypertensive crises.

The Effects of Thoracolumbar Sympathectomy Surgical resection of the thoracolumbar sympathetic trunk, widely used in the 1940s in the treatment of hypertension, has provided the clinician with the only clear-cut examples of extensive injury to the peripheral autonomic nervous system, though in primary orthostatic hypotension (see above) a similar defect has long been suspected. In general it may be said that bilateral thoracolumbar sympathectomy results in surprisingly few physiologic changes. Aside from loss of sweating over the denervated areas of the body, the most pronounced abnormality is an impairment of vasomotor reflexes. In the upright posture, syncope is frequent because of the pooling of blood in the splanchnic bed and lower extremities; there is a steady fall in blood pressure to shock levels and little or no pallor, nausea, vomiting, or sweating—

the usual accompaniments of syncope. Bladder, bowel, and sexual function are preserved, though semen is sometimes ejaculated into the posterior urethra and bladder. No consistent abnormalities of renal or hepatic function have been found.

Disorders of Sweating *Hyperhidrosis* results from overactivity of sudomotor nerve fibers under a variety of conditions. It may occur as an excitatory phase of a peripheral neuropathy and be followed by anhidrosis (e.g., arsenic, thallium) and is one aspect of sympathetic reflex dystrophy. Small nerve fiber lesions, enhancing adrenergic responses, are associated with excessive sweating. Excessive perspiration is also observed as a persistent feature of certain mononeuropathies (e.g., causalgia) and polyneuropathies (''burning foot'' syndrome), in which burning and painful paresthesias and hyperhidrosis are combined. A special type of nonthermoregulatory hyperhidrosis may occur in spinal paraplegics (page 721). Hyperkalemia evokes sweating. Loss of sweating in one part of the body requires compensatory increase in normal parts.

Localized hyperhidrosis may be a troublesome complaint in some patients. One variety, presumably of congenital origin, affects the palms. In some cases, the hyperhidrosis affects mainly the feet and lower extremities. The social embarrassment of a ''succulent hand'' or a ''dripping paw'' is often intolerable. It is taken to be a sign of nervousness, though many persons with this condition disclaim all other neurotic symptoms. Cold, clammy hands are common in individuals with anxiety neurosis, and indeed this has been a useful sign in distinguishing an anxiety state from hyperthyroidism, in which the hands are also moist, but warm. Extirpation of T_2 and T_3 sympathetic ganglia relieves the more severe cases of palmar sweating; a Horner syndrome does not develop if the T_1 ganglion is left intact.

Anhidrosis in restricted skin areas is a frequent and useful finding in peripheral nerve disease. It is due to the interruption of the postganglionic sympathetic fibers. The loss of sweating corresponds to the area of sensory loss. In contrast, sweating is not affected in spinal root disease for the reason that there is much intersegmental mixing of the preganglionic axons, once they enter the sympathetic chain.

Raynaud Phenomenon This disorder, characterized by a painful blanching of the fingers on exposure to cold and emotional stress, was first described by Raynaud in 1862. It occurs in a number of clinical settings. One type, often called secondary, results from any proximal obstruction which reduces intraluminal vascular pressure, and allows protracted vasoconstriction, e.g., cervical rib, brachial atherosclerosis. Local trauma such as using a pneumatic drill or sculling on a cold day may induce the Raynaud phenomenon; it is often associated with connective tissue

disease. Most puzzling of all is why the digital arteries of the hands with a normal intraluminal pressure undergo prolonged vasospasm.

Lafferty et al point out that in contrast to many areas of the body the cutaneous vessels of the hands and feet have only vasoconstrictive fibers. In the pure vasospastic form of the disease there is a defect locally in the histaminergic vasodilating system. Cold or emotional activation of the hypothalamic sympathetic vasoconstrictive mechanism is intact but the neural release of histamine from mast cells in the hands is defective. Mast cells may be injured locally or destroyed by an autoimmune reaction in connective tissue diseases. Since active vasodilatation is under control of the histaminergic system, sympathectomy is usually ineffective. The vasodilating properties of the various prostaglandins have been exploited to good effect in some cases.

Causalgia, the painful syndrome that follows partial interruption of a peripheral nerve, has been ascribed to the cross stimulation of sensory fibers by efferent sympathetic impulses at the point of artificial synapse, where the nerve trunk is injured. The Raynaud phenomenon and causalgia are discussed further on page 176 and page 1068, respectively.

DISTURBANCES OF BLADDER FUNCTION

The familiar functions of the bladder and lower urinary tract—the storage and intermittent evacuation of urine—are served by three structural components: the large detrusor muscle which is the bladder itself, the closely related internal sphincter muscle, and the external sphincter or urogenital diaphragm. The sphincters assure continence during the storage phase, and in the male, the internal sphincter also prevents reflux of semen from the urethra during ejaculation. During micturition the sphincters must relax, allowing the detrusor to expel urine from the bladder into the urethra. This is accomplished by a complex mechanism, involving the sympathetic and parasympathetic nervous systems, the somatic sensorimotor sacral peripheral nerve fibers, the second, third and fourth sacral segments of the spinal cord, the brainstem ''micturition centers,'' and their spinal and suprasegmental connections (Fig. 26-5).

The detrusor (smooth) muscle receives motor innervation from nerve cells in the intermediolateral columns of gray matter, mainly from the third and also from the second and fourth sacral segments of the spinal cord (the ''detrusor center''). These neurons give rise to preganglionic fibers which synapse in parasympathetic ganglia within the bladder wall. Postganglionic fibers end on muscarinic acetylcholine receptors on the smooth muscle fibers. There are also beta-adrenergic receptors in the dome of the bladder and alpha-adrenergic receptors at the base, which are activated by sympathetic fibers of the hypogastric plexus; these fibers arise in the intermediolateral nerve cells of T10, T11, and T12 segments. The internal sphincter and base of the bladder (trigone), consisting of smooth muscle, are also innervated by the sympathetic fibers of the hypogastric nerves; their receptors are mainly of alpha-adrenergic type.

The external urethal (and anal) sphincters are composed of striated muscle fibers and are innervated by a densely packed group of somatomotor neurons in the anterior horns of sacral segments 1, 2, and 3 (nucleus of Onuf), via the pudendal nerves. Cells in the ventrolateral part of Onuf's nucleus innervate the external urethral sphincter, and cells of the medial-dorsal part innervate the anal

sphincter. Close connections exist between the cells of Onuf's nucleus and those of the intermediate lateral column. These muscle fibers respond to the nicotinic effects of acetylcholine.

Afferent fibers from the urethra and external sphincter pass, via pudendal nerves, to the sacral segments of the spinal cord and convey impulses for reflex activities and, through connections with higher centers, for sensation. Some of these fibers probably course through the hypogastric plexus as indicated by the fact that there are vague sensations of discomfort in patients with complete transverse lesions of the spinal cord at T12 and below. The bladder is sensitive to pain and pressure; pain sensation ascends to higher centers in the lateral spinothalamic tracts and pressure, in the posterior columns.

Unlike skeletal striated muscle, the detrusor, because of its postganglionic system, is capable of some contractions, incomplete at best, after complete destruction of the sacral segments of the spinal cord. Isolation of the sacral cord centers (transverse lesions of the cord above the sacral levels) and peripheral nerves permits contractions of the detrusor muscle but they do not empty the bladder com-

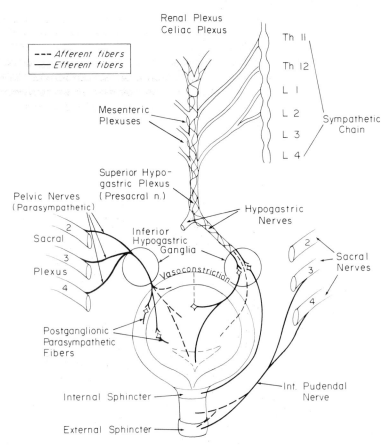

Figure 26-5

Innervation of the urinary bladder and its sphincters.

pletely; patients with such lesions usually develop dyssynergia of the detrusor and external sphincter muscles (see below), indicating that coordination of these muscles occurs at supraspinal levels (Blaivas). With acute transverse lesions of the cord, the function of sacral segments is abolished for several weeks in the same way as the motor neurons of skeletal muscles. This is the state of *spinal shock.*

Efficient emptying of the bladder is possible only when the spinal segments, together with their afferent and efferent nerve fibers, are connected with the so-called micturition centers in the pontomesencephalic tegmentum. These centers receive afferent impulses from the sacral cord segments; their efferent fibers course downward via the reticulospinal tracts in the lateral funiculi of the spinal cord and activate cells in the nucleus of Onuf as well as in the intermediolateral cell groups of the sacral segments (Holstege and Tan). These pontomesencephalic centers also receive descending fibers from anteromedial parts of the frontal cortex, the limbic regions, amygdaloid nuclei, thalamus, hypothalamus and cerebellum. Other fibers, from the motor cortex, descend with the corticospinal fibers to the anterior horn cells (see below) of the sacral cord and innervate the external sphincter. According to Ruch, these descending pathways are both inhibitory (midbrain tegmentum) and facilitatory (pontine tegmentum and posterior hypothalamus). The pathway that descends with the corticospinal tract, from the motor cortex, is inhibitory. Thus the net effect of lesions in the brain and spinal cord on the micturition reflex of animals may be either inhibitory or facilitatory (DeGroat).

Only the perfect integration of this complex neural organization permits the individual to sense fullness of the bladder and the need for emptying; to suppress emptying contractions until the appropriate time and place; to remain continent; to initiate and stop voiding voluntarily; and to empty the bladder completely.

The act of micturition is both reflex and voluntary. When the normal person is asked to void, there is first a voluntary relaxation of the perineum, then an increased tension of the abdominal wall, a slow contraction of the detrusor, and an associated opening of the internal sphincter, and finally a relaxation of the external sphincter (Denny-Brown and Robertson, 1933a). It is useful to think of the detrusor contraction as a spinal stretch reflex, subject to facilitation and inhibition from higher centers. Voluntary closure of the external sphincter and contraction of the perineal muscles causes the detrusor contraction to subside. The abdominal muscles have no power to initiate micturition except when the detrusor muscle is not functioning normally. The voluntary restraint of micturition is a cerebral affair and is mediated by fibers described above—arising in the frontal lobes (paracentral motor region), descending in the spinal cord just anterior and medial to the corticospinal

tracts, and terminating on the cells of the anterior horns and intermediolateral cell columns of the sacral segments, as described above. The integration of detrusor and external sphincteric function depends mainly on the descending pathway from the dorsolateral pontine tegmentum.

These data enable one to understand the effects of the following lesions on bladder function:

1. *Complete destruction of the cord, below T12,* as from trauma, myelodysplasias, tumor, and necrotizing myelitis. The bladder is paralyzed and there is no awareness of the state of fullness; voluntary initiation of micturition is impossible; the tonus of the detrusor muscle is abolished and the bladder distends as urine accumulates until there is overflow incontinence; voiding is possible only by the Crede maneuver of abdominal compression and abdominal straining. Usually the anal sphincter and colon are similarly affected and there is ''saddle'' anesthesia and abolition of the bulbocavernosus and anal reflexes. The cystometrogram shows low pressure and no emptying contractions.

2. *Disease of the motor neurons of the sacral gray matter, the anterior roots, or peripheral nerves,* as in lumbosacral meningomyelocele. This is in effect a lower motor neuron paralysis of the bladder. The disturbance of bladder function is the same as in (1), above, except that sacral and bladder sensation are intact.

It is noteworthy that a hysterical woman can suppress motor function and suffer a similar distention of the bladder.

3. *Interruption of sensory afferent fibers* from the bladder, as in tabes dorsalis, leaving motor nerve fibers unaltered. This is a primary sensory bladder paralysis. Again the disturbance in function is the same as in (1) and (2), above.

Clinically, in the case of a flaccid (atonic) bladder, there may be interruption of both afferent and efferent innervation, or of both, as in cauda equina compression or diabetic neuropathy.

4. *Upper spinal cord lesions.* These result in a *reflex neurogenic (spastic) bladder.* As stated above, if the cord lesion is of sudden onset, the detrusor muscle suffers the effects of spinal shock. At this stage, urine accumulates and distends the bladder to the point of overflow. As the effects of spinal shock subside, the detrusor becomes overactive, and since the patient is unable to inhibit the detrusor and to control the external sphincter, precipitant micturition and incontinence result. In addition, initiation of voluntary micturition is impaired and bladder capacity is reduced. Bladder sensation depends on the extent of

involvement of sensory tracts. Bulbocavernosus and anal reflexes are preserved. The cystometrogram shows uninhibited contractions of the detrusor muscle in response to small volumes of fluid. Of course, if the upper motor neuron lesion evolves slowly, spasticity of the bladder will not be preceded by a flaccid stage.

5. *Mixed type of neurogenic bladder.* In diseases such as multiple sclerosis or syphilitic meningomyelitis, bladder function may be deranged from lesions at multiple levels, i.e., spinal roots, sacral neurons or their fibers of exit, and higher spinal segments. The resultant picture is a combination of sensory, motor, and spastic types of bladder paralysis.

6. *Stretch injury of bladder wall,* as occurs with anatomic obstruction at the bladder neck and occasionally with voluntary retention of urine. Repeated distention of the bladder wall often results in varying degrees of decompensation of the detrusor muscle and permanent atonia or hypotonia. The bladder wall becomes fibrotic. The bladder capacity is greatly increased. Emptying contractions are inadequate, and there is a large residual volume even after the Crede maneuver, and strong contraction of the abdominal muscles. As with motor and sensory paralyses, the patient is subject to cystitis, ureteric reflux, hydronephrosis and pyelonephritis, and calculus formation.

7. *Frontal lobe incontinence.* Often the patient, because of his torpid or confused mental state, ignores the desire to void and the subsequent incontinence. There is also a supranuclear type of hyperactivity of the detrusor and precipitant evacuation. These types of frontal lobe incontinence are considered on page 356.

8. *Nocturnal enuresis, or urinary incontinence during sleep,* due presumably to a delay in acquiring inhibition of micturition, is discussed in Chap. 18.

THERAPY OF DISORDERED MICTURITION

Several drugs are useful in the management of flaccid and spastic disturbances of bladder function. In the case of a flaccid paralysis, bethanacol (Urecholine) produces contraction of the detrusor by direct stimulation of its muscarinic cholinergic receptors. In spastic paralysis, the detrusor can be relaxed by propantheline (Probanthine), which acts as a muscarinic antagonist, and by oxybutine (Ditropan), which acts directly on the smooth muscle and also has a muscarinic antagonist action. Atropine, which is mainly a muscarinic antagonist, only partially inhibits detrusor contraction.

Several other drugs may also be useful in the treatment of neurogenic bladder, but can only be rationally utilized on the basis of sophisticated urodynamic investigation (Krane and Siroky).

Often the patient must resort to intermittent self-catheterization which can be safely carried out with scrupulous attention to sterile technique (washing hands, boiling catheter once a day, etc.). Some forms of antibacterial therapy and acidification of urine with vitamin C (1000 g/ day) are practical aids.

In selected paraplegic patients, the implantation of a sacral anterior root stimulator may prove to be helpful in emptying the bladder and achieving continence (Brindley et al).

DISTURBANCES OF BOWEL FUNCTION

The colon and anal sphincters are obedient to the same principles that govern bladder function. Ileus from spinal shock, reflex neurogenic colon, and sensory and motor paralysis with megacolon are all recognized clinical entities. The colon may be hypotonic and distended and the anal sphincters lax, either from deafferentation (tabes dorsalis) or de-efferentation, or both. The anal and, in the male, the bulbocavernosus reflex may be abolished. Defecation may be urgent and precipitant in higher spinal and cerebral lesions (White et al). Since the same spinal segments and nearly the same spinal tracts subserve bladder and bowel function, meningomyeloceles and other spinal cord diseases often cause so-called double incontinence. However, since the bowel is less often filled and its content is solid, fecal incontinence is usually less troublesome than urinary incontinence.

Systemic diseases may affect the colonic sphincters; examples are myotonic dystrophy and scleroderma, which may weaken the internal sphincter, and polymyositis and myasthenia gravis, which may impair the function of the external sphincter (Schuster). Also, sphincteric damage is frequent after fissurotomy and hemorrhoidectomy.

CONGENITAL MEGACOLON (HIRSCHSPRUNG DISEASE)

This is a rare disease affecting mainly male infants and children. It is due to a congenital absence of ganglion cells in the myenteric plexus. The rectosigmoid and internal sphincter are involved most often, and are the parts affected in restricted Hirschprung disease, but the aganglionosis is sometimes more extensive. The aganglionic segment of the bowel is constricted and cannot relax, thus preventing propagation of peristaltic waves, which in turn produces retention of feces and massive distention of the colon above the aganglionic segment. Some cases of megaloureter are attributed to a similar defect. The treatment is surgical in all cases.

DISTURBANCES OF SEXUAL FUNCTION

Sexual function in the male, which is not infrequently affected in neurologic disease, is conveniently divided into several parts: (1) sexual impulse, drive, or desire, often referred to as *libido;* (2) penile erection, enabling the act of sexual intercourse (potency); and (3) ejaculation of semen by the prostate through the urethra, whereby impregnation of the female may be accomplished.

The arousal of libido in men and women may result from a variety of stimuli, some purely imaginary. Such neocortical influences are transmitted to the limbic system and thence to the hypothalamus and spinal centers. The suprasegmental pathways traverse the lateral funiculi of the spinal cord near the corticospinal tracts to reach sympathetic and parasympathetic segmental centers. Penile erection is effected through sacral parasympathetic motor neurons (S3 and S4) and the nervi erigentes and pudendal nerves. There is evidence also that an outflow from thoracolumbar segments (originating in T12-L1) via the inferior mesenteric and hypogastric plexuses can mediate psychogenic erections in patients with complete sacral cord destruction. Activation from these segmental centers opens vascular channels between arteriolar branches of the pudendal arteries and the vascular spaces of the corpora cavernosa and corpus spongiosum (erectile tissues), resulting in tumescence. Deturgescence occurs when venous channels open widely. Copulation consists of a complex series of rhythmic thrusting movements of pelvic musculature, and ejaculation involves rhythmic contractions of the prostate, the compressor (sphincter) urethrae, and bulbocavernosus and ischiocavernosus muscles, which are partly under the control of both the sympathetic and parasympathetic centers. Afferent segmental influences arise in the glans penis and reach parasympathetic centers at S3 and S4 (reflexogenic erections). The organization of this neural system and the locations of lesions that can abolish normal potency are shown in Fig. 26-6. Similar neural arrangements exist in females.

The different parts of the sexual act may be affected separately. Loss of libido may depend upon both psychic and somatic factors. It may be complete, as in old age or in medical and endocrine diseases, or it may occur only in certain circumstances or in relation to a certain person. In the latter case, which is usually due to psychologic factors, reflexogenic penile erection during REM sleep and even emission of semen may occur, and effective sexual intercourse with another person is possible. Sexual desire can on occasion be altered in the opposite direction, i.e., it may be excessive. This too may be psychologic in origin but sometimes occurs with neurologic disease, such as

encephalitis and tumors affecting the diencephalon, septal region, and temporal lobes.

Sexual desire on the other hand may be present but penile erection impossible to attain or sustain, a condition called *impotence,* in which nocturnal erections are usually preserved. The commonest cause of impotence is a depressive state. It occurs also in patients who suffer disease of the sacral cord segments and their afferent and efferent connections (e.g., cord tumor, tabes, diabetic polyneuropathy), in which case nocturnal erections are absent. The parasympathetic nerves cannot then be activated to cause tumescence of the corpora cavernosa and corpus spongiosum. Diseases of the spinal cord may abolish psychogenic erections, leaving reflexogenic ones intact. In fact, the latter may become overactive, giving rise to sustained painful erections *(priapism).* This is a reminder that all the neural apparatus for the control of sexual function is organized through the lower spinal segments (sacral 3 and 4 and the nervi erigentes and pudendal nerves) and that the mechanism of erection may still be functional, even when completely removed from voluntary control, as in high spinal lesions. Sympathectomy leaves this mechanism for penile erection relatively intact.

Another sexual difficulty may be the premature ejaculation of semen, a common complaint in neurotic individuals, though by no means limited to them. After lumbar sympathectomy the semen may be ejected back into the bladder because of paralysis of the periurethral muscle (prostate) at the verumontanum (colliculus seminalis). Prostatism may have a similar effect.

Finally, diseases of the testes accompanied by insufficient spermatogenesis or diseases of the seminal vesicles which prevent emission of sperm result in *sterility;* in these cases libido and potency may or may not be normal.

Aberrations of sexual function also occur in the female but are more difficult to analyze. Lack of sexual desire or failure to attain orgasm (frigidity) is much more frequent in the female than in the male, occurring in a significant percentage of neurotic women and in others who exhibit no signs of psychic disorder. States of excessive sexual excitability are known in sociopathic individuals and, rarely, in those who suffer disease of the brain. Fecundity and sterility are usually unrelated to the other aspects of sexuality.

The genesis of sexual perversions remains obscure. Endocrine, biochemical, and psychologic studies have failed to clarify the cause and mechanism. Homosexuality appears to be stamped into the limbic-hypothalamic parts of the nervous system in early life; the brain at that time becomes either male or female. Cerebral disorders of sexual function are discussed further in Chap. 25 (page 418) and in Chap. 55, in the section on psychiatry.

AUTONOMIC DISTURBANCES WITH LESIONS OF THE BRAINSTEM

With lesions of any type in the lateral tegmentum of the pons and medulla there may be an ipsilateral paralysis of autonomic function in the arm, trunk, and leg. These parts are warm and dry. In addition there may be a Horner syndrome. Rarely, discrete lesions in higher parts of the brainstem, presumably interrupting the hypothalamotegmental sympathetic pathway, may produce the same effects (Carmel).

Acute medullary lesions, most often due to head injury or massive stroke, may give rise to pulmonary edema of neurogenic type (lungs 2000 g or more at autopsy). The disorder is due to an increase in pulmonary vascular permeability, but little more is known about it. In animals, it can be prevented by transection of the spinal cord at C8, but it is not affected by vagotomy. It can also be prevented by adrenergic blocking agents; hence it is probably mediated by adrenergic centers in either the hypothalamus or medulla.

Figure 26-6

The pathways involved in human penile erection. (From Weiss.)

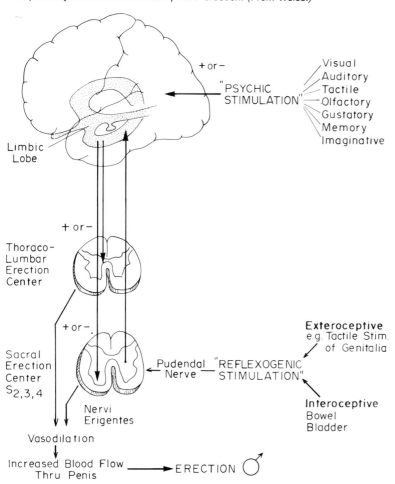

REFERENCES

AGUAYO AJ, NAIR CPV, BRAY GM: Peripheral nerve abnormalities in Riley-Day syndrome. *Arch Neurol* 24:106, 1971.

AHLQUIST RP: A study of adrenotropic receptors. *Am J Physiol* 153:586, 1948.

APPENZELLER O: *The Autonomic Nervous System,* 3rd ed. Amsterdam, North-Holland, 1982.

BLAIVAS JG: The neurophysiology of micturition: a clinical study of 550 patients. *J Urol* 127:958, 1982.

BRINDLEY GS, POLKEY CE, RUSHTON DN, CARDOZO L: Sacral anterior root stimulation for bladder control in paraplegia: The first 50 cases. *J Neurol Neurosurg Pshychiatry* 49:104, 1986.

BURNSTOCK G: Innervation of vascular smooth muscle: Histochemistry and electron microspcopy. *Clin Exp Pharmacol Physiol* 2(suppl):2, 1975.

CANNON WB: *Bodily Changes in Pain, Hunger, Fear and Rage,* 2nd ed. New York, Appleton, 1920.

CARMEL PW: Sympathetic deficits following thalamotomy. *Arch Neurol* 18:378, 1968.

COHEN J, LOW P, FEALEY R et al: Somatic and autonomic function in progressive autonomic failure and multiple system atrophy. *Ann Neurol* 22:692, 1987.

COLLINS KJ: Autonomic failure and the elderly, in Bannister R (ed): *Autonomic Failure.* New York, Oxford Press, 1983, chap 23, pp 489–507.

DEGROAT WC: Nervous control of urinary bladder of the cat. *Brain Res* 87:201, 1975.

DENNY-BROWN D, ROBERTSON EG: On the physiology of micturition. *Brain* 56:149, 1933a.

DENNY-BROWN D, ROBERTSON EG: The state of the bladder and its sphincters in complete transverse lesions of the spinal cord and cauda equina. *Brain* 56:397, 1933b.

DUCHEN LW: Neuropathology of autonomic nervous system in diabetes, in Bannister R. (ed): *Autonomic Failure.* New York, Oxford Press, 1983, chap 21, pp 437–452.

DYCK PJ, KAWAMER Y, LOW PA et al: The number and sizes of reconstituted peripheral, autonomic, sensory, and motor neurons in a case of dysautonomia. *J Neuropathol Exp Neurol* 37:741, 1978.

FALCK B: Observations on the possibilities of the cellular localization of monoamines by a fluorescence method. *Acta Physiol Scand,* vol 56, suppl 197, 1962.

HOLSTEGE G, TAN J: Supraspinal control of motoneurons innervating the striated muscles of the pelvic floor including urethral and anal sphincters in the cat. *Brain* 110:1323, 1987.

JOHNSON RH, SPALDING JMK: *Disorders of the Autonomic Nervous System.* Philadelphia, Davis, 1974.

KAADA B: Brain mechanisms related to aggressive behavior, in Clemente CD, Lindsley DB (eds): *Proceedings of the 5th Conference on Brain Function, November 1965, Aggression and Defense: Neural Mechanisms and Social Patterns.* Berkeley, University of California Press, 1967, pp 95–133.

KEANE JR: Oculosympathetic paresis: Analysis of 100 hospitalized patients. *Arch Neurol* 36:13, 1979.

KIRBY R, FOWLER CV, GOSLING JA et al: Bladder dysfunction in distal autonomic neuropathy of acute onset. *J Neurol Neurosurg Psychiatry* 48:762, 1985.

KRANE RJ, SIROKY MD (eds): *Clinical Neurourology.* Boston, Little, Brown, 1979.

LAFFERTY K, ROBERTS VC, DETRAFFORD JC et al: On the nature of Raynaud's phenomenon: The role of histamine. *Lancet* 2:313, 1983.

LEWIS P: Familial orthostatic hypotension. *Brain* 87:719, 1964.

LEWITT PA: The neurotoxicity of the rat poison Vacor. *N Engl J Med* 302:73, 1980.

LOW PA, DYCK PJ: Splanchnic preganglionic neurons in man. II. Morphometry of myelinated fibers of T7 ventral spinal root. *Acta Neuropathol* 40:219, 1977.

LOW PA, DYCK PJ, LAMBERT EH: Acute panautonomic neuropathy. *Ann Neurol* 13:412, 1983.

LUHAN VA, POLLACK SL: Occlusion of the superior cerebellar artery. *Neurology* 3:77, 1953.

MACMILLAN AL, SPALDING JMK: Human sweating response to electrophoresed acetylcholine: A test of postganglionic sympathetic function. *J Neurol Neurosurg Psychiatry* 32:155, 1969.

MCLEOD JG, TUCK RR: Disorders of the autonomic nervous system. Part I. Pathophysiology and clinical features. Part II. Investigation and treatment. *Ann Neurol* 21:419, 519, 1987.

MANNEN T, IWATA M, TOYOKURA Y, NAGASHIMA K: Preservation of a certain motoneurone group of the sacral cord in amyotrophic lateral sclerosis: Its clinical significance. *J Neurol Neurosurg Psychiatry* 40:464, 1977.

NATHAN PW, SMITH MC: The location of descending fibers to sympathetic neurons supplying the eye and sudomotor neurons supplying the head and neck. *J Neurol Neurosurg Psychiatry* 49:187, 1986.

ONUFROWICZ B: On the arrangement and function of cell groups of the sacral region of the spinal cord of man. *Arch Neurol Psychopathol* 3:387, 1900.

OPPENHEIMER O: Neuropathology of progressive autonomic failure, in Bannister R (ed): *Autonomic Failure.* New York, Oxford Press, 1983, chap 14, pp 267–283.

PALMATIER MA, SCHMIDT RE, PLURAD SB, JOHNSON EM JR: Sympathetic neuronal destruction in macaque monkeys by guanethidine and guanacline. *Ann Neurol* 21:46, 1987.

PETITO CK, BLACK IB: Ultrastructure and biochemistry of sympathetic ganglia in idiopathic orthostatic hypotension. *Ann Neurol* 4:6, 1978.

PICK J: *The Autonomic Nervous System.* Philadelphia, Lippincott, 1970.

RAJPUT AH, ROZDILSKY B: Dysautonomia in parkinsonism: A clinico-pathologic study. *J Neurol Neurosurg Psychiatry* 39:1092, 1976.

RICHARDSON KC: The fine structure of the albino rabbit iris with special reference to the identification of adrenergic and cholinergic nerves and nerve endings in its intrinsic muscles. *Am J Anat* 114:173, 1964.

RUCH T: The urinary bladder, in Ruch TC, Patton HD (eds): *Physiology and Biophysics,* vol 2: *Circulation, Respiration, and Fluid Balance.* Philadelphia, Saunders, 1974, pp 525–546.

SCHUSTER MM: Clinical significance of motor disturbances of the enterocolonic segment. *Am J Dig Dis* 11:320, 1966.

SELYE H: The general adaptation syndrome and the diseases of adaptation. *J Clin Endocrinol Metab* 6:117, 1946.

SHY GM, DRAGER GA: A neurological syndrome associated with orthostatic hypotension: A clinical-pathologic study. *Arch Neurol* 2:511, 1960.

SPOKES EGS, BANNISTER R, OPPENHEIMER DR: Multiple system atrophy with autonomic failure. *J Neurol Sci* 43:59, 1979.

THOMPSON PD, MELMON KL: Clinical assessment of autonomic function. *Anesthesiology* 29:724, 1968.

WEISS HD: The physiology of human penile erection. *Ann Intern Med* 76:792, 1972.

WHITE JC, VERLOT MG, EHRENTHEIL O: Neurogenic disturbances of colon and their investigation by the colonmetrogram. Preliminary report. *Ann Surg* 112:1042, 1940.

WICHSER J, VIJAYAN N, DREYFUS PM: Dysautonomia—its significance in neurologic disease. *Calif Med* 117:28, 1972.

YOUNG RR, ASBURY AK, CORBETT JL, ADAMS RD: Pure pandysautonomia with recovery: Description and discussion of diagnostic criteria. *Brain* 98:613, 1975.

ZIEGLER MG, LAKE R, KOPIN IJ: The sympathetic nervous system defect in primary orthostatic hypotension. *N Engl J Med* 296:293, 1977.

CHAPTER 27

THE HYPOTHALAMUS AND NEUROENDOCRINE DISORDERS

The hypothalamus plays a dual role in the actions of the nervous system. One, that of serving as the "head ganglion" of the autonomic nervous system, was described in the preceding chapter; the other, its function as the head ganglion of the endocrine system, is the subject of this chapter. The activities of these two systems are interdependent and mutually developed; they maintain homeostasis and provide the substructure of emotional behavior and related psychic experience.

The expansion of knowledge of neuroendocrinology during the past few decades stands as one of the most significant achievements in neurobiology. It has been learned that neurons, in addition to transmitting electrical impulses, can synthesize and discharge complex molecules capable of activating or inhibiting glandular cells. This research has led also to the discovery of some 30 or more neurotransmitter peptides, which modulate the activities of other neurons and nonneural cells.

The modern concept of neurotransmission had its beginning with Loewi's discovery, in 1922, of "vagus substance" and "sympathetic substance," obtained by stimulating heart nerves, followed by Dale's discovery of acetylcholine, in 1936. They both obtained indisputable evidence that autonomic and somatic motor neurons synthesized and liberated a substance at their axon terminals, which was necessary for the transmission of a nerve impulse to a muscle cell, thereby causing it to contract. These observations placed neurochemical transmission on solid ground. But even before these discoveries, Speidel, in 1919, and then the Scharrers, in 1929, had described hypothalamic neurons with the morphologic characteristics of glandular cells. Their suggestion that such cells might secrete hormones into the bloodstream was so novel, however, that it was not accepted by most biologists at the time. This seems surprising now that neurosecretion is accepted as a fundamental part of the science of endocrinology and that one hypothalamic releasing factor after another is being isolated and synthesized.

At about the same time it was discovered that certain peptides, secreted by neurons in the central and peripheral nervous systems, were also found in glandular cells of the pancreas and intestines. This seminal observation was made in 1931, by von Euler and Gaddum, who isolated a substance from the intestines that was capable of acting on smooth muscle. But it was not until some 35 years later that Leeman and her associates purified the substance and identified it as substance P (see Aronin et al). Then followed the discovery of somatostatin in 1973, by Brazeau and colleagues, and the endogenous opioids (enkephalin) by Hughes et al, in 1975.

THE HYPOTHALAMUS

This small structure is bounded posteriorly by the mammillary bodies, anteriorly by the optic chiasm and lamina terminalis, superiorly and medially by the hypothalamic sulcus, and inferiorly by the hypophysis. It comprises three main nuclear groups, the standard nomenclature for which was proposed in 1939 by Rioch et al: (1) the anterior group, which includes the supraoptic and paraventricular nuclei; (2) the middle group, which includes the tuberal, arcuate, ventromedial, and dorsomedial nuclei; and (3) the posterior group, which includes the mammillary bodies and the posterior hypothalamic nuclei. The inferior surface of the hypothalamus bulges downward at the site of the tuber cinereum, from the center of which arises the median eminence or infundibulum. The latter stands out because of its vascularity (the hypophysial-portal system of veins courses over the surface). The infundibulum extends into the pituitary stalk, which in turn enters the pars nervosa of the hypophysis.

Nauta and Haymaker subdivided the hypothalamus longitudinally. The *lateral part* lies lateral to the fornix; it is sparsely cellular and its cell groups are traversed by the medial forebrain bundle, which carries finely myelinated and unmyelinated ascending and descending fibers to and from the rostrally placed septal nuclei, substantia innominata, nucleus accumbens, amygdala and piriform cortex, and the caudally placed tegmental reticular formation. The *medial hypothalamus* is rich in cells, some of which are the neurosecretory cells for pituitary regulation and visceral control. It contains two main efferent fiber systems—the mammillothalamic tract of Vicq d'Azyr, which connects the mammillary nucleus with the anterior thalamic nucleus (which in turn projects to the cingulate gyrus), and the mammillotegmental tract. Separate are the stria terminalis, which runs from the amygdala to the ventromedial hypothalamic nucleus, and the fornix, which connects the hippocampus to the mammillary body, septal nuclei, and periventricular hypothalamus. The lateral and medial parts of the hypothalamus are interconnected and their functions are integrated.

The median eminence assumes special importance because of the intimate relation of its cell groups to the anterior lobe of the pituitary gland. It has been subdivided into three zones: the inner ependymal, the inner palisade, and the outer palisade. The ependymal zone is composed of the ependymal cells of the floor of the third ventricle; many of them are of a specialized type, called tanycytes, which show evidence of secretory activity. Their basal processes extend to the outer palisade zone, which contains the unmyelinated nerve fibers of the arcuate and other medial hypothalamic nuclei. The supraopticohypophysial fibers traverse the medial palisade zone, and some terminate on capillaries of the outer palisade zone (Martin and Reichlin). The tuberoinfundibular neurons of the arcuate nucleus and anterior periventricular nuclei synthesize most of the releasing factors now to be described (Fig. 27-1).

THE HYPOPHYSIOTROPIC HORMONES OF THE HYPOTHALAMUS (HYPOTHALAMIC RELEASING FACTORS)

1. *TRH: Thyrotropin-releasing factor.* This was the first of the releasing factors to be identified; its structure was determined in 1969. This hormone is elaborated by the anterior periventricular nuclei, the paraventricular nuclei, the arcuate nuclei, the ventromedial and dorsomedial nuclei,

HYPOTHALAMIC-NEUROHYPOPHYSIAL SYSTEM   HYPOTHALAMIC-ADENOHYPOPHYSIAL SYSTEM

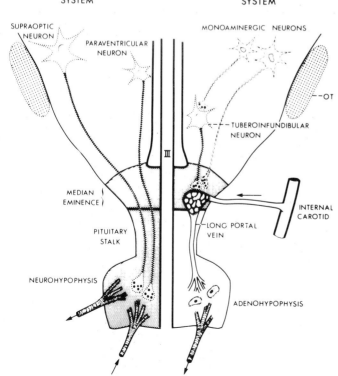

Figure 27-1

Diagram of the hypothalamic-pituitary axis. Indicated on the left is the hypothalamic-neurohypophysial system consisting of supraoptic and paraventricular neurons, axons of which terminate on blood vessels in the posterior pituitary (neurohypophysis). The hypothalamic-adenohypophysial system is illustrated on the right. Tuberoinfundibular neurons, believed to be the source of the hypothalamic regulatory hormones, terminate on the capillary plexus in the median eminence. (Courtesy of Dr. JB Martin.)

but not the posterior hypothalamic or thalamic nuclei. Mainly it stimulates the release of thyroid-stimulating hormone, TSH [which in turn effects the release of T_4 (thyroxine) and T_3 (triiodothyronine)]. Also stimulated are pituitary cells, which release dopamine and somatostatin; the latter has an inhibitory effect on TSH. There is an inhibitory feedback of T_4 and T_3 on TSH and on TRH. About 30 percent of TRH is found outside the hypothalamus in brainstem raphe nuclei, tractus solitarius, and the anterior and lateral horn cells of spinal cord.

2. *GHRF: Growth hormone–releasing factor.* This factor and somatostatin (GH-release-inhibiting factor) are both secreted by specialized tuberoinfundibular neurons and released into the portal system, whence it is carried to somatotrophic cells of the anterior pituitary gland. Immunohistochemical staining has shown the sources of these two hormones to be neurons of the posterior part of the arcuate nuclei and the ventromedian nucleus and other neurons of the premammillary area. Somatostatin is produced more anteriorly by neurons in the periventricular area and small-cell part of the paraventricular nucleus. The amygdala and hippocampus and other limbic structures project to the arcuate nuclei via the medial corticohypothalamic tract (in the stria terminalis) and are believed to account for the sleep- and stress-induced fluctuations of GH and somatostatin. Also it has been demonstrated that all four biogenic amines (dopamine, norepinephrine, epinephrine, and serotonin) influence GH regulation as does acetylcholine, either by direct action on somatotrophic cells or on hypothalamic regulatory neurons. Thyrotropin-releasing hormone also increases GH from somatotropes. Many of the latter contain large eosinophilic granules, but other cells, previously identified incorrectly as chromophobe cells, also contain GH. Somatomedin C, which is synthesized in the liver, exerts feedback control of GH by inhibiting the pituitary somatotropes and the regulatory hypothalamic neurons. Growth hormone enhances skeletal growth by stimulating the proliferation of cartilage and growth of muscle. It also regulates lipolysis, stimulates aminoacid uptake in cells, and has anti-insulin effects. The blood concentrations of GH fluctuate from 1 or 2 to over 60 ng/mL, being highest at the onset of sleep. Both somatostatin and GHRF have been synthesized.

3. *CRF: Corticotropin-releasing factor.* This was first identified in 1981 and has been shown to release ACTH from basophilic cells in the pituitary. These in turn stimulate the synthesis and release of the hormones of the adrenal cortex, mainly glucocorticoids (cortisol or hydrocortisone) but also mineralocorticoids (aldosterone) and androcorticoids. The neurons of origin of CRF lie in a particular part of the paraventricular nucleus, other cells of which form the paraventricular-supraopticohypophysial tract (neurohypophysis) and elaborate vasopressin and oxytocin and several other substances (neurotensin, dynorphin, vasoactive intestinal releasing factor). These hypothalamic cells receive an extensive input from other regions of the nervous system, particularly via the noradrenergic pathways (from medullary reticular, locus ceruleus, and tractus solitarius neurons) and from many of the limbic structures. Presumably, these extrahypothalamic connections provide the mechanism by which stress and pain activate the secretion of ACTH and cortisol. CRF itself is widely distributed in the brain. There is feedback control of CRF and ACTH via glucocorticoid receptors in the hypothalamus and anterior lobe of the pituitary. Serotonin and acetylcholine enhance ACTH secretion and the catecholamines are inhibitory.

4. *GnRH: Gonadotropin-releasing hormone.* This peptide originates in the arcuate nucleus and is present in highest concentration near the median eminence. It effects the release of the two gonadotropic hormones—luteinizing hormone (LH) and follicle-stimulating hormone (FSH). The ovary and the testis, by secreting a peptide called *inhibin*, are able to suppress FSH, as do gonadal steroids, i.e., estrogens. GnRH is normally under the influence of other neuronal systems, which are modulated by catecholamines, serotonin, acetylcholine, and dopamine. Puberty, menstruation, ovulation, lactation, and menopause are all related to GnRH, FSH, LH, and their peripheral effects on the ovaries, uterus, breasts, and testes. Normal levels of blood FSH are 2.5 to 4.9 ng/mL in prepuberty and 7.5 to 11 ng/mL in the adult; levels of blood LH are 2.8 to 9.6 ng/mL in prepuberty and 10 to 18 ng/mL in the adult.

5. *PRF: Prolactin-releasing factor.* This is found in the region of the arcuate nucleus and is able to activate lactotropic cells of the anterior pituitary. However, a number of different peptides—thyroid-releasing factor, vasoactive intestinal peptide, dopamine, peptide-histidine-isoleucine, and oxytocin, among others—all have the capacity to raise the levels of prolactin in the blood. The hypothalamopituitary axis is responsive to input from sensory structures in the nipples, via the spinal cord and brainstem, accounting for the effect of suckling on milk production. The normal blood levels of prolactin are 5 to 25 ng/mL.

6. *The neurohypophysis: Vasopressin and oxytocin.* The supraoptic and paraventricular nuclei are the sources of a neural secretion that is transported, via the axons of these cells, through the stalk of the pituitary, to its posterior lobe. Together they constitute the neurohypophysis, which develops as an evagination of the floor of the third ventricle. The elaborated hormones are vasopressin and oxytocin. Some of the vasopressin-containing endings also terminate

on the capillary plexus of the hypophysial portal system and in other regions of the nervous system. The peptide parts of these two hypothalamic hormones, whose chemical nature was determined by duVigneaud and his colleagues, are almost identical, differing from one another by only two amino acids; but their proteins (neurophysins) are distinctive. Vasopressin, upon reaching the kidney tubules, serves as the antidiuretic hormone and, complemented by thirst mechanisms, maintains the osmolality of the blood. Oxytocin initiates uterine contraction and has milk ejecting effects. Plasma osmolality and circulating blood volume receptors (in the heart and baroreceptors) modify vasopressin secretion by acting on separate osmoreceptors in the hypothalamus. The latter are so exquisitely sensitive that an increase in 1 percent of total body water will cause a fall of 2.8 mosmol/kgH$_2$O (Martin and Reichlin).

From even this brief outline of the hypothalamic releasing factors, it is apparent that the system is extremely complex. The releasing factors that have been identified have overlapping functions. The hypothalamic nuclei act on many parts of the brain in addition to the pituitary. And many parts of the brain influence the hypothalamus through neural connections or modulate its activity and that of the pituitary gland through the action of neurotransmitters and modulators (catecholamines, acetycholine, serotonin, and dopamine). Some of these relationships will emerge in the discussion of syndromes that result from diseases of these parts of the nervous system.

Of particular significance is the role of the hypothalamus in the integration of the endocrine and autonomic nervous systems at both the peripheral and central levels. The best-known example of this interaction is in the adrenal medulla, as indicated in Chap. 26. A similar relationship holds for the pineal gland; release of norepinephrine from postganglionic fibers that end on pineal cells stimulates several enzymes that are involved in the biosynthesis of *melatonin*. Similarly the juxtaglomerular apparatus of the kidney and the islets of Langerhans of the pancreas function as neuroendocrine transducers, since they convert a neural stimulus (in these cases adrenergic) to an endocrine secretion (renin, and glucagon and insulin, respectively).

Finally, as we emphasized in Chap. 26, the hypothalamus regulates both sympathetic and parasympathetic activities. Sympathetic responses are most easily obtained by stimulation of the posterior and lateral regions of the hypothalamus, and parasympathetic ones from the anterior and lateral regions. The course taken by the descending sympathetic pathways is not entirely clear. According to

Carmel, fibers from the lateral hypothalamic area (hypothalamotegmental tract) at first course posteriorly with the medial forebrain bundle into the region of the prerubral field (dorsal and slightly rostral to the red nucleus), the medial tegmentum of the midbrain, and the locus ceruleus; the more medial fibers descend in the dorsal longitudinal fasciculi of Schutz. In the medulla descending sympathetic fibers lie in more compact groups in the retro-olivary region and then descend to synapse with the lateral horn cells of T1-L2 segments. These fiber systems are largely uncrossed and, if interrupted, give rise to a Bernard-Horner syndrome. The pathways of descending parasympathetic fibers are not known.

HYPOTHALAMIC-PITUITARY SYNDROMES

DIABETES INSIPIDUS (DI)

As long ago as 1913, independent pathologic studies of Farini of Venice and von den Velden of Dusseldorf (quoted by Martin and Reichlin) revealed lesions of the hypothalamus in cases of diabetes insipidus. They showed, moreover, that in patients with this disorder the excessive urination could be corrected by injections of extracts of the posterior pituitary. Ranson and his colleagues elucidated the anatomy of the neurohypophysis and traced the posterior pituitary substance to granules in the cells of the supraoptic and paraventricular nuclei and followed their passage to axon terminals in the posterior lobe. DuVigneaud et al determined the chemical structure of the two neurohypophysial peptides, vasopressin and oxytocin, of which these granules were composed. These observations opened up the entire field of neuroendocrinology.

The cause of DI is a lack of vasopressin, also called the antidiuretic hormone (ADH), which normally enters the blood stream and is transported to the kidneys where it acts on the renal tubules to control the absorption of water. As a consequence of this lack, there is diuresis of low-osmolar urine (polyuria), reduction in blood volume, and increased thirst and drinking of water (polydipsia), in an attempt to maintain osmolality. A congenital abnormality or destruction of tubular epithelium has a similar effect—nephrogenic diabetes insipidus.

Martin and Reichlin divide the causes of DI into congenital and idiopathic. A small number of congenital or familial cases have been described in which the disorder exists throughout life, owing to a developmental defect of the supraoptic and paraventricular nuclei and smallness of the posterior lobe of the pituitary. This may be combined with other disorders such as diabetes mellitus, optic atrophy and deafness (Wolfram syndrome), and Friedreich ataxia. In 25 to 50 percent of cases presenting clinically as isolated DI, no cause can be established. In some of the latter there are serum antibodies that react with the supraoptic neurons, raising the question of an autoimmune disorder.

Of the acquired types, tumors and surgical trauma lead the list. In one such series of 41 cases, 29 percent were due to surgery, 26 percent to tumors, 5 percent to head injuries, and 10 percent to histiocytosis X. Sarcoidosis is another known cause of DI. Of the primary tumors, according to Martin and Reichlin, the granular cell tumor (choristoma) is most typical, followed by the infundibuloma and glioma; hamartoma and craniopharyngioma are also well-recognized causes of DI. Pituitary tumors are rarely associated with DI because they do not invade the stalk of the pituitary and the infundibulum. This point has been substantiated by surgical sections of the stalk for metastatic carcinoma and retinitis proliferans; only if the section is high will DI result. Histiocytosis X (eosinophilic granuloma, Letterer-Siwe disease, and Hand-Schuller-Christian disease) is a well-known cause in young patients.

In all these conditions the severity and permanence of the DI are determined by the nature of the lesion. In cases of acute onset, three phases have been delineated: (1) first, a severe DI lasting days; (2) then, as the neurohypophysis degenerates, a reduction in severity of DI due to release of ADH, (3) followed by a persistent pattern. The neurohypophysial axons can regenerate, allowing for some recovery, even after years.

The diagnosis of DI is always suggested by the passage of large quantities of dilute urine. Polydipsia and polyuria will last through the night. The thirst mechanism and drinking usually prevent dehydration and hypovolemia, but if the patient is stuporous or the thirst mechanism is deranged, severe dehydration can occur, leading to stupor, coma, and death. Proof that the patient has DI (and is not a compulsive water drinker) is obtained by injecting five pressor units of Pitressin subcutaneously, which will diminish urine output and increase osmolality. An 8-h dehydration test is another way of increasing urinary osmolality in a person with normal kidneys and neurohypophysis. A radioimmune assay of plasma for ADH is available and will be found reduced to less than 1.0 pg/mL in patients with DI (normal, 2.7 to 1.4 pg/mL).

Vasopressin tannate in oil, synthetic lysin vasopressin nasal spray, and a long-release arginine vasopressin analogue administered by nasal insufflation satisfactorily control chronic DI (see Martin and Reichlin for details of management).

SYNDROME OF INAPPROPRIATE ADH SECRETION (SIADH)

Blood volume and osmolality are normally maintained within narrow limits by the secretion of ADH and by the thirst mechanism. Reduction in osmolality acts via osmo-receptors in the hypothalamus to decrease ADH and to suppress thirst and drinking behavior; increased osmolality and blood volume do the opposite. The normal osmolality is 280 mosmol/kg $\pm$ 1.8, and release of ADH begins when it reaches 287 mosmol/kg (osmotic threshold). At this point plasma ADH levels are 2 pg/mL and increase rapidly as the osmolality rises higher.

Derangement of this delicately regulated mechanism, taking the form of water retention and dilutional hyponatremia, is observed under a variety of clinical circumstances. Instead of suppression of ADH secretion by water retention, the plasma ADH is above normal, presumably because of inappropriate secretion of ADH or ectopic production of the hormone by tumor tissue. In most cases the thirst mechanism is not inhibited by decreased osmolality, and continued drinking further increases blood volume and reduces its solute concentration. The term "inappropriate secretion of antidiuretic hormone" was applied to this syndrome by Schwartz and Bartter, because of its similarity to that produced in animals by the chronic administration of ADH. This condition is observed frequently with a variety of cerebral lesions (infarct, tumor, hemorrhage) that do not involve the hypothalamus directly, and, of course, with many types of hypothalamic disease (trauma, surgery). Neoplasms, particularly lung tumors, may elaborate an ADH-like substance, and certain drugs such as chlorpromazine, carbamazepine, chlorthiazide, and vincristine may have a similar effect.

A fall in serum sodium to 120 to 125 meq/L usually has no effect clinically, although symptoms from an associated neurologic disease may worsen. Sodium levels of 100 to 120 meq/L are usually attended by inattentiveness, drowsiness, and stupor. The rapid restitution of serum sodium to normal or above-normal levels carries a risk of producing central pontine myelinolysis. A safer procedure is to restrict water to 400 to 600 mL/day. If the patient's neurologic condition is serious and the serum sodium is in the range of 100 to 110 meq/L, 3% NaCl should be infused slowly, and if there is adrenal cortical deficiency, glucocorticoids and possibly mineralocorticoids should be given.

Moderate lowering of the serum sodium is a common finding in patients with acute intracranial diseases and postoperatively in neurosurgical patients and is probably due to salt wasting and not to inappropriate ADH secretion.

OTHER DISTURBANCES OF ADH AND THIRST

Conditions have been described in which the osmoreceptor control of ADH and thirst appeared to have been dissociated.

One of our patients, reported by Hayes et al, repeatedly developed severe hypernatremia with levels as high as 180 to 190 meq/L. He appeared to initiate a release of ADH but the thirst mechanism was nonfunctional. Only when compelled to drink water at regular intervals did the serum sodium fall. Robertson has described similar cases and also others with abnormalities of thirst. These cases have been reported under the title of "central" or "essential" hypernatremia.

NEUROENDOCRINE SYNDROMES RELATED TO THE ADRENAL GLANDS

Cushing Disease This disease, first described in a classic monograph by Cushing, in 1932, is now familiar to everyone in medicine. The clinical manifestations are indicative of disturbances in many tissues and organs: truncal obesity with reddish purple cutaneous striae over the abdomen and other parts, dryness and pigmentation of the skin and fragility of skin vessels, excessive facial hair and baldness, cyanosis and mottling of the skin of the extremities, thoracic kyphosis and osteoporosis, generalized muscular weakness, hypertension, glycosuria, and a number of psychologic disturbances. Adrenal hyperplasia secondary to a basophilic adenoma of the pituitary was the established pathology in Cushing's cases. But the same combination of abnormalities may be associated with chronically increased concentrations of cortisol from a primary adrenal tumor, ectopic production of cortisol, or the long-term administration of ACTH or corticosteroids (glucocorticoids). For these latter conditions the term Cushing syndrome is appropriate. Some of its components may be lacking or less conspicuous than in florid Cushing disease, and diagnosis is then facilitated by measurements of ACTH and cortisol in the blood.

In Cushing disease, as was postulated in the initial report, a basophilic adenoma produces a hormone, now called ACTH, that stimulates the adrenals. Unlike the usual pituitary tumors, basophilic adenomas enlarge the sella in only 20 percent of cases. However, by high-resolution CT scanning through the sella, either micro- or macroadenomas can be visualized in about 85 percent of cases of Cushing disease (the other 15 percent have a nonpituitary source). Microadenomas outnumber macroadenomas by 3:1. Many of the small tumors are now being verified by transphenoidal biopsy.

The possibility that excess ACTH production by the pituitary might be due to a disorder of the hypothalamus was conceptualized by Heinbecker in 1944, and the isolation of a corticotropin-releasing factor (CRF) was accomplished by Guillemin and Rosenberg in 1955. However, the proof that Cushing syndrome could be due to an excess of CRF or a lack of hypothalamic inhibitor remains unconvincing. There are at most only a few cases in which a hypothalamic tumor such as a gangliocytoma has caused Cushing disease. More firmly established is the ectopic production of ACTH by a variety of tumors: oat-cell and squamous-cell carcinoma of the lung, carcinoma of the pancreas, thymoma, and many others (pheochromocytoma, medullary carcinoma of the thyroid, islet cell tumors). These types of Cushing syndrome differ from Cushing disease in inducing greater pigmentation, and with the rapid development of hypercorticalism there tends to be more severe hypokalemia, hypertension, and glycosuria. ACTH concentrations may exceed 300 pg/mL and do not change with dexamethasone administration. However, with slow-growing tumors, the ACTH levels and dexamethasone response, as well as the clinical syndrome, may be indistinguishable from Cushing disease due to a pituitary tumor.

For diagnostic purposes, the high ACTH concentration and high blood cortisol levels (over 35 μg/dL in the morning) and lack of diurnal variation are supportive of the diagnosis of Cushing disease. CT scans and MRI of the pituitary and adrenal glands are mandatory. An excess of ACTH is compatible with a pituitary adenoma or the ectopic production of ACTH by a nonpituitary tumor. Suppression of cortisol by high doses of dexamethasone, but not by low doses, is said to indicate primary pituitary disease. (See Martin and Reichlin for details of these testing procedures.)

Treatment is determined by the cause of the syndrome. If due to an adrenal adenoma or to an ectopic tumor, it should be extirpated if possible. If this is not possible, one turns to radiation therapy and the use of drugs to suppress adrenal corticosteroid formation (metyrapone, aminoglutethimide). A basophilic adenoma, if large but not extending out of the sella and encroaching on the optic chiasm, is ideally treated with focused proton beam or focused gamma radiation, but this form of treatment is available in only a few institutions worldwide. The alternative is excision of the tumor by transnasal pituitary microsurgery. Depending on the functional status of the pituitary, replacement therapy may be needed.

Adrenal Cortical Insufficiency (Addison Disease) The classic form of adrenal insufficiency, described by Addison, is due to primary disease of the adrenals. It is characterized by pigmentation of the skin and mucous membranes; nausea, vomiting, and weight loss; and muscle weakness, languor, and a tendency to faint. Following Addison, hypotension, hyperkalemia, hyponatremia, and low serum cortisol concentrations came to be recognized as important clinical features.

In former times, the usual cause of primary adrenal disease was tuberculosis. Now, most cases are designated as idiopathic and are thought to represent an autoimmune disorder, often associated with Hashimoto thryoiditis and diabetes mellitus, and rarely with other endocrine disorders. A hereditary metabolic disease of the adrenals and a demyelinating disease of brain, spinal cord, and nerves, peculiar to males (adrenoleukodystrophy), is known (see page 807). In primary adrenal disease, plasma concentrations of cortisol are low and those of ACTH are elevated. Adrenal insufficiency of whatever cause is a life-threatening condition; always there is a danger of collapse and even death, particularly during periods of infection, surgery, injury, and the like. Lifelong replacement therapy is usually required, with a glucocorticoid (cortisone, 25 to 50 mg, or prednisone, 7.5 to 15 mg daily) and a mineralocorticoid (Florinef, 0.05 to 0.2 mg daily).

Secondary adrenal insufficiency may follow disease of the pituitary. ACTH is low or absent and cortisol secretion is markedly reduced, but aldosterone levels are sustained. Pigmentation is notably absent; it is the elevation of ACTH that causes melanodermia, as occurs, for example, in patients subjected to bilateral adrenalectomy. Hypothalamic lesions, principally involving the paraventricular nuclei, may also cause adrenal insufficiency, but this occurs less frequently than depression of gonadal and thyroid function.

OTHER HYPOTHALAMIC SYNDROMES

Apart from diabetes insipidus and Cushing syndrome, there are a variety of other phenomena attendant upon disease of the hypothalamus. These usually occur not in isolation but in various combinations, comprising a number of rare but widely known syndromes.

Precocious Puberty Neurogenic precocious puberty may occur in males and females and always occasions both a neurologic and endocrine investigation. In the male one searches for evidence of a teratoma of the pineal gland or mediastinum, and an androgenic tumor of the testes or adrenals must be excluded. In the female with early development of secondary sexual characteristics and menstruation, one looks for other evidence of hypothalamic disease as well as an estrogen-secreting tumor. A hamartoma of the hypothalamus (part of von Recklinghausen disease or of polyostotic fibrous dysplasia) has been a frequent lesion in both boys and girls with precocious puberty. In a number of such cases, so-called gelastic seizures have been conjoined (Breningstall). The neurologic study entails CT scans and MR imaging of the hypothalamus, ovaries, and adrenals.

Adiposogenital Dystrophy (Froehlich Syndrome) When Froehlich described this syndrome in 1901,

he related the disorder to a pituitary tumor that had caused both obesity and delayed sexual development. But a few years later Erdheim recognized that the same syndrome could be a manifestation of a lesion (a suprasellar cyst, in his case) that was restricted to the hypothalamus. Later it was determined that obesity and delay in genital development could occur together or separately and were often combined with a loss of vision and unprovoked rage, aggression, and antisocial behavior. Diabetes insipidus may be conjoined. The usual cause of the Froehlich syndrome is a craniopharyngioma, but many other tumors have been reported (pituitary adenoma, cholesteatoma, lipoma, meningioma, glioma, angiosarcoma, and chordoma).

Other Hypothalamic Disorders Associated with Obesity Precise neuroanatomic studies have localized a satiety center in the ventromedial nucleus of the hypothalamus and an appetite center in the lateral hypothalamus. Lesions in the medial hypothalamus result in overeating and obesity; lesions in the lateral hypothalamus, in a failure to eat and thrive. A case that lent itself to close clinicopathologic correlation was described by Reeves and Plum. A hamartoma had destroyed the medial eminence and the ventromedial nuclei bilaterally but had spared the lateral hypothalamus. Hyperphagia and rage were the main clinical features; the associated polydipsia and polyuria were due to extension of the tumor to the anterior hypothalamus.

The biology of appetite, eating behavior, and satiety is extremely complex and cannot be reviewed adequately in a neurology text. Only the most common derangements of these functions can be mentioned here.

Obesity itself can be due to a hypothalamic disturbance, in which the satiety centers are underactive. However, there may be other genetic factors, such as the number of lipocytes that one inherits. Stunkard et al have shown that the body mass (weight in kilograms divided by height in meters) of babies who grow to adulthood in adopted families exhibit the weight class of their biological parents and not of their adopted ones. This applies to thin adults as well. Swedish twin studies have yielded similar results. This, of course, does not eliminate environmental influences; sedentary life in a food-laden society encourages obesity. Since obesity is known to have adverse effects on health, preventive efforts should be directed to children at risk of becoming fat. There are no safe, effective antiobesity medications (or surgical measures), and reliance must still be placed on dieting and educating patients as to the need to change their eating habits.

Extrahypothalamic parts of the brain, if diseased,

may also be associated with increased food-seeking behavior, food ingestion, and weight gain. Examples are involvement of limbic structures, as in the Kluver-Bucy syndrome (page 362) and basal frontal lobe degenerations.

In the Prader-Willi syndrome of hypogenitalism and obesity, hypotonia, mental retardation, and short stature, the early infantile feeding difficulties give way to hyperphagia and a virtually uncontrollable appetite for food. No abnormalities of the hypothalamus were reported in the few autopsied cases.

The association of *anorexia* with disease involving the appetite centers has not been established, though the cases of Lewin et al and of White and Hain are suggestive. Martin and Reichlin, in citing these cases, attribute the anorexia and cachexia to lesions of the lateral hypothalamus.

Abnormalities of Growth Presumably, in most instances of growth retardation, there is a deficiency of growth hormone–releasing factor (GHRF), or of growth hormone (GH) per se. In the Prader-Willi syndrome, Bray et al found the deficiency to be one of GHRF. In certain congenital and developmental diseases the hypothalamus appears to be incapable of releasing GH. For example in the de Morsier septo-optic defect of the brain (median facial cleft, septum pellucidum, optic defect), Stewart et al found a deficiency of GH. In idiopathic hypopituitarism, where stunting of growth is associated with other endocrine abnormalities, about half of the reported cases respond to GHRF but not to hypoglycemia, arginine infusion, and L-dopa. In some dwarfs (Laron dwarf, Seckel bird-headed dwarf) there are extremely high levels of circulating GH, suggesting either a defect in the GH molecule or an unresponsiveness of target organs.

In *gigantism*, most of the reported cases have been due to pituitary tumors (micro- or macroadenomas), which secrete an excess of GH. This must occur prior to closure of the epiphyses. The notion of a purely hypothalamic form of gigantism or acromegaly (hypothalamic acromegaly) has been affirmed by Asa et al, who described six patients with hypothalamic gangliocytomas that produced GHRF. An ectopic source of GH must also be considered.

The mental retardates with gigantism, described by Sotos et al, were found to have no abnormalities of GHRF, GH, or somatomedin.

Disturbances of Temperature Regulation Lesions in the more anterior parts of the hypothalamus may result in hyperthermia. The heat-dissipating mechanisms of the body are impaired. This often has followed operations, or other trauma, in the region of the floor of the third ventricle. The temperature rises to 41°C (106°F) and remains at that level until death some hours or days later, or drops abruptly with recovery. Icy coldness of the extremities, dry skin, tachycardia, and tachypnea—all intended to conserve heat—accompany the hyperthermia. Acetylsalicylic acid has little effect on central hyperthermia; the only way to control it is to cool the body while administering phenobarbital.

Hyperthermia is also part of the malignant hyperthermia syndrome, in which there is an abnormal reaction to muscle relaxants (see page 1113), and of the malignant neuroleptic syndrome, which is based on an idiosyncratic reaction to neuroleptic drugs (page 901). Wolff and his colleagues have described a syndrome of periodic hyperthermia, in which a patient had episodes of fever, vomiting, hypertension, and weight loss, accompanied by an excessive excretion of glucocorticoids. The syndrome has no apparent explanation, although there was a symptomatic response to chlorpromazine.

Lesions in the posterior part of the hypothalamus often have had a different effect; i.e., they often produce hypothermia or poikilothermia (equilibration of body and environmental temperatures). The latter may pass unnoticed unless the patient's temperature is taken after lowering and raising the room temperature. Somnolence, confusion, and hypotension are often associated. *Periodic hypothermia*, believed by Martin and Reichlin to have been first described by Gowers, has been found in association with a cholesteatoma of the third ventricle (Penfield) and with agenesis of the corpus callosum (Noel et al). Periodically the rectal temperature falls to 30°C and seizures may occur.

Chronic hypothermia is a more familiar state than hyperthermia, sometimes recorded in hypothyroidism, in hypoglycemia, and in patients intoxicated with barbiturates or alcohol. It tends to be more frequent in the elderly, who are found to have a defective thermoregulatory mechanism.

Cardiovascular Disorders with Hypothalamic Lesions Ranson and his colleagues demonstrated autonomic effects from stimulating the hypothalamus; the cardiac response was an auricular tachycardia. This and hypertension were recorded in Penfield's case of so-called diencephalic epilepsy (page 419). Acute vascular lesions of the brain, e.g., subarachnoid hemorrhage, may be accompanied by supraventricular tachycardia, ectopic ventricular beats, and ventricular fibrillation; a variety of acute changes in the myocardium have been reported, but the interpretation of such alterations is still under discussion.

Gastric Hemorrhage and Other Disorders In experimental animals, lesions placed in or near the tuberal nuclei appear to induce superficial erosions or ulcerations of the gastric mucosa (Cushing ulcers), sometimes with massive hemmorhage. Gastric lesions of similar type are not infrequently seen in humans with all manner of intracranial diseases (subdural hematoma, lobar hemorrhages, and tumors) and may have been the cause of death. One examines in vain the various hypothalamic nuclei, seeking causative lesions, even though a functional disorder in this region is suspected.

Diencephalic Syndrome   Poor feeding, weight loss, slow psychomotor development, and failure to thrive, sometimes with impaired vision, constitute a syndrome that emerges in the first few months of postnatal life and ends fatally at 1 or 2 years of age. Most of the lesions have been gliomas of the third ventricle, involving the anterior part of the hypothalamus (Burr et al).

Disorders of Consciousness and Personality   From the time of Ranson and of Hess, it has been appreciated that acute lesions in the posterior and lateral part of the hypothalamus could induce stupor or coma, but always it was difficult to determine precisely which structures were involved. And, well before this time, it was known that a mesencephalitis was the basis of the "sleeping sickness" (encephalitis lethargica), described by von Economo. However, one could not say that the lesions in this disease were strictly hypothalamic or that they had interrupted the hypothalamic-mesencephalic connections in the medial forebrain bundle, or the more superiorly placed thalamic reticular activating system. One can be certain that coma from small lesions may occur in the absence of any changes in the hypothalamus and, conversely, that chronic hypothalamic lesions may be accompanied by no more than drowsiness or confusion or no change at all. In one of our early cases with a lesion entirely confined to the hypothalamus, the patient lay for weeks in a state of torpor, and was drowsy and confused. His blood pressure was low, his body temperature was 34 to 35°C, and he had diabetes insipidus. When aroused he was aggressive, like the patient of Reeves and Plum (see above).

Periodic Somnolence and Bulimia (Kleine-Levin Syndrome)   Kleine, in 1925, and Levin, in 1936, described an episodic disorder characterized by somnolence and overeating. For days or weeks, the patients, mostly adolescent boys, would sleep 18 or more hours a day, awakening only long enough to eat and attend to toilet activities. They appeared dull, often confused, restless, and sometimes troubled by hallucinations. In the series of 18 cases later collected by Critchley, the age range was from puberty to 45 years. The episodes varied from 2 days to 12 weeks and in frequency from 2 to 12 yearly. The condition has been seen in females. The somnolence has been well studied by modern laboratory methods and the sleep cycle is normal (see also page 313).

The cause of the condition is disputed. The hyperphagia has suggested a hypothalamic disorder, but anatomical verification is lacking. The case reported by Carpenter et al, in which an acute and chronic inflammation in the medial thalamus and hypothalamus was found, must be questioned as representative of the condition. The patient was a man aged 40 who had diurnal drowsiness, hyperphagia (intermittently relieved by methylphenidate), and hypersexuality over a period of months. In some of the patients, schizophrenia and sociopathic symptoms have been recorded between attacks, raising doubt as to whether all the reported cases are of the same type.

In most instances the disease is self-limited and disappears by early adult life.

NEUROPEPTIDES AND NEUROREGULATION

As was remarked in the introduction to this chapter, any consideration of hypothalamic release factors invites scrutiny of a burgeoning literature on neurotransmitters and neuromodulators. It becomes clear that processes are involved which are far more complex than the relatively simple neuronal synthesis, transmission, and release of hormones. Martin and Reichlin, in their scholarly review of this literature, point out that each of the physiotropic hypothalamic hormones is influenced by many of the neuropeptides such as acetylcholine, serotonin, adrenalin, noradrenalin, dopamine, γ-aminobutyric acid, substance P, enkephalins, and others to be discovered.

At present it is impossible to provide a complete account of these interactions. This is probably the most rapidly advancing field of neurobiology. And what is being discovered will find wide application to the elucidation of many obscure neurologic and psychiatric disease. Some of these new data will be introduced in later chapters.

BIBLIOGRAPHY

Aronin N, diFiglea M, Leeman SE: Substance P, in Krieger DT, Brownstein NJ, Martin JB (eds): *Brain Peptides.* New York, Wiley, 1983, pp 783–804.

Asa SL, Scheithauer BW, Bilbau J et al: A case of hypothalamic acromegaly. A clinico-pathologic study of 6 patients with hypothalamus gangliocytomas producing growth hormone releasing factor. *J Clin Endocrinol Metab* 58:796, 1984.

Bray GA, Gallagher TF: Manifestations of hypothalamic obesity in man. A comprehensive investigation of 8 cases and a review of the literature. *Medicine* 54:301, 1975.

BRAZEAU P, VALE W, BARGUS R et al: Hypothalamic polypeptide that inhibits the secretion of immunoreactive pituitary growth hormone. *Science* 179:77, 1973.

BRENINGSTALL GN: Gelastic seizures, precocious puberty and hypothalamic hamartoma. *Neurology* 35:1180, 1985.

BURR IM, SLONIM AE, DANISH RK: Diencephalic syndrome revisited. *J Pediatr* 88:429, 1976.

CARMEL PW: Sympathetic deficits following thalamotomy. *Arch Neurol* 18:378, 1968.

CARPENTER S, YASSA R, OCHS R: A pathologic basis for Kleine-Levin syndrome. *Arch Neurol* 39:25, 1982.

CRITCHLEY M: Periodic hypersomnia and megaphagia in adolescent males. *Brain* 85:627, 1962.

DALE HH: Transmission of nervous effects by acetylcholine. *Bull NY Acad Med* 13:379, 1937.

DUVIGNEAUD V: Hormones of the posterior pituitary gland: oxytocin and vasopressin. *Harvey Lect* 50:1, 1954–1955.

ERDHEIM J: Ueber Hypophysengangs geschwulste und hirn Cholesteatome. Sitzungs DK Akad d Wissensch. *Math Natur WC Wien* 113:537, 1904.

FROEHLICH A: Ein Fall von Tumor der Hypophysis cerebri ohne Akromegalie. *Wien Klin Wochenschr* 15:883, 1901.

GILBERT GJ: Periodic hypersomnia and bulimia. *Neurology* 141:844, 1964.

GUILLEMIN R, ROSENBERG B: Humeral hypothalamic control of anterior pituitary. A study with combined tissue cultures. *Endocrinol* 57:599, 1955.

HAYES R, MCHUGH PR, WILLIAMS H: Absence of thirst in hydrocephalus. *N Engl J Med* 269:277, 1963.

HEINBECKER P: The pathogenesis of Cushing's disease. *Medicine* 23:225, 1944.

LEWIN K, MATTINGLY D, MILLS RR: Anorexia nervosa associated with hypothalamic tumour. *Br Med J,* 2:629, 1972.

HUGHES IT, SMITH W, KOSTERLITZ HW et al: Identification of two related pentapeptides from the brain with potent opiate agonist activity. *Nature* 258:577, 1975.

KLEIN E W: Periodische Schlafsucht. *Mschr Psychiatry Neurol* 57:285, 1925.

KRIEGLER DT, MARTIN JB: Brain peptides. *N Engl J Med* 304:876, 1981.

LEVIN M: Periodic somnolence and morbid hunger. *Brain* 62:494, 1936.

LEWIN K, MATTINGLY D, MILLS RR: Anorexia nervosa associated with hypothalamic tumour. *Br Med J* 2:629, 1972.

LOEWI A: Ueber humorale uebertragbarkeit der Herznervenwirkung *Arch ges Physiol* 189:239, 1921.

MARTIN JB, REICHLIN S: *Clinical Neuroendocrinology,* 2nd ed. Philadelphia, Davis, 1987.

NAUTA W JH, HAYMAKER W: Hypothalamic nuclei and fiber connections, in Haymaker W, Anderson E, Nauta WJH (eds.): *The Hypothalamus.* Springfield, IL, Charles C Thomas, 1969, pp 136–209.

NOEL P, HUBERT JP, ECTORS M et al: Agenesis of the corpus callosum associated with relapsing hypothermia. *Brain* 96:359, 1973.

PENFIELD W: Diencephalic autonomic epilepsy. *Arch Neurol Psychiatry* 22:358, 1929.

RANSON SW: Somnolence caused by hypothalamic lesions in the monkey. *Arch Neurol Psychiatry* 41:1, 1939.

REEVES AG, PLUM F: Hyperphagia, rage and dementia accompanying a ventromedial hypothalamic neoplasm. *Arch Neurol* 20:616, 1969.

RIOCH D McK, WISLOCKI GB, O'LEARY JL: A precis of preoptic hypothalamic and hypophysial terminology with atlas, in *The Hypothalamus,* vol 20. Baltimore, Williams & Wilkins, 1940.

ROBERTSON GL: Posterior pituitary, in *Endocrinology and Metabolism.* New York, McGraw-Hill, 1987.

SCHARRER E, SCHARRER B: Secretory cells within the hypothalamus, in *The Hypothalamus.* New York, Haffner, 1940.

SCHWARTZ WB, BARTTER FC: The syndrome of inappropriate secretion of antidiuretic hormone. *Am J Med* 42:790, 1967.

SOTOS JF, DODGE PR, MUIRHEAD D et al: Cerebral gigantism in childhood. *N Engl J Med* 271:109, 1964.

SPEIDEL CG: *Carnegie Inst Wash Publ* 13:1, 1919.

STEWART C, CASTRO-MAGANA M, SHERMAN J et al: Septo-optic dysplasia and median cleft face syndrome in a patient with isolated growth hormone deficiency and hyperprotaclomenia. *Am J Dis Child* 137:484, 1983.

STUNKARD AJ, SORENSEN TIA, HANIS C et al: An adoption study of human obesity. *N Engl J Med* 314:193, 1986.

VON EULER US, GADDUM JH: An unidentified depressor substance in certain tissue extracts. *J Physiol* 72:74, 1931.

WHITE LF, HAIN RF: Anorexia in association with a destructive lesion of the hypothalamus. *Arch Pathol* 68:275, 1959.

WOLF SM, ADLER RC, BUSKIRK ER et al: A syndrome of periodic hypothalamic discharge. *Am J Med* 36:1956, 1964.

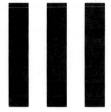

GROWTH AND DEVELOPMENT OF THE NERVOUS
SYSTEM AND THE NEUROLOGY OF AGING

CHAPTER 28

NORMAL DEVELOPMENT AND DEVIATIONS IN DEVELOPMENT OF THE NERVOUS SYSTEM

TIME-LINKED SEQUENCES OF NORMAL DEVELOPMENT

The establishment of a biologic time scale of human development requires observation, under standardized conditions, of a large number of normal individuals of known ages and the testing of them for measurable items of behavior. Because of individual variations in the tempo of development, it is equally important to study the growth and development of any *one* individual for a prolonged period. If these observations are to be correlated with stages of neuroanatomic development, the clinical and morphologic data must be expressed in units that are comparable. Early in life, age periods are difficult to ascertain because of the special difficulty in fixing the time of conception. The average human gestational period is 40 weeks (280 days), but to take birth as zero is obviously fallacious, since it may occur with survival as early as 28 or as late as 49 weeks, a time span of almost 5 months. Conception is the only time when chronological and developmental age correspond, but in practice this can rarely be determined.

After birth, any given item of behavior or structural differentiation must always have two reference points: (1) to some item of behavior already achieved, and (2) to units of chronological time or duration of the life of the organism. The former, or biologic scale, assumes special significance in early prenatal life when development is proceeding at such a rapid pace that small units of time weigh heavily, the organism appearing to change literally day by day; in infancy the tempo of development is somewhat slower, but still very rapid in comparison with later childhood.

The neurologist finds it advantageous to organize knowledge of normal development and disease around each of the time periods given in Tables 28-1 and 28-2.

NEUROANATOMIC BASES OF NORMAL DEVELOPMENT

A large body of knowledge has accumulated concerning the functional and structural status of the nervous system during each of the epochs of life (listed below), and the reader will find it recorded in the references at the end of this chapter. A summary of this information is given in Table 28-2.

EMBRYONAL AND FETAL PERIODS

Knowledge of the nervous system in the germinal and embryonal periods has been derived from the study of a relatively small number of abortuses that have fallen into the hands of anatomists.

Neuroblastic differentiation, migration, and neuronal multiplication are already well under way in the first three weeks of embryonic life. The chemical control of each of these phases (and later, connectivity) originates in the genome of the organism. Primitive cells destined to become neurons originate in or close to the ventricular lining of the neural tube. These cells proliferate at an astonishingly rapid rate (250,000 per minute, according to Cowan) for a circumscribed period (several days to weeks). They become transformed into bipolar neuroblasts, which migrate, in a series of waves, toward the marginal layer of what is to become the cortex of the cerebral hemispheres. The first glial cells also appear very early and presumably provide the scaffolding along which the presumptive neuroblasts move. Each step in the differentiation and migration of the neuroblasts proceeds in an orderly fashion, and one stage progresses to the next with remarkable precision. This process of migration is completed by the end of the fifth fetal month; since most migrations of neurons involve the movement of postmitotic cells, the cerebral cortex by this time has presumably acquired its full complement of nerve cells, estimated variously at 50 to 100 billion (Cowan).

Actually we have little idea of how many nerve cells are to be found in the cerebral or cerebellar cortices at different ages. More are formed than survive, for neuronal death constitutes an important phase of development. To obtain quantitative data of this type is one of the most pressing needs in neuroanatomy.

Within a few months of midfetal life, the cerebrum, which begins as a small bihemisphered organ with hardly a trace of surface indentation, evolves into a deeply sulcated structure. Every step in the folding of the surface to form fissures and sulci is obedient to order, following a temporal pattern of such precision as to permit a reasonably accurate estimation of age by this criterion alone. The major sylvian, rolandic, and calcarine fissures, for example, take on the adult configuration during the fifth month of fetal life, the secondary sulci in the sixth and seventh months, and the tertiary sulci in the eighth and ninth months (see Table 28-2).

Table 28-1
**Time scale of stages in human growth
and development**

Growth period	Approximate age
Prenatal	From 0 to 280 days
Ovum	From 0 to 14 days
Embryo	From 14 days to 9 weeks
Fetus	From 9 weeks to birth
Premature infant	From 27 to 37 weeks
Birth	Average 280 days
Neonate	First 4 weeks after birth
Infancy	First year
Early childhood (preschool)	From 1 to 6 years
Later childhood (prepubertal)	From 6 to 10 years
Adolescence	Girls, 8 or 10 to 18 years Boys, 10 or 12 to 20 years
Puberty (average)	Girls, 13 years Boys, 15 years

Source: GH Lowrey, *Growth and Development of Children*, 8th ed. Chicago, Year Book, 1986.

Table 28-2
**Timetable of growth and nervous system development
in the normal embryo and fetus**

Age, days	Size (crown-rump length), mm	Nervous system development
18	1.5	Neural groove and tube
21	3.0	Optic vesicles
26	3.0	Closure of anterior neuropore
27	3.3	Closure of posterior neuropore; ventral horn cells appear
31	4.3	Anterior and posterior roots
35	5.0	Five cerebral vesicles
42	13.0	Primordium of cerebellum
56	25.0	Differentiation of cerebral cortex and meninges
150	225.0	Primary cerebral fissures appear
180	230.0	Secondary cerebral sulci and first myelination appear in brain
180		Further myelination and growth of brain (see text)

Concomitantly, subtle changes in neuronal organization are occurring in the cerebral cortex and central ganglionic masses. Involved here are synaptogenesis and axonal pathfinding. Neurons become more widely separated as differentiation proceeds, owing to an increase in the size and complexity of dendrites and axons and enlargement of synaptic surfaces (Figs. 28-1 and 28-2). The familiar cytoarchitectural patterns which demarcate one part of the cerebral cortex from another are already in evidence by the thirtieth week of fetal life, and become definitive at birth and in succeeding months.

Myelination provides another index of the development and maturation of the nervous system and is believed to be related to the functional activity of the fiber systems. The acquisition of myelin sheaths by the spinal nerves and roots by the tenth week of fetal life is associated with the beginning of reflex motor activities. Segmental and intersegmental fiber systems in the spinal cord myelinate soon afterward, followed by ascending and descending fibers to and from the brainstem (reticulospinal, vestibulospinal). The acoustic and labyrinthine systems stand out with singular clarity in myelin-stained preparations by the twenty-eighth to thirtieth weeks, and the spinocerebellar and dentatorubral systems by the thirty-seventh week (Fig. 28-3).

NEONATAL PERIOD AND INFANCY

After birth, the brain continues to grow dramatically. From an average weight of 375 to 400 g at birth it reaches about 1000 g by the end of the first postnatal year. Glial cells derived from the matrix zones continue to divide and multiply during the first 6 months of postnatal life. The visual system begins to myelinate about the fortieth week,

and its myelination cycle proceeds rapidly, being nearly complete a few months after birth. The corticospinal tracts are not fully myelinated until halfway through the second postnatal year. Most of the principal tracts are myelinated by the end of this period. In the cerebrum the first myelin is seen at birth, in the posterior frontal and parietal lobes, and the occipital lobes (geniculocalcarine system) myelinate soon thereafter. The myelination of the frontal and temporal lobes proceeds during the first year of postnatal life. Most of the myelination of the cerebrum is completed by the end of the second year (Fig. 28-3).

Figure 28-1

Cox-Golgi preparations of the leg area of the motor cortex (area 4). Upper row, left to right: *8 months premature; newborn at term; 1 month; 3 months;* and *6 months.* Lower row, left to right: *15 months; 2 years; 4 years; 6 years. Magnification, 100×; apical dendrites of Betz cells have been shortened, all to the same degree. (Courtesy of Th Rabinowicz, University of Lausanne.)*

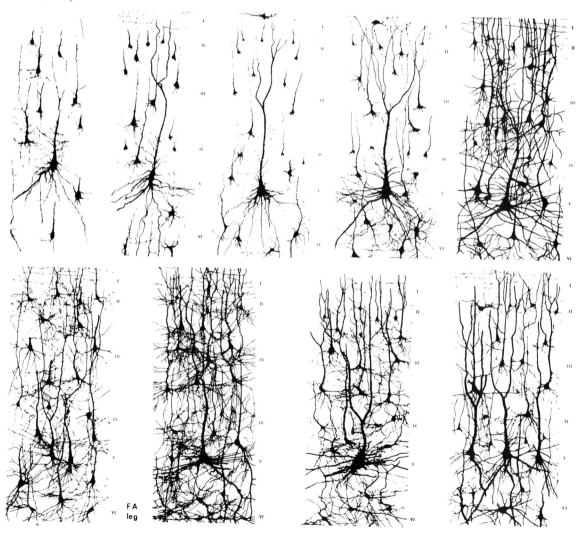

CHILDHOOD, PUBERTY, AND ADOLESCENCE

Growth of the brain continues, at a much slower rate than before, until 12 to 15 years, when the average adult weight of 1230 to 1275 g in females and 1350 to 1410 g in males is attained. Myelination also continues during this period, but much more slowly. Yakovlev and Lecours, who re-examined Flechsig's findings on the ontogeny of myelination, traced the progressive myelination of the middle cerebellar peduncle, acoustic radiation, and bundle of Vicq d'Azyr (mammillothalamic tract) beyond the third postnatal year; the nonspecific thalamic radiations beyond the seventh year; and the fibers of the reticular formation, the great cerebral commissures, and the intracortical association neurons to the tenth year and beyond (Fig. 28-3). They noted that there was an increasing complexity of fiber systems through late childhood and adolescence and perhaps even into middle adult life. Similarly, in the classic studies of Conel, depicting the cortical architecture at each year from birth to the tenth year of life, the dendritic arborizations and cortical interneuronal connections were observed to increase progressively in complexity, thus reducing the "packing density" of neurons, i.e., the number in any given volume (see Fig. 28-1).

Interesting questions are (1) whether neurons begin to function only when their axons have acquired a myelin sheath, (2) whether myelination is under the control of the cell body or the axon, or both, and (3) whether a myelin stain yields sufficient information as to the time of onset and degree of the myelination process. At best these correlations can be only approximate. It seems likely that systems of neurons begin to function before the first appearance of myelin as shown in conventional myelin stains. These correlations need to be restudied, using more delicate measures of function and finer staining techniques, as well as the techniques of phase and electron microscopy.

PHYSIOLOGIC AND PSYCHOLOGIC DEVELOPMENT

The human fetus is capable of an amazingly complex series of reflex activities, some of which appear as early as five weeks of postconceptional age. Cutaneous and proprioceptive stimuli evoke slow, generalized, patterned movements of the head, trunk, and extremities. Individual movements appear to differentiate from these generalized activities. Reflexes subserving blinking, sucking, grasping, and visceral functions, as well as tendon and plantar reflexes, are all elicitable in late fetal life. They seem to develop *pari passu* with the myelination of peripheral nerves, spinal roots, spinal cord, and brainstem. By the twenty-fourth

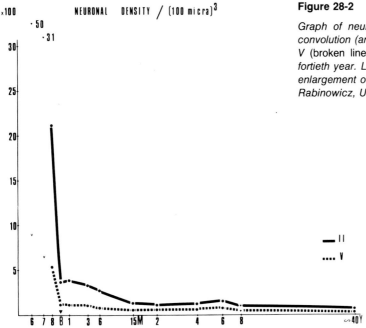

Figure 28-2

Graph of neuronal density in leg area of the precentral convolution (area 4), in cortical layer II (solid line) *and layer V* (broken line), *from the eighth month of fetal life to the fortieth year. Lessening neuronal population coincides with enlargement of cells and dendritic growth. (Courtesy of Th Rabinowicz, University of Lausanne.)*

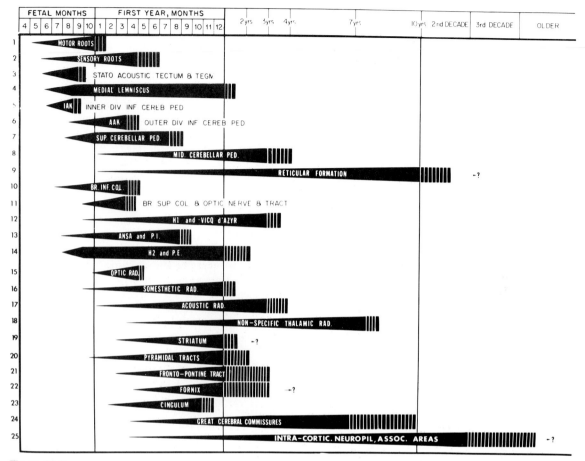

Figure 28-3

The myelogenetic chronology. (From Yakovlev and Lecours.)

week of gestation, the neural apparatus is functioning sufficiently well to give the fetus some chance of survival, should birth occur at this time. The failure of most infants to survive birth at this age is due usually to an inadequacy of pulmonary function. Thereafter, the basic neural equipment matures so rapidly that by the thirtieth week postnatal viability is relatively frequent. It seems that nature prepares the fetus for the contingency of premature birth by hastening to establish the vital functions necessary for extrauterine existence.

It is in the last trimester of pregnancy that a complete timetable of fetal movements, posture, and reflexes would be of the greatest value, for only during this period does the need for a full clinical evaluation arise. That there are recognizable differences between infants born in the sixth, seventh, eighth, and ninth months of fetal life is stated by Saint-Anne Dargassies, who has applied the neurologic

tests earlier devised by André-Thomas and herself. Her observations are in reference to prevailing postures; control and attitude of head, neck, and limbs; muscular tonus; and grasp and sucking reflexes. These findings are of interest and may well prove to be a means of determining exact age, but many more observations are needed with follow-up data on later development before they can be fully accepted as having predictive value. Part of the difficulty here is the extreme variability of the premature infant's neurologic functions, which may change literally from hour to hour.

Even at term, however, there is variability in neurologic functions from one day to the next. These reflect more the traumatic effects of parturition and the effects of drugs and anesthesia given to the mother than the developmental status of the brain.

At term, vital functions are quickly stabilized, and

effective sucking, rooting, and grasping reactions are present. The infant is able to swallow and to cry, and the startle reaction (Moro reflex) can be evoked by sound and by extending the neck suddenly. Support and steppage movements can be demonstrated by placing the infant on his or her feet, and incurvation of the trunk on stroking the back. The placing reaction, whereby the dorsal surface of the foot or hand, brought passively into contact with the edge of a table, is lifted automatically and placed on the flat surface, is also present at birth. These neonatal automatisms depend essentially on the functioning of the spinal cord, brainstem, and possibly diencephalon and pallidum. In effect, the *Apgar score* is really a numerical rating of brainstem-spinal mechanisms (breathing, pulse, color of skin, tone, and responsivity).

Behavior during the neonatal period, infancy, and early childhood is also the subject of a substantial literature, contributed more by psychologists than neurologists. They have explored particularly the sensorimotor performances of the first year and the language and social development in early childhood. In the first 6 years of life the infant and child traverse far more ground developmentally than they ever will again in a similar period. From the newborn state, when the infant is little more than an amorphous mass of protoplasm with a few postural reflexes, there are acquired, within a few months, laughter and head and hand-eye control; by 6 months, the ability to sit; by 10 months, the strength to stand; by 12 months, the coordination to walk; by 2 years, the agility to run; and by 6 years, mastery of the rudiments of a game of baseball or a musical skill. On the perceptual side the neonate progresses, in less than 3 months, from a state in which ocular control is tentative and tonic deviation of the eyes occurs only in response to labyrinthine stimulation, to one in which he or she is able to fixate and follow an object. (The latter corresponds to the development of the macula.) Much later the child is able to make fine discriminations of color, form, and size. As Gesell has remarked in his graphic summarization of the variety, range, and developmental sweep of a child's behavior: ''At birth the child reflexly grasps the examiner's finger, with eyes crudely wandering or vacantly transfixed . . . and by the sixth year the child adaptively scans the perimeter of a square or triangle, reproducing each form with directed crayon. The birth cry, scant in modulation and social meaning, marks the low level of language, which in two years passes from babbling to word formation that soon is integrated into sentence structure, and in six years to elaborated syntactic speech with questions and even primitive ideas of causality. In personality makeup . . . the

school beginner is already so highly organized, both socially and biologically, that he foreshadows the sort of individual he will be in later years.''

The studies of Gesell and Amatruda and of others represent attempts to establish age-linked standards of behavioral development, but the difficulties of using such a rating scale are considerable. The components of behavior that have been chosen as a frame of reference are not likely to be of uniform physiologic value or of comparable complexity, and they have seldom been standardized on large populations of different cultures. Also, the examinations at specified ages are cross-sectional assessments which give little idea of the dynamics of behavioral development. As already stated, temporal patterns of behavior reveal an extraordinary degree of change, emergence, increment, and decrement, and marked variation from one individual to another.

The predictive value of developmental assessment has been the subject of a lively dispute. Gesell has taken the position that the careful observation of a large number of infants, with accurate recording of the age at which various skills are acquired, permits the establishment of norms or averages. From such a framework one can determine the level of developmental attainment, expressed as the development quotient (DQ = developmental age/chronological age) and thus ascertain whether any given child is superior, average, or inferior.

After examining 10,000 infants over a period of 40 years, Gesell concluded that ''attained growth is an indicator of past growth processes and a foreteller of growth yet to be achieved.'' In other words the DQ predicts potential attainment. The other position, taken by Anderson, Kirman, and others is that developmental attainments are of no real value in predicting the level of intelligence but are measures of completely different functions. Illingworth and most clinicians, including the authors, have taken an intermediate position, that the developmental scale in early life is a useful source of information, but it needs always to be combined with a full clinical assessment. When this is done, the clinician has a reasonably certain means of detecting mental retardation and other forms of neurologic impairment.

The trajectory of rapid growth and maturation continues in late childhood and adolescence, though at a slower pace than before. Motor skills attain their maximal precision in the performances of athletes, artists, and musicians, whose peak development is at maturity (age 18 to 21). Capacity for reflective thought and the manipulation of mathematical symbols becomes possible only in adolescence and later. Emotional control, precarious in the school age and all through adolescence, stabilizes in adulthood. We tend to think of all these phenomena as being achieved through the stresses of human relations, which are conditioned and habituated by the powerful influences of social approval. In this extensive and pervasive penetration of the individual by the environment, which is the preoccupation of the child psychiatrist, it is well to remember that the processes of extrinsic and intrinsic organization can be separated only for the purpose of analytical discussion. There is always *interdependence* rather than conflict between them.

MOTOR DEVELOPMENT

As indicated above (and in Table 28-3) the wide variety and seemingly random movements displayed by the healthy neonate are from birth, and certainly within days, firmly organized into reflexive-instinctual patterns called *automatisms*. The most testable of the automatisms are blinking in response to light, tonic deviation of the eyes in response to labyrinthine stimulation (turning of the head), prehensile and sucking movements of the lips in response to labial contact, swallowing, avoidance movements of the head and neck, startle reaction (Moro response) in response to loud noise or dropping of the head into an extended position, grasp reflexes, and support, stepping, and placing movements. As has been remarked, this repertoire of movements depends on reflexes organized at the spinal and brainstem levels. Only the placing reactions, ocular fixation, and following movements (the latter are established by the third month) are thought to depend on emerging cortical connections, but even this is debatable. At this early age, when little of the cerebrum has begun to function, extensive cerebral lesions may cause no derangement of motor function and may pass unnoticed, and many serious cerebral diseases cannot be diagnosed unless special ancillary methods (sensory evoked potentials, EEG, CT scans, MRI) are used. Of testable neurologic functions, disturbances of ocular movement, seizures, tremulousness of the arms, impaired arousal reactions and muscular tone—all of which relate essentially to upper brainstem and diencephalic mechanisms—provide the most reliable clues to neurologic diseases in the neonatal period. Prechtl and his associates have documented the importance of neurologic abnormalities in the neonatal period as predictors of retarded development.

During early infancy the motor system undergoes a variety of differentiations as visual, auditory, and tactile-motor mechanisms develop. Bodily postures are modified to accommodate these complex sensorimotor acquisitions. In the normal infant these emerging motor differentiations and elaborations follow a time schedule prescribed by the maturation of neural connections. Normalcy is expressed by the age of the organism when each and every one of these appear, as shown in Table 28-3.

It is evident from this table that reflex and instinctual

motor activities are of maximal importance in the evaluation of early development. Further, in the normally developing organism, some of these activities disappear as others appear. For example, extension of the limbs without a flexor phase, Moro response, tonic neck reflexes, and crossed adduction in response to knee jerk gradually become less prominent and are usually not elicitable by the sixth month. In contrast, neck-righting reflexes, support reactions, Landau reaction (extending neck and legs when held prone), parachute maneuver, and pincer grasp, which are absent in the first 6 months, begin to appear by the seventh to eighth month and are present in all normal infants by the twelfth month.

Since many functions that are classified as mental at a later period of life have a different anatomic basis than motor functions, it is not surprising that early motor achievements do not correlate closely with childhood intelligence. The converse does not apply, however; delay in the acquisition of motor milestones often correlates with mental retardation. Most severely retarded children sit, stand, walk, and run at a much later age than normal children, and deviations from this rule are exceptional.

In the period of early childhood, the reflexive-instinctual activities are no longer of help in evaluating cerebral development and one must turn to the examination of language functions and learned sensory and motor skills. These are outlined in Tables 28-4 and 28-5.

In later childhood, other acquisitions—such as hopping on one foot, kicking a ball, jumping over a line, walking gracefully, dancing, certain skills in sports—are linked to age. Ozeretzkii has combined these in a scale that often discloses arrests in motor development in the mentally retarded.

SENSORY DEVELOPMENT

Under normal circumstances, sensory development keeps pace with motor development, and at every age sensorimotor interactions are apparent. However, under conditions of disease there are many instances where this generalization does not hold, i.e., motor development remains relatively normal in the face of sensory defects, or vice versa.

The sense organs are fully formed at birth. Although crudely aware of visual, auditory, tactile, and olfactory stimuli, the newborn cannot interpret them. Moreover, any stimulus-related response is only to the immediate situation; there is no evidence that previous experience with the stimulus has influenced the response, i.e., that the newborn

Table 28-3
Neurologic functions and disturbances in infancy

Age	Normal functions	Pathologic signs
Newborn period	Blinking, tonic deviation of eyes on turning head, sucking, rooting, swallowing, yawning, grasping, brief extension of neck in prone position, incurvation response, Moro response, flexion postures of limbs Biceps reflexes present and others variable; infantile type of flexor plantar reflex; stable temperature, respirations and blood pressure; periods of sleep and arousal; vigorous cry	Lack of arousal (stupor or coma) High-pitched or weak cry Abnormal (incomplete or absent) Moro response Opisthotonus Flaccidity or hypertonia Convulsions Tremulous limbs Failure of tonic deviation of eyes on passive movement of head or of head and body
2–3 months	Supports head Smiles Makes vowel sounds Adopts tonic asymmetric neck postures (tonic neck reflexes) Large range of movements of limbs, tendon reflexes usually present Fixates on and follows a dangling toy Suckles vigorously Period of sleep sharply differentiated from awake periods Support and stepping unelicitable Vertical suspension—legs flex, head up Optokinetic nystagmus elicitable	Absence of any or all of the normal functions Convulsions Hypotonia or hypertonia of neck and limbs Vertical suspension—legs extend and adduct
4 months	Good head support, minimal head lag Coos and chuckles Inspects hands Tone of limbs moderate or diminished Turns to sounds Rolls over from prone to supine Grasping, sucking, and tonic neck reflexes subservient to volition	No head support Motor deficits Hypertonia No social reactions Tonic neck reflexes present Strong Moro response Absence of symmetric attitude
5–6 months	Babbles Reaches and grasps Vocalizes in social play Discriminates between family and strangers Moro and grasp disappear Tries to recover loss object Begins to sit; no head lag on pull to sit Positive support reaction Tonic neck reflexes gone Landau (holds head above horizontal and arches back when held horizontally) Begins to grasp objects with one hand; holds bottle	Altered tone Obligatory postures Cannot sit or roll over Hypo- or hypertonia Persistent Moro and grasp Persistent tonic neck reflexes No Landau response

Table 28-3 *(continued)*
Neurologic functions and disturbances in infancy

Age	Normal functions	Pathologic signs
9 months	Creeps and pulls to stand; stands holding on Sits securely Babbles "Mama," "Dada," or equivalent Sociable; plays "pat-a-cake," seeks attention Drinks from cup Landau present Parachute response present Grasps with thumb to forefinger	Fails to attain these motor, verbal, and social milestones Persistent automatisms and tonic neck reflexes or hypo- or hypertonia
12 months	Stands alone May walk, or walks if led Tries to feed self May say several single words, echoes sounds Plantar reflexes definitely flexor Throws objects	Retardation in attaining these milestones Functions at earlier level Persistence of automatisms
15 months	Walks independently (9–16 months), falls easily Moves arms steadily Says several words; scribbles with crayon Requests by pointing Interest in sounds, music, pictures, and animal toys	Retardation at earlier age level Persistent abnormalities of tone and posture Sensory discriminations defective
18 months	Says at least 6 words Feeds self; uses spoon well May obey commands Runs stiffly; seats self in chair Hand dominance Throws ball Plays several nursery games Uses simple tools in imitation Removes shoes and stockings Points to two or three parts of body, common objects, and pictures in book	Cannot walk No words
24 months	Says 2- or 3-word sentences Scribbles Runs well; climbs stairs one at a time Bends over and picks up objects Kicks ball; turns knob Organized play Builds tower of 6 blocks Sometimes toilet trained	Retarded in all motor, linguistic, and social adaptive skills

Source: Modified from Gesell et al.

Table 28-4
**Developmental achievements of the
normal preschool child**

Age	Observed items	Useful clinical tests
2 years	Runs well Goes up and down stairs, one step at a time Climbs on furniture Opens doors Helps to undress Feeds well with spoon Puts three words together Listens to stories with pictures	Pencil-paper test: scribbles, imitates horizontal stroke Folds paper once Builds tower of six blocks
2½ years	Jumps on both feet; walks on tiptoes if asked Knows full name; asks questions Refers to self as "I" Helps put away toys and clothes Names animals in book, knows 1 to 3 colors Can complete three-piece form board	Pencil-paper test: copies horizontal and vertical line Builds tower of eight blocks
3 years	Climbs stairs, alternating feet Talks constantly; recites nursery rhymes Rides tricycle Stands on one foot momentarily Plays simple games Helps in dressing Washes hands Identifies five colors	Builds nine-cube tower Builds bridge with three cubes Imitates circle and cross with pencil
4 years	Climbs well; hops and skips on one foot; throws ball overhand; kicks ball Cuts out pictures with scissors Counts four pennies Tells a story; plays with other children Goes to toilet alone	Copies cross and circle Builds gate with five cubes Builds a bridge from model Draws a human figure with two to four parts other than head Distinguishes short and long line

Table 28-4 (continued)

Age	Observed items	Useful clinical tests
5 years	Skips Names four colors; counts ten pennies Dresses and undresses Asks questions about meaning of words	Copies square and triangle Distinguishes heavier of two weights More detailed drawing of a human figure

can learn and remember. The capacity to attend to a stimulus, to fixate upon it for any period of time, also comes later. Indeed, the length of fixation time is a quantifiable index of perceptual development in infancy.

Information is available about the time at which the infant makes the first interpretable responses to each of the different modes of stimulation. The most nearly perfect senses in the newborn are those of touch and pain. A series of pinpricks causes distress, whereas an abrasion of the skin seems not to do so. The sense of touch clearly plays a role in feeding behavior. Newborn infants react vigorously to irritating odors such as ammonia and acetic acid, but discrimination between olfactory stimuli is not evident until much later. Sugar solutions initiate and maintain sucking from birth on, whereas quinine solutions seldom do, and later the latter stimulus elicits avoidance behavior. Hearing in the newborn is manifest within the first few postnatal days. Sharp, quick sounds elicit responsive blinking and sometimes startle. In some infants, the human voice appears to cause similar reactions by the second week. Strong light and objects held before the face evoke reactions in the neonate, and later visual searching is an integrating factor in most projected motor activities.

Although sensation in the newborn infant must be judged largely by motor reactions, so that sensory and motor developments seem to run in parallel, there are discernible maturational stages that constitute sensory milestones, so to speak. This is most apparent in the visual system, which is more easily studied than some of the other senses. Sustained ocular fixation on an object is observable at birth and even preterm; at this time it is essentially a reflexive phototropic reaction. However, it has been observed that the neonate will consistently gaze at some stimuli more often than at others, suggesting that there must already be some elements of perception and differentiation (Fantz). This type of selective attention to stimuli is spoken of as "differential fixation." So-called voluntary fixation (i.e., following a moving object) is a later development. Horizontal following occurs at about 50 days, and vertical following at 55 days, and following an object that is moving in a circle, at 2.5 months. Preference for a colored stimulus over a gray one was recorded by Staples by the end of the third month. By 6 months the infant discriminates between colors, and saturated colors can be matched at 30 months. Perception of form, judged by the length of time spent in looking at different visual presentations, is evident at 2 or 3 months of age (Fantz). At this time infants are attracted more to certain patterns than to colors. At 3 months, most infants have discovered their hands and spend considerable time watching their movements. Details concerning the ages at which infants observe color, size, shape, and number are available in the Terman-Merrill and the Stutzman Intelligence Tests (see Gibson and Olum). Perception of size becomes increasingly accurate in the preschool years. An 18-month-old child discriminates among pictures of familiar animals and recognizes them equally well if they are upside down.

Visual discriminations are reflected in manual reactions just as auditory discriminations are reflected in vocal responses. Much of early development (first year) involves peering at objects, judging their position, reaching for them, and seizing and manipulating them. The inseparability of

Table 28-5
Useful tests for evaluating learning disabilities in children*

Deficit	Test
Development	Denver Developmental Test; Vineland Social Maturity Test; Leiter International Performance Scale; Otis Group Intelligence Test
Achievement	Wide Range Achievement Test; Gates Primary Reading Test
Vocabulary	Peabody Picture Vocabulary
Developmental Gerstmann syndrome (finger agnosia, right-left disorientation)	Finger Order Tests; Benton Right-Left Discrimination Test
Figure copying	Visual-Motor Integration Test
Visual memory	Benton Visual Retention Test
Error patterns	Boder Test of Reading-Spelling Patterns
Impulsiveness	Matching Familiar Figures Test

*For descriptions of individual tests, see Kinsbourne, 1985.

sensory and motor functions is never more obvious. Sensory deprivation impedes not only the natural sequences of perceptual awareness of the world about but of all motor activities.

Auditory discrimination, reflected in vocalizations such as babbling and later in word formation, is discussed further on in connection with language development.

THE DEVELOPMENT OF INTELLIGENCE

The subject of intellectual endowment and development has already been touched upon in Chap. 20. There it was pointed out that while intelligence is modifiable by training, practice, and schooling, it is much more a matter of native endowment. Intelligent parents tend to beget intelligent children, and stupid ones, stupid children, and this seems to be not simply a question of environment and stimulus to learn. It is evident early in life that some individuals have a superior intelligence and maintain this superiority all through life and that others are the opposite.

Much of the uncertainty about the relative influence of heredity and environment relates to our imprecise definitions of intelligence. Intelligence has been defined variously as the capacity to acquire new knowledge; to solve problems; to perfect through experience new and more efficient modes of social adaptation; and as the totality of capacities of observing, understanding, thinking, and remembering as means of learning and of acting purposefully and rationally.

Even a superficial analysis of these definitions discloses that they include a multiplicity of functions, which probably accounts for a lack of consensus about the mechanism(s) of intelligence. Kurt Goldstein argued that intelligence is a unitary mental capacity, impairment of which gives rise to a fundamental disorder (*Grundstörung*)— a loss of ''abstract attitude.'' By this he meant an incapacity to deal with objects at a conceptual level and an undue tendency to respond to their immediate, concrete attributes. Everyday experience, however, teaches us that people regarded as intelligent are not all alike. As a corollary, it is not always abstract tasks that suffer most when intelligence is impaired. Indeed, as Zangwill has pointed out, even abstraction may not be a unitary function. Other theoreticians, like Carl Spearman, believed that intelligence comprises a general (*g*), or core, factor and a series of special (*s*) factors, such as drive and curiosity, verbal and arithmetic ability, memory, capacity for abstract thinking, practical skills in manipulating objects, geographic or spatial sense, and certain social adaptations (see Chap. 20). Still others think of intelligence as a mosaic of specific abilities. Not only do individuals appear to vary in these special native abilities, but the superior ones are found to use them with greater speed and efficiency. According to this view, individuals gifted in only one ability would not be considered intelligent, only talented in the particular field. Physicians tend to accept this latter view of intelligence as consisting of a series of special abilities, and to recognize among their patients wide individual differences, manifest in their daily activities, what they have already learned and accomplished, their capacity to give a history, and to follow instructions.

The origins of the development of intelligence are difficult to detect. The first hints of something beyond simple sensorimotor reactions and reflex patterns emerge at 8 to 9 months of life when infants begin to crawl and explore. For the first time they separate themselves from the mother. Now, learning proceeds rapidly, as the mother attaches names to objects and helps the baby manipulate them. At about 14 to 15 months the child begins to declare its independence as a social organism by saying ''no'' to every request. Gradually the child acquires verbal facility (learning what words mean), memory, color and spatial perception, a concept of number, and the practical use of tools, each at a particular time according to a schedule set largely by the maturational state of the brain. In these early achievements individuals differ greatly, and they are much influenced by their parents and others around them. The rate of learning, adaptability, understanding, and tolerance of restrictions, and, later, the acquisition of knowledge, capacity to work, and personality structure vary enormously, as will be pointed out below. Neurologists who need a quick and practical method of ascertaining whether an infant or preschool child is measuring up to normal standards for a particular age will find Tables 28-4 and 28-5 useful. The main items are drawn from Gesell and Amatruda and from the Denver Developmental Test.

A variety of intelligence tests, designed to measure special abilities (see Table 28-5), demonstrate the child's increasing success in learning with age. Starting at 6 to 7 years there is a steady improvement in scores that parallels chronological age up to about 13 years, and thereafter the rate of advance diminishes. By 16 to 17 years performance reaches a plateau and remains more or less constant through early adult life. From about the thirtieth year, test scores diminish slowly throughout the remainder of life. Individuals with high or low IQs at 6 years of age tend to maintain their rank at 10, 15, and 20 years, unless the early scores were impaired by anxiety, poor motivation, or a gross lack of opportunity to acquire the necessary skills to take such tests (language skill in particular). Even then, performance tasks, which largely eliminate verbal and mathematical skills, will disclose similar individual differences. Effective performance on tests of whatever type obviously requires interest and motivation on the part of the subject.

The reliability of intelligence tests and their validity as predictive measures of scholastic success and quality of work performance have been heatedly debated for many years. These tests are said by critics to be only measures of achievement, which in themselves are dependent on the child's cultural experiences and opportunities for learning. While no one would disagree that environmental factors may enhance or hinder intellectual development and that a factor of achievement enters into intelligence tests, the most persuasive argument for them as tests of native abilities is that individuals drawn from a fairly homogeneous environment tend to maintain the same position on the intelligence scale throughout their lifetime. Native endowment appears to set the limits of learning and achievement; opportunity and other factors determine how nearly the individual's full potential is realized.

THE DEVELOPMENT OF LANGUAGE

Closely tied to the development of intelligence is the acquisition of language. Indeed, facility with language is one of the best indices of intelligence (Lenneberg). The acquisition of speech and language by the infant and child has been observed methodically by a number of eminent investigators, and their findings provide a background for the understanding of a number of derangements in the development of these functions (Ingram; Rutter and Martin; Minifie and Lloyd).

First, there is the *babbling* and *lalling stage*, during which the infant a few weeks old emits a variety of cooing and then babbling sounds in the form of vowel-consonant (labial and nasoguttural) combinations. At first this appears to be a purely self-initiated activity, being the same in normal and deaf infants. However, a study of the latter shows that auditory modifications begin within a period of 2 to 3 months; without an auditory sense the babblers do not produce the variety of random sounds of the normal infant, nor do they begin to imitate the sounds made by the mother. Thus motor speech activity is stimulated and reinforced mainly by auditory sensations, which become linked to the kinesthetic ones arising from the speech musculature. It is not clear whether the capacity to hear and understand the spoken word precedes or follows the first motor speech. Possibly it varies from one infant to another, but the dependence of motor speech development on hearing is undeniable. Comprehension seems to postdate the first verbal utterance in most infants.

Soon babbling merges with *echo speech,* in which short sounds are repeated parrot-like; gradually longer syllable groups are repeated correctly as the praxic function of the speech apparatus develops. By the end of 12 months the first recognizable words appear. Initially these are attached directly to persons and objects and are used increasingly to designate an object. The word then becomes the symbol, and this substitution greatly facilitates speaking and later thinking about people and objects. To learn to say a spoken name, it is necessary to form a link between the auditory association (Wernicke's) area in the superior temporal gyrus of the dominant hemisphere and the center for motor patterns of speech (Broca's area). Similarly, to learn the name of a seen object requires the formation of a link between the visual association region of the occipital lobe and Wernicke's area. Nouns are learned first, then verbs and other parts of speech. Through exposure to and correction by parents and siblings vocal behavior is gradually shaped to conform to that of the social group in which the child is raised.

During the second year of life, word combinations are learned. They form the propositions which, according to Hughlings Jackson, are the very essence of language. At 18 months the child can combine an average of 1½ words and at 2 years, 2 words; at 2½ years, 3 words, and at 3 years, 4 words. Pronunciation of words undergoes a similar progression; 90 percent of children can articulate all vowel sounds by the age of 3 years. At a slightly later age the consonants *p, b, m, h, w, d, n, t,* and *k* are enunciated; *ng* by the age of 4 years; *y, j, zh,* and *wh* by 5 to 6 years; and *f, l, v, sh, ch, s, v,* and *th* by 7 years. Girls acquire articulatory facility somewhat earlier than boys. The vocabulary increases, so that at 18 months the young child knows 6 to 20 words; by 24 months, 50 to 200 words; by 3 years, 200 to 400 words; and by 4 years, the child is normally capable of telling stories, but with little distinction between fact and fancy. By 6 years, the average child knows several thousand words. Also by that age he or she can indicate spatial and temporal relationships and starts to inquire about causality. The understanding of spoken language always exceeds the child's speaking vocabulary; that is to say, most children understand more than they say.

The next stage of language development is reading. Here there must be an association of graphic symbols with the auditory, visual, and kinesthetic images of words already acquired. Usually the written word is learned by associating it with the spoken word rather than with the seen object. The superior gyrus of the temporal lobe (Wernicke's area) and contiguous parieto-occipital areas of the dominant hemisphere are essential to the establishment of these *cross-modal associations.* Writing is learned soon after reading, the auditory-visual symbols of words being linked to cursive movements of the hand. The tradition of beginning grade

school instruction at 6 years is based not on an arbitrary decision but on the empirically determined age at which the nervous system of the average child is ready to learn and execute the tasks of reading, writing, and soon thereafter, of calculating.

Once language is fully acquired it is integrated into all aspects of complex action and behavior. Every movement of volitional type is activated by a spoken command or the individual's inner phrasing of an intended action. Every plan for the solution of a problem must be cast into language, and the final result is analyzed in verbal terms. Thinking and language are inseparable.

Anthropologists see in all this a grander scheme wherein the individual recapitulates the language development of the human race. They point out that in primitive peoples, language consisted of gestures and the utterance of simple sounds expressing emotion, and that over periods of time, movements and sounds became the conventional signs and verbal symbols of objects and then of the abstract qualities of objects. Historically, signs and spoken language were the first means of human communication; graphic records appeared much later. The American Indian, for instance, never reached the level of syllabic written language. Writing commenced as pictorial representation, and only much later were alphabets devised. The reading and writing of words are comparatively late achievements.

For further details concerning communicative and cognitive abilities and methods of assessment, the reader should consult the monograph by Minifie and Lloyd.

THE DEVELOPMENT OF PERSONALITY

Personality is the most inclusive of all psychologic terms. It encompasses all the physical and psychologic traits that distinguish one individual from every other one. The notion that one's physical characteristics are determined by inheritance is a fundamental tenet of neurobiology. One has but to observe the resemblances between parent and child to confirm this view. Only the extent of human variation occasions surprise. Just as no two persons are physically identical, not even monozygotic twins, so too do they differ in body chemistry or any other quality one chooses to measure. These differences, together with certain predilections to disease, explain why any one person may have an unpredictable reaction to a pathogenic agent. Strictly speaking, the normal person is an abstraction, just as is a typical example of any disease.

However, it is in other, seemingly nonphysical

attributes that individuals display the greatest differences. Here reference is made to their variable place on a scale of energy, capacity for effective work, intellectual power (which largely determine their capacity to learn), sensitivity, temperament, emotional responsivity, aggressivity or passivity, character, and tolerance to stress. The composite of these qualities constitutes the human personality.

According to Freudian theory, the most powerful force in the development of personality is a series of predictable modifications of the sexual instinct. The energy of the sexual impulse, called libido, is traced back to the earliest sensory pleasures that attend the activities of the oral and genital parts of the body. Successively the sexuality of the child expands to include many of the relationships to the mother, to other members of the same sex, and finally to the opposite sex. Powerful forces, such as social custom, repress the sexual impulse, but always with the risk, so it is argued, that the energy of the sexual drive may be displaced into other channels of thought and action, with unwholesome alterations of behavior. Development of personality is thus regarded as a process of sexual maturation, the final purpose of which is to ensure procreation and the installment of the individual as an integral part of a new family unit.

There are many who believe that the Freudian emphasis on sexuality provides far too restricted a theory of personality development. While the tie to the mother can be conceived as deriving from the nursing act, it is likely that body contact with the mother soon becomes less important than touch, smell, sight, and sound as determinative factors in the infant's behavior. Further, many others in the infant's environment, e.g., siblings, father, teacher, begin to figure in special nonsexual ways in the child's development.

In the formation of personality, especially the part concerned with feeling and emotional sensitivity, basic temperament surely plays a part. By nature, some children, from the beginning, seem to be happy, cheerful, and unconcerned about immediate frustrations, and others are the opposite. By the third month of life, Birch and his associates recognized individual differences in activity-passivity, regularity-irregularity, intensity of action, approach-withdrawal, adaptivity-unadaptivity, high-low threshold of response to stimulation, positive-negative mood, high-low selectivity, and high-low distractibility. Ratings on these qualities at this early age were found by these authors to correlate with the results of examinations made at 5 years. Not all psychologists agree with these observations; some insist that the mother's behavior

is of crucial importance in teaching such patterns. The problem is made even more complicated by the possibility that the character of the infant may influence the mother's reactions. One may presume that the more common aspects of personality, i.e., worry about one's health and other matters, anxiety or serenity, timidity or boldness, the power of instinctual drives and need of satisfaction, sympathy for others, sensitivity to criticism, and degree of disorganization resulting from adverse circumstances, are genetically determined. Identical twins raised apart are remarkably alike in many personality traits and have the same IQs, within a few points (Moser et al). The strong genetic influence in personality development has also been demonstrated by Scarr and her associates.

SOCIAL ADAPTATION

Social behavior, like neurologic and psychologic functions in general, depends to a great extent on the development and maturation of the brain. Involved also are genetic factors. Obviously, environment plays a role, for one cannot adapt to society except in the presence of other people; i.e., social interaction is necessary for the emergence of many basic biologic traits. One must think of personality as a series of intrinsic forces continuously emerging and being altered by maturation of the nervous system and by the forces of social demands.

The roots of social behavior are traceable to certain instinctive patterns, and the progressive elaboration of one's social attributes is induced by conditioned emotional reactions. Pleasure accompanies behavior demanded by evolution (e.g., the sexual act, necessary for reproduction, and eating, for health and nutrition). Anxiety and fear protect the organism against conditions that lead to maladaptation.

In the long series of human interactions, first with parents, then siblings, other children, and finally a widening circle of individuals in the classroom and community, the capacity to cooperate, to subjugate one's own egocentric needs to those of the group, and to lead or be led appear as secondary modes of response, i.e., secondary to some of the basic impulses of anger, fear, self-protection, love, and pleasure already described.

The sources of these social reactions are even more obscure than those of temperament, character, and intelligence. The ubiquity of aggressive behavior in children, for example, is often cited as an argument for an innate aggressive instinct. But to a large extent this is a derived mode of behavior. The ascription of aggressive behavior to instinct alone is an example of a common tendency to explain infantile behavior by a prior assignment of adult motives. To elaborate the point, in a normal child aggression usually originates in innate curiosity or takes the form of a defense reaction to frustration and failure. In both instances, aggression is an appropriate reaction. Its frequency in an abnormal child may be related to defects in the germ plasm, as in the case of brain malformations, and also to environmental factors, which expose the infant and child to faulty identification models. Moreover, the display of aggressive behavior is a function of the culture in which the child is reared. While aggression is encouraged in some cultures as a desirable manifestation of energetic and vigorous action, becoming unacceptable only if assaultive and violent, it may not be condoned at all in other cultures. The capacity for aggression is indeed inherent in human impulse, as it is in all animals, but the frequency of its evocation and display are determined by other factors.

The greatest demands and frustrations in social development are likely to occur in late childhood and adolescence. In children, difficulties in social adaptation tend first to be manifest by an inability to take their places in a classroom. Adolescents, half emancipated from family ties, have trouble as they seek the recognition and respect of their peers. For the first time they think seriously of what they are and what they will be. In search of personal identity they become more critical of their parents and turn increasingly to interaction with larger social groups. If the relationship with their parents is firmly established and if the parents respond to their doubts and criticisms with sympathetic understanding, this unsettled state is temporary and is followed by a resynthesis of their relations with the family on a firm and lasting basis. The development of adult gonadal function and the further evolution of psychosexual impulses cause a bewildering array of new sensations. These lead to a surge of interest in physical sex and psychologic sensitization to new aspects of interpersonal relations. An increasing capacity for abstract thought paves the way for advanced education and creativity and for increasing concern about the meaning and value of human existence.

These types of social adjustment continue as long as life continues. As social roles change, as intellectual and physical capacities first advance and later recede, new challenges demand new adaptations. The success of these adaptations is enhanced if started from a solid base of accomplishment as a student and worker, and from a position as a member of a stable family unit, with a religion or a philosophy of life. Conditions that thwart the development of proper attitudes toward family, work, and health often become major causes of maladjustment in later life.

At the highest level of social interaction between an individual and the family unit and community, we see more clearly the workings of another principle—that biologic evolution merges with, and is finally superseded by, cultural evolution. The latter is uniquely human. Only human beings are able to alter their environment in a systematic fashion.

The future can be anticipated and planned. Of the primate family only human beings are able to think and communicate by symbols. Language enables us to think through the consequences of an action before attempting it, to abstract from the concrete to the general situation, and to analyze the relationship between the elements of a problem without the necessity of actually manipulating the elements. Language is also the agency whereby the experiences of the past are made available for understanding current problems. Thus we build continuously on our cultural heritage.

FAILURES AND DISHARMONIES OF NORMAL NEUROLOGIC DEVELOPMENT

DELAY IN MOTOR DEVELOPMENT AND CEREBRAL PALSY

Delay in motor development often accompanies mental retardation, in which case it is part of a developmental lag or immaturity of the entire cerebrum. The most severe forms of delayed motor development, associated with spasticity and athetosis, are invariably manifestations of particular prenatal and paranatal diseases of the brain.

In assessing developmental abnormalities of the motor system in the neonate and young infant several maneuvers, which elicit certain postures and reflexive movements, are helpful. Some of the most useful are the following:

1. The *Moro response* is the infant's reaction to startle and can be evoked by suddenly withdrawing support of the head and allowing the neck to extend. A loud noise, slapping the bed, or jerking one leg will have the same effect, causing an elevation and abduction of the arms followed by a clasping movement to the midline. Present in all newborns and infants up to 4 or 5 months of age, its absence indicates a profound disorder of the motor system. An absent or inadequate Moro response on one side is found in hemiplegia, brachial plexus palsy, and fractured clavicle. Persistence of the Moro response beyond 4 or 5 months of age is noted only in infants with severe neurologic defects.

2. The asymmetric *tonic neck reflex* (extension of the arm and leg on the side to which the head is passively turned and flexion of the opposite limbs), if obligatory and sustained, is a sign of pyramidal or extrapyramidal motor abnormality at any age. Fragments of the reflex, such as a brief extension of one arm, may be elicited in 60 percent of normal infants at 1 to 2 months of age and may be adopted spontaneously up to 6 months. Barlow reports

having obtained this reflex in 25 percent of mentally retarded infants at 9 to 10 months of age.

3. The *placing reaction* (described above, under Psychophysiologic Development) is present in all normal newborns. Its absence or asymmetry under 6 months of age indicates a motor abnormality.

4. The *"parachute response"*—dropping the infant held prone in the horizontal position toward the bed to evoke extension of the arms as if to break the fall—is elicitable in most 9-month-old infants. If asymmetrical, it indicates a unilateral motor abnormality.

5. In the *Landau maneuver* the infant, if suspended horizontally in the prone position, will extend the neck and trunk and will break the trunk extension when the neck is passively flexed. This reaction is present by 6 months; delay in a hypotonic child is indicative of a fault in the motor apparatus.

The detection of gross delays or abnormalities of motor development in the neonatal or early infantile period of life is little aided by tests of tendon and plantar reflexes. Arm reflexes are always rather difficult to obtain in infants, and a normal neonate may have a few beats of ankle clonus. The plantar response is always wavering and uncertain in pattern. A consistent extension of the great toe and fanning of the toes on stroking the side of the foot is abnormal at any age.

The early discovery of cerebral palsy is hampered by the fact that the corticospinal tract is not myelinated until 18 months of age, allowing at best only quasivoluntary movements. A *congenital hemiparesis,* for example, may not be evident until many months have passed. It then becomes manifest by subtle signs such as holding the hand in a fisted posture or inefficiency in reaching for objects and in transferring them from one hand to the other. Later the leg is seen to be less active as the infant crawls, steps, and places the foot. Early hand dominance should always raise the suspicion of a motor defect. Spasticity is most evident in passive abduction of the arm, extension of the elbow, dorsiflexion of the wrist, and supination of the forearm. In the leg, passive flexion of the knee is the best maneuver to elicit the characteristic catch and yielding resistance, but the time of appearance and degree of spasticity are variable from patient to patient. The stretch reflexes are hyperactive, and the plantar reflex may be extensor on the affected side. With *bilateral hemiplegia* the same abnormalities are detectable, but there is greater likelihood of pseudobulbar manifestations, with delayed, poorly enunciated speech. Also, intelligence is more likely

to be impaired (in 40 percent of hemiplegias and 70 percent of quadriplegias). In *diparesis* or *diplegia,* hypotonia gives way to spasticity and the same delay in motor development, except that it is confined to the legs. Aside from the hereditary spastic paraplegias, which may become evident in the second and third years, a common cause of weak spastic legs is prematurity and matrix hemorrhages.

Developmental motor delay and other abnormalities occur in a large proportion of infants with *hypotonia.* Lifting the infant and passive manipulation of the limbs encounter little muscle reactivity. In the lower limbs, the laxity results in a frog-leg posture, along with an increased mobility of the ankles and hips. Hypotonia, if generalized and accompanied by an absence of tendon reflexes, will usually be due to Werdnig-Hoffmann disease (see Chap. 52). Infants who will later manifest a central motor defect can sometimes be recognized by the assumed postures of the limbs, when the infant is lifted. In the normal infant the legs are flexed, slightly rotated externally, and there are vigorous kicking movements; the hypotonic infant with a defect of the motor projection pathways may extend the legs or rotate them internally with dorsiflexion of the feet and toes. Exceptionally the legs are firmly flexed, but in either instance relatively few movements are made.

When hypotonia is a forerunner of an extrapyramidal motor disorder, the first hint of abnormality may be an opisthotonic posturing of the head and neck. However, the irregular involuntary movements of chorea do not appear in the upper extremities before 5 to 6 months of age, and often are so slight as to be overlooked. They increase as the infant matures and by 12 months assume a more athetotic character, often combined with tremor. Tone in the affected limbs is by then increased but may be interrupted by passive manipulation.

When hypotonia is a prelude to a cerebellar motor defect, the ataxia becomes apparent only in the first reaching movements. Tremulous irregular movements of the trunk and head are seen with attempts to sit without support. Still later, in attempting to stand, there is unsteadiness of the entire body.

The other common causes of hypotonia (muscular dystrophies and congenital myopathies, polyneuropathy, Down syndrome, Praeder-Willi syndrome, and spinal cord injuries) are described in their appropriate chapters.

Systemic diseases in infancy pose special problems in evaluation of the motor system. The achievement of motor milestones is delayed by illnesses such as congenital heart disease (especially cyanotic forms), cystic fibrosis, renal and hepatic diseases, infections, and surgical procedures. Under such conditions one does well to deal with the immediate illnesses and defer pronouncements about the status of cerebral function. The brain proves to be simultaneously affected in 25 percent of patients with congenital heart disease and an even higher proportion of patients with rubella and Coxsackie B infections. In a disease such as cystic fibrosis, where the brain is not affected, it is advisable to depend more on the analysis of language development than of locomotion, because muscular activity may be enfeebled.

DELAYS IN SENSORY DEVELOPMENT

Failure to see and to hear are the most important sensory defects that may affect the infant and child. When both senses are affected, the usual cause is a severe cerebral defect. Only at a later age, when the child is more testable, does it become apparent that the trouble is not with the sensory apparatus per se but with the central integrating mechanisms of the brain.

Failure of development of visual function is usually revealed in a disorder of ocular movements. Any defect of the refractive apparatus or visual acuity results in wandering, jerky movements of the eyes. The retinas may be abnormal in such cases, as in congenital hypoplasia of the optic nerves (optic discs are extremely small). The optic discs may be atrophic, but it should be pointed out that the discs in infants tend naturally to be paler than those of an older child. Faulty vision becomes increasingly apparent in older infants when the normal sequences of hand inspection and visuomanual coordination fail to emerge. Retention of pupillary light reflexes in a sightless child signifies a defect in the geniculocalcarine tracts or occipital lobes, or in both, conditions that may be confirmed by testing visual evoked responses.

With respect to hearing, again there is the difficulty in evaluating this function in an infant. Normally, after a few weeks of life, alert parents notice a brisk startle to loud noises, and a response to other sounds. During examination, a tinkling bell brought from behind the infant usually results in head turning and visual searching, but a lack of these responses warns only of the most severe hearing defects. Slight degrees of deafness, enough to interfere with auditory learning, require special testing for their elicitation. To make the problem more difficult, a peripheral as well as a central disorder may be present in some conditions, such as kernicterus. Computerized auditory-evoked responses are particularly helpful in confirming such abnormalities, but we are just now acquiring experience with the test. After the first few months impaired hearing becomes more obvious and interferes with language development, as will be described further on.

MENTAL RETARDATION

The symptom complex of incomplete or insufficient development of mental capacities and associated behavioral abnormalities (variously referred to as *mental retardation,* *subnormality,* or *deficiency,* or as *amentia* or *oligophrenia*) stands as the single largest neuropsychiatric disorder in every civilized society, estimated to affect 2.5 to 3 percent of the total population. Using any one of a number of indices of social and psychologic failure, two somewhat overlapping groups are recognized: (1) The severely impaired, corresponding to the categories of idiot (IQ < 20) and low-grade imbecile (IQ = 20 to 45) in older classifications. This group is also called the *pathologic mentally retarded,* and makes up approximately 10 percent of the subnormal population. (2) The less severely impaired (IQ = 45 to 70), corresponding to the old categories of high-grade imbecile or "feeble-minded." This second group is referred to as the *subcultural, physiological, or familial mentally retarded* and is much larger than the first. In addition there are the simpletons (morons or "debiles") and "borderline" defectives, who are not generally classified as mentally retarded. The American Association on Mental Deficiency has suggested yet another grouping of mental retardation: *profound* (IQ < 25), *severe* (IQ = 25 to 39), *moderate* (IQ = 40 to 54), and *mild* (IQ = 55 to 69). The group of pathologically retarded overlaps the group of subculturally retarded as shown in Fig. 28-4.

There has been much criticism of the use of the IQ and similar tests in defining such groups, for the reasons discussed above. Certainly such scores are meaningless for the idiots who have no language and lack altogether the capacity to reason, but their status is so obvious that there is no problem in diagnosis. Nonetheless, for the others, if drawn from a fairly homogeneous population, the scores have a 0.8 correlation with other indices of subnormality.

Each of the two groups of the mentally retarded exhibits several distinctive features. Members of the pathologic mentally retarded (approximately 600,000 in the United States) require constant care, and the majority are found in special institutions, whereas only about 3 percent (180,000) of the less severely retarded are institutionalized. Males predominate in the pathologic group; females, in the subcultural group. The former often show other neurologic signs, while the latter do not. The pathologic retardates differ also in being physically subnormal and infertile. The parents of the pathologic retardates are usually normal, but siblings may be defective, whereas in the subcultural group parents and siblings are often subnormal in varying degrees (hence the older term "familial mentally retarded").

The pathologic type of subnormality, often consequent to major developmental derailment, chromosomal abnormality, or an exogenous factor, is discussed more fully in Chap. 44. The remainder of this discussion will be confined to the larger subcultural form of mental retardation.

MENTAL RETARDATION WITHOUT EVIDENT CEREBRAL DISEASE (SUBCULTURAL OR FAMILIAL MENTAL RETARDATION)

Clinical Features Two clinical types can be recognized. In one, the essential characteristic is that almost from birth the infant is backward in all aspects of development. There is a tendency to sleep more, to be less demanding of nourishment, to suck poorly and regurgitate, and to move less. Parents often comment on how good the baby is, how little he or she troubles them by crying. As the months pass every achievement is late. The baby is more hypotonic and turns over, sits unsupported, and walks later than the normal infant. Yet despite these obvious motor delays, there is later no sign of paralysis, ataxia, chorea, or athetosis. These babies do not smile at the usual time, and take little notice of the mother or other persons or objects in their environment. They are inattentive to visual and often to auditory stimuli, to the point where questions are raised about blindness or deafness. Certain phases of normal development such as hand-regard may persist beyond the sixth month, when it normally is replaced by other activities. Mouthing (putting everything in the mouth) and slobbering, which should end by 1 year of age, persist. There are only fleeting signs of interest in toys, and the impersistence of attention becomes increasingly prominent. Vocalizations are scant, often guttural, piercing, or high-pitched and feeble.

In the second type, early motor milestones (supporting the head, rolling over, sitting, standing, and walking) may be attained at their normal times, yet the infant is later inattentive and slow in learning. It seems as though motor development had somehow escaped the disordered developmental process. Aimless overactivity may also occur and, like the persistence of rhythmic movements, grinding of the teeth (bruxism), hypotonia, and microcephaly, should raise the suspicion of mental backwardness.

Because the developmental sequence of motor function may be normal, even to the point where the baby acquires a few words by the end of the first year, the examiner may be misled into thinking that the mentally retarded infant was at first normal and then deteriorated. In such infants it can even be shown that various test procedures yield lower scores with progressing age (from 3 years onward), but this is due not to a decline in ability but to the fact that the tests are not comparable. In the first 3 years the tests are weighted toward sensorimotor functions and after that toward perception, memory, and concept formation. Interestingly, the development of language depends upon both groups of functions, needing a certain maturation of the auditory and motor apparatus at the start and highly specialized cognitive skills for continued development. These and other aspects of development of speech and language are considered further on in this chapter.

Members of both groups of subcultural retardates exhibit a number of noteworthy features that have medical and social implications (Reissman). They tend to be sickly, and the more severely retarded among them have poor physiques and are often undersized. Deviant behavior is frequent (6.6 percent incidence in nonretarded children, 28.6 percent in the retarded, and 58.3 percent in the epileptic retarded, according to Rutter et al). Most often deviant behavior takes the form of aggressivity, especially

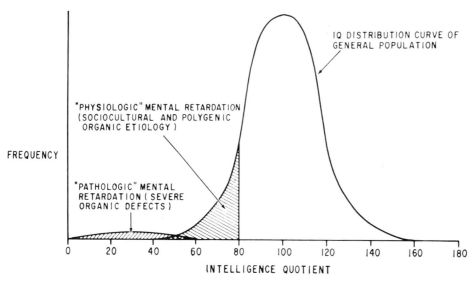

Figure 28-4

Gaussian curve of intelligence and its skewing by the group of mental retardates with diseases of the brain. The shaded areas indicate the two groups of mentally retarded. (See text for discussion.)

in the temporal lobe epileptics. Other behavioral disturbances that prove to be sources of medical complaint are restlessness, repetitive activity, explosive rage reactions and tantrums, stereotyped play, and the seeking of sensory experiences in unusual ways (Chess and Hassibi). The parents of a large proportion of children with deviant behavior fall into the lowest segment of the population socially and economically; in other words, the parents may be incompetent to maintain stable homes and to find work. Abandonment, neglect, and child abuse (battered-child syndrome) are frequent in this group. The majority of afflicted children must be put in special classes or schools, and special measures must be taken to reduce the tendency to truancy, pauperism, sociopathy, and criminality.

An endless debate is centered on matters of causation—whether the so-called subcultural or physiologic retardates are products of a faulty germ plasm which prevents successful competition, or of societal discrimination and lack of training and education, coupled with the effects of malnutrition, infections, or other exogenous factors. Surely both environmental factors and genetic causes are at work, although the relative importance of each has proved difficult to measure (Moser et al).

Pathologic Features The cerebra of the subcultural group of mental retardates have defied interpretation. No visible lesions have been discerned, unlike the pathologic group, in which malformations and a variety of destructive lesions are fairly obvious (see Chap. 44). Even in the severely retarded group, 5 to 10 percent of the cerebra do not differ from normal by gross and microscopic criteria. Admittedly, a few such specimens are underweight by approximately 10 percent, but one cannot presently interpret what this means.

It is certain that a new methodology will be needed if the cerebra of the subcultural retardates and the subnormal extreme of the general population (the part that falls more than 2 SD below the mean) are to be differentiated from the cerebra of highly superior individuals (more than 2 SD above the mean). Differences might be expected in terms of number of neurons in thalamic nuclei and cortex, in dendritic-axonal connectivity, or in synaptic surfaces, elements that are not being assayed by the conventional techniques of tissue neuropathology. The observations of Huttenlocher, who finds a marked sparsity of dendritic arborization in Golgi-Cox preparations, and of Purpura, who finds an absence of short, thick spines on dendrites of cortical neurons and other abnormalities of dendritic spines, are the first steps in this new direction.

Diagnosis Infants should be considered at risk for mental subnormality when there is a family history of mental deficiency, low birth weight in proportion to length of gestation (small-for-date babies), marked prematurity, maternal infection early in pregnancy (especially rubella), and toxemia of pregnancy.

In early life, certain behavioral characteristics are of greater predictive value than psychologic tests. Prechtl and his associates have found that a low Apgar score, flaccidity, underactivity, and asymmetrical neurologic signs are the earliest indices of subnormality in the infant. Slow habituation of orienting reactions to novel auditory and visual stimuli is an early warning of mental retardation.

In the first year or two of life, suspicion of mental retardation is based largely on clinical impression, but it should always be validated by psychometric procedures. Most pediatric neurologists utilize some of the tests described by Gesell and Amatruda or the Denver Developmental Screening Scale from which a developmental quotient (DQ) is calculated.

For testing of preschool children, the Wechsler Preschool and Primary Scale of Intelligence are used, and for school-age children, the Wechsler Intelligence Scale for Children. Normal scores for age eliminate mental retardation as a cause of poor achievement, and special cognitive defects may be revealed by low scores on a particular subtest. Retarded children not only have low scores but exhibit more scatter of subtest scores. They also achieve greater success with performance than with verbal items. The physician must know the conditions of testing, for poor scores may be due to fright, inadequate motivation, lapses in attention, or a subtle sensory defect (auditory or visual) rather than a developmental lag.

The EEG, in addition to exposing asymptomatic seizures, shows a high incidence of other abnormalities in the mentally retarded. Presumably this is due to a greater degree of immaturity of the cerebrum at any given age. However, a normal EEG is of relatively little help. CT scanning has been singularly unhelpful in revealing abnormalities in this group of children.

Always to be considered in the diagnosis of milder grades of retardation are the possible effects of severe malnutrition, neglect and deprivation, chronic systemic disease, deafness, blindness, and possibly childhood psychosis. Of particular importance is the differentiation of a group of patients who are normal for a variable period after birth and then manifest a progressive disease of the nervous system. This type of disorder is representative of a group of hereditary metabolic diseases that will be discussed in Chap. 38. Of importance also is a seizure disorder (and anticonvulsant medications), which can impair cerebral function (see Chap. 15).

Management Since there is little or no possibility of

treating the condition(s) underlying mental retardation and since there is no way of restoring function to a nervous system that is developmentally subnormal, the medical objective is to assist in planning for the patient's training, education, and social and occupational adjustments. The parents must be guided in forming realistic attitudes and expectations. Psychiatric counseling may help the family to maintain gentle but firm support of the patient so that he or she learns all the self-help skills, and acquires self-control, good work habits, and a congenial personality.

Most individuals with an IQ over 60 and no other handicaps can be trained to live an independent life. Special schooling may enable such patients to realize their full potential. Social factors that cause underachievement must be sought and eliminated, if possible. Later there is need of advice about possible occupational attainments.

If the IQ is below 20, institutionalization is almost inevitable, for few families can provide long-term custodial care. Well-run institutions are usually better than community homes because they offer many more facilities (medical, educational, recreational). Often institutionalization is necessary even when the IQ is between 20 and 50. Patients in the latter group, if stable in temperament and relatively well adjusted socially, may work under supervision, but rarely do they become vocationally independent. For the more severely retarded, special training in the basics of hygiene and self-care are the most that can be expected.

Great care must be exercised in deciding about institutionalization. Whereas the severe degrees of retardation are all too apparent by the first or second year, the less severe ones are difficult to recognize early. As was said above, psychologic tests alone are not trustworthy. The method of assessment suggested many years ago by Fernald still has a ring of soundness: (1) physical examination, (2) family background, (3) developmental history, (4) school progress, (5) examination in schoolwork, (6) practical knowledge, (7) social behavior, (8) industrial efficiency, (9) moral reactions, and (10) intelligence as measured by psychologic tests. All these data except (5) and (10) can be obtained by a skillful physician during the initial medical and neurologic examination.

RESTRICTED OR SELECTIVE DEVELOPMENTAL ABNORMALITIES

DISORDERS IN THE DEVELOPMENT OF SPEECH AND LANGUAGE

In the pediatric age period, and extending into adult life, one encounters an interesting assortment of developmental disorders of speech and language. A high percentage of patients with such disorders come from families in which similar speech defects, ambidexterity, and left-handedness are frequent. Males predominate; in some series, male-to-female ratios as high as 10:1 have been reported.

Developmental disorders of speech and language are far more frequent than acquired disorders, i.e., aphasia. The former include developmental speech delay, congenital deafness with speech delay, cleft-palate speech, developmental word deafness, dyslexia (special reading disability), cluttered speech, infantilisms of speech, and stuttering. In these disorders the various stages of language development, described in an earlier section of this chapter, often are not attained at the usual age and may not be achieved even by adult life. Disorders of this type are probably due to slowness in the normal processes of maturation rather than to an acquired disease. Visible lesions are probably not to be expected in most cases, though it must be admitted that the brains of such individuals have rarely been studied by proper methods. Of particular interest in this regard are the cases of developmental dyslexia described by Galaburda and colleagues, in which whole-brain serial sections showed a wider left cerebral hemisphere, an area of polymicrogyria in the left temporal language zones, and a mild dysplasia in the limbic and association cortices of the left hemisphere. The same uncertainty surrounds the anatomic bases of stuttering and other articulatory disorders. These conditions are often misunderstood by parents, teachers, and physicians. The unfortunate child or adult may be judged feebleminded or lazy. Another frequent error is to assume that the condition is due to psychologic factors, since nervousness, depression, poor sleep, and headaches frequently appear in such persons. Many of these emotional disturbances are probably secondary (Baker et al).

Some of the developmental speech disorders to be described below are based on pure sensory defects, others are purely motor. In between are abnormalities that resemble the aphasias of adults and have mixed receptive and expressive elements. In the following pages, we have adopted the more conventional classification.

Developmental Speech Delay   More than 95 percent of infants say their first words at 10 to 12 months and their first phrases before their second birthday, and when this does not happen, it becomes a cause of parental concern. In clinics where speech delay or retarded speech development (no words by 18 months, no phrases by 30 months) is studied systematically, 35 to 50 percent of cases are found to occur in children with mental retardation or "cerebral palsy." Hearing deficit explains many of the other cases, and the remainder represent what appears to be a slowness in the maturation of the motor speech areas or, rarely, an acquired lesion in these parts. Only in this small latter group is it appropriate to refer to the language disorder as aphasia, a term that is customarily reserved for a derangement or loss of language due to cerebral disease.

In one group of children with delayed speech there is no clear evidence of an acquired lesion in the motor speech areas. It is this group, which comprises otherwise normal children who talk late (they deviate from their age norm well beyond 2 SD), that proves the most puzzling. Here it is virtually impossible to draw the line between normal and abnormal. Prelanguage speech continues into the period when words and phrases should normally be used in propositional speech. The combinations of sounds are close to the standard of normal vowel-consonant combinations of the 1- to 2-year-old, and they may even be strung together as in a sentence. Yet as time passes, only a few understandable words may be uttered, even by the third or fourth years. Often one discovers a family history of delayed speech, and three out of four such patients will be boys. When speech does begin, as always happens, it may overlap the early stages of spoken language, and the child progresses rapidly to speaking in full sentences and to develop fluent speech and language. Not infrequently, however, articulation is infantile and the content of speech impoverished semantically and syntactically. With a smaller subgroup, as they begin to speak, they express themselves fluently but with many word distortions and omissions. Clustering of words and excess rapidity make their speech difficult to understand. Such patients usually recover.

During the period of speech delay, the understanding of words and general intelligence develop normally, and communication by gestures may be remarkably facile. In such children, motor speech delay does not presage mental backwardness. (It is said that Albert Einstein did not speak until the age of 4 and lacked fluency at 9.) However, some patients with this type of delayed speech are later found to have dyslexia and dysgraphia, a combination that is inherited as an autosomal dominant trait, again more frequently in boys than girls. In others, reading and writing are acquired at the usual time, even before the first words are spoken.

Aphasia, when it occurs as the result of an acquired lesion (vascular, traumatic) is essentially motor and lasts but a few months. It may be accompanied by a right-sided hemiplegia. An interesting example of acquired aphasia, possibly encephalitic, has been described by Landau and Kleffner in association with seizures and bitemporal focal discharges in the EEG (see page 255).

Congenital Deafness Motor speech delay due to congenital deafness, whether peripheral (loss of pure-tone acuity) or central (pure-tone threshold normal by audiogram) may at first be difficult to discern. One suspects that faulty hearing is causal when there is a history of congenital rubella, erythroblastosis fetalis, meningitis, or bilateral ear infections—the well-known antecedents of deafness, accounting for 75 percent of cases. (It is estimated that 3 million American children have hearing defects; 0.1 percent of the school population is deaf and 1.5 percent hard of hearing.) The parents' attention may be drawn to a defect in hearing when the infant fails to heed loud noises, to turn the eyes to sound sources outside the immediate visual fields, and to react to music, but in other instances it is the delay in speech that calls attention to it.

The deaf child makes the transition from crying to cooing and babbling at the usual age of 3 to 5 months. After the sixth month, however, the child becomes much quieter, and the usual repertoire of babbling sounds becomes stereotyped and unchanging, though still uttered with pleasant voice. A more conspicuous failure comes somewhat later, when babbling fails to give way to word formation. Should deafness develop within the first few years of life, the child gradually loses such speech as had been acquired, but can be retaught by the lip-reading method. The speech, however, is harsh, poorly modulated, and unpleasant and accompanied by many peculiar throat noises of a snorting or grunting kind. Unlike the mentally retarded child, social and other acquisitions appear at the expected times in the congenitally deaf child, who seems eager to communicate and makes known all needs by gesture or pantomime—often very cleverly. In fact, the deaf child may attract attention by vivid facial expressions, motions of the lips, nodding, or head shaking. The Leiter performance scale, which makes no use of sounds, will show that intelligence is normal. Deafness can be demonstrated at an early age by careful observation of the child's responses to sounds and by free-field audiometry, but the full range of hearing cannot be accurately tested before the age of 3 or 4 years. Recording of auditory-evoked brainstem potentials, testing the reaction to sounds by the psychogalvanic reflex technique, and testing of the labyrinths, which are frequently unresponsive in deaf-mutes, may be helpful. Early diagnosis is important in order to obtain possible hearing aids and appropriate language training.

In contrast to the child in whom deafness is the only abnormality, the imbecile or moron is generally defective and talks little because he or she has nothing to say. Autistic children may also be mute, and if they speak, echolalia is prominent and the personal "I" is avoided. Blind children of normal intelligence tend to speak slowly and fail to acquire imitative gestures.

Congenital Word Deafness This disorder, also called *developmental receptive dysphasia, verbal auditory agnosia,* or *central deafness* is rare and may be difficult to distinguish from peripheral deafness. Usually the parents have noted that the word-deaf child responds to loud noises and music, but obviously this does not assure perfect hearing, particularly for high tones. The word-deaf child does not understand what is said, and delay and distortion of speech are evident.

Presumably, in this disorder, the auditory apparatus of the dominant temporal lobe fails to discriminate between the complex acoustic patterns of words and to associate them with visual images of people and objects—a theory that can be neither affirmed nor refuted at this time. One observation stands out—that the child, despite intact pure-tone hearing, does not seem to hear word patterns properly and fails to reproduce them in natural speech. In other ways the child may be bright, but more often than not this auditory imperception of words is associated with hyper-activity, inattentiveness, bizarre behavior, or other perceptual defects incident to focal brain damage, particularly in the temporal lobes. Word-deaf children may chatter incessantly. Often they adopt a language of their own design, which the parents come to understand. This peculiar type of speech is known as *idioglossia*. It is also observed in children with marked articulatory defects.

Speech habilitation of the bright word-deaf child should follow along the same lines as that of the congenitally deaf one. Such a child learns to lip-read quickly and is clever at acting out his or her own ideas.

Congenital Inarticulation In this developmental defect the child seems unable to coordinate the vocal, articulatory, and respiratory apparatus for the purpose of speaking. It too occurs more often in boys than girls, and again there is often a family history of the disorder, although the data are not quite sufficient to establish the pattern of inheritance. The incidence is 1 in every 200 children. The motor, sensory, emotional, and social attainments correspond to the norms for age, although in a few of the cases, a minority in the authors' opinion, there has been some indication of cranial nerve abnormality in the first months of life (ptosis, facial asymmetry, strange neonatal cry, and altered phonation).

In children with congenital inarticulation, the "pre-language" sounds are probably abnormal, but this aspect of the speech disorder has not been well studied. Babbling tends to be deficient, and, in the second year, in attempting to say something, the child makes noises that do not sound at all like language; in this way the child is unlike the late talker already described. Again the understanding of language is entirely normal; the comprehension vocabulary is average for age, and the child can appreciate syntax as indicated by correct responses to questions by nodding or head shaking and by the execution of complex spoken commands. Usually such patients are shy but otherwise quick in response, cheerful, and without behavior disorder. While some of these children are bright, a combination of congenital inarticulation and mild mental dullness is not uncommon. Speech correction should be attempted (by a trained therapist) if many of the spontaneous utterances are intelligible. However, if the child makes no sounds that resemble words, the therapeutic effort should be directed toward a modified school program and mental hygiene, and speech habilitation should wait until some words are acquired.

Studies of the cerebra of such patients are not available, and it is doubtful if they would show any abnormality by the usual techniques of neuropathologic examination. Occasionally, suspicion of a lesion is raised by focal changes in the EEG or a slight widening of the temporal horn of the left ventricle. Delayed speech is often attributed to "tongue-tie," i.e., a short lingual frenulum, but we have never been convinced of this. Also psychologists have attributed speech retardation to overprotectiveness or excessive pressure by the parents. We are inclined to believe that these are the results rather than the cause of the delay.

This subject is well reviewed in the monograph *The Child with Delayed Speech*, edited by Rutter and Martin.

Other Articulatory Defects These are most common in preschool children, having an incidence of 15 percent. There are several varieties. One is *lisping*, in which the *s* sound is replaced by *th*, e.g., *thimple* for *simple*. Another common condition, *lallation*, or *dyslalia*, is characterized by multiple substitutions or omissions of consonants. Milder degrees consist of difficulty in pronouncing one or two consonants. For example, the letter *r* may be incorrectly pronounced, so that it sounds like *w* or *y; running a race* becomes *wunning a wace* or *yunning a yace*. In severe forms speech may be almost unintelligible. The child seems to be unaware that his or her speech differs from that of others and is distressed at not being understood. These and similar abnormalities of speech are often present in normal children and are referred to as "infantilisms." But why do they persist in some individuals? It has been suggested that the development of language is so rapid that there is sometimes a partial failure of the corrective mechanisms of both hearing and imitation.

Of importance is the fact that in more than 90 percent of cases these articulatory abnormalities disappear by the age of 8 years, either spontaneously or in response to speech therapy. The latter is best started if these conditions persist into the fifth year. Presumably the natural cycle of motor speech acquisition has been only delayed, not arrested. Such abnormalities are more frequent among the feebleminded than in normal children; with mental defect many consonants are persistently mispronounced. Worster-Drought has described a congenital form of spastic bulbar speech in which words are spoken slowly, with stiff labial and lingual movements, hyperactive jaw and facial reflexes, and sometimes mild dysphagia and dysphonia. The limbs may be unaffected, in contrast to most children with "cerebral palsy."

The speech disorder resulting from *cleft palate* is easily recognized. Many of these patients also have a harelip; the two abnormalities together interfere with sucking and later in life with the enunciation of labial and guttural consonants. The voice has an unpleasant nasality, and often, if the defect is severe, there is an audible escape of air through the nose.

Aside from these special types of developmental speech disorder, there are many other common speech defects that handicap individuals throughout their lives. *Word blocking, multiple substitution of words, inability to complete spoken sentences*, and *word cluttering* are observed in many adults and make their speech inefficient and unpleasant to hear. These abnormalities are often associated with specific language defects.

The aforementioned developmental abnormalities of speech are often associated with disturbances of higher order language processing. Rapin and Allen have described a number of such disturbances. In one, which they call the "semantic pragmatic syndrome," a failure to comprehend complex phrases and sentences is combined with fluent speech and well-formed sentences but is lacking in content. The syndrome resembles Wernicke or transcortical sensory aphasia (Chap. 22). In another, "semantic retrieval-organization syndrome," a severe anomia blocks word finding in spontaneous speech. A mixed expressive-receptive disorder may also be seen as a developmental abnormality; it contains many of the elements of acquired Broca aphasia (pages 382 and 383).

Congenital Word Blindness (Developmental Dyslexia)

This is a condition that becomes manifest in an older child who fails in the first grade to master the written or printed word. Several excellent books and articles have been written on the subject, to which the interested reader is referred for a detailed account (Orton; Critchley and Critchley; Rutter and Martin; and Kinsbourne).

The main problem is an inability to read words, and also to spell and to write them despite the ability to see and recognize letters. There is no loss of the ability to recognize the meaning of objects, pictures, and diagrams. Often the reading failure can be anticipated before the child enters school, by difficulty in copying, color naming, and formation of number concepts, and by the persistent reversal of letters. The writing appears to be defective because of faulty perception of form and a kind of constructional and directional apraxia. Not infrequently there is an associated

vagueness about the serial order of letters in the alphabet and months in the year, as well as difficulty with numbers (acalculia) and an inability to spell and to read music. Some dyslexic children have had a delay in learning to speak and trouble in acquiring clear articulation. For this reason Ingram sees all these motor and perceptual speech difficulties as parts of a complex of congenital language defect.

Lesser degrees of dyslexia are more common than the severe ones and are found in a large segment of the school population. Some 10 percent of school children have some degree of this disability, but the problem is complex, because the condition is unquestionably influenced by the way reading is taught. However, only a few children are unable to read at all after many years in school.

This form of language disorder, unattended by other neurologic signs, is strongly familial, being almost in conformity with an autosomal dominant or sex-linked recessive pattern. There is a statistically higher incidence of left-handedness among these persons and members of their families.

The steady drill of a cooperative child by a skillful teacher over an extended period (many hours per week) slowly overcomes the handicap and enables an otherwise intelligent child to follow successfully a regular program of education.

In the study of dyslexic and dysgraphic children (and of some whose language function is essentially normal), a number of other apparently congenital developmental abnormalities have been documented, such as (1) inadequate perception of space and form (poor performance on form boards and in tasks requiring construction), (2) inadequate perception of size, distance, and temporal sequences and rhythms, and (3) inability to imitate sequences of movements gracefully, and extreme degrees of clumsiness and reduced proficiency in all motor tasks and games (the *clumsy-child syndrome* described by Gubbay et al). Less fully studied than other developmental disorders, they represent, nonetheless, in the child with normal intelligence, an inordinate delay in one phase of neurologic development. These disorders may also occur in brain-injured children; hence there may be considerable difficulty in separating simple delay or arrest in development from a pathologic process in the brain. As noted above, Galaburda and his associates have studied the brains of four men (ages 14 to 32 years) with this form of developmental dyslexia. In each of them there were developmental anomalies of the cerebral cortex, consisting of neuronal ectopias and architectonic dysplasias, located mainly in the perisylvian regions of the left hemisphere.

Probably all that has been said about dyslexia applies to the kindred states of *acalculia,* where no amount of classroom work helps the child learn arithmetic, and to hyperactivity and attentional defects (Denckla et al). Often these are associated with dyslexia.

Precocious Reading and Calculating

In contrast to the foregoing disorders, precocious reading and calculation abilities have also been identified. A child 2 or 3 years old may read with the skill of an average adult. Extraordinary facility with numbers (mathematical prodigies) and vivid memory capacity (eidetic imagery) are similar traits. Here one observes a remarkable overdevelopment of these single faculties. Occasionally one of these special abilities will be observed in a child with a mild form of autism (Asperger syndrome, page 482). He may exhibit great skill in performing a mathematical trick but be unable to solve simple mathematical problems or to understand the meaning of numbers (a kind of ''idiot savant'').

Stuttering and Stammering

These difficulties occur in an estimated 1 to 2 percent of the school population. Often such conditions disappear in late childhood and adolescence; only about 1 in every 300 individuals suffers from a persistent stammer or stutter. Mild degrees are to some extent cultivated and permit a pause in speech for collecting one's thoughts. And it tends to be imitated in certain social circles (educated Englishmen).

Stammering and stuttering are difficult to classify. In some respects they belong to and are customarily included in the developmental language disorders, but differ in being largely centered in articulation. Essentially they take the form of a disorder of rhythm of speech—an involuntary, repetitive prolongation of speech—due to spasm of the articulatory muscles. The spasm may be tonic and result in a complete blocking of speech (sometimes referred to as stammering) or clonic, i.e., a series of spasms interrupting the emission of consonants, usually the first letter or syllable of a word (stuttering). There is no valid reason to distinguish between these two forms of the disorder, since they are intermingled, and the terms *stammer* and *stutter* are now used synonymously. Certain sounds, particularly *p* and *b,* offer greater difficulty than others; *paper boy* comes out *p-p-paper b-b-boy.* The severity of the stutter is increased by excitement and stress, as when speaking before others, and is reduced when the stutterer is relaxed and alone or when singing. When severe, the spasms may overflow into other groups of muscles such as those of the face, neck, arms. The muscles involved in stuttering show no fault in nonlin-

guistic actions, and all gnostic and semantic aspects of receptive language are intact.

Males are affected four times as often as females. The time of onset of stuttering is mainly at two periods in life—between 2 and 4 years, when speech is beginning, and between 6 and 8 years, when language extends to reciting, reading aloud, and writing in the classroom. However, there may be a later onset. Many afflicted children have an associated difficulty in reading and writing. If stuttering is mild, it tends to develop or to be present only during periods of emotional stress, and in four out of five children it disappears during adolescent or early adult years (Andrews and Harris). If severe, it persists throughout life, regardless of treatment, but tends to improve as the patient grows older.

Theories of causation are legion. Slowness in developing hand and eye preference, ambidexterity, or an enforced change from left- to right-hand use have been popular explanations, of which Orton and Travis were leading advocates. According to this theory, stuttering results from a lack of the necessary degree of unilateral control in the synchronization of bilaterally innervated speech mechanisms. However, these associations seem to apply to only a minority of stutterers (Hécaen and de Ajuriaguerra). The disappearance of mild stuttering with maturation has been attributed incorrectly to all manner of treatment (hypnosis, progressive relaxation, speaking in rhythms, etc.) and used to bolster particular theories of causation. Since stuttering may reappear at times of emotional strain, a psychogenesis has been proposed, but, as Orton points out, if there are any neurotic tendencies in the stutterer, they are secondary rather than primary. We have observed that many stutterers, probably as a result of this impediment to free social intercourse, do become increasingly fearful of talking and develop feelings of inferiority. By the time adolescence and adulthood are reached, emotional factors are so prominent that many physicians have mistaken stuttering for neurosis. Usually there is little or no evidence of any personality deviation before the onset of stuttering, and psychotherapy, though helpful in relieving emotional tension and assisting the patient's adjustment to the condition, has not in our experience had a consistent effect on the underlying defect. A strong family history in many cases and male dominance point to a genetic origin, but the inheritance does not follow a readily discernible pattern.

The nature of stuttering has been difficult to define in physiologic terms. There is no detectable weakness or ataxia of the speech musculature, which functions normally in all acts other than speaking. Stuttering differs from an apraxia in that the muscles of speech, when called upon to perform the specific act of speaking, go into spasm. The spasms are not invoked by other actions (which may not be as complex or voluntary as speaking), differing in this way from the intention spasm of athetosis. A distinction should also be drawn between palilalia and stuttering. Palilalia is a condition in which a word or phrase, usually the last one in a sentence, is repeated. In fact, stuttering appears to represent a special category of movement disorder, much like writer's cramp (page 90). We regard both as restricted extapyramidal motor disorders, bearing some of the characteristics of dystonia.

Rarely, in adults as well as in children, stuttering may appear as a result of a lesion in the motor speech areas, which disturbs the balance between the two cerebral hemispheres. A distinction has been drawn between developmental and acquired stuttering. The latter is said to interfere with the enunciation of any syllable of a word (not just the first), to involve grammatical and substantive words, and to be unaccompanied by anxiety and facial grimacing. Such differences in semiology may be ephemeral. Lesion sites in acquired stuttering are so variable (right frontal, corpus striatum, left temporal, left parietal) as to be difficult to reconcile with proposed theories of developmental stuttering (Fleet and Heilman).

Another form of acquired stuttering is manifestly an expression of extrapyramidal disorder. Here there occurs a prolonged repetition of syllables (vowel and consonant) which the patient cannot easily interrupt. The abnormality involves throat-clearing and other vocalizations. We have observed it in some patients with parkinsonism and progressive supranuclear palsy.

The therapy of stuttering is difficult to evaluate. As remarked above, all speech-fluency disturbances are modifiable by environmental circumstances. Thus a certain proportion of stutterers will become more fluent under certain conditions, such as reading aloud; others will stutter more severely at this time. Again, a majority of stutterers will be adversely affected by talking on the telephone; a minority are helped by this device. Some stutterers are more fluent under conditions of mild alcohol intoxication. Nearly every stutterer is fluent while singing.

On the whole, the therapy of speech-fluency disorders has been a frustrating effort. Schemes such as the encouragement of associated muscular movements ("penciling," etc.) and the adoption of a "theatrical" approach to speaking have been advocated. Common to all such efforts has been the difficulty of achieving carry-over into the natural speaking environment. Progressive relaxation, hypnosis, delayed auditory feedback, loud noise that masks speech sounds, and tranquilization help temporarily. A few controlled studies with antidopaminergic drugs, particularly haloperidol, have shown promising results in a minority of severe stutterers.

Another special developmental disorder, *cluttering, or cluttered, speech,* is characterized by uncontrollable speed of speech, which results in truncated, dysrhythmic, and often incoherent utterances. It is as though the child is too hurried to take the trouble to pronounce each word carefully and to compose sentences. Omissions of consonants, elisions, improper phrasing, and inadequate intonation occur. It is frequently associated with other motor speech impediments. Speech therapy (elocutionary) and maturation are attended by a restoration of more normal rhythms.

AUTISM AND CHILDHOOD PSYCHOSIS

The term *autism,* introduced by Kanner in 1943, refers to another remarkable disharmony of development wherein children, despite excellent motor skill (normal motor milestones and facile use of hands) and retentive memory, fail to mature socially, i.e., to form any emotional bonds with parents and other individuals, and often to learn to speak. It is the discrepancy between their excellent motor skill on the one hand and the global asociality, lack of or restricted communicative speech, and certain other eccentricities of behavior on the other that sets them apart from the more common mental retardates. Severely autistic children cannot be disciplined. They do not heed words or react to other human beings; hence they are uneducable. A minority acquire some language but use it little in communication. The mildest degree of the disease allows an uneven development of cognitive and social abilities.

When the biographies of a group of autistic children are examined, two courses of development are perceived. In one group the child appears to be entirely normal until 18 to 24 months of age, at which time an alarming regression begins, sometimes in temporal relation to an injury or an upsetting experience. In the second group the child appears to be abnormal from the first months of life. The level of activity is reduced, the child cries little and is indifferent to his or her surroundings. Toys are ignored or are held tenaciously. In contrast motor development proceeds normally or is even precocious. Later an unusual sensitivity to all modes of sensory stimulation may be displayed.

Regardless of the mode of onset, older autistic children exhibit a striking disregard for other persons; they make no eye contact and are no more interested in another person than in an article of furniture. Proferred toys are either manipulated cleverly or are ignored. Insistence on constancy of the environment may reach a point where such patients become distraught if even a single object in their room has been moved in their absence. If speech does develop, it is highly automatic and words are spoken without feeling. Reading capacity and calculation may greatly exceed expressive speech. A repertoire of elaborate stereotypic movements, such as a whirling of the body, spinning of objects, and toe walking, are frequent. Certain objects such as spinning toys or running water have a strange fascination for these children.

The outcome of childhood autism is discouraging, according to Eisenberg, who has observed a large number of such patients through adolescence into adulthood. One-third of the patients never speak, another third acquire a rudimentary language devoid of communicative value, and only in the remainder does an affected, stilted, colorless speech develop. As many as a third of all such patients, as they grow older, begin to manifest other visuoperceptive and auditory defects, indicative of a variety of cerebral diseases. This is not surprising, since autism is a rather imprecise syndrome. Hence any group of such patients is contaminated with a variety of other encephalopathic states. Yet in purest form it probably represents a unique metabolic (or other) disease. Moreover, we have the impression that many patients show milder degrees of this disorder, evolving as eccentric, mirthless, flat personalities unable to adapt socially but possessing certain unusual aptitudes (arithmetic ability, factual knowledge of history or science well beyond age norms). They may be called autistic adults. These milder cases were probably described by Asperger.

The basis of childhood autism is as much a mystery today as it was when Kanner described it. Most of these children are physically normal, have a head of average size, and have no somatic defects or other neurologic abnormalities. The EEG may be normal or show slight immaturity. The CT scan reveals ventricles of average size and no atrophy of the brain, and this holds true for autistic adults, whose illness began in childhood. In a few the temporal horn of the left lateral ventricle is enlarged. Using MRI, Courchesne and his colleagues found a hypoplasia of the neocerebellar vermis (lobules VI and VII) in some autistic children and adults, but this finding, even if confirmed, would hardly explain the profound emotional-behavioral disorder. An increased concentration of blood serotonin is found in many but not all patients with autism (Schain and Freedman); the biologic significance of this finding is also unclear.

There is usually no familial tendency, though we have seen the disease in identical twins and in brothers and a small familial subgroup is known to exist. DeMyer found that 4 of 11 monozygotic twins were concordant for autism and that siblings have a 50 times greater risk of developing the disorder. But still, the genetic factor is not strong (prevalence of 20 per 10,000 vs. 4.5 per 10,000 in the general population). In the only careful whole-brain histologic study, Bauman and Kemper found a reduction in size and an increased "packing density" of neurons in the hippocampus, entorrhinal cortex, septal nuclei, mammillary bodies, amygdala, and cerebellum, in comparison with control cases. These findings need to be verified.

The implication that these children or adults are truly autistic, i.e., have a rich inner psychic life or dream world that is out of relation to reality, is an assumption totally without foundation. Despite many claims to the contrary, there is no evidence of psychogenesis. Although this disorder has been referred to as "childhood schizophrenia," the afflicted individuals do not resemble schizophrenics when they reach adolescent and adult years. The very early age of onset, the lack of delusional thinking, and the absence of a family history of psychosis are other points against this being childhood schizophrenia.

Whether there is, quite apart from autism, a form of schizophrenia that affects infants and young children has been difficult to decide. Schizophrenic parents have been known to beget children who from the beginning are aloof, impersonal, withdrawn, and asocial in their daily contact. They may be rigid, resistive, and show abnormal reactions to stimuli (overreaction, avoidance, unnatural fear), inexplicable anxiety, hallucinations, mutism and bizarre postures, hyperactivity, rocking, and spinning. Such states, called *childhood psychosis* or childhood schizophrenia, have been well described by Lauretta Bender.

Psychotherapy is of no proven value. Currently there is interest in determining whether behavior-modification methods have anything to offer. Lithium carbonate, phenytoin, dextroamphetamine, and other of the antipsychotic drugs sometimes result in improvement in behavior. Fenfluramine hydrochloride is said to hold the most promise and is under study.

"MINIMAL BRAIN DYSFUNCTION" SYNDROMES

A large portion of ambulatory pediatric neurology consists of children who are referred because of failure in school. The question asked is whether they have a brain disease or the sequelae of some brain injury that has altered behavior, interfered with learning, or caused clumsiness.

When a large number of such cases is analyzed, fully 80 to 85 percent prove to have no major signs of neurologic disease (Barlow). Perhaps 5 percent are mentally retarded, and another 5 percent show some evidence of cerebral palsy. In the group without neurologic signs, the IQ is normal, though there is a larger number of borderline cases than in the general population. Boys are found to be more hyperactive and inattentive than girls and to have more trouble in learning to read and write. Many are clumsy. Girls tend to have more trouble with numbers and arithmetic.

Dyslexia has already been discussed. The other causes of school failure are grouped under the hyperactivity and the learning disability syndromes, which are discussed below.

HYPERACTIVITY SYNDROME

Human infants exhibit astonishing differences in amount of activity almost from the first days of life. Some babies are constantly on the move, wiry, and hard to hold, and others are placid and as slack as a sack of meal. Irwin, who studied motility in the neonate, found a difference of 290 times between the most and least active in terms of amount of movement per 24 h.

Once walking and running begin, children normally enter a period when they are extremely active, more so than at any other period of life. The degree of activity, which again varies widely from one child to another, seems not to be correlated with the age of achieving motor milestones or with great motor skill at a later time. The male is more active than the female, and the black child tends to be more precocious in motor development and more active than the white. Children with cerebral defects tend to exhibit hyperactivity more often than normal children.

Again, two groups can be discerned: In one the infants are overactive from birth, sleeping less and feeding poorly, and by the age of 2 years the syndrome is obvious. In the other group, an inability to sit quietly becomes apparent at the preschool age (4 to 6 years). Seldom do such children remain in one position for more than a few seconds, even when watching television. They cannot attend to any task no matter how interesting, hence the term "attention deficit disorder." As a rule there is also an abnormal impulsivity and often an intolerance of all measures to control the activity.

Once in school, such children are disruptive. They cannot stay at their desks, take turns in reciting, be quiet, or control their own impulses. The teacher finds it impossible to discipline them and often insists that the parents seek medical consultation. Sometimes it is discovered that one or more males in a previous generation had the same problem. Some children are so hyperactive that they cannot attend regular school. Their behavior verges on the "organic drivenness" that has been known to occur in children whose brains have been injured by encephalitis. Most are less active and can be managed in special ways.

In the majority of patients, the hyperactivity subsides gradually by puberty or soon thereafter, but some of them remain hyperactive to a varying degree as adults. Mild degrees of mental retardation and epilepsy and other special disabilities are conjoined in some patients. Dislocation in educational and social adjustment may render the child prone to truancy and a variety of sociopathic trends in late childhood and adolescence.

There has been a tendency in recent years to consider children with the hyperkinetic syndrome as having minimal brain disease. "Soft neurologic signs" such as right-left confusion, mirror movements, minimal "choreic" instability, awkwardness, finger agnosia, tremor, and borderline hyperreflexia are said to be more frequent. These signs, however, are seen so often in normal children that their attribution to disease is invalid. Schain and others have therefore substituted the term *minimal brain dysfunction*, which in essence does no more than restate the problem. Lacking altogether are accurate clinicoanatomic and clinicopathologic correlative data.

The treatment of the hyperactive child can proceed intelligently only after medical and psychologic explorations have elucidated the context in which the hyperactivity occurs. If the child is hyperactive and inattentive mainly in school and less so in an unstructured environment, it may be that mental retardation or dyslexia, which prevents scholastic success, is a source of frustration and anger. The child then turns to other activities and becomes occupied in ways that disturb the classroom. The hyperactive child may have failed to acquire self-control because of a disorganized home life, and the overactivity is but one manifestation of anxiety or intolerance of constraint. Clearly problems such as these require a modification of the educational program.

For overactive children of normal intelligence who have failed to control their impulses even with parental assistance and who at all times have boundless energy, require little sleep, exhibit a wriggling restlessness (the choreiform syndrome of Prechtl and Stemmer) and incessant exploratory activity that repeatedly gets them into mischief, even to their own dismay, medical therapy is in order—dextroamphetamine in doses of 2.5 to 5 mg tid or methylphenidate, 5 to 10 mg tid. Paradoxically, these two drugs, which are stimulants, have a quieting effect on these children and phenobarbital has the opposite effect. If these agents control the activity and improve school performance (they can be continued for a number of years), there is no need to alter the child's school program. If the child is not helped, lithium, chlorpromazine, or phenytoin should be tried. Psychotherapy may be needed over brief periods for the child and the child's family. Remedial education should be reserved for recalcitrant cases.

LEARNING DISABILITY

School is obviously the most challenging event in the child's life and, since it is compulsory, serves to evince in many children dramatic behavioral disorders. Timid and easily frightened children, despite attempts at kindergarten attendance, may not tolerate separation from their mothers and may refuse to go to school. In others this first step may be achieved, but from the beginning there is failure in all scholastic tasks, even when the child has an apparently normal intelligence. Neuropsychiatric opinion is then sought to ascertain whether the child cannot or will not learn. If the former is evidenced, it must be decided whether the disability is due to a limitation of cognitive functions, a specific reading or calculating disability, or an inattentiveness and overactivity syndrome. Seizures and anticonvulsive medications often are an additional source of trouble. In other words, the role of the child neurologist is to help decide whether the difficulty reflects a general or a restricted cerebral impairment. Reading and writing failure are singled out most often because they are among the first scholastic tasks that the child must master and are of fundamental importance in all later schoolwork.

Often, upon clinical analysis, it is discovered for the first time that mental retardation has been present since birth or early life but ignored by unobservant parents. In others intelligence is normal, and a specific dyslexia or other language problem becomes unmasked when the child is confronted for the first time by demanding tasks. The language problems need to be corrected by special educational methods.

The study of such children should be supplemented by a number of tests of intelligence, language, memory, perception, attention, visual memory, and auditory-visual integration. Kinsbourne (1980) has listed those which are most useful (Table 28-5).

ENURESIS

Voluntary sphincteric control develops according to a predetermined time scale. Usually normal children stop soiling themselves before they can remain dry, and day control precedes night control. Some children are toilet-trained by their second birthday, but many have not acquired full sphincteric control until the fourth year. Constant dribbling usually indicates spina bifida, but in the boy one must look also for obstruction of the bladder neck and in the girl for an ectopic ureter entering the vagina.

When a child of 5 years or older wets the bed nearly every night and is dry by day, the child is said to have *nocturnal enuresis*. This condition afflicts approximately 10 percent of children between 4 and 14 years of age, boys more than girls, and continues in many cases to be a problem even into adolescence and adulthood. Although mentally retarded children are notably late in acquiring sphincter control (some never do), the majority of enuretic individuals are normal in other respects.

The cause of this condition is disputed. Often there is a family history of the same complaint. Some psychiatrists have insisted that overzealous parents "pressure" the child until he develops a complex about his bedwetting. Punishment, shaming, rewards, etc., doubtless have this effect, but the underlying condition is believed by most neurologists to be a delay in the maturation of higher control of spinal reflex centers during sleep. As indicated on page 318, Gastaut and Broughton have uncovered a number of abnormalities of bladder function in the enuretic child. These and other aspects of this disorder are discussed in Chap. 18.

SOCIOPATHY AND NEUROSIS

During the formative years, when children or adolescents seek tribe approval, every blemish, every physical abnormality becomes a cross to bear. On the neurologic side, a stammer or stutter, dyslexia, hyperactivity, etc., not only place them apart but also interfere with the training and education to which their intelligence entitles them. When forced in their schoolwork beyond their capacities in language and speech, they may become rebellious and aggressive or give up completely and divert themselves in other ways. Not infrequently, social development, which may revolve more around classmates than family, is thwarted or misguided.

Extremes of egocentricity, lack of understanding of the feelings, needs, and actions of other members of one's social group, and an inability to judge one's own strengths and weaknesses stand as the central issues in the development of neurosis. Such difficulties usually become manifest by adolescence. Indeed *neurosis* may be defined in such terms. In later life neurotic persons habitually attempt to preserve their egocentric ways in each newly formed social circle. If socially rejected for this or other reasons, anxiety and unhappiness often result. The complete detachment of the child with psychosis, the amorality of the constitutional sociopath, the major disturbances in thinking of the schizophrenic, and the mood swings of the manic-depressive have also expressed themselves in many instances by adolescence. Here one confronts a key problem in psychiatry—the extent to which neurosis, sociopathy, and psychosis have their roots in derangements in the affective and social life of the individual during the processes of personality development. In other words, in what measure are the neuroses and other psychiatric disorders determined by early life experiences, and to what extent are they genetically determined?

The answers to these questions cannot be given with finality. Experienced clinicians tend to believe that genetic factors are more important than environmental ones. The discovery that unusually tall males with severe acne vulgaris and aggressive sociopathic behavior may have a karyotype of XYY chromosomes is an example of a possible genetic relationship. Further, there is no critical evidence to show that deliberate alteration of the familial and social environment or mental hygienic measures now so popular have ever prevented a neurosis, psychosis, or sociopathy. Admittedly, counseling of parents is helpful in managing behavior and adjustment problems of adolescents, but children identified as high-risk individuals because of early truancy, conflict with the law, and general maladjustment, if transferred to a more stable and supportive environment, have as a group not turned out much better than others left alone. Here data are meager, however, and a completely controlled study has probably never been attempted. For this reason the mental hygiene movement continues to be supported in the United States.

Many patients concern the physician, other than those who develop frank neurosis or psychosis, for civilized society is filled with countless unhappy, maladjusted individuals who cannot be called either neurotic or psychotic. It is with reference to these persons that one seeks explanations in terms of psychogenesis and looks for early sociopathic trends. Adolescent turmoil often seems to stem from parental neglect, poor child-parent relationships, or an unstable home environment that has engendered either defiance or excessive dependency. The result may be either a failure of emancipation or an early rupture of family ties, both with a lasting effect on social maturation. Similarly, sexual deviations of the adolescent and young adult are often ascribed to lack of early guidance and instruction. Certainly, the adolescent is not helped by the ambivalence of Western society, which evinces interest in sex but then imposes sanctions on its expression. Actually, little is known about the early conditioning that inculcates traits of masculinity and femininity (see page 1201). Hormonal factors play but a minor part. Whether sexual perversions are due to early patterning of the brain is unsettled. Ignorance of sex and impoverishment of human relations also seem to account for many sexual misadventures.

The sensitivity of adolescents to the good opinion of their peers obviously renders them psychologically vulnerable. If in addition they happen to be endowed with limited intelligence and a physical defect, the grounds for persistent and indomitable feelings of inferiority are laid, especially if there is repeated failure in competition. The individualization of education and vocational training for such adolescents is essential, to permit the talented to exploit their abilities and those with handicaps to be directed into activities that constructively develop personality.

It is during the period of late childhood and adolescence, when the personality is least stable, that transient symptoms, many resembling the psychopathologic states of adult life, are frequent and difficult to interpret. Some of these disorders represent the early signs of schizophrenia or manic-depressive disease, but many borderline personality traits have a way of disappearing as adult years are reached, so that one can only surmise that they were but expressions of adolescent turmoil (see Chap. 55).

REFERENCES

ANDERSON LD: The predictive value of infancy tests in relation to intelligence at five years. *Child Dev* 10:203, 1939

ANDRÉ-THOMAS, CHESNI Y, DARGASSIES ST-ANNE S: *The Neurological Examination of the Infant.* London, Medical Advisory Committee, National Spastics Society, 1960.

ANDREWS G, HARRIS M: *Clinics in Developmental Medicine,* no. 17: *The Syndrome of Stuttering.* London, Heinemann, 1964.

ASPERGER H: Die autistischen Psychopathie in Kindesalter. *Arch Psychiatr Nervenkr* 117:76, 1944.

BAKER L, DENNIS PC, MATTISON RE: Behavior problems in children with pure speech disorders and in children with combined speech and language disorders. *J Abnorm Child Psychol* 8:245, 1980.

BARLOW C: *Mental Retardation and Related Disorders.* Philadelphia, Davis, 1977.

BAUMAN M, KEMPER TL: Histoanatomic observations of the brain in early infantile autism. *Neurology* 35:866, 1985.

BAYLEY H: Comparisons of mental and motor test scores for age 1–15 months by sex, birth order, race, geographic location and education of parents. *Child Dev* 36:379, 1965.

BENDER L: *A Visual-Motor Gestalt Test and Its Use.* New York, American Orthopsychiatric Association, 1938.

BENDER L: The life course of schizophrenic children. *Biol Psychiatry* 2:165, 1970.

BENTON AL: *Revised Visual Retention Test.* New York, Psychological Corporation, 1974.

BENTON AL: Right-left discrimination. *Pediatr Clin North Am* 15:747, 1968.

BIRCH HG, BELMONT L: Auditory-visual integration in normal and retarded readers. *Am J Orthopsychiatry* 34:852, 1964.

BRECKENRIDGE ME, MURPHY MN: *Growth and Development of the Young Child.* New York, Saunders, 1963.

CHESS S: Diagnosis and treatment of the hyperactive child. *NY State J Med* 60:2379, 1960.

CHESS S, HASSIBI M: Behavioral deviations in mentally retarded children. *J Am Acad Child Psychiatry* 9:282, 1970.

CONEL J: *The Postnatal Development of the Human Cerebral Cortex,* vols 1–8. Cambridge, MA, Harvard, 1939–1967.

COURCHESNE E, YEUNG-COURCHESNE R, PRESS GA et al: Hypoplasia of cerebellar vermal lobules VI and VII in autism. *N Engl J Med* 318:1349, 1988.

COWAN WM: The development of the brain. *Sci Am* 241:112, 1979.

CRITCHLEY M, CRITCHLEY EA: *Dyslexia Defined.* Springfield, IL, Charles C Thomas, 1978.

DELONG GR: A neuropsychological interpretation of infantile autism, in Rutter M, Schopler E (eds): *Autism.* New York, Plenum Press, 1978.

DEMYER MK: Infantile autism: Patients and their families. *Curr Probl Pediatr* 12:1, 1982.

DENCKLA MB: Autism, in Asbury AK, McKhann GM, McDonald WI (eds): *Diseases of the Nervous System.* Philadelphia, Saunders, 1986, chap 73.

DENCKLA MB, RUDEL RG, CHAPMAN C et al: Motor proficiency in dyslexic children with and without attentional disorders. *Arch Neurol* 42:228, 1985.

EISENBERG L: The autistic child in adolescence. *Am J Psychiatry* 112:607, 1965.

ELLINGSON RG: The incidence of EEG abnormality among children with mental disorder of apparently nonorganic origin. *Am J Psychiatry* 111:263, 1954.

FANTZ RL: The origin of form perception. *Sci Am* 204:66, 1961.

FERNALD WE: Standardized fields of inquiry for clinical studies of borderline defectives. *Ment Hyg* 1:211, 1917.

FLEET WS, HEILMAN KM: Acquired stuttering from a right hemisphere lesion in a right hander. *Neurology* 35:1343, 1985.

FRANKENBERG WK, DODDS JB, FANDAL AW: *Denver Developmental Screening Test,* rev ed. Denver, University of Colorado Medical Center, 1970.

GALABURDA AM, SHERMAN CF, ROSEN GD et al: Development dyslexia: Four consecutive patients with cortical anomalies. *Ann Neurol* 18:222, 1985.

GESELL A, AMATRUDA CS: *Developmental Diagnosis: Normal and Abnormal Child Development,* 2nd ed. New York, Hoeber-Harper, 1954.

GESELL A (ed): *The First Five Years of Life: A Guide to the Study of the Pre-School Child.* New York, Harper & Row, 1940.

GIBSON EJ, OLUM V: Experimental methods of studying perception in children, in Mussen P (ed): *Handbook of Research Methods in Child Development.* New York, Wiley, 1960, chap 8, pp 311–373.

GOLDSTEIN K: *Language and Language Disturbances: Aphasic Symptom Complexes and Their Significance for Medicine and Theory of Language.* New York, Grune & Stratton, 1948.

GUBBAY SS, ELLIS E, WALTER JN, COURT SDM: Clumsy children: A study of apraxic and agnosic defects in 21 children. *Brain* 88:295, 1965.

HÉCAEN N, DE AJURIAGUERRA J: *Left-handedness.* New York, Grune & Stratton, 1964.

HIER DB, LEMAY M, ROSENBERGER PB: Autism and unfavorable left-right asymetries of the brain. *J Autism Dev. Disord* 9:153, 1979.

HIER DB, LEMAY M, ROSENBERGER PB: Autism and unfavorable left-right asymmetries of the brain. *J Autism Dev. Disord* 9:153, 1979.

HUTTENLOCHER PR: Dendritic development in neocortex of children with mental defect and infantile spasms. *Neurology* 24:203, 1974.

ILLINGWORTH RS: *The Development of the Infant and Young Child, Normal and Abnormal,* 3rd ed. Edinburgh, Churchill Livingstone, 1966.

INGRAM TTS: Developmental disorders of speech, in Vinken PJ, Bruyn W (eds): *Handbook of Clinical Neurology,* vol 4: *Disorders of Speech, Perception and Symbolic Behavior.* Amsterdam, North-Holland, 1969, chap 22, pp 407–442.

IRWIN OC: Can infants have IQ's? *Psychol Rev* 49:69, 1942.

KAGAN J, MOSS HA: *Birth to Maturity: A Study of Psychological Development.* New York, Wiley, 1962.

KANNER I: Early infantile autism. *J Pediatr* 25:211, 1944.

KINSBOURNE M: Developmental Gerstmann's syndrome: A disorder of sequencing. *Pediatr Clin North Am* 15:771, 1968.

KINSBOURNE M: Disorders of mental development, in Menkes JH (ed): *Textbook of Child Neurology,* 3rd ed. Philadelphia, Lea & Febiger, 1985, chap 15, pp 764–801.

LANDAU WM, KLEFFNER FR: Syndrome of acquired aphasia with convulsive disorder in children. *Neurology* 7:523, 1957.

LENNEBERG EH: *Biological Foundations of Language.* New York, Wiley, 1967.

LOWREY GH: *Growth and Development of Children,* 8th ed. Chicago, Year Book, 1986.

MINIFIE FD, LLOYD LL: *Communicative and Cognitive Abilities—Early Behavioral Assessment.* Baltimore, University Park Press, 1978.

MOSER HW, RAMEY CT, LEONARD CO: Mental retardation, in Emery AE, Rimoin DL (eds): *Principles and Practice of Medical Genetics.* Edinburgh, Churchill Livingstone, 1984, chap 29, pp 352–366.

ORTON ST: *Reading, Writing and Speech Problems in Children.* New York, Norton, 1937.

OZERETZKII NI: Technique of investigating motor function, in Gurevich M, Ozeretzkii NI (eds): *Psychomotor Function.* Moscow, 1930. Quoted by Luria AR: *Higher Cortical Functions in Man.* New York, Basic Books, 1966.

PEIPER A: *Cerebral Function in Infancy and Childhood.* New York, Consultants Bureau, 1963.

PHILLIPS JL JR: *The Origins of Intellect. Piaget's Theory,* 2nd ed. San Francisco, Freeman, 1975.

PRECHTL HFR: Prognostic value of neurological signs in the newborn. *Proc R Soc Med* 58:3, 1965.

PRECHTL HFR, BEINTEMA D: *Little Club Clinics in Developmental Medicine,* no 12: *The Neurological Examination of the Full Term Newborn Infant.* London, Heinemann, 1964.

PRECHTL HFR, STEMMER CJ: The choreiform syndrome in children. *Dev Med Child Neurol* 4:119, 1962.

PURPURA DP: Dendritic spine ''dysgenesis'' and mental retardation. *Science* 186:1126, 1974.

RAPIN I, ALLEN DA: Developmental language disorders. Nosologic considerations, in Kirk U (ed): *Neuropsychology of Language, Reading and Spelling.* New York, Academic Press, 1983, pp 155–184.

Raven's Colored Progressive Matrices. New York, Psychological Corporation, 1947–1963.

RENZI E, VIGNOLA LA: Token test: A sensitive test to detect receptive disturbances in aphasics. *Brain* 85:665, 1962.

REISSMAN F: *The Culturally Deprived Child.* New York, Harper & Row, 1962.

RIMLAND B: *Infantile Autism.* New York, Appleton-Century-Crofts, 1964.

RUTTER M, MARTIN JAM (eds): *Clinics in Developmental Medicine, no 43: The Child with Delayed Speech.* London, Heinemann, 1972.

RUTTER M, GRAHAM P, YULE W: *Clinics in Developmental Medicine, nos 35, 36: A Neuropsychiatric Study in Childhood.* London, Heinemann, 1970.

SCARR S, WEBBER RA, CUTTING MA: Personality resemblance among adolescents and their parents in biologically related and adoptive families. *J Pers Soc Psychol* 40:885, 1981.

SCHAIN RJ: *Neurology of Childhood Learning Disorders,* 2nd ed. Baltimore, Williams & Wilkins, 1977.

SCHAIN RJ, FREEDMAN DX: Studies on 5-hydroxyindole metabolism in autistic and other mentally retarded children. *J Pediatr* 58:315, 1961.

SPEARMAN C: *Psychology Down the Ages.* London, Macmillan, 1937.

STAPLES R: Responses of infants to color. *J Exp Psychol* 15:119, 1932.

TIZARD J, O'CONNOR N: The employability of high-grade mentally defectives. *Am J Ment Defic* 54:563, 1950.

TRAVIS LE: *Speech Pathology.* New York, Appleton-Century, 1931.

VOLKMAR FR, COHEN DJ: Neurobiologic aspects of autism. *N Engl J Med* 318:1390, 1988.

WORSTER-DROUGHT C: Congenital suprabulbar paresis. *J Laryngol Otol* 70:453, 1956.

YAKOVLEV PI, LECOURS AR: The myelogenetic cycles of regional maturation of the brain, in Minkowski A (ed): *Regional Development of the Brain in Early Life.* Oxford, Blackwell, 1967, pp 3–70.

ZANGWILL OL: *Cerebral Dominance and Its Psychological Function.* Springfield, IL, Charles C. Thomas, 1960.

CHAPTER 29

THE NEUROLOGY OF AGING

As was remarked in the preceding chapter, standards of growth, development, and maturation are recognized as providing a frame of reference against which every pathologic process in early life must be viewed. However, it has been less appreciated that at the other end of the life cycle neurologic deficits must be judged in a similar way, against a background of normal aging changes. The earliest of these changes begins long before the acknowledged period of senescence and continues throughout the remainder of life. For some reason, perhaps because of man's yearning for lifelong youthfulness and immortality, there has been an unwillingness to accept aging and involution as normal and inevitable phases of life. Not a few medical scientists and physicians believe that all changes in senescence are but the cumulative effects of injury and disease.

As a first generalization, it may be said that the length of life itself, the span of the natural life cycle, is one of the organism's most integral characteristics, genetically programmed in some mysterious way by some kind of biologic death clock. Each species has a characteristic average life span. For the mouse this is 2 years; for the rhesus monkey, 20 to 25 years; for the African elephant, 70 to 75 years; for the Galapagos tortoise, 100 years; and for human beings, about 85 years. Many years ago the German physiologist Max Rubner pointed out that the total number of calories burned per gram of body weight and the total number of heartbeats in the lifetime of each of these mammals and of humans are about the same, despite the great differences in their size and life span. Further, the span of animal and human life correlates roughly with the size of the brain. These observations are intriguing, but their relevance to the aging process is not clear.

The common belief that medical science has greatly lengthened life is a misconception, arising from a failure to distinguish between life span and life expectancy. *Life span* is the average age at which a person would die if he or she had avoided all disease and accidents (i.e., "natural death"). As stated above, this age is fixed biologically and

has been so for millennia. For most persons the clock inevitably runs down by the 85th year, and it seems to make little difference whether one inhabits a luxurious urban apartment or a primitive hut. Only a very small proportion of individuals survive beyond this period. Popular tales about people who are tucked away in the remote regions of the Himalayas, Ecuador, or the Caucasus and live active lives for as long as 120 years or more have proved to be mythical. Actually, by 1988, only one person in the world is known to have lived for 120 years, and survival beyond 112 years has been documented in only three others (two died at 114 years and one at 113 years).

Life expectancy refers to the number of years of life that any individual may statistically expect from birth onward. In contrast to the more or less fixed life span, life expectancy has increased remarkably in the past century. Mainly this has come about through the elimination of fatal infectious diseases in infancy and childhood, allowing an ever increasing number of individuals to attain adult life. Thus, in the United States, the life expectancy of a newborn infant has increased from 50 years in 1900 to 74 years in 1978, and to 77.8 years in the case of a newborn (white) female—a figure approaching the life span. Nevertheless, life expectancy must always fall short of the ideal life span because of the fact that with advancing age there is a steadily increasing susceptibility to fatal disease. The death rate doubles about every 8 years, as we grow older. It has been estimated that if the major causes of death in late adult life and the senium—coronary occlusion and stroke—were eliminated, life expectancy would be extended about 10 years (Preston); if cancer were eliminated completely, life expectancy would be extended only 2 more years.

That the incidence of death increases with age hardly needs to be mentioned, but the particular relationship of one to the other was first recognized in 1825 by the English actuary Benjamin Gompertz. His formulation—that the mortality rate increases exponentially with aging—has been found to apply to many species and is conventionally displayed as a survival curve, in which cumulative survival (percentage of the population remaining alive) is plotted against the age of death. Figure 29-1, taken from Fries and Crapo, displays several such curves—an "ideal" curve, representing the estimated survival if death were due only to trauma and physiologic aging, and the life expectancy curves for 1900 and 1980, based on U.S. Bureau of Health statistics. The figure portrays the dramatic increase in life expectancy in this century. The changing configuration of the life expectancy curve, as it comes to approximate the ideal curve, is spoken of as "rectangularization of the survival curve."

To the biologist and physician, death is not the main consideration. What is more meaningful are indexes of vitality, of resistance to disease, and of organ efficiency. In fact, *senescence* is defined in just such terms, i.e., the progressive diminution of biologic efficiency and capacity of the organism to maintain itself as an efficient machine. A semantic distinction is drawn between the process of aging, or senescence, and the state of being aged, or *senility*. The process of decline or decay that occurs in all organ systems of the body after middle life is called *involution;* unexpected, premature decay of any given tissue or cell population has been termed *abiotrophy*.

The composite of bodily changes due to senescence, such as the cessation of bodily growth, wrinkling of the skin, graying of the hair, loss of teeth, atrophy of gonads, blunting of sensory acuity, stooped posture, loss of muscular strength and endurance, rigidity of mind, and forgetfulness are known to every observant person. Biologists have measured many of these changes. Estimates of structural and functional decline that accompany aging, from 30 to

80 years, are given in Table 29-1. It appears that all structures and functions share in the aging process. It is equally evident, however, that senescence and waning vitality have different times of manifestation and rates of progress in different organs, and that there are wide individual variations as well.

AGING IN THE NERVOUS SYSTEM

Of all the age-related changes, those in the nervous system are of paramount importance. Actors portray old people as feeble, idle, obstinate, given to reminiscing, and walking slowly with a stoop and shuffling steps, with tremulous hands and a soft and quavering voice. In doing so they have selected some of the principal effects of aging on the nervous system. The lay as well as the medical observer is inclined to interpret the changes of advanced age as a kind of second childhood. "Old men are boys again," said Aristophanes. While roughly correct, this view of old age comes largely from certain resemblances, superficial at best, of the senile dement and the helpless young child.

The most consistent neurologic changes in octogenarians, according to Critchley and others, are presbyopia, presbycusis (especially for high tones), diminution in the sense of smell, reduced rate and amount of motor activity,

Figure 29-1

Correlation of mortality rate and age. For details see text. (From Fries and Crapo: Vitality and Aging, Copyright © 1981. All rights reserved.)

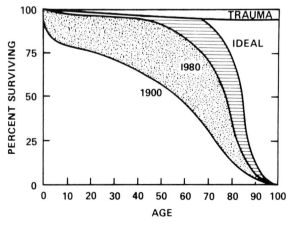

Table 29-1
Physiologic and anatomic deterioration with age

	Percent decrease
Brain weight	15
Blood flow to brain	20
Speed of return of blood acidity to equilibrium after exercise	83
Cardiac output at rest	35
Number of glomeruli in kidney	44
Glomerular filtration rate	31
Number of fibers in nerves	37
Nerve-conduction velocity	10
Number of taste buds	64
Maximum O_2 utilization wth exercise	60
Maximum ventilation volume	47
Maximum breathing capacity	44
Power of hand grip	45
Maximum work rate	30
Basal metabolic rate	16
Body water content	18
Body weight (males)	12

Source: Shock.

slowed reaction time, slowness and narrowed compass of perception (inapperception of the aged), small pupils with restricted pupillary reflexes, limited range of upward gaze, tendency to flexed posture of the trunk and limbs, diminution of vibratory sense in the toes and feet, impairment of fine coordination and agility, reduced muscular power, thinness of the leg muscles, and reduced or absent Achilles reflexes. The most notable of these aging changes, those affecting stance and gait, are described further on in this chapter.

Probably the most detailed information as to the effects of age on the nervous system comes from the measurement of cognitive functions. Cross-sectional studies of large samples of the population, in the course of standardization of the Wechsler Adult Intelligence Scale (1955), indicated that there was a steady decline in cognitive function, starting at 30 years of age and progressing into the senium. Apparently all forms of cognitive function partook of this decline, although, in general, certain elements of the verbal scale (vocabulary, fund of information, and comprehension) withstood the effects of aging better than those of the performance scale (block design, reversal of digits, picture arrangement, object assembly, and the digit symbol task).

This concept of a linear regression of cognitive function with aging has had to be modified in the light of more recent longitudinal studies. If the same individual is examined over a period of many years, there is virtually no decline in his or her performance as measured by tests of verbal function until 70 years of age or more. However, performance on tests of abstraction (e.g., digit symbol substitution) and on tests measuring reaction time or speed in processing information, does decline slowly throughout adult life. And it hardly needs to be pointed out that the ability to memorize and learn, to retain newly acquired information, and to recall names, becomes impaired in elderly individuals, particularly in those more than 70 years of age. These changes, common to most elderly individuals, pose an interesting clinical problem—how to decide whether they are part of the aging process per se or manifestations of Alzheimer disease. The differentiation can usually be made by careful mental status testing, along the lines already described in Chap. 20. Several abbreviated tests of mental status have been developed and are of practical value (Kokmen et al; Folstein et al), in that they can be given at the bedside in 5 min or so. Items such as repetition of auditorily presented digits, orientation as to place and time, capacity to learn and to retain several items, tests of arithmetic and calculation, etc., reveal that the normal aging person scores twice as well as the Alzheimer patient.

The foregoing effects of age on mental abilities are extremely variable. Some 70-year-olds perform better on psychologic testing than some "normal" 20-year-olds. And a few individuals retain exceptional mental power and perform creative work until late life. Verdi, for example, composed *Otello* at the age of 73 years and *Falstaff* at 79. Humboldt wrote the five volumes of his *Kosmos* between the ages of 76 and 89 years; Goethe produced the second part of *Faust* when he was more than 70 years old; and Galileo, Laplace, and Sherrington continued to make scientific contributions in their eighth decades. It must be pointed out, however, that these accomplishments were essentially continuations of lines of endeavor that had been initiated in early adult life. Indeed, little that is new and original is started after the fortieth year. High intelligence, well-organized work habits, and sound judgment compensate for many of the progressive deficiencies of old age.

Personality Changes in the Aged These are less easily measured, but nevertheless certain trends are observable and may seriously disturb the lives of aged persons and those around them. Many old people become opinionated, self-centered, rigid, and conservative; the opposite qualities—undue pliancy, vacillation, and the uncritical acceptance of ideas—are observed in a few. Often these changes are recognized as exaggerations of lifelong personality traits. Many elderly persons seem to lack self-confidence and require a strong probability of success before undertaking certain tasks. Whereas environment plays a part in molding these traits, Kallman's studies of senescent monozygotic twins suggest that genetic factors are more important. Aggressive individuals with much energy and a diversity of interests, leading to a wide range of social interactions, appear to resist the ravages of age better than those with the opposite tendencies. But this may be effect rather than cause. Those with depressive tendencies are more easily overwhelmed by the prospects of the senium and adopt an attitude of hopelessness, fear, suspicion, and worry. This may explain the threefold increase in suicides in late middle life and old age. Certainly an agitated depression is the most frequent psychiatric disease of these periods of life.

One of the weaknesses of all studies of the aged has been the bias of population selection. Many of the reported observations have been restricted to decrepit individuals in homes for the aged. Examination of functionally intact old people of comparable age, such as that of Kokmen and his colleagues, reveals fewer deficits, limited mainly to forgetfulness of names, diminished vibratory sense in the feet, diminished ankle jerks, and slight loss of agility.

Morphologic Basis of Involutional Changes in the Nervous System This has never been fully established. From the third decade of life to the beginning of the tenth decade, the weight of the average male brain declines from 1394 to 1161 g, a loss of 233 g. This is based presumably on a degeneration of neurons and replacement gliosis. The loss amounts to about 25 percent for lumbosacral anterior horn cells, sensory ganglion cells, putaminal and Purkinje cells. Not all neuronal groups are equally susceptible. The locus ceruleus and substantia nigra lose about 35 percent of their neurons between youth and old age, whereas the vestibular nuclei and inferior olives maintain a fairly constant number of cells throughout life. A progressive loss, decade by decade, of certain systems of myelinated fibers of the spinal cord has been convincingly demonstrated by Morrison.

The neuronal population in the neocortex is progressively depleted in the seventh, eighth, and ninth decades. The greatest loss appears to be among the small neurons of the second and fourth layers (external and internal granular laminae) in the frontal and superior temporal regions where it approaches 50 percent by the ninth decade. Cell loss in the limbic system (cingulate, hippocampal and parahippocampal gyri) is of special interest. Ball has measured the neuronal loss in the hippocampus and records a linear decrease of over 25 percent between 45 and 95 years of age. Neuronal loss and replacement gliosis, which we regard as the primary aging changes, proceed without relationship to Alzheimer neurofibrillary changes and senile plaques (Kemper).

In addition to the cell loss, Scheibel et al have described a loss of neuronal dendrites in the aging brain, particularly the horizontal dendrites of the third and fifth layers of the neocortex. However, the careful morphometric studies of Buell and Coleman have shown that the surviving neurons exhibit expanded dendritic trees, suggesting that even aging neurons have the capacity to react to cell loss by growing new synapses.

With advancing age, there is an increasing tendency for "senile plaques" to appear in the inferomedial parts of the temporal lobes (hippocampus and parahippocampus). These are loose aggregates of amorphous argentophilic material containing amyloid. They occur in increasing numbers in the senile, and by the ninth decade of life few cerebra are without them. However, as shown by Tomlinson and his colleagues, relatively few plaques are present in the cerebra of mentally intact old people, in contrast to the large numbers in the Alzheimer disease–senile dementia group. More impressively, only very small numbers of neurons showing neurofibrillary and granulovacuolar changes, essentially confined to the hippocampus and adjacent temporal cortex, may be found in mentally sound individuals, whereas these changes are frequent in the Alzheimer cases.

Several investigators cite the senile plaques and Alzheimer type of fibrillary change as the principal alterations of the aging process in the human nervous system. Roth et al determined a correlation of 0.8 between the

incidence of these changes and the presence as well as degree of dementia. These authors and others have used this finding to support the argument that the Alzheimer disease–senile dementia complex simply represents an acceleration of the natural aging process in the brain. We are more inclined to the idea that these changes represent an *acquired age-linked disease*, analogous to certain cerebrovascular diseases. In support of this latter view are the observations that (1) *Homo sapiens* is the only animal species in which Alzheimer fibrillary changes and senile plaques are found regularly in the aging brain (a few plaque-like structures, but no neurofibrillary changes, have been seen occasionally in old dogs or monkeys); it seems to us unbiologic that human aging should differ from that of all other animal species. (2) Some of the most severe forms of Alzheimer disease occur in middle adult life, long before the senium. (3) These histopathologic changes in variable form occur in a number of other human diseases, such as dementia pugilistica or the punch-drunk state, Down syndrome, postencephalitic Parkinson disease, and progressive supranuclear palsy. (4) Neurofibrillary tangles can be reproduced in the experimental animal by such toxins as aluminum, vincristine, vinblastine, and colchicine. We decided, therefore, that Alzheimer disease is more appropriately considered under degenerative diseases (see Chap. 43), where the entire subject will be discussed further.

Increasing accumulation of lipofuscin granules (see below), sometimes extreme in degree, accompanies advancing age, being especially prominent in the inferior olivary, thalamic and certain other neurons. Amyloid bodies, formed by astrocytes, increase in number. Granulovacuolar changes are a regular finding in the aging hippocampi regardless of the mental state of the individual. Clearly these are aging effects. In addition, slight thickening and hyalinization of the walls of small blood vessels and pericapillary fibrosis also become more evident in the aging brain, and there is a natural inclination to assume this to be the basis of the reduced blood flow that has been reported by several investigators. Many of the small arteries contain amyloid in their walls. Such changes are probably not primary but secondary to reduced circulatory need (the so-called vascular atrophy of involuting organs). There is no evidence that the aforementioned aging changes, which are often loosely referred to as arteriosclerotic, depend on any recognized form of vascular disease.

Many biochemical studies have been made of the effects of aging on cerebral tissues. As would be expected, the substances found in neurons and their medullated fibers diminish in proportion to the loss of these cellular components. DNA, RNA, cerebrosides, and other components of myelin diminish in the brains of aged, mentally intact humans and old animals; intracellular enzymes also diminish. In the intact organism the cerebral uptake of oxygen and glucose are reduced in advanced age, while the cerebral blood flow is essentially unchanged (Dastur et al). The problems raised by all these studies is whether the changes reflect a primary effect of aging or merely the loss of neurons and gliosis.

With respect to the neurotransmitters, it is generally agreed that the amount of striatal dopamine declines in the course of normal aging. However, an accurate assessment of other neurotransmitters has not been possible, because of their marked lability in postmortem material. Choline acetyltransferase, the synthesizing enzyme of acetylcholine, is stable in autopsied brain and has been found to decrease in the aging hippocampus and temporal neocortex (Bowen et al, Davies). Again, the significance of this change is difficult to judge. It may simply reflect the depletion of cells that occurs with aging. The cells of origin of the cholinergic neurotransmitters—the nucleus of Meynert and other nuclei of the basal forebrain (substantia innominata) have not been counted in normal aged individuals but are greatly reduced in number in Alzheimer disease (Whitehouse et al).

AGING CHANGES IN MUSCLES AND NERVES

With advancing age, skeletal muscles lose cells (fibers), and undergo a gradual reduction in their weight more or less parallel to that of the brain. Atrophy of muscle and diminution in peak power and endurance are the clinical expressions of these changes. Our own studies indicate that the wasting involves several processes, some principally myopathic, others denervative from loss of motor neurons. The muscle fibers that are lost are gradually replaced by endomysial connective tissue and fat cells. The surviving fibers are generally thinner than normal (possibly disuse atrophy), but some enlarge, resulting in a wider range of fiber size. Groups of fibers all at the same stage of atrophy undoubtedly relate to loss of motor innervation. The reduction in conduction velocity of motor nerves and, to a greater extent, of sensory nerves in the aged may be taken as another index of loss of motor and sensory axons. All these changes are more marked in the legs than elsewhere.

CHANGES IN LUNGS, HEART, KIDNEYS, SKIN AND SUPPORTING TISSUES, AND ENDOCRINE GLANDS

A textbook of neurology is not the place to itemize these age-linked alterations. It need only be pointed out that each system undergoes a significant regression that seems to be due to age alone and not to any known disease. In many instances the effects of aging in these organs have not been as well studied as those in the nervous system; apparently the diseases in these other organs are so much more dramatic and interesting than the biologic changes due to aging that the latter have been ignored to a large extent. Moreover, little is known of the extent to which these extracerebral changes are determinative of those in the nervous system, either the neuronal aging or the age-linked degenerative diseases.

THE CELLULAR BASIS OF AGING

Many mechanisms are presumed to be involved in the aging process of the cellular constituents and the structural protein (collagen) of the various bodily organs. Recent investigative efforts have been directed along these lines: (1) the decline in functional efficiency and finally the deterioration and death of highly specialized nondividing cells such as the neuron and to some extent the muscle fiber; (2) the failure of cell multiplication and of mitosis in tissues composed of dividing cells; and (3) the progressive alteration of the structural protein collagen, which constitutes about 40 percent of the body protein and serves as the binding substance of the skin, muscle, bones, and blood vessels.

LIFE SPAN AND AGING OF SPECIALIZED CELLS

As was said, nerve and muscle cells, which cease early to divide and are in near-maximum number at birth, must last the lifetime of the individual. Once destroyed, whether by aging or disease, they are never replaced. Obviously the life span is not the same for every cell; some survive longer than others. If a significant number die early, functional deficits result. It seems that the outfall of neurons begins soon after the end of the period of growth and maturation, and it accelerates in the last decades of life. The point at which functional deficits appear varies for each system, depending upon its "safety factor," i.e., the protective excess of cells that must be lost before symptoms appear. Whether cells falter functionally before their final disintegration is unknown. It seems likely that they do, in view of the shrinkage of their dendritic surface, noted by Scheibel et al.

The cytologic events that lead to the death of nondividing cells are little understood. In humans as well as in animals, accumulation of lipofuscin in the cytoplasm is a phenomenon of such constancy that it can be used as a reliable cytologic index of aging. Called "wear and tear" or "age" pigment, these yellow granules of lipochrome, or lipofuscin, form in the cytoplasm of both nerve and muscle cells, in close relation to lysosomes. Simultaneously, the cell diminishes in volume, due presumably to the loss of other cytoplasmic components such as Nissl bodies (the main cytoplasmic RNA of neurons) and mitochondria. The nucleus becomes smaller with infolding of the nuclear membrane and alteration of the nucleolus. Histochemical stains reveal a depletion of oxidative as well as phosphorylative and presumably other enzymes. Neurons are said to lose dendrites and thereby reduce their synaptic surface (Scheibel et al). All these changes have been observed in cultured cells.

Considering the ubiquitous nature of these morphologic changes, it is remarkable that we know so little of their pathogenesis. They have been attributed to progressive exhaustion of cell catalysts (enzymes and coenzymes), but this explanation only restates the problem in rather speculative biochemical terms. It is generally believed that the accumulation of lipofuscin is the result of oxidation of lipids, polymerized with protein and unsaturated peptides, which are released when a cell ages or undergoes necrosis for any reason. According to this view, any factor (e.g., hemorrhage into fatty tissue) which increases the ratio of tissue oxidant to antioxidant favors the accumulation of lipofuscin. Biologic antioxidants such as vitamins C and E, glutathione, cysteine, and sulfhydryl proteins are said to counteract the process.

The concept of lipoidal degeneration of neurons, long a favorite topic of neuropathologists, has its advocates and opponents. The older idea was that the accumulation of lipofuscin was a stage in a degenerative process. An equally tenable view, now with more proponents, is that the sequestration of lysosomes and lipofuscin is a protective mechanism against neuronal degeneration.

LOSS OF CAPACITY FOR CELL MULTIPLICATION AND AGING OF COLLAGEN

The studies of Hayflick and his colleagues on the innate capacity of cells to divide in tissue culture may shed light on this problem. They found that fibroblasts can divide only a finite number of times (contrary to Alexis Carrel's original claim that chicken heart cells, nourished in tissue culture, could continue to live and divide forever). Fibroblasts of a human infant divide about 50 times, those of a 20-year-old about 30 times, and those of an 80-year-old about 20 times. Probably glial cells, leukocytes, and liver cells also possess a limited, genetically determined capacity for mitosis. Toward the end of the life cycle of cultured cells, chromosomal aberrations and peculiarities of cell division appear in some cells. Whether or not these types of cell abnormalities are a characteristic feature of human aging has not been settled. Only if neoplastic transformation takes place (the normal 46-chromosome diploid cell becomes "mixoploid," with 50 to 350 abnormal chromosomes) do cells approach the immortality postulated by Carrel.

Hayflick sees in this aging process and finite lifetime of normal cells a deterioration of the genetic program that "orchestrates" the development of cells. He has postulated that with increasing age the DNA protein-synthesizing apparatus of the dividing cells falls prey to an ever-increasing number of copying errors (as might occur with radiation). The faulty templates serve as faulty models for the production of more faulty enzymes, leading eventually to death of the cell.

Finally, it should be noted that tissue collagen, like nondividing cells, undergoes aging changes in its molecular structure, which progressively diminishes its elasticity and contractility.

AGE-RELATED DISEASES

The fundamental processes of aging, outlined above, operate during all of adult life, and if the person survives long enough, he or she will succumb to the ultimate failure of normal cells to divide or function. However, few people die of old age alone. Most of them die of diseases, to which they are rendered increasingly susceptible by the aging processes. The most common of these are neoplasia, vascular diseases of the heart and brain, fractures of the hip, infections (chiefly pulmonary), and in our opinion, Alzheimer disease. Not only do these diseases increase in frequency with advancing age, but they do so exponentially, like death itself.

Cerebral atherosclerosis is, of course, a frequent finding in the elderly. It does not parallel age with any degree of precision, being severe in some 30- to 40-year-old individuals and practically absent in some octogenarians. In the normotensive it tends to occur in scattered, discrete plaques mostly in the cervical arteries and basal parts of the cerebral arterial system. In the hypertensive it is more diffuse and extends into finer branches of the cerebral and cerebellar arteries. Superficial cerebral softenings (thrombotic and embolic, old and recent) have been found in about half of all individuals over 70 years who have been examined post-mortem. Even without atherosclerosis, which is obviously a disease, the basal arteries undergo other changes in the aged, being somewhat larger and more tortuous and much more opaque than the arteries of a younger person.

While the skull thickens with age, the condition known as *hyperostosis frontalis interna* (Stewart-Morel-Morgagni syndrome) is exclusively a disease of older women. It is said to be joined frequently with obesity and hirsutism. Its neurologic implications are vague, and there has always been a temptation to ascribe more to it than it deserves. At autopsy, aside from close attachment of the dura and opacity of the underlying pia-arachnoid (milk spots), we have observed no consistent neuropathologic lesion.

Likewise, most tumors occur with increasing frequency in early and middle adult life. Only in the most advanced age period does the incidence tend to fall. The cytoplasmic events leading to neoplasia must relate to the process of cell division; postmitotic neurons rarely give rise to tumors. One evidence of this relationship is the tendency of tumors to develop, in many organs, in experimental animals exposed to gamma radiation, and the linear relationship between the intensity of exposure and frequency of tumor formation. One class of endocrine tumors appears to form during periods of intensified functional demands, e.g., hypophysial adenomas with atrophy of gonads and adrenals during late adult life. Reference has already been made to the chromosomal aberrations that appear in older dividing cells. An example is the trisomy of the Down syndrome, which occurs with increasing frequency as the oocyte ages in the later part of reproductive life.

As to the older person's intolerance of infection, it may well relate to failure of the aging organism to adapt to change, rather than to any failure of the inflammatory process. Older people are slower in adjusting to high and low atmospheric temperatures, but their levels of antibodies, production of leukocytes, and vigor of cellular immune response are all suprisingly well maintained. Nonetheless, with age, changes of immune function may result in the synthesis of abnormal immune products that contribute to neurologic disease or increase the susceptibility to infection; or, possibly, age-dependent changes in the nervous system may in some way impair immune regulation (Stefansson et al).

The high incidence of adverse drug reactions in the elderly is related to several factors—the increased duration and severity of disease, the frequent failure to adjust drug dosage to diminished body weight, a reduction in renal clearance, and an increased sensitivity to certain agents, notably heparin and sedatives, such as the benzodiazepine derivatives.

In every major illness in the elderly, the exigencies of disease cannot be met efficiently because of a combination of organ inadequacies, no single one of which is of sufficient severity to be manifest clinically. The sum total of these organ deficits constitutes a kind of gestalt of senility. The long list of diseases found in the elderly at autopsy reflects the increasing susceptibility to disease with aging. However, the contributing effects of the aging processes are relatively

inapparent, which is the reason the student so often asks, after the autopsy of the elderly person, "But what was the cause of death?"

DEGENERATIVE DISEASES OF THE NERVOUS SYSTEM IN THE AGED

GENERALIZED DEGENERATIVE DISEASE— ALZHEIMER–SENILE DEMENTIA COMPLEX

To be distinguished from the slight shrinkage and loss of weight of the brain that occurs in the majority of older people are the severe degrees of diffuse cerebral atrophy that evolve relatively rapidly in the senile or presenile periods. The latter states are invariably associated with dementia and the underlying pathologic changes prove most frequently to be those of *Alzheimer disease*. For reasons that have been given (see above, under "Aging in the Nervous System"), this disease and other age-linked degenerative diseases will be described in Chap. 43.

RESTRICTED DEGENERATIVE DISORDERS

Abnormalities of Gait Human motor agility actually begins to decline in early adult life, even by the thirtieth year, and it seems to be related to a gradual decrease in neuromuscular control as well as to changes in joints and other structures. The reality of this motor decrement is best appreciated by professional baseball or tennis players who retire at 35 or soon thereafter because their legs give out and cannot be restored to their maximal condition by training. They cannot run as well as younger colleagues even though the coordination of their arms in hitting a ball may still be preserved. The older person becomes less confident in walking; touching the handrail in descending stairs is now needed to prevent a misstep. Putting on pants (standing on one leg) becomes difficult. Handwriting tends to worsen, and choking on food is more frequent. Doubtless this complex of motor impairments is based on the aforementioned neuronal losses in the spinal cord, cerebellum, and cerebrum.

A small proportion of the aging population suffers an inordinate deterioration of gait while remaining relatively competent in other ways. In all likelihood, this is an age-linked degenerative disorder of the brain, since most instances of it are sooner or later accompanied by mental changes. As indicated in Chap. 6, gait in the elderly is shorter of step, slower, and more guarded. All the movements are less graceful, more inelastic. The patient looks to the ground and finds it difficult to walk and converse at the same time. The posture of the body is more flexed. The old soldier must now remind himself repeatedly to maintain his bearing. Gradually as the steps shorten, the feet barely clear the ground and finally are merely shuffled forward, a state referred to as *marche à petit pas* (the short-stepped gait). In some instances the patient upon arising from a chair finds it difficult to initiate the first step even though while lying in bed there is no difficulty in moving the legs. After a tremulous pause the first step is finally taken, and the next ones proceed in the customary shuffle. Taking a patient's arm, and walking alongside and urging him or her to keep step with a marching cadence may improve the gait disorder at this stage. Other patients may ascribe the trouble to a loss of confidence or a fright from a bad fall and may ask for gait training, which will not help them. The inexperienced physician may suspect a functional disorder.

In the clinical analysis of such patients one should search for evidence of posterior column or cerebellar ataxia and the spastic ataxia of cervical spondylosis, all of which may unbalance the patient. One recognizes, in several features of the gait disorder, elements of the Parkinson syndrome. Obesity and hypertrophic arthritis of hips and knees or an old hip fracture add to any gait difficulty. Normal-pressure hydrocephalus, correctable by a ventriculoperitoneal shunt, accounts for the gait disorder of some of these senile patients.

The basis of this peculiar gait is probably a combined frontal lobe–basal ganglionic degeneration, the anatomy of which has never been fully clarified. It has been speculated that age-related loss of neurons in the substantia nigra and alterations in the nigrostriatal dopaminergic system may be responsible for the gait disorder, but it does not respond to the administration of L-dopa or to any other therapeutic measures. In its most advanced form the capacity for upright stance and walking is completely lost, and the patient eventually lies curled up in bed in a state of *cerebral paraplegia in flexion* (Fig. 6-1).

Other Restricted Motor Abnormalities in the Aged These are too numerous to be more than cataloged. They inform us of the many ways in which the motor system can deteriorate. *Compulsive, repetitive movements* are the most frequent: mouthing movements, stereotyped grimacing, protrusion of the tongue, side-to-side or to-and-fro tremor of the head, odd vocalizations such as sniffing, snorting, and bleating. In some respects these disorders resemble tics (voluntary movements to relieve tension), but careful observation shows that they are not really voluntary. Haloperidol and other drugs of this class have an unpredictable therapeutic effect, seeming at times to benefit the patient only by the superimposition of a drug-induced rigidity. The differential diagnosis must raise for consideration one of the phenothiazine-induced faciolingual dyskinesias.

Old age is thought always to carry a liability to tremulousness, and, indeed, one sees such patients from

time to time in the clinic. The head, the chin, or the hands tremble and the voice quavers, yet there is not the usual slowness of movement, immobility, facial impassivity, or flexed posture that would stamp the condition as parkinsonian. Some instances are clearly familial, having appeared or worsened only late in life. Cessation of fast-frequency action tremors in response to alcohol and beta-adrenergic blocking agents also support the idea that certain cases are familial in nature (see page 81). The relation to senility is always open to doubt. Charcot, in a review of over 2000 elderly inhabitants at the Salpetrière, could find only about 30 with tremor.

Spastic dysphonia, a disorder of middle and late life characterized by spasm of all the throat muscles on attempted speech, has been discussed on page 392. *Blepharoclonus* or *blepharospasm,* a somewhat similar involuntary movement of the eyelids, is described on page 88.

GERONTOLOGIC NEUROLOGY

This is the branch of medicine that deals with all of the effects of aging upon the nervous system—both of aging itself and of the age-related diseases—as well as with the medical care of the elderly *(geriatrics)*. Unlike pediatric neurology, these disciplines have not aroused much interest. The young physician is more excited by disease than by the seemingly immutable changes due to aging and questions whether medicine has a significant role to play in the care of the neurologic disorders of the elderly.

The authors would answer this question affirmatively and would point out that the majority of all neurologic patients seen in practice are elderly, especially if one includes those with vascular diseases of the brain. Furthermore, many of their diseases are preventable or therapeutically controllable. Since aging changes do not involve all organs and tissues simultaneously, patients need help and advice about certain of these effects at a time when most of their organs are functionally intact. Some of the age-related chemical deficiencies (vitamin B_{12} deficiency, diabetes mellitus) and many of the common restricted involutional changes (presbyopia, etc.) can be corrected. Others can even be turned into assets; the forgetfulness of the aged and their deafness may serve to excuse many of their shortcomings and to spare them effort and annoyance.

Some physicians hesitate to interpret any change as involutional until the patient is past the biblical three score years and ten or may avoid the diagnosis altogether because it implies an incurable condition. Their reasoning is faulty in both instances. Many involutional changes such as presbyopia can be demonstrated in their larval stages in the twenties, and by the mid-forties failing visual accommodation is almost universal. The disorder of uric acid metabolism causing gout is manifested before the age of 40 years in an appreciable percentage of all those afflicted. Many restricted forms of involution or abiotrophy, after rapid progress for a few years, become arrested or progress very slowly and are compensated for in many ways.

In a more general way, geriatric medicine should present the physician's view of what is needed for the ideal care of the elderly. Obviously the primary concern of the physician is with the diagnosis and management of the patient's illness(es). But once this has been accomplished, attention should turn to the multitude of functional impairments that afflict the elderly patient—the simple matters of dressing, bathing, shopping, cooking, management of money, and so forth. In the end it is upon these functional incapacities that the physician must focus, to decide what help the patient requires and to involve the appropriate social agencies in providing this help. The disposition of a patient to the independence of an apartment or to dependency on a nursing home may depend on so mundane a matter as to whether he or she can get from bed to bathroom.

In the past, when America's population was predominantly rural, elderly individuals were cared for by their relatives in their own homes, but this is often impossible or undesirable in present-day urban society. Also, in the past, the younger generation was spared much of the responsibility for the care of their parents because of the high incidence among the elderly of vascular disease, neoplasia, and particularly infection. In the nineteenth century, when pneumonia was more frequently lethal than now, Osler referred to it as the "old man's friend," for, as in Ecclesiastes, he considered death as a kindness to the old and feeble. As medical science and public health measures brought these and other diseases under control, the number of elderly persons increased, and will continue to do so. The census bureau has estimated that by the year 2000 there will be 31 million persons over the age of 65 in the United States, and that 13 million of them will be over 75 years. As the number of elderly increases, the need for looking after them will occupy more and more of the energies of physicians and of society at large.

REFERENCES

BALL MJ: Neuronal loss, neurofibrillary tangles and granulovacuolar degeneration in the hippocampus with aging and dementia. *Acta Neuropathol* 27:111, 1977.

BEHNKE JA, FINCH CE, MOMENT BG (eds): *The Biology of Aging.* New York, Plenum, 1978.

BLESSED G, TOMLINSON BE, ROTH M: The association between quantitative measures of dementia and of senile change in the cerebral grey matter of elderly subjects. *Br J Psychiatry* 114:797, 1968.

BOWEN DM, WHITE P, SPILLANE JA et al: Accelerated aging or selective neuronal loss as an important cause of dementia. *Lancet* 1:11, 1979.

BUELL SJ, COLEMAN PD: Dendritic growth in the aged human brain and failure of growth in senile dementia. *Science* 206:854, 1979.

CARREL A: On the permanent life of tissues outside of the organism. *J Exp Med* 15:516, 1912.

COMFORT A: *The Biology of Senescence,* 3rd ed. New York, Elsevier, 1979.

CRITCHLEY M: Neurologic changes in the aged. *J Chron Dis* 3:459, 1956.

DASTUR DK, LANE MH, HANSEN DB et al: Effects of aging on cerebral circulation and metabolism in man, in Birren JE, Butler RN, Greenhouse SW et al (eds): *Human Aging.* Public Health Service Publication No. 986, 1963, pp 59–76.

DAVIES P: The neurochemistry of Alzheimer's disease and senile dementia. *Med Res Rev* 3:221, 1983.

FOLSTEIN MF, FOLSTEIN SE, MCHUGH PR: "Mini-mental state": A practical method for grading the cognitive state of patients for the clinician. *J Psychiatry Res* 12:189, 1975.

FRIES JF: Aging, natural death, and the compression of morbidity. *N Engl J Med* 303:130, 1980.

FRIES JF, CRAPO LM: *Vitality and Aging.* San Francisco, Freeman, 1981.

HARTROFT WS, PORTA EA: Ceroid. *Am J Med Sci* 250:324, 1965.

HAYFLICK L: The cell biology of human aging. *N Engl J Med* 295:1302, 1976.

KALLMANN FJ: Genetic factors in aging: Comparative and longitudinal observations on a senescent twin population, in Hoch PH, Zubin J (eds): *Psychopathology of Aging.* New York, Grune & Stratton, 1961.

KATZMAN R, TERRY RD: *The Neurology of Aging.* Philadelphia, Davis, 1983.

KAY DWK, BEAMISH P, ROTH M: Old age mental disorder in Newcastle-upon-Tyne. I: A study of prevalence. *Br J Psychiatry* 110:146, 1964.

KEMPER T: Neuroanatomical and neuropathological changes in normal aging and in dementia, in Albert ML (ed): *Clinical Neurology of Aging.* New York, Oxford University Press, 1984, pp 9–52.

KOKMEN E, BOSSEMEYER RW Jr, BARNEY J, WILLIAMS WJ: Neurologic manifestations of aging. *J Gerontol* 32:411, 1977.

KOKMEN E, NAESSENS JM, OFFORD KP: A short test of mental status: Description and preliminary results. *Mayo Clin Proc* 62:281, 1987.

MCFARLAND D: The aged in the 21st century: A demographer's view, in Jarvik LF (ed): *Aging into the 21st Century: Middle-agers Today.* New York, Gardner Press, 1978, chap 1, pp 5–22.

MEDAWAR PB: The definition and measurement of senescence, in Wolstenholme GEW, Cameron MP (eds): *Ciba Foundation*

Colloquia on Aging, vol 1. Boston, Little, Brown, 1955, pp 4–15.

MORRISON LR: *The Effect of Advancing Age upon the Human Spinal Cord.* Cambridge, MA, Harvard, 1959.

OBRIST WD: The EEG of normal aged adults. *Electroencephalogr Clin Neurophysiol* 6:235, 1954.

PRESTON SH: *Mortality Patterns in National Populations.* New York, Academic Press, 1976.

ROTH M, TOMLINSON BE, BLESSED G: Correlation between scores for dementia and counts of senile plaques in cerebral grey matter of elderly subjects. *Nature* 209:109, 1966.

SAMORAJSKI T, ORDY JM: The neurochemistry of aging, in Gaitz CM (ed): *Aging and the Brain.* New York, Plenum Press, 1976, pp 41–63.

SCHEIBEL M, LINDSAY RD, TOMIYASU U, SCHEIBEL AB: Progressive dendritic changes in aging human cortex. *Exp Neurol* 47:392, 1975.

SHOCK NW: The physiology of aging. *Sci Am* 206:100, 1962.

STEFANSSON K, ANTEL J, ARNASON BGW: Neuroimmunology of Aging, in Albert ML (ed): *Clinical Neurology of Aging.* New York, Oxford University Press, 1984, pp 76–94.

TOMLINSON BE, BLESSED G, ROTH M: Observations on the brains of nondemented old people. *J Neurol Sci* 7:331, 1968.

VERZAR F: The aging of collagen. *Sci Am* 208:104, 1963.

WECHSLER D: *Manual for the Wechsler Adult Intelligence Scale.* New York, The Psychological Corporation, 1955.

WELLS CE: *Dementia,* 2nd ed, *Contemporary Neurology Series.* Philadelphia, Davis, 1977.

WHITEHOUSE PJ, CLARK AW, PRICE DL et al: Alzheimer's disease (AD): Loss of cholinergic neurons in the nucleus basalis. *J Neuropathol Exp Neurol* 40:323, 1981.

THE MAJOR CATEGORIES OF NEUROLOGIC DISEASE

CHAPTER 30

DISTURBANCES OF CEREBROSPINAL FLUID CIRCULATION, INCLUDING HYDROCEPHALUS AND MENINGEAL REACTIONS

Examination of the cerebrospinal fluid (CSF) as a diagnostic aid in neurology was discussed in Chap. 2, and the primary inflammatory diseases of the pia-arachnoid (leptomeninges) and ependyma of the ventricles will be considered in Chap. 32. Further, in many chapters to follow, the ways in which the CSF reflects the basic pathologic processes in a wide variety of metabolic, neoplastic, and degenerative diseases will be considered. The latter raise so many interesting and important problems that we considered it advantageous to discuss in one place the mechanisms involved in the formation, circulation, and absorption of the CSF, as well as the disturbances of CSF circulation, particularly increased intracranial pressure (ICP), hydrocephalus, and meningeal hydrops. Also, it is appropriate to discuss in this chapter some of the basic reactions of the ependyma and meninges to bacterial infections and to other infectious and chemical agents.

A few historical points will call to mind how recent is our knowledge of the physiology, chemistry, and cytology of the CSF. Although the lumbar puncture was introduced by Quincke in 1891, it was not until 1912 that Mestrazat made the first correlations between various diseases and the cellular and chemical changes in the CSF, and only in 1937 did Merritt and Fremont-Smith publish their classic monograph on the CSF changes in all types of disease. Most of our detailed knowledge of CSF cytology has accumulated in the last 20 years, since the introduction of the Millipore filter. The studies of Dandy in 1919 and of Weed in 1935 provide the basis of our knowledge of CSF formation, circulation, and absorption; and the studies of Pappenheimer and of Ames and their colleagues and the monographs of Fishman and of Davson and coworkers are the most important recent contributions.

PHYSIOLOGY OF THE CSF

The CSF occupies somewhat less than 10 percent of the intracranial and intraspinal spaces. In the adult, the average intracranial volume is 1700 mL; the volume of the brain is approximately 1400 mL, CSF volume is 150 mL, and blood volume is 150 mL. The proportion of CSF in the ventricles and cisternae and in the subarachnoid spaces between the cerebral hemispheres and in the sulci varies with age. These variations have been plotted in CT scans by Meese et al; the distance between the lateral ventricles gradually widens from 1.0 to 1.5 cm, and the width of the third ventricle increases from 3 to 6 mm (by age 60).

FORMATION

The introduction of the ventriculocisternal perfusion technique by Pappenheimer and his colleagues made possible the accurate measurement of the rates of formation and absorption of the CSF. It is now well established that the mean rate of CSF formation is between 14 and 36 mL/h. Since the volume of CSF is approximately 150 mL, the CSF as a whole is renewed four or five times daily.

The choroid plexuses are the source of about 80 percent of the CSF (some CSF is formed even after the choroid plexuses are removed). The thin-walled vessels of the plexuses allow passive diffusion of substances from the blood plasma into the extracellular space surrounding choroid cells. Also, the choroidal epithelial cells, like other secretory epithelia, contain organelles, indicating their capacity for secretory function, i.e., "active transport." The blood vessels in the subependymal regions and the pia also contribute to the CSF, and some substances enter the

CSF as readily from the meninges as from the choroid plexuses. Thus, electrolytes equilibrate with the CSF at all points in the ventricular and subarachnoid spaces, and the same is true of glucose. The transport of sodium, the main cation of the CSF, is under the influence of a sodium-potassium–activated pump in the choroid plexus cells; and drugs that inhibit this system reduce CSF formation (Cutler and Spertell). Electrolytes enter the ventricles more readily than the subarachnoid space (water does the opposite). The penetration of certain other drugs and metabolites is in direct relation to their lipid solubility. Ionized compounds, such as the amino acids, being relatively insoluble in lipids, enter the CSF slowly, unless facilitated by a membrane transport system. The latter is influenced by the small difference in pH between blood and CSF. Certain hydrophilic molecules, such as sugars, are able to enter the CSF and the intercellular fluid only if they have a molecular configuration that conforms to that of a stereospecific carrier transport system.

Diffusion gradients appear to determine the entry of serum proteins into the CSF and also the exchanges of CO_2. Water diffuses as readily from blood to CSF and intercellular spaces as in the reverse direction. This explains the rapid effects of intravenously injected hypotonic and hypertonic fluids.

Studies using radioisotopic tracer techniques have shown that the various constituents of the CSF (see Table 2-1) are in dynamic equilibrium with the blood. Similarly, CSF in the ventricles and subarachnoid spaces is in equilibrium with the intercellular fluid of the brain, spinal cord, and olfactory and optic nerves. The terms *blood-CSF barrier* and *blood-brain barrier* are used to indicate the relative or absolute exclusion of many substances in the blood from the CSF and from the intercellular fluid of the brain and spinal cord. The site of the barrier varies for the different plasma constituents. One is the endothelium of the choroidal and brain capillaries; another is the plasma membrane and the adventitia (Rouget cells) of the vessels; a third is pericapillary, the foot processes of astrocytes. Large molecules such as albumin (molecular weight of 69,000) are prevented from entry by the capillary endothelium, and this is the barrier also for such molecules as are bound to albumin, e.g., aniline dyes (trypan blue) and bilirubin. Thus it is that aniline dyes injected into the blood will not penetrate nervous tissues but will do so if injected into the subarachnoid space (the barriers are thus circumvented). Metallic ions attached to serum proteins tend to deposit on the plasma membrane and in the perithelium. The various substances formed in the nervous system during its metabolic

activity diffuse rapidly into the CSF. Thus the CSF has a kind of "sink action," to use Davson's term, by which the products of brain metabolism are removed to the blood stream as CSF is absorbed.

ABSORPTION

The absorption of CSF is through the arachnoid villi. These structures are most numerous over the superior surfaces of the cerebral hemispheres (the large ones in the adult are called pacchionian granulations) but are also present at the base of the brain and around the spinal nerve roots. These arachnoid villi penetrate meningeal veins and dural sinus walls, and have been thought to act as functional valves that permit "bulk flow" of CSF into the vascular lumen unidirectionally. However, electron microscopic studies have shown that the arachnoid villi have a continuous membranous covering. The latter is extremely thin, and CSF passes through the villi at a linearly increasing rate with CSF pressures above 68 mmH₂O. Tripathi and Tripathi, in serial electron micrographs, found that the mesothelial cells of the arachnoid villus continually form giant cytoplasmic vacuoles capable of transcellular bulk transport. Certain substances such as penicillin and organic acids and bases are also absorbed by the choroid plexus; the bidirectional action of these cells is like that of the tubule cells of the kidneys. Some substances have been shown in pathologic specimens to pass between the ependymal cells of the ventricles and to enter subependymal capillaries and venules.

CIRCULATION

Harvey Cushing aptly termed the CSF the "third circulation," comparable to that of the blood and lymph. The pathways it traverses are well known. From the principal site of CSF formation in the ventricles it flows downward through the foramens of Magendie and Luschka, to the perimedullary and perispinal subarachnoid spaces, and thence up over the brainstem to the cisternae basalis and ambiens, and finally to the superior and lateral surfaces of the cerebral hemispheres, where most of it is absorbed. The gradient of pressure is highest in the ventricles and diminishes successively along the subarachnoid pathways. Arterial pulsations of the choroid plexuses help drive the fluid from the ventricular system. Strain-gauge manometer recordings have shown the arterial pulse pressure to be 60 mmH₂O in the lateral ventricle, 50 mmH₂O in the cisterna magna, and 30 mmH₂O in the lumbar subarachnoid space.

The periventricular tissues offer resistance to the entrance of CSF and although this so-called transmantle pressure is only slightly above zero, the open ventricular-foraminal-subarachnoid conduit directs the bulk flow of CSF in this direction. Only if this conduit is obstructed, does the transmantle pressure rise and compress the periventricular tissues.

VOLUME AND PRESSURE

Systemic circulatory factors maintain the volume and pressure of the CSF. When the heart stops, the CSF pressure falls to zero. Normally the CSF pressure is in equilibrium with the capillary pressure, which is influenced only by circulatory changes that alter arteriolar tone. Rises in arterial pressure cause little or no increase of pressure at the capillary level and hence no increase in CSF pressure. The inhalation of CO_2, which raises the blood P_{CO_2} and decreases pH and arteriolar resistance, increases the CSF pressure by increasing cerebral blood flow and volume and capillary pressure; and hyperventilation, which reduces P_{CO_2}, has the opposite effect of increasing the pH and vascular resistance, thereby decreasing CSF pressure. Here CSF pressures clearly relate to blood flow and blood volume.

In contrast to arterial blood pressure, venous pressure exerts an immediate effect on CSF pressure by increasing the volume of blood in the veins, venules, and dural sinuses. Jugular compression, as indicated in Chap. 2, causes an immediate rise of intracranial CSF pressure, and this is rapidly transmitted to the lumbar subarachnoid space (Queckenstedt test), unless there is a spinal subarachnoid block. The Valsalva maneuver, as well as coughing, sneezing, and straining all cause an increased intrathoracic pressure, which is transmitted to the jugular and then to the cerebral veins. Abdominal compression distends the lower spinal veins and will increase the lumbar CSF pressure below the point of subarachnoid block. The intracranial pressure rises in heart failure, when venous pressure becomes elevated. Mediastinal tumors, by obstructing the superior vena cava, have the same effect. Removal of CSF causes a temporary lowering of intracranial pressure, and this may persist for days after a lumbar puncture that has resulted in a CSF leak.

FUNCTION

The primary function of the CSF appears to be a mechanical one; it serves as a kind of water jacket for the spinal cord and brain, protecting them from potentially injurious blows to the spinal column and skull and acute changes in venous pressure. As pointed out by Fishman, the 1500-g brain, which has a water content of 80 percent, weighs only 50 g when suspended in CSF, and so the brain virtually floats in its CSF jacket. It is to maintain the relatively constant volume-pressure relationships of the CSF that many of the

physiologic and chemical mechanisms described above are committed. Since the brain and spinal cord have no lymphatic channels, the CSF through its "sink action" (see above) serves to remove the waste products of cerebral metabolism, the main ones being CO_2, lactate, and hydrogen ions. The composition of the CSF is maintained within narrow limits, despite major alterations in the blood; thus the CSF, along with the intercellular fluid of the brain, helps to preserve a stable chemical environment for neurons and their medullated fibers. There is no reason to believe that the CSF is actively involved in the metabolism of the cells of the brain and spinal cord.

DISTURBANCES OF CSF PRESSURE, VOLUME, AND CIRCULATION

MECHANISMS OF INCREASED INTRACRANIAL PRESSURE

The intact cranium and vertebral canal together with the relatively inelastic dura form a rigid container, and an increase in volume of any of its contents, viz., brain, blood, or CSF, will elevate the intracranial pressure. Further, if one of these three elements increases in volume, it must be at the expense of the other two. This is known as the Monro-Kellie hypothesis (Fig. 30-1). Of the three intracranial components—brain tissue, blood, and CSF—the first is the least compressible. A relatively small increment in brain volume does not immediately raise the ICP, because the increased volume can be accommodated for a time by displacement of CSF from the cranial cavity into the spinal canal, and to a lesser extent, by stretching of the dura and by the inherent plasticity of the brain. Further increments in brain volume reduce the volume of intracranial blood, particularly that in the veins and dural sinuses. Also there is evidence that the CSF is formed more slowly in these circumstances. These accommodative pressure-volume relationships are subsumed under the term *compliance*. As the brain, blood, or CSF volumes continue to increase, these accommodative mechanisms fail and ICP then rises exponentially.

There are several recognized mechanisms of elevated ICP: (1) An increased intracranial volume, due to a cerebral tumor, massive infarction or trauma, hemorrhage, or abscess, to an extracerebral hematoma, or to acute brain swelling, as occurs in anoxic states and the Reye syndrome. Here the increase in pressure is both local, because of the dural compartmentalization of the cranial cavity, and also generalized. (2) High venous pressure from heart failure or a superior mediastinal obstruction. This not only increases the volume of blood in pial veins and dural sinuses, but interferes with CSF absorption, which depends on a decreasing gradient of pressure from the subarachnoid space to the dural sinuses. (3) Obstruction to the flow and absorption of CSF. If the obstruction is within the ventricles or in the subarachnoid space around the base of the brain, a tension hydrocephalus results. If the block is at the absorptive sites, a pseudotumor state develops, with the ventricles remaining normal in size and undeformed. Of course, these mechanisms are not mutually exclusive. For example, Van Crevel has observed that with cerebral tumors

increased ICP and papilledema correlate more closely with interference of the CSF flow to absorptive sites than with the size and location of the tumor.

Conditions are somewhat different in infants and small children, whose cranial sutures have not closed. Here, increased ICP is manifested by enlargement of the head, and hydrocephalus, the most common cause, has to be distinguished from constitutional macrocrania, subdural hematoma or hygroma, neonatal hemorrhage, and cysts or tumors.

Each of these many types of increased ICP has its special mechanism(s) and clinical and pathologic features, as outlined below.

ELEVATED ICP DUE TO INTRACRANIAL MASSES AND ACUTE BRAIN SWELLING

Cranial trauma, massive cerebral hemorrhage, infarction, and tumor, hypoxic and ischemic states, and acute brain

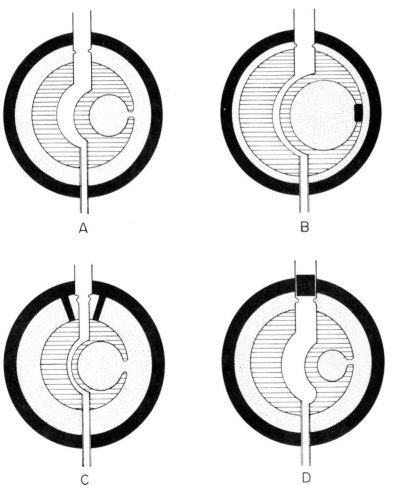

A   B

C   D

Figure 30-1

A. *Schematic representation of the three components of the intracranial contents: the incompressible brain tissue* (shaded); *the vascular system, open to the atmosphere; and the CSF* (dotted). B. *With ventricular obstruction.* C. *With obstruction at or near the points of outlet of the CSF.* D. *With obstruction of the venous outflow. (Redrawn from Foley.)*

swelling (Reye syndrome) are regularly associated with a greatly elevated ICP. Once this complication occurs, unless recognized or treated, death or permanent cerebral damage is almost inevitable. It has been demonstrated repeatedly that the high mortality and morbidity of these intracranial catastrophes is related to uncontrolled or uncontrollable rises in ICP, and that only by aggressive intervention can they be forestalled. Therefore, the clinical features and mechanisms of raised ICP and the measures that reduce it should be part of the working knowledge of neurologists and neurosurgeons.

The standard clinical manifestations of increased intracranial pressure in children and adults are headache, nausea and vomiting, drowsiness, ocular and gaze palsies, papilledema, visual obscurations, and eventual blindness. The practice of monitoring ICP with a pressure device screwed into the skull has permitted correlations to be made between the clinical signs and the levels of ICP. In a normal adult, reclining with the head and trunk elevated to 45°, the ICP is between 2 and 5 mmHg. During coughing it rises to 20 mmHg, but it falls immediately afterward to 10 mmHg. Levels up to 15 mmHg are considered harmless; adequate cerebral perfusion can be maintained even at an ICP of 40 mmHg, provided that blood pressure (BP) remains normal. Higher ICP or lower BP may combine to cause ischemic damage.

Ropper finds that pupillary dilatation, abducens palsies, drowsiness, and the Cushing response (raised systolic pressure and bradycardia, supposedly from medullary compression) do not bear a strict relationship to ICP. Not until the ICP reached 28 to 34 mmHg did the ipsilateral pupil begin to dilate, except with medial temporal lesions and threatening herniation, in which case it could happen at much lower pressures. Likewise, unilateral or bilateral abducens palsies did not bear a close relationship to ICP, being more frequent with bihemispheral lesions and pseudotumor states. In Ropper's series, patients retained normal mental function with pressures of 25 to 40 mmHg, unless there was a lateral shift of diencephalic-mesencephalic structures, with or without temporal lobe herniation. Only with ICP higher than the 40-to-50 mmHg range was cerebral blood flow diminished. When this happened, ischemia and brain death usually followed in a short time. It is with monitored high ICP (25 to 40 mmHg) that Lundberg's plateau (A) waves began to appear, during which the ICP may rise by 5 mmHg, or more (see footnote, page 508). Brain death often occurs during a plateau wave.

Treatment of Raised ICP. Considerable evidence has accumulated that the outcome of these intracranial catastrophes is more favorable if ICP is kept at 15 to 20 mmHg, or less, and if treatment is begun before the ICP has reached this level. The following measures should be

applied even if ICP is not being monitored. The head and body should be elevated 15 to 30 degrees. Since both the cerebral volume and blood flow increase with fever, body temperature must be kept as low as possible. Fluids should be restricted to around 1000 mL per 24 h in order to reduce cerebral edema. Intravenous fluids should be in the form of normal saline and serum osmolality maintained at 305 to 315 mosmol/L. Higher osmolality may lead to hypovolemia and azotemia.

Hyperosmolar agents such as mannitol can be given as an intravenous bolus in a dose of 0.25 g/kg every 3 to 4 h. Some neurosurgeons prefer to use furosemide, glycerol, and ethacrynic acid, especially in the operating room.

With respiration under mechanical control, one can, by increasing the ventilatory rate, reduce P_{CO_2} and thereby lower ICP. In patients who fail to respond to hyperosmolar agents and hyperventilation, large doses of barbiturate are often given to suppress brain metabolism. The usual method is to administer 3 to 5 mg/kg of pentobarbital intravenously, followed by 1 to 3 mg/kg/h.

TENSION HYDROCEPHALUS

Essentially this is a condition in which there is an obstruction to the flow of CSF at some point between its principal site of origin, in the lateral ventricles, and the cerebral subarachnoid space, where most of it is absorbed. Because of the obstruction, CSF accumulates within the ventricles under increasing pressure, enlarging the ventricles and expanding the hemispheres. As stated above, in the infant or small child the head increases in size because of separation of the sutures of the cranial bones. This is called *manifest* or *overt hydrocephalus*.

Unfortunately, the term hydrocephalus (literally, "water head") is frequently applied to the passive enlargement of the ventricles consequent to cerebral atrophy, i.e., *hydrocephalus ex vacuo*, and to the ventricular enlargement in undeveloped brains, a state known as *colpencephaly*. Reference to these conditions as hydrocephalic is such common practice that it is unlikely to change; hence the authors believe it preferable to use the term *tension hydrocephalus* for the obstructive types in which the CSF is or has been under increased pressure.

Dandy introduced the unfortunate terms *communicating* and *noncommunicating (obstructive) hydrocephalus*. The concept of a communicating hydrocephalus was based on the findings that dye injected into a lateral ventricle would diffuse readily into the lumbar subarachnoid space and that air injected into the lumbar subarachnoid space would pass into the ventricular system; in other words, the ventricles are in communication with the spinal subarachnoid space. In noncommunicating or obstructive hydrocephalus, it was assumed, they are not. The distinction between these two types is not fundamental. All forms of tension hydrocephalus are obstructive, and the obstruction is never complete. Complete aqueductal occlusion is incompatible with survival for more than 1 to 2 days. The authors suggest that a more appropriate terminology is one in which a prefix indicates the site of the presumed obstruction, i.e., *meningeal-obstructive, aqueductal-obstructive,* or *third ventricular-obstructive tension hydrocephalus.*

There are several sites of predilection of obstruction to the flow of CSF. One foramen of Monro may be blocked by a tumor with expansion of one lateral ventricle. If the obstruction is in the aqueduct of Sylvius, the third and both lateral ventricles dilate, and if it is in the fourth ventricle, the dilatation includes the aqueduct of Sylvius. Occlusion of the basilar foramens of Magendie and Luschka or of the subarachnoid space around the medulla, pons, and midbrain results in enlargement of the entire ventricular system, including the fourth ventricle. However, if the obstruction is in the subarachnoid space at the mesencephalic level, the accumulation of CSF around the brainstem may prevent the fourth ventricle from enlarging as much as the other ventricles.

A matter of considerable practical as well as theoretical interest is whether a meningeal obstruction over the cerebral hemispheres, at the site of the arachnoidal villi, or a blockage of the dural sinuses into which the CSF is absorbed can result in tension hydrocephalus. Russell, in her large neuropathologic material and in her review of the world's literature, could not find a single well-documented example, and the authors' experience has been similar. Moreover, experiments in animals in which all draining veins had been occluded resulted in a tension hydrocephalus with enlarging lateral ventricles in only a few cases, and in these the investigator could not be sure that a basilar meningeal obstruction or brain atrophy from ischemic necrosis had not been produced inadvertently. Yet Gilles and Davidson believe that tension hydrocephalus in children may be due to a congenital absence or deficient number of arachnoidal villi, and Rosman and Shands have reported an instance that they attributed to increased intracranial venous pressure. Our hesitancy in accepting such examples stems from the difficulty that the pathologist has in judging the patency of the basilar subarachnoid space. The latter is much more reliably

visualized by radiologic than by neuropathologic means. Theoretically, if the obstruction is high, near the superior sagittal sinus, the CSF should accumulate under pressure outside as well as inside the brain, and the ventricles should not enlarge at all or only slightly and very late. The authors remain skeptical of any exceptions to this concept. The radiologic picture of enlarged subarachnoid spaces over and between the cerebral hemispheres, coupled with modest enlargement of the lateral ventricles, has been referred to as an *external hydrocephalus,* but many of the cases so designated have proved to be cases of sporadic or familial megalencephaly.

An increase in the rate of formation or decrease in the rate of absorption would be expected to cause an accumulation of CSF and increased intracranial pressure. The only known cause of overproduction of CSF is a papilloma of the choroid plexus, but even in this circumstance there is usually an associated ventricular obstruction, either of the third or fourth ventricle or of one lateral ventricle. Characteristically, in the latter case, there is both a generalized dilatation of the ventricular system and basal cisterns (due to increased CSF volume?) and an asymmetrical enlargement of the lateral ventricles, due to obstruction of one foramen of Monro.

Lorenzo et al, using the ventricular perfusion technique, have shown that in patients with tension hydrocephalus the rate of formation of CSF is somewhat lower than in persons with normal ventricles. Also in these patients, both adults and children, there is an impairment of CSF absorption. Two types of absorptive difficulty were recognized: in one type, a higher pressure than normal was required to open the absorptive channels, after which CSF was absorbed at a normal rate; in the second type, absorption began at a normal pressure and then proceeded at a much slower rate than normal. The relation of these absorptive defects to a possible abnormality of the arachnoid villi remains to be determined.

Clinical Picture of Hydrocephalus This varies with the age of onset. As remarked above, two major syndromes are recognized, one in which the head enlarges (*overt* hydrocephalus), the other in which the head remains of normal size (*occult* hydrocephalus).

Congenital or Infantile Hydrocephalus of Overt Type The cranial bones fuse by the end of the second year, and for the head to enlarge, the tension hydrocephalus must develop before this time, sometimes in utero, usually in the first few months of life. Up to 5 years of age (and very rarely beyond this time) an increase of intracranial pressure, particularly if it evolves rapidly, will separate the sutures (diastasis). Tension hydrocephalus of mild degree also molds the shape of the skull in early life, and in radiographs the inner table is unevenly thinned, an appearance referred to as "beaten silver" or as convolutional or digital markings. The frontal regions are unusually prominent (bossed) and the skull tends to be brachicephalic, except in the Dandy-Walker syndrome, where, because of bossing of the occiput from enlargement of the posterior fossa, the head is dolichocephalic. With marked enlargement of the skull the face looks relatively small and pinched and the skin over the cranial bones is tight and thin, revealing prominent distended veins.

The usual causes of this disorder are (1) matrix hemorrhages in premature infants, (2) fetal and neonatal infections, (3) Arnold-Chiari malformation, (4) aqueductal stenosis and atresia, and (5) the Dandy-Walker syndrome.

Usually, in this type of hydrocephalus, the head enlarges rapidly and soon surpasses the 97th percentile. The anterior and posterior fontanels are tense, even when the patient is in the upright position. The infant is fretful, feeds poorly, and may vomit. With continued enlargement of the brain, torpor sets in and the infant appears languid, uninterested in the immediate surroundings, and unable to sustain activity. Later it is noticed that the upper eyelids are retracted and the eyes tend to turn down; there is paralysis of upward gaze, and the scleras above the irises are visible. This is the so-called *setting-sun sign* and has been incorrectly attributed to downward pressure of the frontal lobes on the roofs of the orbits. The fact that it disappears on shunting the lateral and third ventricles indicates that it is due to hydrocephalic pressure on the mesencephalic tegmentum. Gradually the infant adopts a posture of flexed arms and flexed or extended legs. Signs of corticospinal tract affection are usually elicitable. Movements are feeble and sometimes the arms are tremulous. There is no papilledema, but later the optic discs become pale and vision is reduced. If the hydrocephalus becomes arrested, the infant or child is retarded but often surprisingly verbal. The head may be so large that the child cannot hold it up and must remain in bed. If the head is only moderately enlarged, the child may be able to sit but not stand, or can stand but not walk. If ambulatory, the child is clumsy. Acute exacerbations of hydrocephalus, or an intercurrent febrile illness, may cause vomiting, stupor, or coma.

The special features of congenital hydrocephalus with Arnold-Chiari malformation, aqueductal stenosis and atresia, and the Dandy-Walker syndrome will be discussed in Chap. 44.

Occult Tension Hydrocephalus In this form of hydrocephalus the increased intracranial pressure is evenly transmitted throughout the subarachnoid spaces and causes papilledema. Bifrontal and bioccipital head-

aches are prominent, but not invariable. Mental and physical activity are gradually reduced. The clinical picture is predominantly one of bilateral frontal lobe disorder. Slowness of response, inattentiveness, distractibility, inability to plan activity or to sustain any type of complex mental function, and perseveration are characteristic. The immediate responses to verbal and other stimuli are normal, though memory may be slightly impaired. Conspicuous by their absence are apraxia, agnosia, or aphasia. The gait deteriorates early in the course of hydrocephalus. At first the gait is only slightly uncertain, with reduced speed and range of movement; later there is a shortening of step and a mild clumsiness that sometimes looks suspiciously parkinsonian or, if more incoordinate, like cerebellar ataxia. Yet rigidity, tremor, or ataxia of leg movements is absent. Later still, the patient cannot walk at all without assistance. There is continuous activity in antigravity muscles. Eventually, help is needed even in standing. Lastly there is sphincteric incontinence. A suck reflex and grasp reflexes of the hand and foot are variably present; plantar reflexes are sometimes extensor.

Occult hydrocephalus due to tumor growth will be discussed further in Chap. 31.

Normal-Pressure Hydrocephalus In nonprogressive meningeal and ependymal diseases the hydrocephalus may stabilize or "compensate," meaning that the formation of CSF equilibrates with absorption. Formation diminishes slightly, perhaps because of compression of the choroid plexus, and absorption increases in proportion to the CSF pressure, but beginning at a higher threshold. Once equilibrium is attained, the intracranial pressure gradually falls, though it maintains a higher but still a diminishing gradient from ventricle to basal cistern to cerebral subarachnoid space. A stage is reached where the pressure reaches a normal level of 150 to 180 mmH_2O while the patient still manifests the cerebral effects of the hydrocephalic state. The name given to this condition by Hakim, Adams, and Fisher is *normal-pressure hydrocephalus* (NPH). With the large ventricles the lower presure continues to exert a force against the tracts in the cerebral white matter that exceeds the effects of a higher pressure with small ventricles.

A triad of clinical findings is characteristic of NPH— a slowly progressive gait disorder, sphincteric incontinence, and impairment of mental function. Grasp relexes in the feet and falling attacks may occur. Headaches are no longer a complaint and may never have been present, and there is no papilledema.

The *gait disturbance* usually takes the form of unsteadiness and impairment of balance, with the greatest difficulty on stairs and curbs (Fisher). Weakness and tiredness of the legs are also frequent complaints, although exmination may disclose no abnormalities. Untreated, the steps become shorter and shuffling and falls are frequent, and eventually standing, sitting, and turning over in bed are impossible. Fisher refers to this advanced disorder of stance and gait as "hydrocephalic astasia-abasia." *Urinary symptoms* in the beginning consist of urgency and frequency. Later, the urgency is associated with incontinence, and ultimately there is "frontal lobe incontinence," in which the patient is indifferent to his or her lapses of continence. The mental symptoms, when they occur, are difficult to distinguish from those of Alzheimer disease.

This syndrome of NPH may follow subarachnoid hemorrhage from ruptured aneurysm or head trauma, chronic meningitis (tubercular, syphilitic, or other), Paget disease of the base of the skull, and mucopolysaccharidosis of the meninges and achondroplasia, but in at least a third of our cases it is due presumably to an asymptomatic fibrosing meningitis of unknown etiology.

The verification of the diagnosis of NPH and the selection of patients for ventriculoperitoneal shunt has presented difficulties. The CT scan (enlarged ventricles without convolutional atrophy) and radionuclide cisternography (reflux into ventricles and delayed pericerebral diffusion) have been the most helpful ancillary examinations. According to Katzman and Hussey the infusion of normal saline into the lumbar subarachnoid space at a rate of 0.76 mL/min for 30 to 60 min provokes a rise in pressure (300 to 600 mmH$_2$O) that is not observed in normal individuals. Theoretically, this test should quantitate the adequacy of CSF absorption, but it has yielded unpredictable results. Drainage of large amounts of CSF may result in clinical improvement for a few days. Pneumoencephalography, with air entering the ventricles but not the cerebral subarachnoid space, was a helpful test but often worsened the clinical state. It is seldom used since the advent of the CT scan. The measurement of CSF pressure over a prolonged period may show intermittent rises of pressure, possibly corresponding to the A waves of Lundberg[1]. The cerebral blood flow is diminished.

The authors have obtained gratifying success, often a complete restoration of mental function and gait, in more than a hundred patients, by effecting a ventriculoatrial or ventriculoperitoneal shunt. As a group these patients all had the first two elements of the clinical triad described above (only half of our patients were incontinent), and their lateral ventricular span at the level of the anterior horns was in excess of 50 mm. Deviations from this syndrome—such as the occurrence of dementia without gait disorder, or the presence of apraxias, aphasias, and other focal cerebral signs—should all lead one to a diagnosis other than NPH. Fisher, after analyzing our cases in which a successful result was obtained, noted that in all except one of them the gait disturbance had been an early and prominent symptom. The most consistent improvement has been attained in those NPH patients in whom a cause could be established (subarachnoid hemorrhage, chronic meningitis, or third ventricular tumor). Uncertainties of diagnosis increase with advancing age owing to the frequent association of senile dementia and the vascular lesions.

Neuropathologic effects of tension hydrocephalus
These have been described by Adams and Sidman and by Penfield and Elvidge. Ventricular expansion is maximal in the frontal horns, explaining the hydrocephalic impairment of frontal lobe functions. The central white matter yields to pressure while the cortical gray matter, thalami, basal ganglia, and brainstem structures remain normal. There is an increase in the content of interstitial fluid in the tissue adjacent to the lateral ventricles. Medullated fibers and axons are injured, but not to the extent that one might expect from the degree of compression; minor degrees of astrocytic gliosis and loss of oligodendrocytes in the affected tissue are present to a decreasing extent away from the ventricles, and represent a hydrocephalic atrophy of the brain, which is permanent. In acute (1 to 2 weeks) experimentally produced hydrocephalus in rabbits, Torvik et al observed no breaks or denuding of the ependyma; but in humans such changes are characteristic, and the choroid plexuses are flattened and fibrotic. The lumens of cerebral capillaries in biopsy preparations are said to be narrowed.

Treatment   The development of sterilizable one-way valves has opened the way to successful treatment of tension hydrocephalus. The valve can be set at a desired pressure, allowing the CSF to escape directly into the blood stream or peritoneal cavity whenever the pressure level is exceeded. Although relatively simple as a surgical procedure, there

---

[1] Lundberg (1960) recorded intraventricular pressures over long periods of time in patients with brain tumors. He described three types of pressure waves, which he designated as A, B, and C, all separable from arterial and respiratory pulsations. Only the A waves were considered to be clinically significant; they consisted of rhythmic rises of pressure occurring every 15 to 30 min, or more protracted fluctuations in pressure. Their physiologic basis is obscure.

are complications, the main ones being a postoperative subdural hygroma or hematoma (if the ventricular pressure is reduced too rapidly, allowing the bridging dural veins to stretch and rupture); infection of the valve and catheter, sometimes with septicemia; and occlusion of the tip of the catheter in the ventricle. The authors have found that the complication rate can be considerably reduced by placing the catheter in the anterior horn of the right ventricle, where there is no choroid plexus, and by using the sterilizable Hakim valve. Meticulous aseptic technique and the preoperative and postoperative administration of oxycillin and gentamycin have reduced the incidence of shunt infections. Once the CSF is shunted, the ventricles diminish in size within 3 or 4 days, even when the hydrocephalus has been present for a year or more. This indicates that the so-called hydrocephalic compression of the cerebrum is largely reversible. Indeed, in Black's series, in only one of his 11 shunted patients did the ventricles fail to return to normal, and in this one patient there was no clinical improvement. Clinical improvement occurs within a few weeks, the gait disturbance being slower to reverse than the mental disorder. Cerebral atrophy from Alzheimer disease and related conditions is not altered by ventriculoatrial shunting. Of course, if the hydrocephalus is caused by an operable tumor, surgical removal is the procedure of choice.

In the treatment of infantile and childhood hydrocephalus one encounters more difficult problems than in the adult. The ventricular catheter may wander or be obstructed and require revision. Peritoneal pseudocysts may form (most shunts in children are ventriculoperitoneal). Whether or not to shunt all hydrocephalic infants soon after birth has not been settled. In several large series of cases that have been treated in this way, the number surviving with superior mental function has been small. As noted by Dennis et al, who examined 78 treated hydrocephalic children, mental functions develop unevenly; nonverbal intelligence lags more than verbal. Fifty-six (i.e., 72 percent) had global IQs falling between 70 and 100, but only three fell below 70; in 22 the IQ was 100 to 115, and in three it was higher. Performance scores were lower than verbal at all levels. The use of diamox to inhibit CSF formation by suppressing the enzyme carbonic anhydrase has not been successful in our hands.

INCREASED ICP DUE TO VENOUS OBSTRUCTION

Occlusion of the major dural sinuses (superior longitudinal and lateral) results in increased intracranial pressure. This is not surprising, in view of the direct effect of venous obstruction on CSF pressure. One form of such intracranial hypertension, due to lateral sinus thrombosis, was referred to by Symonds as "otitic hydrocephalus"—an inappropriate name insofar as the ventricles are not enlarged in this clinical circumstance. As indicated above, venous congestion that complicates heart failure and superior mediastinal obstruction also raises the CSF pressure, again without enlargement of the ventricles. This may also happen with large, high-flow arteriovenous malformations of the brain.

BENIGN INTRACRANIAL HYPERTENSION (PSEUDOTUMOR CEREBRI, MENINGEAL HYDROPS)

This is a syndrome of obscure origin, first described by Quincke in 1897. It is particularly frequent in fat adolescent girls and young women, in whom increased ICP develops over a period of weeks or months. Headache is the usual symptom; others complain of blurred vision, a vague dizziness, diplopia, transient visual obscurations, or a trifling numbness of the face on one side. It is then discovered that they have flagrant papilledema, which immediately raises the specter of a brain tumor. The CSF pressure is elevated, usually in the range of 250 to 450 mmH$_2$O. When the CSF pressure is monitored for many hours it can be seen to fluctuate. There are periods lasting 20 to 30 min when it rises and then abruptly falls nearly to normal, as though an increased volume of CSF were vented. The headache does not correspond to the elevations of pressure (Johnston and Patterson). Aside from the papilledema, there is remarkably little to be found on neurologic examination—perhaps a unilateral or bilateral abducens palsy, fine nystagmus on far lateral gaze, or a minor sensory change. Exceptionally, in children, an otherwise typical Bell's palsy may be associated (Chutorian et al). Visual field testing usually shows slight peripheral constriction with enlargement of the blind spots. With visual loss, more severe constriction of the fields with nasal or infranasal loss is the common finding. CT scans and MRI have shown the ventricles to be normal in size or small. Mentation and alertness are preserved, and the patient seems surprisingly well.

As was remarked above, most of the patients are young women, but the condition may occur in children and in men (Digre et al). Practically all of the women with this disease are obese and so are the men, but to a lesser degree (Durcan et al). An endocrine factor has been postulated on the basis of female predominance and obesity but has never been substantiated. The plasma steroid levels are normal.

If the intracranial hypertension is left untreated or fails to respond to the measures outlined below, the one real danger is loss of vision. This complication has occurred in only a small proportion of our patients, but Corbett et al, who followed a group of 57 patients for 5 to 41 years, found severe visual impairment in 14 of them. Wall and George, using highly refined perimetric methods, have reported an even higher incidence of visual loss. Moreover, children with pseudotumor share the same visual risks as adults (Lessell and Rosman). Sequential quantitative perimetry has been particularly informative in detecting impending visual loss, although this is difficult to carry out in young children. Sometimes vision is lost abruptly, either without warning or following one or more episodes of visual obscuration.

The mechanism of increased CSF pressure in this disorder (and some cases of Guillain-Barré disease) remains elusive. Using the method of constant infusion manometrics, Mann et al studied a group of patients with pseudotumor and demonstrated an increased resistance to CSF outflow, due presumably to an impaired absorptive function of the arachnoid villi. They showed also that CSF production was reduced in these patients. But except for the few cases with dural venous obstruction (see above), the cause of malabsorption is obscure. Using a similar method, Ropper and Marmarou studied a patient with Guillain-Barré disease and found a similar abnormality, i.e., an increased resistance to CSF outflow. However, they discounted the importance of this finding and interpreted their data to indicate that there was an increase in intracranial venous pressure at sites of CSF absorption, and that this was reflected as a raised CSF pressure. Others have attributed benign intracranial hypertension to an increase in brain volume, secondary to an increase in blood or extracellular fluid (Sahs and Joynt, Raichle et al).

Treatment   The first step is to make sure that there is no underlying tumor or other nontumorous cause of raised ICP (see below). Formerly, when reliance was placed on pneumoencephalography and arteriography, the authors observed an occasional patient whose illness had been diagnosed as benign intracranial hypertension because of negative radiologic findings, only to find, after some months or a year had passed, that the ventricles were enlarging and there was an aqueductal stenosis, an astrocytoma, a ventricular cysticercosis, or metastatic tumor. These errors in diagnosis are less frequent since the advent of CT scanning. However, chronic meningeal reactions (e.g., those due to sarcoidosis or to tuberculous or carcinomatous meningitis), which give rise to headache and papilledema, may elude detection by CT scanning and require lumbar puncture for diagnosis.

The diagnosis of pseudotumor cerebri should never be made in the absence of a normal spinal fluid.

At least a third of our patients with pseudotumor cerebri have recovered after repeated lumbar punctures and drainage of sufficient CSF to maintain the pressure at normal or near normal levels (200 to 250 mmH$_2$O). The lumbar punctures were repeated daily at first and then at increasing intervals according to the level of pressure. Evidently this was sufficient to restore the balance between CSF formation and absorption within 6 months. In a smaller group of patients, the CSF pressure remains elevated month after month, and the papilledema becomes chronic. It is the management of this group of patients that is most controversial. Weight reduction is always advised but is difficult to accomplish. Prednisone (40 to 60 mg/day) or oral hyperosmotic agents such as glycerol (15 to 60 mg four to six times daily) or acetazolamide (a 500-mg capsule twice daily) to reduce CSF formation all have their advocates. We have observed a gradual recession of papilledema and a lowering of CSF pressure with administration of glycerol and/or prednisone, but it was always difficult to decide whether this represented the effects of treatment or the natural course of the disease. Greer, who has reported on 110 patients, 11 of whom were treated with these agents, decided that they were of no value. Moreover, in patients whose papilledema seems to recede under the influence of corticosteroids, there is always a danger that papilledema will recur when the drug is tapered. In Greer's series, 12 percent continued to have raised intracranial pressure 5 months after the diagnosis was made.

In patients with protracted high intracranial pressure and papilledema, especially in those with a measurable impairment of vision that does not respond to the usual therapeutic measures, a lumbar thecoperitoneal shunt should be performed. Not more than 10 percent of our patients have needed this surgical procedure. It is quite safe and effective, although in very obese patients there is a tendency for the shunt to close. In the past 30 years, we have not had the need to perform a single subtemporal decompression, the procedure that was formerly used when vision was threatened. In patients who are threatened with visual loss, despite a shunt and use of the aforementioned medical measures, Corbett recommends optic nerve sheath decompression.

OTHER NONTUMOROUS CAUSES OF RAISED INTRACRANIAL PRESSURE

In children, as they are withdrawn from corticosteroid therapy, there may be a period of headache, papilledema, and elevated intracranial pressure with only modest enlargement of the lateral ventricles. As was mentioned earlier, an ear or systemic infection may lead to thrombosis of the lateral or superior sagittal sinus with intracranial hypertension ("otitic hydrocephalus"). Excessive doses of tetracycline and vitamin A (particularly in the form of isotretinoin, an oral vitamin A derivative for the treatment of severe acne) have also been shown to cause a benign intracranial hypertension in children and adolescents. Isolated instances of hypo- or hyperadrenalism, myxedema, and hypoparathyroidism have developed increased CSF pressure and papilledema, and occasionally the administration of estrogens, tetracycline, and phenothiazines has the same effect, for reasons not known.

In patients of any age, an extremely high CSF protein level, which by colloid-osmotic pressure increases the volume of CSF, will raise intracranial pressure without enlargment of the ventricle. This has happened most often in cases of Guillain-Barré disease with protein levels of 500 to 1500 mg/dL. Possibly the same mechanism is operative in rare instances of spinal cord tumors that are accompanied by increased ICP.

VENTRICULAR DILATATION WITHOUT RAISED PRESSURE OR BRAIN ATROPHY

The wide application of CT scanning and MRI is revealing cases of ventricular enlargement where there is no evidence of parenchymal lesions of the cerebrum. This has been reported in patients with anorexia nervosa and Cushing disease and in those receiving corticosteroids for a long period of time. It has also been observed in some schizophrenics and in chronic alcoholics, often in the latter, with no associated neurologic or mental abnormality. Surprisingly, after a prolonged period without steroids or of abstinence from alcohol, the ventricles become smaller. This change in ventricular size is probably related to a shift in fluid volume of cerebral tissue, but this remains speculative.

INTRACRANIAL HYPOTENSION

"Lumbar Puncture Headache" (see also page 137) This is a well-known phenomenon, attributable to lowering of the ICP by leakage of CSF through the needle tract into the paravertebral muscles and other tissues. Actually the syndrome includes more than headache. There may be pain at the base of the skull posteriorly and in the neck and upper thoracic spine, stiffness of the neck, and nausea and vomiting. At times the signs of meningeal irritation are so prominent as to raise the question of postlumbar puncture meningitis, although lack of fever usually excludes this possibility. In the infant or child, stiffness of the neck may be accompanied by irritability, unwillingness to move, and refusal of food. Most characteristic is the relation of the headache to upright posture and its relief within a few minutes after assuming the recumbent position. The use of a 22- to 24-gauge needle and the performance of a single clean tap reduce the likelihood of the headache. A period of enforced recumbency, though widely practiced as a means of preventing lumbar puncture headache, probably does not lessen the incidence or the duration of the headache (Carbaat and Van Crevel). Once started, the headache may last for days or even a week or more. The CSF pressure is in the range of 0 to 50 mmH$_2$O. Forcing fluids and intravenous infusion of hypotonic fluids (1000 to 2000 mL of 5% glucose) may be helpful. Analgesic medication is required only if the patient must get up to care for him- or herself or to travel.

Aside from this condition there are few adverse effects of lumbar puncture and these are relatively rare: transient cranial nerve palsy (usually the sixth), bacterial meningitis, spinal subdural or epidural abscess or hematoma, injury of a lumbar root and sciatic pain, damage to an intervertebral disc, and inadvertent injection of air or a chemical contaminant, with aseptic pleocytosis.

Less well known is a syndrome of *spontaneous intracranial hypotension*. The authors have observed several patients in whom the same syndrome as that which follows lumbar puncture occurred after straining, a nonhurtful fall, or for no known reason. The CSF pressure is low or not measurable, and the fluid may contain 20 to 50 mononuclear cells per milliliter. Presumably there has been a tear in the delicate arachnoid surrounding a nerve root, with continuous leakage of CSF. The site of the leak usually cannot be ascertained, except for the one into the paranasal sinuses (CSF rhinorrhea). Recumbency for a few days permits the pressure to build up, and there has been no recurrence in the cases that we have encountered.

The use of a one-way valve and a ventriculoatrial or ventriculoperitoneal shunt may also result in a low-pressure syndrome. Usually the valve setting is too low, and readjustment to maintain a higher pressure corrects this. Unexplained is a peculiar state of ventricular collapse in shunted patients ("slit ventricles"), in conjunction with a blocked catheter, high intracranial pressure, and papilledema. This has usually occurred in children treated for hydrocephalus.

MENINGEAL AND EPENDYMAL REACTIONS

The anatomy of the pia-arachnoid (which forms the double membrane surrounding the brain, optic nerves, and spinal cord) and the ependyma of the ventricles, and their communication via the foramens of Luschka and Magendie, account for the fact that whatever foreign agent enters the subarachnoid space (SAS) or the ventricles has free access to the other spaces containing CSF. The pia provides a relative barrier, at least to bacteria, between the SAS and the brain and spinal cord. The arachnoidal membrane is a bacterial barrier between the SAS and the subdural space. The dura is tightly adherent to the inner periosteum of the cranial bones, so that there is no cranial

epidural space, and the inner side of the dura has no true endothelial lining. There is, however, a wide space between the dura that surrounds the spinal cord and the vertebral bodies. Because of these barriers, the subarachnoid, subdural, and epidural spaces can be affected separately by disease. The subarachnoid-ventricular spaces are the ones most frequently involved.

PIA-ARACHNOID–EPENDYMAL–CHOROIDAL REACTIONS TO INFECTION

Various bacteria and other infectious agents may gain entrance to the ventricles and SAS, and having done so,

Table 30-1
Pathologic-clinical correlations in acute, subacute, and chronic meningitis

I. In acute meningitis:

   A. *Pure pia-arachnoiditis*: headache, stiff neck, Kernig and Brudzinski signs. These signs depend on the activation of protective reflexes which shorten the spine and immobilize it. Extension of the neck and flexion of the hips and knees reduce stretch on inflamed spinal structures; resistance to forward flexion of the neck and extension of the legs involves maneuvers that oppose these protective reflexes.

   B. *Subpial encephalopathy*: confusion, stupor, coma, and convulsions are related to this lesion. The tissue beneath the pia is not penetrated by bacteria; hence the change is probably toxic. Cerebral infarction due to cortical vein thrombosis may underlie these symptoms in some cases.

   C. *Inflammatory or vascular involvement of cranial nerve roots*: ocular palsies, facial weakness, and deafness are the main clinical signs. *Note*: Deafness may also be due to middle ear infection, to extension of meningeal infection to the inner ear, or to toxic effects of antimicrobial agents.

   D. *Thrombosis of meningeal veins*: focal convulsions, focal cerebral defects such as hemiparesis, aphasia (rarely prominent), etc., may appear on the third or fourth day after the onset of meningeal infection, but more often after the first week.

   E. *Ependymitis, choroidal plexitis*: it is doubtful if there are any recognizable clinical effects aside from those of the associated meningitis and hydrocephalus.

II. In more subacute and chronic forms of meningitis:

   A. *Tension hydrocephalus*, due at first to purulent exudate around the base of the brain, later to meningeal fibrosis, and rarely to aqueductal stenosis. *In adults*, there are variable degrees of impairment of consciousness, decorticate postures (arms flexed, legs

extended), grasp and suck reflexes, and sphincteric incontinence. CSF pressure may at first be elevated; as the ventricles enlarge and the choroid plexuses are compressed, it may fall to within limits of normal (normal-pressure hydrocephalus). *In infants and young children*, the main signs are enlarging head, inability to look upward (eyes turn down and lids retract on effort to look up—"sunset" sign); in mildest form, there are only psychomotor retardation, unsteadiness of gait, and incontinence.

   B. *Subdural effusion*: impaired alertness, refusal to eat, vomiting, immobility, bulging fontanels, and persistence of fever despite clearing of CSF. In infants, the effusion causes an exaggerated transillumination. If fever is present but CSF pressure is normal, and if one-sided cerebral signs are clearly in evidence, thrombophlebitis with infarction of underlying brain is the leading possibility.

   C. *Extensive venous or arterial infarction*: unilateral or bilateral hemiplegia, decorticate or decerebrate rigidity, cortical blindness, stupor or coma with or without seizures.

III. Late effects or sequelae:

   A. *Meningeal fibrosis around optic nerves or around spinal cord and roots*: blindness and optic atrophy, and spastic paraparesis with sensory loss in the lower segments of the body (opticochiasmatic arachnoiditis and meningomyelitis, respectively).

   B. *Chronic meningoencephalitis with hydrocephalus*: dementia, stupor or coma, and paralysis (e.g., general paralysis of the insane). If lumbosacral posterior roots are chronically damaged, a tabetic syndrome results.

   C. *Persistent hydrocephalus in the child*: blindness, arrest of all mental activity, bilateral spastic hemiplegia.

they diffuse readily throughout all of the compartments containing CSF. They excite a chemical and cellular reaction that is mediated mainly through the capillaries and venules of the vascular pia and choroid plexuses. The blood-CSF barrier becomes more permeable, and neutrophilic leukocytes, lymphocytes, plasma cells, and other mononuclear cells enter the subarachnoid space. Foreign substances are phagocytized by histiocytes (macrophages) and may be isolated in granulomas by foreign-body giant cells. The more chronic of these reactions lead to fibroblastic proliferation, often with obliteration of the subarachnoid spaces and the development of hydrocephalus. The delicate lining of the ventricles and the fronds of the choroid plexuses, composed of a single layer of cuboidal cells, are regularly damaged. Bacteria or chemical agents may penetrate the tissue beneath the ependyma and excite a focal histiocytic-microglial reaction that erupts into the ventricle. The ependymal cells are shed or are overgrown by subependymal microgliacytes and astrocytes, and the end stage of the process is a granular ependymitis. The aqueduct may become stenotic as part of this subependymal gliosis, and the choroid plexuses may become fibrotic. Some foreign materials drain from the ventricles into subependymal veins.

Structures lying within and next to the cerebrospinal SAS are vulnerable to these reactions. The roots of cranial and spinal nerves, which have no true perineurium, may be injured. The subpial cerebral and cerebellar cortices, the subpial tracts of the spinal cord, and the subpial fibers of the optic nerves, although protected against ingress of bacteria, are nevertheless susceptible to their toxins. The histologic changes in these structures are more subtle, but no less real, than those in the SAS, and are reflected in the encephalopathy and myelopathy that may accompany chronic meningitis. Pial veins may become thrombosed, and cerebral and spinal cord infarction may result. Later, the walls of meningeal arteries become thickened and their lumens narrowed. The thin arachnoidal membrane may be transgressed, particularly in children, and the subdural space is invaded; subdural exudates and vascular and fibroblastic reactions result.

The clinical correlates of these reactions, exemplified best by bacterial meningitis, are shown in Table 30-1.

CHEMICAL REACTIONS OF THE MENINGES

The instillation of chemical agents into the CSF always carries the risk of inducing some of the reactions described above. If the substance diffuses rapidly into the blood, as occurs with spinal anesthetic, no harm is done. Agents such as *Pantopaque*, which were used extensively to visualize the subarachnoid space, often caused meningeal reactions and even granuloma formation, and always had to be removed after the test. We have observed rare cases of arachnoiditis with spinal cord compression and fatal hydrocephalus as a reaction to Pantopaque that had not been removed.

Chemical contaminants of spinal anesthetics have had deleterious effects on spinal roots and meninges, optic nerves, and meninges at the base of the brain. The authors have seen more than 40 cases of serious *neurologic damage from spinal anesthesia* when the latter was dispensed from vials that were kept in sterilizing detergent solutions. Usually, in these cases, the anesthetic effect was inadequate, and immediately following the instillation of the anesthetic agent there was back pain and a rapidly progressive lumbosacral root syndrome (areflexic paralysis and anesthesia of legs and paralysis of sphincters). The CSF protein rose rapidly with slight pleocytosis.

Another delayed, chronic effect—a postspinal anesthesia myeloencephalopathy—may occur. Months or even years after spinal anesthesia there is a gradual onset of spastic-ataxic paraparesis and sensory disturbance, hydrocephalus, and blindness. When care is taken to avoid contamination of the spinal anesthetic, these complications can be prevented.

Recurrent hemorrhage into the ventricles or subarachnoid space gives rise to two other interesting clinical-pathologic syndromes: *postmeningeal hemorrhage hydrocephalus* and *meningeal hemosiderosis*. The former has been described in the preceding section, in relation to normal-pressure hydrocephalus. With reference to the latter, as blood hemolyzes, iron-containing compounds are liberated into the subarachnoid and intraventricualr spaces. The blood products, particularly hematin, are toxic. In the adventitia of the meningeal arteries they may possibly induce spasm and ischemia of the brain. A cerebellar degeneration is added to the hydrocephalus.

REFERENCES

Adams RD, Fisher CM, Hakim S et al: Symptomatic occult hydrocephalus with ''normal'' cerebrospinal fluid pressure: A treatable syndrome. *N Engl J Med* 273:117, 1965.

ADAMS RD, SIDMAN R: *Introduction to Neuropathology*. New York, McGraw-Hill, 1968, pp 85–86.

AMES A, SAKANOUE M, ENDO S: Na, K, Ca, Mg and Cl concentrations in choroid plexus fluid and cisternal fluid compared with plasma ultrafiltrate. *J Neurophysiol* 27:672, 1964.

BARROWS LJ, HUNTER FT, BANKER BQ: The nature and clinical significance of pigments in the cerebrospinal fluid. *Brain* 78:59, 1955.

BLACK PM: Idiopathic normal pressure hydrocephalus. Results of shunting in 62 patients. *J Neurosurg* 53:371, 1980.

CARBAAT P, VAN CREVEL H: Lumbar puncture headache: Controlled study on the preventive effect of 24 hours' bed rest. *Lancet* 2:1133, 1981.

CHUTORIAN AM, GOLD AP, BRAUN CW: Benign intracranial hypertension and Bell's palsy. *N Engl J Med* 296:1214, 1977.

CORBETT JJ: Problems in the diagnosis and treatment of pseudotumor cerebri. *Can J Neurol Sci* 10:221, 1983.

CORBETT JJ, SAVINO PJ, THOMPSON HS et al: Visual loss in pseudotumor cerebri. *Arch Neurol* 39:461, 1982.

CUTLER, RWP, SPERTELL RB: Cerebrospinal fluid: A selective review. *Ann Neurol* 11:1, 1982.

DANDY WE: Experimental hydrocephalus. *Ann Surg* 70:129, 1919.

DAVSON H, WELCH K, SEGAL MB: *Physiology and Pathophysiology of the Cerebrospinal Fluid*. New York, Churchill Livingstone, 1987.

DENNIS M, FRITZ CR, NETLEY CT et al: The intelligence of hydrocephalic children. *Arch Neurol* 38:607, 1981.

DIGRE KB, CORBETT JJ: Pseudotumor cerebri in men. *Arch Neurol* 45:866, 1988.

DURCAN FJ, CORBETT JJ, WALL M: The incidence of pseudotumor cerebri. *Arch Neurol* 45:875, 1988.

FISHER CM: Hydrocephalus as a cause of disturbances of gait in the elderly. *Neurology* 32:1358, 1982.

FISHMAN RA: *Cerebrospinal Fluid in Diseases of the Nervous System*. Philadelphia, Saunders, 1980.

FISHMAN RA: The pathophysiology of pseudotumor cerebri: An unsolved puzzle (editorial). *Arch Neurol* 41:257, 1984.

FOLEY J: Benign forms of intracranial hypertension—''toxic'' and ''otitic'' hydrocephalus. *Brain* 78:1, 1955.

GILLES FH, DAVIDSON RI: Communicating hydrocephalus associated with deficient dysplastic parasagittal arachnoid granulations. *J Neurosurg* 35:421, 1971.

GREER M: Benign intracranial hypertension, in Vinken PJ, Bruyn GW (eds): *Handbook of Clinical Neurology*, vol 16. Amsterdam, North-Holland, 1974, chap 4, pp 150–166.

HAKIM S, ADAMS RD: The special clinical problem of symptomatic hydrocephalus with normal cerebrospinal fluid pressure. *J Neurol Sci* 2:307, 1965.

HUSSEY F, SCHANZER B, KATZMAN R: A simple constant-infusion

manometric test for measurement of CSF absorption: II. Clinical studies. *Neurology* 20:665, 1970.

JOHNSTON I, PATERSON A: Benign intracranial hypertension. *Brain* 97:289, 301, 1974.

KATZMAN R, HUSSEY F: A simple constant-infusion manometric test for measurement of CSF absorption: I. Rationale and method. *Neurology* 20:534, 1970.

LESSELL S, ROSMAN P: Permanent visual impairment in childhood pseudotumor cerebri. *Arch Neurol* 43:801, 1986.

LORENZO AV, PAGE KK, WATTERS GV: Relationship between cerebrospinal fluid formation, absorption and pressure in human hydrocephalus. *Brain* 93:679, 1970.

LUNDBERG N: Continuous recording and control of ventricular fluid pressure in neurosurgical practice. *Acta Psychiatry Scand* 36(suppl 149):1960.

MANN JD, JOHNSON RN, BUTLER AB, BASS NH: Impairment of cerebrospinal fluid circulatory dynamics in pseudotumor cerebri and response to steroid treatment. *Neurology* 29:550, 1979.

MARSHALL L, SMITH R: The outcome of aggressive treatment of head injuries. *J Neurosurg* 50:20, 1979.

MEESE W, KLUGE W, GRUMME T, HOPFENMULLER W: CT evaluation of the CSF spaces in healthy persons. *Neuroradiology* 19:131, 1980.

MERRITT HH, FREMONT-SMITH F: *The Cerebrospinal Fluid*. Philadelphia, Saunders, 1937.

MESTREZAT W: *Le Liquide céphalo-rachidien normal et pathologique: Valeur clinique de l'examen chimique; Syndromes humoraux dans les diverses affections*. Paris, A. Maloine, 1912.

MILHORAT TH: *Pediatric Neurosurgery*. Philadelphia, Davis, 1978.

PAPPENHEIMER JR, HEISEY SR, JORDAN EF, DOWNER J: Perfusion of the cerebral ventricular system in unanesthetized goats. *Am J Physiol* 203:763, 1962.

PENFIELD W, ELVIDGE AR: Hydrocephalus and the atrophy of cerebral compression, in Penfield W (ed): *Cytology and Cellular Pathology of the Nervous System*. New York, Hoeber, 1932, pp 1203–1217.

QUINCKE H: Die Lumbarpunktion des Hydrocephalus. *Klin Wochenschr* 28:929, 965, 1891.

RAICHLE ME, GRUBB RL, PHELPS ME et al: Cerebral hemodynamics and metabolism in pseudotumor cerebri. *Ann Neurol* 4:104, 1978.

ROPPER AH: Raised intracranial pressure in neurologic disease. *Seminars Neurol* 4:397, 1984.

ROPPER AH, MARMAROU A: Mechanism of pseudotumor in Guillain-Barré syndrome. *Arch Neurol* 41:259, 1984.

ROSMAN NP, SHANDS KN: Hydrocephalus caused by increased intracranial venous pressure: A clinicopathological study. *Ann Neurology* 3:445, 1978.

RUSSELL DS: *Observations on the Pathology of Hydrocephalus*. London, HM Stationery Office, 1949.

SAHS A, JOYNT RJ: Brain swelling of unknown cause. *Neurology* 6:791, 1956.

SYMONDS CP: Otitic hydrocephalus. *Brain* 54:55, 1931.

TRIPATHI BS, TRIPATHI RC: Vacuolar transcellular channels as a drainage pathway for CSF. *J Physiol* (Lond) 239:195, 1974.

TORVIK A, STENWIG AE, FINSETH I: The pathology of experimental obstructive hydrocephalus. *Acta Neuropathol* 54:143, 1981.

VAN CREVEL H: Papilledema, CSF pressure, and CSF flow in cerebral tumours. *J Neurol Neurosurg Psychiatry* 42:493, 1979.

WALL M, GEORGE D: Visual loss in pseudotumor cerebri. *Arch Neurol* 44:170, 1987.

WEED LH: Certain anatomical and physiological aspects of the meninges and cerebrospinal fluid. *Brain* 58:383, 1935.

CHAPTER 31

INTRACRANIAL NEOPLASMS

Speaking generally, tumors of the central nervous system constitute a bleak but vitally important chapter of neurologic medicine. Also, in general, it may be said of them that they occur in great variety; produce neurologic symptoms because of their size, location, and invasive qualities; usually destroy the tissues in which they are situated and displace those around them; are a frequent cause of increased intracranial pressure; and are often lethal. This dismal state of affairs is beginning to change, however, thanks to advances in anesthesiology, stereotactic and microneurosurgical techniques, radiation therapy, and the use of antineoplastic agents.

For the student of medicine the most important facts to assimilate are that (1) many types of tumor occur in the cranial cavity and spinal canal, and that certain ones are much more frequent than others (see Table 31-1); (2) some of these tumors, such as the craniopharyngioma, meningioma, and schwannoma, have a disposition to grow in particular parts of the cranial cavity, thereby evincing certain syndromes; (3) growth rates and invasiveness of tumors vary, some like the glioblastoma being highly malignant, invasive, and rapidly progressive and others like the meningioma being benign, slowly progressive, and compressive. These pathologic peculiarities are important, for they have valuable clinical implications—frequently providing the explanation of slowly or rapidly evolving clinical states, and determining a good or poor prognosis after surgical excision.

INCIDENCE OF CNS TUMORS AND THEIR TYPES

In 1983 there were an estimated 400,000 deaths from cancer in the United States. Of these the number of patients who died of primary tumors of the brain seems comparatively small (ca. 12,000), but in another 70,000 to 80,000 patients the brain was affected (mainly by metastases) at the time

of death. Thus, in somewhat more than 20 percent of all the patients with cancer, the brain and its coverings were involved by neoplasm at some time in the course of the illness. Among causes of death from intracranial disease, tumor is exceeded in frequency only by stroke. In children, primary tumors of the brain represent 20 percent of all childhood cancers. In the United States, the yearly incidence rate of all brain tumors is 46 per 100,000, and of primary tumors, 15 per 100,000.

It is difficult to obtain accurate statistics of the types of intracranial tumors, for most of them have been obtained from university hospitals and specialized neurosurgical centers, which attract the more easily diagnosed and treatable forms. From the figures of Posner and Chernick one can infer that secondary tumors of the brain greatly outnumber primary ones, yet in the large series reported in the past (those of Zülch, Cushing, Olivecrona, and Zimmerman) only 3 to 6 percent are of this type. In the autopsy statistics of municipal hospitals, where one would expect a more natural selection of cases, the figures for metastatic growths vary widely (4 to 37 percent); probably they err on the low side since the brain is frequently not examined in cancer patients, and many of the patients with more benign tumors may have found their way to specialized neurosurgical services.

With these reservations concerning frequency, the figures in Table 31-1 might be taken as representative.

BIOLOGY OF NERVOUS SYSTEM TUMORS

In considering the biology of primary nervous system tumors, one of the first problems is the definition of neoplasia. It is well known that a number of lesions may simulate brain tumors in their clinical manifestations and histologic appearance, but they are really hamartomas and not true tumors. A hamartoma is a "tumor-like formation that has its basis in maldevelopment" (Russell) and undergoes little change during the life of the host. The difficulty one encounters in distinguishing it from a true neoplasm, which is an evolving blastomatous lesion whose constituent cells multiply without restraint, is well illustrated by tuberous sclerosis and von Recklinghausen neurofibromatosis. In these diseases both types of lesion are found. In a number of mass lesions such as certain cerebellar astrocytomas, bipolar astrocytomas of the pons and optic nerves, von Hippel-Lindau cerebellar cysts, and pineal teratomas, a clear distinction between neoplasms and hamartomas is often not possible.

The many thoughtful studies of brain tumors have shed little light on their origin. Certainly an analysis of case records has yielded no clue as to why a tumor should begin to grow in the brain during adult life. Antecedent head injury, infection, metabolic and other systemic disease, and exposure to toxins and radiation have all been invoked as causative factors; however, with the exception of radiation and possibly of viral infection, there is no conclusive evidence that any of them play a part in the causation of cerebral neoplasms in humans.

Table 31-1
Types of intracranial tumor in the combined series of Zülch, Cushing, and Olivecrona, expressed in percentage of total (approximately 15,000 cases)*

Tumor	Percent of total
Gliomas†	
Glioblastoma multiforme	20
Astrocytoma	10
Ependymoma	6
Medulloblastoma	4
Oligodendrocytoma	5
Meningioma	15
Pituitary adenoma	7
Neurinoma (schwannoma)	7
Metastatic carcinoma	6
Craniopharyngioma, dermoid, epidermoid, teratoma	4
Angiomas	4
Sarcomas	4
Unclassified (mostly gliomas)	5
Miscellaneous (pinealoma, chordoma, granuloma)	3
Total	100

*In the large Latin American series reported by Polak, the frequency of tumor types is much the same, except for a somewhat higher proportion of metastatic tumors.
†In *children*, the proportions differ: astrocytoma, 48 percent; medulloblastoma, 44 percent; ependymoma, 8 percent.

Johannes Müller (1838), in his atlas *Structure and Function of Neoplasms,* first enunciated the appealing idea that tumors might originate in embryonic cells left in the brain during development. This idea was elaborated by Cohnheim (1878), who postulated that the cause of tumors was an anomaly of the embryonic anlage. Tumors would be expected to form, he stated, at sites where there are rapid differentiations of germ layers and complex migrations of cells. How easy it would be for a defective or incomplete migration to leave embryonic cells in the wrong place; and their unnatural environment might encourage neoplasia. Ribbert, in 1918, extended this hypothesis by postulating that the multipotentiality of some of these embryonic cells would favor blastomatous growth. Also implicit in this histogenetic theory is the idea that the degree of anaplasia, or its opposite, differentiation, depends on the status of the cell rests.

This Cohnheim-Ribbert theory seems most applicable to tumors that arise from vestigial tissues, such as craniopharyngiomas, teratomas, lipomas, and chordomas, some of which are more like hamartomas than neoplasms. Ostertag (1936) suggested that gliomas might have a similar dysontogenetic origin (i.e., from rests of glioblasts), but such rests have never been identified in the normal brain. Possibly this embryonic rest theory might account for cerebral gliomas that arise in the course of certain genetic diseases, as with von Recklinghausen neurofibromatosis, tuberous sclerosis, or hemangioblastomatosis; or it might account for certain midline tumors at sites of closure of the neural tube (polar spongioblastoma; retinoblastoma; gliomas of optic nerve, hypothalamus, periaqueductal region, cerebellum, and spinal cord). However, even in the case of the medulloblastoma, where this embryonic rest theory is invoked most often, one cannot be sure that the neoplasm arises from primitive neuroblasts of the posterior medullary velum.

The factor of age is important in the biology of brain tumors. Medulloblastomas, polar spongioblastomas (piloid astrocytomas), and pinealomas occur mainly before the age of 20 years, and meningiomas and glioblastomas are most frequent around the age of 50 years. Heredity figures importantly in retinoblastomas, neurofibromas, and hemangioblastomas. The rare familial disorders of multiple endocrine neoplasia and multiple hamartomas are associated with an increased incidence of anterior pituitary tumors and meningiomas, respectively. Gliomas have also been reported occasionally in more than one member of a family, but the study of such families has not disclosed the operation of a genetic factor. Only in the gliomas associated with neurofibromatosis and tuberous sclerosis and in the cerebellar hemangioblastoma of von Hippel-Lindau disease is there significant evidence of a hereditary determinant. Martuza has traced the embryogenesis of these tumor types and the retinoblastomas to mutations of normal genes (see further on and also Chap. 44 for details).

The discovery that carcinogens, notably hydrocarbons and nitrosamines, could cause gliomas in animals (certain viruses have similar effects in animals and man; see page 526) cast serious doubt on the validity of the dysontogenetic theory. Examining the origins of the experimental tumors, Zimmerman and others found that the proliferating tumor cells were well-differentiated adult elements, not embryonic remnants. Kernohan and Sayre, on the basis of their studies in humans, came to the same conclusion.

These observations have led to two main concepts of pathogenesis of primary tumors of the CNS: (1) a histogenic theory (Bailey and Cushing, 1926), which is based on the known or assumed embryology of nerve and glial cells. This has remained the basis of most classifications of tumors of central neurogenic origin; and (2) the dedifferentiation theory, now generally accepted, that the tumors arise from neoplastic transformation of adult elements. A normal astrocyte, oligodendrocyte, microgliocyte, or ependymocyte is transformed into a neoplastic cell, and as it multiplies, the daughter cells become variably anaplastic, the more so as the degree of malignancy increases. (Anaplasia refers to the primitive undifferentiated state of the constituent cells.)

PATHOPHYSIOLOGY

Certain principles of physics and physiology govern the production of symptoms by tumor growth. As pointed out in Chap. 30, the cranial cavity has a restricted volume, and the three elements contained therein—the brain (about 1400 mL), CSF (150 mL), and blood (150 mL)—are relatively incompressible. According to the Monro-Kellie hypothesis, the total bulk of the three elements is at all times constant, and any increase in the volume of one of them must be at the expense of one or both of the others; a diminished volume of one is met with a compensatory increase in the others (see Fig. 30-1). A tumor growing in one part of the brain compresses and destroys brain tissue and displaces CSF and blood; once the limit of this accommodation is reached, the intracranial pressure (ICP) rises. The elevation of the ICP and perioptic pressure impairs axonal transport in the optic nerve and the venous drainage from the optic

nerve head and retina, which manifests itself by papilledema ("choked disc," see page 199).

It needs to be pointed out, however, that only some brain tumors cause papilledema and that many others—often quite as large—do not. Thus one may question whether the Monro-Kellie hypothesis and its simple implied relationships of intracranial volume and CSF pressure adequately explain the development of raised CSF pressure and papilledema with brain tumors. In fact, in a slow process such as tumor growth, brain tissue is compressible, as one might suspect from the large indentations of brain produced by meningomas. The studies of van Crevel, using radionuclide cisternography, indicate that in such cases the main factor in the production of papilledema is not the tumor volume but the obstruction of CSF flow, whereby the CSF fails to reach and be absorbed at the superior sagittal sinus.

Presumably, with tumor growth, the venules in the cerebral tissue adjacent to the tumor are compressed, with resulting elevation of capillary pressure, particularly in the cerebral white matter. Microvascular transudative factors, such as proteases released by tumor cells, cause a weakening of the blood-brain barrier and also contribute to vasogenic edema (see below). The small protein fragments that are generated by this protease activity exert osmotic effects as they spread through the white matter of the brain. This is the postulated basis of the regional swelling, also called *localized cerebral edema,* that surrounds the tumor (see further on).

Any general increase in venous pressure retards the absorption of CSF and results in an increase in the volume of the latter. The pressure in the subarachnoid space must always be maintained at a level above that in the venous sinuses in order for CSF absorption to occur. If the increase in venous and CSF pressure occurs slowly, it is compensated at least partially by dilatation of arteries and arterioles; if the increase is rapid, the arterial blood pressure must rise also—usually the systolic more than the diastolic. As a rule this is accompanied by bradycardia (carotid sinus reflex); the combination of increased blood pressure and bradycardia is spoken of as the Cushing effect. These circulatory adjustments are initiated by venous stasis and the accumulation of CO_2 in the vasomotor centers of the medulla and carotid bodies. The respiratory centers also become affected; increases in intracranial pressure usually cause an irregularity and, finally, an arrest of respiration.

BRAIN EDEMA

This is a most important aspect of tumor growth, but it also assumes importance in cerebral trauma, infarction, abscess, and hypoxia—as well as in certain toxic and metabolic states. Brain edema is such a prominent feature of cerebral neoplasm that this is a suitable place to summarize what is known about it.

For a long time it has been recognized that conditions leading to peripheral edema, such as hypoalbuminemia and increased systemic venous pressure, do not have a similar effect on the brain. In contrast, lesions that alter the blood-brain barrier cause rapid swelling of brain tissue. Klatzo specifies two categories, *vasogenic* edema and *cytotoxic* edema; Fishman accepts these two categories but adds a third, which he calls *interstitial*. An example of the latter is said to be obstructive hydrocephalus, in which CSF seeps into the periventricular tissues and occupies the space between cells. Most neuropathologists use the term *interstitial* to refer to any increase in the extravascular intercellular compartment of the brain. This would include vasogenic edema.

Vasogenic edema is the type seen in the vicinity of tumor growths and other localized processes as well as in toxic injury to the blood vessels (e.g., lead encephalopathy). It is practically limited to the white matter and is evidenced by decreased attenuation on CT scanning and increased protein levels in the CSF. Presumably there is increased permeability of the capillary endothelial cells so that plasma enters the extracellular spaces (Fig. 31-1A). The heightened permeability has been attributed to a defect in the tight endothelial cell junctions, but current evidence indicates that increased vesicular transport across the endothelial cells is a more important factor. Experimentally, the increase in permeability has been shown to vary inversely with the molecular weight of various markers; inulin (molecular weight 5000) enters the intercellular space more readily than albumin (molecular weight 70,000). The particular vulnerability of white matter to vasogenic edema is not well understood; probably it is related to a lower capillary density and lower blood flow in white matter than in the cortical gray matter. The accumulation of plasma filtrate, with its high protein content, in the extracellular spaces and between layers of the myelin sheaths would be expected to alter the ionic balance of nerve fibers, impairing their function.

Cytotoxic edema is exemplified by hypoxic injury, in which all the cellular elements (neurons, glia, and endothelial cells) imbibe fluid and swell, with a corresponding reduction in the extracellular-fluid space. The effect of oxygen deprivation is to cause a failure of the ATP-dependent sodium pump within cells; sodium accumulates in the cells, and water follows (Fig. 31-1B). Interesting, however, is the fact that several of the most frequent metabolic and nutritional encephalopathies such as normotensive uremia, and thiamine and vitamin B_{12} deficiencies are not attended by either vasogenic or cytotoxic edema. The term *cellular edema* is preferable to cytotoxic edema because it emphasizes the cellular swelling rather

than a toxic factor in the genesis of the brain edema. As indicated above, it is most often due to hypoxia, but it may also complicate acute hypo-osmolality of the plasma, as occurs with dilutional hyponatremia, inappropriate secretion of antidiuretic hormone, or an osmotic disequilibrium syndrome (page 857). *Interstitial (hydrocephalic) edema* is a recognizable condition but in our view is of little clinical significance, since the edema extends for only 2 to 3 mm from the ventricular wall; we would refer to this state as periventricular interstitial edema in association with tension hydrocephalus.

Most patients with brain tumors have regional swelling of tissue of the vasogenic type, apparently secondary to the elaboration of a transudative factor and high-protein interstitial fluid and to the compressive effects of the mass on surrounding veins. Once pressure is raised in a particular region of the brain, it begins to cause displacement and herniation which allow other vascular and pressure factors to come into play; if respiratory difficulty and secondary hypotension occur, cytotoxic edema is added.

BRAIN HERNIATIONS

The problem of brain herniations is of great importance in all mass lesions, and the underlying principles must be understood. Such phenomena become possible because the cranial cavity is subdivided into several compartments by sheets of relatively rigid dura (the falx cerebri which divides the supratentorial space into right and left halves, and the tentorium which separates the cerebellum from the occipital lobes). The pressure from a mass within any one compartment, therefore, is not evenly distributed. This causes shifts or herniations of brain tissue from one compartment where the pressure is high to another where it is lower. There are three well-known herniations, the *subfalcial, temporal lobe–tentorial,* and *cerebellar–foramen magnum* (Fig. 31-2), and several less familiar ones (cerebellar-tentorial, diencephalic–sella turcica, and orbital frontal–middle cranial fossa). Herniation of swollen brain through an opening in the calvarium, in relation to craniocerebral injury or operation, is yet another (transcalvarial) type.

Subfalcial herniation, in which the cingulate gyrus is pushed under the falx, occurs frequently, but little is known of its clinical manifestations. The most important herniation is the *temporal lobe–tentorial* one, which was described originally by Adolf Meyer, and the clinical significance of which was first appreciated by Kernohan and Woltman and by Jefferson. Here the medial part of one temporal lobe (usually the uncus) is forced into the oval-shaped tentorial opening through which the midbrain passes. The uncal hernia pushes the midbrain and subthalamus to the opposite side and against the opposite free edge of the tentorial opening, exerting great pressure on the midbrain and subthalamus and on the vessels that encircle and enter these structures. The hemiparesis that results from compression of the cerebral peduncle by the tentorium is ipsilateral to the cerebral lesion and thus constitutes a false localizing sign (crus phenomenon or syndrome). This and other features of transtentorial herniation are considered in Chap. 16 and are summarized in Table 31-2. The extent to which the clinical disturbances attributed to uncal herniation are due to the actual hernia or to a lateral shift of central (diencephalic-mesencephalic) structures is controversial. In our observations of pathologic specimens we have noted that early symptoms, particularly impaired consciousness, may occur with a lateral displacement and that frank herniation may occur later—a sequence that Ropper has been able to demonstrate by CT scanning and MRI.

The *cerebellar–foramen magnum herniation* or *pressure cone*, first described by Cushing in 1917, consists of downward displacement of the inferior mesial parts of the cerebellar hemispheres (mainly the ventral paraflocculi or tonsillae) through the foramen magnum, behind the cervical

Figure 31-1

A. *Schematic representation of the astrocytes and endothelial cells of the capillary wall in the normal state* (above) *and in vasogenic edema* (below). *Heightened permeability in vasogenic edema is due partly to a defect in tight endothelial junctions but mainly to active vesicular transport across endothelial cells.* B. *Cellular (cytotoxic) edema, showing swelling of the endothelial, glial, and neuronal cells, at the expense of the extracellular fluid space of the brain. (From Fishman.)*

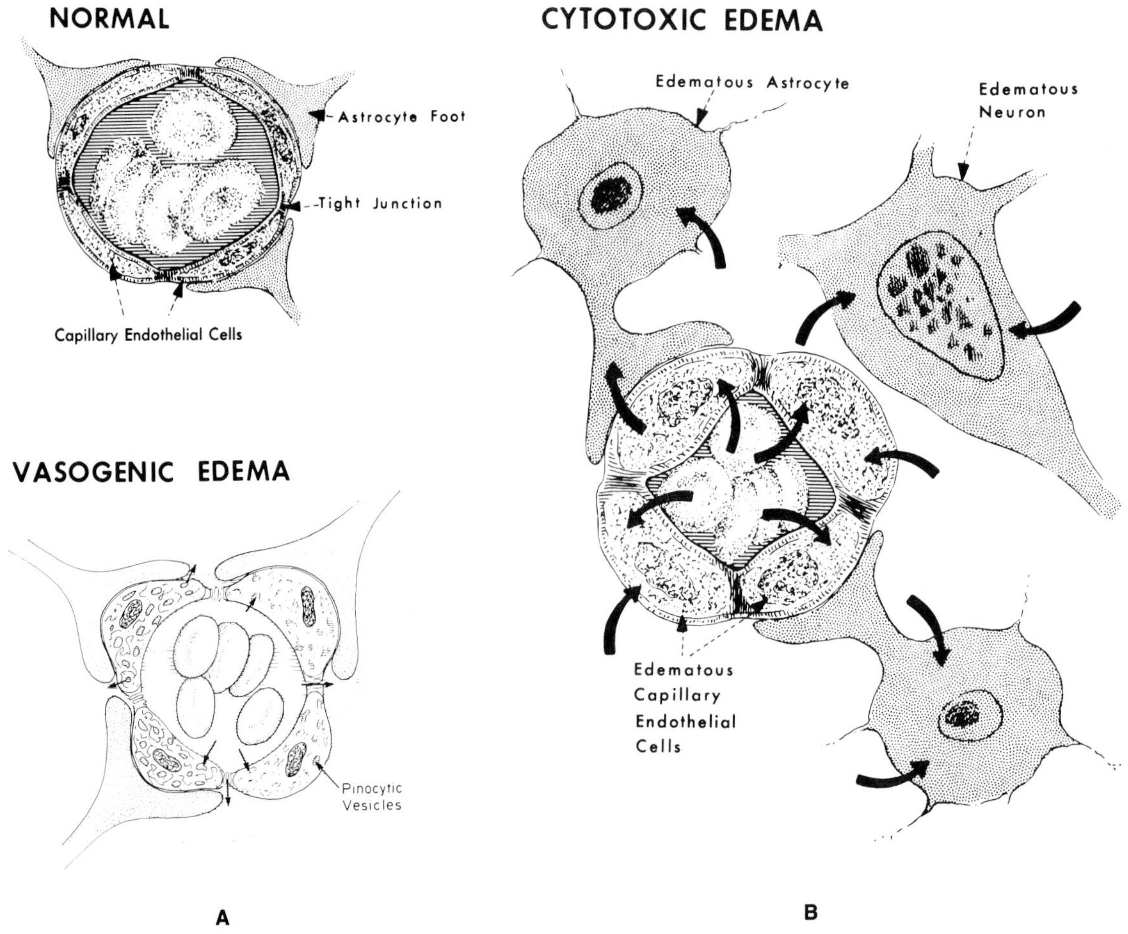

Table 31-2
Temporal lobe–tentorial (uncal) herniation

Pathologic change	Mechanism	Clinical disorders
Injury to outer fibers of ipsilateral oculomotor nerve	Strangulation of nerve between herniating tissue and medial petroclinoid ligament; less often, downward pressure and entrapment of nerve between posterior cerebral and superior cerebellar arteries	Ptosis and pupillary dilatation (Hutchinson pupil), ophthalmoplegia later
Creasing of contralateral cerebral peduncle (Kernohan's notch)	Pressure of laterally displaced midbrain against sharp edge of tentorium	Hemiplegia ipsilateral to herniation (*false localizing sign*) and bilateral corticospinal tract signs
Lateral flattening of midbrain and zones of necrosis and secondary hemorrhages in tegmentum and base of subthalamus, midbrain, and upper pons (Duret hemorrhages)	Crushing of midbrain between herniating temporal lobe and opposite leaf of tentorium and vascular occlusion (hemorrhages around arterioles and veins)	Cheyne-Stokes respirations; stupor-coma; bipyramidal signs; decerebration; dilated, fixed pupils and alterations of gaze (facilitated oculocephalic reflex movement giving way to loss of all response to head movement and labyrinthine stimulation)
Unilateral or bilateral infarction (hemorrhagic) of occipital lobes	Compression of posterior cerebral artery against the tentorium by herniating temporal lobe	Usually none detectable during coma; homonymous hemianopia (unilateral or bilateral) with recovery
Rising intracranial pressure and hydrocephalus	Lateral flattening of aqueduct and blockage of perimesencephalic subarachnoid space	Increasing coma, rising blood pressure, bradycardia

Figure 31-2

Mass shifts associated with a parietal lobe tumor. Top. *The cingulate gyrus is displaced under the falx, toward the opposite side.* Middle. *The inferomedial parts of the temporal lobe are forced into the posterior fossa through the tentorial hiatus, alongside the brainstem (temporal lobe–tentorial herniation or pressure cone).* Bottom. *The cerebellar tonsils are pressed into the foramen magnum, displacing the medulla caudally. The gyri overlying the tumor are flattened. (From Zülch.)*

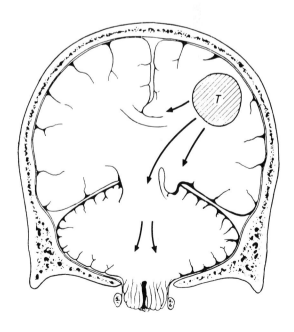

cord. The displacement may be bilateral or unilateral, in the case of a one-sided cerebellar lesion. Bilateral displacement may result from a centrally placed frontal tumor or from general swelling of the brain. It may also accompany temporal lobe–tentorial herniation, which is usually caused by laterally placed cerebral hemispheric or surface lesions (particularly in the temporal region). The herniating cerebellar tissue may swell and become infarcted; but whether it does or not, the lethal effects of this herniation are the result of medullary compression.

The clinical manifestations are less well delineated than those of the temporal lobe–tentorial herniation. Cushing considered the typical signs of cerebellar herniation to be episodes of tonic extension and arching of the neck and back and extension and internal rotation of the limbs, with respiratory disturbances, cardiac irregularity (bradycardia or tachycardia), and loss of consciousness. Other signs include pain in the neck, stiff neck, head tilt, paresthesias in the shoulders, dysphagia, loss of tendon reflexes, and autonomic effects (cardiac dysrhythmia and respiratory arrest). It is important to determine which signs are due to the cerebellar herniation per se and which to the attendant intracranial pressure effects and hydrocephalus. We would suggest that head tilt, stiff neck, arching of the neck, and paresthesias over the shoulders are attributable to the herniation, and that tonic extensor spasms of the limbs and body (so-called cerebellar fits) and coma are due to the compressive effects of the cerebellar lesion or hydrocephalus on upper brain-stem structures. Respiratory arrest is the most feared and often a fatal effect of medullary compression.

The elevation of intracranial pressure from a mass lesion or hydrocephalus, if severe, causes a depression of cerebral function. This is manifested clinically by reduced speed of psychocerebral activities, apathy, drowsiness, inattentiveness, and impaired ability to register information—and electrically by a diffuse decrease in the frequency of brain waves. The rate of cerebral blood flow also is slowed.

A knowledge of the effects of elevated intracranial pressure, localized vasogenic edema, and herniations and displacements of tissue are absolutely essential to understanding the clinical behavior of intracranial growths. The symptoms of intracranial tumors are more often related to these effects than to direct invasion of neurologic structures, and many false localizing signs (unilateral or bilateral abducens palsy, ipsilateral or bilateral corticospinal tract signs, etc.) are due to these mechanical changes.

CLINICAL AND PATHOLOGIC CHARACTERISTICS OF BRAIN TUMORS

It should be stated at the outset that tumors of the brain may exist with hardly any symptoms. Often a slight bewilderment, slowness in comprehension, or loss of capacity to sustain continuous mental activity is the only deviation from normal function, and signs of focal cerebral disease are wholly lacking. In some patients, on the other hand, there is early indication of cerebral disease in the form of a seizure or other dramatic symptom, but the evidence for a time may

not be clear enough to warrant the diagnosis of a cerebral tumor. In a third group, the existence of a brain tumor can be assumed because of the presence of increased intracranial pressure, with or without localizing signs of the tumor. In a fourth group, the symptoms are so definite as to make it probable that not only is there an intracranial neoplasm, but that it is located in a particular region. In fact, these localized growths may create certain syndromes seldom caused by any other disease.

In the further exposition of this subject, intracranial tumors are considered in relation to the common clinical circumstances in which they are likely to be found, as follows:

1. Patients who present with general impairment of cerebral function, headaches, or seizures.

2. Patients who present with evidence of increased intracranial pressure.

3. Patients who present with specific intracranial tumor syndromes.

PATIENTS WHO PRESENT WITH GENERAL IMPAIRMENT OF CEREBRAL FUNCTION, HEADACHES, OR SEIZURES

These are the patients who give the greatest difficulty in diagnosis and about whom decisions are often made with a great degree of uncertainty. Their initial symptoms are vague, and not until some time has elapsed will signs of focal brain disease appear; when they do, they are not always of accurate localizing value. Altered mental function, headache, dizziness, and seizures are the usual manifestations in this group of patients.

Changes in Mental Function   Practically every patient in this group will show some alteration of mental function, but in order to learn of it one must often obtain the observations of a person who knows the patient intimately. A lack of persistent application to the tasks of the day, an undue irritability, emotional lability, mental inertia, faulty insight, forgetfulness, reduced range of mental activity, indifference to common social practices, lack of initiative and spontaneity—all of which may incorrectly be attributed to worry, anxiety, or depression—are the usual abnormalities. We have sought a convenient term for this complex of symptoms, which is the most common type of mental disturbance encountered with neurologic disease, but none seems entirely appropriate. There is both a reduction in the amount of thought and action, and a slowing of reaction time. MacCabe refers to this condition as "mental asthenia," which has the merit of distinguishing it from depression. We prefer to call it *psychomotor asthenia*. Much of this change in behavior is accepted by the patient with forbearance; if any complaint is made, it is of being weak, tired, or dizzy (nonrotational). Inordinate drowsiness, apathy, equanimity, or stoicism may be prominent features of this state. Within a few weeks or months these symptoms become more prominent. When questioned, a long pause precedes each reply, and at times the patient may not bother to respond at all. Or at the moment the examiner decides that the patient has not heard the question and prepares to repeat it, an appropriate answer is given, usually in few words. Moreover, the responses are often more intelligent than one would expect, considering the torpid mental state. There are, in addition, patients who are overtly confused or demented (see Chaps. 19 and 20). The dullness and somnolence increase gradually and finally, as increased intracranial pressure supervenes, they progress to stupor or coma.

Mental symptoms of this type cannot be ascribed to disease in any particular part of the brain, but the tumors most likely to cause them are the ones that interfere with long association fiber systems of the cerebral white matter (frontal, temporal, and corpus callosum gliomas); growths that are limited to the cortex and subcortical white matter are less likely to affect the mind. Much of the drowsiness, torpor, inertia, lack of spontaneity, and general restriction of mental horizon is related to increased intracranial pressure and is unrelated to the site and nature of the lesion.

Headaches These are an early symptom in about one-third of "tumor patients," and are variable in nature. In some the pain is slight, dull in character, and episodic; in others it is severe and either dull or sharp, but also transitory or intermittent. If there are any characteristic features of the headache, they would be its nocturnal occurrence or presence on first awakening, and perhaps its deep nonpulsatile quality. However, these are not specific attributes, since migraine, hypertensive vascular headaches, etc., may also begin in the early morning hours or on awakening. Tumor patients do not always complain of the pain even when it is present but may betray its existence by placing their hands to their heads and looking distressed. When headache appears in the course of the psychomotor asthenia syndrome, it serves to clarify the diagnosis, but not nearly as much as does the occurrence of a seizure.

The mechanism of the headache is not fully understood. In the majority of instances, the CSF pressure is normal during the first weeks when the headache is present, and one can attribute it only to local swelling of tissues and to distortion of blood vessels in or around the tumor. Later the headache appears to be related to generalized rises in intracranial pressure. Tumors above the tentorium cause headache on the side and in the vicinity of the tumor, in the orbital-frontal, temporal, or parietal region; those in the posterior fossa usually cause ipsilateral retroauricular or occipital headache. With elevated intracranial pressure, bifrontal and bioccipital headache is the rule, regardless of the location of the tumor.

Vomiting This symptom appears in about one-third of the patients with a tumor syndrome of this type and usually accompanies the headache. It is more frequent with tumors of the posterior fossa. The most persistent vomiting that we have observed was in a patient with a low brainstem glioma and in another with a subtentorial meningioma. Some patients may vomit unexpectedly and forcibly, without preceding nausea (projectile vomiting), but others suffer both nausea and great pain. Usually the vomiting is not related to the ingestion of food; often it occurs before breakfast.

No less frequent is the complaint of *giddiness* or *dizziness*. As a rule it is not described with accuracy and consists of an unnatural sensation in the head, coupled with feelings of strangeness and insecurity when the position of the head is altered. Frank positional vertigo may be a symptom of a tumor in the posterior fossa (see Chap. 14).

Seizures The occurrence of focal or generalized seizures is the other major manifestation of cerebral tumor. They have been observed, in various series, in 20 to 50 percent of all patients with cerebral tumors. The occurrence of a seizure for the first time during adult years and the existence of a localizing aura are always suggestive of tumor. The localizing significance of seizure patterns has already been discussed (see page 253). There may be one seizure or many, and they may follow the other symptoms or precede them by weeks or months or, exceptionally, by several years in patients with astrocytoma, oligodendroglioma, or meningioma.

Management The management of patients who present any of the aforementioned symptoms requires brief discussion. Any impairment of intellectual function—especially if accompanied by recurrent headaches that are different from the patient's customary headaches or by a seizure, appearing for the first time—justifies a careful review of the patient's general medical status. In obtaining further data, one must rely heavily on the observations of other members of the family. A thorough neurologic examination must follow, with careful inspection of optic fundi, and with testing of visual fields, motor, reflex, and sensory functions in the limbs, alertness, memory, visuospatial orientation, facility in language (speaking, reading, writing, and understanding the spoken word), and calculation.

Sooner or later, regional or localizing symptoms and signs will be discovered, but nearly always they are slight and subtle; it is only by repeated examinations that one will note the earliest stages of a hemiparesis, aphasia, visual field defect, hemianesthesia, etc. Signs of increased intracranial pressure may become manifest and establish the diagnosis of tumor with reasonable certainty even before focal or lateralizing signs are detectable.

Choosing the appropriate time for performing diagnostic tests requires balanced clinical judgment. Since many of the symptoms described above could be due to any number of diseases, it is wise to observe the patient for a time with repeated examinations and not to proceed precipitously with a series of expensive and difficult procedures. As the clinical picture begins to unfold, a CT or MR scan and plain films of the chest should always be obtained (to help exclude metastatic carcinoma), and if the scans are unrevealing, a lumbar puncture and EEG should be performed, preferably after admitting the patient to a hospital. Perimetry, audiograms, radionuclide scans, evoked potential studies, and vestibular and psychometric tests are also helpful in the study of certain patients. Arteriography should be reserved for those in whom the clinical syndrome is already strongly suggestive of tumor and then only if the CT scan has not clarified the problem sufficiently.

The cerebral tumors which are most likely to produce the syndrome described above are glioblastoma multiforme, astrocytoma, oligodendroglioma, ependymoma, metastatic carcinoma, meningioma, and primary lymphoma of the brain.

Glioblastoma multiforme The glioblastoma multiforme accounts for about 20 percent of all intracranial tumors, for about 55 percent of all tumors of the glioma group, and for more than 90 percent of gliomas of the cerebral hemispheres in adults. Although predominantly cerebral in location, similar tumors may be observed in the brainstem, cerebellum, or spinal cord. The peak incidence is in middle adult life, but no age group is exempt. According to Zülch and to Rubinstein, the incidence in men is twice that in women.

The glioblastoma has been known since the time of Virchow and was definitively recognized as a glioma by Bailey and Cushing in their histogenetic classification. It is highly malignant, infiltrates the brain extensively, and may attain enormous size before attracting medical attention. It may extend to the meningeal surface or the ventricular wall, which probably accounts for the increase in CSF protein (more than 100 mg/dL in many cases), as well as

for an occasional pleocytosis of 10 to 100 cells or more, mostly lymphocytes. Malignant cells, carried in the CSF, may form distant foci on spinal roots or cause a widespread meningeal gliomatosis. Extraneural metastases are very rare; usually they involve bone and lymph nodes, after craniotomy. About 50 percent of glioblastomas are bilateral or occupy more than one lobe of a hemisphere; between 3 and 6 percent show multicentric foci of growth.

The tumor has a variegated appearance, being a mottled gray, red, orange, or brown, depending on the degree of necrosis and presence of hemorrhage, recent or old. It is highly vascular, and in an arteriogram one can often see a network of abnormal vessels, mistaken at times for a hemangioma, and displacement of normal vessels as an effect of the tumor mass (*mass lesion*). Some part of one lateral ventricle is often distorted, and both lateral and third ventricles may be displaced contralaterally, features that are demonstrated by CT scan (Fig. 31-3).

The characteristic histologic findings are great cellularity with pleomorphism of cells and hyperchromatism of nuclei; identifiable astrocytes with fibrils in combination with astroblasts in many cases; tumor giant cells and cells in mitosis; hyperplasia of endothelial cells of small vessels; and necrosis, hemorrhage, and thrombosis of vessels. Originally regarded as derived from and composed of primitive embryonal cells, this tumor is now generally thought to arise through anaplasia of mature astrocytes. For this reason, Kernohan and Sayre suggested that the term *glioblastoma* be replaced by *malignant astrocytoma, grade 3 or 4*. Currently, the terms that are favored are glioblastoma multiforme and anaplastic astrocytoma; these terms probably correspond to astrocytomas grade 4 and 3, respectively. The two tumors differ in age of onset and response to treatment. The mean age of patients with glioblastoma is 56 years, and with anaplastic astrocytoma, 46 years. In a recent large series, the 18-month postoperative survival was 15 percent in patients with glioblastoma and 62 percent in those with anaplastic astrocytoma.

Clinically, the diffuse cerebral symptoms and seizures (present in 30 to 40 percent of cases) usually give way in a few weeks or months to a more definite frontal, temporal, parieto-occipital, or callosal syndrome. Seldom, however, do the symptoms and signs point to one lobe, and often one is satisfied to be able to specify the general region of the hemisphere which is involved. MacCabe's observation that 10 percent of glioblastomas begin with mental symptoms matches our own experience.

In a minority of patients (4 percent, according to Frankel and German) the onset of symptoms may be sudden. This is usually attributed to hemorrhage or the rapid expansion of a cyst within the tumor. The CSF is occasionally bloody under these circumstances. We have also observed patients in whom the clinical picture evolved within 2 to 3 weeks and, with unsuccessful surgery, ended fatally soon afterward. However, in most cases, symptoms have been present for 3 to 6 months before the diagnosis is established. The rapid development of focal cerebral symptoms is usually related to cerebral edema, hemorrhage, and necrosis rather than tumor infiltration. Indeed, it is remarkable how large and extensive the tumor may become before it deranges cerebral function.

The natural history of glioblastoma is well known. Less than a fifth of all patients survive for 1 year after the onset of symptoms, and only about 10 percent beyond 2 years. Cerebral edema, increased intracranial pressure, and temporal lobe–tentorial herniation are the immediate causes of death.

The treatment of glioblastomas is rather unsatisfactory. At operation only part of the tumor can be removed. The multicentricity and diffusely infiltrative character of these tumors defy the scalpel. Following a maximally feasible resection, without the addition of radiation and chemotherapy, there is a median survival of only 14 weeks, but very few patients survive beyond a year. Radiation therapy, in doses up to 5000 rads over a period of 3 to 4 weeks, increases survival by 5 months. The addition of the chemotherapeutic agent BCNU increases survival only modestly. Dexamethasone improves neurologic functioning. Survival beyond 2 years occurs but is exceptional; most of the patients die in approximately 12 months (Shapiro).

An unusual variant of this tumor is *gliomatosis cerebri*, in which an entire hemisphere or the entire brain is diffusely infiltrated, without a discrete tumor mass being seen. Many small series of such cases have been reported since Nevin introduced this term in 1938, but no distinctive clinical picture has emerged (Dunn and Kernohan). Impairment of intellect, headache, seizures, and papilledema are the major manifestations and do not set these cases apart from the usual forms of glioblastoma where the tumor may also be more widespread than the macroscopic picture suggests. The CT scan shows small ventricles and multiple areas of diminished density, despite the diffuse nature of the tumor.

Astrocytoma Grade 1 and 2 astrocytomas, which constitute between 25 and 30 percent of cerebral gliomas,

Figure 31-3

Glioblastoma multiforme. A. *Unenhanced CT scan showing a large lesion of the hemisphere encroaching on the lateral ventricle.* B. *Enhanced view.*

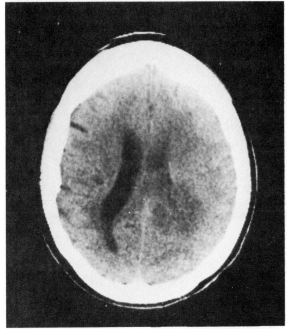

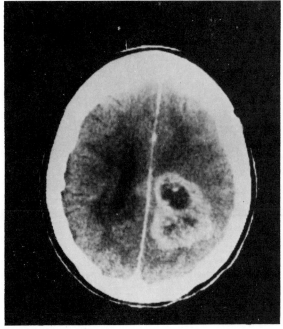

A

B

may occur anywhere in the brain or spinal cord. Favored sites are the cerebrum, cerebellum, hypothalamus, optic nerve and chiasm, and pons. The cerebral hemisphere astrocytomas generally occur in adults in their third and fourth decades; astrocytomas in other parts are more frequent in children and adolescents.

Cerebral astrocytoma is a slowly growing tumor of infiltrative character with a tendency to form large cavities or pseudocysts. Other tumors of this category are noncavitating, grayish white, firm, and relatively avascular, almost indistinguishable from normal white matter, with which they merge imperceptibly. Calcium may be deposited in parts of the tumor and be seen in CT scans. The CSF is acellular, and the only abnormalities are the increased pressure and protein content in some cases. The tumor may distort the lateral and third ventricles and displace the anterior and middle cerebral arteries (seen in CT scans and arteriograms; see Fig. 31-4). Microscopically the tumor is composed of well-differentiated astrocytes of fibrillary, protoplasmic, or transitional type. Many cerebral astrocytomas eventually undergo malignant degeneration and present as mixed astrocytomas and glioblastomas.

In about half the patients with astrocytoma, the opening symptom is a focal or generalized seizure, and between 60 and 75 percent of patients have recurrent seizures in the course of their illness. The onset of focal seizures in individuals 20 to 60 years of age should always arouse suspicion of a cerebral astrocytoma. Other subtle cerebral symptoms follow after months, sometimes after years. Headaches and signs of increased intracranial pressure are relatively late occurrences.

Temporal lobe gliomas in which mental symptoms precede seizures give rise to particular difficulty in diagnosis. Slight character and personality changes, moodiness, pseudoneurotic symptoms, and episodes suggestive of schizophrenia may precede or follow the onset of temporal lobe seizures. Hemiparesis, in frontal gliomas, may present only as a slight drift of the outstretched arm, a mild limp, and enhanced tendon reflexes, and may remain slight in degree for a long time. Language difficulties and sensory changes are also frequently slight and subtle.

Seizures, headaches, and the mental symptoms described above may be present for several years, in some instances for 10 years or even longer, before the diagnosis is made. In contrast to glioblastoma, the average survival period after the first symptom is 67 months in cases of cerebral astrocytoma, and 89 months in cerebellar ones.

Excision of a part of the cerebral astrocytoma and particularly removing the cystic part may allow survival in a functional state for many years. Radiation therapy is said to improve survival, but no prospective controlled studies have been carried out. The cystic astrocytoma of the cerebellum is particularly benign. It declares itself in children by some combination of gait unsteadiness, unilateral cerebellar signs, and increased intracranial pressure (headaches, vomiting), and about 10 percent of patients are alive and well as long as 20 to 30 years after excision of the cyst. In such cases, of course, accuracy of the original diagnosis of neoplasm is always open to question. The astrocytomas of the pons, hypothalamus, optic nerves, and chiasm are discussed in more detail further on in this chapter.

Oligodendroglioma This tumor was first identified by Bailey and Cushing in 1926, and described more fully by Bailey and Bucy in 1929. The tumor is derived from oligodendrocytes and may be identified at any age, most often in the third and fourth decades, with an earlier

Figure 31-4

Enhanced CT scan showing a deep parietal astrocytoma and edema of the surrounding white matter. The tumor encroaches upon the opposite hemisphere. The large area of diminished attenuation within the tumor represents a cyst. Mental symptoms and recurrent generalized seizures had been present for many years before the diagnosis was made.

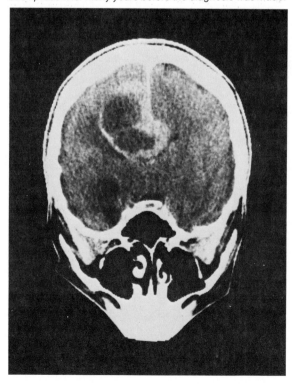

peak at 6 to 12 years. It is relatively infrequent, constituting about 5 to 7 percent of all intracranial gliomas. Males outnumber females 2:1. In some cases the tumor may be recognized macroscopically because of its pink-gray color and multilobular form, its relative avascularity and firmness (slightly tougher than surrounding brain), and its tendency to encapsulate and to form calcium and small cysts. Most oligodendrogliomas, however, are indistinguishable grossly from other gliomas. The type cell has a small, round nucleus and halo of unstained cytoplasm. The cell processes are few and stubby, and are visualized only with silver carbonate stains. Microscopic calcifications are observed frequently, mainly in relation to zones of necrosis. Probably half the tumors generally classified as oligodendrogliomas are in fact mixed types (oligodendroglioma-astrocytoma).

The most common sites of this tumor are the frontal lobes (40 to 70 percent), often deep in the white matter with little or no surrounding edema. Sometimes it presents as an intraventricular tumor and rarely it occurs in other parts of the cerebrum, third ventricle, brainstem, cerebellum, and spinal cord. By extending to the pial surface or ependymal wall, the tumor may metastasize distantly in ventriculosubarachnoid spaces, accounting for 11 percent of the Polmeteer and Kernohan series of gliomas with meningeal dissemination (less frequent than medulloblastoma and glioblastoma; see also Yung et al). Malignant degeneration (evidenced by greater cellularity and by numerous and abnormal mitoses) occurs in about a third of cases.

The typical oligodendroglioma grows slowly, and the interval between the first symptom and surgical intervention varies from 28 to 70 months. As with astrocytomas, the first symptom in more than half the patients is a focal or generalized seizure; seizures often persist for many years before other symptoms develop. Approximately 15 percent of patients enter the hospital with early symptoms and signs of increased intracranial pressure; but even by the time surgery is performed, only about half of all cases have increased intracranial pressure, and only about one-third have focal cerebral signs (hemiparesis). Much less frequent findings are unilateral extrapyramidal rigidity, cerebellar ataxia, Parinaud syndrome, intratumoral hemorrhage, and meningeal oligodendrogliosis (cranial-spinal nerve palsies, hydrocephalus, lymphocytes in CSF). Calcium is seen in CT scans in more than half the cases.

Surgical excision followed by radiation therapy is the usual treatment. However, because of the uncertainty as to the histologic classification of many of the reported cases, it is not clear whether radiation therapy is attended by longer survival. Well-differentiated oligodendrogliomas should probably not receive radiation. Mixed oligodendrogliomas and astrocytomas should be treated like astrocytomas. Postoperative survival time is governed mainly by the histologic grade of the tumor. In the very large series of Ludwig and coworkers (323 patients) the 5-year survival ranged from 0 to 71 percent, depending upon the histologic grade of the tumor.

Ependymoma This tumor proves to be more complex and variable than other gliomas. Correctly diagnosed by Virchow as early as 1863, its origin from ependymal cells was suggested by Mallory, who found the typical blepharoplasts (small, darkly staining dots, related to ciliation of these cells) in a sacral tumor. Two types were recognized by Bailey and Cushing: one was the ependymoma, and the other, with more malignant and invasive properties, was the ependymoblastoma. More recently a myxopapillomatous type, localized exclusively in the filum terminale of the spinal cord, has been identified (see Chap. 36).

Ependymomas are derived from differentiated ependymal cells, i.e., the cells lining the ventricles of the brain and the central canal of the spinal cord. As one might expect, the tumors either grow into the ventricle or adjacent brain tissue. The most common cerebral site is the fourth ventricle; in the spinal cord most ependymomas originate in the lumbosacral regions, many from the conus or filum terminale. Grossly, those in the fourth ventricle are grayish pink, firm, cauliflower-like growths; those in the cerebrum, arising from the wall of the lateral ventricle, may be large (several centimeters in diameter), reddish gray, and softer and more clearly demarcated from adjacent tissue than astrocytomas, but they are not encapsulated. The tumor cells tend to form canals (rosettes) or circular arrangements (pseudorosettes). Some ependymomas, called epithelial, are densely cellular and anaplastic; others are better differentiated and form papillae. Some of the well-differentiated fourth ventricular tumors are probably derived from subependymal astrocytes.

Approximately 5 percent of all intracranial gliomas are of this type; the percentage is higher in children (8 percent). About 40 percent of the infratentorial ependymomas occur in the first decade of life, a few as early as the first year. The supratentorial ones are more evenly distributed among all age groups.

The *symptomatology* depends on the location of the growth. The clinical manifestations of fourth ventricular tumors (the most common intracranial site) will be described later in this chapter. Cerebral ependymomas resemble the other gliomas in their clinical expression. Seizures occur in approximately one-third of the cases. The interval between the first symptom to operation ranges from 4 weeks, in the most malignant types, to 7 to 8 years. In a follow-up study of 101 cases in Norway, where ependymomas comprised 1.2 percent of all primary intracranial tumors (and 32 percent of intraspinal tumors), the postoperative survival was poor. Within a year, 47 percent had died, but 13 percent were alive after 10 years. Doubtless the prognosis differs depending on the degree of anaplasia. Postoperative irradiation extended the survival period (Mørk and Løken). Antitumor drugs are often used in combination with radiation therapy for cerebral ependymoblastomas.

Meningioma This is a benign tumor, first illustrated by Matthew Bailie, in his *Morbid Anatomy* (1787), and first recognized by Bright, in 1831, as originating from the dura mater or arachnoid. It was analyzed from every point of view by Harvey Cushing and was the subject of one of his most important monographs. Meningiomas comprise about 15 percent of all primary intracranial tumors; they are more common in women than in men (2:1) and have their highest incidence in the seventh decade. There is evidence that persons who have undergone radiation therapy to the scalp or cranium are particularly vulnerable to the development of meningiomas, and that the meningiomas in these patients occur at an earlier age than in nonirradiated persons (Rubinstein et al). Many meningiomas are associated with a karyotype abnormality—a loss of one chromosome 22 or a deletion of part of 22. Also some meningiomas, like many other neoplasms, contain estrogen receptors. The implications of these findings are not yet clear.

The precise origin of meningiomas is still not settled. According to Rubinstein, they may arise from dural fibroblasts, or, more commonly, from arachnoidal cells, in particular from those packing the arachnoid villi. Since these clusters of arachnoidal cells penetrate the dura in largest number in the vicinity of venous sinuses, these are the sites of predilection. Grossly the tumor is firm, gray, and sharply circumscribed, and it takes the shape of the space in which it grows; i.e., some tumors are flat and plaque-like, others are round and lobulated. They may indent the brain and acquire the pia-arachnoid as part of their capsule, but always they are sharply demarcated from the brain tissue. Rarely, they arise from arachnoidal cells within the choroid plexus, forming intraventricular meningiomas. Microscopically the cells are relatively uniform with round or elongated nuclei, visible cytoplasmic membrane, and a characteristic tendency to encircle one another, forming whorls and *psammoma bodies*. Cushing and Eisenhardt divided meningiomas into many subtypes depending

on the character of the stroma and their relative vascularity, but the validity of such a classification is debatable.

The most common sites are the sylvian region, superior parasagittal surface of frontal and parietal lobes, olfactory groove, lesser wing of the sphenoid bones, tuberculum sellae, superior surface of cerebellum, cerebellopontine angle, and spinal canal. Inasmuch as they extend to the dural surface, they often invade and erode the cranial bones or excite an osteoblastic reaction. Sometimes they give rise to an exostosis on the external surface of the skull. Some meningiomas, such as those of the olfactory groove, sphenoid wing, and tuberculum sellae, may express themselves by highly distinctive syndromes that are diagnostic in themselves; these will be described further on in this chapter. The following remarks apply only to meningiomas of the parasagittal, sylvian, and other surface areas.

Small meningiomas, less than 2.0 cm in diameter, are often found at autopsy in middle-aged and elderly persons, without having caused symptoms. Only when they exceed a certain size and indent the brain do they alter function. The size that must be reached before symptoms appear varies with the size of the space in which they grow and the surrounding anatomic arrangements. Small tumors under the floor of the third ventricle are more likely to be symptomatic than small ones that lie over the cerebrum. Focal seizures are often an early sign. The parasagittal frontal-parietal meningioma may cause a slowly progressive spastic weakness and/or numbness of one leg, and later of both legs. The sylvian tumors are manifested by a variety of signs in accord with their location.

Meningiomas may give rise to neurologic signs for 10 to 15 years before the diagnosis is established, attesting to their slow rate of growth. Some tumors reach enormous size before coming to medical attention. A few may be detected in plain films or in CT scans in individuals with unrelated neurologic diseases. Increased intracranial pressure eventually occurs, but it is less frequent with meningiomas than with gliomas.

Diagnosis is greatly facilitated by the ready visualization of meningiomas with isotopic and contrast-enhanced CT scanning (Fig. 31-5) and MRI (Fig. 31-13), and by arteriography, which reveals the prominent vascularity as a "blush." The CSF protein is usually elevated.

Surgical excision should afford permanent cure in all accessible surface tumors. A few show malignant, invasive qualities. Recurrence is likely if removal is incomplete. The most difficult ones to remove surgically lie beneath the hypothalamus, along the medial part of the sphenoid bone and parasellar region, or anterior to the brainstem. By invading adjacent bone they become inoperable. Carefully planned radiation therapy is beneficial both in cases that are inoperable and in those in which the tumor is incompletely removed (Leibel et al).

Primary cerebral lymphoma For many years it was taught that this tumor is a histiocytic sarcoma, originating in the reticuloendothelial system and that the meningeal and perivascular histiocytes and the microgliocytes, the representatives of this system in the brain, are its natural sources. Hence the older terms reticulum cell sarcoma and microglioblastoma. Now it is known, on the basis of immunocytochemical studies, that the cells of the tumor react like B lymphocytes, and that the tumor corresponds histologically to what Rappaport called the large cell or histiocytic type of malignant lymphoma. Large series of cases have been reported by Schaumburg, by Henry, and by Helle and their colleagues.

The tumor may arise primarily in any part of the cerebrum, cerebellum, or brainstem and may be either monofocal or multifocal. It forms a pinkish gray, soft, ill-defined, infiltrative mass, difficult at times to distinguish from a malignant glioma. Perivascular and meningeal spread results in shedding of cells into the CSF. The tumor is highly cellular, with little tendency to necrosis. The nuclei are oval or bean-shaped with scant cytoplasm. Mitotic figures are numerous. The stainability of reticulum and microglial cells, the latter by silver carbonate, serves to distinguish this tumor microscopically.

This tumor pursues much the same clinical course as the glioblastoma, and the interval between the first symptom and operation has been approximately 3 months. Behavioral and personality changes and focal cerebral signs predominate over headache and other signs of increased intracranial pressure as presenting manifestations. Most cases occur in adult life, but some occur in children in whom the tumor may simulate the cerebellar symptomatology of medulloblastoma. The finding, on CT scan, of one or more dense, homogeneously enhancing periventricular masses, is characteristic. Lymphocytic and mononuclear pleocytosis is more frequent than with gliomas, and tumor cells may be seen. The immunohistochemical demonstration of monoclonal lymphocytes or an elevated beta microglobulin indicates leptomeningeal spread of the tumor (Li et al).

Patients with AIDS and less common immunodeficiency states such as the Wiskott-Aldrich syndrome and ataxia-telangiectasia, and patients receiving immunosuppressive drugs for long periods, such as those undergoing renal transplantation, are particularly liable to develop this

Figure 31-5

Contrast-enhanced CT scans. A. *Falx meningioma.* B. *Sphenoid wing meningioma.*

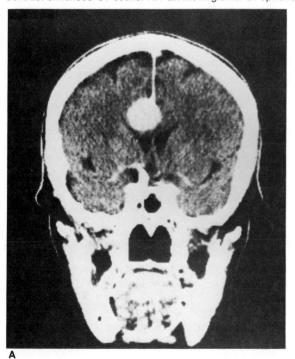

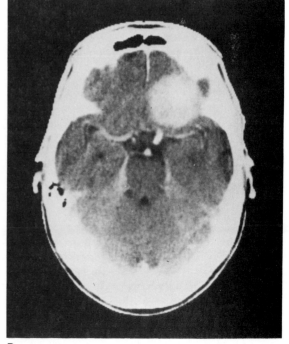

A

B

type of primary cerebral lymphoma. Hochberg and his colleagues have studied five patients with primary cerebral lymphoma in whom there was serologic evidence of a recent infection with Epstein-Barr (EB) virus. Moreover, the EB virus genome was incorporated in tumor cells but not in neighboring nerve cells. The neoplasms in these patients developed in the absence of immunosuppression or systemic lymphoma, suggesting that the tumor was induced by the EB virus. Sometimes this tumor appears as a complication of obscure medical conditions such as salivary and lacrimal gland enlargement (Mikulicz syndrome). Its frequency appears to be increasing.

Because the tumors are deep and often multicentric, surgical resection is ineffective, except in rare instances. Stereotactic needle biopsy is the preferred method of establishing the histologic diagnosis. Radiation and steroid therapy are highly effective. Posner has summarized the response to treatment in a large number of patients. Despite an impressive initial response, most patients relapse within a year. Median survival is less than 24 months, although individual patients may live longer.

Metastatic carcinoma Of the secondary intracranial tumors only metastatic carcinoma occurs with high frequency. Occasionally one encounters a rhabdomyosarcoma, Ewing tumor, lymphoma, carcinoid, etc., but these tumors occur so infrequently that their cerebral metastases seldom become a matter of diagnostic concern. Intracranial metastases assume three main patterns—those to the skull and dura, those to the brain itself, and those of the craniospinal meninges (meningeal carcinomatosis).

Metastases to the skull and dura can occur with any tumor that metastasizes to bone, but are particularly common with carcinoma of the breast and prostate and with multiple myeloma. These secondary deposits often occur without metastases to the brain itself and are believed to reach the skull via Batson's vertebral venous plexus—a valveless system of veins that runs the length of the vertebral column from the pelvic veins to the large venous sinuses of the skull, bypassing the systemic circulation. Metastatic tumors of the convexity of the skull are usually asymptomatic (only rarely do they extend to the brain), but those of the base may involve the cranial nerve roots or the pituitary body. Bony metastases are readily recognized on bone and CT scans. Occasionally, a carcinoma metastasizes to the subdural surface and compresses the brain, like a subdural hematoma.

Carcinomas reach the brain by hematogenous spread. About a third of them originate in the lung, and half this number in the breast; melanoma is the third most frequent source, and the gastrointestinal tract (particularly the colon and rectum) and kidney are the next most common. Carcinoma of the gallbladder, liver, thyroid, testicle, uterus, ovary, pancreas, etc., account for the remainder. Carcinoma of the prostate, esophagus, oropharynx, and skin (except for melanocarcinoma) rarely metastasize to the brain. From a somewhat different point of view, certain neoplasms are particularly prone to metastasize to the brain—75 percent of melanomas do so, 57 percent of testicular tumors, and 35 percent of bronchial carcinomas (Posner and Chernick). According to these authors the cerebral metastasis is solitary in 47 percent of cases, a figure that is somewhat higher than that reported by others (see Henson and Urich).

Generally the cerebral metastasis has all the gross and microscopic features of any carcinomatous implant; it forms a circumscribed mass, usually solid but sometimes cystic, and excites rather little glial reaction but much regional vasogenic edema (Fig. 31-6). Metastases from chorioepithelioma and melanoma and some from the lung and kidney are likely to be hemorrhagic.

The usual clinical picture in metastatic carcinoma of the brain does not differ from that of glioblastoma multiforme. Headache, focal weakness, mental and behavioral abnormalities, seizures, ataxia, aphasia, and signs of increased intracranial pressure—all inexorably progressive—

Figure 31-6

Contrast-enhanced CT scan showing a large solitary metastasis (choriocarcinoma) with surrounding edema.

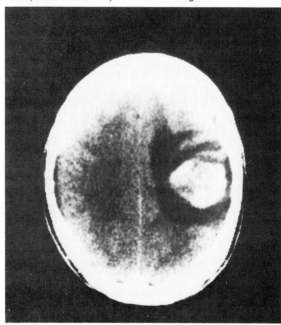

are the common clinical manifestations. However, a number of unusual syndromes also occur. One that presents particular difficulty in diagnosis is a syndrome of diffuse cerebral disturbance with headache, nervousness, depressed mood, trembling, mental confusion, and forgetfulness, a picture very much like that of general paresis. *Carcinomatosis of the cerebellum* with headache, dizziness, and ataxia (the latter being brought out only by having the patient walk) is another condition that is difficult to diagnose during life. Sometimes the onset of neurologic symptoms is abrupt rather than insidious. Some cases of sudden onset can be explained by bleeding into the tumor, and others perhaps by tumor embolism, causing cerebral infarction and leaving a metastasis in its wake. Also, marantic endocarditis with cerebral embolism must be suspected when stroke occurs in a tumor patient.

When the several clinical syndromes due to metastatic tumor are fully developed, diagnosis is relatively easy. If only headache and vomiting are present, a common error is to explain these symptoms on a psychologic basis. One should invoke such an explanation only if the patient has the standard symptoms of some psychiatric illness. CT and particularly MRI, before and after the injection of a contrast agent, are the most sensitive tests for the presence of intracerebral metastases (Fig. 31-6). They have been positive in practically all of our cases. Metastatic disease must be distinguished from a primary tumor of the brain and from certain neurologic syndromes that sometimes accompany carcinoma but which are not due to the invasion or compression of the nervous system by tumor, i.e., polyneuropathy (especially with carcinoma of the lung), polymyositis, spinocerebellar degeneration (ovarian and other carcinomas), and certain cerebral disorders (multifocal leukoencephalopathy, "limbic encephalitis"). These latter syndromes are discussed further on, under "Remote Effects of Neoplasia on the Nervous System."

The treatment of secondary tumor of the nervous system is undergoing change. Several clinical trials suggest that prophylactic irradiation of the neuraxis delays occurrence of metastases and prolongs the ultimate survival of patients with small cell carcinoma of the lung (Nugent et al). Also, CT and MRI are disclosing an increasing number of solitary parenchymatous metastases. If the growth of the primary tumor and its systemic metastases is under good control, and if the cerebral metastasis is accessible to the surgeon and is not located in a strategic motor or language area of the brain, then surgical excision followed by radiation therapy can be undertaken. Patchell and coworkers have shown that the survival and the interval between treatment and recurrence were longer in patients treated in this way than in comparable patients treated with radiation alone. However, these authors say little about the quality of life of the surgical survivors, and frequently this is the most

important consideration in deciding about surgery. In patients with multiple metastases, radiation therapy and steroids nearly always result in some symptomatic improvement. Heretofore, systemic chemotherapy has been thought to be ineffective against cerebral metastases. There is, however, growing evidence that some metastatic brain tumors are quite sensitive to conventional chemotherapeutic agents given intravenously or intra-arterially, provided that the primary tumor is also sensitive. The data from one study suggested that systemic chemotherapy was effective in controlling brain metastases from breast carcinoma in 50 percent of the treated patients (Rosner et al). Intrathecal and intraventricular chemotherapy have no role in the treatment of parenchymal metastases. Immunotherapy has not yet been widely employed.

Despite these therapeutic measures, survival is only slightly prolonged. The average period of survival, even with therapy, is about 6 months. Between 15 and 30 percent of patients live for a year and 5 to 10 percent for 2 years. The patients with bone metastases live longer than those with parenchymatous and meningeal metastases.

Widespread dissemination of tumor cells throughout the meninges and ventricles (*meningeal carcinomatosis*) has been the pattern in about 4 percent of neurologic metastases in our cases of adenocarcinoma of breast, lung, and gastrointestinal tract, melanoma, and childhood leukemia. Headache, backache, radiculopathies (particularly of the cauda equina), cranial nerve palsies, and dementia have been the principal manifestations. Half the patients develop hydrocephalus. Tumor cells can be identified by cytocentrifugation and Millipore filtering in the large majority of cases, providing that more than one examination is done. Increased pressure, elevation of protein and low glucose levels, and lymphocytic pleocytosis are other common CSF findings. In 40 percent of cases there was evidence of one or more parenchymal lesions by CT scan, and in some cases CT scan showed enhancement of the cerebral cortex in addition. Treatment consists of radiation therapy to the symptomatic areas, followed by the intraventricular administration of methotrexate, but these measures rarely stabilize neurologic symptoms for more than a few weeks. The median duration of survival after diagnosis of meningeal carcinomatosis was 5.8 months in the large series reported by Wasserstrom et al, but only 43 days in the series of Sorenson et al.

Involvement of the nervous system in leukemia and systemic lymphoma Almost one-third of all leukemic patients have evidence of diffuse infiltration of the leptomeninges and cranial and spinal nerve roots at autopsy (Barcos et al). The incidence is greater in acute than in chronic leukemia, and greater in lymphocytic than in myelocytic leukemia, and much greater in children than in adults. The highest incidence is in children with acute lymphocytic (lymphoblastic) leukemia who relapse after treatment with combination chemotherapy (60 to 70 percent at time of death). The clinical and CSF picture of meningeal leukemia is much the same as that of meningeal carcinomatosis, discussed above. The treatment of the two disorders is also the same.

The studies of Price and Johnson have demonstrated that CNS leukemia is primarily an arachnoidal disease. The earliest evidence of leukemia is detected in the walls of superficial arachnoid veins, with or without cells in the CSF. The leukemic infiltrate then extends to the deep perivascular spaces, where it is confined, at least for a time, by the pia-glial membrane; at this stage the CSF consistently contains leukemic cells. Depending on the severity of arachnoidal involvement, transgression of the pia-glial membrane then occurs with varying degrees of parenchymal infiltration by collections of leukemic cells. Hemorrhages of varying sizes are common complications and sometimes lethal. *Chloroma*, a solid mass of myelogenous leukemic cells in the brain, is distinctly uncommon.

Cranial irradiation, combined with methotrexate given intrathecally or intravenously, has been effective in the prevention and treatment of meningeal involvement in childhood leukemia. However, it has been associated, in a significant number of patients, with a distinctive necrotizing leukoencephalopathy. This neurologic complication may appear within several days or months after the last administration of the drug, and several months after completion of radiotherapy (Robain et al). Leukoencephalopathy occurs most frequently when all three modalities of treatment, i.e., cranial irradiation and intrathecal and intravenous methotrexate, are used. It is less frequent when two modalities are used and least frequent when only one is used. The initial symptoms, consisting of apathy, drowsiness, depression, and behavioral disorders, evolve over a few weeks to include cerebellar ataxia, spasticity, pseudobulbar palsy, extrapyramidal motor abnormalities, and akinetic mutism. Hypodense areas of varying size appear in the CT scan. In some patients the disease stabilizes, with severe persistent sequelae, but in most death occurs within several weeks or months of onset. Throughout the cerebral white matter and to a lesser extent in the brainstem, there are foci of coagulation necrosis of varying size and severity. In the smaller lesions, a perivascular topography of the tissue

disintegration is evident. The pathogenesis of this disorder is unclear. Radiation injury seems to be the most important factor, coupled with the age of the patient (most patients are under 5 years). It has been speculated that radiation breaks down the blood-brain barrier, allowing methotrexate to injure myelin.

Extradural compression of the spinal cord or cauda equina is the most common neurologic complication of lymphoma, the result of extension from vertebrae or paravertebral lymph nodes. Treatment is radiation or, if a tissue diagnosis is lacking, surgical decompression. Systemic lymphoma rarely metastasizes to the brain. In our large series of cases and in a review of over 10,000 autopsies, we observed only a half-dozen instances where patients with Hodgkin disease had deposits of tumor cells in the brain, and there were no intracerebral metastases of multiple myeloma or plasmacytoma. In a more recent clinical series of 592 patients with non-Hodgkin lymphoma, there were only eight with intracerebral metastases (Levitt et al). Much more common is meningeal dissemination of lymphoma, the clinical and CSF pictures of which are similar to those of meningeal leukemia and carcinomatosis. The optimum treatment has not yet been ascertained. Systemic and intraventricular chemotherapy and radiotherapy have all met with some degree of success. Leukemic conversion (''blast crisis'') undoubtedly favors leptomeningeal dissemination.

So-called *malignant angioendotheliomatosis* is a rare and generally fatal disease, characterized by the proliferation of neoplastic mononuclear cells within the lumens of many small blood vessels, mainly of the skin and CNS. Formerly thought to represent a malignant proliferation of endothelial cells or a widespread dissemination of unrecognized primary carcinoma, it now appears, on the basis of antigenic phenotyping of neoplastic lymphoid cells, to be an angiotropic (intravascular) large-cell lymphoma (Sheibani et al).

Sarcomas of the brain These are malignant tumors composed of cells derived from connective tissue elements (fibroblasts, rhabdomyocytes, lipocytes, osteoblasts, smooth muscle cells). They take their names from their histogenetic derivation, viz., fibrosarcoma, rhabdomyosarcoma, osteogenic sarcoma, and sometimes from the tissue of which the cells are a part, viz., adventitial sarcomas, hemangiopericytoma.

All these tumors are rare. They constitute from 1 to 3 percent of intracranial tumors, depending on how wide a range of neoplasms one chooses to include in this group (see below). Occasionally one or more deposits of these types of tumors will occur as a metastasis from a sarcoma in another organ. Others are primary in the cranial cavity and exhibit as one of their unique properties a tendency to metastasize to nonneural tissues, which happens infrequently in primary glial tumors. It is a disturbing fact that a few sarcomas have developed 5 to 10 years after gamma irradiation, or, in one instance, after proton beam irradiation of the brain.

A number of other cerebral tumors, described in the literature as sarcomas, are probably tumors of other types. The rapidly growing, highly malignant "monstrocellular sarcoma" of Zülch or "giant cell fibrosarcoma" of Kernohan and Uihlein, so named for their multinucleated giant cells, have been reinterpreted by Rubinstein as a form of giant cell glioblastoma or mixed glioblastoma and fibrosarcoma. The "hemangiopericytoma of the leptomeninges," also classified by Kernohan and Uihlein as a form of cerebral sarcoma is considered by Rubinstein to be a variant of the angioblastic meningioma of Bailey and Cushing.

PATIENTS WHO PRESENT WITH SIGNS OF INCREASED INTRACRANIAL PRESSURE

A certain number of patients when first seen show the characteristic symptoms and signs of increased intracranial pressure (periodic bifrontal and biooccipital headaches which awaken the patient during the night or are present upon awakening, projectile vomiting, mental torpor, unsteady gait, sphincteric incontinence, and papilledema). The physician confronted with this clinical problem is forced to take immediate action because a critical rise in intracranial pressure may occur at any time and result in coma, respiratory arrest, and death. Admission to a hospital with a neurosurgical service is mandatory; nevertheless all the medical aspects of the patient's problem should be explored first.

Three questions demand immediate answers: (1) Does the patient have a space-occupying intracranial lesion? (2) Where in the cranial cavity is it situated? (3) What is its nature? With respect to the first question, it is well to keep in mind that a number of medical conditions, which are discussed in other parts of this text, may simulate an intracranial growth that causes only the general symptoms of increased intracranial pressure. These are (1) benign intracranial hypertension or pseudotumor cerebri (page 509), (2) hypertensive encephalopathy (page 676), (3) chronic pulmonary disease with hypercapnia and hypoxia (page 850), (4) chronic meningitis or adhesive arachnoiditis and/or aqueductal stenosis (page 513), (5) thrombosis of cerebral veins and dural sinuses (page 565), (6) some endocrinopathies (adrenal tumor, Addison disease, or hypoparathyroidism; page 858), (7) excessive vitamin A and tetracycline therapy in children, (8) withdrawal from corticosteroid therapy in children, (9) pseudotumor from intoxication with chlordecone or Kepone (Sanborn et al), and sometimes (10) corticosteroid therapy.

Another condition that can simulate intracranial neoplasm is a *supratentorial* or *infratentorial arachnoid cyst* (localized pseudotumor). This lesion, which is probably congenital, presents clinically at all ages but may only become evident in adult life, when it gives rise to symptoms of increased intracranial pressure and sometimes to focal cerebral signs as well. In infants and young children, macrocrania and extensive unilateral transillumination are characteristic features. Usually these cysts overlie the sylvian fissure, less often other parts of the cerebral convexity; occasionally they are interhemispheric or lie under the cerebellum. They may attain a large size, to the point of enlarging the middle fossa and elevating the lesser wing of the sphenoid, but they do not communicate with the ventricle. The cysts are readily recognized on the nonenhanced CT scan or MRI, which shows a circumscribed tissue defect with the density of CSF (Gandy and Heier). Such patients should also be studied by angiography, so as not to overlook a chronic subdural hematoma, which is often associated and which may not be visualized on the CT scan.

True and False Localizing Signs If the clinical findings permit the exclusion of the aforementioned causes of increased intracranial pressure, there is reasonable certainty that the patient has an intracranial growth. The problem then is to search for signs that will localize the lesion. In doing this, several pitfalls must be avoided. One common source of error is to place undue reliance on a sign which proves to have no localizing value whatsoever. One should distrust any symptom or sign that develops late, after headache and increased intracranial pressure have been established, for it often turns out to be a *false localizing sign*. Under these circumstances drowsiness, slowness in response, inattentiveness, and emotional blunting can be found as often with cerebellar as with cerebral growths. Unsteadiness of gait, urinary incontinence, and psychomotor asthenia may occur as part of hydrocephalus from any cause. Unilateral or bilateral abducens palsy [due to stretching of the sixth nerve(s)] is a common false localizing sign, and reference has already been made to the ptosis, dilated pupil, ipsilateral hemiparesis, and bilateral Babinski signs that result from temporal lobe herniation. Jacksonian and generalized seizures and ipsilateral or bilateral corticospinal signs may be observed in the advanced stages of a cerebellar tumor.

Early and sometimes relatively slight focal signs that may be easily overlooked are sometimes the most reliable guides to localization of the tumor. Examples of useful early signs are a mild weakness or stiffness and hyperreflexia of an arm and leg in a frontal tumor; ataxia of gait (but not of limbs) and head tilt in midline cerebellar tumors; paralysis of upward gaze and Argyll-Robertson pupillary phenomenon in pinealomas; pale optic discs and chiasmal field defects in craniopharyngiomas; and homonymous visual inattention and sensory extinction in posterior cerebral tumors (see page 365). The problem of localization is usually settled by the CT scan, which should be obtained in all patients with symptoms of increased intracranial pressure, with or without focal signs.

The tumors most likely to cause increased intracranial pressure without conspicuous focal or lateralizing signs are medulloblastoma, ependymoma of the fourth ventricle, hemangioblastoma of the cerebellum, pinealoma, colloid cyst of the third ventricle, and craniopharyngioma. In addition, in some of the cerebral gliomas discussed in the preceding section, particularly those of the corpus callosum and frontal lobes, increased intracranial pressure may occasionally precede focal cerebral signs.

Medulloblastoma

This is a rapidly growing embryonic tumor that arises in the posterior part of the cerebellar vermis and neuroepithelial roof of the fourth ventricle of children, and rarely in the cerebellum of adults.

The origin of this tumor has never been settled. One theory is that it is derived from the fetal remnants of the external granular layer of the cerebellum; another, that it arises from cell rests in the posterior medullary velum. Bailey and Cushing introduced the name *medulloblastoma*, although medulloblasts have never been identified in the fetal or adult human brain; nevertheless the term is retained for no reason other than its familiarity.

The tumor frequently fills the fourth ventricle and infiltrates its floor. Seeding of the tumor may occur on the meningeal surfaces of the cisterna magna, and around the spinal cord. The tumor is solid, gray-pink in color, and fairly well demarcated from the adjacent brain tissue. It is very cellular, and the cells are small and closely packed with hyperchromatic nuclei, little cytoplasm, many mitoses, and a tendency to form clusters or pseudorosettes.

The majority of the patients are children 4 to 8 years of age, and males outnumber females 3:2 or 3:1 in the many reported series. As a rule, symptoms have been present for 1 to 5 months before the diagnosis is made. The clinical picture is distinctive. Typically, the child becomes listless, vomits repeatedly, and has a morning headache. The first diagnosis that suggests itself may be gastrointestinal disease or abdominal migraine. Soon, however, a stumbling gait, frequent falls, and a squint lead to

a neurologic examination and the discovery of papilledema. The latter is present in all except a small number of patients by the time they come to the attention of a neurologist, except when the tumor is located laterally in the cerebellum, as it usually is in adults. Dizziness (positional) and nystagmus are frequent. A small proportion of patients have a slight sensory loss on one side of the face, and a mild facial weakness; bilateral abducens palsies are frequent. Head tilt, the occiput being tilted back and away from the side of the tumor, indicates the presence of cerebellar herniation. Rarely, signs of spinal root and subarachnoid metastases precede cerebellar signs. Extraneural metastases (cervical lymph nodes, lung, liver, bone) may occur, usually after craniotomy which allows tumor cells to reach scalp lymphatics. Decerebrate attacks (''cerebellar fits'') may appear in the late stages of the disease.

The tumor is highly radiosensitive. Chemotherapy has been shown to be of marginal value (Allen et al). With surgery, radiation of the entire neuraxis, and chemotherapy, there is a 5-year survival in more than two-thirds of cases. Brainstem invasion, incomplete removal, and later age of onset reduce the period of survival.

The *neuroblastoma* of childhood is a tumor of nearly identical histologic type, arising in the adrenals and metastasizing widely. Usually it remains extradural if it invades the cranial and spinal cavities. Polymyoclonia with opsoclonus may complicate the disease. The rare cerebral neuroblastomas in adults are more benign (Rubinstein).

Ependymoma and papilloma of the fourth ventricle

Ependymomas, as pointed out earlier in this chapter, arise from the walls of the ventricles. About 70 percent of them originate in the fourth ventricle, according to Fokes and Earle (Fig. 31-7). Whereas supratentorial ependymomas are spread evenly throughout life, fourth ventricular ependymomas occur mostly in childhood, less often in adult life. In the large Fokes and Earle series of 83 cases, 33 occurred in the first decade, 6 in the second, and 44 after the age of 20 years. Males have been affected almost twice as often as females.

The tumor usually arises from the floor of the fourth ventricle, extends through the foramina of Luschka and Magendie and may invade the medulla. These tumors produce a clinical syndrome much like that of the medulloblastoma except for their more protracted course and lack of early cerebellar signs. Symptoms may be present for 1 or 2 years before diagnosis and operation. About two-thirds of the patients come to notice because of increased intracranial pressure; in the rest, vomiting, difficulty in swallowing, paresthesias of extremities, abdominal pain, vertigo, and head tilt are prominent manifestations. Surgical removal offers the only hope of survival. As indicated earlier, the addition of radiation therapy prolongs survival. Prolongation of life is sometimes attained through ventriculoperitoneal shunting of CSF.

Papillomas of the choroid plexus are about one-fifth as frequent as ependymomas. They arise mainly in the lateral and fourth ventricles, occasionally in the third. The two most authoritative studies (by Laurence et al and by Matson and Crofton) give the ratios of lateral/third/fourth ventricular locations as 50:10:40. The tumor, which takes the form of a giant choroid plexus, has as its cellular element the plexus epithelium, which is closely related embryologically to the ependyma.

Essentially these are tumors of childhood. Fully 50 percent cause symptoms in the first year of life and 75 percent in the first decade. In the younger patients hydrocephalus proves to be the presenting syndrome, often aggravated acutely by hemorrhage; there may be papilledema, an unusual finding in a hydrocephalic child. Headaches, lethargy, stupor, spastic weakness of legs, unsteadiness of gait, and diplopia are more frequent in the older child. Sometimes patients present with a syndrome of the cerebellopontine angle (see further on), where the tumor presumably arises from choroid plexus that projects into the lateral recess. One consequence of the tumor is said to

be increased CSF formation, which contributes to the hydrocephalus (see page 503). Treatment is by surgical excision, but palliative shunting may be needed first if the patient's condition does not permit surgery.

Hemangioblastoma of the cerebellum This tumor is also referred to in connection with von Hippel–Lindau disease (page 987). Dizziness, ataxia of gait or of the limbs on one side, symptoms and signs of increased intracranial pressure, and in some instances an associated retinal angioma constitute the neurologic syndrome. Many patients have polycythemia due to elaboration of an erythropoietic factor by the tumor. Dominant inheritance is well known. The angiographic picture is characteristic: a tightly packed cluster of small vessels forming a mass 1.0 to 2.0 cm in diameter. Craniotomy with opening of the cerebellar cyst and excision of the mural hemangioblastomatous nodule may be curative. Those in the spinal cord are frequently associated with a syringomyelic lesion (greater than 70

Figure 31-7

Ependymoma of the fourth ventricle. A. Contrast-enhanced CT scan in a 4-year-old girl who presented with signs of increased intracranial pressure. Note hydrocephalus and end of shunt tube in left lateral ventricle. B. An ependymoma growing out of the fourth ventricle.

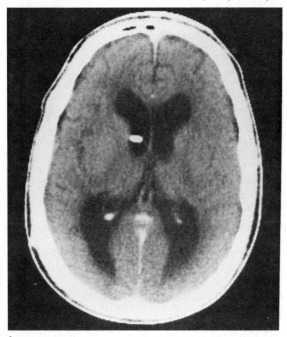

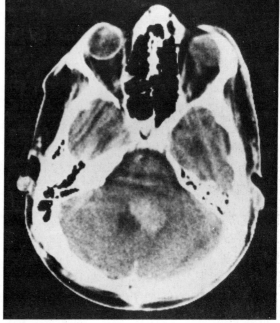

A

B

percent of cases); they may be multiple and are located mainly in the posterior columns. A retinal hemangioblastoma may be the initial finding and may lead to blindness if not treated by laser beam. The children of a parent with a hemangioblastoma of the cerebellum should be examined regularly for an ocular lesion and renal cell carcinoma (another complication).

Pinealoma There has been much uncertainty as to the proper classification of pineal tumors. Originally they were all thought to be composed of pineal cells, hence true pinealomas, a term suggested by Krabbe. Globus and Silbert believed that the tumors originated from embryonic pineal cells. But later Russell repudiated these ideas of histogenesis and declared the majority to be atypical teratomas, resembling seminoma of the testicle. Today several types are recognized—the germinoma (atypical teratoma), the pinealoma (pineocytoma and pineoblastoma), the true teratoma with cellular derivatives of all three germ layers, and the glioma.

The *germinoma* is a firm, discrete mass that usually reaches 3 to 4 cm in greatest diameter. It compresses the superior colliculi and sometimes the superior surface of the cerebellum, and narrows the aqueduct of Sylvius. Often it extends anteriorly into the third ventricle and may then compress the hypothalamus. A germinoma may also arise in the floor of the third ventricle; this has been referred to as an ectopic pinealoma or *suprasellar germinoma*. Microscopically, these tumors are composed of large, spherical epithelial cells separated by a network of reticular connective tissue, which contains many lymphocytes.

The pineocytoma and pineoblastoma reproduce the normal structure of the pineal gland. They enlarge the gland, are locally invasive, and may extend into the third ventricle and seed along the neuraxis. Their growth characteristics resemble those of the germinoma. The teratoma and dermoid and epidermoid cysts have no special features— some are quite benign. The gliomas have the usual morphologic characteristics of an astrocytoma of varying degrees of malignancy. Of the four groups, approximately 50 percent of all pineal tumors are germinomas. True teratomas and gliomas are relatively infrequent. Children, adolescents, and young adults—males more than females—are affected. Only rarely does one see a patient with a pineal tumor that has developed after the thirtieth year of life.

In some cases the clinical syndrome of the several types of pineal tumors consists solely of symptoms and signs of increased intracranial pressure. Beyond this, the most characteristic localizing signs are an inability to look

upward (Parinaud syndrome) and slightly dilated pupils that react on accommodation but not to light. These signs are related to hydrocephalus (dilatation of the posterior part of the third ventricle compressing the tegmentum of the upper midbrain) and not to the local pressure effects of the tumor. Sometimes ataxia of the limbs, choreic movements, or spastic weakness appear in the later stages of the illness, but it is uncertain whether such symptoms are due to neoplastic compression of the brachia conjunctiva and other midbrain structures, or to hydrocephalus. Precocious puberty occurs in males who harbor a germinoma. Diagnosis is made by CT scan (Fig. 31-8) and MRI. The CSF may contain tumor cells and lymphocytes.

Formerly judged to be inoperable, the use of the operating microscope now makes excision by a supracerebellar or transtentorial approach feasible. Operation for purposes of excision and histologic diagnosis is advised because each type of pineal tumor needs to be managed differently. Moreover, one may occasionally find an arachnoidal cyst that needs only excision. The germinomas should be removed insofar as possible and the whole neuraxis irradiated. The use of chemotherapy in addition to or instead of cranial irradiation is being evaluated (Allen et al; Jennings et al). Several of our patients survived more than 5 years after the removal of pineal gliomas. A combination of ventricular shunting and radiation of the tumor is favored in some clinics because of the high risk of surgery. If the tumor rapidly decreases in size, one can assume that it is

Figure 31-8

Contrast-enhanced CT scan showing a pineal germinoma.

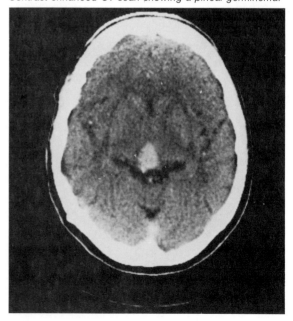

a germinoma. Stereotaxic biopsy is being used to an increasing degree and may obviate surgical exploration which carries a significant mortality (Pecker et al). A ventriculojugular or ventriculoperitoneal shunt is required in the majority of cases.

Colloid (paraphysial) cyst and other tumors of the third ventricle The most important of these is the colloid tumor, which is derived, it is generally believed, from ependymal cells of a vestigial third ventricular structure known as the paraphysis. The cysts that form in this structure are always situated in the anterior portion of the third ventricle between the interventricular foramens and are attached to the roof of the ventricle. The cysts vary in size from 1 to 4 cm in diameter, are oval or round with a smooth external surface, and are filled with a glary, gelatinous material containing a variety of mucopolysaccharides. The wall is composed of a layer of epithelial cells, some ciliated, surrounded by a capsule of fibrous connective tissue. Although congenital, these cysts practically never declare themselves clinically until adult life, when they block the third ventricle and produce an obstructive hydrocephalus.

This tumor should be suspected in patients who present with intermittent severe bifrontal-bioccipital headaches, sometimes modified by posture ("ball valve" obstruction of the third ventricle), or with crises of headache and obtundation, incontinence, unsteadiness of gait, bilateral paresthesias, dim vision, and weakness of the legs with sudden falls but no loss of consciousness ("drop attacks," see page 298). Stooping has resulted in an increase or onset of headache and loss of balance in several of our patients. Some of the patients have no headache and present with the symptoms of normal-pressure hydrocephalus. The treatment for many years has been surgical excision, but more recently satisfactory results have been obtained by ventriculoperitoneal shunt of the CSF, leaving the benign growth untouched. Decompression of the cyst by aspiration under stereotaxic control has also been effective in some cases.

Other tumors found in the third ventricle and giving rise mainly to obstructive symptoms are craniopharyngiomas (see below), papillomas of the choroid plexus, and ependymomas (pages 534, 535).

Craniopharyngioma (suprasellar epidermoid cyst, Rathke pouch or hypophysial duct tumor, adamantinoma, ameloblastoma) These are congenital tumors, generally believed to originate from *cell rests* (remnants of Rathke's pouch) at the junction of the infundibular stem and pituitary. By the time the tumor has attained a diameter of 3 to 4 cm, it is almost always cystic. Usually it lies above the sella turcica, depressing the optic chiasm and extending up into the third ventricle. Less often

it is subdiaphragmatic, i.e., within the sella, where it compresses the pituitary body and erodes one part of the wall of the sella or a clinoid process; but seldom does it balloon the sella like a pituitary adenoma. Large tumors may obstruct the flow of CSF. The tumor is oval, round, or lobulated and has a smooth surface. The wall of the cyst and the solid parts of the tumor consist of cords and whorls of epithelial cells (often with intercellular bridges and keratohyalin) separated by a loose network of stellate cells. The cyst contains dark albuminous fluid, cholesterol crystals, and calcium deposits; the calcium can be seen in plain films or CT scans of the suprasellar region in 70 to 80 percent of cases. The sella beneath the tumor tends to be flattened and enlarged. The majority of the subjects are children, but the tumor is not infrequent in adults, and some of our patients have been up to 60 years of age.

The presenting syndrome may be one of increased intracranial pressure, but more often it takes the form of a combined pituitary-hypothalamic-chiasmal derangement. The symptoms are often subtle and long-standing. In children, adiposity, delayed physical and mental development (Froehlich or Lorain syndrome—see page 451), headaches, vomiting, dim vision with chiasmal field defects, optic atrophy, and papilledema are the main clinical features. In adults, waning libido, amenorrhea, slight spastic weakness of one or both legs, headache without papilledema, failing vision, and mental dullness and confusion are the usual manifestations. Later, drowsiness, ocular palsies, diabetes insipidus, and disturbance of temperature regulation—indicating hypothalamic involvement—may occur.

In the *differential diagnosis* of the several tumor syndromes described in this section, a careful clinical analysis is often more important than laboratory procedures. The procedures that are likely to give the most useful information are the CT scan (Fig. 31-9) and MRI. Modern neurosurgical techniques reinforced by corticosteroid therapy before and after surgery, and careful control of temperature and water balance postoperatively permit successful excision of all or part of the tumor in the majority of cases. The mortality rate in the best neurosurgical clinics ranges from 5 to 8 percent. Stereotaxic aspiration is sometimes a useful palliative procedure as are radiation therapy and ventricular shunting in patients with solid, nonresectable tumors.

PATIENTS WHO PRESENT WITH SPECIFIC INTRACRANIAL TUMOR SYNDROMES

In this group of tumors general cerebral symptoms and signs of increased intracranial pressure occur late or not at all. The physician arrives at the correct diagnosis by localizing the lesion accurately from a set of neurologic findings and by reasoning that the etiology must be neoplastic because of the afebrile, steadily progressive nature of the illness. CT scanning, MRI, and other special studies will usually confirm the clinical impression.

Tumors that produce these unique intracranial syndromes are craniopharyngioma (described above), acoustic neuroma and other tumors of the cerebellopontine angle, pituitary adenomas and nonneoplastic enlargements of the sella, meningiomas of the sphenoid ridge and olfactory groove, glioma of the optic nerve and chiasm, pontine glioma, and chordoma and other erosive tumors at the base of the skull.

Acoustic Neuroma (Schwannoma, Neurofibroma)
This tumor was first described as a pathologic entity by Sandifort in 1777, first diagnosed clinically by Oppenheim in 1890, and first recognized as a surgically treatable disease

Figure 31-9

Contrast-enhanced mass, which proved to be a craniopharyngioma, filling the entire suprasellar cistern. The patient was a 50-year-old man with a 10-month history of headaches and a chiasmal–optic nerve defect.

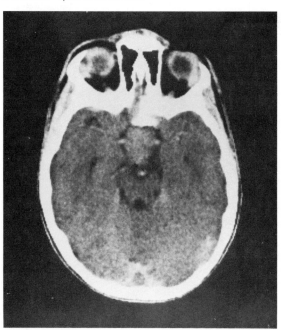

around the turn of the century. Cushing's monograph (1917) was a milestone, and the papers of House and Hitselberger and of Ojemann et al provide excellent descriptions of the modern diagnostic tests and surgical treatment, as well as comprehensive bibliographies.

Acoustic neuroma occurs occasionally as part of von Recklinghausen neurofibromatosis, in which case it takes one of two forms. In classic von Recklinghausen disease (peripheral, or type 1, neurofibromatosis, see page 985) a schwannoma may sporadically involve the eighth nerve, usually in adult life, just as it may involve any other nerve in the body. Rarely, if ever, do bilateral acoustic neuromas occur in this form of the disease. Bilateral acoustic neuromas are the hallmark of the genetically distinct neurofibromatosis 2, in which they practically always occur before the age of 21 and show a strong (autosomal dominant) heredity.

The usual acoustic neuroma in adults presents as a solitary tumor. Being a schwannoma, it originates in nerve. The examination of small tumors reveals that they practically always originate on the vestibular division of the eighth nerve just within the internal auditory canal; as they grow, they extend into the posterior fossa to occupy the angle between the cerebellum and pons (cerebellopontine angle). In their lateral position they are so situated as to compress the seventh, fifth, and less often the ninth and tenth cranial nerves which are implicated in various combinations. Later they displace and compress the pons and lateral medulla and obstruct the CSF circulation.

Certain biologic data assume clinical importance. The highest incidence is in the fifth and sixth decades, and the sexes are equally affected. Familial occurrence marks only the tumors which are a part of von Recklinghausen disease.

The earliest symptom reported by the patients in the series of Ojemann et al was loss of hearing (33 of 46 patients), headache (4 of 46), disturbed sense of balance (3 of 46), unsteadiness of gait (3 of 46), and facial pain, tinnitus, and facial weakness—each in a single case. Some patients sought medical advice soon after the appearance of the initial symptom, some late, after other symptoms had occurred. Usually, by the time of the first neurologic examination, the clinical picture was quite complex. One-third of the patients were troubled by vertigo associated with nausea, vomiting, and pressure in the ear. The vertiginous symptoms resembled those of Ménière disease, but differed in that discrete attacks separated by normalcy were rare. The vertigo coincided more or less with hearing loss and tinnitus (most often a unilateral high-pitched ringing, sometimes a machinery-like roaring or hissing sound, like a kettle). By then, many of the patients were also complaining of unsteadiness, especially on rapid changes of position (e.g., in turning), and this may have interfered with work and other activities. A few of our patients ignored their deafness for many months or years, or attributed it to some other disorder; in them the presenting syndrome consisted of impaired mentation (psychomotor asthenia), imbalance, and sphincteric incontinence. Hearing loss, slight facial weakness, and numbness of a cheek were then the only clinical findings that permitted an acoustic neuroma to be distinguished from some other cause of normal-pressure hydrocephalus.

The *neurologic findings* at the time of examination in the above-mentioned series of 46 patients were as follows: eighth nerve involvement (auditory and vestibular) in 45 of 46, facial weakness including disturbance of taste (26 of 46), sensory loss over face (26 of 46), gait abnormality (19 of 46), and unilateral ataxia of limbs (9 of 46). Inequality of reflexes and eleventh and twelfth nerve palsies were present in only a few patients. Signs of increased intracranial pressure appeared late, and were present in not more than 25 percent of our patients. These findings are comparable to those reported by House and Hitselberger and more recently by Harner and Laws.

Audiologic and vestibular evaluation includes the tuning fork tests, pure tone and speech audiometry, auditory fatigue and recruitment tests, brainstem evoked responses, and vestibular tests, all of which have been described in Chap. 14. In combination, they permit localization of the deafness and vestibular disturbance to the cochlear and vestibular nerves rather than their end organs in practically all cases. Radiographs of the internal auditory meatus show enlargement on the affected side in most. The CSF protein is raised in two-thirds of the patients (over 100 mg/dL in one-third). The contrast-enhanced CT scan (Fig. 31-10*A*) will detect practically all acoustic neuromas that are larger than 2.0 cm in diameter and that project further than 1.5 cm into the cerebellopontine angle, although even smaller intracanalicular tumors can reliably be detected by MRI (Fig. 31-10*B*).

The tumor is usually 2 to 3.5 cm in greatest diameter and oval in shape, conforming to the shape of the space in which it grows; its surface is smooth, firm, and whitish in color. It is always encapsulated. The spindle-shaped cells of which it is composed, arranged in bundles and palisades, allow ready identification. Mononuclear giant cells and hyperchromatism may suggest malignant change, but mitoses are not present. Hemorrhage and necrosis occur frequently.

The treatment is surgical excision. Neurosurgeons who have had the largest experience with these tumors favor the microsurgical suboccipital transmeatal operation (Martuza and Ojemann). In most instances the facial nerve can be preserved, and in some, the cochlear nerve as well. In the hands of a skillful otologic surgeon, small tumors can be removed safely by the translabyrinthine approach, if no attempt is to be made to save hearing. In older patients

with small tumors, one may safely delay operation or treat them with focused gamma or proton radiation.

Neurinoma or schwannoma of the trigeminal or gasserian ganglion or neighboring cranial nerves, and meningioma of the cerebellopontine angle may in some instances be indistinguishable from an acoustic neuroma. They should always be considered if early deafness, tinnitus, and lack of response to caloric stimulation ("dead labyrinth") are not the initial symptoms of the cerebellopontine angle syndrome. A true *cholesteatoma (epidermoid cyst)* is a relatively rare tumor that is located most often in the cerebellopontine angle, where it may simulate an acoustic neuroma. Other disorders that enter into the differential diagnosis are glomus jugulare tumor (see below), metastatic cancer, syphilitic meningitis, arachnoid cyst, vascular malformations, and plasmacytoma of the petrous bone. All these disorders may produce a cerebellopontine angle syndrome, but are more likely to cause only unilateral lower cranial nerve palsies and their temporal course tends to differ from that of acoustic neuroma. Occasionally, a tumor that originates in the pons or in the fourth ventricle (ependymoma, astrocytoma, papilloma, medulloblastoma) but grows eccentrically may present as a cerebellopontine angle syndrome.

The *glomus jugulare tumor* is of particular interest. It is a purplish red, highly vascular tumor composed of large epithelioid cells in an alveolar pattern and an abundant capillary network. The tumor is believed to be derived from minute clusters of nonchromaffin paraganglioma cells (glomus bodies) found mainly in the adventitia of the dome of the jugular bulb (*glomus jugulare*) immediately below the floor of the middle ear, but also in multiple other sites in and around the temporal bone. These clusters of cells are part of the chemoreceptor system that includes also the carotid, vagal, ciliary, and aortic bodies. The typical syndrome consists of partial deafness, facial palsy, dysphagia, and unilateral atrophy of the tongue, combined with a vascular polyp in the external auditory meatus and a palpable mass below and anterior to the mastoid eminence, often with a bruit. Other neurologic manifestations are phrenic nerve palsy, numbness of the face, a Horner syndrome, cerebellar ataxia, and temporal lobe epilepsy. The jugular foramen is eroded (visible in basilar skull films), and the CSF protein may be elevated. Women are affected more than men, and the peak incidence is during middle adult life. The tumor grows slowly over a period of many years, sometimes 10 to 20 or more. Treatment consists of radical mastoidectomy and removal of as much tumor as possible, followed by radiation. The combined intracranial and extracranial two-stage operation has resulted in cure of many cases (Gardner et al). A detailed account of this tumor will be found in the article by Kramer.

Carotid Body Tumor This is a benign but potentially malignant tumor originating in a small aggregate of cells of neuroectodermal type. The normal carotid body is small (4 mm in greatest diameter and 10 mg in weight) and is located at the bifurcation of the common carotid artery. The cells are of uniform size, have abundant cytoplasm, are rich in substance P, and are sensitive to changes in P_{O_2}, P_{CO_2}, and pH (i.e., they are chemoreceptors, not to be confused with baroreceptors). The tumors that arise from these cells are identical in appearance with the paraganglioma. Interestingly, they are 12 times more frequent in individuals living at high altitudes.

Clinically the usual presentation is of a painless mass at the side of the neck below the angle of the jaw; thus it needs to be differentiated from branchial cleft cysts, mixed tumors of the salivary gland, and carcinomas and aneurysms in this region. As the tumor grows (at an estimated rate of 2.0 cm every 5 years) it may implicate the sympathetic, glossopharyngeal, vagus, spinal accessory, and hypoglossal nerves. Hearing loss, tinnitus, and vertigo are present in some cases. Tumors of the carotid body have been a source of transient ischemic attacks in 5 to 15 percent of the 600 or more reported cases. There are only 35 reported cases in which malignant transformation has occurred.

The tumor is not associated with the glomus jugulare tumor but has been seen in combination with von Recklinghausen neurofibromatosis. Familial cases are known, especially with bilateral carotid body tumors (about 5 percent of these tumors are bilateral). The treatment should be surgical excision with or without prior embolization; radiation therapy is not advised.

Pituitary Adenomas Tumors arising in the anterior pituitary are of considerable interest to neurologists because they often cause visual and other symptoms related to involvement of structures bordering upon the sella turcica. Pituitary tumors are age-linked; they become increasingly numerous with each decade and by the eightieth year, small adenomas are found in more than 20 percent of pituitary glands. Only a small proportion enlarge the sella and these

Figure 31-10

A. Contrast-enhanced CT scan showing a large acoustic neuroma that had produced an obstructive hydrocephalus. B. T1-weighted axial MR image, after gadolinium. Arrow points to an intracanalicular schwannoma.

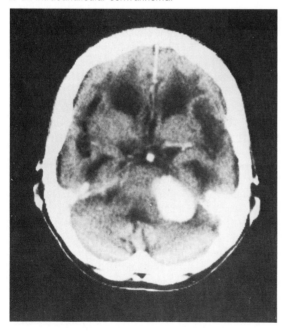
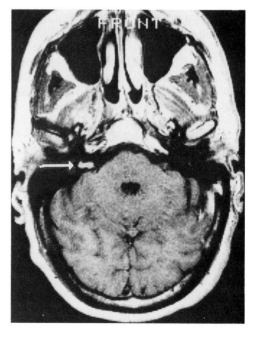

account for the 6 to 8 percent of pituitary tumors listed in all series of intracranial neoplasms.

On the basis of conventional staining methods, cells of the normal pituitary gland were for many years classified as chromophobe, acidophil, and basophil, these types being present in a ratio of 5:4:1. Adenomas of the pituitary are most often composed of chromophobe cells (4 to 20 times as common as acidophil cell adenomas); the incidence of basophil cell adenomas is uncertain. Histologic study is now based on immunoperoxidase staining techniques and is concerned with defining the nature of the hormones within the pituitary cells—both of the normal gland and of pituitary adenomas. These methods have shown that either a chromophobe or an acidophil cell may produce prolactin, growth hormone (GH), or thyroid-stimulating hormone (TSH), whereas the basophil cells produce ACTH, β-lipotropin, luteinizing hormone (LH), and follicle-stimulating hormone (FSH). The prolactinomas account for nearly 30 percent of all pituitary tumors.

Pituitary tumors usually arise as discrete nodules in the anterior part of the gland (adenohypophysis). The tumors are reddish gray, soft (almost gelatinous), and often partly cystic, with a rim of calcium in some instances. Most often the adenomatous cells are arranged diffusely, with little stroma and few blood vessels; less frequently the architecture is sinusoidal or papillary in type. Variability of nuclear structure, hyperchromatism, cellular pleomorphism, and mitotic figures are interpreted as signs of malignancy. Tumors of less than 1 cm in diameter are referred to as "microadenomas," and are at first confined to the sella. As the tumor grows, it first compresses the pituitary gland; then, as it extends upward and out of the sella, it compresses the optic chiasm; and later, with continued growth, it may extend into the cavernous sinus, third ventricle, temporal lobes, or posterior fossa. Recognition of an adenoma when it is still confined to the sella is of considerable practical importance, since total surgical removal of the tumor or proton-beam therapy are possible at this stage, with prevention of further damage to normal glandular structure and the chiasm. Penetration of the diaphragma sellae by the tumor and invasion of the surrounding structures make treatment more difficult.

Pituitary adenomas come to medical attention because of endocrine abnormalities or visual disorder; headaches are present in nearly one-half of the macroadenomas. The visual disorder usually proves to be a *complete or partial bitemporal hemianopia* which has developed gradually. Early, the upper parts of the visual fields may be affected predominantly. A small number of patients will be almost blind in one eye and have a temporal hemianopia in the other. Bitemporal central hemianopic scotomata are a less frequent finding. A postfixed chiasm may be compressed n such a way that there is an interrupution of some of the

nasal retinal fibers, which, as they decussate, project into the base of the opposite optic nerve (Wilbrand's knee). This results in a central scotoma on one or both sides (junctional syndrome) as well as a temporal field defect (see Fig. 12-2). If the visual disorder is of long standing, the optic nerve heads are visibly atrophic. *Bitemporal hemianopia with a normal sella* usually means that the causative lesion is a saccular aneurysm of the circle of Willis or a meningioma of the tuberculum sellae. In 5 to 10 percent of cases, compression of the cavernous sinus causes some combination of ocular palsies. Other neurologic abnormalities, rare to be sure, are seizures from indentation of the temporal lobe, CSF rhinorrhea, and diabetes insipidus, hypothermia, and somnolence from hypothalamic compression.

The development of sensitive (radioimmunoassay) methods for the measurement of pituitary hormones in the serum has made possible the detection of adenomas at an early stage of their development and the designation of several types of pituitary adenomas on the basis of the endocrine disturbance. Between 60 and 70 percent of tumors, both in men and women, are prolactin-secreting. About 10 to 15 percent secrete growth hormone and a smaller number secrete ACTH. Tumors that secrete gonadotropins and TSH are quite rare, and a small number of pituitary tumors produce no hormone (stem cell or undifferentiated cell adenomas). The major endocrine syndromes are discussed below.

Amenorrhea-galactorrhea syndrome As a rule, this syndrome becomes manifest during the child-bearing years. The history usually discloses that menarche had occurred at the appropriate age; primary amenorrhea is rare. A common history is that the patient took birth control pills, only to find, when she stopped, that the menstrual cycle did not re-establish itself. On examination, there may be no abnormalities other than galactorrhea. Serum prolactin levels are increased (usually in excess of 100 ng/mL). In general, the longer the duration of amenorrhea and the higher the serum prolactin level, the larger will be the tumor. The elevated prolactin levels distinguish this disorder from idiopathic galactorrhea, in which serum prolactin levels are normal.

Males with prolactin-secreting tumors rarely have galactorrhea and usually present with a larger tumor and complaints such as headache, impotence, and visual abnormalities. In normal persons, the serum prolactin level rises markedly in response to the administration of chlorpromazine or a 200-μg dose of thyrotropin-releasing hormone (TRH); patients with a prolactin-secreting tumor fail to show such a response. With large tumors that compress normal pituitary tissue, thyroid and adrenal function will also be impaired.

Acromegaly This disorder is due to an overproduction of growth hormone (GH) occurring after puberty; prior to puberty, an oversecretion of GH produces gigantism. In a small number of acromegalic patients, there is an excess secretion of both GH and prolactin, derived apparently from two distinct populations of tumor cells. The diagnosis of this disorder, which is often long delayed, is made on the basis of the characteristic clinical changes, the finding of elevated serum GH values (> 10 ng/ml), and the failure of the GH level to rise in response to the administration of glucose or TRH.

Cushing disease Described in 1932 by Harvey Cushing, this condition is only about one-fourth as frequent as acromegaly. A distinction needs to be made between Cushing disease and Cushing syndrome. The disease is due to oversecretion of ACTH by a pituitary adenoma, whereas the syndrome refers to the effects of glucocorticoid excess from any one of several sources—iatrogenic steroid administration, adenoma of the adrenal cortex, ACTH-producing bronchial carcinoma (rarely), as well as a pituitary tumor. The clinical effects are the same in all of these disorders and include truncal obesity, hypertension, muscle weakness, amenorrhea, hirsutism, abdominal striae, glycosuria, osteoporosis, and in some cases a characteristic psychosis (page 1233).

Although Cushing originally attributed the disease to basophil adenomata, the pathologic change may consist only of hyperplasia of basophilic cells or a nonbasophilic adenoma. Seldom is the sella turcica enlarged, and visual symptoms or signs of cavernous sinus compression are therefore rare. The diagnosis of Cushing disease is made by demonstrating an increased level of plasma and urinary cortisol; these levels are not suppressed by the administration of relatively small doses of dexamethasone (0.5 mg four times daily), but they are suppressed by high doses of dexamethasone (8 mg daily). A low level of ACTH in the blood, increased cortisol in the blood and increased free cortisol in the urine, and nonsuppression of adrenal function after administration of high doses of dexamethasone are evidence of an adrenal source of the Cushing syndrome—usually an adrenal tumor, less often a micronodular hyperplasia.

Diagnosis of pituitary adenoma This is likely when a chiasmal syndrome is combined with an endocrine syndrome of either hypopituitary or hyperpituitary type. Laboratory data confirmatory of an endocrine disorder, as described above, and a ballooned sella turcica in plain films of the skull make diagnosis virtually certain. Patients who are suspected of harboring a pituitary adenoma, but in whom the plain films are normal, should have high-resolution CT scans with thin slice techniques, preferably in the coronal plane. MRI is even more effective and is replacing CT scanning. This procedure will demonstrate pituitary adenomas as small as three mm in diameter, and is a means of following the response of the tumor to therapy.

Tumors other than pituitary adenomas may sometimes expand the sella. Enlargement may be due to an intrasellar craniopharyngioma, carotid aneurysm, or a cyst of the pituitary gland. Intrasellar, epithelial-lined cysts are rare lesions. They originate from the apical extremity of Rathke's pouch, which may persist as a cleft between the anterior and posterior lobes of the hypophysis. Rarer still are intrasellar cysts that have no epithelial lining and contain thick, dark brown fluid, the product of intermittent hemorrhages. Both of these types of intrasellar cyst may compress the pituitary gland and mimic the effects of pituitary adenomas.

Far more common than the aforementioned conditions is a *nontumorous enlargement of the sella* ("*empty sella*"). This results from a defect in the dural diaphragm, which may occur without obvious cause or may follow surgical excision of a pituitary adenoma or pituitary apoplexy (see below). The arachnoid over the defective diaphragma sellae will bulge through the hole, and the sella then enlarges gradually, apparently as a result of the pressure and pulsations of the CSF acting on the walls of the sella turcica. In the process, the pituitary gland becomes flattened, sometimes to an extreme degree, but the functions of the gland are usually unimpaired. Downward herniation of the optic chiasm occurs occasionally, and may cause visual disturbances simulating those of a pituitary adenoma.

All radiographic changes associated with nontumorous enlargement of the sella occur below the plane of the diaphragma sellae. High-resolution CT scanning and MRI are usually the only diagnostic procedures that are necessary.

Treatment of intrasellar pituitary adenomas This varies with the type and size of the tumor and the status of the endocrine and visual systems. There is not yet complete agreement as to the most effective approach. The administration of the dopamine agonist bromocriptine, which acts as a prolactin inhibitor, may be the only therapy needed for small or even large prolactinomas and is a useful adjunct in the treatment of the amenorrhea-galactorrhea syndrome and some cases of acromegaly. Under the influence of bromocriptine, the tumor decreases in size within days, the prolactin level falls, and the visual field defect improves. Treatment must be continuous to prevent relapse.

An alternative treatment, if vision is not being threatened, is proton beam radiation. This form of radiation can be focused precisely on the tumor and will destroy it. At the time of writing, Kjellberg had treated over 1000 patients at the Massachusetts General Hospital without a single fatality and, in recent years, with no complications. A single brief transcranial exposure is all that is necessary. The endocrine abnormalities must be corrected by hormone replacement therapy. Unfortunately, proton beam therapy is available in only very few centers worldwide.

If proton beam therapy is unavailable or if the patient is intolerant of bromocriptine, the treatment is surgical, using a transsphenoidal microsurgical approach, with an attempt at total removal of the tumor and preservation of normal pituitary function. This is followed by conventional radiation therapy and such hormonal supplementation as is necessary.

The treatment of pituitary adenomas is considered further in Chap. 27.

Large extrasellar extensions of a pituitary growth must be removed by craniotomy, using a transfrontal approach, followed by radiation therapy.

The *pituitary apoplexy syndrome,* described by one of the authors (R.D.A.) with Brougham and Heusner, occurs as a result of infarction of an adenoma that has outgrown its blood supply. It is characterized by the acute onset of headache, ophthalmoplegia, bilateral amaurosis, and drowsiness or coma, with either subarachnoid hemorrhage or pleocytosis and elevated protein in the CSF. The CT scan shows infarction of tumor, often with hemorrhage, in and above an enlarged sella. Pituitary apoplexy may threaten life, and needs to be treated by dexamethasone (6 to 12 mg every 6 h) and, if there is no improvement after 24 to 48 h, by transnasal decompression of the sella. Some pituitary adenomas are cured by this accident.

Meningioma of the Sphenoid Ridge This tumor is situated over the lesser wing of the sphenoid bone (Fig. 31-5). As it grows, it may expand medially to involve structures in the wall of the cavernous sinus, anteriorly into the orbit, or laterally into the temporal bone. Fully 75 percent are in women and the average age at the time of onset is 50 years. Most prominent among the symptoms are a slowly developing unilateral exophthalmos, slight bulging of the bone in the temporal region, and radiologic evidence of thickening or erosion of the lesser wing of the sphenoid bone. Variants of the clinical syndrome include anosmia, oculomotor palsy, the Tolosa-Hunt syndrome (see Table 47-2), blindness and optic atrophy in one eye, sometimes with papilledema of the other eye (Foster Ken-

nedy syndrome), mental changes, uncinate fits, and increased intracranial pressure. Sarcomas arising from the skull bones, metastatic carcinoma, orbitoethmoidal osteoma, benign giant cell bone cyst, tumors of the optic nerve, and angiomas of the orbit must be considered in the differential diagnosis. Auscultation of the skull, plain skull films with laminography, bone scans, and carotid arteriography in addition to CT scanning, are helpful in differentiating these lesions. The tumor is resectable without further injury to the optic nerve, if the bone has not been invaded and the operating microscope is used during the dissection.

Meningioma of the Olfactory Groove This tumor originates in arachnoidal cells along the cribriform plate. The diagnosis depends on the finding of ipsilateral or bilateral anosmia, ipsilateral or bilateral blindness, often with optic atrophy on one side and papilledema on the other (Kennedy syndrome), and mental changes. The tumors may reach enormous size before coming to the attention of the physician. The anosmia, if unilateral, is rarely if ever reported by the patient. The unilateral visual disturbance may consist of a slowly developing central scotoma. Abulia, confusion, forgetfulness, and inappropriate jocularity (witzelsucht) are the usual psychic disturbances (see page 358). The patient may be indifferent to or joke about his or her blindness. Usually there are radiographic changes along the cribriform plate, and often an extremely high CSF protein level (200 to 400 mg/dL). Except for the largest tumors, extirpation is possible.

Meningioma of the Tuberculum Sellae Harvey Cushing was the first to delineate the syndrome caused by this tumor. Of his 23 cases, all were female. The presenting symptoms were visual failure—a slowly advancing bitemporal hemanopia with a sella of normal size. Often the field defects were asymmetrical, indicating a combined chiasm–optic nerve involvement. Usually there are no hypothalamic or pituitary deficits. If the tumor is not too large, complete excision is possible. If removal is incomplete, or if the tumor recurs or undergoes malignant changes, radiation therapy is indicated.

Glioma of the Brainstem Astrocytomas of the brainstem (formerly called *bipolar spongioblastomas*) are relatively slow growing tumors that infiltrate tracts and nuclei. They produce a variable clinical picture, depending on their location in the medulla, pons, or midbrain. As a rule this tumor begins in childhood (peak age of onset is 7 years, and 80 percent appear before the twenty-first year), and symptoms have usually been present for 3 to 5 months before coming to medical notice. In most patients the initial manifestation is a palsy of one or more cranial nerves, most often the sixth and seventh on one side, followed by long tract signs—hemiparesis, unilateral ataxia, ataxia of gait, paraparesis, hemisensory syndromes, and gaze disorders. In the remaining patients the symptoms occur in the reverse order, i.e., long tract signs precede the cranial nerve abnormalities. The duration of survival is longer in this group of patients than in those whose illness begins with cranial nerve palsies. The combination of cranial nerve palsy or palsies on one side and motor and/or sensory tract signs on the other always indicates brainstem disease. Headache, vomiting, and papilledema usually occur late in the course of the illness. The course is slowly progressive over several years unless some part of the tumor becomes more malignant (glioblastoma multiforme) or spreads to the meninges (meningeal gliomatosis), in which instance the illness may terminate fatally within months. In some 50 or more fatal cases at the Massachusetts General Hospital, more than half were glioblastomas and had resulted in death within a few months. Patients with pontine astrocytoma may survive for 5 or more years. The main clinical problem is to differentiate this disease from a pontine form of multiple sclerosis, a vascular malformation of the pons, and a brainstem encephalitis. MRI, which visualizes posterior fossa structures better than CT, is the most helpful procedure in diagnosis and sometimes in prognosis—the course being relatively benign in those with an isodense, enhancing CT picture (Stroink et al). In a few instances surgical exploration is necessary to establish the diagnosis (inspection and possibly biopsy). The treatment is radiation, and if intracranial pressure is increased, ventricular shunting of CSF becomes necessary. Trials of adjuvant chemotherapy have not shown any benefit (Allen et al).

Glioma of the Optic Nerves and Chiasm This tumor, like the brainstem glioma, occurs most frequently during childhood and adolescence. In 85 percent of cases the tumor appears before the age of 15 years (average 3.5) and is twice as frequent in girls as in boys (see Cogan). The initial symptoms are dimness of vision with constricted fields, followed by bilateral field defects of homonymous, heteronymous, and sometimes bitemporal type, blindness, and optic atrophy with or without papilledema. Ocular proptosis is the other main symptom. Hypothalamic signs (infantilism, adiposity, polyuria, somnolence, and genital atrophy) occur occasionally. MRI and CT scans (Fig. 31-12) and ultrasound

examination will usually reveal the tumor, and radiographs will show an enlargement of the optic foramen (greater than 7.0 mm). With this finding and the lack of ballooning of the sella or suprasellar calcification, one can exclude pituitary adenoma, Hand-Schüller-Christian disease, and craniopharyngioma. In adolescents and young adults, the medial sphenoid, olfactory groove, and intraorbital meningiomas (optic nerve sheath meningioma) are other tumors that cause blindness and proptosis. The treatment is surgical excision or radiation, depending on the exact location. Both gliomas and nontumorous gliotic (hamartomatous) lesions of the optic nerves may occur in von Recklinghausen disease; the latter are sometimes impossible to distinguish from optic nerve gliomas.

Chordoma This is a soft, jelly-like, gray-pink growth that arises from remnants of the primitive notochord, most often along the clivus (from dorsum sellae to foramen magnum) and in the sacrococcygeal region. It affects males more than females, usually in early or middle adult years, and should always be suspected in syndromes involving multiple cranial nerves or the cauda equina. About 40

Figure 31-11

T1-weighted coronal MR image, after gadolinium, showing a pontine glioma.

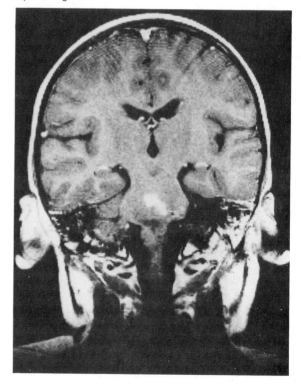

percent of chordomas occur in each of these two extremes of the neuraxis, and the rest are found at any point in between. The tumor is made up of cords or masses of large cells with granules of glycogen in their cytoplasm, and often with multiple nuclei and intracellular mucoid material. They are locally invasive, especially of surrounding bone, but do not metastasize. The neurologic syndrome is remarkable in that all or any combination of cranial nerves from the second to twelfth on one or both sides may be involved. Associated signs in the series of Kendell and Lee were facial pain, conductive deafness, and cerebellar ataxia, the result of pontomedullary and cerebellar compression. The tumors at the base of the skull may destroy the clivus and bulge into the nasopharynx, causing nasal obstruction and discharge, and sometimes dysphagia. Thus, chordoma is one of the lesions that may present both as an intracranial and extracranial mass, the others being meningioma, neurofibroma, glomus jugulare tumor, and carcinoma of sinuses or pharynx. Plain films of the base of the skull in addition to MRI are important in diagnosis. Midline (Wegener) granulomas must be differentiated. The treatment of the chordoma is surgical excision and radiation.

Nasopharyngeal Growths Which Erode the Base of the Skull   These are rather common in a general hospital, and they arise from the mucous membrane of the paranasal sinuses or the nasopharynx near the eustachian tube, i.e., the fossa of Rosenmueller (*transitional cell carcinoma, Schmincke tumor*). In addition to symptoms of nasopharyngeal or sinus disease, which may not be prominent, facial pain and numbness (trigeminal), abducens palsy, and other cranial nerve palsies may occur. Diagnosis depends on inspection and biopsy of a nasopharyngeal mass, biopsy of an involved cervical lymph node, and radiologic evidence of erosion of the base of the skull. Bone scan and CT scan are helpful in diagnosis. The treatment is radiation. Carcinoma of the ethmoid or sphenoid sinuses and postradiation neuropathy, coming on years after the treatment of a nasopharyngeal tumor, may produce a similar clinical picture.

Other Tumors of the Base of the Skull   There exist a large number and variety of tumors, rather rare to be sure, that derive from tissues at the base of the skull, paranasal sinuses, ears, etc., and which give rise to certain distinctive syndromes. Included in this category are osteomas, chondromas, chordomas, ossifying fibromas, giant cell tumors of bone, lipomas, epidermoids, teratomas, glomus tumors, mixed tumors of the parotid gland, and hemangiomas and cylindromas of the sinuses and orbit. Most of these tumors are benign, but some have a potential for malignant change. To the group must be added well-known malignant tumors that metastasize to basal skull

bones or involve them as part of a multicentric neoplasia, e.g., primary lymphoma, Ewing sarcoma, plasmacytoma, and leukemic deposits.

Suprasellar arachnoid cysts also occur in this region. CSF flows upward from the interpeduncular cistern but is trapped above the sella by thickened arachnoid (membrane of Liliequist). As the CSF accumulates it forms a cyst that invaginates the third ventricle; the dome of the cyst may intermittently block the foramina of Monro and cause hydrocephalus (Fox and Al-Mefty). Children with this condition exhibit a curious to-and-fro, bobbing and nodding of the head, like a doll with a weighted head resting on a coiled spring. This has been referred to as the "bobble-headed doll syndrome" by Benton and his colleagues; it can be cured by emptying the cyst.

Details of pathology, embryogenesis, and symptomatology of these various tumors are far too numerous to include in a textbook devoted to principles of neurology. Table 31-3, adapted from Bingas' large neurosurgical

Figure 31-12

Glioma of the optic chiasm. The contrast-enhanced CT scan shows the tumor directly above the dorsum sellae. The patient was a 7-year-old girl with neurofibromatosis who presented with severe visual loss and bilateral optic atrophy.

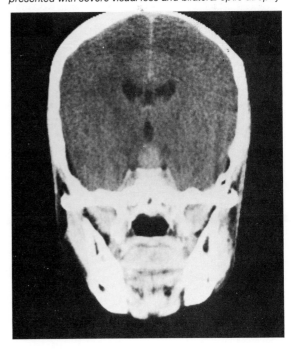

Table 31-3
The most important clinical syndromes caused by tumors at the base of the skull

Site of lesion	Eponym	Clinical symptoms	Etiology
Anterior part of the base of the skull		Olfactory disturbances (uni- or bilateral anosmia), possibly psychiatric disturbances, seizures.	Tumors which have invaded the anterior part of the base of the skull from the frontal sinus or the ethmoid bone, osteomas. Meningiomas of the olfactory groove.
Superior orbital fissure	Rochon-Duvigneau; syndrome of the pterygopalatine fossa (Behr) and the base of the orbit (DeJean) commencing with a lesion of the maxillary and pterygoid rami and evolving into the superior orbital fissure syndrome.	Lesions of the third, fourth, sixth, and first division of the fifth nerves with ophthalmoplegia, pain and sensory disturbances in the area of V_1; often exophthalmos, some vegetative disturbances.	Tumors: meningiomas, osteomas, dermoid cysts, giant cell tumors, tumors of the orbit, nasopharyngeal tumors, more rarely optic nerve gliomas; eosinophilic granulomas, angiomas, local or neighboring infections, trauma.
Apex of the orbit	Jacod-Rollet (often combined with the syndrome of the superior orbital fissure); infraclinoid syndrome of Dandy.	Visual disturbances, central scotoma, papilledema, optic nerve atrophy; occasional exophthalmos, chemosis.	Optic nerve glioma, infraclinoid aneurysm of the internal carotid artery, trauma, orbital tumors, Paget disease.
Cavernous sinus	Foix-Jefferson; syndrome of the sphenopetrosal fissure (Bonnet and Bonnet) corresponding in part to the cavernous sinus syndrome of Raeder.	Ophthalmoplegia due to lesions of the third, fourth, sixth, and often fifth nerves, exophthalmos, vegetative disturbances. Jefferson distinguished three syndromes: (1) the anterior-superior, corresponding to the superior orbital fissure syndrome; (2) the middle, causing ophthalmoplegia and lesions of V_1 and V_2; (3) the caudal, in addition affecting the whole trigeminal nerve.	Tumors of the sellar and parasellar area, infraclinoid aneurysms of the internal carotid artery, nasopharyngeal tumors, fistulae of the sinus cavernosus and the carotid artery (traumatic), tumors of the middle cranial fossa, e.g. chondromas, meningiomas, and neurinomas.
Apex of the petrous temporal bone	Gradenigo-Lannois	Lesions of the fifth and sixth nerves with neuralgia, sensory and motor disturbances, diplopia.	Inflammatory processes (otitis), tumors such as cholesteatomas, chondromas, meningiomas, neurinomas of the gasserian ganglion and trigeminal root, primary and secondary sarcomas at the base of the skull.

Table 31-3 (*continued*)
The most important clinical syndromes caused by tumors at the base of the skull

Site of lesion	Eponym	Clinical symptoms	Etiology
Sphenoid and petrosal bones, (petrosphenoidal syndrome)	Jacod	Ophthalmoplegia due to loss of function of the third, fourth, and sixth nerves, amaurosis, trigeminal neuralgia possibly with sensory signs.	Tumors of the sphenoid and petrosal bones and middle cranial fossa, nasopharyngeal tumors, metastases.
Jugular foramen	Vernet	Lesions of ninth, tenth, and eleventh nerves with disturbance of deglutition, curtain phenomenon, sensory disturbances of the tongue, soft palate, pharynx and larynx, hoarseness, weakness of the sternocleidomastoid and trapezius.	Tumors of the glomus jugulare; neurinomas of eighth, ninth, tenth, and eleventh nerves; chondromas, cholesteatomas, meningiomas, nasopharyngeal and ear tumors; infections, angiomas, rarely trauma.
Anterior occipital condyles	Sicard-Collet (Vernet-Sargnon)	Loss of twelfth nerve function (loss of normal tongue mobility) in addition to the symptoms of the jugular foramen.	Tumors of the base of the skull, ear, parotid; leukemic infiltrates; aneurysms, angiomas, and inflammations.
Retroparotid space (retropharyngeal syndrome)	Villaret	Lesions of the lower group of nerves (Sicard-Collet) and Bernard-Horner syndrome with ptosis and miosis.	Tumors of the retroparotid space (carcinomas, sarcomas), trauma, inflammations.
Half of the base of the skull	Garcin (Guillain-Alajouanine-Garcin); also described by Hartmann in 1904.	Loss of function of all twelve cranial nerves of one side; in many cases, isolated cranial nerves spared; rarely signs of raised intracranial pressure or pyramidal tract symptoms.	Nasopharyngeal tumors, primary tumors at the base of the skull, leukemic infiltrates of basal meninges, trauma, metastases.
Cerebellopontine angle		Loss of function of eighth nerve (hearing loss, vertigo, nystagmus), cerebellar disturbances, lesions of the fifth, seventh, and possibly ninth and twelfth cranial nerves. Signs of raised intracranial pressure, brainstem symptoms.	Acoustic neuromas (raised protein in CSF), meningiomas, cholesteatomas, metastases, cerebellar tumors, neurinomas of the caudal group of nerves and the trigeminal nerve, vascular processes such as angiomas, basilar aneurysms.

Source: Adapted from Bingas.

service in Berlin, summarizes the known facts about each of these tumors, and his authoritative article in the *Handbook of Clinical Neurology* is recommended as a reference and bibliographic source.

Modern radiologic technology serves now to clarify many of the diagnostic problems posed by these tumors. MRI is particularly helpful in delineating structures at the base of the brain and upper cervical region. CT scan is capable also of determining the absorptive values of the tumor itself, and when the lesion is analyzed in this way, an etiologic diagnosis sometimes becomes possible. For example, the absorptive value of lipomatous tissue is different from that of brain tissue, glioma, blood, and calcium. Bone scans (technetium and gallium) display active destructive lesions with remarkable fidelity, but even when these are seen it may be difficult to obtain a satisfactory biopsy in some cases.

Tumors of the Foramen Magnum Tumors in the region of the foramen magnum are of particular importance because of the difficulties in differentiation from diseases such as multiple sclerosis, Arnold-Chiari malformation, syringomyelia, and bony abnormalities of the craniocervical junction. Erroneous diagnosis is a serious matter since the majority of such tumors are benign and extramedullary, i.e., potentially resectable and curable. If unrecognized, they terminate fatally by causing medullary-spinal compression.

Although not numerous (about 1 percent of all intracranial and intraspinal tumors), sizable series have been collected by several investigators (see Meyer et al for a complete bibliography). In all series neurofibromas (schwannomas or neurilemmomas) and meningiomas are the most common types; others, all rare, are teratomas, dermoids, granulomas, cavernous hemangiomas, hemangioblastomas, lipomas, and epidural carcinomas.

Pain in the suboccipital or posterior cervical region, mostly on the side of the tumor, is usually the first and by far the most prominent complaint. In some instances the pain may extend into the shoulder and even the arm. The latter distribution is more frequent with tumors arising in the spinal canal and extending intracranially than the reverse. For uncertain reasons the pain may radiate down the back, even to the lower spine. Both spine and root pain can be distinguished, the latter due to involvement of either the C_2 or C_3 root or of both. Weakness of one shoulder and arm progressing to the ipsilateral leg and then to the opposite leg and arm is a relatively characteristic sequence of events, caused by the encroachment of tumor upon corticospinal

tracts. Occasionally both upper limbs are involved alone; surprisingly, there may be atrophic weakness of the hand or forearm or even intercostal muscles with diminished tendon reflexes well below the level of the tumor, an observation made originally by Oppenheim. Whether these latter findings are due to compromise of circulation (descending spinal artery or venous obstruction) or hydromyelia is unsettled. Involvement of sensory tracts also occurs; more often it is posterior column sensibility that is impaired on one or both sides with patterns of progression similar to the motor paralysis. Sensation of intense cold in the neck and shoulders has been another unexpected complaint and also "bands" of hyperesthesia round the neck and back of head. Segmental bibrachial sensory loss has been demonstrated in a few of the cases and a Lhermitte sign (electric-like sensations down the spine and limbs on neck flexion) has been reported frequently. Cranial nerve signs most frequently seen, and indicative of cranial extensions, are: dysphagia, dysphonia, dysarthria, and drooping shoulder (due to vagal, hypoglossal, and spinal accessory involvement); nystagmus and episodic diplopia; sensory loss over

Figure 31-13

T1-weighted sagittal MR image demonstrating a meningioma just below the foramen magnum.

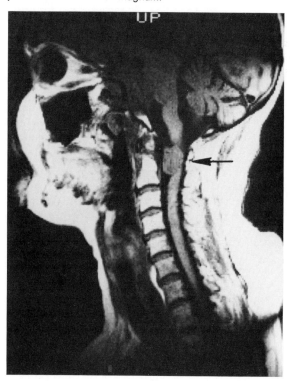

the face and unilateral or bilateral facial weakness; and a Horner syndrome.

The clinical course of such lesions often extends for two years or longer, with deceptive and unexplained fluctuations. With *dermoid cysts* of the upper cervical region, as in the case reported by Adams and Wegner, complete and prolonged remissions from quadriparesis may occur. The important diagnostic measure is MRI (Fig. 31-13) and, if unavailable, Pantopaque or metrizamide myelography.

Tumors of the foramen magnum should be suspected in patients with persistent occipital neuralgia, or those who carry a diagnosis of spinal or brainstem-cerebellar multiple sclerosis, Arnold-Chiari malformation, and chronic adhesive arachnoiditis. Treatment is surgical excision (see Hakuba et al).

REMOTE EFFECTS OF NEOPLASIA ON THE NERVOUS SYSTEM

In the past 35 years there has been delineated a group of neurologic disorders that occur in patients with carcinoma or some other type of neoplasia, even though the nervous system has not been directly invaded or compressed by the tumor. These so-called *paraneoplastic disorders* are not specific or confined to cancer, but the two conditions are linked far more frequently than could be accounted for by coincidence. Some of the paraneoplastic disorders, namely polyneuropathy, polymyositis, and the myasthenic-myopathic syndrome of Lambert-Eaton, are described on pages 1049, 1107, and 1159, respectively. Here a few remarks will be made about several other degenerative and inflammatory lesions that involve the spinal cord, cerebellum, brainstem, and cerebral hemispheres.

CARCINOMATOUS CEREBELLAR DEGENERATION

This nonmetastatic effect of carcinoma is quite uncommon. In reviewing this subject in 1970, we were able to find only 41 pathologically verified cases, and in a subsequent review (Henson and Urich, 1982) only a few more cases were added. The actual incidence is obviously higher than these figures indicate. At the Cleveland Metropolitan General Hospital, in a series of 1700 consecutive autopsies in adults, there were five instances of cerebellar degeneration associated with neoplasm. In the experience of Henson and Urich, about half of all patients with nonfamilial, late onset, cortical cerebellar degeneration proved sooner or later to be harboring a neoplasm.

In most of the reported cases, the underlying carcinoma has been in the lung (44 percent), a figure that reflects the high incidence of this tumor. However, the association

of ovarian carcinoma and lymphoma, particularly Hodgkin disease (17 and 14 percent, respectively), is higher than would be expected on the basis of the frequency of these malignancies. Carcinomas of the breast, uterus, bowel, and other viscera have accounted for the remaining cases.

Characteristically, the cerebellar symptoms have an insidious onset and steady progression over a period of weeks to months; in about half the cases, the cerebellar signs are recognized before those of the associated neoplasm. Ataxia of gait and of the limbs, affecting arms and legs more or less equally, dysarthria, and nystagmus are the usual manifestations. In addition, there are certain symptoms and signs not ordinarily considered to be cerebellar in nature, notably diplopia, vertigo, and disorders of ocular motility—findings that serve to distinguish carcinomatous from alcoholic and other varieties of cerebellar degeneration. Occasionally myoclonus and opsoclonus may be associated. The CSF may show a mild pleocytosis and increase of protein, or it may be entirely normal.

Pathologically there are diffuse degenerative changes of the cerebellar cortex and deep cerebellar nuclei. Purkinje cells are affected predominantly and all parts of the cerebellar cortex are involved more or less equally. Rarely there are associated degenerative changes in the spinal cord, involving the posterior columns and spinocerebellar tracts. The cerebellar lesions are frequently associated with perivascular and meningeal clusters of inflammatory cells. Henson and Urich regard the inflammatory changes as an independent process, part of a subacute paraneoplastic encephalomyelitis.

Little can be done to modify the cerebellar symptoms, although there are on record several cases in which there was a partial or complete remission of symptoms after removal of the primary tumor (Paone and Jeyasingham). The disorder is probably autoimmune. A number of studies have documented the presence of antibodies to Purkinje cell cytoplasmic protein antigen. Greenlee and Brashear found that sera from patients with ovarian carcinoma and pathologically confirmed cerebellar degeneration, when applied to frozen sections of human cerebellum, caused bright cytoplasmic staining of Purkinje cells and neurons of the deep cerebellar nuclei. Moreover, sera from neurologically normal patients with ovarian carcinoma reacted in the same way, indicating that development of antibodies to Purkinje cells may precede the onset of clinically evident cerebellar degeneration. These sera did not react with any other nervous tissue or viscera. Anti-Purkinje cell antibodies have now been identified in the sera of patients with carcinoma of the lung and breast and Hodgkin disease (Cunningham et al).

The subject of the autoimmune pathogenesis of paraneoplastic neurologic syndrome has been reviewed in detail by Anderson et al.

PROGRESSIVE MULTIFOCAL LEUKOENCEPHALOPATHY

This is a rare, subacutely evolving, fatal disease of the brain, occurring mainly in adults with chronic lymphoproliferative or myeloproliferative disease, less frequently with tuberculosis, sarcoid, and other nonneoplastic granulomatous disorders. Since it now seems certain that this neurologic complication of neoplasm has a viral etiology, it is considered with other viral infections, on page 608.

ENCEPHALOMYELITIS ASSOCIATED WITH CARCINOMA

The occurrence of encephalomyelitic changes in association with carcinoma has been described by several authors (Corsellis et al, Dorfman and Forno, Henson and Urich). In most of the reported cases (53 of 69 reviewed by Henson and Urich) the encephalomyelitis was associated with carcinoma of the bronchus, usually of the oat-cell type. Histologically, this group of paraneoplastic disorders is characterized by an extensive loss of nerve cells, accompanied by microglial proliferation, small patches of necrosis, and a marked perivascular cuffing by lymphocytes. Foci of lymphocytic infiltration have been observed in the leptomeninges as well. These pathologic changes may involve the brain and spinal cord diffusely, but more often they predominate in a particular part of the nervous system, notably in the limbic lobes ("limbic encephalitis"), brainstem (particularly in the medulla), cerebellum (see above), and gray matter of the spinal cord. The symptoms will of course depend on the location and severity of the inflammatory changes. Anxiety and depression, a confusional-agitated state, hallucinations, retentive memory defect (Korsakoff psychosis), and dementia—singly or in various combinations—are the usual manifestations of so-called limbic encephalitis. Vertigo, nystagmus, ataxia, nausea and vomiting, and a variety of ocular and gaze palsies reflect the presence of brainstem encephalitis; as indicated above, these symptoms are frequently joined with cerebellar ataxia. There may be a slowly progressive, symmetric or asymmetric amyotrophy of the arms, less often of the legs, related to inflammatory changes in the anterior horns of the spinal gray matter. Sensory symptoms may be related to neuronal loss in the posterior horns, but degeneration of the posterior columns can usually be traced to loss of neurons in the dorsal root ganglia, i.e., a sensory neuropathy.

It is noteworthy that in some patients no pathologic changes are demonstrable in the brain, even though there had been a prominent dementia during life. Contrariwise, widespread inflammatory changes may be found at autopsy, without clinical abnormalities having been recorded during life.

CARCINOMATOUS MYELOPATHY

In addition to the rare instances of subacute degeneration of spinal cord tracts that may occur with cerebellar degeneration (see above) there has been described, in association with neoplasm elsewhere in the body, a rapidly progressive form of degeneration that affects the spinal cord primarily (Mancall and Rosales). The latter disorder has been characterized by a rapidly ascending sensorimotor deficit that terminates fatally in a matter of days or weeks and by a roughly symmetrical necrosis of both the gray and white matter of most of the cord. This form of necrotizing myelopathy is distinctly rare, and its status as a remote effect of carcinoma is uncertain.

Henson and Urich have drawn attention to yet another rare spinal cord disorder, usually associated with carcinoma of the lung. This takes the form of large wedge-shaped necrotic lesions scattered throughout the cord and affecting mainly the white matter of the posterior and lateral columns. The clinical correlates of this disorder are unclear.

Yet another spinal cord disorder is a *subacute motor neuronopathy* that occurs as a remote effect of Hodgkin disease and other lymphomas (Schold et al). Clinically it takes the form of a relatively benign, purely motor weakness of the limbs, the course and severity of which are independent of the underlying neoplasm. The basic neuropathologic change is a depletion of anterior horn cells. In addition, the few autopsied cases have shown a gliosis of the posterior columns, pointing to an asymptomatic affection of the primary sensory neuron.

OTHER PARANEOPLASTIC DISORDERS

Mention has already been made of a syndrome of myoclonus-opsoclonus-ataxia that occurs in children with neuroblastoma (page 534). The neurologic disorder usually subsides spontaneously, which is why its pathologic basis is not known. We have seen an instance of opsoclonus-myoclonus in a middle-aged woman with bronchial carcinoma who showed a marked degeneration of the dentate nuclei. A presumed association between amyotrophic lateral sclerosis and carcinoma has not been verified. Isolated case reports relating neuromyelitis optica and optic neuritis to neoplasm cannot presently be evaluated.

Radiation treatment of cerebral neoplasm, the pituitary gland, or neighboring structures of the head and neck, infrequently gives rise to the delayed development of coagulation necrosis of the white matter of the brain and occasionally of the brainstem. In some areas, the tissue undergoes softening and liquefaction, with cyst formation. With lesser degrees of injury, the process is predominantly a demyelinating one, with partial preservation of axons. The primary damage is believed to occur in the walls of blood vessels, in the form of hyaline thickening and fibrinoid necrosis, with thrombosis.

The symptoms, coming on 3 months to 3 years after radiation therapy, are those of cerebral tumor—subacutely evolving focal abnormalities, depending on the site of the lesion; focal or generalized seizures; impairment of mental function; and eventually increased intracranial pressure. Whole brain radiation, for tumor or acute lymphoblastic leukemia, can lead to diffuse cerebral atrophy, enlarged ventricles, and panhypopituitarism (particularly in children who suffer growth retardation).

In the production of radiation necrosis, the total and fractional doses of radiation and the time over which treatment is administered are obviously important factors, but the exact amounts that produce such damage cannot be stated. Other elements, still undefined, must play a part, since similar courses of radiation treatment may damage one patient and leave another patient unaffected. CT scans show a low-density, contrast-enhancing lesion, and angiography shows an avascular mass. MRI is even more sensitive in distinguishing radiation necrosis from tumor and peritumor products, but histologic proof is still necessary to differentiate the mass from cerebral tumor and to prevent further radiotherapy. Treatment has consisted of surgical resection, if feasible, supplemented with corticosteroids.

CONCLUDING REMARKS

The physician's responsibilities in this field of intracranial tumors are (1) to provide a diagnosis (tumor cases must be distinguished from all others); (2) to exclude the possibility that the intracranial mass is part of a general disease that would contraindicate surgery, i.e., metastatic carcinoma, syphilis, tuberculosis, etc.; (3) to exclude the several pseudotumor syndromes; (4) to maintain the patient in the best possible condition, until surgery can be undertaken (fluids, electrolytes, corticosteroid therapy, etc.); and (5) to assist the surgeon in the postoperative medical management.

Tumors of the spinal cord and peripheral nerves are discussed in Chaps. 36 and 46, respectively.

REFERENCES

Adams RD, Wegner W: Congenital cyst of the spinal meninges as cause of intermittent compression of the spinal cord. *Arch Neurol Psychiatry* 58:57, 1947.

Allen JC, Bloom J, Ertel I et al: Brain tumors in children: Current cooperative and institutional chemotherapy trials in newly diagnosed and recurrent disease. *Semin Oncol* 13:110, 1986.

Allen JC, Kim JH, Packer RJ: Neoadjuvant chemotherapy for newly diagnosed germ-cell tumors of the central nervous system. *J Neurosurg* 67:65, 1987.

Anderson NE, Cunningham JM, Posner JB: Autoimmune pathogenesis of paraneoplastic neurological syndromes. *CRC Crit Rev Neurobiol* 3:245, 1987.

Antunes JL, Housepian EM, Frantz AG et al: Prolactin-secreting pituitary tumors. *Ann Neurol* 2:148, 1977.

Bailey P, Bucy PC: Oligodendrogliomas of the brain. *J Pathol Bacteriol* 32:735, 1929.

Bailey P, Cushing H: *A Classification of Tumors of the Glioma Group on a Histogenetic Basis with a Correlated Study of Prognosis*. Philadelphia, Lippincott, 1926.

Barcos M, Lane W, Gomez GA et al: An autopsy study of 1,206 acute and chronic leukemias (1958–1982). *Cancer* 60:827, 1987.

Bellur SN, Chandra V, McDonald LW: Association of meningiomas with extraneural primary malignancy. *Neurology* 29:1165, 1979.

Benton JW, Nellhaus G, Huttenlocher PR et al: The bobble-head doll syndrome. *Neurology* 16:725, 1966.

Bingas B: Tumors of the base of the skull, in Vinken PJ, Bruyn GW (eds): *Handbook of Clinical Neurology*, vol 17. Amsterdam, North-Holland, 1974, chap 4, pp 136–233.

Brougham M, Heusner AP, Adams RD: Acute degenerative changes in adenomas of the pituitary body—with special reference to pituitary apoplexy. *J Neurosurg* 7:421, 1950.

Burger PC: Malignant astrocytic neoplasms: Classification, pathologic anatomy and response to treatment. *Semin Oncol* 13:16, 1986.

Cogan DG: Tumors of the optic nerve, in Vinken PJ, Bruyn GW (eds): *Handbook of Clinical Neurology*, vol 17. Amsterdam, North-Holland, 1974, chap 9, pp 350–374.

Coppeto JR, Roberts M: Fibrosarcoma after proton-beam pituitary ablation. *Arch Neurol* 36:380, 1979.

Corsellis JAN, Goldberg GJ, Norton AR: Limbic encephalitis and its association with carcinoma. *Brain* 91:481, 1968.

Cunningham J, Graus F, Anderson N, Posner JB: Partial characterization of the Purkinje cell antigens in paraneoplastic cerebellar degeneration. *Neurology* 36:1163, 1986.

Cushing H: Some experimental and clinical observations concerning states of increased intracranial tension. *Am J Med Sci* 124:375, 1902.

Cushing H: *The Pituitary Body and Its Diseases*. Philadelphia, Lippincott, 1912.

Cushing H: *Tumors of the Nervus Acusticus and Syndrome of the Cerebellopontine Angle*. Philadelphia, Saunders, 1917.

CUSHING H: *Intracranial Tumors: Notes Upon a Series of 2000 Verified Cases with Surgical-Mortality Percentages Pertaining Thereto.* Springfield, IL, Charles C Thomas, 1932.

CUSHING H, EISENHARDT L: *Meningiomas.* New York, Hafner, 1962.

DORFMAN LJ, FORNO LS: Paraneoplastic encephalomyelitis. *Acta Neurol Scand* 48:556, 1972.

DRAYER B, KATTAH J, ROSENBAUM A et al: Diagnostic approaches to pituitary adenomas. *Neurology* 29:161, 1979.

DUFFNER PK, COHEN ME, MYERS MH, HEISE HW: Survival of children with brain tumors: SEER program, 1973–1980. *Neurology* 36:597, 1986.

DUNN J, KERNOHAN JW: Gliomatosis cerebri. *Arch Pathol* 64:82, 1957.

FISHMAN RA: *Cerebrospinal Fluid in Diseases of the Nervous System.* Philadelphia, Saunders, 1980.

FOKES EC JR, EARLE KM: Ependymomas: Clinical and pathological aspects. *J Neurosurg* 30:585, 1969.

FOX JL, AL-MEFTY O: Suprasellar arachnoid cysts: An extension of the membrane of Liliequist. *Neurosurgery* 7:615, 1980.

FRANKEL SA, GERMAN WJ: Glioblastoma multiforme: A review of 219 cases with regard to natural history, pathology, diagnostic methods and history. *J Neurosurg* 15:489, 1958.

GANDY SE, HEIER LA: Clinical and magnetic resonance features of primary intracranial arachnoid cysts. *Ann Neurol* 21:342, 1987.

GARDNER G, COCKE EW JR, ROBERTSON JT et al: Combined approach surgery for removal of glomus jugulare tumors. *Laryngoscope* 87:665, 1977.

GREENLEE JE, BRASHEAR HR: Antibodies to cerebellar Purkinje cells in patients with paraneoplastic cerebellar degeneration and ovarian carcinoma. *Ann Neurol* 14:609, 1983.

HAKUBA A, HASHI K, FUJITANI K et al: Jugular foramen neurinomas. *Surg Neurol* 11:83, 1979.

HARNER SG, LAWS ER: Clinical findings in patients with acoustic neurinoma. *Mayo Clin Proc* 58:721, 1983.

HARPER CG, STEWART-WYNNE EG: Malignant gliomas in adults. *Arch Neurol* 35:731, 1978.

HASEGALOA H, ALLEN JC, MEHTA BM et al: Enhancement of CNS penetration of methotrexate by hyperosmolar intracarotid mannitol in carcinomatous meningitis. *Neurology* 29:1280, 1979.

HELLE T, BRITT RH, COLBY TV: Primary lymphoma of the central nervous system. *J Neurosurg* 60:94, 1984.

HENRY JM, HEFFNER RR JR, DILLARD SH et al: Primary malignant lymphomas of the central nervous system. *Cancer* 34:1293, 1974.

HENSON RA, URICH H: *Cancer and the Nervous System.* Oxford, Blackwell, 1982.

HOCHBERG FH, MILLER G, SCHOOLEY RT et al: Central nervous system lymphoma related to Epstein-Barr virus. *N Engl J Med* 309:745, 1983.

HOUSE WF, HITSELBERGER WE: Acoustic tumors, in Vinken PJ, Bruyn GW (eds): *Handbook of Clinical Neurology,* vol 17. Amsterdam, North-Holland, 1974, chap 18, pp 666–692.

JEFFERSON G: The tentorial pressure cone. *Arch Neurol Psychiatry* 40:837, 1938.

JENNINGS MT, GELMAN R, HOCHBERG F: Intracranial germ-cell tumors: Natural history and pathogenesis. *J Neurosurg* 63:155, 1985.

KAUFMAN B, PEARSON OH, CHAMBERLIN WB: Radiographic features of intrasellar masses and progressive, asymmetrical non-tumorous enlargement of the sella turcica, the "empty" sella, in *Diagnosis and Treatment of Pituitary Tumors,* International Congress Series no. 303. Amsterdam, Excerpta Medica, 1973, pp 100–129.

KENDELL BE, LEE BCP: Cranial chordomas. *Br J Radiol* 50:687, 1977.

KERNOHAN JW, SAYRE GP: *Tumors of the Central Nervous System. Fascicle 35, Atlas of Tumor Pathology.* Washington. Armed Forces Institute of Pathology, 1952.

KERNOHAN JW, UIHLEIN A: *Sarcomas of the Brain.* Springfield, IL, Charles C Thomas, 1962.

KERNOHAN JW, WOLTMAN HW: Incisura of the crus due to contralateral brain tumor. *Arch Neurol Psychiatry* 21:274, 1929.

KJELLBERG RN: A system of therapy of pituitary tumors: Bragg peak proton hypophysectomy, in Seydel HG (ed): *Tumors of the Nervous System.* New York, Wiley, 1975, pp 145–174.

KLATZO I: Neuropathological aspects of brain edema. *J Neuropathol Exp Neurol* 26:1, 1967.

KRAMER W: Glomus jugulare tumors, in Vinken PJ, Bruyn GW (eds): *Handbook of Clinical Neurology,* vol. 18. Amsterdam, North-Holland, 1975, chap 19, pp 435–455.

LASSMAN LP: Tumors of the pons and medulla, in Vinken PJ, Bruyn GW (eds): *Handbook of Clinical Neurology,* vol 17. Amsterdam, North-Holland, 1974, chap 19, pp 693–706.

LAURENCE KM, HOARE RD, TILL K: The diagnosis of choroid plexus papilloma of the lateral ventricle. *Brain* 84:628, 1961.

LEIBEL SA, WARA WM, SHELINE GE et al: The treatment of meningiomas in childhood. *Cancer* 37:2709, 1976.

LEVITT LJ, DAWSON DM, ROSENTHAL DS, MOLONEY WC: CNS involvement in the non-Hodgkin's lymphomas. *Cancer* 45: 545, 1980.

LI C-Y, WITZIG TE, PHYLIKY RL et al: Diagnosis of B-cell non-Hodgkin's lymphoma of the central nervous system by immunocytochemical analysis of cerebrospinal fluid lymphocytes. *Cancer* 57:737, 1986.

LUDWIG CL, SMITH MT, GODFREY AD, ARMBRUSTMACHER VW: A clinicopathological study of 323 patients with oligodendrogliomas. *Ann Neurol* 19:15, 1986.

MACCABE JJ: Glioblastoma, in Vinken PJ, Bruyn GW (eds): *Handbook of Clinical Neurology,* vol 18. Amsterdam, North-Holland, 1975, chap 2, pp 49–71.

MANCALL EL, ROSALES RK: Necrotizing melopathy associated with visceral carcinoma. *Brain* 87:639, 1964.

MARTUZA RI: Genetics of neuro-oncology. *Clin Neurosurg* 21:417, 1984.

MARTUZA RL, OJEMANN RG: Bilateral acoustic neuromas: Clinical aspects, pathogenesis and treatment. *Neurosurgery* 10:1, 1982.

MATSON DD, CROFTON FDL: Papilloma of choroid plexus in childhood. *J Neurosurg* 17:1002, 1960.

MEYER A: Herniation of the brain. *Arch Neurol Psychiatry* 4:387, 1920.

MEYER FB, EBERSOLD MJ, REESE DF: Benign tumors of the foramen magnum. *J. Neurosurg* 61:136, 1984.

MØRK SJ, LØKEN AC: Ependymoma—a followup study of 101 cases. *Cancer* 40:907, 1977.

NEVIN S: Gliomatosis cerebri. *Brain* 61:170, 1938.

NUGENT JL, BUNN PA, MATTHEWS MJ et al: CNS metastases in small cell bronchogenic carcinoma. *Cancer* 44:1885, 1979.

OJEMANN RG, MONTGOMERY W, WEISS L: Evaluation and Surgical treatment of acoustic neuroma. *N Engl J Med* 287:895, 1972.

OLIVECRONA H: The surgical treatment of intracranial tumors, in *Handbuch der Neurochirurgie,* vol IV. Berlin, Springer-Verlag, 1967, pt 4, pp 1–301.

PAONE JF, JEYASINGHAM K: Remission of cerebellar dysfunction after pneumonectomy for bronchogenic carcinoma. *N Engl J Med* 302:156, 1980.

PATCHELL RA, CIRRINCIONE C, THALER HT et al: Single brain metastasis: Surgery plus radiation or radiation alone. *Neurology* 36:447, 1986.

PECKER J, SCARABIN JM, BRUCHER JM, VALLEE B: Apport des techniques stéréotaxiques au diagnostic et au traitement des tumeurs de la région pinéale. *Rev Neurol* (Paris) 134:287, 1978 (Eng abstr).

POLAK M: Registro latino americano de tumores del sistemo nerviosa. Clasificacion sinonimia y estadistica. *Rev Neurol Argentina* 11:97, 1985.

POLMETEER FE, KERNOHAN JW: Meningeal gliomatosis. *Arch Neurol Psychiatry* 57:593, 1947.

POSNER JB: Primary lymphoma of the CNS. *Neurology Alert* 5:21, 1987.

POSNER J, CHERNICK NL: Intracranial metastases from systemic cancer. *Adv Neurol* 19:575, 1978.

PRICE RA, JOHNSON WW: The central nervous system in childhood leukemia: I. The arachnoid. *Cancer* 31:520, 1973.

RIBBERT H: *Geschwulstlehre.* Bonn, Verlag Cohen, 1904.

ROBAIN O, DULAC O, DOMMERGUES JP et al: Necrotising leukoencephalopathy complicating treatment of childhood leukaemia. *J Neurol Neurosurg Psychiatry* 47:65, 1984.

ROPPER AH: Lateral displacement of the brain and level of consciousness in patients with an acute hemispheral mass. *N Engl J Med* 314:953, 1986.

ROSNER D, NEMOTO T, LANE WW: Chemotherapy induces regression of brain metastases in breast carcinoma. *Cancer* 58:832, 1986.

RUBINSTEIN AB, SHALIT MN, COHEN ML et al: Radiation-induced cerebral meningioma: a recognizable entity. *J Neurosurg* 61:966, 1984.

RUBINSTEIN LJ: *Tumors of the Central Nervous System,* fasc. 6, 2nd series, Atlas of Tumor Pathology. Washington, Armed Forces Institute of Pathology, 1972.

RUBINSTEIN LJ: Embryonal central neuroepithelial tumors and their differentiating potential. *J Neurosurg* 62:795, 1985.

RUSSELL DS: The pinealoma: Its relationship to teratoma. *J Pathol Bacteriol* 56:145, 1944.

RUSSELL DS: Cellular changes and patterns of neoplasia, in Haymaker W, Adams RD (eds): *Histology and Histopathology of the Nervous System.* Springfield, IL, Charles C Thomas, chap 14.

RUSSELL DS, RUBINSTEIN LJ: *Pathology of Tumours of the Nervous System,* 4th ed. London, E Arnold, 1977.

SANBORN GE, SELHORST GB, CALABRESE VP, TAYLOR, GR: Pseudotumor cerebri and insecticide intoxication. *Neurology* 29:1222, 1979.

SCHAUMBURG HH, PLANK CR, ADAMS RD: The reticulum cell sarcoma: Microglioma group of brain tumors. *Brain* 95:199, 1972.

SCHOLD SC, CHO E-S, SOMASUNDARAM M, POSNER JB: Subacute motor neuronopathy: A remote effect of lymphoma. *Ann Neurol* 5:271, 1979.

SHAPIRO WR: Therapy of adult malignant brain tumors: What have the clinical trials taught us? *Semin Oncol* 13:38, 1986.

SHEIBANI K, BATTIFORA H, WINBERG CD et al: Further evidence that "malignant angioendotheliomatosis" is an angiotropic large-cell lymphoma. *N Engl J Med* 314:943, 1986.

SORENSON SC, EAGAN RT, SCOTT M: Meningeal carcinomatosis in patients with primary breast or lung cancer. *Mayo Clin Proc* 59:91, 1984.

STROINK AR, HOFFMAN HJ, HENDRICK EB, HUMPHREYS RP: Diagnosis and management of pediatric brainstem gliomas. *J Neurosurg* 65:745, 1986.

TOMLINSON BE, PERRY RH, STEWART-WYNNE EG: Influence of site of origin of lung carcinomas on clinical presentation and central nervous system metastases. *J Neurol Neurosurg Psychiatry* 42:82, 1979.

VICTOR M, FERRENDELLI JA: The nutritional and metabolic diseases of the cerebellum: Clinical and pathological aspects, in Fields WS, Willis WD Jr (eds): *The Cerebellum in Health and Disease.* St Louis, Warren H Green, 1970, chap 16, pp 412–449.

WAGA S, MORIKAWA A, SAKAKURA M: Craniopharyngioma with midbrain involvement. *Arch Neurol* 36:319, 1979.

WALKER RW, POSNER JB: Central nervous system neoplasms, in Appel SH (ed): *Current Neurology,* vol 5. New York, Wiley, 1984, chap 9, pp 285–322.

WASSERSTROM WR, GLASS JP, POSNER JB: Diagnosis and treatment of leptomeningeal metastases from solid tumors: Experience with 90 patients. *Cancer* 49:759, 1982.

YUNG WA, HORTEN BC, SHAPIRO WR: Meningeal gliomatosis: A review of 12 cases. *Ann Neurol* 8:605, 1980.

ZIMMERMAN HM: Brain tumors: Their incidence and classification in man and their experimental production. *Ann NY Acad Sci* 159:337, 1969.

ZÜLCH KJ: *Brain Tumors, Their Biology and Pathology,* 3rd ed. New York, Springer, 1986.

CHAPTER 32

NONVIRAL INFECTIONS OF THE NERVOUS SYSTEM

This chapter is concerned mainly with the pyogenic or bacterial infections of the central nervous system (CNS), i.e., bacterial meningitis, intracranial thrombophlebitis, brain abscess, epidural abscess, and subdural empyema. The granulomatous infections of the CNS, notably tuberculosis, syphilis and other spirochetal infections, and certain fungus infections, will also be discussed in some detail. In addition, brief consideration will be given to sarcoid, a granulomatous disease of uncertain etiology, and to the CNS effects of certain rickettsias, protozoa, and worms.

A number of other infectious diseases of the nervous system are more appropriately discussed elsewhere in this book. Diseases due to bacterial exotoxins—diphtheria, tetanus, botulism—are considered with other toxins of the nervous system (Chap. 42). Leprosy, which is essentially a disease of the peripheral nerves, is considered in Chap. 46. Viral infections of the nervous system, because of their frequency and importance, have been allotted a chapter of their own (Chap. 33).

PYOGENIC INFECTIONS OF THE CENTRAL NERVOUS SYSTEM

The pyogenic infections of the cranial contents originate in one of two ways, either by hematogenous spread (emboli of bacteria or infected thrombi) or by extension from cranial structures (ears, paranasal sinuses, osteomyelitic foci in the skull, penetrating cranial injuries, or congenital sinus tracts). In a small number of cases, infection is iatrogenic, being introduced by a lumbar puncture needle, cerebral surgery, or a shunting device. In animals with experimentally produced bacteremia, a needle placed in the subarachnoid space may cause localization of bacteria at the site of injury. Whether or not this occurs in bacterial infections of humans is not known.

Concerning the hematogenous pathway surprisingly little is known, for human autopsy material seldom divulges information on this point, and animal experiments involving the injection of virulent bacteria into the blood stream have yielded somewhat contradictory results. In most instances of bacteremia or septicemia, the nervous system seems not to be infected; yet in certain cases, a bacteremia due to pneumonia is the only apparent forerunner of meningitis. This reflects the differences in virulence of the common meningeal pathogens. In chronic pulmonary diseases, septic emboli have been seen in the pulmonary veins, from which they may reach the cerebral arteries; and in acute and subacute bacterial endocarditis, bacterial emboli are found in cerebral and meningeal arteries. The ideal site of lodgment of these emboli for the production of meningitis—whether in choroid plexuses or in meningeal or superficial cerebral vessels—has not been ascertained.

With respect to the formation of brain abscess, the notable feature is the resistance of cerebral tissue to infection. Direct injection of virulent bacteria into the brain of an animal seldom results in abscess formation. In fact, this condition has been produced consistently only by injecting culture medium along with the bacteria or by causing necrosis of the tissue at the time it is inoculated with bacteria. In humans, infarction of brain tissue by arterial occlusion (embolism) or venous occlusion (thrombophlebitis) appears to be the common and perhaps necessary antecedent.

The cranial epidural and subdural spaces are notably invulnerable to blood-borne infective agents, in contrast to the spinal epidural space, which is a more frequent site of suppuration. Furthermore, the cranial bones and the dura mater (which essentially constitutes the inner periosteum of the skull) protect the cranial cavity against the ingress of bacteria. This protective mechanism may fail if suppuration occurs in the middle ear, mastoid cells, or frontal, ethmoid, and sphenoid sinuses. Two pathways from these sources have been demonstrated: (1) infected thrombi may form in diploic veins and spread along these vessels into the dural sinuses (into which the diploic veins flow) and from there, in retrograde fashion, along the meningeal veins into the brain; and (2) an osteomyelitic focus may form, with erosion of the inner table of bone and invasion of the dura, subdural space, pia-arachnoid, and even the brain substance. Each of these pathways has been observed in some fatal cases of epidural abscess, subdural empyema, leptomeningitis, cranial venous sinusitis and meningeal thrombophlebitis, and brain abscess. However, in many cases coming to autopsy, the pathway of infection cannot be determined.

A hematogenous infection in the course of a bacteremia usually permits a single type of virulent organism to gain entry to the cranial cavity. In the adult the most common pathogenic organisms are pneumococcus, meningococcus, *Haemophilus influenzae*, *Listeria monocytogenes*, staphylococcus, and streptococcus; in the neonate, *Escherichia coli* and group B streptococcus; in the infant and child, *H. influenzae*. In contrast, when septic material embolizes from infected lungs or congenital heart lesions, or extends directly from ears or sinuses, more than one type of bacterial flora common to these organs may be transmitted. Such "mixed infections" pose difficult problems in therapy. Occasionally, in these latter conditions, when active suppuration has occurred, the demonstration of the causative organisms may be unsuccessful, even from the pus of an abscess.

BACTERIAL MENINGITIS (LEPTOMENINGITIS)

This condition consists essentially of an infection of the pia and arachnoid and the fluid in the space that they enclose. Since the subarachnoid space is continuous around the brain, spinal cord, and the optic nerves, an infective agent (or tumor cells or blood) gaining entry to any one part of the space may spread rapidly to all of it, even its most remote recesses; in other words, meningitis is always *cerebrospinal*. Infection also reaches the ventricles of the brain, either directly from the choroid plexuses or by reflux through the foramina of Magendie and Luschka.

Bacterial Meningitis as a Biologic Phenomenon The effect of bacteria or other microorganisms in the subarachnoid space is to cause an inflammatory reaction in the pia and arachnoid, in the cerebrospinal fluid (CSF), and in the ventricles, involving all the structures that lie within or adjacent to these spaces.

The first effect is hyperemia of the meningeal vessels; very shortly thereafter there occurs a migration of neutrophils into the subarachnoid space. The subarachnoid exudate increases rapidly, particularly over the base of the brain, and extends into the sheaths of cranial and spinal nerves and, for a very short distance, into the perivascular spaces of the cortex. During the first few days, neutrophils, many of them containing phagocytized bacteria, are the predominant cells. Within a few days lymphocytes and histiocytes increase gradually in relative and absolute numbers. During all this time there is exudation of fibrinogen and other blood proteins. In the latter part of the second week plasma cells appear and subsequently increase in number. At about the same time the cellular exudate is disposed in two layers— an outer one, just beneath the arachnoid membrane, made up of neutrophils and fibrin, and an inner one, next to the pia, composed largely of lymphocytes, plasma cells, and macrophages. Although fibroblasts begin to proliferate early, they are not conspicuous until later, when they take part in the organization of the exudate, resulting in fibrosis of the arachnoid and loculation of pockets of exudate.

During the process of resolution the inflammatory cells disappear in almost the same order as they appear. Neutrophils begin to disintegrate by the fourth to fifth day, and soon no new ones appear. Lymphocytes, plasma cells, and macrophages disappear more slowly and may remain in small numbers for several months. The completeness of resolution depends to a large extent on the stage at which the infection is arrested. If controlled in the very early stages, there may not be any residual change in the arachnoid; following an infection of several weeks' duration there is a permanent fibrous overgrowth of the meninges resulting in a thickened, cloudy, or opaque arachnoid and often in adhesions between the pia and arachnoid and even between arachnoid and dura.

The pathogenesis of the exudative reaction in the subarachnoid space does not differ from that caused by pyogenic organisms in other tissues. Bacteria or their toxins act as an irritant and induce vascular congestion and increased permeability of venules and capillaries (the first visible cellular exudate is around small meningeal veins). Leukocytosis and migration of neutrophils are probably related to the formation in the meninges of chemical substances, which attract these cells in order to destroy the bacteria and toxic substances. Fibrinogen appears very early and is converted to fibrin after a few days. Lymphocytes migrate from the blood vessels and are probably the source of the plasma cells that appear later; the latter cells react with the capsular antigens of bacteria and produce antibodies. The conversion of meningeal histiocytes to macrophages is evidently a response to degeneration of other cellular elements, such as neutrophils and lymphocytes. Productive fibrosis, at first cellular and later fibrous, is the result of subacute and chronic inflammation.

From the earliest stages of the meningitis, changes are found in the small- and medium-sized subarachnoid arteries. The endothelial cells swell, multiply, and crowd into the lumen. This reaction appears within 48 to 72 h and increases in the following days. The adventitial connective tissue sheath becomes infiltrated by neutrophils. Foci of necrosis of the arterial wall sometimes occur. Neutrophils and lymphocytes migrate to the subintimal region, often forming a conspicuous layer. Later there is subintimal fibrosis. This is a striking feature of nearly all types of subacute and chronic infections of the meninges, but most notably of tuberculous meningitis.

In the veins, swelling of the endothelial cells and infiltration of the adventitia also occur. Subintimal layering, as occurs in arterioles, is not observed, but there may be a diffuse infiltration of the entire wall. It is in veins so affected that focal necrosis of the vessel wall and mural thrombi are most often found. Thrombophlebitis does not usually develop before the end of the second week of the infection.

The unusual prominence of the vascular changes may be related to their anatomic peculiarities. The adventitia of the subarachnoid vessels, both arterioles and venules, is actually formed by an investment of the arachnoid membrane, which is invariably involved by the infectious process. Thus in a sense the vessel wall is affected from the beginning by an inflammatory process arising within itself. The much more frequent occurrence of thrombosis in veins than in arteries is probably accounted for by the thinner walls and the slower current (possibly stagnation) of blood in the former.

Although the spinal and cranial nerves are surrounded by purulent exudate from the beginning of the infection, the perineurial sheaths become infiltrated by inflammatory cells only after several days. Exceptionally, in some nerves, there is infiltration of the endoneurium, and degenerating myelinated fibers with fatty macrophages and proliferating Schwann cells and fibroblasts can be demonstrated. More often there is little or no damage to nerve fibers. Occasionally cellular infiltrations may be found in the optic nerves or olfactory bulbs, but the more common finding is a proliferation of glial cells beneath the pia, similar to that in brain tissue.

The outer arachnoid membrane tends to serve as an effective barrier to the spread of infection, but some reaction in the subdural space may occur nevertheless. This happens more often in infants (subdural effusions) than in adults. As a rule there are no large quantities of subdural pus, but small amounts of fibrinous exudate are found frequently in microscopic sections that include the cranial and particularly the spinal dura.

When fibrinopurulent exudate accumulates in large quantities around the spinal cord, it blocks off the spinal subarachnoid space. Hydrocephalus is produced by exudate in the foramina of Magendie and Luschka or in the subarachnoid space around the pons and midbrain, interfering with the flow of CSF from the cisterna magna and lateral recesses to the basal cisterns and convexities. In the later stages, fibrous subarachnoid adhesions are an additional and sometimes the most important factor interfering with the circulation of CSF. An infrequent late sequela of bacterial meningitis is *chronic adhesive arachnoiditis* or *chronic meningomyelitis*.

In the early stages of meningitis very little change in the substance of the brain can be detected. After several days microglia and astrocytes increase in number, at first in the outer zone and later in all layers of the cortex. The associated nerve cell changes may be very slight. Obviously some disorder of the cortical neurons must be present from the beginning of the infection to account for the stupor or coma and convulsions so often observed, but several days must elapse before any change can be demonstrated microscopically. It is uncertain whether these cortical changes are due to the diffusion of toxins from the meninges, to a circulatory disturbance, or to some other factor. The changes are not due to the presence of bacteria in the substance of the brain, and should therefore be regarded as a noninfectious encephalopathy. Impaired cerebral perfusion is probably an important factor. Cerebral angiography, performed in children with meningitis, shows a leakage of contrast material into the cortex, a change that is rapidly reversed with treatment (Kroll and Moxon). Also, in cases of septic shock, the fall in blood pressure, coupled with a rise in intracranial pressure, reduces cerebral perfusion pressure (Scheld). Ischemic necrosis of the cerebral cortex is in some cases the result of cerebral thrombophlebitis, but in others, with quite extensive cortical necrosis, no thrombosed veins are found.

In the early stages of meningitis there may be little change in the ependyma and the subependymal tissues, but in the later stages conspicuous changes are invariably found. The most prominent finding is infiltration of the subependymal perivascular spaces and often of the tissues with neutrophilic leukocytes, and later with lymphocytes and plasma cells. There may be desquamation of ependymal cells. Microglia and astrocytes proliferate, the latter sometimes overgrowing and burying remnants of the ependymal lining. We believe that the bacteria pass through the ependymal lining and set up this inflammatory reaction. This sequence of events is favored by a developing hydrocephalus, which stretches and breaks the ependymal lining. The glial changes are secondary to damage of subependymal tissues.

The choroid plexus is at first congested, but within

a few days becomes infiltrated with neutrophils and lymphocytes, and eventually may be covered with exudate. As in the case of the meningeal exudate, lymphocytes, plasma cells, and macrophages later predominate. Eventually there is organization of the exudate covering the plexus.

The reader may question this long digression into matters that are more pathologic than clinical, but only by consideration of the morphologic features of meningitis can one understand the basis of the clinical state. The meningeal and ependymal reactions to bacterial infection and the clinical correlates of these reactions have been summarized in Table 30-1.

Types of Bacterial Meningitis Almost any bacterium gaining entrance to the body may produce meningitis, but by far the most common are *Haemophilus influenzae*, *Neisseria meningitidis*, and *Streptococcus pneumoniae*, which account for about 75 percent of cases. Infection with *Listeria monocytogenes* is now the fourth most common type of nontraumatic or nonpostsurgical bacterial meningitis in adults. The following are less frequent causes: *Staphylococcus aureus* and group A streptococci, usually in association with brain abscess, epidural abscess, head trauma, neurosurgical procedures, or cranial thrombophlebitis; *Escherichia coli;* group B streptococci, in newborns; and the other Enterobacteriaceae such as *Klebsiella, Proteus,* and *Pseudomonas,* which are usually a consequence of lumbar puncture, spinal anesthesia, or shunting procedures to relieve hydrocephalus. Rarer meningeal pathogens include *Salmonella, Shigella, Clostridium, Neisseria gonorrhoeae,* and *Acinetobacter calcoaceticus*–biotype lwoffi (formerly called *Mima polymorpha*), which may be difficult to distinguish from *Haemophilus* and *Neisseria.*

Epidemiology Pneumococcal, *H. influenzae,* and meningococcal meningitis have a worldwide distribution, occurring mainly during the fall, winter, and spring, and predominating in males. Each has a relatively constant seasonal incidence, although epidemics of meningococcal meningitis seem to occur roughly in 10-year cycles. Drug-resistant strains appear with varying frequency, and such information, gleaned from national surveillance, is of practical importance. *H. influenzae* meningitis, which was formerly encountered almost exclusively in children between 2 months and 7 years of age, is now being reported with increasing frequency in adults over 50 years of age (in the United States there are between 12,000 and 15,000 cases each year). Meningococcal meningitis occurs most often in children and adolescents, but is also encountered throughout much of adult life, with a sharp decline in incidence after the age of 50. Pneumococcal meningitis predominates in the very young and in adults over 40 years of age.

Pathogenesis The three most common meningeal pathogens are all inhabitants of the nasopharynx in a significant part of the population and depend upon antiphagocytic capsular or surface antigens for survival in the tissues of the infected host; all express their pathogenicity largely in the form of extracellular proliferation. It is evident from the frequency with which the carrier state is detected that nasal colonization is not a sufficient explanation of infection of the meninges. Factors that predispose the colonized patient to blood stream invasion, which is the usual route by which bacteria reach the meninges, are obscure but include antecedent viral infections of the upper respiratory passages or, in the case of the pneumococcus, infections in the lung. Once blood-borne, the factors that lead to meningeal localization of bacteria are unknown, but it is evident that pneumococci, *H. influenzae,* and meningococci possess a unique predilection for the meninges. Whether the organisms enter the CSF via the choroid plexus or meningeal vessels is unknown. It has been postulated that the entry of bacteria into the subarachnoid space is facilitated by disruption of the blood-CSF barrier by trauma, circulating endotoxin, or an initial viral infection of the meninges.

Avenues other than the blood stream by which bacteria can gain access to the meninges include congenital neuroectodermal defects, craniotomy sites, diseases of the middle ear and paranasal sinuses, skull fractures, and, in cases of recurrent infection, dural tears from remote minor or major trauma. Occasionally a brain abscess may rupture into the subarachnoid space or ventricles, thus infecting the meninges. The isolation of anaerobic streptococci, *Bacteroides,* or *Actinomyces,* or a mixture of microorganisms from the CSF, should suggest the possibility of a brain abscess with an associated meningitis.

In most patients the precise route by which bacteria infect the meninges cannot be determined.

Clinical Features *Adults and older children* The early clinical effects of acute pyogenic meningitis are fever, severe headache, generalized convulsions, a disorder of consciousness (i.e., drowsiness, confusion, stupor, and coma), and stiffness of the neck (resistance to passive movement) on forward bending. Flexion at the hip and knee in response to forward flexion of the neck (Brudzinski sign) and inability to completely extend the legs (Kernig sign) are of the same nature as stiff neck, but less reliable. Diagnosis may be difficult when the initial manifestations are pain in the neck or abdomen, or a confusional state or delirium.

Any circumstance that prolongs the meningitis increases the risk of injury to the many structures enumerated above; this fact accounts for many of the clinical features in the subacute and chronic varieties of meningeal infection. The potential pathologic-clinical relations of acute, subacute, and chronic meningitis are summarized in Table 30-1.

The symptoms that comprise the meningitic syndrome are common to the three main types of bacterial meningitis, but certain clinical features correlate more closely with particular types of meningitis. *Meningococcus meningitis* should always be suspected during epidemics of meningitis; when the evolution is extremely rapid; when the onset is attended by a petechial or purpuric rash or by large ecchymoses and lividity of the skin of lower parts of the body; and when circulatory collapse occurs. Since a petechial rash accompanies approximately 50 percent of meningococcus infections, its presence dictates immediate institution of therapy for a neisserian infection, even though similar rashes may be observed with certain viral and occasionally with other bacterial meningitides. (ECHO-9 and *Staph. aureus* infections). *Pneumococcus meningitis* is usually preceded by an infection in the lungs, ears, or sinuses, and the heart valves may be affected. In addition, a pneumococcus etiology should be suspected in alcoholics, splenectomized patients, and in those with recurrent bacterial meningitis, dermal sinus tracts, sickle-cell anemia, and basilar skull fracture. *H. influenzae* meningitis usually follows upper respiratory and ear infections in the child.

Other specific bacterial etiologies are also suggested by particular clinical settings. Meningitis in the presence of furunculosis or following a neurosurgical procedure should raise the possibility of a coagulase-positive staphylococcal infection. Ventriculovenous shunts, inserted for the control of hydrocephalus, are particularly prone to infection with coagulase-negative staphylococci. Brain abscess, myeloproliferative or lymphoproliferative disorders, defects in cranial bones (tumor, osteomyelitis), collagen diseases, metastatic cancer, and therapy with immunosuppressive agents are clinical conditions which favor the invasion of the craniospinal cavities by such pathogens as Enterobacteriaceae, *Listeria, Herellea* (now called *Acinetobacter calcoaceticus,* biotype anitratus), and *Pseudomonas.*

The signs of meningeal irritation—stiff neck, Kernig sign, and Brudzinski sign—may be absent in the very young or the deeply stuporous or comatose patient. Focal cerebral signs in the early stages of the disease, although seldom prominent, are most frequent in pneumococcal and influenzal meningitis. Some of the transitory focal cerebral signs

may represent postictal phenomena (Todd's paralysis); others may be related to an unusually intense focal meningitis. Seizures are encountered most often with *H. influenzae* meningitis, but it is difficult to judge their significance, since young children may convulse with fever of any cause. Persistent focal cerebral lesions, which develop most often in the second week of the meningeal infection, are consequent to vasculitis—usually occlusion of cerebral veins—and infarction of cerebral tissue. Cranial nerve abnormalities are particularly frequent with pneumococcal meningitis, the result of invasion of the nerve by purulent exudate as it traverses the subarachnoid space.

Infants and newborns Acute bacterial meningitis during the first month of life is said to be more frequent than in any subsequent 30-day period of life. It poses a number of special problems. Infants, of course, cannot complain of headache, stiff neck may be absent and one has only the nonspecific signs of a systemic illness—fever, irritability, drowsiness, vomiting, convulsions, and a bulging fontanel—to suggest the presence of meningeal infection. Signs of meningeal irritation do occur, but only late in the course of the illness. A high index of suspicion and liberal use of the lumbar puncture needle are the keys to early diagnosis. Lumbar puncture is crucial, and it must be performed before any antibiotics are administered for other neonatal infections. An antibiotic regimen sufficient to control a septicemia may allow a meningeal infection to smolder and to flare up after antibiotic therapy has been discontinued.

A number of other facts about the natural history of neonatal meningitis are noteworthy. It is more common in males than in females, in a ratio of about 3:1. Obstetrical abnormalities in the third trimester (premature birth, prolonged labor, premature rupture of fetal membranes) occur frequently in mothers of infants who develop meningitis in the first weeks of life. The most significant factor in the pathogenesis of the meningitis is maternal infection (usually a urinary tract infection or perinatal fever of unknown cause). The infection in both mother and infant is most often due to gram-negative enterobacteria, particularly *E. coli,* and group B streptococci, and less often to *Pseudomonas, Listeria, Staphylococcus aureus* or *epidermidis* (formerly *albus*), and group A streptococci. Analysis of postmortem material indicates that in most cases infection occurs at or near the time of birth, although clinical signs of infection may not become evident until several days or a week later.

Spinal Fluid Examination As has already been indicated, the lumbar puncture is an indispensable part of the examination of patients with the symptoms and signs of meningitis, or of any patient in whom this diagnosis is suspected. Bacteremia is not a contraindication to lumbar puncture. If the patient has a bleeding disease or evidence of increased intracranial pressure, then a CT scan or MRI should be done first, looking for a mass lesion.

Pleocytosis of the spinal fluid is diagnostic. The number of leukocytes in the CSF ranges from 1000 to 100,000 per cubic millimeter, but the usual number is from 1000 to 10,000. Occasionally, in pneumococcal and influenzal meningitis, the CSF may contain a large number of bacteria but few if any neutrophils for the first few hours. Cell counts above 50,000 per cubic millimeter raise the possibility of a brain abscess having ruptured into the ventricles. Neutrophilic leukocytes predominate (85 to 95 percent of the total), but an increasing proportion of mononuclear cells is found as the infection continues, especially in partially treated meningitis. In the early stages, careful cytologic examination may disclose that some of the mononuclear cells are myelocytes or young neutrophils. Later, as treatment takes effect, the proportions of lymphocytes, plasma cells, and histiocytes steadily increase.

The spinal fluid *pressure* is so consistently elevated (above 180 mmH$_2$O) that a normal or low pressure on the initial lumbar puncture in a patient with suspected bacterial meningitis should raise the possibility that the needle is partially occluded or the spinal subarachnoid space is blocked. Pressures over 400 mmH$_2$O always suggest brain swelling and potential cerebellar herniation.

The *protein* levels are higher than 45 mg/dL in 90 percent of the cases, and most fall in the range of 100 to 500 mg/dL. The *glucose* content is depressed, usually to a level lower than 40 mg/dL, or less than 40 percent of the blood glucose concentration (measured concomitantly), provided the latter is less than 250 mg/dL. However, in atypical or *culture-negative cases*, other conditions associated with a depressed CSF glucose should be considered. These include hypoglycemia from any cause; sarcoidosis of the central nervous system; fungal or tuberculous meningitis; and some cases of subarachnoid hemorrhage, meningeal carcinomatosis, or gliomatosis. Chloride levels in the CSF are usually low (less than 700 mg/dL), reflecting dehydration and low serum chloride levels.

Gram stain of the spinal fluid sediment permits identification of the causative agent in most cases of bacterial meningitis; pneumococci and *H. influenzae* are identified more readily than meningococci. Small numbers of gram-negative diplococci in leukocytes may be indistinguishable from fragmented nuclear material, which may also be gram-negative and of the same shape. In such cases, a thin film of uncentrifuged CSF may lend itself more readily to morphologic interpretation than a smear of the sediment. The commonest error in reading Gram-stained smears of CSF is misinterpretation of precipitated dye or debris as gram-positive cocci, or a confusion of pneumococci with

H. influenzae. The latter organisms may stain heavily at the poles so that they resemble gram-positive diplococci, and older pneumococci often lose their capacity to take a gram-positive stain.

Cultures of the spinal fluid are best obtained by collecting the fluid in a sterile tube, and immediately inoculating plates of blood, chocolate, and MacConkey agar, and tubes of thioglycolate (for anaerobes) and at least one other broth; the advantage of using broth media is that large amounts of CSF can be cultured. Cultures are positive in 70 to 90 percent of cases of bacterial meningitis.

During the past 15 years counterimmunoelectrophoresis (CIE) has proved to be a valuable adjunct in the diagnosis of bacterial meningitis. This is a sensitive technique that permits the detection of bacterial antigens in the CSF in a matter of 30 to 60 min. It is particularly useful in patients with partially treated meningitis, in whom the CSF still contains bacterial antigens but in whom no organisms can be detected on a smear or grown in culture. Two more recently developed serologic methods, radioimmunoassay (RIA) and latex particle agglutination (LPA), and an enzyme-linked immunosorbent assay (ELISA) may be even more sensitive than CIE.

Measurements of CSF lactic dehydrogenase (LDH) appear to be of prognostic and diagnostic value in bacterial meningitis. A rise in total LDH activity is consistently observed in patients with bacterial meningitis; most of this is due to fractions 4 and 5, which are derived from granulocytes. LDH fractions 1 and 2, which are presumably derived from brain tissue, are only slightly elevated in bacterial meningitis, but rise sharply in patients who die or who develop neurologic sequelae. Thus the test may be helpful in singling out the patient who is most at risk. CSF lysozymal enzymes, derived from leukocytes, meningeal cells, or plasma, may also be increased in meningitis, but the clinical significance of this observation is unknown. CSF levels of lactic acid (determined by either gas chromatography or enzymatic analysis) are also consistently elevated in bacterial and fungal meningitides (above 35 mg/dL) and may be helpful in distinguishing these disorders from viral meningitides, in which lactic acid levels remain normal.

Other Laboratory Findings In addition to CSF cultures, blood cultures should always be obtained because they are positive in 40 to 60 percent of patients with *H. influenzae*, meningococcal, and pneumococcal meningitis, and they may provide the only definite clue as to the causative agent (if CSF cultures are negative). Routine cultures of the oropharynx are as often misleading as they are helpful because pneumococci, *H. influenzae,* and meningococci are such common inhabitants of healthy persons. In contrast, *cultures of the nasopharynx* may be helpful in diagnosis; the finding of typable, encapsulated *H. influenzae* or groupable meningococci may provide the clue to the etiology of the meningeal infection. Contrariwise, the absence of such findings makes an *H. influenzae* and meningococcus etiology unlikely. The *leukocyte count* in the blood is generally elevated, and usually there is a shift to the left. Blood urea nitrogen and serum electrolytes may be abnormal because of severe dehydration. In addition, inappropriate secretion of antidiuretic hormone (ADH) with resultant severe hyponatremia and water intoxication may occur.

Radiologic Studies Patients with bacterial meningitis should have radiographs of the chest, skull, and sinuses as soon as possible after admission to the hospital. Chest films are particularly important because they may disclose a silent area of pneumonitis or abscess. Sinus and skull films may provide clues to the presence of cranial osteomyelitis, paranasal sinusitis, and mastoiditis. If there is a suspicion of enlargement of the ventricles, or of a brain abscess or subdural empyema (or hygroma), a CT scan will settle the matter.

Recurrent Bacterial Meningitis This is probably observed most frequently in patients who have had some type of ventriculovenous shunting procedure for the treatment of hydrocephalus. The patient with recurrent bacterial meningitis of inapparent origin should always be suspected of having a congenital neuroectodermal sinus or a fistulous connection between the nasal sinuses and the subarachnoid space. The fistula in these latter cases is more often traumatic than congenital in origin (a previous basilar skull fracture), although the interval between injury and the initial bout of meningitis may be several years. The site of trauma is in the frontal or ethmoid sinuses or the cribriform plate, and *Streptococcus pneumoniae* is the usual pathogen. Often it proves to be one of the higher serologic types, reflecting the predominance of such strains in nasal carriers. These cases have a good prognosis; mortality is much lower than in ordinary cases of pneumococcal meningitis.

Cerebrospinal fluid rhinorrhea is present in most of the cases of posttraumatic meningitis, but it may be transient and difficult to find. Suspicion of its presence is raised by the occurrence of a watery nasal discharge that increases when the head is dependent and is salty to the taste or by

the recent onset of anosmia. The presence and site of a CSF leak can be demonstrated by injecting a dye (such as carmine red), radioactive albumin, or metrizamide into the spinal subarachnoid space and watching for its appearance in nasal secretions. Another method of detecting CSF rhinorrhea is to measure the glucose concentration of nasal secretions. The usual mucous secretions contain little glucose, but in CSF rhinorrhea the amount of glucose approximates that in CSF. Attempts to demonstrate CSF rhinorrhea should be made only after the acute infection has subsided; if evidence of a fistula is found, and it persists for several weeks, surgical repair should be considered.

Differential Diagnosis The diagnosis of bacterial meningitis is not difficult, providing a high index of suspicion is maintained. All febrile patients with lethargy, headache, or confusion of sudden onset, even if only low-grade fever is present, should be subjected to lumbar puncture. It is particularly important to think of meningitis in febrile, confused alcoholic patients. Too often one incorrectly ascribes the symptoms to intoxication, delirium tremens, or hepatic encephalopathy until examination of the CSF reveals a meningitis. This practice may result in many negative spinal fluid examinations, but this is acceptable, in the authors' view, because the penalty for overlooking a bacterial meningitis is so great.

It needs to be re-emphasized that bacterial meningitis can be diagnosed definitively only by examination of the CSF. Spontaneous subarachnoid hemorrhage, chemical meningitis (following lumbar puncture, spinal anesthesia, or myelography), and viral, tuberculous, leptospiral, and fungal meningoencephalitis often enter into the differential diagnosis.

A number of nonbacterial meningitides must also be considered in the differential diagnosis when the meningitis recurs repeatedly and all cultures are negative. Included in this group are E-B virus infections, Behçet disease, which is characterized by recurrent oral-pharyngeal mucosal ulceration, uveitis, orchitis, and meningitis; so-called Mollaret meningitis, which consists of recurrent episodes of fever and headache, in addition to signs of meningeal irritation; and the Vogt-Koyanagi-Harada syndrome, in which the recurrent meningitis is associated with iridocyclitis and depigmentation of the hair and skin. The CSF in these recurrent types of meningitis may contain large numbers of polymorphonuclear leukocytes, but no bacteria, and the glucose content is not reduced (see also page 601).

The other intracranial suppurative diseases and their differentiation from bacterial meningitis are considered later in this chapter.

Treatment Bacterial meningitis is a medical emergency. The first therapeutic measures are directed to sustaining blood pressure and counteracting septic shock (volume replacement, pressor therapy) and choosing an antibiotic known to be bactericidal for the established or suspected organism and to enter the CSF in effective amounts. Treatment should begin while awaiting diagnostic laboratory tests and should be changed later in accordance with the findings. The following therapeutic regimens are recommended:

1. For adults with pneumococcal or meningococcal meningitis, penicillin G, at least 12 to 15 million units intravenously each day in four to six divided doses; for children the daily dose of penicillin G should be 200,000 to 300,000 units per kilogram of body weight. For children over 2 months of age with *H. influenzae* or uncomplicated meningitis of unknown etiology, chloramphenicol is the drug of choice, because of the emergence of ampicillin-resistant strains, worldwide. Chloramphenicol should be given in doses of 100 mg/kg per day intravenously in a continuous infusion or in divided doses for 2 or 3 days, then 50 mg/kg by the same route. Alternatively, ampicillin may be used (400 mg/kg intravenously in divided doses; adults should receive 12 g/day), but only when the organisms have been shown to be susceptible to this drug. A few strains of ampicillin- and chloromycetin-resistant *H. influenzae* infections have been reported. "Third-generation" cephalosporins (cefotaxime, cefaperazone, and ceftizoxime) have been used successfully in such cases.

In adult patients with any of the three major types of bacterial meningitis who are allergic to the penicillins, chloramphenicol in a dosage of 6 g/day intravenously may be used. Older cephalosporins are not recommended for the treatment of meningitis.

2. For meningitis due to Enterobacteriaceae, the drug of choice is ampicillin or gentamicin, the latter in a dosage of 5 mg/kg per day, administered intravenously in divided dosages at 6-h intervals. However, except in infants, therapeutic success with gentamicin may depend upon intrathecal administration, since adequate CSF concentrations are obtained only by this route. For this reason, ampicillin is preferred, if the offending organism proves to be sensitive to this drug. *Pseudomonas* meningitis should also be treated with gentamicin, as outlined above, with the addition of carbenicillin in large doses intravenously. Third-generation cephalosporins are now considered to be the drugs of choice for the treatment of ampicillin-resistant gram-negative bacterial infections, especially *Pseudomonas*.

3. Meningitis due to *Staph. aureus* should be treated with a penicillinase-resistant penicillin (oxacillin or nafcillin, in a dosage of 10 to 12 g/day), or methicillin, in a dosage of 18 to 20 g/day, intravenously.

Foci of infection in the paranasal sinuses or mastoids, an infected ventriculovenous shunt, or a cranial osteomye-litis should be identified, so that appropriate surgical treatment may be carried out when the acute episode of meningitis has subsided.

Duration of therapy Most cases of bacterial meningitis should be treated for a period of 10 to 14 days except when there is a persistent parameningeal focus of infection. Antibiotics should be administered in full doses parenterally (preferably intravenously) throughout the period of treatment. Treatment failures with several drugs, notably ampicillin, may be attributable to oral or intramuscular administration, resulting in inadequate concentrations in the CSF. Repeated lumbar punctures are not necessary to assess the effects of therapy as long as there is progressive clinical improvement. The CSF glucose may remain low for many days after other signs of infection have subsided, and should occasion concern only if bacteria are present and the patient remains febrile and ill.

Prolongation of fever is due usually to subdural effusion(s), sinus thrombosis, mastoiditis, intercurrent infection, phlebitis, or rarely to abscess of the brain; and it requires continuation of therapy for a longer period. Bacteriologic relapse, after treatment is discontinued, requires immediate reinstitution of therapy.

Adrenocortical steroids The few controlled studies available have demonstrated that steroids exert no beneficial effects in pyogenic meningitis. These drugs should not be used except possibly in overwhelming meningococcal sepsis and cerebral edema.

Other forms of therapy The intrathecal administration of enzymes, which is intended to lyse excessive subarachnoid cellular exudate causing spinal block or hydrocephalus in the subacute stages of bacterial meningitis, is not of proven value. There is also no evidence that repeated drainage of CSF is therapeutically effective. In fact, increased CSF pressure in the acute phases of bacterial meningitis is largely a consequence of cerebral edema, and the lumbar puncture may predispose to cerebellar herniation and death. Mannitol and urea have been employed with apparent success in some cases of severe brain swelling with unusually high initial CSF pressures (over 400 mmH$_2$O). Acting as osmotic diuretics, these agents enter cerebral tissue slowly, and their net effect is to decrease brain water and sodium. The administration of these agents may be associated to some extent with the occurrence of a late rebound phenomenon. Neither agent has been studied in controlled fashion. An adequate but not excessive amount of parenteral fluids should be given, and anticonvulsants should be prescribed when seizures are present. In children, care should be taken to avoid hyponatremia and water intoxication—causes of brain swelling.

Prophylaxis All household contacts of patients with bacterial meningitis should be protected. The risk of secondary cases is small for adolescents and adults but ranges from 2 to 4 percent for those less than 5 years of age. A daily dose of rifampin, 20 mg/kg orally for 4 days, suffices. If 2 weeks or more have elapsed since the index case was found, no prophylaxis is needed.

Prognosis Untreated, bacterial meningitis is usually fatal. The overall mortality rate of treated *H. influenzae* and meningococcal meningitis has remained fixed at 5 to 15 percent for many years; in pneumococcal meningitis the rate is considerably higher (15 to 30 percent). Fulminant meningococcemia, with or without meningitis, also has a high mortality rate because of the associated vasomotor collapse and infective shock, associated with adrenocortical hemorrhages (Waterhouse-Friderichsen syndrome). A disproportionate number of deaths occur in infants and in the aged. The mortality rate is highest in neonates, from 40 to 75 percent in reported series; at least half of those who recover show serious neurologic sequelae. The presence of bacteremia, coma, seizures, and a variety of concomitant diseases, including alcoholism, diabetes mellitus, multiple myeloma, and head trauma, all worsen the prognosis. The triad of pneumococcal meningitis, pneumonia, and endocarditis has a particularly high fatality rate.

It is often impossible to explain the death of the patient, or at least to trace it to a single specific mechanism. The effects of overwhelming infection, with bacteremia and hypotension or brain swelling and cerebellar herniation, are clearly implicated in the deaths of some patients during the initial 48 h. These events may occur in bacterial meningitis of any etiology; however, they are more frequent in meningococcal infection (Waterhouse-Friderichsen syndrome). Some of the deaths occurring later in the course of the illness are attributable to respiratory failure, often consequent to aspiration pneumonia.

Relatively few patients who recover from meningococcal meningitis show residual neurologic defects, whereas such defects are encountered in at least 25 percent of children with *H. influenzae* meningitis and up to 30 percent of patients with pneumococcal meningitis. Ferry et al, in a prospective study of 50 infants who survived *H. influenzae* meningitis, found that about 50 percent were normal,

whereas 9 percent had behavioral problems and about 30 percent had neurologic deficits (seizures, impairment of hearing, language, mentation, and motor function). Dodge and his colleagues found that 31 percent of children with pneumococcal meningitis were left with persistent sensorineural hearing loss; for meningococcal and *H. influenzae* meningitis, the figures were 10.5 and 6 percent, respectively. The acute complications of bacterial meningitis, the intermediate and late neurologic sequelae, and the pathologic basis of these effects are summarized in Table 30-1.

BACTERIAL ENCEPHALITIS

Quite apart from acute and subacute bacterial endocarditis, which may give rise to cerebral embolism and characteristic inflammatory reactions in the brain (see further on), there are several systemic bacterial infections that are commonly complicated by an encephalitis or meningoencephalitis. Three of them, recently recognized, are Legionnaires' disease, *Mycoplasma pneumoniae* infections, and *Listeria monocytogenes* meningoencephalitis.

Legionnaires' disease is an infectious, potentially fatal disease, caused by the gram-negative bacillus *Legionella pneumophila*. It first came to medical notice in July 1976 when a large number of members of the American Legion fell ill at their annual convention in Philadelphia. The fatality rate was high. In addition to the obvious pulmonary infection, extrapulmonary manifestations referable to the CNS and other organs were observed. Lees and Tyrrell described patients with severe and diffuse cerebral involvement and Baker et al and Shetty et al described others with cerebellar and brainstem affection. The clinical syndromes have varied. One consisted of headache, obtundation, acute confusion or delirium with high fever, and evidence of pulmonary distress; another took the form of tremor, nystagmus, cerebellar ataxia, ocular and gaze palsies, and dysarthria. Other neurologic abnormalities have been observed, such as inappropriate ADH secretion, or a syndrome of encephalomyelitis or transverse myelitis. The CSF is entirely normal, and CT scans of the brain are negative, a circumstance that makes diagnosis difficult. The neuropathologic abnormality has not been studied. Suspicion of the disease should prompt tests for serum antibodies to the bacillus, which rise to high levels in a week to 10 days. In most patients the signs of CNS disorder resolve rapidly and completely, although residual impairment of memory and cerebellar ataxia have been recorded. Treatment in adults consists of erythromycin, 0.5 to 1.0 g intravenously, every 6 h for a 3-week period.

Mycoplasma infections of the lung are associated with a number of neurologic syndromes. Some of these are difficult to interpret because the frequency of this upper or lower respiratory infection is so high (20 to 50 percent of all pneumonias) that coincidental involvement of the lungs and nervous system is always possible. Polyneuritis, cranial neuritis, acute myositis, aseptic meningitis, transverse myelitis, acute disseminated (postinfectious) encephalomyelitis and acute hemorrhagic leukoencephalitis (of Hurst) have all been reported in association with mycoplasmal pneumonias (Westenfelder et al; Fisher et al; Rothstein and Kenny). We have observed several patients with a striking brainstem syndrome incurred during a mycoplasmal pneumonia. The organism has only once been cultured from the brain in fatal cases. The mechanism of the cerebral damage has not been established, but the nature of the neurologic complications (particularly postinfectious encephalomyelitis and acute hemorrhagic leukoencephalitis) and their temporal relationship to the mycoplasmal infection suggest that immune factors are operative (see Chap. 37). Most of the patients have recovered with few or no sequelae, but rare fatalities occur.

The diagnosis is usually established by culture of the organism from the respiratory tract, rising serum titers of complement fixing and cold agglutinin antibodies, and complement fixing antibodies in the CSF. The CSF usually contains small numbers of lymphocytes and other mononuclear cells and an increased protein. At the time of onset of the neurologic symptoms there may be no sign of pneumonia.

Listeria monocytogenes meningoencephalitis is most likely to occur in immunosuppressed and debilitated individuals and is a well-known and often fatal cause of meningitis in the newborn. Meningitis is the usual neurologic manifestation, but there are numerous recorded instances of a focal encephalitis, sometimes with a normal CSF. Between 1929, when the organism was discovered, and 1962, when Gray collected all the reported cases, it was noted that 35 percent of 467 patients had either meningitis or meningoencephalitis as the primary manifestation. One of the patients described by Lechtenberg et al had a proven brain abscess. The organism can be cultured from the blood and CSF. The treatment is ampicillin (1 g intravenously every 4 h) in combination with tobramycin (5 to 6 mg/kg intravenously in three divided doses daily). If the condition of the host is compromised the outcome is often fatal. A number of our patients without serious medical disease have made a full and prompt recovery.

SUBDURAL EMPYEMA

Subdural empyema is an intracranial suppurative process, usually on one side, between the inner surface of the dura and the outer surface of the arachnoid. The term subdural abscess, among others, has been applied to this condition, but the proper name is *empyema,* indicating suppuration in a preformed space. Contrary to prevailing opinion, subdural

empyema is not a rarity (about one-fifth as frequent as cerebral abscess). It is distinctly more common in males, a feature for which there is no plausible explanation.

Source of Infection The infection usually originates in the frontal or ethmoid sinuses, or, less often, in the sphenoid and maxillary sinuses and in the middle ear and mastoid cells. Infection gains entry to the subdural space by direct extension through bone and dura, or as a result of thrombophlebitis involving the venous sinuses, particularly the superior longitudinal sinus. Rarely the subdural infection is metastatic, from infected lungs; hardly ever is it secondary to bacteremia or septicemia. Occasionally it extends from a brain abscess.

It is of interest that cases of sinus origin predominate in adolescent and young adult men (Kaufman et al). In such cases, streptococci (nonhemolytic and viridans) are the most common organisms, followed by anaerobic streptococci or *Bacteroides.* Less often *Staph. aureus, E. coli, Proteus,* and *Pseudomonas* are causative. In about half the cases, no organisms can be cultured or seen on Gram stain. The factors that lead to a subdural empyema rather than to a cerebral abscess are not understood.

Pathology A collection of subdural pus, in quantities of a few milliliters to 100 to 200 mL, lies over the cerebral hemisphere. Pus may spread into the interhemispheric fissure or be confined there, and occasionally it is found in the posterior fossa, covering the cerebellum. It is often mistaken for meningitis. The arachnoid, when cleared of exudate, is cloudy, and thrombosis of meningeal veins may be seen. The underlying cerebral hemisphere is depressed, as in subdural hematoma, and in fatal cases there is often an ipsilateral temporal lobe pressure cone. Microscopic examination discloses various degrees of organization of the exudate on the inner surface of the dura, and infiltration of the underlying arachnoid with small numbers of neutrophilic leukocytes, lymphocytes, and mononuclear cells. The thrombi in cerebral veins seem to begin on the sides of the veins nearest the subdural exudate. The superficial layers of the cerebral cortex undergo ischemic necrosis, which probably accounts for the unilateral seizures and other signs of disordered cerebral function.

Symptomatology and Laboratory Findings Usually the history includes reference to chronic sinusitis or mastoiditis with a recent flare-up, causing local pain and increase in purulent nasal or aural discharge. In sinus cases, the pain is usually over the brow or between the eyes, and it is associated with tenderness on pressure over these parts, and sometimes orbital swelling. General malaise, fever, and headache—at first localized, then severe and generalized and associated with vomiting—are the first indications of intracranial spread. They are followed in a few days by drowsiness and increasing stupor, rapidly progressing to coma. At about the same time, focal neurologic signs appear, the most important of which are unilateral motor seizures, hemiplegia, hemianesthesia, aphasia, and paralysis of lateral conjugate gaze. Fever and leukocytosis are always present and the neck is stiff.

The usual CSF findings are an increased pressure, pleocytosis in the range of 50 to 1000 per cubic millimeter, polymorphonuclear cells predominating, elevated protein concentration (75 to 300 mg/dL) and normal glucose values. If the patient is stuporous or comatose, there is risk in performing a lumbar puncture because it may aggravate a threatening pressure cone of the temporal lobe. Instead, one should proceed with other diagnostic procedures (see below).

Diagnosis Skull films usually demonstrate a sinus infection or mastoiditis, and in addition may reveal an osteomyelitis of the frontal bone. The single most useful procedure is the CT scan. If this is not immediately available, carotid arteriography, which discloses inward displacement of meningeal vessels and contralateral shift of the anterior cerebral arteries, is useful. A lateral frontal burr hole with exposure of the dura reveals pus under increased pressure.

Several conditions need to be distinguished clinically from subdural empyema, particularly cerebral thrombophlebitis and brain abscess (see below), acute herpes simplex encephalitis (page 603), acute necrotizing hemorrhagic leukoencephalopathy (page 771), and focal embolic encephalomalacia due to bacterial endocarditis (see further on in this chapter).

Treatment By the time they are recognized, most subdural empyemas require immediate drainage through enlarged multiple frontal burr holes, or through an osteoplastic flap in cases of interhemispheric or posterior fossa empyema. The surgical procedure should be coupled with appropriate antibiotic therapy, which consists of the intravenous administration of 20 to 24 million units of penicillin per day plus chloramphenicol, 2 to 4 g/day. Bacteriologic findings may dictate a change to more appropriate drugs. Without such massive antimicrobial therapy and surgery, most patients will die, usually within 7 to 14 days, often while the unsuspecting physician and surgeon are waiting for better

localization of an assumed cerebral abscess, the most common mistaken diagnosis. On the other hand, patients who are treated promptly may make a surprisingly good recovery, including full or partial resolution of their focal neurologic deficits within a few months.

As with certain brain abscesses, small subdural collections of pus, which are recognized by CT scanning before stupor and coma have supervened, may respond to treatment with heavy doses of antibiotic alone. The resolution or lack of resolution of the empyema can be followed readily by repeated CT or MR scanning (Leys et al).

EXTRADURAL ABSCESS

This condition is almost invariably associated with osteomyelitis in a cranial bone and originates from an infection in the ear or paranasal sinuses, or from a surgical procedure, particularly if the frontal sinus or mastoid had been opened or a foreign body had been used (e.g., dural graft, tantalum button over a burr hole, or Crutchfield tongs). Rarely, the infection is metastatic or spreads outward from a dural sinus thrombophlebitis. Pus and granulation tissue accumulate on the outer surface of the dura, separating it from the cranial bone. The symptoms are those of a local inflammatory process: frontal or auricular pain, purulent discharge from sinuses or ear, and fever and local tenderness. Sometimes the neck is slightly stiff. Localizing neurologic signs are usually absent. Rarely, a focal seizure may occur, or the fifth and sixth cranial nerves are involved with infections of the petrous part of the temporal bone, producing an abducens palsy, pain in the eye and temple, and impaired sensation in the face (Gradenigo syndrome). The CSF is usually clear and under normal pressure but may contain a few lymphocytes and neutrophils (20 to 100 per milliliter) and a slightly increased amount of protein. Treatment consists of antibiotics aimed at the appropriate pathogen(s)—often *Staph. aureus*. Later, the diseased bone in the frontal sinus or the mastoid, from which the extradural infection had arisen, may have to be removed and the wound packed to ensure adequate drainage. Results of treatment are usually good.

Spinal Epidural Abscess This type of abscess possesses unique clinical features and constitutes an important neurologic and neurosurgical emergency. It is discussed in Chap. 36.

INTRACRANIAL THROMBOPHLEBITIS

The dural sinuses drain blood from all of the brain into the jugular veins. The largest and most important of these channels, and the ones usually involved by infection, are the lateral (transverse), cavernous, petrous, and with lesser frequency, the longitudinal sinuses. A complex system of lesser sinuses and cerebral veins connects these large sinuses to one another as well as to the diploic and meningeal veins, and veins of the face and scalp. The basilar venous sinuses are contiguous to several of the paranasal sinuses and mastoid cells.

Usually there is evidence that thrombophlebitis of the large dural sinuses has extended from a manifest infection of the middle ear and mastoid cells, the paranasal sinuses, or skin around the upper lip, nose, and eyes. These cases are frequently complicated by other forms of intracranial suppuration, including meningitis, extradural abscess and subdural empyema, and brain abscess. Occasionally infection may be introduced by direct trauma to large veins or dural sinuses. A variety of organisms, including all the ones that ordinarily inhabit the paranasal sinuses and skin of the nose and face, may give rise to intracranial thrombophlebitis. Streptococci and staphylococci are the ones most often incriminated.

Lateral (Transverse) Sinus Thrombophlebitis In lateral sinus thrombophlebitis, which usually follows chronic infection of the middle ear, mastoid, or petrous bone, earache and mastoid tenderness are succeeded, after a period of a few days to weeks, by generalized headache and, in some instances, papilledema. If the thrombophlebitis remains confined to the transverse sinus, there are no other neurologic signs. Spread to the jugular bulb may give rise to the syndrome of the jugular foramen (see Table 47-1) and involvement of the superior sagittal sinus, to seizures and focal cerebral signs. Fever, as in all forms of intracranial thrombophlebitis, tends to be high and intermittent, and other signs of toxemia may be prominent. Infected emboli may be released into the blood stream, causing petechiae in the skin and mucous membranes, and pulmonary sepsis. The CSF is usually normal, but may show a small number of cells and a modest elevation of protein content.

As a diagnostic aid, compression of each jugular vein during the Queckenstedt maneuver will demonstrate failure of the CSF pressure to rise when the vein ipsilateral to the involved lateral sinus is compressed (Tobey-Ayer test). If compression of the jugular vein causes swelling of the veins of the face and retina, it indicates obstruction of the opposite jugular vein or its transverse sinus (Crowe test). Neither of these tests is entirely reliable because anatomic anomalies of the large veins are frequent. Also, some danger attaches to compression of the jugular vein in the face of increased intracranial pressure. For these reasons, one usually resorts to jugular venography as the definitive diagnostic procedure. When the intracranial pressure is greatly elevated, the suspicion of cerebellar abscess is raised, but this process is usually characterized by other neurologic signs—especially nystagmus to the side of the

lesion, and ipsilateral ataxia of the arm and leg. CT and MR scans will exclude abscess and hydrocephalus.

Cavernous Sinus Thrombophlebitis This condition is usually secondary to infections of the ethmoid, sphenoid, or maxillary sinuses or the skin around the eyes and nose. Occasionally, no antecedent infection can be recognized. In addition to headache, high fluctuating fever, and signs of toxemia, there are characteristic local effects. Obstruction of the ophthalmic veins leads to chemosis, proptosis, and edema of the ipsilateral eyelids, the forehead, and the nose. The retinal veins become engorged and this may be followed by retinal hemorrhages and papilledema. Involvement of the third, fourth, sixth, and ophthalmic division of the fifth cranial nerves, which lie in the lateral wall of the cavernous sinus, leads to ptosis, varying degrees of ocular palsy, and pain and sensory loss around the eye and in the forehead. Within a few days, spread through the circular sinus to the opposite cavernous sinus results in bilateral symptoms. The posterior part of the cavernous sinus may be infected via the superior and inferior petrosal veins without the occurrence of orbital edema or ophthalmoplegia. The CSF is usually normal unless there is an associated meningitis or subdural empyema. The only effective therapy in the fulminant variety, associated with thrombosis of the anterior portion of the sinus, has been antimicrobial therapy aimed at coagulase-positive staphylococci, and occasionally gram-negative pathogens as well. Anticoagulants have been used occasionally, but their value has not been proved. Cavernous sinus thrombosis must be differentiated from mucormycosis and orbital cellulitis, which usually occur in uncontrolled diabetics (described later in this chapter), other fungus infections (aspergillus), carcinomatous invasion of the sphenoid bone, and sphenoid wing meningioma.

Thrombophlebitis of the Superior Longitudinal Sinus Occasionally this may be asymptomatic, but more often there is a clinical syndrome of unilateral convulsions and hemiplegia, first on one side of the body, then on the other, due to extension of the thrombophlebitis into the superior cerebral veins. Because of the localization of function in the cortex that is drained by the sinus, the paralysis takes the form of a crural monoplegia, or, less often, of a paraplegia. A cortical sensory loss may occur in the same distribution. Homonymous hemianopia or quadrantanopia, aphasia, paralysis of conjugate gaze, and urinary incontinence (in bilateral cases) have also been observed. Headache, papilledema, and increased intracranial pressure may accompany these signs. The diagnosis can be corroborated by direct jugular venography or by demonstrating a failure of the superior sagittal sinus to fill during the late venous phase of the carotid arteriogram. Treatment consists of large doses of antibiotics and temporization until the thrombus recanalizes. Recovery from paralysis may be complete, or the patient may be left with seizures and varying degrees of spasticity in the legs.

It should be reiterated that all types of thrombophlebitis, especially those related to ear and paranasal sinus infection, may be associated with other forms of intracranial suppuration, namely bacterial meningitis, subdural empyema, or brain abscess. Therapy in these complicated forms of infection must be individualized. As a rule, the best plan is to institute antibiotic treatment of the intracranial disease and to decide, after it has been brought under control, whether surgery on the offending ear or sinus is necessary. To operate on the primary focus before medical treatment has taken hold is to court disaster. In cases complicated by bacterial meningitis, treatment of the latter usually takes precedence over the surgical treatment of complications, such as brain abscess and subdural empyema.

Aseptic Thrombosis of Intracranial Venous Sinuses This may develop after sinus and ear infections, and may lead to an obscure increase in intracranial pressure because of the occlusion of the superior sagittal or a lateral sinus. The most common type occurs in children and adolescents with otitis media. The symptoms include headache, vomiting, papilledema, and bilateral sixth nerve palsies. There is no fever; there are no signs of toxemia; CSF is normal except for raised pressure. Symonds referred to this condition as "otitic hydrocephalus," but pointed out later that hydrocephalus is a misnomer, as there is no dilatation of the ventricles. Conditions that predispose to aseptic thrombosis are postpartum and postoperative states, which are often characterized by thrombocytosis and hyperfibrinogenemia; congenital heart disease and marasmus in infants; sickle-cell disease; and primary or secondary polycythemia. The diagnosis of aseptic venous or sinus thrombosis in the absence of one of these conditions usually proves to be incorrect.

BRAIN ABSCESS

Pathogenesis With the exception of a small proportion of cases (about 10 percent) in which infection may be introduced from the outside (compound fractures of the skull, intracranial operations), brain abscess is always

secondary to a focus of suppuration elsewhere in the body. Approximately 40 percent of all brain abscesses are secondary to disease of the paranasal sinuses, middle ear, and mastoid cells. Of those originating in the ear, about one-third lie in the anterolateral part of the cerebellar hemisphere, and the remainder lie in the middle and inferior parts of the temporal lobe, above the tegmen tympani. The sinuses most frequently implicated are the frontal and sphenoid, and the abscesses derived from them are in the frontal and temporal lobes, respectively. Suppurative pulmonary infections (abscess, bronchiectasis) account for a considerable number of brain abscesses.

Otogenic and rhinogenic abscesses reach the nervous system in one of two ways. One is by direct extension, in which the bone of the middle ear or nasal sinuses becomes the seat of an osteomyelitis, with subsequent inflammation and penetration of the dura and leptomeninges by infected material, and the creation of a suppurative tract into the brain. Alternately (or concomitantly), infection may spread along the walls of veins. Also, thrombophlebitis of the pial veins and dural sinuses, by infarcting brain tissue, renders the latter more vulnerable to invasion by infectious material. The close anatomic relationship of the lateral (transverse) sinus to the cerebellum explains the frequency with which this portion of the brain is infected via the venous route. The spread along venous channels also explains how an abscess may sometimes form at a considerable distance from the primary focus in the middle ear or paranasal sinuses.

About one-third of all brain abscesses are metastatic, i.e., hematogenous. The majority of these are traceable to a primary septic focus in the lungs or pleura (bronchiectasis, empyema, lung abscess, or bronchopleural fistula). Other metastatic abscesses are traceable to a cardiac abnormality—either infected valves or a congenital defect that permits infected emboli to short-circuit the pulmonary circulation and reach the brain. Occasional cases are associated with infected pelvic organs, skin, tonsils, abscessed teeth, and osteomyelitis of noncranial bones.

In about 20 percent of all cases of brain abscess, the source cannot be ascertained (Murphy et al). Brain abscess is almost never a consequence of bacterial meningitis. Metastatic abscesses are most likely to occur in the distal territory of the middle cerebral arteries, and they are frequently multiple, in contrast to otogenic and rhinogenic abscesses (Fig. 32-1).

A careful distinction should be made between the neuropathologic effects of subacute and acute bacterial endocarditis. *Subacute bacterial endocarditis* (SBE), i.e., the type caused by the implantation of streptococci of low virulence (alpha and gamma streptococci) on valves previously damaged by rheumatic fever, or on a patent ductus arteriosus or ventricular septal defect, seldom if ever gives rise to brain abscess. The cerebral lesions of SBE, which may be the initial clinical manifestations, are due to the embolic occlusion of vessels by fragments of vegetations and bacteria, which cause infarction of brain tissue and a restricted inflammatory response around the involved blood vessels and in the overlying meninges. The CSF contains a moderate number of polymorphonuclear leukocytes and frequently red cells as well, but the glucose content is never lowered and suppuration in the brain or in the subarachnoid space does not occur. It is theorized that the chronicity of the streptococcal infection allows the body to develop an immunity to the organisms. The meningeal pleocytosis is associated with headache, stiff neck, and alterations of consciousness.

In contrast to SBE, the more fulminant, *acute bacterial* (*ulcerative*) *endocarditis*—i.e., the type caused by *Staph. aureus*, hemolytic streptococcus, or the pneumococcus—organisms that may involve previously normal valves—frequently gives rise to multiple small abscesses in the brain (and in other organs of the body). Purulent meningitis may also develop, or there may be infarcts or meningocerebral hemorrhages, secondary to ruptured mycotic aneurysms. Rarely do the miliary abscesses progress to large ones, however. Rapidly evolving cerebral signs in

patients with acute endocarditis (delirium, confusional state, mild focal cerebral signs) are nearly always caused by embolic infarction or hemorrhage.

It is estimated that about 5 percent of cases of congenital heart disease are complicated by brain abscess (Cohen, Newton). In children, more than 60 percent of cerebral abscesses are associated with congenital heart disease (Matson). The abscess is usually solitary; this fact, coupled with the potential correctability of the underlying cardiac abnormality, makes the recognition of brain abscess in congenital heart disease a matter of considerable practical importance. For some unknown reason, brain abscess associated with congenital heart disease is rarely seen before the third year of life; infarction of the brain due to thrombosis of arteries or veins is the usual neurologic complication in the first 2 years of life. The tetralogy of Fallot is by far the most common anomaly associated with brain abscess, but the latter may occur with any type of right-to-left shunt which allows venous blood returning to the heart to enter the systemic circulation, without first passing through the

Figure 32-1

A. *Multiple brain abscesses associated with bacterial endocarditis (Staphylococcus aureus) in a 55-year-old man. The large abscess in the left hemisphere shows a characteristic ring enhancement. B. Contrast-enhanced CT scan 4 months after institution of antibiotic treatment. The abscesses have resolved.*

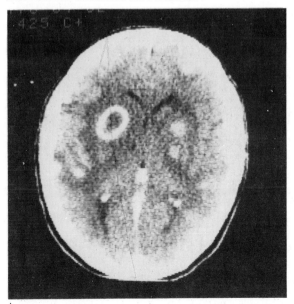

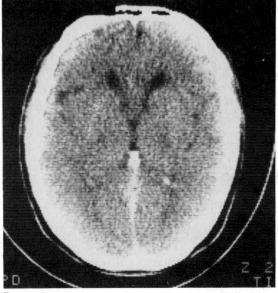

A   B

lungs. A pulmonary arteriovenous malformation, in a patient with familial telangiectasis, has a similar effect. The filtering effect of the lungs is thus prevented, and pyogenic bacteria or infected emboli from a variety of sources may gain access to the brain, where, aided by the effects of venous stasis and perhaps of infarction, an abscess is established. At least this is the current theory of its mechanism.

Etiology The most common organisms causing brain abscess are streptococci, many of which are anaerobic or microaerophilic. These organisms are often found in combination with other anaerobes, notably *Bacteroides* and *Propionibacterium* (diphtheroids), and may be combined with Enterobacteriaceae, such as *E. coli* and *Proteus*. Staphylococci are also a common cause of brain abscess, but pneumococci, meningococci, and *H. influenzae* are rarely so. In addition the gram-positive higher bacteria *Actinomyces* and *Nocardia*, and certain fungi, notably *Candida*, have been isolated in some cases. The bacterial species varies with the source of the abscess; staphylococcal abscesses are usually a consequence of accidental or surgical trauma; enteric organisms are almost always associated with otitic infections; and anaerobic streptococci are commonly metastatic from the lung. An important condition predisposing to nocardial brain abscess is pulmonary nocardial infection associated with alveolar proteinosis. Thus knowledge of the site of the abscess and the antecedent history enables one to start appropriate therapy while awaiting the result of culture.

Pathology Localized inflammatory exudate, septic thrombosis of vessels, and aggregates of degenerating leukocytes represent the early reaction to bacterial invasion of the brain. Surrounding the necrotic tissue is edema and macrophages, astroglia, microglia, and many small veins—some of which show endothelial hyperplasia and contain fibrin and are cuffed with polymorphonuclear leukocytes. At this stage, which is rarely observed postmortem, the necrotic tissue is poorly circumscribed and tends to spread by a coalescence of inflammatory foci. The term *cerebritis* is loosely applied to this local suppurative encephalitis or immature abscess.

Within several days, the intensity of the reaction begins to subside, and the infection tends to become delimited. The center of the abscess takes on the character of pus; at the periphery, fibroblasts proliferate from the adventitia of newly formed blood vessels to form a wall of granulation tissue, which is readily identified within 2 weeks of the onset of the infection. As the abscess becomes more

chronic, the granulation tissue is replaced by collagenous connective tissue. The inner layer of this wall is made up of degenerating neutrophils and fibrin, and the outer layer merges with a zone of altered tissue in which the white matter is edematous and contains lymphocytes and plasma cells, some lying free and others cuffing the vessels, thrombosed small vessels, and small foci of necrosis. Thus, the abscess appears to be delimited and in a reparative phase, but there is still evidence of infection around it. Occlusion of the more peripheral vessels could conceivably result in extension of the abscess toward the satellite necrotic zones. It has also been noted, in both experimental animals and humans, that the capsule of the abscess is not of uniform thickness, frequently being thinner in its deeper portions. All these factors account for the propensity of cerebral abscesses to spread deeply into the white matter, to produce daughter abscesses or a chain of abscesses, extensive cerebral edema, and in some instances to culminate in a catastrophic rupture into the ventricles.

Clinical Manifestations Headache is the most frequent initial symptom of intracranial abscess. Other presenting symptoms, roughly in order of their frequency, are drowsiness and confusion; focal or generalized seizures; and focal motor, sensory, or speech disorders. In patients who harbor chronic ear, sinus, or pulmonary infections, a recent activation of the infection frequently precedes the onset of cerebral symptoms. In patients without an obvious focus of infection, headache or other cerebral symptoms may appear abruptly on a background of mild, general ill health or congenital heart disease. In some patients, bacterial invasion of the brain may be asymptomatic or may be attended only by a transitory focal neurologic disorder, as may happen when a septic embolus lodges in a brain artery. Sometimes stiff neck accompanies generalized headache, suggesting the diagnosis of meningitis (especially a partially treated one).

These early symptoms may improve in response to antimicrobial agents, but within a few days or weeks, recurrent headache, slowness in mentation, focal or generalized convulsions, and obvious signs of increased intracranial pressure provide evidence of an inflammatory mass in the brain. Localizing neurologic signs become evident sooner or later, but like papilledema, they occur relatively late in the course of the illness; as stated above, some patients present with focal neurologic signs.

The nature of the focal neurologic signs will, of course, depend on the location of the abscess. In *temporal lobe abscess,* headache in the early stages is usually on the same side as the abscess and is localized to the frontotemporal region. If the abscess lies in the dominant temporal lobe, there is characteristically an anomic aphasia (page 387). An upper homonymous quadrantanopia may be demonstrable, due to interruption of the inferior portion of the optic radiation; this may be the only sign of abscess of the right temporal lobe. Contralateral motor or sensory defects in the limbs tend to be minimal, though weakness of the lower face is often observed.

In *cerebellar abscess,* headache in the postauricular or suboccipital region is usually the first symptom and may at first be ascribed to the infection in the mastoid cells. Coarse nystagmus, weakness of conjugate gaze to the side of the lesion, and a cerebellar ataxia of the ipsilateral arm and leg are present. The ataxia may be difficult to demonstrate if the patient is very ill. As a general rule, the signs of increased intracranial pressure are more prominent with cerebellar abscesses than with cerebral ones. Mild contralateral or bilateral corticospinal tract signs are evidence of brainstem compression; in the late stages, consciousness becomes impaired and is an ominous sign.

In *frontal lobe abscess,* headache, drowsiness, inattention, and general impairment of mental function are prominent. Hemiparesis with unilateral motor seizures and a motor disorder of speech are the most frequent neurologic signs. An abscess of the *parietal lobe* will give a series of characteristic focal disturbances (page 363). The main manifestation of an *occipital lobe lesion* is a homonymous hemianopia. All of the aforementioned focal signs may be obscured by drowsiness, stupor, and inattentiveness, and one must be persistent in searching for them.

While *fever* is characteristic of the invasive phase of cerebral abscess (suppurative encephalitis), the temperature may return to normal as the abscess becomes encapsulated. The same is true of leukocytosis. In the early stages of abscess formation, the CSF pressure is moderately increased, the cell count ranges from 20 to 300 per cubic millimeter, occasionally higher or lower, with 10 to 80 percent neutrophils, and the protein content is only modestly elevated, rarely more than 100 mg/dL. Glucose values are not lowered and the fluid is sterile, unless there is a concomitant suppurative meningitis. Later, the CSF pressure rises markedly. In a small number of cases there are no spinal fluid abnormalities.

It is apparent from this review of the clinical features that the picture of brain abscess is far from stereotyped. Whereas headache may be the most prominent feature in most patients, seizures or certain focal signs may predominate in others, and a considerable number of patients will present with the signs of increased intracranial pressure. Attempts have been made by some authors to divide the clinical course of brain abscess into three or four distinct stages, with the implication that these follow one another in a predictable sequence. Such a concept does not coincide with our experience. In many instances the symptoms evolve swiftly, new ones being added day by day. In patients with metastatic brain abscesses, the duration of the

illness, from the first symptom to the time of death, is 5 to 14 days in half the cases (Gates et al). In others, the invasive stage of cerebral infection is inconspicuous, and the course is so indolent that the entire clinical picture does not differ from that of brain tumor. Another impressive feature of cerebral abscess is the unpredictability with which the symptoms may evolve, particularly in children. Thus, a patient whose clinical condition seems to have stabilized, may be found, in a matter of hours or a day or two, to be in an advanced or irreversible state of coma.

Diagnosis The diagnosis of brain abscess depends on (1) a demonstrated source of infection in the middle ear, mastoid, sinuses, lungs or heart, or the presence of a right-to-left cardiac shunt; (2) evidence of increased intracranial pressure; (3) focal cerebral or cerebellar signs; and (4) a characteristic CSF reaction in most cases (see above). Lumbar puncture may be dangerous when intracranial pressure is obviously elevated, in which case one depends mainly on the information provided by the CT scan or MRI.

The CT scan is the most important ancillary procedure in the diagnosis of brain abscess. Suppurative encephalitis appears as an area of decreased density and the fully formed abscess appears as a low-density core and a contrast-enhanced regular or irregular capsule (Fig. 32-1). Practically all abscesses larger than 1 cm produce positive scans. There is practically no likelihood of cerebral abscess if the CT and MRI scans are negative.

Plain films of the chest and skull should always be obtained in order to exclude a possible pulmonary or paracranial source of infection. The EEG usually demonstrates a focus of high-voltage slow (delta) activity over a cerebral abscess and may be used to follow its development or regression after therapy. Arteriography has been largely supplanted by scanning procedures.

When the classic clinical picture is present and when the CT scans and other diagnostic procedures corroborate the presence of a mass lesion, the diagnosis is easy. If there is no apparent source of infection and there are only signs and symptoms of a mass lesion, the diagnosis includes glioma, metastatic carcinoma, subdural hematoma, and cerebral hemorrhage. Sometimes only surgical exploration will settle the issue. Once the inflammatory nature of the intracranial mass has been established, brain abscess must be distinguished from subdural empyema and intracranial thrombophlebitis with hemorrhage and infarction of brain (see earlier section in this chapter), herpes simplex encephalitis (page 603), and acute hemorrhagic leukoencephalitis (page 771).

Treatment During the stage of acute suppurative encephalitis, intracranial operation accomplishes little, and probably causes only additional traumatization and swelling of brain tissue and dissemination of the infection. Some cases of acute intracranial suppuration can be cured at this stage by the adequate administration of antibiotics. Even without bacteriologic examination of the intracerebral mass, certain antibiotics can be used—20 to 24 million units of penicillin G and 4 to 6 g chloramphenicol, each drug being given intravenously in divided daily doses. This choice of antimicrobial agents is based on the fact that anaerobic streptococci and *Bacteroides* are the preponderant causative organisms. If there is evidence of staphylococcal infection, adequate amounts of penicillinase-resistant penicillin should be added. The initial elevation of intracranial pressure and threatening temporal lobe or cerebellar herniation should be managed by intravenous injection of mannitol followed by dexamethasone, 6 to 12 mg every 6 h. If improvement does not begin promptly and progress steadily, it becomes necessary to needle the abscess for precise etiologic diagnosis (using Gram stain and culture).

Persistence or progression of high intracranial pressure manifested by deepening stupor and threat of herniation indicates the need for surgical intervention, regardless of the stage of the abscess. Likewise, clear-cut evidence of a mass lesion that is not improving with antimicrobial therapy is an indication for surgery. The usual methods of treatment are aspiration of the abscess or unroofing of the abscess and drainage. If superficial and well capsulated, total excision should be attempted; if deep, aspiration and the injection of antimicrobial agents into the abscess are the only treatment, which may have to be repeated. The combination of antimicrobial therapy and surgery has greatly reduced the mortality from brain abscess. The least satisfactory results are obtained in multiple metastatic abscesses, but even these may respond (see Fig. 32-1). Neurologic residua occur in about 30 percent of surviving patients. Of these, focal epilepsy is one of the most troublesome. Following successful treatment of a cerebral abscess in a patient with congenital heart disease, correction of the cardiac anomaly is indicated to prevent recurrence.

TUBERCULOUS MENINGITIS

In the United States the incidence of tuberculous meningitis, which reflects the incidence of tuberculosis in general (22,000 new cases in 1984), has decreased sharply in recent decades. At the Cleveland Metropolitan General Hospital, for example, the incidence of tuberculous meningitis during the years 1959–1963 was between 4.4 and 8.4 per 10,000 admissions (a decade earlier it was 5.8 to 12.9 per 10,000 admissions). By contrast, at the K. E. M. Hospital in Bombay, during the period 1961 to 1964, the incidence of this disease (in children) was 400 per 10,000 admissions, and similar figures have been reported from other parts of India. In the past two decades there has been a further reduction in the incidence of tuberculosis and tuberculous meningitis. We only see one or two new cases of tuberculous meningitis each year, and lately, practically all of them have been in adults. Nevertheless, in the economically depressed countries, tuberculosis remains a medical problem of very serious proportions.

PATHOGENESIS

Tuberculous meningitis is usually caused by the acid-fast organism *Mycobacterium tuberculosis* and exceptionally by *Mycobacterium bovis*. Rich described two stages in the pathogenesis of the meningitis—first a bacterial seeding of the meninges and subpial regions of the brain with the formation of tubercles, followed by the rupture of one or more of the foci and the discharge of bacteria into the subarachnoid space. The meningitis may occur as a terminal event in cases of miliary tuberculosis or as part of generalized tuberculosis with a single focus (tuberculoma) in the brain.

PATHOLOGIC FINDINGS

Small discrete white tubercles are scattered over the convexities and base of the cerebral hemispheres. The brunt of the pathologic process falls on the basal meninges, where a thick, gelatinous exudate accumulates, obliterating the pontine and interpeduncular cisterns and extending to the meninges around the medulla, the floor of the third ventricle and subthalamic region, the optic chiasm, and the under surfaces of the temporal lobes. By comparison, the convexities are little involved. Microscopically, the meningeal tubercles are like those in other parts of the body, consisting of a central zone of caseation, surrounded by epithelioid cells and some giant cells, lymphocytes, plasma cells, and connective tissue. The exudate is composed of fibrin, lymphocytes, plasma cells, and other mononuclear cells, some polymorphonuclear leukocytes, and areas of caseation necrosis. The ependyma and choroid plexus are studded with minute glistening tubercles. The exudate also surrounds the spinal cord. Unlike the pyogenic meningitides, the inflammatory exudate is not confined to the subarachnoid space but frequently spreads along the pial vessels and invades the underlying brain, so that the process is truly a meningoencephalitis.

Other pathologic changes depend upon the chronicity of the pathologic process and recapitulate the changes that occur in the subacute and chronic forms of the pyogenic meningitides (Table 30-1). Cranial nerves are involved by the inflammatory exudate as they traverse the subarachnoid space. Arteries become inflamed and occluded, with infarction of brain. Blockage of the basal cisterns frequently results in a meningeal obstructive type of hydrocephalus. So-called noncommunicating hydrocephalus, due to marked ependymitis with blocking of the CSF in the aqueduct or fourth ventricle, is a less common occurrence.

CLINICAL FEATURES

Tuberculous meningitis occurs in persons of all ages. Formerly it was more frequent in young children than in other age groups, but now it is more frequent in the adult, at least in the United States. The early manifestations are usually headache (more than one-half the cases), lethargy, confusion, and fever associated with stiff neck (75 percent of cases) and Kernig and Brudzinski signs. In young children and in infants, apathy, hyperirritability, vomiting, and seizures are the usual symptoms, and stiff neck may not be prominent or may be absent altogether.

Characteristically, these symptoms evolve less rapidly in tuberculous than in pyogenic meningitis, usually over a period of a week or two, sometimes longer. Because of the inherent chronicity of the disease, signs of cranial nerve involvement (usually ocular palsies, less often facial palsies or deafness) may be present at the time of admission to the hospital (in 20 percent of the cases). Occasionally the disease may present with a focal neurologic deficit, due to hemorrhagic infarction, or with signs of raised intracranial pressure, and rarely with symptoms referable to the spinal cord and nerve roots.

In most patients with tuberculous meningitis there is evidence of active tuberculosis elsewhere, usually in the lungs, occasionally in bone or kidney. In some patients only inactive pulmonary lesions are found, and in others there is no evidence of tuberculosis outside of the nervous system. In the previously mentioned Cleveland series, which comprised 35 patients, active pulmonary tuberculosis was found in 19, inactive in 6, and involvement of the nervous system alone in 9; only 2 of the 35 patients had nonreactive tuberculin tests (Hinman). Among our adult patients alcohol abuse is common; rather few are immunosuppressed.

The course of the illness, if untreated, is characterized by confusion and progressively deepening stupor and coma, coupled with cranial nerve palsies, pupillary abnormalities, focal neurologic deficits, raised intracranial pressure and decerebrate postures, and an invariably fatal outcome within 4 to 8 weeks of the onset.

LABORATORY STUDIES

Again, the most important is the lumbar puncture, which should be performed before the administration of antibiotics.

The CSF is usually under increased pressure and contains between 50 and 500 white cells per cubic millimeter, rarely more. Early in the disease there may be a more or less equal number of polymorphonuclear leukocytes and lymphocytes, but after several days, lymphocytes predominate. Protein content of the CSF is always elevated, between 100 to 200 mg/dL in most cases, but much higher if CSF blockage occurs around the spinal cord. Glucose is reduced to levels below 40 mg/dL, but rarely to the very low values observed in pyogenic meningitis; the glucose falls slowly and a reduction may only become manifest several days after the patient has been admitted to the hospital. The serum sodium and chloride and CSF chloride are often reduced, in most instances because of inappropriate ADH secretion or tuberculosis of the adrenals.

The demonstration of tubercle bacilli in smears of CSF sediment, stained by the Ziehl-Neelsen method, is a function not only of their number but also of the persistence with which they are sought. There are effective means of culturing the tubercle bacilli; but since their quantity is usually small, attention needs to be paid to proper technique. The amount of CSF submitted to the laboratory is critical; the more that is cultured, the greater the chances of recovering the organism. Usually growth in culture media is not recognized for 3 to 4 weeks. For this reason, if a presumptive diagnosis of tuberculous meningitis has been made, and cryptococcosis and other fungal infections and meningeal neoplasia can be excluded, treatment should be instituted immediately, without waiting for the results of bacteriologic study.

Other diagnostic procedures (CT scans, MRI, arteriography) may be necessary in patients who present with or develop raised intracranial pressure, hydrocephalus, or focal neurologic deficits. The CT scan will demonstrate hydrocephalus. As mentioned earlier this is usually of the meningeal obstructive variety in which case infusion of contrast material may show an enhancement pattern in the basal cisterns, subpial cortex, and subependymal regions, findings that suggest a CSF block at or below the tentorium. One or more tuberculomas may also be visualized. Angiography may demonstrate major vascular occlusive disease.

OTHER FORMS OF CNS TUBERCULOSIS

Tuberculous serous meningitis This condition, which is essentially a self-limited meningitis, is observed with some frequency in countries where tuberculosis is prevalent. The CSF shows a modest pleocytosis in some but not all cases, a normal or elevated protein content, and normal glucose levels. Headache, lethargy, and confusion are present in some cases and there are mild meningeal signs. Lincoln, who was the first to call attention to the syndrome, believed it to be a meningeal reaction to an adjacent tuberculous focus that did not progress to a frank meningitis. This form of meningitis is not always self-limited. In two of our patients who presented with a brainstem tuberculoma, there was a serous meningitis that progressed finally to a fatal generalized tuberculous meningitis.

Tuberculomas   These are tumor-like masses of tuberculous granulation tissue which form in the parenchyma of the brain. The larger ones may produce symptoms of a space-occupying lesion, but many are unaccompanied by symptoms of focal cerebral disease. In the United States and other affluent countries, tuberculomas are rarities; but in underdeveloped countries they constitute from 5 to 30 percent of all intracranial mass lesions. Because of their proximity to the meninges, the CSF often contains a small number of lymphocytes and increased protein, but the glucose level is not reduced. Tuberculomas may be multiple.

Myeloradiculitis   The spinal cord may be affected in a number of ways in the course of tuberculous infection. In addition to causing spinal block, the inflammatory meningeal exudate may invade the underlying parenchyma, producing signs of posterior and lateral column and spinal root disease. Spinal cord symptoms may also accompany vertebral caries (Pott's paraplegia) and are then due to compression by an epidural mass of granulation tissue, and, less frequently, to the mechanical effects of angulation of the vertebral column.

TREATMENT

The treatment of tuberculous meningitis consists of the administration of a combination of drugs—isoniazid (INH), rifampin (RMP), and a third drug, which may be ethambutal (EMB), ethionamide (ETA), or pyrazinamide (PZA). All of these drugs have the capacity to penetrate the CNS, with INH, ETA, and PZA ranked higher than the other two in this respect. These drugs need to be given for a prolonged period, 18 to 24 months as a general rule (although it may not be necessary to give all three drugs for the entire period).

INH is the single most effective drug. It can be given in a single daily dose of 5 mg/kg in adults and 10 mg/kg in children. Its most important adverse effects are neuropathy (see page 1043) and hepatitis, particularly in alcoholics. The former can be prevented by the administration of 50 mg pyridoxine daily. In patients who develop the symptoms of hepatitis or abnormal liver function tests, INH should be discontinued. The usual dose of RMP is 600 mg daily for adults, 15 mg/kg for children. EMB is given in a single daily dose of 15 mg/kg. The dosage of ETA is 750 to 1000 mg daily for adults; because of its tendency to produce gastric irritation, it is given in divided doses, after meals. Rarely, this drug causes optic neuropathy, so that patients taking this drug should have regular examinations of visual acuity and red-green color discrimination. PZA is given once daily in doses of 30 to 50 mg/kg. Rash, gastrointestinal disturbances, and hepatitis are the main adverse effects. Except for INH, these drugs can only be given orally or by stomach tube. INH may be given parenterally, in the same dosage as with oral use. *Corticosteroids* should be used only in patients whose lives are threatened by the effects of subarachnoid block, and only in conjunction with antituberculous drugs.

Intracranial tuberculoma calls for a course of chemotherapy, as outlined above. Under the influence of these drugs, the tuberculoma(s) may decrease in size and small ones ultimately disappear or calcify as judged by CT scan; if they do not, and especially if there is "mass effect," excision may be necessary. Patients with Pott's paraplegia, or localized granulomas with spinal cord compression, should also be explored surgically after an initial course of chemotherapy, and an attempt should be made to excise the tuberculous focus.

The overall mortality of patients with CNS tuberculosis is still significant (about 10 percent), infants and the elderly being at greatest risk. Early diagnosis, as one might expect, enhances the chances of survival. In patients who are treated late in the disease, when coma has supervened, the mortality rate is nearly 50 percent. Between 20 and 30 percent of survivors manifest a variety of neurologic sequelae, the most important of which are retarded intellectual development, psychiatric disturbances, recurrent seizures, visual and oculomotor disorders, deafness, and hemiparesis. A detailed account of these has been given by Wasz-Höckert and Donner.

SARCOIDOSIS (Besnier-Boeck-Schaumann Disease)

The infectious etiology of sarcoidosis has never been established, but the disease may suitably be considered at this point because of its close resemblance pathologically and clinically to tuberculosis and other granulomatous infections. The essential lesion in sarcoidosis consists of focal collections of epithelioid cells surrounded by a rim of lymphocytes; frequently there are giant cells, but caseation is lacking. The sarcoid tubercles may be found in all organs and tissues including the nervous system, but the most frequently involved are the mediastinal and peripheral lymph nodes, lungs, liver, skin, phalangeal bones, eyes, and parotid glands.

Sarcoidosis is accompanied by nervous system involvement in approximately 5 percent of cases, according to the worldwide surveys of Delaney and of Siltzbach et al. It may take any one of several forms. As indicated on page 1048, isolated sarcoid granulomas may involve peripheral or cranial nerves, giving rise to a subacute or chronic neuropathy of asymmetric type (Jefferson). Polyneuropathy may occur, but is rare. Of the cranial nerves, the facial is the most frequently involved, usually as part of the uveoparotid syndrome. Central nervous system sarcoidosis is infrequent; it includes several syndromes due to localized involvement of the meninges, brain, and spinal cord. In Scadding's series of 275 patients, for example, only 3 developed central nervous system (CNS) lesions; in other large series the incidence of CNS involvement was greater [10 of 145 patients studied by Mayock et al (see below)]. Delaney, in a review of the literature, found the overall frequency of neurologic involvement in cases of sarcoidosis to be 5 percent, about equally divided between involvement of the peripheral and central nervous systems.

In the CNS, sarcoidosis takes the form of a granulomatous infiltration of the meninges and underlying parenchyma, most prominent at the base of the brain. The disease process is subacute or chronic in nature, mimicking other granulomatous lesions and neoplasms. Visual disturbances, due to lesions in and around the optic nerves and chiasm, and polydipsia, polyuria, somnolence, or obesity, due to involvement of the pituitary and hypothalamus, are the usual features. Hydrocephalus, seizures, cranial nerve palsies, and corticospinal and cerebellar signs are other common manifestations. In rare cases, the spinal meninges and cord are infiltrated, imparting a picture of adhesive arachnoiditis; in others, focal cerebral signs, including seizures, due presumably to large focal deposits of sarcoid in the brain, are observed. The spinal fluid shows a slight lymphocytic pleocytosis (10 to 200 cells per cubic millimeter, mostly lymphocytes) and moderate increase in protein content and gamma globulin. The glucose content is reduced in some patients. The spinal form may be associated with CSF block.

As to the relative frequency of affection of different parts of the nervous system, Mayock and his associates, in a personal series of 145 cases of sarcoidosis, observed neurologic signs in 23 cases (16 percent); as indicated above, the CNS was involved in 10 cases; in the remainder

the signs were indicative of cranial or peripheral nerve involvement.

The diagnosis of CNS sarcoidosis is made on the basis of the clinical features together with clinical and biopsy evidence of sarcoid granulomas in other tissues (uveal tract, skin, lungs, bones). The contrast-enhanced CT scan is a useful means of detecting meningeal involvement, and MR imaging may disclose periventricular and white matter lesions, although the latter pattern is not specific. Test material for the Kveim reaction is not generally available, although this diagnostic test is still under investigation in several centers. Delayed hypersensitivity skin reactions are frequently depressed. Mild anemia, lymphocytopenia (occasional eosinophilia), elevated sedimentation rate, hyperglobulinemia, and an elevated level of angiotensin-converting enzyme are the common findings in active disease. Differential diagnosis includes epidemic parotitis, leprosy, cryptococcosis, syphilis, and tuberculosis.

Administration of corticosteroids is the only known effective therapy. The major problem is knowing when to treat the patient, because the disease remits spontaneously in about half the cases. The recent onset of neurologic symptoms, indicating an active phase of the disease, is the most certain indication for steroid therapy. Prednisone, in divided daily doses of 40 mg, is given for 2 weeks, followed by 2-week periods in which the dose is reduced by 5 mg until a maintenance dose of 20 to 10 mg is reached. Therapy should be continued for at least 6 months, and in many cases for several years.

NEUROSYPHILIS

The incidence of neurosyphilis, like that of CNS tuberculosis, has declined dramatically in the past three decades. In the United States, for instance, the rate of first admissions to mental hospitals because of neurosyphilis fell from 4.3 per 100,000 population (in 1946) to 0.4 per 100,000 (in 1960). Nevertheless, new cases of neurosyphilis and incompletely treated old ones are still being seen from time to time. The number of reported cases of early syphilis has actually increased in the last decade, mainly because of the high incidence in the homosexual population, so that one may logically anticipate an increase in late syphilis, including neurosyphilis. Recently we have observed a number of AIDS patients with active forms of neurosyphilis.

ETIOLOGY AND PATHOGENESIS

Syphilis is caused by a slender, spiral, motile organism, the *Treponema pallidum*. The biologic characteristics of this organism and the natural history of the disease which it produces are described in *Harrison's Principles of Internal Medicine,* which should be read as an introduction to the following discussion. In this chapter, only some basic facts regarding the neurosyphilitic infection will be considered. These facts have been reasonably well established by clinical and postmortem observation, and without knowledge of them it is not possible to treat patients with syphilis intelligently.

1. *The treponeme usually invades the CNS within 3 to 18 months of inoculation with the organism.* If the nervous system is not involved by the end of the second year, as shown by completely negative CSF, there is only 1 chance in 20 that the patient will develop neurosyphilis as a result of the original infection; and if the CSF is negative at the end of 5 years, the likelihood of developing neurosyphilis falls to 1.0 percent.

2. *The initial event in the neurosyphilitic infection is a meningitis which occurs in about 25 percent of all cases of syphilis.* Usually this meningitis is asymptomatic and can only be discovered by lumbar puncture. Exceptionally, it is more intense and causes cranial nerve palsies, seizures, apoplectic phenomena (due to associated vascular lesions), and symptoms of increased intracranial pressure. As a corollary, the occurrence of these symptoms in a young adult should always suggest the possibility of neurosyphilis and requires examination of the CSF.

3. *This meningitis may persist in an asymptomatic state and ultimately, after a period of years, cause parenchymal damage.* In some cases, however, there may be a natural subsidence of the meningitis—a spontaneous cure.

4. *All forms of neurosyphilis begin as a meningitis, and a more or less active meningeal inflammation is the invariable accompaniment of all forms of neurosyphilis.* The early clinical syndromes are meningitis and meningovascular syphilis; the late ones are vascular syphilis (1 to 12 years) followed by general paresis, tabes dorsalis, optic atrophy, and meningomyelitis. *These latter are pathologic sequences which result from chronic syphilitic meningitis.* These sequences and their interrelationships are illustrated in Fig. 32-2.

The intermediate pathologic stages in the transformation of asymptomatic syphilitic meningitis to the late forms of parenchymal neurosyphilis are unknown. Syphilis is by far the most chronic form of meningitis affecting human beings, and many of the pathologic changes thought to be peculiar to syphilis of the nervous system are simply due to the chronicity of the meningeal reaction. Confirmation

of this view comes from the study of the brain and spinal cord in the more chronic cases of tuberculous and cryptococcal meningitis. Inflammation and thrombosis of subarachnoid arteries, meningoencephalitis, ependymitis, and meningomyelitis, resembling closely the lesions of neurosyphilis, can be found in all these chronic forms of meningitis.

5. From a clinical point of view, *asymptomatic neurosyphilis is the most important form of neurosyphilis.* If all cases of asymptomatic neurosyphilis were discovered and adequately treated, the symptomatic varieties of neurosyphilis could be prevented. Conversely, if not treated or inadequately treated, a certain proportion of patients with asymptomatic neurosyphilis will develop meningovascular syphilis, general paresis, tabes, etc. Since asymptomatic neurosyphilis can be recognized only by the changes in the CSF, it is axiomatic that all patients with late syphilis must have a lumbar puncture and spinal fluid examination.

6. *So-called vascular syphilis is usually, if not always, meningovascular syphilis.* In all types of meningitis—that is, bacterial, fungal, treponemal—it is common to find an inflammatory reaction in the walls of subarachnoid arteries. In the more chronic stages of meningitis, fibrous thickening of the vessel wall occurs with narrowing of the lumen and thrombotic occlusion.

7. Clinical syndromes such as syphilitic meningitis, meningovascular syphilis, general paresis, tabes dorsalis, optic atrophy, and meningomyelitis are abstractions, which at autopsy seldom exist in pure form. Since all of them have a common origin in a meningitis there is usually a combination of two or more syndromes, e.g., meningitis and vascular syphilis, taboparesis, etc. Just why the most intense meningeal reaction and consequent parenchymal damage is in the cerebral hemispheres in one case, and around the optic nerves or spinal cord in another, is not known. Even though the patient's symptoms may have been referable to only one part of the nervous system, postmortem examination usually discloses diffuse changes in both brain and spinal cord, which were of insufficient severity to be detected clinically.

8. *The CSF is a sensitive indicator of the presence of active neurosyphilitic infection.* It reflects the presence of meningeal inflammation. The finding of pleocytosis and an increased total protein in the CSF corresponds to the infiltration of the pia-arachnoid with lymphocytes and plasma cells at autopsy. Occasionally postmortem examination shows a slight to moderate cellular infiltration of the meninges in patients whose CSF during life contained no cells; in such cases the total protein is usually elevated.

The *abnormalities of the CSF which are commonly found in neurosyphilis are* (a) 200 to 300 cells per cubic millimeter, mostly lymphocytes and a few plasma cells and other mononuclear cells, (*b*) elevation of the total protein, from 40 to 200 mg/dL, (*c*) an increase in gamma globulin, and (*d*) positive serologic tests. The glucose content is usually normal.

The serologic diagnosis of syphilis depends on the demonstration of one of two types of antibodies—nonspecific or nontreponemal (reagin) antibodies and specific treponemal antibodies. The common tests for reagin are the Kolmer, which uses a complement fixation technique, and the Venereal Disease Research Laboratory (VDRL) slide test, which uses a flocculation technique. These reagin tests in the CSF, if positive, are diagnostic of neurosyphilis. However, these tests are negative in a significant proportion of patients with late syphilis and in those with neurosyphilis in particular (*seronegative syphilis*). In such patients (and in patients with suspected false positive reagin tests) it is essential to employ tests for specific treponemal antibodies, which are positive in practically every instance of neurosyphilis. The fluorescent treponemal antibody absorption (FTA-ABS) test is the one in common use. The *T. pallidum* immobilization (TPI) test is highly reliable but expensive

and difficult to perform, and for these reasons it is no longer used as a routine laboratory procedure.

The earliest changes in the CSF consist of pleocytosis and an elevation of protein. These may occur in the first few weeks of the infection before the serologic tests become positive. Later, the CSF changes may vary. With either spontaneous or therapeutic remission of the disease, the cells disappear first; next the total protein returns to normal; and then the gamma globulin levels are reduced. The positive serologic tests are the last to revert to normal. Frequently the CSF serology remains positive, despite repeated courses of therapy and the subsidence of all signs of inflammatory activity (see below). The *blood serology* is positive if there is an abnormal CSF, but exceptions to this rule have been recorded.

9. *The CSF is an almost infallible guide, probably even more than the clinical symptomatology, in the diag-*

Figure 32-2

Diagram of the evolution of neurosyphilis.

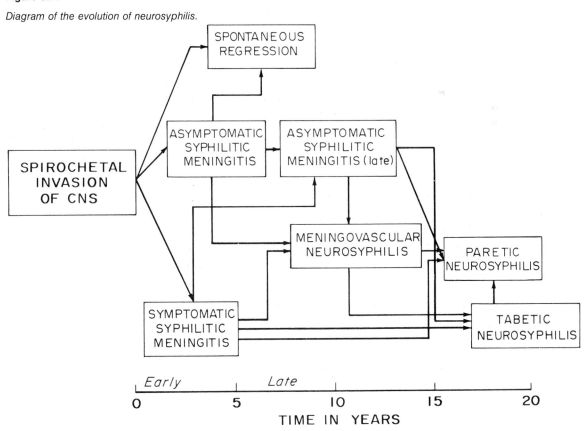

nosis, treatment, and prognosis of the disease. If the CSF is negative in a patient with manifestations of neurosyphilis, it may be safely concluded that the syphilitic inflammation in the nervous system is burned out and that further progression of the disease probably will not occur. In cases with progressive neurologic symptoms and a completely negative CSF, postmortem examination usually discloses a nonsyphilitic neurologic disease. If treatment restores the CSF to normal, particularly the cell count and protein, arrest of the clinical symptoms almost always occurs. A return of cells and elevation of protein precedes or accompanies the clinical relapse.

10. *The clinical syndromes and pathologic reactions of congenital syphilis are similar to those of the acquired forms, differing only in the age at which they occur.* All the aforementioned biologic events are equally applicable to congenital and acquired neurosyphilis (see page 997).

PRINCIPAL TYPES OF NEUROSYPHILIS

Asymptomatic Neurosyphilis In this condition, there are no symptoms or physical signs except, in some cases, abnormal pupils (see page 223). The diagnosis is based entirely on the CSF findings without which the case would be regarded as latent syphilis, or if other viscera are affected, as cardiovascular syphilis, gumma, etc. The abnormality in the CSF varies, as mentioned in paragraph 8 above. Cases coming accidentally to autopsy have shown only lymphocytic, plasma cell, and mononuclear infiltrates of the pia, a sparse granular ependymitis, and slight infiltrations of meningeal vessels.

Meningeal Syphilis Symptoms of meningeal involvement may occur at any time after inoculation, but most often within the first 2 years. The commonest symptoms are headache, stiff neck, cranial nerve palsies, convulsions, and mental confusion. Occasionally the symptoms consist of headache, papilledema, nausea, and vomiting, due to the presence of increased intracranial pressure. The patient is afebrile, unlike the one with tuberculous meningitis. The CSF is always abnormal, often more so than in asymptomatic neurosyphilis. Obviously the meningitis is more intense in this type and may be associated with hydrocephalus. The prognosis, with adequate treatment, is good. The symptoms usually disappear within days to weeks, but if the CSF remains abnormal, it is likely that some other form of neurosyphilis will subsequently develop.

Meningovascular Syphilis This form of neurosyphilis should always be considered when a young person has one or several cerebrovascular accidents, i.e., a sudden development of hemiplegia, aphasia, sensory loss, visual disturbance, or mental confusion. The commonest time of occurrence of meningovascular syphilis is 6 to 7 years after the original infection, but it may be as early as 6 months or as late as 10 to 12 years. The CSF almost always shows some abnormality, usually an increase in cells, protein content, and gamma globulin, as well as a positive serologic test. Patients in middle or late life with stroke and a positive serologic test in the CSF will usually be found at autopsy to have atherothrombotic or embolic infarction, rather than meningovascular syphilis. The changes in the latter disorder consist not only of meningeal infiltrates but also inflammation of arteries as well as productive fibrosis that leads to narrowing and finally occlusion. The vascular lesion was first described by Heubner, hence *Heubner arteritis*. In some cases of vascular syphilis there is a meningoencephalitis as well.

The neurologic signs that remain after 6 months will usually be permanent, but adequate treatment will prevent further apoplectic episodes. If repeated cerebrovascular accidents occur despite adequate therapy, one must always consider the possibility of nonsyphilitic vascular disease of the brain.

Paretic Neurosyphilis (General Paresis, General Paralysis of the Insane, Dementia Paralytica, Syphilitic Meningoencephalitis) The general setting of this form of cerebral syphilis is a long-standing meningitis; as was remarked above, some 15 to 20 years usually separate the onset of paresis from the original infection.

The history of the disease is entwined with some of the major developments of neuropsychiatry. Haslam in 1798 and Esquirol at about the same time first delineated the clinical state. Bayle in 1822 commented on the arachnitis and meningitis, and Calmeil, on the encephalitic lesion. Nissl and Alzheimer added details to the pathologic descriptions. The syphilitic nature of the disease was suspected by Lasègue and others long before Schaudinn's discovery of the spirochete and was finally affirmed by Noguchi in 1913. Kraepelin's monograph, *General Paresis* (1913), is one of the classic reviews (see Merritt et al for these and other historical references).

Once a major cause of insanity, accounting for some 4 to 10 percent of admissions to asylums, general paresis is now a rarity. The discovery of penicillin has provided the means of eradicating the disease. The famous dictum of Krafft-Ebing that general paresis is a product of syphilization and civilization is no longer applicable. Blacks are as susceptible as whites except for the West Indian natives, who are notoriously resistant. Pregnancy appears to protect the female, but the incidence in women who have never been pregnant is nearly the same as in men. Since syphilis is acquired mainly in late adolescence and early adult life, the middle years (30 to 50) are the usual time of onset of the paretic symptoms. Congenital paresis blights early mental development in half the cases, and results in late childhood and adolescent regression in both normal and mentally retarded children.

Symptomatology The clinical picture, in its fully developed form, is one of progressive mental and physical dissolution, and includes dementia, dysarthria, myoclonic jerks, action tremor, seizures, hyperreflexia, Babinski signs, and Argyll-Robertson pupils. However, more importance attaches to diagnosis at an earlier stage when few of these manifestations are conspicuous. The insidious onset of memory defect, impairment of reasoning, and reduction in critical faculties, along with minor oddities of deportment and conduct, irritability, and lack of interest in personal appearance are not too different from the syndrome of dementia already outlined in Chap. 20. One can appreciate how elusive the disease may be, at any one point in its early evolution. Indeed, with the currently low index of suspicion of the disease, diagnosis at this *preparalytic stage* is more often accidental than deliberate.

Classical writings have stressed the development of delusional systems, most dramatically in the direction of megalomania, which are evident to family and friends and not at all to the individual involved. Typically, the patient conceives ambitious schemes to aggrandize a fortune or to enhance social prestige. The delusions are viewed by the patient in an uncritical fashion that obscures their extravagance and worthlessness. When thwarted, the patient may become quarrelsome and obstinate. Another warning of imminent dissolution is an obvious disregard for social conventions and moral standards.

In the authors' experience, flagrant and elaborate delusional systems are altogether exceptional in the early or preparalytic phase. More usual has been a simple dementia with weakening of intellectual capacities, forgetfulness, disorders of speaking and writing, and vague concerns about health. The first hint of a syphilitic encephalitis may be facial quivering, tremulousness of the hands, indistinct hurried speech, myoclonus, and seizures, reminiscent of delirium or acute viral encephalitis. As the deterioration continues into the *paralytic stage,* intellectual function decays completely, and aphasias, agnosias, and apraxias intrude themselves. Wilson (quoting Kraepelin) estimated that two-thirds of the patients at this stage become psychotic, either with expansive-grandiose or depressive-hypochondriacal delusions, and one-third continue with a simple dementia. Even in the past, however, the much-discussed megalomania with its release of boundless energies, extreme

boastfulness, ridiculous claims of supernatural power, of being King, Emperor, or God never appeared in more than 30 percent of the cases.

Physical dissolution progresses concomitantly—poor carriage, debility, muscular hypotonia, unsteadiness, dysarthria, and tremor of the tongue and hands. All these disabilities lead eventually to a bedridden state; hence, the term paretic is quite applicable. Other symptoms are hemiplegia, hemianopia, aphasia, cranial nerve palsies, seizures with prominent focal signs of unilateral frontal or temporal lobe disease, also known as Lissauer's cerebral sclerosis. Normal-pressure hydrocephalus is probably the basis of some of the cerebral symptoms. Agitated, delirious, depressive, and schizoid psychoses were special psychiatric syndromes that could be differentiated from the so-called functional psychoses by the mental decline, the neurologic signs, and the CSF findings.

We have elaborated the neuropsychiatric features of this disease, even though rare nowadays, because they manifest so uniquely a chronic frontotemporoparietal encephalitis and create a picture unlike that of most of the degenerative diseases discussed in Chap. 43. Also it is well to remember that many of our ideas about the brain and the mind were shaped historically by this disease.

The blood serology is positive in nearly all cases. The CSF is invariably abnormal, usually with 10 to 200 lymphocytes, plasma cells, and other mononuclear cells per cubic millimeter, a total protein of 40 to 200 mg/dl, an elevated gamma globulin, and strongly positive serologic tests. The elevated gamma globulin in the CSF is produced intrathecally and has been shown to be absorbed to the *Treponema pallidum* (Vardtal et al). Hence the gamma globulin (oligoclonal IgG) represents a specific antibody response to this organism.

The pathologic changes consist of meningeal thickening, brain atrophy, ventricular enlargement, and granular ependymitis. Microscopically, the perivascular spaces are filled with lymphocytes, plasma cells, and mononuclears; nerve cells have disappeared; there are numerous rod-shaped microgliacytes and plump astrocytes in parts of the cortex devastated by neuronal loss; iron is deposited in mononuclear cells; and with special stains spirochetes are visible in the cortex. The changes are most pronounced in the frontal and temporal lobes. Meningeal fibrosis with obstructive hydrocephalus is probably present in many cases.

The prognosis in early cases is fairly good; 35 to 40 percent will make some occupational readjustment, and the disease will be arrested but leave the patient economically dependent in another 40 to 50 percent. Without treatment there is progressive mental enfeeblement, and death occurs within 3 to 4 years.

Tabetic Neurosyphilis (Tabes Dorsalis) This type of neurosyphilis, described by Duchenne in his classic monograph *L'Ataxie locomotrice progressive* (1858), usually develops 15 to 20 years after the onset of the infection. The major symptoms are lightning pains, ataxia, and urinary incontinence; the chief signs are absent knee and ankle reflexes, impaired vibratory and position sense in feet and legs, and a Romberg sign. The ataxia is due purely to the sensory defect. Muscular power, by contrast, is fully retained in most cases. The pupils are abnormal in over 90 percent of cases, usually Argyll-Robertson in type, and the majority of patients show ptosis or some degree of ophthalmoplegia. Optic atrophy is frequent. The lancinating or lightning pains (present in over 90 percent of cases) are, as their name implies, sharp, stabbing, and brief, like a flash. They are more frequent in the legs than elsewhere, but roam over the body from face to feet, sometimes playing persistently on one spot "like the repeated twanging of a fiddle string," as Wilson remarked. They may come in bouts lasting several hours or days. "Pins and needles" feelings, coldness, numbness, tingling, and other paresthesias are also present and are associated with variable impairment of tactile, pain, and thermal sensation. The bladder is insensitive and hypotonic, resulting in unpredictable overflow incontinence. Constipation and megacolon as well as impotence are other expressions of dysfunction of the sacral roots and cord.

In the established phase of the disease, now seldom seen, ataxia is the most prominent feature. The patient totters and staggers while standing and walking. In mild form it is best seen as the patient tries to walk between obstacles, attempts to walk a straight line, turns suddenly, or halts. To correct the instability the patient places the feet wide apart, flexes the body slightly and repeatedly contracts the extensor muscles of the feet as he or she sways (*la danse des tendons*). In moving forward, the patient flings the leg abruptly in a piece, and the foot strikes the floor with a resounding thump. The patient clatters along in this way with eyes glued to the floor. If vision is blocked, the patient is rendered helpless. When the ataxia is severe, walking becomes impossible despite relatively normal strength of the leg muscles. Trophic lesions, perforating ulcers of feet, and Charcot joints are characteristic complications of the tabetic state.

With regard to Charcot joints, they occur in 1 to 10 percent of tabetics. Most often they affect the hips, knees,

and ankles but sometimes they are seen in the lumbar spine or upper limbs. The process generally begins as an osteoarthritis which, with repeated injury to the insensitive joint, progresses to destruction of the articular surfaces. Osseous architecture disintegrates, with fractures, dislocations, and subluxations, some of which occasion discomfort. We have observed the arthropathy to occur as frequently in the burned-out as in the active phase of tabes; hence it is only indirectly related to the syphilitic process. Although the basic abnormality appears to be repeated injury to an anesthetic joint, the process need not be painless. Presumably a deep and incomplete hypalgesia is enough to interfere with protective mechanisms.

Visceral crises represent another interesting manifestation of this disease. The gastric ones are the best known. The tabetic is seized abruptly with epigastric pain that spreads around the body or up over the chest. There may be a sense of thoracic constriction, and nausea and vomiting—the latter repeated until nothing but blood-tinged mucus and bile are raised. The symptoms may last for several days; a barium swallow sometimes demonstrates pylorospasm. The attack subsides as quickly as it came, leaving the patient exhausted, with a soreness of the epigastric skin. Intestinal crises with colic and diarrhea, pharyngeal and laryngeal crises with gulping movements and dyspneic attacks, rectal crises with painful tenesmus, and genitourinary crises with strangury and dysuria are all less frequent but well-documented types.

In 5 to 10 percent of cases the CSF is normal when the patient is first examined (so-called burned-out tabes). In the others it is abnormal, but often less so than in general paresis.

Pathologic study reveals a striking thinning and grayness of the posterior roots, principally lumbosacral, and a thinness of the spinal cord due mainly to the degeneration of the posterior columns. Only a slight outfall of neurons is observed in the dorsal root ganglia, and the peripheral nerves are essentially normal. For many years there was an argument as to whether the spirochete first attacked the posterior columns of the spinal cord (Spielmeyer), or the posterior root as it pierced the pia (Obersteiner and Redlich), or the more distal part of the radicular nerve where it acquires its arachnoid and dural sheaths (Nageotte), or the dorsal root ganglion cell. Our observations of rare "active cases" have shown the inflammation to be all along the root, and the dorsal ganglion cell loss and posterior column degeneration to be secondary.

The hypotonia, areflexia, and ataxia relate to destruction of proprioceptive fibers in the sensory roots, and the ataxia is also purely sensory. The hypotonia and insensitivity of the bladder are due to deafferentation at S2 and S3 levels, and the same is true of the impotence and obstipation. Lightning pains and visceral crises cannot be fully explained but are probably attributable to incomplete posterior root lesions at different levels. Analgesia and joint insensitivity relate to the partial loss of A-δ and C fibers in the roots.

If the CSF is negative and there is no evidence of cardiovascular or other types of syphilis, no further antisyphilitic treatment is necessary. If positive, the patient should be treated with penicillin as described below. Residual symptoms in the form of lightning pains, gastric crises, Charcot joints, or urinary incontinence frequently continue long after all signs of active neurosyphilitic infection have disappeared. These should be treated symptomatically rather than by antisyphilitic drugs (see below under "Treatment").

Syphilitic Optic Atrophy   This takes the form of progressive blindness beginning in one eye and then involving the other. The usual finding is a constriction of the visual fields but scotomata may occur in rare cases. The optic discs are gray-white. Other forms of neurosyphilis, particularly tabes dorsalis, not infrequently coexist. The CSF is almost invariably positive though the degree of abnormality may be slight in some cases. The prognosis is poor if vision in both eyes is greatly reduced. If only one eye is badly affected, sight in the other eye can usually be saved. In exceptional cases visual impairment may progress, even after the CSF becomes negative. The pathologic changes consist of a perioptic meningitis with subpial gliosis and fibrosis replacing degenerated optic nerve fibers. Exceptionally there are vascular lesions with infarction of central parts of the nerve.

Spinal Syphilis   There are several types of spinal syphilis other than tabes. Two of them, syphilitic meningomyelitis (sometimes called Erb's spastic paraplegia, because of the predominance of bilateral corticospinal tract signs) and spinal meningovascular syphilis, are observed from time to time, though less often than tabes. Spinal meningovascular syphilis may occasionally take the form of an anterior spinal artery syndrome. In meningomyelitis there occurs a subpial loss of myelinated fibers and gliosis, as a direct result of the chronic fibrosing meningitis. Gumma of the spinal meninges and cord also occurs, but is rare. Progressive muscular atrophy (syphilitic amyotrophy) is a very rare disease of questionable syphilitic etiology. The same is true of syphilitic hypertrophic pachymeningitis or arachnoiditis, which allegedly gives rise to radicular pain and amyotrophy of the hands, and signs of long tract involvement in the legs (syphilitic amyotrophy with spastic-ataxic paraparesis). In all these syndromes there is an abnormal CSF, unless of course the neurosyphilitic infection is burned out.

The prognosis in spinal neurosyphilis is uncertain. There is improvement or at least an arrest of the disease process in most instances, though a few may progress

slightly after the treatment is begun. A steady advance of the disease in the face of a negative CSF usually means that the original diagnosis was incorrect and that the patient suffers from some other disease, e.g., a spinal form of multiple sclerosis.

Syphilitic Nerve Deafness   This may occur in either early or late syphilitic meningitis and may be combined with other syphilitic syndromes. We have had little experience with this disorder.

TREATMENT

Penicillin is the drug of choice for all varieties of neurosyphilis, both asymptomatic and symptomatic. The dosage recommended by the United States Public Health Service is 6.0 to 9.0 million units, either as benzathine penicillin G (3.0 million units at intervals of 7 days) or crystalline penicillin G (600,000 units daily for 15 days). However, there is considerable uncertainty about these recommendations. Several reports have documented the failure of benzanthine penicillin G to cure neurosyphilis, and the adequacy of the above-mentioned dosages has been questioned. For these reasons the authors favor the use of crystalline penicillin G, given intravenously in much higher dosage—18 to 24 million units daily (3 to 4 million units every 4 h) for 14 days. Erythromycin and tetracycline, in doses of 0.5 g every 6 h for 20 to 30 days, are suitable substitutes in patients who are sensitive to penicillin. The so-called Jarisch-Herxheimer reaction, which occurs after the first dose of penicillin and is a matter of concern in the treatment of primary syphilis, is usually of little consequence in neurosyphilis; it consists usually of no more than a mild temperature elevation and leukocytosis.

Certain symptoms of neurosyphilis, especially tabetic neurosyphilis, are unpredictable and often little influenced by treatment with penicillin and require other measures. Lightning pains may respond to phenytoin or to carbamazepine. Analgesics may be helpful, but opiates must be avoided. Neuropathic (Charcot) joints require bracing or fusion. Atropine and phenothiazine derivatives are said to be useful in the treatment of visceral crises.

In all forms of neurosyphilis, the patient should be re-examined every 3 months and the CSF should be retested after a 6-month interval. If after 6 months the patient is free of symptoms and the CSF abnormalities have been reversed (disappearance of cells, reduction in protein, gamma globulin, and serology titers), no further treatment is indicated. Further follow-up should include another clinical examination at 9 and 12 months and another lumbar puncture at the end of a year. Satisfactory progress is judged by absence of symptoms and further improvement in the CSF. These procedures should be repeated every 6 months until the CSF becomes completely negative. In the opinion of most syphilologists, a persistent weakly positive serologic (VDRL) test after the cells and protein levels have returned to normal does not constitute an indication for further treatment. According to the Dattner-Thomas concept of neurosyphilitic activity, such a CSF assures that the disease is quiescent or arrested. Others are not convinced of the reliability of this concept and prefer to give more penicillin. If at the end of 6 months there are still an increased number of cells and an elevated protein in the fluid, another full course of penicillin should be given. Clinical relapse is almost invariably attended by recurrence of cells and increase in protein levels. Rapid clinical progression in the face of a negative CSF suggests the presence of a nonsyphilitic disease of the brain or cord.

Finally it may be said that the neurologist finds the various forms of neurosyphilis of more theoretical than practical importance. No other disease portrays more vividly the effects of a chronic, continuously active cerebrospinal meningitis on the entire neuraxis.

OTHER SPIROCHETAL DISEASES (LYME DISEASE AND ERYTHEMA CHRONICUM MIGRANS)

Until comparatively recent times the nonvenereal treponematoses were of little interest to neurologists of the western world. Yaws, pinta, and endemic syphilis rarely if ever affected the nervous system. Leptospirosis was essentially an acute liver disease with only one variant causing a nonicteric lymphocytic meningitis; and tick- and louse-borne relapsing fevers were medical curiosities that did not involve neurologists.

However, in the last few years, a tick-borne multisystem disease with prominent neurologic features cropped up in western Europe, under the name of erythema chronicum migrans (ECM), and in the eastern United States, as Lyme disease, named after the Connecticut town where it was first recognized. The identity of the two diseases has been established as well as their close relationship to relapsing fever—a disease that is also caused by spirochetes of the genus *Borrelia* and is also transmitted by ticks and lice. The entire group is now classed as the borrelioses.

All these spirochetoses induce in humans a chronic illness, which, like syphilis, evolves in stages, with early

spirochetemia, vascular damage in many organs, and a high level of neurotropism. Also, as in syphilis, the nervous system is invaded early in the form of an asymptomatic meningitis. Later on manifest neurologic abnormalities appear, but only in a proportion of such cases. As with syphilis, the neurologic complications are mainly derivations of chronic meningitis; unlike syphilis, peripheral nerves may be implicated. Immune factors may be important in the termination of the latent periods and the development of the neurologic syndromes.

Lyme disease is less acute than leptospirosis (Weil disease) and less chronic than syphilis. It successively involves the skin, the nervous system, the heart, and articular structures over a period of a year and then burns out. The infective organism is the spirochete *Borrelia burgdorferi*, and the vectors in the United States are the common ixodid ticks. Antibodies from humans with Lyme disease cross-react with those from ticks. The precise roles of the infecting spirochete, the antibodies it induces, and other features of the human host response in the production of clinical symptoms and signs are not fully understood.

In Europe and the United States, the skin lesion at the site of a tick bite is the initial manifestation, occurring within 30 days of exposure. It is a solitary enlarging ring-like erythematous lesion that may be surrounded by satellites or undergo wider dissemination. There are associated influenza-like symptoms. Weeks to months later neurologic or cardiac symptoms appear in 15 and 8 percent of the cases, respectively. Still later arthritis or, more precisely, synovitis, develops in about two-thirds of the cases. None of the infected patients have died, so little is known of the pathology, but a long period of disability is to be expected if the disease is not recognized and treated. Diagnosis is not difficult during the summer and autumn seasons in regions where the disease is endemic and when all the clinical manifestations are present. But in many cases the skin lesion is forgotten, or there were only a few or no secondary ones and the patient is seen in the neurologic phase of the illness. Then diagnosis may be difficult.

The usual pattern of neurologic involvement is in the form of a fluctuating meningoencephalitis with cranial or peripheral neuritis, enduring for months (Reik). By the time the neurologic disturbances appear the systemic symptoms and skin lesions have long since vanished. The cardiac disorder takes the form of myocarditis, a pericarditis, or an atrioventricular block.

The nervous system affection, consisting of headache, stiff neck, nausea and vomiting, malaise and chronic fatigue and fluctuating over a period of weeks to months, is rather nonspecific. These symptoms relate to meningitis. There is a CSF lymphocytosis with cell counts as high as 3000/mL and protein levels up to 400 mg/dL. Usually the glucose level is normal. Somnolence, irritability, faulty memory, depressed mood, and behavioral changes have been interpreted as marks of encephalitis but are difficult to separate from the effects of meningitis. Seizures, choreic movements, cerebellar ataxia, and dementia are recorded. A myelitic syndrome, causing quadriparesis, is also documented. In about half the cases, cranial neuropathies become manifest; the most frequent is facial palsy but combinations of all the others including the optic nerve have been observed, usually in association with meningitis. One-third to one-half of the patients with meningitis have multiple radicular or peripheral nerve lesions in various combinations (Finkel).

Laboratory tests are of help. The most valuable are the indirect immunofluorescence assay and the enzyme-linked immunosorbent assay (ELISA); they are positive in about 50 percent of patients in the early stage of Lyme disease and in 100 percent of those in the later stage. False-positive tests do occur, in some of the conditions that react to syphilitic reagin. *B. burgdorferi*–specific antibodies can be demonstrated in the CSF.

The recommended treatment in the first stage of the disease is oral penicillin, tetracycline, or erythromycin. CNS cardiac and arthritic disease can thereby be prevented. Once the meninges are implicated, high-dose penicillin, 20 million units daily for 10 days, must be given intravenously. Prednisone is said also to be beneficial. Tetracycline, 500 mg four times a day for 30 days, is recommended by Reik. For late abnormalities no treatment has proved to be effective. Most of the symptoms tend to regress regardless of the type of treatment given.

FUNGAL INFECTIONS OF THE NERVOUS SYSTEM

Fungal infections of the CNS are much less common than bacterial ones, although their pathologic and clinical effects are not unalike. Fungi may give rise to meningitis and meningoencephalitis, intracranial thrombophlebitis, brain abscess, and rarely mycotic aneurysms. A large number of fungal diseases may involve the nervous system, but only a few do so with any regularity. Of 57 cases studied by Walsh et al, there were 27 cases of candidiasis, 16 of aspergillosis, and 14 of cryptococcosis. Mucormycosis and coccidioidomycosis are less frequent, and blastomycosis and actinomycosis occur in isolated instances.

GENERAL FEATURES

Fungal infections of the CNS may arise without obvious predisposing cause (community-acquired), but frequently they complicate some other disease process, such as organ transplantation, leukemia, lymphoma or other malignancy, diabetes, collagen vascular disease, prolonged corticosteroid therapy (often hosptial-acquired). The mechanisms that are operative in the latter situation are not fully understood, but the most obvious factors are interference with the body's normal flora and impaired immunologic responses. Thus fungal infections tend to occur in patients with leukopenia or insufficient antibodies, particularly in those being treated for prolonged periods with antibiotics, corticosteroids, and other immunosuppressant drugs, cytotoxic agents, and antimetabolites. Infections that are related to impairment of the body's protective mechanisms are referred to as *opportunistic*, and include not only fungal infections, but those due to certain bacteria (*Pseudomonas* and other gram-negative organisms, *Listeria monocytogenes*), *viruses* (*cytomegalovirus*, *H. simplex*, varicella-zoster, and HIV), and protozoa (*Toxoplasma*). It follows that these types of infection should always be considered and sought in the aforementioned clinical situations.

Fungal meningitis develops insidiously as a rule, over a period of several days or weeks, like tuberculous meningitis, and the symptoms and signs are also much the same. Involvement of several cranial nerves, arteritis with thrombosis and infarction of brain, multiple cortical and subcortical microabscesses, and communicating or obstructive hydrocephalus frequently complicate the course of fungal meningitis, as they do all chronic meningitides. Often the patient is afebrile.

The spinal fluid changes in fungal meningitis are also like those of tuberculous meningitis. Pressure is elevated to a varying extent, pleocytosis is moderate, usually less than 1000 cells per cubic millimeter, and lymphocytes predominate. Exceptionally, in acute cases, more than 1000 cells per cubic millimeter and a predominant polymorphonuclear response are observed. Glucose is subnormal, and protein is elevated—sometimes to very high levels.

Specific diagnosis can best be made from smears of the CSF sediment and from cultures, and also by demonstrating specific antigens by immunodiffusion, latex particle aggregation, or comparable antigen-recognition tests. The CSF examination should also include a search for tubercle bacilli and abnormal white cells, because of the frequent concurrence of fungal infection and tuberculosis, leukemia, or lymphoma.

Some of the special features of the more common fungal infections are indicated below.

CRYPTOCOCCOSIS (TORULOSIS, EUROPEAN BLASTOMYCOSIS)

Cryptococcosis (formerly called *torulosis*) is one of the most frequent fungal infections of the CNS. The cryptococcus is a common soil fungus, found in the roosting sites of birds, especially pigeons. Usually the respiratory tract is the portal of entry, less often skin and mucous membranes. The pathologic changes are those of a granulomatous meningitis; in addition, there may be small granulomas and cysts within the cerebral cortex, and sometimes large granulomas and cystic nodules form deep in the brain. The cortical cysts contain a gelatinous material and large numbers of organisms; the solid granulomatous nodules are composed of fibroblasts, giant cells, aggregates of organisms, and areas of necrosis.

Cryptococcus meningitis has a number of distinctive clinical features as well. Most cases are acquired outside of the hospital and evolve subacutely, like other fungal infections or tuberculosis. The disease may be fatal within a few weeks if untreated. In the majority of patients early complaints are headache, nausea, and vomiting; mental changes are present in about half of them. In other cases, however, headaches, fever, and stiff neck are lacking altogether, and the patient presents with symptoms of gradually increasing intracranial pressure due to hydrocephalus (papilledema is present in half) or with a confusional state, dementia, cerebellar ataxia, or spastic paraparesis, usually without other focal neurologic deficit. Cranial nerve palsies are infrequent findings. Rarely, a granulomatous lesion forms in one part of the brain, and the only clue to the etiology of the cerebral tumor is a lung lesion and CSF abnormality. Meningovascular lesions, presenting as strokes, may be superimposed on the clinical picture. As a rule, the course is steadily progressive over a period of several weeks or months, but in a few patients it may be remarkably indolent, lasting for years, during which there may be periods of clinical improvement and normalization of the CSF. Lymphoma, Hodgkin disease, leukemia, carcinoma, tuberculosis, and other debilitating diseases that alter the immune responses are predisposing factors in as many as half the patients.

The principal diseases to be considered in differential diagnosis are tuberculous meningitis (distinguished by fever, pulmonary lesions, low serum sodium due to inappropriate secretion of ADH, and organisms in CSF); granulomatous cerebral vasculitis (normal glucose values in CSF); multifocal leukoencephalopathy (negative CSF); unidentifiable forms of viral meningoencephalitis (normal CSF glucose values); and lymphomatosis or carcinomatosis of meninges (neoplastic cells in CSF).

Specific diagnosis depends upon finding *Cryptococcus neoformans* in the CSF. These are spherical cells, 5 to 15 μm in diameter, which retain the Gram stain and are surrounded by a thick refractile capsule. Large volumes of CSF (20 to 40 ML) may be needed to find the organism. India-ink preparations are distinctive and diagnostic in

experienced hands. The carbon particles fail to penetrate the capsule, producing a wide halo around the doubly refractile wall of the yeast. In the patients reviewed by Stockstill and Kauffman; the India-ink preparations were positive in 9 of 16 cases. In most cases the organisms grow readily in Sabouraud glucose agar at room temperature and at 37C, but in some cases they cannot be identified by smear or culture, and the only evidence for infection is a positive latex agglutination test for the cryptococcal polysaccharide antigen in the CSF. The latter test, if negative, excludes cryptococcus meningitis with a 95 percent reliability.

Treatment This consists of the intravenous administration of amphotericin B, beginning with 5 mg daily, and increasing this dose by increments to 1.0 mg/kg, at which point the drug may be given every second day, to a total of 2.0 to 3.0 g. An alternate method, and the one we advocate, is to give the full dosage of amphotericin after just a single test dose of 5 mg. The intrathecal administration of the drug, in addition to the intravenous route, is not essential. Renal tubular acidosis frequently complicates amphotericin B therapy. Administration of the drug should be discontinued if the blood urea nitrogen reaches 40 mg/dL, and resumed when it approaches normal levels. Mortality rate, even in the absence of other disease, is about 40 percent. A recent prospective collaborative study has shown that the addition of flucytosine (150 mg/kg daily) to amphotericin B results in fewer failures or relapses, more rapid sterilization of the CSF, and less nephrotoxicity than the use of amphotericin B alone (Bennett et al).

MUCORMYCOSIS (ZYGOMYCOSIS, PHYCOMYCOSIS)

This is a malignant infection of cerebral vessels with one of the *Mucorales*. It occurs as a rare complication of diabetic acidosis, in drug addicts, and in patients with leukemia and lymphoma, particularly those treated with corticosteroids and cytotoxic agents.

The cerebral infection begins in the nasal turbinates and paranasal sinuses, spreads from there along infected vessels to the retro-orbital tissues (where it results in proptosis, ophthalmoplegia, and edema of the lids and retina), and then to the brain, causing hemorrhagic infarction at various sites. Numerous hyphae are present within the thrombi and vessel wall, often extending into the surrounding parenchyma. Usually the cerebral form of mucormycosis is rapidly fatal. Rapid correction of hyperglycemia and acidosis, and treatment with amphotericin B have resulted in recovery in some patients.

CANDIDIASIS (MONILIASIS)

Candidiasis is probably the most frequent type of opportunistic fungus infection. The commonest antecedents of candida sepsis are severe burns and total parenteral nutrition, particularly in children. Urine, blood, skin, and particularly the heart (myocardium and valves) and lungs (alveolar proteinosis) are the usual sites of primary infection. Lipton and his colleagues, who reviewed 2631 autopsy records at the Peter Bent Brigham Hospital (1973 to 1980), found evidence of candida infection in 28 cases and in half of the latter the CNS was infected. The CNS infections took the form of scattered intraparenchymal microabscesses, noncaseating granulomas, large abscesses, and meningitis and ependymitis, in that order of frequency. In most of their cases, the diagnosis had not been made during life, possibly because of the difficulty of obtaining the organism from the CSF. Even with treatment (intravenous amphotericin B) the prognosis is extremely grave. No special features distinguish this fungal infection from others; meningitis, meningoencephalitis and cerebral abscess, usually multiple, are the modes of clinical presentation. Diagnosis depends on identification of the specific organism in the CSF.

ASPERGILLOSIS

In most instances, this fungal infection has presented as a chronic sinusitis (particularly sphenoidal) with osteomyelitis at the base of the skull, or as a complication of otitis and mastoiditis. Cranial nerves adjacent to the infected bone or sinus may be involved. We have also observed brain abscesses and cranial and spinal dural granulomas. It does not present as a meningitis. In some cases the infection is acquired in the hospital, and an antecedent may be a pulmonary infection that is unresponsive to antibiotics. Diagnosis is often made by seeing the organism in a biopsy specimen or culturing it. Also, specific antibodies are detectable. Amphotericin B, in combination with 5-fluorocytosine and imidazole drugs, is of questionable value. If given after surgical removal of the infected material, a few patients recover.

COCCIDIOIDOMYCOSIS

This is a common infection in the southwestern United States. Usually it causes only a benign, influenza-like illness with pulmonary infiltrates that mimic those of nonbacterial pneumonia, but in a few individuals (0.05 to 0.2 percent) it progresses to the disseminated form of the disease, of which meningitis may be a part. The pathologic reactions in the meninges and CSF and the clinical features are very much like those of tuberculous meningitis. *Coccidioides immitis* is recovered with difficulty from the CSF, but readily from the lungs, lymph nodes, and ulcerating skin lesions.

Treatment consists of the intravenous administration of amphotericin B, coupled with a device implanted into the lateral ventricle which permits injection of the drug for a period of years (Ommaya reservoir). Even with the most diligent treatment, only about half the patients with meningeal infections survive.

A similar type of meningitis may occasionally complicate *histoplasmosis, blastomycosis,* and *actinomycosis.* None of these chronic meningitides possesses any specific features. Patients with chronic meningitis in whom no cause can be discovered should have their CSF tested for antibodies to *Sporothrix schenkii,* an uncommon fungus that is difficult to culture. Several even rarer fungi that need to be considered in the diagnosis of chronic meningitis have recently been discussed by Swartz. Penicillin is the drug of choice in actinomycosis and amphotericin B in the others.

INFECTIONS CAUSED BY RICKETTSIAS, PROTOZOA, AND WORMS

RICKETTSIAL DISEASES

Rickettsias are obligate intracellular parasites that appear microscopically as pleomorphic coccobacilli. They are maintained in nature by a cycle involving an animal reservoir, an insect vector (lice, fleas, mites, and ticks), and humans. Epidemic typhus is an exception, involving only lice and human beings. At the time of the First World War, and before, the rickettsial diseases, typhus in particular, were remarkably prevalent and of the utmost gravity. In eastern Europe, between 1915 and 1922, there were an estimated 30 million cases of typhus, with 3 million deaths. Now the rickettsial diseases are of minor importance, the result of insect control by DDT and other chemicals and the therapeutic effectiveness of broad-spectrum antibiotics. In the United States these diseases are quite rare. About 200 cases of spotted fever (the most common rickettsial disease) occur each year, with a mortality of 5 percent or less. Neurologic manifestations occur in only a small portion of these cases, and neurologists may not encounter a single instance in a lifetime of practice. For this reason, the rickettsial diseases are discussed here only briefly. (A comprehensive account will be found in *Harrison's Principles of Internal Medicine.*)

The following are the major rickettsial diseases:

1. *Epidemic typhus,* small pockets of which are present in many underdeveloped parts of the world. It is transmitted from lice to humans and from person to person.

2. *Murine (endemic) typhus,* which is present in the same areas as Rocky Mountain spotted fever (see below). It is transmitted from rats to humans by rat fleas.

3. *Scrub typhus* or *tsutsugamushi fever*, which is confined to eastern and southeastern Asia. It is transmitted by mites from infected rodents or humans.

4. *Rocky Mountain spotted fever*, first described in Montana, is most common in Long Island, Tennessee, Virginia, North Carolina, and Maryland. It is transmitted by special varieties of ticks.

5. *Q fever*, which has a worldwide distribution (except for the Scandinavian countries and the tropics). It is transmitted in nature by ticks but also by inhalation of dust and handling of materials infected by the causative organism, *Coxiella burnetii*.

With the exception of Q fever, the clinical manifestations and pathologic effects of the rickettsial diseases are much the same, varying only in severity. Typhus may be taken as the prototype. The incubation period varies from 3 to 18 days. The onset is usually abrupt with fever that rises to extreme levels over several days, and with headache and prostration. A macular rash, which resembles that of measles and involves the trunk and extremities, appears on the fourth or fifth febrile day. An important diagnostic sign in scrub typhus is the necrotic ulcer and eschar at the site of attachment of the infected mite. Delirium, followed by progressive stupor and coma, sustained fever, and occasionally focal neurologic signs and optic neuritis, characterize the untreated cases. Stiffness of the neck is noted only rarely, and the CSF may be entirely normal or show only a modest lymphocytic pleocytosis. Q fever, unlike the other rickettsioses, is not associated with an exanthem or agglutinins for the *Proteus* bacteria (Felix-Weil reaction), and the main symptoms are those of a low-grade meningitis. Patients who survive the illness usually recover completely; a few are left with residual neurologic signs.

The rickettsial lesions are scattered diffusely throughout the brain, affecting gray and white matter alike. The changes consist of swelling and proliferation of endothelial cells of small vessels and a microglial reaction, with the formation of microglial or so-called typhus nodules.

Treatment This consists of the administration of chloramphenicol or tetracycline, which are highly effective in all rickettsial diseases. If these drugs are given early, coincident with the appearance of the rash, symptoms abate dramatically and little further therapy is required. Cases that are recognized late in the course of the disease require considerable supportive care, including the administration of corticosteroids, whole-blood transfusions, and intravenous albumin, to overcome the effects of toxemia, anemia, and hypoproteinemia.

AMEBIC MENINGOENCEPHALITIS

This disease is caused by free-living flagellate amebas, usually of the genus *Naegleria*. It is acquired by swimming in ponds or lakes, although a large outbreak in Czechoslovakia followed swimming in a chlorinated indoor swimming pool. Most of the cases in this country have occurred in the southeastern states. In 1978, the Centers for Disease Control recorded 123 cases worldwide with only three survivors.

The onset of the illness is abrupt, with severe headache, fever, nausea and vomiting, and stiff neck. The course of the illness is inexorably progressive—with seizures, increasing stupor and coma and focal neurologic signs—and the outcome is practically always fatal, usually within a week of onset. The reaction in the CSF is like that in acute bacterial meningitis—increased pressure, a large number of polymorphonuclear leukocytes, and an increased protein and decreased glucose content. The diagnosis depends on eliciting a history of swimming in fresh warm water, particularly of swimming underwater for sustained periods, and on finding viable trophozoites in a wet preparation of unspun spinal fluid. Gram stains and ordinary cultures do not reveal the organism.

Autopsy discloses a purulent meningitis and numerous microabscesses in the underlying cortex. Chronic amebic meningoencephalitis is not a recognized disease in humans, although such an instance, due to *Hartmannella rhysodes*, has been reported from Nigeria (Cleland et al). The organism was cultured from the CSF during periods of recurrent seizures and confusion.

Treatment with the usual antiprotozoal agents is ineffective. Because of the in vitro sensitivity of *Naegleria* to amphotericin B, this drug should be used, as for cryptococcal meningitis. With such a regimen, recovery is sometimes possible.

TOXOPLASMOSIS

This disease is caused by *Toxoplasma gondii,* a tiny (2 to 5 μm) obligate intracellular parasite that is readily recognized in Wright- or Giemsa-stained preparations. Infection in humans is either congenital or acquired. Congenital infection is the result of parasitemia in the mother, who happens to be pregnant at the time of her initial (asymptomatic) toxoplasma infection. (Mothers can be assured, therefore, that there is no risk of producing a second infected infant.) Several modes of transmission of the acquired form have been described—the eating of raw beef, contact with cat feces, and the handling of uncooked mutton (in western Europe).

The congenital infection has attracted more attention, because of the severe destructive effects upon the neonatal brain. Signs of active infection—fever, rash, seizures, hepatosplenomegaly—may be present at birth. More often, chorioretinitis, hydrocephalus or microcephaly, cerebral calcification, and psychomotor retardation are the major manifestations. These may become evident soon after birth, or only several weeks or months later. Most infants succumb, others survive with varying degrees of the aforementioned abnormalities.

Although serologic surveys indicate that toxoplasma infection is widespread and frequent (about one-third of American city dwellers have specific antibodies), cases of clinically evident active infection are rare.

In 1975 the medical literature contained only 45 well-documented cases of acquired toxoplasmosis (Townsend et al). It is noteworthy that in half of them there was an underlying systemic disease (malignant neoplasms, renal transplants, collagen vascular disease) that had been treated intensively with immunosuppressive agents. Many cases of acquired toxoplasmosis are now being seen because of its frequent occurrence in patients with AIDS (see Chap. 33). Frequently the neurologic manifestations of toxoplasma are misinterpreted as being related to the disease with which toxoplasmosis is associated and an opportunity for effective therapy is missed.

The clinical picture varies. There may be a fulminating, widely disseminated infection with a rickettsia-like rash, encephalitis, myocarditis, and polymyositis. The neurologic signs may consist only of myoclonus and asterixis, suggesting a metabolic encephalopathy; more often, there are the signs of a meningoencephalitis, i.e., seizures, mental confusion, signs of meningeal irritation, coma, and a lymphocytic pleocytosis and increased protein in the CSF. The brain in such cases shows necrotic lesions with free and encysted *T. gondii,* scattered throughout the white and gray matter. Rarely, large areas of necrosis manifest themselves as one or more mass lesions.

Specific diagnosis depends of the finding of organisms in CSF sediment and occasionally in biopsy specimens of muscle or lymph node. A presumptive diagnosis can be made on the basis of a Sabin-Feldman dye test titer of 1:512 or more, a rise in titer, or a positive IgM indirect fluorescent antibody test. Patients with a presumptive diagnosis should be treated with sulfadiazine (4 g initially, then 2 to 6 g daily) and pyrimethamine (100 to 200 mg initially, then 25 mg daily). Leucovorin, 2 to 10 mg daily, should be given to counteract the antifolate action of pyrimethamine. Treatment should be continued for at least 4 weeks. In patients with AIDS, treatment needs to be lifelong, in order to prevent relapses.

OTHER DISEASES DUE TO PROTOZOA

A number of these are of importance in tropical countries. One is *cerebral malaria,* which complicates about 2 percent of cases of *falciparum malaria;* this is a rapidly fatal disease, characterized by headache, seizures, and coma, and rarely by hemiplegia, aphasia, hemianopia, cerebellar ataxia, and other focal neurologic signs. Capillaries are filled with malarial parasites, and the brain is dotted with small foci of necrosis surrounded by glia (Durck nodes). Usually the neurologic symptoms occur in the second or third week of the infection, but they may occur as the initial manifestation. Children in hyperendemic regions are the ones most susceptible to cerebral malaria. Among the adults only pregnant women and nonimmune individuals who discontinue prophylactic medication are liable to CNS involvement (Toro and Roman). Useful laboratory findings are anemia and parasitized RBCs. The CSF may be under increased pressure and sometimes contains a few white blood cells. The glucose content is normal. With *Plasmodium vivax* infections there may be drowsiness, confusion, and seizures, without invasion of brain by the parasite. Quinine, chloroquine, and related drugs are curative if the cerebral symptoms are not pronounced, but once coma and convulsions supervene, 20 to 30 percent of patients do not survive. Toro and Roman state that the administration of large doses of dexamethasone administered as soon as cerebral symptoms appear, may be life-saving. CSF pressure should be relieved by appropriate measures.

Trypanosomiasis is a common disease in equatorial Africa and in Central and South America. The African type (''sleeping sickness'') is caused by *Trypanosoma brucei* and is transmitted by several species of the tsetse fly. The infection begins with a chancre at the site of inoculation and localized lymphadenopathy. Later, episodes of parasitemia occur, and at some time during this stage of dissemination, usually in the second year of the infection, the trypanosomes give rise to a diffuse meningoencephalitis. The latter expresses itself clinically as a chronic progressive neurologic syndrome, consisting of a vacant facial expression, ptosis and ophthalmoplegia, dysarthria and then muteness, seizures, progressive apathy, stupor, and coma.

The South American variety of trypanosomiasis (Chagas disease) is caused by *Trypanosoma cruzi,* and is transmitted from infected animals to humans by the bite of reduviid bugs. The sequence of local lymphadenopathy, hematogenous dissemination, and chronic meningoencephalitis is like that of African trypanosomiasis.

Treatment is with pentavalent arsenicals, which are more effective in the African form of the disease.

TRICHINOSIS

This disease is caused by the intestinal nematode *Trichinella spiralis.* Infection in humans results from the ingestion of uncooked or undercooked pork (occasionally bear meat) containing the encysted larvae of *T. spiralis*. The larvae are liberated from their cysts by the gastric juices and develop into adult male and female worms in the duodenum and jejunum. After fertilization, the female burrows into the intestinal mucosa, where she deposits several successive batches of larvae. These make their way via the lymphatics, regional lymph nodes, thoracic duct, and blood stream into all parts of the body. The new larvae penetrate all tissues, but survive only in muscle, where they become encysted and eventually calcify. Animals are infected in the same way as humans, and the cycle can be repeated only if a new host ingests the encysted larvae. The most authoritative review of this subject is that of Gould.

The early symptoms of the disease, beginning a day or two after the ingestion of pork, are those of a mild gastroenteritis. These are followed by symptoms attributable to invasion of muscle by larvae. The latter symptoms begin about the end of the first week and may last for 4 to 6 weeks. Low-grade fever, pain and tenderness of muscles, edema of the conjunctivae and eyelids, and fatigue are the usual manifestations. Muscle weakness may be present, and if severe, the tendon reflexes may be lost. The weakness may be generalized or limited to certain groups of muscles, e.g., ocular muscles (with diplopia and strabismus), tongue muscles (with dysarthria). The diaphragm is most susceptible to invasion, followed by the extraocular, tongue, laryngeal, jaw, intercostal, neck, back, abdominal, and limb muscles, in that order.

Heavy infestation may be associated with central nervous system disorder. Headache, stiff neck, and a mild confusional state are the usual symptoms. Delirium, coma, hemiplegia, and aphasia occur occasionally. The spinal fluid is usually normal, but may contain a moderate number of lymphocytes and rarely, parasites.

An eosinophilic leukocytosis usually appears when the muscles are invaded. Serologic (precipitin) test and skin test become positive early in the third week. The heart is often involved, manifested by tachycardia and electrocardiographic changes. These findings may aid in the diagnosis, which can be confirmed by finding the larvae in muscle biopsy, using the technique of low-power scan of wet tissue pressed between two glass slides.

Trichinosis is seldom fatal. Most cases recover completely, although myalgia may persist for several months. Once recurrent seizures and focal neurologic deficits appear, they may persist indefinitely. The latter are based on a trichina encephalitis (the filiform larvae may be seen in cerebral capillaries and in cerebral parenchyma) and emboli from mural thrombi arising in infected heart muscle.

In the treatment of trichinosis, thiabendazole, an antihelminthic agent, and corticosteroids are of particular value. Thiabendazole, 25 mg/kg twice daily for 5 to 7 days, is effective in both the enteral and parenteral phases of the disease, preventing larvae reproduction (therefore useful in patients known to have ingested trichinous meat) and interfering with the metabolism of muscle-dwelling larvae. Fever, myalgia, and eosinophilia respond well to the anti-inflammatory and immunosuppressant effects of prednisone (40 to 60 mg daily), and a salutary effect has been noted on the cardiac and neurologic complications as well.

CYSTICERCOSIS

Cysticercosis is the larval or intermediate stage of infection with the pork tapeworm, *Taenia solium*. In Central and South American countries, cysticercosis is a leading cause of epilepsy and other neurologic disturbances. Because of the massive emigration from these endemic areas, patients with cysticercosis are now being seen with some regularity in countries where the disease had previously been unknown. Usually the disease is recognized by the presence of multiple calcified lesions in the thigh, leg, and shoulder muscles and in the cerebrum (Fig. 32-3).

Figure 32-3

Unenhanced CT scan from a 12-year-old girl, recently from Central America, with recurrent seizures of several years duration. The calcified spheres, scattered throughout the cerebral hemispheres, probably represent a remote infection with cysticercosis (similar calcific lesions were found in her muscles).

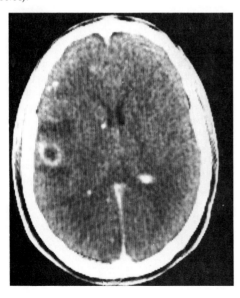

The cerebral manifestations of cysticercosis are diverse, related to the encystment and subsequent calcification of the larvae in the cerebral parenchyma, subarachnoid space, and ventricles. Most often the neurologic disease presents with seizures, although many patients are asymptomatic, the cysts being discovered radiologically. The therapy of this disorder has been greatly enhanced in recent years by the serial use of CT scans and the administration of praziquantel, an antihelminthic agent that is also active against all species of schistosomes. The usual dose of praziquantel is 50 mg per kilogram of body weight, given daily for 15 to 30 days, depending upon the number and size of the cysts. Initially, treatment may seem to exacerbate neurologic symptoms, with an increase in cells and protein in the CSF, but then the patients improve and many become asymptomatic, with a striking decrease in the size and number of cysts on CT scanning. In some patients, a large subarachnoid or intraventricular cyst may obstruct the flow of CSF, in which case surgical removal of the cyst or a shunt procedure becomes necessary.

In a smaller and more malignant form of the disease, the cysticerci are located in the basilar subarachnoid space, where they induce an intense inflammatory reaction, leading to hydrocephalus, vasculitis, cranial nerve palsies, and brainstem damage. This form of the illness is little altered by the use of praziquantel or any other form of therapy (Estañol et al).

SCHISTOSOMIASIS

The ova of trematodes seldom involve the nervous system, but when they do, the infecting organism is usually *Schistosoma japonicum* or, less often, *S. haematobium* or *S. mansoni*. *S. japonicum* has a tendency to localize in the cerebral hemispheres and *S. mansoni* in the spinal cord. The cerebral lesions form in relation to invaded blood vessels and take the form of necrotizing parenchymal foci infiltrated by eosinophils and giant cells with deposits of calcium.

Schistosomiasis is widespread in tropical regions, especially in Egypt, and North American neurologists have little contact with it. An estimated 3 to 5 percent of patients develop neurologic symptoms several months after exposure and early gastrointestinal symptoms. Headaches, convulsions (either focal or generalized), and other cerebral signs appear and with numerous lesions of larger size, papilledema may develop.

Some types of *Schistosoma* (also called *Bilharzia*) tend to localize in the spinal cord, causing an acute or subacute myelitis with the clinical picture of a transverse cord lesion. This is one of the most frequent forms of myelitis in Brazil and other parts of South America. Unless treated immediately, there may be permanent paralysis.

In the CSF, there is a pleocytosis, often with an increase in eosinophils, increased protein content, and sometimes increased pressure. Biopsy of liver and rectal mucosa, skin tests, and complement fixation tests confirm the diagnosis. *Treatment* consists of praziquantel orally in a dosage of 20 mg/kg tid. Eight of nine patients with epilepsy due to cerebral schistosomiasis became seizure-free after treatment with praziquantel. Surgical excision of granulomatous tumors is sometimes indicated.

Other Helminthic Infections Infection with *Echinococcus* may occasionally affect the brain. The usual sources of infection are water and vegetables contaminated by canine feces. After ingestion, the ova hatch and the freed embryos migrate, primarily to lung and liver, but sometimes to brain (approximately 2 percent of cases), where a large solitary (hydatid) cyst may be formed. Treatment with the drug mebendazole is recommended when surgery is not feasible.

Cerebral coenuriasis (*Coenurus cerebralis*) is an uncommon infestation by larvae of the tapeworm *Multiceps multiceps*. It occurs mainly in sheep-raising areas where there are many dogs, the latter being the definitive hosts. The larvae form grape-like cysts, most often in the posterior fossa, which obstruct the spinal fluid pathways and cause signs of increased intracranial pressure.

The nervous system may also be invaded directly by certain worms (ascaris, filaria) and flukes (schistosoma, paragonimus). These diseases are virtually nonexistent in the United States.

REFERENCES

Adams RD, Kubik CS, Bonner FJ: The clinical and pathological aspects of influenzal meningitis. *Arch Pediatr* 65:354, 1948.

Baker P, Price T, Allen CD: Brainstem and cerebellar dysfunction with Legionnaires' disease. *J Neurol Neurosurg Psychiatry* 44:1054, 1981.

Bennett JE, Dismukes WE, Duma RJ et al: A comparison of amphotericin B alone and combined with flucytosine in the treatment of cryptococcal meningitis. *N Engl J Med* 301:126, 1979.

Berman PH, Banker BQ: Neonatal meningitis: A clinical and pathological study of 29 cases. *Pediatrics* 38:6, 1966.

Bhandari YS, Sarkari NBS: Subdural empyema: A review of 37 cases. *J Neurosurg* 32:35, 1970.

Brewer NS, MacCarty CS, Wellman WE: Brain abscess: A review of recent experience. *Ann Intern Med* 82:571, 1975.

Cleland PG, Lawande RG, Onyemelukwe G, Whittle HC: Chronic amebic meningoencephalitis. *Arch Neurol* 39:56, 1982.

COHEN MM: The central nervous system in congenital heart disease. *Neurology* 10:452, 1960.

COONROD JD, DANS PE: Subdural empyema. *Am J Med* 53:85, 1972.

DELANEY P: Neurologic manifestations in sarcoidosis. Review of the literature, with a report of 23 cases. *Ann Intern Med* 87:336, 1977.

DE LOUVOIS J, GORTVAI P, HURLEY R: Bacteriology of abscesses of the central nervous system: A multicentre prospective study. *Br Med J* 2:981, 1977.

DODGE PR, DAVIS H, FEIGIN RD et al: Prospective evaluation of hearing impairment as a sequela of acute bacterial meningitis. *N Engl J Med* 311:869, 1984.

ESTAÑOL B, CORONA T, ABAD P: A prognostic classification of cerebral cysticercosis: Therapeutic implications. *J Neurol Neurosurg Psychiatry* 49: 1131, 1986.

FERRY PC, CULBERTSON JL, COOPER JA et al: Sequelae of *Haemophilus influenzae* meningitis: Preliminary report of a long-term follow-up study, in Sell SH, Wright PF (eds): *Haemophilus Influenzae—Epidemiology, Immunology and Prevention of Disease.* New York, Elsevier, 1982, sec 3, pp 111–116.

FINKEL M: Lyme disease and its neurologic complications. *Arch Neurol* 45:99, 1988.

FISHER RS, CLARK AW, WOLINSKY JS et al: Post infectious leukoencephalitis complicating *Mycoplasma pneumoniae* infection. *Arch Neurol* 40:109, 1983.

GALBRAITH JG, BARR VW: Epidural abscess and subdural empyema, in Thompson RA, Green JR (eds): *Advances in Neurology,* vol 6. New York, Raven Press, 1974, pp 257–267.

GARFIELD J: Management of supratentorial intracranial abscess: A review of 200 cases. *Br Med J* 2:7, 1968.

GATES EM, KERNOHAN JW, CRAIG W McK: Metastatic brain abscess. *Medicine* 29:71, 1950.

GOULD SE: *Trichinosis in Man and Animals.* Springfield, IL, Charles C Thomas, 1970.

GRAY ML, KILLINGER AH: *Listeria monocytogenes* and listeria infections. *Bacteriol Rev* 30:309, 1966.

HAND LW, SANFORD JP: Posttraumatic bacterial meningitis. *Ann Intern Med* 72:869, 1970.

HEINEMAN HS, BRAUDE AI, OSTERHOLM JL: Intracranial suppurative disease. *JAMA* 218:1542, 1971.

HINMAN AR: Tuberculous meningitis at Cleveland Metropolitan General Hospital. *Am Rev Respir Dis* 94:465, 1966.

HOOPER DC, PRUITT AA, RUBIN RH: Central nervous system infections in the chronically immunosuppressed. *Medicine* 61:166, 1982.

JEFFERSON M: Sarcoidosis of the nervous system. *Brain* 80:540, 1957.

KANE CH, MOST H: Schistosomiasis of the central nervous system. *Arch Neurol Psychiatry* 59:141, 1948.

KAUFMAN DM, LITMAN N, MILLER MH: Sinusitis induced subdural empyema. *Neurology* 33:123, 1983.

KROLL JS, MOXON ER: Acute bacterial meningitis, in Kennedy PGE, Johnson RT (eds): *Infections of the Nervous System.* Boston, Butterworth, 1987, chap 2.

KUBIK CS, ADAMS RD: Subdural empyema. *Brain* 66:18, 1943.

LECHTENBERG R, STERRA MF, PRINGLE GF et al: Listeria monocytogenes: Brain abscess or meningoencephalitis? *Neurology* 29:86, 1979.

LEES AW, TYRRELL WF: Severe cerebral disturbance in Legionnaires' disease. *Lancet* 2:1331, 1978.

LEWIS JL, RABINOVICH S: The wide spectrum of cryptococcal infection. *Am J Med* 53:315, 1972.

LEYS, D, DESTEE A, PETIT H, WAROT P: Management of subdural intracranial empyemas should not always require surgery. *J Neurol Neurosurg Psychiatry* 49:635, 1986.

LINCOLN EM: Tuberculous meningitis in children: Serous meningitis. *Am Rev Tuberculosis* 56:95, 1947.

LIPTON SA, HICKEY WF, MORRIS JH, LOSCALZO J: Candidal infection in the central nervous system. *Am J Med* 76:101, 1984.

MATHIES AW: Penicillins in the treatment of bacterial meningitis. *J R Coll Physicians* 6:139, 1972.

MATSON DD: *Neurosurgery of Infancy and Childhood.* Springfield, IL, Charles C Thomas, 1969, p 716.

MAYOCK RL, BERTRAND P, MORRISON CE, SCOTT JH: Manifestations of sarcoidosis. *Am J Med* 35:67, 1963.

MERRITT HH, ADAMS RD, SOLOMON H: *Neurosyphilis.* New York, Oxford, 1946.

MURPHY FK, MACKOWIAK P, LUBY J: Management of infections affecting the nervous system, in Rosenberg RN (ed): *The Treatment of Neurological Diseases.* New York, Spectrum, 1979, pp 249–376.

NAGEOTTE J: Pathogénie du tabes dorsale. *Presse Med* 2:1179, 1902.

NEWTON EM: Hematogenous brain abscess in cyanotic congenital heart disease. *Q J Med* 25:201, 1956.

OBERSTEINER H, REDLICH E: Über das Wesen und Pathogenese der tabetischen hinterstrang Degeneration. *Arb Hirnanatomischen Institut* 2:158, 1894; 3:192, 1895.

REIK L: Spirochetal infections of the nervous system, in Kennedy PGE, Johnson RT (eds): *Infections of the Nervous System.* Boston, Butterworth, 1987, chap 4.

RICH AR: *The Pathogenesis of Tuberculosis,* 2nd ed. Oxford, Blackwell, 1951.

ROTHSTEIN TL, KENNY GE: Cranial neuropathy, myeloradiculopathy, and myositis. Complications of *Mycoplasma pneumoniae* infection. *Arch Neurol* 36:476, 1979.

SCADDING JG: *Sarcoidosis.* London, Eyre and Spottiswoode, 1967.

SCHELD WM: Pathogenesis and pathophysiology of pneumococcal meningitis, in Sande MA, Smith AL, Root RK (eds): *Bacterial Meningitis.* New York, Churchill Livingstone, 1985.

SCHMIDT RP, GONYEA EF: Neurosyphilis, in Baker AB, Baker LH (eds): *Clinical Neurology,* vol 2. New York, Harper & Row, 1980, chap. 28.

SEIDEL JS, HARMATZ P, VISVESVARA GS et al: Successful treatment of primary amebic meningoencephalitis. *N Engl J Med* 306:346, 1982.

SHETTY KR, CILVO CL, STARR BD, HARTER DH: Legionnaires' disease with profound cerebellar involvement. *Arch Neurol* 37:379, 1980.

SILTZBACH LE, JAMES DG, NEVILLE E et al: Course and prognosis of sarcoidosis around the world. *Amer J Med* 57:847, 1974.

SOTELO J, ESCOBEDO F, RODRIGUEZ-CARBAJAL J et al: Therapy of parenchymal brain cysticercosis with praziquantel. *N Engl J Med* 310:1001, 1984.

SPIELMEYER W: Zur Pathogenese der Tabes. *Z Ges Neurol Psychiatr* 84:257, 1923; 91:672, 1924; 97:287, 1925.

STOCKSTILL MT, KAUFFMAN CA: Comparison of cryptococcal and tuberculous meningitis. *Arch Neurol* 40:81, 1983.

SWARTZ MN: ''Chronic meningitis''—many causes to consider. *N Engl J Med* 317:957, 1987.

SWARTZ MN, DODGE PR: Bacterial meningitis: A review of selected aspects. *N Engl J Med* 272: 725, 779, 842, 898, 1965.

SYMONDS CP: Otitic hydrocephalus. *Brain* 54:55, 1931.

SYPHILIS: CENTERS FOR DISEASE CONTROL recommended treatment schedules, Venereal Disease Control Advisory Committee. *Morbid Mortal Week Rep* 25:101, 1976.

TANDON PN, PATHAK SN: Tuberculosis of the central nervous system, in Spillane JD (ed): *Tropical Neurology*. London, Oxford, 1973, pp 37–62.

THOMPSON RA: Clinical features of central nervous system fungus infection, in Thompson RA, Green JR (eds): *Advances in Neurology,* vol 6. New York, Raven Press, 1974, pp 93–100.

TORO G, ROMAN G: Cerebral malaria. *Arch Neurol* 35:271, 1978.

TOWNSEND JJ, WOLINSKY JS, BARINGER JR, JOHNSON PC: Acquired toxoplasmosis. *Arch Neurol* 32:335, 1975.

VARTDAL F, VANDVIK B, MICHAELSEN TE et al: Neurosyphilis: Intrathecal synthesis of oligoclonal antibodies to treponema pallidum. *Ann Neurol* 11:35, 1982.

WALSH TJ, HIER DB, CAPLAN LR: Fungal infections of the central nervous system: Comparative analysis of risk factors and clinical signs in 57 patients. *Neurology* 35:1654, 1985.

WASZ-HÖCKERT O, DONNER M: Results of the treatment of 191 children with tuberculous meningitis. *Acta Paediatr* 51(suppl 141):7, 1962.

WATT G, LONG GW, RENOA CP: Praziquantel in treatment of cerebral schistosomiasis. *Lancet* 11:529, 1986.

WEISS W, FIGUEROA W, SHAPIRO WH, FLIPPIN HF: Prognostic factors in pneumococcal meningitis. *Arch Intern Med* 120:517, 1967.

WESTENFELDER GO, AKEY DT, CORWIN SJ, VICK NA: Acute transverse myelitis due to mycoplasma pneumoniae infection. *Arch Neurol* 38:317, 1981.

WILSON SAK: *Neurology*. London, William Woods, 1940.

YOSHIKAWA TT, CHOW AW, GUZE LB: Role of anaerobic bacteria in subdural hematoma. *Am J Med* 58:99, 1975.

CHAPTER 33

VIRAL INFECTIONS OF THE NERVOUS SYSTEM

The notion that certain viruses are neurotropic, i.e., have a selective affinity for the nervous system, is no longer tenable. With the possible exception of rabies, viral infections of the nervous system are invariably complications of generalized viral infections. Considering the frequency of the latter, invasion of the nervous system is a relatively uncommon occurrence; nevertheless, it may be of overriding clinical importance. Many of the common viruses (herpes simplex, measles, varicella, for example), which cause only insignificant systemic illnesses, can have a devastating effect upon the nervous system. In other words, the neural aspects of viral infection may assume a clinical importance that is quite disproportionate to the systemic illnesses of which they are a part, and the term *neurotropic* should be used only in this qualified sense.

A detailed discussion of viral morphology and cell-virus interactions is beyond the scope of a textbook of neurology. An authoritative overview of this subject, by Tyler and Fields, can be found in the eleventh edition of *Harrison's Principles of Internal Medicine* (Chap. 128) and the introductory sections of R. T. Johnson's monograph on *Viral Infections of the Nervous System.*

PATHWAYS OF INFECTION

Viruses gain entrance to the body by one of several pathways. The most common viruses—mumps, measles, varicella—enter via the respiratory passages. Polioviruses and other enteroviruses enter by the oral-intestinal route; herpes simplex enters mainly via the oral or genital mucosal route. Other viruses are acquired by inoculation, as a result of the bites of animals (e.g., rabies) or mosquitoes (*arthropod-bo*rne or arbovirus infections). The fetus may be infected transplacentally by the rubella virus and cytomegalovirus.

Following entry into the body, the virus multiplies locally and in secondary sites, and usually gives rise to a viremia. Most viral particles are cleared from the blood by monocytes and other elements of the reticuloendothelial system, but if the viremia is massive or other factors are favorable, they will invade the CNS via the cerebral capillaries and the choroid plexus. Clearance of virus from CNS tissues is accomplished by humoral immune globulins and secretory IgA antibodies produced by thymus-derived lymphocytes.

Another pathway of infection is along peripheral nerves; centripetal movement of virus is accomplished by retrograde axoplasmic flow. Herpes simplex and rabies viruses and possibly herpes zoster virus utilize this peripheral nerve pathway, which explains why the initial symptoms of rabies and the rare B virus infection of monkeys (*herpes simiae*) occur locally, at a segmental level that corresponds to the animal bite. Experimentally it has been shown that viruses may spread to the CNS by penetrating the olfactory mucosa, but the role of this pathway in human infection is not certain. Of these different routes of infection, the hematogenous one is by far the most important. The steps in the hematogenous spread of infection are illustrated diagramatically in Fig. 33-1.

MECHANISMS OF VIRAL INFECTIONS

Viruses, once they invade the nervous system, have diverse clinical and pathologic effects. One reason for this diversity is that different cell populations within the CNS vary in their susceptibility to infection with different viruses. To be susceptible to a viral infection the host cell must have specific receptor sites on its cytoplasmic membrane, to which the virus attaches. Thus, some infections are confined

Figure 33-1

Steps in the hematogenous spread of virus to the central nervous system. (Courtesy of RT Johnson.)

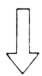

ENTRY INTO HOST
 Inoculation
 Respiratory
 Enteric

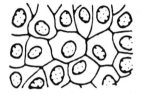

GROWTH IN EXTRANEURAL TISSUES
 Primary sites
  subcutaneous tissue and muscle, lymph
  nodes, respiratory or gastrointestinal
  tracts
 Secondary sites
  muscle, vascular endothelium, bone
  marrow, liver, spleen, etc.

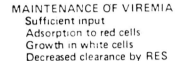

MAINTENANCE OF VIREMIA
 Sufficient input
 Adsorption to red cells
 Growth in white cells
 Decreased clearance by RES

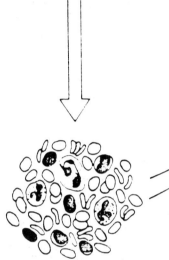

Normally phagocytozed by
reticuloendothelial system

CROSSING FROM BLOOD TO BRAIN

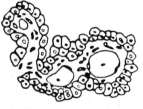

CHOROID PLEXUS TO CSF
 Growth in choroid plexus
 Passage through choroid plexus

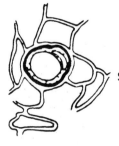

SMALL VESSELS TO BRAIN
 Transport by infected leukocytes
 Infection of vascular endothelium
 Diffusion across normal cells and
  membranes
 Passage through areas of permeability

591

to meningeal cells, in which case the clinical manifestations will be those of a benign aseptic meningitis. Other viruses will involve parenchymal cells of the brain or spinal cord, giving rise to the more serious disorders of encephalitis and poliomyelitis, respectively. In some viral infections the susceptibility of particular cell groups is even more specific. In poliomyelitis, for example, there is a particular vulnerability of motor neurons of cranial and spinal nerves, and in rabies, of neurons of the trigeminal ganglia, cerebellum, and limbic lobes. The susceptible cell must be capable of initiating penetration by the virus or its nucleocapsid, mainly by the process of endocytosis, and of releasing the nucleoprotein protective coating of the virus. For virus reproduction the cell must have the metabolic capacity to transcribe and translate virus-coated proteins, to replicate viral nucleic acid, and, under the direction of the virus genome, to assemble virions.

The pathologic effects of viruses upon susceptible cells vary greatly. In acute encephalitis, susceptible neurons are invaded directly by virus, and the cells undergo lysis, with an appropriate glial and inflammatory reaction. In the disease known as progressive multifocal leukoencephalopathy (PML), there appears to be a selective lysis of oligodendrocytes, resulting in foci of demyelination. In acute disseminated (postinfectious) encephalomyelitis, the destruction of myelin has a different mechanism, probably an immune response focused on viral antigens on the surfaces of oligodendrocytes. In herpes zoster and in certain instances of herpes simplex, the virus remains latent in cells for long periods until immunity falls, particularly in old age, or some other factor may trigger an outbreak of acute infection. In certain congenital infections, e.g., rubella and cytomegalovirus, the virus persists in nervous tissue for months or years. Differentiating cells of the fetal brain have particular vulnerabilities, and viral incorporation may give rise to malformations and to hydrocephalus (e.g., mumps virus with ependymal destruction and aqueductal stenosis). In experimental animals, cerebral neoplasms can be induced when the viral genome is incorporated into the host cell DNA. This latter mechanism has not been convincingly demonstrated in humans (Johnson). In still other circumstances, a protracted viral infection simulating degenerative disease occurs only after a long incubation period (*slow virus*) and excites little or no inflammatory reaction.

CLINICAL SYNDROMES

The number of viruses that affect the nervous system is legion. Among the enteroviruses alone, almost 70 distinct serologic types have been associated with CNS disease, and additional types from this family of viruses and others are still being discovered. There is no need to consider these viruses individually, since there are only a limited number of ways in which they express themselves clinically. Six syndromes recur with regularity and should be familiar to all neurologists: (1) acute anterior poliomyelitis; (2) herpes zoster ganglionitis; (3) acute aseptic (nonsuppurative or ''lymphocytic'') meningitis; (4) acute encephalitis or meningoencephalitis; and (5) chronic infections due to ''slow viruses'' and unconventional agents, simulating degenerative disease; and (6) immunosuppression by retroviruses, i.e., the acquired immune-deficiency syndrome (AIDS).

SYNDROME OF ACUTE ANTERIOR POLIOMYELITIS

In the past, this syndrome was almost invariably the result of infection by one of the three types of poliovirus. Illnesses that are clinically indistinguishable from poliovirus infections can be caused by other enteroviruses, such as Coxsackie viruses, groups A and B, and echoviruses, and in countries with successful vaccine programs, these are now the most common causes of the anterior poliomyelitis syndrome. The illnesses caused by these latter viruses are generally benign and the associated paralysis is rarely significant. Epidemics of hemorrhagic conjunctivitis (which are caused by enterovirus 70 and which are common in Asia and Africa) are, in a small percentage of cases, associated with a lower motor neuron paralysis, resembling poliomyelitis (Wadia et al). However, the important (paralytic) disease in this category is poliomyelitis, and the remainder of the discussion will be concerned with it alone.

Poliomyelitis has ceased to be a scourge in areas where vaccination is common, but its lethal and crippling effects are still fresh in memory. As recently as the summer of 1955, when New England experienced its last epidemic, 3950 cases of acute poliomyelitis were reported in Massachusetts alone, and 2771 of these were paralytic. Now paralytic poliomyelitis is a rarity in the United States; the authors have not seen a bona fide instance for many years. Nevertheless small outbreaks have occurred among religious groups that do not practice immunization and in parts of the world where a vaccination program has not been started or sustained. In the United States, approximately 15 cases of paralytic poliomyelitis are reported each year—about equally divided among unvaccinated children and adults exposed to a vaccinated child. And, of course, the paralytic residua of previous epidemics are everywhere around us. It is necessary, therefore, to review the main features of the disease, and also for the reason that it stands as a prototype of a neurotropic viral infection.

ETIOLOGY AND EPIDEMIOLOGY

The disease is caused by small RNA viruses that are members of the enterovirus group of the picornavirus family. Three antigenically distinct types have been defined, and infection with one does not protect against the others. The disease has a worldwide distribution, but epidemics, when they occurred, were more frequent in the north temperate zone, in regions of excellent sanitation, than elsewhere. The peak incidence of infection in the northern hemisphere was in the months of July through September.

Poliomyelitis is a highly communicable disease. The main reservoir of infection is the human intestinal tract (humans are the only known natural hosts), and the main route of infection is fecal-oral, i.e., hand to mouth, as with other enteric pathogens. The virus multiplies in the pharynx and intestinal tract, and during the incubation period, which is from 1 to 3 weeks, virus can be recovered from both of these sites. The virus penetrates the intestinal wall and is borne in the blood to all parts of the body. In only a small fraction of infected patients is the nervous system invaded. It is estimated that between 95 to 99 percent of infected patients are asymptomatic or experience a nonspecific illness. It is the latter type of patient—the carrier with inapparent infection—that is most important in the spread of the virus from one person to another.

CLINICAL MANIFESTATIONS

As indicated above, the large majority of infections are unaccompanied by any symptoms (*inapparent infection*), or there may be only mild systemic symptoms with pharyngitis or gastroenteritis or flu-like symptoms (so-called *minor illness* or *abortive poliomyelitis*). These mild symptoms of poliomyelitis correspond to the period of viremia and dissemination of the virus, and in most cases they give rise to an effective immune response, which accounts for their failure to cause meningitis or poliomyelitis. In the relatively small proportion of patients in whom the nervous system is invaded, the illness still has a wide range of severity, from a mild attack of aseptic meningitis (*nonparalytic* or *preparalytic poliomyelitis*) to the most severe forms of paralytic disease (*paralytic poliomyelitis*).

Nonparalytic or Preparalytic Poliomyelitis The prodromal symptoms are those of the minor illness, mentioned above. Listlessness, generalized, nonthrobbing headache, fever of 38 to 40°C, stiffness and aching in the muscles, sore throat in the absence of upper respiratory infection, anorexia, nausea, and vomiting are the usual manifestations. These symptoms may subside to a varying extent, to be followed after 3 to 4 days by recrudescence of headache and fever and by symptoms of nervous system involvement (so-called dromedary or biphasic form). More often the second phase of the illness blends with the first. Tenderness and pain in the muscles, tightness of the hamstrings (*spasm*), and pain in the neck and back become increasingly prominent. Other manifestations of nervous system involvement include irritability, restlessness, and emotional instability. The occurrence of the latter symptoms is frequently a prelude to paralysis. Added to these symptoms are stiffness of the neck on forward flexion, Kernig and Brudzinski signs, and the characteristic CSF findings of *aseptic meningitis*. The cell count is between 25 and 500 per cubic millimeter, occasionally higher; neutrophils predominate in the first few days of the illness, then lymphocytes; protein is elevated, rarely to more than 150 mg/dL; and the glucose content is normal.

The symptoms described above may constitute the entire illness. In such instances, fever and other systemic manifestations subside in a matter of days, although the signs of meningeal irritation may persist for a week or two. Alternatively, the preparalytic symptoms may be followed by paralytic ones. The weakness becomes manifest while the fever is at its height, or, just as frequently, as the temperature is falling and the general clinical picture seems to be improving.

The clinical patterns of preparalytic and paralytic poliomyelitis vary to some extent, depending upon the age of the patient. The diphasic or dromedary course is common in children, but unusual in patients over 15 years of age. Symptoms tend to develop more rapidly in younger patients, and the interval between onset of symptoms and paralysis tends also to be shorter in this group. Pain in the muscles is a more prominent feature in adolescents and adults than in young children.

Paralytic Poliomyelitis The conventional division of paralytic poliomyelitis into spinal, bulbar, and encephalitic types is a convenient descriptive device, but it has no valid pathologic basis, as will be indicated further on. Clinically, one or other of these forms may predominate, but more often they occur in combination.

Muscle weakness may develop rapidly, attaining its maximum severity in 48 h or even less, or more slowly, or in stuttering fashion, for a week or longer. As a general rule, there is no progression of weakness after the temperature has been normal for 48 h. The distribution of spinal paralysis is quite variable. In children under 5 years of age, the most common but by no means the only form is a weakness of one leg; in older children, weakness of an arm or both legs is usual, and in the 16- to 65-year-old group, an asymmetric weakness of all four limbs. The most widespread weakness occurs in infants. Rarely there may be an acute symmetrical paralysis of the muscles of the trunk and limbs, as occurs in the Guillain-Barré syndrome. Certain host factors, such as excessive physical activity and local injections during the period of asymptomatic infection, are thought to favor the development of paralysis of the exercised muscles or injected limbs.

Coarse fasciculations are frequently seen as the muscles weaken; they are transient as a rule, but occasionally they persist. Abdominal, cremasteric, and tendon reflexes are diminished and lost as the weakness of abdominal and limb muscles evolves. Patients frequently complain of paresthesias in the affected limbs, but objective sensory loss is not demonstrable. Retention of urine is a common occurrence in adult patients, but does not persist. Atrophy of muscle can be detected within 3 weeks of onset of paralysis, and is permanent.

More or less pure bulbar affection may be seen in children, particularly in those in whom tonsils and adenoids had been removed. Adults with bulbar symptoms almost always have spinal involvement as well. Any of the cranial muscles may be weakened, but the most frequently involved are the muscles of deglutition, because of affection of the nucleus ambiguus. The other great hazards of bulbar disease are the disturbances of respiration and vasomotor control—hiccough, shallowness and progressive slowing of respiration, cyanosis, hypertension, and ultimately hypotension and circulatory collapse. When these symptoms are added to paralysis of phrenic and intercostal musculature, the fatality rate is between 25 and 75 percent. Restlessness and agitation, anxiety and fear of death, somnolence, confusion, stupor, and coma are the symptoms usually referred to as encephalitic.

Immune reactions to the virus may arrest the infection at any stage (systemic, meningeal, paralytic). Individuals whose immune reactions are suppressed by neoplasms, corticosteroids, or other drugs may develop a slowly progressive motor paralysis that extends over a period of months or a year or more (chronic poliomyelitis).

PATHOLOGIC CHANGES AND CLINICOPATHOLOGIC CORRELATIONS

In fatal infections, nonparalytic as well as paralytic, lesions are found in the cerebral cortex, brainstem, and spinal cord. As far as the pathologist is concerned, therefore, all cases of poliomyelitis are also encephalitic. The cerebral cortical lesions, however, are confined to the precentral gyrus and are usually of insufficient severity to cause symptoms. The

brunt of the disease is borne by the hypothalamus, thalamus, motor nuclei of the brainstem and surrounding reticular formation, vestibular nuclei and roof nuclei of the cerebellum, and the neurons of the anterior and intermediate columns. In these areas, nerve cells are destroyed and phagocytized (neuronophagia). A leukocytic reaction is present for only a few days but mononuclear cells and microglia persist as perivascular accumulations for many months. The initial inflammatory response may at times be so severe as to cause small foci of tissue necrosis and petechial hemorrhages.

The nature of the histopathologic changes and their relationship to the clinical findings have been studied most carefully by Bodian, both in experimental animals and in humans, and the following account is based largely on his observations.

The earliest visible alterations, in response to invasion of the CNS by virus, is central chromatolysis of the cytoplasmic Nissl substance of the nerve cells, along with an inflammatory reaction. These changes are accompanied by a multiplication of virus in the CNS, and both precede the onset of paralysis by a day or by several days. Changes in the nerve cells proceed rapidly; progressive dissolution of cytoplasmic Nissl substance is followed by disintegration of the nucleus and then by complete lysis or necrosis of the cell.

The infected motor neurons continue to function until the stage of severe chromatolysis is reached. Furthermore, if damage to the cell has attained only the stage of central chromatolysis, complete morphologic recovery can be expected. Cells are either destroyed quickly in the first few days of the disease, or are restored to morphologic normality—a process that takes a month or longer. After this time the degree of paralysis and atrophy is closely correlated with the number of motor nerve cells that have been destroyed; where limbs remain atrophic and paralyzed, less than 10 percent of neurons survive in corresponding cord segments.

The variability of the clinical signs and symptoms depends mainly on the variation in severity of the nerve cell injury and inflammatory response in different regions. Only when the pathologic changes reach a certain threshold of severity, exceeding the margin of safety of the particular cell population involved, is a clinical effect observed.

The nerve cell changes and inflammatory reaction in the cerebral cortex are of insufficient severity to cause the so-called encephalitic changes (restlessness, anxiety, confusion, stupor, etc.). The latter seem to be related to the presence of severe brainstem lesions, including those in the hypothalamus. Also, hypotension and hypoxia may be responsible for these symptoms.

Lesions in the motor nuclei of the brainstem may be associated with paralysis in corresponding muscles, but only if the lesions are severe in degree. In fatal cases it is usual to find lesions in all brainstem nuclei (except those of the basis pontis and inferior olives); yet paralytic symptoms in corresponding muscles are rarely recorded, except in those of the face, larynx, and pharynx. This testifies to the wide margin of safety in the oculomotor, motor trigeminal, and hypoglossal nuclei. The nuclei of the vestibular complex and reticular formation are the most severely affected brainstem nuclei, along with the roof nuclei of the cerebellum. Vertigo, nystagmus, ataxia, and tremor are probably related to the latter lesions, but these clinical manifestations are distinctly uncommon. Symptoms of nausea and vomiting may also be due to lesions in these nuclei. The disturbances of swallowing, respiration, and vasomotor control are related to lesions in the medullary reticular formation, including the region of the nucleus ambiguus.

Atrophic, areflexic paralysis of muscles of the trunk and limbs relates, of course, to destruction of neurons in the corresponding segments of the spinal cord gray matter, more specifically those in the anterior and intermediate horns. Impairment of sensation can practically never be detected in poliomyelitis, although mild, spotty lesions are observed frequently in the dorsal horns. The common symptoms of stiffness and pain in the neck and back are usually attributed to "meningeal irritation"; probably they are related to the mild inflammatory exudate in the meninges and to lesions of varying severity in the dorsal root ganglia and dorsal horns. Also it is likely that these lesions account for the muscle pain and paresthesias in parts that later become paralyzed. Abnormalities of autonomic function are probably attributable to lesions of autonomic pathways in the reticular substance of the brainstem and in the lateral horn cells in the spinal cord.

It is of interest that while poliovirus has been readily isolated from CNS tissue of fatal cases, it can rarely be recovered from the CSF during clinical disease. This is in contrast to the closely related Coxsackie and echo picornaviruses which have been isolated frequently from the CSF during neurologic illnesses.

TREATMENT

Patients with suspected acute poliomyelitis should be kept in bed and hospitalized if signs of nervous system involvement are detected. Careful observation of swallowing function, vital capacity, pulse, and blood pressure is necessary in anticipation of respiratory and circulatory complications.

If the neurologic signs are limited to those of meningeal irritation and muscle pain, the administration of aspirin or other mild analgesics and the application of hot packs provide relief. With paralysis of limb muscles, foot

boards, hand and arm splints, and knee and trochanter rolls prevent foot drop and other deformities. Passive movement prevents contractures and ankylosis.

Respiratory failure may be caused by paralysis of the intercostal and diaphragmatic muscles or by depression of the respiratory centers in the brainstem. Either type calls for the use of a positive-pressure respirator, and this also requires a tracheotomy. The management of the respirator patient and of the pulmonary and circulatory complications does not differ from that of patients with other neurologic diseases, such as myasthenia gravis or acute ascending polyneuropathy, and is best carried out in special respiratory care units.

The authors know of no systematic study of the potency of the new antiviral agents in this disease.

PROGNOSIS

The overall mortality rate of acute paralytic poliomyelitis is between 5 and 10 percent, higher in adults and with increasing age, and higher in very young children and infants. If the patient survives the acute stage, paralysis of respiration and deglutition usually recover completely; in only a small fraction of such patients is chronic respirator care necessary. Many patients also recover completely from muscular weakness, and most of them improve to some extent. The return of muscle strength occurs mainly in the first 3 to 4 months and is the result of morphologic restitution of partially damaged nerve cells. Branching of axons of intact motor cells with reinnervation of muscle fibers of denervated motor units may also play a part. Slow recovery of slight degree may then continue for a year or more, the result of hypertrophy of undamaged muscle.

PREVENTION

This, of course, has proved to be the most significant aspect of treatment, and one of the outstanding accomplishments of modern medicine. The cultivation of poliovirus in cultures of human embryonic tissues—the achievement of Enders and his associates—made possible the development of vaccines that offer effective and long-lasting immunity. The first of these was the injectable Salk vaccine, containing formalin-inactivated virulent strains of the three viral serotypes. This has been replaced by the Sabin vaccine, which consists of attenuated live virus, administered orally in two doses 8 weeks apart; boosters are required at 1 year of age and before starting school. Since 1965, the reported annual incidence rate of poliomyelitis has been less than 0.01 per

100,000 (compared to a rate of 24 cases per 100,000 during the years 1951 to 1955). Very rarely, poliomyelitis may follow vaccination (0.02 to 0.04 cases per million doses). Equally rare are instances of postvaccinal encephalomyelitis. The only obstacle to complete prevention of the disease is inadequate utilization of the vaccine. Significant segments of the population in areas with low public-health standards are not being immunized. Conceivably, with an increasing lack of immunity, outbreaks of poliomyelitis could occur once again.

A delayed progression of muscle weakness has been observed in late adult life (see page 956).

SYNDROME OF HERPES ZOSTER

Herpes zoster (zona, ''shingles'') is a common viral infection of the nervous system, occuring at an overall rate of 3 to 5 cases per 1000 persons per year, and at a much higher rate with advancing age. It is characterized clinically by radicular pain, a vesicular cutaneous eruption, and, less often, by segmental sensory and motor loss. The pathologic changes consist of an acute inflammatory reaction in isolated spinal or cranial sensory ganglia, the posterior gray matter of the spinal cord, and the adjacent leptomeninges. The neurologic implications of the segmental distribution of the rash were recognized by Richard Bright, as long ago as 1831. The inflammatory changes in the corresponding ganglia and related portions of the spinal nerves were first described by von Barensprung in 1862 and were later studied extensively by Head and Campbell. The concept that varicella and zoster are caused by the same agent was introduced by von Bokay, in 1909, and was established more recently by Weller and his associates (1954, 1958). The common agent, referred to as varicella or varicella-zoster (VZ) virus, is a DNA virus that is similar in structure to the virus of herpes simplex. These and other historical features of herpes zoster are reviewed by Denny-Brown and by Weller and their colleagues.

PATHOLOGY AND PATHOGENESIS

The pathologic changes in herpes zoster are unique and consist of (1) an inflammatory reaction in several unilateral adjacent sensory ganglia of the spinal or cranial nerves, frequently of such intensity as to cause necrosis of all or part of the ganglion, with or without hemorrhage; (2) an inflammatory reaction in the spinal roots and peripheral nerve contiguous to the involved ganglion; (3) a poliomyelitis which closely resembles acute anterior poliomyelitis,

but is readily distinguished by its unilaterality, segmental localization, and greater involvement of the posterior horn, posterior root, and dorsal root ganglion; and (4) a relatively mild leptomeningitis, largely limited to the involved spinal or cranial segments and nerve roots. These pathologic changes are the substratum of the neuralgic pains, the pleocytosis, and the local palsies that may attend and follow the zoster infection.

The pathogenesis of herpes zoster is not fully understood, but the most widely accepted hypothesis is that it represents a spontaneous reactivation of varicella virus infection, which becomes latent in the sensory ganglia following a primary infection with chickenpox (Hope-Simpson). This hypothesis is consistent with the differences in the clinical manifestations of chickenpox and herpes zoster, even though both are caused by the same virus. Chickenpox is highly contagious, has a well-marked seasonal incidence (winter and spring) and a tendency to occur in epidemics. Zoster, on the other hand, is not communicable (except to a person who has not had chickenpox), occurs sporadically throughout the year, and shows no increase in incidence during epidemics of chickenpox. In patients with zoster, there is practically always a past history of chickenpox. In rare instances of herpes zoster in infants such a history may be lacking, but in these latter cases there usually has been prenatal maternal contact with the VZ virus.

Although the VZ virus has not been cultured from sensory ganglia of asymptomatic individuals, its nucleic acid has been demonstrated, indicating the presence of the virus. Also the closely related viruses of herpes simplex have been obtained from human trigeminal and sacral ganglia (Baringer). The supposition is that in both varicella and zoster infections the virus makes its way from the cutaneous vesicles, along the sensory nerves to the ganglion, where it remains latent until activated, at which time it progresses down the axon to the skin. Multiplication of the virus in epidermal cells causes swelling, vacuolization, and lysis of cell boundaries, leading to the formation of vesicles and Lipschutz inclusion bodies. Alternatively, the ganglia could be infected during the viremia of chickenpox, but then one would have to explain why only one or a few sensory ganglia become infected. Reactivation of virus is attributed to waning immunity, which would explain the increasing incidence of zoster with aging (increasing lack of exposure to children with chickenpox) and with lymphomas, administration of immunosuppressive drugs, and radiation therapy.

CLINICAL FEATURES

As has been indicated, the incidence of herpes zoster rises with age. Hope-Simpson has estimated that if a cohort of

1000 people lived to 85 years of age, half would have had one attack of zoster and 10 would have had two attacks. The notion that one attack of zoster provides lifelong immunity is incorrect, although recurrent attacks of herpes are usually due to the simplex virus. The sexes are equally affected as are both sides of the body. Zoster occurs in about 10 percent of patients with lymphoma and 25 percent of patients with Hodgkin disease—particularly in those who have undergone splenectomy and received radiotherapy. Conversely, about 5 percent of patients who present with herpes zoster are found to have a concurrent malignancy (about twice the number that would be expected).

The vesicular eruption is usually preceded for several days by itching, tingling, or burning sensations in the involved dermatome(s), and sometimes by malaise and fever as well. Or there is severe localized pain that may be mistaken for pleurisy, appendicitis, or cholecystitis until the diagnosis is clarified by the appearance of vesicles (nearly always within 72 to 96 h). The rash consists of tense clear vesicles on an erythematous base, the contents of which becomes cloudy after a few days (due to accumulation of inflammatory cells) and dry, crusted, and scaly after 5 to 10 days. In a small number of patients the vesicles are confluent and hemorrhagic, and healing is delayed for several weeks. In most cases, pain and dysesthesia last for 1 to 4 weeks; but in the others (7 to 33 percent of cases, in different series) the pain persists for months or, in different forms, even for years, and presents a difficult problem in management. Impairment of superficial sensation in the affected dermatome(s) is common and, in about 5 percent of patients, segmental weakness and atrophy are added. In the majority of patients the rash and sensorimotor signs are limited to the territory of a single dermatome, but in some, particularly those with cranial or limb involvement, two or more contiguous nerves are involved. Rarely (and usually in association with malignancy) the rash is generalized, like that of chickenpox. The CSF frequently shows a mild increase in cells, mainly lymphocytes, and a modest increase in protein content. The diagnosis can be confirmed by direct immunofluorescence of a biopsied skin lesion, using antibody to VZ virus.

Virtually any dermatome may be involved in herpes zoster, but some regions are far more frequently involved than others. The thoracic dermatomes, particularly T5 to T10, are the most common sites, accounting for more than two-thirds of all cases, followed by the craniocervical regions. In the latter cases the disease tends to be more severe, with greater pain, more frequent meningeal signs, and involvement of the mucous membranes.

There are two rather characteristic cranial herpetic syndromes—so-called ophthalmic herpes and geniculate herpes. In *ophthalmic herpes,* which accounts for 10 to 15 percent of all cases of herpes zoster, the rash and pain are in the distribution of the first division of the trigeminal nerve, and the pathologic changes are centered in the gasserian ganglion. The main hazard in this form of the disease is herpetic involvement of the cornea and conjunctiva, with corneal anesthesia and residual scarring. Palsies of extraocular muscles, ptosis, and mydriasis are frequently associated, indicating that the third, fourth, and sixth cranial nerves are affected in addition to the gasserian ganglion.

A less common cranial nerve syndrome consists of a facial palsy in combination with a herpetic eruption of the external auditory meatus, with or without tinnitus, vertigo, and deafness. Ramsay Hunt attributed this syndrome to herpes of the geniculate ganglion, despite the fact that pathologic confirmation of such a lesion has not been forthcoming, either in Hunt's time or since then. One of the authors (R.D.A.) found the geniculate ganglion to be only slightly affected in a man who died 64 days after the onset of a so-called Ramsay Hunt syndrome (during which time he had recovered from the facial palsy); there was, however, a neuritis of the facial nerve, a finding that provided an explanation for the facial palsy.

Herpes zoster of the palate, pharynx, neck, and retroauricular region (herpes occipitocollaris) depends upon herpetic infection of the upper cervical roots and the ganglia of the vagus and glossopharyngeal nerves. Herpes zoster in this distribution may be associated with the Ramsay Hunt syndrome.

Encephalitis and *myelitis* are rare but well-described complications of cervicocranial zoster. *Cerebral angiitis,* histologically similar to granulomatous angiitis, is another rare complication of herpes zoster in these locations. Typically, in these latter patients, the resolution of the cutaneous lesions is followed by the acute onset of hemiparesis, hemianesthesia, aphasia, or other focal neurologic or retinal deficits, associated with a mononuclear pleocytosis and elevated IgG indices in the CSF. CT scans have demonstrated small deep infarcts in the hemisphere ipsilateral to the zoster infection. Whether the angiitis results from direct spread of viral infection from neighboring nerves or represents an allergic reaction during convalescence from zoster has not been established. These complications of herpes zoster have been reviewed by Jamsek and by Hilt and their associates.

The notion that a facial palsy or pain in the distribution of a trigeminal or intercostal nerve, without subsequent rash, is due to herpetic ganglionitis without spread to the skin (zoster sine herpete) is purely speculative. In a few such cases an antibody response to the VZ virus has been found, but the vast majority of cases of Bell's palsy, tic douloureux, and intercostal neuralgia are not associated with serologic evidence of activation of the VZ virus or with any other viral infection.

TREATMENT

During the acute stage analgesics and lotions or powders applied to the skin lesions help to blunt the pain. The administration of corticosteroids has been shown to decrease the incidence of postherpetic neuralgia, though it does not shorten the period of acute pain, and probably carries no hazard in patients with uncomplicated zoster. Corticosteroids are contraindicated in patients with neoplasms or other immunodeficient states because of the increased danger of dissemination of the lesions. In the latter patients a course of adenine arabinoside (vidarabine) may be worthwhile; immunosuppressed patients who receive this drug in the first 6 days of the disease have a more rapid clearance of virus from vesicles and less pain than nontreated controls (Whitley et al). Acyclovir (800 mg five times daily for 7 days) also shortens the duration of acute pain and speeds the healing of vesicles, provided that treatment is begun within 48 h of the appearance of the rash (McKendrick et al). However, neither vidarabine nor acyclovir decreases the incidence of postherpetic neuralgia. All patients with ophthalmic zoster should receive acyclovir orally; in addition, topically applied acyclovir or idoxuridine (IDU) to the eye, either in a 0.1% solution every hour or a 0.5% ointment four or five times a day, is recommended by some ophthalmologists.

The management of postherpetic pain and dysesthesia can be a trying matter for both the patient and the physician. It would appear that incomplete interruption of nerves results in a hyperpathic state, in which every stimulus excites pain. Sometimes, a course of carbamazepine moderates the pain, particularly if it is of lancinating type. It should be emphasized that postherpetic neuralgia eventually subsides even in the most severe and persistent cases. Until this happens, the physician must exercise skill and patience in the medical management of chronic pain (see page 115), and avoid the temptation of subjecting the patient to one of the many surgical measures that have been advocated for this disorder. Excision or undercutting the involved region of skin, section of the spinal nerves or roots, and chordotomy have generally proved to be ineffective, or at best given only temporary relief. Many of the patients with the most persistent complaints have all the symptoms of a depressive state and will be helped by appropriate antidepressive medications.

THE SYNDROME OF ASEPTIC MENINGITIS

The term *aseptic meningitis* was first introduced to designate what was thought to be a specific disease, but it is now applied to a symptom complex that can be produced by any one of numerous infective agents, the majority of which are viral. Since aseptic meningitis is rarely fatal, the precise CNS changes are uncertain, but are presumably limited to the meninges. Conceivably, there may be some minor changes in the brain itself, but these are of insufficient severity to cause neurologic symptoms and signs.

In outline, *the clinical syndrome of aseptic meningitis consists of fever, headache, and other signs of meningeal irritation, and a predominantly lymphocytic pleocytosis with normal CSF glucose.* Usually the onset is acute and the temperature is elevated, from 38 to 40°C. Headache, perhaps more severe than that associated with other febrile states, is the most frequent symptom. A variable degree of lethargy, irritability, and drowsiness may occur; confusion, stupor, and coma are decidedly rare. Photophobia and pain on movement of the eyes are common complaints. Stiffness of the neck and spine on forward bending attests to the presence of meningeal irritation, but at first it may be so slight as to pass unnoticed. Here the Kernig and Brudzinski signs help very little, for they are often absent in the presence of a manifest viral meningitis. Other symptoms and signs are infrequent; these include sore throat, nausea and vomiting, vague weakness, pain in the back and neck, paresthesias in an extremity, isolated strabismus and diplopia, a slight inequality of reflexes, or a wavering Babinski sign. In general, then, the symptoms are mild, and at times the meningitis is entirely asymptomatic. An erythematous papulomacular, nonpruritic rash, confined to the head and neck or generalized, may be a prominent feature (particularly in children) of the aseptic meningitis caused by certain echoviruses and Coxsackie viruses. An enanthem, taking the form of grayish-white spots on the buccal mucosa, may occur with echovirus infections.

The CSF findings consist of a pleocytosis (mainly mononuclear, except in the first day of the illness, when more than half the cells may be neutrophils), and a small and variable increase in protein. Micro-organisms cannot be demonstrated, either by smear or bacterial culture. As a rule, the glucose content of the CSF is normal; this is important because a low glucose concentration, in conjunction with a lymphocytic or mononuclear pleocytosis, usually signifies tuberculous or fungal meningitis, or certain noninfectious disorders such as metastatic carcinoma, lymphoma, or sarcoid of the meninges. Very rarely, a mild depression of the CSF glucose (never below 25 mg/dL) occurs with the meningitis caused by mumps, type 2 herpes simplex, lymphocytic choriomeningitis, or VZ virus. Since the CSF glucose level may be normal or near normal in the early stages of tuberculous or cryptococcal meningitis, this determination should be repeated at intervals until the diagnosis is established or the patient is definitely convalescent.

CAUSES OF ASEPTIC MENINGITIS

Aseptic meningitis is a common occurrence, with an annual incidence rate of 11 to 27 cases per 100,000 population (Beghi et al, Ponka and Pettersson). *The majority of cases of aseptic meningitis are due to viral infections.* Of these the most common are the enteroviral infections—echovirus, Coxsackie, and nonparalytic poliomyelitis, which make up 80 percent of cases in which a specific viral cause can be established. Mumps is the next most common, followed by herpes simplex (type 2), lymphocytic choriomeningitis (LCM), and adenovirus infections. The California virus, which is an arthropod-borne (arbo) virus, is responsible for a small number of cases (usually the arboviruses cause frank encephalitis or meningoencephalitis). All these viral infections, together with leptospirosis, comprise about 95 percent of cases of aseptic meningitis of established etiology. Rarely, the icteric stage of infectious hepatitis is preceded by mild meningitis, the nature of which becomes evident when the jaundice appears. Infectious mononucleosis (Epstein-Barr virus) and rarely a pneumonia caused by *Mycoplasma pneumoniae* may produce what appears to be a primary meningitis.

Recently it has been recognized that infection with human immunodeficiency virus (HIV) may present as an acute, self-limited aseptic meningitis with an infectious mononucleosis-like clinical picture. HIV has been obtained from the CSF in the acute phase of the illness, but seroconversion occurs only later, during convalescence (see further on in this chapter).

Also, recently, and for the first time, herpes simplex virus type 1 (HSV-1) has been isolated from the CSF of a patient with so-called Mollaret meningitis (Steel et al). This is a rare syndrome consisting of recurrent bouts of fever and the signs and symptoms of aseptic meningitis, from which the patient recovers rapidly and spontaneously and for which no cause had been found heretofore. Whether HSV-1 is responsible for all cases of Mollaret meningitis remains to be determined.

It should be noted that in every published series of cases from virus isolation centers, a specific cause cannot be established in a third or more of cases of presumed viral origin.

DIFFERENTIAL DIAGNOSIS OF VIRAL MENINGITIS

Clinical distinctions between the many viral forms of aseptic meningitis cannot be made with a high degree of reliability,

but useful leads can be obtained by attention to certain details of the clinical history and physical examination. It is important to inquire about immunizations, past history of infectious disease, family outbreaks, insect bites, contact with animals, and areas of recent travel. The presence or absence of an epidemic, the season during which the illness occurs, and the geographic location are other helpful data.

The enteroviruses (polioviruses, echoviruses, and Coxsackie viruses) are by far the commonest causes of viral meningitis. Because they grow in the intestinal tract and are spread mainly by the fecal-oral route, family outbreaks are usual and the infections are most common among children. A number of echovirus and Coxsackie virus infections are associated with exanthemata, and group A Coxsackie viruses may in addition be associated with the grayish vesicular lesions of herpangina of the pharyngeal mucosa. Pleurodynia, brachial neuritis, pericarditis, and orchitis are characteristic of group B Coxsackie virus infections. Pain in the back and neck and in the muscles should always suggest poliomyelitis. As has been stated, lower motor neuron weakness may occur with echovirus and Coxsackie virus infections, but it is mild and transient in nature. The peak incidence of enteroviral infections is in August and September. This is true also of infections due to arboviruses, but as a rule the latter cause encephalitis rather than meningitis.

Mumps meningitis occurs sporadically throughout the year, but the highest incidence is in late winter and spring. Males are affected three times more frequently than females. Other manifestations of mumps infection—parotitis, orchitis, oophoritis, and pancreatitis—may or may not be present. It should be noted that orchitis is not specific for mumps but occurs occasionally with group B Coxsackie virus infections, infectious mononucleosis, and lymphocytic choriomeningitis. A definite past history of mumps aids in excluding the disease, since an attack confers lifelong immunity.

The natural host of the LCM virus is the common house mouse, *Mus musculus*. Humans acquire the infection by contact with infected hamsters or with food or dust that is contaminated by mouse excreta. The meningitis may be preceded by respiratory symptoms (sometimes with pulmonary infiltrates) of a week's duration. The infection is particularly common in late fall and winter, presumably because mice enter dwellings at that time.

The infectious agent in leptospirosis is a spirochete, but the clinical syndrome which it produces is indistinguishable from viral meningitis. Infection is acquired by contact with soil or water contaminated by the urine of rats, and also of dogs, swine, and cattle. Although leptospirosis may appear in any season, its incidence in the United States shows a striking peak in August. The presence of conjunctival suffusion, a transient blotchy erythema, severe leg and back pain, and pulmonary infiltrates should suggest leptospiral infection (and also Borreliosis).

Wild rodents may also be the source of encephalomyocarditis virus infection, and cats, of course, of cat-scratch disease. The latter has been found to induce a localized cranial arteritis (Selby and Walker).

The presence of sore throat, generalized lymphadenopathy, transient rash, and mild icterus are suggestive of infectious mononucleosis. Icterus is a prominent manifestation of viral hepatitis.

A mononucleosis type infection (fever, rash, arthralgias, lymphadenopathy) in an individual with recent sexual exposure to a known or potentially infected partner or contaminated blood should always raise the possibility of HIV infection.

Aside from viral isolation and serologic tests, few laboratory examinations are helpful. The peripheral white cell count is usually normal but may sometimes be slightly elevated or depressed. Eosinophilia should suggest a parasitic infection. Most cases of infectious mononucleosis can be identified by the blood smear and specific serologic tests. LCM may produce an intense pleocytosis. Counts above 1000 mononuclear cells per cubic millimeter are most often due to LCM, but may occur occasionally with mumps and with echovirus 9; in the latter, neutrophils may predominate in the CSF for a week or longer. Serologic reactions of CSF should be interpreted with caution because inflammation of many types can produce a false positive reaction; infectious mononucleosis and lupus erythematosus often evoke false positive serum reactions for syphilis. Liver function tests are abnormal in many patients with infectious mononucleosis, leptospiral infections, and anicteric hepatitis; hepatic abnormalities are not regularly present in the other entities under consideration. In the majority of patients with *Mycoplasma pneumoniae* infections, cold agglutinins appear in the serum toward the end of the first week of the illness.

NONVIRAL FORMS OF ASEPTIC MENINGITIS

Four other categories of disease may cause an apparently sterile, predominantly lymphocytic or mononuclear reaction in the leptomeninges: (1) bacterial infections lying adjacent to the meninges, (2) specific meningeal infections or parainfectious diseases in which the organism is difficult or

impossible to isolate, (3) neoplastic invasion (usually lymphoma or carcinoma), and (4) recurrent inflammatory meningitides of obscure origin. The recognition of these is of great importance, since they require vigorous antibiotic therapy or some other form of treatment.

In respect to the first category, a smoldering paranasal sinusitis or mastoiditis may produce a CSF picture of aseptic meningitis because of intracranial extension (epidural or subdural infection). Or a brain abscess, the localizing signs of which are minimal or absent, may deceive the clinician into making a diagnosis of aseptic meningitis (see Chap. 32). Also it must be remembered that antibiotic therapy given for a systemic or pulmonary infection may suppress a coexistent meningitis to the point where mononuclear cells predominate, glucose is near normal, and organisms are not detected in the CSF. A mistaken diagnosis of aseptic meningitis may then be made on the basis of the CSF examination. The true state of affairs becomes evident only when the illness worsens and bacteria again appear in the CSF. Careful attention to the history of recent antimicrobial therapy sometimes permits recognition of these cases before symptoms recur.

Syphilis, cryptococcosis, and tuberculosis are the important members of the second group. Acute syphilitic meningitis may be asymptomatic or symptomatic; in the latter case there will be both the clinical and CSF picture of aseptic meningitis except that the patient is usually afebrile. In former times acute syphilitic meningitis was likely to develop as a neurorecurrence after inadequate arsenic therapy, but now it may be the first manifestation of a florid syphilitic infection (see page 574). Tuberculous meningitis, in its initial stages, may occasionally masquerade as an innocent aseptic meningitis; the diagnosis may be delayed because the tubercle bacillus is frequently difficult to find in stained smears, and cultures require several weeks. Similarly, the diagnosis of cryptococcus is missed occasionally because the organisms may be present in such low numbers as to be overlooked in smears. Brucellosis (Mediterranean fever, Malta fever) is a rare disease, practically confined to the Middle East, that may present as an acute meningitis or meningoencephalitis, with the CSF findings of an aseptic meningitis. Brucella melitensis can rarely be cultured from blood or CSF and diagnosis depends upon the detection of high serum antibody titers and *brucella*-specific immunoglobulins on the enzyme-linked immunosorbent assay (ELISA). Lymphocytic meningitis may occur as a complication of Q fever, a rickettsial disease.

Rarely, children with scarlet fever or streptococcus pharyngitis have been noted to develop meningeal signs and pleocytosis, the result of a sterile serous inflammation that does not involve invasion of the meninges by organisms. The same may occur in subacute bacterial endocarditis.

In the third (neoplastic) group, leukemias and lymphomas are the most common sources of meningeal reactions. In children, a leukemic "meningitis" with cells (lymphoblasts or myeloblasts) in the CSF numbering in the thousands occurs frequently in the late stages of the illness. In adults, a pleocytosis with lymphocyte or lymphoblast counts reaching as high as 4000 per cubic millimeter may complicate lymphomas with or without leukemia. In these disorders and in meningeal carcinomatosis (from lung, breast, melanoma, or other source) great numbers of neoplastic cells may extend through the leptomeninges, involving cranial and spinal nerve roots, and produce a picture of meningoradiculitis with normal or low CSF glucose values. Infiltration of the meninges by a glioma or pinealoma may have the same effect. Millipore filter preparations usually permit identification of the tumor cells. These diseases are discussed in detail in Chap. 31.

Finally, in a number of other chronic or acutely recurring diseases of obscure origin, the CSF formula corresponds to that of aseptic meningitis: (1) The Vogt-Koyanagi-Harada syndrome, which is characterized by various combinations of iridocyclitis, depigmentation of the hair and skin around the eyes, loss of eyelashes, dysacusis, and deafness. The course is quite benign, and the pathologic basis of the syndrome is not known. (2) Mollaret recurrent meningitis, for which there may now be a known viral cause (see above). (3) Allergic or hypersensitivity meningitis, occurring in the course of serum sickness and diseases of connective tissue, such as lupus erythematosus. (4) Behçet disease.

Behçet disease is the most important member of these recurrent inflammatory CNS diseases. It is most common in Japan, the Near East, and the Mediterranean region. Men are affected far more often than women. Originally, the disease was distinguished by the clinical triad of relapsing iridocyclitis, meningitis, and ulcers of mouth and genitalia, but it is now known to be a systemic disease with a much wider range of symptoms, including erythema nodosum, thrombophlebitis, polyarthritis, ulcerative colitis, and a number of neurologic manifestations. The latter occur in about 30 percent of patients (Chajek and Fainaru) and include recurrent meningoencephalitis, cranial nerve (particularly abducens) palsies, cerebellar ataxia, and corticospinal tract signs. There may be episodes of diencephalic and brainstem dysfunction, resembling minor strokes. A few postmortem examinations have related these stroke-like episodes to small, appropriately placed foci of necrosis, along with perivascular and meningeal infiltration with lymphocytes. The neurologic symptoms usually have an abrupt onset and are accompanied by a brisk pleocytosis (lymphocytes or neutrophils may predominate), along with elevated protein but normal glucose values (one of our cases had 3000 neutrophils per cubic millimeter at the onset

of an acute meningitis). As a rule, neurologic symptoms clear completely in several weeks, but they have a tendency to recur, and some patients are left with persistent neurologic deficits. Rarely the clinical picture is that of a progressive confusional state and dementia (see the reviews of Alema and of Lehner and Barnes for detailed accounts of the clinical and immunologic features).

In summary, the history of the illness, the associated clinical findings, and the laboratory tests usually provide the clues to the diagnosis of nonviral forms of aseptic meningitis. Most important is to keep in mind the possibility of tuberculosis, cryptococcosis, syphilis, inadequately treated pyogenic meningitis, and Borreliosis—all of which may simulate aseptic meningitis. These diseases present urgent diagnostic problems, for they may take the life of the patient if they are not recognized and treated. In contrast, the various viral forms of aseptic meningitis are usually self-limited and benign.

THE SYNDROME OF ACUTE ENCEPHALITIS

From the foregoing discussion it is evident that the separation of the clinical syndrome of aseptic meningitis and encephalitis is not always easy. In some patients with aseptic meningitis, drowsiness or confusion may be present. Conversely, in some patients with encephalitis the cerebral symptoms may be mild or inapparent, and only the meningeal symptoms and CSF abnormalities may be manifest. These facts make it difficult to place complete reliance on statistical data from various virus laboratories about the relative incidence of meningitis and encephalitis. Although the same spectrum of viruses causes both meningitis and encephalitis, some cause only benign disease. It is our impression that many cases of enteroviral infection and practically all cases of mumps and LCM are little more than examples of intense meningitis. Rarely have they caused death with postmortem demonstration of cerebral lesions, and surviving patients seldom have residual neurologic signs.

The core of the encephalitis syndrome consists of an acute febrile illness with evidence of meningeal involvement, added to which are various combinations of the following symptoms and signs: convulsions, delirium, confusion, stupor, or coma; aphasia or mutism; hemiparesis with asymmetry of tendon reflexes and Babinski signs; involuntary movements, ataxia, and myoclonic jerks; nystagmus, ocular palsies, and facial weakness. Some one or other of these groups of findings predominates in certain types of encephalitis, as will be pointed out below, but always the clinical diagnosis, in the setting of a febrile aseptic meningitis, rests on the demonstration of derangement of the function of the cerebrum, brainstem, or cerebellum. Death occurs in 5 to 20 percent of patients with acute viral encephalitis and residual signs such as mental deterioration, amnesic defect, personality change, and hemiparesis are seen in about another 20 percent. However, these overall figures fail to reflect the widely varying incidence of mortality and residual neurologic abnormalities that follow infection by different viruses. In herpes simplex encephalitis, for example, the mortality is about 50 percent, and in eastern equine encephalitis, between 20 and 40 percent; and about half of the survivors of these encephalitides have serious neurologic sequelae. On the other hand, neurologic sequelae have been observed in only 5 to 10 percent of those with western equine infections.

ETIOLOGY

Whereas numerous viral, bacterial, fungal, and parasitic agents are listed as causes of the encephalitis syndrome, only the viral ones are considered here, for it is to these that one usually refers when the term *encephalitis* is used. The nonviral forms of encephalitis are considered in Chap. 32.

As with aseptic meningitis, the number of viruses that can cause an encephalitis or a postinfectious allergic reaction is large, and one might suppose that the clinical problems would be infinitely complex. However, the types of viral encephalitis that occur with sufficient frequency to be of diagnostic importance are relatively few, and many of them have a characteristic geographic and seasonal incidence. In the United States, *eastern equine encephalitis*, as the name implies, has been observed mainly in the eastern states; there have been only two recognized outbreaks of this disease in New England, each in the early autumn. *Western equine encephalitis* is fairly uniformly distributed west of the Mississippi. *St. Louis encephalitis*, another arthropod-borne late-summer encephalitis, occurs nationwide but especially along the Mississippi River. *Venezuelan equine encephalitis*, which is common in South and Central America, is practically confined to the southwestern part of the United States and Florida. *California virus encephalitis* predominates in the northern midwest and northeastern states. *Rabies* infections occur nationwide, but mostly in the Middle West and along the West Coast. Japanese B encephalitis, Russian spring-summer encepha-

litis, Murray Valley encephalitis (Australian X disease), and many other viral encephalitides are unknown in the United States.

In a prospective virologic study of all children examined at the Mayo Clinic during the years 1974 to 1976, a diagnosis of aseptic meningitis, meningoencephalitis, or encephalitis was entertained in 42 cases and an infectious agent was identified in 30 of them. (Donat et al). The California virus was isolated in 19 cases, one of the enteroviruses (echovirus types 19, 16, 21 or Coxsackie virus), in 8, and the remainder of the group included mumps, rubeola, herpes simplex, adenovirus 3, and *M. pneumoniae* (several patients had combined infections). The results were similar to other reported series. Only two patients died (one with simplex encephalitis), and the rest recovered without sequelae.

Infectious mononucleosis, which is a primary infection with the Epstein-Barr (E-B) virus, may be complicated by meningitis, encephalitis, facial palsy, or polyneuritis of the Guillain-Barré type. Or, each of these neurologic complications can occur in the absence of the characteristic fever, pharyngitis, and lymphadenopathy. The frequency of the neurologic complications is impossible to state because of the great difficulty in recovering virus from the CSF or nervous tissue and in proving the diagnosis by serologic testing.

Herpes simplex encephalitis, like E-B virus infection, has no particular seasonal incidence or geographic distribution (see below). Definite cases of epidemic (lethargic) encephalitis have seldom been observed in acute form since 1930, though patients with residual symptoms (Parkinson syndrome) are still to be seen in neurology clinics.

Encephalitis or encephalomyelitis that follows measles, rubella, chickenpox, or rabies vaccination by a few days to a week represents a disordered immune reaction of nervous tissue to a preceding viral infection, and is considered with the demyelinative diseases, in Chap. 37.

ARTHROPOD-BORNE (ARBO) VIRUS ENCEPHALITIS

The arbovirus infections that occur in the United States and their geographic range have been listed above. There are alternating cycles of viral infection in mosquitoes and vertebrate hosts; the uninfected mosquito may become infected by taking a blood meal from a viremic host (horse or bird) or, if infected, will inject virus into the host, including humans. The seasonal incidence of these infections is limited to the summer and early fall, when mosquitoes are biting. In the equine encephalitides, regional deaths in horses usually precede human epidemics. In St. Louis encephalitis, the urban bird or animal or possibly the human becomes the intermediate host. These encephalitides occur in epidemics that appear to be related to the migration of infected birds. California virus infections are endemic because of the cycle of infection in small rodents.

The clinical manifestations of the various arbovirus infections are indistinguishable one from the other, although they do vary with the age of the patient. In infants, there may be only an abrupt onset of fever and convulsions. In older children the onset is usually less abrupt, with complaints of headache, listlessness, nausea or vomiting, drowsiness, and fever for several days before medical attention is sought. Convulsions, confusion and stupor, and stiff neck then become prominent. Photophobia, diffuse myalgia, and tremor (sometimes of the intention type) may be observed in this age group and in adults. Reflex asymmetry, hemiparesis, extensor plantar signs, and sucking and grasping reflexes may also occur.

The CSF findings are much the same as in aseptic meningitis. The fever and neurologic signs subside after 4 to 14 days, unless death supervenes or destructive CNS changes have occurred.

The pathologic changes consist of widespread degeneration of single nerve cells with neuronophagia as well as scattered foci of inflammatory necrosis involving both the gray and white matter. The brainstem is relatively spared. In eastern equine encephalitis the destructive lesions may be massive, involving the major part of a lobe or hemisphere, but in the other arbovirus infections the foci are microscopic in size. Perivascular cuffing by lymphocytes and other mononuclear leukocytes and plasma cells, and a patchy infiltration of the meninges with similar cells are the other histopathologic hallmarks of viral encephalitis.

Of the arbovirus infections in the United States, eastern equine encephalitis is the most serious since a large proportion of those infected develop encephalitis, and of the latter, about two-thirds die or are left with severe disabling abnormalities—mental retardation, emotional disorders, recurrent seizures, blindness, deafness, hemiplegia, and speech disorders. Fortunately, eastern equine encephalitis is also the least frequent of the arbovirus infections. The mortality rate in other arbovirus infections varies from 2 to 12 percent in different outbreaks, and the incidence of serious sequelae is about the same.

HERPES SIMPLEX ENCEPHALITIS (ACUTE INCLUSION BODY ENCEPHALITIS)

This is the commonest and gravest form of acute encephalitis. About 2000 cases occur yearly in the United States; between 30 and 70 percent of these are fatal, and the majority of patients who survive are left with serious neurologic abnormalities. It is the only common form of encephalitis that occurs sporadically throughout the year and in patients of all ages and in all parts of the world. It

is due almost always to the type 1 herpes simplex virus which is also the cause of the common herpetic lesions of the oral mucosa; rarely, however, are the oral lesions associated with encephalitis. The type 2 virus may also cause acute encephalitis, but only in the neonate and in relation to genital herpetic infection in the mother. Occasionally, the localized adult type of encephalitis is caused by the type 2 virus and the diffuse neonatal encephalitis by type 1. Type 2 infection in the adult may cause an aseptic meningitis, and sometimes a polyradiculitis or myelitis, again in association with a recent genital herpes infection.

The symptoms, which evolve over several days, are in most cases like those of any other acute encephalitis, viz., fever, headache, seizures, confusion, stupor, and coma. In some patients these manifestations are preceded by symptoms and findings that betray the propensity of this disease to involve the inferomedial portions of the frontal and temporal lobes. These latter manifestations include olfactory or gustatory hallucinations, anosmia, temporal lobe seizures, a brief period of personality change, bizarre or psychotic behavior, aphasia, and hemiparesis. Very rarely an affection of memory can be recognized, but usually this only becomes evident later, in the convalescent stage of the illness. Swelling and herniation of one or both temporal lobes through the tentorium may occur, leading to deep coma and respiratory arrest during the first 24 to 72 h.

The CSF is often under increased pressure, and almost invariably shows a pleocytosis (range 10 to 500 cells per cubic millimeter, usually less than 200). Mainly the cells are lymphocytes, but occasionally there is a significant number of neutrophils. Red cells, sometimes numbering in the thousands, and xanthochromia are found in some cases, reflecting the hemorrhagic nature of the lesions. The protein content is increased in most cases. Rarely, the CSF glucose levels may be reduced to slightly less than 40 mg/dL, creating confusion with tuberculous and fungal meningitides. The herpes simplex virus can rarely be isolated from the CSF.

The lesions take the form of an intense hemorrhagic necrosis of the inferior and medial parts of the temporal lobes and the orbital parts of the frontal lobes. This distribution of lesions is so characteristic that the diagnosis can be made by simple inspection. Cases described in past years as *acute necrotizing encephalitis* were probably instances of herpes simplex encephalitis. In the acute stages of the disease, intranuclear eosinophilic inclusions are found in neurons and glial cells, in addition to the usual microscopic abnormalities of acute encephalitis.

The unique localization of the lesions in this disease

could possibly be explained by the route(s) of virus entry into the CNS. Two such routes have been suggested (Davis and Johnson). The virus is thought to be latent in the trigeminal ganglia and, with reactivation, to infect the nose and then the olfactory tract. Alternatively, with activation in the trigeminal ganglia, the infection may spread along fibers that innervate the leptomeninges of the anterior and middle fossae. The lack of lesions in the olfactory bulbs in as many as 40 percent of fatal cases (Esiri) is a point in favor of the second pathway.

The *diagnosis* may be difficult. Acute herpes simplex encephalitis must be distinguished from other types of viral encephalitis, acute hemorrhagic leukoencephalitis (page 767) and from subdural empyema, cerebral abscess, thrombophlebitis, and septic embolism (Chap. 32). The EEG changes, consisting of periodic high-voltage sharp waves in the temporal regions, and slow-wave complexes at regular 2 to 3 per second intervals are suggestive though not specific for the disease. The CT scan is helpful in 50 to 60 percent of cases (Fig. 33-2); low-density, nonenhancing areas with surrounding edema and sometimes with scattered areas of hemorrhage occupy the inferior parts of the frontal and

Figure 33-2

Herpes simplex encephalitis. Contrast-enhanced scan showing asymmetrical areas of inflammation and necrosis involving inferior portions of the frontal and temporal lobes.

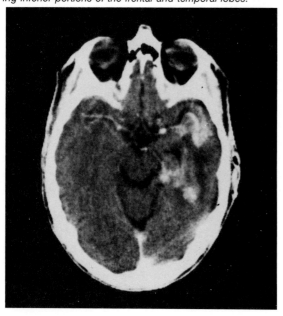

temporal lobes. A rising titer of neutralizing antibodies can be demonstrated from the acute to the convalescent stage, but this is not of diagnostic help in the acutely ill patient and may not be etiologically significant in patients with recurrent herpes infections of the oral mucosa. At present, the only certain way to establish the diagnosis of acute herpes simplex encephalitis is by fluorescent antibody study and by viral culture of cerebral tissue obtained by brain biopsy.

Until recently there has been no specific *treatment* for herpes simplex encephalitis. A collaborative study, sponsored by the National Institutes of Health, has indicated that the antiviral agent, adenine arabinoside (vidarabine), significantly reduces both the mortality and morbidity from herpes simplex encephalitis; moreover, early treatment (when the patient is only lethargic and not stuporous or comatose) with this drug increases the chances of survival (Whitley et al, 1977, 1981). Vidarabine is given intravenously, 15 mg/kg daily for 10 days. The drug is relatively nontoxic, but its administration requires a large amount of fluid; the judicious use of diuretics as well as corticosteroids for brief periods helps to control brain swelling and prevent herniation. Subsequently it was shown by Skoldenberg et al and by Whitley et al that acyclovir (30 mg/kg per day for 10 days) is significantly more effective than vidarabine in terms of both mortality and morbidity. Recent observations indicate that a longer course of the drug (14 days) is necessary to prevent relapse (Whitley). In some instances it is feasible to do a brain biopsy in order to confirm the diagnosis, but the authors do not consider this procedure to be necessary in every suspected case. If the diagnosis is reasonably certain, it is preferable to proceed at once with treatment than to lose the time required to obtain a brain biopsy and to find appropriate laboratory facilities for immunocytochemical and electron microscopic studies.

The *outcome* of this disease, both the mortality and morbidity, is governed to a large extent by the patient's age and state of consciousness at the time of institution of vidarabine therapy. Lethargic patients under 30 years of age have a mortality of about 25 percent, compared to more than 50 percent for semicomatose or comatose patients over 30 years of age. More importantly, only 10 percent or less of survivors escape neurologic sequelae if treatment is initiated after the onset of coma. The neurologic sequelae are of the most serious type, consisting of a Korsakoff amnesic defect or global dementia, seizures, and dysphasia.

ENCEPHALITIS LETHARGICA (VON ECONOMO DISEASE, SLEEPING SICKNESS)

Although examples of a somnolent-ophthalmoplegic encephalitis dot the early medical literature (e.g., nona, febre lethargica, schlafkrankheit), it was in the wake of the influenza pandemic of World War I that this disease burst on the medical horizon and continued to occur for about 10 years. No disease just like it had been recorded before 1914. Although the viral agent was never identified, the clinical and pathologic features were typical of viral infection. The unique symptoms were ophthalmoplegia and pronounced somnolence, from which the disease took its name. A small proportion of the patients were overly active rather than somnolent, and a third group had manifested a disorder of movement in the form of bradykinesia, catalepsy, mutism, chorea or myoclonus. Headache, dizziness, fatigability, and frank confusional psychosis were common features. In contrast, paralysis (hemiplegia), cortical sensory loss, aphasia, disorders of hearing and vision, and convulsions were notably infrequent. The onset was acute or subacute, and the symptoms persisted for several weeks. Lymphocytic pleocytosis was found in half the patients, together with variable elevation of the CSF protein content. More than 20 percent of the victims died within a few weeks, and many survivors were left with varying degrees of impairment of mental function. Also, after an interval of months or years (occasionally as long as 25 years) a high proportion of survivors developed the syndrome of parkinsonism, as described on page 938. In fact, this is the only form of encephalitis known to cause an immediate or delayed extrapyramidal syndrome of this type (a similar though not identical syndrome may follow Japanese B encephalitis). Myoclonus, dystonia, oculogyric crises (page 210) and other muscle spasms, bulimia, obesity, reversal of the sleep pattern, and, in children, a change in personality with compulsive behavior, were other distressing sequelae.

The pathology was typical of a viral infection (nerve cell destruction and neuronophagia, perivascular cuffing with lymphocytes and other mononuclear cells, and meningeal infiltrations of similar cells), localized principally to regions of the midbrain, subthalamus, and hypothalamus. In the patients who died years later with a Parkinson syndrome, depigmentation of the substantia nigra and locus ceruleus due to nerve cell destruction, fibrillary changes in the nerve cells of the substantia nigra, oculomotor and adjacent nuclei, and gliosis were the only findings.

Few new cases have been seen in the United States and western Europe since 1930. Sporadic cases such as the four reported by Howard and Lees may be examples of this disease, but there is no way of proving their identity. The only treatment available for the few survivors consists of administration of L-dopa and other antiparkinsonian drugs, as outlined on page 941.

The importance of encephalitis lethargica relates to (1) the unique clinical syndromes and sequelae (Parkinson syndrome, tics, sleep disorder, oculogyric crises, psychopathic behavioral states), and (2) its place as the first

recognized slow virus infection of the nervous system in human beings.

RABIES

This disease stands apart from other acute viral infections by virtue of the long latent period that follows inoculation with the virus and its distinctive clinical and pathologic features. Human cases of this disease are rare: since 1960 there have never been more than five reported cases yearly in the United States, and in some areas (Australia, Hawaii, Great Britain, and the Scandinavian peninsula) no indigenous cases have ever been reported. The importance of this disease derives from two facts: it is almost invariably fatal once the characteristic clinical features appear, and the survival of the inoculated individual depends upon the institution of specific therapeutic measures before the infection becomes clinically evident. Furthermore, each year 20,000 to 30,000 individuals are treated with rabies vaccine because of contacts with animals that might have been rabid, and although the incidence of complications of rabies vaccination is much lower than before, serious reactions continue to be encountered (see below and also Chap. 37).

Etiology   Practically all cases of rabies are the result of inoculation of the virus through the skin by an animal bite. In underdeveloped countries, where rabies is relatively common, the most frequent source is the rabid dog. In western Europe and the United States the most common rabid species are skunks, foxes, bats, and racoons, among wild animals, and dogs and cats among domestic ones. Because rabid animals commonly bite without provocation, the nature of the attack should be determined. Also, the prevalence of animal rabies virus varies widely in the United States, and local presence of the disease should be assessed. As indicated earlier, the virus spreads along peripheral nerves to reach the nervous system.

Clinical Features   The incubation period is usually 20 to 60 days, but may be as short as 14 days, especially in cases with multiple deep bites around the face and neck. The initial neurologic symptoms (following a 2- to 4-day prodromal period of fever, headache, and malaise) consist of severe anxiety and speech and psychomotor overactivity, followed by dysphagia (hence salivation and "frothing at the mouth"), spasms of throat muscles induced by attempts to swallow water (hence hydrophobia), dysarthria, numbness of the face, and spasms of facial muscles—to which are added generalized seizures and a confusional psychosis.

This localization indicates the intensive involvement of the tegmental medullary nuclei in the *rabid* form of the disease. A less common *paralytic form,* due to spinal cord affection, may accompany or replace the state of excitement. Coma gradually follows the acute neurologic symptoms and death ensues within 4 to 10 days.

Pathologic Features   The disease is distinguished by the presence of cytoplasmic eosinophilic inclusions, the Negri bodies. They are most prominent in the pyramidal cells of the hippocampus and the Purkinje cells, but have been seen in nerve cells throughout the CNS. In addition there may be widespread perivascular cuffing and meningeal infiltration with lymphocytes and mononuclear cells and small foci of inflammatory necrosis, as one sees in other viral infections. The focal collections of microglia in this disease are referred to as *Babes nodules.*

Treatment   Bites and scratches should be thoroughly washed with soap and water and, after all soap has been removed, cleansed with benzyl ammonium chloride (Zephiran), which has been shown to inactivate the virus. Wounds that have broken the skin require tetanus prophylaxis, as described on page 908.

After a bite by a seemingly healthy animal, surveillance of the animal for a 10-day period is necessary. Should signs of illness appear in the animal, it should be killed and the brain sent, under refrigeration, to a government-designated laboratory for appropriate diagnostic tests. Wild animals, if captured, should be killed and the brain examined in the same way.

If the animal is found by fluorescent-antibody or other tests to be rabid or if the patient was bitten by a wild animal that escaped, the patient should receive *postexposure prophylaxis.* Human rabies immune globulin (HRIG), which avoids the complications of equine antirabies serum, should be given in a dose of 20 units per kilogram of body weight (one-half infiltrated around the wound and one-half intramuscularly). This provides passive immunization for 10 to 20 days, allowing time for active immunization. In the recent past, duck embryo vaccine (DEV) was used for the latter purpose and greatly reduced the danger of serious allergic reactions in the CNS (encephalomyelitis) from about 1 in 1000 cases to 1 in 20,000 cases. A more recently developed rabies vaccine, grown on a human diploid cell line (HDCV), has reduced the doses needed to just five (from the 23 needed with DEV); these are given as 1-mL injections on the day of exposure and then on days 3, 7, 14, and 28 after the first dose. The new vaccine has

increased the rate of antibody response and reduced even further the allergic reactions by practically eliminating foreign protein. Recent improvements in the intensive care of respiratory and other vital functions have resulted in survival of proven cases of rabies encephalitis. A thorough trial of the new antiviral agents on patients already symptomatic has not been undertaken.

Persons at risk for rabies, such as animal handlers and laboratory workers, should receive pre-exposure vaccination with HDCV.

SUBACUTE AND CHRONIC VIRAL INFECTIONS SIMULATING DEGENERATIVE DISEASE

The idea that viral infections may lead to chronic disease, especially of the nervous system, has been entertained for more than half a century, but only in relatively recent years has it been firmly established. The following indirect and direct evidence supports this view: (1) the demonstration of a slowly progressive noninflammatory degeneration of nigral neurons long after an attack of encephalitis lethargica; (2) the finding of inclusion bodies in cases of subacute and chronic sclerosing encephalitis; (3) the discovery of chronic degenerative diseases in sheep caused by a virus-like agent (scrapie) and by a conventional RNA virus (visna); both are transmissible. It was in relation to these diseases in sheep that Sigurdsson first used the term *slow infection,* to indicate long incubation periods, during which the animals appeared well; (4) the demonstration by electron microscopy of viral particles in the lesions of multifocal leukoencephalopathy and, later, isolation of the virus from the lesions; and (5) the transmission of kuru and subacute spongiform encephalopathy (*Creutzfeldt-Jakob* disease) to chimpanzees and from one chimpanzee to another. It has been suggested that the late onset of motor system disease after poliomyelitis may represent a slow infection (Mulder et al), but such a relationship has never been established. Claims have also been made by several Soviet scientists for a viral causation of multiple sclerosis, amyotrophic lateral sclerosis, and other degenerative diseases, but the evidence is questionable.

The slow infections of the nervous system are of two general types: (1) those due to conventional viruses, viz., subacute sclerosing panencephalitis, progressive rubella panencephalitis, and progressive multifocal leukoencephalopathy (and visna in sheep), and (2) those due to unconventional agents, viz., kuru and subacute spongiform encephalopathy (and mink encephalopathy and scrapie in sheep). Although the agents producing these latter disorders are transmissible and capable of replication, they are insensitive to the various forms of physicochemical treatment that inactivate conventional viruses, they do not cause an immune response, and viral particles have not been seen in infected tissue. These unconventional agents have been referred to as *subacute spongiform encephalopathy agents* and as *slow viruses,* but they probably represent a new type of transmissible agent.

The aforementioned slow infections so perfectly simulate degenerative disease that notions about many other diseases of white and gray matter of the brain, presently classified as degenerative, are being altered. One of the most exciting prospects in medical neurology is thus unfolding before us.

SUBACUTE SCLEROSING PANENCEPHALITIS (SSPE)

This disease was first described by Dawson in 1934, under the title "inclusion body encephalitis," and extensively studied by Van Bogaert, who named it *subacute sclerosing leukoencephalitis.* The condition is rare, about one case per million children per year. In the United States, measles vaccination has greatly reduced the incidence, but the National SSPE Registry continues to record 10 to 20 new cases each year (some of which may be vaccine-induced).

SSPE affects children and adolescents for the most part, rarely appearing beyond the age of 18 years. Typically there is a history of primary measles infection at a very early age, often before 2 years, followed by a 6- to 8-year asymptomatic period. The illness evolves in several stages. Initially there is a decline in proficiency at school, temper outbursts and other changes in personality, difficulty with language, and loss of interest in usual activities. These soon give way to the second stage, in which there occurs a severe and progressive intellectual deterioration, in association with focal or generalized seizures, widespread myoclonus, ataxia, and sometimes visual disturbances due to progressive chorioretinitis. As the disease advances, rigidity, hyperactive reflexes, Babinski signs, progressive unresponsiveness, and signs of autonomic dysfunction appear. In the final stage the child lies insensate, virtually "decorticated." The course is usually steadily progressive, death occurring within 1 to 3 years. In about 10 percent of cases the course is more prolonged, with one or more remissions. In a similar number the course is fulminating, leading to death within 3 months.

The EEG shows a characteristic abnormality consisting of periodic (every 5 to 8 s) bursts of 2 to 3 per second high-voltage waves, followed by a relatively flat pattern. The CSF contains few or no cells, but the protein is increased, particularly the gamma globulin. In addition, agarose gel electrophoresis shows oligoclonal bands of IgG. These have been shown to represent measles-virus specific antibody (Mehta et al). High levels of neutralizing antibody

to measles (rubeola) virus have been found in serum and CSF, but the virus has been recovered from the brain tissue only with difficulty in a few instances.

The *lesions* involve the cerebral cortex and white matter of both hemispheres and the brainstem. The cerebellum is usually spared. Destruction of nerve cells, neuronophagia, and perivenous cuffing by lymphocytes and mononuclear cells indicate the viral nature of the infection. In the white matter there is degeneration of medullated fibers (myelin and axis cylinders), accompanied by perivascular cuffing with mononuclear cells and fibrous gliosis (sclerosing encephalitis). Eosinophilic inclusions, the histopathologic hallmark of the disease, are found in the cytoplasm and nuclei of neurons and glial cells. Virions, thought to be measles nucleocapsids, have been observed in inclusion-bearing cells examined with the electron microscope.

How a ubiquitous and transient viral infection in a seemingly normal young child allows the development, many years later, of a relatively rare encephalitis is a matter of speculation. Sever believes that there is a delay in the development of immune responses during the initial infection, with the subsequent development of immune responses that are imperfect and incapable of clearing the suppressed infection. An alternative explanation (Hall et al) is that certain brain cells fail to synthesize a so-called M protein, which is essential for the assembly of the viral membrane, and that this limitation of host cell capability is related to the extent of viral seeding of the brain during the initial infection.

The *differential diagnosis* includes the childhood and adolescent dementing diseases such as lipid storage diseases (Chap. 38) and Schilder disease (page 764). In presumptive cases of SSPE, the findings of periodic complexes in the EEG, elevated gamma globulin in the CSF, and elevated measles-antibody titers in the serum and CSF are sufficient to make the diagnosis. To date, no effective treatment has been available, although the administration of the antiviral drug inosiplex has been found by some authors to cause improvement and to prolong survival (Robertson et al, Dyken et al). Other authors have not corroborated these effects (Haddad and Risk). The therapeutic value of alpha interferon is still under investigation.

SUBACUTE MEASLES ENCEPHALITIS WITH IMMUNOSUPPRESSION

Whereas SSPE occurs in children who were previously normal, another type of measles encephalitis develops both in children and adults with defective cell-mediated immune responses (Wolinsky et al). In this latter type, measles, or exposure to measles, precedes the encephalitis by 1 to 6 months. Seizures (often epilepsia partialis continua), focal neurologic signs, stupor, and coma are the main features of the neurologic illness and lead to death within a few days to a few weeks. The CSF may be normal, and levels of measles antibodies do not increase. Aicardi et al have isolated measles virus from the brain of such a patient. The lesions are similar to those of SSPE (eosinophilic inclusions in neurons and glia, with varying degrees of necrosis) except that inflammatory changes are lacking. In a sense this subacute measles encephalitis is an opportunistic infection of the brain in an immunodeficient patient. The short interval between exposure and onset of neurologic disease, the rapid course, and lack of antibodies distinguish subacute measles encephalitis from both SSPE and post-measles encephalomyelitis (Chap. 37).

PROGRESSIVE RUBELLA PANENCEPHALITIS

Generally the deficits associated with congenital rubella infection are nonprogressive at least after the second or third year of life (page 996). There are however, descriptions of children with the congenital rubella syndrome in whom a progressive neurologic deterioration occurred after a stable period of 8 to 19 years (Townsend et al, Weil et al). In 1978, Wolinsky described 10 cases of this syndrome, a few of them apparently related to acquired rather than to congenital rubella. Since then, this late-appearing, progressive syndrome seems to have disappeared, no new cases having been reported in the past decade.

The clinical syndrome in these cases has been quite uniform. On a background of the fixed stigmata of congenital rubella, there occurs a deterioration in behavior and school performance, often associated with seizures, and soon thereafter, a progressive impairment of mental function (dementia). Clumsiness of gait is an early symptom, followed by a frank ataxia of gait and then of the limbs. Spasticity and other corticospinal tract signs, dysarthria, and dysphagia ensue. Pallor of the optic discs, ophthalmoplegia, spastic quadriplegia, and mutism mark the final phase of the illness.

The CSF shows a mild increase in cells (lymphocytes), a modest elevation of protein, and a marked increase in the proportion of gamma globulin (35 to 52 percent of the total protein), which assumes an oligoclonal pattern when analyzed by agarose gel electrophoresis. The CSF and serum rubella-antibody titers are elevated.

Pathologic examination of the brain has shown a widespread, progressive subacute panencephalitis mainly affecting the white matter. No inclusion-bearing cells were seen. Thus it appears that rubella virus infection, acquired in utero or in the postnatal period, may persist in the nervous system for years, before rekindling a chronic active infection.

Analogies have been drawn between this disorder and the chronic encephalitis associated with the rubeola virus (SSPE). The latter disorder has not been associated with maternal infection, however; furthermore, myoclonus and EEG abnormalities are not as prominent as in SSPE, and inclusion bodies, which characterize SSPE, have not been observed in the patients with progressive rubella panencephalitis.

PROGRESSIVE MULTIFOCAL LEUKOENCEPHALOPATHY (PML)

This disorder, observed originally by the authors in 1952, has been fully described morphologically by Åström and his colleagues and by Richardson. It is characterized by widespread demyelinative lesions, mainly of the cerebral hemispheres, but also of the brainstem and cerebellum, and rarely of the spinal cord. The lesions vary greatly in size and severity—from microscopic foci of demyelination to massive zones of destruction of both myelin and axis cylinders involving the major part of a cerebral hemisphere. There are distinctive abnormalities of the glial cells. Many of the reactive astrocytes in the lesions are gigantic and contain deformed and bizarre-shaped nuclei and mitotic figures, changes that are seen otherwise only in malignant glial tumors. Also, at the periphery of the lesions, the nuclei of oligodendrocytes are greatly enlarged and contain abnormal inclusions. Vascular changes are lacking, and inflammatory changes are usually insignificant.

Clinical Features An uncommon disease of late adult life, PML rarely occurs independently. Usually it is associated with chronic neoplastic disease (mainly chronic lymphocytic leukemia, Hodgkin disease, lymphosarcoma, myeloproliferative disease) and less often with nonneoplastic granulomatosis, such as tuberculosis or sarcoid. A number of cases have occurred in patients with AIDS (see further on) and in those receiving immunosuppressive drugs for renal transplantation and for other reasons. The neurologic disorder evolves over a period of several days to weeks. Hemiparesis progressing to quadriparesis, visual field defects, cortical blindness, aphasia, ataxia, dysarthria, dementia, confusional states, and coma are the typical manifestations. Seizures and cerebellar ataxia are rare. In most cases death occurs in 3 to 6 months from the onset of neurologic symptoms. The CSF is usually normal. The

CT scan in several personally observed cases has localized the lesions (which appear as low-density, nonenhancing areas) with striking accuracy.

Pathogenesis Waksman's original suggestion (quoted by Richardson) that PML could be due to viral infection of the CNS in patients with impaired immunologic responses, proved to be correct. ZuRhein and Chou (1965), in an electron microscopic study of cerebral lesions from a patient with PML, demonstrated crystalline arrays of particles resembling papovaviruses in the inclusion-bearing oligodendrocytes. Since then, a human polyoma virus, designated ''JC virus'' or JCV, has been implicated as the causative agent (Padgett et al). A related virus, simian virus 40 (SV 40), has been found in two cases (Johnson et al).

Treatment The disease is generally believed to be untreatable and to end fatally in 3 to 20 months. Several anecdotal reports of the efficacy of cytosine arabinoside have appeared, but an equal number of reports have denied such an effect. Vidarabine, a less toxic drug, has been used in several patients with PML without success.

THE SUBACUTE SPONGIFORM ENCEPHALOPATHIES

This category of diseases, as indicated earlier, includes scrapie in sheep, and kuru and so-called Creutzfeldt-Jakob disease in humans.

Kuru, first recognized among the Fore natives of the New Guinea highlands, was the first slow infection documented in human beings. Clinically the disease takes the form of an afebrile, progressive cerebellar ataxia, with abnormalities of extraocular movements, weakness progressing to immobility, incontinence in the late stages, and death within 3 to 6 months of onset. The remarkable epidemiologic and pathologic similarities between kuru and scrapie were pointed out by Hadlow (1959), who suggested that it might be possible to transmit kuru to subhuman primates. This was accomplished in 1966 by Gajdusek, Gibbs, and Alpers; a kuru-like syndrome was transmitted to chimpanzees after a latency of 18 to 36 months. Since then the disease has been transmitted from one chimpanzee to another, and to other primates, by both neural and nonneural tissues. The transmissible agent has not been visualized, however.

The incidence of kuru has decreased markedly in recent years, probably because of the cessation of ritual cannibalism, by which the disease had been transmitted. In this ritual, infected tissue was ingested and rubbed over the body of the victim's kin (women and young children of either sex) permitting absorption of the infective agent through conjunctivae, mucous membranes, and abrasions in the skin.

Subacute Spongiform Encephalopathy (Heidenhain Disease, Creutzfeldt-Jackob Disease) These terms refer to a distinctive cerebral disease, in which a rapidly progressive and profound dementia is associated with cerebellar ataxia and diffuse myoclonic jerks. The major neuropathologic changes are in the cerebral and cerebellar cortices; the outstanding features of the lesions are widespread neuronal loss and gliosis accompanied by a striking vacuolation or spongy state of the affected regions—hence the designation *subacute spongiform encephalopathy* (SSE). Less severe changes in a patchy distribution are found in cases with a brief clinical course.

These changes, both clinical and pathologic, occur with such uniformity from case to case that they doubtless form a nosologic entity. It is frequently referred to as Creutzfeldt-Jakob disease, an inappropriate term in the authors' opinion, since it seems to us unlikely that SSE and the somewhat ill-defined syndrome(s) described by Creutzfeldt and Jakob are truly the same disease. Pending further knowledge, at any rate, we believe that they should be kept distinct from one another, or at least, whenever one speaks of Creutzfeldt-Jakob disease, it should be specified what is meant—either subacute spongiform encephalopathy or the slower progressive dementia with signs of pyramidal and extrapyramidal affection originally described by Creutzfeldt and Jakob (the latter condition is discussed on page 935). Precision in definition of these states is of greater importance now than before, since it was shown by Gibbs et al that brain tissue from patients with SSE, injected into chimpanzees, can transmit the disease after an incubation period of a year or longer. These workers have recently developed a much more rapid means of diagnosis of SSE as well as of kuru and the Gerstmann-Straussler syndrome (see below). Preparations of brain tissue from such patients (but not from patients with other degenerative diseases) were found to react against an antiserum to a similar fraction made from scrapie-infected hamster brain (Brown et al).

Pathology As already indicated, the disease affects principally the cerebral and cerebellar cortices, generally in a diffuse fashion, although in some cases the occipitoparietal regions are almost exclusively involved, as in those described by Heidenhain. The degeneration and disappearance of nerve cells is associated with extensive astroglial proliferation; ultrastructural studies have shown that the microscopic vacuoles, which give the tissue its typically spongy appearance, are located within the cytoplasmic processes of glial cells and dendrites of nerve cells. Despite the fact that the disease is due to a transmissible agent, possibly a virus, the lesions show no evidence of an inflammatory reaction.

Epidemiology and pathogenesis The disease appears in all parts of the world and in all seasons, with an annual incidence of 0.45 case per million of population. (Matthews). In Israelis of Libyan origin and in immigrants to France from North Africa, the incidence is much higher, for reasons that are not understood. Although the reported incidence of SSE is somewhat higher in urban than in rural areas, temporospatial clustering of cases has not been observed, at least in the United States. A small proportion of all series of cases is familial—varying from 5 percent reported by Cathala et al to 15 percent of 1435 cases analyzed by Masters et al. The occurrence of familial cases suggests a genetic susceptibility to infection, although the possibility of common exposure to the transmissible agent cannot be dismissed. The only clearly demonstrated mechanism of spread of SSE is iatrogenic, having occurred in a few cases after corneal transplantation, after implantation of infected depth electrodes, and after the injection of human growth hormone that had been prepared from pooled cadaveric pituitary glands (Gibbs et al). Individuals exposed to scrapie-infected sheep and to patients with SSE are not disproportionately affected by the disease.

Clinical features Transmissible SSE is in most cases a disease of late middle age, although it can occur in young adults. The sexes are affected equally. In the large series reported by Brown and by Bernoulli and their colleagues, prodromal symptoms, consisting of fatigue, depression, weight loss, and disorders of sleep and appetite and lasting for several weeks, were observed in about one-third of the patients.

The early stages of the disease are characterized by a great variety of clinical manifestations, but the most frequent are changes in behavior, emotional response, and intellectual function, together with abnormalities of cerebellar function and vision, such as distortions of the shape and alignment of objects or actual impairment of visual acuity. In some instances cerebellar ataxia precedes the mental changes. In many instances the early phase of the disease is dominated by symptoms of delirium—hallucinations, delusions, confusion, and agitation. Characteristically, the disease progresses rapidly, so that obvious deterioration may be seen from week to week and even day

to day. Sooner or later, in almost all cases, myoclonic contractions of various muscle groups appear, perhaps unilaterally at first, but later becoming generalized. These are associated with a striking startle response, mainly to a loud noise. In general, the myoclonic jerks are evocable by sensory stimuli of all sorts, but they occur spontaneously as well. Twitches of individual fingers are typical. Ataxia and dysarthria are likewise prominent. These changes gradually give way to stupor and coma, but the myoclonic contractions may continue to the end. In many but not all the patients, the EEG pattern is distinctive, changing over the course of the disease from one of diffuse and nonspecific slowing to one of stereotyped high-voltage slow and sharp wave complexes on an increasingly flat background ("burst suppression"). The high-voltage sharp waves are synchronous with the myoclonus but persist in its absence. Blood and CSF are normal.

The disease is invariably fatal, usually in less than a year from the onset. In about 10 percent of patients, the illness begins with almost stroke-like suddenness and runs its course rapidly, in a matter of a few weeks or months. A small number of patients have reportedly survived for 2 to 10 years, but these cases should be accepted with caution; in some of them, SSE appears to have been superimposed on Alzheimer or Parkinson or other chronic disease.

Masters et al first reported the production of a spongiform encephalopathy in chimpanzees inoculated with brain tissue from three of seven patients with the so-called *Gerstmann-Sträussler-Scheinker syndrome*. This is a rare, strongly familial disease of insidious onset and chronic course (mean duration 5 years). It is characterized by a progressive cerebellar ataxia, often with dementia, and by diffuse neuronal loss and deposition of amyloid plaques in the cerebral and cerebellar cortices, with relatively mild but characteristic spongy changes (page 937). This syndrome probably represents a familial form of Creutzfeldt-Jakob disease, of slowly progressive type.

Differential diagnosis The diagnosis of most cases of SSE presents no difficulty. Not infrequently, however, we have been surprised by a "typical" case that proves to be some other disease. The early stages of lithium intoxication, metabolic-encephalopathy, carcinomatous meningitis, or even Schilder disease may mimic SSE. Contrariwise, the early mental changes of SSE may be misinterpreted as an atypical or unusually intense emotional reaction to environmental factors or as one of the major psychoses. Patients presenting in the later stages of SSE may for a time be taken to have Alzheimer disease with myoclonus or the Parkinson–amyotrophic lateral sclerosis–dementia syndrome, until the rapidly evolving clinical picture clarifies the issue. SSPE (see above) in its fully developed form resembles SSE, but the former is chiefly a disease of children or young adults, and the CSF shows elevation of gamma globulin (IgG), whereas the latter is essentially a disease of middle age and the presenile period, and the CSF is normal. Cerebral lipidosis in children or young adults can result in a similar combination of myoclonus and dementia, but the clinical course in such cases is extremely chronic, and there are retinal changes that do not occur in SSE.

Management No specific treatment is known. The antiviral agents amantadine, vidarabine, and acyclovir have been ineffective. In view of the transmissibility of the disease from humans to primates and iatrogenically from patient to patient, certain precautions should be taken in the medical care of and handling of materials from patients with SSE. The precautions are similar to those recommended for patients with hepatitis B. Special isolation rooms are not necessary. The transmissible agent is resistant to boiling, formalin, alcohol, and ultraviolet radiation, but can be inactivated by autoclaving at 132°C and 15 lb/in^2 for 1 h or by immersion for 1 h in 5% sodium hypochlorite (household bleach). Workers exposed to infected materials should wash thoroughly with ordinary soap. Needles, glassware, needle electrodes, and other instruments should be handled with great care and immersed in appropriate disinfectants or incinerated. Possible contact with blood or urine requires that gloves be worn. The performance of a brain biopsy or autopsy does not carry a special risk. Obviously such patients or any others known to have been demented should not be donors of organs for transplantation.

All aspects of the slow transmissible diseases of the nervous system are discussed in a two-volume publication, edited by Prusiner and Hadlow, and in a recent review by Matthews.

THE ACQUIRED IMMUNE-DEFICIENCY SYNDROME (AIDS)

In the late 1970s physicians became aware of the frequent occurrence of otherwise rare opportunistic infections and neoplasms—notably pneumocystis carinii pneumonia and Kaposi sarcoma—in urban homosexual men and drug abusers. The study of these patients led to the recognition of a new viral disease. As the name indicates, it is characterized by an acquired and usually profound depression of cell-mediated immunity (cutaneous anergy, lymphopenia, reversal of the T-helper/T-suppressor cell ratio, and depressed in vitro lymphoproliferative response to various antigens and mitogens). It is this that explains the development of a wide range of opportunistic infections and unusual neoplasms. Virtually all organ systems are vulnerable, including the central and peripheral nervous

systems and muscle. Moreover, the nervous system is susceptible not only to diseases that are due to immunosuppression but also to the AIDS virus per se.

EPIDEMIOLOGY

In less than a decade AIDS has spread nearly worldwide and has attained epidemic proportions. By early 1987, more than 1 million persons in the United States were seropositive for the virus. By August 1988, more than 70,000 cases of AIDS had been reported in the United States (reporting began in 1981), and more than 40,000 of these patients had died. By all accounts, the incidence will continue to increase in the immediate future. It has been estimated by the Centers for Disease Control that, barring any foreseeable changes in epidemiology and treatment, 250,000 persons in the United States will have acquired the disease by 1991. The disease is now the subject of intense public interest and laboratory investigation. Comprehensive and authoritative reviews of the neurologic aspects of AIDS have recently been published by Rosenblum and by Brew and their colleagues; these are listed in the references.

AIDS affects mainly homosexual and bisexual males (72 percent of all cases) and male and female drug users (17 percent). A much smaller group at risk consists of hemophiliacs and other patients who receive infected blood or blood products, and the disease has occurred in infants born of mothers with AIDS or at risk for AIDS. Moreover, this virus may be transmitted by asymptomatic, still immunologically competent mothers to their offspring. Gradually, the number of affected heterosexuals is increasing, mainly through the activities of bisexual men and prostitutes. Four-fifths of all the reported cases in the United States have been from New York, California, New Jersey, and Florida. The means of transmission of HIV are narrowly restricted—sexual intercourse, direct inoculation of infected blood or body fluids into the blood stream or across epithelial barriers, or mother to child infection in utero and possibly through breast milk. In central African countries the incidence of this viral infection is even greater than in the western world, and a heterosexual transmission appears to predominate.

The AIDS virus was first isolated by French workers from the lymph nodes of an infected individual (lymphadenopathy-associated virus or LAV), and at about the same time a human T-cell lymphotropic virus (HTLV), identical to LAV, was discovered in patients in the United States. The designation now being used is human immunodeficiency virus (HIV-1 or HIV); it is the etiologic agent in AIDS and not simply a newly recognized opportunistic infection. On the basis of its structure and biology, HIV is classified as a retrovirus, subfamily lentivirus, which includes a number of other viruses that cause chronic nervous system disease (notably visna in sheep).

HIV infection produces a spectrum of disorders, ranging from *clinically inevident seroconversion* (the most common) to widespread lymphadenopathy and other relatively benign systemic manifestations, such as diarrhea, malaise, and weight loss (the so-called *AIDS-related complex or ARC*), to full-blown AIDS, which comprises the direct effects of the virus on all organ systems as well as the complicating effects of a multiplicity of neoplasms and parasitic, fungal, viral, and bacterial infections (all of which require cell-mediated immunity for containment).

HIV INFECTION OF THE NERVOUS SYSTEM

All parts of the CNS (meninges, brain, and spinal cord), the peripheral nerves and roots, and muscle may be involved in the course of HIV infection. This involvement may be the result of primary infection with the virus or secondary to immunosuppression, or both. Clinically, neurologic abnormalities are noted in only about one-third of patients with AIDS, but at autopsy the nervous system is affected in nearly all of them. The infections and neoplastic lesions that complicate AIDS are listed in Table 33-1, and their pathology is discussed by Gray et al.

It has already been mentioned that HIV infection may present as an acute *asymptomatic meningitis,* with a mild lymphocytic pleocytosis and modest elevation of CSF protein. The acute illness may also take the form of a *meningoencephalitis* or even a *myelopathy* or *neuropathy* (see below). Most patients recover from the acute illnesses; the relationship to AIDS may pass unrecognized, since these illnesses are quite nonspecific clinically and may precede seroconversion. Once seroconversion has occurred, during either the acute illness or convalescence, the patient becomes vulnerable to all the late complications of HIV infection. In adults, the mean latency of HIV infection is 8 years (1 year or less in infants), and it is now believed that practically all seropositive individuals will sooner or later develop AIDS.

In the later stages of HIV infection, the commonest neurologic complication is a particular form of subacute or chronic HIV encephalitis presenting as a kind of dementia; formerly it was called AIDS encephalopathy or encephalitis and now is generally referred to as the *AIDS dementia complex* or *ADC* (Navia and Price). This disorder, which may be the major or sole manifestation of the disease, takes the form of a slowly or rapidly progressive dementia,

accompanied by apathy and abnormalities of motor function. Incoordination of the limbs, ataxia of gait, and impairment of smooth pursuit and saccadic eye movements are usually early accompaniments of the dementia. Heightened tendon reflexes, Babinski signs, grasp and suck reflexes, weakness of the legs progressing to paraplegia, bladder and bowel incontinence reflecting spinal cord or cerebral involvement, and mutism are prominent in the later stages of the disease. According to Brew and his colleagues, the AIDS dementia complex is present in one-third of AIDS patients early in the course of the illness and in two-thirds of them late in the disease.

Table 33-1
Neurologic complications in HIV-1 infected patients

Brain
  Predominantly nonfocal
    AIDS dementia complex (subacute-chronic HIV encephalitis)
    Acute HIV-related encephalitis
    Cytomegalovirus encephalitis
    Herpes simplex virus encephalitis
    Metabolic encephalopathies
  Predominantly focal
    Cerebral toxoplasmosis
    Progressive multifocal leukoencephalopathy
    Cryptococcoma
    Varicella-zoster virus encephalitis
    Tuberculous brain abscess/tuberculoma
    Neurosyphilis (meningovascular)
    Vascular disorders—notably nonbacterial endocarditis and cerebral hemorrhages associated with thrombocytopenia
    Primary CNS lymphoma
Spinal cord
  Vacuolar myelopathy
  Herpes simplex or zoster myelitis
Meninges
  Aseptic meningitis (HIV)
  Cryptococcal meningitis
  Tuberculous meningitis
  Syphilitic meningitis
  Metastatic lymphomatous meningitis
Peripheral nerve and root
  Infectious
    Herpes zoster
    Cytomegalovirus polyradiculopathy
  Virus or immune related
    Acute and chronic inflammatory HIV polyneuritis
    Mononeuritis multiplex
    Sensorimotor demyelinating polyneuropathy
    Distal painful sensory polyneuritis
  Muscle
    Polymyositis and other myopathies

Source: Brew et al.

The pathologic basis of the dementia is a diffuse and multifocal rarefaction of the cerebral white matter, accompained by scanty perivascular infiltrates of lymphocytes and clusters of a few foamy macrophages and multinucleated cells (Navia et al). Cytomegalovirus infection may be added, but accumulating virologic evidence indicates that the AIDS dementia complex is due to direct infection with HIV. Epstein and his colleagues have described a similar disorder in children, who develop a progressive encephalopathy as the primary manifestation of AIDS. The disease in children is characterized by spastic weakness and impairment of cognitive functions, and secondarily by an impairment of brain growth.

The CSF in uncomplicated demented patients may be normal or may manifest the infection by a mild elevation of protein content and, less frequently, a mild lymphocytosis. HIV can be isolated from the CSF and can be used to assess viral antigens. The CT scan, which shows widened sulci and enlarged ventricles, and MRI, which shows patchy or diffuse white matter changes, are particularly useful in diagnosis.

A *myelopathy,* taking the form of a vacuolar degeneration that bears some resemblance to subacute combined degeneration, is frequently associated with the AIDS dementia complex, or it may occur in isolation, as the leading manifestation of the disease (Petito et al). The spinal cord disorder is discussed further on page 746.

AIDS may also be complicated by an *affection of the peripheral nerves.* Eight of 50 patients reported by Snider et al had a distal symmetrical neuropathy, predominantly sensory and dysesthetic in type. The HIV virus has been isolated from the peripheral nerves, and it stands as the first proven viral polyneuritis. In other patients, a painful mononeuropathy multiplex or a progressive cauda equina syndrome occurs, seemingly related to a focal vasculitis and cytomegalovirus infection (Eidelberg et al). Cornblath and his colleagues have documented the occurrence of inflammatory demyelinating peripheral neuropathy, both of the acute (Guillain-Barré) and chronic types, in otherwise asymptomatic patients with HIV infection; all of these patients had a mild pleocytosis, in addition to an elevated CSF protein content. Also, all of the latter patients with inflammatory demyelinating neuropathy recovered—either spontaneously or in response to corticosteroids or plasmapheresis—suggesting an immunopathogenesis. Cornblath et al have suggested that all patients with inflammatory demyelinating polyneuropathies now be tested for the presence of HIV infection. Probably some instances of polyneuropathy in AIDS patients are due to the nutritional depletion that characterizes advanced instances of the disease and to the effects of therapeutic agents such as vincristine and isoniazid.

A primary affection of muscle, taking the form of an *inflammatory polymyositis,* has been described in AIDS, occurring at any stage of the disease (Simpson and Bender). In some of these cases, the myopathy has improved with corticosteroid therapy.

OTHER CNS COMPLICATIONS OF AIDS

In addition to the direct neurologic effects of HIV infection, a variety of opportunistic disorders, both focal and nonfocal, occur in such patients, as outlined in Table 33-1. Interestingly there appears to be a predilection for certain ones such as toxoplasmosis, cytomegalic inclusion disease, cryptococcosis, herpes simplex and zoster, and unusual types of tuberculosis. Some are complications of venereal infections. Usually *Pneumocystis carinii* infection and Kaposi sarcoma do not spread to the nervous system.

Of the focal complications, *cerebral toxoplasmosis* is the most frequent (and treatable), followed by primary CNS lymphoma (page 529), progressive multifocal leukoencephalopathy (page 608), and the focal encephalitis and vasculitis of varicella-zoster infection, which was considered earlier in this chapter. In an autopsy series of AIDS reported by Navia et al, toxoplasma abscesses were found in approximately 13 percent. Lumbar puncture, double-dose contrast-enhanced CT scanning and MRI are essential in diagnosis. Since the disease represents reactivation of a prior toxoplasma infection, it is important to identify seropositive patients early in the course of AIDS and to treat them vigorously with pyrithiamine (25 mg daily by mouth) and a sulfonamide (2 to 6 g daily in four divided doses).

About 5 percent of AIDS patients develop a *primary CNS lymphoma,* which may be difficult to distinguish from toxoplasmosis clinically or radiologically. If the cytologic study of the CSF is negative, brain biopsy may be necessary for diagnosis. The prognosis in such patients is poor; the response to radiation therapy and corticosteroids is short-lived and survival is measured in months.

Varicella-zoster virus infections are relatively rare complications of AIDS but are usually severe in nature. They take the form of multifocal lesions of the cerebral white matter, like those of progressive multifocal leukoencephalopathy, or a cerebral vasculitis with hemiplegia (usually in association with ophthalmic zoster), and rarely a myelitis. Herpes simplex virus, types 1 and 2, have also been identified in the brains of AIDS patients, but their clinical correlates are unclear. There is no evidence that acyclovir or other antiviral agents are effective in any of these viral infections.

Two particular types of mycobacterial infection tend to complicate AIDS—*M tuberculosis* and *M avium intracellulare*. Tuberculosis infection predominates among drug abusers and AIDS patients in underdeveloped countries. Diagnosis and treatment are along the same lines as in non-AIDS patients. Atypical mycobacterial infections are usually associated with other destructive cerebral lesions and do not respond to therapy. Responses of such cases to antituberculous therapy are difficult to interpret.

Syphilitic meningitis and *meningovascular syphilis* appear to have an increased incidence in AIDS patients. CSF cell counts are unreliable as signs of luetic activity, and diagnosis depends entirely upon serologic tests. It seems unlikely that AIDS causes false-positive tests for syphilis, but this remains to be established.

Among the nonfocal neurologic complications of AIDS, the most common are opportunistic infections with *cytomegalovirus (CMV)* and *cryptococcus*. At autopsy, about one-third of AIDS patients are found to be infected with CMV. However, the contribution of this infection to the clinical picture is uncertain. An encephalitis with seizures and clouding of consciousness and a myeloradiculitis have been attributed to CMV infection. The diagnosis of CMV infection during life is also uncertain. CSF cultures are usually negative and antibody titers are nonspecifically elevated. Where the diagnosis is strongly suspected, treatment with a new antiviral agent (ganciclovir) has been recommended (Brew et al).

Cryptococcal meningitis and *solitary cryptococcoma* are the most frequent fungal complications of HIV infection. Flagrant symptoms of meningitis or meningoencephalitis may be lacking, however, and the CSF may show little abnormality with reference to cells, protein, and glucose. For these reasons evidence of cryptococcal infection of the spinal fluid should be actively sought with India ink preparations and fungal cultures. Treatment is along the lines outlined in Chap. 32.

DIAGNOSTIC TESTS FOR HIV INFECTION

Many screening tests are now available for the detection of antibodies to HIV. All of them are based on an enzyme-linked immunoassay (ELISA or EIA), which has proved to be highly sensitive. However, there is a high incidence of false-positive reactions, particularly when these tests are used to screen persons at low risk for HIV infection. All positive EIA tests should therefore be repeated.

The *Western blot test*, which identifies antibodies to specific viral proteins, is more specific than EIA tests and should be used to confirm a positive screening test. Indeterminate Western blot tests should be repeated monthly for several months to detect a rising concentration of antibodies. An immunofluorescence assay (IFA) can also be used to confirm a positive screening test but remains to be licensed by the FDA. Newer tests, using purified antigens, are being developed and should be more specific than those currently available.

Finally, it should be repeated that specific agents for the treatment of HIV infection are not available and that the management of AIDS continues to be purely symptomatic, i.e., managing each of the infections and neoplastic complications as they are recognized, using the most suitable measures currently available. Preliminary observations suggest that the nucleoside analogue azidothymidine (AZT or zidovudine) may be beneficial in controlling pneumocystis carinii infection and possibly HIV infection, but this requires further evaluation.

OTHER SUBACUTE FORMS OF ENCEPHALITIS (PRESUMABLY VIRAL)

Increasingly, in patients who harbor malignant tumors, particularly those receiving complex forms of therapy, we are being confronted by patients with subacute forms of encephalitis. In some of these infections, the limbic parts of the brain (limbic encephalitis) are involved in a topographic pattern similar to herpes simplex encephalitis. In others the lesions are concentrated in the brainstem (brainstem encephalitis) and cerebellum. To date all attempts to identify the viruses by serologic tests and virus isolation have been unsuccessful. Because of the frequent association of these types of encephalitis with neoplasms we have chosen to discuss them in Chap. 31.

VIRAL INFECTIONS OF THE DEVELOPING NERVOUS SYSTEM

Viral infections of the fetus, notably rubella and cytomegalovirus, and herpes simplex infection of the newborn are important causes of CNS abnormalities. They are considered in Chap. 44, under "Developmental Diseases of Infancy and Childhood."

REFERENCES

ADAMS H, MILLER D: Herpes simplex encephalitis: A clinical and pathological analysis of twenty-two cases. *Postgrad Med J* 49:393, 1973.

AICARDI J, GOUTIERES F, ARSENIO-NUNES HL, LEBON P: Acute measles encephalitis in children with immunosuppression. *Pediatrics* 55:232, 1977.

ALEMA G: Behçet's disease, in Vinken PJ, Bruyn GW (eds):

Handbook of Clinical Neurology, Infections of the Nervous System, Part II, vol 34. Amsterdam, North-Holland, 1978, chap 24, pp 475–512.

ÅSTRÖM KE, MANCALL EL, RICHARDSON EP JR: Progressive multifocal leukoencephalopathy. *Brain* 81:93, 1958.

BARINGER JR: Human herpes simplex virus infections, in Thompson RA, Green JR (eds): *Advances in Neurology*, vol 6. New York, Raven Press, 1974, pp 41–51.

BEGHI E. NICOLOSI A, KURLAND LT et al: Encephalitis and aseptic meningitis, Olmstead County, Minnesota, 1950–1981. Epidemiology. *Ann Neurol* 16:283–294, 1984.

BERNOULLI CC, MASTERS CL, GAJDUSEK DC et al: Early clinical features of Creutzfeldt-Jakob disease (subacute spongiform encephalopathy), in Prusiner SB, Hadlow WS (eds): *Slow Transmissible Diseases of the Nervous System*. New York, Academic Press, 1979, vol 1, pp 229–251.

BODIAN D: Histopathologic basis of clinical findings in poliomyelitis. *Am J Med* 6:563, 1949.

BREW B, SIDTIS J, PETITO CK, PRICE RW: The neurologic complications of AIDS and human immunodeficiency virus infection, in Plum F (ed): *Advances in Contemporary Neurology*. Philadelphia, FA Davis, 1988, Chap 1.

BROWN P, COKER-VANN M, POMEROY K et al: Diagnosis of Creutzfeldt-Jakob disease by Western blot identification of marker protein in human brain tissue. *N Engl J Med* 314:347, 1986.

CATHALA F, BROWN P, CHATELAIN J et al: Maladie de Creutzfeldt-Jacob en France. Interet des formes familiales. *Presse Med* 15:379, 1986.

CHAJEK T, FAINARU M: Behçet's disease: Report of 41 cases and a review of the literature. *Medicine* 54:179, 1975.

CORNBLATH DR, MCARTHUR JC, KENNEDY PGE et al: Inflammatory demyelinating peripheral neuropathies associated with human T-cell lymphotropic virus type III infection. *Ann Neurol* 21:32, 1987.

DAVIS LE, JOHNSON RT: An explanation for the localization of herpes simplex encephalitis. *Ann Neurol* 5:2, 1979.

DENNY-BROWN D, ADAMS RD, FITZGERALD PJ: Pathologic features of herpes zoster: A note on "geniculate herpes." *Arch Neurol Psychiatry* 51:216, 1944.

DONAT JF, RHODES KH, GROOVER RV et al: Etiology and outcome in 42 children with acute nonbacterial encephalitis. *Mayo Clin Proc* 55:156, 1980.

DYKEN PR, SWIFT A, DURANT MA: Long-term follow-up of patients with subacute sclerosing panencephalitis treated with inosiplex. *Ann Neurol* 11:359, 1982.

EIDELBERG D, SOTREL A, VOGEL H et al: Progressive polyradiculopathy in acquired immune deficiency syndrome. *Neurology* 36:912, 1986.

ENDERS JF, WELLER TH, ROBBINS FC: Cultivation of Lansing strain of poliomyelitis virus in cultures of various human embryonic tissues. *Science* 109:85, 1949.

EPSTEIN LG, SHARER LR, CHOE S et al: HTLV-III/LAV-like retrovirus particles in the brains of patients with AIDS encephalopathy. *AIDS Res* 1:447, 1985.

ESIRI MM: Herpes simplex encephalitis. An immunohistological study of the distribution of viral antigen within the brain. *J Neurol Sci* 54:209, 1982.

GAJDUSEK DC, GIBBS CJ JR, ALPERS M: Experimental transmission of a kuru-like syndrome to chimpanzees. *Nature* 209:794, 1966.

GIBBS CJ JR, GAJDUSEK DC, ASHER DM, ALPERS MP: Creutzfeldt-Jakob disease (spongiform encephalopathy): Transmission to the chimpanzee. *Science* 161:388, 1968.

GIBBS CV, JOY A, HEFFNER R et al: Clinical and pathological features and laboratory confirmation of Creutzfeldt-Jakob disease in a recipient of pituitary derived growth hormone. *N Engl J Med* 313:734, 1985.

GRAY F, GHERARDI R, SCARAVILLI F: The neuropathology of the acquired immunodeficiency syndrome (AIDS): A review. *Brain* 111:245, 1988.

HADDAD FS, RISK WS: Isoprinosine treatment in 18 patients with subacute sclerosing panencephalitis: A controlled study. *Ann Neurol* 7:185–188, 1980.

HADLOW WJ: Scrapie and kuru. *Lancet* 2:289, 1959.

HALL WW, LAMB RA, CHOPPIN PW: Measles and SSPE virus proteins: Lack of antibodies to the M protein in patients with subacute sclerosing panencephalitis. *Proc Natl Acad Sci USA* 76:2047, 1979.

HEIDENHAIN A: Klinische und anatomische Untersuchungen über eine eigenartige organische Erkrankung des Zentralnervensystems im Praesenium. *Z Gesamte Neurol Psychiatry* 118:49, 1929.

HILT DC, BUCHHOLZ D, KRUMHOLZ A et al: Herpes zoster ophthalmicus and delayed contralateral hemiparesis caused by cerebral angiitis: Diagnosis and management approaches. *Ann Neurol* 14:543, 1983.

HOPE-SIMPSON RE: The nature of herpes zoster: A long-term study and a new hypothesis. *Proc R Soc Med* 58:9, 1965.

HOWARD RS, LEES AJ: Encephalitis lethargica: A report of four cases, *Brain* 110:19, 1987.

JAMSEK J, GREENBERG SB, TABER L et al: Herpes zoster associated encephalitis: Clinicopatholic report of 12 cases and review of the literature. *Medicine* 62:81, 1983.

JOHNSON KP (ed): *Neurovirology*. Neurologic Clinics. Philadelphia, WB Saunders 2 (May), 1984.

JOHNSON RT: Selective vulnerability of neural cells to viral infections. *Brain* 103:447, 1980.

JOHNSON RT: *Viral Infections of the Nervous System*. New York, Raven Press, 1982.

JOHNSON RT, NARAYAN O, WEINER LP: The relationship of SV 40-related viruses to progressive multifocal leukoencephalopathy, in Robinson WS, Fox CF (eds): *Mechanisms of Virus Disease*. Menlo Park, CA, WA Benjamin, 1974, pp 187–197.

LEHNER T, BARNES CG (eds): *Behçet's Syndrome: Clinical and Immunological Features*. New York, Academic Press, 1980.

LEPOW ML, CARVER DH, WRIGHT HT JR et al: A clinical, epidemiologic, and laboratory investigation of aseptic meningitis during the four-year period 1955–1958. *N Engl J Med* 266:1181, 1188, 1962.

LINNEMANN CC JR, ALVIRA MM: Pathogenesis of varicella-zoster angiitis in the CNS. *Arch Neurol* 37:239, 1980.

MASTERS CL, HARRIS JO, GAJDUSEK C et al: Creutzfeldt-Jakob

disease: Patterns of worldwide occurrence and the significance of familial and sporadic clustering. *Ann Neurol* 5:177, 1979.

MASTERS CL, GAJDUSEK DC, GIBBS CJ JR: Creutzfeldt-Jakob disease virus isolations from the Gerstmann-Sträussler syndrome. *Brain* 104:559, 1981.

MATTHEWS WB: Slow infections, in Kennedy PGE, Johnson RT (eds): *Infections of the Nervous System.* London, Butterworths, 1987, pp 227–247.

McKENDRICK NW, McGILL JI, WHITE JE, WOOD MJ: Oral acyclovir in acute herpes zoster. *Br Med J* 293:1529, 1986.

MEHTA PD, PATRICK BA, THORMAR H: Identification of virus-specific oligoclonal bands in subacute sclerosing panencephalitis by immunofixation after isoelectric focusing and peroxidase staining. *J Clin Microbiol* 16:985, 1982.

MOLLARET MP: La méningite endothelio-leucocytaire multi-récurrente bénigne. Syndrome nouveau ou maladie nouvelle? *Rev Neurol (Paris)* 76:57–76, 1944.

MULDER DW, ROSENBAUM RA, LAYTON DP: Late progression of poliomyelitis or forme fruste amyotrophic lateral sclerosis? *Mayo Clin Proc* 47:756, 1972.

NAVIA BA, PETITO CK, GOLD JWM et al: Cerebral toxoplasmosis complicating the acquired immune deficiency syndrome: Clinical and neuropathological findings in 27 patients. *Ann Neurol* 19:224, 1986.

NAVIA BA, JORDAN BD, PRICE RW: The AIDS dementia complex. I. Clinical features. *Ann Neurol* 19:517, 1986.

NAVIA BA, CHO E-S, PETITO CK et al: The AIDS dementia complex. II. Neuropathology. *Ann Neurol* 19:525, 1986.

NAVIA BA, PRICE RW: The acquired immunodeficiency syndrome dementia complex as the presenting or sole manifestation of human immunodeficiency virus infection. *Arch Neurol* 44:65, 1987.

PADGETT BL, WALKER DL, ZURHEIN GM, ECKROADE RJ: Cultivation of papova-like virus from human brain with progressive multifocal leukoencephalopathy. *Lancet* 1:1257, 1971.

PETITO CK, NAVIA BA, CHO E-S et al: Vacuolar myelopathy pathologically resembling subacute combined degeneration in patients with acquired immunodeficiency syndrome (AIDS). *N Engl J Med* 312:874, 1985.

PONKA A, PETTERSSON T: The incidence and aetiology of central nervous system infections in Helsinki in 1980. *Acta Neurol Scand* 66:529–535, 1982.

PRUSINER SB, HADLOW WJ (eds): *Slow Transmissible Diseases of the Nervous System.* New York, Academic Press, 1979.

RICHARDSON EP JR: Progressive multifocal leukoencephalopathy. *N Engl J Med* 265:815, 1961.

ROBERTSON WC JR, CLARK DB, MARKESBERY WR: Review of 38 cases of subacute sclerosing panencephalitis: Effect of amantadine on the natural course of the disease. *Ann Neurol* 8:422, 1980.

ROSENBLUM ML, LEVY RM, BREDESEN DE (eds): *AIDS and the Nervous System.* New York, Raven Press, 1988.

SELBY G, WALKER GL: Cerebral arteritis in cat-scratch fever. *Neurology* 29:1413, 1979.

SEVER JL: Persistent measles infection in the central nervous system. *Rev Infect Dis* 5:467, 1983.

SIMPSON DM, BENDER AN: HTLV-III associated myopathy (abstr). *Neurology* 37(suppl):319, 1987.

SKOLDENBERG B, FORSGREN M, ALESTIG K et al: Acyclovir versus vidarabine in herpes simplex encephalitis: Randomized multi-center study in consecutive Swedish patients. *Lancet* 2:707, 1984.

SNIDER WD, SIMPSON DM, NIELSEN S et al: Neurological complications of acquired immune deficiency syndrome. Analysis of 50 patients. *Ann Neurol* 14:403, 1983.

STEEL JG, DIX RD, BARINGER JR: Isolation of herpes simplex virus type I in recurrent Mollaret meningitis. *Ann Neurol* 11:17, 1982.

TOWSEND JJ, BARINGER JR, WOLINSKY JS et al: Progressive rubella panencephalitis: Late onset after congenital rubella. *N Engl J Med* 292:990, 1975.

VON ECONOMO C: *Encephalitis Lethargica.* New York, Oxford, 1931.

WADIA NH, KATRAK SM, MISRA VP et al: Polio-like motor paralysis associated with acute hemorrhagic conjunctivitis in an outbreak in 1981 in Bombay, India: Clinical and serologic studies. *J Infect Dis* 147:660, 1983.

WEIL ML, ITABASHI HH, CREMER NE et al: Chronic progressive panencephalitis due to rubella virus simulating subacute sclerosing panencephalitis. *N Engl J Med* 292:994, 1975.

WELLER TH, WITTON HM, BELL EJ: Etiologic agents of varicella and herpes zoster. *J Exp Med* 108:843, 1958.

WHITLEY RJ, SOONG S-J, DOLIN R et al: Adenine arabinoside therapy of biopsy-proved herpes simplex encephalitis. *N Engl J Med* 297:289, 1977

WHITLEY RJ: The frustrations of treating herpes simplex virus infections of the central nervous system. *JAMA* 259:1067, 1988.

WHITLEY RH, SOONG SJ, HIRSCH MS et al: Herpes simplex encephalitis: Vidarabine therapy and diagnostic problems. *N Engl J Med* 304:313, 1981.

WHITLEY RV, ALFORD CA, HIRSCH MS et al: Vidarabine versus acyclovir therapy in herpes simplex encephalitis. *N Engl J Med* 314:144, 1986.

WOLINSKY JS: Progressive rubella panencephalitis, in Vinken PJ, Bruyn GW (eds): *Handbook of Clinical Neurology,* vol 34. Amsterdam, North-Holland, 1978, pp 331–342.

WOLINSKY JS, SWOVELAND P, JOHNSON KP, BARINGER JR: Subacute measles encephalitis complicating Hodgkin's disease in an adult. *Ann Neurol* 1:452, 1977.

ZURHEIN GM, CHOU SM: Particles resembling papova-viruses in human cerebral demyelinative disease. *Science* 148:1477, 1965.

CHAPTER 34

CEREBROVASCULAR DISEASES

Among all the neurologic diseases of adult life, the cerebrovascular ones clearly rank first in frequency and importance. At least 50 percent of the neurologic disorders in a general hospital are of this type. At some time or other every physician will be required to examine patients with cerebrovascular disease and should at least know something of the common types—particularly those in which there is a reasonable prospect of successful medical or surgical intervention. There is another advantage to be gained from the study of this group of diseases, namely that they have traditionally provided one of the most instructive approaches to neurology. As our colleague C. M. Fisher has remarked, house officers and students literally learn neurology "stroke by stroke." The focal ischemic lesion has divulged some of the most important ideas about the function of the human brain.

INCIDENCE OF CEREBROVASCULAR DISEASES

Stroke, after heart disease and cancer, is the third commonest cause of death in the United States. Every year there are 85,000 or more fatalities from this cause; in addition about 1 million persons survive strokes, but are left disabled. Interestingly the incidence has been falling for the past 30 to 35 years. In Rochester, Minnesota, Garraway et al found a reduction of 54 percent in cerebral infarction and hemorrhage when the period 1975–1979 was compared with 1945–1949 and Nicholls and Johnson reported a 20 percent decline in the United States between 1968 and 1976. Both sexes shared in the reduced incidence. The incidence of coronary heart disease and malignant hypertension has also fallen. There has been no change in the frequency of aneurysmal rupture, however. Probably this diminution in the incidence of stroke is related to a reduced incidence of cerebral embolism from heart disease and the improved control of hypertension.

DEFINITION OF TERMS

The term *cerebrovascular disease* designates any abnormality of the brain resulting from a pathologic process of the blood vessels. *Pathologic process* is given an inclusive meaning, viz., any lesion of the vessel wall, occlusion of the lumen by thrombus or embolus, rupture of the vessel, altered permeability of the vascular wall, and increased viscosity or other change in the quality of the blood. The pathologic change may be considered not only in its grosser aspects—thrombosis, embolism, rupture of a vessel—but also in terms of the more basic or primary disorder, i.e., the genesis of atherosclerosis, hypertensive arteriosclerotic change, arteritis, aneurysmal dilation, and developmental malformation. Equal importance attaches to the secondary parenchymal changes in the brain. These are of two types—ischemia, with or without infarction, and hemorrhage—and unless they occur, the vascular lesion usually remains silent. The only exceptions to this statement are the local pressure effects of an aneurysm, vascular headache (migraine, hypertension, temporal arteritis), multiple small vessel disease with progressive encephalopathy (as in malignant hypertension or cerebral giant cell arteritis), and increased intracranial pressure (as occurs occasionally in hypertensive encephalopathy and venous sinus thrombosis). The many types of cerebrovascular diseases are listed in Table 34-1.

More than any other organ, the brain depends from minute to minute on an adequate supply of oxygenated blood. Constancy of the cerebral circulation is assured by a series of baroreceptors and vasomotor reflexes under the control of centers in the lower brainstem. In Stokes-Adams attacks, for example, unconsciousness occurs within 10 s of the beginning of asystole, and in animal experiments the complete stoppage of blood flow for longer than 4 to 5 min produces irreversible damage. Brain tissue deprived of blood undergoes *ischemic necrosis or infarction* (also referred to as a zone of *softening* or *encephalomalacia*). Obstruction of an artery by thrombus or embolus is the usual cause of focal ischemic damage, but failure of the circulation and hypotension from cardiac decompensation or shock, if severe and prolonged, can produce focal as well as diffuse ischemic changes.

Cerebral infarcts vary greatly in the amount of congestion and hemorrhage that are found within the softened tissue. Some infarcts are devoid of blood and therefore pallid (*pale infarction*); others show mild congestion (dilatation of blood vessels and escape of red blood cells), especially at their margins; still others show an extensive extravasation of blood from many small vessels in the infarcted tissue (red or *hemorrhagic infarction*). Some infarcts are all of one type, either pale or hemorrhagic; others are mixed. The reason for the occurrence of red infarction—always, it seems, in cases of cerebral embolism—is not fully understood. The explanation most consistent with our observations is that embolic material, after occluding an artery and causing ischemic necrosis of brain tissue, then fragments and migrates distally from its original site. This allows at least partial restoration of the circulation to the infarcted zone, and blood seeps through the damaged vessels (Fisher and Adams). In such cases, one usually cannot find the embolus by arteriography or postmortem examination, or one finds only a few fragments proximal to the pale ischemic zones.

In hemorrhage, blood leaks from the vessel (usually a small artery) directly into the brain, one of the ventricles, or the subarachnoid space. Once the leakage is arrested, the blood slowly disintegrates and is absorbed over a period of weeks and months. The mass of clotted blood causes physical disruption of the tissue and pressure on the surrounding brain.

THE STROKE SYNDROME

So distinctive is the mode of presentation of cerebrovascular disease that the diagnosis is seldom in doubt. The common mode of expression is the *stroke*, defined as a sudden, nonconvulsive, focal neurologic deficit. In its most severe form the patient becomes hemiplegic and even comatose, an event so dramatic that it has been given its own designation, namely *apoplexy, stroke, shock,* or *cerebrovascular accident (CVA)*. In its mildest form it may consist of a trivial neurologic disorder insufficient even to arouse concern or demand medical attention. There are all gradations of severity between these two extremes, but in all forms of stroke the denominative feature is the *temporal*

Table 34-1
Causes of cerebral abnormalities from disease of cerebral arteries and viens

1. Atherosclerotic thrombosis
2. Transient ischemic attacks
3. Embolism
4. Ruptured or unruptured saccular aneurysm or AVM
5. Arteritis
   a. Menigovascular syphilis, arteritis secondary to pyogenic and tuberculous meningitis, rare infective types (typhus, schistosomiasis, malaria, trichinosis, mucormycosis, etc.)
   b. Connective tissue diseases (polyarteritis nodosa, lupus erythematosus), necrotizing arteritis, Wegener arteritis, temporal arteritis, Takayasu disease, granulomatous or giant cell arteritis of the aorta, and giant cell granulomatous angiitis of cerebral arteries
6. Cerebral thrombophlebitis: secondary to infection of ear, paranasal sinus, face, etc.; with meningitis and subdural empyema; debilitating states, postpartum, postoperative, cardiac failure, hematologic disease (polycythemia, sickle-cell disease), and of undetermined cause
7. Hematologic disorders: polycythemia, sickle-cell disease, thrombotic thrombocytopenic purpura, thrombocytosis, etc.
8. Trauma to carotid artery
9. Dissecting aortic aneurysm
10. Systemic hypotension with arterial stenoses: "simple faint," acute blood loss, myocardial infarction, Stokes-Adams syndrome, traumatic and surgical shock, sensitive carotid sinus, severe postural hypotension
11. Complications of arteriography
12. Neurologic migraine with persistent deficit
13. With tentorial, foramen magnum, and subfalcial herniations
14. Miscellaneous types: fibromuscular dysplasia, radioactive or x-irradiation, lateral pressure of intracerebral hematoma, unexplained middle cerebral infarction in closed head injury, pressure of unruptured saccular aneurysm, local dissection of carotid or middle cerebral artery, complication of oral contraceptives
15. Undetermined cause as in children and young adults: moyamoya; multiple, progressive intracranial arterial occlusions (Taveras).

profile of neurologic events. It is the abruptness with which the neurologic deficit develops—a matter of seconds, minutes, hours, or at most a few days—that stamps the disorder as vascular. Embolic strokes characteristically begin suddenly and the deficit reaches its peak almost at once.

Thrombotic strokes may have the same abrupt onset, but in many the onset is somewhat slower, over a period of several minutes or hours, and occasionally days, and usually in a saltatory fashion, i.e., in a series of steps, rather than smoothly. Stenosis of multiple arteries (extracranial and middle cerebral) may result in a chronic marginal low blood flow, which by fluctuating during activity may diminish vision or induce a movement abnormality (Yanagihara et al). In hypertensive cerebral hemorrhage, the deficit, from the moment of onset, is steadily progressive over a period of minutes or hours. The other important aspect of the temporal profile is the arrest and then regression of the neurologic deficit in all except the fatal strokes. Not infrequently an extensive deficit from embolism reverses itself dramatically within a few hours or days. More often, and this is the case in most thrombotic strokes, improvement occurs gradually over weeks and months, and the residual disability is considerable. A gradual downhill course over a period of several days or weeks will usually be traced to a nonvascular disease. The only exceptions are multiple arteriolar and venular occlusions (platelet thrombosis, arteritis, lupus erythematosus, and hypertensive arteriolar sclerosis).

The neurologic deficit reflects both the location and size of the infarct or hemorrhage. Hemiplegia stands as the classic sign of all cerebrovascular diseases, whether in the cerebral hemisphere or brainstem, but there are many other manifestations as well, occurring in an almost infinite number of combinations. These include mental confusion, numbness and sensory deficits of many types, aphasia, visual field defects, diplopia, dizziness, dysarthria, and so forth. The neurovascular syndromes that they form enable the physician to locate the lesion—sometimes so precisely that the affected arterial branch can be specified—and to indicate whether the lesion is an infarct or hemorrhage. The many neurovascular syndromes will be described in the section that follows.

It would be incorrect to assume that every cerebrovascular illness expresses itself as a clearly delineated stroke. Sometimes neither the patient nor the family can date the onset of the illness. Certain effects of vascular disease may be so mild as to pass unnoticed, and are presented as complaints only when their cumulative effects become manifest. Furthermore, certain dominant hemispheric lesions cause aphasic disturbances, which hamper history taking, and nondominant ones may cause anosognosia, which leaves the patient unaware of any deficits.

New laboratory methods for the demonstration of both the cerebral lesion and the offending vessel(s) have revolutionized the clinical study of stroke patients. Computerized tomography (CT) scanning demonstrates and accurately localizes small hemorrhages, hemorrhagic infarcts, subarachnoid blood, clots in and around aneurysms,

regions of infarct necrosis, arteriovenous malformations, and ventricular deformities. Magnetic resonance imaging (MRI) also demonstrates these lesions and in addition reveals flow voids and hemosiderin as well as the alterations resulting from ischemic necrosis and gliosis. Radionuclide scanning visualizes many hematomas and some infarcts in their early stages (days to weeks), although not in their late ones. Atheromatous plaques and stenoses of large vessels, particularly the carotid arteries, can frequently be detected by the use of ultrasound and Doppler flow studies. Arteriography demonstrates stenoses and occlusions of the larger vessels (both thrombotic and in some instances embolic) as well as aneurysms, vascular malformations, and other rare blood vessel diseases. This technique may also demonstrate hematomas, but only the larger ones, and then by displacement of vessels (mass effect). Digital subtraction angiography (DSA) visualizes cervical and basal intracranial arteries and has the advantage of safety (see further on). Lumbar puncture indicates whether blood has entered the subarachnoid space (aneurysm, vascular malformation, hypertensive hemorrhage, and some instances of hemorrhagic infarction), but the CSF is clear in pale infarction from thrombosis and embolism. In many stroke cases the CT scan, which entails no risk to the patient, precludes the need for arteriography and lumbar puncture, both of which are sometimes hazardous.

RISK FACTORS

Several factors are known to increase the patient's liability to stroke. The most important of these are hypertension and diabetes. Diabetes hastens the atherosclerotic process in both large and small arteries; Weinberger et al and Roehmholdt et al have found diabetic patients to be twice as liable to stroke as age-matched nondiabetic groups. Hypertension does the same, in addition to being the most readily recognized factor in the genesis of primary intracerebral hemorrhage. Furthermore, it appears that systolic blood pressure is as important as diastolic pressure in producing these adverse effects (Rabkin et al). The cooperative study of the Veterans Administration has convincingly demonstrated that the long-term control of hypertension decreases the incidence of both atherothrombotic infarction and intracerebral hemorrhage. Heart disease, particularly congestive failure and coronary atherosclerosis, greatly increase the probability of stroke. It is also likely that smoking, obesity, and hyperlipidemia constitute risk factors. As for embolic strokes, the most important risk factors are structural cardiac disease and arrhythmias, particularly auricular fibrillation. The interactions between diabetes and hypertension on the one hand and intracerebral hemorrhage and atherothrombotic infarction on the other, and the association of cardiac disease and cerebral embolism are considered further on in this chapter, in relation to each of these categories of cerebrovascular disease.

Public health measures designed to detect and eliminate these risk factors provide the most intelligent, long-range approach to the treatment of cerebral vascular disease.

THE ISCHEMIC STROKE

Focal cerebral ischemia differs from global ischemia. In the latter state there is no collateral flow and irreversible destruction of neurons occurs within 4 to 8 min at normal body temperature. In focal ischemia there is nearly always some degree of circulation (via collateral vessels), permitting the delivery of glucose and other substances, which cannot be properly metabolized under anaerobic conditions.

The effects of arterial occlusion on brain tissue vary, depending upon the location of the occlusion in relation to available collateral and anastomotic channels. If the obstruction lies proximal to the circle of Willis (toward the heart), the anterior and posterior communicating arteries of the circle often are adequate to prevent infarction. In occlusion of the internal carotid artery in the neck, there may be retrograde anastomotic flow from the external carotid artery through the ophthalmic artery or via smaller external-internal connections (Figs. 34-1 and 34-2). With blockage of the vertebral artery the anastomotic flow may be via the deep cervical, thyrocervical, or occipital artery, or retrograde from the other vertebral artery. If the occlusion is in the stem portion of one of the cerebellar arteries or one of the cerebral arteries, i.e., distal to the circle of Willis, then a series of meningeal interarterial anastomoses may carry sufficient blood into the compromised territory to lessen (rarely to prevent) ischemic damage. (see Figs. 34-1 and 34-3). Also there is a capillary anastomotic system between adjacent arterial branches, and although it may reduce the size of the ischemic field, particularly of the penetrating arteries, it is probably inconsequential in preventing infarction. Thus in the event of occlusion of a major arterial trunk, the extent of infarction ranges from none at all to the entire vascular territory of that vessel. Between these two extremes are countless variations in the extent of infarction and its degree of completeness.

Additional *ischemia-modifying factors* are operative in determining the extent of necrosis. The speed of occlusion assumes importance; gradual narrowing of a vessel allows time for collateral channels to open. The level of blood pressure may influence the result; hypotension at a critical moment may render anastomotic channels ineffective. Hypoxia and hypocapnia would obviously have a deleterious effect. Altered viscosity and osmolality of the blood and hyperglycemia are potentially important factors, but difficult to evaluate. Finally, anomalies of vascular arrangement (of neck vessels, circle of Willis, and surface arteries) and the existence of previous vascular occlusions must influence the outcome.

The specific neurologic deficit obviously relates to the location and size of the infarct or focus of ischemia. The territory of any artery, large or small, deep or superficial, may be involved. When an infarction lies in the territory of a carotid artery, unilateral signs predominate, as would be expected: hemiplegia, hemianesthesia, hemianopia, aphasia, and agnosias of certain types are the usual consequences. In the territory of the basilar artery the signs of infarction are frequently bilateral; quadriparesis, hemiparesis, or hemisensory or bilateral sensory impairment occur in conjunction with cranial nerve palsies and other segmental brainstem or cerebellar signs.

PATHOPHYSIOLOGY OF FUNCTIONAL PARALYSIS AND TISSUE NECROSIS UNDER CONDITIONS OF ISCHEMIA

As mentioned above, certain vessels (carotid, vertebral, and sometimes a cerebral artery at its origin) can be occluded with little or no disturbance of neurologic functions, and at autopsy there may be complete integrity of the tissue in the territory of the occluded vessel. Moreover, if infarction has occurred, it usually involves a zone that is smaller than the one normally supplied by the artery in question. The margins of the infarct are hyperemic, being nourished by meningeal collaterals, and here there is no necrosis or only minimal parenchymal damage. The necrotic tissue swells rapidly, mainly because of excessive intracellular and intercellular water content. Since cerebral anoxia also causes necrosis and swelling (although in a different distribution), oxygen lack must be a factor common to both infarction and anoxic encephalopathy. Obviously the effects of ischemia, whether functional and reversible or structural and irreversible, depend on its degree and its duration, as was discussed by Vander Eecken and Adams (1953) and by Adams (1954).

If the brain is observed at the time of arterial occlusion, the venous blood is first seen to darken, owing to an increase in reduced hemoglobin. The viscosity of the blood and resistance of flow increase and there is sludging of formed elements within vessels. The tissue becomes pale. Arteries and arterioles constrict, especially in the pale areas. Upon opening the occluded artery the sequence is reversed and there may be a slight hyperemia. If the

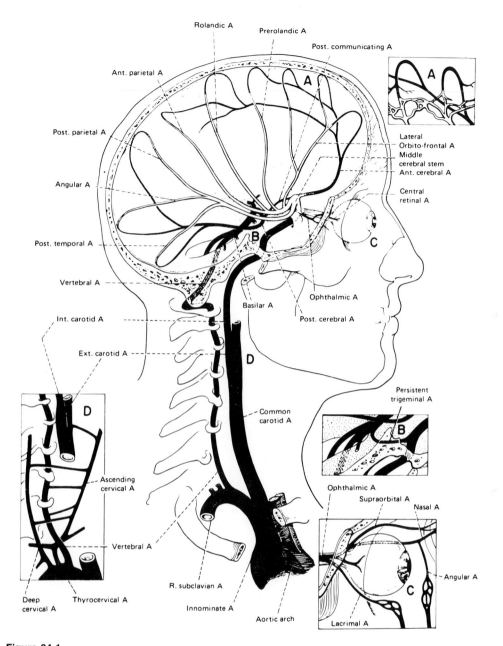

Figure 34-1

Arrangement of the major arteries on the right side carrying blood from the heart to the brain. Also shown are collateral vessels that may modify the effects of cerebral ischemia. For example, the posterior communicating artery connects the internal carotid and the posterior cerebral arteries, and may provide anastomosis between the carotid and basilar systems. Over the convexity, the subarachnoid interarterial anastomoses linking the middle, anterior, and posterior cerebral arteries are shown, with insert A illustrating that these anastomoses are a continuous network of tiny arteries forming a border zone between the major cerebral arterial territories. Occasionally a persistent trigeminal artery connects the internal carotid and basilar arteries proximal to the circle of Willis, as shown in insert B. Anastomoses between the internal and external carotid arteries via the orbit are illustrated in insert C. Wholly extracranial anastomoses from muscular branches of the cervical arteries to vertebral and external carotid arteries are indicated by insert D.

ischemia is prolonged, the sludging and endothelial damage prevents normal reflow.

These flow factors have been examined in detail in experimental animals by Heiss and by Siesjo and their colleagues. They have determined the critical threshold of cerebral blood flow (CBF), measured by xenon clearance, below which functional impairment occurs. In several animal species, including macaque monkeys and gerbils, the critical level was 23 mL/100 g/min (normal 55 mL); and if, after short periods of time, CBF was restored to levels above 23 mL, the impairment of function was reversed. Reduction of CBF below 8.0 to 9.0 mL/100 g/min caused infarction, regardless of its duration. The state of hypoperfusion of the brain (CBF between 8 and 23 mL/100 g/min) has been called the "ischemic penumbra." At this level of blood flow the EEG was slowed, and below this level it was isoelectric. In the ischemic penumbra the K level increased (efflux from injured depolarized cells) and the ATP and creatine phosphate were depleted, but these biochemical abnormalities, if not too severe, returned to normal when the circulation was increased. Disturbance of calcium ion homeostasis and accumulation of free fatty acids interfered with full recovery. Marked ATP depletion, increase in extracellular K, increase in intracellular Ca. and

cellular acidosis with a CBF of 6.0 to 8.0 mL/100 g/min was invariably associated with histologic signs of necrosis, though these did not become apparent for several hours. It was found that biogenic amines (norepinephrine and serotonin) and substance P are reduced in zones of ischemic necrosis (Zivin and Stashak). Also free fatty acids (appearing as phospholipases) are activated and destroy the phospholipids of membranes. Prostaglandins, leukotrienes, and free radicals accumulate. Intracellular proteins and enzymes are denatured. Cells swell (cellular edema). In marginally perfused adjacent areas serotonin declines transiently and then returns to normal.

Morphologic changes may also occur in the ischemic penumbra but are time dependent; that is to say, they vary with the duration of the ischemia. In this partial ischemic state, between upper and lower thresholds, the critical factor is not a particular CBF value, but the combination of residual flow and its duration and other factors. The curve expressing the two functions—the CBF and duration—tends toward infinity at 18 mL/100 g/min. Also of interest is the fact that not all neurons in marginally necrotic areas are destroyed. Why some are selectively vulnerable is not understood.

Olsen and his colleagues have studied CBF in patients with middle cerebral artery occlusion; they confirmed the presence of hypoperfusion in zones shown to be infarcted by CT scan and of hyperperfusion in the border zones. In some hypoperfused regions, in patients with impaired

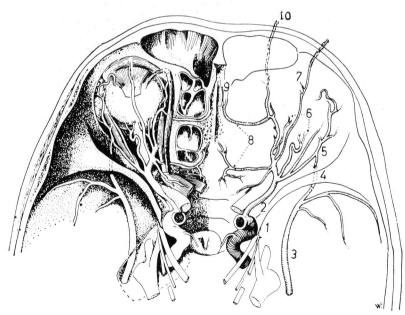

Figure 34-2

Diagram of orbital arteries: (1) internal carotid; (2) ophthalmic; (3) middle meningeal; (4) anastomosis; (5) lacrimal; (6) ocular (including central retinal); (7) supraorbital; (8) anterior and posterior ethmoidal; (9) anterior meningeal; (10) supratrochlear. (From Krayenbühl and Yasargil.)

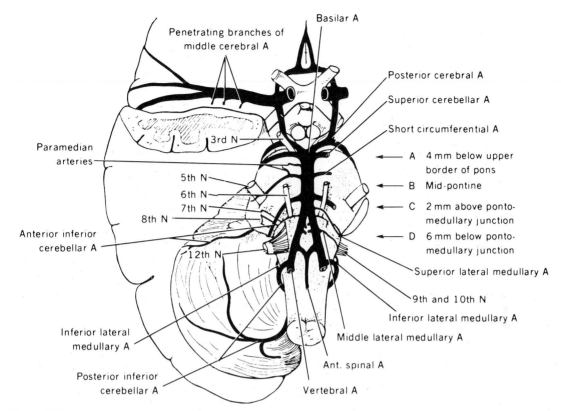

Figure 34-3

Diagram of the brainstem showing the principal vessels of the vertebral-basilar system. The letters and arrows on the right indicate the levels of the four cross sections which follow: A = Fig. 34-16; B = Fig. 34-15; C = Fig 34-14; D = Fig. 34-13.

Although vascular syndromes of the pons and medulla have been designated by sharply outlined shaded areas, one must appreciate that since satisfactory clinicopathologic studies are scarce, the diagrams do not always represent established fact. The frequency with which infarcts fail to produce a well-recognized syndrome and the special tendency for syndromes to merge with one another must be emphasized.

function, the blood flow measurements fell in the ischemic penumbra. "Steal" phenomena from surrounding normal brain, claimed to occur upon CO_2 inhalation in cases of infarction, was not demonstrable. Blood flow through collaterals was increased when CO_2 was inhaled and the blood pressure raised 30 to 40 mm systolic.

Ames and Nesbett have studied the rabbit retina in an immersion chamber in which O_2 and various substrates could be altered directly rather than through the vasculature. They found that cells could withstand a complete absence of O_2 of 20-min duration. After 30 min of anoxia, there was extensive irreversible damage, reflected by an inability of the tissue to utilize glucose and to synthesize protein. Hypoglycemia further reduced the tolerance to hypoxia, whereas tolerance of hypoxia could be prolonged by reducing the energy requirements of cells (increasing Mg in the medium). The long period of tolerance of retinal neurons to complete ischemia in vitro, in comparison to that in vivo, probably is related to what Ames has called the no-reflow phenomenom (swelling of capillary endothelial cells which prevents the restoration of circulation).

The relevance of these findings to stroke relates to the possibility of salvaging brain tissue by maintaining blood flow within the hypoperfused (ischemic penumbra) zone. In fact we know that under conditions of partial ischemia, cerebral tissue may survive for periods of 5 to 6 h or even longer. Body temperature is an important factor. A reduction of even 2 to 3°C, by reducing the metabolic requirements of neurons, increases their tolerance to hypoxia by 25 to 30 percent.

The accumulation of lactic acid in cerebral tissue (and the biochemical changes subsequent to the cellular acidosis) appears to be of particular importance in determining the extent of cell damage under conditions of ischemia (see reviews of Raichle and of Plum). Myers and Yamaguchi first showed that monkeys infused with glucose before the induction of cardiac arrest suffered more brain damage than did either fasted or saline-infused animals. They suggested that the high cerebral glucose level under anaerobic conditions led to increased glycolysis during the ischemic episode and that the accumulated lactate was neurotoxic. Plum and his colleagues have provided experimental evidence that with high lactate levels (approximately 16 mmol/kg or higher) ischemia produces infarction of cerebral tissue, and, with lower levels, a more selective neuronal injury. On the basis of such observations, Plum has suggested that scrupulous control of the blood glucose might reduce the risk of cerebral infarction in the diabetic and otherwise stroke-prone patients and during conditions of potential hyperglycemia.

NEUROVASCULAR SYNDROMES

For reasons already given, the clinical picture that results from an occlusion of any one artery differs in minor ways from one patient to another. There is sufficient uniformity, however, to justify a study of the typical syndrome related to each major artery. The following descriptions apply particularly to infarction and ischemia due to embolism and thrombosis. Although hemorrhage within a specific vascular territory may give rise to many of the same effects, the total clinical picture is apt to differ because in its deep extension and pressure effects the hemorrhage involves the territory of more than one artery.

THE CAROTID ARTERY

The territory supplied by this vessel and its main branches is shown in Figs. 34-4 and 34-6. The clinical manifestations of atherosclerotic thrombotic disease of this artery are the most variable of any cerebrovascular syndrome, as one might infer from what was said above. Occlusion, which occurs most frequently in the first part of the internal carotid artery (immediately beyond the carotid bifurcation), is not infrequently silent, owing to the efficacy of the external orbital-internal carotid and willisian collaterals; but in other instances it may cause a massive infarction involving the anterior two-thirds or all of the cerebral hemisphere, including the basal ganglia, and lead to death in a few days. Two mechanisms of cerebral ischemia have been identified: vascular occlusion from an embolism or propagating thrombus and perfusion failure from distal insufficiency. The former leads to branch occlusions of the anterior and middle cerebral arteries: the latter leads to distal field (watershed or border-zone) ischemia. Failure of distal perfusion may involve all or part of the middle cerebral territory; and when the anterior communicating artery is very small, the ipsilateral anterior cerebral territory is affected as well. If the two anterior cerebral arteries arise from a common stem on one side, infarction may occur in the territories of both vessels. The territory supplied by the posterior cerebral artery will also be included in the infarction when this vessel receives its main supply from the internal carotid rather than the basilar artery. Not infrequently the territory of the anterior choroidal artery is also affected. If one internal carotid artery had been occluded at an earlier time, occlusion of the other one may cause bilateral cerebral infarction. The clinical effects in such cases may include coma with quadriplegia and continuous horizontal "metronomic" conjugate eye movements.

Symptomatic occlusion of the internal carotid artery usually produces a picture resembling that of middle cerebral artery occlusion—contralateral hemiplegia, hemihypesthesia, and aphasia (with involvement of the dominant hemisphere). When the anterior cerebral territory is included, there will be added some or all of the clinical features of the latter (see further on). Such patients are usually stuporous or semicomatose, because of the sheer mass of swollen, necrotic brain. Headache, usually located above the eyebrow, may also occur with thrombosis or embolism of the carotid artery. The headache associated with occlusion of the middle cerebral artery is usually more lateral, at the temple, and that of posterior cerebral occlusion is in or behind the eye.

When the circulation of one carotid artery has been compromised and the most distal parts of the middle and anterior cerebral territories come to lie in the zone of maximal ischemia (this zone is situated between the two vascular territories rather than in the center of each one) the greater involvement tends to fall in the distal territory of the middle cerebral artery. The zone of damage forms an elongated sickle-shaped strip of variable width from the frontal to the occipital poles. This tendency for a certain number of carotid infarcts to occupy the distal rather than central part of the sylvian region is a product of vascular arrangements that alter the pattern of ischemia. The distal zone also proves to be the most vulnerable in transient ischemic attacks with stenosis of the carotid artery. These attacks usually take the form of weakness or paresthesias of the arm, and only when the ischemia is more extensive do they include the face and tongue. If the perfusion failure is prolonged, the ischemic stroke that results takes the form of a sensorimotor deficit in the arm with relative sparing of the face and leg, an aphasic syndrome if the dominant

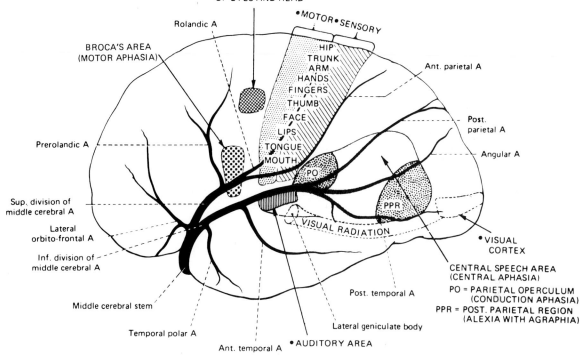

Figure 34-4

Diagram of a cerebral hemisphere, lateral aspect, showing the branches and distribution of the middle cerebral artery and the principal regions of cerebral localization. Below is a list of the clinical manifestations of infarction in the territory of this artery and the corresponding regions of cerebral damage.

Signs and symptoms	Structures involved
Paralysis of the contralateral face, arm, and leg	Somatic motor area for face and arm and the fibers descending from the leg area to enter the corona radiata
Sensory impairment over the contralateral face, arm, and leg (pinprick, cotton touch, vibration, position, two-point discrimination, stereognosis, tactile localization, barognosis, cutaneographia)	Somatic sensory area for face and arm and thalamoparietal projections
Motor speech disorder	Broca's area of the dominant hemisphere
"Central" aphasia, word deafness, anomia, jargon speech, alexia, agraphia, acalculia, finger agnosia, right-left confusion (the last four comprise the Gerstmann syndrome)	Central language area and parietoccipital cortex of the dominant hemisphere
Apractagnosia (amorphosynthesis), anosognosia, hemiasomatognosia, unilateral neglect, agnosia for the left half of external space, "dressing apraxia," "constructional apraxia," distortion of visual coordinates, inaccurate localization in the half field, impaired ability to judge distance, upside-down reading, visual illusions	Usually nondominant parietal lobe. Loss of topographic memory is usually due to a nondominant lesion, occasionally to a dominant one.

Figure 34-4 (*continued*)

Signs and symptoms	Structures involved
Homonymous hemianopia (often superior homonymous quadrantanopia)	Optic radiation deep to second temporal convolution
Paralysis of conjugate gaze to the opposite side	Frontal contraversive field or fibers projecting therefrom
Avoidance reaction of opposite limbs	Parietal lobe
Miscellaneous:	
Ataxia of contralateral limb(s)	Parietal lobe
So-called Bruns ataxia or apraxia of gait	Frontal lobes (bilateral)
Loss or impairment of optokinetic nystagmus	Supramarginal or angular gyrus
Limb-kinetic apraxia	Premotor or parietal cortical damage
Mirror movements	Precise location of responsible lesions not known
Cheyne-Stokes respiration, contralateral hyperhidrosis, mydriasis (occasionally)	Precise location of responsible lesions not known
Pure motor hemiplegia	Upper portion of the posterior limb of the internal capsule and the adjacent corona radiata

hemisphere is involved, and unilateral neglect if the non-dominant hemisphere is involved (Mohr and Pessin). The frequent sparing of the posterior part of the hemisphere is reflected in a low incidence of posterior types of aphasia and persistent homonymous hemianopia.

The internal carotid artery nourishes the optic nerve and retina as well as the brain (Figs. 34-1 and 34-2). Transient monocular blindness occurs as an intermittent symptom prior to the onset of stroke in approximately 25 percent of cases of symptomatic carotid occlusion. Yet central retinal artery ischemia is relatively rare in this condition, presumably because of efficient collateral supply.

Whereas most cerebral arteries can be evaluated only indirectly, by analysis of the clinical effects of occlusion, more direct means are available for the evaluation of the common and internal carotid arteries in the neck. With severe atherosclerotic stenosis at the level of the carotid sinus, with or without a superimposed thrombus, stethoscopy frequently discloses a *bruit*. Occasionally the bruit is due to stenosis at the origin of the external carotid artery and can then be misleading. If the bruit is heard at the angle of the jaw, the stenosis usually lies in the carotid sinus; if heard lower in the neck, it is in the common carotid or subclavian artery. The duration and quality of the bruit are important—bruits that extend into diastole and are high-pitched are almost invariably associated with a tight stenosis (lumen< 1.5 mm). One must be careful to distinguish bruits in the neck from transmitted aortic valve murmurs or a jugular vein obstruction. An additional sign of carotid occlusion is the presence of a bruit on the opposite side, heard best by placing the bell of the stethoscope over the eyeball; presumably the murmur is due to augmented circulation through the patent but irregularly narrowed

vessel. *Pulsation* may be palpably reduced or absent in the common carotid artery in the neck, in the external carotid artery in front of the ear, and in the internal carotid artery in the lateral wall of the pharynx. In the presence of a unilateral internal carotid occlusion, compression of the normal common carotid should be avoided because it may precipitate unconsciousness, seizures, or an EEG change. *Central retinal artery pressure* is reduced on the side of a carotid occlusion or severe stenosis. A diastolic retinal pressure (determined by ophthalmic dynamometry) of less than 20 mmHg usually means that the common or internal carotid artery is occluded. The state of the arterial channels over the face may also suggest carotid occlusion. The supraorbital and supratrochlear pulses (on the upper orbital rim) become prominent as these vessels dilate to carry blood through the orbit via the ophthalmic artery into the upper carotid. Noninvasive methods for measuring carotid flow are now available in most hospitals, i.e., continuous-wave Doppler or range-gated pulsed Doppler, and oculoplethysmography. The occurrence of *retinal emboli*, either shining or plain reddish in appearance, is another sign of carotid disease (crystalline cholesterol may be sloughed from an atherosclerotic ulcer).

Other neurologic and nonneurologic signs of carotid occlusion include pulseless arms (as in pulseless disease, see below); faintness in arising from the horizontal position or recurrent loss of consciousness when walking; headache and sometimes ocular, retro-orbital, and neck pain; transient blindness, either unilateral or bilateral; unilateral visual loss or dimness of vision with exercise, in bright light, or on assuming an upright position; premature cataracts; retinal atrophy and pigmentation; atrophy of the iris; leukomas; peripapillary arteriovenous anastomoses in the retinae; optic atrophy; claudication of jaw muscles; perforation of the nasal septum; saddle nose deformity; facial atrophy (unilateral or bilateral); indolent infections of the face; abnormal facial pigmentation; and loss of hair.

Stenoses and ulcerations of the internal carotid artery near its origin from the common carotid artery (the bulb) may be a source of fibrin platelet emboli or a fluctuant reduction in blood flow, resulting in transient ischemic attacks. These are discussed further on.

MIDDLE CEREBRAL ARTERY

This artery through its *cortical branches* supplies the lateral part of the cerebral hemisphere (Fig. 34-4). Its territory encompasses (1) the cortex and white matter of the lateral and inferior aspects of the frontal lobe including motor areas 4 and 6, contraversive centers for lateral gaze, and motor speech area of Broca (dominant hemisphere); (2) cortex and white matter of the parietal lobe including the

sensory cortex and the angular and supramarginal convolutions; and (3) superior parts of the temporal lobe and insula, including the sensory language areas of Wernicke. The *penetrating branches* of the middle cerebral artery supply the putamen, part of the head and body of the caudate nucleus, the outer globus pallidus, the posterior limb of the internal capsule, and the corona radiata (Fig. 34-5). Both the size of the middle cerebral artery and the territory that it supplies are longer than those of the anterior and posterior cerebral arteries.

The middle cerebral artery may be occluded in its stem, blocking the flow in deep penetrating as well as the superficial cortical branches, or each of the two divisions in the sylvian sulcus and their major branches may be occluded separately. The classic picture of total occlusion

Figure 34-5

Diagram of a cerebral hemisphere, coronal section, showing the territories of the major cerebral vessels.

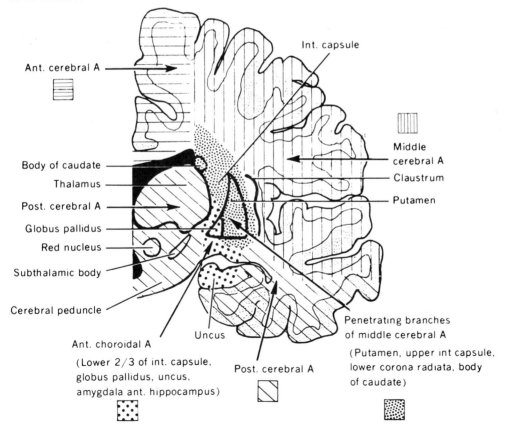

is contralateral hemiplegia, hemianesthesia, and homonymous hemianopia, with deviation of the head and eyes toward the side of the lesion; in addition there is a global aphasia with left hemispheric lesions (Fig. 34-4) and amorphosynthesis with right-sided ones (see page 365). In the beginning the patient is dull or stuporous. Once established, the motor, sensory, and language deficits remain static or improve very little as months and years pass. If globally aphasic, seldom does the patient ever again communicate effectively. Occlusion of branches of the middle cerebral artery give rise to only parts of the symptom complex.

Occlusion of the stem of the middle cerebral artery by a thrombus, contrary to former teaching, is relatively infrequent (2 to 5 percent of middle cerebral artery occlusions). Pathologic studies have shown that most carotid occlusions are thrombotic, whereas most middle cerebral occlusions, particularly of the cortical branches, are embolic (Fisher, 1975). Most emboli tend to drift into superficial cortical branches; not more than 1 in 20 will enter penetrating basal branches. The distal territory of the middle cerebral artery may also be rendered ischemic by failure of the systemic circulation, especially if the carotid artery is stenotic; this may simulate embolic branch occlusions.

An embolus entering the middle cerebral artery often lodges in one of its two main divisions, the superior (supplying the rolandic and prerolandic areas) or inferior (supplying the inferior parietal and lateral temporal lobes). Major infarction in the territory of the superior division causes a dense sensorimotor deficit in the contralateral face, arm, and leg and ipsilateral deviation of head and eyes, and mimics the syndrome of stem occlusion, except that there is less impairment of alertness. If the occlusion is lasting (not merely transient ischemia with disintegration of the embolus), there will be slow improvement, and after a few months the patient will be able to walk with a spastic leg, while the motor deficits of the arm and face remain severe. The sensory deficit may be profound, resembling that of a thalamic infarct (pseudothalamic syndrome of Foix). Lesser degrees take the form of stereoagnosia, impaired position sense, graphesthesia, tactile localization, and two-point discrimination, and variable changes in touch, pain, and temperature sense. A pseudoradicular pattern of sensory loss in the hand and forearm (radial or ulnar half) from a parietal infarct was originally described by Dejerine. With left-sided lesions there is initially a global aphasia, which changes to a predominantly motor aphasia, with improvement in the comprehension of spoken and written words and the emergence of an effortful, hesitant, gram-matically simplified, dysmelodic speech. Embolic occlusion, limited to one of the branches of the superior division, produces a highly circumscribed infarct that further fractionates the syndrome. With occlusion of the ascending frontal branch the motor deficit is limited to the face and arm with little affection of the leg, and the latter, if weakened at all, soon improves; and with left-sided lesions an initial mutism and mild comprehension defect give way, within days to weeks, to grammatically appropriate speech, slightly dysmelodic, with normal comprehension (see Chap. 22). Embolic occlusion of the rolandic branches results in sensorimotor paresis with severe dysarthria but little evidence of aphasia. It resembles a pure motor stroke from lacunar infarction (see further on). Embolic occlusion of ascending parietal and other posterior branches of the superior division may cause no sensorimotor deficit, but only a conduction aphasia (page 385) and bilateral ideomotor apraxia. Improvement can be expected within a few weeks to months.

The inferior division of the middle cerebral artery is occluded less often than the superior one, but again nearly always due to cardiogenic embolism. The usual result in left-sided lesions is a Wernicke aphasia (see page 383). After remaining static for weeks to months, improvement can be expected. In less extensive infarcts from branch occlusions (superior parietal, angular, or posterior temporal), the deficit in comprehension of spoken and written language may be especially severe. Again, after a few months the deficits usually improve, often to the point where they are evident only in self-generated efforts to read and copy visually presented material. With either right or left hemisphere lesions there is usually a homonymous hemianopia and with right-sided ones, a left visual neglect and other signs of amorphosynthesis; an agitated delirium, presumably from temporal lobe damage, may be a prominent feature in these latter patients.

Foix and Levy described the clinical effects of deep capsular–basal ganglionic lesions and superficial cortical-subcortical ones. There were few important differences in the degree and pattern of the hemiplegia and sensory disorder. Homonymous hemianopia can occur with posterior capsular lesions, but it may be simulated by visual hemi-neglect of contralateral space.

The middle cerebral artery may become stenotic rather than occluded. In the series of Feldmeyer et al and of Day, many of the permanent deficiencies were preceded by transient ischemic attacks, giving a picture that resembles carotid stenosis.

ANTERIOR CEREBRAL ARTERY

This artery, through its cortical branches, supplies the anterior three-quarters of the medial surface of the cerebral

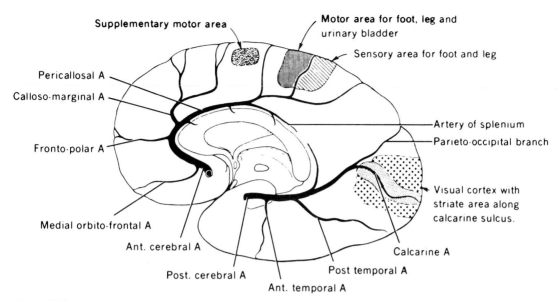

Figure 34-6

Diagram of a cerebral hemisphere, medial aspect, showing the branches and distribution of the anterior cerebral artery and the principal regions of cerebral localization. Below is a list of the clinical manifestations of infarction in the territory of this artery and the corresponding regions of cerebral damage.

Signs and symptoms	Structures involved
Paralysis of opposite foot and leg	Motor leg area
A lesser degree of paresis of opposite arm	Involvement of arm area of cortex or fibers descending therefrom to corona radiata
Cortical sensory loss over toes, foot, and leg	Sensory area for foot and leg
Urinary incontinence	Posteromedial part of superior frontal gyrus (bilateral)
Contralateral grasp reflex, sucking reflex, gegenhalten (paratonic rigidity), "frontal tremor"	Medial surface of the posterior frontal lobe (?)
Abulia (akinetic mutism), slowness, delay, lack of spontaneity, whispering, motor inaction, reflex distraction to sights and sounds	Uncertain localization—probably superomedial lesion near subcallosum
Impairment of gait and stance (gait "apraxia")	Inferomedial frontal–striatal (?)
Mental impairment (perseveration and amnesia)	Localization unknown
Miscellaneous: dyspraxia of left limbs	Corpus callosum
Tactile aphasia in left limbs	Corpus callosum
Cerebral paraplegia	Motor leg area bilaterally (due to bilateral occlusion of anterior cerebral arteries)

Note: Hemianopia does not occur; transcortical aphasia occurs rarely (page 388).

hemisphere, including the medial-orbital surface of the frontal lobe, the frontal pole, a strip of the lateral surface of the cerebral hemisphere along the superior border, and the anterior four-fifths of the corpus callosum. Deep branches, arising near the circle of Willis (proximal or distal to the anterior communicating artery), supply the anterior limb of the internal capsule and the inferior part of the head of the caudate nucleus (Figs. 34-5 to 34-7). The largest of these is Heubner's artery, which supplies the head of the caudate, anterior limb of the internal capsule, and anterior part of the globus pallidus.

Again the clinical picture will depend on the location and size of the infarct, which in turn relates to the site of the occlusion, the pattern of the circle of Willis, and the other ischemia-modifying factors mentioned above. Well-studied cases of infarction in the territory of this artery are not numerous; hence the syndromes are imperfectly known (see Brust for a review of recent literature and description of developmental abnormalities).

Occlusion of the stem of the outer cerebral artery proximal to its connection with the anterior communicating

Figure 34-7

Corrosion preparations with plastics demonstrating penetrating branches of the anterior and middle cerebral arteries. (1) Lateral lenticulostriate arteries. (2) Heubner artery and medial lenticulostriate arteries. (3) Anterior cerebral artery. (4) Internal carotid artery. (5) Middle cerebral artery. (From Krayenbühl and Yasargil.)

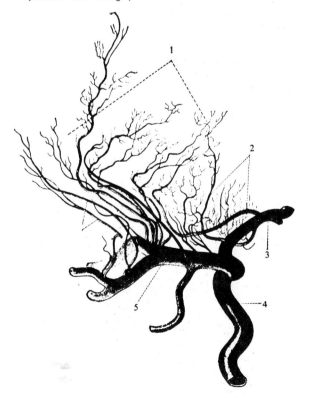

artery is usually well tolerated since adequate collateral flow will come from the artery of the opposite side. Maximal disturbance occurs when both arteries arise from one anterior cerebral stem, in which case there will be infarction of the medial parts of both cerebral hemispheres. This results in paraplegia, incontinence, and abulic and aphasic symptoms.

Complete infarction due to occlusion of one anterior cerebral artery distal to the anterior communicating artery results in a sensorimotor deficit of the opposite foot and leg, and a lesser degree of paresis of the arm, and sparing of the face. The motor disorder is more in the foot and leg than in the thigh. Sensory loss is mainly of the discriminative modalities and is mild or absent in some cases. The head and eyes may deviate to the side of the lesion. Urinary incontinence, contralateral grasp and sucking reflexes, and paratonic rigidity (gegenhalten) may be evident. With a left-sided occlusion there may be a sympathetic apraxia of the left arm and leg. Also, transcortical motor aphasia may occur with occlusions of Heubner's branch of the left anterior cerebral artery. Alexander and Schmitt cite cases in which a right hemiplegia (predominant in leg) with grasping and groping responses of the right hand and buccofacial apraxia are accompanied by a diminution or absence of spontaneous speech, agraphia, labored tele-graphic speech, and a limited ability to name objects and to compose word lists, but a striking preservation of the ability to repeat spoken and written sentences (transcortical motor aphasia). Disorders of behavior that may be overlooked are abulia, presenting as a slowness and lack of spontaneity in all reactions; a tendency to speak in whispers; and distractibility. Branch occlusions of the anterior cerebral artery produce only fragments of the total syndrome, usually a spastic weakness or cortical sensory loss in the opposite foot and leg. Bilateral occlusion of the anterior cerebral arteries, embolic or surgical (following operations on anterior communicating aneurysms), results in akinetic mutism and frontal lobe personality changes (see Chap. 21).

ANTERIOR CHOROIDAL ARTERY

This is a long narrow artery that springs from the internal carotid, just above the origin of the posterior communicating artery. It supplies the internal segment of the globus pallidus and posterior limb of the internal capsule and various contiguous structures, and penetrates the temporal horn of the lateral ventricle, where it supplies the choroid plexus and anastamoses with the posterior choroidal artery.

Only a few complete clinicopathologic studies form the basis of our knowledge of the syndrome caused by occlusion of this artery. It was found by Foix et al to consist of contralateral hemiplegia, hemihypesthesia, and homonymous hemianopia due to involvement of the posterior limb of the internal capsule and white matter posterolateral to it, through which the geniculocalcarine tract passes. Cognitive function is notably spared. Decroix and his colleagues have reported 16 cases in which the lesion was verified by CT scan and thought to lie in the vascular territory of this artery. In most of these cases the clinical syndrome has fallen short of what is expected on anatomic grounds. With right-sided lesions there may be left spatial neglect and constructional apraxia, and slight disorders of speech and language may accompany left-sided lesions. Of course the lesion may have extended beyond the territory of this artery, since postmortem confirmation was lacking. It should be remembered that for a time the anterior choroidal artery was being surgically ligated, for the purpose of abolishing the tremor and rigidity of unilateral Parkinson disease, without these ischemic effects having occurred.

VERTEBRAL-BASILAR AND POSTERIOR CEREBRAL ARTERIES

Posterior Cerebral Artery In about 70 percent of cases both posterior cerebral arteries arise from the basilar, and only thin posterior communicating arteries join this system to the internal carotids. In 20 to 25 percent, one posterior cerebral artery comes from the basilar and the other from the internal carotid; in the remainder both come from the carotids.

The configuration and branches of the *circular or proximal segment of the posterior cerebral* artery are illustrated in Figs. 34-8 and 34-9. *The interpeduncular branches* arising just above the basilar bifurcation supply the red nuclei, substantiae nigrae, medial parts of the cerebral peduncles, oculomotor and trochlear nuclei and nerves, reticular substance of the upper brainstem, decussation of the brachia conjunctiva (superior cerebellar peduncles), medial longitudinal fasciculi, and medial lemnisci. The portion of the posterior cerebral artery giving rise to the interpeduncular branches (the portion between the bifurcation of the basilar artery and the ostium of the posterior communicating artery) is also referred to as the *mesencephalic artery* or the *basilar communicating artery*.

The thalamoperforant branches (also referred to as *paramedian thalamic arteries*) arise more distally, near the junction of the posterior cerebral and posterior communicating arteries, and supply the inferior, medial, and anterior parts of the thalamus. As pointed out by Percheron, the arterial configuration of these arteries varies: In some cases, the paramedian thalamic arteries arise symmetrically, one from each side; in other cases, both arteries arise from the same posterior cerebral stem, either separately or by a common trunk which then bifurcates. In the latter case, one posterior cerebral stem (basilar communicating artery) supplies the medial thalamic territories on both sides, and an

occlusion of this artery or one paramedian thalamic artery produces a bilateral butterfly-shaped lesion in the medial parts of the diencephalon.

The thalamogeniculate branches arise still more distally, opposite the lateral geniculate body, and supply the geniculate body and the central and posterior parts of the thalamus. Medial branches from the posterior cerebral, as it encircles the midbrain, supply the lateral part of the cerebral peduncle, lateral tegmentum and corpora quadrigemina, and pineal gland. Posterior choroidal branches run to the posterosuperior thalamus, choroid plexus, hippocampus, and psalterium (decussation of fornices).

The terminal or *cortical branches of the posterior cerebral artery* supply the inferomedial part of the temporal lobe and the medial occipital lobe, including the lingula, cuneus, precuneus, and visual areas 17, 18, and 19 (see Figs. 34-6, 34-8, and 34-9).

Potentially, occlusion of the posterior cerebral artery can produce a greater variety of clinical effects than occlusion of any other artery, because both the upper brainstem, which is crowded with important structures, and the inferior parts of the temporal and medial parts of the occipital lobes lie within its domain. Obviously the site of the occlusion and arrangement of the circle of Willis will in large measure determine the location and extent of the resulting infarct. For example, occlusion proximal to the posterior communicating artery may be asymptomatic if the collateral flow is adequate (A, Fig. 34-8; see also Fig. 34-9). Even distal to the posterior communicating artery, an occlusion may cause relatively little damage if the collateral flow through border zone collaterals from anterior and middle cerebral arteries is sufficient.

For convenience of exposition it is helpful to divide the various posterior cerebral artery syndromes into three groups: (1) anterior and proximal (involving interpeduncular, thalamic perforant, and thalamogeniculate branches), (2) cortical (inferior temporal and medial occipital), and (3) bilateral.

Anterior and proximal syndromes (*Figs. 34-9 and 34-10*) The *thalamic syndrome of Déjerine and Roussy* (see also page 114) follows infarction of the sensory relay nuclei in the thalamus, the result of occlusion of thalamogeniculate branches. There is both a deep and cutaneous sensory loss, usually severe in degree, of the opposite side of the body, accompanied by a transitory hemiparesis. A homonymous hemianopia may be conjoined. In some instances there is a dissociated sensory loss, pain and thermal sensation being more affected than touch, vibration, and position, or only one part of the body may be anesthetic. After an interval, sensation begins to return and the patient may then be afflicted with pain, paresthesia, and hyperpathia in the affected parts. There may also be distortion of taste, athetotic posturing of the hand, and depression of mood. Such conditions may persist for years.

Central midbrain and subthalamic syndromes are due to occlusion of the interpeduncular branches. The clinical changes include the Weber syndrome (oculomotor palsy with contralateral hemiplegia), paralysis of vertical gaze, stupor or coma, and movement disorders, most often an ataxic tremor that may be contralateral, i.e., on the side of hemiparesis (see below). A persistent hemiplegia from infarction of the cerebral peduncle is relatively rare.

Anteromedial-inferior thalamic syndromes follow occlusion of the thalamoperforant branches. Here the most common effect is an extrapyramidal movement disorder (hemiballismus or hemichoreoathetosis). Deep sensory loss, hemiataxia, or tremor may be added in various combinations. Hemiballismus is due usually to occlusion of a small branch to the corpus Luysii or its connections with the pallidum. Occlusion of the paramedian thalamic branch(es) to the medial dorsal nuclei or to the dominant medial dorsal nucleus gives rise to an amnesic (Korsakoff) syndrome.

Cortical syndromes Classically, occlusion of branches to the temporal and occipital lobes gives rise to a homonymous hemianopia because of involvement of the primary visual receptive area (calcarine or striate cortex), or of the converging geniculocalcarine fibers. It may be incomplete and then involves the upper quadrants of the visual fields more than the lower ones (see Chap. 12). Macular or central vision may be spared because of collateralization of the occipital pole from distal branches of the middle (or anterior) cerebral arteries. There may be visual hallucinations in the blind parts of the visual fields (Cogan) or metamorphopsia and palinopsia (Brust and Behrens). Posterior cortical infarcts of the dominant hemisphere cause alexia (with or without agraphia), anomia (amnesic aphasia), a variety of visual agnosias, and rarely an impairment of memory (see pages 386 and 370). The anomias (dysnomias) are most severe for colors, but the naming of other visually presented material such as pictures, musical notes, mathematical symbols, and manipulable objects may also be impaired. The patient may treat objects as familiar, that is, describe their functions and use them correctly, but be unable to name them. Color dysnomia and amnesic aphasia are more often present in this syndrome than is alexia. The defect in retentive memory is of varying severity and may or may not improve with the passage of time. Bilateral inferomesial occipitoparietal lesions may be accompanied by topographic disorientation and lack of recognition of faces (prosopagnosia).

A complete proximal arterial occlusion leads to a syndrome that combines cortical and anterior-proximal syndromes in part or totally. The vascular lesion may be either an embolus or an atherosclerotic thrombus.

Bilateral cortical syndrome This may occur as a result of successive infarctions or from a single embolic

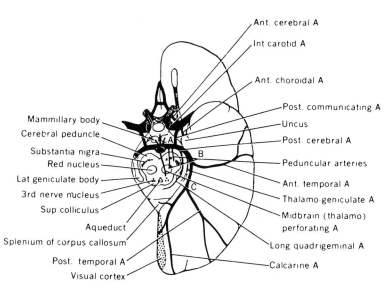

Ant. cerebral A
Int carotid A
Ant. choroidal A
Post. communicating A
Uncus
Post. cerebral A
Peduncular arteries
Ant. temporal A
Thalamo-geniculate A
Midbrain (thalamo) perforating A
Long quadrigeminal A
Calcarine A

Mammillary body
Cerebral peduncle
Substantia nigra
Red nucleus
Lat geniculate body
3rd nerve nucleus
Sup colliculus
Aqueduct
Splenium of corpus callosum
Post. temporal A
Visual cortex

Figure 34-8

Inferior aspect of the brain showing the branches and distribution of the posterior cerebral artery and the principal anatomic structures supplied. On the next page are listed the clinical manifestations produced by infarction in its territory and the corresponding regions of damage.

Figure 34-8 (*continued*)

Signs and symptoms	Structures involved
Peripheral territory	
Homonymous hemianopia	Calcarine cortex or optic radiation; hemiachromatopsia may be present. Macular or central vision is preserved if striate area is spared.
Bilateral homonymous hemianopia, cortical blindness, unawareness or denial of blindness; achromatopsia, failure to see to-and-fro movements, inability to perceive objects not centrally located, apraxia of ocular movements, inability to count or enumerate objects	Bilateral occipital lobe possibly with involvement of parietooccipital region
Dyslexia without agraphia, color anomia	Dominant calcarine lesion and posterior part of corpus callosum
Memory defect	Lesion of inferomedial portions of temporal lobe bilaterally or on the dominant side only
Topographic disorientation and prosopagnosia	Nondominant calcarine and lingual gyri, usually bilateral
Simultagnosia	Dominant visual cortex, sometimes bilateral
Unformed visual hallucinations, metamorphopsia, teleopsia, illusory visual spread, palinopsia, distortion of outlines, photophobia	Calcarine cortex
Central territory	
Thalamic syndrome: sensory loss (all modalities), spontaneous pain and dysesthesias, choreoathetosis, intention tremor, spasms of hand, mild hemiparesis	Ventral posterolateral nucleus of thalamus in territory of thalamogeniculate artery. Involvement of the adjacent subthalamic nucleus or its pallidal connections results in hemiballismus and choreoathetosis.
Thalamoperforate syndrome: (1) superior, crossed cerebellar ataxia; (2) inferior, crossed cerebellar ataxia with ipsilateral third nerve palsy (Claude syndrome)	Dentatothalamic tract and issuing third nerve
Weber syndrome—third nerve palsy and contralateral hemiplegia	Issuing third nerve and cerebral peduncle
Contralateral hemiplegia	Cerebral peduncle
Paralysis or paresis of vertical eye movement, skew deviation, sluggish pupillary responses to light, slight miosis and ptosis (retraction nystagmus and ''tucked-in'' eyelids may be associated)	Supranuclear fibers to third nerve, high midbrain tegmentum ventral to superior colliculus (interstitial nucleus of Cajal, nucleus of Darkschewitsch, and posterior commissure)
Contralateral ataxic or postural tremor	Dentatothalamic tract (?) after decussation. Precise site of lesion unknown.
Decerebrate attacks	Damage to motor tracts between red and vestibular nuclei

Note: Tremor in repose has been omitted because of the uncertainty of its occurrence in the posterior cerebral artery syndrome. Peduncular hallucinosis may occur in thalamic-subthalamic ischemic lesions, but the exact location of the lesion is unknown.

or thrombotic occlusion of the upper basilar artery, especially if the posterior communicating arteries are unusually small.

Bilateral lesions of the occipital lobes, if extensive, cause total blindness of the *cortical* type, i.e., a bilateral homonymous hemianopia, sometimes accompanied by unformed visual hallucinations. The pupillary reflexes are preserved, and funduscopically the optic discs are normal.

Often the patient is unaware of being blind and may in fact deny it, even when it is pointed out. More frequently the lesions are incomplete, and a sector or sectors of the visual fields remain intact. When the intact remnant is small, vision appears to fluctuate from moment to moment, as the patient attempts to capture the image in the island of intact vision. Hysteria may be suspected because of such inconsistencies. In bilateral lesions that are confined to the occipital poles, there may be a loss of only central vision (homonymous central scotomas). With other lesions of the occipital pole there may be homonymous paracentral scotomas, or the occipital poles may be spared, leaving the patient with only central ("gun barrel") vision. Horizontal or altitudinal field defects are usually due to lesions affecting the upper or lower banks of the calcarine sulci (see page 203). The Balint syndrome (page 371) is another effect of bilateral occipital lesions.

With bilateral lesions that involve the inferomedial portions of the temporal lobes, the impairment of memory may be severe (Korsakoff amnesic state). This syndrome and its accompaniments are fully described in Chaps. 20 and 21.

Vertebral Artery   The vertebral arteries are the chief arteries of the medulla; each supplies the lower three-fourths of the pyramid, the medial lemniscus, all or nearly all the retro-olivary (lateral medullary) region, the restiform body, and the posterior inferior part of the cerebellar hemisphere (Figs. 34-11 and 34-12). The relative sizes of the vertebral arteries vary considerably and, in approximately 10 percent of cases, one vessel is so small that the other is essentially the only artery of supply to the brainstem. In the latter cases, if collateral flow from the carotid system via the circle of Willis is unavailable, occlusion of the one functional vertebral artery would be equivalent to occlusion of the basilar artery or both vertebral arteries. The posterior inferior

cerebellar artery is usually a branch of the vertebral artery, but can have a common origin with the anterior inferior cerebellar artery from the basilar artery. It is necessary to keep these anatomic variations in mind when considering the effects of vertebral artery occlusion.

Since the vertebral arteries have a long extracranial course and pass through the transverse processes of C6 to C2 vertebrae before entering the cranial cavity, one might expect them to be subject to trauma, spondylotic compression, and a variety of vascular diseases. In our experience this rarely happens. We have not seen convincing examples of spondylotic occlusion. Neck rotation (chiropractic or other) has been reported to cause brainstem ischemia in more than 50 cases (Caplan). Dissection of the vertebral artery is also well documented, but rare; it declares itself by cervico-occipital headache and deficits of brainstem function, usually bilateral.

The results of vertebral occlusion are quite variable. When there are two good-sized arteries, occlusion of one may cause no recognizable symptoms and signs or pathologic changes. If the subclavian artery is blocked proximal to the origin of the vertebral artery, exercise of the arm on that side may draw blood from the vertebral-basilar system into the arm, sometimes resulting in the symptoms of basilar insufficiency. This phenomenon, described in 1961 by Reivich and his colleagues, was referred to by Fisher as the *subclavian steal*. Its most notable feature is transient weakness of the left arm, on exercise. There may also be headache and claudication of the arm. If the occlusion of the vertebral artery is so situated as to block the branches supplying the *lateral medulla*, a characteristic syndrome may result; this is probably the most frequent consequence

Figure 34-9

The posterior cerebral and basilar arteries. (From Krayenbühl and Yasargil.)

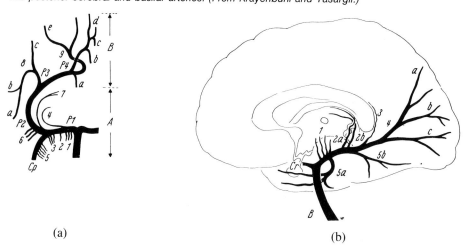

(a)   (b)

Figure 34-9 (*continued*)

Figure 34-9a: Posterior cerebral artery	Regions of vascular supply
A Circular or proximal segment	
(1) Paramedian arteries (interpeduncular, intercrural, perforating)	Substantia nigra, red nucleus, mammillary body, oculomotor nerve, trochlear nerve
(2) Quadrigeminal arteries	Quadrigeminal bodies
(3) Thalamic arteries (medial and lateral)	Central nucleus, medial nucleus, ventrolateral nucleus of the thalamus, pulvinar, lateral geniculate body, internal capsule (posterior portion)
(4) Medial posterior choroidal arteries	
(5) Premammillary arteries (of the posterior communicating artery)	Epithalamus, thalamus, choroid plexus, pineal gland
(6) Peduncular artery	Tuber cinereum, cerebral peduncle, ventral nuclei of the thalamus, nuclei of the hypothalamus, optic chiasm
(7) Lateral posterior choroidal arteries (anterior and posterior)	Hippocampal gyrus, lateral geniculate body, pulvinar, dentate fascia, hippocampus, anterior basal cortex of the temporal lobe, choroid plexus of the temporal horn, trigone, dorsolateral nuclei of the thalamus
B Cortical or distal segment	
(8) Lateral occipital artery	
(a) Anterior temporal arteries	Laterobasal aspects of the temporal and occipital lobe
(b) Middle temporal arteries	
(c) Posterior temporal arteries	
(9) Medial occipital artery	
(a) Dorsal callosal artery	Splenium
(b) Posterior parietal artery	Cuneus, precuneus
(c) Occipitoparietal artery	
(d) Calcarine arteries	Calcarine gyrus, occipital pole
(e) Occipitotemporal artery	Laterobasal occipital lobe

Figure 34-9b: Basilar artery

B   Basilar artery
Cr   Posterior communicating artery
(1)   Thalamic arteries
(2a) Medial posterior choroidal artery
(2b) Lateral posterior choroidal artery
(3)   Dorsal callosal artery
(4)   Medial occipital artery
       (a) Posterior parietal arteries
       (b) Occipitopaietal arteries
       (c) Calcarine arteries
(5a) Anterior and middle temporal arteries
(5b) Posterior temporal artery

of occlusion of one vertebral artery (see below). When the branch to the anterior spinal artery is blocked, flow from the corresponding branch is usually sufficient to prevent infarction of the cervical cord. If the branch to the pyramid is occluded, that part of the pyramidal tract may be infarcted unless collateral flow is adequate. Any of these branches may become occluded in its course as well as at its origin from the vertebral artery, with similar effects.

Rarely, occlusion of the vertebral artery or one of its medial branches produces an infarct that involves the medullary pyramid, the medial lemniscus, and the emergent hypoglossal fibers [causing a contralateral paralysis of arm and leg (with sparing of the face), contralateral loss of position and vibration sense, and ipsilateral paralysis and atrophy of the tongue]. This is the *medial medullary syndrome* (Fig. 34-13). Occlusion of a vertebral artery low in the neck is usually compensated by anastomotic flow to the upper part of the artery via the thyrocervical, deep cervical, and occipital arteries, or influx from the circle of Willis.

The *lateral medullary syndrome* (Fig. 34-13), known as the syndrome of Wallenberg (who described a case in 1895), is produced by infarction of a wedge of lateral medulla lying posterior to the inferior olivary nucleus. The classic syndrome, as outlined by Fisher, Karnes, and Kubik, reflects the involvement of the spinothalamic tract (*contralateral* impairment of pain and thermal sense over half the body, sometimes the face); descending sympathetic tract (*ipsilateral* Horner syndrome of miosis, ptosis, decreased sweating); issuing fibers of the ninth and tenth nerves (hoarseness, dysphagia, ipsilateral paralysis of the palate and vocal cord, diminished gag reflex); vestibular nuclei (nystagmus, oscillopsia, vertigo, nausea, vomiting); olivocerebellar and/or spinocerebellar fibers and, sometimes, restiform body (*ipsilateral* ataxia of limbs, falling to the ipsilateral side); descending tract and nucleus of the fifth nerve (pain, numbness, impaired sensation over ipsilateral half of the face); nucleus and tractus solitarius (loss of taste); and rarely cuneate and gracile nuclei (numbness of *ipsilateral* limbs). This syndrome, one of the most striking in neurology, is almost always due to ischemic necrosis. Although it has traditionally been attributed to occlusion of the posterior inferior cerebellar artery, careful studies have shown that in 8 out of 10 cases it is the vertebral artery that is occluded; in the remainder, either the posterior inferior cerebellar artery or one of the lateral medullary arteries is occluded.

Figure 34-10

Diagram of the vascularization of the diencephalon. Distribution of (1) the anterior cerebral artery, (2) the posterior cerebral artery, (3) the anterior and posterior choroidal arteries, (4) the posterior communicating artery, and (5) the internal carotid artery. (From Krayenbühl and Yasargil.)

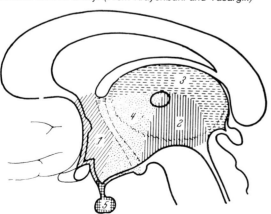

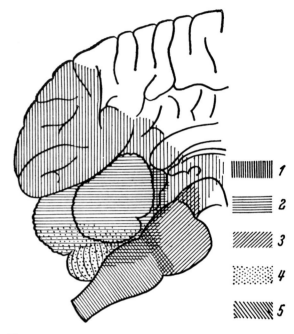

Figure 34-11

Regions of supply by the posterior segment of the circle of Willis, lateral view: (1) posterior cerebral artery; (2) superior cerebellar artery; (3) basilar artery and superior cerebellar artery; (4) posterior inferior cerebellar artery; (5) vertebral artery (posterior inferior cerebellar artery, anterior spinal artery, posterior spinal artery).

Infarction in the *posterior medullary region* causes ipsilateral cerebellar ataxia and, rarely, hiccup. The symptoms associated with isolated infarction of the inferior part of the cerebellum include sudden vertigo, nausea, vomiting, ataxia, and nystagmus—a picture that mimics acute labyrinthine disorder.

Basilar Artery   The branches of the basilar artery may be conveniently grouped as follows: (1) paramedian, 7 to 10 in number, supplying a wedge of pons on either side of the midline; (2) short circumferential, five to seven in number, supplying the lateral two-thirds of the pons and the middle and superior cerebellar peduncles; (3) the long circumferential, two on each side (the superior and anterior inferior cerebellar arteries), which run laterally around the pons to reach the cerebellar hemispheres (Figs. 34-11 and 34-12); and (4) several paramedian (interpeduncular) branches at the bifurcation of the basilar artery supplying the medial subthalamic and high midbrain regions (see above). The other branches of the posterior cerebral artery have also been described above.

The picture of basilar occlusion due to thrombosis may arise in several ways: (1) occlusion of the basilar artery itself, usually in the lower third at the site of an atherosclerotic plaque; (2) occlusion of both vertebral arteries; and (3) occlusion of a single vertebral artery, when it is the only one of adequate size. It needs to be emphasized that thrombosis frequently involves only a branch of the basilar artery rather than the trunk (*basilar branch occlusion*). When the obstruction is embolic, the embolus usually lodges at the upper bifurcation of the basilar or in one of the posterior cerebral arteries, since if it is small enough to pass through the vertebral artery, it easily traverses the length of the basilar artery, which is of greater diameter than either vertebral artery.

The syndrome of *basilar artery occlusion*, as outlined by Kubik and Adams, reflects the involvement of a large number of structures: corticospinal and corticobulbar tracts, cerebellum, middle and superior cerebellar peduncles, medial and lateral lemnisci, spinothalamic tracts, medial longitudinal fasciculi, pontine nuclei, vestibular and cochlear nuclei, descending hypothalamospinal sympathetic fibers, and the third through eighth cranial nerves (the nuclei and their segments within the brainstem).

The *complete basilar syndrome* comprises bilateral long tract signs (sensory and motor) with variable cerebellar, cranial nerve and other segmental abnormalities of the brainstem. Often the patient is comatose because of ischemia of the high midbrain reticular activating system. Others are

Figure 34-12

Regions supplied by the posterior segment of the circle of Willis, basal view: (1) posterior cerebral artery; (2) superior cerebellar artery; (3) paramedian arteries of the basilar artery and spinal artery; (4) posterior inferior cerebellar artery; (5) vertebral artery; (6) anterior inferior cerebellar artery; (7) dorsal spinal artery. (From Krayenbühl and Yasargil.)

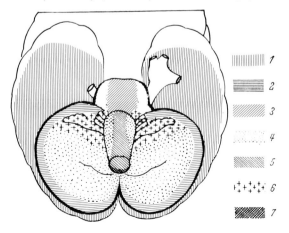

mute and quadriplegic but conscious, due to interruption of motor pathways and sparing of the reticular activating system (pseudocoma or "locked-in" syndrome). In the presence of the full syndrome, it is usually not difficult to make the correct diagnosis. The aim should be, however, to recognize basilar insufficiency long before the stage of total deficit has been reached. The early manifestations (some in the form of transient ischemic attacks) occur in many combinations [vertigo, headache, blurred vision, diplopia, dysarthria, weakness or numbness of the limbs (first on one side, then the other), ataxia, and rarely drop attacks. These are described in detail further on (page 650).

Occlusion of branches at the bifurcation of the basilar artery results in a remarkable number of complex syndromes that include, in various combinations, somnolence, memory defects, visual hallucinations, disorders of ocular movement (convergence spasm, paralysis of vertical gaze, retraction nystagmus, pseudoabducens palsy, retraction of upper eyelids), skew deviation of the eyes, an agitated delirious state, and visual defects. These have been reviewed by Petit et al and Castaigne et al as paramedian thalamic, subthalamic, and midbrain infarctions and by Caplan as "top of the basilar" syndromes.

The main signs of occlusion of the *superior cerebellar artery* are ipsilateral cerebellar ataxia (middle and/or superior cerebellar peduncles); nausea and vomiting; slurred (pseudobulbar) speech; and loss of pain and thermal sensation over the opposite side of the body (spino-thalamic tract). Partial deafness, static tremor of the ipsilateral upper extremity, an ipsilateral Horner syndrome, and palatal myoclonus have also been reported.

With occlusion of the *anterior inferior cerebellar artery* the extent of the infarct is extremely variable. The size of this artery and the territory it supplies vary inversely with the size and territory of supply of the posterior inferior cerebellar artery. The principal findings are vertigo, nausea, vomiting, nystagmus, tinnitus; ipsilateral cerebellar ataxia (inferior cerebellar peduncle or restiform body), an ipsilateral Horner syndrome and paresis of conjugate lateral gaze; and contralateral loss of pain and temperature sense of the arm, trunk, and leg (lateral spinothalamic tract). If the occlusion is close to the origin of the artery, the corticospinal fibers may also be involved, producing a hemiplegia.

Another cardinal manifestation of brainstem involvement is a "crossed" or "alternate" cranial nerve and long tract sensory or motor deficit. These "crossed" syndromes, which may involve cranial nerves III through XII, are listed in Table 47-2. Although the finding of bilateral neurologic signs strongly suggests brainstem involvement, it must be emphasized that in many instances of infarction within the basilar territory the signs are limited to one side of the body, with or without cranial nerve involvement, indicating occlusion of a branch of the basilar artery, not of the main trunk.

It is impossible from motor signs alone to distinguish a hemiplegia of pontine origin from one of cerebral origin. With brainstem lesions, as with cerebral lesions, a flaccid paralysis gives way to spasticity after a few days or weeks, and there is no satisfactory explanation for the variability in this period of delay or for the occurrence in some cases of spasticity from the onset of the stroke. Localization depends upon coexisting neurologic phenomena. With a hemiplegia of lower brainstem origin the eyes may deviate to the side of the paralysis, just the opposite of supratentorial lesions. The pattern of sensory disturbance may be helpful. A dissociated sensory deficit over the face or half the body usually indicates a lesion within the brainstem, while a hemisensory loss involving all modalities indicates a lesion in the upper brainstem, thalamus, or deep in the white matter of the parietal lobe. When position sense, two-point discrimination, and tactile localization are affected relatively

more than pain, temperature, and tactile sense, a cerebral lesion is suggested; the converse suggests a brainstem localization. Bilaterality of both motor and sensory signs is almost certain evidence that the lesion lies infratentorially. When hemiplegia or hemiparesis and sensory loss are coextensive, the lesion lies supratentorially. Additional manifestations that point unequivocally to a brainstem site are rotational dizziness, diplopia, cerebellar ataxia, a Horner syndrome, and deafness. The several brainstem syndromes illustrate the important point that the cerebellar pathways, spinothalamic tract, trigeminal nucleus, and sympathetic fibers can be involved at different levels, and neighborhood phenomena must be used to identify the exact site.

A myriad of proper names have been applied to the brainstem syndromes (see Table 47-2). Most of them were originally described in relation to tumors and other non-vascular diseases. The diagnosis of vascular disorders in this region of the brain is not greatly facilitated by a knowledge of these eponymic syndromes, and it is much more profitable to memorize the anatomy of the brainstem. The principal syndromes to be recognized are the full basilar, vertebral, posterior inferior cerebellar, anterior inferior cerebellar, superior cerebellar, pontomedullary, and those of the medial medullary branches. In Figs. 34-13 to 34-16 we have presented both medial and lateral syndromes at four levels of the medulla and pons. Other syndromes can usually be identified as fragments of the major ones.

Figure 34-13

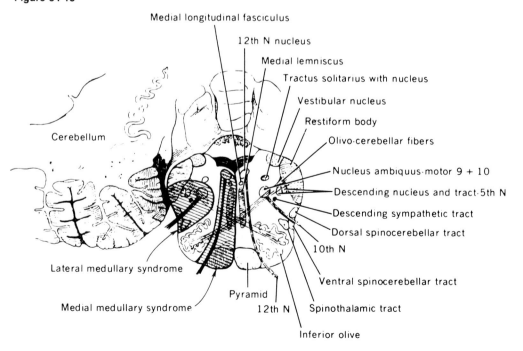

- Medial longitudinal fasciculus
- 12th N nucleus
- Medial lemniscus
- Tractus solitarius with nucleus
- Vestibular nucleus
- Restiform body
- Cerebellum
- Olivo-cerebellar fibers
- Nucleus ambiguus-motor 9 + 10
- Descending nucleus and tract-5th N
- Descending sympathetic tract
- Dorsal spinocerebellar tract
- 10th N
- Lateral medullary syndrome
- Ventral spinocerebellar tract
- Medial medullary syndrome
- Pyramid
- 12th N
- Spinothalamic tract
- Inferior olive

Figure 34-13 (*continued*)

Signs and symptoms	Structures involved
1. Medial medullary syndrome (occlusion of vertebral artery or branch of vertebral or lower basilar artery)	
a. On side of lesion	
(1) Paralysis with atrophy of half the tongue	Issuing twelfth nerve
b. On side opposite lesion	
(1) Paralysis of arm and leg sparing face	Pyramidal tract
(2) Impaired tactile and proprioceptive sense over half the body	Medial lemniscus
2. Lateral medullary syndrome (occlusion of any of five vessels may be responsible—vertebral, posterior inferior cerebellar, or superior, middle, or inferior lateral medullary arteries)	
a. On side of lesion	
(1) Pain, numbness, impaired sensation over half the face	Descending tract and nucleus of fifth nerve
(2) Ataxia of limbs, falling to side of lesion	Uncertain—restiform body, cerebellar hemisphere, olivocerebellar fibers, spinocerebellar tract (?)
(3) Vertigo, nausea, vomiting	Vestibular nuclei and connections
(4) Nystagmus, diplopia, oscillopsia	Vestibular nuclei and connections
(5) Horner syndrome (miosis, ptosis, decreased sweating)	Descending sympathetic tract
(6) Dysphagia, hoarseness, paralysis of vocal cord, diminished gag reflex	Issuing fibers ninth and tenth nerves
(7) Loss of taste (rare)	Nucleus and tractus solitarius
(8) Numbness of ipsilateral arm, trunk, or leg	Cuneate and gracile nuclei
(9) Hiccup	Uncertain
b. On side opposite lesion	
(1) Impaired pain and thermal sense over half the body, sometimes face	Spinothalamic tract
3. Total unilateral medullary syndrome (occlusion of vertebral artery); combination of medial and lateral syndromes	
4. Lateral pontomedullary syndrome (occlusion of vertebral artery); combination of medial and lateral syndromes	
5. Basilar artery syndrome (the syndrome of the lone vertebral artery is equivalent); a combination of the various brainstem syndromes plus those arising in the posterior cerebral artery distribution. The clinical picture comprises bilateral long-tract signs (sensory and motor) with cerebellar and cranial nerve abnormalities.	
a. Paralysis or weakness of all extremities, plus all bulbar musculature	Corticobulbar and corticospinal tracts bilaterally
b. Diplopia, paralysis of conjugate lateral and/or vertical gaze, internuclear ophthalmoplegia, horizontal and/or vertical nystagmus	Ocular motor nerves, apparatus for conjugate gaze, medial longitudinal fasciculus, vestibular apparatus
c. Blindness, impaired vision, various visual field defects	Visual cortex
d. Bilateral cerebellar ataxia	Cerebellar peduncles and the cerebellar hemispheres
e. Coma	Tegmentum of midbrain, thalami
f. Sensation may be strikingly intact in the presence of almost total paralysis. Sensory loss may be syringomyelic or the reverse or involve all modalities	Medial lemniscus, spinothalamic tracts or thalamic nuclei

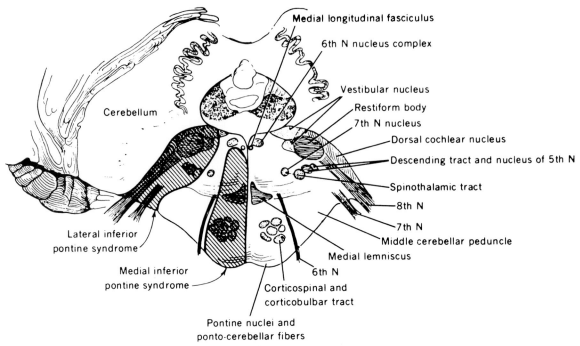

Medial longitudinal fasciculus

6th N nucleus complex

Vestibular nucleus

Restiform body

7th N nucleus

Dorsal cochlear nucleus

Descending tract and nucleus of 5th N

Spinothalamic tract

8th N

7th N

Middle cerebellar peduncle

Medial lemniscus

6th N

Corticospinal and corticobulbar tract

Pontine nuclei and ponto-cerebellar fibers

Cerebellum

Lateral inferior pontine syndrome

Medial inferior pontine syndrome

Figure 34-14

Signs and symptoms	Structures involved
1. Medial inferior pontine syndrome (occlusion of paramedian branch of basilar artery)	
a. On side of lesion	
(1) Paralysis of conjugate gaze to side of lesion (preservation of convergence)	Pontine "center" for lateral gaze (PPRF)
(2) Nystagmus	Vestibular nuclei and connections
(3) Ataxia of limbs and gait	Middle cerebellar peduncle (?)
(4) Diplopia on lateral gaze	Abducens nerve or nucleus
b. On side opposite lesion	
(1) Paralysis of face, arm, and leg	Corticobulbar and corticospinal tract in lower pons
(2) Impaired tactile and proprioceptive sense over half of the body	Medial lemniscus
2. Lateral inferior pontine syndrome (occlusion of anterior inferior cerebellar artery)	
a. On side of lesion	
(1) Horizontal and vertical nystagmus, vertigo, nausea, vomiting, oscillopsia	Vestibular nerve or nucleus
(2) Facial paralysis	Seventh nerve or nucleus
(3) Paralysis of conjugate gaze to side of lesion	Pontine "center" for lateral gaze (PPRF)
(4) Deafness, tinnitus	Auditory nerve or cochlear nucleus
(5) Ataxia	Middle cerebellar peduncle and cerebellar hemisphere
(6) Impaired sensation over face	Descending tract and nucleus fifth nerve
b. On side opposite lesion	
(1) Impaired pain and thermal sense over half the body (may include face)	Spinothalamic tract
3. Total unilateral inferior pontine syndrome (occlusion of anterior inferior cerebellar artery); lateral and medial syndromes combined	

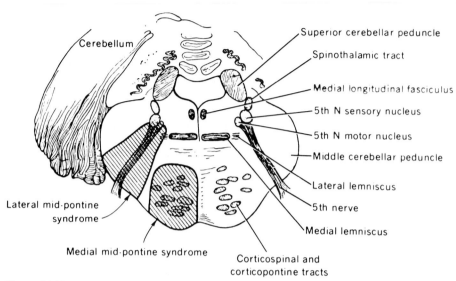

Figure 34-15

Signs and symptoms	Structures involved
1. Medial midpontine syndrome (paramedian branch of midbasilar artery)	
a. On side of lesion	
(1) Ataxia of limbs and gait (more prominent in bilateral involvement)	Middle cerebellar peduncle
b. On side opposite lesion	
(1) Paralysis of face, arm, and leg	Corticobulbar and corticospinal tract
(2) Deviation of eyes	
(3) Variably impaired touch and proprioception when lesion extends posteriorly. Usually the syndrome is purely motor.	Medial lemniscus
2. Lateral midpontine syndrome (short circumferential artery)	
a. On side of lesion	
(1) Ataxia of limbs	Middle cerebellar peduncle
(2) Paralysis of muscles of mastication	Motor fibers or nucleus of fifth nerve
(3) Impaired sensation over side of face	Sensory fibers or nucleus of fifth nerve

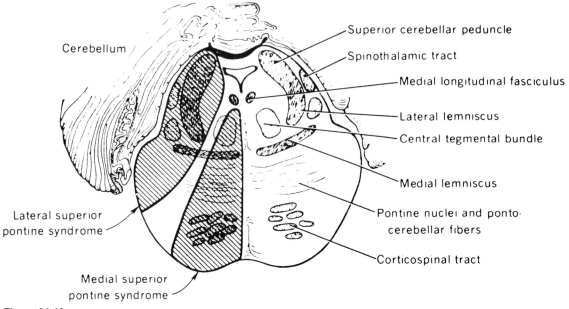

Cerebellum

Superior cerebellar peduncle

Spinothalamic tract

Medial longitudinal fasciculus

Lateral lemniscus

Central tegmental bundle

Medial lemniscus

Pontine nuclei and ponto-cerebellar fibers

Corticospinal tract

Lateral superior pontine syndrome

Medial superior pontine syndrome

Figure 34-16

Signs and symptoms	Structures involved
1. Medial superior pontine syndrome (paramedian branches of upper basilar artery) *a.* On side of lesion	
(1) Cerebellar ataxia	Superior and/or middle cerebellar peduncle
(2) Internuclear ophthalmoplegia	Medial longitudinal fasciculus
(3) Rhythmic myoclonus of palate, pharynx, vocal cords, respiratory apparatus, face, oculomotor apparatus, etc.	Central tegmental bundle
b. On side opposite lesion	
(1) Paralysis of face, arm, and leg	Corticobulbar and corticospinal tract
(2) Rarely touch, vibration, and position senses are affected	Medial lemniscus
2. Lateral superior pontine syndrome (syndrome of superior cerebellar artery) *a.* On side of lesion	
(1) Ataxia of limbs and gait, falling to side of lesion	Middle and superior cerebellar peduncles, superior surface of cerebellum, dentate nucleus
(2) Dizziness, nausea, vomiting	Vestibular nuclei ⎤ Territory of
(3) Horizontal nystagmus	Vestibular nuclei ⎟ descending branch to
(4) Paresis of conjugate gaze (ipsilateral)	Uncertain ⎬ middle cerebellar
(5) Loss of optokinetic nystagmus	Uncertain ⎟ peduncle from superior
(6) Skew deviation	Uncertain ⎦ cerebellar artery
(7) Miosis, ptosis, decreased sweating over face (Horner syndrome)	Descending sympathetic fibers
b. On side opposite lesion	
(1) Impaired pain and thermal sense on face, limbs, and trunk	Spinothalamic tract
(2) Impaired touch, vibration, and position sense, more in leg than arm (there is a tendency to incongruity of pain and touch deficits)	Medial lemniscus (lateral portion)

As one might surmise, small penetrating branches of the cerebral arteries may become occluded, and the resulting infarcts may be so small or so situated as to cause no symptoms whatsoever. As the softened tissue is removed it leaves a small cavity or lacune. Early in the twentieth century, Pierre Marie confirmed the occurrence of multiple small cavities of this type first described by Durant-Fardel in 1843, and referred to the condition as *état lacunaire*. He distinguished them from a fine loosening of tissue around thickened vessels that enter the anterior and posterior perforated spaces, an appearance to which he referred as *état criblé*. Pathologists have not always agreed on these distinctions, but Fisher and Adams have taken the position that the lacunar state is due always to occlusion of small arteries, 50 to 150 μm in diameter, and the cribriform state to mere thickening of vessels.

In our pathologic material, there has always been a strong correlation of the lacunar state with a combination of hypertension and atherosclerosis, and to a lesser degree with diabetes. One may hypothesize that the basis of the lacunar state is unusually severe atherosclerosis that has involved not just the large arteries, as it usually does, but has extended into their finest branches.

When Fisher examined a series of such lesions in serial section, from a basal parent artery up to and through the lacune, he found atheroma and thrombosis to be the basic abnormality in some and a lipohyalin degeneration and occlusion of small vessels in others. In some instances the latter changes had resulted in false aneurysm formation, resembling the Charcot-Bouchard aneurysms of brain hemorrhage (see further on). Usually 4 to 6, sometimes up to 10 to 15 lacunes are found in any given specimen. They are situated, in descending order of frequency, in the putamen, caudate, thalamus, basis pontis, internal capsule, and convolutional white matter. The cavities range from 3 to 15 mm in diameter, and whether they cause symptoms depends entirely on their location. In a series of 1042 consecutive adults, whose brains were examined post mortem, Fisher observed one or more lacunes in 11 percent.

Fisher has delineated some of the more frequent symptomatic forms. If the lacune lies in the territory of a lenticulostriate artery, i.e., in the internal capsule or adjacent corona radiata, it may cause a *pure motor hemiplegia* or a *pure hemisensory syndrome*. In some instances (10 of 34 lacunar syndromes, according to Weisberg) the neurologic deficit evolves in a relatively leisurely fashion over as long a period as 2 to 3 days, raising the possibility of a small hemorrhage. The CT scan shows the lesion in about two-thirds of the cases and MRI in probably a higher proportion. The weakness in pure motor hemiplegia involves the face, arm, and leg. Sometimes the motor disorder takes the form of a pure dysarthria. Recovery, which may begin within hours, days, or weeks, is often nearly complete. Similarly, with a lacune of the thalamus or parietal white matter, presenting as a pure *hemisensory* defect, no other neurologic abnormalities coexist. The course and outcome are much the same as in a pure hemiplegia. In the basis pontis the syndrome may be one of pure motor hemiplegia, mimicking that of internal capsular infarction except for sparing of the face and ipsilateral paresis of conjugate gaze; or a combination of dysarthria and clumsiness of one hand may occur. Occasionally a lacunar infarction of the pons, midbrain, capsule, or parietal white matter gives rise to a hemiparesis with ataxia on the same side as the weakness (Sage and Lepore). Surely other syndromes are occurring but have yet to be defined. Some of the brainstem syndromes may blend with basilar branch syndromes, and these, too, are in need of precise definition. Multiple lacunar infarcts, involving the corticospinal and corticobulbar tracts, are by far the most common cause of pseudobulbar palsy.

CLASSIFICATION OF CEREBROVASCULAR DISEASES

In classifying the cerebrovascular diseases it is most practical, from the clinical viewpoint, to preserve the classic division into thrombosis, embolism, and hemorrhage; our descriptions will follow this scheme. The causes of each of the "big three," along with the criteria for diagnosis and the confirmatory laboratory tests for each of them, will be considered in separate sections. This plan has the disadvantage of not providing a niche for disorders such as reversible ischemia, hypertensive encephalopathy, and venous thrombosis; these will be considered in separate sections.

The frequency of the different types of cerebrovascular disease has been difficult to ascertain. Obviously clinical diagnosis is not always correct, and clinical services are heavily weighted with acute strokes and nonfatal cases. An autopsy series inevitably includes many old vascular lesions, particularly infarcts, whose exact nature cannot always be determined, and there is a bias also toward large fatal lesions (usually hemorrhages).

Table 34-2 summarizes the findings of the Harvard Cooperative Stroke Registry, comprising 756 successive patients, each of whom was examined by a physician knowledgeable about strokes and subjected when necessary to all appropriate ancillary examinations (four-vessel arteriography, CT scan, lumbar puncture). For comparison, we have included an autopsy series of 179 successive cases of cerebral vascular disease, examined during the year 1949 by Fisher and Adams. Interestingly, in both series the ratio of infarcts to hemorrhages was 4:1 and embolism accounted for approximately one-third of all strokes.

ATHEROTHROMBOTIC INFARCTION

Most cerebrovascular disease can be attributed to atherosclerosis and hypertension; until ways are found to prevent or control them, vascular disease of the brain will not cease to be a major cause of morbidity.

Hypertension and atherosclerosis interact in a variety of ways. Atherosclerosis, by reducing the resilience of large arteries, induces hypertension. Atherosclerotic stenosis of the renal arteries, by causing ischemia of the kidneys, does the same. In turn, sustained hypertension worsens atherosclerosis, seemingly "driving" it into the walls of small arteries. Also, it leads to a disorganization of the walls of small branch arteries (0.5 mm or less) in which all the coats of the vessel become impregnated with a kind of hyaline-lipid material, a process that Fisher has called *lipohyalinosis*.

Table 34-2
Major types of cerebrovascular diseases and their frequency

	Harvard stroke series† (756 successive cases)	BCH autopsy series† (179 cases)
Atherosclerotic thrombosis	244 (32%)	21 (12%)
Lacunes	129 (18%)	34 (18.5%)
Embolism	244 (32%)	57 (32%)
Hypertensive hemorrhage	84 (11%)	28 (15.5%)
Ruptured aneurysms and vascular malformations	55 (7%)	8 (4.5%)
Indeterminate		17 (9.5%)
Other‡		14 (8%)

*Compiled by J Mohr, L Caplan, D Pessin, P Kistler, and G Duncan at Massachusetts General Hospital and Beth Israel Hospital, Boston.
†Compiled by CM Fisher and RD Adams in an examination of 740 brains during the year 1949 at Mallory Institute of Pathology, Boston City Hospital.
‡Hypertensive encephalopathy, cerebral vein thrombosis, meningovascular syphilis, and polyarteritis nodosa.

The segment so affected may weaken and allow the formation of a small dissecting aneurysm (Charcot-Bouchard aneurysm) which some neuropathologists hold responsible for the hypertensive brain hemorrhage. Lipohyalinosis also results in thrombosis of small penetrating arteries, leading to the aforementioned lacunar state.

The atheromatous process in brain arteries is identical to that in the aorta, coronary, and other arteries. In general the process in the cerebral arteries runs parallel to but is somewhat less severe than that in the aorta, heart, and lower limbs. There are many exceptions to this rule, however, and not infrequently a brain artery becomes occluded when there is not the slightest clinical evidence of coronary or peripheral vascular disease. Although atheromatosis is known to have its onset in childhood and adolescence, only in the middle and late years of life is it likely to have clinical effects. Hypertension, hyperlipemia, and diabetes aggravate the process. As with coronary and peripheral atherosclerosis, individuals with low blood levels of high density lipoprotein (HDL) and high levels of low-density lipoprotein (LDL) cholesterol are particularly disposed to cerebral atherosclerosis (Nubiola et al). HDL is the major acceptor of cholesterol from cells and is therefore antiatherogenic. Cigarette smoking, another risk factor, decreases HDL cholesterol and reduces cerebral blood flow (Kubota et al).

There is a tendency for atheromatous plaques to form at branchings and curves of the cerebral arteries. The most frequent sites are in the internal carotid artery at the carotid sinus, in the cervical part of the vertebral arteries and at their junction to form the basilar, at the main bifurcation of the middle cerebral arteries, in the posterior cerebral arteries as they wind around the midbrain, and in the anterior cerebral arteries as they curve over the corpus callosum. It is rare for the cerebral arteries to develop plaques beyond their first major branching. Also it is rare for the cerebellar and ophthalmic arteries to show atheromatous involvement, except in conjunction with hypertension. The common carotid and vertebral arteries, at their origins from the aorta, are frequent sites of atheromatous deposits. However, because of abundant collateral arterial pathways, occlusions at these sites are not commonly associated with cerebral ischemia.

The atheromatous lesions develop and grow silently for 20 or 30 or more years, and only in the event of a thrombotic complication do they become symptomatic. Although atheromatous plaques may narrow the lumen of an artery, causing stenosis, complete occlusion is nearly always the consequence of thrombosis. In general, the more severe the atheromatosis the more likely the thrombotic complication, but the two phenomena do not always run in parallel. A patient with only scattered atheromatous plaques may thrombose a vessel, whereas another with marked atherosclerosis may have few thrombosed vessels or none at all. Atheromatous lesions may regress to some extent under the influence of diet and certain drugs. Hennerici et al followed a series of patients with carotid stenoses for a period of 18 months and observed regression in nearly 20 percent of the lesions. In the large majority of cases atherosclerosis is a progressive disease.

Degeneration or hemorrhage into the wall of a sclerotic vessel (from rupture of vasa vasorum) may damage the endothelium. Platelets and fibrin then adhere to the damaged part of the wall and form delicate, friable clots, or a subintimal atheromatous deposit may slough, spewing crystalline cholesterol emboli into the lumen and occluding small distal vessels. Presumably a thrombus does not occlude the lumen completely from the first moment of its formation; total blockage may occur only after several hours. In some instances thrombotic particles may form and break off repeatedly, thus becoming an important source of cerebral embolism. Once the lumen of the artery has been completely occluded, the thrombus may propagate distally and proximally to the next branching points and block an anastomotic channel.

These several events in the atherosclerotic-thrombotic process probably account for the prodromal ischemic attacks—intermittent blockage of the circulation and variable impairment of function in the vascular territory often proceeding to permanent ischemic effects and later progression (after several days). Not infrequently several arteries are affected by stenosis and thrombosis over a period of months or years; then it becomes difficult to decipher the interplay of factors that lead to symptoms both transitory or persistent. Some of the possibilities have been outlined by Adams, Torvik, and Fisher. The evolution of the thrombotic process is sufficiently prolonged to explain the clinical state known as *stroke in evolution*; and when the hemodynamic disturbance stabilizes, the stage of *completed stroke* is reached. These different stages acquire significance in relation to therapy and prognosis.

Since atherosclerotic thrombosis involves the deposition of fibrin and platelets, these blood elements have been studied extensively, without throwing much light on the subject. Measurements of platelet agglutination have yielded contradictory results, as have studies of platelet number and fibrinogen levels. A platelet-specific protein, β-thromboglobulin, is said to be increased immediately after an ischemic event. The metabolic disturbances in homocystinuria and Fabry disease favor thrombosis.

CLINICAL PICTURE

In general, the evolution of the clinical phenomena in relation to thrombosis is more variable than that of embolism and hemorrhage. In approximately 75 percent of our patients the main part of the stroke (paralysis or other deficit) is preceded by minor signs or one or more transient attacks of focal neurologic dysfunction (Table 34-3). In a sense, these herald the oncoming vascular catastrophe. *A history of such prodromal episodes is of paramount importance in establishing the diagnosis of cerebral thrombosis.* (Only rarely and for unclear reasons are embolism and cerebral hemorrhage preceded by a transient neurologic disorder.) In carotid and middle cerebral artery disease the transient warning attacks consist of monocular blindness, hemiplegia, hemianesthesia, disturbances of speech and language, confusion, etc. In the vertebral-basilar system, the prodromata most often take the form of episodes of dizziness, diplopia, numbness, impaired vision in one or both visual fields, and dysarthria. These will be described more fully further on, under "transient ischemic attacks" (TIAs). Such attacks last from a few minutes to several hours; in most instances the duration is less than 10 min. Those of several hours' duration are usually due to embolism. The final stroke may be preceded by one or two attacks or a hundred or more, and it may follow the onset of the attacks by hours, weeks, or months. When there are no prodromal ischemic attacks, one must use other criteria to establish the diagnosis of atherosclerotic thrombosis.

The main part of the thrombotic stroke, whether or not it is preceded by warning attacks, develops in one of several ways. Most often there is a single attack, and the

Table 34-3
Development of the clinical picture in 125 cases of cerebral thrombosis (C. M. Fisher)

Clinical development	No. of cases	Percent
Transient ischemic attacks progressing to a major or minor persistent neurologic deficit	53	42
Stepwise development of a stroke, with or without transient ischemic attacks	23	18
Stroke developing as a single event: Abrupt (hours), with or without fluctuations	14	11
Slow, gradual (a few days), with or without minor fluctuations	7	6
Transient ischemic attacks only	17	14
Development of a limited stroke followed by transient ischemic attacks	11	9

whole illness evolves within a few hours. More telling diagnostically is a "stuttering" or intermittent progression of neurologic deficits extending over several hours or a day or longer. Again, a partial stroke may occur, and even recede temporarily for several hours, after which there is rapid progression to the completed stroke. Several fleeting episodes may be followed by a longer one and hours or a day or two later by a major stroke. Several parts of the body may be involved at once, or only one part, such as a limb or one side of the face, the other parts becoming involved serially in steplike fashion until the stroke is fully developed. More perplexing diagnostically is a "slow stroke" that evolves over a period of weeks and is due to chronic hypoperfusion. Sometimes the deficit is episodic; involuntary movements of a hand or arm or dimness of vision, lasting 5 to 10 min, is brought on by standing or walking. We have several times observed these episodic phenomena in patients with bilateral carotid stenosis or occlusion. In this group of patients there is a reduction in regional blood flow and slowing of the EEG. All these modes of development indicate cerebral thrombosis, and their temporal dispersion reflects *thrombosis in evolution.* It might be commented that each of the transient attacks and the abrupt episodes of progression reproduce the profile of the stroke in miniature. The principle of intermittency seems to characterize the thrombotic process from beginning to end.

Even more frequent than the modes of onset outlined above is the occurrence of the thrombotic stroke during sleep; the patient awakens paralyzed, either during the night or in the morning. Unaware of any difficulty, he or she may arise and fall helplessly to the floor with the first step. This is the story in fully 60 percent of our patients with thrombotic strokes and in a certain number with embolic ones as well.

Most deceptive of all are the patients in whom the neurologic disorder has evolved over 1 to 2 weeks in a slow, gradual fashion. One's first impulse is to make a diagnosis of brain tumor, abscess, or subdural hematoma. Some patients of this type have even come to surgery only to show infarct necrosis of the brain. This error can usually be avoided by a minute analysis of the course of the illness, which will disclose an uneven, saltatory progression; and if the clinical data are incomplete, observation for a few days or weeks will reveal the stroke profile more clearly. Actually there are very few cases—and these are usually instances of pure motor hemiplegia—in which the evolution of a thrombotic stroke was evenly progressive over a period of days.

Arterial thrombosis is not usually accompanied by headache, but the latter does occur in some cases. Usually the pain is located on one side of the head in carotid occlusion (see page 136), at the back of the head or simultaneously in forehead and occiput in basilar occlusion, and behind the ipsilateral ear in vertebral occlusion. The headache is not as violent as in intracerebral or subarachnoid hemorrhage, and there is no stiffness of the neck. The mechanism is unclear. Presumably it is related to the disease process within the vessel since it may antedate the other manifestations of the stroke by days or even weeks.

Hypertension is more often present than not in patients with atherothrombotic infarction. Diabetes mellitus is common also. Often there is evidence of vascular disease in other parts of the body: a history of coronary occlusion or angina pectoris, an ECG abnormality, intermittent claudication, or an absence of one or several pulses in the lower limbs. The retinal arteries may show uniform or focal narrowing, increase and irregularity of the light reflex, and arteriovenous "nicking," but these findings are to be correlated with hypertension rather than atherosclerosis. The same is true of retinal hemorrhages and exudates. The patient is more often elderly, but may be in the fourth decade or younger when stricken.

LABORATORY FINDINGS

The CSF pressure is normal in patients with atherothrombotic infarction unless the infarct is massive and the damaged tissue swells. Then it may, exceptionally, lead to a greatly increased intracranial pressure and fatal temporal lobe or cerebellar herniation. Cerebral thrombosis never causes blood to enter the CSF. Frequently the CSF protein is elevated (usually 50 to 100 mg/dL). Rarely is the total protein in excess of 100 mg/dL; when it is, a faint xanthochromia (1 to 2 on a scale of 10) may be perceived and some other diagnosis must be considered. A small number of polymorphonuclear leukocytes (3 to 8 per cubic millimeter) is common in the first few days. Rarely, and for unexplained reasons, a brisk, transient pleocytosis (400 to 2000 polymorphonuclear leukocytes per cubic millimeter) occurs on about the third day. A persistent pleocytosis, however, suggests a chronic meningitis (syphilis, tuberculosis, cryptococcosis), granulomatous arteritis, septic embolism, thrombophlebitis, or a nonvascular process. Occasionally, the serologic test for syphilis may be positive. Meningovascular syphilis occurring during the first few years of a syphilitic infection is an uncommon but well-recognized entity. Nearly always in such cases there are increased protein, pleocytosis, and a positive VDRL or other serologic test in both blood and CSF (see page 575). If the CSF is bloody, a positive serologic test is not valid since the reagin may have been carried into the CSF by the contaminated blood.

Serum cholesterol or triglycerides, or both, are elevated in some cases, but normal values are not helpful. The EEG is only of limited value in indicating infarction or distinguishing it from hemorrhage. In extensive cerebral infarction the brain waves in overlying leads may be of slightly lower frequency and lower voltage than normal. High-voltage slow waves (3 to 5 per second) favor hemorrhage. Arteriography is the definitive diagnostic procedure for the demonstration of arterial thrombosis or stenosis and also provides information about collateral flow. Injection of radiopaque fluid into the major cervicocerebral arteries via a catheter introduced into the femoral artery is preferred to direct puncture of the common carotid artery. Arteriography carries a slight risk of serious complications (0.5 percent), and in patients with vessels narrowed by atherosclerosis the infarction may be extended (6 to 7 percent). It should be only used, therefore, when the diagnosis of vascular disease is uncertain or when surgery or anticoagulant therapy is being contemplated in an indefinite case. Digital subtraction angiography (DSA), in which the major arteries of the neck and brain are visualized after the injection of a large bolus of radiopaque material in the

antecubital vein, has to a large extent replaced connventional arteriography because of the low risk. The disadvantages are that the cerebral vessels are less well visualized and that the large volume of infused material may precipitate cardiac decompensation in patients with heart disease. MRI demonstrates ischemic zones within a few hours after the stroke. Also radionuclide scans and positron emission techniques often show the infarct before it becomes visible in CT scans. Scintillation counting over the two sides of the skull after the intravenous injection of radioactive material may provide a comparative index of circulation in the two carotid systems. CT scanning usually shows the necrotic tissue within a few days and later demonstrates cavitation (Figs. 34-17 and 34-18). Lacunar infarcts are too small to be seen in one-third of the patients.

COURSE AND PROGNOSIS

When the patient is seen early in the course of cerebral thrombosis, it is difficult to give an accurate prognosis.

Figure 34-17

Ischemic infarction of the midbrain due to basilar artery occlusion. Unenhanced CT scan, 72 h after onset, shows a large area of decreased attenuation (necrotic tissue) sparing only the colliculi.

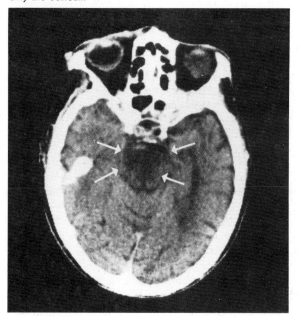

Figure 34-18

Large hemispheric ischemic infarct with prominent gyral enhancement ("luxury perfusion") 2 weeks after stroke.

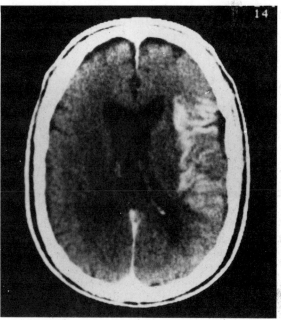

One must ask where the patient stands in the stroke process at the time of the examination. Is worsening to be anticipated or not? No rules have yet been formulated which allow one to predict the course with confidence. A mild paralysis today may become a disastrous hemiplegia tomorrow, or the patient's condition may only worsen temporarily for a day or two. In basilar artery occlusion, dizziness and dysphagia may progress in a few days to total paralysis and deep coma. The course of cerebral thrombosis is so often progressive that a cautious attitude on the part of the physician is justified in what first appears to be a mild stroke.

As indicated above, progression of the stroke is due most often to increasing stenosis of the involved artery by mural thrombus. In some instances, extension of the thrombus along the vessel may block side branches and hinder anastomotic flow. In the basilar artery, thrombus may gradually build up along its entire length. In the carotid system, thrombus at times propagates distally from the site of origin in the neck to the supraclinoid portion, and possibly into the anterior cerebral artery, preventing collateral flow from the opposite side. In middle cerebral occlusion, retrograde thrombosis may extend back to the mouth of the anterior cerebral, perhaps secondarily infarcting the territory of that vessel. Embolic particles from the site of an incompletely thrombosed artery may precipitate an abrupt change. Sometimes a completely thrombosed artery can be the source of an embolus to more distal branches after a period of several days (Barnett).

Several other circumstances influence the *immediate prognosis* in cerebral thrombosis. In the case of large infarcts, swelling of the infarcted tissue may occur, followed by displacement of central structures, tentorial herniation, and death of the patient in several days. Even smaller infarcts of the inferior surface of the cerebellum may cause foramen magnum herniation. Milder degrees of swelling and increased intracranial pressure, though causing an apparent progression for 2 to 3 days, do not prove fatal. In extensive basilar infarction associated with deep coma, the mortality rate approaches 40 percent. If coma or stupor is present from the beginning, survival is largely determined by the success in keeping the airway clear, controlling brain edema, preventing aspiration pneumonia, and maintaining fluid and electrolyte balance. Respiratory and urinary infections are constant dangers, and once they begin, there is usually a rapid decline in the patient's condition as body temperature rises. With smaller thrombotic infarcts the mortality is 3 to 6 percent.

As for the *eventual or long-term prognosis* of the neurologic deficit, there are many possibilities. Improvement is the rule if the patient survives. The patient with a lacunar infarct and pure motor hemiparesis fares well. Recovery from small infarcts may start within a day or two, and restoration may be complete or nearly complete within a week. In cases of severe deficit there may be no significant recovery, and after months of assiduous efforts at rehabilitation, the patient may remain bereft of speech and understanding, with the upper extremity still useless and the lower extremity serving only as an uncertain prop in attempting to walk. Between these two extremes there is every gradation of recovery. In general, the longer the delay in onset of recovery, the poorer the prognosis. If recovery does not begin in 1 or 2 weeks, the outlook is gloomy both for motor and language function. Constructional apraxia, uninhibited anger (with temporal lesions), nonsensical logorrhea and placidity, unawareness of the paralysis and neglect (with nondominant lesions), all tend to diminish and may disappear within a few weeks. A hemianopia that has not cleared in a few weeks will usually be permanent, although reading and color discrimination may continue to improve. In lateral medullary infarction, difficulty in swallowing may be protracted, lasting 4 to 8 weeks or longer; yet relatively normal function is finally restored in nearly every instance. Aphasia, dysarthria, cerebellar ataxia, and walking may improve for a year or longer, but for all practical purposes it may be said that whatever motor and language deficits remain after 5 to 6 months will be permanent.

Characteristically, the paralyzed muscles are flaccid in the first days or weeks following a stroke, and the tendon reflexes are usually unchanged, but may be slightly increased or decreased. Gradually spasticity develops, and the tendon reflexes become brisker. The arm tends to assume a flexed adducted posture, whereas the leg is usually extended. Function is rarely if ever restored after the slow evolution of spasticity. Conversely, the early development of spasticity in the arm, or the early appearance of a grasp reflex may presage a favorable outcome. In some patients with extensive temporoparietal lesions the hemiplegia remains flaccid; the arm dangles and the slack leg must be braced to stand. If the internal capsule is not interrupted completely in a stroke that involves the lenticular nucleus or thalamus, the paralysis may give way to hemichoreoathetosis, hemitremor, or hemiataxia, depending upon the particular anatomy of the lesion. Bowel and bladder control usually returns; sphincteric disorders persist in only a few cases. Often the hemiplegic limbs are at first tender and ache on manipulation. Nevertheless, physiotherapy should be initiated early in order to prevent pseudocontracture of muscles and periarthritis at the shoulder, elbow, wrist, knuckles, knee, and ankle. These are frequent complications and often the source of pain and added disability, particularly in relation to the shoulder. Occasionally, atrophy of bone and pain in the hand may accompany the shoulder pain (shoulder-hand syndrome). An annoying feeling of dizziness and unsteadiness often persists after damage to the vestibular system in brainstem infarcts.

Recurrent convulsive (epileptic) seizures are relatively uncommon sequelae of thrombotic strokes, in comparison to embolic cortical infarcts, which are followed by recurrent focal or generalized seizures in more than 20 percent of patients.

Many patients complain of fatigability and are depressed, particularly after strokes that involve the left frontal lobe (Starkstein et al). The explanation of these symptoms is uncertain; some are expressions of a reactive depression. Only a few patients develop serious *behavior problems* or are psychotic after a stroke, but paranoid trends, ill temper, stubbornness, and peevishness are common.

Finally, in regard to prognosis, it must be mentioned that having had one thrombotic stroke, the patient is at risk in the ensuing months and years of having a stroke at the same or another site, especially if there is hypertension or diabetes mellitus. When multiple infarcts occur over a period of months or years, a dementia may develop, in addition to focal cerebral deficits. As a group these cases are referred to as *multi-infarct dementia* (see page 338). In some of these cases the major lesions involve the white matter with relative sparing of the cortex and basal ganglia. This type of lesion is often referred to as *Binswanger's subcortical encephalopathy*, which we equate with multiple white matter infarcts and lacunes (see Nichols and Mohr). The parts of the white matter that are destroyed have been shown to lie in the border zones between the penetrating cortical and basal ganglionic arteries.

In Rochester, Minnesota, during the period of 1970 to 1974, 94 percent of patients with ischemic strokes survived for 5 days and 84 percent for 1 month (Garraway and colleagues). The survival was 54 percent at 3 years and 40 percent at 7 years. In each of these groups, survival was significantly greater than it had been during the period 1965 to 1969. Among long-term survivors, heart disease is a more frequent cause of death than further stroke.

TRANSIENT ISCHEMIC ATTACKS OF CEREBRAL ORIGIN

It has already been pointed out that when transient ischemic attacks (TIAs) precede a stroke, they almost always stamp the process as thrombotic. Furthermore, neuropathologic studies inform us that these attacks are linked almost exclusively to atherosclerotic thrombosis. There would seem to be little doubt that these attacks are due to transient focal

ischemia, and they might be referred to as temporary strokes which fortunately reverse themselves. They belong, therefore, under the heading of atherosclerotic thrombotic disease, but are discussed separately here because of their clinical importance. In a prospective study of 390 patients with focal TIAs caused by atherosclerotic vascular disease, the 5-year cumulative rate of fatal or nonfatal cerebral infarction was 22.7 percent (Heyman et al). Interestingly, the rate of myocardial infarction in this group of patients, particularly in those with carotid lesions, was almost as high (21 percent). Thus TIAs caused by carotid atherosclerosis is a predictor not only of cerebral infarction but also of myocardial infarction. About two-thirds of all patients with TIAs are men or hypertensive, or both, reflecting the higher incidence of atherosclerosis in hypertensives and in males. Occasionally, in younger adults, TIAs may occur as a benign phenomenon, without recognizable features of or risk factors for atherosclerosis.

CLINICAL PICTURE

TIAs can reflect the involvement of virtually any cerebral or cerebellar artery, deep or superficial: common carotid, internal carotid, middle cerebral, anterior cerebral, ophthalmic, vertebral, basilar, posterior cerebral, a cerebellar artery or a penetrating branch to the basal ganglia and brainstem. If the posterior cerebral arteries are included in the vertebral-basilar system, ischemic episodes are slightly more common in that system than in the carotid. TIAs may precede, accompany, or follow the development of a stroke, or they can occur by themselves without leading to a stroke, a fact that makes any form of therapy difficult to evaluate.

TIAs may last a few seconds up to 12 to 24 h; most of them last 2 to 15 min, and an attack of more than 30 min is uncommon. There may be only a few attacks or several hundred. Between attacks, the neurologic examination may disclose no abnormalities. A stroke may occur after the first or second episode or only after hundreds of attacks have occurred over a period of weeks or months. Not infrequently the attacks gradually cease and no important paralysis occurs. So far it has not been possible to distinguish the cases in which a stroke will not develop from those in which it will, except in a general way. About 20 percent of infarcts that follow TIAs occur within a month after the first attack, and about 50 percent within a year (Whisnant et al, 1973).

The neurologic features of the transient episode indicate the territory or artery involved and are fragments borrowed from the stroke which may be approaching. In the *carotid system,* attacks reflect involvement of cerebral hemisphere and eye. The visual disturbance is ipsilateral; the sensorimotor disturbance is contralateral. Individual attacks tend to involve either the eye or the brain. It is almost unknown for the eye and the brain to be involved simultaneously. Usually the initial attacks are ocular and the later ones are hemispheric. In the hemispheric attacks, ischemia occurs foremost in the distal territory of the middle cerebral artery and adjacent border zone, producing weakness or numbness of the opposite hand and arm. However, many different combinations may be seen: face and lips, or lips and fingers, fingers alone, hand and foot, etc. Less common manifestations include headache, confusion, aphasia and difficulty in calculation (when the dominant hemisphere is involved), and other temporoparietal disturbances. In ocular attacks, transient monocular blindness is the usual symptom. (amaurosis fugax). Many of the latter episodes evolve swiftly and are described as a shade falling smoothly over the visual field until the eye is completely but painlessly blind. The attack clears slowly and uniformly. Uncommonly, it may take the form of a wedge of visual loss, sudden generalized blurring, or rarely, a bright light. Transient attacks of monocular blindness are usually more stereotyped than hemispheric attacks. TIAs consisting of a homonymous hemianopia and/or paresthesias of the hand and arm should suggest a stenosis of the posterior cerebral artery. The implications of amaurosis fugax have been evaluated by Poole and Russell. They observed a group of 110 medically treated patients for periods of 6 to 19 years following an episode of amaurosis fugax (exclusive of the type caused by cholesteral emboli). At the end of 6 years, the mortality rate (due mainly to heart disease) had risen to 21 percent and the incidence of stroke to 13 percent (compared to expected figures of 15 and 4 percent, respectively, in an age-matched population). Of the patients who were alive at the end of the obsevation period, 43 percent had no attacks of amaurosis fugax following the initial episode.

The clinical picture of transient attacks in the vertebral-basilar system is diverse, since such varied motor-sensory traffic is sustained by the blood carried in these vessels. Dizziness, diplopia (vertical or horizontal), dysarthria, bifacial numbness, and weakness or numbness of part or all of one or both sides of the body (i.e., a disturbance of the long motor or sensory tracts bilaterally) are the hallmarks of vertebral-basilar involvement. Transient vertigo or diplopia (or headache), occurring as solitary symptoms, should not be interpreted as a TIA. Also, in some patients, the complaint of dizziness will prove to be part of carotid TIAs; hence this symptom is not a reliable indicator of the vascular circuit that is involved, according to Ueda et al. Abnormalities of brainstem auditory evoked potentials may persist for several days after a vertebrobasilar TIA and help to distinguish an attack in this vascular territory (Factor and Dentinger). Other manifestations, in their approximate order of frequency, include headache, staggering, veering to one side, a feeling of cross-eyedness, dark vision, blurred vision, tunnel vision, partial or complete blindness, pupillary change, ptosis, paralysis of gaze, dysarthria, and dysphagia. Less common symptoms include noise or pounding in the ear or in the head, pain in the head or face or other peculiar head sensations, vomiting, hiccups, memory lapse, confused behavior, drowsiness, transient unconsciousness (rare), impaired hearing, deafness, a feeling of movement of a part, hemiballismus, peduncular hallucinosis, and forced deviation of the eyes. Drop attacks, according to Russell, have been recorded in 10 to 15 percent of patients with vertebral-basilar insufficiency. They may also occur with bilateral anterior cerebral artery ischemia if both hemispheres are supplied by one anterior cerebral artery, the other being hypoplastic, as it is in 4 percent of brains.

TIAs may be identical or they may vary in detail, although maintaining the same basic pattern. For example, weakness or numbness may involve fingers and face in some episodes, and only the fingers in others; or dizziness and ataxia may occur in some attacks, while in others diplopia is added to the picture. In basilar artery disease each side of the body may be affected alternately. All the involved parts may be affected simultaneously, or a march or spread from one region to another occurs over a period of 10 s to a minute or a few minutes—much slower than the spread of a seizure. The individual attack may cease abruptly or fade gradually.

MECHANISM

Ophthalmoscopic observations of the retinal vessels made during episodes of transient monocular blindness show either arrest of the blood flow in the retinal arteries and breaking up of the venous columns to form a "boxcar" pattern, or scattered bits of white material temporarily blocking the retinal arteries. This indicates that in ischemic attacks a temporary, complete or relatively complete cessation of blood flow occurs locally, sometimes associated with microembolism.

TIAs have been attributed to cerebral vasospasm or to transient episodes of systemic arterial hypotension with resulting compromise of the intracranial circulation, but neither of these mechanisms has been established. Although dropping the blood pressure to 80 mmHg or less by tilting the patient from a horizontal to an upright position may cause EEG changes, it has not in the authors' experience reproduced the attacks. Nevertheless, the onset of attacks in a small proportion of patients has been clearly related to standing up after lying or sitting. In the majority of cases, attacks bear no relation to position or activity, although in general they are likely to occur when the patient is up and around rather than lying down. They have been encountered rarely in relation to exercise, outbursts of anger or joy, and bouts of coughing, and in states of anemia, polycythemia, and hypoglycemia. Transient symptoms present on awakening from sleep usually indicate that a stroke is in the offing.

There is good evidence that the attacks can be abolished by anticoagulant drugs, but the mechanism of this effect is not known. Whatever the exact cause of TIAs, they are intimately related to vascular stenosis and ulceration due to atherosclerosis and thrombus formation in the majority of cases.

Embolization of fibrin-platelet material from atherosclerotic sites is frequently suggested as an explanation of TIAs. This may indeed be the cause of attacks in many cases, but it is difficult to understand, in attacks of identical pattern, how successive emboli from a distance would enter the same arterial branch each time. Moreover, one would expect the involved cerebral tissue to be at least partially damaged, leaving some residual signs. When a single transient episode has occurred, the factor of recurrence does not assist in the diagnosis, and cerebral embolism must then be strongly considered. In some cases of documented embolism, the deficit fluctuates from normal to abnormal repeatedly for as long as 36 h, giving the appearance of TIAs; in others, a deficit of several hours' duration occurs, fulfilling the traditional criterion of TIAs. These cases should be considered as symptomatically short-lived strokes when the ipsilateral carotid artery territory is found normal arteriographically. A single transitory episode, especially if it lasts longer than 1 h, and *multiple episodes of different pattern* suggest embolism and must be clearly distinguished from brief (2 to 10 min) *recurrent attacks of the same pattern*, which suggest atherosclerosis and thrombosis. Recurrent seizures and attacks of migraine, syncope and vertigo must also be clearly distinguished from TIAs, using the criteria outlined in Chaps. 15, 9, 17, and 14, respectively.

The routine of four-vessel arteriography has shed some light on the problem. Usually the internal or common carotid or vertebral-basilar arteries are stenotic and sometimes an atheromatous ulcer is seen. In some instances the TIAs begin after the artery has been occluded by thrombus. As shown by Barnett, emboli may arise from the distal end of the thrombus or by way of a collateral artery. However, almost a fifth of the 95 patients with ''carotid TIAs'' in the Massachusetts General Hospital series (Pessin et al), and a

somewhat larger proportion of the Winston-Salem series (Ueda et al) had open carotid arteries with neither stenosis nor ulceration. In most of the cases with arteriographically normal carotids the ischemic attacks exceeded 1 h in duration, suggesting embolism from the heart or great vessels; but there was also a small number of brief ischemic attacks that were unexplained by arteriography. Of course a small atheromatous ulceration may not be seen in the arteriogram. The majority of those with bruits had stenoses with more than 50 percent reduction in the lumen.

TREATMENT OF ATHEROTHROMBOTIC INFARCTION AND TRANSIENT ISCHEMIC ATTACKS

The main objective of medical therapy is the prevention of stroke. Ideally this should be accomplished by finding patients in the asymptomatic stage of atherosclerosis. Practically speaking, since the medical profession has no efficient, cost-effective methods of screening large populations at risk of developing stroke, one must direct treatment to patients who have already begun to have symptoms, either TIAs or ischemic lesions that are reversible to some extent. Another approach, not yet explored, would be to select patients with only coronary heart disease and attempt to prevent cerebral vascular disease.

The treatment of atherothrombotic disease may be divided into four parts: (1) management in the acute phase, (2) measures to restore the circulation and arrest the pathologic process, (3) physical therapy and rehabilitation, and (4) measures to prevent further strokes and progression of vascular disease.

MANAGEMENT IN THE ACUTE PHASE

Surgical Revascularization Rarely is the patient who has had a stroke brought to medical attention within a few minutes of onset. This may happen when a patient is in the hospital for another reason. If the common or internal carotid artery has just become thrombosed, immediate surgical removal of the clot or the performance of a bypass procedure may restore function. Ojemann and Crowell have operated on 55 such cases as an emergency procedure; 26 of them had stenotic vessels and 29 acutely thrombosed vessels. Of the latter, circulation was restored in 21 with an excellent or good result in 16. In 19 of the 26 cases with stenotic carotid arteries an excellent or good result was obtained. Usually several hours will have elapsed before the diagnosis is established; if the interval is longer than 12 h, opening the occluded vessel is of little value. Nor is the intracarotid injection of urokinase or streptokinase (to dissolve the clot) of any value after this interval.

MEASURES TO RESTORE THE CIRCULATION AND ARREST THE PATHOLOGIC PROCESS

Once a thrombotic stroke has developed fully, no therapy so far devised is of any value in restoring the damaged cerebral tissue or its function. One's efforts, therefore, must be directed to making a diagnosis of thrombosis at the earliest possible stage and circumventing the full catastrophe by all means presently available. These measures are instituted at various stages of the process, when only transient ischemic attacks are occurring, or at any point in the progression of a thrombosis-in-evolution, or when almost the full neurologic deficit has appeared. Even when persistent signs and symptoms have appeared, it is conceivable that some of the tissue affected, particularly at the edges of the infarct (the "ischemic penumbra"), has not been irreversibly damaged and will survive if blood flow can be increased.

The following therapeutic methods are being used at present or have been tried in the recent past.

Medical Therapy If the patient is deeply stuporous or comatose, care follows along the lines indicated in Chap. 16.

On the assumption that a decrease in the cerebral circulation might result from assuming the upright position and thereby aggravate cerebral ischemia, patients with a major stroke as the result of ischemic infarction should remain horizontal in bed for the first few days. When sitting and walking begins, special attention should be given to maintenance of the systemic circulation (avoid standing quietly for prolonged periods, sitting with the feet up, etc.). The treatment of previously unappreciated hypertension is preferably deferred until later, when the neurologic deficit has stabilized. It is of great importance that the blood pressure be maintained [correction of blood loss, use of metaraminol bitartrate (Aramine) or levarterenol bitartrate (Levophed) in myocardial infarction with vascular collapse, avoidance of autonomic blocking agents, etc.]. Injections of epinephrine have been recommended as a means of raising the systemic blood pressure above the usual levels. Although this enhances cerebral blood flow and might be beneficial, a systematic trial in thrombotic cases has not been undertaken. One would fear that it might increase the edema or cause hemorrhage into the infarcted tissue. Certainly it is reasonable to maintain a slightly elevated blood pressure with colloids, but one should avoid intravenous glucose. Anemia must be corrected. Polycythemia, if severe, should be reduced, for it may slow the circulation locally.

Therapy for Cerebral Edema In the first few days following major cerebral infarction, cerebral edema, both cellular and vasogenic, may threaten life. In such instances, dexamethasone in intramuscular doses of 4 to 6 mg every 4 to 6 h together with controlled ventilation may be useful. Intravenous mannitol, in doses of 1½ g/kg, then 50 g every 2 to 3 h, and glycerol, in oral doses of 30 mL every 4 to 6 h or daily intravenous doses of 50 g dissolved in 500 mL of 2.5 percent saline solution, are other available forms of therapy. Apart from their effects on edema, the value of these agents in improving the neurologic deficit is questionable.

Cerebral Vasodilators and Thrombolytic Agents Despite experimental evidence that some vasodilators such as CO_2 inhalation and papaverine increase cerebral blood flow, none of them has proved beneficial in carefully studied human stroke cases at the stage of transient ischemic attacks or thrombosis-in-evolution or with established strokes. Vasodilators may actually be harmful rather than beneficial, at least on theoretical grounds, since by lowering the systemic blood pressure or by dilating vessels to normal brain tissue (the autoregulatory mechanisms are lost in vessels within the infarct), they may reduce the intracranial anastomotic flow. Moreover, the vessels in the margin of the infarct (border zone) are already maximally dilated. Also, the thrombolytic agents, fibrinolysin and tissue plasminogen activator, have not proved helpful in patients with transient ischemia, thrombosis-in-evolution, and established stroke. There have been claims of benefit from the use of prostacyclin and naloxone, but these remain to be validated.

Anticoagulant Drugs These have been said to prevent transient ischemic attacks and an impending stroke. Anticoagulants also may halt the advance of a progressive thrombotic stroke, but not in all cases. In deciding whether to use anticoagulants, one faces the question of where in the course of the stroke the patient stands when first examined. Will the course be benign or disastrous? As was stated above, there are no reliable rules for predicting this at the present time. One fact seems definite—that anticoagulants are not of value in the fully developed stroke, whether this be in the patient with a lacunar infarct or in the patient with a devastating thrombosis with hemiplegia. Whether anticoagulants prevent the recurrence of a thrombotic stroke when given for a prolonged period is a question that has never been answered satisfactorily, and the incidence of complicating hemorrhage probably outweighs the value of anticoagulants in these cases (see further on).

The effectiveness of anticoagulant therapy in preventing strokes in patients with TIAs is equivocal. Whisnant et al have calculated that the incidence of stroke in an untreated group of patients with TIAs is 10 percent in the first 6 months; in contrast, only 1 percent of normal individuals in the same group would be expected to have a stroke each year.

Weksler and Lewin have reviewed the results obtained with oral anticoagulant therapy in four prospective randomized studies. The combined numbers were 93 treated patients and 85 untreated controls. They found no evidence of stroke prevention. There were 15 deaths in the treated group (six from hemorrhage) and 10 deaths in the untreated group (one from hemorrhage).

The problem that continues to plague all attempts to use anticoagulants is the risk of hemorrhage, which approaches 20 percent with a mortality of 1 percent. The risk of intracranial hemorrhage is estimated by Whisnant et al to be 5 percent and is more frequent in elderly patients who had been treated for more than 1 year. Again, it would appear that with long-term administration of anticoagulant, the risk of hemorrhage outweighs the benefit from prevention of stroke or myocardial infarct.

The planned use of anticoagulant drugs makes an accurate diagnosis imperative. Intracranial hemorrhage must be ruled out by CT scan. It must be remembered that a clear CSF does not necessarily exclude hemorrhage. Estimation of prothrombin activity and coagulation time are desirable before therapy is started, but if this is not feasible, the initial doses of anticoagulant drugs can usually be given safely if there is no evidence of bleeding anywhere in the body. Severe hypertension is not necessarily a contraindication to anticoagulant therapy. There is no reliable evidence that complications are more frequent in the presence of hypertension if the prothrombin time is not allowed to exceed one and one-half times normal, and therefore the authors have not withheld anticoagulant therapy in these patients; however, when the blood pressure is greater than 220/120 mmHg, an attempt is made at the same time to lower the pressure gradually. It is preferable to avoid reduction of the blood pressure in the 2-week period immediately following a thrombotic stroke. Other contraindications to anticoagulant therapy are bleeding peptic ulcer, uremia, hepatic failure, and the prospect of poor compliance by the patient.

When anticoagulant therapy is instituted in the prodromal or early phase of a stroke, heparin is administered intravenously by continuous drip (1000 units/h). Heparin therapy is maintained for 1 to 2 weeks while warfarin (Coumadin) therapy is being instituted, and the latter may

be continued for several months (see below). Coumadin can be used alone from the beginning when transient ischemic attacks occur less than once every few days.

Coumadin therapy is relatively safe, provided the prothrombin activity is maintained at 15 to 17 s (normal 12 s) and the level is determined regularly (once a day, for the first 10 days, then three times a week, and finally once every 1 or 2 weeks). Therapy can be prolonged for months and years, but the tendency now is not to give Coumadin for indefinite lengths of time. There are data to suggest that the greatest usefulness of Coumadin is in the first 2 to 4 months following the onset of the ischemic attack(s); after that the risk of intracranial hemorrhage increases greatly and the benefits of anticoagulant therapy are less clear (Sandok et al). Coumadin overdosage may cause hemorrhage into the brain or subdural space or into the kidney, nose, bowel, skin, or muscle; fresh plasma and vitamin K_1 should be administered immediately.

Antiplatelet Drugs Several other drugs which prevent clotting by reducing platelet adhesiveness are under study and show promise of preventing thrombotic and embolic strokes. Aspirin (600 mg twice daily) can be substituted for Coumadin. Dipyridamole (Persantine) in doses of 50 mg every 8 h and sulfinpyrazone (Anturane), in doses of 200 mg every 8 h, may also prove to be useful. Aspirin inhibits platelet aggregation and reduces thromboxane (A_2), a vasoconstricting prostaglandin, and also prostacyclin, a vasodilating prostaglandin. Dipyridamole acts by inhibiting platelet phosphodiesterase so that cyclic AMP is not catabolized, and sulfinpyrazole is believed to inhibit the "platelet release reaction," interfering with platelet adherence to endothelial cells.

Aspirin and sulfinpyrazone have been evaluated by the Canadian Cooperative Study Group in 585 patients with threatened stroke, followed for an average period of 26 months. All the patients had had at least one cerebral or retinal ischemic attack in the previous 3 months. The cases were randomized and the trials were double-blind. Aspirin reduced the risk of recurrent ischemic attacks, stroke, or death by 19 percent and the risk of stroke or death by 31 percent, but this latter effect was sex-dependent: in men the risk of stroke or death was reduced 48 percent, whereas no significant trend was observed among women. Sulfinpyrazone did not reduce ischemic attacks and diminished the risk of strokes or death by only 10 percent. Because of the small sample size of this trial and other considerations, several epidemiologists (Lilienfeld, Kurtzke) have not accepted the major conclusions of the Canadian study and believe that the therapeutic efficacy of aspirin remains to be proved.

Two other randomized series have been reported, one by a Danish group headed by Sorenson et al and the other by a French group (Bousser et al). The first series consisted of 203 patients who had had reversible TIAs. After a period of 25 months, no significant differences were found between the aspirin- and placebo-treated groups with respect to stroke or death. The French series comprised 604 patients with transient or completed strokes, who were followed for 3 years. Strokes occurred in 10.5 percent of patients treated with aspirin or aspirin and dipyridamole and in 18 percent of a placebo group. Myocardial infarction was less frequent in the two treated groups.

Other Forms of Medical Treatment Hemodilution has been shown to increase microcirculatory flow in experimental infarction. Dextran 60 or albumin is given intravenously with or without preceding venesection. The hematocrit is reduced to 30 to 35 percent and central venous pressure raised to 8 to 12 cmH$_2$O. The clinical efficacy of this method remains to be proven.

Barbituates have also been advocated because they prolong survival of neurons in experimental anoxia and ischemia. But they have not received wide approval because they make the neurologic status difficult to follow and may depress respiration. Also hypothermia, which by reducing metabolism facilitates survival of brain tissue, has not had sufficient beneficial value to justify its use. Calcium blockers, which reduce the incidence of neuronal death and counteract vasoconstriction, have been used in experimental animals and in stroke patients. Cerebral blood flow was much improved and lactic acidosis was much less when nimodipine (0.5 mg/kg) was infused. Gelmers gave either 15 or 30 μg/kg in an intracarotid infusion to five patients and obtained a dose-related increase in cerebral blood flow.

Of recent interest has been the development of a series of new tissue plasminogen activators. When administered intravenously these enzymes convert plasminogen to plasmin, which is a proteolytic enzyme capable of hydrolyzing fibrin, fibrinogen, and other coagulation proteins. These drugs have been effective in venous, but not in arterial, thromboses (Hirsh). Recently there has also been interest in drugs that inhibit excitatory amino acid transmitters, but none has been successfully applied to humans.

Surgery Arterial stenosis or an ulcerating arterial plaque in the neck and thorax of patients with recurrent ischemic attacks is frequently amenable to surgical management, employing thromboendarterectomy or bypass grafts. Most often it is the carotid sinus region that lends itself to such therapy. Other sites suitable for surgical management include the common carotid, innominate, and subclavian arteries. Operation on the vertebral artery at its origin has not proved beneficial.

Before operation the existence of the lesion and its extent must be determined by arteriography, a procedure that carries a risk of worsening the stroke or producing focal signs (see above). If the patient is in good medical condition, has normal vessels on the contralateral side, and normal cardiac function, these lesions can usually be dealt with safely by endarterectomy. The overall morbidity and mortality should not exceed 3 percent. In the series of Ojemann and Crowell, in 304 elective carotid endarterectomies, the operative mortality was 1 percent; major and minor strokes each occurred in 1 percent in relation to the operation. For internal carotid thrombi that extended into the siphon and stem of the middle cerebral, a transcranial (superficial temporal-middle cerebral) anastomosis was devised. Though technically feasible, the therapeutic value of this operation has been discredited by the careful worldwide study of Barnett and his many collaborators; the transcranial operation produced no reduction in TIAs, strokes, or death.

Concerning the relative value of anticoagulants and surgery in the treatment of patients with TIAs, there is still a wide divergence of opinion. In fact, currently available data have not completely settled the question as to whether any specific treatment is worthwhile. Toole and his colleagues reported on 225 patients who had been observed for 3 to 14 years (average 5.5 years). During this period, 82 patients had died—21 of cerebral infarction, 52 of heart disease, and 9 of other causes. Of 56 untreated patients, 11 (19 percent) had cerebral infarctions of which 4 were fatal. Of the 45 patients treated medically, 10 (24 percent) had cerebral infarctions of which 3 were fatal. Of 124 patients treated surgically, 27 (21 percent) had postoperative cerebral infarctions of which 7 were fatal. About the same number of patients in the medical and surgical groups continued to have TIAs.

Whisnant and his colleagues observed 199 patients with TIAs, some of whom were untreated and the rest treated with anticoagulants. The survival rate in the two groups was approximately the same, which is not surprising, since the primary cause of death in all patients with TIAs was myocardial infarction. The group receiving anticoagulants had fewer strokes than the untreated group but the difference was small and not significant statistically. Among patients with vertebral-basilar TIAs, those treated with anticoagulants had definitely fewer strokes, starting at 3 months after the onset of attacks. However, the risk of intracranial hemorrhage was at least four times greater in the anticoagulant-treated group.

In another series from the Mayo Clinic reported by Whisnant et al, 151 patients with TIAs referable to one carotid system were subjected to endarterectomy. As with the series of Ojemann and Crowell the mortality was less than 1 percent and morbidity from an operation-related stroke was 3 percent. After the first month the incidence of further ischemic strokes was 2 percent per year and long-term mortality was 3 percent per year. They concluded that the frequency of cerebral vascular complications was significantly reduced by endarterectomy. In a group of 70 symptomatic patients who underwent carotid endarterectomy, carotid stenosis and occlusion recurred in 9 percent within 3 years of the operation (Turnipseed et al); progression of disease in the unoperated carotid artery occurred in more than 20 percent.

Surgical therapy, in our opinion, is as yet applicable only to the group of carotid artery cases with extracranial stenosis and ulcerated plaques. This group constitutes less than 20 percent of all patients with TIAs (Marshall). Despite the equivocal nature of the data quoted above, the authors have the distinct impression that well-executed surgery in appropriately chosen cases stops the TIAs, and that the prognosis is better than if no treatment is given. We continue to use anticoagulants in patients with nonsurgical carotid and all vertebrobasilar TIAs.

Some of the problems in the management of patients with TIAs are discussed further in the final section of this chapter.

PHYSICAL THERAPY AND REHABILITATION

Beginning within a few days, the paralyzed limbs should at intervals be carried through a full range of passive movement many times a day. The purpose is to avoid contracture (and periarthritis), especially at the shoulder, elbow, hip, and ankle. Soreness and aching in the paralyzed limbs should not be allowed to interfere with exercises. Patients should be moved from bed to chair as soon as the illness permits. Nearly all hemiplegics regain the ability to walk to some extent, usually within a 3- to 6-month period, and this should be a primary aim in rehabilitation. The presence of deep sensory loss, in addition to hemiplegia, is the main limiting factor. A short or long leg brace is often required. Speech therapy should be given in appropriate cases, if for no reason other than to improve the morale of the patient and family (see Chap. 22). Physical therapy seems not to benefit patients with cerebellar ataxia. As motor function improves, and if mentality is preserved, instruction in the activities of daily living and the use of

various special devices can assist the patient in becoming at least partly independent in the home.

PREVENTIVE MEASURES

Since the primary objective in the treatment of atherothrombotic disease is prevention, efforts to control the risk factors must continue. Large populations need to be screened for the presence of hypertension, diabetes, hyperlipidemia, and coronary artery disease in the period of life when strokes are frequent. The carotid vessels, being readily accessible, need always to be studied for the presence of a bruit; the latter quite reliably indicates a stenosis though not all stenoses cause a bruit. A self-audible bruit has been associated with an enlarged, superiorly displaced jugular bulb—a benign anatomical variant that can be discerned on CT scan (Adler and Ropper). However, there is still uncertainty as to how to proceed in patients with asymptomatic carotid bruits. The population study by Heyman et al has shed some light on this problem. These authors found that cervical bruits in men constituted a risk for death from ischemic heart disease. They also found that the presence of asymptomatic bruits in men (but not in women) does carry a slightly increased risk of stroke but, more importantly, that the subsequent stroke often fails to correlate in its angioanatomic locus and laterality with the cervical bruit. Similar findings have been reported by Ford et al and by Chambers and Norris. One may conclude that asymptomatic cervical bruits do not in themselves justify invasive diagnostic procedures or surgical correction of underlying extracranial arterial lesions. Our practice has been to perform noninvasive studies of the carotid vessels (Doppler flow, DSA), and only if the lumen is decreasing in size and becomes narrowed to less than 2.0 mm is surgery considered. In a series of 41 such cases (Ojemann and Crowell) there were no surgical complications. In some instances the carotid endarterectomy followed coronary by-pass surgery and in others the two operations were combined.

For patients who have had a stroke and are functional, preventive measures consist of avoiding situations in which strokes are likely to occur: (1) particular care should be taken to maintain the systemic blood pressure, oxygenation, and intracranial blood flow during surgical procedures, especially in elderly patients; (2) hypotensive agents, whether given therapeutically or for diagnostic procedures, should be administered with caution; (3) in the elderly patient, in whom deep sleep might contribute to a state of cerebral ischemia, oversedation should be avoided; (4) systemic hypotension, severe anemia, and polycythemia should be treated promptly; and (5) rapid diuresis may be contra-indicated.

The ultimate solution of the problems of ischemic infarction and TIAs lies in more fundamental fields, namely the prevention or alleviation of hypertension and athero-sclerosis.

EMBOLIC INFARCTION

In most cases of cerebral embolism, the embolic material consists of a fragment that has broken away from a thrombus within the heart. Less frequently the source is intra-arterial, from an atheromatous plaque that has damaged the endo-thelium or ulcerated into the lumen of the carotid sinus, or from the distal (intracranial) end of a thrombus in the internal carotid artery. Embolism due to fat, tumor cells, or air is a rare occurrence and seldom enters into the differential diagnosis of stroke. The embolus usually be-comes arrested at a bifurcation or other site of narrowing of the lumen, and ischemic infarction follows. The infarction is pale, hemorrhagic, or mixed; hemorrhagic infarction, as pointed out earlier, nearly always indicates embolism, though most embolic infarcts are pale. Any region of the brain may be affected, the territory of the middle cerebral artery, particularly the upper division, being the most frequently involved. The two hemispheres are approximately equally affected. Large embolic masses can block large vessels (sometimes the carotids in the neck), while tiny fragments may reach vessels as small as 0.2 mm in diameter. The embolic material may remain arrested and plug the lumen solidly, but more often it breaks into fragments that enter smaller vessels and disappear completely, so that careful pathologic examination fails to reveal their final location. In the latter case, the clinical effects may clear in a few days. The anatomic diagnosis must then be made by inference, e.g., absence of a vascular occlusion at the proper site to explain the infarct, absence of atherosclerosis or other cause of occlusion in the cerebral vessel, presence of a source of emboli and infarcts in other organs such as kidneys and spleen, the occurrence of hemorrhagic infarc-tion, and finally, the clinical history.

Because of the rapidity with which embolic occlusion develops, there is not much time for collateral influx to become established. Thus, sparing of territory distal to the site of occlusion is not as evident as in thrombosis. However, the *ischemia-modifying factors* mentioned above under ''The

Ischemic Stroke'' are still operative and influence the size and severity of the infarct.

Brain embolism is essentially a manifestation of heart disease, and fully 75 percent of cardiogenic emboli lodge in the brain. The commonest cause is *chronic atrial fibrillation* due to atherosclerotic or rheumatic heart disease, the source of the embolus being a mural thrombus within the atrial appendage (Table 34-4). Atrial fibrillation due to other types of heart disease (e.g., hypertensive or syphilitic) can, of course, act in the same way. Embolism occurs also during paroxysmal atrial fibrillation or flutter. Patients with chronic arteriosclerotic and rheumatic atrial fibrillation are, respectively, 5 and 17 times more liable to stroke than an age-matched population with normal cardiac rhythm (Wolf et al). *Mural thrombus* deposited on the damaged endo-cardium overlying a myocardial infarct is an important source of cerebral emboli, as is a thrombus associated with severe mitral stenosis without atrial fibrillation. *Cardiac catheterization or surgery*, especially valvuloplasty, may disseminate fragments of thrombus or a calcified valve. *Mitral and aortic valve prostheses* are presently asso-ciated with embolism in 70 percent of cases. *Paradoxic embolism* can occur when an abnormal communication exists between the right and left sides of the heart (particu-larly a patent foramen ovale), or when both ventricles

Table 34-4
Causes of cerebral embolism

1. Cardiac origin
    a. Atrial fibrillation and other arrhythmias (with rheu-matic, atherosclerotic, hypertensive, congenital or syphilitic heart disease)
    b. Myocardial infarction with mural thrombus
    c. Acute and subacute bacterial endocarditis
    d. Heart disease without arrhythmia or mural thrombus (mitral stenosis, myocarditis, etc.)
    e. Complications of cardiac surgery
    f. Valve prostheses
    g. Nonbacterial thrombotic (marantic) endocardial veg-etations
    h. Prolapsed mitral valve
    i. Paradoxical embolism with congenital heart disease
    j. Trichinosis

2. Noncardiac origin
    a. Atherosclerosis of aorta and carotid arteries (mural thrombus, atheromatous material)
    b. From sites of cerebral artery thrombosis (basilar, vertebral, middle cerebral)
    c. Thrombus in pulmonary veins
    d. Fat, tumor, or air
    e. Complications of neck and thoracic surgery

3. Undetermined origin

communicate with the aorta; thus embolic material arising in the veins of the lower extremity or anywhere in the systemic venous tree can bypass the pulmonary circulation and reach the cerebral vessels. Pulmonary hypertension (often from previous pulmonary embolism) favors the occurrence of paradoxic embolism. Subendocardial fibroelastosis, idiopathic myocardial hypertrophy, cardiac myxomas, and cardiac lesions in trichinosis are rare causes of embolism.

The *vegetations of acute and subacute bacterial endocarditis* give rise to several different lesions in the brain (see page 566). Mycotic aneurysm is a rare complication of septic embolism and may be a source of intracerebral or subarachnoid hemorrhage. *Marantic* or *nonbacterial endocarditis* is a frequently overlooked cause of cerebral embolism and at times produces a baffling clinical picture, especially when associated, as it often is, with carcinomatosis.

The following sources of embolic material are more difficult to prove or are less frequently seen than those mentioned above: (1) Mural thrombus, deposited upon ulcerated atheroma in the arch of the aorta or in the carotid arteries, may break loose and find its way into brain arteries. Massage of the carotid sinus, a favorite site for atherosclerosis, may dislodge mural thrombus, with the production of a hemiplegia. This is why carotid massage should not be done in the elderly and only with caution in others. (2) Atheromatous material may be washed out of a large plaque in the aorta or carotid arteries (possibly during arteriography) and carried distally into the branches of the cerebral tree. (3) A mitral valve prolapse (MVP) may be a source of emboli, especially in young patients. The importance of MVP as a source of cerebral embolism is uncertain. In a group of 60 patients who had TIAs or partial stroke and were under 45 years of age, (MVP) was detected (by echocardiography and a characteristic midsystolic click) in 24 patients, but in only 5 of 60 age-matched controls (Barnett et al). On the other hand, in a group of 438 cases of MVP, Sandok and Giuliani found only 40 patients with a prior history of focal cerebrovascular ischemic events (26 with no identifiable mechanism other than MVP). In another large series of 760 cases of MVP, followed for 5 years by cardiologists, only one had an ischemic stroke (Jones et al). And among 54 young adults admitted to the Toronto stroke unit, Hachinski and Norris found only one case of cerebral embolism possibly due to MVP. Rice and his colleagues have described a familial syndrome of premature stroke in association with mitral valve prolapse. (4) The pulmonary veins are a source of cerebral emboli, as indicated by the occurrence of cerebral abscesses in association with pulmonary suppurative disease and by the high incidence of cerebral deposits secondary to pulmonary carcinoma. (5) Surgery of the neck and thorax can be complicated by cerebral embolism. A rare type is that which follows thyroidectomy, in which thrombosis in the stump of the superior thyroid artery extends proximally until a section of it, protruding into the lumen of the carotid, is carried into the cerebral arteries. (6) During arteriography emboli may arise from the tip of the catheter and account for some of the arteriographic accidents.

Cerebral embolism must always have occurred when secondary tumor is deposited in the brain, and cerebral embolism regularly accompanies septicemia. Embolism in the course of septicemia usually indicates the presence of an endocarditis with thrombus formation. A mass of tumor cells or bacteria is seldom large enough to occlude a cerebral artery and produce the picture of stroke. Nevertheless, tumor embolism with stroke has been reported, secondary to cardiac myxomas and occasionally with other tumors. It must be distinguished from marantic endocarditis and embolism that occasionally complicate neoplasm. Cerebral fat embolism is related to trauma. As a rule, the emboli are minute and widely dispersed, giving rise first to pulmonary symptoms and then to multiple cerebral petechial hemorrhages; accordingly the clinical picture is not strictly focal, as it is in a stroke although in some instances it may have focal features. Cerebral air embolism is a rare complication of criminal abortion or of cervical and thoracic operations, and was formerly encountered as a complication of pneumothorax therapy. This condition is usually difficult to separate on clinical grounds from the deficits following hypotension or hypoxia, which frequently coexist.

Not infrequently the diagnosis of cerebral embolism is made at autopsy without finding a source. Possibly the search for a thrombotic nidus had not been sufficiently thorough in these cases, and small thrombi in the atrial appendage, endocardium (between the papillary muscles of the heart), aorta and its branches, or pulmonary veins were overlooked. Nevertheless, in some cases studied most carefully no source of embolic material has been discovered.

CLINICAL PICTURE

Of all strokes, those due to cerebral embolism develop most rapidly, "like a bolt out of the blue." As a rule, the full-blown picture evolves within several seconds or a minute, exemplifying most strikingly the temporal profile of a stroke. With rare exceptions, there are no warning episodes. The embolus strikes at any time of the day or night. Getting up to go to the bathroom is a time of danger. Only occasionally, and for unclear reasons, the clinical picture unfolds more gradually, over many hours, with some fluctuation of symptoms. Possibly the embolus initiates a thrombotic process in the occluded vessel.

The neurologic picture will depend on the artery involved and the site of obstruction. The syndromes related to each angioanatomic territory are the same as those outlined above, under "Neurovascular Syndromes." A large embolus may plug the internal carotid artery or the stem of the middle cerebral artery, producing the full-blown syndromes referable to occlusion of these arteries. More often the embolus is smaller and passes into one of the branches of the middle cerebral artery, producing a strikingly focal disorder, such as a motor aphasia, a monoplegia, or a receptive type of aphasia with little or no motor paralysis. In fact, most patients with a diagnosis of middle cerebral artery thrombosis prove to have embolic occlusion of the middle cerebral artery (or an atherosclerotic thrombosis of the internal carotid artery).

Embolic material entering the vertebral-basilar system occasionally is arrested in the vertebral artery just below its union with the basilar; more often it traverses the vertebral and also the basilar artery, which is larger, and is not arrested until it reaches the upper bifurcation. If arrested here, it abruptly produces deep coma and total paralysis. More often the embolus enters one or both of the posterior cerebral arteries and, by infarcting the visual cortex, causes a unilateral or bilateral homonymous hemianopia. Occasionally it will enter one of the small branches to the subthalamus; one of the "top of the basilar" syndromes results (see above). Embolic infarction of the undersurface of the cerebellum is common, and the resulting swelling of necrotic brain may cause acute, fatal brainstem compression within a few days of the vascular occlusion. Embolic material rarely enters the penetrating branches of the pons.

It is important to emphasize that an embolus in its passage along an artery may produce a severe neurologic deficit that is only temporary; symptoms disappear as the embolus fragments. In other words, *embolism is a common cause of a single evanescent stroke.* Also, as has already been pointed out, it can give rise to multiple transient attacks of almost identical or differing pattern.

Although the abruptness with which the stroke develops and the lack of prodromal symptoms point strongly to embolism, it is the total clinical picture upon which the diagnosis is based. If hemorrhage is ruled out, particularly by the use of the CT scan, only thrombosis and dissecting arterial occlusion remain to be excluded. The presence of atrial fibrillation, a history of myocardial infarction (recent or in the preceding months), or the occurrence of embolism

to other regions of the body all support the diagnosis of embolism. This diagnosis merits careful consideration in young persons in whom atherosclerosis is unlikely. Not infrequently the first sign of myocardial infarction is the occurrence of embolism; therefore, it is advisable that an *electrocardiogram (ECG) be made in all patients with stroke of uncertain origin,* particularly since about 20 percent of myocardial infarctions are of the "silent" variety; and if the ECG does not yield relevant information, Holter monitoring for 24 to 48 h or echocardiographic study of heart valves should be undertaken.

LABORATORY FINDINGS

The findings described above, under "Atherothrombotic Infarction," apply also to embolism, except for hemorrhagic infarction and septic embolism (focal embolic encephalitis). In some 30 percent of cases, cerebral embolism produces a hemorrhagic infarct, but only in a minority of these do red cells enter the CSF (rarely as high as 10,000 red cells per cubic millimeter). In the milder cases of hemorrhagic infarction, a slight xanthochromia may appear after a few days. CT scan may be helpful in showing hemorrhagic infarction, particularly if the scan is repeated once or twice after the second or third day of onset (Fig. 34-19). The

Figure 34-19

Contrast-enhanced CT scan showing a large occipital and several small embolic (hemorrhagic) infarcts, 2 days after the onset of cerebral symptoms.

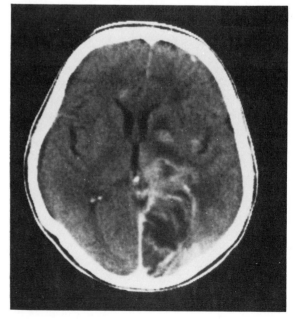

possibility that an embolic infarct is bloody underlines the danger of administering anticoagulants routinely, without a careful examination of the CSF. Also, it is the single exception to the rule that the presence of blood in the CSF of the stroke patient is due to an intracerebral hemorrhage, aneurysm, or vascular malformation.

In septic embolism resulting from subacute bacterial endocarditis the white blood cells in the CSF may be increased, usually up to 200 per cubic millimeter, but occasionally much higher; the proportion of lymphocytes and polymorphonuclears varies with the acuteness of the septic process. There may also be an equal number of red blood cells and a faint xanthochromia. The protein content is elevated, but the glucose content is within normal limits. No bacteria are seen or obtained by culture. The CSF formula in acute bacterial endocarditis may be that of a subacute endocarditis or a purulent meningitis.

COURSE AND PROGNOSIS

The remarks made concerning the *immediate prognosis* of atherothrombotic infarction apply here as well. Massive brainstem infarction as a result of basilar embolism is almost always fatal. Most other patients survive the initial insult, and in many of them the neurologic deficit may recede relatively rapidly, as indicated above. The *eventual prognosis* is determined by the occurrence of further emboli and the gravity of the underlying illness—cardiac failure, myocardial infarction, bacterial endocarditis, malignancy, etc. In about 80 percent of cases, the first episode of cerebral embolism will be followed by another, frequently with severe damage. Furthermore, there is no certain way of predicting when the second embolus will strike; 10 to 20 percent of patients will have their second embolus within 10 days after the initial one, thus imparting an element of urgency to the institution of anticoagulant therapy.

TREATMENT

Three phases of therapy—(1) general medical management in the acute phase, (2) measures directed to restoring the circulation, and (3) physical therapy and rehabilitation—are much the same as described above under "Atherothrombotic Infarction." Attempted embolectomy at the bifurcation of the common carotid artery has usually failed, but should be considered. If pulsation in the temporal artery in front of the ear is present, the embolus has passed beyond that bifurcation, into the internal carotid system, and embolectomy will be unsuccessful. Embolectomy of the middle cerebral artery, a procedure made possible by the development of microvascular surgical techniques, may be successful in some cases. Fibrinolysin therapy has not been systematically evaluated.

Of prime importance is the *prevention of cerebral embolism*, and this applies both to patients who have had an episode of embolism and to those who have not but are at risk to do so. The long-term use of anticoagulants has proved to be effective in the prevention of embolism in cases of atrial fibrillation, myocardial infarction, and valve prosthesis. In patients with atrial fibrillation of recent onset, an attempt should be made to restore normal sinus rhythm by the use of electrical cardioversion, but failing in this attempt, prophylactic anticoagulant therapy is recommended.

After cerebral embolism has occurred, the question arises as to the advisability of delaying anticoagulation therapy for several days, in order to avoid bleeding into a potentially hemorrhagic infarct. Hemorrhage into the infarct occurs in approximately 30 percent of all embolic cerebral infarcts and may require 3 or 4 days or longer to become apparent (Irino et al). For this reason it is our practice to perform a CT scan and lumbar puncture 3 to 4 days following cerebral embolism. If these procedures disclose no evidence of hemorrhage, we proceed with intravenous heparin followed by Coumadin. Care must be taken to avoid excessive anticoagulation as this may increase the risk of frank hemorrhage into the infarct. We recommend that large loading doses of intravenous heparin be avoided and that the anticoagulant be introduced gradually by continuous intravenous infusion. In patients with large cerebral infarcts, especially those who are also hypertensive, there is a distinct risk of anticoagulant-related hemorrhage into the acute infarct (Shields et al). In these patients, anticoagulation therapy should be avoided in the acute setting. Indications are that these guidelines are safe but exceptions to this statement may be expected.

Also, in our opinion, the use of anticoagulant therapy in patients with acute myocardial infarction, including those judged to be in the "good risk" category, is advisable. In cerebral embolism associated with subacute bacterial endocarditis, anticoagulant therapy is contraindicated because of the danger of intracranial bleeding, and it is preferable to rely on rapid sterilization of the blood stream.

Valvuloplasty, removal of valvular verrucous lesions in endocarditis, and amputation of the atrial appendage have substantially reduced the incidence of embolism in rheumatic heart disease. The need for special care in preventing emboli from entering the carotid arteries during the performance of valvuloplasty is appreciated by all cardiac surgeons.

OTHER OCCLUSIVE CEREBROVASCULAR DISEASES

FIBROMUSCULAR DYSPLASIA

This is a segmental, nonatheromatous, noninflammatory arterial disease of unknown etiology. The disease is uncommon (0.5 percent of 61000 arteriograms in the series of So et al), but it is being reported with increasing frequency because of improved diagnostic arteriography.

First described in the renal artery by Leadbetter and Burkland (1938), fibromuscular dysplasia is now known to affect other vessels including cervicocerebral ones. Of the latter, the internal carotid artery is involved most frequently followed by the vertebral and cerebral arteries. The radiologic alteration consists of a series of transverse constrictions, giving the appearance of an irregular string of beads or a tubular narrowing and is observed bilaterally in 75 percent of cases. Usually only the extracranial part of the artery is involved. In the series of Houser et al, 42 of 44 patients were women, and 75 percent were over 50 years of age. All of the patients reported by So et al were women, ranging in age from 41 to 70 years. Cerebral ischemia is the regular consequence of the lesion, but 20 to 30 percent have intracranial saccular aneurysms (rarely a giant aneurysm), which may be a source of subarachnoid hemorrhage.

The pathology of this disease is poorly defined. In the narrowed arterial segments there are degeneration of elastic tissue, disruption and loss of the muscular coat, and increase in fibrous tissue. The dilatations are due to atrophy of the vessel wall. Some patients have had atherosclerosis in addition. Usually vascular occlusion is not present, though there may be marked stenosis; hence the cause of the ischemic lesion in the brain is unsettled. Possibly emboli form in the pouches or in relation to intraluminal septae. So and his colleagues recommend excision of the affected segments if the neurologic symptoms are related to them, and conservative therapy if the fibromuscular dysplasia is a chance arteriographic finding in an asymptomatic patient. In one group of 75 untreated asymptomatic patients followed for more than 4 years, 3 had an infarct 4 to 18 years later (Corrin et al). Ojemann and Crowell have successfully dilated the constricted segments by exposing the vessel and inserting a dilator. Associated saccular aneurysms should be surgically obliterated.

SPONTANEOUS DISSECTION OF THE INTERNAL CAROTID ARTERY

It is well known that Erdheim's medionecrosis aortica cystica may extend into the common carotid arteries,

occluding them and causing massive infarction of the cerebral hemispheres. Weisman and Adams cited examples of this in their study of the neurology of dissecting aneurysms of the aorta, in 1944. But in more recent years, attention has been drawn to the occurrence of spontaneous dissection of the internal carotid artery and the fact that it is an important cause of hemiplegia in young adults. Several large series of such cases have been reported by Ojemann, by Mokri, and by Bogousslavsky, and their colleagues.

Spontaneous carotid dissection is a not uncommon vascular accident. Bogousslavsky et al found 30 instances in 1200 consecutive patients with a first stroke (2.5 percent). Clinically it is of interest that most of the patients have had warning attacks of unilateral cranial or facial pain, followed, within minutes to days, by signs of ischemia in the internal carotid artery territory. The pain is nonthrobbing in nature and centered most often in and around the eye, less often in the frontal or temporal regions, angle of the mandible, or high neck. The ischemic manifestations consist of transient attacks in the territory of the internal carotid, followed frequently by the signs of hemispheric stroke, which may evolve smoothly over a period of a few minutes to hours or in stepwise fashion. A unilateral Horner syndrome may be conjoined. A new cervical bruit, amaurosis fugax, faintness and syncope, and facial numbness are less common symptoms. Most of the patients described by Mokri et al presented with one of two distinct syndromes: (1) unilateral headache associated with an ipsilateral Horner syndrome; and (2) unilateral headache and delayed focal cerebral ischemic symptoms.

Arteriography reveals an elongated, irregular, narrow column of dye, beginning 1.5 to 3 cm above the carotid bifurcation and extending to the base of the skull, a picture which Fisher has called the *string sign*. There may be a tapered occlusion or an outpouching at the end of the string. Less often the aneurysm is located in the midcervical region, and occasionally the dissection extends into the middle cerebral artery or involves the opposite carotid artery or the vertebral and basilar arteries. In several cases the dissecting hemorrhage of the internal carotid artery has been detected by MR imaging; further studies will determine whether this procedure will obviate the need for angiography.

The usual treatment has been anticoagulation to prevent embolism. Whether surgical measures are of value is uncertain. The important datum to emerge from the study of Mokri et al is that a complete or excellent recovery occurs in 85 percent of patients with the angiographic signs of dissection; mainly these were patients without stroke. The outcome in patients with stroke is far less benign. About one-quarter such patients succumb and one-half of the survivors are seriously impaired (Bogousslavsky et al). In the remainder, early reopening of the occluded artery occurs (as determined by Doppler ultrasonography), with good functional recovery.

The pathogenesis of the dissection is undetermined. Although the lesion may develop spontaneously, it has been found in relation to trauma to the head and neck and to carotid puncture for angiography. In most of the recently reported cases, cystic medial necrosis has not been found on microscopic examination of the involved artery. In some there was a disorganization of the media and internal elastic lamina, but its specificity is in doubt, since Ojemann and his colleagues noted a similar change in some of their control cases. A small proportion of cases show the changes of fibromuscular dysplasia. A more thorough study of these vessels in routine autopsy material is needed.

MOYAMOYA DISEASE AND MULTIPLE PROGRESSIVE INTRACRANIAL ARTERIAL OCCLUSIONS

The term *moyamoya* is a Japanese word for a *cloud of smoke* or *haze,* and it has been used in recent years to refer to an *extensive basal cerebral rete mirabile*—a network of small anastomotic vessels at the base of the brain around and distal to the circle of Willis, seen in carotid arteriograms, along with segmental stenosis or occlusion of the terminal parts of both internal carotid arteries.

Nishimoto and Takeuchi collected 111 cases, selected on the basis of these two radiologic criteria. The condition was observed mainly in infants, children, and adolescents (more than half the cases were less than 10 years of age, and only 4 of 111 cases were older than 40 years). All their patients were Japanese; both males and females were affected, and eight were siblings. The symptom that led to medical examination was usually weakness of an arm or leg or both on one side. The weakness tended to clear rapidly but recurred in some instances. Headache, convulsions, impaired mental development, visual disturbance, and nystagmus were less frequent. In older patients, subarachnoid hemorrhage was the most common initial manifestation. Other symptoms and signs were speech disturbance, sensory impairment, involuntary movements, and unsteady gait. Only six of the entire series became worse after the initial illness, and four died. Postmortem examination of these cases has not yielded a clear picture of the carotid lesion. The adventitia, media, and internal elastic lamina of the stenotic or occluded arteries were normal, and only the intima was thickened by fibrous tissue. No inflammatory cells or atheromata were seen. In a few cases, hypoplasia of the vessel with absent muscularis has been described. The rete mirabile consists of a fine network of vessels over the basal surface (in the pia-arachnoid) which, according to Yamashita et al, reveal microaneurysm formation due to weakness of the internal elastic lamina and thinness of the vessel wall. The latter lesion may be the source of subarachnoid hemorrhage. Thus one part of the symptomatology is traced to the carotid stenosis and another to the rupture of the vascular network.

This form of cerebrovascular disease is not limited to the Japanese. The authors have observed several such patients, as have many others in the United States, western Europe, and Australia. Opinion is divided as to whether the basal rete mirabile represents a congenital vascular malformation (i.e., a persistence of the embryonal network) or a rich collateral vascularization, secondary to a congenital hypoplasia or acquired stenosis or occlusion of the internal carotid arteries early in life. The association between moyamoya and certain HLA types favors an hereditary basis (Kitahara et al).

The condition described in non-Orientals by Taveras as *multiple progressive intracranial arterial occlusion* occurs in the same age period as moyamoya and has many of the clinical characteristics of the latter. It lacks only the cloud of fine anastomotic channels. It is probable, also, that the diffuse meningeal angiomatosis described by Divry and Van Bogaert is a form of moyamoya. Snedden's syndrome of familial livedo reticularis with multiple vascular lesions may prove to be another variant. Since the vascular pathology of all these diseases is incompletely studied, their exact relationships cannot be stated at this time.

STROKES IN CHILDREN AND YOUNG ADULTS

The occurrence of acute hemiplegia in infants and children is a well-recognized phenomenon. In a series of 555 consecutive postmortem examinations at the Children's Medical Center in Boston, there were 48 cases (8.7 percent) of occlusive vascular disease of the brain (Banker). The occlusions were both embolic (mainly associated with *congenital heart disease*) and thrombotic, and the latter were actually more common in veins than in arteries.

Similarly, stroke is not an uncommon event in young adults (15 to 45 years). This group accounts for an estimated 3 percent of cerebral infarctions. In terms of causation, this group is remarkably heterogeneous. In a series of 144 such patients, more than 40 possible etiologies were identified (H.P. Adams et al). Nevertheless, 78 percent of the group could be accounted for by three categories of disease, more or less equal in size—atherosclerotic infarction (usually with a recognized risk factor), cardiogenic embolism (particularly in association with rheumatic heart disease, bacterial and verrucous endocarditis, paradoxical embolism, prosthetic valves), and nonatherosclerotic vasculopathies (arterial trauma, "spontaneous" dissection of the carotid artery, moyamoya, lupus erythematosus, drug-induced, etc.). Hematologically related disorders—use of oral contraceptives (see below), postpartum state, acute alcoholic intoxication, hypercoagulable states—were the probable causes in 15 percent of the series of 144 patients.

Persistent cerebral ischemia and infarction may occasionally complicate migraine in young persons (page 142). The combination of migraine and "the pill" is particularly hazardous. In a similar vein, despite the commonality of mitral valve prolapse in young adults, it is probably only rarely a cause of stroke (see above). Stroke due to either arterial or venous occlusion occurs occasionally in association with ulcerative colitis and regional enteritis. Evidence points to a hypercoagulable state during exacerbations of the inflammatory bowel disease, but a precise defect in coagulation has not been defined. Meningovascular syphilis should always be a diagnositc consideration in this age group.

Sickle-cell anemia is an important cause of stroke in black children; acute hemiplegia is the most common manifestation, but all types of focal cerebral disorder have been observed. The pathologic findings are those of infarction, large and small, and their basis is assumed to be vascular obstruction associated with the sickling process. Intracranial bleeding (subdural, subarachnoid, and intracerebral) may also complicate sickle-cell anemia, and for some reason there is an increased incidence of pneumococcal meningitis in this disease. Plasma C-protein deficiency, *homocystinuria* and *Fabry's angiokeratosis,* hereditary metabolic diseases described in Chap. 38, may give rise to strokes in children or young adults.

Oral Contraceptives and Cerebral Infarction

Episodes of transient or prolonged cerebral ischemia are common occurrences during pregnancy and the puerperium as well as during estrogen therapy and the administration of the contraceptive pill (which contains both estrogen and progestin). Fisher has reviewed the literature and has himself analyzed 12 postpartum, 9 puerperal, and 14 contraceptive cases, and 9 cases in which estrogen therapy was being given; arterial thrombosis was demonstrated in half of the group.

It now seems clear that women who take oral contraceptives in the child-bearing years, particularly if they are over 35 years of age and also smoke, are hypertensive and have migraine, are at increased risk of developing cerebral infarction as well as ischemic heart disease, and subarachnoid hemorrhage (Longstreth and Swanson, Vessey et al). The cerebral infarction in these cases is due to arterial occlusion, occurring in both the carotid-middle cerebral and vertebral-basilar territories. In most of the

reported fatal cases, the thrombosed artery has been free of atheroma or other disease. This has been taken to indicate that embolism is responsible for the strokes; no source of embolism has been demonstrated, however. Noncerebral venous thrombosis is another, relatively rare complication of "the pill." These observations, coupled with evidence that estrogen alters the coagulability of the blood, suggest that a state of hypercoagulability is an important factor in the genesis of contraceptive-associated infarction. The increased plasma concentrations of LDL cholesterol and decreased concentrations of HDL cholesterol that are associated with the more potent progestins may be another factor.

The vascular lesion underlying cerebral thrombosis in women taking oral contraceptives has been studied by Irey and his colleagues. It consists of intimal hyperplasia of nodular eccentric topography with increased acid mucopolysaccharides and replication of the internal elastic lamina. Similar changes have been found in pregnancy and in humans and animals receiving exogenous steroids, including estrogens.

Stroke in Pregnancy Pregnancy also increases the incidence of cerebrovascular events. Most of the focal vascular lesions during pregnancy are due to arterial occlusion, occurring in the second and third trimesters and first week after delivery. Venous occlusion tends to occur 1 to 4 weeks postpartum. In Glasgow, one-third of 65 women with stroke (15 to 45 years of age) were pregnant or puerperal. In Rochester, the incidence rate of stroke during pregnancy was 6.2 per 100,000, but doubled with each advance in age from 25 to 29, 30 to 39, and 40 to 49 years. Included in most series are cases of cardiac disease, particularly valve-related embolism.

STROKE WITH CARDIAC SURGERY

Incident to cardiac arrest and by-pass surgery there is risk of both generalized and focal hypoxia-ischemia of the brain. Improved operative techniques have lessened the incidence of these complications, but they are still distressingly frequent. Fortunately most of these cerebral disorders are transient. In a prospective study of 42 patients undergoing coronary by-pass surgery, at the Cleveland Clinic, Breuer et al found that 5.2 percent had strokes, but they were severe in only 2 percent.

Mohr examined 100 consecutive cases pre- and postoperatively at the Massachusetts General Hospital and observed two types of complications—one occurring immediately after the operation and the other after an interval of days or weeks. The immediate neurologic disorder consisted of a delay in awakening from the anesthesia, a slowness in thinking, disorientation, agitation, combative-ness, visual hallucinations, and poor registration and recall of what was happening. These symptoms, sometimes verging on delirium or psychosis, usually cleared within 5 to 7 days, although some patients were not entirely normal mentally some weeks later. As the confusion cleared, about half of the patients were found to have small visual field defects, dyscalculia, oculomanual ataxia, alexia, and other perceptive defects suggestive of lesions in the parieto-occipital regions. The immediate disorders were attributed to hypotension and various types of embolism (air, silicon, fat, platelet). The delayed effects were more clearly embolic and were especially frequent in patients having prosthetic valve placements, but they also occurred subsequent to arterial homografts. In one series the incidence of embolism was calculated to be 4.6 percent per month in the valve replacement group and 1 percent per month with vascular homografts over a 4-year period.

In another study of 100 consecutive patients who underwent open heart surgery for valve replacement, evidence of cerebral damage was found in 37, and in seven of them residual neurologic signs were still present at the end of a year (Sotaniemi). Long perfusion time was the most significant risk factor, whereas age and moderate operative hypotension proved to be unimportant.

INTRACRANIAL HEMORRHAGE

This is the third most frequent cause of stroke. Although more than a dozen causes of intracranial hemorrhage are listed in Table 34-5, primary or hypertensive ("spontaneous") intracerebral hemorrhage, ruptured saccular aneurysm and vascular malformation, and hemorrhage associated with bleeding disorders account for almost all of the hemorrhages that present as strokes. Duret hemorrhages, hypertensive encephalopathy, and brain purpura will not simulate a stroke and are included only for the sake of completeness.

PRIMARY (HYPERTENSIVE) INTRACEREBRAL HEMORRHAGE

This is the common, well-known "spontaneous" brain hemorrhage. Although it occurs rarely with levels of blood pressure in the normal range and sometimes with levels of only 150/90 to 170/90, in most cases the levels are much higher. Hypertensive hemorrhage occurs within brain tissue, and rupture of arteries lying in the subarachnoid space is practically unknown, apart from aneurysm. The extravasation forms a roughly circular or oval mass that disrupts the tissue and grows in volume as the bleeding continues. Adjacent brain tissue is displaced and compressed. If the hemorrhage is large, midline structures are displaced to the opposite side and vital centers are compromised, leading to coma and death. Rupture or seepage into the ventricular system usually occurs, and the CSF becomes bloody in more than 90 percent of cases. A hemorrhage of this type almost never ruptures through the cerebral cortex, the blood reaching the subarachnoid space via the ventricular system. When the hemorrhage is small and located at a distance from the ventricles, the CSF may remain clear even on repeated examination. And one can see in unenhanced CT scans that the blood clot is remote from the ventricles and cisterns of the subarachnoid space.

Extravasated blood undergoes a series of changes beginning with the collection of phagocytes at the outer rim and followed within 5 or 6 days by the formation of a brown-orange peripheral zone of hemosiderin-filled macrophages. The mass gradually decreases in size, and after

Table 34-5
Causes of intracranial hemorrhage (including intracerebral, subarachnoid, ventricular, and subdural)

1. Primary (hypertensive) intracerebral hemorrhage
2. Ruptured saccular aneurysm
3. Ruptured AVM
4. Undetermined cause (normal blood pressure, no aneurysm or AVM)
5. Trauma including postraumatic delayed apoplexy
6. Hemorrhagic disorders: leukemia, aplastic anemia, thrombocytopenic purpura, liver disease, complication of anticoagulant therapy, hyperfibrinolysis, hypofibrinogenemia, hemophilia, Christmas disease, etc.
7. Hemorrhage into primary and secondary brain tumors
8. Septic embolism, mycotic aneurysm
9. With hemorrhagic infarction, arterial or venous
10. With inflammatory disease of the arteries and veins
11. With arterial amyloidosis
12. Miscellaneous rare types: after vasopressor drugs, upon exertion, during arteriography, during painful urologic examination, as a late complication of early-life carotid occlusion, complication of carotid-cavernous AV fistula, with anoxemia, migraine, teratomatous malformations. Herpes simplex encephalitis and acute necrotizing hemorrhagic encephalopathy may be associated with up to 2000 red blood cells or more per cubic millimeter in the CSF; tularemia, anthrax, and pseudomonas meningitis and snake venom poisoning may cause bloody CSF.

a period of some 2 to 6 months, only an orange-stained cleft is left at the site of the hemorrhage.

Hemorrhages may be described as massive, small, slit, and petechial. *Massive* refers to hemorrhages several centimeters in diameter; *small* applies to those 1 to 2 cm in diameter. *Slit* refers to a hypertensive hemorrhage that lies subcortically at the junction of white and gray matter.

In order of frequency, the most common sites of hypertensive hemorrhage are (1) the putamen and adjacent internal capsule (50 percent of cases), (2) various parts of the central white matter of the temporal, parietal, or frontal lobes (lobar hemorrhages) sometimes extending from the putamen, (3) thalamus, (4) cerebellar hemisphere, and (5) pons. The vessel involved is usually a penetrating artery. The nature of the vascular lesion that leads to arterial rupture is not fully known, but in the few cases studied by serial sections, the hemorrhage appeared to arise from an arterial wall altered by the effects of hypertension, i.e., the change referred to in a preceding section as segmental lipohyalinosis and the false aneurysm of Charcot-Bouchard. Russell has affirmed the relationship of these aneurysms to hypertension and their frequent localization on penetrating small arteries and arterioles of the basal ganglia, thalamus, pons, and subcortical white matter. An increasing number of our patients are found to have amyloidosis of intracerebral arteries, and Regli et al have actually found the site of rupture in one or two cases to be through an arterial wall heavily impregnated with amyloid. When the amyloidosis is severe there may occur a succession of cerebral hemorrhages, many of them lobar (Tyler et al).

Clinical Picture Of all the cerebrovascular diseases, brain hemorrhage is the most dramatic and from ancient times has been surrounded by "an aura of mystery and inevitability." It has been given its own name, "apoplexy." The prototype is an obese, plethoric, hypertensive male who, "while sane and sound, falls senseless to the ground, impervious to shouts, shaking, and pinching, breathes stertorously, and dies in a few hours." A massive blood clot escapes from the brain as it is removed post mortem. With smaller hemorrhages, the clinical picture conforms closely to the temporal profile of a stroke, i.e., an abrupt onset of symptoms that evolve gradually and steadily over minutes, hours, or occasionally days (usually 1 to 24 h), depending on the size of the ruptured artery and the speed of bleeding. Hemorrhages that complicate the administration of anticoagulants may evolve at a slower pace. Usually there are no warnings or prodromal symptoms. Headache, dizziness, epistaxis, or other symptoms do not occur with

any consistency, and many patients have felt entirely well up to the moment of vessel rupture. There is no age predilection except that the average age of occurrence is lower than in thrombotic infarction and neither sex is more disposed. The incidence of hypertensive cerebral hemorrhage is higher in blacks than in whites, and seems recently to have been reported with increasing frequency in Japanese. In the majority of cases, the hemorrhage has its onset while the patient is up and active; onset during sleep is a rarity. The level of blood pressure is elevated in 75 to 80 percent of cases and is maintained early in the course of the stroke or may even rise, so that the existence of hypertension is readily established when the patient is first examined. Hypertension is usually of the "essential" type, but other causes must always be considered—renal disease, renal artery occlusion, toxemia of pregnancy, pheochromocytoma, aldosteronism, ACTH or corticosteroid overdosage, and, rarely, violent exertion or intense excitement. Cardiomegaly is often present.

There is ordinarily only one episode of hemorrhage, and recurrent bleeding from the same site, as happens with saccular aneurysm and arteriovenous malformation, is not encountered. Blood that has extravasated into cerebral tissue is removed slowly, over a period of weeks and months, during which time symptoms and signs persist. Hence the neurologic deficit is never transitory in intracerebral hemorrhage, as it so often is in thrombosis and embolism; for the same reason, one should not expect rapid improvement in the neurologic deficit from one examination to another.

The neurologic symptoms and signs vary with the site and size of the extravasation. The most common syndrome is the one due to *putaminal hemorrhage*, with implication of the adjacent internal capsule (Fig. 34-20). With large hemorrhages patients lapse almost immediately into stupor and coma with hemiplegia, and their condition visibly deteriorates as the hours pass. More often, however, the patient complains of headache or of some other abnormal cephalic sensation. Within a few minutes the face sags on one side, speech becomes slurred or aphasic, the arm and leg gradually weaken and the eyes tend to deviate away from the side of the paretic limbs. These events occur gradually over a period of 5 to 30 min; this type of evolution is strongly suggestive of intracerebral bleeding. Gradually the paralysis worsens, a Babinski sign appears, the affected limbs become flaccid, painful stimuli are not appreciated, speaking becomes impossible, and confusion gives way to stupor. In the most advanced stages, signs of upper brainstem compression appear—coma, bilateral Babinski signs, deep, irregular, or intermittent respiration, dilated fixed pupils, and, occasionally, decerebrate rigidity. The pulse is bounding at first and weakens as the coma deepens.

The use of CT scanning has revealed many small putaminal hemorrhages, some causing no headache and only a slight motor deficit. In former times these would have been misdiagnosed as an embolic or thrombotic ischemic stroke, especially if the CSF was clear. Hier et al remark that the size of the hemorrhage is a reliable indicator of prognosis. Many with small hemorrhages survive. In their series of 24 successive cases, which included many small hemorrhages, the mortality rate was 37 percent. Waga and Yamamoto, in a review of 74 cases, also noted a low mortality (13 to 20 percent) in patients who showed small hemorrhages and were conscious or only slightly drowsy.

Thalamic hemorrhage of moderate size also produces a hemiplegia or hemiparesis by compression of the adjacent internal capsule. The sensory deficit equals or outstrips the motor weakness. Aphasia may be present with lesions of the dominant side, and amorphosynthesis and contralateral neglect with nondominant lesions. A homonymous field defect, if present, usually clears in a few days. Thalamic hemorrhage, by virtue of its extension into the subthalamus, causes a series of ocular disturbances—palsies of vertical and lateral gaze, forced deviation of the eyes downward, inequality of pupils with absence of light reaction, skew deviation with the eye opposite the hemorrhage being displaced downward and medially, ipsilateral ptosis and miosis, absence of convergence, retraction nystagmus, and tucking in of the eyelids. Retraction of the neck may be prominent. Again the prognosis for survival and return to

Figure 34-20

An unenhanced CT scan showing the typical picture of a massive primary (hypertensive) hemorrhage in the basal ganglia. The third ventricle and opposite lateral ventricle are compressed by the expanding mass (12 h after onset of stroke).

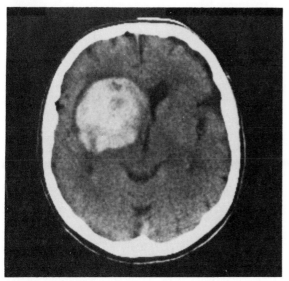

an independent life relates to the size of the hemorrhage, as reflected in the state of consciousness and bilaterality of neurologic signs (Kwak et al).

In *pontine hemorrhage,* deep coma usually ensues in a few minutes, and the clinical picture includes total paralysis, prominent decerebrate rigidity, and small (1 mm) pupils that react to light. Lateral eye movements, evoked by head turning or caloric testing, are impaired or absent. Death usually occurs within a few hours, but there are rare exceptions in which consciousness is retained and the clinical manifestations indicate a smaller lesion in the tegmentum of the pons, e.g., disturbances of lateral ocular movements, crossed sensory or motor disturbances, small pupils, and cranial nerve palsies, in addition to signs of bilateral corticospinal tract involvement. We have seen patients with small tegmental hemorrhages survive with good functional recovery. In the series of 60 patients with pontine hemorrhage reviewed by Nakajima, 19 survived (eight of these had remained alert). Usually the hemorrhage was smaller than 1.0 cm in the nonfatal cases.

Cerebellar hemorrhage usually develops over a period of several hours, and loss of consciousness at the onset is unusual. Repeated vomiting is a prominent feature, along with occipital headache, vertigo, and inability to sit, stand, or walk. There is a paresis of conjugate lateral gaze to the side of the hemorrhage, forced deviation of the eyes to the opposite side, or an ipsilateral sixth nerve weakness. Vertical eye movements are retained. Other ocular signs include blepharospasm, involuntary closure of one eye, skew deviation, "ocular bobbing," and small, often unequal pupils that continue to react until very late in the illness. In the early phase of the illness there may be little or no evidence of cerebellar disease; only a minority of cases show nystagmus or cerebellar ataxia of the limbs, although these signs must always be sought. A mild ipsilateral facial weakness and a diminished corneal reflex are common. Dysarthria and dysphagia may be prominent. Contralateral hemiplegia and facial weakness do not occur. At the onset there is occasionally a spastic paraparesis or a quadriplegia with preservation of consciousness. The plantar reflexes are flexor in the early stages, but extensor later. As the hours pass, and occasionally with unanticipated suddenness, the patient becomes stuporous and then comatose as a result of brainstem compression, at which point reversal of the syndrome, even by surgical therapy, is seldom successful.

In a summary of the findings in 26 cases of *lobar hemorrhage,* Ropper and Davis found 11 to lie within the occipital lobe (with pain around the ipsilateral eye and a dense homonymous hemianopia); seven in the temporal lobe (with pain in or anterior to the ear, a partial hemianopia, and a fluent aphasia); four in the frontal lobe (with contralateral hemiplegia, mainly of the arm, and frontal headache; and three in the parietal lobe (with anterior temporal headache and hemisensory deficit contralaterally). The occurrence of a progressively worsening headache, vomiting, and drowsiness in conjunction with one of these syndromes was said to be diagnostic, and, of course, the presence of lobar hemorrhage is readily corroborated by the CT scan. Fourteen of the 26 patients had had normal blood pressure and in several of the fatal cases there was amyloidosis of the affected vessels. Two patients were receiving anticoagulants; two had an arteriovenous malformation and one had a metastatic tumor. In a series of 22 patients reported by Kase et al, 55 percent were normotensive; metastatic tumors, arteriovenous malformations, and blood dyscrasias were noted in 14, 9, and 5 percent of the patients, respectively.

It will be noted that in the localization of intracerebral hemorrhages, *ocular signs* are important. In putaminal hemorrhage the eyes are deviated to the side opposite the paralysis; in thalamic hemorrhage the commonest ocular abnormality is downward deviation of the eyes, and the pupils may be unreactive; in pontine hemorrhage the eyeballs are fixed and the pupils tiny but reactive; and in cerebellar hemorrhage the eyes are deviated laterally to the side opposite the lesion.

A *severe headache* is generally considered to be an accompaniment of intracerebral hemorrhage, and in many cases it is a prominent and helpful diagnostic point. Nevertheless, in almost 50 percent of our cases headache has been absent or mild in degree. *Nuchal rigidity* is found frequently but again, it is so often absent that failure to find it should by no means detract from the diagnosis. Stiffness of the neck characteristically disappears as coma deepens. *Vomiting* at the onset of intracerebral hemorrhage occurs much more frequently than with infarction. It is important to note that often the patient is alert and responding accurately when first seen. This is true even when the CSF is grossly bloody; thus the adage that hemorrhage into the ventricular system always precipitates coma is quite incorrect. Only if bleeding into the ventricles is massive will coma result. *Cerebral seizures,* usually focal, occur in some 10 percent of cases of supratentorial hemorrhage in the first few days, especially in association with subcortical *slit* hemorrhages. The fundi often show hypertensive changes in the arterioles. Rarely, white-centered retinal hemorrhages (Roth spots) or fresh preretinal (subhyaloid) hemorrhages occur, but the latter are much more common with ruptured aneurysm, or arteriovenous malformation, or severe trauma.

Many of the less precisely localizing neurologic manifestations of ischemic and embolic infarction are also encountered in intracerebral hemorrhage, including coma, stupor, drowsiness, confusion, Cheyne-Stokes respiration, bilateral or contralateral grasping and sucking reflexes, incontinence of bowel and bladder, and unilateral and bilateral extensor rigidity.

Although the proper interpretation of this array of clinical data allows the correct diagnosis to be established in most cases, the ancillary examinations described below are helpful, especially in the diagnosis of small hemorrhages.

Laboratory Findings Among laboratory methods for the diagnosis of intracerebral hemorrhage, the CT scan occupies the foremost position. This procedure has proved totally reliable in the detection of hemorrhages that are 1.0 to 1.5 cm or more in diameter and situated in the cerebral or cerebellar hemispheres. Small pontine hemorrhages are visualized with less certainty. The CT scan is particularly useful in the diagnosis of brain hemorrhages that do not spill blood into the CSF and were heretofore clinically unrecognizable. At the same time coexisting hydrocephalus, tumor, cerebral swelling, and displacement of the intracranial contents are readily appreciated. MRI is particularly useful for demonstrating brainstem hemorrhages and residual hemorrhages, which remain visible long after they cannot be seen by the CT scan (after 4 to 5 weeks). Hemosiderin has its own characteristic appearance.

Before the introduction of CT scanning the examination of the CSF was the most dependable method for the diagnosis of hemorrhage. In cases of massive hemorrhage, the CSF is often under increased pressure; but in almost half our cases, readings under 200 mmH$_2$0 have been obtained. The fluid is usually grossly bloody, although the count may vary from a few thousand cells up to one million per cubic millimeter. With smaller hemorrhages in central structures, the CSF contains a lesser amount of blood; in some cases of intracerebral hemorrhage, particularly the *slit* type, it may be entirely clear. In these latter cases, slight xanthochromia may appear after a few days. At times the CSF may be clear grossly, but contains some 200 to 400 red cells per cubic millimeter; it is then difficult to decide if this represents a primary cerebral hemorrhage or a traumatic tap. These details are mentioned because if a CT scan is unavailable they are critical in making an accurate diagnosis of the type of stroke, prior to the use of therapeutic measures such as anticoagulant drugs or surgical exploration. A traumatic tap, which may greatly complicate the diagnostic problem, can be distinguished from preexisting bleeding by the criteria outlined in Chap. 2.

Lumbar puncture is not always innocuous; temporal lobe herniation may be aggravated in cases of massive supratentorial hemorrhage or softening. Despite this danger, the procedure is necessary when CT scanning is not available, if specific therapeutic measures are contemplated, or if any suspicion exists about the presence of meningitis. Skull films early in the course of cerebral hemorrhage may show a shift of the calcified pineal gland, a change rarely seen in infarction. The EEG is not diagnostic, but high-voltage, slow waves are the most common finding with hemorrhage into the cerebral hemisphere. Films of the chest will often show cardiomegaly. Urinary abnormalities usually reflect coexisting renal disease, although transient glucosuria has been reported to result specifically from intracranial hemorrhage. The white cell count in the peripheral blood often rises to 15,000 to 20,000 per cubic millimeter, a higher figure than in thrombosis. The sedimentation rate also is elevated.

Course and Prognosis The immediate prognosis is grave; some 30 to 35 percent of patients die in 1 to 30 days. Either the hemorrhage extends into the ventricular system, or the temporal lobe herniates and compresses the midbrain; usually both occur. Sometimes the hemorrhage itself seeps into vital centers. Gastric erosion and gastrointestinal hemorrhage of neurogenic origin may occur at any time within the first week or so. In patients who survive, i.e., in those with smaller hemorrhages, there can be a surprisingly adequate restitution of function, since, in contrast to infarction, the hemorrhage has to some extent pushed brain tissue aside instead of destroying it. Function may be slow to return, however, because extravasated blood is slow to be removed from the tissues. Since rebleeding from the same site is unlikely, the patient may live for many years. In some instances of medium-sized cerebral and cerebellar hemorrhages, the patient survives and his or her condition gradually stabilizes, but papilledema appears after several days of increased intracranial pressure. This does not mean that the hemorrhage is increasing in size or swelling—only that papilledema is slow to develop. Failure to appreciate this fact has in many instances dictated unnecessary attempts to evacuate the clot. Healed scars impinging on the cortex are liable to be epileptogenic.

Treatment *The general medical management of the comatose patient with intracerebral hemorrhage* is the same as for the patients with ischemic infarction and has been outlined on page 652. The management of patients with large intracerebral hemorrhages includes maintaining adequate ventilation, controlled hyperventilation to a Pco_2 of 25 to 30 mmHg, and tissue dehydration by the use of mannitol or furosemide (osmolality kept at 305 to 315 mosmol/L and Na at 150 meq), and limiting fluid intake to 1200 mL/day, given as intravenous infusions of normal saline.

Surgical removal of the clot in the acute stage, either by evacuation or aspiration, may occasionally be life-saving, and we have referred a number of our patients who had hemorrhages over 3.0 cm in diameter and whose clinical state was deteriorating for surgical treatment. The best surgical results have been in patients with lobar or putaminal hemorrhages. Also a number of patients with cerebellar hematomas seem to have been helped by evacuation of the clot, preferably before coma has supervened. Once the patient becomes deeply comatose, with dilated fixed pupils, nothing can be done to help.

Ropper and King find that in comatose patients with large hemorrhages the placement of a subarachnoid screw device for constant monitoring of intracranial pressure enables the clinician to more intelligently use medical measures, as outlined in Chap. 16. If the intracranial pressure is not controllable, it may be an indication for surgical removal of clot. In general, however, the surgical results have not been better than those obtained by medical measures (see also Waga).

Attempts to halt the hemorrhage by lowering the systemic blood pressure through the use of autonomic blocking agents have not been effective, and in many instances the inadvertent occurrence of hypotension has seriously complicated the illness. Artificial hypothermia has been used sporadically, but there are insufficient data to permit appraisal of this procedure.

The *most important preventive measures* are the use of antihypertensive drugs in cases of essential hypertension and the early detection of toxemia of pregnancy.

RUPTURED SACCULAR ANEURYSM

This is the fourth most frequent cerebrovascular disorder—following atherothrombosis, embolism, and hypertensive intracerebral hemorrhage. Saccular aneurysms, or berry aneurysms, as they are called, take the form of small, thin-walled blisters protruding from the arteries of the circle of Willis or its major branches. As a rule, the aneurysms are located at bifurcations and branchings (Fig. 34-17) and are generally presumed to result from developmental defects in the media and elastica. An alternate theory holds that the aneurysmal process is initiated by focal destruction of the internal elastic membrane, which is produced by hemodynamic forces at the apices of bifurcations (Ferguson). Owing to the local weakness, the intima bulges outward, covered only by adventitia; the sac gradually enlarges and finally rupture occurs. Saccular aneurysms vary in size from 2 mm up to 2 or 3 cm in diameter, averaging 8 to 10 mm. They vary greatly in form. Some are round and connected to the parent artery by a narrow stalk; others are broad-based without a stalk; still others are narrow cylinders. The site of rupture is usually at the dome of the aneurysm, which may present one or more secondary sacculations.

In routine autopsies the incidence of ruptured aneurysms is 1.8 percent; of unruptured ones, 2.0 percent, excluding minor outpouchings of 3 mm or less. It has been estimated that 400,000 Americans harbor unruptured aneurysms and that there are 26,000 subarachnoid hemorrhages from them per year (Sahs). Rupture of saccular aneurysm is rare in childhood, and they are seldom found at routine postmortem examination; they increase in frequency to reach their peak incidence between 35 and 65 years of age. Therefore, they are not congenitally formed anomalies but develop over the years on the basis of the developmental or acquired arterial defect. There is an increased incidence of congenital polycystic kidney, fibromuscular dysplasia, moyamoya, and coarctation of the aorta among persons with saccular aneurysm. A saccular aneurysm is seen in about 1 of 20 arteriovenous malformations. Hypertension is more frequently present than in the general population, but aneurysms frequently occur in persons with normal blood pressure. Cigarette smoking may increase the risk of subarachroid hemorrhage (Fogelholm and Murros). Preg-

nancy is not associated with an increased incidence of aneurysmal rupture. Atherosclerosis, though present in the walls of some saccular aneurysms, probably plays no part in their formation or enlargement.

Approximately 90 to 95 percent of saccular aneurysms lie on the anterior part of the circle of Willis (Fig. 34-21). The four most common sites are (1) in relation to the anterior communicating artery, (2) at the origin of the posterior communicating artery from the stem of the internal carotid, (3) at the first major bifurcation of the middle cerebral artery, and (4) at the bifurcation of the internal carotid into middle and anterior cerebral arteries. Other sites include the internal carotid artery in the cavernous sinus, the origin of the ophthalmic artery, the junction of the posterior communicating and posterior cerebral arteries, the bifurcation of the basilar artery, and the origins of the three cerebellar arteries. Aneurysms are multiple in 20 percent of patients, and they may be situated unilaterally or bilaterally.

There are several types of aneurysm other than saccular, e.g., mycotic, fusiform, diffuse, and globular. The mycotic aneurysm is caused by a septic embolus that weakens the wall of the vessel in which it lodges; and the last three are named for their predominant morphologic characteristics and consist of enlargement or dilatation of the entire circumference of the involved vessels, usually

Figure 34-21

Diagram of the circle of Willis to show the principal sites of saccular aneurysms. Approximately 90 percent of aneurysms are on the anterior half of the circle.

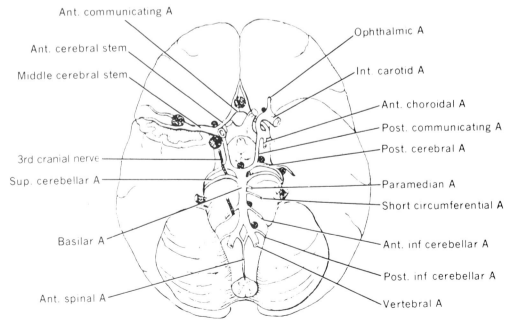

Ant. communicating A

Ant. cerebral stem

Middle cerebral stem

3rd cranial nerve

Sup. cerebellar A

Basilar A

Ant. spinal A

Ophthalmic A

Int. carotid A

Ant. choroidal A

Post. communicating A

Post. cerebral A

Paramedian A

Short circumferential A

Ant. inf cerebellar A

Post. inf cerebellar A

Vertebral A

the internal carotid, vertebral, or basilar arteries. They are often referred to as arteriosclerotic aneurysms, since they frequently show atheromatous deposition in their walls, but it is likely that they are at least partly developmental in nature. Some are gigantic and press on neighboring structures or become occluded by thrombus and rupture only infrequently.

Clinical Picture Prior to rupture, saccular aneurysms are usually asymptomatic. Stewart et al have described patients in whom transient ischemic attacks had occurred in the vascular field supplied by an unruptured aneurysm, but this is exceedingly rare; thromboembolism originating in the aneurysm was the postulated mechanism. Occasionally, large aneurysms immediately distal to the cavernous sinus may compress the optic nerves or chiasm, third nerve, hypothalamus, or pituitary gland. In the cavernous sinus they may press on the third, fourth, sixth, or ophthalmic division of the fifth cranial nerve (see page 215 and also Fig. 34-22). In the posterior fossa, one or more of the lower cranial nerves may be compressed adjacent to the brainstem. Rarely they cause headache, but by then other signs will usually have appeared.

When rupture occurs, blood under high pressure is forced into the subarachnoid space (the circle of Willis lies in the subarachnoid space), and the resulting clinical events assume one of three patterns: (1) the patient may be stricken with an excruciating generalized headache and fall unconscious almost immediately; (2) headache may develop as in (1), but the patient remains relatively lucid; (3) rarely, consciousness may be lost quickly without any preceding complaint. Decerebrate rigidity may occur at the onset of hemorrhage in association with unconsciousness. If the hemorrhage is massive, death may ensue in a matter of minutes, hours, or a day or two, so that ruptured aneurysm

must be considered in the differential diagnosis of sudden death. A considerable proportion of patients never reach a hospital. Persistent deep coma is accompanied by irregular respirations, attacks of extensor rigidity, and finally respiratory arrest and circulatory collapse. In these rapidly fatal cases, the subarachnoid blood has greatly increased the intracranial pressure and in some instances has dissected intracerebrally and entered the ventricular system (meningocerebral-ventricular hemorrhage).

In milder cases, consciousness, if lost, may be regained within a few minutes or hours, but a residuum of drowsiness, confusion, and amnesia, accompanied by severe headache and stiff neck persists for several days. It is not uncommon for the drowsiness and confusion to last 10 days or longer. If the hemorrhage is confined to the subarachnoid space, there are few or no lateralizing neurologic signs.

In most patients there are no warning symptoms; some, however, will have had an episode of headache, or perhaps a transitory unilateral weakness, numbness and tingling, or speech disturbance in the days or weeks preceding the major event. These prodromal symptoms are generally attributed to minor leakage from the aneurysm, but occasionally severe prodromal headache may occur without evidence of bleeding. Rupture of the aneurysm usually occurs while the patient is active rather than during sleep, and in many instances sexual intercourse or other exertion precipitates the ictus.

Gross lateralizing signs in the form of hemiplegia, hemiparesis, homonymous hemianopia, or aphasia are absent in the majority of cases, but can occur; in the acute stages these disturbances are due to an intracerebral clot or

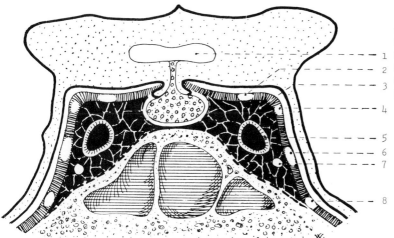

Figure 34-22

Diagram of the cavernous sinus: (1) optic chiasm; (2) oculomotor nerve; (3) cavernous sinus; (4) trochlear nerve; (5) internal carotid artery; (6) ophthalmic nerve; (7) abducens nerve; (8) maxillary nerve. (From Krayenbühl and Yasargil.)

ischemia in the territory of the aneurysm-bearing artery. The initial neurologic deficits may clear in a matter of days, indicating that hemorrhage into brain tissue was not responsible for them. The pathogenesis of such manifestations is not fully understood, but a transitory fall in pressure in the circulation distal to the aneurysm is postulated. Transient deficits, still more evanescent, are not uncommon and constitute reliable telltales of the site of the ruptured aneurysm (see below).

A *delayed hemiplegia* or other deficit may occur 4 to 12 days after rupture and rarely before or after this period. These delayed accidents and the focal narrowing of a large artery or arteries, seen on angiography, are loosely referred to as "cerebral vasospasm." Fisher et al have shown that spasm is most frequent in arteries surrounded by the largest collection of subarachnoid blood. The cause of the vasospasm appears to be a direct effect of blood or some blood product, possibly hematin, in the adventitia of the artery. Areas of ischemic necrosis of tissue in the territory of the vessel bearing the aneurysm, usually without atherosclerosis or thrombosis of the vessel, is the usual finding in such cases at autopsy. These ischemic lesions are often multiple and occur with great frequency, according to Hijdra et al (57 of 176 prospectively studied patients with aneurysmal subarachnoid hemorrhage). After a few days, arteries in chronic spasm undergo a series of morphologic changes. The smooth muscle cells of the media become necrotic, and the adventitia is infiltrated with neutrophilic leukocytes, mast cells, and red blood corpuscles, some of which migrate to a subendothelial position (Chyatte and Sundt). A *subacute hydrocephalus* due to blockage of the CSF pathways by blood may appear after 2 to 4 weeks.

In most patients the neurologic manifestations do not point to the exact site of the aneurysm, but in many instances they do provide clues to the localization, as follows: (1) Third nerve palsy (ptosis, diplopia, dilatation of pupil, and divergent strabismus) usually indicates an aneurysm at the junction of the posterior communicating artery and the internal carotid stem; the third nerve passes immediately lateral to this point. (2) Transient paresis of one or both of the lower limbs at the onset of the hemorrhage suggests an anterior communicating aneurysm which has interfered with the circulation in the anterior cerebral arteries. (3) Hemiparesis or aphasia points to an aneurysm at the first major bifurcation of the middle cerebral artery. (4) Unilateral blindness indicates an aneurysm which lies anteromedially in the circle of Willis (at the origin of the ophthalmic artery, or at the bifurcation of the internal carotid artery). (5) A state of retained consciousness with akinetic mutism or

abulia (sometimes associated with paraparesis) favors a location on the anterior communicating artery, with ischemia of or hemorrhage into one or both of the frontal lobes or hypothalamus. (6) The side on which the aneurysm lies may be indicated by a unilateral preponderance of headache or preretinal hemorrhages, occurrence of monocular pain, or, rarely, lateralization of an intracranial sound heard at the time of rupture of the aneurysm. Sixth nerve palsy, unilateral or bilateral, is usually attributable to raised intracranial pressure and is seldom of localizing value.

Other neurologic signs, which have relatively little localizing value, include sucking and grasping reflexes, a Korsakoff type of amnesia that usually clears in 4 to 6 weeks (occasionally it persists), choreoathetosis, and extensor rigidity. *Seizures*, usually brief and generalized, occur commonly (10 to 26 percent of cases, according to Hart et al) in relation to acute bleeding (or rebleeding). These early seizures do not correlate with the location of the aneurysm and do not appear to alter the prognosis.

In summary, the clinical sequence of sudden violent headache, collapse, relative preservation of consciousness, and a paucity of lateralizing signs in the face of massive subarachnoid hemorrhage is diagnostic of a ruptured saccular aneurysm.

Other clinical data may be of assistance in reaching a correct diagnosis. Nuchal rigidity is usually present, but occasionally it is absent, and the main complaint of pain may be referable to the interscapular region or even the low back rather than to the head. Examination of the fundi frequently reveals smooth-surfaced, sharply outlined collections of blood that cover the retinal vessels—the so-called preretinal or subhyaloid hemorrhages; Roth spots are seen occasionally. Bilateral Babinski signs are found in the first few days following rupture. Fever to 39°C is common in the first week. Escaping blood occasionally enters the subdural space and produces a hematoma, evacuation of which may be life-saving. Spontaneous intracranial bleeding with normal blood pressure should always suggest ruptured aneurysm or arteriovenous malformation, a bleeding diathesis, and rarely hemorrhage into a cerebral tumor.

Laboratory Findings Carotid and vertebral angiography is the only certain means of demonstrating an aneurysm and does so in some 85 percent of patients in whom aneurysm appears to be the correct diagnosis on clinical grounds, i.e., in cases of so-called spontaneous subarachnoid hemorrhage.

A CT scan will detect blood within the brain or ventricular system or locally or diffusely in the subarachnoid spaces (Fig. 34-23). When two or more aneurysms are visualized by arteriography, the CT scan may identify the one that had ruptured by the clot that surrounds it. Also a coexistent hydrocephalus will be demonstrable.

Usually the CSF is grossly bloody, with red cell

counts up to 1 million per cubic millimeter or even higher. With a relatively mild hemorrhage, there may be only a few thousand cells. It is unlikely that an aneurysm can rupture entirely into brain tissue without some leakage of blood into the subarachnoid fluid, so that the diagnosis of ruptured saccular aneurysm should never be made unless blood is present in the CSF. Usually deep xanthochromia is found after centrifugation. The CSF is under greatly increased pressure, as high as 1000 mmH$_2$O, an important finding in differentiating spontaneous subarachnoid hemorrhage from a traumatic tap. The level of CSF pressure correlates with the initial level of consciousness. The proportion of white to red blood cells in the CSF is usually the same as in the circulating blood, but in some patients a brisk CSF leukocytosis appears within 48 h, reaching 2000 to 3000 cells per cubic millimeter. The protein is elevated, and in some instances glucose is abnormally low.

In general, skull films yield so little information that they are hardly worthwhile, unless a head injury and skull fracture cannot be excluded. In a few patients they may show erosion of one or both of the anterior clinoid processes from the pressure of an adjacent aneurysm, or calcification in the region of a previous hemorrhage. A calcified pineal gland may be displaced by an intracerebral or subdural clot.

An albuminuria and glycosuria may be present for a few days. Rarely diabetes insipidus occurs. A leukocytosis of 15,000 to 18,000 cells per cubic millimeter is common.

Figure 34-23

Unenhanced CT scan from patient with ruptured saccular aneurysm. Blood fills the subarachnoid space over the cerebral hemispheres as well as entering the sulci and interhemispheric fissure.

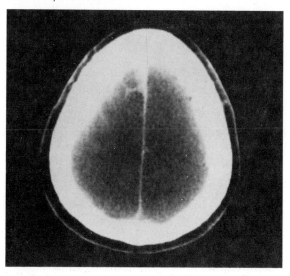

Acute subarachnoid hemorrhage may be associated with ECG abnormalities suggestive of myocardial ischemia. The EEG is of little help in localizing the lesion unless a gross neurologic deficit is present, in which case the localization is probably evident clinically.

Course and Prognosis The outstanding characteristic of this condition is the tendency for the hemorrhage to recur. This threat colors all prognostications, and unfortunately there appears to be no way of determining reliably which cases will bleed again. The cause of recurrent bleeding is not understood, but may be related to naturally occurring mechanisms of clot formation and lysis.

Patients with the typical clinical picture of spontaneous subarachnoid hemorrhage, in whom an aneurysm or arteriovenous malformation cannot be demonstrated angiographically, have a distinctly better prognosis than those in whom the lesion is visualized (Nishioka et al). In the former patients, it is usually advisable to repeat the arteriogram in 2 weeks, because vascular spasm may have obscured the aneurysm originally.

McKissock and his colleagues found that the patient's state of consciousness at the time of arteriography was the single best index of prognosis. Their data, representative of most large series, indicate that of every 100 patients reaching a hospital and coming to arteriography, 17 will be stuporous or comatose, and 83 will appear to be recovering from the ictus. At the end of the next 6 months, 7 of the first 17 patients will have died from the original hemorrhage, and 7 more will have had a fatal recurrence. Of the other 83, 1 will have died of the original hemorrhage and 52 will have had a recurrence, of whom 33 will have died. Thus, of the entire 100 patients, at the end of 6 months, 8 will have died of the original hemorrhage, 59 will have had a recurrence, with 40 deaths, making a total of 48 deaths and 52 survivors. Of the survivors, 36 will have returned to full work, 12 will be partly disabled, and 4 totally disabled. The disability is due to paralysis, mental deterioration, or epilepsy.

In regard to the recurrence of bleeding, it was found that of 50 patients seen on the first day of the illness, 5 rebled in the first week (all fatal), 8 in the second week (5 fatal), 6 in the third and fourth weeks (4 fatal), and 2 in the next 4 weeks (2 fatal), making a total of 21 recurrences (16 fatal) in 8 weeks. In this particular series, rerupture did not occur in the first 2 days; thereafter, it occurred at a steady rate for the next 19 days and tapered off abruptly. However, in our experience, rerupture in the first 2 days certainly occurs. These figures have changed very little in recent years (Aoyagi and Hayakawa); bleeding occurs within

2 weeks in 20 percent of patients, with a peak incidence in the 24 h after the initial bleed.

The most comprehensive information about the *long-term prognosis in patients treated only by a conservative medical program* is contained in the report of the Cooperative Study of Intracranial Aneurysms and Subarachnoid Hemorrhage (Sahs et al). There were 568 patients whose aneurysmal bleed had occurred betwen 1958 and 1965 and who were selected for conservative management. A follow-up search in 1981 and 1982 disclosed that 378 or two-thirds of the patients had died (40 percent of the deaths had occurred within 6 months of the original bleed). For the patients who survived the original hemorrhage for 6 months, the chances of survival during the next two decades were significantly worse than those of a matched population. Rebleeding occurred in 2.2 percent per year during the first decade and 0.86 percent per year during the second decade. Rebleeding episodes were fatal in 78 percent of cases.

Treatment This is influenced by the clinical status of the patient. Ideally all patients should have the aneurysmal sac surgically obliterated, but the mortality is unacceptably high if the patient is stuporous or comatose (grade IV or V, see below). It is now common practice to assess the patient with reference to the scale introduced by Botterell and by Hunt and Hess, as follows:

Grade I. Asymptomatic or with slight headache and stiff neck

Grade II. Moderate to severe headache and nuchal rigidity but no focal or lateralizing neurologic signs

Grade III. Drowsiness, confusion, and mild focal deficit

Grade IV. Persistent stupor or semicoma, early decerebrate rigidity and vegetative disturbances

Grade V. Deep coma and decerebrate rigidity

CT scan should be the initial diagnostic study, and if positive, it precludes the need for a CSF examination. The scan may indicate which of several aneurysms had bled, as well as the presence of cerebral hemorrhage or infarction and hydrocephalus. A large localized collection of subarachnoid blood may indicate the region of subsequent vasospasm. Patients in grades I and II should have four-vessel arteriography as soon as possible.

The general medical management in the acute stage includes the following, all or in part: strict bed rest in a darkened room, fluid administration to maintain normal circulating volume and venous pressure, use of elastic stockings, stool softeners, and anticonvulsant medication (phenytoin, 300 to 400 mg daily); administration of aminocaproic acid (loading dose of 5g followed by 1 to 1.5 g/h intravenously) or tranexamic acid (6 to 12 mg/day); hydralazine (5 to 20 mg intramuscularly every 3 h), propranolol or intravenous nitroprusside—to maintain systolic blood pressure at 150 mmHg or less; and codeine for headache.

No drug has proved to be effective in preventing rebleeding or relieving vascular spasm.

The antifibrinolytic agents, tranexamic and aminocaproic acid appear to impede lysis of the clot at the site of aneurysmal rupture. In our hands, the drugs, if given from the onset of bleeding to the time of operation, but not longer than 3 weeks, seem to have been effective in reducing the incidence of rebleeding. The studies of Vermeulen and of Kassell et al have corroborated this impression. These authors have pointed out, however, that the reduction in recurrent bleeding with antifibrinolytic drugs is largely offset by an increased incidence of cerebral infarction. The most important measure for the prevention of delayed cerebral ischemia is thought to be intravascular volume expansion (Solomon and Fink). This form of treatment carries the risk of rerupture of an unclipped aneurysm, so that it should be reserved for the postoperative period.

Repeated drainage of the CSF by lumbar puncture is no longer practiced. One lumbar puncture is carried out for diagnostic purposes if the CT scan is inconclusive, and thereafter it is performed only for the relief of intractable headache, to detect recurrence of bleeding, or to measure the intracranial pressure prior to surgery.

Surgical Therapy Apart from occasionally evacuating an associated intracerebral clot or placing a ventriculoatrial shunt to relieve the stupor and tension hydrocephalus that sometimes develop after aneurysmal rupture (see above), surgical treatment is directed to the prevention of recurrence of hemorrhage. The procedures are either *extracranial* (ligation of the common carotid in the neck) or *intracranial* (clipping or ligating the neck of the aneurysm; wrapping or tamponade of the aneurysmal sac by muscle, fascia, plastic coating, or arterial graft; trapping the aneurysm; ligation of the main feeding vessel proximal to the aneurysm). Occasionally extracranial and intracranial procedures are combined. Because of the aforementioned high mortality if surgery is undertaken early, some surgeons choose to delay surgery for 1 to 2 weeks after rupture, allowing the patient's condition to stabilize. Before treatment is undertaken, the site, size, and form of the aneurysm must be determined by angiography. At the same time the pattern of the anterior half of the circle of Willis is noted, as it may influence the choice of operative procedure. It has been demonstrated that in patients with ruptured saccular aneurysms, whose condition stabilizes to the point where they can be operated upon, do better than those treated conservatively. In the hands of specialized anesthetists and cerebrovascular surgeons using microdissection instrumentation the operative mortality, even in grade III and IV patients, has now been reduced to 2 to 3 percent.

Even with an estimated operative mortality of 5 percent, surgically treated patients would fare better than patients treated conservatively (see above, and also Richardson and Jane). Presently it is our practice to refer all patients whose condition has stabilized to our neurosurgical colleagues for direct ligation. For a detailed discussion of the operative approach to each of the major classes of saccular aneurysm, the reader is referred to the monograph by Ojemann and Crowell.

Unruptured Intracranial Aneurysms Not infrequently, cerebral angiography or CT scanning discloses the presence of an unruptured saccular aneurysm, invariably raising the problem of management. There is only limited information about the natural history of these lesions. Wiebers et al observed 65 patients with one or more unruptured aneurysms for at least 5 years after their detection. The only clinical feature of significance, relative to rupture, was aneurysm size, which was noted in 73 instances. None of 44 aneurysms smaller than 1 cm in diameter ruptured, whereas 8 of 29 aneurysms 1 cm or larger eventually did rupture, with a fatal outcome in seven of them. In the Cooperative Study of Intracranial Aneurysms (reported by Locksley) none of the aneurysms less than 7 mm in diameter "had further trouble." On the basis of these observations and his own experience Ojemann recommends that patients with asymptomatic unruptured aneurysms be subjected to angiography at regular intervals and that surgical treatment be advised when an aneurysm is shown to be larger than 7 mm in diameter.

Giant Aneurysms As has been stated, these are believed to be congenital anomalies even when there is considerable atherosclerosis in their walls. They may become enormous in size, by definition greater than 2.5 cm in diameter. Most are located on the carotid, basilar, anterior, or middle cerebral arteries. They slowly expand and grow by accretion of blood clot within their lumens or by the organization of surface blood from small leaks. At a certain point they compress adjacent structures, e.g., those in the cavernous sinus, optic nerve, or lower cranial nerves. Clotting within the aneurysm may cause ischemia of tissue in their territory. Some of them rupture and cause subarachnoid hemorrhage but not with the frequency of saccular aneurysms.

Treatment is surgical. Some can be ligated at their neck, others by trapping or by the use of an intravascular detachable balloon. Drake has summarized his experience in the treatment of 174 such cases.

ARTERIOVENOUS MALFORMATIONS OF THE BRAIN

An arteriovenous malformation (AVM) consists of a tangle of dilated vessels, which form an abnormal communication between the arterial and venous systems, really an arteriovenous fistula. It is a developmental abnormality, representing persistence of an embryonic pattern of blood vessels, and not a neoplasm, but the constituent vessels may proliferate with the passage of time. AVMs have been designated by a number of other terms, such as angioma and arteriovenous aneurysm, but these are less appropriate; *angioma* suggests a tumor and *aneurysm* is generally reserved for the lesions that have been described above.

Vascular malformations vary in size from a small blemish, a few millimeters in diameter, lying in the cortex or white matter, to a huge mass of tortuous channels comprising an AV shunt of sufficient magnitude, in rare instances, to raise cardiac output. Hypertrophic dilated *arterial feeders* approach the main lesion, disappear below the cortex, and break up into a network of thin-walled blood vessels that connect directly with draining veins. The latter often form greatly dilated, pulsating channels, carrying away arterial blood. The tangled blood vessels interposed between arteries and veins are abnormally thin and do not have the structure of either normal arteries or veins. AVMs occur in all parts of the brain, brainstem, and spinal cord, but the larger ones are more frequently found in the central part of the cerebral hemispheres, commonly forming a wedge-shaped lesion extending from the cortex to the ventricular lining.

AVMs are about one-tenth as common as saccular aneurysms and about equally frequent in males than females. AVMs and saccular aneurysms (on the main feeding artery of the AVM) are associated in 3 to 17 percent of cases; the frequency increases with the size of the AVM and age of the patient (Miyasaka et al). Rarely, AVMs occur in more than one member of a family in the same or successive generations. The natural history of AVMs has been studied by Crawford et al. From a group of 343 patients, 217 were managed without surgery and observed for many years (mean, 10.4 years). Hemorrhage occurred in 42 percent and seizures in 18 percent. By 20 years after diagnosis, 29 percent had died and 27 percent had a neurologic handicap. Although the lesion is present from birth, onset of symptoms is most common between 10 and 30 years of age; occasionally it is delayed to as late as age 50 or beyond. In about half the patients, the first clinical manifestation is a cerebral-subarachnoid hemorrhage; in 30 percent, a seizure is the first and only manifestation; and in 20 percent, headache. Progressive hemiparesis or other focal neurologic deficit is present in about 10 percent of patients. Seizures, when focal motor in type, may be followed by a temporary postictal paralysis. When hemorrhage occurs, blood may enter the subarachnoid space almost exclusively, producing a picture identical with that of ruptured saccular aneurysm, but since the AVM lies within the cerebral tissue, bleeding is more likely to be partly intracerebral, causing a hemiparesis, hemiplegia, etc., or even death.

Before rupture, chronic nondescript headache is a frequent complaint. Occasionally typical migraine is associated. Huge AVMs may produce a slowly progressive neurologic deficit because of compression of neighboring structures by the enlarging mass of vessels and shunting of blood through greatly dilated vascular channels ("intracerebral steal") with hypoperfusion of the surrounding structurally normal brain (Homan et al). When the vein of Galen is involved, hydrocephalus may result, but more often this is caused by the meningeal fibrosing effect of subarachnoid hemorrhage in the posterior fossa. Not infrequently one or both carotid arteries pulsate unusually forcefully in the neck. A systolic bruit heard over the carotid in the neck, or over the mastoid process or the eyeballs in a young adult, is almost pathognomonic of AVM. The patient should be exercised to bring out a bruit if none is present at rest. The blood pressure may be elevated or normal; it is axiomatic that the occurrence of intracranial bleeding with normal blood pressure should raise the suspicion of an AVM, ruptured saccular aneurysm, a bleeding diathesis, cerebral vessel amyloidosis, or hemorrhage into a tumor. Rarely, inspection of the eye grounds discloses a retinal vascular malformation, which is coextensive with a similar lesion of the optic nerve and basal portions of the brain. Cutaneous, orbital, and nasopharyngeal AVMs may occasionally be conjoined. Rarely skull films show crescentic linear calcifications in the territory of larger malformations. Fully 95 percent of AVMs are disclosed by CT scan if a contrast study is done (Fig. 34-24). Arteriography establishes the diagnosis with certainty, and will demonstrate AVMs larger than 5 mm in diameter. Small ones may be obscured by hemorrhage, and even at autopsy a careful search under the dissecting microscope may be necessary to find them.

Most AVMs are clinically silent for a long time, but sooner or later they bleed. The first hemorrhage may be fatal, but in more than 90 percent of cases the bleeding stops and the patient survives. The rate of rebleeding is about 6 percent in the first year after a hemorrhage and 2 to 3 percent per year thereafter, if no treatment is given; if

there has been no previous hemorrhage, the risk is somewhat less, perhaps 2 to 3 percent per year (Graf et al). The preferred treatment is surgical excision by a neurovascular surgeon. Twenty to 40 percent of AVMs are amenable to block dissection, with an operative mortality rate of 2 to 5 percent and a morbidity of 5 to 25 percent. In the others, attempts have been made to obliterate the malformed vessels by ligation of feeding arteries and the use of artificial embolization and rapidly setting plastics; the latter are injected via a balloon that has navigated a feeding vessel. Complete obliteration of large AVMs is often impossible by these methods. Kjellberg et al have treated more than 1050 AVMs with low-dose (subnecrotizing) focused proton beam. A single treatment is given, and the patient is sent home the following day. After 2 years, 75 to 80 percent of AVMs less than 2.5 cm in diameter will virtually have disappeared or be reduced in size by more than 50 percent (Fig. 34-25). Of the larger ones the majority are shrunken or appear less dense. The rest have shown no change. The clinical results of proton therapy have been reported by Kjellberg et al. There has been no recurrence of hemorrhage in up to 5 years in those patients whose AVM has disappeared. The frequency and severity of hemorrhage has been significantly reduced in the last 1000 cases. We must follow the cases for several more years to completely evaluate this method of therapy.

Figure 34-24

Contrast-enhanced CT scan showing an AVM of the temporal lobe.

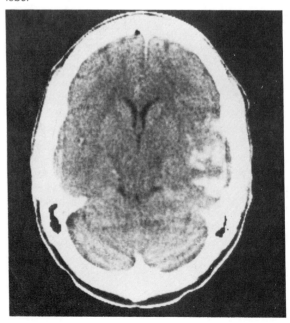

Cavernous and venous vascular malformations (5 percent of Kjellberg's series) are often multiple and familial. Many of them cannot be seen by CT scans or even by angiography. By MRI they present as a central low-flow void surrounded by a dark border of hemosiderin. They can be excised or, if deep, can be treated by focused gamma or proton radiotherapy.

OTHER CAUSES OF INTRACRANIAL BLEEDING

Acute extradural and *acute subdural hemorrhage* must always be considered in the patient who, under unknown circumstances, has rather abruptly developed a neurologic deficit such as hemiparesis or confusion, with or without bloody CSF. In *chronic subdural hemorrhage,* which can occur without known trauma, the indefinite picture of drowsiness, confusion, and mild hemiparesis may erroneously be attributed to a stroke, especially in elderly persons. Failure to make the correct diagnosis deprives the patient of lifesaving surgical intervention. There should be no hesitation in subjecting patients to CT scanning whenever the diagnosis of subdural hemorrhage cannot be excluded on clinical grounds. If the patient falls and strikes the head at the onset of a stroke, it may be difficult or impossible to decide if the blood in the CSF is due to the stroke or to *cerebral contusion.* Trauma may also cause *acute or delayed intracerebral hemorrhage, acute intracerebellar or infratentorial subdural hemorrhage, acute brain swelling,* and on rare occasions, extensive *focal infarction* of undetermined pathogenesis (see Chap. 34).

Several *hematologic disorders* are commonly complicated by hemorrhage into the brain. The most frequent of these are leukemia, aplastic anemia, and thrombocytopenic purpura. As a rule this complication signals a fatal issue. Other less common causes of intracerebral bleeding are advanced *liver disease* and *lymphoma.* Usually several factors are operative in these cases: reduction in prothrombin or other clotting elements (fibrinogen, factor V), bone marrow suppression by antineoplastic drugs, and disseminated intravascular coagulation. Any part of the brain may be involved, and the hemorrhagic lesions are usually multiple. Frequently also there is evidence of abnormal bleeding elsewhere (skin, mucous membranes, kidney) by the time cerebral hemorrhage occurs. As has been pointed out repeatedly, intracranial bleeding is an important com-

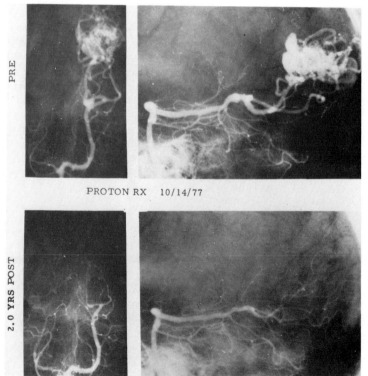

PRE

PROTON RX   10/14/77

2.0 YRS POST

Figure 34-25

Top. *Parieto-occipital AVM, fed by the posterior cerebral artery, in a 50-year-old woman. The AVM had bled and caused small intracerebral and subdural hematomas, with a visual field defect.* Bottom. *Arteriograms taken 2 years after proton beam treatment. The patient was asymptomatic.*

plication of *anticoagulant therapy*; the hemorrhages that develop, though sometimes situated in the sites of predilection of hypertensive hemorrhage, are more likely to occur elsewhere. When the bleeding is precipitated by warfarin therapy, treatment with fresh-frozen plasma and vitamin K is recommended; when associated with aspirin therapy or other agents that affect platelet function, fresh platelet infusions, often in massive amounts, are required to control the hemorrhage.

Occasionally the origin of intracranial hemorrhage cannot be determined clinically or pathologically. In some postmortem cases a careful search under the dissecting microscope discloses a small AVM; this is the basis for suspecting that an overlooked AVM may be the cause of cerebral hemorrhage in other cases. *Primary intraventricular hemorrhage*, a rare event, can sometimes be traced to a vascular malformation or neoplasm of the choroid plexus; more often, such a hemorrhage is the result of paraventricular bleeding, in which blood enters the ventricle immediately, without producing a large parenchymal clot.

Hemorrhage into primary and secondary brain tumors is not rare, and when this is the first clinical manifestation of the neoplasm, diagnosis may be extremely difficult. Choriocarcinoma, melanotic, renal cell, and bronchogenic carcinoma, pituitary adenoma, glioblastoma multiforme, and medulloblastoma may present in this way. Careful inquiry will usually disclose that neurologic symptoms, compatible with intracranial tumor growth, had preceded the onset of hemorrhage. Needless to say, a thorough search should be made in these circumstances for evidence of intracranial tumor or of secondary tumor deposits in other organs, particularly the lungs.

Mycotic aneurysms, a term introduced by Osler in 1875, designates an aneurysm caused by a localized bacterial or fungal inflammation of an artery. With the introduction of antibiotics, mycotic aneurysms have become less frequent but are still being seen in patients with bacterial endocarditis and in intravenous drug abusers. Peripheral arteries are involved more often than intracranial ones, and about two-thirds of the latter are associated with subacute bacterial endocarditis due to streptococcus infections. Recently the number of mycotic aneurysms due to staphylococcal infections has increased.

The usual pathogenic sequence is an embolic occlusion of a small artery, which may announce itself clinically by an ischemic stroke, with cells in the CSF. Later, or as the first manifestation, the weakened vessel wall gives way and causes a subarachnoid or a brain hemorrhage. The mycotic aneurysm may appear on only one or several arteries and the hemorrhage may recur.

A consensus regarding treatment has not been reached. The underlying endocarditis or septicemia mandates appropriate antibiotic therapy and in at least 30 percent of cases healing can be observed in multiple angiograms. The treatment should continue for 6 weeks. Our neurosurgical colleagues have made a practice of excising an accessible one if it is solitary and the systemic infection is under control. Some mycotic aneurysms do not bleed, and in our view medical therapy always takes precedence over surgical therapy.

Brain purpura, incorrectly referred to as hemorrhagic encephalitis, consists of multiple petechial hemorrhages scattered throughout the white matter of the brain. This disorder is described on pages 772 and 913. The clinical picture is that of a diffuse cerebral disease. Blood does not appear in the CSF, and the condition should not be confused with a stroke. *Brainstem hemorrhages* secondary to temporal lobe herniation, though extremely common, do not present as a cerebrovascular accident.

Inflammatory diseases of arteries and veins, especially polyarteritis nodosa and lupus erythematosus, are sometimes associated with hemorrhage into the nervous system. In these disorders, rupture of a vessel may occur on the basis of hypertension or local vascular disease. Bleeding nearly always occurs into the brain tissue rather than the subarachnoid space.

The other rare types of hemorrhage, listed in Table 34-5, are self-explanatory.

Hemorrhages of *intraspinal* origin may be the result of trauma, AVM (the usual cause of nontraumatic hematomyelia), or bleeding into tumors. Spinal subarachnoid hemorrhage from an AVM may simulate an intracranial subarachnoid hemorrhage, causing headache, stiff neck, and even subhyaloid hemorrhages. Extradural and subdural spinal extravasations may be *spontaneous* (often in relation to rheumatoid arthritis), but much more often are due to trauma or anticoagulants, or both. Extradural spinal hemorrhage causes the rapid evolution of paraplegia, and diagnosis must be prompt if function is to be salvaged by surgical drainage.

HYPERTENSIVE ENCEPHALOPATHY

This term refers to a relatively rapidly evolving syndrome in which severe hypertension is associated with headache, nausea and vomiting, visual disturbances, convulsions, confusion, stupor, and coma. These symptoms of diffuse cerebral disturbance may be accompanied by focal or lateralizing neurologic signs, either transitory or lasting, which should always suggest that cerebral hemorrhage or infarction, i.e., the more common cerebrovascular complications of severe chronic hypertension has been added. Multiple microinfarcts and petechial hemorrhages in one region may rarely result in a mild hemiparesis, aphasic disorder, or rapid failure of vision (usually due to retinal lesions). By the time the neurologic manifestations appear, the hypertension has usually reached the malignant stage, with retinal hemorrhages, exudates, and papilledema (*hypertensive retinopathy* grade IV), and with evidence of renal and cardiac disease. In many but not all the cases, the CSF pressure and protein values are elevated, the latter to more than 100 mg/dL in some cases. Lowering of the blood pressure with hypotensive drugs may reverse the picture in a day or two. If the hypertension cannot be controlled, the outcome is usually fatal.

Hypertensive encephalopathy may complicate hypertension from any cause (chronic renal disease, acute glomerulonephritis, acute toxemia of pregnancy, pheochromocytoma, Cushing syndrome, ACTH toxicity) but occurs most often in patients with "essential" hypertension. Blacks are disproportionately affected, at least in our experience (Chester et al). Three clinical stages in the development of the disease can usually be recognized. For the first 3 to 6 years after the discovery of hypertension the patient is generally asymptomatic and the hypertension is modest in degree. The second or accelerated phase is heralded by an increase of the diastolic pressure to about 130 mmHg and the appearance of extravascular retinal lesions. Headache is a persistent complaint, and transient episodes of blurred vision, drowsiness, and confusion occur frequently. These symptoms respond to a variable degree to antihypertensive drugs, as does the blood pressure, but over a period of 2 to 4 years most patients develop signs of cardiac and renal disease and of cerebral infarction. In the third phase multiple hospitalizations become necessary because of the encephalopathic symptoms, described above. Blood pressure reaches extreme levels (diastolic well above 130 mmHg), and papilledema and uremia are practically always present. Intensive antihypertensive therapy may initially be effective, but remissions become progressively shorter and less complete and are ultimately followed by a refractory period and death. In eclampsia and acute renal disease, particularly of children, encephalopathic symptoms may develop at blood pressure levels that are considerably lower than the ones which characterize hypertensive encephalopathy of "essential" type.

Neuropathologic examination may reveal a rather normal-looking brain, but occasionally cerebral swelling or hemorrhages of various sizes, or both, will be found. A cerebellar pressure cone reflects increased volume of tissue and increased pressure in the posterior fossa, and in some instances lumbar puncture may have precipitated a fatality. Microscopically there are widespread minute infarcts in the brain (with a predilection for the basis pontis), the result of fibrinoid necrosis of the walls of arterioles and capillaries, and occlusion of their lumens by fibrin thrombi. Similar vascular changes are found in other organs, particularly the retinae and the kidneys.

Volhard originally attributed the symptoms of hypertensive encephalopathy to vasospasm. This notion was reinforced by Byrom, who demonstrated, in rats, a segmental constriction and dilatation of cerebral and retinal arterioles in response to severe hypertension. However, the observations of Byrom, and of others, indicate that overdistension of the arterioles, rather than excessive constriction, may be responsible for the necrosis of the vessel wall (see reviews of Auer and of Chester et al).

The term *hypertensive encephalopathy* should be reserved for the above syndrome and should not be used to refer to chronic recurrent headaches, dizziness, epileptic seizures, transient ischemic attacks, or strokes that often occur in association with high blood pressure.

The standard treatment consists of measures that promptly reduce arterial blood pressure, but they must be used cautiously since a 40 percent reduction in the mean pressure from hypertensive levels may result in hypoperfusion of the brain and border-zone infarction. A safe target would be 150/100. Intravenous sodium nitroprusside, 0.5 to 0.8 mg/kg/min, is given in 15 to 30 s. A head-up position helps. MgSO$_4$ intravenously is still recommended by many obstetricians for eclampsia. If there is evidence of brain edema and increased intracranial pressure, dexamethasone, 4 to 6 mg every 6 h, is added. Because of the convulsive nature of the syndrome a loading dose of phenytoin is advisable. Once the desired level of blood pressure is attained, oral hypotensive medication can be substituted.

INFLAMMATORY DISEASES OF BRAIN ARTERIES

Inflammatory diseases of the blood vessels of infectious origin, and their effects upon the nervous system, are considered in detail in Chap. 32. There it is pointed out that *meningovascular syphilis, tuberculous meningitis, fungal meningitis,* and the *subacute (untreated or partially treated forms) of bacterial meningitis (H. influenzae,* staphylococcal, pneumococcal) may be accompanied by inflammatory changes and occlusion of either the cerebral arteries or veins. Occasionally in syphilitic and tuberculous meningitis a stroke may be the first clinical sign of meningitis; more often it develops well after the meningeal symptoms are established.

Typhus, schistosomiasis, mucormycosis, malaria, and trichinosis are rare types of infective diseases of the arteries which, unlike the above, are not secondary to meningeal inflammation. In *typhus and other rickettsial diseases,* capillary and arteriolar changes and perivascular inflammatory cells are found in the brain, and presumably they underlie the convulsions, acute psychoses, and coma that characterize the neurologic disorder in these diseases. The internal carotid artery may be occluded in diabetic patients as part of the orbital and cavernous sinus infections with *mucormycosis*. In *trichinosis*, the cause of the cerebral symptoms has not been established. Parasites have been found in the brain; in one of our cases the cerebral lesions were produced by bland emboli arising in the heart and related to a severe myocarditis. In *cerebral malaria* convulsions, coma, and sometimes focal symptoms appear to be due to the blockage of capillaries and precapillaries by masses of parasitized red blood corpuscles. *Schistosomiasis* may implicate cerebral or spinal arteries. These diseases are discussed further in Chap. 32.

OTHER INFLAMMATORY DISEASES OF CRANIAL ARTERIES

Included under this heading is a diverse group of arteritides that have little in common with one another, except their tendency to involve the cerebral vasculature: the giant-cell arteritides, polyarteritis nodosa, systemic lupus erythematosus, and Wegener granulomatosis.

Three *giant-cell arteritides* may affect cranial-cervical-cerebral arteries: (1) extracranial (temporal) arteritis; (2) intracranial (granulomatous) arteritis; and (3) aortic branch arteritis, one form which is known as Takayasu disease.

A second group of inflammatory diseases of the cranial arteries includes *polyarteritis nodosa, the Wegener type of granulomatous arteritis, and systemic lupus erythematosis*. Immunologic studies have shown that in these diseases there is an abnormal deposit of complement-fixing immune complex on the endothelium, leading to inflammation, vascular occlusion, or rupture with hemorrhage. The initial event is thought to be evoked by a virus, bacterium, or drug. This applies particularly to lupus erythematosus and polyarteritis nodosa. It is postulated by some immunologists that in the granulomatous arteritides a different mechanism is operative—an exogenous antigen induces antibodies that attach to the primary target (the vessel wall) as immune complexes, damage it, and attract lymphocytes and mononuclear cells. The giant cells form around remnants of the vessel wall (elastic tissue, etc).

Recently, an association between ulcerative colitis and a necrotizing cerebral angiitis has been reported (Nelson et al).

Extracranial or Temporal Arteritis (Giant-Cell Arteritis, Cranial Arteritis; see also pages 146 and 175) This is an uncommon affliction of elderly persons in which arteries of the external carotid system, particularly the temporal branches, are the seat of a subacute granulomatous inflammatory exudate consisting of lymphocytes and other mononuclear cells, neutrophilic leukocytes, and giant cells. The most severely affected parts of the artery usually become thrombosed.

Headache or head pain is the chief complaint, and there may be severe pain, aching, and stiffness in the proximal muscles of the limbs, associated with a markedly elevated sedimentation rate. Thus the clinical picture overlaps that of *polymyalgia rheumatica*. Other less frequent systemic manifestations include fever, anorexia and loss of weight, malaise, anemia, and a mild leukocytosis.

Occlusion of branches of the ophthalmic artery, resulting in blindness, occurs in one or both eyes in over 25 percent of patients. Occasionally the arteries of the ocular nerves are involved, causing an ophthalmoplegia. An arteritis of the aorta and its major branches, including carotid, subclavian, coronary, and femoral arteries, is found at postmortem examination. Significant inflammatory involvement of intracranial arteries is rare, perhaps because of a relative lack of elastic tissue, but strokes do occur occasionally on the basis of occlusion of the internal carotid and vertebral arteries. The diagnosis should be suspected in elderly patients who develop severe, persistent headache, and depends on finding a tender thrombosed or thickened cranial artery and demonstration of the lesion in a biopsy. The administration of prednisolone provides striking relief of the headache and polymyalgic symptoms and also prevents blindness. Prednisolone, 50 to 75 mg/day, needs to be given in very gradually diminishing doses for several months or longer in some cases.

Intracranial Granulomatous Arteritis Scattered examples of a small vessel, giant-cell arteritis of undetermined etiology, in which only brain vessels are affected, have come to our notice over the years. The clinical state has taken diverse forms, sometimes presenting as a low-grade, nonfebrile meningitis with sterile CSF, followed by infarction of one or several parts of the cerebrum or cerebellum. In other cases it has masqueraded as a cerebral tumor evolving over a period of weeks, or as a viral encephalitis. Severe headaches, focal cerebral or cerebellar signs of gradual evolution (seldom stroke-like), CSF pleocytosis and elevated protein, and papilledema (in about half the cases) as a result of increased intracranial pressure have constituted the most frequently encountered syndrome. In some patients the diagnosis was made from tissue excised during an operation for a suspected brain tumor, and in others the diagnosis was made only at autopsy, the findings coming as a distinct surprise.

The affected vessels are in the 100- to 500-μm range and are surrounded and infiltrated by lymphocytes, plasma cells, and other mononuclear cells; giant cells are distributed in small numbers in the media, adventitia, or perivascular connective tissue. Infarction of tissue relates to thrombosis. The meninges are variably infiltrated with inflammatory cells. Usually only a part of the brain has been affected—in one instance the cerebellum, in another one frontal lobe and the opposite parietal lobe. The disease raises questions of sarcoidosis, which is believed at times to be limited to the nervous system, or of the special type of polyarteritis (allergic granulomatous angiitis) described by Churg and Strauss. Unlike the latter disease, however, the lungs and other organs are spared; there is no eosinophilia, increase in sedimentation rate, or anemia. We have the impression that some patients suspected of this disease (those presenting as an aseptic meningitis with multiple infarcts) have responded dramatically to corticosteroid therapy.

Aortic Branch Disease (Occlusive Thromboaortopathy, Takayasu Disease)

This is a nonspecific arteritis involving mainly the aorta and the large arteries arising from its arch. Most of the patients have been young Oriental females. The exact etiology has never been ascertained but an autoimmune mechanism has been suspected.

Constitutional symptoms such as malaise, fever, anorexia, weight loss, and night sweats usually introduce the disease. The erythrocyte sedimentation rate is elevated in the early and active stages. Later there occurs evidence of occlusion of the innominate, subclavian, carotid, vertebral, and other arteries. The affected arteries no longer pulsate, hence the alternate term "pulseless disease." However, it should be noted that the Occidental pulseless disease is usually due to atherosclerosis. When renal arteries are involved, hypertension may result and coronary occlusion is often fatal. Involvement of the pulmonary artery may lead to pulmonary hypertension. Blurred vision, especially upon activity, dizziness, hemiparetic and hemisensory syndromes are the usual neurologic findings (Lupi-Herrera et al).

Pathologic studies disclose a periarteritis, often with giant cells and reparative fibrosis. Many of the patients die in 3 to 5 years. According to Ishikawa et al, the administration of corticosteroids in the acute inflammatory stage of the disease improves the prognosis. Reconstructive vascular surgery has helped some of the patients in the later stages of the disease.

Polyarteritis (Periarteritis) Nodosa

In this disorder there is an inflammatory necrosis of arteries and arterioles throughout the body. The lungs are usually spared, which

is the basis of distinguishing this form of vasculitis from allergic granulomatous angiitis, mentioned above. The vasa nervorum are involved frequently by the lesions of polyarteritis, giving rise to a *mononeuropathy multiplex* or to a symmetrical polyneuropathy (see page 1047). Involvement of the central nervous system is unusual and takes the form of widespread microinfarcts; macroscopic infarction is a rarity.

There is also another type of small vessel arteritis occurring as a hypersensitivity phenomenon. Often it is associated with an allergic skin lesion. The clinical picture does not resemble that of polyarteritis nodosa; the response to corticosteroids is excellent.

Wegener Granulomatosis

This is a rare disease of unknown causation, affecting adults as a rule and predominating in males in a ratio of 2:1. Subacutely evolving necrotizing granulomas of the upper and lower respiratory tracts, followed by necrotizing glomerulonephritis and systemic vasculitis are its main features. Neurologic complications come later in approximately 50 percent of cases and take two forms: (1) a peripheral neuropathy in 20 to 30 percent of cases, about equally divided between a pattern of polyneuropathy and of mononeuropathy multiplex; (2) multiple cranial neuropathies as a result of direct extension of the nasal and sinus granulomas to upper cranial nerves and of pharyngeal lesions to the lower nerves. The basilar parts of the skull may be eroded with spread of granuloma to the cranial cavity and more remote parts.

The vasculitis implicates both small arteries and veins. There is a fibrinoid necrosis of their walls and an infiltration by neutrophils and histiocytes. The sedimentation rate is elevated as are the rheumatoid and antiglobulin factors.

Spectacular therapeutic success in this formerly fatal disease has been achieved by the use of cyclophosphamide, chlorambucil, and azathiaprine. Cyclophosphamide in oral doses of 1 to 2 mg/kg/day has cured 90 to 95 percent of the cases. In acute cases, rapidly acting steroids—prednisolone, 50 to 75 mg/day, should be given in conjunction with the immunosuppressant drug(s).

Systemic Lupus Erythematosus

Involvement of the nervous system is an important aspect of this disease. In the series reported by Johnson and Richardson, the central nervous system was involved in 75 percent of cases. Cerebral seizures, disturbances of mental function and of consciousness, and signs referable to cranial nerves are the usual neurologic manifestations; most often they develop in the late stages of the disease, but they may occur early and may be mild and transient. Hemiparesis, paraparesis, aphasia, homonymous hemianopia, movement disorders, and derangements of hypothalamic function are less common. In some instances the CNS manifestations resemble multiple sclerosis, especially when there is only optic neuritis. Rarely there is a vacuolar myelopathy, similar to that of AIDS. The presence of serum antinuclear antibodies is of help in the diagnosis of lupus erythematosus. The CSF is entirely normal or shows only a mild lymphocytic pleocytosis and increase in protein content—although in some patients, primarily those with myelopathy and peripheral neuropathy, which are rare complications of systemic lupus erythematosus, the protein content may be greatly increased.

Most of the neurologic manifestations can be accounted for by widespread microinfarcts in the cerebral cortex and brainstem, and these in turn are related to destructive and proliferative changes in arterioles and capillaries. The acute lesion is subtle; it is not a typical fibrinoid necrosis of the vessel wall, like that in hypertensive encephalopathy, and there is no cellular infiltration. Thus, the changes do not represent a vasculitis in the strict sense of the word. Other neurologic manifestations are related to hypertension, which frequently accompanies the disease and may precipitate cerebral hemorrhage; to endocarditis, which may give rise to cerebral embolism; to thrombolic thrombocytopensic purpura, which commonly complicates the terminal phase of the disease (Devinsky et al); and to treatment with corticosteroids, which may precipitate or accentuate muscle weakness, seizures, and psychosis. In other cases, steroids appear to improve these neurologic manifestations.

OTHER LESS COMMON FORMS OF CEREBROVASCULAR DISEASE

Marantic Endocarditis and Cerebral Embolism

Sterile vegetations, referred to also as *terminal or nonbacterial thrombotic endocarditis,* consist of fibrin and platelets and are loosely attached to the mitral and aortic valves and contiguous endocardium. They are a common source of cerebral embolism (almost 10 percent of all instances of cerebral embolism, according to Barron et al). In almost half the patients, the vegetations are associated with a malignant neoplasm; the remainder occur in patients debilitated by other diseases (Biller et al). Except for the setting in which it occurs, marantic embolism has no distinctive clinical features that permit differentiation from cerebral

embolism of other types. The apoplectic nature of marantic embolism distinguishes it from tumor metastases. The hazards of anticoagulants in gravely ill patients with widespread malignant disease probably outweigh the benefits to be derived from this form of treatment.

The lesions of small cerebral arteries observed in patients with rheumatic heart disease and referred to as *rheumatic arteritis* have not been well characterized, clinically or pathologically.

Venous Thrombosis
Cerebral thrombophlebitis of bacterial origin and its main clinical features are described in Chap. 32. There occurs, in addition, bland occlusion of cerebral veins (phlebothrombosis), taking the form of an infarctive stroke. Diagnosis is difficult except in certain clinical settings known to favor the occurrence of venous thrombosis, such as cyanotic congenital heart disease, the puerperium and possibly the postoperative period, sickle-cell anemia, hypercoagulative states of the blood, antithrombin III deficiency, Behçet disease, disseminated intravascular coagulation, and polycythemia. A stroke in patients suffering from any one of these conditions should suggest venous thrombosis though in some instances—e.g., postpartum strokes—arteries are occluded as often as veins. The somewhat slower evolution of the clinical syndrome and its greater epileptogenic and hemorrhagic tendency favor venous over arterial thrombosis. Averback, who reported seven cases of venous thrombosis in young adults, has emphasized the diversity of the clinical state. Two of his patients had carcinoma of the breast, and one, ulcerative colitis.

Nevertheless, certain syndromes occur with sufficient regularity to suggest thrombosis of a particular vein or sinus. As pointed out in Chap. 12, marked chemosis and proptosis, with affection of cranial nerves III, IV, VI, and ophthalmic division of V, are indicative of anterior cavernous sinus thrombophlebitis. Seizures and hemiparesis, predominantly of the leg, first on one side and then the other, are suggestive of sagittal sinus and cerebral vein thrombosis; headache is usually present. Ocular apraxia with bifrontal lesions was a feature in one of our patients. Posterior cavernous sinus thrombosis, spreading to the inferior petrosal sinus, may cause palsies of cranial nerves VI, IX, X, and XI, without proptosis. And involvement of the superior petrosal sinus may be accompanied by a fifth nerve palsy. Increased intracranial pressure without ventricular dilatation attends thrombosis of the main jugular vein and lateral sinus or torcula.

The CSF pressure is usually increased and may be clear or sanguineous. The enhanced CT scan and arteriography (venous phase) greatly facilitate diagnosis. Anticoagulant therapy, combined with antibiotics if the vein occlusion is inflammatory, has been life-saving in some cases. The overall mortality rate is 20 to 30 percent.

Thrombotic Thrombocytopenic Purpura (TTP, Thrombotic Microangiopathy, Moschcowitz Syndrome) This is yet another uncommon but serious disease of the small blood vessels, observed mainly in young adults. It is characterized pathologically by widespread occlusions of arterioles and capillaries involving practically all organs of the body, including the brain. The nature of the occluding material has not been completely defined. Fibrin components have been identified by immunofluorescent techniques; some investigators have demonstrated disseminated intravascular platelet aggregation, rather than fibrin thrombi.

Clinically, the patients have fever, anemia, symptoms of renal and hepatic disease, and thrombocytopenia—the latter giving rise to the common hemorrhagic manifestations (petechiae and ecchymoses of the skin, retinal hemorrhages, hematuria, gastrointestinal bleeding, etc.). Neurologic symptoms are practically always present, and are the initial manifestation of the disease in about half the cases. Confusion, delirium, seizures, and altered states of consciousness—sometimes remittent or fluctuating in nature—are the usual signs of nervous system disorder and are readily explained by the widespread microscopic ischemic lesions in the brain. Gross infarction is rarely observed.

Thrombocytosis and Thrombocythemia These terms refer to an increase of platelets above 800,000 per cubic millimeter. The condition is generally considered to be a form of myeloproliferative disease. In some patients there is an enlarged spleen, polycythemia, chronic myelogenous leukemia, or myelosclerosis. In several of our patients explanation of the thrombocytosis was found. They presented with recurrent thrombotic episodes, often of minor degree and transient. Plasmapheresis, to reduce the platelets, and antimitotic drugs, to suppress megakaryocyte formation, relieved the neurologic symptoms.

Thromboangiitis Obliterans of Cerebral Vessels (Winiwarter-Buerger Disease) Despite the large volume of literature on this subject, there is little evidence that it is a recognizable entity. Thin, thread-like, white leptomeningeal arteries and border-zone infarction of the brain have been considered characteristic, but as C. M. Fisher has convincingly demonstrated, these lesions are simply the result of atherosclerosis or embolic occlusion of the carotid or cerebral arteries with *stasis thrombosis* and organization of the more distant cerebral branches. Buerger disease of the legs has an equally dubious status.

STROKE AS A COMPLICATION OF HEMATOLOGIC DISEASE

The brain is involved in the course of many hematologic disorders, some of which have already been mentioned.

Sickle-cell anemia is an inherited disease that is related to the presence of an abnormal hemoglobin—hemoglobin S—in the red corpuscles. Clinical abnormalities occur only in patients with sickle-cell disease, i.e., with the homozygous state, and not in those with the sickle-cell trait, which represents the heterozygous state. The disease, which is practically limited to blacks, begins early in life and is characterized by "crises" of infections (particularly pneumococcal meningitis), pain in the limbs and abdomen, chronic leg ulcers, and infarctions of bones and visceral organs. Ischemic infarctions of the brain, both large and small, are the most common neurologic complications but cerebral, subarachnoid, and subdural hemorrhage may also occur.

Similar thrombotic and hemorrhagic accidents are common complications of *polycythemia vera*. This is a myeloproliferative disorder of unknown cause, characterized by a marked increase in red cell mass (7 to 11 million per cubic millimeter) and blood volume, and often by an increase in white cells and platelets as well. This condition needs to be distinguished from the many secondary or symptomatic forms of polycythemia (erythrocytosis), in which the platelets and white cells remain normal. The high incidence of thrombosis in polycythemia vera is attributed to the high blood viscosity, engorgement of vessels, and reduced rate of blood flow. The cause of cerebral hemorrhage in this disease is less clear although a number of abnormalities of platelet function and of coagulation have been described (see Davies-Jones et al).

Rarely the myeloproliferative disorder is more or less limited to the megakaryocyte-platelet line, in which case it is referred to as *essential thrombocythemia*. Its main features are a persistent thrombocytosis (>1 million per cubic millimeter), splenomegaly, severe hemorrhagic manifestations, and thrombo-occlusive events involving the retina, brain, and distal arteries of the extremities. The opposite disorder, *thrombotic thrombocytopenia*, has been mentioned above. A wide variety of bleeding disorders such as *leukemia, aplastic anemia, thrombocytopenic purpura, and hemophilia* may give rise to cerebral hemorrhage and are discussed on page 676. Many rare forms of bleeding disease may be complicated by hemorrhagic manifestations; these have been reviewed by Davies-Jones and his colleagues.

THE DIAGNOSIS OF CEREBROVASCULAR DISEASE

Perhaps the commonest and most serious disorder of coagulation affecting the nervous system is *disseminated intravascular coagulation* (DIC). This process depends on the release of thromboplastic substances from damaged tissue, resulting in the activation of the coagulation system and the formation of fibrin, in the course of which clotting factors and platelets are consumed. Any mechanism that produces tissue damage will result in release of tissue thromboplastins into the circulation. Thus, DIC complicates a wide variety of clinical conditions such as trauma, cardiothoracic surgery, heat stroke, burns, severe infections, incompatible blood transfusions and other immune complex disorders, diabetic ketoacidosis, leukemia, obstetric complications, cyanotic congenital heart disease, and shock from many causes.

The essential pathologic change in DIC is the occurrence of widespread fibrin thrombi in small vessels, resulting in numerous small infarctions of many organs, including the brain. Sometimes DIC is manifested by a hemorrhagic diathesis in which petechial hemorrhages are situated around small penetrating vessels. In some cases the cerebral hemorrhage is quite extensive, similar to a primary hypertensive hemorrhage. The main reason for the hemorrhage is the consumption of platelets and various clotting factors that occur during fibrin formation; in addition, fibrin degradation products have anticoagulant properties of their own. Although DIC can result from brain damage itself (the brain is the richest source of tissue thromboplastin), it is far more often a complication of severe systemic disease of the types mentioned above. The diffuse nature of the neurologic damage may suggest a metabolic rather than a structural disorder of the brain. In the absence of a clear metabolic, infective, or neoplastic cause of an encephalopathy, the onset of acute and fluctuating focal neurologic abnormalities or a generalized and sometimes terminal neurologic deterioration during the course of a severe illness should arouse the suspicion of DIC, and coagulation factors should be measured. Platelet counts are invariably depressed and there is evidence of consumption of fibrinogen and other clotting factors, indicated by prolonged thrombin, prothrombin, and partial thromboplastin times.

Many other hemotologic disorders that may affect the nervous system are considered in other parts of this text. The neurologic complications of vitamin B_{12} deficiency are described in Chap. 39, kernicterus (hemolytic disease of the newborn) in Chap. 44, leukemia and lymphoma in Chap. 31, and myeloma, paraproteinemia, and porphyria in Chap. 46.

There are two separate aspects of the problem of differential diagnosis: (1) vascular disease must be distinguished from other neurologic illnesses, and (2) the different kinds of vascular disease must be separated from one another. In the following paragraphs many of the important points discussed in the body of the chapter will be summarized.

DIFFERENTIATION OF VASCULAR DISEASE FROM OTHER NEUROLOGIC ILLNESSES

The diagnosis of a vascular lesion rests essentially on recognition of the stroke syndrome, and without evidence of this the diagnosis must always be in doubt. The three criteria by which the stroke is identified should be re-emphasized: (1) the temporal profile of the clinical syndrome, (2) evidence of focal brain disease, and (3) the clinical setting. Definition of the temporal profile requires a clear history of the premonitory phenomena, the mode of onset, and the evolution of the neurologic disturbance in relationship to the patient's medical status. If these data are lacking, the stroke profile may still be determined by extending the period of observation for a few days or weeks, thus resorting to the clinical rule that the physician's best diagnostic tool is the second and third examination. An inadequate history is the most frequent cause of diagnostic error.

There are few categories of neurologic disease whose temporal profile mimics that of the cerebrovascular disorders. Migraine may do so, but the history usually provides the diagnosis. Tumor, infection, inflammation, degeneration, and nutritional disease are not likely to manifest themselves precipitously. Trauma, of course, occurs abruptly, but usually the cause is readily discerned. In multiple sclerosis and other demyelinative diseases, there may be a relatively abrupt onset or exacerbation of symptoms, but for the most part they occur in a different age group and clinical setting. A stroke developing over a period of several days usually progresses in a stepwise fashion, increments of deficit being added from time to time. A slow, gradual downhill course over a period of 2 weeks or more indicates that the lesion is probably not vascular, but rather a tumor, abscess, granuloma, or subdural hematoma.

Many thrombotic strokes are preceded by transient ischemic attacks (TIAs) which, if recognized, are diagnostic of this form of vascular disease. It is essential that TIAs be differentiated from cerebral seizures, syncopal attacks, neurologic migraine, and attacks of labyrinthine vertigo, since a failure to do so may result in unnecessary arteriographic studies and even a surgical operation.

In regard to the focal neurologic deficit of cerebrovascular diseases, many nonvascular diseases (tumor, abscess, multiple sclerosis, multifocal leukoencephalitis, etc.) may produce symptoms that are much the same, and the diagnosis cannot rest solely on this aspect of the clinical picture. Nonetheless, certain combinations of neurologic signs, which conform to a neurovascular pattern, e.g., the lateral medullary syndrome, are seen almost exclusively in occlusive vascular disease.

With very few exceptions, the presence of *blood in the CSF* points to a cerebrovascular lesion, provided that trauma and a *traumatic tap* can be excluded. *Headache* is common in cerebrovascular disease; it occurs not only in hemorrhage but also in thrombosis and embolism. *Cerebral seizures* are almost never the premonitory, first, or only manifestation of a stroke but can occur in the first few hours after infarction or intracranial bleeding. *Brief unconsciousness* (5 to 10 min) is rare in stroke, being seen only in ruptured aneurysm and basilar artery insufficiency. Certain neurologic disturbances are hardly ever attributable to stroke, e.g., diabetes insipidus, bitemporal hemianopia, parkinsonism, generalized myoclonus, and isolated cranial nerve palsies, and their presence may be of help in ruling out vascular disease.

Finally, the diagnosis of cerebrovascular disease should always be made on positive data, and not by exclusion.

A *few conditions are so often confused with cerebrovascular diseases that they merit further consideration.* When a history of trauma is absent, the headache, drowsiness, mild confusion, and hemiparesis of *subdural hematoma* may be ascribed to a "small stroke," and the patient may fail to receive immediate surgical therapy. In subdural hematoma the symptoms and signs usually develop gradually over a period of days or weeks. The degree of headache, obtundation, and confusion is disproportionately greater than the focal neurologic deficit, which tends to be indefinite and variable. There may be episodes in which hemiparesis and aphasia worsen. The CSF may be blood-tinged or xanthochromic when the type of stroke under suspicion would not be expected to show this. Occasionally the EEG is strikingly silent over a subdural hematoma. If the patient has fallen and injured his or her head at the onset of the stroke, it may be impossible to rule out a complicating subdural hematoma on clinical grounds alone, in which case the CT scan should be diagnostic.

The reverse diagnostic error will not be made if one remembers that patients with subdural hematoma rarely exhibit a total hemiplegia, monoplegia, hemianesthesia, homonymous hemianopia, or aphasia. If such focal signs are present and particularly if they developed suddenly, subdural hematoma is not likely to be the explanation.

A *brain tumor*—especially a rapidly growing glioblastoma multiforme, which may produce a severe hemiplegia within a week or two—can be mistaken for a stroke. Also, the neurologic deficit due to secondary carcinoma may evolve rapidly. However, in both conditions, a detailed history will indicate that the evolution of symptoms was gradual; and if they progressed in saltatory fashion, seizures will usually have occurred. Standard ancillary examinations should never be omitted in these circumstances. A chest film frequently discloses a primary or secondary tumor, and an increased blood sedimentation rate suggests that a concealed systemic disease process is at work. A lack of detailed history may also be responsible for the opposite diagnostic error, i.e., mistaking a relatively slowly evolving stroke (usually due to internal carotid artery occlusion) for a tumor. Arteriography and CT scanning will usually settle the problem. Rarely a *brain abscess* develops without an evident focus of infection and may escape consideration, especially if the patient is elderly.

Senile dementia is often ascribed, on insufficient grounds, to the occurrence of multiple small strokes. If vascular lesions are responsible, evidence of an apoplectic episode or episodes and of focal neurologic deficit, to account for at least part of the syndrome, will almost invariably be disclosed by history and examination. In the absence of a history of episodic development or of focal neurologic signs, it is unwarranted to attribute senile dementia to cerebral vascular disease—in particular, to small strokes in silent areas. *Cerebral arteriosclerosis* is another term that is used carelessly to explain such mental changes, the implication being that arteriosclerosis itself causes ischemic damage to the nervous system, producing loss of intellectual function but no other focal neurologic signs. If cerebral arteriosclerosis (atherosclerosis) is actually responsible, there should be evidence of it in the form of strokes at some time in the course of the illness, and also in the heart (myocardial infarction, angina pectoris) or legs (intermittent claudication, loss of pulses). Frequently both vascular lesions and Alzheimer disease are present, in which case there may be difficulty in determining to what extent each of them is responsible for the neurologic deficit.

Recurrent cerebral seizures as the result of stroke occur in some 20 percent of cases (*postinfarction epilepsy*). When evidence, by history or examination, of the original stroke is lacking, as it often is, or if the seizures are not observed or leave behind a temporary increase in the neurologic deficit (Todd's paralysis), the diagnosis of another stroke or of a tumor may be made in error.

Fear, anxiety, and depression in patients who have had one stroke may lead to additional symptoms, such as generalized weakness, paresthesias, headache, or disequilibrium, and suggest to the patient and physician that further vascular lesions have occurred or threaten.

Miscellaneous conditions that are occasionally taken to be a stroke are Bell's palsy, Stokes-Adams attacks, a severe attack of labyrinthine vertigo, diabetic ophthalmoplegia, acute ulnar, radial, or peroneal palsy, embolism to a limb, and temporal arteritis associated with blindness.

Contrariwise, certain manifestations of stroke may be incorrectly interpreted to indicate some other neurologic disorder. In lateral medullary infarction, *dysphagia* may be the outstanding feature, and if the syndrome is not kept in mind, a fruitless radiologic investigation may be undertaken, looking for an esophageal neoplasm. *Headache*, at times severe, occurs as a prodrome of a thrombotic stroke or subarachnoid hemorrhage; unless this is appreciated a diagnosis of migraine may be made. *Dizzy spells or brief lapses or intermittent loss of equilibrium* due to vascular disease of the brainstem may be ascribed to Ménière disease, Stokes-Adams syncope, or paroxysmal tachycardia. A detailed account of the attack will usually avert this error. A strikingly *focal monoplegia of cerebral origin*, causing only weakness of the hand or arm, or only foot drop, is not infrequently misdiagnosed as a peripheral lesion.

The differentiation of vascular from other neurologic diseases in the presence of coma offers special problems. If the patient is comatose when first seen and an adequate history is not available, cerebrovascular lesions have to be differentiated from all the other causes of coma described in Chap. 16. In most cases there will be some history to assist in the series of necessary diagnostic deductions.

Differentiation of Thrombosis, Embolism, Hypertensive Hemorrhage, and Ruptured Saccular Aneurysm

Although it is difficult to lay down simple, hard-and-fast rules, it is usually possible to distinguish these four conditions at the bedside.

The most important diagnostic criteria of *atherothrombotic infarction* are (1) a history of prodromal TIAs, (2) an intermittent or stepwise evolution of the neurologic deficit, with recovery or improvement between worsenings, rather than a steady progression, (3) relative preservation of consciousness unless the upper part of the basilar territory is infarcted, (4) normal CSF, except for modest elevation of protein and occasionally a pleocytosis with massive infarction, (5) onset during sleep or on arising or during a period of hypotension, (6) evidence of atherosclerosis in the coronary and peripheral vessels and the aorta, (7) the advanced age of the patient and the presence of disorders usually associated with atherosclerosis (hypertension, diabetes mellitus, and xanthomatosis), (8) headache (either as a prodromal warning or accompanying the stroke), (9) carotid bruit in the neck, indicating carotid stenosis, and (10) occlusion or severe stenosis of the internal carotid artery in the neck as determined by palpation, auscultation, and DSA.

Cerebral embolism is characterized by (1) abrupt development of the completed stroke—within a few seconds or minutes; (2) absence of prodromal TIAs (*rarely*, one or two transitory episodes occur in the hours before the stroke, especially if the embolus lodges in the carotid artery); (3) a source of emboli, usually in the heart, i.e., atrial fibrillation or other arrhythmia, myocardial infarction, subacute bacterial endocarditis, mitral stenosis, prolapsed mitral valve, valvulotomy or prosthetic valve, or marantic endocarditis associated with carcinoma; (4) evidence of recent embolism in other organs, i.e., spleen, kidney, extremities, gastrointestinal tract, or lungs; (5) evidence of recent strokes in different cerebrovascular territories; (6) clear CSF except in a small proportion of cases with extensive hemorrhagic infarction; (7) rapid improvement (many embolic strokes produce persistent deficits, but it is not uncommon for an extensive focal deficit to reverse itself in minutes, hours, or days); (8) relative preservation of consciousness in the presence of extensive neurologic deficit, unless the upper part of the basilar territory is involved or massive brain swelling has occurred with temporal lobe–tentorial herniation; (9) occurrence at an age when atherosclerosis is usually not a factor and in the absence of hypertension, diabetes, or arteritis; and (10) localized headache of moderate severity.

The diagnosis of arteritis as a cause of infarction is justifiable only in the following circumstances: (1) evidence of arteritis elsewhere; (2) in young individuals who manifest neither hypertension nor signs of cardiovascular disease; and (3) in individuals with an infection which could affect the meningeal vessels (syphilis, tuberculosis, etc.).

Venous thrombosis with infarction should be considered when focal neurologic signs develop in the period following parturition or an operation, in the course of meningeal infection, ear or sinus suppuration, and in patients with cachexia, congenital heart disease, polycythemia, or sickle-cell disease.

In *hypertensive cerebral hemorrhage* the diagnosis rests on (1) presence of hypertension; (2) absence of prodromal phenomena; (3) frequent but not invariable occurrence of headache; (4) gradual development of a neurologic deficit over a period of several minutes to hours (sometimes the onset is more abrupt); (5) presence of hemorrhage in CT scan or, if not available, grossly bloody

CSF (rarely the hemorrhage does not extend to the ventricular system and thus does not reach the CSF); (6) deepening stupor or coma (generally speaking, a patient with an extensive paralysis due to hemorrhage will be stuporous, whereas a hemiplegic stroke that leaves the patient alert and the mind relatively clear proves far more often to be due to an infarct); (7) onset during waking hours rather than in sleep; and (8) nuchal rigidity, except when deep coma supervenes.

The chief clinical features of *ruptured saccular aneurysms* are (1) sudden onset of severe headache; (2) brief or prolonged loss of consciousness at onset (in the most severe cases coma persists, and the patient dies within a few hours); (3) grossly bloody CSF under increased pressure; (4) relative alertness (after initial episode) and absence of focal neurologic signs (except for third or sixth nerve palsies); (5) preretinal (subhyaloid) hemorrhages (these suggest ruptured aneurysm or AVM, although they can occur in massive intracerebral hemorrhage and after trauma); (6) stiff neck on forward flexion, Kernig and Brudzinski signs (these also are not invariable); (7) transient weakness, numbness, aphasia, or seizure at onset; (8) usually an absence of warning attacks, although there may be a history of one or more transient episodes of headache (''leaks''?); (9) onset during exertion, sexual intercourse, etc.; (10) absence of hypertension in many cases; and (11) presence of coarctation of the aorta and polycystic disease of the kidneys in some cases.

Saccular aneurysm is likely to produce diffuse subarachnoid hemorrhage without causing significant damage to the cerebral hemispheres. If the CSF is bloody and the patient retains mental clarity or is only mildly confused, aneurysm or cerebellar hemorrhage is the likely diagnosis. If the aneurysm also bleeds into the brain tissue or into the ventricular system, focal neurologic signs and coma ensue, as in intracerebral hemorrhage. Cerebral infarction in the 4- to 10-day period following aneurysmal rupture is another cause of focal neurologic deficit.

Intracranial hemorrhage from a vascular malformation is a tenable diagnosis under the following circumstances: (1) stroke in a young patient with bloody CSF in the absence of hypertension; (2) antecedent epilepsy, often with transient postictal paralysis; (3) presence of a cervical or cranial bruit sometimes heard by the patient; (4) repeated subarachnoid hemorrhages (sometimes five or more); (5) calcification in the lesion in the skull films; and (6) lateralizing neurologic signs which are more frequent than with aneurysm.

In all forms of intracranial hemorrhage—primary (hypertensive) cerebral hemorrhage, ruptured saccular aneurysm, and AVM—the unenhanced CT scan will disclose the bleeding from the moment of its occurrence.

THE COMMON CLINICAL PROBLEMS CREATED BY CEREBROVASCULAR DISEASES

The perceptive physician realizes at once that the diagnosis of cerebrovascular diseases may be ridiculously simple or incredibly difficult. The welter of details that have accumulated about cerebrovascular diseases is hardly reassuring to one who seeks a confident clinical approach to this category of disease. Yet experience teaches that certain diagnostic problems recur with impressive consistency and a planned approach to each of them enables the physician to make a correct diagnosis in 80 to 90 percent of cases, and to take proper action.

THE PATIENT ARRIVING COMATOSE

The most common vascular cause of coma is intracranial hemorrhage, usually one deep in the substance of the brain, in a setting of hypertension. Less often it results from the meningocerebral or subarachnoid hemorrhage of a ruptured aneurysm or AVM or from occlusion of the basilar or carotid artery.

The comatose state from hypertensive hemorrhage or from aneurysmal meningocerebral hemorrhage probably reflects disordered function of the upper brainstem. This may be the result of a major shift of central structures by a mass lesion and transtentorial-temporal herniation, disruption from pontine hemorrhage, or compression from upward cerebellar herniation in the case of a cerebellar hemorrhage. When temporal lobe–transtentorial herniation has occurred, the brainstem dysfunction may be so complete as to mask the unilateral signs of the basal ganglionic–capsular hemorrhage. The coma is then accompanied by decerebration and bilateral signs. Then the larger pupil, which is usually ipsilateral to the involved hemisphere, may provide the only clue as to the side of the lesion. In these circumstances the CSF will be bloody virtually without exception, but to do a lumbar puncture may worsen the patient's condition. Whenever possible, immediate CT scanning or MRI is the preferred diagnostic step and lumbar puncture should be deferred. Urgency of action is no longer of importance, for in coma from all the foregoing causes, the outlook is rather hopeless. Surgical evacuation of the hematoma, to be effective, must be undertaken before the stage of coma and fixed dilated pupils is reached. Even with early craniotomy, however, the chances of survival and functional restoration are increased very little.

Coma due to ruptured aneurysm may occur without bleeding into the brain (probably the effects of presure and diffuse cerebral hypoperfusion). Initially all cerebral and upper brainstem function may be abolished, with respiratory arrest, bradycardia and hypotension. In some instances the patient is thought to be dying and may be given artificial resuscitation. This state of deep coma, flaccid limbs, immobile eyes, and fixed pupils may prove fatal or it may persist for only a few moments, following which more vigorous heart action, rising blood pressure, and spontaneous respirations emerge, along with restoration of tone, reflexes, and eye movements; the coma gradually diminishes and is replaced by stupor and an improving state of consciousness over several hours. This continuously improving state is typical of ruptured aneurysm and is usually well under way by the time such patients reach a hospital. On examination, subhyaloid hemorrhages are occasionally seen and are highly characteristic of ruptured aneurysm. Stiff neck can usually be elicited as the patient begins to awaken, but not when he or she is comatose or stuporous. The CT scan is most helpful for it may show the aneurysm or at least the pattern of the subarachnoid hemorrhage. If hemorrhage is not seen, the lumbar puncture should suffice as the next diagnostic step. If the patient regains full alertness and has only headache and stiff neck, four-vessel arteriography is undertaken. If stuporous or semicomatose or severely hypertensive, arteriography should be deferred for a few days so that hypertension can be reduced and other later complications of ruptured aneurysm, such as spasm and hydrocephalus, can be sought at the same time as one attempts to visualize the aneurysm.

Coma from ischemic disease alone occurs in three circumstances, each highly lethal: basilar artery occlusion, internal carotid occlusion with massive infarction and transtentorial herniation, and bilateral carotid occlusion. In the latter circumstance, a unilateral carotid occlusion occurs on a background of a previous (sometimes asymptomatic) carotid occlusion on the other side. The result is bihemispheral cerebral infarction, which leaves the patient deeply comatose, bilaterally paralyzed, with almost unique, continuous, side-to-side ("metronomic") conjugate horizontal eye movements, only transiently interrupted by caloric stimulation or doll's-head maneuver. The diagnosis of basilar artery occlusion poses little problem when the brainstem is severely but incompletely damaged, as evidenced by ocular and other segmental brainstem abnormalities in combination with long tract signs. When there is nearly complete destruction of the brainstem, coma is accompanied by motor signs so symmetric and ocular motility so impaired that it may be difficult on clinical grounds alone to differentiate this state from severe drug intoxication. In the latter state, ice-water caloric stimulation and brisk rotation of the head from side to side usually evoke ocular motility. In basilar and carotid artery occlusion the CSF is clear, and arteriography is currently the most direct corroborative diagnostic step. If lumbar puncture is delayed for several days after the onset of a large embolic or thrombotic infarction, a brisk leukocytosis is occasionally found, reflecting the cellular response to the massive necrosis; in the case of embolism the presence of red cells may reflect a hemorrhagic infarction. CT scanning in this setting should suffice to settle any worries of occult abscess in a patient whose ictus had not been witnessed.

Myocardial infarction with cardiac arrest and generalized cerebral hypoxia and ischemia is another cause of profound coma.

There is usually little that can be done for the persistently comatose stroke patients, other than to provide general supportive measures.

THE NONCOMATOSE PATIENT WHO PRESENTS WITH A NEUROLOGIC DISORDER OF RECENT ONSET

There are several characteristic patterns of evolution within the group of stroke illnesses that help the physician to decide whether embolus, thrombosis, parenchymal hemorrhage, or ruptured aneurysm is responsible. A clear history is absolutely essential in differentiating these types of stroke. Their differentiating characteristics and the methods of investigation and management have been outlined in the preceding section of this chapter.

THE PATIENT WHO PRESENTS WITH A TRANSIENT ISCHEMIC ATTACK

As has been remarked, no reliable means have yet been developed to predict the outcome at any stage of the evolving stroke process, and a significant percentage of patients develops massive infarction following what seemed initially to be a trivial transient attack. Once it has been determined that the focal neurologic disorder represents a transient ischemic attack, the patient should be subjected to an arteriogram, preferably DSA. The more recent the attack, the more urgent the need for angiography. In carotid artery disease, endarterectomy appears to halt the symptomatic progress and is warranted at the stage of TIAs or a minor persisting deficit, if it can be determined that the disease is principally located in the carotid artery in the neck. Cases in which the disease falls heaviest on the intracranial portion of the artery, e.g., at the carotid siphon, and all cases of basilar disease, can only be treated with anticoagulants (transcranial anastomosis appears not to be beneficial). It might be argued that arteriography be deferred in patients whose TIAs suggest disease of the basilar territory, since the arteriographic findings presumably would not modify the treatment plan. However, TIAs attributed on clinical grounds to basilar ischemia sometimes prove to be associated with carotid disease.

The routine investigation of TIAs by arteriography raises a number of problems. Symptomatic atherothrombosis involving the carotid or basilar artery is sometimes worsened drastically by this procedure. It is for this reason that DSA is a welcome innovation (see page 17). Increasing use is also being made of noninvasive methods, such as Doppler flow studies and ultrasound imaging of the carotid arteries. These methods yield data that have a fair correlation with angiographic findings in atherothrombotic carotid disease and are proving useful in the investigation of asymptomatic bruits and other forms of cerebrovascular disease. However, when accurate information is needed urgently for possible carotid surgery, it is our practice to proceed directly to angiography, despite the slight risk involved.

Ischemic disease of the *lacunar type* warrants anticoagulation only in the stage when it simulates TIAs and is better withheld once the stroke is under way or completed, lest the damaged arterial wall that set the stage for the lacunar stroke yields and gives rise to hemorrhage. Many such cases continue to progress over a 2- to 3-day period, often to a total deficit in the affected modality, sensory or motor. This progress is usually smooth, raising fears of a deep hemorrhage, yet the expected coinvolvement of the other modality (sensory with motor or vice versa) does not develop; the issue is easily settled by a normal CT scan, since even small hematomas are easily detected by this method.

THE PATIENT WITH THE INOBVIOUS STROKE

Although hemiplegia is the classic sign of stroke, cerebrovascular disease may present with signs that spare the motor pathways, yet carry the same prognostic and therapeutic implications. Fortunately, only five such inobvious stroke syndromes occur regularly. The first is a *leaking aneurysm* presenting as a sudden, generalized headache (unlike any experienced in the past), often having developed during exertion, and persisting for hours or days. Examination may disclose no abnormalities, except for a slightly stiff neck. Casual urinary and less often fecal incontinence, vague recollection for recent events, and unaccountable delays in answering simple questions may also be present and reflect emerging hydrocephalus in the days after the onset of headache. Subdural hematoma, anticoagulant-induced frontal pole hemorrhage, brain tumor, and other entities must be included in the differential diagnosis.

A second type of inobvious stroke is *cerebellar hemorrhage*. Sudden onset of dizziness, repeated uncontrollable vomiting, inability to stand and walk, ipsilateral gaze palsy, ipsilateral facial paresis, and, less often, ipsilateral cerebellar ataxia are often incompletely detected and fail to be assembled into the diagnostic syndrome by the examining physician. Considerate of the patient's misery, the physician often defers testing the patient's ability to stand and walk, and, finding no obvious hemiparesis, he may also defer testing ocular movements fully; the mild facial asymmetry easily escapes notice in the setting of vomiting and dizziness. Labyrinthitis, Ménière disease, alcoholic or drug intoxication, even viral gastroenteritis, are some of the labels that have been applied to this syndrome, and little thought is given to impending disaster because the patient seems so alert—until brainstem compression suddenly intervenes, with fatal results. MRI, CT scan, or lumbar puncture is an essential diagnostic step in the evaluation of all such cases. Evacuation of the hematoma in the acute phase has proved to be the only reliable therapeutic step.

A third inobvious stroke involves the *posterior cerebral artery territory*. Homonymous hemianopia is often not implicitly appreciated by the patient, whose complaints, if any, center on the need for new eyeglasses, or vague descriptions of blurring of vision. Accompanying deficits in higher cerebral function, including reading, naming of colors, manipulable objects or faces, description or tracing of routes, require testing despite the patient's seeming normalcy during conversation. Headache that may accompany embolism in the posterior cerebral artery is often referred to the outer edge of the ipsilateral eyebrow.

The fourth common inobvious stroke is an episode of mild paraphasic speech and slightly impaired auditory comprehension that characterizes certain instances of *Wernicke's aphasia due to embolism*. The patient is often thought to be confused. Most of them perform satisfactorily at a superficial level in making socially appropriate greetings and gestures, and they may approve readily of the examiner's efforts to shorten the interview by posing questions to be answered yes or no. Scrutiny of their remarks and behavior during history-taking will elicit the deficit.

Finally, it should be mentioned that a *confusional, amnesic, or even a psychotic* state may occasionally be the sole clinical manifestation of a stroke. Only the abruptness of onset of the mental symptoms and appropriate CT changes in one frontal lobe or in the medial diencephalic or inferomedial temporal region on the dominant side (or both sides) betray the vascular nature of the event. Careful examination of the amnesic patient may disclose subtle evidence of a dysphasia (alexia, anomia, achromatopsia).

In a similar vein, a searching past history may reveal the fact that a degree of general intellectual impairment had preceded the acute confusional or psychotic episode.

THE PATIENT WITH A HISTORY OF A RECENT NEUROLOGIC DEFICIT OF VASCULAR TYPE

This is the time when the identification of the patient at risk becomes an important matter, for it offers the best opportunity for medical intercession. Excluding a postconvulsive state, any deficit in neurologic function involving a cerebral or brainstem location that has persisted over a few hours should be taken as evidence of a destructive vascular lesion in the brain even though the deficit appears to have disappeared. Electrolyte disturbance, fever, intoxication with drugs, etc., may cause an apparent relapse, and knowledge of such a prior lesion is of immeasurable value in assessing the significance of any focal cerebral disorder that emerges during a general metabolic derangement. A history of the brief episodic focal deficit compels consideration of TIAs. In such a setting, migraine, seizure, depression, cerebral hypoperfusion states, and other entities arise in the differential diagnosis. Search for extracranial vascular abnormalities including a carotid bruit is useful. If the episodes are recurrent, the similarities between episodes, the arterial territory implicated by the symptoms, and their duration are all important features to be studied. TIAs that warn of disaster frequently last only seconds to a few minutes, and are often shrugged off by the patient as insignificant. Although some patients experience hundreds of attacks over months before a stroke, most experience few, often only one; and the last and sometimes the only such attack tends to occur within the day(s) before the stroke. The more recent the last attack, the more expeditious should be the attempt to find the source of the prior deficit.

REFERENCES

ABU-ZEID HAH, CHOI NW, HSU P-H, MAINI KK: Prognostic factors in the survival of 1,484 stroke cases observed for 30 to 48 months. *Arch Neurol* 35:121, 1978.

ADAMS HP JR, BUTLER MJ, BILLER J, TOFFOL GN: Nonhemorrhagic cerebral infarction in young adults. *Arch Neurol* 43:793, 1986.

ADAMS RD: Mechanisms of apoplexy as determined by clinical and pathological correlation. *J Neuropathol Exp Neurol* 13:1, 1954.

ADAMS RD, VANDER EECKEN HM: Vascular disease of the brain. *Annu Rev Med* 4:213, 1953.

ADAMS RD, TORVIK A, FISHER CM: Progressing stroke: Patho-

genesis, in Siekert RG, Whisnant JP (eds): *Cerebral Vascular Diseases, Third Conference.* New York, Grune & Stratton, 1961, pp 133–150.

ADLER JR, ROPPER AH: Self-audible venous bruits and high jugular bulb. *Arch Neurol* 43:257, 1986.

ALEXANDER MP, SCHMITT MA: The aphasia syndrome of stroke in the left anterior cerebral artery territory. *Arch Neurol* 37:97, 1980.

AMEEN AA, ILLINGSWORTH R: Anti-fibrinolytic treatment in the pre-operative management of subarachnoid hemorrhage caused by ruptured intracranial aneurysm. *J Neurol Neurosurg Psychiatry* 44:220, 1981.

AMES A, NESBETT FB: Pathophysiology of ischemic cell death. I: Time of onset of irreversible damage; importance of the different components of the ischemic insult. *Stroke* 14:219, 1983.

AMES A, NESBETT FB: Pathophysiology of ischemic cell death. II: Changes in plasma membrane permeability and cell volume. *Stroke* 14:227, 1983.

AMES A, NESBETT FB: Pathophysiology of ischemic cell death. III: Role of extracellular factors. *Stroke* 14:233, 1983.

AMES A, WRIGHT RL, KOWADA M et al: Cerebral ischemia. II: The no-reflow phenomenon. *Am J Pathol* 52:437, 1968.

AOYAGI N, HAYAKAWA I: Analysis of 223 ruptured intracranial aneurysms with special reference to rupture. *Surg Neurol* 21:445, 1984.

AUER LM: The pathogenesis of hypertensive encephalopathy. *Acta Neurochir,* suppl 27, 1978.

AVERBACK P: Primary cerebral venous thrombosis in young adults: The diverse manifestations of an unrecognized disease. *Ann Neurol* 3:81, 1978.

BANKER BQ: Cerebral vascular disease in infancy and childhood. I: Occlusive vascular disease. *J Neuropathol Exp Neurol* 20:127, 1961.

BARNETT HJM: The EC/IC bypass study group. Failure of extracranial-intracranial arterial bypass to reduce the risk of ischemic stroke. Results of an international randomized trial. *N Engl J Med* 313:1191, 1985.

BARNETT HJM, BOUGHNER GR, COOPER PF: Further evidence relating mitral-valve prolapse to cerebral ischemic events. *N Engl J Med* 302:139, 1980.

BARRON KD, SIQUEIRA E, HIRANO A: Cerebral embolism caused by nonbacterial thrombotic endocarditis. *Neurology* 10:391, 1960.

BILLER J, CHALLA VR, TOOLE JF, HOWARD VJ: Nonbacterial thrombotic endocarditis. *Arch Neurol* 39:95, 1982.

BOTTERELL EH, LOUGHEED WM, SCOTT JW, VANDEWATER SL: Hypothermia, and interruption of carotid or carotid and vertebral circulation, in the surgical management of intracranial aneurysms. *J Neurosurg* 13:1, 1956.

BOGOUSSLAVSKY J, DESPLANT P-A, REGLI F: Spontaneous carotid dissection with acute stroke. *Arch Neurol* 44:137, 1987.

BOUSSER MG, ESCHWEGE E, HAGUENAU M et al: "AICLA" controlled trial of aspirin and dipyridamole in the secondary prevention of atherothrombotic cerebral ischemia. *Stroke* 14:5, 1983.

BREUER AC, FURLAN AJ, HANSON MR et al: Central nervous system complications of coronary bypass graft surgery: Prospective analysis of 421 patients. *Stroke* 14:682, 1983.

BRUST JCM: Anterior cerebral artery, in Barnett HJM, Mohr JP, Stein BM, Yalsu FM (eds): *Stroke*. New York, Churchill Livingstone, 1986, chap 23.

BRUST JCM, BEHRENS MM: "Release hallucinations" as the major symptom of posterior cerebral artery occlusion: A report of 2 cases. *Ann Neurol* 2:432, 1977.

BYROM FB: The pathogenesis of hypertensive encephalopathy. *Lancet* 2:201, 1954.

CANADIAN COOPERATIVE STUDY GROUP: Randomized trial of aspirin and sulfinpyrazone in threatened stroke. *N Engl J Med* 299:53, 1978.

CAPLAN LR: "Top of the basilar" syndrome. *Neurology* 30:72, 1980.

CAPLAN LR: Vertebrobasilar occlusive disease, in Barnett HJM, Stein BM, Mohr JP, Yatsu FM (eds): *Stroke*, vol 1. New York, Churchill Livingstone, 1986, p 560.

CASTAIGNE P, LHERMITTE F, BUGE A et al: Paramedian thalamic and midbrain infarcts: Clinical and neuropathological study. *Ann Neurol* 10:127, 1981.

CELESIA GG, STROTHER CM, TURSKI PA et al: Digital subtraction angiography. *Arch Neurol* 40:70, 1983.

CHAMBERS BR, NORRIS JW: Outcome in patients with asymptomatic neck bruits. *N Engl J Med* 315:860, 1986.

CHESTER EM, AGAMANOLIS DP, BANKER BQ, VICTOR M: Hypertensive encephalopathy: A clinicopathologic study of 20 cases. *Neurology* 28:928, 1978.

CHURG J, STRAUSS L: Allergic granulomatosis, allergic angiitis and periarteritis nodosa. *Am J Pathol* 27:277, 1951.

CHYATTE W, SUNDT TM: Cerebral vasospasm after subarachnoid hemorrhage. *Mayo Clin Proc* 59:498, 1984.

COGAN DG: Visual hallucinations as release phenomena. *Albrecht von Graefe Arch Klin Ophthalmol* 188:139, 1973.

CONIN LS, SANDOK BA, HOUSER W: Cerebral ischemic events in patients with carotid artery fibromuscular dysplasia. *Arch Neurol* 38:616, 1981.

CORRIN LS, SANDOK BA, HAUSER OW: Cerebral ischemic events in patients with fibromuscular dysplasia. *Arch Neurol* 38:616, 1981.

CRAWFORD PM, WEST CR, CHADWICK DW et al: Arteriovenous malformations of the brain; natural history in unoperated patients. *J Neurol Neurosurg Psychiatry* 49:1, 1986.

DAVIES-JONES GAB, PRESTON FE, TIMPERLEY WR: *Neurological Complications in Clinical Haematology*. Oxford, Blackwell Scientific Publications, 1980.

DAY AL: Anatomy of extracranial vessels, in Smith RR (ed): *Stroke and Extracranial Vessels*. New York, Raven Press, 1984, pp 9–22.

DECROIX JP, GRAVELEAU R, MASSON M, CAMBIER J: Infarction in the territory of the anterior choroidal artery. *Brain* 109:1071, 1986.

DEJERINE J: *Semiologie d'Affections du Systeme Nerveux*. Paris, Masson, 1914.

DEVINSKY O, PETITO CK, ALONSO DR: Clinical and neuropathological findings in systemic lupus erythematosus: The role of vasculitis, heart emboli, and thrombotic thrombocytopenic purbura. *Ann Neurol* 23:380, 1988.

DIVRY P, VAN BOGAERT L: Une maladie familiale caractérisée par une angiomatose diffuse cortico-méningée noncalcifiante et une démyélinisation progressive de la substance blanche. *J Neurol Neurosurg Psychiatry* 9:41, 1946.

DRAKE CG: Giant intracranial aneurysms: Experience with surgical treatment of 174 patients. *Clin Neurosurg* 26:12, 1979.

FACTOR SA, DENTINGER MP: Early brain-stem auditory evoked responses in vertebrobasilar transient ischemic attacks. *Arch Neurol* 44:544, 1987.

FAUGHT E, TRADER SD, HANNA GR: Cerebral complications of arteriography for transient ischemia and stroke. *Neurology* 29:4, 1979.

FELDMEYER JJ, MERENDEZ G, REGLI F: Stenoses symptomatiques de l'artere cerebrale moyenne. *Rev Neurol* 139:725, 1983.

FERGUSON GG: Physical factors in the initiation, growth, and rupture of human intracranial saccular aneurysms. *J Neurosurg* 37:666, 1972.

FIELDS WS: *Pathogenesis and Treatment of Cerebrovascular Disease*. Springfield, IL, Charles C Thomas, 1961.

FISHER CM: Cerebral thromboangiitis obliterans. *Medicine* 36:169, 1957.

FISHER CM: The pathologic and clinical aspects of thalamic hemorrhage. *Trans Am Neurol Assoc* 84:56, 1959.

FISHER CM: A lacunar stroke: The dysarthria–clumsy hand syndrome. *Neurology* 17:614, 1967.

FISHER CM: Cerebral ischemia—less familiar types. *Clin Neurosurg* 18:267, 1971.

FISHER CM: The anatomy and pathology of the cerebral vasculature, in Meyer JS (ed): *Modern Concepts of Cerebrovascular Disease*. New York, Spectrum, 1975, pp 1–41.

FISHER CM: Capsular infarct: The underlying vascular lesions. *Arch Neurol* 36:65, 1979.

FISHER CM: Late-life migraine accompaniments as a cause of unexplained transient ischemic attacks. *Can J Neurol Sci* 7:9, 1980.

FISHER CM: Lacunar strokes and infarcts: A review. *Neurology* 32:871, 1982.

FISHER CM, ADAMS RD: Observations on brain embolism with special reference to the mechanism of hemorrhagic infarction. *J Neuropathol Exp Neurol* 10:92, 1951.

FISHER CM, KARNES WE, KUBIK CS: Lateral medullary infarction—the pattern of vascular occlusion. *J Neuropathol Exp Neurol* 20:323, 1961.

FISHER CM, KISTLER JP, DAVIS JM: Relation of cerebral vasospasm to subarachnoid hemorrhage visualized by CT scanning. *Neurosurgery* 6:1, 1980.

FOGELHOLM R, MURROS K: Cigarette smoking and subarachnoid hemorrhage: A population-based case-control study. *J Neurol Neurosurg Psychiatry* 50:78, 1987.

FOIX C, CHAVANY JA, LEVY M: Syndrome pseudothalamique d'origine parietale. *Rev Neurol* 35:68, 1927.

FOIX C, LEVY M: Les ramollisement sylvien. *Rev Neurol* 11:51, 1927.

FORD CS, FRYE JL, TOOLE JF, LEFKOWITZ D: Asymptomatic carotid bruit and stenosis. *Arch Neurol* 43:219, 1986.

Garraway WM, Whisnant JP, Drury I: The continuing decline in the incidence of stroke. *Mayo Clin Proc* 58:520, 1983.

Garraway WM, Whisnant JP, Drury I: The changing pattern of survival following stroke. *Stroke* 14:699, 1983.

Gelmers HJ: Effect of nimodipine on postischemic cerebrovascular reactivity, as revealed by measuring regional cerebral blood flow. *Acta Neurochir (Wien)* 63:283, 1982.

Graf CJ, Perret GE, Torner JC: Bleeding from cerebral arteriovenous malformations as part of their natural history. *J Neurosurg* 58:331, 1983.

Hachinski V, Norris JW: *The Acute Stroke*. Philadelphia, FA Davis, 1985.

Hart RG, Byer JA, Slaughter JR et al: Occurrence and implications of seizures in subarachnoid hemorrhage due to ruptured intracranial aneurysms. *Neurosurgery* 8:417, 1981.

Hart RG, Coull BM, Hart D: Early recurrent embolism associated with nonvalvular atrial fibrillation: A retrospective study. *Stroke* 14:688, 1983.

Heiss WD: Flow thresholds of functional and morphological damage of brain tissue. *Stroke* 14:329, 1983.

Hennerici M, Trockel U, Rautenberg W et al: Spontaneous progression and regression of carotid atheroma. *Lancet* 1:1415, 1985.

Heyman A, Wilkinson WE, Heyden S et al: Risk of stroke in asymptomatic persons with cervical arterial bruits. *N Engl J Med* 302:838, 1980.

Heyman A, Wilkinson WE, Hurwitz BJ et al: Risk of ischemic heart disease in patients with TIA. *Neurology* 34:626, 1984.

Hier DB, Davis KR, Richardson EP, Mohr JP: Hypertensive putaminal hemorrhage. *Ann Neurol* 1:152, 1977.

Hijdra A, Van Gijn, Stefanko S et al: Delayed cerebral ischemia after aneurysmal subarachnoid hemorrhage. Clinicoanatomic correlations. *Neurology* 36:329, 1986.

Hirsh J: Anticoagulant and platelet antiaggregant agents, in Barnett HJM, Mohr JP, Stein BM, Yatsu FM (eds): *Stroke*. New York, Churchill Livingstone, 1986, chap 48.

Homan RW, Devous MD, Stokely EM, Bonte FJ: Quantification of intracerebral steal in patients with arteriovenous malformation. *Arch Neurol* 43:779, 1986.

Houser OW, Baker HL Jr, Sandok BA, Holley KE: Fibromuscular dysplasia of the cephalic arterial system, in Vinken PJ, Bruyn GW (eds): *Handbook of Clinical Neurology*, vol 11: *Vascular Disease of the Nervous System*, pt 1. Amsterdam, North-Holland, 1972, chap 14, pp 366–385.

Hunt WE, Hess RM: Surgical risk as related to time of intervention in the repair of intracranial aneurysms. *J Neurosurg* 28:14, 1968.

Irey NS, McAllister HA, Henry JM: Oral contraceptives and stroke in young women: A clinicopathologic correlation. *Neurology* 28:1216, 1978.

Irino T, Taneda M, Minami T: Sanguineous cerebrospinal fluid in recanalized cerebral infarction. *Stroke* 8:22, 1977.

Ishikawa K, Uyama M, Asayama K: Occlusive thromboaortopathy (Takayasu's disease): Cervical arterial stenoses, retinal

arterial pressure, retinal microaneurysms and prognosis. *Stroke* 14:730, 1983.

Johnson RT, Richardson EP: The neurological manifestations of systemic lupus erythematosus. *Medicine* 47:337, 1968.

Jones HR, Naggar CZ, Seljan MP, Downing LL: Mitral valve prolapse and cerebral ischemic events: A comparison between a neurology population with stroke and a cardiology population with mitral valve prolapse observed for five years. *Stroke* 13:451, 1982.

Kase CS, Williams JP, Wyatt DA, Mohr JP: Lobar intracerebral hematomas: Clinical and CT analysis of 22 cases. *Neurology* 32:1146, 1982.

Kassel NF, Torner JC, Adams HP: Antifibrinolytic therapy in the acute period following aneurysmal subarachnoid hemorrhage. Preliminary observations from the Cooperative Aneurysm Study. *J Neurosurg* 61:225, 1984.

Kitahara T, Okumura K, Semba A et al: Genetic and immunologic analysis on moya-moya. *J Neurol Neurosurg Psychiatry* 45:1048, 1982.

Kjellberg RN, Hanamura T, Davis KR et al: Bragg-peak proton-beam therapy for arteriovenous malformations of the brain. *N Engl J Med* 309:269, 1983.

Krayenbühl H, Yasargil MG: Radiological anatomy and topography of the cerebral arteries, in Vinken PJ, Bruyn GW (eds): *Handbook of Clinical Neurology*, vol 11: *Vascular Diseases of the Nervous System*, pt 1. Amsterdam, North-Holland, 1972, chap 4, pp 65–101.

Kubik CS, Adams RD: Occlusion of the basilar artery—a clinical and pathological study. *Brain* 69:73, 1946.

Kubota K, Yamaguchi T, Abe Y et al: Effects of smoking on regional cerebral blood flow in neurologically normal subjects. *Stroke* 14:720, 1983.

Kurtzke JF: Critique of the Canadian "TIA" study, in Price TR, Nelson E (eds): *Cerebrovascular Diseases*. New York, Raven Press, 1979, pp 243–250.

Kwak R, Kadoya S, Suzuki T: Factors affecting the prognosis in thalamic hemorrhage. *Stroke* 14:493, 1983.

Lilienfeld AM: Critique of "A randomized trial of aspirin and sulfinpyrazone in threatened stroke," in Price TR, Nelson E (eds): *Cerebrovascular Diseases*. New York, Raven Press, 1979, pp 239–241.

Locksley HB: Report on the Cooperative Study of Intracranial Aneurysms and Subarachnoid Hemorrhage. *J. Neurosurg* 25:321, 1966.

Lodder J, van der Lugt PJM: Evaluation of the risk of immediate anticoagulant treatment in patients with embolic stroke of cardiac origin. *Stroke* 14:42, 1983.

Longstreth WT, Swanson PD: Oral contraceptives and stroke. *Stroke* 15:747, 1984.

Lupi-Herrera E, Sanchez-Torres G, Marcushamer J et al: Takayasu's arteritis: Clinical study of 107 cases. *Am Heart J* 93:94, 1977.

Marshall J: Angiography in the investigation of ischemic episodes in the territory of the internal carotid artery. *Lancet* 1:719, 1971.

McKissock W, Paine KW, Walsh LS: An analysis of the results of treatment of ruptured intracranial aneurysms: A report of 722 consecutive cases. *J Neurosurg* 17:762, 1960.

McKissock W, Richardson A, Walsh L: Middle cerebral

aneurysms: Further results in the controlled trial of conservative and surgical treatment of ruptured intracranial aneurysms. *Lancet* 2:417, 1962.

McKissock W, Richardson A, Walsh L: Anterior communicating aneurysms: A trial of conservative and surgical treatment. *Lancet* 1:873, 1965.

Miyasaka K, Wolpert SM, Prager RJ: The association of cerebral aneurysms, infundibula, and intracranial arteriovenous malformations. *Stroke* 13:196, 1982.

Mohr JP, Caplan LR, Melski JW et al: The Harvard Cooperative Stroke Registry: A prospective registry of patients hospitalized with stroke. *Neurology* 28:754, 1978.

Mohr JP, Pessin MS: Extracranial carotid artery disease, in Barnett HJM, Mohr JP, Stein BM, Yatsu FM (eds): *Stroke.* New York, Churchill Livingstone, 1986, chap 21.

Mokri B, Sundt TM Jr, Houser W, Piepgras DG: Spontaneous dissection of the cervical internal carotid artery. *Ann Neurol* 19:126, 1986.

Moore PM, Cupps TR: Neurological complications of vasculitis. *Ann Neurol* 14:155, 1983.

Myers RE, Yamaguchi S: Nervous system effects of cardiac arrest in monkeys. *Arch Neurol* 34:65, 1977.

Nakajima K: Clinicopathological study of pontine hemorrhage. *Stroke* 14:485, 1983.

Nelson J, Barron MM, Riggs JE et al: Cerebral vasculitis and ulcerative colitis. *Neurology* 36:719, 1986.

Nicholls ES, Johansen HL: Implications of changing trends in cerebrovascular and ischemic heart disease mortality. *Stroke* 14:153, 1983.

Nichols FT, Mohr JP: Binswanger's subacute arteriosclerotic encephalopathy, in Barnett HJM et al (eds): *Stroke,* vol 2, New York, Churchill-Livingstone, 1986, pp 875–885.

Nishimoto A, Takeuchi S: Moyamoya disease, in Vinken PJ, Bruyn GW (eds): *Handbook of Clinical Neurology,* vol 12: *Vascular Diseases of the Nervous System,* pt 2. Amsterdam, North-Holland, 1972, chap 11, pp 352–383.

Nishioka H, Torner JC, Graf CJ et al: Cooperative study of intracranial aneurysms and subarachnoid hemorrhage: A long-term prognostic study. II. Ruptured intracranial aneurysms managed conservatively. *Arch Neurol* 41:1142, 1984.

Nubiola AR, Masana L, Masdeu S et al: High-density lipoprotein cholesterol in cerebrovascular disease. *Arch Neurol* 38:468, 1981.

Ojemann RG: Management of the unruptured intracranial aneurysm. *N Engl J Med* 304:725, 1981.

Ojemann RG, Crowell RM: *Surgical Management of Cerebrovascular Disease.* Baltimore, Williams & Wilkins, 1983.

Ojemann RG, Fisher CM, Rich JC: Spontaneous dissecting aneurysms of the internal carotid artery. *Stroke* 3:434, 1972.

Olsen TS, Larsen B, Herning M et al: Blood flow and vascular reactivity in collaterally perfused brain tissue. *Stroke* 14:332, 1983.

Percheron G: Les artères du thalamus humain. II: Artères et territoires thalamiques paramédians de l'artère basilaire communicante. *Rev Neurol* 132:309, 1976.

Pessin MS, Duncan GW, Mohr JP, Poskanzer DC: Clinical and angiographic features of carotid transient ischemic attacks. *N Engl J Med* 296:358, 1977.

Pessin MS, Hinton RC, Davis KR et al: Mechanisms of acute carotid stroke. *Ann Neurol* 6:245, 1979.

Petit H, Rousseaux M, Clarisse J, Delafosse A: Troubles oculo-céphalomoteurs et infarctus thalamo-sous-thalamique bilatéral. *Rev Neurol* 137:709, 1981.

Plum F: What causes infarction in ischemic brain? The Robert Wartenberg lecture. *Neurology* 33:222, 1983.

Poole CMJ, Russell RWR: Mortality and stroke after amaurosis fugax. *J Neurol Neurosurg Psychiatry* 48:902, 1985.

Rabkin SW, Mathewson FAL, Tate RB: Long-term changes in blood pressure and risk of cerebrovascular disease. *Stroke* 9:319, 1978.

Raichle ME: The pathophysiology of brain ischemia. *Ann Neurol* 13:2, 1983.

Rebollo M, Val JF, Garijo F, Quintana F, Berciano J: Livedo reticularis and cerebrovascular lesions (Sneddon's syndrome). *Brain* 106:965, 1983.

Regli F, Vonsattel GP, Perentes E, Assal G: Cerebral amyloid angioplasty. A clinicopathological study. *Rev Neurol* (Paris) 137: 181, 1981.

Reivich M, Holling HE, Roberts B, Toole JF: Reversal of blood flow through the vertebral artery and its effect on cerebral circulation. *N Engl J Med* 265:878, 1961.

Rice GPA, Boughner DR, Stiller C, Ebers GC: Familial stroke syndrome associated with mitral valve prolapse. *Ann Neurol* 7:130, 1980.

Richardson AE, Jane JA: Long-term prognosis in untreated cerebral aneurysms. I: Incidence of late hemorrhage in cerebral aneurysm: Ten-year evaluation of 364 patients. *Ann Neurol* 1:358, 1977.

Roehmholdt ME, Palumbo PJ, Whisnant JP, Elveback LR: Transient ischemic attack and stroke in a community-based diabetic cohort. *Mayo Clin Proc* 58:56, 1983.

Ropper AH, Davis KR: Lobar cerebral hemorrhages: Acute clinical syndromes in 26 cases. *Ann Neurol* 8:141, 1980.

Ropper AH, King RB: Intracranial pressure monitoring in comatose patients with cerebral hemorrhage. *Arch Neurol* 41:725–728, 1984.

Russell RWR: *Vascular Diseases of the Nervous System,* 2nd ed. Edinburgh, Churchill Livingstone, 1983, pp 206–207.

Sage JI, Lepore FE: Ataxic hemiparesis from lesions of the corona radiata. *Arch Neurol* 40:449, 1983.

Sahs AL, Nibbelin KDW, Torner JC (eds): *Aneurysmal Subarachnoid Hemorrhage.* Baltimore, Urban & Schwarzenberg, 1981.

Sahs AL et al: Cooperative study of intracranial aneurysms and subarachnoid hemorrhage: A long term prognostic study. *Arch Neurol* 41:1140, 1142, 1147, 1984.

Sandok BA, Furlan AJ, Whisnant JP, Sundt TM Jr: Guidelines for the management of transient ischemic attacks. *Mayo Clin Proc* 53:665, 1978.

Sandok BA, Giuliani ER: Cerebral ischemic events in patients with mitral valve prolapse. *Stroke* 13:448, 1982.

Sharma SS, Vijayan GP, Seth HN, Suri ML: Platelet adhesiveness, plasma fibrinogen, and fibrinolytic activity in young patients with ischaemic stroke. *J Neurol Neurosurg Psychiatry* 41:118, 1978.

SHIELDS RW JR, LAURENO R, LACHMAN T, VICTOR M: Anticoagulant-related hemorrhage in acute cerebral embolism. *Stroke* 15:426, 1984.

SIESJO BK: Historical overview. Calcium, ischemia, and death of brain cells. *Ann NY Acad Sci* 522:638, 1988.

SIGSBEE B, DECK MDF, POSNER JB: Nonmetastatic superior sagittal sinus thrombosis complicating systemic cancer. *Neurology* 29:139, 1979.

SNEDDEN JB: Cerebrovascular lesions and livedo reticularis. *Br J Dermatol* 77:180, 1965.

So EL, TOOLE JF, DALAL P, MOODY DM: Cephalic fibromuscular dysplasia in 32 patients: Clinical findings and radiologic features. *Arch Neurol* 38:619, 1981.

TOOLE JF, YUSON CP, JANEWAY R: Transient ischemic attacks: A study of 225 patients. *Neurology* 28:746, 1978.

TURNIPSEED WD, BERKOFF HA, CRUMMY A: Postoperative occlusion after carotid endarterectomy. *Arch Surg* 115:573, 1980.

TYLER KL, POLETTI CE, HEROS RC: Cerebral amyloid angiopathy with multiple intracerebral hemorrhages: Case report. *J Neurosurg* 57:286, 1982.

UEDA K, TOOLE JF, MCHENRY LC: Carotid and vertebral transient ischemic attacks: Clinical and angiographic correlation. *Neurology* 29:1094, 1978.

VANDER EECKEN HM, ADAMS RD: Anatomy and functional significance of meningeal arterial anastomoses of human brain. *J Neuropathol Exp Neurol* 12:132, 1953.

VERMEULEN M, LINDSAY KW, MURRAY GD et al: Antifibrinolytic treatment in subarachnoid hemorrhage. *N Engl J Med* 311:432, 1984.

SOLOMON RA, FINK ME: Current strategies for the management of aneurysmal subarachnoid hemorrhage. *Arch Neurol* 44:769, 1987.

SORENSEN PS, PEDERSEN H, MARQUARDSEN J et al: Acetylsalicylic acid in the prevention of stroke in patients with reversible cerebral ischemic attacks: A Danish Cooperative Study. *Stroke* 14:15, 1983.

SOTANIEMI KA: Brain damage and neurological outcome after open-heart surgery. *J Neurol Neurosurg Psychiatry* 43:127, 1980.

STARKSTEIN SE, ROBINSON RG, PRICE TR: Comparison of cortical and subcortical lesions in the production of post-stroke mood disorders. *Brain* 110:1045, 1987.

STEWART RM, SAMSON D, DIEHL J et al: Unruptured cerebral aneurysms presenting as recurrent transient neurologic deficits. *Neurology* 30:47, 1980.

STRAND T, ASPLUND K, ERIKSSON S et al: A randomized control trial of hemodilution therapy in acute ischemic stroke. *Stroke* 15:980, 1984.

SUSAC JO, HARDMAN JM, SELHORST JB: Microangiopathy of the brain and retina. *Neurology* 29:313, 1979.

TAKAYASU M: A case with peculiar changes of the central retinal vessels. *Acta Soc Ophthalmol Jpn* 12:554, 1908.

TAVERAS JM: Multiple progressive intracranial arterial occlusions: A syndrome of children and young adults. *Am J Roentgenol* 106:235, 1969.

TAOMOTO K, ASADA M, KAMAZAWA Y, MATSUMOTO S: Usefulness of the measurement of plasma β-thromboglobulin (β-TG) in cerebrovascular disease. *Stroke* 14:518, 1983.

VESSEY MP, LAWLESS M, YEATES D: Oral contraceptives and stroke. Findings in a large prospective study. *Br Med J* 289:530, 1984.

VOLHARD F: Clinical aspects of Bright's disease, in Berglund H et al (eds): *The Kidney in Health and Disease.* Philadelphia, Lea & Febiger, 1935, pp 665–688.

WAGA S, YAMAMOTO Y: Hypertensive putaminal hemorrhage: Treatment and results. Is surgical treatment superior to conservative? *Stroke* 14:486, 1983.

WEINBERGER J, BISCARRA V, WEISBERG MK: Factors contributing to stroke in patients with atherosclerotic disease of the great vessels: The role of diabetes. *Stroke* 14:709, 1983.

WEISBERG LA: Lacunar infarcts. *Arch Neurol* 39:37, 1982.

WEISMAN AD, ADAMS RD: The neurological complications of dissecting aortic aneurysm. *Brain* 67:69, 1944.

WEKSLER BB, LEWIN M: Progress in cerebrovascular disease: Anticoagulation in cerebral ischemia. *Stroke* 14:658, 1983.

WHISNANT JP: The role of the neurologist in the decline of stroke. *Ann Neurol* 14:1, 1983.

WHISNANT JP, CARTLIDGE NEF, ELVEBACH LR: Carotid and vertebral-basilar transient ischemic attacks: Effects of anticoagulants, hypertension and cardiac disorders on survival and stroke occurrence—a population study. *Ann Neurol* 3:107, 1978.

WHISNANT JP, MATSUMOTO N, ELVEBACK LR: Transient cerebral ischemic attacks in a community: Rochester, Minnesota, 1955 through 1969. *Mayo Clin Proc* 48:194, 1973.

WHISNANT JP, SANDOK BA, SUNDT TM: Carotid endarterectomy for unilateral carotid system transient cerebral ischemia. *Mayo Clin Proc* 58:171, 1983.

WIEBERS DO, WHISNANT JP, O'FALLON WM: The natural history of unruptured intracranial aneurysms. *N Engl J Med* 304:696, 1981.

WIEBERS DO: Ischemic cerebrovascular complications of pregnancy. *Arch Neurol* 42:1106, 1985.

WOLF PA, KANNEL WB, MCGEE DL et al: Duration of atrial fibrillation and imminence of stroke: The Framingham Study. *Stroke* 14:664, 1983.

WOOD JH, FLEISCHER AS: Observations during hypervolemic hemodilution of patients with acute focal cerebral ischemia. *JAMA* 248:2999, 1982.

YAMASHITA M, OKA K, TANAKA K: Histopathology of the brain vascular network in Moyamoya disease. *Stroke* 14:50, 1983.

YANAGIHARA P, PIEPGRAS DG, KLASS DW: Repetitive involuntary movement associated with episodic cerebral ischemia. *Ann Neurol* 18:244, 1985.

ZIVIN JA, STASHAK J: The effect of ischemia on biogenic amine concentrations in the central nervous system. *Stroke* 14:556, 1983.

CHAPTER 35

CRANIOCEREBRAL TRAUMA

Among the vast array of neurologic diseases, cerebral trauma ranks high in order of frequency and gravity. The basic process is at once both simple and complex—simple because there is usually no problem about etiologic diagnosis, viz., a blow to the head—and complex because of uncertainty about the pathogenesis of the immediate cerebral disorder and a number of delayed effects that may complicate the injury. About the trauma itself, nothing medical can be done, for it is finished before the physician arrives on the scene. At most there can be an assessment of the factors conducive to further injury and the institution of measures to avoid them. But of the disastrous intracranial phenomena that are initiated by head injury, several fall within the purview of the physician, for they evolve during the period of medical observation, offering possibilities of both prevention and treatment.

It is a common misconception that craniocerebral injuries are matters that concern only the neurosurgeon and not the general physician or neurologist. Actually, some 80 percent of head injuries are first seen by a general physician, and probably fewer than 20 percent ever require neurosurgical intervention of any kind—and even this number is decreasing. Often neurologists must take charge of the head-injured patient, or their opinion is sought in consultation. To enact their role effectively they must be familiar with the clinical manifestations and the natural course of the primary brain injury and its complications, and have a sound grasp of the underlying physiologic mechanisms. Such knowledge must be up-to-date and immediately applicable. Matters pertaining to spinal injury are considered in Chap. 36. The present chapter undertakes to review the salient facts concerning injuries to the brain and to outline a clinical approach that the authors have found useful over the years.

DEFINITIONS AND MECHANISMS

The very language that one uses to discuss certain types of head injury divulges a number of misconceptions that have been inherited from previous generations of physicians. Words have crept into the medical vocabulary and have often been retained long after the ideas for which they stood have been refuted—attesting to the disadvantage of premature adoption of explanatory rather than descriptive terms. The word *concussion,* for example, implies a violent shaking and agitation of the brain and the transient functional impairment resulting therefrom. Yet despite numerous experiments to demonstrate physical changes within the nerve cells, axons, or myelin sheaths (vibration effects, formation of intracellular vacuoles, etc.), no convincing confirmation of their existence has been possible. Similarly the word *contusion,* meaning a bruising of tissue without interruption of physical continuity, is applied rather indiscriminately to a variety of clinical states, some of which could not depend on a pathologic change of this type, e.g., "minor contusion state or syndrome"—an expression introduced by Wilfred Trotter, who was himself most critical of words that "embalm a fallacious theory."

In all attempts to analyze the mechanism(s) of cerebral trauma one fact stands pre-eminent—that there must be the sudden application of a physical force of considerable magnitude to the head. Unless the head is struck, the brain suffers no injury—except in the rare instances of violent flexion-extension (whiplash) of the neck and somewhat controversial cases of crush injury to the chest or explosive injury with raised intrapulmonary pressure.

A second factor of particular importance in brain injury is the mobility of the head and brain. As will be pointed out below, all concussive injuries relate to a physical force (large blunt object) that imparts motion to the stationary head or a hard surface that arrests the motion of the moving head. These constitute the common civilian head injuries. Termed *blunt or nonpenetrating head injuries,* they are remarkable in two respects: (1) they frequently induce at least a temporary loss of consciousness; (2) even though the skull is not penetrated and fragments of bone are not driven into its cavity, the brain may suffer gross damage, i.e., contusion, laceration, hemorrhage, swelling, and herniation. A theory that would bring into plausible form these gross neuropathologic changes and the transient loss of consciousness (concussion) or prolonged coma has yet to be formulated.

By contrast, high-velocity missiles may penetrate the skull and cranial cavity or, rarely, the skull is compressed between two converging forces crushing the brain, without causing significant displacement of the head and brain. In these circumstances the patient may suffer severe and often fatal injury without immediate loss of consciousness. Hemorrhage, destruction of brain tissue, and, if the patient survives for a time, meningitis or abscess, are the principal pathologic changes created by injuries of these types. They offer little difficulty in understanding. The various types of head injuries are illustrated in Fig. 35-1.

The relation of skull fracture to brain injury has been viewed in changing perspective throughout the history of this subject. In early times, fractures dominated the thinking of the medical profession, and cerebral lesions were regarded as secondary. Later it became known that the skull, though rigid, is still flexible enough to yield to a blow that could injure the brain without causing fracture. Therefore, the presence of a fracture, although a rough measure of the violence to which the brain has been exposed, is no longer considered an infallible index of the presence of cerebral injury. Even in fatal head injuries, autopsy reveals an intact skull in some 20 to 30 percent of cases. Contrariwise many patients suffer skull fractures without serious or prolonged disorder of cerebral function.

The modern trend is to be concerned primarily with the presence or absence of brain injury rather than with the

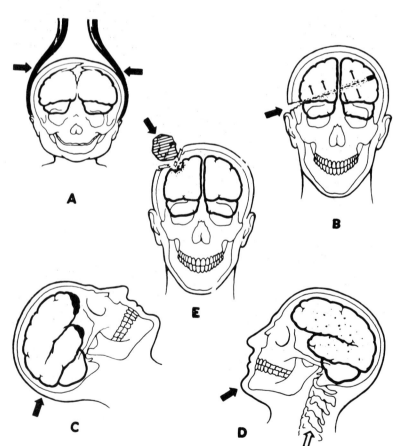

Figure 35-1

Mechanisms of craniocerebral injury. A. Cranium distorted by forceps (birth injury). B. Gunshot wound of the brain. C. Falls (also traffic accidents). D. Blows on the chin ("punch drunk"). E. Injury to skull and brain by falling objects. [From Courville (a study based upon a survey of lesions found in a series of 15,000 autopsies).]

fracture of the skull itself. Nevertheless, fractures cannot be dismissed without further comment, for several reasons. The presence of a fracture always warns of the possibility of cerebral injury (estimated to be 20 times more frequent with skull fracture than without). Moreover, fractures assume importance in indicating the site and possible severity of brain damage, in providing an explanation for cranial nerve palsies, and in creating potential pathways for the ingress of bacteria and air or the egress of cerebrospinal fluid (CSF). Some of the major sites and directions of basilar skull fractures are indicated in Fig. 35-2. One can readily perceive the possibilities of injury to cranial nerves in relation to such fractures.

INJURY OF CRANIAL NERVES AND OTHER BASILAR STRUCTURES BY FRACTURES

Basilar fractures of the skull are often difficult to detect in plain skull films, but their presence may be disclosed by a number of characteristic clinical signs. Fracture of the petrous pyramid often deforms the external auditory canal or tears the tympanic membrane, with leakage of spinal fluid (otorrhea); or, blood may collect behind an intact tympanic membrane and discolor it. If the fracture extends more posteriorly, damaging the sigmoid sinus, the tissue behind the ear and over the mastoid process becomes boggy and discolored (Battle sign). Basilar fracture of the anterior skull may cause blood to leak into the periorbital tissues, imparting a characteristic "raccoon" or "panda bear" appearance.

Commonly the existence of a basilar fracture is indicated by signs of cranial nerve damage. Nerves that are particularly liable to trauma are the olfactory, optic, oculomotor, trochlear, facial, auditory, and the first and second branches of the trigeminal. Anosmia and an apparent loss of taste (actually a loss of perception of aromatic flavors, since the elementary modalities of taste—salt, sweet, bitter, sour—are unimpaired) are frequent sequelae of head injury, especially falls on the back of the head. In the majority of cases the anosmia is permanent. If unilateral, it will not be noticed by the patient. The mechanism of these disturbances is believed to be displacement of the brain and tearing of the olfactory nerve filaments in or near the cribriform plate, through which they course.

A fracture in or near the sella may tear the stalk of the pituitary gland, with resulting diabetes insipidus, impotence and reduced libido, and amenorrhea. A fracture of the sphenoid bone may lacerate the optic nerve, with blindness from the beginning. The pupil is dilated and unreactive to a direct light stimulus but still reacts to a light stimulus to the opposite eye (consensual reflex). The optic disc becomes pale, i.e., atrophic, after an interval of several weeks. Partial injuries may result in a troublesome blurring of vision due to scotomas.

Injury to the eighth cranial nerve with petrous fractures causes a loss of hearing and/or postural vertigo and nystagmus immediately after the trauma. Deafness due to nerve injury must be distinguished from the deafness caused by bleeding into the middle ear, with disruption of the

Figure 35-2

The course of fracture lines through the base of the skull. Arrows indicate point of application and direction of force. (From Courville.)

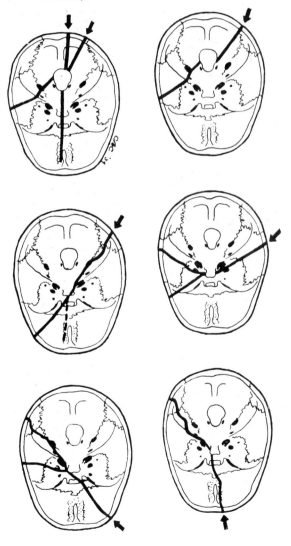

ossicular chain (conduction deafness), and the high tone hearing loss due to cochlear concussion. Vertigo needs to be distinguished from posttraumatic nervous giddiness.

In oculomotor nerve injury there is a divergent squint, with loss of internal and vertical movement of the eye and a fixed, dilated pupil. Diplopia—worse on looking down—and compensatory tilting of the head suggest trochlear nerve injury. These ocular nerve disorders must be distinguished from ocular displacement due to direct injury to the eye and its attached muscles. Injury of the facial nerve by a basilar fracture may be present immediately after the injury or delayed for several days. The delayed form is usually transitory, and its mechanism is not known. It may be misinterpreted as an important progression of the intracranial traumatic lesion. Injury to the ophthalmic or maxillary divisions of the trigeminal nerve may be the result of either a basilar fracture across the middle cranial fossa or a direct extracranial injury to the branches of the nerves. Numbness and paresthesias of the skin supplied by the nerve(s) or a troublesome neuralgia are the sequelae of these injuries.

CAROTID-CAVERNOUS FISTULA

A basilar fracture through the sphenoid and petrous bones may lacerate the internal carotid artery where it lies in the cavernous sinus. Within hours or a day or two a severe and disfiguring pulsating exophthalmos develops as arterial blood enters and distends the orbital veins that empty into the sinus. Usually the orbit feels tight and is painful. The eye may become partially or completely immobile because of pressure on the ocular nerves. The sixth nerve is affected most often and the third and fourth less frequently. Also, there may be a loss of vision, due to involvement of the optic nerve; congestion of the retinal veins and glaucoma are additional factors in the visual failure. Surgical therapy is indicated; the several techniques include embolization via a catheter in the internal carotid artery, trapping the torn carotid segment, and ligating the carotid artery in the neck (see review by Stern).

Not all carotid-cavernous fistulae are traumatic. They may occur occasionally with rupture of an intracavernous saccular aneurysm or in Danlos-Ehlers disease, where the connective tissue is defective; or the cause may be unexplained.

PNEUMOCELE AND RHINORRHEA

If the skin over a skull fracture is lacerated and the underlying meninges are torn, or if the fracture passes through the inner wall of a nasal sinus, bacteria or air may enter the cranial cavity with resulting meningitis, abscess, and aerocele (air in the ventricles). Also, CSF may leak into the sinus and present as a watery discharge from the nose (*CSF rhinorrhea*). The nasal discharge can be identified as CSF by testing it for glucose with diabetic test tape (mucus has no glucose) or for the presence of fluorescein or metrizamide that had been injected into the lumbar subarachnoid space and absorbed by pledgets placed in the nasal cavity. Persistence of the rhinorrhea or the occurrence of repeated episodes of meningitis is an indication for repair of the torn dura mater over the fissure. Depressed fractures are of significance only if the underlying dura is lacerated or the brain is compressed by indentation of bone. They should then be surgically repaired within the first 24 to 48 h.

CEREBRAL CONCUSSION

Much has been written about the mechanisms of concussion and coma in closed or blunt head injury. Certain facts concerning these conditions stand out. (1) Concussion, meaning a *usually reversible traumatic paralysis of nervous function,* is always immediate (not delayed even by seconds). (2) The effects of concussion on brain function may last for a variable time (seconds, minutes, hours, or longer). To set arbitrary limits on the duration of loss of consciousness, i.e., to consider a brief loss as indicative of concussion and a prolonged loss as indicative of contusion or other traumatic cerebral lesion—as proposed in some medical writings—is illogical and unsound physiologically, as pointed out by Symonds. Any such difference is quantitative, not qualitative. Admittedly, in the more prolonged states of coma there is a greater chance of finding hemorrhage and contusion, which undoubtedly contribute to the persistence of coma and the likelihood of irreversible change. (3) The optimal condition for the production of concussive paralysis of brain function, demonstrated originally by Denny-Brown and Russell, is a change in the momentum of the head; i.e., either movement is imparted to the head by a blow, or movement of the head is arrested by a hard, unyielding surface. These two types of blunt (nonpenetrating) head injury are called accelerative and decelerative, respectively.

The mechanism of concussive cerebral paralysis has been interpreted in various ways throughout medical history, in the light of scientific knowledge available at a particular time. The favored hypotheses for the better part of a century was vasoparalysis (suggested by Fischer in 1870) or an arrest of circulation by an instantaneous rise in intracranial pressure (which was proposed by Strohmeyer in 1864 and popularized by Trotter in 1932). The latter asserted that the brief period of cerebral anemia induced an immediate paralysis of cerebral function with a tendency to rapid and spontaneous recovery, usually leaving no visible sign of damage to the brain. More prolonged periods of concussive coma were attributed by Trotter to contusion, a proposition for which he adduced no pathologic evidence. Jefferson, in his essay on the nature of concussion, convincingly refuted these vascular hypotheses; later, Shatsky et al, by the use of high-speed cineangiography (1000 frames per second), showed displacement of vessels but no arrest of circulation immediately after impact.

Beginning with the work of Denny-Brown and Russell, the physical factors involved in head and brain injury have been subjected to careful analysis. As indicated above, these investigators determined that the change in momentum of the head is critical in the genesis of concussion. They demonstrated, in the monkey and cat, that concussion resulted when the head was struck by a heavy mass, as large as or larger than the head, with a velocity greater than 28 ft/s (energy of 17.83 ft-lb). If the head was prevented from moving at the moment of impact, this degree of force invariably failed to produce concussion.

Holbourn, in 1943, attempted to solve the paradox of why coma occurs when a freely moving head is struck but does not occur when the head is stationary. From the study of gelatin models under conditions simulating head trauma he deduced that when the head is struck, movement of the round, partly tethered but suspended brain always lags (inertia); but inevitably the brain moves also, and when it does it must rotate, for it occupies a round skull whose motions (because of attachment to the neck) usually describe an arc. Pudenz and Sheldon and later Ommaya et al (1964) proved the correctness of this assumption by photographing the brain through a lucite calvarium at the moment of impact. The brain is thus subjected to shearing stresses set up by rotational forces. Such motions of the brain could explain the immediate loss of consciousness (see below). Also, they provide a reasonable explanation for the occurrence of surface injuries in certain places, i.e., where the swirling brain comes into contact with bony prominences on the inner surface of the skull (petrous and orbital ridges, sphenoid wings), and of injuries to the corpus callosum where it comes in contact with the falx. However, the precise mechanism(s) involved in the genesis of concussion are still not fully explained; explanations in terms such as "molecular commotion," direct injury of neurons (Denny-Brown and Russell), neuronal chromatolysis (Groat et al), rupture of axons (see below), and "synaptic breaks" in the gray matter, remain to be verified.

Strich, in 1956, studied the brains of five patients who died between 5 and 15 months after severe closed head injuries that had caused protracted coma. Using the Marchi staining method, she observed an uneven, multifocal degeneration of the cerebral white matter. In these cases, in which there was said to have been "no skull fracture, raised

intracranial pressure or gross subarachnoid hemorrhage," the clinical state had been attributed to midbrain and subthalamic hemorrhages or softenings, but these changes were not found at autopsy. A shearing of myelin or axons was postulated. Strich later extended her observations to 20 cases. In patients with more recent lesions she observed ballooning of axis cylinders (end bulbs), a finding that was confirmed by Nevin and others and more recently by J. H. Adams and his colleagues. Symonds saw in these pathologic changes a possible explanation of concussion, i.e., an effect of Holbourn's shearing stresses, which distort and stretch axis cylinders.

Much interest in recent years has centered on the *anatomic site of the concussive injury*. Once it became known that the reticular formation of the upper brainstem served as a nonspecific activating system for the cerebral cortex, the possibility suggested itself that it was the site of concussive injury. Foltz and Schmidt showed that in the concussed monkey lemniscal sensory transmission through the brainstem was unaltered, but its effect in activating the high reticular formation was blocked. They also demonstrated that the electrical activity of the medial reticular formation was depressed for a longer time and more severely than that of the cerebral cortex. These effects on the reticular formation were thought to be analogous to the ones produced by ether and barbiturate anesthesia. It has been suggested that maximal shearing stress occurs at the point where the cerebral hemispheres could most easily rotate on the relatively fixed brainstem, i.e., at the midbrain-subthalamic level. Using the fluorescein technique, Ommaya et al (1964) found selective changes of the blood-brain barrier in the lower brainstem and spinal cord of concussed animals, i.e., lower than the level of injury postulated by Foltz and Schmidt. Meyer and Denny-Brown believe the cerebral cortex to be directly involved because of the finding in monkeys of a change in the cortical DC potentials immediately after concussive injury.

Formerly it was thought that the initial effect of a blunt concussive injury was to excite the nervous system, with evocation of a massive discharge. The "stars" that one sees with a minor blow to the head and the gasp of the injured animal were cited as expressions of this effect. However, continuous electrical monitoring through implanted cortical electrodes at the time of impact and for 10 s afterward offered no support for this suggestion. There was no increase in electrical activity and nothing resembling a seizure discharge; instead, cortical activity was briefly suppressed and relatively little altered thereafter.

The *clinical effects of concussion* are invariable:

immediate abolition of consciousness, suppression of reflexes (falling to the ground if standing), transient arrest of respiration, a brief period of bradycardia and fall in blood pressure following a momentary rise at the time of impact. If sufficiently intense, death may occur at this moment, presumably from respiratory arrest. Usually the vital signs return to normal and stabilize within a few seconds while the patient remains unconscious. The plantar reflexes are extensor. Then, after a variable period of time, the patient begins to stir, opens the eyes, but is unseeing. Corneal, pharyngeal, and cutaneous reflexes, originally depressed, begin to return; and the limbs are withdrawn from painful stimuli. Gradually contact is made with the environment, and the patient passes successively through stages of obeying only simple commands and of responding slowly and inadequately to simple questions. Memories are not formed during this period; the patient may carry on a conversation which, later on, cannot be recalled. Finally there is full recovery corresponding to the time when the patient can form consecutive memories of current experiences. The time required for the patient to pass through these stages of recovery may be a few minutes or several hours or days, but again, between these extremes Symonds sees only quantitative differences, varying with the intensity of the process. The sequences which he believes to represent lower levels of brain function return first and higher levels, later. To the observer such patients are comatose only from the moment of injury until they open their eyes and begin to speak; for the patient, the period of unconsciousness extends from a point before the injury occurred (*retrograde amnesia*) until the time when he or she is able to form consecutive memories, viz., at the end of the period of *anterograde amnesia*. The duration of the amnesic period, particularly of anterograde amnesia, is the most reliable index of the severity of the concussive injury.

After simple concussion of short duration there are probably no gross or microscopic changes. The CSF is normal and the EEG discloses no abnormalities. However, certain biochemical and ultrastructural alterations have been described in experimental animals. There is depletion of mitochondrial ATP, and sometimes a disruption of the blood-brain barrier near the point of impact. A diffuse axonal injury is also reported.

In severe craniocerebral injury there are other biochemical changes, but their significance is uncertain. Acetylcholine and lactate are elevated in the CSF during the first 3 to 4 days after the injury (leakage from damaged brain) and then gradually return to normal. Serum lactate is also raised, presumably because of the ready diffusibility of lactic acid from brain and CSF to blood. Also during the first few days there is sodium retention, followed by sodium diuresis. However, during the phase of sodium retention there is actually a mild hyponatremia, due to simultaneous water retention. Potassium, in contrast, remains in balance throughout this period. Nitrogen loss— amounting to about 10 g/day—is a consistent finding in all types of serious head injury during the first days following trauma.

In fatal cases of head injury, where these concussive effects must have existed, the brain is often bruised, swollen, and lacerated, and there may be hemorrhage, either meningeal or intracerebral. The prominence of these gross pathologic findings led to the prevalent view that cerebral injuries are largely matters of bruises and hemorrhages and urgent operations. That this can hardly be the case is suggested by the fact that some patients survive head injuries that are clinically as severe or almost as severe as the fatal ones and make an excellent recovery. Years later, postmortem examinations disclose old contusions (plaques jaunes) and hemorrhages of approximately the same distribution and extent as those observed in some of the immediately fatal cases. One can only conclude, therefore, that most of the immediate symptoms of severe head injury, both general and localized, depend on invisible and highly reversible changes, probably of the same nature as the changes that underlie concussion.

Nevertheless, bruises, lacerations, hemorrhages, localized swellings, and herniations of tissue cannot be disregarded, because they are probably responsible for or contribute to many of the fatalities that occur 12 to 72 h or more after the injury. Of these lesions the most important are bruising of the surface of the brain beneath the point of impact (*coup lesion*) and the more extensive lacerations and contusions on the side opposite the site of impact (*contrecoup lesion*). The usual sites are shown in Fig. 35-3. Blows to the front of the head produce mainly coup lesions, whereas blows to the back of the head cause mainly contrecoup lesions (sometimes coup lesions as well). Blows to the side of the head produce coup or contrecoup lesions, or both. Irrespective of the site of the impact, the common sites of cerebral contusions are in the frontal and temporal lobes, as illustrated in Fig. 35-4. The inertia of the malleable brain, which causes it to be flung against the side of the skull that was struck, to be pulled away from the contralateral side, and to rotate against bony promontories within the cranial cavity explain these coup-contrecoup contusions. The experimental studies of Ommaya and his colleagues indicate that the effects of linear acceleration of the head are of much less significance than those due to rotation. Relative sparing of the occipital lobes in coup-contrecoup injury is explained by the smooth inner surface of the occipital bones and tentorium.

In addition to contusions there are intracerebral hemorrhages and variable degrees of vasogenic edema, which increase in the first 24 to 48 h. Later, zones of infarction may appear, probably due to vascular spasm, like those of aneurysmal subarachnoid hemorrhage.

CLINICAL MANIFESTATIONS OF HEAD INJURY

The physician first called upon to see a patient who has had a closed (blunt) head injury will generally find the patient in one of three clinical conditions, each of which must be dealt with differently. Usually it is possible to categorize such a patient in this way, by assessing his mental and general neurologic status when first seen and at intervals after the accident.

PATIENTS WHO ARE CONSCIOUS OR ARE RAPIDLY REGAINING CONSCIOUSNESS WHEN FIRST SEEN (MINOR HEAD INJURY)

This is the most frequently encountered form of head injury. Roughly two degrees of disturbed function can be recognized. In one, the patient was not unconscious at all, but only stunned or "saw stars." This injury is insignificant when judged in terms of life and death and brain damage—though as we shall point out further on, there is always the possibility of skull fracture or the later development of an epidural or subdural hematoma. Moreover, the patient is still liable to troublesome posttraumatic symptoms, particularly posttraumatic nervous instability (headache, giddiness, fatigability, insomnia, and nervousness) which may appear soon after or within a few days of the injury. In the second instance, consciousness was temporarily abolished for a few seconds or minutes, viz., the patient was concussed. When such patients are first seen, recovery may already be complete, or they may be in one of the stages of recovery described above. Even though mentally clear these patients may have an amnesia for events immediately preceding and following the injury. Thereafter, as in the first group of patients, headache and other symptoms of posttraumatic nervous instability may develop and hysterical reactions may occur in high-strung individuals.

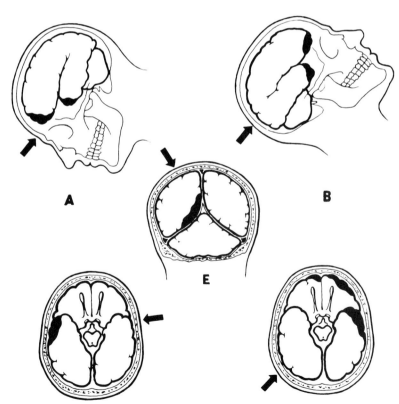

Figure 35-3

Mechanisms of cerebral contusion. Arrows indicate point of application and direction of force; black areas indicate location of contusion. A. Frontotemporal contusion consequent to frontal injury. B. Frontotemporal contusion following occipital injury. C. Contusion of temporal lobe due to contralateral injury. D. Frontotemporal contusion due to injury to opposite temporo-occipital region. E. Diffuse mesial temporo-occipital contusion due to blow on vertex. (From Courville)

In cases of this type, there is little need of a neurologic consultation and hospitalization is not required, providing that a responsible family member is available to report any change in the clinical state. Whether to obtain films of the head and neck is an unresolved problem. In our litigious society, the physician is inclined to do so. If there is no fracture and the patient is mentally clear, Jennett estimates there is only 1 chance in 1,000 of developing an intracranial hemorrhage. This increases to 1 in 30 in patients with a fracture.

These minor and seemingly trivial head injuries may sometimes be followed by a number of puzzling and worrisome clinical phenomena, some insignificant, others serious and indicative of a pathologic process other than concussion. The latter are described below. When they occur, a neurologic or neurosurgical consultation is indicated.

Delayed Collapse after Head Injury Following an accident the injured person, after walking about and seeming to be normal, may turn pale and fall unconscious to the ground. Recovery occurs within a few seconds or minutes. This is a vasodepressor syncopal attack, related to pain and emotional upset, and differs in no way from syncope that follows pain and fright without injury. Such syncopal attacks also occur with injuries that spare the head, but with head injury they become more difficult to interpret.

Denny-Brown has described a more severe type of delayed posttraumatic collapse. The patient appears to be recovering from a blow to the head, which may simply have dazed him or caused a brief period of unconsciousness, when suddenly, after a period of several minutes to hours, he collapses and becomes unresponsive. The most disquieting feature of this clinical state is a marked bradycardia, which, coupled with the lucid interval, raises the specter of an evolving epidural hemorrhage (actually, bradycardia is a late and inconstant sign of epidural bleeding). However, intracranial pressure is not raised, the disorder fails to develop further, and following a brief period of restlessness, vomiting, and headache, the patient recovers completely over a period of several days. Denny-Brown has suggested that this form of delayed posttraumatic collapse is due to a contusion of the medulla, but how this explains the sequence of clinical events is not clear. The authors believe it to be a severe form of vagal syncope.

Drowsiness, Headache, and Confusion This syndrome occurs most often in children who after a concussive or nonconcussive head injury seem not to be themselves. They lie down, are drowsy, complain of headache, and may vomit—symptoms that raise the suspicion of an epidural hemorrhage. There may be minor alterations in the EEG. The intravenous administration of 5 percent glucose and water is particularly dangerous in children with this type

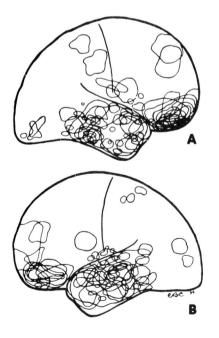

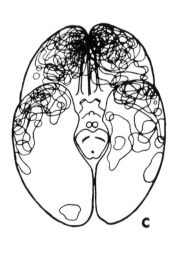

Figure 35-4

Composite drawing showing size and location of contusions found in a series of 40 consecutive cases. The tendency to localize in the subfrontal and temporal regions is clearly indicated. (From Courville.)

of injury and in more serious ones, because it may induce water intoxication and diffuse cerebral edema. Under these circumstances, there is an excessive excretion of antidiuretic hormone causing retention of water. These symptoms subside after a few hours, attesting to the benign nature of the condition.

Occasionally a migraine attack may be induced by a blow to the head, and this can be perplexing for a few hours, especially if it is the first attack of migraine in a child.

Transient Traumatic Paraplegia or Blindness With falls or blows on top of the head, both legs may become temporarily weak and numb with bilateral Babinski signs and possibly sphincteric incontinence. Blows to the occiput may cause temporary blindness. The symptoms disappear after a few hours. It seems unlikely that these transient symptoms represent a direct localized concussive effect, caused either by indentation of skull against the brain or movement of these parts of the brain against the inner table of the skull. A concussion of the cervical portion of the spinal cord is another suggested but improbable mechanism of transient paraplegia. Possibly the blindness and the paraplegia, which are usually followed by a throbbing vascular type of headache, represent a migrainous type of vascular change provoked by the trauma.

Delayed Hemiplegia or Coma Most of the examples we have seen were male adolescents or young adults who some hours after a relatively minor athletic or road injury developed a massive hemiplegia, hemianesthesia, homonymous hemianopia, or aphasia (with left-sided lesions). Arteriography may reveal a dissecting aneurysm of the internal carotid artery. In other instances, particularly after a blow to the neck, a mural thrombus forms in the carotid, which, in turn, may shed an embolus to the anterior or middle cerebral artery. In yet other instances, the hemiplegia has no explanation other than the blow to the head. The other causes of delayed hemiplegia and coma are an acute epidural or subdural hematoma, and in more severe injuries, an intracerebral hemorrhage (occasionally from a preexistent AVM) or cerebral venous thrombosis. With fractures of large bones there may be, after 24 to 72 h, an acute onset of pulmonary symptoms (dyspnea and hyperpnea) followed by coma with or without focal signs; this sequence is due to cerebral fat embolism, first of the lungs and then of the brain.

Posttraumatic Nervous Instability See further on, under "Sequelae of Severe Head Injury."

Concussion Complicated by Serious Cerebral Damage In the purely concussive syndrome one is jus-

tified in assuming that the patient has suffered no serious cerebral contusion, no subarachnoid or intracerebral hemorrhage, or brain swelling. The EEG, if taken when the patient is first seen, is normal, as is the CSF. The skull is fractured in only a small proportion of such cases. If the fracture is in the calvarium it is of little significance. Fractures at the base are associated with damage to cranial nerves and other structures, as described earlier in this chapter.

On rare occasions, a patient who is regaining consciousness when first seen, and who seems at first to belong in the category of minor head injury, will prove to have more serious cerebral damage. While under observation such a patient may speak or respond to commands to some extent, but later slip back into coma. Here the resemblance to a pure concussive state ends, for the period of initial coma in such cases is usually prolonged (more than 5 min), and mental clarity is not fully regained. Moreover, the CSF may be bloody and under increased pressure. Contusions, swelling of brain tissue, and hemorrhage may be demonstrated by CT and MRI. For these reasons, this type of case falls into the category of head injury described below.

PATIENTS WHO ARE AND HAVE BEEN COMATOSE FROM THE TIME OF HEAD INJURY

Here the central problem, so ably set forth by Symonds, is the relationship between concussion and contusion. Since consciousness is abolished immediately upon receipt of the head injury, one can hardly doubt the existence of concussion in such cases, but when hours and days pass without consciousness being regained, the other half of the definition of concussion, viz., that the paralysis of cerebral function be transitory, is abnegated. Moreover, when the pathologic data in such cases are examined carefully, there is almost invariably evidence of increased intracranial pressure, and of cerebral bruises, lacerations, subarachnoid hemorrhage, zones of infarction, and scattered intracerebral hemorrhages, both at the point of injury (coup) and on the opposite side (contrecoup), in the corpus callosum, and between these points, along the *line of force* of the injury. Hemorrhages and foci of necrosis are found in the midbrain and upper pons. The tissue around the contusions is swollen, and later the white matter in these regions appears pale in myelin stains. Some blood in the subdural space is not unusual. A major shift of the thalamus and midbrain and a temporal lobe–tentorial pressure cone are frequently present, the latter with creasing of the opposite cerebral peduncle by the free margin of the tentorium and secondary midbrain hemorrhages and zones of necrosis (page 515). The conclusion that prolongation of coma and death are due to the contusive complications seems quite logical. Surely they are not part of pure concussion in which obvious and irreversible lesions do not occur.

There may be even greater difficulty in separating the effects of concussion and contusion on the basis of the clinical facts. We have already pointed out that patients with craniocerebral injuries that have caused prolonged coma, bloody CSF, unilateral or focal cerebral signs, and EEG abnormalities may hover on the brink of death for a time and then slowly recover. Moreover, such patients may sometimes be restored to a level of normal or near normal neurologic function. The question then is how the patient could have recovered from seemingly irreversible cerebral contusions. Symonds interprets the prolonged coma as a manifestation of a particularly severe concussion and questions whether rapid reversibility is a valid criterion of the concussive state. While agreeing that there must be different degrees of concussive paralysis of cerebral function and that there is no way of deciding at what point concussive coma ceases and gives way to contusive coma, the authors would point out that the pathologic processes of contusion and hemorrhage also have a certain reversibility. If the latter are not too extensive, and if there are no hypoxic-hypotensive effects, and if the upper brainstem is not damaged by direct injury or secondarily by a temporal lobe pressure cone, a few surface lesions would not be expected to cause severe and lasting cerebral defects. We prefer to believe that in states of protracted cerebral disorder the injury has produced not only a prolonged concussive effect, but also contusion(s) of the brain. In our opinion it is the latter, with subsequent swelling of tissue, bleeding, herniation and displacement of brainstem, and respiratory disturbances leading to hypoxia and hypotension, that usually account for the fatal effects of head injury and, with survival, for the persistent neurologic deficits.

In this category of serious head injury, where the patient is in coma when first seen by the physician and has been so from the onset, one must always assume that gross pathologic changes in a state of evolution have been superimposed on concussion. Further, the very acuteness of both processes (concussion and contusion) offers promise of reversibility if life-threatening complications can be averted.

Three clinical subgroups can be recognized: one in which cerebral damage and other bodily injuries are incompatible with survival; a second in which improvement sets in within a few days or a week or two, followed by recovery but leaving the patient with residual signs; and a third and relatively small group in which the patients remain permanently comatose, stuporous, or profoundly reduced in their cerebral capacities. Of course there are many degrees of injury that fall between these three arbitrary subgroups.

The first subgroup comprises patients who are so severely injured that life is obviously endangered. When first seen, such a patient may be in a state of shock with subnormal blood pressure, hypothermia, fast, thready pulse, and pale, moist skin. If this state persists along with deep coma, widely dilated fixed pupils, absent eye movements and corneal and pharyngeal reflexes, flaccid limbs, stertorous and irregular respirations or respiratory failure, death usually follows in short order. Once respiration ceases and the EEG becomes isoelectric, the clinical state corresponds to *brain death* as described on page 276. In some of these patients, the blood pressure and respirations regularize, and the degree of cerebral injury can then be evaluated over a period of hours and days by observing the depth of coma, and the temperature, pulse, and blood pressure. Deep coma with subnormal temperature and rising pulse rate are grave prognostic signs as are a rapidly rising temperature and pulse rate with rapid and irregular respirations. In some fatal cases the temperature continues to rise until the end when there is circulatory collapse.

One form of severe cerebral injury consists of direct midbrain-subthalamic hemorrhages without temporal lobe–tehtorial herniation. Clinically the patient is immediately comatose with midposition or enlarged unreactive pupils, impaired or absent oculocephalic reflexes, extensor posturing on painful stimulation, and flaccid limbs. Small linear or rounded hemorrhages are seen in a nonenhanced scan. Evidently these hemorrhages are consequent upon rotational forces in the upper brainstem.

In this category of cerebral injury, where the patients survive for only a few hours or days, postmortem examination almost invariably discloses cerebral contusion, focal brain swelling, hemorrhage, and necrosis of tissue. Tearing of bridging veins allows blood to seep into the subdural space. In 50 consecutive autopsies of such cases summarized in Rowbotham's excellent monograph, all but two showed macroscopic changes. The lesions in these cases consisted of surface contusions (48 percent), lacerations of the cerebral cortex (28 percent), subarachnoid hemorrhage (72 percent), subdural hematoma (15 percent), extradural hemorrhage (20 percent), and skull fractures (72 percent). As a rule, several of these changes are found in the same patient. Moreover, trauma of extracranial organs and tissues is frequent. In one series of 50 fatal head injuries, there were associated fractures of the limbs in 21 percent, chest injuries in 19 percent, abdominal injuries in 13 percent, and ruptured viscera in a few patients. These extracerebral injuries obviously contribute to the fatal outcome. Widespread axonal injury, manifested in silver stained sections by torn fibers, end bulbs, microglial stars, and wallerian degeneration, may be found in places in the central and subcortical white matter. Strich, who made the early observation of these changes, considers them to be of basic importance and the explanation of immediate and prolonged coma. They were confirmed by Adams et al and Gennarelli et al, the latter group working with subhuman primates. In the authors' pathologic material such changes are readily verified but they tend to be focal, in regions near hemorrhages, contusions, and ischemic lesions. The latter are frequent in the brains of patients who survive for several days in coma (Graham et al).

In respect to the second subgroup, i.e., the relatively less severe and seldom fatal head injuries, all gradations in tempo and degree of recovery may be observed. In the least severely injured of this group, recovery of consciousness begins in a few hours, although there may be a relapse within the first day or two as the contused brain tissue swells. The CSF is usually bloody. Eventually recovery may be complete, but the period of traumatic amnesia covers a span of several days or weeks. Regarding the duration of the concussive effects, it should be repeated that penetrating types of injuries and depressed fractures may occasionally injure the brain without causing concussion at all, but here we are considering only the blunt, nonpenetrating head injuries.

In the more severely injured of this group, the temperature, pulse, and respirations, although slightly elevated, tend to become stable within a few days, and not long thereafter the level of awareness and responsiveness improves slightly. Still there is danger of a rapid and fatal rise in temperature even after the second and third day. Once the patient begins to speak, there is reasonable certainty of progressive improvement. However, improvement may be distressingly slow, and the patient may remain stuporous or barely arousable for days on end or even several weeks. A substantial risk of developing aspiration pneumonia, gastric hemorrhage, and epidural and subdural hemorrhage continues for 2 to 3 weeks.

In this foregoing group, the sequence of clinical events is the same as that described under concussion, except that their duration is more protracted. Stupor gives way to a confusional state that may last for weeks, and it may for a variable period be associated with aggressive behavior and uncooperativeness (traumatic delirium). The period of traumatic amnesia is proportionately longer than in the less severely injured. It is during the period of recovering consciousness that focal neurologic signs (hemiparesis, aphasia, abulia, etc.) become most obvious, though some of these signs may have been discerned in the comatose state. Once the patient improves to the point of being able to converse, he or she is slow in thinking, unstable in

emotional reactions, and faulty in judgment—a state sometimes called "traumatic psychosis" or "traumatic dementia."

Finally there is that relatively small, distressing group of severely brain-injured patients in whom the vital signs become normal, but who never regain consciousness. As the weeks pass, the prospects become more bleak. Such a patient may still emerge from coma after 6 to 8 weeks and make a surprisingly good though usually incomplete recovery, but such instances are very rare. Some of those who survive for long periods may open their eyes, but they betray no evidence of seeing or recognizing even the closest members of their family. They do not speak, or they say only a few words; emotional reactions are inappropriate; food placed in the mouth may be chewed and swallowed ("persistent vegetative state," see page 276). Hemiplegia or quadriplegia with varying degrees of decerebrate or decorticate postures are usually demonstrable. Finally, life is mercifully terminated by some medical complication. In 10 or more such cases that have come to autopsy, the authors have found old contusions and hemorrhages and a few scattered focal cerebral lesions with wallerian degeneration in appropriate regions of the brain; but most importantly, there has been damage to one or other cerebral peduncle and old hemorrhages and zones of necrosis in the subthalamus and tegmentum of the upper brainstem. The latter changes may be primary, or secondary to temporal lobe–tentorial herniation. If primary (due to impact and without increased intracranial pressure) the signs of brainstem lesions are present immediately after the injury.

Among the patients who remained unconscious from the moment of injury, J. H. Adams and his colleagues, and Strich, Nevin, and others before them, have attributed the protracted coma to hemorrhagic necrosis of the corpus callosum and the dorsolateral quadrant (tegmentum) of the rostral brainstem, in the region of the superior cerebellar peduncles, along with diffuse damage to axons in the descending tracts in the lower brainstem and in parts of the cerebral white matter. These abnormalities are thought to be the direct consequence of trauma (shearing effect) and not secondary effects from brain swelling, anoxia, or temporal lobe herniation and brainstem compression. This contention is supported by the recent experimental observations of Gennarelli et al, who produced coma in monkeys by intense acceleration of the head, followed by abrupt deceleration. In animals subjected to a single episode of head motion in the sagittal or oblique direction, the coma was of short duration (<15 min) and the neuropathologic changes insignificant. However, lateral or coronal head motion resulted in prolonged coma (>6 h) and severe neurologic disability; neuropathologic abnormalities were found in 18 of 26 laterally injured animals and consisted of focal lesions in the corpus callosum and tegmentum of the upper brainstem in the region of the superior cerebellar peduncle, as well as diffuse axonal damage in the cerebral white matter. It is noteworthy that in all of the cases of protracted coma there were lesions in the upper brainstem reticular formation, which the authors believe to be the site of the lesions that cause concussion.

In generalizing about this category of head injury, i.e., patients who are and have been comatose from the time of injury, we have the impression that the effects of contusion, hemorrhage, and brain swelling are most severe about 18 to 36 h after the injury; and, if the patients survive this period, the chances of dying from the complications of craniocerebral trauma (contusions, intracerebral hemorrhage, localized cerebral edema, herniations of the temporal lobe, subdural hemorrhage, hypoxia, and pneumonia) are greatly reduced. The mortality rate of those who reach the hospital in coma is about 20 percent, and most of the deaths occur in the first 12 to 24 h as a result of direct injury to the brain in combination with other nonneurologic injuries. Of those alive at 24 h, the overall mortality falls to 7 to 8 percent; after 48 h, only 1 to 2 percent succumb. As will be emphasized further on, there is evidence that immediate transfer to a critical care unit of a neurosurgical service, where intracranial pressure, cerebral blood flow, and oxygenation are carefully monitored, will improve the chances of survival and of returning to useful life (Ropper et al).

PATIENTS WHO ARE UNCONSCIOUS WHEN FIRST SEEN BUT ARE SAID TO HAVE REGAINED CONSCIOUSNESS AFTER THE ACCIDENT (LUCID INTERVAL)

This group is smaller than the other two, but is of great importance because it includes many patients who are in urgent need of surgical treatment. The initial coma may have lasted only a few minutes, and exceptionally there may have been none at all—in which instance one might wrongly conclude that since there was no concussion there is no possibility of traumatic hemorrhage or other type of brain injury. In other cases there may be a more protracted coma that deepens progressively as the lesions evolve (no lucid interval). The following conditions must be considered in every case of this type.

Acute Epidural Hemorrhage   As a rule, this condition is due to a temporal or parietal fracture with laceration of

the middle meningeal artery and vein. Less often there is a tear in a dural venous sinus. The injury, even when it fractures the skull, may not have produced coma. A typical example is that of a child who has fallen from a bicycle or swing or has suffered some other hard blow to the head and was only momentarily unconscious. A few hours or a day later (exceptionally, with venous bleeding, the interval may be several days or a week), headache of increasing severity develops, with vomiting, drowsiness, confusion, aphasia, seizures (which may be one-sided), hemiparesis with slightly increased tendon reflexes, and a Babinski sign. As coma develops, the hemiparesis may give way to bilateral spasticity of the limbs and Babinski signs. Respirations become deeper and stertorous, then shallow and irregular, and finally cease. The pulse is often slow (below 60 beats per minute) and bounding, with a concomitant rise in systolic blood pressure (Cushing effect). The pupil may dilate on the side of the hematoma. The CSF is usually under increased pressure, though normal pressures do not exclude the possibility of an epidural hematoma. The fluid may be clear or bloody, depending on whether or not there is an associated cerebral contusion or laceration, or subarachnoid hemorrhage. Death, which is almost invariable if the clot is not removed surgically, comes at the end of a comatose period, rarely if ever in a conscious patient, and is due to respiratory arrest. The visualization of a fracture line across the groove of the middle meningeal artery and knowledge of which side of the head was struck (the clot is usually on that side) are of aid in diagnosis and lateralization of the lesion. The CT scan reveals a lens-shaped clot with a smooth inner margin and inward displacement of surface arteries is seen by carotid arteriography (Fig. 35-5). The surgical procedure consists of placement of several burr holes (a single one may miss the clot), drainage, identification of the bleeding vessel, and ligation. The operative results are excellent, except in the cases with extended fractures and laceration of the dural venous sinuses, in which the epidural hematoma may be bilateral rather than unilateral, as it ordinarily is. If coma, bilateral Babinski signs, spasticity, or decerebrate rigidity supervene before operation, the prognosis for life becomes poor. This usually means that temporal lobe herniation and crushing of the midbrain have already occurred.

Acute and Chronic Subdural Hematoma   The problems created by acute and chronic subdural hematomas are so different that they need to be discussed separately. In *acute subdural hematoma*, which may be unilateral or bilateral, there may be a brief lucid interval between the blow to the head and the advent of coma. Or, more often, the patient is comatose from the time of the injury. Frequently the acute subdural hematoma is combined with cerebral contusion and laceration, and the clinical effects of these several lesions are difficult to distinguish; there are

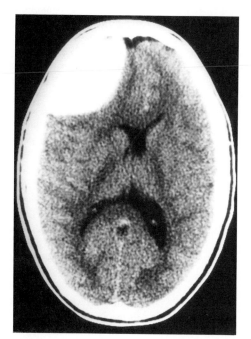

Figure 35-5

Unenhanced CT scan showing acute epidural hematoma with shift of lateral ventricles to opposite side.

some patients in whom it is impossible to state before operation whether the clot is epidural or subdural in location. The CT scan visualizes the clot accurately in about 90 percent of cases. In less acute hematomas the fluid is isodense with the cortex, and its presence is betrayed by a ventricular shift. If bilateral, there is no shift (see Figs. 35-6 and 35-7). Arteriography shows displacement of cerebral arteries inward from the skull. Treatment consists of wide craniotomy to permit control of the bleeding and removal of the clot. The surgical results are less certain than in chronic subdural hematoma. If the clot is too small to explain the coma or other symptoms, there is probably extensive contusion and laceration of the cerebrum. Exceptionally the subdural hematoma forms in the posterior fossa and gives rise to headache, vomiting, pupillary inequality, dysphagia, cranial nerve palsies, and, rarely, stiff neck and ataxia of the trunk and gait, in some combination.

In *chronic subdural hematoma,* the traumatic etiology is less clear. The head injury, especially in elderly persons and in those taking anticoagulant drugs, may be trivial (striking the head against the branch of a tree, or on the mantel of a fireplace during a faint, etc.), and it may have been forgotten. A period of weeks then follows when headaches (not invariable), giddiness, slowness in thinking, confusion, apathy and drowsiness, and rarely a seizure or two are the main symptoms. The initial impression may be that the patient has a vascular lesion or brain tumor or

suffers from drug intoxication or a depressive, senile, or other type of psychosis. As with acute subdural hematoma, the disturbances of mentation and consciousness (drowsiness, inattentiveness, incoherence of thinking and confusion) are more prominent than focal or lateralizing signs, and they may fluctuate. The focal signs usually consist of hemiparesis and rarely of an aphasic disturbance. Homonymous hemianopia, hemiplegia, and hemianesthesia are seldom observed, probably because the geniculocalcarine pathway is deep and not easily compressed; hemiplegia, i.e., complete paralysis of one arm and leg, is usually indicative of a lesion within the cerebral hemisphere, rather than a compressive lesion on its surface, and sensory changes are likely to be overlooked in a stuporous confused patient. An important feature of the hemiparesis is that it may be contralateral or ipsilateral, depending on whether the temporal lobe has herniated through the notch of the tentorium and compressed the contralateral cerebral peduncle against the free edge of the tentorium (false localizing sign; see page 520). As the condition progresses, the patient becomes comatose but often with striking fluctuations of

Figure 35-6

Contrast-enhanced CT scan showing a large, right frontal subdural hematoma of 10 days' duration. Presence of the clot, which is isodense with the cerebral cortex, is betrayed by the marked ventricular shift.

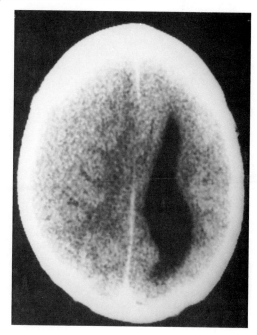

awareness. The ipsilateral pupil dilates (Hutchinson pupillary sign), owing, it is believed, to direct pressure of the herniating temporal lobe upon the oculomotor nerve. The dilated pupil and ptotic eyelid are more reliable indicators of the side of the hematoma than the hemiparesis, though they too may be misleading in certain cases. Convulsions are seen occasionally, most often in alcoholics or in patients with cerebral contusions, but cannot be regarded as a cardinal sign of subdural hematoma. In infants and children, enlargement of the head, vomiting, and convulsions are prominent manifestations of subdural hematoma.

Skull films are seldom helpful and then only when there is a shift of a calcified pineal to one side or an unexpected fracture line. The EEG is usually abnormal bilaterally, sometimes with reduced voltage or electrical silence over the hematoma and high-voltage slow waves over the opposite side, because of the damping effects of the clot and displacement of the brain, respectively. The cortical branches of the middle cerebral artery are separated from the inner surface of skull, and the anterior cerebral artery may be displaced contralaterally in an arteriogram. The CSF may be clear and acellular, bloody, or xantho-

Figure 35-7

Chronic subdural hematomas over both frontal lobes, without shift of the ventricular system. Chronicity results in hypodense appearance.

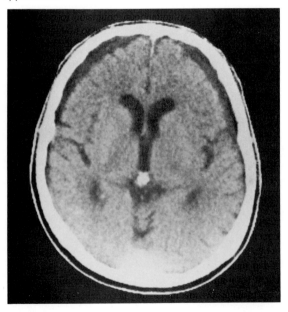

chromic, depending on the presence or absence of recent or old contusions and subarachnoid hemorrhage; the pressure may be elevated, normal, or subnormal. A xanthochromic fluid with relatively low protein content should always raise the suspicion of chronic subdural hematoma. Of all these diagnostic procedures, arteriography and CT scan are the most reliable (Fig. 35-7).

Acute, rapidly evolving subdural hematomas are due to tearing of bridging veins, and symptoms are caused by direct compression of the brain by an expanding clot of fresh blood. Unlike epidural arterial hemorrhage, which is steadily progressive, venous bleeding is usually arrested by the rising intracranial pressure.

The chronic subdural hematoma becomes encysted by fibrous membranes (pseudomembranes) which grow from the dura. Some hematomas—probably the ones in which the initial bleeding was slight (see below)—resorb spontaneously. Others expand slowly and act as space-occupying masses. In 1932, Gardner proposed that the gradual enlargement of the hematoma is due to the accession of fluid, particularly CSF, which is drawn into the hemorrhagic cyst by its increasing osmotic tension, as red blood cells hemolyse and protein is liberated. This hypothesis, which came to be widely accepted, is not supported by the available data. Rabe and his colleagues have demonstrated convincingly that red cell breakdown contributes little, if at all, to the accumulation of fluid in the subdural space. More recently, Weir has shown that there is no significant difference in the osmolalities of fluid samples taken simultaneously from the subdural hematoma, venous blood, and CSF. Why somewhat less than one-half of all subdural hematomas remain solid and nonenlarging and the remainder liquefy and then enlarge, is not known. The experimental observations of Labadie and Glover suggest that the volume of the original clot is a critical factor: the larger its initial size, the more likely that it will enlarge. An inflammatory reaction, triggered by the breakdown products of blood elements in the clot, appears to be an additional stimulus for growth as well as for neomembrane formation. According to Rabe et al, the most important factor in the accumulation of subdural fluid is a pathologic permeability of the capillaries in the outer pseudomembrane. The CSF plays no discernible role in this process, contrary to the original view of Munro and Merritt. In any event, as the hematoma enlarges, the compressive effects increase. Severe cerebral compression and displacement with temporal lobe–tentorial herniation are the usual causes of death.

Treatment consists of placing burr holes and evacuating the clot before deep coma has developed.

Subdural hygroma (a collection of blood and CSF in the subdural space) may form after an injury, as well as after meningitis (in an infant or young child). It is said that a tear of the arachnoid permits bacteria to enter and excite a serous reaction in the subdural space. Subdural hygromas may appear without infection, presumably due to a ball-valve effect of the arachnoidal tear. In the past, subdural hygroma also occurred as a complication of pneumoencephalography. Drowsiness, confusion, irritability, and fever are relieved when the subdural fluid is aspirated or drained. Shrinkage of the hydrocephalic brain after ventriculoperitoneal shunting is also conducive to the formation of a subdural hematoma or hygroma.

Acute Contusional Swelling This complication is observed in patients who had suffered a moderately severe injury and were unconscious for more than 5 min at the onset. They then improve to the point where they are capable of purposive movements of a protective kind though still confused, mute, and often unresponsive to command; or they may even have begun to respond to forceful commands or to answer a few simple questions when they rapidly relapse into stupor or light coma, raising the suspicion of brain compression from an epidural hemorrhage. Actually, a true lucid interval of normal consciousness has not occurred. However, in the patient with uncomplicated contusion, relapse is seldom profound, and the stupor or light coma can be reversed by the use of dehydrating measures, suggesting that brain swelling is an important pathogenetic factor. The plantar reflex may be extensor on one or both sides and, if unilateral, is always on the side of a hemiparesis. When the abnormal plantar reflexes are not part of a unilateral or bilateral hemiparesis, they usually become flexor by the time the traumatic confusion clears. Pulse and temperature may be slightly elevated for several days. The CSF is often bloody and under increased pressure. [In a series of 200 head injuries, half of which were of a mild type, Russell found 32 with more than 1000 red cells per cubic millimeter. All of the latter had some stiffness of the neck on forward flexion. If there was much blood (more than 100,000 red cells per cubic millimeter), the patient was either comatose or stuporous.]

If improvement resumes after hours or a day or two, one can be assured that serious cerebral compression from dural clots or a delayed cerebral hemorrhage (see below) has not occurred. The threat of temporal lobe–tentorial herniation continues for some days and should this happen the outlook is bleak.

Traumatic Cerebral Hemorrhage Acute, massive brain hemorrhage may develop as late as a week or more after a moderate to severe head injury (spätapoplexie), but seldom is there a true lucid interval. This condition, the pathogenesis of which is not well understood, occurs mainly in the elderly. The clinical picture is similar to that of hypertensive brain hemorrhage (deepening coma with hemiplegia, a

dilating pupil, bilateral Babinski signs, stertorous and irregular respirations). The problem that sometimes cannot be solved, even at postmortem examination, is whether there had been a fall, followed after an interval by the common variety of primary intracerebral hemorrhage, or whether a *delayed hemorrhage* into traumatized brain tissue occurred. Of course, slow venous bleeding might permit a relatively lucid interval of 2 to 3 days between injury and the symptoms of the cerebral hemorrhage, but this is not the explanation of most of the cases. Coma or confusion, if present from the time of the injury, may obscure the signs of the intracerebral hemorrhage. Craniotomy with evacuation of the clot has given a successful result in a few cases. The wider application of CT scans at intervals after the injury should help elucidate the pathogenesis and, of course, facilitate diagnosis.

"PUNCH-DRUNK ENCEPHALOPATHY" (DEMENTIA PUGILISTICA)

The cumulative effects of repeated cerebral injuries, observed in boxers who had engaged in many contests over a long period of time, constitute a type of head injury that is difficult to classify. What is referred to is the development, after many years in the ring (sometimes toward the end of the boxer's career, more often a number of years after retirement), of a state of forgetfulness, slowness in thinking and other signs of dementia, and dysarthric speech. Movements are slow, stiff and uncertain, especially those involving the legs, and there is a shuffling, wide-based, unsteady gait. Often there is a parkinsonian syndrome (found in 20 of the 52 cases that Roberts abstracted from the literature up to 1969), and sometimes a moderately disabling ataxia. The plantar reflexes may be extensor on one or both sides. The EEG shows slow waves of theta and sometimes of delta type. Pneumoencephalograms in these patients had shown dilated lateral ventricles and also, according to Spillane, a cavum septi pellucidi, a finding that distinguished the punch-drunk state from other forms of cerebral atrophy. The clinical syndrome has been analyzed by Roberts, who found it present to some degree in 37 of 224 professional boxers whom he had examined. More recent studies have shown that about one-half of all professional boxers, both active and retired, have CT changes (ventricular dilatation and or sulcal widening, cavum septi pellucidi) and that these abnormalities are related to the number of bouts (Ross et al; Casson et al).

A thorough pathologic study of this disorder has been made by Corsellis and his associates. They examined the brains of 15 retired boxers who had shown the punch-drunk syndrome and identified a group of cerebral changes that appear to explain the clinical findings. Mild to moderate enlargement of the lateral ventricles and thinning of the corpus callosum were found in all cases. Also, practically all of them showed a greatly widened cavum septi pellucidi and the septal leaves were grossly fenestrated. Readily identified areas of glial scarring were situated on the inferior surface of the cerebellar cortex, most marked in the folia around the groove formed by the sloping edge of the foramen magnum. In these areas, and well beyond them, Purkinje cells were lost and the granule cell layer was somewhat thinned. Surprisingly, cerebral cortical contusions were found in only a few cases. Notably absent, also, was evidence of previous hemorrhage. Eleven of the 15 cases showed varying degrees of loss of pigmented cells of the substantia nigra and locus ceruleus, and many of the cells that remained showed the Alzheimer neurofibrillary change; Lewy bodies were not observed, however. The neurofibrillary changes were scattered diffusely through the cerebral cortex and brainstem, but were most prominent in the medial temporal gray matter. Noteworthy was the absence or almost complete absence of senile plaques.

The pathogenesis of the punch-drunk state remains unclear. Meningeal fibrosis and hydrocephalus from repeated small subarachnoid hemorrhages is an unlikely explanation but cannot be excluded.

PENETRATING WOUNDS OF THE HEAD (Missiles and Fragments)

All the descriptions in the preceding pages apply to blunt, nonpenetrating injuries of the skull and their effects on the brain. The disorders included in this section are more the concern of the neurosurgeon than the neurologist. In the past, most injuries of penetrating type were the preoccupation of the military surgeon, but with the increasing amount of violent crime in Western society they have become commonplace on the emergency wards of general hospitals.

Missile injuries, in civilian life, refer essentially to injuries caused by bullets fired from rifles or handguns at high velocities. Air is compressed in front of the bullet so that it has an explosive effect upon entering tissue and causes damage for a considerable distance around the missile tract. *Fragments* or *shrapnel* are pieces of exploding shells, grenades, or bombs, and are the usual causes of penetrating cranial injuries in wartime. The cranial wounds that result from missiles and shrapnel have been classified by Purvis as (1) tangential injuries, with scalp lacerations, depressed skull fractures, and meningeal and cerebral lacerations, (2) penetrating injuries with indriven metal particles and hair, skin, and bone fragments, and (3) through-and-through wounds.

If the brain is penetrated at the lower levels of the brainstem, death is instantaneous from respiratory and cardiac arrest. Fully 80 percent of patients with through-and-through injuries die at once or within a few minutes. If vital centers are untouched, the immediate problem is intracranial bleeding and rising intracranial pressure from swelling of the traumatized brain tissue. There is also bleeding from the scalp wound, but this can be staunched without difficulty, and circulatory collapse can be counteracted if the patient reaches the emergency ward alive.

Once the initial complications are dealt with, the surgical problems, as outlined by Meirowsky, are reduced to three: (1) prevention of infection by rapid and radical (definitive) debridement, followed by the administration of broad spectrum antibiotics, (2) control of increased intracranial pressure and shift of midline structures by removal of clots of blood and the vigorous administration of mannitol or other dehydrating agents and dexamethasone, and (3) the prevention of life-threatening systemic complications.

When first seen, the majority of patients with penetrating cerebral lesions are comatose. Despite the fact that a small metal fragment may penetrate the skull without causing concussion, this is not true of high-velocity missiles. In a series of 132 cases of the latter type, analyzed by Frazier and Ingham, consciousness was retained at the time of injury in only 22; of those patients who were unconscious, the depth and duration of coma seemed to depend upon the degree of cerebral necrosis, edema, and hemorrhage. Upon emerging from coma the patient passes through states of stupor, confusion, and amnesia, as do patients with severe closed head injuries. Headache, vomiting, vertigo, pallor, sweating, slowness of pulse, and elevation of blood pressure are other common findings. Focal or focal and generalized seizures occur in the early phase of the injury in some 15 to 20 percent of cases.

Recovery may take many months. Frazier and Ingham comment on the "loss of memory, slow cerebration, indifference, mild depression, inability to concentrate, fatigability, nervous irritability, vasomotor and cardiac instability, frequent seizures, headaches and giddiness," all reminiscent of the contusion syndrome of blunt head injury. Every possible combination of focal cerebral symptoms may be caused by such lesions, and there is no point in detailing them further. Useful references are the articles by Feiring and Davidoff, and also those of Russell, and of Teuber, listed at the end of this chapter.

Epilepsy is the most troublesome sequela. Ascroft

and Caviness, in reviewing World War II cases, found that approximately half of all patients with wounds that had penetrated the dura eventually developed epilepsy, most often focal in nature; the figures of Caveness, for Korean War veterans, are about the same.

CSF rhinorrhea may occur as an acute manifestation of a penetrating injury that produces a fracture through the frontal, ethmoid, or sphenoid bones. Cairns listed these acute cases as a separate group in his classification of CSF rhinorrheas, the others being (1) a delayed form after craniocerebral injury, (2) a form that follows sinus and cranial surgery, and (3) a spontaneous variety.

Pneumoencephalocele (aerocele), i.e., air entering the cerebral subarachnoid space or ventricles spontaneously or as a result of sneezing or blowing the nose, indicates an opening from the paranasal sinus through the dura. Feiring and Davidoff cite cases where the air actually entered the cerebral tissue and produced focal signs. This the authors have never seen.

CRUSHING INJURIES OF THE SKULL

Aside from the absence of concussion, these relatively rare cerebral lesions present no special clinical features or neurologic problems not already discussed.

BIRTH INJURIES

These involve a unique combination of physical forces and circulatory-oxygenation factors and are discussed separately in Chap. 44.

SEQUELAE OF SEVERE HEAD INJURY

The signs of focal brain disease, whether due to closed head injuries or to open and penetrating ones, tend always to ameliorate as the months pass. A hemiplegia is often reduced to a minimal hemiparesis or to an ineptitude of voluntary motor function with exaggerated reflexes and an equivocal Babinski sign on that side, and an aphasia to a stuttering or hesitant paraphasia or dysnomia that is not disabling except to a professional person, speaker, or writer. Many of the signs of brainstem disease (cranial nerve dysfunction and ataxia) improve also, usually within the first 6 months after injury (Jennett and Bond), and often to a surprising extent. Most of the patients who were in coma for many hours or days, i.e., those with severe brain injuries, are left with memory impairment and other cognitive defects and with personality changes. These may be the only lasting sequelae. According to Jennett and Bond, these mental and personality changes are a greater handicap than focal neurologic ones in social adjustment. In open head wounds and penetrating brain injuries, Grafman found

that the magnitude of tissue loss and location of the lesion both affected the outcome.

POSTTRAUMATIC EPILEPSY

Epilepsy is the most common sequela of craniocerebral trauma, with an overall incidence of about 5 percent in patients with closed head injuries and of 50 percent in patients who had sustained a compound skull fracture and wound of the brain. The basis is nearly always a contusion or laceration of the cortex. As one might expect, the risk of developing posttraumatic epilepsy is related to the severity of the head injury. In the cohort of 2747 head-injured patients described by Annegers et al, the risk of seizures after severe head injury was 7 percent within 1 year and 11.5 percent in 5 years; after moderate injury (skull fracture or $\frac{1}{2}$ to 24 h of unconsciousness or amnesia) the risk fell to 0.7 and 1.6 percent. After mild injury the incidence of seizures was not significantly greater than in the general population. The likelihood of epilepsy is said to be greater in parietal and posterior frontal lesions, but it may arise from lesions in any area of the cerebral cortex.

The interval between the head injury and the first seizure varies greatly. A small number of patients have a generalized seizure within moments of the injury ("immediate epilepsy"). Four to 5 percent of hospitalized head-injured individuals have one or more seizures within the first week of their injury ("early epilepsy"). Immediate seizures have a good prognosis as far as recurrence is concerned; on the other hand, late epilepsy is significantly more common in patients who experienced early epilepsy (Jennett). In medical writings the term posttraumatic epilepsy usually refers to *late epilepsy*, i.e., to seizures that develop several weeks or months after the head injury (1 to 3 months in most cases). Approximately 6 months after injury, half the patients who will develop epilepsy have had their first attack, and by the end of 2 years the figure rises to 80 percent (Walker). The interval between head injury and development of seizures is said to be longer in children. The longer the interval, the less certain one is of its relation to the traumatic incident. Data derived from a 15-year study of military personnel with severe (penetrating) brain wounds indicate that patients who escape seizures for 1 year after injury can be 75 percent certain of remaining seizure-free; patients without seizures for 2 years can be 90 percent certain, and for 3 years, 95 percent certain. For the less severely injured (mainly closed-head injuries) the corresponding times of assurance are 2 to 6 months, 12 to 17 months, and 21 to 25 months (Weiss et al).

Posttraumatic seizures are either focal in type or generalized with loss of consciousness (grand mal); petit mal is rarely if ever due to trauma. The significance of the different patterns of focal seizures, which vary according to the location of the lesion, has been worked out in detail by Penfield and his associates (page 253). The frequency of seizures in any given patient varies widely; some patients have only a few, others many, with occasional flurries of status epilepticus. The EEG is of value in diagnosis; a focus of spike or sharp waves is the characteristic finding.

Posttraumatic seizures tend to decrease in frequency as the years pass, and some patients (10 to 30 percent, according to Caveness) eventually stop having them. Individuals who have early attacks (within a week of injury) are more likely to have a complete remission of their seizures than those whose attacks begin a year or so after injury. A low frequency of attacks is another favorable prognostic sign. Alcoholism has an adverse effect on this seizure state. We have observed some 25 patients with posttraumatic epilepsy, in whom seizures had ceased altogether for several years, but then recurred, only in relation to drinking. In these patients the seizures were precipitated by a weekend or only one evening of heavy drinking, and occurred as a rule not when the patient was intoxicated but in the sobering-up period.

Usually the seizures can be controlled by anticonvulsant medications, and relatively few are recalcitrant to the point of requiring excision of the epileptic focus. The surgical results vary according to the methods of selection and techniques of operation. Under the best of neurosurgical conditions, with careful selection of cases, Rasmussen (and Penfield) have been able to eradicate seizures in approximately 50 percent of cases by excision of the focus.

The use of phenytoin or other anticonvulsant drug to prevent the first seizure and subsequent epilepsy has its proponents and opponents. In one study, fewer patients taking phenytoin had developed seizures at the end of the first year than a placebo group, but a year after medication was discontinued the incidence was the same in the two groups. In the United Kingdom, severe head injury is a contraindication to driving for a year because of the risk of a first seizure.

POSTTRAUMATIC NERVOUS INSTABILITY

This troublesome and frequent sequela of head injury has been alluded to above as well as in Chap. 9, on headache. This disorder has also been called the *postconcussion syndrome*, *posttraumatic headache*, *traumatic neurasthenia* (Symonds), and *traumatic psychasthenia* (Mapother). Headache is the central symptom, either generalized or localized to the part that had been struck. It is variously described as an aching, throbbing, pounding, stabbing, pressing, or band-like pain and is remarkable for its variability. The intensification of the headache and other symptoms by mental and physical effort, straining, stooping, and emotional excitement has already been mentioned; rest and quiet tend to relieve them. Such headaches may present a major obstacle to convalescence. Dizziness, another prominent symptom, is usually not a true vertigo but a giddiness or light-headedness. The patient may feel unsteady, dazed, weak, or faint. However, a certain number of patients describe symptoms that are consonant with labyrinthine disorder. They report that objects in the environment move momentarily, and that looking upward or to the side may cause a sense of unbalance; labyrinthine tests may show either hyporeactivity, or the results may be normal. McHugh finds a high incidence of minor abnormalities by electronystagmography both in concussed patients and in those suffering from whiplash injuries of the neck, but some of the data we find difficult to interpret. Exceptionally, vertigo is accompanied by diminished excitability of both the labyrinth and the cochlea (deafness), and one may assume the existence of direct injury to the nerve or end organ.

The patient with posttraumatic nervous instability is intolerant of noise, emotional excitement, and crowds. Tenseness, restlessness, inability to concentrate, a feeling of nervousness, fatigue, worry, apprehension, and an inability to tolerate the usual amount of alcohol complete the clinical picture. In contrast to this multiplicity of subjective symptoms, memory and other intellectual functions show little or no impairment on detailed testing. The resemblance of these symptoms to those of anxiety and depression is at once apparent. The syndrome, once established, may persist for months or even years, but usually the symptoms lessen as time passes. Strangely, it is almost unknown in children. Its intensity and duration are augmented by compensation problems and litigation, suggesting a psychopathologic factor.

EXTRAPYRAMIDAL AND CEREBELLAR DISORDERS

The question of *posttraumatic Parkinson syndrome* has been discussed many times, usually with the conclusion that it does not exist. Most such patients probably had paralysis agitans or postencephalitic parkinsonism that was brought to light by the head injury. Cerebellar ataxia and extrapyramidal signs are rare consequences of cranial trauma unless the latter was complicated by cerebral anoxia. When cerebellar ataxia is due to the trauma itself, it is frequently unilateral and the result of injury to the superior cerebellar peduncle. An ataxia of gait may reflect the presence of a communicating hydrocephalus. The one exception to these statements is the punch-drunk syndrome.

POSTTRAUMATIC HYDROCEPHALUS

This is a not uncommon complication of severe head injury. Intermittent headaches, vomiting, confusion, and drowsiness are the initial manifestations. Later there are mental dullness, apathy, and psychomotor retardation, by which time the CSF pressure may have fallen to a normal level (normal-pressure hydrocephalus). Postmortem examinations have demonstrated an adhesive basilar arachnoiditis. Since a similar syndrome is observed occasionally after the rupture of a saccular aneurysm with massive subarachnoid hemorrhage, the same mechanisms, i.e., blocking of the aqueduct and fourth ventricle by blood clot and basilar meningeal fibrosis, may also be operative in traumatic hydrocephalus. Response to ventriculoperitoneal shunt may be dramatic. Zander and Foroglou have had extensive experience with this condition and have written informatively about it.

POSTTRAUMATIC PSYCHIATRIC DISORDERS

In all patients with cerebral concussive injury there will be a gap in memory (traumatic amnesia) spanning a variable period from before the accident to some point following it. This gap is permanent and is filled in only by what the patient is told. In addition, as has been stated, in the introduction to this section, some degree of impairment of higher cortical function may persist for weeks (or be permanent) after moderate to severe head injuries, even after the patient has reached the stage of forming continuous memories. During the period of deranged mentation, the memory disorder is the most prominent feature so that the state resembles the alcoholic form of Korsakoff psychosis. Pfeifer-Nietleben asserts that this amnesic state is a constant feature of one phase of every prolonged traumatic mental disorder, but to the authors it merely emphasizes the ease with which memory can be tested. Such patients rarely confabulate and usually have an inability to register events and information, an abnormality not ordinarily observed in the pure amnesic-confabulatory syndrome. Apart from disorientation in place and time there is also a defect in perception and in the ability to synthesize perceptual data. Judgment is impaired, sometimes severely. A perseverative tendency interferes with action and thought.

These difficulties of obvious organic type were described in detail by Schilder and by Goldstein. The latter author, in his search for underlying psychologic mechanisms, settled on the following factors: (1) a raised threshold of sensory excitation (defective perception), (2) a persistence or perseveration of response to any stimulus that surpasses the threshold and causes excitation, (3) undue influence on the organism by all external factors, i.e., distractibility, and (4) difficulty in separating figure from background. The latter failure, according to Goldstein, is the most important, for in every perception and every thought process, there must be the selection of a "figure" and the exclusion of all other elements. The authors find this formulation to be an interesting way of phrasing the distractibility, perseveration, and defects in perception, but fail to see the reason for reducing all mental activity to disturbance in figure-background relationships or (in another favorite Goldstein idiom) for reversion from an abstract (higher level) mode of thinking to a lower and more concrete level.

There are other mental and behavioral abnormalities of a more subtle type that remain as sequelae to cerebral injury. As the stage of posttraumatic dementia recedes, the patient may find it impossible to work or to adjust to the family situation. Such patients continue to be abnormally abrupt, argumentative, stubborn, opinionated, and suspicious. Unlike the traumatic mental disorder described above, in which there is a certain uniformity, these traits vary with the patient's age, constitution, past experience, and environmental stress. Extremes of age are important. The most prominent behavioral abnormality in children, described by Bowman et al and by Black et al, is a change in character. They become impulsive, heedless of the consequences of their actions, and lacking in moral sense—much like those who have recovered from encephalitis lethargica. Some adolescents or young adults show the general lack of inhibition and impulsivity of frontal lobe disease. In the older person it is the impairment of intellectual functions that assumes prominence. Even more important is the constitution of the patient. Stable, athletic, tough-fibered individuals take a concussive injury in stride while the sensitive, nervous, complaining types may be so overwhelmed by such an accident that they are unable to expel the incident from their minds. Environmental stress assumes importance as well, for if too much is demanded of the patient soon after injury, irritability, insomnia, and anxiety are enhanced. A calm, supportive environment that does not tax mental energies is conducive to a smooth convalescence.

The tendency is for all such symptoms to subside slowly, though not always completely, even in those in whom an accident has provoked a frank outburst of psychosis, as may happen to a manic-depressive, a paranoid schizophrenic, or a neurotic. These forms of "traumatic insanity" were carefully analyzed for the first time by Adolf Meyer.

TREATMENT

PATIENTS WHO WERE ONLY CONCUSSED

Patients with an uncomplicated concussive injury, who have already regained consciousness by the time they are seen in hospital, pose few difficulties in management. They should be detained in hospital until appropriate examinations (CT scans, skull films, etc.) have been made and proved to be negative, until the capacity to make consecutive memories has been regained, and arrangements have been made for observation by the family of signs of possible delayed complications (subdural and epidural hemorrhage, intracerebral bleeding, and edema).

The patients with persistent complaints of headache, dizziness, and nervousness, the syndrome that we have designated as *posttraumatic nervous instability*, are most difficult to manage. Three subgroups can be discerned:

1. A group in which the accident has provoked anxiety or an anxious-depressive reaction. Compensation factors loom large in this group especially for the patient whose circumstances are marginal and who is uncertain of a job and must care for dependents. Such a person is often willing to persist in illness even if compensated at a level considerably below his or her earning capacity, if it provides a modicum of security. Obviously, we are dealing here with matters that have little relation to the physical factors involved in cerebral trauma.

2. A group of patients in whom the *premorbid personality* was of a neurotic or depressive type. The injury to the brain is but one more factor in decompensating a tenuous social and occupational adjustment.

3. A small number of patients, obviously the more severely injured, who upon close examination are found to be *still suffering from a personality change* and *subtle impairments of cognitive function,* i.e., traumatic psychosis or dementia. The anxiety and depression reflect an awareness of their inability to cope with environmental stress.

A rational therapeutic program must be planned in accordance with the basic problem. If there is mainly an anxiety state or anxious depression, the use of drugs, such as meprobamate, chlordiazepoxide, or diazepam are useful for the former, and amitriptyline or imipramine for the latter. Simple analgesics, such as aspirin or aspirin-codeine compounds, should be prescribed for the headache and flurazepam or chloral hydrate for insomnia. Litigation should be settled as soon as possible. To delay settlement usually works to the disadvantage of the patient. Long periods of observation and waiting only reinforce the patient's worries and fears and reduce the motivation to return to work.

THE CONCUSSIVE-CONTUSIONAL INJURY

If the physician arrives at the scene of the accident and finds an unconscious patient, a quick examination should be made before the patient is moved. First it must be determined whether the patient is breathing and has a clear airway and obtainable pulse and blood pressure, and whether there is dangerous hemorrhage from a scalp laceration. Severe head injuries that arrest respiration are soon followed by cessation of cardiac function. Injuries of this magnitude are usually fatal and if resuscitative measures do not restore and sustain cardiopulmonary function within 4 to 5 min, the brain is irreparably damaged. The likelihood of a cervical fracture-dislocation, which is occasionally associated with head injury, is the reason for taking the precautions, outlined on page 718, in moving the patient. Bleeding from the scalp can usually be controlled by a pressure bandage, unless an artery is divided, and then a suture becomes necessary. Resuscitative measures (artificial respiration and cardiac compression) should be continued until taken over by ambulance personnel. All such patients should be taken to a hospital and specifically to one that has an emergency and intensive care facility prepared to deal with all aspects of serious trauma.

In the hospital the first step is to clear the airway and ensure adequate ventilation by endotracheal intubation, if necessary. Shock, if present, should be controlled by the application of warm blankets, keeping the head low, and leaving the patient undisturbed for a few minutes. The shock usually comes under control in a few minutes with or without vasopressor drugs or transfusions. Persistent shock is rare in head injury and always should raise the suspicion of a ruptured viscus with internal bleeding, extensive fractures, or trauma to the cervical cord. Cervical spine films and a CT scan should be obtained en route to the intensive care unit, once vital functions are stable. If films of the cervical spine are negative there is no longer a need to immobilize the neck.

A rapid survey can now be made, with attention to the depth of coma, size of the pupils and their reaction to light, ocular movements, corneal reflexes, facial movements during grimace, swallowing, vocalization, gag reflexes, tone and movements of the limbs, predominant postures, reactions to pinch, and reflexes. The scalp should be carefully inspected and any wound probed with a sterile gloved finger. The hair should be cut away from any scalp wounds. Bogginess of the temporal or postauricular area (Battle sign), bleeding from the nose or ear, and extensive conjunctival edema and hemorrhage are useful signs of an underlying skull fracture. However, it should be remembered that rupture of an eardrum or a blow to the nose may also cause bleeding from these parts. Fracture of the orbital bones may displace the eye, with resulting strabismus; fracture of the jaw results in malocclusion and discomfort on attempting to open the mouth. If urine is retained and the bladder is distended, a catheter should be inserted and kept there. Temperature, pulse, respiration, blood pressure, and state of consciousness should be checked and charted every hour.

Teasdale and Jennett have proposed a practical rating scale by which the state of impaired consciousness can be evaluated hour by hour (Glasgow coma scale). It registers three aspects of neurologic functions: (1) eye opening (spontaneously, in response to command, and to pain); (2) verbal responsiveness (in terms of orientation, confusion, inappropriateness, and incomprehensibility); (3) motor responsiveness (to command, to a localized stimulus, flexion and extension). This scale, reproduced in Table 35-1, requires little training of ward personnel. It is useful in predicting the outcome of severe head injuries and in defining the duration of prolonged coma and stupor. A deteriorating scale dictates a change in management.

CT scanning is of importance at this juncture. A sizable epidural, subdural, or intracerebral blood clot is an indication for immediate surgery. The presence of contusions, brain edema, and displacement of central structures calls for the institution of measures to control intracranial pressure. It is now common practice to install a monitoring device through the skull to the subarachnoid space or ventricle, which allows continuous recording of intracranial pressure. No longer is the pressure measured through a lumbar puncture needle since such measurements do not accurately reflect intracranial pressure and may increase the risk of a cerebellar or temporal lobe herniation. The first step in lowering a presumptively high intracranial pressure (ICP) is to control the factors that are known to raise the ICP, such as hypoxia, hypocarbia, hyperthermia, awkward head positions, and high mean airway pressures (Ropper). Elevating the head and trunk about 60° will also help lower the ICP in some patients. If the intracranial pressure exceeds 15 to 20 mmHg, other measures should be used, such as increasing the hypocarbia by controlled ventilation (maintain P_{CO_2} at 28 to 33 mmHg) and hyperosmolar dehydration (0.25 to 1.0 g of 20% mannitol every 3 to 6 h and 1.0 mg of furosemide per kilogram to hold serum osmolality at 305 to 315 mosmol/L). If the ICP does not respond to these measures, the outlook for survival is bleak. Hypothermia and barbiturate anesthesia to reduce brain metabolism are being used, but relatively few patients have responded. Barbiturates may lower the blood pressure, which worsens the situation, though Marshall et al claim a high rate of good survival in cases where ICP exceeded 40 mmHg. Hypertension secondary to elevation of ICP appears

to increase the edema. Corticosteroids, according to Gudeman et al, have no beneficial effect in head trauma, but there are exceptions and many neurosurgeons still give them. The ideal mean blood pressure is 100 to 120 mmHg. If higher, there are plateau waves, and it should be lowered by diuretics and beta adrenergic blocking drugs; if lower, vasopressor agents should be used.

If coma persists for more than 48 h, an oral gastric tube should be passed and fluids and nourishment given by this route. Intravenous fluids should be administered, slowly and parsimoniously (no more than 1000 mL of normal saline or Ringer's lactate in 24 h). An excess of fluid may result in pulmonary edema and in further cerebral edema. The liability to the latter is especially dangerous in children who, because of inappropriate ADH secretion, easily become water-intoxicated. Cimetidine (300 mg intravenously every 4 h or antacids by stomach tube) to keep gastric acidity at a pH above 3.5 is of value in preventing gastric hemorrhage. Phenobarbital or phenytoin is recommended for the prevention of seizures.

Table 35-1
Glasgow coma scale
Circle the apropriate number and compute the total.

Eyes open	
Never	1
To pain	2
To verbal stimuli	3
Spontaneously	4

Best verbal response	
No response	1
Incomprehensible sounds	2
Inappropriate words	3
Disoriented and converses	4
Oriented and converses	5

Best motor response	
No response	1
Extension (decerebrate rigidity)	2
Flexion abnormal (decorticate rigidity)	3
Flexion withdrawal	4
Localizes pain	5
Obeys	6
Total	3–15

Radiographs of the skull and other parts can usually be postponed for a day or two, unless there is a suspicion of an epidural hemorrhage, in which case they should be done at once, to visualize a crack across the course of the middle meningeal artery. CT scan is obtained on admission and at later intervals, depending on the clinical problem. Restlessness is controlled by diazepam, chlordiazepoxide, or similar sedative, but only if careful nursing fails to quiet the patient and provide sleep for a few hours at a time. Fever is counteracted by antipyretics such as acetaminophen, and, if necessary, by a cooling blanket.

Once the patient has regained consciousness, the danger of suffocation, aspiration pneumonia, thrombophlebitis, and pulmonary embolism has usually passed. There follows a period of close medical observation, the various proximate and chronic complications being managed if and when they arise, along the lines described earlier in this chapter.

Death from head injury in the first few hours probably cannot be prevented. Eighty-five percent of patients with a Glasgow coma scale rating of 3 to 4 die within the first 24 h. The advisability of any surgical procedure during this period is much debated. If the patient survives for 1 or 2 days but remains in coma, the control of brain swelling and hemorrhage by surgical means must be considered. Should the condition of the patient then begin to deteriorate (pulse rising, temperature rising or falling below normal, state of consciousness worsening, hemiplegia more obvious, plantar reflexes more clearly extensor), a decision must be made concerning an epidural or subdural hemorrhage and increasing brain edema with temporal lobe herniation. Rowbotham, who has had extensive experience with cases of this type, recommends a right-sided temporal decompression and two inspection burr holes in the left, one at the sylvian point and one at the parietal eminence, for some of these patients. In his opinion the indications for surgery are (1) retrogression following a period of improvement, which cannot be controlled by intravenous dehydration measures; (2) decerebrate rigidity that has its onset after an interval of 24 h (early decerebrate rigidity implies primary brainstem injury), if meningitis is ruled out; (3) persistent coma with a dilated fixed pupil on one side, with no improvement after 12 h; and (4) prolonged unconsciousness associated with persistently high ICP. Not all neurologists and neurosurgeons agree on this plan and would insist on diagnostic CT scans and arteriography as guides. Kjellberg and Prieto found that bifrontal craniectomy for massive traumatic cerebral edema was not consistently effective, and this is the impression of most neurosurgeons. Certainly the removal of a large epidural or subdural hemorrhage, which cannot be diagnosed easily in the comatose patient, may be a lifesaving procedure.

In recent years a striking reduction in the mortality from acute head injuries has been achieved by the application of intensive care together with the free use of tracheostomy. Brain swelling may respond to controlled ventilation, and many of the comatose patients who would otherwise have succumbed to respiratory obstruction, pulmonary infections, or dehydration are thereby saved. Also, greater efforts to evacuate intracranial hematomas as soon as possible seem to have helped. The mortality rate of a group of patients in a state of decerebrate rigidity has been reduced by 50 percent, and the total mortality rate of all hospitalized patients has fallen from about 10 to 3.5 percent. Unfortunately many of the survivors are left permanently disabled.

The treatment of other problems attendant upon protracted coma has been outlined on pages 289 and 290. Every patient presents special problems that must be dealt with individually.

SUBDURAL AND EPIDURAL HEMORRHAGES

Treatment of these disorders has been discussed in relation to their descriptions in an earlier part of this chapter.

GENERAL PRINCIPLES OF MANAGEMENT

A head injury has special significance to most persons. Often victims of head injury fear for their sanity and are concerned about their capacity to resume their place in society. In former times, the management of head-injured persons involved long discussions of the seriousness of the injury, protracted bed rest, and inactivity, all of which served only to engender greater anxiety. Even worse, these measures were not of proved value. It is now widely acknowledged that the patient does better if the physician minimizes the seriousness of the head injury and reassures the patient about the prognosis. Early rehabilitation should be encouraged. It may safely begin as soon as the CSF becomes clear, usually within a few weeks except, of course, in the relatively rare cases of protracted coma.

Rehabilitation centers are of great help in restoring morale and re-educating the patient. Rusk and his associates in the New York Rehabilitation Institute were able to return about half of a group of severely head-injured to an independent existence within a year and most of these maintained their improved status after 5 years.

PROGNOSIS

The prognosis of head injury is influenced by several factors. The *age of the patient* is one. Increasing age reduces the chances of survival and of good recovery. Older patients often remain disabled, especially when compensation is involved. Young and middle-aged adults do better, particularly if they are not entitled to compensation. Russell has pointed out that the severity of the injury as measured by the duration of *traumatic amnesia* is a useful prognostic index. In patients with a period of amnesia of less than 1 h, 95 percent of patients were back at work within 2 months; if longer than 24 h, only 80 percent had returned to work within 6 months. About 60 percent of the patients in his series, however, still had symptoms at the end of 2 months, and 40 percent at the end of 18 months. Of the most severely injured (those comatose for several days), many remain permanently disabled. However, the degree of recovery is often better than one expects; the motor impairment, aphasia, and dementia tend to lessen and may clear. Improvement can continue over a period of 3 or more years. Children seem to recover more completely than adults.

For discussion of trauma of spinal cord, nerve roots, and peripheral nerves, see Chaps. 36 and 46.

REFERENCES

ADAMS JH, MITCHELL DE, GRAHAM DI, DOYLE D: Diffuse brain damage of immediate impact type. *Brain* 100:489, 1977.

ADAMS JH, GRAHAM DI, MURRAY LS, SCOTT G: Diffuse axonal injury due to nonmissile head injury in humans: An analysis of 45 cases. *Ann Neurol* 12:557, 1982.

ANNEGERS JF, GRABOW JD, GROOVER RV et al: Seizures after head trauma: A population study. *Neurology* 30:683, 1980.

ASCROFT PB: Traumatic epilepsy after gunshot wounds of the head. *Br Med J* 1:739, 1941.

BLACK P, JEFFRIES J, BLUMER D et al: The post-traumatic syndrome in children, in Walker AE, Caveness WF, Critchley M (eds): *The Late Effects of Head Injury.* Springfield, IL, Charles C Thomas, 1969, chap 14, pp 142–194.

BOWMAN KM, BLAU A, REICH R: Psychiatric states following head injury in adults and children, in Feiring EH (ed): *Brock's Injuries of the Brain and Spinal Cord and Their Coverings,* 5th ed. New York, Springer, 1974, chap 18, pp 570–613.

British Medical Journal: A Group of Neurosurgeons: Guidelines for initial management after head injury in adults. *Br Med J* 288:983, 1984.

CAIRNS H: Injuries of frontal and ethmoid sinuses with special reference to CSF rhinorrhea and aerocele. *J Laryngol Otol* 52:289, 1937.

CASSON IR, SHAM RAJ, CAMPBELL EA et al: Neurological and CT evaluation of knocked-out boxers. *J Neurol Neurosurg Psychiatry* 45:170, 1982.

CAVENESS WF: Onset and cessation of fits following craniocerebral trauma. *J Neurosurg* 20:570, 1963.

CAVENESS WF: Post traumatic sequelae, in Caveness WF, Walker AE (eds): *Head Injury.* Philadelphia, Lippincott, 1966, chap 17, pp 209–219.

CAVENESS VS JR: Epilepsy and craniocerebral injury of warfare, in Caveness WF, Walker AE (eds): *Head Injury.* Philadelphia, Lippincott, 1966, chap 18, pp 220–234.

CORSELLIS JAN, BRUTON CJ, FREEMAN-BROWNE D: The aftermath of boxing. *Psychol Med* 3:270, 1973.

COURVILLE CB: *Pathology of the Central Nervous System,* pt 4. Mountain View, CA, Pacific, 1937.

CRITCHLEY M: Medical aspects of boxing. *Br Med J* 1:357, 1957.

DENNY-BROWN D: Delayed collapse after head injury. *Lancet* 1:371, 1941.

DENNY-BROWN D, RUSSELL WR: Experimental cerebral concussion. *Brain* 64:93, 1941.

FEIRING EH, DAVIDOFF LM: Gunshot wounds of the brain and their complications, in Feiring EH (ed): *Brock's Injuries of the Brain and Spinal Cord and Their Coverings,* 5th ed. New York, Springer, 1974, chap 9, pp 283–335.

FOLTZ EL, SCHMIDT RP: The role of reticular formation in the coma of head injury. *J Neurosurg* 13:145, 1956.

FRAZIER CH, INGHAM SD: A review of the effects of gunshot wounds of the head based on the observation of 200 cases at U.S. Army General Hospital, No. 11, Cape May, N.J. *Trans Am Neurol Assoc* 45:59, 1919.

GARDNER WJ: Traumatic subdural hematoma with particular reference to the latent interval. *Arch Neurol Psychiatry* 27:847, 1932.

GENNARELLI TA, THIBAULT LE, ADAMS JH et al: Diffuse axonal injury and traumatic coma in the primate. *Ann Neurol* 12:564, 1982.

GOLDSTEIN K: *After-Effects of Brain Injuries in War.* New York, Grune & Stratton, 1942.

GRAHAM DI, ADAMS JH, DOYLE D: Ischemic brain damage in fatal nonmissile injuries. *J Neurol Sci* 39:213, 1978.

GRAFMAN J, JONES BS, MARTIN A et al: Intellectual function following penetrating head injury in Vietnam veterans. *Brain* 3:169, 1988.

GROAT RA, WINDLE WF, MAGOUN HW: Functional and structural changes in the monkey's brain during and after concussion. *J Neurosurg* 2:26, 1945.

GUDEMAN JK, MULLA JD, BECKER DP: Failure of high-dose steroid therapy to influence intracranial pressure in patients with severe head injury. *J Neurosurg* 51:301, 1979.

HOLBOURN AHS: Mechanics of head injury. *Lancet* 2:438, 1943.

JEFFERSON G: The nature of concussion. *Br Med J* 1:1, 1944.

JENNETT B: *Epilepsy after Non-missile Head Injuries,* 2nd ed. London, Heinemann, 1975.

JENNETT B: Anticonvulsant drugs and advice about epilepsy after head injury and intracranial surgery. *Br Med J* 286:627, 1973.

JENNETT B, BOND M: Assessment of outcome after severe brain damage. *Lancet* 480, 1975.

JENNETT B, TEASDALE G: *Management of Head Injuries: Contemporary Neurology,* no 20. Philadelphia, Davis, 1981.

KJELLBERG RN, PRIETO A: Bilateral craniectomy for massive cerebral edema. *J Neurosurg* 34:488, 1971.

LABADIE EL, GLOVER D: Physiopathogenesis of subdural hematomas. *J Neurosurg* 45:382, 393, 1976.

MAPOTHER E: Mental symptoms associated with head injury: The psychiatric aspect. *Br Med J* 2:1055, 1937.

MARSHALL LF, SMITH RW, SHAPIRO HM: The outcome with aggressive treatment in severe head injury. Part II: Acute and chronic barbiturate administration in the management of head injury. *J Neurosurg* 50:26, 1979.

McHUGH HE: Auditory and vestibular disorders in head injury, in Caveness WF, Walker AE (eds): *Head Injury*. Philadelphia, Lippincott, 1966, chap 8, pp 97–105.

MEIROWSKY AM: Penetrating craniocerebral trauma, in Caveness WF, Walker AE (eds): *Head Injury*. Philadelphia, Lippincott, 1966, chap 15, pp 195–202.

MEYER A: The anatomical facts and clinical varieties of traumatic insanity. *Am J Insanity* 60:373, 1904.

MEYER JS, DENNY-BROWN D: Studies of cerebral circulation in brain injury: II. Cerebral concussion. *Electroencephalogr Clin Neurophysiol* 7:529, 1955.

MILLER JD, BUTTERWORTH JF, GUDEMAN SK et al: Further experience in the management of severe head injury. *J. Neurosurg* 54:209, 1981.

MUNRO D: The diagnosis, treatment and immediate prognosis of cerebral trauma. *N Engl J Med* 210:287, 1934.

MUNRO D, MERRITT HH: Surgical pathology of subdural hematoma based on a study of 105 cases. *Arch Neurol Psychiatry* 35:64, 1936.

NEVIN NC: Neuropathological changes in the white matter following head injury. *J Neuropathol Exp Neurol* 26:77, 1967.

OMMAYA AK, GRUBB RL, NAUMANN RA: Coup and contre-coup injury: Observations on the mechanics of visible brain injuries in the rhesus monkey. *J Neurosurg* 35:503, 1971.

OMMAYA AK, ROCKOFF LD, BALDWIN M: Experimental concussion. *J Neurosurg* 21:249, 1964.

PENFIELD W, JASPER HH: *Epilepsy and Functional Anatomy of the Human Brain*. Boston, Little, Brown, 1954.

PFEIFER-NIETLEBEN B: Die psychischen Störungen nach Hirnverletzungen, in Bumke O (ed): *Handbuch der Geisteskrankheiten*. 1928, band 7, teil 3, p 415.

PUDENZ RH, SHELDON CH: The lucite calvarium—method for direct observation of the brain. *J Neurosurg* 3:487, 1946.

PURVIS JT: Craniocerebral injuries due to missiles and fragments, in Caveness WF, Walker AE (eds): *Head Injury*. Philadelphia, Lippincott, 1966, chap 10, pp 133–141.

RABE EF, FLYNN RE, DODGE PR: A study of subdural effusions in an infant. *Neurology* 12:79, 1962.

RABE EF, YOUNG GF, DODGE PR: The distribution and fate of subdurally instilled human serum albumin in infants with subdural collections of fluid. *Neurology* 14:1020, 1964.

RASMUSSEN T: Surgical therapy of post-traumatic epilepsy, in Walker AE, Caveness WF, Critchley M (eds): *Late Effects of Head Injury*. Springfield, IL, Charles C Thomas, 1969, chap 26, pp 277–305.

ROBERTS AH: *Brain Damage in Boxers: A Study of Prevalence of Traumatic Encephalopathy among Ex-professional Boxers*. London, Pitman, 1969.

ROPPER AH: Trauma of the head and spinal cord, in Braunwald E, Isselbacher KJ, Petersdorf RG, Wilson JD, Martin JB, Fauci AS (eds): *Harrison's Principles of Internal Medicine*, 11th ed. New York, McGraw-Hill, 1987, chap 344.

ROPPER AH, KENNEDY SK, ZERVAS NT (eds): *Neurological and Neurosurgical Intensive Care*. Baltimore, University Park Press, 1983.

ROPPER AH, MILLER D: Acute traumatic midbrain hemorrhage. *Ann Neurol* 18:80, 1985.

ROSS RJ, COLE M, THOMPSON JS, KIM KH: Boxers—computed tomography, EEG, and neurological evaluation. *JAMA* 249:211, 1983.

ROWBOTHAM GF: *Acute Injuries of the Head*, 4th ed. Baltimore, Williams & Wilkins, 1964.

RUSK HA, BLOCK JM, LOWMAN EW: Rehabilitation of the brain-injured patient. A report of 157 cases with long-term follow-up of 118, in Walker AE, Caveness WF, Critchley M (eds): *Late Effects of Head Injury*. Springfield, IL, Charles C Thomas, 1969, chap 29, pp 327–329.

RUSSELL WR: Cerebral involvement in head injury: A study based on the examination of 200 cases. *Brain* 55:549, 1932.

RUSSELL WR: *The Traumatic Amnesias*. London, Oxford, 1971.

SCHILDER P: Psychic disturbances after head injuries. *Am J Psychiatry* 9:155, 1934.

SHATSKY SA, EVANS DE, MILLER F, MARTINS AN: High speed angiography of experimental head injury. *J Neurosurg* 41:523, 1974.

SPILLANE JD: Brain injuries in boxers, in Feiring EH (ed): *Brock's Injuries of the Brain and Spinal Cord and Their Coverings*, 5th ed. New York, Springer, 1974, chap 16, pp 529–543.

STERN WE: Carotid-cavernous fistula, in Vinken PJ, Bruyn GW (eds): *Handbook of Clinical Neurology*, vol 24. Amsterdam, North-Holland, 1975, chap 22, pp 399–440.

STRICH SJ: The pathology of severe head injury. *J Neurol Neurosurg Psychiatry* 19:163, 1956.

STRICH SJ: The pathology of severe head injury. *Lancet* 2:443, 1961.

SWANN KW: Management of severe head injury, in Ropper AH et al (eds): *Neurological and Neurosurgical Intensive Care*. Baltimore, University Park Press, 1983, pp 207–230.

SYMONDS CP: Concussion and its sequelae. *Lancet* 1:1, 1962.

SYMONDS CP: Concussion and contusion of the brain and their sequelae, in Feiring EH (ed): *Brock's Injuries of the Brain and Spinal Cord and Their Coverings*, 5th ed. New York, Springer, 1974, chap 4, pp 100–161.

TEASDALE G, JENNETT B: Assessment of coma and impaired consciousness. A practical scale. *Lancet* 2:81, 1974.

TEUBER H-L: Effects of brain wounds implicating right or left hemisphere in man, in Mountcastle VB (ed): *Interhemispheric Relations and Cerebral Dominance*. Baltimore, Johns Hopkins, 1962, pp 131–157.

TOGLIA JU: Dizziness after whiplash injury of the neck and closed head injury: Electronystagmographic correlations, in Walker AE, Caveness WF, Critchley M (eds): *Late Effects of Head Injury*. Springfield, IL, Charles C Thomas, 1969, chap 6, pp 72–83.

TROTTER W: Certain minor injuries of the brain. *Lancet* 1:935, 1924.

TROTTER W: Injuries of the skull and brain, in *Choyce's System of Surgery.* London, Cassell, 1932, vol 3, p 358.

VAN DER ZWAN A: Late results from prolonged traumatic unconsciousness, in Walker AE, Caveness WF, Critchley M (eds): *Late Effects of Head Injury.* Springfield, IL, Charles C Thomas, 1969, chap 13, pp 138–141.

WALKER AE: Post-traumatic epilepsy, in Rowbotham GF (ed): *Acute Injuries of the Head,* 4th ed. Baltimore, Williams & Wilkins, 1964, chap 15, pp 486–509.

WEIR B: The osmolality of subdural hematoma fluid. *J Neurosurg* 34:528, 1971.

WEISS GH, SALAZAR AM, VANCE SC et al: Predicting posttraumatic epilepsy in penetrating head injury. *Arch Neurol* 43:771, 1986.

ZANDER E, FOROGLOU G: Post-traumatic hydrocephalus, in Vinken PJ, Bruyn GW (eds): *Handbook of Clinical Neurology,* vol 24. Amsterdam, North-Holland, 1976, chap 12, pp 231–253.

CHAPTER 36

DISEASES OF THE SPINAL CORD

Diseases of the nervous system may be confined to the spinal cord, where they produce a number of distinctive syndromes. The latter relate to special physiologic and anatomic features of the cord, such as its prominent function in nervous conduction and in relatively primitive reflex activity; its long cylindrical shape; its tight envelopment by meninges; the peripheral location of medullated fibers, next to the pia; the special arrangement of its blood vessels; and its particular relationships to the vertebral column. Because of the frequency and gravity of spinal cord disorders, and the special problems that they raise in diagnosis, we have allotted a separate chapter to them.

In keeping with the general plan of this book, the disorders of the spinal cord are grouped into relatively common syndromes. Some of the anatomic and physiologic considerations pertinent to an understanding of disorders of the cord (and of the spine) will be found in Chaps. 3, 8, and 10; others will be discussed in relation to particular spinal cord syndromes.

PARAPLEGIA OR QUADRIPLEGIA DUE TO COMPLETE TRANSVERSE LESIONS OF THE SPINAL CORD

This syndrome is best considered in relation to trauma, its most frequent cause, but it occurs also as a result of infarction or hemorrhage and with rapidly advancing compressive, necrotizing, demyelinative, or inflammatory lesions.

TRAUMA TO THE SPINE AND SPINAL CORD

Throughout recorded medical history, signal advances in the understanding of the physiology of the spinal cord have coincided with periods of warfare. The first thoroughly documented study of the effects of sudden total cord transection was that of Theodor Kocher in 1896, based on his observations of 15 patients. During World War I, Riddoch—and later, Head and Riddoch—gave the classic descriptions of spinal transection in humans; in France, Lhermitte and Guillain and Barré made additional observations. World War II marked a turning point in the understanding and management of spinal cord injuries. The advent of antibiotics and of rapid and efficient means of transportation permitted the survival of unprecedented numbers of soldiers with spinal cord injuries, and incidentally provided the opportunity for their long-term observation. In special centers, exemplified by the Long Beach, Hines, and West Roxbury Veterans Administration Hospitals in the United States and the Stoke Mandeville National Spinal Injuries Centre in England, the care and rehabilitation of the paraplegic has been perfected. Studies conducted in these centers have greatly enhanced our knowledge of the functional capacity of the spinal cord chronically isolated from the human brain. Kuhn, Munro, Comarr, Martin and Davis, Guttmann, and Pollock, listed in the references, have made particularly important contributions to this subject.

MECHANISMS OF INJURY

Although trauma may involve the spinal cord alone, it is seldom that the vertebral column is not injured at the same time. Often there is an associated head injury as well, as pointed out in Chap. 35.

A useful classification of spinal injuries is one that divides them into fracture-dislocations, pure fractures, and pure dislocations. The relative frequency of these types is about 3:1:1. Except for bullet, shrapnel, and stab wounds, a direct blow to the spine is a relatively uncommon cause of serious vertebral injury. In civilian life, most spinal injuries are the result of *force applied at a distance*. All three types of injury mentioned above are produced by a similar mechanism, usually a vertical compression of the spinal column to which anteroflexion is almost immediately added (anterohyperflexion injury); or, in the neck, the mechanism may be one of vertical compression and retro-hyperflexion (commonly referred to as hyperextension). The most important variables in the mechanics of vertebral injury are *the nature of the bones, and the intensity, direction, and point of impact of the force.*

If the cranium is struck by a hard object at high velocity, a skull fracture occurs, the force of the injury being absorbed mainly by the elastic quality of the skull. If the traumatizing force is relatively soft yet unyielding, the spine, and particularly its most mobile (cervical) portion, will be the part injured. If the neck happens to be rigid and straight and the force is applied quickly to the head, the atlas and the odontoid process of the axis may break. If the force is applied less quickly, an element of flexion or retroflexion is added.

When the cervical spine is sharply retroflexed, the spinous and articular processes of the midcervical vertebrae (C4 to C6) are forced together, and these, now acting as a fulcrum, cause a separation between the vertebral body and the adjacent lower intervertebral disc. This results in dislocation, and the cord is caught between the laminae of the lower vertebra and the body of the higher one. Depending upon the intensity of the driving force, the separation may continue, with rupture of the anterior ligament. The posterior ligament may become dislodged from the vertebra below and may then buckle and squeeze the spinal cord backward against the lower vertebra. Hyperextension injury to the spinal cord may occur without apparent damage to the spine, being caused by an inward bulge of the ligamentum flavum.

In the case of severe forward flexion of the head and neck, the adjacent vertebrae are forced together at the level of maximum stress. The anterior-inferior edge of the upper vertebral body is driven into the one below, sometimes splitting it in two. The posterior part of the fractured body is displaced backward and compresses the cord. Less severe degrees of anteroflexion injury produce only dislocation. Vulnerability to the effects of anteroflexion and retroflexion injuries is increased by the presence of cervical spondylosis or ankylosing spondylitis or a congenital stenosis of the spinal canal.

The spinal cord may be damaged without radiologic evidence of fracture or dislocation, particularly in children, and sometimes one cannot determine the full extent of spinal injury even at autopsy, because of the difficulty in examining the vertebrae. MRI or lateral spine films are by far the most satisfactory means of demonstrating the degree of vertebral injury and the tearing of ligaments with dislocation, but one must be careful to avoid full flexion or extension of the neck in order to prevent further injury to the spinal cord.

Another mechanism of cord and root injury, involving extremes of extension and flexion of the neck, is so-called *whiplash* or *recoil injury*. This type of injury is most often the result of an automobile accident. A vehicle struck sharply from behind causes the passenger's head to be whipped back; or if the vehicle stops abruptly, there is sudden forward flexion of the neck, followed by retroflexion. Occipitonuchal muscles and other supporting structures of the neck and head are affected much more often than spinal cord or roots. Nevertheless, in rare instances, quadriplegia, temporary or permanent, results from a violent whiplash injury. The exact mechanism of neural injury in these circumstances is not clear; perhaps there is a transient posterior dislocation, or momentary retropulsion of the intervertebral disc into the spinal canal. Again, the presence of cervical spondylosis adds to the hazard of damage to the cord or roots. Also there are examples of spinal cord trauma that result from the persistent hyperextension of the cervical spine during a protracted period of coma. Arterial hypotension is probably an added factor. This combination accounts for some of the cases of quadriplegia in opiate or other drug addicts (Ell et al).

A special type of spinal cord injury, occurring most often in wartime, is one in which a high-velocity missile passes through the vertebral canal and damages the spinal cord directly. In some cases the missile strikes the vertebral column without entering the spinal canal but virtually shatters the contents of the dural tube or produces lesser degrees of impairment of spinal cord function. Rarely, a vertebral injury of this type will cause a paralysis of spinal cord function that is completely reversible in a day or two (*spinal cord concussion*). This latter condition may also be produced by forceful falls flat on the back. Little is known of the underlying pathologic changes. The term *concussion,* as applied to spinal cord injury, has led to much confusion because it has been applied indiscriminately to a variety of minor or partial spinal cord injuries in addition to the completely and rapidly reversible form of spinal cord paralysis.

Acute traumatic paralysis may also be the consequence of a vascular mechanism. Fibrocartilaginous emboli from a ruptured nucleus pulposus into arteries and/or veins of the spinal cord may cause infarction (see below). Or, a traumatic dissecting aneurysm of the aorta may occlude the segmental arteries of the spinal cord, as in the case reported by Kneisley.

An analysis of 2000 cases of spinal injury, collected from the medical literature by Jefferson, showed that most vertebral injuries occurred at the levels of the first and second cervical, fourth to sixth cervical, and eleventh thoracic to second lumbar vertebrae. Industrial accidents most often involved the dorsolumbar vertebrae; accidents in which the individual fell with head down, as in diving into shallow water, affected the cervical region. These are not only the most mobile portions of the vertebral column, but also the regions in which the cervical and lumbar enlargements of the cord greatly reduce the space between neural and bony structures. The thoracic portion of the cord is relatively small and the canal is roomy, and additional protection is provided by the high articular facets (making dislocation difficult) and limitations in anterior movement imposed by the thoracic cage.

In the authors' experience, the usual circumstances of spinal cord injury have been motor vehicle accidents, falls during a state of alcoholic intoxication, diving accidents, gunshot or stab wounds, crushing industrial injuries, and birth injury, in that order of frequency. The majority of the fatal cases had fracture dislocations or dislocations of the upper cervical spine. Respiration is paralyzed by lesions at C1, C2, and C3. Among those who survive, fracture-dislocation of the lower cervical spine is the most frequent established mechanism of spinal cord injury in civilian life. The annual incidence nationwide is 2.5 to 5.0 cases per 100,000 population.

PATHOLOGY OF SPINAL CORD INJURY

As a result of squeezing or shearing of the spinal cord, there is destruction of gray and white matter and a variable amount of hemorrhage, chiefly in the more vascular parts. These changes are maximal at the level of injury and one or two segments above and below it. Rarely is the cord cut in two, and seldom is the pia-arachnoid lacerated. The condition is best designated as *traumatic necrosis of the spinal cord.* Separation of such pathologic entities as hematomyelia, concussion, contusion, and hematorrhachis (bleeding into the spinal canal) is of little value either clinically or pathologically. As a lesion heals, it results in a gliotic focus or cavitation. Progressive meningeal fibrosis and a tension hydromyelia will sometimes lead to a delayed syndrome of progressive traumatic syringomyelia.

In most traumatic lesions the central part of the spinal cord with its vascular gray matter suffers greater injury than the peripheral parts. And in some instances, the lesion is virtually restricted to the anterior and posterior gray matter. This has been called the *central cervical cord syndrome* (Schneider et al).

As with most lesions, the total clinical effect is compounded of an irreversible structural component and a disorder of function, each of which may vary in degree. The extent and permanence of the clinical manifestations are determined by the relative proportions of these two elements.

CLINICAL EFFECTS OF SPINAL CORD INJURY

When the spinal cord is suddenly and completely severed, three disorders of function are at once evident: (1) all voluntary movement in parts of the body below the lesion is immediately and permanently lost; (2) all sensation from the lower (aboral) parts is abolished; and (3) reflex function in all segments of the isolated spinal cord is suspended. The last effect, called *spinal shock,* involves tendon as well as autonomic reflexes; it lasts for weeks to months and is so dramatic that Riddoch used it as a basis for dividing the clinical effects into two stages: (1) spinal shock or areflexia and (2) heightened reflex activity. The separation of these two stages is not as sharp as this clinical division might imply but is nevertheless fundamental. Less complete lesions of the spinal cord may result in little or no spinal shock, and the same is true of lesions that develop slowly.

Stage of Spinal Shock or Areflexia The loss of motor function at the time of injury—quadriplegia (better termed tetraplegia) with lesions of the fourth to fifth cervical segments, paraplegia with lesions of the thoracic cord—is accompanied by atonic paralysis of bladder and bowel, gastric atony, loss of sensation below the level corresponding to the spinal cord lesion, muscular flaccidity, and complete or almost complete suppression of all spinal segmental reflex activity below the lesion. This condition, in which the neural elements below the lesion fail to perform their normal function because of their separation from higher levels, involves all skeletal muscles, bladder, bowel, and sexual function, and autonomic control. Vasomotor tone, sweating, and piloerection in the lower parts of the body are temporarily lost. The lower extremities lose heat if left uncovered, and they swell if dependent. The skin is dry and pale, and ulcerations may develop over bony prominences. The sphincters of the bladder and the rectum remain contracted (due to loss of inhibitory influence of higher CNS centers), but the detrusor and smooth muscles are atonic. Urine accumulates until the intravesicular pressure is sufficient to overcome the sphincter; then driblets escape (overflow incontinence). There is also passive distention of the bowel, retention of feces, and absence of peristalsis (paralytic ileus). Genital reflexes (penile erection, bulbo-cavernosus reflex, contraction of dartos muscle) are abolished or profoundly depressed.

The duration of the state of complete areflexia varies greatly. In a small number (5 of Kuhn's 29 patients, for example) it is permanent, or only fragmentary reflex activity is regained many months or years after the injury. Presumably in such patients the spinal segments below the lesion have themselves been injured—perhaps by a vascular mechanism, although this explanation is unproven. In others, minimal genital and flexor reflex activity can be detected within a few days of the injury. In the majority of patients, this *minimal reflex activity* appears within a period of 1 to 6 weeks. Noxious stimulation of the plantar surfaces evokes a tremulous twitching and brief flexion or extension movements of the great toes. Contraction of the sphincter ani is elicited by plantar or perianal stimulation, and the genital reflexes reappear at about the same time.

The explanation of spinal shock, which is brief in submammalian forms and more lasting in higher mammals and especially in primates, is believed to be the sudden interruption of suprasegmental descending fiber systems that normally keep the spinal motor neurons in a continuous state of subliminal depolarization (ready to respond). Fulton found that in the cat and monkey the facilitatory tracts in question are the reticulospinal and vestibulospinal. Subsequent studies showed that in monkeys some degree of spinal shock can result from a limited sectioning of the corticospinal tracts. This cannot be the complete explanation, however, at least in humans, for spinal shock may be very mild or inevident as a result of cerebral and brainstem lesions that interrupt the corticospinal tracts. Interest in recent years has focused on a possible role for neurotransmitters (catecholamines, endorphins, substance P, and 5-hydroxytryptamine). There is some evidence, according to Mathias and Frankel, that naloxone and the endogenous opiate antagonist thyrotropic releasing factor have a beneficial effect in reversing the circulatory collapse and possibly reducing the extent of an acute spinal cord lesion.

Stage of Heightened Reflex Activity Usually, after a few weeks, the reflex responses to stimulation, which are initially minimal and transient, become stronger and more easily elicitable, and come to include additional and more proximal muscles. Gradually the typical pattern of flexion reflexes emerges: dorsiflexion of the big toe (Babinski sign); fanning of the other toes; and later, flexion or slow withdrawal movements of the foot, leg, and thigh (triple flexion). Tactile stimulation of the foot may suffice as a stimulus, but a painful stimulus is more effective. The Achilles reflexes and then the patellar reflexes return. Retention of urine becomes less complete, and at irregular intervals urine is expelled by active contraction of the detrusor muscle. Reflex defecation also begins. After several months the withdrawal reflexes become greatly exaggerated to the point of flexor spasms and may be accompanied by profuse sweating, piloerection, and automatic emptying of bladder (occasionally of the rectum). This is the "mass

reflex," which is evoked by stimulation of the skin of the legs or by some interoceptive stimulus, such as a full bladder. Varying degrees of heightened flexor reflex activity may last for years, especially if sepsis of the bladder or skin intervenes. Heat-induced sweating is defective, but reflex-evoked ("spinal") sweating may be profuse (see Kneisley). Presumably, in such cases, the lateral horn cells in much of the thoracic cord are still viable and disinhibited. *Above* the level of the lesion, thermoregulatory sweating may be exaggerated and is accompanied by cutaneous flushing, pounding headache, hypertension, and reflex bradycardia. This latter syndrome ("autonomic dysreflexia") is episodic and occurs in response to a specific stimulus, such as a distended bladder or rectum. It has been ascribed to the reflex release of noradrenalin from the disinhibited sympathetic terminals and of adrenalin from the adrenal medulla.

Extensor reflexes eventually develop in most cases (18 of 22 of Kuhn's patients who survived more than 2 years), *but they do not lead to the abolition of the flexor reflexes.* The overactivity of extensor muscles may appear as early as 6 months after the injury, but only do so, as a rule, after the flexor responses are fully developed. Extensor responses are at first manifest in certain muscles of the hip and thigh, and later of the leg. In a few patients extensor reflexes are organized into support reactions sufficient to permit *spinal standing.* Kuhn observed that extensor movements were at first provoked most readily by a sudden shift from a sitting to a supine position, and later by proprioceptive stimuli (squeezing thigh muscles) and tactile stimuli from wide areas. Marshall, in a study of 44 patients with chronic spastic paraplegia of spinal origin, found all possible combinations of flexor and extensor reflexes; the type of reflex obtained was determined by the intensity and duration of the stimulus (a mild prolonged noxious stimulus evoked an ipsilateral extensor reflex; an intense brief stimulus, a flexor response).

From these observations one would suspect that the ultimate posture of the legs—flexion or extension—does not depend solely on the completeness or incompleteness of the spinal cord lesion, as originally postulated by Riddoch. The development of paraplegia in flexion relates also to the level of the lesion, being seen most often with cervical lesions and progressively less often with more caudal ones. Repeated flexor spasms, which are more frequent with higher lesions, and the ensuing contractures ultimately determine a fixed flexor posture. Conversely, reduction of flexor spasms by elimination of nociceptive stimuli (infected bladder, decubiti, etc.) favors an extensor posture of the legs. According to Guttmann, the positioning of the limbs during the early stages of paraplegia greatly influences their ultimate posture. Thus, prolonged fixation of the paralyzed limbs in adduction and semiflexion favors subsequent paraplegia in flexion. Placing the patient prone, or placing the limbs in abduction and extension facilitates the development of predominantly extensor postures. Nevertheless, strong and persistent extensor postures are observed only with partial lesions of the spinal cord.

Of some interest is the fact that many patients report subjective sensation below the level of their transection. A variety of paresthesias is described, but the most common is a dull, burning pain in the lower back and abdomen, buttocks, and perineum. The pain may be intense and last for a year or longer, after which it gradually subsides. It may persist after rhizotomy but can be abolished by anesthetizing the stump of the proximal (upper) segment of the spinal cord, according to Pollock and his collaborators. Transmission of sensation over splanchnic afferents to levels of the spinal cord above the lesion, the conventional explanation, is therefore not the most plausible one.

The overactivity of neurons in the isolated segments of the spinal cord is not fully understood. One assumes that suprasegmental inhibitory influences have been removed by the transection so that afferent sensory impulses evoke exaggerated nocifensive and phasic and tonic myotatic reflexes. But isolated neurons also become hypersensitive to neurotransmitters. Since the early experiments of Cannon and Rosenblueth it has been known that section of sympathetic motor fibers leaves the denervated structures hypersensitive to adrenalin; these authors also found the motor neurons in the isolated spinal segments to be abnormally sensitive to acetylcholine.

Various combinations of residual deficits (lower and upper motor neuron and sensory) may be expected. Complete or incomplete voluntary motor paralysis, a flaccid atrophic paralysis (if appropriate segments of gray matter are destroyed), a spastic weakness of the legs, paraplegia in flexion or extension, and a partial or complete Brown-Séquard syndrome, all with variable sensory impairment in the legs and arms, are some of the resulting clinical pictures. High cervical lesions may result in extreme and prolonged tonic spasms of the legs due to release of tonic myotatic reflexes. Under these circumstances, attempted voluntary movement may excite intense contraction of all flexor and extensor muscles lasting for several minutes. Segmental damage in low cervical or lumbar gray matter, destroying inhibitory Renshaw neurons, may release activity of anterior horn cells leading to spinal segmental spasticity. Any

residual symptoms persisting after 6 months are likely to be permanent, although in a small proportion of patients some return of function (particularly sensation) is possible after this time. Loss of motor and sensory function above the lesion, coming on years after the trauma, occurs occasionally and is due to cavitation in the proximal segment of the cord (see further on, under "Syringomyelia").

The level of the spinal cord and vertebral lesions can be determined from the clinical findings. A complete paralysis of the arms and legs usually indicates a fracture or dislocation at the fourth to fifth cervical vertebrae. If the legs are paralyzed and the arms can still be abducted and flexed, the lesion is likely to be at the fifth to sixth cervical vertebrae. Paralysis of the legs and only the hands indicates a lesion at the sixth to seventh cervical level. Below the cervical region, the spinal cord segments and roots are not opposite their similarly numbered vertebrae (Fig. 36-1). The spinal cord ends opposite the first lumbar interspace. Vertebral lesions below this point give rise predominantly to cauda equina syndromes; these carry a better prognosis than injuries to the lower thoracic vertebrae, which involve both cord and multiple roots. In all cases of spinal cord and cauda equina injury the prognosis for recovery is favorable if any movement or sensation is elicitable during the first 48 to 72 h.

The acute central spinal cord syndrome characteristically affects motor function in the upper limbs more than in the lower ones; bladder dysfunction with urinary retention occurs in some of the cases and sensory loss may be slight (hyperpathia over the shoulders and arms may be the only sensory abnormality). The destruction of gray matter (motor and sensory neurons) may leave an atrophic, areflexive paralysis, and a segmental analgesia and thermohypalgesia. Retroflexion injuries of the head and neck are the ones most often associated with this central cord syndrome, but hematomyelia, necrotizing myelitis, fibrocartilagenous embolism, and possibly infarction due to compression of the vertebral artery at the medullary-cervical region are other causes (Morse).

Treatment In general, the treatment of spinal injuries is conservative and symptomatic. In all cases of suspected spinal injury, the immediate concern is that there be no movement (especially flexion) of the cervical spine from the moment of the accident. The patient should be placed prone or supine on a firm flat surface (with one person assigned to keeping the head immobile) and should be transported by a vehicle that can accept the litter. Heavy sandbags or similar objects should be placed on each side of the head and neck, and a small hard roll under the nape of the neck.

Once it has been determined that the spinal cord has been injured, corticosteroids may be given, as for brain

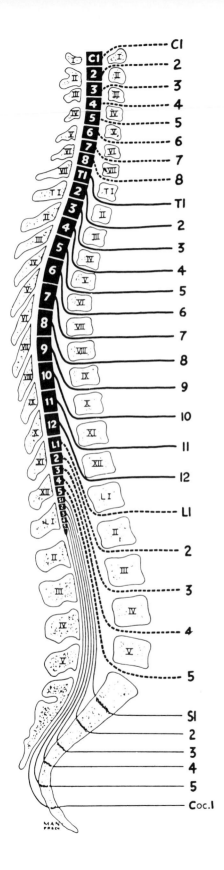

swelling (page 709), to reduce spinal cord edema. If the spinal cord injury is associated with dislocation of the vertebrae, traction on the neck is necessary to secure proper alignment. This is accomplished by a head halter attached through the head of the bed, over a pulley, to a weight of 10 to 25 lb, or even better, by the use of Crutchfield tongs that fasten onto the skull. In thoracic crush injuries, hyperextension can be maintained by placing a narrow pillow under the affected area. Traction should be continued for 4 to 6 weeks, and then a brace may be substituted.

There are two schools of thought concerning the early management of spinal cord injury. One, represented by Guttmann and others, advocates reduction of the dislocated vertebras by traction and immobilization until skeletal immobility is obtained, and then rehabilitation. The other school, represented by Munro and more recently by Collins and Chehrazi, proposes early surgical decompression, correction of bony displacements, removal of herniated disc tissue and intra- and extramedullary hemorrhage; often the spine is fixed at the same time by a bone graft or wiring. Other American neurosurgeons take a less aggressive stance, delaying operation or operating only when the spinal canal is narrowed by more than one-third of its diameter (as shown by MRI or a metrizamide-CT myelogram through a lateral C1-C2 puncture). With complete spinal cord lesions, most surgeons do not favor myelography and surgery. The results of the conservative and aggressive surgical plans of management have been difficult to compare. Collins, a participant in the NIH study of acute management of spinal cord injury, concludes that the survival rate has increased as a result of early stabilization of fractures, and orthopedic fixation of the spine, prevention of respiratory, urinary, and cutaneous complications, and the early institution of rehabilitation measures, but as recently as 1982 there was no evidence that the degree of neurologic disability had been reduced.

The greatest risk to the patient with spinal cord injury is in the first week or 10 days when gastric dilatation, ileus, shock, and infection are the main problems. According to Messard et al, the mortality rate falls rapidly after the first 3 months, and beyond this time 86 percent of paraplegics

Figure 36-1

The relationship of spinal segments and roots to the vertebral bodies and spinous processes. The cervical roots (except C8) exit through foramina above their respective vertebral bodies, and the other roots issue below these bodies. (From W Haymaker, B Woodhall, Peripheral Nerve Injuries, 2nd ed, Philadelphia, Saunders, 1953.)

and 80 percent of quadriplegics will survive for 10 years or longer. In children, the survival rate is even higher (De Vivo et al). The latter authors found that the cumulative 7-year survival rate in spinal cord–injured patients (who had survived at least 24 h after injury) was 87 percent. Poor prognostic factors were advancing age at the time of injury and being rendered completely quadriplegic.

The aftercare of patients with paraplegia is concerned with management of bladder and bowel disturbances, care of the skin, and maintenance of nutrition. Decubitus ulcers can be prevented by special skin care. At first continual catheterization is necessary, and then, after several weeks, one turns to intermittent catheterization once or twice daily by the "no touch" technique. Close watch is kept for bladder infection, and this is treated promptly should it occur. Morning suppositories and enemas are usually the most effective means of controlling fecal incontinence. Spasticity and flexor spasms may be troublesome. Oral baclofen may provide some relief. In permanent spastic paraplegia with severe stiffness and adduction and flexor spasms, intrathecal baclofen, delivered by self-administered pump in doses of 12 to 400 mg/day, has reportedly been helpful. The drug is believed to act on spinal synaptic reflexes (Penn and Kroin). Physiotherapy, muscle re-education, and the proper use of braces are all important in the rehabilitation of the patient. All this is best carried out in special centers for rehabilitation of spinal cord injuries.

Guttmann's monograph provides a comprehensive account of the modern management of spinal cord injuries, as well as many other aspects of the subject.

SPINAL CORD INJURY DUE TO ELECTRIC CURRENTS AND LIGHTNING

Among the physical agents that may injure the spinal cord acutely, electric currents and lightning should be mentioned. These agents also injure the brain and peripheral nerves, and their effects will be noted briefly. It is the spinal cord, however, that is involved most frequently and severely.

Electrical Injuries In the United States, inadvertent contact with an electric current causes about 1000 deaths annually and many more nonfatal but serious injuries. About one-third of the fatal accidents results from contact with household currents, indicating the vulnerability of most of the population to this type of injury.

The factor that contributes most significantly to damage of the nervous system is the strength of the current

or amperage with which the victim comes in contact, and not the voltage, as is generally believed. The former is derived from the formula:

$$\text{Current strength (amperage)} = \frac{\text{tension (volts)}}{\text{resistance (ohms)}}$$

In any particular case, the duration of contact with the current and the resistance offered by the skin (this is greatly reduced if the skin is moist or immersed in water) may be of critical importance. The physics of electrical injuries is much more complex than these brief remarks indicate (for full discussion see review by Panse).

Any part of the peripheral or central nervous system may be injured by electric currents and lightning. The effects may be immediate, which is understandable, but of greater interest are the rare instances of neurologic damage that occur many days or months after the accident. The immediate effects are apparently the result of direct heating of the nervous tissue, but the pathogenesis of the delayed effects is not well understood. Most likely they are secondary to vascular occlusive changes induced by the electric current, a mechanism that also seems to underlie the delayed effects of radiation therapy (see below).

The sequelae of electrical injuries are most often referable to the spinal cord and occur when the path of the current is from arm to arm or arm to leg. Initially there are pain and paresthesias immediately in the involved limb, but these symptoms are transient. A delayed spinal cord syndrome has been described, most often taking the form of segmental muscular atrophy, occasionally of a syndrome simulating that of amyotrophic lateral sclerosis or transverse myelopathy. Unlike the delayed cerebral symptoms (see below), the spinal cord ones may be of gradual onset and slow progression.

When the head is one of the contact points, the patient may become unconscious, or suffer tinnitus, deafness, or headache for a short period following the injury. In a small number of surviving patients, after an asymptomatic interval of days to months, there has been an apoplectic onset of hemiplegia, with or without aphasia, or a striatal or brainstem syndrome, presumably due to thrombotic occlusion of cerebral vessels with infarction of tissue.

Lightning The factors involved in injuries from lightning are less well defined than those from electric currents, but the effects are much the same. The risk of being struck by lightning is about 30 times greater in rural areas than in cities. Lightning prefers prominences such as trees and hills, so these should be avoided; a person caught in the open should curl up on the ground, lying on one side, with legs close together.

Arborescent red lines or burns on the skin indicate

the point of contact of lightning, but the path through the body can be deduced only approximately, from the clinical sequelae. Lightning that strikes the head is particularly dangerous, proving fatal in 30 percent of cases. Death is due to ventricular fibrillation or to the effects of intense desiccating heat on the brain. Persons struck by lightning are initially unconscious, irrespective of where they are struck. In those who survive, consciousness is usually regained rapidly and completely. Rarely, unconsciousness or an agitated-confusional state may persist for a week or two. There is usually a disturbance of motor-sensory function of a limb or all the limbs, which may be pale and cold or cyanotic. As a rule, these signs are also evanescent, but in some instances they persist, or an atrophic paralysis of a limb or part of a limb makes its appearance after a symptom-free interval of several months. Persistent seizures are surprisingly rare.

RADIATION INJURY OF THE SPINAL CORD

Delayed necrosis of the spinal cord and brain is a well-recognized sequela of radiation therapy for tumors in these regions. The peripheral nerves are more resistant to this adverse effect, although we have observed, as have others, an early reversible and a late progressive and permanent sensorimotor disorder coming on several months or years after irradiation. In addition, there is a delayed neuropathy in the distribution of the brachial plexus after radiation therapy for breast carcinoma. Finally, a lower motor neuron lesion, presumably due to injury to anterior horn cells, may also follow radiation therapy.

Transient Myelopathy. The early type of radiation myelopathy (appearing 3 to 6 months after radiotherapy) is characterized by paresthesias in the extremities. The paresthesias may be evoked or exacerbated by neck flexion (Lhermitte sign). In one of our patients there was impairment of vibratory and position sense in the legs but no weakness. The sensory abnormalities disappear after a few months and, according to Jones, are not followed by the delayed progressive radiation myelopathy (see below). The pathology has not been fully demonstrated, buth there is a spongy appearance of the white matter with demyelination and depletion of oligodendrocytes. The authors have not studied this lesion.

Delayed Progressive Radiation Myelopathy This, the most common complication of radiation therapy, is a progressive myelopathy that follows, after a characteristic latent period, the irradiation of malignant tissues in the vicinity of the spinal cord. The incidence of this complication is difficult to determine because many patients die of their malignant disease before the cord lesion matures, but is

estimated to be between 2 and 3 percent (Palmer). At the Massachusetts General Hospital, seven cases have been observed in 15 years. Patients who have undergone hyperthermia as a treatment for cancer are particularly vulnerable to radiation myelopathy (Douglas et al).

The neurologic disorder first appears many months after the course of radiation therapy, practically always after 6 months and usually between 12 and 15 months (latent periods as long as 60 months or even longer have been reported). The onset is insidious, usually with sensory symptoms—paresthesias and dysesthesias of the feet or a Lhermitte sign, and similar symptoms in the hands in cases of cervical cord damage. Weakness of one or both legs usually follows the sensory loss. Initially, local pain is notably absent, in distinction to spinal metastases. In some cases, one cannot predict whether the sensory abnormalities will be transitory, or persistent; more often additional signs make their appearance and progress, at first rapidly and then more slowly and irregularly, over a period of several weeks or months, with involvement of the corticospinal and spinothalamic pathways. Originally, the neurologic disturbance may take the form of a Brown-Séquard syndrome, but later the syndrome is that of a transverse myelopathy, with a spastic paraplegia, sensory level on the trunk, and sphincteric disturbance.

Reagan et al, who have had a large experience with radiation myelopathy at the Mayo Clinic (1 percent of all cases of myelopathy were of this type), describe yet another myelopathic radiation syndrome, namely, a slowly evolving amyotrophy, with paresis, atrophy of muscles, and areflexia in parts of the body supplied by anterior horn cells of the irradiated spinal segments. Most patients with this form of the disease die within a year of onset. Knowledge of the pathology is incomplete.

The CSF in the delayed progressive radiation myelopathy is normal except for a slight elevation of protein content in some cases. Also, myelography usually discloses no abnormalities, though in a few instances the spinal cord may be swollen. This is an important point to establish, because a mistaken diagnosis of intraspinal tumor may lead to another operation or further irradiation of an already damaged cord.

In the spinal cord, corresponding with the level of the irradiated area and extending over several segments, is an irregular zone of coagulation necrosis, involving both white and gray matter, the former to a greater extent than the latter. Varying degrees of secondary degeneration involve the ascending and descending tracts. Vascular changes—necrosis of arterioles or hyaline thickening of their walls, with thrombotic occlusion of their lumens—are prominent in the most severely damaged portions of the cord. Most authors have attributed the parenchymal lesion to the blood vessel changes; others believe that the degree of vascular change is insufficient to explain the parenchymal change (Malamud et al, Burns et al). Certainly the most severe parenchymal changes in the cord are typical of infarction; but the insidious onset and slow, steady progression of the clinical disorder would then need to be explained by a succession of vascular occlusions. Exceptionally, in patients in whom a transverse myelopathy has developed within a few hours (as described by Reagan et al), a larger spinal artery must have become thrombosed.

It needs to be stressed that radiation myelopathy is an iatrogenic disease and is therefore preventable. The tolerance of the adult human spinal cord to radiation, taking into account the volume of tissue irradiated, the duration of the irradiation, and total dose, has been determined by Kagan and his colleagues. These authors reviewed all of the cases in the literature up to 1980 and concluded that radiation injury could be avoided if the total dose was kept below 6000 rads and given over a period of 30 to 70 days—providing the daily fractions were below 200 rads and the rate was not much above 900 rads per week. It is noteworthy that in the cases reported by Sanyal et al the amount of radiation exceeded these limits. We have the impression that the incidence of this tragic complication is decreasing.

A number of case reports remark on temporary improvement in neurologic function after the administration of steroids. This therapy should be tried because in some patients the disease process after a time appears to be arrested short of complete transection of all sensory and motor tracts. Claims have also been made of regression of early symptoms in response to the administration of split heparin products.

Neurologists attached to tumor treatment centers are sometimes confronted with the late development (up to 10 to 15 years) of a slowly progressive sensorimotor paralysis. The condition raises questions of recurrent tumor, but absence of a mass lesion and of pain (motor weakness predominates) and the signs on neurologic examination are most consistent with a regional fibrosing neuropathy. Examples we have seen are multiple cranial neuropathies after radiation of nasopharyngeal tumors, cervical and brachial neuropathies after laryngeal and breast cancers, and lumbosacral plexopathies with pelvic tumors. Operations to extricate nerves are unsuccessful. Eventually the neurologic deficit is arrested (see also page 1066).

MYELITIS

In the nineteenth century, almost every disease of the spinal cord was labeled myelitis. Morton Prince, writing in Dercum's *Textbook of Nervous Diseases* in 1895, referred to traumatic myelitis, compressive myelitis, etc., obviously giving a rather imprecise meaning to the term. Gradually, however, as knowledge of neuropathology advanced, one disease after another was removed from this category until only the truly inflammatory ones remain. Yet at the same time some of the relationships between inflammation and infection have become more obscure. Some slow and unconventional viruses can destroy neural tissue without the appearance of inflammatory cells.

Today the spinal cord is known to be the locus of a limited number of infective and noninfective inflammatory processes, some causing selective destruction of neurons, others involving the meninges and white matter or leading to a necrosis of both gray and white matter. The currently accepted term for all these diseases is *myelitis*. A distinction is usually drawn between the *acute* variety, in which symptoms develop rapidly and reach their peak of severity within days; the *subacute,* in which the disease evolves over a period of 2 to 6 weeks; and the *chronic,* in which more than 6 weeks elapse between the onset and full development of the clinical picture. Of course there is no sharp division between these classes; but in general, the more acute the evolution, the greater the possibility of reversibility, viz., the impermanence of structural change.

Other special terms are used to indicate more precisely the distribution of the inflammatory process: if confined to gray matter, the proper expression is *poliomyelitis;* if to the white matter, *leukomyelitis.* If the whole thickness of the cord is involved, the myelitis is said to be ''transverse'' if the lesions are multiple and widespread over a long vertical extent, the modifying adjectives *diffuse* or *disseminated* are used. The term *meningomyelitis* refers to combined inflammation of meninges and spinal cord, and *meningoradiculitis,* to combined meningeal and root involvement. An inflammatory process limited to the spinal dura is called *pachymeningitis;* and if infected material collects in the epidural space, it is called *epidural abscess* or *granuloma.*

CLASSIFICATION OF INFLAMMATORY DISEASES OF THE SPINAL CORD

I. Myelitis due to filterable viruses
   A. Poliomyelitis, groups A and B Coxsackie virus, echovirus
   B. Herpes zoster
   C. Rabies
   D. B virus
   E. HTLV-1 and HTLV-3

II. Myelitis secondary to bacterial, fungal, and parasitic diseases of the meninges and spinal cord
    A. Syphilitic myelitis
       1. Chronic meningoradiculitis (tabes dorsalis)
       2. Chronic meningomyelitis
       3. Meningovascular syphilis
       4. Gummatous meningitis including chronic spinal pachymeningitis
    B. Pyogenic or suppurative myelitis
       1. Subacute meningomyelitis
       2. Acute epidural abscess and granuloma
       3. Abscess of spinal cord
    C. Tuberculous myelitis
       1. Pott's disease with spinal cord compression
       2. Tuberculous meningomyelitis
       3. Tuberculoma of spinal cord
    D. Parasitic and fungal infections producing epidural granuloma, localized meningitis, or meningomyelitis and abscess
III. Myelitis (myelopathy) of unknown etiology
    A. Postinfectious and postvaccinal
    B. Acute and chronic relapsing multiple sclerosis
    C. Necrotic or degenerative

From this outline it is evident that many different and totally unrelated diseases are under consideration and that a general description cannot possibly encompass such a diversity of pathologic processes. Many of the myelitides are considered elsewhere in this volume in relation to the diseases of which they are a part. Here it is only necessary to comment on the three principal categories and to describe a few of the common subtypes.

MYELITIS DUE TO FILTERABLE VIRUSES

Poliomyelitis and herpes zoster are the important members of this category. The viruses of poliomyelitis have an affinity for neurons of the anterior horn, and those of herpes zoster for the dorsal root ganglia; hence the disturbance of function is in terms of motor and sensory neurons respectively, and not of spinal tracts. Their onset is acute, and although there are systemic symptoms and cutaneous ones (in the case of zoster), it is the nervous system disorder that is most significant. The patient suffers the immediate effects of nerve cell destruction, and improvement nearly always follows as altered nerve cells recover. Later in life, as the neuronal loss of aging occurs in anterior horn cells and dorsal root ganglia, there may be a slow deterioration referable to the depleted system of neurons.

There are other forms of poliomyelitic reactions of unknown, presumably viral etiology (see further on, under spinal myoclonus). Affection of the white matter, with sensory and motor paralysis below the level of a lesion, has only been reported in so-called dumb rabies (in contrast

to the usual form of "mad" or "furious" rabies encephalitis), zoster and simplex myelitis, and an infection transmitted by the bite of a monkey, called the *B virus*, each of which is very rare and more recently in HTLV virus infections. As a generalization one may say that any myelitis that expresses itself by dysfunction of motor and sensory tracts will usually prove not to be viral in origin, but due rather to one of the disease processes in category II or III. The common types of viral myelitis are described in Chap. 33.

MYELITIS SECONDARY TO BACTERIAL, FUNGAL, AND PARASITIC DISEASES OF THE MENINGES AND SPINAL CORD TISSUE

This class of spinal cord disease seldom offers any difficulty in diagnosis. The CSF often holds the clue to causation. The inflammatory reaction of the spinal meninges is only one manifestation of a generalized disease process. The spinal lesion may involve primarily the pia-arachnoid (leptomeningitis), the dura (pachymeningitis), or the epidural space, e.g., abscess or granuloma; in the latter circumstance, damage to the spinal cord is due to compression and ischemia. In some acute diseases both the spinal cord and meninges are simultaneously affected or the cord lesions may predominate. Chronic spinal meningitis may involve the pial arteries, and as the inflamed vessels become thrombosed, infarction (myelomalacia) of the spinal cord results. Chronic meningeal inflammation may provoke a progressive constrictive pial fibrosis that virtually strangulates the spinal cord. Spinal roots may in certain instances become progressively damaged, especially the lumbosacral ones that have a long meningeal course. Posterior roots that enter the subarachnoid space near arachnoidal villi (where CSF is resorbed) tend to suffer greater injury than anterior ones (e.g., tabes dorsalis). Interestingly there are many types of chronic spinal or cerebrospinal meningitis that remain entirely asymptomatic until the spinal cord or roots become involved.

Syphilitic myelitis is discussed on page 579. *Abscess of the spinal cord* (acute bacterial myelitis) is exceedingly rare and probably undiagnosable. At times it is a single pyogenic metastasis. *Acute spinal epidural abscess and granuloma* are the more important representatives of this group.

Spinal Epidural Abscess Children or adults may be affected. An injury to the back, often trivial, at the time of a furunculosis or other skin or wound infection or a bacteremia, may permit seeding of the spinal epidural space or of a vertebral body. The latter gives rise to osteomyelitis with extension to the epidural space. *Staphylococcus aureus* is the most frequent etiologic agent, followed by streptococci, gram-negative bacilli, and anaerobic organisms.

At first, the suppurative process is accompanied only by fever and pain in the back, followed within a day or several days by radicular pain. Headache and nuchal rigidity are frequently present. After several more days there is the onset of a rapidly progressive paraparesis and paraplegia, associated with sensory loss in the lower parts of the body, sphincteric paralysis, and urinary and fecal retention. Percussion of the spine elicits tenderness over the site of the infection. Examination reveals all the signs of a transverse cord lesion with elements of spinal shock if paralysis has evolved rapidly. The CSF contains a small number of white cells (usually fewer than 100 per cubic millimeter), both polymorphonuclear leukocytes and lymphocytes—unless the needle penetrates the abscess, when pure pus is obtained. The protein content is relatively high (100 to 400 mg per 100 ml, or more), but the glucose is normal. More importantly, there is a dynamic block (positive Queckenstedt test).

There are other circumstances in which an acute spinal epidural abscess may develop. It may occur in a patient with chronic medical disease(s), in which a septicemia develops. Here the spinal symptoms may be minimal until the onset of the signs of spinal cord compression some days or weeks later. In other cases organisms may be introduced into the epidural space via a lumbar puncture needle, during epidural or spinal anesthesia, or during a laminectomy for a ruptured lumbar disc. The localization is then over lumbar and sacral roots. In these cases of *cauda equina epidural abscess,* pain may be severe and neurologic symptomatology minimal unless the infection extends upward to the upper lumbar and thoracic segments of the spinal cord.

The foregoing clinical and spinal fluid findings call for immediate myelography, to determine the level of block and the operative site. If not treated surgically by laminectomy and drainage at the earliest possible moment, the spinal cord lesion, which is due in part to ischemia (compression mainly of veins), becomes more or less irreversible. Antibiotic therapy must also be given. The cauda equina epidural abscess without neurologic signs should be treated with appropriate antibiotics. If osteomyelitis develops, it may require drainage. When osteomyelitis of a vertebral body is the primary abnormality, the epidural

extension may implicate only a few spinal sensory and motor roots, leaving long tracts intact. In the cases described by Messer and Litvinoff, stiff neck, fever, and deltoid-biceps weakness were the main neurologic abnormalities.

Subdural bacterial infections also occur and are virtually indistinguishable from epidural ones. A clue may be provided by the myelogram in which the obstructive lesion has a less sharp margin and a greater vertical extent.

Subacute pyogenic infections and granulomatous infections (tuberculous, fungal) may also arise in the spinal epidural space. The clinical picture is less dramatic, and local and radicular pain is slight or absent; the diagnosis depends on the demonstration, in a patient with weakness and sensory loss below a certain level on the trunk, of a partial or complete block by contrast myelography. Osteomyelitis may not be seen for a time in plain films, but bone scans and MRI are revealing. Treatment depends on the nature of the underlying disease and the general condition of the patient.

SPINAL CORD ABSCESS

This entity was first described by Chiari in 1900, and, while rare, it occurs often enough to have been the subject of some 40 reports. In some instances the patient was known to have had a systemic bacterial infection, a septicemia or endocarditis. The symptoms are indistinguishable from those of epidural abscess, namely spine and radicular pain followed by sensory and motor paralysis; the CSF findings are also the same. A myelographic block may not be present, but this is not a reliable criterion for excluding the diagnosis of spinal cord abscess. Woltman and Adson have described a patient in whom surgical drainage of an encapsulated intramedullary abscess led to recovery, and Morrison et al reported a similar case, caused by *Listeria monocytogenes*, which was successfully drained and the meningeal infection suppressed by ampicillin and chloramphenicol. Acute transverse myelitis has been observed several times in the course of a typical pneumonitis due to *Mycoplasma pneumoniae*. In the patient reported by Westenfelder et al, the CSF contained 80 lymphocytes per cubic millimeter, an elevated protein, and normal glucose, and there was a high titer of antibodies to *M. pneumoniae* in both serum and CSF. Spinal cord abscess may be a rare complication of spinal dysraphism.

Tuberculous Myelitis Solitary tuberculoma of the spinal cord as part of a generalized infection is an extreme rarity. Tuberculous osteitis of the spine with kyphosis (Pott's disease) is more frequent; pus or caseous granulation tissue may extrude from an infected vertebra and gives rise to an epidural abscess that compresses the cord (Pott's paraplegia). Occasionally a tuberculous meningitis may result in pial arteritis and spinal cord infarction. The paraplegia may appear before the tuberculous meningitis is diagnosed.

All these forms of tuberculosis have become infrequent in the United States and Western Europe. Additional comments will be found on pages 570 to 572.

Meningomyelitis Due to Fungus and Parasitic Diseases A wide variety of fungal and parasitic agents may involve the spinal meninges. They are rare and some do not occur at all in the United States or are limited to certain geographic areas. *Actinomyces, Blastomyces, Coccidioides,* and *Aspergillus* may invade the spinal epidural space via intervertebral foramens or by extension from a vertebral osteomyelitic focus. *Cryptococcus,* which causes meningoencephalitis and rarely a cerebral granuloma, seldom leads to spinal lesions. Hematogenous metastases to the spinal cord or meninges may occur in both blastomycosis and coccidioidomycosis. Occasionally echinococcus infection of the posterior mediastinum may extend to the spinal canal (epidural space) via intervertebral foramina and compress the spinal cord.

Schistosomiasis (bilharziasis) is a recognized cause of myelitis in the Far East, Africa, and South America; occasionally, it is complicated by compression and necrosis of the spinal cord. The spinal cord is a target for all three common forms of *Schistosoma* (*S. haematobium, S. mansoni,* and *S. japonicum*). We have studied two patients in whom the spinal cord in the low thoracic and lumbar region was infected approximately 3 weeks after swimming in contaminated water. The CSF showed only a slight elevation of protein, and there was no abnormality in the myelogram. The administration of praziquantel arrested the course of the illness, but the patients were left disabled. The lesions in such cases are destructive of gray and white matter with ova in arteries and veins leading to obstruction and ischemia. The devastating character of the cord lesion is documented in the report of Queiroz et al.

MYELITIS (MYELOPATHY) OF UNDETERMINED ETIOLOGY

These disorders take the form of a leukomyelitis based either on demyelination or necrosis of the tracts in the spinal cord. Varied clinical syndromes are induced, and the basic disease is classified in most textbooks under headings such as postinfectious myelitis, postvaccinal myelitis, acute multiple sclerosis, chronic relapsing multiple sclerosis, necrotizing myelitis, and neuromyelitis optica (Devic disease). While each of these conditions may affect other parts of the central nervous system (most often the optic nerves) as well as the spinal cord, not infrequently the only manifestations are spinal. The distinctions between the aforementioned myelitides are sufficient to justify their

separate classification, for in most cases they run true to form; but transitional cases, sharing the attributes of more than one disease, are encountered in any large clinical and pathologic material.

Postinfectious and Postvaccinal Myelitis The characteristic features of these diseases are (1) their temporal relationship to a viral infection (usually one with exanthematous manifestations such as rubeola, varicella, variola, and rarely rubella, influenza, mumps) or a vaccination (antirabies, cowpox); (2) the development of neurologic signs over the period of a few days; and (3) a monophasic temporal course, i.e., a single attack of several weeks' duration with variable degrees of recovery and no recurrence. In most cases these diseases involve the brain as well as the spinal cord (i.e., they are encephalomyelitic); in others the spinal cord is affected predominantly or exclusively.

The usual history in the latter cases is for weakness and numbness of the feet and legs (less often of the hands and arms) and difficulty in voiding to develop over a few days, as the skin rash is fading. Recrudescence of fever may precede or coincide with the onset of neurologic symptoms. Headache and stiff neck may or may not be present. The neurologic symptoms progress for several days after which they remain stationary and then recede slowly. Almost invariably the CSF contains lymphocytes and other mononuclear cells in the range of 20 to 200 (rarely higher) per cubic millimeter with normal or slightly raised protein and normal glucose values. In most cases there are other neurologic signs pointing to lesions in the optic nerves, brainstem, cerebellum, and cerebrum. In some of the cases that followed antirabies inoculation, the peripheral nerves were affected more than the spinal cord; this happens rarely in the postexanthem cases. Myelitic symptoms that follow antirabies inoculation begin 10 to 20 days after the first treatment and once started, worsen with each subsequent injection. Use of the new vaccine that is grown on human tissue cultures, rather than myelinated spinal cord, has almost eliminated this complication.

Most puzzling are autopsy-verified instances of postinfectious myelitis in which the disease developed without an apparent antecedent infection or after one that could not be identified (influenza?). Clinical diagnosis in such cases must be based on the time course of the illness and the clinical and CSF findings. There is always uncertainty in such cases as to whether the illness is the opening phase of multiple sclerosis.

The pathologic changes take the form of myriads of

subpial and perivenular zones of demyelination, with perivascular and meningeal infiltrations of lymphocytes and other mononuclear cells, and para-adventitial pleomorphic histiocytes and microgliacytes (see page 769).

Once symptoms begin, it is doubtful if any except supportive therapy is of value. One's first impulse, assuming the mechanism to be an autoimmune disorder, is to administer ACTH or prednisone as soon as the diagnosis is made. Perhaps it is advisable to do so, but there is no evidence that this practice alters the natural course of the illness.

The prognosis must be guarded. Improvement of the purely myelitic disease occurs invariably, sometimes to an astonishing degree, but there are examples in which the sequelae have been severe and permanent. The authors have several times given a good prognosis for long-term recovery and assurance of no subsequent relapse only to witness a recrudescence of symptoms at a later date, proving the original illness to have been multiple sclerosis.

Demyelinative Myelitis   The lesions of acute multiple sclerosis, presenting as a myelitis, share many of the properties of the postinfectious type, except that the clinical manifestations tend to evolve more slowly, over a period of 1 to 3 weeks or longer. Also, their relation to inoculation or infection is less certain, and in most recorded examples these antecedent events were lacking. Yet as Uchimura and Shiraki have shown in their study of postrabies inoculation in Japan, where the myelitis took the form of acute multiple sclerosis, the disease does have the monophasic character and some of the pathologic attributes of the postinfectious variety. However, other cases declare, by subsequent attacks, that the basic illness is one of chronic recurrent demyelination, identical to the usual type of multiple sclerosis.

The most typical mode of clinical expression is by numbness that spreads over one or both sides of the body from the sacral segments to the feet, anterior thighs, and up over the trunk, with coincident weakness and then paralysis of the legs. As the latter becomes complete, the bladder is also paralyzed. The sensorimotor disturbance may extend to involve the arms. Depending on the speed and intensity of the paralysis, elements of spinal shock may supervene. The CSF usually shows a pleocytosis, as in the postinfectious variety, but may be normal. The condition is painless and without fever, and the patient recovers with variable residual signs.

There may be difficulty in separating this disease (a severe myelitis of acute multiple sclerosis type with spinal shock) from the ascending Landry-Guillain-Barré polyneuritis, from spinal epidural abscess, and from an infective meningomyelitis. The most helpful finding is a sensory and motor level on the trunk below which all function is abolished; this never really happens in polyneuritis. Spine ache and tenderness and root pain are features of epidural abscess, along with fever, leukocytosis, increased sedimentation rate, and often a positive bone scan; myelographic block is invariable. Rarely, however, a demyelinative myelitis causes some pain, and the cord may swell sufficiently to interfere with the flow of contrast media. In a few such cases, because of the danger of leaving an epidural abscess undrained, or in the mistaken belief that the swollen cord represented an intramedullary tumor, laminectomy has been performed with negative results.

Treatment with ACTH or corticosteroids, as outlined for multiple sclerosis (page 766), may lead to a regression of symptoms, sometimes with relapse when the injections are discontinued too soon (after 1 to 2 weeks). Other patients, however, show no apparent response, and a few have even continued to worsen while the hormones are being given.

The episode of evolving myelitis in what proves later to have been the first phase of a chronic (polyphasic) multiple sclerosis has virtually the same pattern and course as the episode of acute (monophasic) multiple sclerosis. (See Chap. 37 for the description of other clinical variants of acute multiple sclerosis.)

Acute Necrotizing Myelitis   In every large medical center, occasional examples of this disorder are to be found among the many patients who present with an acute onset of paraplegia or quadriplegia, sensory loss, and sphincter paralysis. The neurologic signs may erupt in hours, with such precipitancy as to suggest a vascular lesion (myelomalacia from extra- or intravertebral arterial occlusion or hematomyelia from a vascular malformation or bleeding diathesis). In other cases the disease evolves at a somewhat slower pace, over several days, and some, but not all, are attended by unilateral or bilateral optic neuritis. In the series of cases reported by Bassoe and Hassin, Greenfield and Turner, Kahle and Schaltenbrand (see references in Hughes), and most recently by Hughes, patients of all ages and both sexes were affected. Sensory disturbance tends to precede motor, and the latter, at first of upper motor neuron type, later gives way to a flaccid, areflexic paralysis. A few or several hundred mononuclear cells per cubic millimeter and increased protein may be found in the CSF. Survival is the rule, but the neurologic deficits tend to be lasting.

In several cases coming to postmortem examination at variable intervals after the onset, the acute lesion has proved to be a necrotizing hemorrhagic leukomyelitis, not essentially different from the hemorrhagic leukoencephalitis described on page 771. For this reason the authors agree with Hughes in classifying it with the demyelinative diseases. Perivenous demyelination and diffuse necrosis of all tissue elements appear related to the deposit of immune complexes and injury of walls of small vessels, leading to fibrin thrombi and fibrin exudation. Older lesions will have left the spinal cord cavitated or collapsed for a vertical extent of 5 to 20 cm. The optic nerve lesions tend usually to be of demyelinative type, in fact are much the same as those of multiple sclerosis. This combination of spinal cord necrosis and optic neuritis appears to correspond to the syndrome described by Devic in 1894 and named neuro-myelitis optica. But nearly all neurologists agree that a similar clinical syndrome involving the optic nerve and spinal cord (usually without necrosis) may be caused by postinfectious encephalomyelitis and by multiple sclerosis. In one of the authors' cases, in which death occurred many years after the onset of the myelitis, there was an old necrotizing myelitic lesion and many cerebral ones, the latter typical of multiple sclerosis. Cases of this type show the overlapping relationship between the necrotizing and demyelinative processes.

Under the title of *subacute necrotic myelitis* Foix and Alajouanine and later Greenfield and Turner described a disorder of adult males, characterized by an amyotrophic paraplegia that ran a progressive course over several months. An early spastic state evolved into a flaccid, areflexive paralysis. Sensory loss, at first dissociated and then complete, and loss of sphincteric control came on after the paresis. The CSF protein was considerably elevated but there were no cells. Postmortem examinations in their cases and in others have shown the lumbosacral segments to be the most severely involved, with progressively less severe affection of the thoracic segments. In the affected areas there was severe necrosis of both gray and white matter with appropriate macrophage and astrocytic reactions. The walls of small vessels, which seemed to be increased in number, were thickened, cellular, and fibrotic. Yet their lumens were not occluded. The veins were also thickened and surrounded by lymphocytes, mononuclear cells, and macrophages. These findings have been difficult to interpret. The importance of spinal phlebothrombosis in the pathogenesis has been emphasized, but in the case of Mair and Folkerts only one thrombosed anterior spinal vein was seen; and in the cases of Foix and Alajouanine no thrombosed vessels were found. The authors believe the evidence of venous occlusion to be unconvincing, but concede that there is a rare clinical entity of spinal thrombophlebitis (cf. Antoni).

Paraneoplastic Myelitis A subacute necrotic myelitis, developing in conjunction with a bronchogenic carcinoma, was first brought to medical notice by Mancall and Rosales, in 1964. Several dozen cases have since been recorded, some in association with solid visceral lymphomas. The clinical syndrome, as we have seen it, consists of a rapidly progressive loss of motor and then sensory tract function,

usually with sphincter disorder. It is usually painless and the myelogram is normal, in distinction to extradural metastatic disease with cord compression. The CSF may contain a few mononuclear cells and a slightly increased protein or it may be normal. The lesions are essentially of necrotic type and respect neither gray nor white matter, but the latter is more affected. There is no evidence of an infective-inflammatory or ischemic lesion, for the blood vessels, apart from a modest mononuclear cuffing, are normal. No tumor cells are visible in the CSF, meninges, or spinal cord tissue, and no virus has been isolated. Even more puzzling is the fact that lesions of the same type have been reported in patients who at autopsy harbored no tumor.

In some cases of paraneoplastic myelopathy, the degenerative changes are more chronic, confined to the posterior and lateral funiculi, and often associated with a diffuse loss of Purkinje cells. This latter syndrome has a disproportionately high association with ovarian carcinoma, but has been observed with carcinoma of other types and with Hodgkin disease. All of the reported cases of these types have ended fatally; steroids and plasmapheresis were of no value.

Reference has already been made to an entirely different, but equally obscure type of paraneoplastic syndrome, characterized by an apparently primary loss of anterior horn cells.

As to the etiology of paraneoplastic spinal cord disease, an intriguing finding has been reported by Arnason and more recently by Babikian et al. In the serum of such patients, they have found an IgG antibody that cross-reacts with the tumor cells and some component of the neural tissue. In the case of Babikian et al, in which there was both an axonal neuropathy and a myelopathy with a small-cell carcinoma of the lung, the cord receptor was a neuron-specific enolase. The cord lesion resembled an anterior-posterior poliomyelitis, a lesion that we have seen in two patients, one with Hodgkin disease, the other with bronchogenic carcinoma. A viral etiology must still be ruled out in cases of the latter type and probably of necrotizing myelitis as well.

OTHER MYELITIDES OF INDETERMINATE CAUSE

The older medical literature contains numerous references to bacterial infections (pneumonia, gonorrhea, and other) that resulted in some type of myelopathy. However, the descriptions are inexact and pathologic verification is lacking so that it is difficult to interpret them. The same is true of myelopathies that follow intravenous injections of contaminated heroin and other drugs. The authors have the impression that some type of ischemia or angiitis may underlie them. Their rarity does not promise a quick solution to the problem.

Whitely et al have drawn attention to a rare but distinctive form of *encephalomyelitis of unknown cause*, characterized clinically by tonic rigidity and intermittent myoclonic jerking of the trunk and limb muscles and by painful spasms evoked by sensory or emotional stimuli. Signs of brainstem involvement occur in the late stages of the disease, which is usually progressive over a period of several weeks, months, or a year or longer; consciousness is preserved, however. The CSF may be normal or show a mild lymphocytosis and increase in protein content. This is probably the same disorder that had been described earlier by Campbell and Garland under the title of *subacute myoclonic spinal neuronitis*, and more recently by Howell et al. The disorder under discussion needs to be differentiated clinically from the syndrome of *continuous muscle fiber activity* of Isaacs and the *"stiff man" syndrome* of Moersch and Woltman (see Chap. 54).

The brunt of the pathologic process falls on the cervical portion of the spinal cord. Widespread loss of internuncial neurons with relative sparing of the anterior horn cells, neuronophagia of internuncial neurons, reactive gliosis and microglial proliferation, conspicuous lymphocytic cuffing of small blood vessels, and scanty meningeal inflammation are the main findings. Involvement of the white matter is less conspicuous.

The pathophysiology of the rigidity in these cases is not well understood, but may be due to the impaired function (or destruction) of Renshaw cells, with the release of tonic myotatic reflexes (Penry et al). The painful spasms and dysesthesias relate in some way to neuronal lesions in the posterior horns of the spinal cord and dorsal root ganglia. We agree with Whitely and with Lhermitte and their coworkers that the cases in which rigidity, painful spasms, and myoclonus progress over a few weeks or months, associated with pleocytosis and a normal myelogram, probably suffer from a rare and obscure form of viral myelitis and encephalitis. As has been indicated on page 86, myoclonic jerking of the trunk and limbs may be due to neuronal damage that is limited to the spinal cord.

VASCULAR DISEASES OF THE SPINAL CORD

In comparison to the brain, the spinal cord is an uncommon site of vascular disease. Blackwood, in a review of 3737

necropsies at the National Hospital for Nervous Diseases, London, in the period 1903 to 1958, found only nine cases, but in general hospitals such as ours, they are much more frequent. The spinal arteries are not susceptible to atherosclerosis, and emboli rarely lodge there. As was stated above, in relation to chronic meningeal infections, an endarteritis or phlebitis involving vessels on the surface of the cord may lead to thrombosis and infarction. Polyarteritis nodosa may rarely have a similar effect, although this disease is more often localized to the peripheral than to the central nervous system. Very rarely the spinal cord is affected in lupus erythematosus; a vascular basis is likely but has not been established. Transient or lasting ischemia of the cervical segments has been observed by the authors as a complication of vertebral angiography and aortography. Occlusion of vertebrospinal branches results in lesions of the upper cervical segments; occlusion of thyrocervical branches of the carotid, in lesions of the middle cervical segments; and of costocervical branches of the carotid in lesions of lower cervical segments. Most but not all cases recover after several days. Fibrocartilaginous emboli in spinal arteries and veins after trauma is another documented cause of infarction (see further on).

Of all the vascular disorders of the spinal cord, infarction and bleeding are the only ones that occur with any regularity. An understanding of these disorders requires some knowledge of the blood supply of the spinal cord.

VASCULAR ANATOMY OF THE SPINAL CORD

The blood supply of the spinal cord is derived from a paired series of segmental vessels arising from the aorta and from branches of the subclavian and internal iliac arteries (Fig. 36-2). The most important branches of the subclavian are the vertebral arteries, the segmental branches of which form the rostral origins of the anterior median and posterior and lateral spinal arteries and constitute the major blood supply to the cervical cord. The thoracic and lumbar cord are nourished by segmental arteries arising from the aorta and internal iliac arteries; segmental branches of the lateral sacral arteries supply the sacral cord.

A typical segmental artery divides into an anterior and posterior ramus (Fig. 36-3). Each posterior ramus gives rise to a spinal artery which enters the vertebral foramen, pierces the dura, and supplies the spinal ganglion and roots through its anterior and posterior radicular branches. Most anterior radicular arteries are small, but a variable number (four to nine), arising at irregular intervals, are much larger and supply most of the blood to the spinal cord.

Lazorthes, in his excellent review of the circulation of the spinal cord, divides the radiculomedullary arteries into three groups: (1) upper or cervicothoracic which are derived from the anterior spinal arteries, branches of

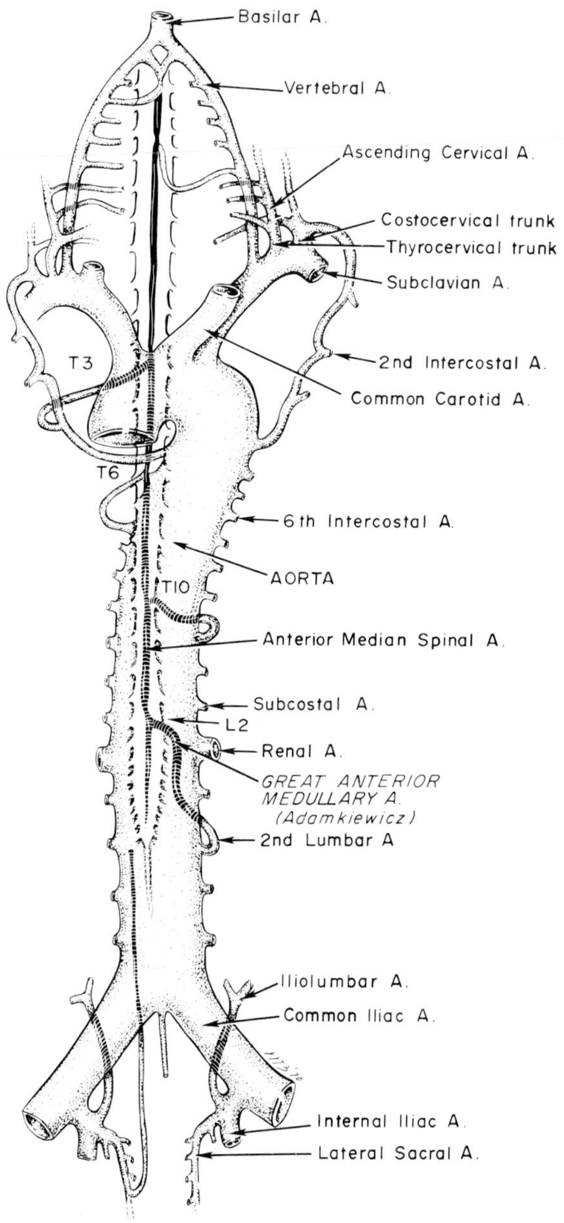
Basilar A.
Vertebral A.
Ascending Cervical A.
Costocervical trunk
Thyrocervical trunk
Subclavian A.
2nd Intercostal A.
Common Carotid A.
T3
T6
6th Intercostal A.
AORTA
T10
Anterior Median Spinal A.
Subcostal A.
L2
Renal A.
GREAT ANTERIOR
MEDULLARY A.
(Adamkiewicz)
2nd Lumbar A
Iliolumbar A.
Common Iliac A.
Internal Iliac A.
Lateral Sacral A.

Figure 36-2

Anterior view of spinal cord with its segmental blood supply from the aorta. See text for details. (From Herrick and Mills.)

thyrocervical and costoverbral arteries; (2) intermediate or middle thoracic (T4 to T8 cord segments), usually from a single T7 radicular artery; and (3) lower or thoracolumbar from the T10 or T11 anterior radicular artery (of Adamkiewicz) also called the *arteria radicularis magna.* The latter may supply the lower two-thirds of the cord, but in any individual one cannot predict the precise area supplied by this or any other anterior radiculomedullary artery, or what proportion of cord will be infarcted if one of these vessels is occluded.

The anterior medullary arteries form the single anterior median spinal artery, which runs the full length of the cord in the anterior sulcus and gives off direct penetrating branches via the central (sulcocommissural) arteries. These penetrating branches supply most of the anterior gray columns and the ventral portions of the dorsal gray columns of neurons (Fig. 36-3). The peripheral rim of white matter of the anterior two-thirds of the cord is supplied from a pial radial network, which also originates from the anterior median spinal artery. Thus, the branches of the anterior median spinal artery supply roughly the ventral two-thirds of the spinal cord. The posterior medullary arteries form the paired posterior spinal arteries that supply the dorsal third of the cord by means of direct penetrating vessels and a plexus of pial vessels (similar to that of the ventral cord, with which it anastomoses freely). Within the cord substance, then, there is a ''watershed'' area of capillaries where the penetrating branches of the anterior median spinal artery (via the central arteries) meet the penetrating branches of the posterior spinal arteries and the branches of the circumferential pial network. All spinal segments, because of the variable size of collateral arteries, do not have the same abundance of circulatory protection. Hence a hypotensive crisis, as in diabetic acidosis, anesthesia, etc., may result in ischemic necrosis of certain segments, usually the upper thoracic, leading to interruption of sensorimotor tracts.

Normally there are 8 to 12 anterior medullary veins and a greater number of posterior medullary veins arranged fairly close to one another at every segmental level.

INFARCTION OF SPINAL CORD (MYELOMALACIA)

Ischemic softening of the spinal cord usually involves the territory of the anterior spinal artery, i.e., a variable vertical extent of the ventral two-thirds of the spinal cord. The resulting clinical abnormalities are generally referred to as the *anterior spinal artery syndrome,* first described by Spiller in 1909. Atherosclerosis and thrombotic occlusion of the anterior spinal artery itself is not common, however, and infarction in the territory of this artery is more often secondary to disease of important medullary arteries (see above) or to disease of the aorta—either advanced atherosclerosis or a dissecting aneurysm, which occludes or shears off the important segmental spinal arteries at their origins. Nonetheless, we have seen a number of possible instances in adolescents and young adults in whom no aortic or spinal arterial disease could be demonstrated. Cardiac surgery, which requires clamping of the aorta for more than 30 min, and aortic arteriography may occasionally be complicated by infarction in the territory of the anterior spinal artery. Occasionally, polyarteritis nodosa or emboli arising from a severely atheromatous aorta may occlude a spinal medullary artery. Infarction may be associated with a vascular mal-

formation of the spinal cord, but more often this lesion gives rise to hemorrhage.

The clinical manifestations of arterial occlusion will of course vary with the level of infarction, but common to all cases is the *development of motor paralysis and dissociated sensory loss* below the level of the lesion, accompanied by paralysis of sphincteric function. The symptoms may develop instantaneously or over an hour or two, surely much more rapidly than in the myelitides. Pain is sometimes a complaint, either diffuse in a segment of the body (e.g., legs) or more often radicular, corresponding to the upper level of the lesion. Paralysis is usually bilateral, occasionally unilateral, and is rarely complete. Except in high cervical lesions, the sensory changes are dissociated; i.e., pain and temperature sensations are lost (due to interruption of the spinothalamic tracts), but vibration and position sense are unimpaired (sparing of posterior columns). In this respect the syndrome differs from the transverse cord syndrome of trauma. Initially the limbs are flaccid and areflexic, as in spinal shock from transverse traumatic lesions, followed after several weeks by the development of spasticity,

Figure 36-3

Representative cross section of lumbar vertebra and spinal cord with its blood supply at level of an anterior medullary artery. The shaded zones in the posterior part of the cord, ventral part of the cord, and margins of the ventral cord represent the regions of blood supply of the posterior spinal arteries, central (sulcal) arteries, and pial plexus, respectively. Borders of these three zones, appearing as white in the diagram, represent watershed areas. (From Herrick and Mills.)

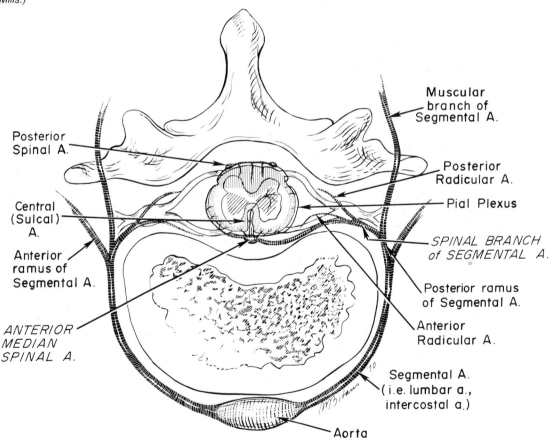

hyperactive tendon reflexes, clonus and Babinski signs, and some degree of voluntary bladder control (unless sacral segments have been infarcted). Dissecting aneurysm of the aorta—which announces itself by intense interscapular and/or chest pain (occasionally it is painless), widening of the aorta, and circulatory obstruction to the legs or arms and various organs—gives rise to a number of neurologic syndromes. The most common of these syndromes are (1) paralysis of the sphincters and both legs with sensory loss usually below T6 (Weisman and Adams), (2) obstruction of a brachial artery with sensorimotor neuropathy in the limb, and (3) obstruction of a common carotid artery with hemiplegia. Rarely, ischemic infarction of the cord is confined to the gray matter. In these cases there is also an abrupt onset of muscle weakness in the legs, but no pain or sensory loss.

In the past, aortography was sometimes complicated by an acute myelopathy, and the authors have observed a number of such cases. Killen and Foster, in 1966, reviewed 43 examples of this accident. The onset of sensorimotor paralysis is immediate, and the effects are often permanent. The syndrome of painful segmental spasms, spinal myoclonus, and rigidity has also been observed under these conditions (page 732). Vascular spasm and occlusion result in infarct necrosis. The frequency of this complication has been greatly reduced by the introduction of less toxic contrast media.

Treatment of all forms of spinal cord infarction can only be symptomatic, with attention in the acute stage to the care of bladder, bowel, and skin; after 10 to 14 days, more active rehabilitation measures can be started.

HEMORRHAGE INTO THE SPINAL CORD (HEMATOMYELIA) AND SPINAL CANAL (HEMATORRHACHIS)

Hemorrhage into the spinal cord is also rare, compared to the frequency of cerebral hemorrhage. The apoplectic onset of symptoms that involve tracts (motor or sensory or both) in the spinal cord, associated with blood and xanthochromia in the spinal fluid, are the identifying features of hematomyelia. Aside from trauma, *hematomyelia is usually traceable to a vascular malformation or bleeding disease, and particularly to the administration of anticoagulants.* Bleeding into the epidural or subdural space may have the same causes and give rise to a rapidly evolving compressive myelopathy. Like epidural abscess, this represents a neurologic emergency and calls for immediate myelographic localization and surgical evacuation.

Advances in the techniques of selective spinal angiography and microsurgery have permitted the visualization and treatment of vascular lesions with a precision not imaginable a few decades ago (see Djindjian). These angiographic procedures make it possible to distinguish between the several types of vascular malformations and hemangioblastomas and to localize them accurately to the spinal cord, epidural, or subdural space, or the vertebral bodies.

VASCULAR MALFORMATIONS

These are well-known lesions, occurring not infrequently, and causing both ischemic and hemorrhagic lesions. One of the most clearly delineated types is the *venous angioma* (angioma racemosum venosum) which is located on the dorsal surface of the lower half of the spinal cord, and occurs most often in middle aged and elderly men (23 of 25 of Logue's cases were male). In only a few has there been an associated dermatomal nevus. The clinical picture has been well described by Wyburn-Mason. Acute pain (cramp-like, lancinating), most often in a sciatic distribution, is a prominent early feature. It may occur in a series of episodes over a period of several days or weeks, sometimes worse in recumbency. Almost always it is associated with weakness or paralysis of one or both legs and numbness and paresthesias in the same distribution. Wasting and weakness of legs may introduce the disease in some instances, with uneven progression, sometimes in a series of apoplectic episodes. Severe disability of gait is usually present within 6 months and half of Logue's cases were chair-bound within 3 years; the life span is 5 to 6 years. Diagnosis is now confirmed by selective arteriography, CT scan with contrast, and myelography.

When viewed pathologically the dorsal surface of the lower cord is covered with a tangle of veins, some involving roots and penetrating the surface of the cord. These lesions rarely bleed. The saltatory progression of symptoms is due presumably to occlusion of vessels, or their enlargement and compression of the spinal cord. Logue, who reported the operative results in 24 patients, believes that raised intravascular pressure causes compression of tracts in the spinal cord. By occluding the feeding artery, which is often single, and eliminating the pressure in veins and capillaries (stripping veins from the cord), he arrested the course of disease in all of his patients and reduced their pain. In some of our cases, there was improvement in the neurologic state over a few weeks or months. Embolization is also recommended by some radiologists.

In contrast, the *arteriovenous angiomas* tend to involve the posterior parts of the lower thoracic and upper lumbar segments or the anterior parts of the cervical enlargement. The patients are often younger, and the sexes are equally affected. The clinical syndrome may take the form of slow spinal cord compression, sometimes with a sudden exacerbation; or the initial symptoms may be apoplectic in nature, due either to thrombosis of a vessel or a hemorrhage (hematomyelia and subarachnoid hemorrhage); the latter complication occurred in 7 of 30 cases reported by Wyburn-Mason.

In the Klippel-Trénaunay-Weber syndrome, a vascular malformation of the spinal cord is associated with a cutaneous vascular nevus; when the malformation lies in the low cervical region, there may be enlargement of finger, hand, or arm (the hemangiectatic hypertrophy of Parkes Weber). Some of these vascular lesions have been treated by defining and ligating their feeding vessels. In other cases it has been possible to extirpate the entire lesion.

Other vascular anomalies of the spinal cord include: aneurysm of a spinal artery with coarctation of the aorta (rare); multiple cavernous hemangiomas with angiomas of brain, kidney, and pancreas (distinct from Von Hippel-Lindau disease); and telangiectasia, which may or may not be associated with the hereditary hemorrhagic telangiectasia of Osler-Rendu-Weber. The authors have had under their care several patients with the latter disease, who developed acute hemorrhagic lesions of the spinal cord. The cord lesions cause partial syndromes and are usually followed by considerable recovery of function. The CSF may or may not be sanguineous. Rarely, the same disease is responsible for a hemorrhagic lesion of the brain. Its association with arteriovenous fistulas of the lung is a rare source of brain abscess.

CAISSON DISEASE

Decompression sickness, the disorder observed in persons who are subjected to high underwater pressure, affects mainly the upper thoracic spinal cord, as a result of nitrogen bubbles forming and being trapped in spinal vessels. There may be little or no involvement of the brain. Haymaker, who has provided the most complete account of the neuropathologic changes, observed lesions of ischemic type mainly in the white matter of the upper thoracic cord; the posterior columns were more affected than lateral and anterior ones.

FIBROCARTILAGINOUS EMBOLISM

In 1961 Naiman et al first described the case of an adolescent boy who died of sudden paralysis after an athletic injury and was found to have extensive myelomalacia due to numerous occlusions of spinal vessels by emboli of nucleus pulposus. More than 30 such cases have now been reported. Bots and his colleagues encountered three cases in one year. The clinical picture is essentially one of spinal apoplexy—a healthy adult suddenly experiences pain in the back or neck accompanied by a transverse cord lesion affecting all sensory, motor, and sphincteric functions within minutes. In most reported instances the patient had not and was not engaged in any unusual activity; only three had fallen and injured themselves, and one had been loading goods when affected. Survival ranged from hours to months. The CSF was normal. At autopsy numerous small arteries and/or veins within the spinal cord were occluded by typical fibrocartilage; there was infarct necrosis of the spinal cord, and, in four cases, of the medulla oblongata. Bots et al believe that this condition accounts for some cases of inexplicable spinal apoplexy. No clue is available to explain how nucleus pulposus enters the vessels of the vascularized annular ligament and vertebral marrow. Ruptured disc of the usual type was not evident in these patients.

THE SYNDROME OF SUBACUTE OR CHRONIC SPINAL PARAPARESIS WITH OR WITHOUT ATAXIA

The gradual development of weakness of the legs is the common manifestation of several diseases. A syndrome of this type, which begins insidiously in late childhood or adolescence and progresses steadily over many years, is usually indicative of spinocerebellar degeneration (Friedreich ataxia) or one of its variants; we have also observed several cases of non-Friedreich cerebellar or spinocerebellar ataxia that begins in childhood and progresses through adolescence (see Chap. 44). In early adult life, multiple sclerosis is the most frequent cause; syphilitic meningomyelitis and spinal arachnoiditis are uncommon causes. In middle and late adult life, subacute combined degeneration of the cord (vitamin B_{12} deficiency), combined system disease of the nonpernicious anemia type, a late demyelinative myelopathy, cervical spondylosis, spinal arachnoiditis, and tumor are the important diagnostic considerations. In most forms of subacute and chronic spinal cord disease, spastic paraparesis is much more prominent than posterior column ataxia (Friedreich ataxia and vitamin B_{12} deficiency myelopathy are notable exceptions).

HEREDITARY SPINAL (FRIEDREICH) ATAXIA AND SPASTIC PARAPARESIS

See Chap. 43.

Ataxic paraparesis is probably the most common manifestation of multiple sclerosis. Asymmetric affection of the limbs, and signs of cerebral, optic nerve, brainstem, and cerebellar involvement usually provide the confirmatory evidence for the diagnosis of this disease. Nevertheless, purely spinal involvement may occur, no lesions being found outside the spinal cord, even at autopsy. A frequent problem in diagnosis is posed by the older adult patient who is not known to have had multiple sclerosis in earlier life (previous episodes having been asymptomatic or forgotten). Such cases must be differentiated from cervical spondylosis and tumor. Of aid in the diagnosis are the CSF findings, particularly the IgG abnormalities, the demonstration by evoked potential studies of lesions in the optic nerves and in the auditory and tactile tracts of the brainstem, and the enhanced CT and MR studies, which may disclose unsuspected cerebral white matter lesions (see Chap. 37).

SYPHILITIC MENINGOMYELITIS

Here, as in multiple sclerosis, the degree of ataxia and spastic weakness is variable. A few patients have an almost pure state of spastic weakness of the legs, requiring differentiation from motor system disease and familial spastic paraplegia. Such a syndrome, formerly called Erb's spastic paraplegia and attributed to meningovascular syphilis, is now recognized as being nonspecific. In a minority of patients, sensory ataxia and other posterior column signs predominate, and ventral roots are involved in the chronic meningeal inflammation. There may be signs of segmental amyotrophy, hence the term *syphilitic amyotrophy of the upper extremities with spastic paraplegia*. Confirmation of this diagnosis depends on finding a lymphocytic pleocytosis, an elevated protein and gamma globulin, and a positive serologic reaction in the CSF. Other aspects of this disease and treatment are discussed on page 579.

SUBACUTE COMBINED DEGENERATION (SCD) OF THE SPINAL CORD

This form of spinal cord disease, due to vitamin B_{12} deficiency, is fully described in Chap. 39. Almost invariably it begins with symptoms and signs of posterior column involvement, followed within a matter of several weeks or months by affection of the corticospinal tracts. Of particular importance is the fact that SCD is a treatable disease and that the degree of reversibility is dependent upon the duration of symptoms before specific treatment is begun. There is a premium, therefore, on early diagnosis.

COMBINED SYSTEM DISEASE OF NONPERNICIOUS ANEMIA TYPE

An intrinsic disease of the spinal cord, more common than SCD and affecting the posterior and lateral columns (in this sense, *a combined system disease*), is not associated with pernicious anemia. In this syndrome, in distinction to SCD, signs of corticospinal tract disease precede those of the posterior columns and are more prominent throughout the illness, which is slowly and chronically progressive. Little is known of its pathologic basis or cause.

Progressive spastic or spastic-ataxic paraparesis of a chronic, irreversible type may also develop *in conjunction with chronic, decompensated liver disease* (see page 962); in certain cases of *adrenoleukodystrophy*, particularly in the symptomatic heterozygote, i.e., the female carrier (page 812); and in *adhesive spinal arachnoiditis*, which is discussed below.

SPINAL ARACHNOIDITIS (CHRONIC ADHESIVE ARACHNOIDITIS, MENINGITIS CIRCUMSCRIPTA SPINALIS)

This is a relatively uncommon spinal cord disorder (about one-eighth as frequent as intraspinal tumors, according to Lombardi et al). It is characterized clinically by a combination of root and spinal cord symptoms which may mimic intraspinal tumor. Pathologically there is opacification and thickening of the arachnoidal membranes and adhesions between the arachnoid and dura—the result of proliferation of connective tissue. The subarachnoid space is obliterated. In this sense, the term arachnoiditis is not entirely appropriate, although it seems likely that the connective tissue overgrowth is a reaction to an antecedent arachnoidal inflammation. Some forms of arachnoiditis can be traced to syphilis or to a subacute therapeutically resistant meningitis of other type. Still others apparently follow the introduction of a variety of substances into the subarachnoid space for diagnostic or therapeutic purposes. These include penicillin and other antibiotics, Pantopaque and other contrast media, and (formerly) spinal anesthetics. Repeated corticosteroid injections have also been incriminated. A syndrome of increasing frequency is that which complicates repeated Pantopaque myelography and surgery for lumbar discs (lumbar arachnoiditis). Less convincing are cases attributed to closed spinal injuries. In many cases no antecedent event can be recognized.

Pathologic Features   Arachnoiditis is usually a diffuse process with a predilection for the thoracic segments. In advanced cases the subarachnoid space is completely obliterated, and the roots and cord are strangulated by the thickened connective tissue. Peripherally placed fibers of the cord are destroyed to a varying extent, and the posterior and lateral columns undergo secondary degeneration. In a few cases the pathologic process is confined to relatively circumscribed portions of the cord, and the subarachnoid space is occupied by loculated collections of fluid (meningitis serosa circumscripta). The rare association of spinal arachnoiditis and syringomyelic cavitation of the cord is considered later in this chapter.

Clinical Manifestations Spinal arachnoiditis may occur at any age, although the highest incidence of onset of symptoms is between 40 and 60 years; it is rare below the age of 20. Symptoms may occur in close temporal relationship to an acute arachnoidal inflammation or be delayed for weeks, months, or even years. The commonest mode of onset is with pain in the distribution of one or more sensory nerve roots, first on one side, then on both. The pain has a burning, stinging, or aching quality and is persistent. Impaired reflexes are common, but weakness and atrophy, the results of damage to anterior roots, are less frequent findings, and tend to occur in cases involving the cauda equina. In thoracic lesions, symptoms of root involvement may antedate those of cord compression by months or years. Sooner or later, however, there is involvement of the spinal cord manifested by a slowly progressive spastic ataxia with sphincter disturbances.

The localized lumbar arachnoiditis associated with repeated disc surgery and myelography (the common variety being seen in chronic pain clinics) is characterized by back and/or leg pain with other inconstant signs of radiculopathy (loss of tendon reflexes, weakness and variable degrees of sensory loss), usually bilateral (see page 165).

Formerly, many examples of adhesive arachnoiditis were observed following spinal anesthesia (occurring soon afterward or after an interval of weeks, months, or even years). This complication was eventually traced to a detergent that had contaminated vials of procaine. If enough of the contaminant was injected, an areflexic paralysis and sensory loss in the legs and sphincteric paralysis developed within a few days, along with considerable pain. Recovery, complete or partial, usually occurred within a year or two. More pernicious, however, was a delayed meningomyelopathy that developed within a few months to a few years, causing a spastic paralysis, sensory loss, incontinence of sphincters, and decubiti. Some of the patients died later of blindness and hydrocephalus. There was no effective treatment. This remarkable chemical meningitis has virtually disappeared since anesthetists began to prepare their spinal anesthetic from crystals.

The spinal fluid is abnormal in practically all cases of adhesive arachnoiditis. In some there is a moderate lymphocytic pleocytosis, but the striking findings are those of partial or complete block (positive Queckenstedt test) and elevated protein content, sometimes extreme in degree. In the localized lumbar arachnoiditis, referred to above, the CSF may be normal or show only a slight increase in protein content. The myelographic appearance of arachnoiditis is characteristic (patchy holdup and dispersion of the column of dye and "candle-guttering" appearance) and allows one to make the diagnosis with certainty.

Treatment In the early stages of arachnoiditis, corticosteroids have been given to control the inflammatory reaction and to prevent progress of the disease, but their value is questionable. Surgery may be effective in the rare case of localized "cyst" formation and cord compression and posterior rhizotomy may be useful in relieving severe radicular pain. For chronic adhesive lumbar arachnoiditis, there is no effective surgical or medical treatment. Administration of corticosteroids, systemic and epidural, have usually not been beneficial.

CERVICAL SPONDYLOSIS WITH MYELOPATHY

It has been stated, correctly in our opinion, that this is the most frequently observed myelopathy in general hospitals. Basically a degenerative disease of the spine, involving the lower cervical vertebrae, it narrows the spinal canal and intervertebral foramina and causes progressive injury of the spinal cord or roots, or both.

Historical Note Key, in 1838, probably gave the first description of a spondylotic bar. In two cases of compressive myelopathy with paraplegia, he found "a projection of the intervertebral substance, or rather the posterior ligament of the spine, which was thickened and presented a firm ridge which had lessened the diameter of the canal by nearly a third. The ligament, where it passes over the posterior surface of the intervertebral substance, was found to be ossified." In 1892, Horsley performed a cervical laminectomy in such a patient, in whom a subacutely evolving paraplegia had been precipitated by trauma: a "transverse ridge of bone" was found to be compressing the spinal cord at the level of the sixth cervical vertebra. Thereafter, operations were performed in many cases of this sort, and the tissues removed at operation were repeatedly misidentified as benign cartilaginous tumors or "chondromata." In 1928, Stookey described in detail the pathologic effects upon the spinal cord and roots of these "ventral extradural chondromas."

Also of historical importance is Gowers' original account, in 1892, of *vertebral exostoses,* in which he described osteophytes that protrude from the posterior surfaces of the vertebral bodies and encroach upon the spinal canal, causing slow compression of the cord, as well as bony overgrowth in the intervertebral foramina, giving rise to radicular pain. Gowers correctly predicted that these lesions would offer a more promising field for the surgeon than other kinds of vertebral tumors.

Schmorl and his associates, beginning in 1929, drew attention to the rupture of the nucleus pulposus into the adjacent vertebral body (Schmorl nodules) and into the spinal canal, but little clinical significance was attributed to these lesions. Peet and Echols, in 1934, were probably the first to suggest that the so-called chondromata represented protrusions of intervertebral disc material. This idea gained wide credence after the publication, in the same year, of the classic article on ruptured intervertebral disc by Mixter and Barr. Although the latter names are usually associated with the lumbar disc syndrome, 4 of their original 19 cases were instances of cervical disc disease.

For some reason, there was little awareness of the frequency and importance of spondylotic myelopathy for many years after these basic observations were made. All the interest was in the acute ruptured disc. Finally it was Russell Brain, in 1948, who put cervical spondylosis on the neurologic map, so to speak. He drew a distinction between acute rupture and protrusion of the cervical disc (often traumatic and more likely to compress the nerve roots than the spinal cord), and chronic spinal cord and root compression, consequent upon disc degeneration and associated osteophytic outgrowths (*hard disc*) and changes in joints, ligaments, and bones. In 1957, Payne and Spillane documented the importance of a smaller-than-normal spinal canal in the genesis of myelopathy in patients with cervical spondylosis. These reports were followed by a flood of writings on the subject (see Wilkinson), yet few of our standard textbooks of neurology contain adequate accounts of it. Nurick's review of the natural history of cervical spondylosis and the results of surgical therapy is a useful modern reference.

Symptomatology In outline, the most characteristic syndrome consists of a triad of (1) painful, stiff neck, (2) brachialgia, and (3) spastic weakness with variable ataxia of the legs. Each of these components may occur separately or they may occur in several combinations and sequences.

With reference to the first of these symptoms, in any sizable group of patients beyond 50 years of age, about 40 percent will be found to have some clinical abnormality of the neck, usually crepitus or pain, with restriction of lateral flexion and rotation (less often of extension). Pallis et al, in a survey of 50 patients, all of them over 50 years of age

and none with neurologic complaints, found that 75 percent showed radiologic evidence of narrowing of the cervical spinal canal due to posterior osteophytosis or narrowing of the intervertebral foramina due to osteoarthropathy at the neurocentral and apophyseal joints; about half of the patients with radiologic abnormalities showed physical signs of root or cord involvement (changes in the tendon reflexes in the arms, briskness of reflexes and impairment of vibratory sense in the legs, and occasional Babinski signs). The occasional occurrence of a Babinski sign in older individuals who had never complained of neurologic symptoms may be explained by an otherwise silent osteophyte. Thus, Savitsky and Madonick found a Babinski sign in 4.3 percent of 2500 nonneurologic hospital patients; this sign was four times more frequent in persons over 50 years of age than in those under 50.

In patients with only shoulder and arm symptoms as well as patients in whom these symptoms are combined with a disorder of the legs, pain is the most frequent symptom. It is centered in the back of the neck, often radiating to an area above the scapula. When brachialgia is also present it takes several forms: a stabbing pain in the pre- or postaxial border of the limb, extending to the elbow, wrist, or fingers; or a persistent dull ache in the forearm or wrist, sometimes with burning. In rare instances the pain is referred substernally. Some patients also complain of paresthesias, most often in one or two digits, a part of the palm, or in a longitudinal band along the forearm. Slight clumsiness or weakness of the hand is another complaint. The biceps and supinator reflexes may be depressed, sometimes in association with an increase in the triceps reflex. The hand or forearm muscles undergo slight atrophy if chronically weakened. In patients with sensory loss, pain and thermal sensation appear to be affected more than tactile sense.

The third part of the triad, the myelopathy, most often presents as a complaint of weakness of one leg and a slight unsteadiness of gait. The whole leg feels stiff and heavy and gives out quickly after exercise. Mobility of the ankle is often reduced, and the advancing toes and lateral border of the shoe scrape the floor. On examination spasticity is more evident than weakness, and the tendon reflexes are increased (ankle jerks may not share in this change in the elderly). Although the patient may believe only one leg to be affected, it is commonly found that both plantar reflexes are extensor, the one on the side of the stiffest leg being more clearly so. Less often both legs are equally affected. As to the sensory disorders, numbness, tingling, and prickling of the soles of the feet and around the ankles are the most frequent complaints. Impaired vibratory sensation, pattern recognition, tactile sense from the hip down, and postural sense in the toes and feet (all indicating a lesion of the posterior columns), are the most conspicuous sensory findings. Less often there is loss of pain and thermal sense. These sensorimotor defects tend also to be asymmetrical. Rarely the pattern takes the form of a Brown-Séquard syndrome (page 129). Neck flexion may induce electrical feelings down the spine (Lhermitte sign). Paresthesias and dysesthesias in the lower extremities and trunk may be the principal symptoms.

As the myelopathy progresses, both legs weaken further and become more spastic. Sphincteric control may then be altered; slight hesitancy or precipitancy of micturition are the usual complaints, and frank incontinence is infrequent. In its more advanced form walking must be aided by cane(s) or walker, and in some cases all locomotion ultimately becomes impossible, especially in the senile patient.

Pathogenesis   The particular vulnerability of the lower cervical spine to degenerative change has no ready explanation. Perhaps it is related in some way to the high degree of mobility of the lower cervical vertebrae, which is accentuated by their situation next to the relatively immobile thoracic spine.

The mechanism of spinal cord injury would seem to be simple compression. When the spinal canal is diminished in its anterior-posterior dimension at one or several points to less than 9 to 10 mm, the available space for the spinal cord is insufficient. However, the presence and degree of cord injury correlates poorly with the anteroposterior dimensions of the spinal canal. The range of the latter in symptomatic cervical spondylosis is from 8 to 15 mm (normal, 17 to 18 mm). One must consider, therefore, the effects of the natural motions of the spinal cord during flexion and extension of the neck. Adams and Logue confirmed the observation of O'Connell that during full flexion and extension of the neck the cervical cord and dura move up and down. The spinal cord is dragged over protruding osteophytes, and conceivably this type of intermittent trauma progressively injures the spinal cord. Also it has been shown that the spinal cord, displaced posteriorly by osteophytes, will be compressed by the infolding ligamentum flavum each time the neck is extended (Stoltmann and Blackwood). Segmental ischemic necrosis resulting from intermittent compression of arteries to the spinal cord or from compression (spasm?) of the anterior spinal artery has also been postulated. Most neuropathologists favor the idea of intermittent cord compression between osteophytes anteriorly and ligamentum flavum posteriorly, with an added vascular element accounting for the scattered lesions deep in the cord. Trauma from sudden extreme extension, as in a fall or chiropractic manipulation, or from a lesser degree of retraction of the head during myelography, a tooth extraction, or a tonsillectomy, may be an additional factor—particularly in patients with congenitally narrow canals.

Pathologic Changes   The fundamental lesion is a tearing of the annulus fibrosus, with extrusion of disc material into the spinal canal. The disc becomes covered with fibrous tissue, partly calcified, or covered with bone. Another common lesion is bulging of the annulus without extrusion of nuclear material. This may also be associated with the formation of osteophytes and transverse bony ridges. The latter, unlike ruptured discs that occur chiefly at the C5-C6 or C6-C7 interspace, may extend two or three interspaces higher and occur at several levels. The adjacent dura mater may be thickened and adherent to the posterior longitudinal ligament. The underlying pia-arachnoid is also thickened. This series of pathologic changes is frequently ascribed to hypertrophic osteoarthritis. However, in lesser degree, the osteophyte formation and ridging are so frequently observed in patients who have no other signs of arthritic disease that this explanation is surely incorrect. Subclinical trauma is far more likely, in the authors' opinion.

When the root is compressed by osteophytic overgrowth, the dural sleeve is thickened, and the root fibers are damaged. Usually the fifth, sixth, or seventh cervical roots are affected in this way, both the anterior and posterior, or only the anterior. A small neuroma may appear proximal to the site of anterior root compression.

The spinal cord is flattened and the dura ridged. The root lesions may lead to secondary wedge-shaped areas of degeneration in the lateral parts of the posterior columns at higher levels. The most marked changes in the spinal cord are at the level(s) of compression. There may be zones of demyelination or focal necrosis at the points of attachment of the dentate ligaments (which tether the spinal cord to the dura) and zones of necrosis in the posterior and lateral columns, as well as loss of nerve cells. It is the latter lesions, often asymmetrical, that are attributed by Hughes to ischemia.

Differential Diagnosis   When pain and stiffness in the neck, brachialgia, and sensorimotor-reflex changes in the arms are combined with signs of myelopathy, there is little difficulty in diagnosis. When the neck and arm changes are inconspicuous or absent, the diagnosis becomes difficult. The myelopathy must then be distinguished from the late, progressive form of spinal multiple sclerosis (page 765). Since posterior osteophytes and other bony alterations are frequent in the sixth and seventh decades, the question that must be answered is whether the vertebral changes bear any relationship to the neurologic abnormality. The problem is resolved by finding some degree of sensorimotor or reflex change corresponding only to the level of the spinal abnormalities, a point that always favors spondylotic myelopathy. A lack of such corresponding changes, an elevation of CSF gamma globulin, and signs of lesions in the optic nerves and brainstem argue for demyelinative myelopathy. Myelography becomes critical in such cases. MRI and metrizamide myelography combined with CT scanning are the most helpful diagnostic procedures. Contrast myelography with the patient supine and lateral views taken during flexion and extension of the neck are also useful in settling the problem.

It is said that spondylotic myelopathy may simulate amyotrophic lateral sclerosis (amyotrophy of arms and spastic weakness of the legs). This has seldom been a diagnostic problem in our experience. We have observed only a few patients with spondylotic myelopathy who exhibited an absolutely pure motor syndrome, i.e., one in which there was no cervical or brachial pain and no sensory symptoms in the arms or impairment of vibratory or position sense in the legs. A pure spastic paraparesis may also occur in multiple sclerosis, liver failure, hereditary spastic paraplegia with or without dementia, and adrenoleukodystrophy.

Subacute combined degeneration of the spinal cord due to vitamin B_{12} deficiency (page 833), *combined system disease* of nonpernicious anemia type (see above), and spinal cord tumor (discussed later in this chapter) are always listed among the conditions that might be confused with spondylotic myelopathy. Adherence to the diagnostic criteria for each of these disorders should eliminate the possibility of error in most instances.

The special problems attendant upon spondylotic radiculopathy are discussed on pages 167 and 172.

Treatment   The slow, intermittently progressive course of cervical myelopathy with long periods of relatively unchanging symptomatology makes it difficult to evaluate therapy. Assuming that the prevailing opinions of the mechanisms of the cord and root injury are correct, then the use of a soft collar to restrict anterior-posterior motions of the neck seems reasonable. This form of treatment alone may be sufficient to control the discomfort in the neck and arms. Rarely in our experience has brachialgia alone been sufficiently severe and persistent to require radicular decompression.

Many of our patients have been dissatisfied with this passive approach and dislike or refuse to wear a collar continuously. If posterior osteophytes have narrowed the spinal canal at several interspaces, a posterior decompressive laminectomy with severance of the dentate ligaments, to untether the spinal cord, helps to prevent further injury. The results of such a procedure are fairly satisfactory. In fully two-thirds of the patients, improvement in the function of the legs occurs; in most of the others, progression of the myelopathy is halted. The operation carries some risk, and rarely an acute quadriplegia—due, presumably, to manipulation of the spinal cord and damage to nutrient spinal arteries—has followed the surgical procedure. When one or two interspaces are the site of osteophytic overgrowths, their removal by an anterior approach has given even better results and carries less risk.

OTHER SPINAL ABNORMALITIES WITH MYELOPATHY

The spinal cord is obviously vulnerable to any vertebral maldevelopment or disease that encroaches upon the spinal canal or compresses its nutrient arteries. Some of the common ones are listed below.

Anomalies at the Craniocervical Junction   Of these, congenital *fusion of the atlas and foramen magnum* is the most common. McCrae, who reviewed the radiologic findings in over 100 patients with bony abnormalities at the craniocervical junction, found a partial or complete bony union of atlas and foramen magnum in 28 cases. He found also that whenever the anteroposterior diameter of the canal behind the odontoid process was less than 19.0 mm, there were signs of spinal cord compression. Fusion of the second and third cervical vertebras is a common anomaly as well, but does not seem to be of clinical significance.

Platybasia and basilar invagination   Platybasia refers to a flattening of the base of the skull (the angle formed by intersection of the plane of the clivus and the plane of the anterior fossa is greater than 135°). Basilar impression or invagination means an upward bulging of the margins of the foramen magnum; if the occipital condyles, which bear the thrust of the spine, are displaced above the plane of the foramen magnum, basilar invagination is present. Each of these abnormalities may be congenital or acquired (as in Paget disease), and frequently they are conjoined. They give rise to a characteristic shortness of the neck and a combination of cerebellar and spinal signs.

Abnormalities of the odontoid process   These were found in 17 of McCrae's series. There may be complete separation of the odontoid from the axis or chronic *atlantoaxial dislocation* (atlas displaced anteriorly in relation to the axis). These abnormalities may be congenital or the result of injury, and are known causes of acute or chronic spinal cord compression.

Rheumatoid arthritis is another cause of atlantoaxial dislocation. The ligaments that attach the odontoid to the atlas and to the skull are weakened by the destructive inflammatory process. The subsequent dislocation of the atlas on the axis may remain mobile or become fixed and give rise to an intermittent or persistent mild to moderate paraparesis or quadriparesis. Similar effects may result from a forward subluxation of C4 on C5 (see Nakano et al).

In all the congenital anomalies of the foramen magnum and the high cervical spine there is a high incidence of syringomyelia. McCrae found, at the Montreal Neurological Institute, that 38 percent of all patients with syringomeylia and syringobulbia showed such bony anomalies. All patients whose symptoms might be explained by a lesion in the cervicocranial region (particularly where multiple sclerosis and foramen magnum tumor are suspected) should have careful radiologic examination.

In mucopolysaccharidosis IV, or the Morquio syndrome, a nearly invariable feature is the absence or severe hypoplasia of the odontoid process. This abnormality, combined with laxity or redundancy of the ligaments, results in atlantoaxial subluxation and compression of the spinal cord. Affected children refuse to walk or develop spastic weakness of the limbs. Early in life they excrete an excess of keratan sulfate (Chap. 38), but this may no longer be detectable in adult life. In certain mucopolysaccharidoses, we have also seen a true pachymeningiopathy, with great thickening of the basal cisternal and high cervical dura and spinal cord compression. Surgical decompression and spinal immobilization may be curative.

Achondroplasia occasionally results in great thickening of the vertebral bodies, neural arches, laminae, and pedicles because of increased periosteal bone formation. The spinal canal is narrowed in the thoracolumbar region, often with kyphosis and sometimes leading to a progressive spinal cord or cauda equina syndrome.

Ankylosing spondylitis of the lumbar spine may be associated with a cauda equina syndrome. Bartleson et al described 14 patients and referred to 30 others culled from medical journals, who, years after the onset of spondylitis, developed sensory, motor, reflex, and sphincteric disorders referrable to the L4, L5, and sacral roots. Surprisingly, the spinal canal was not narrowed and the caudal sac was actually dilated. There were usually diverticulae of the posterior root sleeves. No explanation can be given for the radicular symptoms and signs, which can be verified by

electromyography. Surgical decompression has not benefitted the patients, nor has corticosteroid therapy. We have observed similar symptoms in the cervical region, also with root-sleeve diverticulae. Compression of the cord itself does not occur in ankylosing spondylitis, except as a complication of trauma. Multiple arachnoid cysts in the thoracic region have been associated with a spinal cord syndrome in *Marfan disease*.

Paget Disease (Osteitis Deformans) Enlargement of the vertebral bodies, pedicles, and laminae in Paget disease may result in narrowing of the spinal canal and a clinical picture of spinal cord compression. It is of interest that Paget disease and fibrous dysplasia are the only diseases known to enlarge the spine. In Paget disease alkaline phosphatase values are high and the typical bone changes are seen in radiographs. Usually several adjacent vertebrae of the thoracic spine are involved. Other parts of the skeleton are also involved (see below),which facilitates diagnosis. The level of the lesion is determined by myelography. Posterior surgical decompression, leaving the pedicles intact, is indicated if there is sufficient stability of the vertebral bodies to prevent collapse. Calcitonin should be administered. Neurologic disturbances in Paget disease and the results obtained by the use of daily injections of porcine or synthetic salmon calcitonin over a 6- to 12-month period are described by Chen et al. Addition of ascorbic acid may be helpful.

Paget disease of the skull may cause neurosensory deafness, occasionally compression of an optic nerve, with loss of sight, and lower cranial neuropathies (weak, atrophic tongue; dysphagia; dysphonia; pain at base of occiput). The latter effects may be combined with spinal and cerebellar abnormalities, due to basilar invagination. Several patients with normal-pressure hydrocephalus related to basilar impression have been seen in our clinics. They were completely relieved by ventriculoperitoneal shunts.

INTRASPINAL TUMORS

Tumors of the spinal cord are considerably less frequent than tumors that involve the brain; in the Mayo Clinic series of 8784 primary tumors of the central nervous system, only 15 percent were intraspinal (Sloof et al). In distinction to brain tumors, the majority of intraspinal ones are benign and produce their effects mainly by compression of the spinal cord, rather than by invasion. Thus, a large proportion of intraspinal tumors are amenable to surgical removal, and their early recognition, before irreversible neurologic changes have occurred, becomes a matter of utmost importance.

Anatomic Considerations Neoplasms and other space-occupying lesions within the spinal canal can be conveniently divided into two groups: (1) those that arise within the substance of the spinal cord and invade and destroy tracts and central gray structures (*intramedullary*), and (2) those arising outside the spinal cord (*extramedullary*), either in the vertebral bodies and epidural tissues (extradural), or in the leptomeninges or roots (intradural). In a general hospital, the relative frequency of spinal tumors in these different locations is about 5 percent intramedullary, 40 percent intradural-extramedullary, and 55 percent extradural. This percentage of extradural lesions is higher than that encountered in more specialized neurosurgical clinics (e.g., Elsberg's figures of 7, 64, and 29 percent, respectively), probably because the latter do not include as many patients with extradural lymphomas, metastatic carcinomas, etc., seen in general hospitals.

The commonest *extramedullary tumors* are the neurofibromas and meningiomas, which together constitute about 55 percent of all intraspinal neoplasms. They are more often intradural than extradural. Neurofibromas have a predilection for the thoracic region, whereas meningiomas are more evenly distributed over the vertical extent of the cord. The other extramedullary tumors are sarcomas, vascular tumors, chordomas, and epidermoid and similar tumors, in that order of frequency.

Intramedullary tumors of the spinal cord have the same cellular origins as those arising in the brain (Chap. 31), although the proportions of particular cell types differ. Ependymomas (many of which arise from the filum terminale) make up about 60 percent of the spinal cord cases, and astrocytomas about 25 percent. The latter is the commonest intramedullary tumor, if one excludes the filum terminale. Oligodendrogliomas are much less common. The remainder (about 10 percent) consists of a diverse group of nongliomatous tumors: lipomas, epidermoids, dermoids, teratomas, hemangiomas, hemangioblastomas, and metastatic carcinomas. The hemangioma may be a source of spontaneous hematomyelia. As will be indicated further-on there is a frequent association between intramedullary tumors (both gliomatous and nongliomatous) and syringomyelia. The basis of this relationship remains obscure.

Intramedullary growths invade as well as compress and distort fasciculi in the adjacent white matter. As the cord enlarges from the tumor growing within it or is compressed by a tumor from without, the free space around the cord is consumed, and the CSF below the lesion becomes isolated or loculated from the remainder of the circulating fluid above the lesion. This is indicated eventually by a Froin syndrome (xanthochromia and clotting of CSF), a positive Queckenstedt test, and an interruption of flow of contrast medium in the subarachnoid space (myelogram).

Secondary spinal cord tumors can also be subdivided into intramedullary and extramedullary types. Intramedullary metastases are not as rare as is generally believed. In a retrospective autopsy study of 627 patients with systemic cancer, Costigan and Winkelman found 153 cases with CNS metastases, 13 of which had metastases within the cord. In 9 of the 13 cases, the metastasis was deep in the cord, unassociated with leptomeningeal carcinomatosis; in four cases the neoplasm seemed to extend from the pia. Bronchogenic carcinoma was the main source. Diagnosis is difficult; differentiation is from meningeal carcinomatosis, radiation myelopathy, and paraneoplastic necrotizing myelopathy. Treatment is ineffective, unless radiation therapy is begun before paraplegia supervenes (Winkelman et al).

Extramedullary tumor growth is far more often extradural than intradural. The latter takes the form of a meningeal carcinomatosis or lymphomatosis and has been considered in Chap. 31. Extradural metastases (carcinoma, lymphoma, myeloma) are probably the most common of all spinal tumors. They arise from hematogenous deposits or extend from tumors of the vertebral bodies or from extraspinal deposits via the intervertebral foramina.

Symptomatology Patients with spinal cord tumors are likely to manifest one of three clinical pictures, either (1) a purely sensorimotor spinal tract syndrome, or (2) a painful radicular–spinal cord syndrome, or (3) rarely, a syringomyelic syndrome.

Sensorimotor spinal tract syndromes The predominant clinical picture relates to compression and less often to invasion and destruction of spinal cord tracts. The onset of the compressive symptoms is usually gradual and the course progressive over a period of weeks and months. The initial disturbance is likely to be motor, and the distribution asymmetric. With cervical lesions, a common sequence of motor impairment is first an arm, followed by the ipsilateral leg, contralateral leg, and finally the remaining arm. With thoracic lesions, one leg usually becomes weak and stiff before the other one. Subjective sensory symptoms of the dorsal column type (tingling paresthesias) assume the same pattern. Pain and thermal senses are more likely to be affected than tactile, vibration, and position senses, and initially the sensory disturbance is contralateral to the maximum motor weakness (Brown-Séquard syndrome). Nevertheless the posterior columns are also frequently involved. The bladder and bowel usually become paralyzed coincident with paralysis of the legs. If the compression is relieved, there is recovery from these sensory and motor symptoms, often in the reverse order of their affection; the first part affected is the last to recover, and sensory symptoms tend to disappear before motor ones.

Radicular-spinal cord syndrome The syndrome of spinal cord compression is often combined with radicular pain, i.e., pain in the distribution of a sensory nerve root. It is described as knife-like or as a dull ache with superimposed sharp stabs of pain, which are intensified by coughing, sneezing, or straining, and which radiate in a distal direction, i.e., away from the spine. Segmental sensory changes (paresthesias, impaired perception of pin-prick and touch) and/or motor disturbances (cramp, atrophy, fascicular twitching, and loss of tendon reflex) and an ache in the spine, in addition to the radicular pain, are the usual manifestations of a cord compressive–irritative root lesion. Tenderness of spinous processes over the growth is found

Figure 36-4

MR imaging of the cervical region in a 14-year-old boy. The spinal canal is widened. Within the cervical spinal cord there is an area of increased signal (light area), representing a cyst, bordered by areas of relatively decreased signal (dark areas), representing the spinal cord. At operation, the lesion proved to be a cystic astrocytoma.

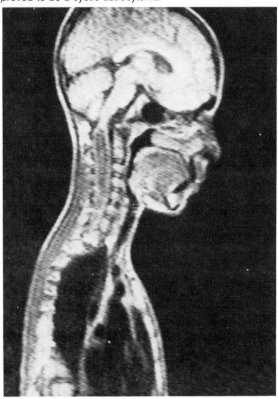

in about half the patients. These segmental changes, particularly the sensory ones, often precede the signs of spinal cord compression by months or years if the lesion is benign. The latter consist of (1) an asymmetric spastic weakness of the legs with thoracolumbar lesions and of the arms and legs with cervical lesions, (2) a sensory level on the trunk below which perception of pain and temperature is reduced or lost, (3) posterior column signs, and (4) a spastic bladder under weak voluntary control.

No single symptom is unique to *intramedullary tumors*. Pain is the most common symptom and is almost invariably present with tumors of the filum terminale. Ependymomas and astrocytomas, the two most common intramedullary tumors, usually give rise to a mixed sensorimotor tract syndrome. When the intramedullary tumor involves the central gray matter, a third *syringomyelic syndrome* may result. Theoretically, intramedullary tumors that destroy mainly the gray matter should cause a central cord syndrome, with segmental or dissociated sensory loss, amyotrophy, early incontinence, and late corticospinal weakness. But in our experience this distinction between intra- and extramedullary lesions is seldom dependable. Rarely, for reasons that are difficult to understand, an extramedullary tumor may give rise to a syringomyelic syndrome.

The diagnosis is established by radiographs of the spine (erosion of vertebrae, widened spinal canal), lumbar puncture (elevated CSF protein and signs of block), and electromyography, which demonstrates the fasciculations and denervation resulting from involvement of motor roots. The most important diagnostic procedures are MRI and contrast myelography with CT scanning, which permit precise localization of the lesion. No doubt, MRI and CT scanning will assume increasing importance and replace myelography as a diagnostic method, as techniques for visualizing the spinal cord improve. MRI can show an intramedullary tumor with great clarity (Fig. 36-4).

Special spinal syndromes Unusual clinical syndromes may be found in patients with *tumors near the foramen magnum*. They may produce a quadriparesis with pain in the back of the head and stiff neck, weakness and atrophy of the hands and dorsal neck muscles, and variable sensory changes, or, if spread occurs intracranially, there may be signs of cerebellar and lower cranial nerve involvement. These types of tumor are described fully in Chap. 31. Lesions at the level of the lowermost thoracic and the first lumbar vertebrae may result in *mixed cauda equina and spinal cord symptoms*. A Babinski sign means that the spinal cord is involved, above the fifth lumbar segment. *Lesions of the cauda equina* alone, always difficult to separate from those of the lumbosacral plexuses and multiple nerves, are usually attended in the early stages by pain which is variously combined with an asymmetric, atrophic, areflexic paralysis, radicular sensory loss, and sphincteric disorder. These must be distinguished from *lesions of the conus medullaris* (lower sacral segments of the spinal cord) in which there are early disturbances of the bladder and bowel (urinary retention and constipation), back pain, hypesthesia or anesthesia over the sacral dermatomes, a lax anal sphincter with loss of anal and bulbocavernosus reflexes, impotence, and sometimes weakness of leg muscles. Sensory abnormalities may precede motor and reflex changes by many months. *Pain and stiffness of the back* may antedate signs of spinal cord disease or dominate the clinical picture in some cases of extramedullary tumor. The back pain is usually worse when the patient lies down, or may become worse after several hours in the recumbent position and be improved by sitting up. Very rarely, for reasons that are quite unclear, tumors of the thoracolumbar cord (extramedullary, as a rule) are associated with dementia and communicating hydrocephalus; these symptoms respond to shunting and removal of the spinal tumor (Feldman et al). *In children,* severe back pain associated with spasm of paravertebral muscles is often prominent initially; scoliosis and spastic weakness of the legs come later. Because of this somewhat unusual clinical presentation and the rarity of intraspinal lesions in childhood, spinal cord tumors in this age group may be overlooked.

Differential Diagnosis Several problems may arise in the diagnosis of spinal cord tumors, in addition to the ones mentioned above. In their early stages they must be distinguished from other diseases which cause pain over certain segments of the body, i.e., those affecting the gallbladder, kidney, stomach and intestinal tract, pleura, etc. The localization of the pain to a dermatome, its intensification by sneezing, coughing, and straining, the finding of segmental sensory changes and minor alterations of motor, reflex, or sensory function in the legs will usually provide the clues to the presence of a spinal cord–radicular lesion. Examination of the CSF, spine films, MRI, and myelography with CT scanning will settle the diagnosis in most instances.

If symptoms and signs of disorder of sensorimotor tracts are present, there is still the problem of locating the segmental level of the lesion. At first the sensory and motor deficits may be most pronounced in those parts of the body farthest removed from the lesion, i.e., in feet or lumbosacral segments. Later the levels of the sensory and motor deficits ascend, but they may continue to be below the lesion. In determining the level of the lesion, the location of the root pain and atrophic paralysis is of greater help than the upper level of hypalgesia.

Once vertebral and segmental levels of the lesion are settled, there remains the necessity of determining whether the lesion is extradural, intradural-extramedullary, or intra-

medullary, and whether the lesion is neoplastic. This is important from the standpoint of etiologic diagnosis. If there is a visible or palpable spinal deformity or radiographic evidence of vertebral destruction, one may confidently assume an extradural localization. Even without these changes one still suspects an extradural lesion if root pain developed early and is bilateral, if pain and aching in the spine are prominent and percussion tenderness is marked, if motor symptoms below the lesion precede sensory ones, and sphincter disturbances are late. However, to distinguish between intradural-extramedullary lesions and intramedullary lesions on clinical grounds alone may be impossible. The presence of radicular pain and early CSF block (positive Queckenstedt test and high protein) favor an extramedullary localization. The findings of segmental amyotrophy and sensory loss of dissociated type (loss of pain and temperature and preservation of tactile sensation) point to an intramedullary lesion.

Extradural tumors, both primary and secondary, need to be differentiated from cervical spondylosis; from tuberculous granuloma and other chronic pyogenic or fungal granulomatous lesions; and from the rare necrotizing myelopathy associated with occult tumors. In the region of the lower back, i.e., over the cauda equina, one must distinguish between tumor and protruded intervertebral disc. Here, an extradural tumor may produce mainly sciatic and low back pain with little or no motor, sensory, reflex, or sphincteric disturbances. In this situation, the most important diagnostic measure is myelography. With intradural-extramedullary lesions the important diagnostic considerations are meningioma, neurofibroma, meningeal carcinomatosis, cholesteatoma, and teratomatous cyst, a meningomyelitic process or adhesive arachnoiditis. Contrast myelography with CT scanning and the study of cells in the CSF by Milliporefilter techniques are the most useful laboratory aids. Intramedullary lesions are usually gliomas or vascular malformations. The definition of the latter lesions by means of selective spinal angiography has been discussed in an earlier section of this chapter. In general, a negative Queckenstedt test, normal or relatively low protein in the CSF, and a negative myelogram will serve to rule out intraspinal tumors or granulomatous lesions.

Treatment This varies with the nature of the lesion and the clinical condition of the patient. Intradural-extramedullary tumors should be removed as soon as possible after diagnostic myelography, and this applies to benign extradural tumors as well. Laminectomy, decompression, excision under the operating microscope, and radiotherapy constitute the treatment of intramedullary gliomas. Such patients may improve and lead useful lives for a decade or longer.

Epidural growths of carcinoma and lymphoma are best managed by the use of radiation therapy, endocrine therapy (for carcinoma of breast and prostate), the administration of antineoplastic drugs (for certain lymphomas and myelomas), and the use of high-dose steroids and analgesics for pain. Sometimes laminectomy and decompression are necessary for diagnosis and, with a rapidly growing tumor, to prevent irreversible compressive effects and infarction of the spinal cord. Rarely is operation necessary, however; Gilbert and his associates have presented convincing evidence that patients who receive high-dose corticosteroids and fractionated radiation (500 rads on each of the first 3 days and then spaced radiation up to 3000 rads) do as well as the surgically treated ones. The main consideration in the management of epidural metastases is the need for early diagnosis, at a stage when only back pain is present, before neurologic symptoms and signs have appeared. Once neurologic signs appear, the results of treatment are poor. Thus, patients with back pain and vertebral metastases should have MRI and myelography, and be treated aggressively with radiation (Rodichok et al, Portenoy et al).

With tuberculous caries, immobilization of the spine in hyperextension and appropriate chemotherapy are indicated, and laminectomy should be reserved for exceptional cases with complete and irreversible spinal block. The management of other forms of spinal cord and cauda equina compression are considered in relation to the specific compressive lesions.

OTHER RARE CAUSES OF SPINAL CORD COMPRESSION

Intraspinal (intra- or extradural) lipoma should be suspected when there is a particularly protracted clinical course, a palpable subcutaneous soft tissue mass, an associated bony abnormality, and myelographic and MR evidence of a large dural sac and low-lying conus medullaris. Thomas and Miller found 60 such cases (over a period of 40 years) in the files of the Mayo Clinic. Epidural lipomatosis with cauda equina compression has been reported several times in Cushing disease and after long-term use of corticosteroids. This has been attributed to fat deposition. Copious amounts of normal adipose tissue are found at laminectomy, and removal of this tissue relieves the symptoms. Lowering the dose of steroid and caloric restriction will also mobilize the fat and result in clinical recovery. The clinical picture may suggest discogenic disease (Lipson et al).

Arachnoid diverticula—intra- or extradural outpouchings from the posterior nerve root—are very rare causes of a radicular-spinal cord syndrome. They tend to occur in younger patients, mainly in the thoracic region. The symptoms, in order of decreasing frequency, are pain, weakness, gait disorder, and sensory and sphincteric disturbances (Cilluffo et al).

Spinal cord compression with paraplegia has also been caused by extramedullary hematopoiesis in cases of myelosclerosis, thalassemia, cyanotic heart disease, myelogenous leukemia, sideropenic anemia, and polycythemia vera (Oustwani et al).

Solitary osteochondromas of vertebral bodies and multiple exostoses of hereditary type are other reported causes of spinal cord compression. In the case reported by Buur and Morch the clinical syndrome was one of pure spastic paraparesis of several months' progression.

VACUOLAR MYELOPATHY WITH AIDS

As the neurology of AIDS has been elucidated, this new clinical and pathologic entity has emerged. Its frequency is impressive—20 of 89 successive cases of AIDS on whom a postmortem examination was performed (Petito et al). Often the clinical symptoms and signs of spinal cord disease are obscured by a neuropathy or one or more of the central nervous system disorders that complicate AIDS—due either to HIV-1 or an opportunistic infection (cytomegalic inclusion virus disease, toxoplasmosis, etc.). In five severe cases of vacuolar myopathy in Petito's series, there was leg weakness or leg and arm weakness (often asymmetrical and developing over a period of weeks, to which the signs of sensory tract involvement and sphincteric disorder were added). The interval between the onset of spinal cord symptoms and death was 4 to 6 months. The white matter of the spinal cord is vacuolated, most severely in thoracic segments. Posterior and lateral funiculi are affected without reference to sensory or motor systems. Axons are involved to a lesser degree. Lipid-laden macrophages are present in abundance. Similar vacuolar lesions may be seen in the brain in some cases.

Although the lesions in the spinal cord resemble those of pernicious anemia, their distribution is somewhat different and serum B_{12} and folic acid levels have been normal. A similar lesion was seen in one of our cases of chronic lupus erythematosus.

TROPICAL SPASTIC PARAPARESIS DUE TO HUMAN T-LYMPHOTROPIC VIRUS TYPE 1 (HTLV-1)

Although tropical spastic paraparesis was made known to neurologists 30 years ago through the observations and writings of Cruickshank, it is only since the publication of the last edition of this book that an infective inflammation of chronic nature due to the retrovirus HTLV-1 has been discovered. The clinical implications of these findings are broad and extend even to the etiology of the demyelinative diseases.

Spinal cord diseases of this type have been reported from the Caribbean islands, southern United States, southern Japan, South America, and Africa. The clinical picture is one of a slowly progressive paraparesis with increased tendon reflexes and Babinski signs; disorder of sphincteric control is usually an early finding. Sensory function is variably affected, usually only in the lower extremities. Paresthesias, reduced vibratory and position senses, and ataxia have been reported. A few of the patients have had an associated polyneuropathy, as in Cruikshank's early cases. The upper extremities are usually spared (except for lively tendon reflexes), as are cerebral and brainstem structures.

The cerebrospinal fluid contains small numbers of lymphocytes of T type (10 to 50 per cubic millimeter), normal protein, and glucose levels, and an increase in IgG with antibodies to HTLV-1. MRI reveals a normal brain but a smallness of the spinal cord. A report of the neuropathology of 15 cases documents an inflammatory myelitis with focal spongiform demyelinative and necrotic lesions, perivascular and meningeal infiltrates, and focal destruction of gray matter. The posterior columns and corticospinal tracts are the main sites of disease. Some of the T lymphocytes have a leukemia-like appearance, and the HTLV-1 virus has been identified as a cause of one type of leukemia (Osame et al). The disease tends to cluster, and females of adult age appear to be the most susceptible.

The clinical picture can easily be confused with progressive spastic paraplegia and the chronic phase of multiple sclerosis. Intriguing is the report by Koprowski et al of HTLV-1 antibodies in multiple sclerosis; this finding needs to be corroborated.

LATHYRISM

From the interesting historical review of Dastur one learns that this disease was known to Hippocrates, Pliny, and Galen in Europe, to Avicenna in the Middle East, and to the ancient Hindus. The term ''lathyrism'' was applied to the disease by Cantani, in Italy, because of its recognized relationship to the prolonged consumption of *Lathyrus sativus* (chickling pea). The disease is common in some districts in India and Africa.

During periods of famine, when wheat and other grains are in short supply, the diet may for months consist of flour made of the chickling pea. In such exposed individuals there occurs a gradual weakening of the legs

accompanied by spasticity and cramps. Paresthesias, numbness, and formication of the legs and frequency and urgency of micturition, impotence, and sphincteric spasms are added. The upper extremities may exhibit coarse tremors and involuntary movements. Once these symptoms are installed, they are more or less permanent, most of the patients living out their natural life span.

Only two reports on the neuropathology of this condition were known to Dastur, one by Buzzard and Greenfield in England, the other by Filiminoff in Russia. Both patients had been in a stationary paraplegic state for years. Greenfield noted a loss of ascending and descending tracts in the spinal cord, particularly the corticospinal and direct spinocerebellar. Filiminoff observed a loss of myelinated fibers in the lateral and posterior columns. (Unlike the cases of Spencer et al, there had been a loss of pain and thermal sensation in the upper extremities). The larger Betz cells had disappeared, while anterior horn cells were unaffected. Gliosis and thickening of blood vessels was seen in the degenerated tracts.

The toxic nature of this disease, long suspected, has been confirmed by Spencer and his colleagues. They extracted a neuroexcitatory amino acid, beta-N-oxalylaminoalanine (BOAA), from chickling peas and were able to induce corticospinal dysfunction in monkeys given this substance with a nutritious diet. More recently, Hugon and coworkers have produced a primate model of lathyrism by feeding monkeys a diet composed of *Lathyrus sativus*, in addition to an alcoholic extract of this legume. These findings tend to negate the importance of several other factors that until now had been thought to be causative— namely malnutrition, ergot contamination, and toxins derived from *Vicia sativa*, the common vetch that grows alongside the lathyrus species.

DYSRAPHIC AND CONGENITAL TUMOR SYNDROMES

See Chap. 44.

SYNDROME OF SEGMENTAL SENSORY DISSOCIATION WITH BRACHIAL AMYOTROPHY(Syringomyelic Syndrome)

This syndrome is most often ascribable to syringomyelia (i.e., a central cavitation of the spinal cord of undetermined cause), but a similar clinical syndrome may sometimes be observed in association with other pathologic states, such as intramedullary cord tumors, traumatic myelopathy, post-radiation myelopathy, spinal arachnoiditis, infarction (myelomalacia) and bleeding (hematomyelia), and rarely with extramedullary tumors, cervical spondylosis, and cervical necrotizing myelitis.

SYRINGOMYELIA

Syringomyelia (from the Greek *syrinx*, "pipe" or "tube") may be defined as a chronic progressive degenerative disorder of the spinal cord, characterized clinically by brachial amyotrophy and segmental sensory loss of dissociated type, and pathologically by cavitation of the central parts of the spinal cord, usually in the cervical region but extending upward in some cases into the medulla oblongata and pons (syringobulbia) or downward into the thoracic or even the lumbar segments. Not infrequently there are associated abnormalities of the vertebral column (thoracic scoliosis, fusion of vertebrae, or Klippel-Feil anomaly), base of the skull (platybasia and basilar invagination), and of cerebellum and brainstem (type I Chiari malformation). Approximately 90 percent of cases of syringomyelia have type I Chiari malformation, and of type I Chiari malformations, approximately 50 percent have syringomyelia. In a small number of cases an intramedullary tumor (astrocytoma, hemangioblastoma, ependymoma) or traumatic necrosis of the spinal cord has been found in or near some part of the syrinx.

Historical Note Although pathologic cavitation of the spinal cord was recognized as early as the sixteenth century, the term *syringomyelia* was first used to describe this process in 1827 by Ollivier d'Angers (cited by Ballantine et al). Later, following the recognition of the central canal as a normal structure, it was assumed by Virchow (1863) and by Leyden (1876) that cavitation of the spinal cord had its origin in an abnormal expansion of the central canal, and they renamed the process *hydromyelia*. Cavities in the central portions of the spinal cord, unconnected with the central canal, were recognized by Hallopeau (1870); Simon suggested in 1875 that the term *syringomyelia* be reserved for such cavities and that the term *hydromyelia* be restricted to dilatation of the central canal itself. Thus a century ago the stage was set for an argument about pathogenesis that has not been settled to the present day.

Pathogenesis One theory of pathogenesis, of which Gardner was the most persuasive protagonist, is that normal flow of CSF is prevented by a congenital failure of opening of the outlets of the fourth ventricle. As a result, a pulse wave of CSF pressure, generated by systolic pulsations of the choroid plexuses, is transmitted into the cord from the fourth ventricle through the central canal. According to this theory, the syrinx consists essentially of a greatly dilated central canal with a ramifying diverticulum from the central canal, that dissects along gray matter and fiber tracts. The frequency with which syringomyelia is linked to malformations at the craniocervical junction, i.e., to lesions that could interfere with normal flow of CSF, has lent credence to this theory.

There are many instances, however, where Gardner's hydrodynamic theory does not explain the syringomyelia. In some cases the foramens of Luschka and Magendie are found to be patent, and other abnormalities of the posterior fossa or foramen magnum are also not in evidence. Cases have been observed in which two well-developed cavities, one at a cervical and another at a lumbar level, were unconnected by any patent channel. Furthermore, in many cases, including several of our own, histologic sections of the tissue between the fourth ventricle and the syrinx in the spinal cord have failed to demonstrate any connection (see also Hughes).

Gardner's theory has been questioned on other grounds. Ball and Dayan have calculated the pulse-pressure wave transmitted into the cord to be of so low an order as to be most unlikely to produce a syrinx. These authors have suggested a somewhat different mechanism. In their view, the CSF, under increased pressure because of subarachnoid obstruction at the craniocervical junction, tracks into the spinal cord along the Virchow-Robin spaces. Over a prolonged period of time, small pools of fluid coalesce to form a syrinx, which originally forms independently of the central canal but eventually becomes connected with it. A blastomatous formation in the spinal cord, akin to tuberous sclerosis or central von Recklinghausen disease but with a tendency for the abnormal tissue to cavitate, is another suggested explanation of syrinx formation. Still others have suggested that edema is a major pathogenetic factor, induced by angiomatous malformations, neoplasms, trauma, arachnoiditis, etc. This hardly exhausts the list of hypotheses, but none of them has been confirmed, and there is no point in enumerating all of them here. The authors favor the view that in the most common type of syringomyelia a cervical cord lesion, produced in childhood as part of a Chiari malformation, results in an enlarging cavity and diverticulation of the spinal canal, via a hydrodynamic mechanism within the destructive lesion—as was postulated originally by Gordon Holmes. We are impressed with the relationship between basal cranial, cervical spine, and cerebellospinal malformations and hydrosyringomyelia, and with disturbed hydrodynamics of CSF as important factors in the pathogenesis. Logue and Edwards document several cases where the foramen magnum was obstructed by a lesion other than a Chiari formation—dural cyst, localized arachnoiditis, atlanto-axial fusion, simple cerebeller cyst, and basilar invagination.

Irrespective of its mode of origin, the syrinx first occupies the central gray matter of the *cervical* portion of the spinal cord, where it interrupts the crossing pain and temperature fibers in the anterior commissure at several successive cord segments. As the cavity enlarges it extends symmetrically or asymmetrically into the posterior and anterior horns and eventually into the lateral and posterior funiculi of the cord. It may enlarge the spinal cord and even widen the interpedicular spaces. The cavity is lined with astrocytic glia and a few thick-walled blood vessels, and the fluid in the cavity is clear and has a relatively low protein content, like CSF.

The cavitation is always to be found in the cervical portion of the cord in close relation to the cerebellar hernia and foramen magnum and only reaches the thoracic and lumbar portions by extension from the cervical region. Either a cavity or a glial septum may extend asymmetrically into the medulla oblongata, usually in the vicinity of the descending tract of the fifth cranial nerve (syringobulbia).

Thus, wider experience with the pathology of syringomyelia and better understanding of the postulated mechanisms have led to the following classification, modified from Barnett et al:

Type I Syringomyelia with obstruction of the foramen magnum and dilation of the central canal
   A. With type I Chiari malformation
   B. With other obstructive lesions of the foramen magnum
Type II Syringomyelia without obstruction of foramen magnum (idiopathic type)
Type III Syringomyelia with other diseases of the spinal cord
   A. Spinal cord tumors
   B. Traumatic myelopathy
   C. Spinal arachnoiditis and pachymeningitis
Type IV Pure hydromyelia with or without hydrocephalus

Clinical Features The clinical picture varies in these four pathologic types, the differences depending not only on the extent of the syrinx, but also on the associated pathologic changes, particularly those related to the Chiari formation. Types I to III syringomyelia are sporadic disorders; familial occurrence is very rare. Symptoms usually begin in the adult age period (35 to 45 years). Males and females are equally affected. Rarely there is some abnormality at birth and occasionally the first symptom is in late childhood or adolescence. Usually the onset is insidious, and the course is irregularly progressive. In many instances the symptoms or signs are discovered accidentally (a painless burn or atrophy of the hand), and the patient cannot say

when the disease began. Rarely there is an almost apoplectic onset or worsening; there are cases on record of an aggravation of old symptoms or the appearance of new symptoms after a violent strain or paroxysm of coughing. Once the disease is recognized, some patients remain much the same for years, even decades, but more often there is progression to the point of being chair-bound within 5 to 10 years. This extremely variable course makes it difficult to evaluate therapy.

The precise clinical picture at any given point in the evolution of the disease depends upon the cross-sectional and longitudinal extent of the syrinx, but *certain features are fundamental and the clinical diagnosis can hardly be made without them. These features are segmental weakness and atrophy of the hands and arms with loss of tendon reflexes and segmental anesthesia of the dissociated type* (loss of pain and thermal sense and preservation of the sense of touch) over the neck, shoulders, and arms. Finally there is weakness and ataxia of the legs from involvement of the corticospinal tracts and posterior columns in the cervical region. Kyphoscoliosis is added in many of the cases.

The particular muscle groups that are affected on the two sides may vary. Exceptionally motor function is spared, and the segmental dissociated sensory loss and/or pain are the only marks of the disease. In a few of the cases, especially those with the Chiari malformation, the reflexes in the arms are preserved or even hyperactive as might be expected with upper rather than lower motor neuron involvement. Or the shoulder muscles may be atrophic and the hands spastic. In the lower extremities the weakness, if present, is of a spastic (corticospinal) type.

The characteristic segmental sensory dissociation is usually bilateral but a unilateral pattern is not unknown, and this is true of the amyotrophy as well. The sensory loss has a cape or hemicape distribution, often extending to the face or back of the head and onto the trunk. While tactile sensation is usually preserved, there are cases in which it is impaired, usually in the region of the most dense analgesia. Exceptionally there is no sensory loss in the presence of amyotrophy; such cases have been recorded where only a hydrocephalus and hydromyelia were present (type IV). If tactile sensation is affected in the arms, joint position and vibratory sense tend also to be impaired. In the lower extremities there may be some loss of pain and thermal sensation proximally and over the abdomen, but usually there is a loss of vibratory and position sense which is indicative of posterior column lesions and is the basis of ataxia. A Horner syndrome may result from ipsilateral involvement of the intermediolateral cell column at C8, T1, and T2 levels.

Pain is a symptom in about half of our patients with types I and II syringomyelia. The pain is usually unilateral or more marked on one side and is of a burning, aching quality, mostly in or at the border of areas of sensory impairment. In a few patients it involves the face or trunk. An aching pain at the base of the skull or posterior cervical region, intensified by coughing, sneezing, or stooping (brief exertional pain) is often present in type I cases. But, as Logue and Edwards point out, pain of this type is often a feature of Chiari malformation without syringomyelia and is probably attributable to compression or stretching of cervical roots.

Syringobulbia is the bulbar equivalent of syringomyelia. Usually the two coexist, but occasionally the bulbar manifestations precede the spinal ones or occur independently. The glial cleft or cavity is located most often in the lateral tegmentum of the medulla, but it may extend into the pons and, rarely, even higher. The symptoms and signs are characteristically unilateral and consist of nystagmus, analgesia, and thermoanesthesia of the face (numbness), wasting and weakness of the tongue (dysarthria), and palatal and vocal cord paralysis (dysphagia and hoarseness). Diplopia, episodic vertigo and trigeminal pain, and persistent hiccough are less common symptoms. The clinical and pathologic features of syringobulbia have been described in great detail by Jonesco-Sisesti. A most unusual keyhole–shaped syrinx, which was confined to the upper pons and midbrain and commuicated with the fourth ventricle, has been desribed by de la Monte and her colleagues.

When Chiari malformation is associated with syringomyelia, it may be impossible to distinguish between its compressive effects on the brainstem and downward displacement of the medulla with stretching of lower cranial nerves, and the effects of syringobulbia. Clinical features that favor the diagnosis of type I syringomyelia with Chiari malformation are nystagmus, cerebellar ataxia, exertional head-neck pain, prominent corticospinal and sensory tract involvement in the lower extremities, hydrocephalus, and craniocervical malformations. In type I syringomyelia without Chiari malformation but with some other type of obstructive lesion at the foramen magnum, the clinical picture is much the same, and the diagnosis of the foramen magnum lesion can only be made by MRI, myelography, or surgical exploration.

The association of syringomyelia with an intramedullary tumor (type III) should be suspected when there is a syringomyelic type of sensorimotor abnormality extending over many segments of the body. With Von Hippel-Lindau disease the diagnosis hinges on the finding of the characteristic hereditary retinal and cerebellar vascular malformations. In the posttraumatic cases, a traumatic necrosis of the spinal cord that has been stable for months or years begins to cause pain and spreading sensory or motor loss usually recognizable in segments above the original lesion. This has occurred in approximately 3 percent of the cases of Rossier et al, more in quadriplegics than in paraplegics.

In the few cases of hydromyelia that have come to our attention there has been a long-standing hydrocephalus, often congenital, complicated years later by progressive weakness and atrophy of the muscles of the arms and hands. Segmental sensory loss has been reported in only a few instances. Proof of the existence of this entity in the past has been based on necropsy demonstration of an enormously widened central canal without a true syrinx. Now it should be diagnosable by MRI.

Diagnosis The clinical neurologic picture is so characteristic that diagnosis is seldom in doubt. In the past, Pantopaque myelography performed with the patient in the supine, head-down position revealed the Chiari malformation. Metrizamide myelography and delayed CT scanning usually expose the syrinx; the contrast material fills the syrinx and the central canal directly, probably from the surface of the cord (Ball and Dayan). Recently we have obtained spectacular demonstrations of the syrinx, Chiari malformations, and other foramen magnum lesions by MRI in the sagittal plane of the brain and spinal cord (Fig. 36-5).

Treatment The only therapy of value for type I syringomyelia is surgical decompression of the foramen magnum and upper cervical canal. Radiation therapy, which was formerly recommended, is of no benefit. The reader will find the articles of Hankinson and of Logue and Edwards, who have treated large series of cases, to be the most informative.

The operation advised by Gardner of plugging the connection between the fourth ventricle and the central canal of the cervical cord has been abandoned by most neurosurgeons. There have been complications of the operative procedure, and the results appear to be no better than those obtained from simple decompression. The latter operation also carries some risk, especially if there is an attempt to excise the tonsillar projections of the cerebellum. In the series of Logue and Edwards, comprising 56 cases of type I syringomyelia, the occipitocervical pain was relieved in most patients, but the shoulder-arm pain usually persisted. Upper motor neuron weakness of the legs and sensory ataxia were often improved whereas the segmental sensory and motor manifestations of the syringomyelia were not. Hankinson has reported good results from decompression in 75 percent of type I cases of syringomyelia. Whether the long-term course of these diseases will be altered (10 to 15 years) has not been determined.

Syringostomy or shunting of the cavity has been performed in type I and many of the type II cases, but the results have been unpredictable. Love and Olafson, who performed syringostomy in 40 patients of both types (mainly type II) stated that 30 percent had an excellent outcome. Our experiences with this procedure have not persuaded us of its lasting value; most of our patients, even those who reported some improvement originally, soon relapsed to their preoperative state, and the disease then progressed in the usual way.

Surgery for the relatively rare posttraumatic cases has given more favorable results. With incomplete myelopathy, syringostomy has relieved the pain in all of Shannon's 10 patients. Where he found the myelopathy to be complete, the cord was transected and the upper stump excised.

Figure 36-5

Chiari I malformation associated with hydromyelia. T1-weighted MR image (paramedian view) shows the cerebellar tonsils projecting into the upper cervical canal and a hydromyelic cavity extending from C2 to T2-T3. The patient was a 33-year-old woman with persistent paresthesias and dysesthesias of the right upper limb and loss of sensation over the right neck.

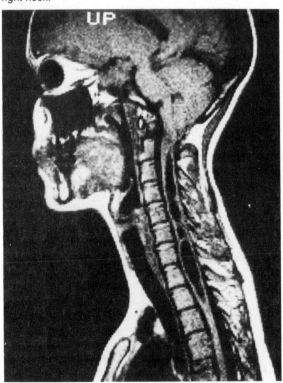

In the cases of syringomyelia with tumor, where the cyst fluid usually is of high protein content and viscid (unlike the low protein fluid of the usual syrinx), it is enough to excise the tumor. This has been done successfully with hemangioblastomas of the posterior columns and occasionally with ependymomas.

The rare hydromyelic cases should benefit from ventriculoperitoneal shunts of the hydrocephaly, and a few excellent results are reported. This procedure has also been attempted in type I cases, with indifferent results, unless there is an associated hydrocephalus. Draining the central canal by amputation of the tip of the sacral cord has been unsuccessful.

CONCLUDING REMARKS

In conclusion, it is always well to remind oneself that of the more than 30 diseases of the spinal cord, effective means of treatment are available for only a few—spondylosis, extramedullary spinal cord tumors, syphilis (meningomyelitis and tabes), epidural abscess, hematoma and granuloma (tuberculous, fungal), and subacute combined degeneration and other forms of nutritional myelopathy. The physician's major responsibility is to determine whether the patient has one of the treatable diseases.

REFERENCES

ADAMS CBT, LOGUE V: Studies in cervical spondylotic myelopathy. *Brain* 94:569, 1971.

ANTONI N: Spinal vascular malformations (angiomas) and myelomalacia. *Neurology* 12:795, 1962.

ARNASON BGW: Paraneoplastic syndromes of muscle, nerve, and brain: Immunologic considerations, in Rose PC (ed): *Clinical Neuroimmunology.* Oxford, Blackwell Scientific, 1979.

BABIKIAN VL, STEFANSSON K, DIEPERINK ME et al: Paraneoplastic myelopathy: Antibodies against protein in normal CSF and underlying neoplasm. *Lancet* 2:49, 1985.

BAKER AS, OJEMANN RG, SWARTZ MN, RICHARDSON EP JR: Spinal epidural abscess. *N Engl J Med* 293:463, 1975.

BALL MJ, DAYAN AD: Pathogenesis of syringomyelia. *Lancet* 2:799, 1972.

BALLANTINE HT, OJEMANN RG, DREW JH: Syringohydromyelia, in Krayenbühl H, Maspes PE, Sweet WH (eds): *Progress in Neurological Surgery*, vol 4. New York, S Karger, 1971, pp 227–245.

BARNETT HJM, FOSTER JB, HUDGSON P: *Syringomyelia.* Philadelphia, Saunders, 1973.

BARTLESON JO, COHEN MD, HARRINGTON TM: Cauda equina

syndrome secondary to long-standing ankylosing spondylitis. *Ann Neurol* 14:662, 1983.

BLACKWOOD W: Discussion of vascular disease of the spinal cord. *Proc R Soc Med* 51:543, 1958.

BOTS TAM, WATTENDORF AR, BURUMA OJS: Acute myelopathy caused by fibrocartilagenous emboli. *Neurology* 31:1250, 1981.

BRAIN WR: Discussion on rupture of the intervertebral disc in the cervical region. *Proc R Soc Med* 41:509, 1948.

BRAIN WR, NORTHFIELD D, WILKINSON M: The neurological manifestations of cervical spondylosis. *Brain* 75:187, 1952.

BURNS RJ, JONES AN, ROBERTSON JS: Pathology of radiation myelopathy. *J Neurol Neurosurg Psychiatry* 35:888, 1972.

BUUR T, MORCH MM: Hereditary multiple exostoses with spinal cord compression. *J Neurol Neurosurg Psychiatry* 46:96, 1983.

BUZZARD EF, GREENFIELD JG: *Pathology of the Nervous System.* London, Constable, 1921.

CAMPBELL AMG, GARLAND H: Subacute myoclonic spinal neuronitis. *J Neurol Neurosurg Psychiatry* 19:268, 1956.

CANNON WB, ROSENBLUETH A: *The Supersensitivity of Denervated Structures.* New York, Macmillan, 1949.

CHEN JR, RHEE RSC, WALLACH S et al: Neurologic disturbances in Paget disease of bone: Response to calcitonin. *Neurology* 29:448, 1979.

CILLUFFO JM, GOMEZ MR, REESE DF et al: Idiopathic ("congenital") spinal arachnoid diverticula. *Mayo Clin Proc* 56:93, 1981.

COLLINS WF, CHEHRAZI B: Concepts of the acute management of spinal cord injury, in Mathews WB, Glaser GH (eds): *Recent Advances in Clinical Neurology.* London, Churchill Livingstone, 1983, chap 3, pp 67–82.

COMARR AE: The practical urological management of the patient with spinal cord injury. *Brit J Urol* 31:1, 1959.

COSTIGAN DA, WINKELMAN MD: Intramedullary spinal cord metastasis. *J Neurosurg* 62:227, 1985.

CRUICKSHANK EK: A neuropathic syndrome of uncertain origin. *West Indian Med* 5:147, 1956.

DASTUR DK: Lathyrism. *World Neur* 3:721, 1962.

DE LA MONTE SM, HOROWITZ SA, LAROCQUE AA, RICHARDSON EP JR: Keyhole aqueduct syndrome. *Arch Neurol* 43:926, 1986.

DEVIVO MJ, KARTUS PT, STOVER SI: Seven-year survival following spinal cord injury. *Arch Neurol* 44:872, 1987.

DJINDJIAN R: Angiomas of the spinal cord, in Vinken PJ, Bruyn GW (eds): *Handbook of Clinical Neurology,* vol 32. Amsterdam, North-Holland, 1978, chap 16, pp 465–510.

DOUGLAS MA, PARKS LC, BEBIN J: Sudden myelopathy secondary to therapeutic total-body hyperthermia after spinal-cord irradiation. *N Engl J Med* 304:583, 1981.

ELKINGTON J ST C: Arachnoiditis, in Feiling A (ed): *Modern Trends in Neurology.* New York, Hoeber-Harper, 1951, pp 149–161.

ELL JJ, UTTLEY D, SILVER JR: Acute myelopathy in association with heroin addiction. *J Neurol Neurosurg Psychiatry* 44:448, 1981.

ELSBERG CA: *Surgical Diseases of the Spinal Cord, Membranes and Nerve Roots: Symptoms, Diagnosis and Treatment.* New York, Hoeber-Harper, 1941.

FELDMAN E, BROMFIELD E, NAVIA B et al: Hydrocephalic dementia and spinal cord tumor. *Arch Neurol* 43:714, 1986.

FILIMINOFF IN: Zur pathologisch-anatomischen Charakteristik des Lathyrismus. *Z Ges Neurol Psychiatry* 105:76, 1926.

FOIX C, ALAJOUANINE T: La myélite nécrotique subaiguë. *Rev Neurol* 2:1, 1926.

FOLLISS AGH, NETZKY MG: Progressive necrotic myelopathy, in Vinken PJ, Bruyn GW (eds): *Handbook of Clinical Neurology,* vol 9. Amsterdam, North-Holland, 1970, chap 16, pp 452–468.

FULTON JF: *Physiology of the Nervous System.* London, Oxford University Press, 1943.

GARDNER WJ: Hydrodynamic mechanism of syringomyelia: Its relationship to myelocele. *J Neurol Neurosurg Psychiatry* 28:247, 1965.

GILBERT RW, KIM J-H, POSNER JB: Epidural spinal cord compression from metastatic tumor: Diagnosis and treatment. *Ann Neurol* 3:40, 1978.

GREENBERG HS, KIM JH, POSNER JB: Epidural spinal cord compression from metastatic tumor. *Ann Neurol* 8:361, 1980.

GREENFIELD JG, TURNER JWA: Acute and subacute necrotic myelitis. *Brain* 62:227, 1939.

GUILLAIN G, BARRÉ JA: Les plaies de la moelle épinière par blessures de guerre. *Presse Med* 24:497, 1916.

GUTTMANN L: *Spinal Cord Injuries: Comprehensive Management and Research.* Oxford, Blackwell, 1976.

HANKINSON J: Syringomyelia and the surgeon, in Williams D (ed): *Modern Trends in Neurology,* vol. 5. London, Butterworth, 1970, chap 7, pp 127–148.

HAYMAKER W: Decompression sickness, in Scholz W (ed): *Handbuch der Speziellen Pathologischen Anatomie und Histologie,* vol XIII/1B. Berlin, Springer, 1957, pp 1600–1672.

HEAD H, RIDDOCH G: The automatic bladder: Excessive sweating and some other reflex conditions in gross injuries of the spinal cord. *Brain* 40:188, 1917.

HERRICK M, MILLS PE JR: Infarction of spinal cord. *Arch Neurol* 24:228, 1971.

HOLMES G: On the spinal injuries of warfare. Goulstonian lectures. *Br Med J* 2:769, 1915.

HOWELL DA, LEES AJ, TOGHILL PJ: Spinal internuncial neurones in progressive encephalomyelitis with rigidity. *J Neurol Neurosurg Psychiatry* 42:773, 1979.

HUGHES JT: *Pathology of the Spinal Cord,* 2nd ed. Philadelphia, Saunders, 1978.

HUGHES JT, BROWNELL B: Cervical spondylosis complicated by anterior spinal artery thrombosis. *Neurology* 14:1073, 1964.

HUGON J, LUDOLPH A, ROY DN et al: Studies on the etiology and pathogenesis of motor neuron diseases. II. Clinical and electrophysiologic features of pyramidal dysfunction in macaques fed *Lathyrus sativus* and IDPN. *Neurology* 38:435, 1988.

JEFFERSON G: Discussion on spinal injuries. *Proc R Soc Med* 21:625, 1927.

JONES A: Transient radiation myelitis. *Br J Radiol* 37:727, 1964.

JONESCO-SISESTI N: *Syringobulbia. A Contribution to the Pathophysiology of the Brainstem.* Translated into English, edited, and annotated by RT Ross. New York, Praeger, 1986.

KAGAN RA, WOLLIN M, GILBERT HA et al: Comparison of the tolerance of the brain and spinal cord to injury by radiation, in Gilbert HA, Kagan RA (eds): *Radiation Damage to the Nervous System.* New York, Raven Press, 1980.

KILLEN DA, FOSTER JH: Spinal cord injury as a complication of contrast angiography. *Surgery* 59:962, 1966.

KNEISLEY LW: Hyperhydrosis in paraplegia. *Arch Neurol* 34:536, 1977.

KOCHER T: Die Wirletzungen der Virbelsäule zugleich als Beitrag zur Physiologie des menschlichen Rückenmarcks. *Mitt Grenzgeb Med Chir* 1:415, 1896.

KOPROWSKI H, DEFREITAS EC, HARPER ME et al: Multiple sclerosis and human lymphotropic retroviruses. *Nature* 318:154, 1985.

KUHN RA: Functional capacity of the isolated human spinal cord. *Brain* 73:1, 1950.

LAZORTHES G: Pathology, classification and clinical aspects of vascular diseases of the spinal cord, in Vinken PJ, Bruyn GW (eds): *Handbook of Clinical Neurology,* vol 12, 1972, chap 19, pp 492–506.

LHERMITTE F, CHAIN F, ESCOUROLLE R et al: Un nouveau cas de contracture tétaniforme distinct du stiff-man syndrome. *Rev Neurol* 128:3, 1973.

LHERMITTE J: *La section totale de la moelle épinière.* Bourges, Imprimerie V Tardy, 1919.

LIPSON SJ, NAHEEDY MH, KAPLAN MH: Spinal stenosis caused by epidural lipomatosis in Cushing's syndrome. *N Engl J Med* 302:36, 1980.

LOGUE V: Angiomas of the spinal cord: Review of the pathogenesis, clinical features, and results of surgery. *J Neurol Neurosurg Psychiatry* 42:1, 1979.

LOGUE V, EDWARDS MR: Syringomyelia and its surgical treatment—an analysis of 75 cases. *J Neurol Neurosurg Psychiatry* 44:273, 1981.

LOMBARDI G, PASSERINI A, MIGLIAVACCA F: Spinal arachnoiditis, *Br J Radiol* 35:314, 1962.

LOVE JG, OLAFSON RA: Syringomyelia: a look at surgical therapy. *J Neurosurg* 24:714, 1966.

MAIR WGP, FOLKERTS JF: Necrosis of spinal cord due to thrombophlebitis (subacute necrotic myelitis). *Brain* 76:563, 1953.

MALAMUD N, BOLDREY EB, WELCH WK, FADELL EJ: Necrosis of brain and spinal cord following x-ray therapy. *J Neurosurg* 11:353, 1954.

MANCALL EL, ROSALES RK: Necrotizing myelopathy associated with visceral carcinoma. *Brain* 87:639, 1964.

MARSHALL J: Observations on reflex changes in the lower limbs in spastic paraplegia in man. *Brain* 77:290, 1954.

MARTIN J, DAVIS L: Studies upon spinal cord injuries; altered reflex activity. *Surg Gynec Obstet* 86:535, 1948.

MATHIAS CJ, FRANKEL HL: Autonomic failure in tetraplegia, in Bannister R (ed): *Autonomic Failure.* Oxford, Oxford University Press, 1983, pp 453–488.

MCCRAE DL: Bony abnormalities in the region of the foramen magnum: Correlation of the anatomic and neurologic findings. *Acta Radiol* 40:335, 1953.

MESSARD L, CARMODY A, MANNARINO E, RUGE D: Survival after spinal cord trauma. A life table analysis. *Arch Neurol* 35:78, 1978.

MESSER HD, LITVINOFF J: Pyogenic cervical osteomyelitis. *Arch Neurol* 33:571, 1976.

MIXTER WJ, BARR JS: Rupture of the intervertebral disc with involvement of the spinal canal. *N Engl J Med* 211:210, 1934.

MORRISON RE, BROWN J, GOODING RS: Spinal cord abscess caused by *listeria monocytogenes. Arch Neurol* 37:243, 1980.

MORSE SD: Acute central cervical spinal cord syndrome. *Ann Emerg Med* 11:436, 1982.

MUNRO D: The rehabilitation of patients totally paralyzed below the waist. *N Engl J Med* 234:207, 1946.

NAIMAN JL, DONAHUE WL, PRITCHARD JS: Fatal nucleus pulposus embolism of spinal cord after trauma. *Neurology* 11:83, 1961.

NAKANO KK, SCHOENE WC, BAKER RA, DAWSON DM: The cervical myelopathy associated with rheumatoid arthritis: Analysis of 32 patients, with 2 postmortem cases. *Ann Neurol* 3:144, 1978.

NURICK S: The cervical spine and paraplegia, in Williams D (ed): *Modern Trends in Neurology,* vol 6. London, Butterworth, 1975, pp 167–182.

OSAME M, MATSUMOTO M, USUKU K et al: Chronic progressive myelopathy associated with elevated antibodies to human T-lymphotropic virus type I and adult T-cell leukemialike cells. *Ann Neurol* 21:117, 1987.

OUSTWANI MB, KURTIDES ES, CHRIST M, CIRIC I: Spinal cord compression with paraplegia in myelofibrosis. *Arch Neurol* 37:389, 1980.

PALLIS C, JONES AM, SPILLANE JD: Cervical spondylosis. *Brain* 77:274, 1954.

PALMER JJ: Radiation myelopathy. *Brain* 95:109, 1972.

PANSE F: Electrical lesions of the nervous system, in Vinken PJ, Bruyn GW (eds): *Handbook of Clinical Neurology,* vol 7. Amsterdam, North-Holland, 1970, chap 13, pp 344–387.

PANT SS, BHARGAVA AN, SINGH MM, DHANDA PC: Myelopathy in hepatic cirrhosis. *Br Med J* 1:1064, 1963.

PAYNE EE, SPILLANE JD: The cervical spine: An anatomicopathological study of 70 specimens (using a special technique) with particular reference to the problem of cervical spondylosis. *Brain* 80:571, 1957.

PEET MM, ECHOLS DH: Herniation of nucleus pulposus; cause of compression of spinal cord. *Arch Neurol Psychiatr* 32:924, 1934.

PENN RD, KROIN JS: Continuous intrathecal baclofen for severe spasticity. *Lancet* 2:125, 1985.

PENRY JK, HOEFNAGEL D, VANDEN NOORT S et al: Muscle spasm and abnormal posture resulting from damage to interneurones in spinal cord. *Arch Neurol* 34:560, 1960.

PETITO CK, NAVIA BA, CHO ES et al: Vacuolar myelopathy pathologically resembling subacute combined degeneration in patients with AIDS. *N Engl J Med* 312:374, 1985.

POLLOCK LJ, BROWN M, BOSHES B et al: Pain below the level of injury of the spinal cord. *Arch Neurol Psychiatry* 65:319, 1951.

POLLOCK LJ: Spasticity, pseudospontaneous spasm, and other reflex activities late after injury to the spinal cord. *Arch Neurol Psychiatry* 66:537, 1951.

PORTENOY RK, LIPTON RB, FOLEY KM: Back pain in the cancer patient: An algorithm for evaluation and management. *Neurology* 37:134, 1987.

QUEIROZ L DE S, NUCCI A, FACURE NO, FACURE JJ: Massive spinal cord necrosis in schistosomasis. *Arch Neurol* 36:517, 1979.

REAGAN TJ, THOMAS JE, COLBY MY: Chronic progressive radiation myelopathy. *JAMA* 203:128, 1968.

RIDDOCH G: The reflex functions of the completely divided spinal cord in man, compared with those associated with less severe lesions. *Brain* 40:264, 1917.

ROBERTSON WB, CRUICKSHANK EK: Jamaican (tropical) myelo-neuropathy, in Minckler J (ed): *Pathology of the Nervous System,* vol 3. New York, McGraw-Hill, 1972.

RODICHOK LD, HARPER GR, RUCKDESCHELL JC et al: Early diagnosis of spinal epidural metastases. *Am J Med* 70:1081, 1981.

ROSSIER AB, FOO D, SHILLITO J: Post-traumatic cervical syringomyelia. *Brain* 108:439, 1985.

SANYAL B, PANT GC, SUBRAHMANIYAM K et al: Radiation myelopathy. *J Neurol Neurosurg Psychiatry* 42:413, 1979.

SAVITSKY N, MADONICK MJ: Statistical control studies in neurology; Babinski sign. *Arch Neurol Psychiatry* 49:272, 1943.

SCHMORL G: Zur pathologischen Anatomie der Wirbelsaule. *Klin Wochenschr* 8:1243, 1929.

SCHNEIDER RC, CHERRY G, PANTEK H: The syndrome of acute central cervical spinal cord injury. *J Neurosurg* 11:546, 1954.

SHAW MDM, RUSSELL JA, GROSSART KW: The changing pattern of arachnoiditis. *J Neurol Neurosurg Psychiatry* 41:97, 1978.

SHANNON N, SIMON L, LOGUE V: Clinical features, investigation, and treatment of post-traumatic syringomyelia. *J Neurol Neurosurg Psychiatry* 44:35, 1981.

SLOOF JH, KERNOHAN JW, MacCARTY CS: *Primary Intramedullary Tumors of the Spinal Cord and Filum Terminale.* Philadelphia, Saunders, 1964.

SPENCER PS, ROY DN, LUDOLPH A et al: Lathyrism: Evidence for role of the neuroexcitatory amino acid BOAA. *Lancet* 2:1066, 1986.

SPILLER WG: Thrombosis of the cervical anterior median spinal artery; syphilitic acute anterior poliomyelitis. *J Nerv Ment Dis* 36:601, 1909.

STOLTMANN HF, BLACKWOOD W: The role of the ligamenta flava in the pathogenesis of myelopathy in cervical spondylosis. *Brain* 87:45, 1964.

STOOKEY B: Compression of the spinal cord due to ventral extradural cervical chondromas. *Arch Neurol Psychiatry* 20:275, 1928.

THOMAS JE, MILLER RH: Lipomatous tumors of the spinal canal. *Mayo Clin Proc* 48:393, 1973.

UCHIMURA I, SHIRAKI H: A contribution to the classification and pathogenesis of demyelinating encephalomyelitis. *J Neuropathol Exp Neurol* 16:139, 1957.

WADIA NH: Myelopathy complicating congenital atlanto-axial dislocation (a study of 28 cases). *Brain* 90:449, 1967.

WEISMAN AD, ADAMS RD: The neurological complications of dissecting aortic aneurysm. *Brain* 67:69, 1944.

WESTENFELDER GO, AKEY DT, CORWIN SJ et al: Acute transverse myelitis due to *Mycoplasma pneumoniae* infection. *Arch Neurol* 38:317,1981.

WHITELY AM, SWASH M, URICH H: Progressive encephalomyelitis with rigidity. *Brain* 99:27, 1976.

WILKINSON M: *Cervical Spondylosis,* 2nd ed. Philadelphia, Saunders, 1971.

WOLTMAN HW, ADSON AW: Abscess of the spinal cord. *Brain* 49:193, 1926.

WINKELMAN MD, ADELSTEIN DJ, KARLINS NL: Intramedullary spinal cord metastases. Diagnostic and therapeutic considerations. *Arch Neurol* 44:526, 1987.

WYBURN-MASON R: *Vascular Abnormalities and Tumors of the Spinal Cord and Its Membranes.* St Louis, Mosby, 1944.

ZIEVE L, MENDELSON DF, GOEPFERT M: Shunt encephalomyelopathy. *Ann Intern Med* 53:53, 1960.

ZÜLCH KL: Mangeldurchblutung an der Grenzzone zweier Gefässgebiete. *Dtsch Z Nervenheilk* 172:1, 1954.

CHAPTER 37

MULTIPLE SCLEROSIS AND ALLIED DEMYELINATIVE DISEASES

It has long been the practice to set apart a group of diseases of the brain and spinal cord in which destruction of myelin (demyelination) is a prominent feature. To define these diseases precisely is difficult, for the simple reason that there is probably no disease in which myelin destruction is the exclusive pathologic change. The idea of a demyelinative disease is, more or less, an abstraction that serves primarily to focus attention on one of the more striking and distinctive features of a pathologic process.

The commonly accepted pathologic criteria of a demyelinative disease are (1) destruction of the myelin sheaths of the nerve fibers, (2) a relative sparing of the other elements of nervous tissue, i.e., of axis cylinders, nerve cells, and supporting structures, (3) an infiltration of inflammatory cells in a perivascular distribution, (4) a particular distribution of lesions, often perivenous and primarily in white matter, either in multiple small disseminated foci or in larger foci spreading from one or more centers, and (5) a relative lack of wallerian, or secondary, degeneration of fiber tracts (an expression of the relative integrity of the axis cylinders in the lesions).

The diseases included in the following classification conform approximately to the above criteria. Like all classifications that are not based on etiology, this one has its shortcomings, in that it is somewhat arbitrary and inconsistent. In some of the diseases here classified as demyelinative, there is a more or less equal affection of both axis cylinders and myelin. Furthermore, a number of diseases in which demyelination is a prominent feature are not included. In some cases of anoxic encephalopathy, for example, the myelin sheaths of the radiating nerve fibers in the deep layers of the cerebral cortex or in ill-defined patches in the convolutional and central white matter are destroyed, while most of the axis cylinders are spared. A relatively selective degeneration of myelin may also occur in some small ischemic foci due to vascular occlusion. In subacute combined degeneration of the cord (SCD), associated with pernicious anemia, myelin may be affected

earlier and to a greater extent than axis cylinders; and the same is true of progressive multifocal leukoencephalopathy (PML), central pontine myelinolysis, and Marchiafava-Bignami disease. Some of these disorders and several others are no longer classified as demyelinative diseases because their etiology has become known. PML has proved to be a viral infection of oligodendrocytes in immune-deficient subjects, and SCD is due to vitamin B_{12} deficiency, so that these disorders are more appropriately included with the viral and nutritional diseases, respectively. Other diseases are not categorized as demyelinative because they lack the characteristic perivascular inflammatory lesion, and exhibit pathologic features that are judged to be more fundamental than the demyelination.

In the language of neurology, therefore, the term *demyelination* has acquired a special meaning; if it is to retain its value, it should be used in the restricted sense indicated above and not as a synonym for complete degeneration of nerve fibers or necrosis of white matter, even though the lesions may look alike in a section stained for myelin. In this latter, more general sense there are few diseases of the central nervous system to which the term *demyelinating* would not apply.

CLASSIFICATION OF THE DEMYELINATIVE DISEASES

I. Multiple sclerosis (disseminated or insular sclerosis)
    A. Chronic relapsing encephalomyelopathic form
    B. Acute multiple sclerosis
    C. Neuromyelitis optica
II. Diffuse cerebral sclerosis (encephalitis periaxalis diffusa) of Schilder and concentric sclerosis of Baló
III. Acute disseminated encephalomyelitis
    A. Following measles, chickenpox, smallpox, and rarely mumps, rubella, and influenza
    B. Following rabies or smallpox vaccination

IV. Acute and subacute necrotizing hemorrhagic encephalitis
  A. Acute encephalopathic form (hemorrhagic leukoencephalitis of Hurst)
  B. Subacute necrotic myelopathy?
  C. Acute brain purpura (acute pericapillary encephalorrhagia)?

MULTIPLE SCLEROSIS

Multiple sclerosis (MS), referred to by the British as *disseminated sclerosis* and by the French as *sclerose en plaques,* is among the most venerable of neurologic diseases and one of the most important, by virtue of its frequency, chronicity, and tendency to attack young adults. It is characterized clinically by episodes of focal disorder of the optic nerves, spinal cord, and brain, which remit to a varying extent and recur over a period of many years. The clinical manifestations are protean, being determined by the varied location and extent of the foci of demyelination; nevertheless, the lesions tend to have a predilection for certain portions of the central nervous system, resulting in characteristic complexes of symptoms and signs that can often be readily recognized.

Classic features include motor weakness, paresthesiae, impaired vision, diplopia, nystagmus, dysarthria, intention tremor, ataxia, impairment of deep sensation, bladder dysfunction, paraparesis, and alteration in emotional responses. Diagnosis may be uncertain at the onset and in the early years of the disease, when symptoms and signs point to a lesion in only one locus of the nervous system. Later, as the disease disseminates through the cerebrospinal axis, diagnostic accuracy approaches 100 percent. A long period of latency (1 to 10 years or longer) between a minor initial symptom, that may not even come to medical attention, and the subsequent development of more characteristic symptoms and signs may delay the diagnosis. In most cases the initial manifestations improve partially or completely, to be followed, after a variable interval, by the recurrence of the same abnormalities or the appearance of new ones, referable to other parts of the nervous system. In as many as half the patients, the disease presents as an intermittently progressive illness, and sometimes as a steadily progressive one. As a general clinical rule, the diagnosis of multiple sclerosis is not secure unless there is a history of remission and relapse and evidence on examination of more than one discrete lesion of the CNS.

PATHOLOGIC FINDINGS

Before being sectioned, the brain generally shows no evidence of disease, but the surface of the spinal cord may feel uneven. Sectioning of the brain and cord discloses numerous scattered lesions that are slightly depressed below the cut surface and stand out from the surrounding white matter by virtue of their pink-gray color (due to loss of myelin). The lesions may vary in diameter from less than a millimeter to several centimeters; they affect principally the white matter of the brain and spinal cord and do not extend beyond the root entry zones of the cranial and spinal nerves. Because of their sharp delineation they are called plaques.

The topography of the lesions is noteworthy. A periventricular localization is characteristic, but only where subependymal veins line the ventricles (mainly the lateral ventricles). Other favorite structures are the optic nerves and chiasm (but not the tracts) and the spinal cord, where pial veins lie next to the white matter. The lesions are distributed randomly through the brainstem, spinal cord, and cerebeller peduncles without reference to particular systems of fibers. In the cerebral cortex the lesions destroy myelin but leave the nerve cells essentially intact.

The histologic appearance of the lesion depends on its age. Relatively recent lesions show a partial or complete destruction and loss of myelin throughout a zone formed by the confluence of many small, predominantly perivenous foci, with sparing of axis cylinders and a variable but slight degeneration of oligodendroglia, a neuroglial (astrocytic) reaction, and perivascular and para-adventitial infiltration with mononuclear cells and lymphocytes. Later, large numbers of microglial phagocytes (macrophages) infiltrate the lesions, and astrocytes in and around the lesions increase in number and size. Long-standing lesions, on the other hand, will show thickly matted, relatively acellular fibroglial tissue, with only occasional perivascular lymphocytes and macrophages; in such lesions intact axis cylinders may still be found. Sparing of axis cylinders prevents wallerian degeneration. However, in old lesions with loss of many axis cylinders there may be descending and ascending degeneration of long fiber tracts in the spinal cord. Partial remyelination is believed to take place on undamaged axons (Prineas and Connell). All gradations of pathologic change between these two extremes may be found in lesions of diverse size, shape, and age, consistent with the extended clinical course.

ETIOLOGY

Cruveilhier (circa 1835), in his classic original description, attributed the disease to suppression of sweat and since that time there has been endless speculation about the etiology. Many of the early theories appear ludicrous in the light of present-day concepts, and others are only of historical interest. There is. no point in enumerating them here; complete accounts are to be found in the reviews of McAlpine and his associates (1972), DeJong (1970), Prineas

(1970), R. T. Johnson (1975, 1978), Portersfield (1977), and McDonald (1983; 1986).

Although the precise cause or causes of multiple sclerosis remain undetermined, a number of epidemiologic facts have been clearly established and will eventually have to be incorporated in any etiologic hypothesis. The disease has a prevalence of less than 1 per 100,000 in equatorial areas; 6 to 14 per 100,000 in southern United States and southern Europe; and 30 to 80 per 100,000 in Canada, northern Europe, and northern United States. A less well-defined gradient exists in the Southern Hemisphere. Kurland's studies indicate that there is a threefold increase in prevalence and a fivefold gradient in mortality rate between New Orleans (30°N latitude) on the one hand, and Boston (42°N) and Winnipeg (50°N) on the other. A similar geographic gradient is less well defined in Japan; however, the prevalence of multiple sclerosis there is much lower than in North America or northern Europe.

The increasing risk of developing multiple sclerosis with increasing latitude has been confirmed by Kurtzke et al, who have studied a series of unprecedented size (5305 undoubted cases of multiple sclerosis and matched controls). Their study showed that in the United States, blacks are at lower risk than whites at all latitudes, but both races show the same south-to-north gradient in risk, indicating the importance of an environmental factor, regardless of race. An "epidemic" of multiple sclerosis has been described by Kurtzke and Hyllested in the Faroe Islands of the North Atlantic. They found a much higher than expected incidence of the disease, occurring as three separate outbreaks of decreasing extent between the years 1943 and 1973. It is their contention that the disease was introduced by British troops who occupied the islands in large numbers in the years immediately preceding the outbreak. Kurtzke and his colleagues have also described a similar postwar epidemic in Iceland.

Several studies indicate that persons who migrate from a high-risk to a low-risk zone carry with them at least part of the risk of their country of origin, even though the disease may not become apparent until 20 years after migration. Such a pattern has been demonstrated both in South Africa and in Israel. Dean determined that the prevalence in native-born white South Africans was 3 to 11 per 100,000, whereas the rate in immigrants from northern Europe was about 50 per 100,000, only slightly less than in the nonimmigrating natives of those countries. The data of Dean and Kurtzke indicate further that in persons who had immigrated before the age of 15 the risk was similar to that of native-born South Africans, whereas in persons who had immigrated after that age, the risk was similar to that of their birthplace. Alter et al found that in the descendants of European immigrants born in Israel the risk of multiple sclerosis was low, similar to that of other native-born Israelis, whereas among recent immigrants the

incidence in each national group approached the incidence in the land of birth. Again the critical age of immigration appeared to be about 15 years. These epidemiologic studies and others have shown that multiple sclerosis is associated with particular localities rather than with a particular ethnic group in those localities, and emphasize the importance of environmental factors in the genesis of the disease.

A familial tendency toward multiple sclerosis is now recognized. McAlpine et al have calculated that for a first-degree relative of a patient with multiple sclerosis the risk of developing the disease is from 5 to 15 times greater than for a member of the general population, and the risk is greater for siblings than for parents. A genetic factor became manifest also in a study of multiple sclerosis in twins (Ebers et al). The diagnosis was verified in both of 7 of 27 monozygotic twins (26 percent) and in only one pair of 43 dizygotic twins (2.3 percent). The concordance rate in dizygotic pairs is similar to that in nontwin siblings. Within families with more than one affected member, no consistent genetic pattern has emerged. There is a tendency to consider all diseases with an increased familial incidence as hereditary, but instances of the same condition in several members of a family may simply reflect an exposure to a common environmental agent. Paralytic poliomyelitis, for example, was about eight times more common in immediate family members than in the population at large.

Also suggestive of a genetic factor in the causation of multiple sclerosis is the finding that certain histocompatibility (HLA) antigens are more frequent in patients with multiple sclerosis than in control subjects. The strongest association is with the D or DR locus on the sixth chromosome. HLA antigens that are overrepresented in multiple sclerosis (HLA-DR2 and, to a lesser extent, -DR3, -B7, and -A3) are thought to be markers for a multiple sclerosis "susceptibility gene"—possibly an immune response gene. These antigens may prove to be related to the frequency, of the disease, but at the moment their exact role remains to be established (see reviews of Whitaker and McDonald).

The low conjugal incidence of multiple sclerosis supports the view that common exposure to this disease occurs early in life. In order to test this hypothesis, Schapira et al determined the periods of common exposure (common habitation periods) among members of families with two or more cases. From this they calculated the mean common exposure to have occurred before 14 years of age, with a latency of about 21 years—figures that are in general agreement with those derived from the migration studies quoted above.

The incidence of multiple sclerosis in children is

very low; only 0.3 to 0.4 percent of all cases occur during the first decade. In an analysis of three childhood-onset cases Hauser et al found no phenotypic differences between childhood and adult cases. Beyond childhood the risk of first developing symptoms of the disease rises steeply with age, reaching a peak at 30 to 35 years, then falling off sharply and becoming low in the sixth decade. It has been pointed out that multiple sclerosis has a unimodal age-specific onset curve, similar to the age-specific onset curves of many infectious diseases.

About two-thirds of cases of multiple sclerosis have their onset between 20 and 40 years of age. In a smaller number the disease appears to develop in late adult life (late fifties and sixties). In the latter patients, early symptoms may have been forgotten or never declared themselves clinically (we have found the typical lesions of multiple sclerosis in autopsied individuals who had no history of neurologic illness). Gilbert and Sadler report five such cases and from their pathologic findings declare that the true incidence of multiple sclerosis may be three times higher than stated figures. The incidence of multiple sclerosis is higher in women than in men (1.7:1), but the significance of this fact is unclear.

Studies in Norway and Sweden have suggested that the risk of developing multiple sclerosis is somewhat greater in farmers than in urban dwellers; studies of American Army personnel have suggested the opposite (Beebe et al). Several surveys in Great Britain have intimated that the disease is more frequent in the higher socioeconomic groups than in the lower ones. Relationships to numerous other environmental factors (surgical operations, anesthesia, exposure to household pets, the fillings in teeth) have been proposed but are unsupported by firm evidence.

All these epidemiologic data indicate that multiple sclerosis is related to some environmental factor, which is encountered in childhood, and, after years of latency, either evokes the disease or contributes to its causation. In recent years, speculation has grown that this factor is an infection, presumably viral. A large body of indirect evidence has been marshaled in support of this idea, based on the demonstration, in patients with multiple sclerosis, of alterations in humoral and cell-mediated immunity to viral agents [see reviews of R. T. Johnson (1975, 1978), Lampert, K. P. Johnson et al, and McFarlin and McFarland]. However, no virus (including any member of the human T-cell lymphotropic retroviruses) has ever been seen in or isolated from the tissues of patients with multiple sclerosis, despite innumerable attempts to do so, and no satisfactory viral model of multiple sclerosis has been produced experimentally.

If the initial insult to the nervous system is a viral or viral-like infection, then some secondary factor must be operative in later life to initiate the neurologic disease and to cause exacerbations. The most popular view is that this secondary mechanism is an autoimmune reaction, attacking myelin, and in its most intense form, destroying all tissue elements, including axis cylinders. An analogy has been drawn between the lesions of multiple sclerosis and those of disseminated encephalomyelitis, which is almost certainly an autoimmune disease of delayed hypersensitivity type (see further on). Elevated levels of antibodies to measles and to other viruses (herpes simplex, varicella-zoster, Epstein-Barr, vaccinia, rubella, and HTLV-1) have been found in the serum and CSF of patients with multiple sclerosis.

Antibodies to specific myelin basic protein (MBP) determinants have also been found in both serum and CSF, and increase with disease activity. MBP and measles virus antibodies cross-react. Multiple sclerosis sera, added to cultures of nervous system tissue, destroy myelin, inhibit myelination, and block axonal conduction. Antibodies to oligodendrocytes are present in the serum of 90 percent of patients with multiple sclerosis. The significance of the aforementioned findings is not entirely clear, but the best evidence suggests that the humoral immune system is overactive both systemically and within the CNS. Certainly multiple sclerosis occurs in patients who have never had an attack of measles and have no antibodies to this disease, and Poskanzer et al found that multiple sclerosis patients have no immunity to measles. Contrariwise, elevated levels of antibodies to measles and other viruses are found in a significant proportion of normal control subjects, and in a variety of diseases other than multiple sclerosis (lupus erythematosus, rheumatoid arthritis, chronic liver disease).

Considerable attention has been focused on the possible pathogenetic role of T lymphocytes, which regulate humoral immune responses either as potentiators (T-helper cells) or inhibitors (T-suppressor cells) of immunoglobulin production by the B lymphocytes. A reduction in the blood of suppressor T lymphocytes was originally thought to characterize clinical relapse but has proved to be an inconstant feature. However, a reduction in T cells, both helper and suppressor subsets, or an increase in helper-suppressor ratios, does appear to be associated with increasing disability in patients with multiple sclerosis. The precise role of the T cells remains to be established, but the findings to date support the idea that an autoimmune mechanism is operative in multiple sclerosis. Nevertheless, it is noteworthy that the prevalence of other disorders of presumed autoimmune origin is no higher in multiple sclerosis patients than in the general population.

Yet another way in which viral infections and autoimmune reactions in the nervous system might be linked has been suggested by R. T. Johnson. He found that several different viruses (rubeola, rubella, varicella) could cause autoimmunization of T lymphocytes against myelin basic protein. This means that the T lymphocyte recognizes an indentical structure in the virus and myelin sheath. Once the autoimmune process is initiated by a virus in childhood, it could later be reactivated by any of the common viral infections to which one is exposed, particularly in the higher northern and southern latitudes.

PRECIPITATING FACTORS

A variety of events occurring immediately before the initial symptoms or exacerbations of multiple sclerosis have been invoked as precipitating factors. The most common are infection, trauma, and pregnancy. However, in our experience none of these has been convincingly related to new attacks of multiple sclerosis, and there are no adequately controlled studies to support this idea. The incidence of influenza or other infections preceding the onset or exacerbations of the disease varies in different series from 5 to 50 percent. The possible role of physical injury in precipitating multiple sclerosis is difficult to assess. McAlpine and Compston found that the incidence of trauma within a 3-month period preceding the onset of multiple sclerosis was slightly greater than in a random control group of hospital patients. Furthermore, there appeared to be a relationship between the site of the injury (e.g., a limb or the jaw, following dental extraction) and the site of initial symptoms, particularly in patients who developed symptoms within a week of injury. We do not find this evidence convincing. Other forms of trauma (including lumbar puncture and general surgical procedures) that occur after the onset of the neurologic disorder have not been shown to have an adverse effect on the course of the illness. On the other hand, direct trauma to CNS tissue, as occurs during neurosurgery, may lead to new demyelinating lesions in the immediate area (Riechert et al). There is a definite increase of exacerbations during the pregnancy year (i.e., in the 9 months of pregnancy and particularly in the 3 months that follow), suggesting that a hormonal change may have a secondary effect on immune function.

CLINICAL MANIFESTATIONS

The conventional view of multiple sclerosis as a disease that strikes young people at a time when they are enjoying perfect health is not altogether correct. Often the history discloses that fatigue, lack of energy, weight loss, and vague muscle and joint pains had been present for several weeks or months before the onset of neurologic symptoms. Nor is it generally appreciated that the neurologic disorder frequently has an acute, almost apoplectic, onset. McAlpine et al (1972), who analyzed the mode of onset in 219 patients, found that in about 20 percent the neurologic

symptoms were fully developed in a matter of minutes, and, in a similar number, in a matter of hours. In about 30 percent the symptoms evolved more slowly, over a period of a day or several days, and in another 20 percent more slowly still, over several weeks to months. In the remaining 10 percent the symptoms had an insidious onset and slow, steady progression over months and years. The latter pattern is more likely to appear in patients over the age of 45 years.

Early Symptoms and Signs Weakness and/or numbness in one or more limbs are the initial symptoms in about one-half the patients. Symptoms of tingling of the extremities and tight band-like sensations around the trunk or limbs are commonly associated and are probably the result of involvement of the posterior columns of the spinal cord. The resulting clinical syndromes vary from mere dragging or poor control of one or both legs to a spastic or ataxic paraparesis, or both. The tendon reflexes later become hyperactive with extensor plantar reflexes, the abdominal reflexes disappear, and varying degrees of deep and superficial sensory loss may be associated. It is a useful adage that the patient with multiple sclerosis presents with symptoms in one leg and signs in both. The patient will complain of weakness, incoordination, or numbness and tingling in one lower extremity and prove to have bilateral Babinski signs and other evidence of bilateral corticospinal and posterior column disease. Passive flexion of the neck may induce a tingling, electric-like feeling down the back and, less commonly, down the anterior thighs. This phenomenon is known as a Lhermitte sign, although it is more a symptom than a sign and was originally described by Babinski in a case of cervical cord trauma. Lhermitte's contribution was to draw attention to this phenomenon as a frequent manifestation of multiple sclerosis.

In about 25 percent of all patients (and in a larger proportion of children) the initial manifestation is an episode of *retrobulbar or optic neuritis*. Characteristically, the syndrome is one of rapid evolution, over a period of several hours to days, of partial or total loss of vision in one eye. Rarely, the visual loss is steadily progressive for several months, mimicking a compressive lesion of the optic nerve (Ormerod and McDonald). Usually a scotoma involving the macular area can be demonstrated, but a wide variety of other field defects may occur, even hemianopic ones, sometimes homonymous (see page 202). In some patients, both optic nerves are involved, either simultaneously or within a few days to weeks of one another, and one in eight patients will have repeated attacks. In about half the patients, if serial examinations are made, some evidence of swelling of the optic nerve head (papillitis) will be observed.

The occurrence of papillitis depends upon the proximity of the demyelinating lesion to the nerve head. Subtle manifestations of optic nerve affection such as atrophy of retinal nerve fibers (page 199) and abnormalities of the visual evoked response (page 27) should always be sought in patients who have no visual symptoms but are suspected of having multiple sclerosis. It will be recalled that the optic nerve is in fact a tract of the brain, and involvement of the optic nerves is therefore consistent with the rule that lesions of multiple sclerosis occur only in the central nervous system.

About one-third of patients with optic neuritis recover completely, and most of the remaining patients improve significantly, even if they show pallor of the optic disc. When improvement occurs, it begins usually within 2 weeks of onset, as is true of most acute manifestations of multiple sclerosis. Once improvement in neurologic function begins, it may continue for several months.

Approximately one-half of the patients who present with optic neuritis alone will eventually develop other signs of multiple sclerosis. The risk is much lower if the initial attack of optic neuritis occurs in childhood (suggesting that the childhood disease is of a different type) and somewhat higher—up to 60 percent of cases—if the attack occurs in adult life (Nikoskelainen and Riekkinen, Landy). The longer the period of observation and the greater the care given to detection of mild cases, the greater will be the proportion of patients who develop other signs of multiple sclerosis; however, most do so within 5 years of the original attack (Ebers; Hely et al). In fact, in many patients with clinically isolated optic neuritis, MRI has disclosed lesions of the cerebral white matter—suggesting that dissemination, albeit asymptomatic, had already occurred (Jacobs et al, Ormerod et al).

It is unclear whether optic neuritis that occurs alone and is not followed by other evidence of demyelinating disease is simply an isolated form of multiple sclerosis or a manifestation of some other disease process, such as postinfectious encephalomyelitis. No pathologic basis for optic neuritis other than demyelinative disease has so far been established, though it is known that a vascular lesion or compression of an optic nerve by a tumor or mucocele will sometimes cause a central scotoma.

Other initial manifestations of multiple sclerosis, in descending order of frequency, are unsteadiness in walking, brainstem symptoms (diplopia, vertigo, vomiting), and disorders of micturition. Onset with discrete manifestations, such as hemiplegia, trigeminal neuralgia or other pain syndromes, facial paralysis, deafness, or seizures occurs in a small proportion of cases. More often than not the disease presents with more than one of the aforementioned symptoms.

Not infrequently the disease begins with nystagmus and ataxia, with or without weakness and spasticity of the limbs, a syndrome that reflects involvement of the cerebellar and corticospinal tracts and their connections. Ataxia of cerebellar type can be recognized by scanning speech, rhythmic instability of the head and trunk, intention tremor of the arms and legs, and incoordination of voluntary movements and gait, as described in Chap. 4. The combination of nystagmus, scanning speech, and intention tremor is known as *Charcot's triad,* and while this group of symptoms is often seen in the advanced stages of the disease, most neurologists would agree that it is a rare mode of presentation. The most severe forms of cerebellar ataxia, in which the slightest attempt to move the trunk or limbs precipitates a violent and uncontrollable ataxic tremor, are observed among patients with multiple sclerosis. The responsible lesion probably lies in the tegmentum of the midbrain and involves the dentatorubrothalamic tracts. and adjacent structures. Cerebellar ataxia may be combined with sensory ataxia, due to involvement of the posterior columns of the spinal cord or medial lemnisci of the brainstem. In many cases of this type the signs of spinal cord involvement ultimately become predominant; in others, the cerebellar signs predominate.

Diplopia is another common presenting complaint. It is due most often to involvement of the medial longitudinal fasciculus, producing an internuclear ophthalmoplegia (see page 216). The latter is characterized by paresis of the medial rectus on attempted lateral gaze, with a coarse nystagmus in the abducting eye; in multiple sclerosis, this abnormality is usually bilateral. As a corollary, the presence of bilateral internuclear ophthalmoplegia in a young adult is virtually diagnostic of multiple sclerosis. Other palsies of gaze, due to interruption of supranuclear connections, or palsies of individual ocular muscles, due to involvement of the third or sixth cranial nerves in their intramedullary course, also occur—but less frequently. Other manifestations of brainstem involvement include myokymia or paralysis of facial muscles, deafness, tinnitus, unformed auditory hallucinations (because of involvement of cochlear connections), and vertigo and vomiting (vestibular connections). The occurrence of transient facial anesthesia or of trigeminal neuralgia in a young adult should always suggest the diagnosis of multiple sclerosis, with involvement of the intramedullary fibers of the fifth cranial nerve. In the most severe forms of the disease, all or some of the aforementioned brainstem symptoms may be combined with quadriplegia, pseudobulbar palsy, and cerebellar ataxia.

Symptoms of bladder dysfunction—including hesitancy, urgency, frequency, and incontinence—occur commonly with spinal cord involvement. Urinary retention, due to affection of sacral segments is less frequent (Fig. 26-6). In males, these symptoms are often associated with impotence, a symptom that the patient may not report unless specifically questioned in this regard.

Traditional teaching has overemphasized the frequency of *euphoria,* a pathologic cheerfulness or elation that seems inappropriate in the face of the obvious neurologic deficit. (Charcot spoke of this phenomenon as "stupid indifference" and Vulpian as "morbid optimism.") Some patients do show this mental abnormality, the result probably of lesions of the white matter of the frontal lobes, always in association with other signs of cerebral impairment. In some instances it is manifestly a part of the syndrome of pseudobulbar palsy. A much larger number of patients, however, are *depressed,* irritable, and short-tempered as a reaction to the disabling features of the disease. Dalos et al, in comparing multiple sclerotic patients with a group of traumatic paraplegics, found a significantly higher incidence of *emotional disturbance* in the former group, especially during periods of relapse. Other mental disturbances, such as a loss of retentive memory, a global *dementia,* or a confusional-psychotic state, also occur with some regularity. About 2 to 3 percent of patients with multiple sclerosis, at some time during the course of their disease, will have a seizure or recurrent *seizures,* presumably as the result of lesions in the cerebral cortex or subjacent white matter.

Dull, aching pain in the low back is a common complaint, but its relation to the lesions of multiple sclerosis is uncertain. Sharp, burning, poorly localized pains in a limb or both legs and girdle pains—presumably caused by demyelinative foci involving the root entry zones—occur but are infrequent. These symptoms may precede the onset of sensory signs or appear at any time in established cases of the disease.

Abrupt attacks of neurologic deficit, lasting a few seconds or minutes and sometimes recurring many times daily, are an infrequent but well-recognized feature of multiple sclerosis. Usually the attacks occur in the course of the illness, rarely as an initial manifestation. The clinical manifestations are referable to any part of the central nervous system but most often consist of dysarthria and ataxia; paroxysmal pain and dysesthesia in a limb; flashing lights; or tonic flexion (dystonia) of the hand, wrist, and elbow with extension of the lower limb. Unusually severe and often transient fatigue is another peculiar symptom of multiple sclerosis. It often appears without warning and is more likely to occur when there is fever or other evidence of disease activity. The cause of these transitory phenomena is uncertain. They have been attributed by Halliday and McDonald to ephaptic ("cross-talk") transmission between adjacent demyelinated axons within a lesion. Carbamazepine is usually effective in controlling the attacks.

These transitory symptoms, sometimes clearly related to fever, high ambient temperature, changes in serum Ca and other electrolytes, and possibly emotional upsets, make it difficult to determine whether or not the symptoms of a given attack in the multiple sclerotic patient represent a new lesion. Years ago, Thygessen pointed out, in an analysis of 105 exacerbations in 60 patients, that there were new symptoms in only 19 percent; in the remainder there was only a recurrence of old symptoms. Another problem is that the original lesion may have been asymptomatic. For example, many of the patients found to have impaired visual evoked responses have never had symptomatic visual changes and body temperature is raised and slows nerve conduction. Symptoms and signs may indicate progression of a given lesion but without the appearance of new plaques (Prineas and Connell). All these factors should be taken into consideration in evaluating the clinical course of the illness and the effects of a therapeutic program (Poser).

Symptoms and Signs in the Established Stage of the Disease When the diagnosis of multiple sclerosis has become virtually certain, a number of clinical syndromes are observed to occur with regularity. Approximately one-half of the patients will manifest a clinical picture of *mixed* or *generalized type* with signs pointing to involvement of the optic nerves, brainstem, cerebellum, and spinal cord. Another 30 to 40 percent will exhibit varying degrees of spastic ataxia and deep sensory changes in the extremities, i.e., essentially a *spinal form of the disease.* A predominantly *cerebellar* or *pontobulbar-cerebellar form* will be noted in only about 5 percent of cases and an *amaurotic form* in a like number. Thus the mixed cerebrospinal and spinal forms together have comprised at least 80 percent of our clinical material.

A number of interesting *variants of multiple sclerosis* have come to our attention over the years and have given rise to difficulties in diagnosis. Several times we have been consulted by a young patient with typical tic douloureux; only their young age, and bilaterality of the pain in some of them, raised the suspicion of multiple sclerosis, confirmed later by sensory loss in the face and other neurologic signs. Brachial, thoracic, or lumbosacral pain consisting mainly of thermal and algesic dysesthesias were sources of puzzlement in several other patients until additional lesions developed. In several patients the abrupt occurrence of a right hemiplegia and aphasia first raised the probability of a cerebrovascular lesion, only to be followed by spinal cord lesions. In still others, a slowly evolving hemiplegia had led to the diagnosis of a cerebral glioma.

Several times we have seen coma during relapse, and in each instance it continued to death. In one case it occurred in a 64-year-old woman who had had two previous episodes of nondisabling spinal multiple sclerosis at 30 and 44 years of age. A confusional psychosis with drowsiness was the reported initial syndrome in another patient whom we later saw with a relapse involving cerebellum and spinal cord. Another unusual syndrome is one of slow intellectual decline with slight cerebellar ataxia. A 10-year, slowly progressive cerebellar ataxia in an adolescent girl who later developed internuclear ophthalmoplegia was another perplexing variant. A rapid onset of ascending paralysis of bladder and bowel, legs, and trunk with severe pain in sacral parts, areflexia, and 1600 mononuclear cells per cubic millimeter of CSF occurred in another of our patients and lasted 2 years before she began to walk; earlier she had had diplopia and retrobulbar neuritis. Repeatedly, seemingly more in recent years, we have observed patients whose illness satisfied all the clinical criteria for the diagnosis of multiple sclerosis, except for the onset of symptoms in the sixth or seventh decade. Presumably we were witnessing the late deteriorative phase of the illness, and the earlier symptoms had been forgotten or were never recognized (see above under ''Etiology'').

Several other variants of multiple sclerosis merit more extended discussion. They are acute multiple sclerosis, neuromyelitis optica, acquired Schilder disease, and the conjunction of multiple sclerosis and polyneuropathy.

Acute Multiple Sclerosis Rarely, multiple sclerosis takes a highly malignant form. A combination of cerebral, brainstem, and spinal manifestations evolve over a few weeks, rendering the patient stuporous or comatose, or decerebrate with prominent cranial nerve and corticospinal abnormalities. Death may end the illness within a few weeks to months without any remission having occurred. At autopsy the lesions (unlike those of acute disseminated encephalomyelitis) are of macroscopic dimensions, typical of the acute plaques of multiple sclerosis. The only difference from the usual form of multiple sclerosis is that many plaques are of the same age and the confluence of many perivenous zones of demyelination is more obvious. Two of our most striking examples of this rapidly fatal form were in a 6-year-old girl and a 16-year-old boy, both of whom died within 5 weeks of the onset of symptoms. Another was a 30-year-old man who lived 2 months. In none of them had there been a preceding exanthem or inoculation or any symptoms suggestive of demyelinative disease.

Nonfatal clinical cases of similar type in children, adolescents, and young adults are admitted to our hospitals once or twice a year. Some have responded to ACTH, and others worsened while receiving this medication. Some have made an astonishing recovery after several months, and a few have then remained well for 25 to 30 years. Others have relapsed and the subsequent clinical course was typical of multiple sclerosis.

It seems to the authors that more than one disease is being included in the clinical category of acute multiple sclerosis. One type conforms in its temporal profile to a rather protracted form of acute disseminated encephalomyelitis—an acute monophasic illness extending over 4 to 8 weeks akin to some of the Japanese postrabies-inoculation cases (Shiraki and Otani). Others subsequently prove to be typical polyphasic multiple sclerosis. Only the clinical course presently separates the two types.

Neuromyelitis Optica The simultaneous or successive involvement of optic nerves and spinal cord has been convincingly documented. The combination was remarked upon by Clifford Albutt in 1870, and Gault (1894), stimulated by his teacher Devic, devoted his thesis to the subject. Devic endeavored to crystallize medical thought about a condition that has come to be known as *neuromyelitis optica*. Its principal features are the acute to subacute onset of blindness in one or both eyes preceded or followed within days or weeks by a transverse or ascending myelitis (Beck). As stated on page 730, the lesions in the spinal cord and sometimes the optic nerves are usually of necrotizing rather than demyelinative type, leading eventually to cavitation; and, as would be expected, the clinical effects are more likely to be permanent than those of demyelination. Many of the patients have been children, and in a number of instances they suffered only a single episode of neurologic illness.

While it is true that cases corresponding to this prototype are seen on occasion in every large medical center, and at all age periods, the isolation of such an entity on clinical grounds alone has been unsatisfactory. Most of our patients have proved by subsequent clinical developments, and in a few instances by autopsy, to have chronic relapsing multiple sclerosis. In one notable example, where hemiplegia and aphasia were followed within 2 weeks by a necrotizing myelitis from which there was no recovery, the patient then developed typical attacks of multiple sclerosis, including retrobulbar neuritis. At autopsy more than 15.0 cm of the spinal cord had been destroyed, reducing it to a collapsed membranous tube. Elsewhere the lesions were typically demyelinative. Also, acute disseminated encephalomyelitis may occasionally present as a neuromyelitis optica.

One must conclude that *neuromyelitis optica* is

usually a form of multiple sclerosis, but other types of demyelinative disease, namely acute disseminated encephalomyelitis, acute multiple sclerosis, and acute necrotizing hemorrhagic leukoencephalitis and leukomyelitis may on occasion present this clinical syndrome.

Acquired Schilder Disease Exceptionally the cerebrum is the site of massive demyelination, occurring in multiple foci or as a single large focus. Such cases are more frequent in childhood and adolescence than in adult life. As with the case reported by Ellison and Barron, the disease may follow the course of multiple sclerosis. This topic is discussed in the next section of this chapter.

Multiple Sclerosis in Conjunction with Peripheral Neuropathy From time to time we observe patients with multiple sclerosis, who also have an unmistakable polyneuropathy or mononeuropathy multiplex. This relationship always invites speculation and controversy. The rarity of the combination suggests a coincidental occurrence of multiple sclerosis and a neuropathy, but often no ready explanation for the latter disorder, in terms of a well-recognized form of neuropathy, is forthcoming. One view is that an autoimmune demyelination has been incited in both peripheral nerve and spinal cord. Of course, radicular and neuropathic symptoms, motor and/or sensory, can result from the involvement of myelinated fibers in the root entry zone of the cord, or of fibers of exit, in the ventral white matter. In the late stages of multiple sclerosis there is always the possibility of vitamin-deficiency polyneuropathy or multiple pressure palsies.

Cerebrospinal Fluid In about one-third of all patients, particularly those with an acute onset or exacerbation, there may be a slight to moderate mononuclear pleocytosis (usually less than 50 cells per cubic millimeter). In rapidly progressive cases of neuromyelitis optica (see above) and in certain instances of severe demyelinative disease of the brainstem, the total cell count may reach or exceed 100 and rarely 1000 cells per cubic millimeter, and with the high cell counts the greater proportion may be polymorphonuclear leukocytes. This pleocytosis is in fact the only measure of activity of the disease. Other laboratory tests (except for myelin basic protein, see below) do not reflect the activity of the disease.

Also, in about 40 percent of patients, the total protein content of the CSF is increased. The increase is slight, however, and a level of more than 100 mg/dL is so unusual that the possibility of another diagnosis should be entertained. More importantly, the proportion of gamma globulin (essentially IgG) is increased (above 10 to 13 percent of the total protein) in about two-thirds of patients. An even more sensitive diagnostic measure is the *IgG index*, which

is obtained by measuring albumin and gamma globulin in both the serum and CSF and using the formula:

$$\frac{\text{CSF IgG/serum IgG}}{\text{CSF alb/serum alb}}$$

A ratio of more than 1.7 indicates the probability of multiple sclerosis. It has been shown that the gamma globulins in the CSF of patients with multiple sclerosis are synthesized in the CNS (Tourtellotte) and that they migrate in agarose electrophoresis as abnormal discrete populations, so-called oligoclonal (IgG) bands. A simple method for demonstrating these bands has been described, using readily available commercial reagents and apparatus (Johnson et al, 1977). The IgG index and the test for oligoclonal IgG bands are readily available clinical laboratory tests and together will show CSF abnormalities in over 90 percent of cases of multiple sclerosis. Such bands also appear in the CSF of patients with syphilis and subacute sclerosing panencephalitis—disorders that should not be difficult to distinguish from multiple sclerosis on clinical grounds. The demonstration of oligoclonal bands in the CSF and not in the blood can be particularly helpful in the diagnosis of early or atypical multiple sclerosis. The presence of such bands in a first attack of multiple sclerosis is predictive of chronic relapsing multiple sclerosis, according to Moulin et al and others.

It has been shown also, by the use of a sensitive radioimmunoassay, that the CSF contains high levels of myelin basic protein during acute exacerbations of multiple sclerosis, and that these levels are lower in slowly progressive multiple sclerosis and normal during remissions of the disease (Cohen et al). Thus the assay is a useful measure of activity of multiple sclerosis; unfortunately, the method is not simple and is being carried out in only a few laboratories.

When cells, total protein, gamma globulin, and oligoclonal bands are all taken into account, some abnormality will be found in almost every patient with multiple sclerosis. At present the measurement of gamma globulins and oligoclonal bands in the CSF are the only reliable chemical tests of multiple sclerosis.

Other Laboratory Tests When the clinical data point to only one lesion in the CNS, as often happens in the early stages of the disease or in the late spinal form, a number of delicate physiologic tests may establish the existence of other asymptomatic lesions. These tests include visual, auditory, and tactile evoked responses, perceptual delay on visual stimulation, electro-oculography to show a lag in contraction of an ocular muscle, altered blink reflexes, and a change in flicker fusion of visual images. Halliday and McDonald report abnormalities in one or more of these tests in 50 to 90 percent of a series of multiple sclerosis patients. At the Massachusetts General Hospital, abnormal visual evoked responses were found in 80 percent of patients with definite multiple sclerosis and 60 percent of patients with probable or possible multiple sclerosis. The corresponding figures for brainstem auditory evoked responses (usually decreased amplitude of wave 5) were 47 percent and 20 percent, and for somatosensory evoked responses, 69 percent and 51 percent, respectively.

CT scans are also useful in demonstrating cerebral lesions during the early stages of evolution. Doubling the dose of contrast material and delaying the scan for an hour postinfusion has been shown to increase the yield of lesions during exacerbations of multiple sclerosis (Sears et al). It is now widely appreciated that MRI is much more reliable than CT scanning in revealing asymptomatic plaques of multiple sclerosis in the cerebrum, brainstem, optic nerves, and spinal cord (Fig. 37-1). Our experience accords with that of Stewart et al, who found multifocal lesions in 80 percent of their cases. In a series of 114 patients with clinically definite multiple sclerosis, Ormerod and his colleagues found periventricular MR abnormalities in all but 2 patients and discrete cerebral white matter lesions in all but 12. The periventricular lesions are characteristically irregular in outline. It should be stressed that periventricular hyperintensity is observed with a variety of pathologic processes and even in normal persons, particularly older ones. In these latter cases, the periventricular changes are usually milder in degree and smoother in outline than the lesions of multiple sclerosis. The discrete cerebral lesions of multiple sclerosis do not impart a specific MR appearance. As with other laboratory procedures, MR changes assume diagnostic significance only if they are consistent with the clinical findings (Paty et al).

PATHOPHYSIOLOGY

The observations of delayed optic nerve conduction of patterned visual stimuli in patients with normal visual acuity and normal fields have reopened the matter of the pathophysiology of demyelination. When the latter process is acute and reversible within a few days, there is obviously a functional block in nerve fiber conduction. In such a brief period recovery could not be due to remyelination. More likely, recovery is due to subsidence of the edema and acute inflammatory changes in and around the lesion.

Remyelination probably does occur, but it is a slower process and partial at best, and its functional effects in the CNS are unknown. A slowing of optic nerve conduction, if it is present in an eye with normal vision, may account for the reduction in flicker fusion and in perception of multiple visual stimuli (Halliday and McDonald).

CLINICAL COURSE AND PROGNOSIS

The intermittency of the clinical manifestations—the disease advancing in a series of attacks each permitting less and less remission—is perhaps the most important clinical attribute of the disease. Some patients will have a complete clinical remission after the initial attack, or rarely there may be a series of exacerbations, each with complete remission; such exacerbations may be severe enough to have caused quadriplegia and pseudobulbar palsy. The relapse rate is 0.3 to 0.4 attacks per year according to the calculations of McAlpine and Compston, and the interval

Figure 37-1

MRI in multiple sclerosis. First echo of a T2-weighted spin-echo sequence, showing multiple areas of increased intensity in a periventricular distribution. The patient was a 47-year-old woman who complained of vertigo and tinnitus and showed only minimal neurologic signs.

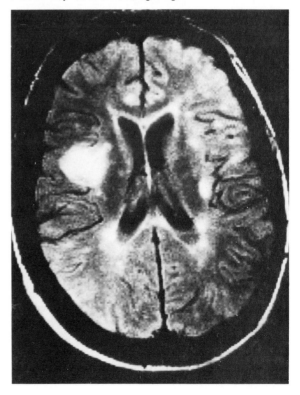

between the opening symptom and the first relapse is highly variable. It was within 1 year in 30 percent of McAlpine's cases and within 2 years in another 20 percent. A further 20 percent relapsed in 5 to 9 years and another 10 percent in 10 to 30 years. Not only is the length of this latent interval remarkable, but also the fact that the pathologic process can remain potentially active for such a long time.

After a number of years there is an increasing tendency for the patient to enter a phase of slow, steady or fluctuating deterioration of neurologic function, attributable to the cumulative effect of increasing numbers of lesions, but in about 10 percent of cases the course of the disease is unevenly progressive from the beginning. In these latter cases the disease usually takes the form of a spastic paraparesis and probably represents the most frequent type of obscure myelopathy observed by the authors, as pointed out on page 737 and below. Examination of the CSF and the use of the other laboratory tests, described above, are essential in such cases.

Few if any factors are known to affect the course of the disease. Contrary to commonly held opinion, pregnancy does not have an adverse effect on multiple sclerosis. In fact, pregnancy may be associated with clinical stability or improvement. However, as noted above, there appears to be an increased risk of exacerbations in the first few months postpartum (Birk and Rudick).

The duration of the disease is exceedingly variable. A small number of patients die within several months or years of the onset, but the average duration is in excess of 30 years. A 60-year appraisal of the resident population of Rochester, Minnesota, disclosed that 74 percent of patients with multiple sclerosis survived 25 years as compared to 86 percent of the general population. At the end of 25 years, one-third of the surviving patients were still working and two-thirds were still ambulatory (Percy et al). Other statistical analyses give a worse prognosis. Patients with mild and quiescent forms of the disease are, of course, less likely to come to the attention of physicians working with chronically ill patients.

DIAGNOSIS

In the usual forms of multiple sclerosis, i.e., in those with a relapsing and remitting course and evidence of disseminated lesions in the CNS, the diagnosis of multiple sclerosis is rarely in doubt. Only meningovascular syphilis, certain rare forms of cerebral arteritis, vascular malformations of the brainstem or spinal cord with multiple bleeds, lupus erythematosus and Behçet disease, could possibly simulate relapsing multiple sclerosis, and each of these has its own characteristic diagnostic features. Difficulties are most likely to arise when the standard clinical criteria for the diagnosis of multiple sclerosis are lacking, as occurs in

the acute initial attack of the disease and in cases with an insidious onset and slow, steady progression.

As has been stated, *the initial attack of multiple sclerosis* may mimic acute labyrinthine vertigo or tic douloureux. Careful neurologic examination of such patients usually discloses the signs of a brainstem lesion; the CSF examination may be particularly helpful in these circumstances. Extensive brainstem demyelination of subacute evolution, involving tracts and cranial nerves sequentially, may be mistaken for a pontine glioma. CT scanning, MRI, and the course of the illness settle the matter; symptoms of brainstem multiple sclerosis remit as a rule, and to a surprisingly complete degree in many cases. During epidemics of poliomyelitis, the acute onset of multiple sclerosis with limb weakness and pleocytosis was sometimes mistaken for paralytic poliomyelitis, but this is no longer a practical consideration.

Disseminated encephalomyelitis (see further on) is an acute illness with widely scattered lesions, but is self-limited and monophasic; furthermore, fever, stupor, and coma, which are characteristic, rarely occur in multiple sclerosis.

In lupus erythematosus the central nervous system may be affected before other organs; and multiple small vascular lesions may give rise to a chronic relapsing-remitting clinical picture simulating multiple sclerosis. We have encountered cases of this type, and Allen et al have reported examples. Usually a careful search for other manifestations of lupus will clarify the problem. The distinguishing features of Behçet disease are recurrent iridocyclitis and meningitis, mucous membrane ulcers of the mouth and genitalia, and symptoms of articular, renal, lung, and multifocal cerebral disease.

The *purely spinal form of multiple sclerosis,* presenting as a progressive spastic paraparesis with varying degrees of posterior column involvement, is a special source of diagnostic difficulty. Such patients require careful evaluation for the presence of spinal cord compression due to neoplasm or cervical spondylosis. Radicular pain at some point in the illness is a frequent manifestation of the latter disorders and is rare in multiple sclerosis. Pain in the neck, immobility of the cervical spine, and severe muscle wasting due to spinal root involvement, as is sometimes seen in spondylosis, are almost unknown in multiple sclerosis. As a general rule, loss of abdominal reflexes, impotence in males, and disturbances of bladder function occur early in the course of demyelinative myelopathy, but late or not at all in cervical spondylosis. The CSF protein in the latter condition is apt to be significantly elevated, but abnormalities of gamma globulin are absent, in distinction to multiple sclerosis. Slowed or altered visual, auditory, and somatic sensory evoked potentials may be demonstrated in many patients with multiple sclerosis, even those without deafness, optic atrophy, or a history of optic neuritis, and provide proof of dissemination of lesions. The highest court of appeal is MRI and myelography, and every patient with progressive spastic paraparesis in whom the neurologic signs are limited to the spinal cord should be investigated by these.

Amyotrophic lateral sclerosis (ALS) and subacute combined degeneration (SCD) of the cord should not be confused with multiple sclerosis. ALS can be identified by the presence of muscle wasting, fasciculations, and the total absence of sensory involvement. SCD is characterized by symmetric involvement of the posterior and then lateral columns of the spinal cord, low serum level of vitamin B_{12}, gastric achlorhydria, megaloblastic marrow and macrocytic anemia in many cases, and defective absorption of vitamin B_{12}, as determined by the Schilling test (page 835).

The presence of *nystagmus*, disorders of ocular movement, such as a mild dysmetria or internuclear ophthalmoplegia, and increased latencies of visual evoked potentials should always be sought in patients with progressive spastic paraparesis, since such an association might establish the diagnosis of multiple sclerosis. One or more such abnormalities are so common in multiple sclerosis that their absence should always suggest the possibility of an alternative diagnosis. It is important to remember that barbiturate and phenytoin toxicity may cause nystagmus and ataxia.

Platybasia and basilar impression of the skull should also be considered in the differential diagnosis, but patients with these conditions have a characteristic shortening of the neck, and careful radiographs of the base of the skull will be diagnostic. Neurologic syndromes resulting from the Arnold-Chiari malformation (without meningomyelocele) and from tumors of the cerebellopontine angle and other parts of the posterior fossa and foramen magnum have been misdiagnosed as multiple sclerosis. In each of these instances, a solitary, strategically placed lesion may give rise to a variety of neurologic symptoms and signs referable to the brainstem, cerebellum, lower cranial nerves, and upper cervical cord, and may give the impression of dissemination of lesions. It is an excellent clinical rule that a diagnosis of multiple sclerosis should not be made when all the patient's symptoms and signs can be explained by a lesion in one region of the neuraxis.

Confusion may occasionally arise with the hereditary ataxias, which are generally distinguished by their familial incidence and other associated genetic traits; by their insidious onset and slow, steady progression; and by their symmetry and stereotyped clinical pattern. Intactness of abdominal reflexes and sphincteric function, and the presence of pes cavus, kyphoscoliosis, and cardiac disease are other features that favor the diagnosis of a heredodegenerative disorder (see Chap. 43).

Careful clinical appraisal will usually lead to accurate diagnosis, but the label of "multiple sclerosis" should not be attached to a patient until the evidence is unequivocal. Once such a label is applied, it tends to stick; and since the diagnosis of multiple sclerosis will explain almost any subsequent neurologic event, attention may be directed away from consideration of another, perhaps treatable, disease.

It is important to establish the diagnosis of multiple sclerosis with certainty and as soon as possible. Most of the patients are young and are confronted with a large number of decisions (education, marriage, children) that would obviously be influenced by a diagnosis of a chronic and possibly disabling disease.

TREATMENT

As one might expect, numerous forms of treatment have been proposed, and many have been thought to be successful because of the remitting nature of the disease. Only ACTH and prednisone have proved to have a beneficial effect on the disease, on the basis of controlled clinical trials. Under the influence of these agents, recovery from acute relapses appears to be hastened, particularly from an attack of optic neuritis. However, a substantial group of patients with acute exacerbations fails to respond to this type of treatment, and in others, benefit is not apparent for a month or longer after the course of ACTH is completed. Also, there is no evidence that ACTH or steroids have a significant effect upon the ultimate degree of improvement, or that they prevent the recurrence of the disease, so there is no justification for treatment over a period of many months or years.

A variety of dosage schedules have been employed. It seems important that a high dose be used initially to be effective. We give ACTH intravenously in a dose of 80 units in 500 mL dextrose and water for 3 days, followed by 40 units of gel intramuscularly every 12 h for 7 days. The dose is then reduced by 10 units every 3 days. Many patients who show improvement on this therapy continue to improve or maintain their previous improvement even though the medication is gradually reduced and discontinued. Other patients have a recurrence of symptoms as the dose is reduced and need to be maintained on small doses of ACTH (20 to 40 units) every other day for a period of several months. Because of the risk of potassium depletion, the patients are given potassium supplements in a daily dose of 60 meq/L. Confusion, euphoria, or depression may be severe enough to require termination of medication, and lithium or a sedative drug may be necessary because of nervousness and insomnia. The occurrence of peripheral edema due to sodium retention can be treated with mild diuretics and salt restriction. Gastrointestinal bleeding and the activation of tuberculosis and diabetes should always be considered as possible complications of treatment. Hirsutism and acne cannot be prevented but disappear when the medication is stopped.

The intravenous administration of methylprednisolone (500 mg daily for 3 to 5 days) is probably as effective as ACTH. When it is impractical to administer parenteral ACTH or methylprednisolone, comparable amounts of oral prednisone may be substituted. The reports concerning the effectiveness of intrathecal prednisolone are conflicting, and this form of treatment is not recommended.

A number of experimental agents that modify immune reactivity have been tried, with limited success. Drugs such as azathiaprine and cyclophosphamide and total lymphoid irradiation have been given to small groups of patients and seem to have improved the clinical course of some of them (Aimard et al, Hauser et al, Cook et al). The positive clinical effects of these measures lend support to the concept that an autoimmune process is responsible for the CNS lesions of multiple sclerosis. However, the risks of prolonged use of immunosuppressive drugs, including a risk of neoplastic change, will probably preclude their widespread use. Moreover, the most careful study to date, by the British and Dutch Multiple Sclerosis Azathiaprine Trial Group, attributed no significant advantage to treatment with this drug [*Neurology* 38 (suppl 2), 1988].

There are no valid control studies to substantiate the claims that have been made for the value of low-fat diets, gluten-free diets, or linoleate supplementation of the diet. The therapeutic value of plasmapheresis, synthetic polypeptides, and hyperbaric oxygen has not been established. Initial clinical trials using systemically administered natural α-interferon (Panitch) and intrathecally injected human fibroblast (β)-interferon (Jacobs et al) indicate that both these agents may decrease the exacerbation rate of multiple sclerosis; on the other hand, the administration of gamma interferon may actually exacerbate the disease (Panitch et al). Many other immunotherapeutic agents are currently being tested, the rationale for which has been reviewed in detail by Weiner and Hafler. The most recent of these is a polymer of myelin basic protein, called copolymer I or Cop I, which has been reported by Bornstein and his colleagues to have a beneficial effect in the exacerbating and remitting form of MS. These authors were careful to point out, however, that the initial salutary results need to be confirmed by more extensive clinical trials.

General measures include the provision of an adequate period of bed rest and convalescence to ensure maximum recovery from the initial attack or exacerbation, prevention of excessive fatigue and infection, the use of all possible rehabilitative measures to postpone the bedridden stage of the disease (braces, chairs, ramps, lifts, cars with manual controls, etc.), and meticulous attention to the prevention of bedsores in the bedridden patient by the use of alternating pressure mattresses, silicone gel pads, and other special devices.

Disorders of bladder function may raise serious problems in management. Where the major disorder is one of urinary retention, bethanacol chloride may be helpful. In patients with a spastic bladder, the use of propantheline (Pro-Banthine) or oxybutine (Ditropan) may serve to relax the detrusor muscle (Chap. 26). Some patients with severe bladder dysfunction, particularly those with urinary retention, benefit from intermittent catheterization, which lessens the constant risk of infection from an indwelling catheter. Antibiotics and acidifying drugs to suppress urinary tract infections should also be employed. Severe constipation is best managed with properly spaced enemas. Often a program of bowel training can be successfully undertaken.

In patients with severe spastic paralysis and painful flexor spasms of the legs, the self-administered, intrathecal injection of baclofen, as in other spastic states, is sometimes of value. Failing this measure, crushing of the obturator nerves may give relief for a prolonged period. Some patients with lesser degrees of spasticity have benefitted from the oral administration of baclofen.

The very severe and disabling tremor that is brought out by the slightest movement of the limbs can, if unilateral, be managed surgically, by ventrolateral thalamic ablation. Recently Hallett and his colleagues have reported that severe postural tremor of this type can be improved by treatment with isoniazid (300 mg daily, increased by increments of 300 mg weekly to a dose of 1200 mg daily) in combination with 100 mg pyridoxine daily. How isoniazid produces its beneficial effects is not known.

The importance of an understanding and sympathetic physician in the care of patients with a chronic incapacitating neurologic disease of this kind cannot be overemphasized. From the beginning, when the patients first inquire about the nature of their disease, they require advice about their daily routine, marriage, pregnancy, the use of drugs, inoculations, etc. The term *multiple sclerosis* should not be introduced unless the diagnosis is certain, and then it should be qualified by a balanced explanation of the symptoms, stressing always the optimistic aspects of the disease. Most patients desire an honest appraisal of their condition and prognosis. Some patients consider the uncertainty of their prognosis worse than the actual disability.

DIFFUSE CEREBRAL SCLEROSIS OF SCHILDER (Schilder Disease, Encephalitis Periaxalis Diffusa)

The term *diffuse sclerosis* was probably first used by Strumpell (1879) to describe the hard texture of the freshly removed brain of an alcoholic; later the term was applied to widespread cerebral gliosis of whatever cause. In 1912, Schilder described an instance of what he considered to be "diffuse sclerosis." This was the case of a 14-year-old girl with progressive mental deterioration and signs of increased intracranial pressure, terminating fatally after 19 weeks. Postmortem examination disclosed the presence of large, well-demarcated areas of demyelination in the white matter of both cerebral hemispheres, as well as a number of smaller demyelinative foci, resembling the common lesions of multiple sclerosis. Because of the similarities of the pathologic changes to those of multiple sclerosis (prominence of the inflammatory reaction and relative sparing of axis cylinders) Schilder called this disease *encephalitis periaxalis diffusa,* bringing it in line with *encephalitis periaxalis scleroticans,* a term that Marburg had used to describe a case of acute multiple sclerosis. Unfortunately, in subsequent publications, Schilder used the same term for two other conditions of different type. One appears to have been a familial leukodystrophy (adrenoleukodystrophy) in a boy, and the other, quite unlike the first two cases, was suggestive of an infiltrative lymphoma. These later reports by Schilder seriously confused the subject for many years. The terms *Schilder's disease* and *diffuse sclerosis* were used to describe these and many different conditions. Some resembled Schilder's original descriptions; others differed with respect to familial occurrence and widespread symmetric destruction and gliosis of the white matter, often with metachromatic or globoid bodies representing catabolic products of myelin; and still others (e.g., subacute encephalitides, vascular encephalopathies) seemed to have no connection with either of these categories.

One group of diseases of the cerebral white matter that can be readily culled from the overall category of diffuse sclerosis is the leukodystrophies, including the adrenoleukodystrophy of boys and young men, the globoid-cell leukodystrophy of Krabbe, sudanophilic leukodystrophy, and the metachromatic leukodystrophy of Greenfield, all of which may involve peripheral nerves as well as central nervous system tissue. These diseases are characterized clinically by progressive visual failure, mental deterioration, and spastic paralysis; and pathologically by massive and more or less symmetrical destruction of the white matter of the cerebral hemispheres. In each of them there is a specific inherited biochemical defect in the metabolism of myelin proteolipids. These inherited metabolic diseases are discussed further in Chap. 38.

If one sets aside these hereditary metabolic leukodystrophies and the varied childhood disorders of cerebral white matter that have indiscriminately been included under the rubric of "Schilder's disease" or "diffuse sclerosis," there remains a characteristic group of cases that does indeed correspond to Schilder's original description. These latter cases are nonfamilial and are most frequently encountered in children or young adults. Clinically they are characterized by a progressive course that may be steady and unremitting or punctuated by a series of episodes of rapid worsening. In rare instances the disease may become arrested for many years, or the patient may even improve for a time. Dementia, homonymous hemianopia, cortical blindness and deafness, varying degrees of hemiplegia and quadriplegia, and pseudobulbar palsy are the usual clinical findings. The CSF may show changes similar to those in chronic relapsing multiple sclerosis. Death occurs in most patients within a few months or years, but some survive for a decade or longer. In the differential diagnosis, cerebral neoplasm is the main consideration.

The characteristic lesion in these cases is a large, sharply outlined, asymmetrical focus of myelin destruction often involving an entire lobe or cerebral hemisphere, typically with extension across the corpus callosum and affection of the opposite hemisphere. In some cases both hemispheres may be symmetrically involved. A careful examination of the optic nerves, brainstem, and spinal cord will often disclose the typical discrete lesions of multiple sclerosis. Histologically, the large single focus as well as the smaller disseminated ones, show the characteristic features of multiple sclerosis.

Poser's review of the literature, in 1957, uncovered 105 cases which could be designated as the Schilder type of diffuse sclerosis, in the original sense of the term. In 33 of these, the only lesions were the extensive areas of demyelination involving the centrum ovale; most of the patients in this group were children, and the disease had a tendency to take an acute or subacute progressive course. In 72 patients, isolated demyelinative plaques were found in other parts of the CNS, in addition to the large foci in the cerebral white matter; the age of onset in this latter group was similar to that of chronic, relapsing multiple sclerosis, and frequently the illness ran a protracted and remitting course. In a second paper, Poser reviewed the literature of the past 30 years (up to 1984) and reported a case with dramatic MRI lesions.

It is apparent that diffuse cerebral sclerosis of this

type must be closely related to multiple sclerosis, and may indeed be a variant of it, as Schilder originally proposed. The treatment of this form of juvenile cerebral multiple sclerosis is the same as that outlined for multiple sclerosis.

The *concentric sclerosis of Baló* is probably a variety of Schilder disease, which it resembles in its clinical aspects and in the overall distribution of its lesions. The distinguishing feature is the occurrence of alternating bands of destruction and preservation of myelin in a series of concentric rings. The occurrence of lesions in this pattern suggests the centrifugal diffusion of some factor that is damaging to myelin. A similar pattern of lesions, although far less extensive, is seen in occasional cases of chronic relapsing multiple sclerosis.

In adrenoleukodystrophy, in which there is a combination of adrenal atrophy, bronzing of the skin, and leukodystrophy, the neurologic picture and the cerebral lesion are indistinguishable from Schilder disease, but the sex-linked male inheritance and the adrenal atrophy are unique to the former (see page 811 for further description of this metabolic disorder).

ACUTE DISSEMINATED ENCEPHALOMYELITIS (Postinfectious, Postexanthem, Postvaccinal Encephalomyelitis; Acute Perivascular Myelinoclasis)

Some of these terms, used originally to refer to the neurologic sequelae of infectious fevers, were introduced into medicine in the late nineteenth century, but it wasn't until about 60 years ago that Perdrau, Greenfield, and others identified a pathologic reaction type common to a number of exanthems and vaccination. The current view of this entity is that it represents an acute demyelinative disease, distinguished pathologically by numerous foci of demyelination that are scattered throughout the brain and spinal cord; these foci vary from 0.1 to 1 mm in diameter and invariably surround small and medium-sized veins. The axons and nerve cells are more or less intact. Equally distinctive is the inflammatory reaction; the reacting cells consist of pleomorphic microglia, corresponding to the zones of demyelination, and of lymphocytes and mononuclear cells, cuffing the vessels. Multifocal meningeal infiltration is another invariable feature but is rarely severe in degree.

The clinical manifestations reflect the diffuse involvement of the brain and spinal cord and the meninges. There is an acute onset of confusion, somnolence, and often convulsions, with headache, fever, and stiffness of the neck. Ataxia, myoclonic movements, and choreoathetosis may be observed. In the more severe cases, stupor, coma, and, at times, decerebrate rigidity may occur in rapid

succession. With spinal cord involvement there is partial or complete paraplegia or quadriplegia, diminution or loss of tendon reflexes, sensory impairment, and varying degrees of paralysis of bladder and bowel.

An acute encephalitic, myelitic, or encephalomyelitic process of this type may occur before (rare), concurrently with, or more often, shortly after the onset of the exanthem of measles, rubella, smallpox, and chickenpox and very rarely with mumps and influenza. A similar illness may follow vaccination against rabies and smallpox and reportedly after the administration of tetanus antitoxin. Some cases, clinically and pathologically indistinguishable from these two categories of acute disseminated encephalomyelitis, appear to develop after banal respiratory infections, *Mycoplasma pneumoniae*, and occasionally without any clearly defined preceding illness, vaccination, or inoculation.

The disease has grave significance because of the substantial death rate and persistent neurologic defects in patients who survive. There may be only a mild spastic paraplegia and impairment of sphincter control. In children, recovery from the acute stage is sometimes followed by a permanent disorder of behavior, mental retardation, or epilepsy. As in most acute diseases of the nervous system, the functional derangement during the acute stage is out of all proportion to the permanent structural damage.

The pathogenesis of disseminated encephalomyelitis is still unclear, despite its obvious association with viral infections. Usually a definite interval separates the onset of disseminated encephalomyelitis from the onset of the rash; also, the pathologic changes are quite different from those of viral infections and virus has never been recovered from the CSF or brains of patients with disseminated encephalomyelitis. For these reasons it is thought that the latter disorder represents an immune-mediated complication of infection, rather than a direct viral infection of the CNS. A laboratory model of the disease, experimental allergic encephalomyelitis (EAE), has been produced by inoculating animals with a combination of sterile brain tissue and adjuvants. The experimental disease appears most commonly between the 8th and 15th day after sensitization (see below) and is characterized by the same perivenular demyelinative and inflammatory lesions that one observes in the human disease. Presumably the lesions are the result of a T-cell-mediated immune reaction to myelin basic proteins.

The notion that postmeasles encephalomyelitis and EAE have a similar pathogenesis has received strong support from the observations of R. T. Johnson and his colleagues. They studied 19 patients with postinfectious encephalomyelitis complicating natural measles-virus infections. Early myelin destruction was demonstrated by the presence of myelin basic protein in the CSF, and lymphocyte proliferative responses to myelin basic protein were found in 8 of 17 patients tested. Similar responses were found in patients with encephalomyelitis after rabies vaccine and after varicella and rubella virus infections, suggesting a common immune-mediated pathogenesis. Moreover, the patients with postmeasles encephalomyelitis showed a lack of intrathecal synthesis of antibody against measles virus, indicating that the neurologic disease was not dependent on virus replication within the CNS.

POSTVACCINAL ENCEPHALOMYELITIS

Since late in the nineteenth century it has been known that a severe form of encephalomyelitis may complicate the injection of rabies vaccine (*neuroparalytic accident*). Until quite recently, the vaccine in common use consisted of killed rabies virus produced in rabbit brain tissue; encephalomyelitis occurred in about 1 in 750 patients inoculated with this vaccine, and in about 25 percent of cases this complication proved fatal. Alternative vaccines, made from embryonated duck eggs (or human diploid cells) infected with fixed viruses, contain very little or no nerve tissue and are almost free of neurologic complications. In underdeveloped countries, where less expensive brain-based vaccines are still in use, neuroparalytic accidents continue to occur. The recent observations of Hemachudha et al indicate that the altered immune mechanism that is operative in the neuroparalytic accident is the same as that in postmeasles encephalomyelitis and experimental allergic encephalomyelitis.

There are numerous recorded instances of rabies vaccine (with neural tissue) inducing an acute multiple sclerosis. Shiraki and Otani reported such examples from Japan. The evolution of symptoms was subacute, over a period of 2 to 4 weeks, and the demyelinative lesions were macroscopic—up to 1 to 2.0 cm in diameter—but composed of confluent perivascular lesions. The disease could be reproduced in dogs, persuasive evidence that acute multiple sclerosis is a variant of acute disseminated encephalomyelitis.

Encephalomyelitis following vaccination against smallpox has been known since 1860, but only isolated instances were recognized until 1922, when the first major outbreak of postvaccinal encephalomyelitis occurred. The disease may appear at any time between the second and twenty-fifth days after vaccination, but usually between the tenth and thirteenth days (end of pustular stage). The disease occurred about once in 4000 vaccinations and about 20

times more frequently after primary vaccination than after revaccination. Encephalomyelitis following smallpox vaccination is now of historical interest only. Smallpox seems to have disappeared as a human illness worldwide. In the United States, there have been no new cases for years, and smallpox vaccination is no longer recommended as part of immunization schedules.

The onset of postvaccinal encephalomyelitis is generally abrupt—with headache, drowsiness, fever, vomiting, and sometimes convulsions. There may be stiffness of the neck and other signs of meningeal irritation. Typically, signs of spinal cord involvement appear soon afterward, with flaccid weakness or paralysis, usually involving all four limbs; occasionally hemiplegia may occur. Tendon reflexes disappear, and the plantar responses become extensor. Sphincter control is often lost, and sensory loss, though variable, may be extensive and severe. Nystagmus, ocular palsies, and pupillary changes indicate brainstem involvement, and stupor and deepening coma point to diencephalic or cerebral lesions; these signs have a serious prognosis. Variations of this clinical picture are common. One patient may suffer a predominantly encephalitic illness with convulsions and coma and little evidence of cord damage; in another, hemiplegia or a pure transverse myelitis may occur, without headache, neck stiffness, or clouding of consciousness. The site of vaccination has no influence on the neurologic syndrome. The CSF almost invariably shows a moderate increase in protein and cells, predominantly lymphocytes, but in rare cases it has been normal.

The association of the neurologic disorder with vaccination usually leaves the diagnosis in little doubt, and the characteristic combination of encephalitic and myelitic features will help to distinguish the condition from meningitis, viral encephalitis, and poliomyelitis. Rarely, an atypical case may mimic any one of these disorders. On occasion, the disease may suggest involvement of nerve roots and peripheral nerves and resemble acute inflammatory polyneuritis (Guillain-Barré syndrome). In fact, the rabies vaccine produced in South America from suckling mouse brain causes this type of peripheral nerve disease more often than it causes encephalomyelitis.

The mortality rate of postvaccinal encephalomyelitis is high, between 30 and 50 percent. If recovery occurs it may be surprisingly complete. However, a significant proportion of patients show residual neurologic signs, intellectual impairment, and behavioral abnormalities.

POSTINFECTIOUS ENCEPHALOMYELITIS

This syndrome occurs most often in association with measles. Clinically evident neurologic complications occur in 1 in 800 to 1 in 2000 cases. Prior to widespread immunization against measles, an epidemic in a large city might have counted 100,000 cases of measles and resulted in a substantial number of neurologic complications. The mortality among patients with such complications ranges from 10 to 20 percent; about an equal number are left with persistent neurologic damage. Patients without clinically apparent neurologic residua may undergo significant and sometimes permanent changes in behavior. The neurologic complications of measles alone provide sufficient justification for immunization against the disease.

The incidence of encephalomyelitis following smallpox was approximately 2.5 cases per 1000. The incidence is much less following chickenpox and rubella. Very rarely, an acute encephalomyelitic reaction may follow mumps. More often, however, mumps is complicated by a true viral meningoencephalitis, which may be difficult to differentiate clinically from a postinfectious process. Mumps virus can usually be cultured from the CSF during the acute stage of the meningoencephalitis.

The encephalomyelitic syndrome generally begins 2 to 4 days after the appearance of the rash. Very rarely it precedes the rash. Usually the rash is fading and other symptoms are improving when the patient suddenly develops a recrudescence of fever, convulsions, stupor, and deepening coma. Less commonly, the patient may develop hemiplegia or evidence of cerebellar disease, and occasionally a transverse myelitis, sphincteric disturbances, or other signs of spinal cord involvement. Choreoathetotic movements are seen infrequently. In many cases the disease is much less severe and the patient suffers a transient encephalitic illness with headaches, confusion, and signs of meningeal irritation. The CSF, as in postvaccinal encephalomyelitis, usually, though not always, shows a lymphocytic pleocytosis and increase in protein content.

Differential Diagnosis It needs to be emphasized that not all the neurologic complications of measles and other exanthems are examples of postinfectious encephalomyelitis. In some cases cerebrovascular disease (particularly thrombophlebitis), hypoxic encephalopathy, or acute toxic hepatoencephalopathy (Reye syndrome) may be responsible. The Reye syndrome is usually not difficult to separate from postinfectious encephalomyelitis, even when it follows chicken pox or viral influenza, because of the normal CSF and high levels of serum NH_3 (see Chap. 40). Infectious mononucleosis, herpes simplex encephalitis, and other forms of encephalitis may all mimic postinfectious encephalomyelitis. In a child the first attack of seizures in what will prove to be idiopathic epilepsy may at first raise suspicion of encephalitis or postinfectious encephalomyelitis.

Prevention and Treatment The incidence of postinfectious and postvaccinal encephalomyelitis has declined significantly in the past 15 years. Paradoxically, this has resulted from the initiation of widespread immunization

against measles and from the discontinuation of immunization against smallpox. The universal use of tissue culture vaccine for rabies prophylaxis may well eliminate the encephalomyelitic complications of rabies vaccination.

The use of high-potency steroids appears to be the treatment of choice, although controlled trials of this treatment have not been carried out. Steroids, given as soon as possible after the appearance of neurologic signs, modify the severity of experimental allergic encephalomyelitis, and this provides the logic for their use in the human counterpart of this disease.

ACUTE NECROTIZING HEMORRHAGIC ENCEPHALOMYELITIS (Acute Hemorrhagic Leukoencephalitis of Weston Hurst)

This, the most fulminant form of demyelinative disease, affects mainly young adults but also children. It is almost invariably preceded by a respiratory infection of variable duration (1 to 14 days), sometimes due to *Mycoplasma pneumoniae* but more often of indeterminate cause. The neurologic symptoms appear abruptly, beginning with headache, fever, stiff neck, and confusion. These are followed in short order by signs of disease of one or both cerebral hemispheres and brainstem—focal seizures, hemiplegia or quadriplegia, pseudobulbar paralysis, and progressively deepening coma. Leukocytosis is usually present, sometimes reaching 30,000 cells per cubic millimeter, and the sedimentation rate is elevated. The CSF is often under increased pressure; cells vary in number from a few lymphocytes to a polymorphonuclear pleocytosis of up to 3000 cells per cubic millimeter; red cells may be present in variable numbers; protein content is increased, but glucose values are normal. Diagnosis is facilitated by the CT scan which reveals the massive lesion in the cerebral white matter (Fig. 37-2). Many cases terminate fatally in 2 to 4 days but some survive somewhat longer. Patients with a similar clinical picture and who are thought to have the same disease on the basis of brain biopsy examinations have recovered with almost no residual symptoms.

Acute encephalitis due to herpes simplex or other viruses, brain abscess, subdural empyema, and focal embolic encephalomalacia are the important considerations in the differential diagnosis.

The pathologic findings are distinctive. On sectioning the brain, the white matter of one or both hemispheres is seen to be destroyed almost to the point of liquefaction. The involved tissue is pink or yellow-gray and flecked with multiple small hemorrhages. Similar changes are often found in the brainstem and cerebellar peduncles and rarely in the spinal cord. On histologic examination one finds widespread necrosis of small blood vessels and brain tissue around the vessels, with intense cellular infiltration, multiple small hemorrhages, and a violent inflammatory reaction in the meninges. The pathologic picture resembles that of disseminated encephalomyelitis in its perivascular distribution, with the added feature of more widespread necrosis and a tendency of lesions to form large foci in the cerebral hemispheres. The vascular alterations account for the exudation of fibrin into the vessel wall and surrounding tissue.

It is probable that certain patients showing an explosive myelitic illness are suffering from a necrotizing lesion of similar type, but pathologic evidence in support of this view has been difficult to obtain (see page 730).

The etiology of this condition remains obscure, but the resemblance to other demyelinating diseases should be emphasized. The similarities of the histologic changes to those of disseminated encephalomyelitis, noted above,

suggest that the two diseases are related forms of the same fundamental process. In fact, cases combining both types of pathologic change have been described (Fisher et al). The observations of Behan and colleagues that the lymphocytes of a patient with postinfectious encephalomyelitis and of another with acute necrotizing hemorrhagic encephalitis underwent transformation to lymphoblasts in response to a pure encephalitogenic myelin basic protein, support the view that delayed hypersensitivity mechanisms are operative in both diseases. Also it is noteworthy that among the small number of patients who have recovered from what appeared to be a typical necrotizing hemorrhagic encephalitis, a few have gone on to develop typical multiple sclerosis. These points of similarity are sufficient to suggest that corticosteroids should be used in the treatment of acute necrotizing hemorrhagic encephalopathy; in several personally observed patients, we have had the impression that they produced a favorable result.

BRAIN PURPURA (PERICAPILLARY ENCEPHALORRHAGIA)

This is another hemorrhagic condition, sometimes confused with acute necrotizing hemorrhagic encephalitis. The lesions in brain purpura are always small, 0.1 to 2.0 mm in diameter, and are confined to the white matter, particularly the corpus callosum, centrum ovale, and middle cerebellar peduncles. Each lesion is situated around a small blood vessel, usually a capillary. In this para-adventitial area both the myelin and axis cylinders are destroyed, and the lesion is usually though not always hemorrhagic. Fibrin exudation, perivascular and meningeal infiltrates of inflammatory cells, and widespread necrosis of tissue are not observed; in these respects brain purpura differs fundamentally from acute necrotizing hemorrhagic encephalitis. Usually the patient has become stuporous and comatose without focal neurologic signs and the CSF is normal. The etiology of brain purpura is quite obscure. It may complicate virus pneumonia and arsenical intoxication, or there may be no associated disease.

Figure 37-2

Acute necrotizing hemorrhagic leukoencephalitis, mainly bifrontal.

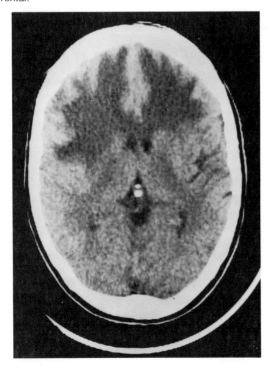

REFERENCES

ADAMS RD, KUBIK CS: The morbid anatomy of the demyelinative diseases. *Am J Med* 12:510, 1952.

ADAMS RD, RICHARDSON EP JR: The demyelinative diseases of the human nervous system: A classification; a review of salient neuropathologic findings; comments on recent biochemical studies, in Folch-Pi J (ed): *Chemical Pathology of the Nervous System.* New York, Pergamon Press, 1961, pp 162–196.

AIMARD G, CONFAVREUX C, VENTRE JJ et al: Étude de 213 cas de sclérose en plaques traités par l'azathiaprine de 1967–1982. *Rev Neurol* 139:509, 1983.

ALLEN IV, MILLER JHD, SHILLINGTON RKA: Systemic lupus erythematosus clinically resembling multiple sclerosis and with unusual pathological ultrastructural features. *J Neurol Neurosurg Psychiatry* 42:392, 1979.

ALTER M, HALPERN L, KURLAND LT et al: Multiple sclerosis in Israel. *Arch Neurol* 7:253, 1962.

BEEBE GW, KURTZKE JF, KURLAND LT et al: Studies on the natural history of multiple sclerosis: 3. Epidemiologic analyses of the Army experience in World War II. *Neurology* 17:1, 1967.

BEHAN PO, GESCHWIND N, LAMARCHE JB et al: Delayed hypersensitivity to encephalitogenic protein in disseminated encephalomyelitis. *Lancet* 2:1009, 1968.

BIRK K, RUDICK R: Pregnancy and multiple sclerosis. *Arch Neurol* 43:719, 1986

BORNSTEIN MB, MILLER A, SLAGLE S et al: A pilot trial of COP I in exacerbating-remitting multiple sclerosis. *N Engl J Med* 317:408, 1987.

COHEN SR, HERNDON RM, McKHANN GM: Radioimmunoassay of myelin basic protein in spinal fluid. *N Engl J Med* 295:1455, 1976.

COOK SD, DEVEREUX C, TROIANO R et al: Effect of total lymphoid irradiation in chronic progressive multiple sclerosis. *Lancet* 1:1405, 1986.

COXE WS, LUSE SA: Acute hemorrhagic leukoencephalitis. *J Neurosurg* 20:584, 1963.

DALOS NP, ROBINS PV, BROOKS BR et al: Disease activity and emotional state in multiple sclerosis. *Ann Neurol* 13:573, 1983.

DEAN G: The multiple sclerosis problem. *Sci Am* 233:40, July 1970.

DEAN G, KURTZKE JF: On the risk of multiple sclerosis according to age at immigration to South Africa. *Br Med J* 3:725, 1971.

DEJONG RN: Multiple sclerosis: History, definition and general considerations, in Vinken PJ, Bruyn GW (eds): *Handbook of Clinical Neurology*, vol 9. Amsterdam, North-Holland, 1970, chap 3, pp 45–62.

DEKEYSER J: Autoimmunity in multiple sclerosis. *Neurology* 38:371, 1988.

EBERS GC: Optic neuritis and multiple sclerosis. *Arch Neurol* 42:702, 1985.

EBERS GC, BULMAN DE, SADOVNICK AD: A population-based study of multiple sclerosis in twins. *N Engl J Med* 315:1638, 1986.

ELLISON PH, BARRON KD: Clinical recovery from Schilder's disease. *Neurology* 29:244, 1979.

FISHER RS, CLARK AW, WOLINSKY JS et al: Post-infectious leukoencephalitis complicating *Mycoplasma pneumoniae* infection. *Arch Neurol* 40:109, 1983.

GILBERT JJ, SADLER M: Unsuspected multiple sclerosis. *Arch Neurol* 40:533, 1983.

HALLETT M, LINDSEY JW, ADELSTEIN BD, RILEY PO: Controlled trial of isoniazid therapy for severe postural cerebellar tremor in multiple sclerosis. *Neurology* 35:1314, 1985.

HALLIDAY AM, McDONALD WI: Pathophysiology of demyelinating disease. *Br Med Bull* 33:21, 1977.

HAUSER SL, BRESNAN MJ, REINHERZ EL, WEINER HL: Childhood multiple sclerosis: Clinical features and demonstration of changes in T-cell subsets with disease activity. *Ann Neurol* 11:463, 1982.

HAUSER SL, DAWSON DM, LEHRICH JR: Intensive immune suppression in progressive multiple sclerosis: A randomized three arm study of high-dose intravenous cyclophosphamide, plasma exchange and ACTH. *N Engl J Med* 308:173, 1983.

HELY MA, McMANIS PG, DORAN TJ et al: Acute optic neuritis: A prospective study of risk factors for multiple sclerosis. *J Neurol Neurosurg Psychiatry* 49:1125, 1986.

HEMACHUDHA T, GRIFFIN DE, GIFFELS JJ et al: Myelin basic protein as an encephalitogen in encephalomyelitis and polyneuritis following rabies vaccination. *N Engl J Med* 316:369, 1987.

JACOBS L, KINKEL PR, KINKEL WR: Silent brain lesions in patients with isolated idiopathic optic neuritis. *Arch Neurol* 43:452, 1986.

JACOBS L, O'MALLEY JA, FREEMAN A et al: Intrathecal interferon in the treatment of multiple sclerosis; patient follow up. *Arch Neurol* 42:841, 1985.

JOHNSON KP, ARRIGO SC, NELSON BS, GINSBERG A: Agarose electrophoresis of cerebrospinal fluid in multiple sclerosis. *Neurology* 27:273, 1977.

JOHNSON KP, LIKOSKY WH, NELSON BJ, FINE G: Comprehensive viral immunology of multiple sclerosis. I: Clinical, epidemiological, and CSF studies. *Arch Neurol* 37:537, 610, 616, 1980.

JOHNSON RT: The possible viral etiology of multiple sclerosis, in Friedlander WJ (ed): *Advances in Neurology*, vol 13. New York, Raven Press, 1975, pp 1–46.

JOHNSON RT: Current knowledge of multiple sclerosis. *South Med J* 71:2, 1978.

JOHNSON RT, GRIFFIN DE, HIRSCH RL et al: Measles encephalomyelitis—clinical and immunologic studies. *N Engl J Med* 310:137, 1984.

KURLAND LT: The frequency and geographic distribution of multiple sclerosis as indicated by mortality statistics and morbidity surveys in the United States and Canada. *Am J Hyg* 55:457, 1952.

KURTZKE JF, HYLLESTED K: Multiple sclerosis in the Faroe Islands. II. Clinical update, transmission, and the nature of MS. *Neurology* 36:307, 1986.

KURTZKE JF, BEEBE GW, NORMAN JE JR: Epidemiology of multiple sclerosis in U.S. veterans. I: Race, sex, and geographic distribution. *Neurology* 29:1228, 1979.

KURTZKE JF, GUDMUNDSSON KR, BERGMANN S: Multiple sclerosis in Iceland. 1: Evidence of a post-war epidemic. *Neurology* 32:143, 1982.

LAMPERT PW: Autoimmune and virus-induced demyelinating diseases. *Am J Pathol* 91:176, 1978.

LANDY PJ: A prospective study of the risk of developing multiple sclerosis in optic neuritis in a tropical and sub-tropical area. *J Neurol Neurosurg Psychiatry* 46:659, 1983.

McALPINE D, COMPSTON MD: Some aspects of the natural history of disseminated sclerosis. *Q J Med* 21:135, 1952.

McALPINE D, LUMSDEN CE, ACHESON ED: *Multiple Sclerosis: A Reappraisal*. Edinburgh, Churchill-Livingstone, 1972.

McDONALD WI: The mystery of the origin of multiple sclerosis. *J Neurol Neurosurg Psychiatry* 49:113, 1986.

McDONALD WI: Attitudes to the treatment of multiple sclerosis. *Arch Neurol* 40:667, 1983.

McDonald WI, Halliday AM: Diagnosis and classification of multiple sclerosis. *Br Med Bull* 33:4, 1977.

McFarlin DE, McFarland HF: Multiple sclerosis. *N Engl J Med* 307:1246, 1982.

Mathews WB, Acheson ED, Batchelor JR, Weller RO (eds): *McAlpine's Multiple Sclerosis.* New York, Churchill Livingstone, 1985.

Moulin D, Paty DW, Ebers GC: The predictive value of CSF electrophoresis in "possible" multiple sclerosis. *Brain* 106:809, 1983.

Nikoskelainen E, Riekkinen P: Optic neuritis—a sign of multiple sclerosis or other diseases of the nervous system. *Acta Neurologica Scand* 50:690, 1974.

Ormerod IEC, McDonald WI: Multiple sclerosis presenting with progressive visual failure. *J Neurol Neurosurg Psychiatry* 47:943, 1984.

Ormerod IEC, McDonald WI, duBoulay GH et al: Disseminated lesions at presentation in patients with optic neuritis. *J Neurol Neurosurg Psychiatry* 49:124, 1986.

Osterman PO, Westerbey CE: Paroxysmal attacks in multiple sclerosis. *Brain* 98:189, 1975.

Panitch HS: Systemic α-interferon in multiple sclerosis. Long-term patient followup. *Arch Neurol* 44:61, 1987.

Panitch HS, Haley AS, Hirsch RLA et al: A trial of gamma interferon in multiple sclerosis. Clinical Results. *Neurology* 36 (suppl 1):285, 1986.

Paty DW, Asbury AK, Herndon RM et al: Use of magnetic resonance imaging in the diagnosis of multiple sclerosis: Policy statement. *Neurology* 36:1575, 1986.

Percy AK, Nobrega FT, Okazaki H: Multiple sclerosis in Rochester, Minnesota: A 60-year appraisal. *Arch Neurol* 25:105, 1971.

Portersfield JS (ed): Multiple sclerosis. *Br Med Bull* 33:1977.

Poser CM, Goutieres F, Carpentier M: Schilder's myelinoclastic diffuse sclerosis. *Pediatrics* 77:107, 1986.

Poser CM: Diffuse-disseminated sclerosis in the adult. *J Neuropathol Exp Neurol* 16:61, 1957.

Poser CM: Exacerbations, activity and progression in multiple sclerosis. *Arch Neurol* 37:471, 1980.

Poser CM, van Bogaert L: Natural history and evolution of the concept of Schilder's diffuse sclerosis. *Acta Psychiatr Neurol Scand* 31:285, 1956.

Poskanzer DC, Schapira K, Miller H: Multiple sclerosis and poliomyelitis. *Lancet* 2:917, 1963.

Prineas JW: The etiology and pathogenesis of multiple sclerosis, in Vinken PJ, Bruyn GW (eds): *Handbook of Clinical Neurology,* vol 9. Amsterdam, North-Holland, 1970, chap 6, pp 107–160.

Prineas JW, Connell F: Remyelination in multiple sclerosis. *Ann Neurol* 5:22, 1979.

Riechert T, Hassler R, Mundinger F et al: Pathologic-anatomic findings and cerebral localization in stereotactic treatment of extrapyramidal motor disturbances in multiple sclerosis. *Confin Neurol* 37:24, 1975.

Schapira K, Poskanzer DC, Miller H: Familial and conjugal multiple sclerosis. *Brain* 86:315, 1963.

Schilder P: Zur Kenntniss der sogennanten diffusen Sklerose. *Z Gesamte Neurol Psychiat* 10:1, 1912.

Sears ES, McCammon A, Bigelow R, Hayman LA: Maximizing the harvest of contrast enhancing lesions in multiple sclerosis. *Neurology* 32:815, 1982.

Shiraki H: The comparative study of rabies post-vaccinal encephalomyelitis and demyelinating encephalomyelitides of unknown origin with special reference to the Japanese cases, in Bailey OT, Smith DE (eds): *The Central Nervous System: Some Experimental Models of Neurological Diseases.* Baltimore, Williams and Wilkins, 1968, pp 87–123.

Shiraki H, Otani S: Clinical and pathological features of rabies postvaccinal encephalomyelitis in man, in Kies MW, Alvord EC Jr (eds): *"Allergic" Encephalomyelitis.* Springfield, IL, Charles C Thomas, 1959, pp 58–129.

Stewart JM, Houser GW, Baker HL: Magnetic resonance imaging and clinical relationships in multiple sclerosis. *Mayo Clin Proc* 62:174, 1987.

Thygessen P: *The Course of Disseminated Sclerosis: A Close-Up of 105 Attacks.* Copenhagen, Rosenkilde and Bagger, 1953.

Tourtellotte WW, Booe IM: Multiple sclerosis: The blood-brain barrier and the measurement of de novo central nervous system IgG synthesis. *Neurology* 28(suppl):76, 1978.

Waksman BH: Current trends in multiple sclerosis research. *Immunology Today* 1981, pp 87–93.

Waksman BH: Rationales of current therapies for multiple sclerosis. *Arch Neurol* 40:671, 1983.

Weiner HL, Hafler DA: Immunotherapy of multiple sclerosis. *Ann Neurol* 23:211, 1988.

Whitaker JN: Current views regarding the etiology and pathogenesis of multiple sclerosis, in Isselbacher KJ (ed): *Update IV, Harrison's Principles of Internal Medicine.* New York, McGraw-Hill, 1983, pp 39–48.

Wilson SAK: Neuromyelitis, in *Neurology,* 2nd ed, vol 1. Baltimore, Williams & Wilkins, 1955, vol 1, pp 233–236.

CHAPTER 38

THE INHERITED METABOLIC DISEASES OF THE NERVOUS SYSTEM

Advances in biochemistry have led to the discovery of such a large number of metabolic diseases of the nervous system that it taxes the mind even to remember their names. Largely this resulted from the application by Dent of a paper chromatographic method for the analysis of amino acids in blood and urine. More recently, high-pressure gas-liquid chromatography, mass spectroscopy, and electron microscopy have continued to reveal previously unknown diseases and to clarify the basic biochemistry of old ones.

Through these innovative methodologies, mass screening and prevention are now practicable, and the physician's role is changing as a consequence. No longer must he or she wait until a disease of the nervous system has declared itself by symptoms and signs, by which time the lesion may have become irreversible. Now it is possible to find patients who, though asymptomatic, are at risk, and to introduce dietary and other measures to prevent injury to the nervous system. To assume this responsibility intelligently requires some knowledge of genetics, of biochemical screening methods, and of public health measures.

Of the 2208 entities itemized in the 1988 edition of McKusick's catalogs of inherited diseases, about 250 are identified as enzymopathies, i.e., mendelian disorders with a demonstrated primary enzyme defect. Enzymopathies constitute one-third of the known recessive (autosomal and X-linked) disorders. Most of them become manifest in infancy and childhood. Only a few appear as late as adolescence or adult life; many damage the nervous system so severely that survival to adult years and reproduction are impossible. As a group, these diseases—along with congenital anomalies (Chap. 44) and birth injuries, epilepsy, disharmonies of development and learning disabilities (Chap. 28)—make up the bulk of the problems with which the pediatric neurologist must contend.

The pathogenesis of the hereditary metabolic diseases, while not fully understood, can be traced in most instances to an inborn enzymatic defect. The cells of all organs are to some extent exposed to the failure of a metabolic pathway, the lack of an essential substrate, or to the accumulation of a harmful metabolite. It is the nervous system, however, that is most consistently affected, perhaps because of its protracted growth and maturation, which extend for years after birth. Although the diseases under discussion are genetic, the pattern of heredity is such that neither parent is clinically abnormal, viz., recessive. Often the heterozygous status of the parents cannot be detected. Moreover, the mother's normal metabolism usually protects the fetus in utero; only after birth does the faulty metabolism induced by the abnormal gene begin to exert its deleterious effects on brain function and structure.

The clinical syndromes by which these metabolic diseases declare themselves vary in accordance with the nature of the biochemical defect and the stage of maturation of the nervous system at which it acts. In phenylketonuria, for example, there is a rather diffuse but specific effect on the cerebral white matter, but only during the period of active myelination. Once the maturational processes are complete, the biochemical abnormality becomes relatively harmless. Even more important is the level of function that has been achieved by the developing nervous system when the disease strikes. A derangement of function in a neonate or infant, in whom much of the cerebrum is functioning poorly, is much less obvious than one in an older child; and, as the disease evolves, the clinical manifestations are influenced always by the continuing maturation of the untouched elements in the nervous system.

Because of the overriding importance of the age factor and the tendency of certain pathologic processes to appear in particular epochs of life, the authors believe that it is logical to group the inherited metabolic diseases not according to their major syndromes of expression, as we have done in other parts of the book, but in relation to the periods of life at which they are most likely to occur: the neonatal period, infancy (1 to 12 months), early childhood

(1 to 4 years), late childhood, adolescence, and adult life. Only in the latter two age periods will we return to a syndromic ordering of diseases. In adopting this chronologic subdivision, it is not to be denied that variants of these diseases sometimes appear at more than one period of life, and these deviations will be remarked upon at appropriate times.

THE NEUROLOGY OF NEONATAL METABOLIC DISEASES

A small number of progressive metabolic diseases become manifest in the first few days of life. The importance of these diseases relates not to their frequency (they constitute only a small fraction of diseases that compromise function of the nervous system in the first weeks of life) but to the fact that they must be recognized promptly if the child is to be prevented from dying or from the worse fate of lifelong idiocy. These threats give a new sense of urgency to medical action in pediatric neurology.

Two approaches to the neonatal metabolic disorders are possible—one, to screen every newborn, using a battery of biochemical tests of blood and urine; the other, to undertake in the days following birth a detailed neurologic assessment that will detect the earliest signs of these diseases. Unfortunately the biochemical tests are costly, and not all have been simplified to the point where they can be adapted to a mass screening program; and many of the commonly used clinical tests at this age have yet to be validated as signs of disease. Moreover, practical issues such as cost-effectiveness insinuate themselves, to the distress of the pediatrician.

THE NEUROLOGIC ASSESSMENT OF NEONATES WITH METABOLIC DISEASE

As was pointed out in Chap. 28, the neonate, in terms of nervous functioning, is essentially a brainstem-spinal preparation. The pallidum and visual-motor cortices are only beginning to be myelinated and their contribution to the totality of neonatal behavior cannot be very great. Neurologic examination, to be informative, must therefore be directed to evaluating diencephalic-midbrain, cerebellar–lower brainstem, and spinal functions. The integrity of these functions in the neonate are most reliably assessed by noting the following:

1. The state of alertness and attention (stimulus responsivity and capacity of the pediatrician to make contact), as well as sleep patterns and EEG—diencephalic mechanisms

2. Movements and postures of the neck, trunk, and limbs such as reactions of support, extension of the neck and trunk, flexion movements and steppage—lower brainstem (reticulospinal), cerebellar, and spinal mechanisms

3. Reflex organization of eye movements—tegmental midbrain and pontine mechanisms

4. Certain reflexive reactions such as the startle (Moro) response and placing reactions of the foot and hand—upper brainstem–spinal mechanisms with cortical facilitation

5. Control of respiration and body temperature; regulation of thirst, fluid balance, and appetite—hypothalamus-brainstem-spinal mechanisms

Derangements of these functions are manifested as impairments of alertness and arousal, disturbances of ocular movement (oscillations of the eyes, nystagmus, loss of tonic conjugate deviation of the eyes in response to vestibular stimulation, i.e., to rotation of the infant), tremors, clonic jerkings, tonic spasms, opisthotonus, diminution or absence of limb movements, irregular or chaotic breathing, hypothermia or poikilothermia, bradycardia, circulatory difficulties, poor color, and seizures.

In most instances of neonatal metabolic disease the pregnancy and delivery had proceeded without mishap. Birth at full term is usual. The infant is of a size and weight expected for the duration of pregnancy, and there are no signs of a developmental abnormality (in a few instances the infant is somewhat small). Furthermore, function continues to be normal in the first few days of life. The first hint of trouble may be the early occurrence of feeding difficulties: food intolerance, diarrhea, and vomiting. The infant becomes fretful and fails to gain weight and thrive—all of which suggest a disorder of amino acid, ammonia, or organic acid metabolism.

The first definite indication of disordered nervous function is likely to be the occurrence of seizures. These usually take the form of unpatterned clonic or tonic contractions of one side of the body, sudden arrest of respiration, turning of the head and eyes to one side, or twitching of the hands and face. Some of the seizures may become generalized. They occur singly or in clusters, and in the latter instance are associated with unresponsiveness, immobility, and arrest of respiration. While seizures are occurring, certain other automatic activities such as sucking, grasping, and steppage, and the Moro and support reactions are suppressed.

The other clinical manifestations, according to authorities such as Prechtl and Beintema, and Joppich and Schulte, can be subdivided roughly into three groups, each of which constitutes a kind of syndrome: (1) hyperkinetic-hypertonic, (2) apathetic-hypotonic, or (3) unilateral or hemisyndromes. Prechtl and Beintema, from a study of more than 1500 newborns, found that if clinical examination consistently disclosed any one of the three syndromes, the chances are two out of three that by the seventh year the child will be abnormal neurologically. They found that neurologic signs, such as facial palsy, grasping, excessive floppiness, and impairment of sucking—while sometimes indicative of serious disease of the nervous system—are less dependable; also, being rare, these signs will identify but few brain-damaged infants. It is not the single neurologic sign but groups of them that are held to be the most reliable indices of brain abnormality, and the three syndromes mentioned above are the important ones, even though their anatomic and physiologic bases are not completely understood.

In our observations of the neonatal metabolic diseases we have endeavored to determine if particular ones consistently manifest themselves by one or other of the three syndromes; this we are able to affirm to some degree. In cases of hypocalcemia-hypomagnesemia, the hyperkinetic-hypertonic syndrome prevails, but most of the other diseases tend to induce the apathetic-hypotonic state. Nonetheless, the hyperactive-hypertonic syndrome may represent the initial phase of the illness and always carries a less ominous prognosis than the apathetic-hypotonic state, which represents a more severe and potentially dangerous condition regardless of cause. We have not been confident in the recognition of the hemi- or unilateral syndromes in any of the metabolic diseases. Even more discouraging has been the frequent overlapping of the three syndromes, and the fact that seizures may occur in all of them. Clearly what is needed is a new neonatal neurologic semiology utilizing every possible type of stimulus-response test including visual, auditory, and somatosensory evoked potentials; also needed are ways of accurately quantifying more of the natural activities of this age period. Even the *brain death syndrome*, in which all brainstem-spinal reflexes are abolished, has not been fully defined in the neonate (Adams et al).

THE NEONATAL METABOLIC DISEASES AND THEIR ESTIMATED FREQUENCY

In Massachusetts, a state-sponsored screening program for all newborns has been in operation for more than 20 years. The data on 16 metabolic diseases have been collated by our colleague H. L. Levy and are summarized in Table 38-1. Some of these disorders can be recognized by simple color reactions in the urine; these are listed in Table 38-2.

To this group should be added other inherited hyperammonemic syndromes and vitamin responsive aminoacidopathies such as pyridoxine dependency, as well as certain nonfamilial metabolic disorders that make their appearance in the neonatal period—hypocalcemia and hypomagnesemia with tetany, hypoglycemia, cretinism, and congenital adrenal hyperplasia.

It is important to note that the three most frequently identified hereditary metabolic diseases—phenylketonuria, hyperphenylalaninemia, and histidinemia—are ones that do not become clinically manifest in the neonatal period. This is fortunate, for it allows time to introduce preventive measures before the first symptoms become manifest. A number of others, which can be recognized either by screening or by early signs, are synopsized below.

Vitamin-Responsive Aminoacidopathies Included under this heading is a group of diseases that respond not to dietary restriction of a specific amino acid but to the oral supplementation of a specific vitamin. Some 25 vitamin-responsive aminoacidopathies are known (the more common ones are listed in Table 39-3) and 14 of them result in injury to the central nervous system. *Pyridoxine dependency* is the classic example. This is a rare disease, inherited as an autosomal recessive trait. It is characterized by the early onset of convulsions, sometimes in utero, failure to thrive, hypertonia-hyperkinesia, irritability, tremulous movements ("jittery baby"), exaggerated auditory startle (*hyperacusis*), and later, if untreated, by psychomotor retardation. The specific laboratory abnormality is an increased excretion of xanthurenic acid in response to a tryptophan load. The neuropathology has been studied in only a few cases. In one of our patients, a 13½-year-old boy with mental retardation, pale optic discs, and spastic legs, the brain weight was 350 g below normal. There was a decreased amount of central white matter in the cerebral hemispheres and a depletion of neurons in the thalamic nuclei and cerebellum, with gliosis (Lott et al). The administration of 50 to 100 mg of vitamin B_6 ablates the seizure state, and daily doses of 40 mg permit normal development.

Galactosemia Inheritance of this disorder is autosomal recessive in type. The biochemical abnormality consists of a defect in galactose-1-phosphate uridyl transferase (G-1-PUT), the enzyme that catalyzes the conversion of galactose-1-phosphate to galactose uridine diphosphate. At least seven forms of galactosemia have been described, based on the degree of completeness of the metabolic block. The onset of symptoms is in the first days of life, after the ingestion of milk; vomiting and diarrhea are followed by a failure to thrive. Drowsiness, inattention, hypotonia, and diminution

Table 38-1
Metabolic disorders and their estimated frequency among newborn infants in Massachusetts

Disorders	Total screened	Total detected	Frequency
Phenylketonuria*	981,361	67	1:15,000
Atypical phenylketonuria†	981,361	57	1:17,000
Iminoglycinuria	332,143	34?‡	1:10,000?‡
Cystinuria†	332,143	21	1:16,000
Hartnup disease	332,143	18	1:18,000
Histidinemia	332,143	18	1:18,000
Galactosemia*	550,000	5	1:110,000
Maple syrup urine disease*	842,004	5	1:170,000
Argininosuccinic acidemia*	332,143	5	1:70,000
Cystathioninemia	332,143	3	1:110,000
Homocystinuria*	449,615	3	1:150,000
Hyperglycinemia (nonketotic)*	332,143	2	1:170,000
Propionic acidemia*	332,143	1	1:300,000
Hyperlysinemia†	332,143	1	1:300,000
Hyperornithinemia†	332,143	1	1:300,000
Fanconi syndrome†	332,143	1	1:300,000

*Disorders with definite clinical complications.

†Disorders that may or may not be associated with clinical disease.

‡Number of cases and incidence for iminoglycinuria may be falsely high since carriers for this disorder who have only hyperglycinemia later in life may have iminoglycinuria as young infants.

Source: Levy.

in the vigor of neonatal automatisms then become evident. The fontanelles may bulge, the liver and spleen enlarge, the skin becomes yellow (in excess of neonatal jaundice), and anemia develops. Cataracts may form due to the accumulation of galactitol in the lens. Surviving infants show retarded psychomotor development, visual impairment, and residual cirrhosis, sometimes with splenomegaly and ascites. In one such patient, who died at 8 years, the main change in the brain was slight microencephaly with fibrous gliosis of the white matter and some loss of Purkinje

Table 38-2
Urinary screening tests for metabolic defects

Disease	Ferric chloride	DNPH*	Benedict's	Nitroprusside reaction
Phenylketonuria	Green	+	−	−
Maple syrup urine disease	Navy blue	+	−	−
Tyrosinemia	Pale green (transient)	+	±	−
Histidinemia	Green-brown	±	−	−
Propionic acidemia	Purple	+	−	−
Methylmalonic aciduria	Purple	+	−	−
Homocystinuria	−	−	−	+
Cystinuria	−	−	−	+
Galactosemia	−	−	+	−
Fructose intolerance	−	−	+	−

* Diaminophenylhydrazine.

and granule cells in the cerebellum, also with gliosis (Crome). The diagnostic laboratory findings are an elevated blood galactose level, low glucose, galactosuria, and deficiency of G-1-PUT in red and white blood cells and in liver cells. The treatment is essentially dietary, using milk substitutes.

Hyperglycinemia Two forms have been delineated: a ketotic and a nonketotic.

Ketotic hyperglycinemia (*propionic acidemia*) is an autosomal recessive disease, expressed clinically by episodes of vomiting, lethargy, coma, convulsions, hypertonia, and respiratory difficulty. The onset is in the neonatal or early infantile period and in time psychomotor retardation becomes evident. Death occurs usually within a few months. Propionic acid, glycine, various forms of fatty acids, and butanone are elevated in the serum. Milk protein and casein hydrolysate induce ketotic attacks.

Ketotic hyperglycinemia can occur with a number of organic acidurias of infancy. The most important of these are methylmalonic acidemia, isovaleric acidemia, and lactic acidemia. Each of these disorders presents in early infancy with profound metabolic acidosis and intermittent lethargy and coma, with early death in about half the patients and developmental retardation in those who survive. Rare subtypes of *methylmalonic acidemia* respond to vitamin B_{12}. In *isovaleric acidemia,* which is characterized by a striking odor of stale perspiration, marked restriction of dietary protein may prevent attacks of ketoacidosis and permit relatively good psychomotor development. Numerous metabolic defects, most commonly of pyruvate decarboxylase and pyruvate dehydrogenase, are responsible for the accumulation of lactic and pyruvic acids. The latter enzymatic defect has also been demonstrated in a recurrent form of cerebellar ataxia and athetosis and in Leigh disease, which are described further on in this chapter, and possibly in some cases of Friedreich ataxia (Chap. 43).

In the *nonketotic form* there are high levels of glycine but no acidosis, and the effects on the nervous system are more devastating. In the 30 or more reported cases (the authors have seen several) the neonate is hypotonic, listless, and dyspneic with dysconjugate eye movement, and seizures. A few survive to infancy but are extremely retarded and helpless. Spongy degeneration of the brain has been reported, both in this disease and in the ketotic form (Shuman et al). There is no treatment.

Inherited Hyperammonemic Syndromes These are a series of diseases caused by inborn deficiencies of the enzymes of the Krebs-Henseleit urea cycle and designated as carbamyl phosphate synthetase deficiency (type I hyperammonemia), ornithine transcarbamylase deficiency (type II hyperammonemia), citrullinemia, argininosuccinic aci-

duria, and hyperargininemia. Hyperornithemia and hyperlysinemia are closely related disorders. A detailed account of these inherited hyperammonemic syndromes is contained in the review by Walser.

The pattern of inheritance of each of these disorders is autosomal recessive except for type II hyperammonemia, which is an X-linked dominant trait. Their clinical manifestations are a common expression of an accumulation of ammonia or of urea cycle intermediates in the brain, and they differ only in severity, in accordance with the degree of completeness of the enzymatic deficiency and with the age of the affected individual.

In the most severe forms of these disorders, the infants are asymptomatic at birth and during the first few days of life, after which they refuse their feedings, vomit, and rapidly become inactive, lethargic, and lapse into an irreversible coma. Profuse sweating, focal or generalized seizures, rigidity with opisthotonus, and respiratory distress have been observed in the course of the illness.

In less severely affected infants, hyperammonemia develops after the onset of protein feeding. There is a failure to thrive, and attempts to enforce feeding or periods of constipation (which increase ammonia production in the bowel) may be accompanied by bouts of vomiting, extreme hyperirritability, and screaming. Diagnosis is established by the finding of hyperammonemia, as high as 1500 µg/dL in types I and II hyperammonemia. The precise biochemical diagnosis requires testing of blood and urine for amino acids or assays for specific enzymes in red cells or liver biopsies. The primary hyperammonemias need to be distinguished from the organic acidurias, including methylmalonic aciduria (see above), in which hyperammonemia can occur as a secondary metabolic abnormality.

In older infants and children, such as those with ornithine transcarbamylase deficiency (Kendall et al), the symptoms are even less severe or partial and are compatible with survival. This is particularly true of symptomatic female carriers (Rowe et al). Alternating hypertonia and hypotonia, seizures, ataxia, and periods of confusion, bizarre behavior, blurred vision, stupor and coma are the other major manifestations. The disease is sex-linked. Males tend to be more severely affected than heterozygous females. During episodes of stupor, brain edema may be seen by CT or MRI; in time, the brain edema gives way to atrophy and appears as symmetrical areas of decreased attenuation in the cerebral white matter. Between attacks, some patients with partial ornithine transcarbamylase deficiency may be normal or show only a slight hyperbilirubinemia (DiMagno et al, Rowe et al). With prolonged survival, signs of motor and mental retardation become evident, and the patient is vulnerable to repeated infections. In about half of the patients with argininosuccinic aciduria, there is an excessive dryness and brittleness of the hair (trichorrhexis nodosa). The diagnosis is established by measuring ornithine trans-carbamylase in the liver or in jejunal biopsy material.

In all the neonatal hyperammonemic diseases, the liver cell appears inadequate in one or more of its many metabolic functions, but how the enzymatic deficiencies or other disorders of amino acid metabolism affect the brain remains uncertain. It must be assumed that in some of them the saturation of the brain by ammonia impairs the oxidative metabolism of cerebral neurons, and when blood levels of ammonium increase (from protein ingestion, constipation, etc.), episodic coma or a more chronic impairment of cerebral functions occurs—as it does in cirrhosis of the liver and in portal-systemic encephalopathy.

The *treatment* of acute hyperammonemic syndromes is directed to the lowering of ammonium (by peritoneal dialysis, exchange transfusions, and administration of amino or keto acids). In more chronic cases treatment consists of decreasing the ammonium load (by dietary protein restriction and by administration of oral antibiotics, enemas, and lactulose). In infants with inborn errors of ureagenesis there is a constant danger of recurrent episodes of hyperammo-nemia and coma, particularly in response to infections. Early diagnosis is essential (plasma ammonium three times normal), and a systematic form of management (as outlined by Brusilow et al and by Msall et al) should be undertaken.

Maple Syrup Urine Disease and Variants These conditions are the result of inborn errors of branched-chain amino acid catabolism. Maple syrup urine disease may be taken as the prototype of the group. The pattern of inheritance is autosomal recessive. The infant appears normal at birth, but begins to feed poorly toward the end of the first week, and this is followed by the appearance of hypotonicity-apathy, diminished neonatal automatisms, convulsions, severe ketoacidosis, and often coma and death toward the end of the second to fourth week. Milder forms of the disease present with feeding difficulties that begin somewhat later in the early infantile period, followed by recurrent infections, episodic acidosis, and coma, and retarded psychomotor development with clumsiness, ataxia, and Babinski signs, or there may be a nonspecific mental retardation. The urine smells like maple syrup and gives a positive 2,4-dinitrophenylhydrazine (DNPH) test.

Other important laboratory findings are elevation of plasma and urine levels of leucine, isoleucine, valine, and keto acids. Secondary accumulation of a derivative of α-hydroxybutyric acid probably accounts for the maple syrup odor. The neuropathologic findings are uncertain; there appears to be a pallor and loss of myelin and gliosis of the cerebral white matter. Treatment by restriction of foods containing branched-chain amino acids (leucine, isoleucine, and valine) allows reasonably normal mental development. A thiamine-responsive variant with a slightly different pattern of ketoacids has been described by Prensky and Moser.

Sulfite Oxidase Deficiency This is an extremely rare disorder of sulfur metabolism, manifested clinically during the neonatal period by seizures, reduced level of responsivity, and spasms with opisthotonus. With survival into infancy, episodic confusion and stupor give way to seizures, mental retardation and ataxia. Shih et al have identified sulfite, thiosulfite, and *S*-sulfocysteine in the urine. Cerebral atrophy with loss and destruction of white matter and gray matter (cerebral cortex, basal ganglia, and cerebellar nuclei) have been observed in one postmortem examination. Increasing the intake of molybdenum or lowering the dietary intake of sulfur amino acids are theoretical therapeutic possibilities, as yet untried.

DIAGNOSIS OF NEONATAL METABOLIC DISEASES

An important clue, of course, is provided by a family history of an earlier neonatal disease or unexplained death in the same sibship or in a male maternal relative.

A history that protein foods are rejected by the infant, or even a history among relatives of dislike of protein or feeding difficulties in infancy, should raise the suspicion of an inherited hyperammonemic disorder. A mass screening program may disclose a biochemical abnormality; this is the optimal state of affairs especially if the information becomes available before symptoms appear.

A number of nonhereditary metabolic diseases must be distinguished from the hereditary ones. *Hypocalcemia* is one of the most frequent causes of neonatal seizures; tetany, spasms, and tremulous movements are usually present. Its cause is unknown, but the disorder is easily corrected, with excellent prognosis. Symptomatic *hypoglycemic reactions* are frequent in neonates. Premature infants are the most susceptible. With blood sugar levels of less than 30 mg/dL in the mature infant, and less than 20 mg/dL in the premature, there are convulsions, tremulousness, and drowsiness. Maternal toxemia and diabetes mellitus are also predisposing factors. Other causes are adrenal insufficiency, galactosemia, and an idiopathic form due to pancreatic islet-cell hyperplasia. The damaging effects of untreated hypoglycemia are well documented in the report of Koivisto and associates. *Cretinism* and *idiopathic hypercalcemia* are also recognizable entities at this age period.

The hereditary metabolic diseases must also be distinguished from a number of other catastrophic disorders that occur at or soon after birth, such as asphyxia, perinatal ventricular hemorrhage with the respiratory distress syndrome of hyaline membrane disease, other hypotensive-hypoxic states, erythroblastosis fetalis with kernicterus, neonatal bacterial meningitis, meningoencephalitis (herpes simplex, cytomegalic inclusion disease, listeriosis, rubella, syphilis, and toxoplasmosis), and hemorrhagic disease of the newborn.

THE HEREDITARY METABOLIC DISEASES OF EARLY INFANCY

The hallmark of all the hereditary metabolic diseases is psychosensorimotor regression. However, those that have their onset in the first year of life pose extraordinary problems in neurologic diagnosis. If the onset is in the first postnatal months, before the infant has had time to develop a complex repertoire of behavior, the first signs of disease may take the form of subtle delays in maturation rather than of psychomotor regression. Departures from normalcy include a lack of interest in surroundings, a lack of visual engagement, continued poor head control, an inability to sit up at the usual time, and poor hand-eye coordination. Of course, embryologic maldevelopment of the brain may have similar effects, and even systemic diseases and other visceral malformations such as cystic fibrosis of the pancreas, renal disease, biliary atresia and congenital heart disease, chronic infection, malnutrition, and seizures (with drug therapy) may appear to impede psychomotor development. Diagnosis becomes somewhat easier in the second half of the first year, especially if development in the first half had proceeded normally. Then an observant mother can perceive loss of certain early acquisitions, attesting to the progressive nature of the disease.

The most distinctive members of this category are the so-called lysosomal storage diseases. Here there is a genetic deficiency of the enzymes (usually one or more acid hydrolases) that are necessary for the degradation of specific glycosidic or peptide linkages in the intracytoplasmic lysosomes, causing them to become engorged with material that they would ordinarily degrade, with eventual damage to the nerve cell or myelin sheath. Most are classed as sphingolipidoses by Brady and his colleagues, who have deciphered the enzyme defect in many of them. A specific lysosomal enzyme is now known to degrade each of the glycoproteins, glycolipids, and mucopolysaccharides, by removing from them a monosaccharide or sulfate moiety.

It is the type of enzyme deficiency and accumulated metabolite, as well as the tissue distribution of the undegradable substrate, that impart a distinctive biochemical and clinical character to the disease. The concept of lysosomal storage diseases, introduced by Hers in 1965, has excited great interest among neurologists because of the potential for prenatal diagnosis and detection of carriers. The diagnosis of this group of diseases has been facilitated by the use of the CT scan and evoked potential techniques, which confirm the existence of the leukodystrophies, and by the electron microscopic examination of biopsies of skin or conjunctiva and circulating lymphocytes. One can see lysosomal storage material in nonneuronal cells as well as in cultured amniotic fluid cells. The activity of most lysosomal enzymes can be determined by the use of artificial chromogenic or fluorogenic substrates.

There are now more than 40 lysosomal "storage" diseases in which the biochemical abnormalities have been determined. They are listed in Table 38-3, which is adapted from the review of Kolodny and Cable. In addition to the sphingolipidoses, which are the lysosomal storage diseases most likely to be encountered in the first year of life, the table includes the storage diseases that are encountered in childhood and adolescence, to be considered later in the chapter.

The more frequent inherited metabolic diseases of infancy are listed below:

1. Tay-Sachs disease (G_{M2} gangliosidosis) and variants such as Sandhoff disease

2. Infantile Gaucher disease

3. Infantile Niemann-Pick disease

4. Infantile G_{M1} generalized gangliosidosis

5. Krabbe globoid-body leukodystrophy

6. Farber lipogranulomatosis

7. Pelizaeus-Merzbacher and other sudanophilic leukodystrophies

8. Spongy degeneration (Canavan–Van Bogaert)

9. Alexander disease

10. Alpers disease

11. Subacute necrotizing encephalomyelopathy

12. Congenital lactic acidosis

13. Zellweger encephalopathy

14. Lowe oculorenalcerebral disease

15. Kinky-hair or steely-hair disease

Table 38-3
Lysosomal storage diseases

	Enzyme deficiency	Accumulated metabolite
	Sphingolipidoses	

G_{M1} gangliosidosis
  Type 1—infantile, generalized
  Type 2—juvenile
	G_{M1} ganglioside β-galactosidase	G_{M1} ganglioside, galactose-containing oligosaccharides

G_{M2} gangliosidosis:		
Tay-Sachs disease	Hexosaminidase A	G_{M2} ganglioside
Sandhoff disease	Hexosaminidases A and B	G_{M2} ganglioside, globoside
AB variant	G_{M2} activator factor	G_{M2} ganglioside
Sulfatidoses		
Metachromatic leukodystrophy	Aryl sulfatase A	Sulfatide
Activator factor deficiency	Cerebroside sulfate sulfatase activator factor	Sulfatide
Mucosulfatidosis (multiple sulfatase deficiency)	Aryl sulfatases A, B, C; steroid sulfatase; iduronate sulfatase, heparan N-sulfatase	Sulfatide, steroid sulfate, heparan sulfate, dermatan sulfate
Krabbe disease	Galactocerebrosidase	Galactocerebroside
Fabry disease	α-Galactosidase A	Ceramide trihexoside
Gaucher disease		
Infantile form	β-Glucosidase	Glucocerebroside
Adult form	β-Glucosidase	Glucocerebroside
Niemann-Pick disease	Sphingomyelinase	Sphingomyelin
Farber disease	Ceramidase	Ceramide
	Mucopolysaccharidoses	
Hurler-Scheie syndrome	α-Iduronidase	Dermatan sulfate, heparan sulfate
Hunter disease	Iduronate sulfatase	Dermatan sulfate, heparan sulfate
Sanfilippo disease		
Type A	Heparan N-sulfatase	Heparan sulfate
Type B	α-N-Acetylglucosaminidase	Heparan sulfate
Type C	Heparan-N-acetyltransferase	Heparan sulfate
Type D	α-N-Glucosamine-6-sulfatase	Heparan sulfate
Morquio disease		
Type A	N-Acetylgalactosamine-6-sulfate sulfatase	Keratan sulfate
Type B	β-Galactosidase	Keratan sulfate
Maroteaux-Lamy disease	Arylsulfatase B	Dermatan sulfate
β-Glucuronidase deficiency (Sly disease)	β-Glucuronidase	Dermatan and heparan sulfate
	Mucolipidoses	
Type I	α-N-Acetylneuraminidase	Sialyloligosaccharides
Type II (I-cell disease)	Cellular deficiency of many lysosomal enzymes; increased levels of same enzymes extracellulary	Mucopolysaccharide, glycolipid
Type III (pseudo-Hurler polydystrophy)		
Type IV	Unknown	Mucopolysaccharide, ganglioside
	Oligosaccharidoses	
Fucosidosis	α-L-Fucosidase	Fucosyl-sphingolipids, oligosaccharides, and glycopeptides
Mannosidosis	α-Mannosidase	Mannosyl-oligosaccharides
Aspartylglucosaminuria	Aspartylglucosamine amide hydrolase	Aspartyl-2-deoxy-2-acetamidoglucosylamine
	Glycogenoses	
Pompe disease	α-Glucosidase	Glycogen
	Other lysosomal storage diseases:	
Wolman disease	Acid lipase	Cholesterol esters, triglycerides
Acid phosphatase deficiency	Lysosomal acid phosphatase	Phosphate esters

In the following descriptions, we have summarized the clinical and pathologic features of each of the diseases listed above, and have italicized the characteristic clinical signs and the corroborative laboratory tests.

TAY-SACHS DISEASE (G$_{M2}$ GANGLIOSIDOSIS)

This is an autosomal recessive disease, mostly of Jewish infants of eastern European background. The onset is in the first weeks and months of life, usually by the fourth month. The first manifestations are an abnormal *startle to acoustic stimuli*, listlessness, and irritability, followed by a *delay in psychomotor development* or regression (4 to 6 months), with loss of ability to roll over and sit. At first *axial hypotonia* is prominent, followed by *spasticity* and other corticospinal tract signs, visual failure, and *cherry-red spots* in the retinas in more than 90 percent of patients. In the second year, there are tonic-clonic or minor motor seizures and an increasing size of the head (diastasis of sutures) with relatively normal ventricles, and in the third year, dementia, decerebration, blindness, and cachexia; death occurs at 3 to 5 years. The EEG becomes abnormal in the early stages (paroxysmal slow waves with multiple spikes). Occasionally one observes basophilic granules in leukocytes and vacuoles in lymphocytes. There are no visceral, skeletal, or bone marrow abnormalities by light microscopy.

The basic enzymatic abnormality is a *deficiency of hexosaminidase A*, which normally cleaves the *N*-acetyl-galactosamine from gangliosides. The accumulation of gangliosides was the first detected abnormality, which explains why the term gangliosidoses was given to this class of disease. The enzyme defect can be found in the serum, white blood cells, and cultured fibroblasts from the amniotic fluid—allowing parents the option of abortion to prevent a presently untreatable disease. Testing for hexosaminidase A also permits the detection of heterozygote carriers of the gene defect.

The brain is large, sometimes twice the normal weight. In addition there is a loss of neurons and a reactive gliosis, and remaining nerve cells throughout the central nervous system are distended with glycolipid. Mucosal biopsies of the rectum disclose glycolipid distention of the ganglion cells. Under the electron microscope the particles of stored material appear as membranous cytoplasmic bodies. Retinal ganglion cells distended with the same material, together with fat-filled histiocytes, cause the whitish gray rings around the fovea, where there are no nerve cells (allowing the vascular choroid to appear as a red spot).

The same neuropathologic process has been found in a few congenital cases in which there was a rapidly progressive decline of a microcephalic infant. Kolodny and Raghavan have discussed two other variants, probably alleles of hexosamine A defect. One presents as a childhood spinocerebellar degeneration, the other as a progressive muscular atrophy in adults (see further on).

In *Sandhoff disease*, which affects non-Jewish infants, there is a deficiency of both hexosaminidase A and B, moderate hepatosplenomegaly, and coarse granulations in bone marrow histiocytes. In a few cases the visceral organs are not enlarged. The clinical and pathologic picture is the same as in Tay-Sachs disease except for the signs of visceral lipid storage.

INFANTILE GAUCHER DISEASE (TYPE II NEUROPATHIC FORM)

This is an autosomal recessive disease, without ethnic predominance. The onset is usually before 6 months and frequently before 3 months, with a more rapid course than Tay-Sachs disease (most patients with infantile Gaucher disease are dead by 1 year and 90 percent by 2 years). There is rapid loss of head control, ability to roll over and sit, and purposeful movements—along with apathy, irritability, frequent crying, and difficulty in sucking and swallowing. Progression is slower in some cases with acquisition of single words by the first year, bilateral corticospinal signs (Babinski signs and hyperactive reflexes), persistent *retroflexion of the neck,* and *strabismus.* Laryngeal stridor and trismus, diminished reaction to stimuli, smallness of the head, rare seizures, normal optic fundi, *enlarged spleen* and slightly enlarged liver, poor nutrition, skin and scleral pigmentation, and sometimes lymphadenopathy complete the clinical picture. The CSF is normal; the EEG is abnormal but nonspecific.

The important laboratory findings are an *increase in serum acid phosphatase and characteristic histiocytes (Gaucher cells) in marrow* smears and liver biopsies. A *deficiency of glucocerebrosidase* in leukocytes and hepatocytes is diagnostic; glucocerebroside accumulates in the involved tissues. The characteristic pathologic features are the Gaucher cells (20 to 60 μm in diameter, with a wrinkled appearance of the cytoplasm and eccentricity of the nucleus) in marrow, lungs, and other viscera; a few of these cells can also be found in the brain, but here the main abnormality is a loss of nerve cells, particularly in the bulbar nuclei, and a reactive gliosis.

Type I Gaucher disease is nonneuropathic. A third type of Gaucher disease expresses itself in late childhood or adolescence by a slowly progressive mental decline, seizures, and ataxia, and later, by spastic weakness. Vision and retinae remain normal. The nucleotide sequence of the cloned glucocerebrosidase of type I Gaucher disease was found by Tsuji et al to be different from that of types II and III.

INFANTILE NIEMANN-PICK DISEASE

This also is an autosomal recessive disease. Two-thirds of the reported cases have been of Ashkenazi Jewish parentage. The onset of symptoms is between 3 and 9 months of age, frequently with marked *enlargement of liver, spleen, and lymph nodes;* rarely there is jaundice and ascites. *Cerebral deterioration* is definite by the end of the first year, often earlier; the usual manifestations are loss of spontaneous movements, lack of interest in the environment, axial hypotonia with bilateral corticospinal signs, *blindness* and *amaurotic nystagmus,* and *a macular red spot* (in about one-quarter of the patients). Seizures occur relatively late. There is no acoustic myoclonus, and head size is normal or slightly reduced. Loss of tendon reflexes and slowed nerve conduction have been reported, but are rare. Protuberant eyes, mild hypertelorism, pigmentation of oral mucosa and dysplasia of dental enamel have also been reported in rare instances. Most patients succumb to intercurrent infection by the end of the second year. *Vacuolated histiocytes ("foam cells") in the bone marrow and vacuolated blood lymphocytes* are the important laboratory findings. A *deficiency of sphingomyelinase* in leukocytes, cultured fibroblasts, and hepatocytes is diagnostic. Neurons are decreased in number and many of those that remain are pale, ballooned, and granular. The most prominent changes may be seen in the midbrain, spinal cord, and cerebellum. The white matter is little affected. The retinal cell changes are similar to those in the brain. The foamy histiocytes (Niemann-Pick cells) that fill the viscera contain sphingomyelin and cholesterol; the distended nerve cells contain mainly sphingomyelin.

The late infantile and juvenile forms of Niemann-Pick disease are discussed in a later section of this chapter (page 796).

INFANTILE, GENERALIZED (TYPE I) G$_{M1}$ GANGLIOSIDOSIS (FAMILIAL NEUROVISCERAL LIPIDOSIS, PSEUDO-HURLER DISEASE)

This is probably an autosomal recessive disease, and is without ethnic predominance. The infants appear abnormal at birth, with *dysmorphic facial features* like those of the

mucopolysaccharidoses (depressed and wide nasal bridge, frontal bossing, hypertelorism, epicanthi, puffy eyelids, long upper lip, gingival and alveolar hypertrophy, macroglossia, low-set ears). Other indications of the disease are an early onset of impaired awareness; reduced responsivity in the first days or weeks of life; *no psychomotor development* after 3 to 6 months; hypotonia and later hypertonia with lively tendon reflexes and Babinski signs. Seizures are frequent. The head size is variable (microcephaly more often than macrocephaly). *Loss of vision, coarse nystagmus and strabismus, macular cherry-red spots* (in half the cases), flexion pseudocontractures of elbows and knees, kyphoscoliosis, and *enlarged liver and sometimes spleen* are the other important clinical findings. Radiographic abnormalities include subperiosteal bone formation, midshaft widening, demineralization, and hypoplasia and beaking of the thoracolumbar vertebras. Vacuoles are seen in 10 to 80 percent of blood lymphocytes, and foam cells in the urinary sediment. A *partial or complete deficiency of β-galactosidase* and accumulation of G$_{M1}$ ganglioside in the brain and viscera are the specific biochemical abnormalities. Neurons and glial cells throughout the CNS are swollen with G$_{M1}$ ganglioside. In addition, the epithelial cells of the renal glomeruli, the histiocytes of the spleen, and the liver cells contain a modified keratan sulfate and a galactose-containing oligosaccharide. The changes in the bone are like those seen in the Hurler form of mucopolysaccharidosis. The disease should be suspected in a child who has the facial features of mucopolysaccharidosis and severe neurologic abnormalities.

A remarkable benign variant, also inherited as an autosomal recessive trait, begins later in childhood but may advance so slowly as to allow attainment of adult life. Dystonia, myoclonus, seizures, and macular red spots featured the two cases described by Goldman et al.

GLOBOID CELL LEUKODYSTROPHY (KRABBE DISEASE)

This is an autosomal recessive disease without ethnic predilection. The onset is usually before the sixth month and often before the third month (10 percent after 1 year). *Generalized rigidity,* loss of head control, diminished alertness, frequent vomiting, hyperirritability and bouts of inexplicable crying, and spasms induced by stimulation are early manifestations. With increasing muscular tone *opisthotonic recurvation* of neck and trunk develop. Later signs are adduction of legs, flexion of arms, clenching of fists, Babinski signs, and hyperactive reflexes. In other cases tendon reflexes are depressed or lost. Blindness and optic atrophy supervene. Convulsions occur but are rare and difficult to distinguish from tonic spasms. The head size is normal or rarely slightly increased. In the last stage, which may occur one to several months after the onset, the child is blind and usually deaf, opisthotonic, irritable, and cachectic. Most patients are dead by the end of the first year, and survival beyond two years is unusual.

The EEG shows nonspecific slowing without spikes, and the *CSF protein is usually elevated* (70 to 450 mg/dL). CT scans show symmetrical nonenhancing areas of increased density in the internal capsules and basal ganglia, with involvement of more of the cerebral white matter and brainstem as the disease advances.

Clinical signs of neuropathy are difficult to detect, except for a decrease or loss of tendon reflexes, but *EMG evidence of denervation and decrease in motor nerve conduction velocity* are frequent findings.

The deficient enzyme in Krabbe disease is *galactocerebrosidase*, resulting in the accumulation of galactocerebroside, particularly in the cerebral white matter. Gross examination of the brain discloses a marked reduction in the cerebral white matter, which feels firm and rubbery. Microscopically, there are widespread myelin degeneration and gliosis in the cerebrum, brainstem, spinal cord, and nerves; the characteristic globoid cells (abnormal, large histiocytes containing accumulated metabolite) and Schwann cells with tubular or crystalloid inclusions are present in electron-microscopic preparations.

About a dozen variant examples of globoid cell leukodystrophy have been reported, in which neurologic regression begins in the 2- to 6-year period. Visual failure with optic atrophy and normal electroretinogram is an early finding. Later there are ataxia, spastic weakness of the legs, mental regression, and finally decerebration. In three personally observed patients, a progressive quadriparesis with mild pseudobulbar signs, slow regression in memory and other mental functions, dystonic posturing of the arms, and preserved sphincteric control constituted the clinical picture. The patients are alive at ages 9, 12, and 16 years. These CNS abnormalities are unaccompanied by any changes in the spinal fluid. The nerve conduction velocities in the late-onset form, unlike those in the infantile form, are normal. Galactocerebrosidase levels are not as much reduced as in the infantile form; possibly the late-onset variant represents a structural mutation of the enzyme (see Farrell and Swedberg).

LIPOGRANULOMATOSIS (FARBER DISEASE)

This is a very rare disorder that is probably genetic, affecting both sexes and without any particular racial predilection. The onset is in the first weeks of life, with a *hoarse cry* (fixation of laryngeal cartilage), respiratory distress, and sensitivity of the joints—followed by characteristic *periarticular* and *subcutaneous swellings* and *progressive arthropathy* leading to ankylosis. Usually there is severe

psychomotor retardation, but a few patients have appeared neurologically normal. Inanition and recurrent infections lead to death in the first 2 years. The diagnostic abnormality is a *deficiency of ceramidase* leading to accumulation of ceramide. There is widespread lipid storage in neurons and in granulomas in the skin, and accumulation of PAS-positive macrophages in periarticular and visceral tissues.

SUDANOPHILIC LEUKODYSTROPHIES AND PELIZAEUS-MERZBACHER DISEASE

These are a heterogeneous group of disorders that have in common a defective myelination of the cerebrum, brainstem, cerebellum, spinal cord, and peripheral nerves. Morphologic peculiarities and genetic features separate a certain group called *Pelizaeus-Merzbacher disease;* other types are artificially delineated, and as a result a relatively meaningless terminology has been introduced.

Pelizaeus-Merzbacher Disease   This is predominantly an X-linked disease of childhood and adolescence and includes other closely related pathologic entities with different modes of inheritance. The onset may be in the first months of life or later in childhood. The first signs are *abnormal movements of the eyes* (rapid, irregular, often asymmetrical pendular nystagmus) and intermittent shaking movements of the head (like spasmus nutans), followed by spastic weakness of the limbs, *ataxia,* intention tremor, choreiform or athetotic movements of arms, and slow psychomotor development with failure to sit, stand, and walk. Seizures occur occasionally. In cases developing later, pendular nystagmus, choreoathetosis, corticospinal signs, dysarthria, cerebellar ataxia, and mental deterioration are the major manifestations. Patients may survive to the second and third decades. One group of cases resembles the Cockayne syndrome with photosensitivity of skin, dwarfism, cerebellar ataxia, corticospinal signs, cataracts, retinitis pigmentosa, and deafness. Pathologically, islands of preserved myelin give a tigroid pattern of degenerated and intact myelin in the cerebrum.

Unclassified Sporadic and Familial Sudanophilic Leukodystrophies   There are two types of disorder, one with early and the other with late onset. In the former, onset is before 3 months with survival of less than 2 years; in the latter type, onset is from 3 to 7 years, and the course is chronic. *Psychomotor regression; spastic paralysis; incoordination; blindness and optic atrophy; seizures (rare); severe microcephaly;* and absence of skeletal, visceral, and hematologic evidence of the metabolic abnormality are the main features. No characteristic laboratory abnormalities are known. Diffuse degeneration of medullated fibers with phagocytosis of sudanophilic-degeneration products of myelin (visible by MRI) and gliosis are the major changes.

SPONGY DEGENERATION OF INFANCY (CANAVAN-VAN BOGAERT-BERTRAND DISEASE)

This is an autosomal recessive disease. Of 48 affected families reported by Banker and Victor, 28 were Jewish. Onset is early, often recognizable in the first 3 months of life. There is either a lack or rapid *regression of psychomotor function, loss of sight and optic atrophy,* lethargy, difficulty in sucking, irritability, reduced motor activity, hypotonia followed by spasticity of the limbs with corticospinal signs, and an *enlarged head* (macrocephaly). There are no visceral or skeletal abnormalities. Seizures occur in some cases. An interesting but unexplored aspect of the disease is the occurrence of blond hair and light complexion in affected members, in contrast to the darker hair and complexion of their normal siblings (Banker and Victor). The CSF is usually normal, but the protein is slightly elevated in some cases; there are no diagnostic biochemical abnormalities. CT scanning reveals a *decreased attenuation of cerebral and cerebellar white matter in an enlarged brain with relatively normal ventricles,* features that are diagnostic of this disease.

The characteristic pathologic changes are an increase in brain volume (and weight), spongy degeneration in the deep layers of the cerebral cortex and subcortical white matter, widespread loss of myelin involving the convolutional more than the central white matter, loss of Purkinje cells, and hyperplasia of Alzheimer type II astrocytes throughout the cerebral cortex and basal ganglia. Adachi et al have demonstrated an abnormal accumulation of fluid in astrocytes and between splitting myelin lamellae, and have suggested that the loss of myelin is secondary to these changes.

The disease has to be distinguished clinically from G_{M2} gangliosidosis, Alexander disease, Krabbe disease, and nonprogressive megalocephaly, and pathologically from a variety of disorders that are characterized by vacuolation of nervous tissue.

ALEXANDER DISEASE

The classification of this rare disease is uncertain. A familial incidence has not been reported, and no metabolic fault has

been defined. It shares certain features with the leukodystrophies and gray matter diseases, both clinically and pathologically. The onset is in infancy with *a failure to thrive, psychomotor retardation, and seizures.* An early and progressive *macrocephaly* has been a consistent feature. Pathologically, there are severe destructive changes in the cerebral white matter, most intense in the frontal lobes. Eosinophilic hyaline bodies, most prominent just below the pia and around blood vessels, are seen throughout the cerebral cortex, brainstem, and spinal cord. These have been identified as *Rosenthal fibers* and probably represent glial degradation products.

ALPERS DISEASE

This is a progressive disease of the cerebral gray matter, known also as progressive cerebral poliodystrophy and diffuse cerebral degeneration in infancy. A familial form (probably autosomal recessive) and some sporadic cases are known, with a certain uniformity of clinical features— *seizures* and *diffuse myoclonic jerks* from early infancy, followed by incoordination of movements; *progressive spasticity* of limb, trunk, and cranial muscles; blindness and optic atrophy; growth retardation and increasing microcephaly; and finally, virtual decortication. In some instances, the late onset of jaundice and fatty degeneration or cirrhosis of the liver have been described; the hepatic changes are distinctive and probably not related to the use of anticonvulsant drugs (Harding et al). The nature of this combined hepatic-cerebral degeneration remains unexplained. EEG changes, progressive atrophy (particularly occipital) on CT scan, loss of visual evoked potentials, and abnormal liver function tests may be diagnostically useful. Neuropathologic examination shows marked atrophy of the cerebral convolutions and cerebellar cortex with loss of nerve cells and fibrous gliosis. Hypoglycemic, hypoxic, and hypotensive encephalopathies need always to be considered in the diagnosis, but can usually be identified by knowledge of the occurrence of such catastrophies.

SUBACUTE NECROTIZING ENCEPHALOMYELOPATHY (SNE, LEIGH DISEASE)

This is a familial disorder of autosomal recessive type with a wide range of clinical manifestations. The onset, in more than half the cases, is in the first year of life, mostly before the sixth month. Loss of head control and other recent motor acquisitions, hypotonia, poor sucking, anorexia and vomiting, irritability and continuous crying, generalized seizures and myoclonic jerks constitute the usual clinical picture. If the onset is in the second year, there are difficulties in walking, ataxia, dysarthria, intellectual regression, tonic spasms, *characteristic respiratory disorders* (episodic hyperventilation, periods of apnea, gasping, quiet sobbing), *external ophthalmoplegia*, nystagmus, and disorders of gaze (like those of Wernicke disease), *paralysis of deglutition*, and abnormal movements of the limbs (jerky, choreiform, ataxic). Peripheral nerves are involved in some cases (areflexia, weakness, atrophy, and slowed conduction velocity). In some children the disease is episodic, in others intermittently progressive and quite protracted, with exacerbation of neurologic symptoms in association with nonspecific infections. CSF is usually normal, but the protein may be elevated.

The pathologic changes take the form of bilaterally symmetric foci of necrosis and spongiform degeneration, vascular proliferation, and gliosis in the thalami, midbrain, pons, medulla, and spinal cord. Also, demyelinative lesions are present in the peripheral nerves. In their distribution and histologic appearance the CNS lesions of SNE resemble those of Wernicke disease, except that the lesions of SNE tend to be more extensive—sometimes involving the striatum—and they tend to spare the mammillary bodies. The lesions may be visible in CT scans and are strikingly demonstrated by MR imaging.

The clinical boundaries of Leigh disease have not been defined precisely. A familial disorder of infancy and early childhood, referred to as bilateral *striatal necrosis* and associated with dystonia, visual failure, and other neurologic defects, may represent a variant of Leigh disease. The same may be true for a distinctive clinical syndrome of mitochondrial myopathy, encephalopathy, lactic acidosis, and stroke-like episodes (MELAS), described by Pavlakis et al.

Leigh disease is characterized by a number of biochemical abnormalities. Pincus and his colleagues described a substance in the patient's urine, blood, and CSF that inhibits thiamine pyrophosphate—ATP phosphoryl transferase, an enzyme that catalyzes the formation of thiamine triphosphate (TTP) from thiamine pyrophosphate. However, this abnormality has not been found consistently. The administration of massive doses of thiamine chloride has reportedly caused an improvement in the neurologic status of some patients, but the effect has not been sustained.

Pyruvate metabolism appears to be altered in this disease, as indicated by the occurrence of lactic acidosis and the elevation of pyruvate, lactate, and α-ketoglutarate in the blood. The original suggestion by Hommes et al, that the cause of SNE is an isolated deficiency of pyruvate carboxylase, has not been substantiated (Sander et al). Moreover, such a deficiency has been identified in a number of infants who showed none of the clinical or pathologic signs of SNE.

Kerr and his colleagues have described a pathologically proven case of SNE that was characterized biochem-

ically by a defect in pyruvate dehydrogenase, but this defect has not been found in other cases of this disease. DeVivo and coworkers have adduced evidence that the fundamental biochemical disturbance is a failure in the activation mechanism of the pyruvate dehydrogenase complex (a group of five enzymes that are involved in the oxidative decarboxylation of pyruvate to acetyl CoA) rather than a defect of individual members of the complex, such as pyruvate carboxylase or pyruvate dehydrogenase.

CONGENITAL LACTIC ACIDOSIS

This is a very rare disease of the neonatal period or early infancy, of unproven genetic etiology. The symptoms have consisted of *psychomotor regression* and *episodic hyperventilation, hypotonia,* and *convulsions,* with intervening periods of normalcy. *Choreoathetosis* has been observed in a few cases. Death usually occurs before the third year. The important laboratory findings are *acidosis with high lactate levels* and hyperalininemia. The defect is probably in the pyruvate dehydrogenase complex of enzymes, which function in the oxidative decarboxylation of pyruvate to acetyl CoA. The few cases that have been examined post mortem have shown necrosis and cavitation of the globus pallidus and cerebral white matter. Possibly this disorder is a variant of Leigh disease. It needs to be distinguished from the several diseases of infancy that are complicated by lactic acidosis.

THE CEREBROHEPATORENAL (ZELLWEGER) SYNDROME

This disease, estimated to occur once in every 100,000 births, is inherited as an autosomal recessive trait. It has its onset in the neonatal period or early infancy, and leads to death usually within a few months. Motor inactivity and hypotonia, *dysmorphic alterations of the skull and face* (high forehead, shallow orbits, hypertelorism, highly arched palate, abnormal helices of ears, retrognathia), poor visual fixation, *multifocal seizures,* swallowing difficulties, flexion fixation of the limbs, *cataracts,* abnormal retinal pigmentation, optic atrophy, cloudy corneas, *hepatomegaly,* and hepatic dysfunction are the usual manifestations. Stippled, irregular calcifications of the patellae and greater trochanters are highly characteristic. There are no distinctive biochemical abnormalities. Pathologically, there are dysgenesis of the cerebral cortex and degeneration of white matter, as well as a number of visceral abnormalities—cortical renal cysts, hepatic fibrosis, intrahepatic biliary dysgenesis, agenesis of the thymus, and iron storage in the reticuloendothelial system.

Neonatal Adrenoleukodystrophy and Zellweger Disease   Recently, A. E. Moser et al have demonstrated a fivefold increase of very long chain fatty acids, particularly hexacosenoic acid, in the plasma and cultured skin fibroblasts from 35 patients with the Zellweger syndrome. A similar abnormality was found in cultured amniocytes of women at risk of bearing a child with the Zellweger syndrome, thus permitting prenatal diagnosis. The findings of Moser et al are in keeping with the current notions about the basic abnormality in the Zellweger syndrome, namely that it is due to a lack of liver peroxisomes (oxidase-containing, membrane-bound cytoplasmic organelles), in which the very long chain fatty acids are normally oxidized (Goldfischer et al). Their proposal is that Zellweger disease, which is inherited as an autosomal recessive trait, and neonatal adrenoleukodystrophy, a sex-linked recessive trait, both belong to a newly recognized class of peroxisomal diseases. However, the pattern of these very long chain fatty acids is different in the two disorders.

In the authors' opinion, this finding does not establish the identity of the two diseases. Nor do Moser et al declare that it does.

THE OCULOCEREBRORENAL (LOWE) SYNDROME

Here the mode of inheritance is probably X-linked recessive, although sporadic cases have been reported in girls. The clinical abnormalities comprise *bilateral cataracts* (which may be present at birth) and *glaucoma,* large eyes with megalocornea and buphthalmos, corneal opacities and blindness, pendular nystagmus, hypotonia and absent or depressed tendon reflexes, corticospinal signs without paralysis, slow movements of the hands, high-pitched cry, occasional seizures, and *psychomotor regression.* Later the frontal bones become prominent and the eyes sunken. The characteristic biochemical abnormality is a renal tubular acidosis and death is usually from *renal failure.* Additional laboratory findings include demineralization of bones and typical rachitic deformities, anemia, metabolic acidosis, and generalized aminoaciduria. The neuropathologic changes are nonspecific; inconstant atrophy and poor myelination have been described in the brain, and tubular abnormalities in the kidneys. Differential diagnosis is from the Zellweger syndrome.

KINKY-HAIR OR STEELY-HAIR DISEASE (MENKES DISEASE)

This is a rare disorder, inherited as a sex-linked recessive trait. In most of our cases, birth was premature. Poor feeding and failure to gain weight, instability of temperature (mainly *hypothermia*), and *seizures* become apparent in early infancy. The hair is normal at birth, but the secondary growth is lusterless and depigmented; strands of hair break easily and feel like steel wool, and under the microscope they appear twisted (*pili torti*). Radiologic examination shows *metaphyseal spurring,* mainly of the femora, and subperiosteal calcifications of the shafts. Arteriography discloses *tortuosity and elongation of the cerebral and systemic arteries,* and occlusion of some of them. There is no discernible neurologic development, and rarely does the child survive beyond the second year. Three of our cases have been examined post mortem (Williams et al). There is diffuse loss of neurons in the relay nuclei of the thalamus, the cerebral cortex and cerebellum (granule and stellate cells), and dendritic arborizations of residual neurons of the motor cortex and Purkinje cells.

The manifestations of this disease are attributable to a profound deficiency of copper. The *basic defect is in the absorption of copper from the gastrointestinal tract* (Danks). Further, since copper fails to cross the placenta, a severe reduction of copper in the brain and liver is evident from birth. In this sense, the abnormality of copper metabolism is the opposite of that in Wilson disease. Parenteral administration of cupric salts restores the serum and hepatic copper, but its effect on the clinical symptoms remains to be determined.

DIAGNOSIS OF INHERITED METABOLIC DISEASES OF INFANCY

It will be recognized, from the foregoing synopses, that many of the neurologic manifestations of the inherited metabolic diseases of infancy are nonspecific and are common to most or all of the diseases in this group. In general, in the early stages of all these diseases there is a loss of postural tone and a paucity of movement, without paralysis or loss of reflexes; later there is spasticity with hyperreflexia and Babinski signs. Equally nonspecific are features such as irritability and prolonged crying; poor feeding, difficulty in swallowing, inanition and retarded growth; failure of fixation of gaze and following (often misinterpreted as blindness); and tonic spasms, clonic jerks, and focal and generalized seizures.

In general terms, the differentiation of the inherited metabolic diseases of infancy rests upon four types of data: (1) a few highly characteristic neurologic and ophthalmic signs; (2) the presence of an enlarged liver and spleen; (3)

special dysmorphic features of the face; and (4) the results of certain relatively simple laboratory tests, such as radiographs of the thoracolumbar spine, hips, and long bones, smears of the peripheral blood and bone marrow, CSF examination, and certain biochemical estimations. Attention to these particular clinical and laboratory features, tabulated below, permits the correct diagnosis in most cases.

Neurologic signs that are more or less specific to certain metabolic diseases include the following:

1. Acousticomotor obligatory startle: Tay-Sachs disease

2. Abolished tendon reflexes with definite Babinski signs: globoid cell (Krabbe) leukodystrophy, occasionally Leigh disease, and (beyond infancy) metachromatic leukodystrophy

3. Peculiar eye movements, pendular nystagmus, and head rolling: Pelizaeus-Merzbacher disease, Leigh disease; later, hyperbilirubinemia and Lesch-Nyhan hyperuricemia (see further on)

4. Marked rigidity, opisthotonus, and tonic spasms: Krabbe, infantile Gaucher, or Alpers disease

5. Intractable seizures and generalized or multifocal myoclonus: Alpers disease

6. Intermittent hyperventilation: Leigh disease and congenital lactic acidosis (also nonprogressive familial agenesis of vermis)

Ocular abnormalities of specific diagnostic value include the following:

1. Rapid pendular nystagmus: Pelizaeus-Merzbacher disease, rarely Krabbe leukodystrophy

2. Macular cherry-red spots: Tay-Sachs disease and Sandhoff variant, some cases of infantile Niemann-Pick disease, and rarely lipofuscinosis

3. Corneal opacification: Lowe disease, infantile G_{M1} gangliosidosis; later, the mucopolysaccharidoses

4. Cataracts: galactosemia, Lowe disease, Zellweger disease (also congenital rubella)

Other medical findings of specific diagnostic value:

1. Dysmorphic facies: generalized G_{M1} gangliosidosis, Lowe and Zellweger syndromes, and some early cases of mucopolysaccharidosis and mucolipidosis

2. Enlarged liver and spleen: infantile Gaucher disease and Niemann-Pick disease; one type of hyperammonemia; Sandhoff disease; later, the mucopolysaccharidoses and mucolipidoses

3. Enlarging head without hydrocephalus (macrocephaly): spongy degeneration of infancy, some cases of Tay-Sachs disease, Alexander disease

4. Beaking of vertebral bodies in radiographs: G_{M1} gangliosidosis (and, at a more advanced age, the mucopolysaccharidoses, fucosidosis, mannosidosis, and the mucolipidoses)

5. Multiple arthropathies and raucous dysphonia: Farber disease

6. Storage granules and vacuolated lymphocytes: Niemann-Pick disease, generalized G_{M1} gangliosidosis

7. Abnormal histiocytes in marrow smears: Gaucher cells, foamy histiocytes in Niemann-Pick disease, generalized G_{M1} gangliosidosis and closely related diseases, Farber disease

8. Colorless, friable hair: Menkes disease

INHERITED METABOLIC DISEASES OF LATE INFANCY AND EARLY CHILDHOOD

Included here are the diseases that become manifest between the ages of 1 and 4 years. Diagnosis is less difficult than in the neonate and young infant. A morbid process in the nervous system is reliably ascertained by the obvious progression of a neurologic disorder, such as a loss of ability to walk and to speak, which usually parallels a regression in other high-level (quasi-intellectual) functions. Embryologic anomalies, prenatal diseases, and birth injuries can be excluded with relative certainty if psychomotor development was normal in the first year or two. Diseases characterized by seizures and myoclonus may prove more difficult to interpret, for the seizures may occur at any age from a variety of antecedent or immediate neurologic causes, and, if frequent, may cause a significant impairment of psychomotor function. The effects of anticonvulsant medications may add to the impairment of diencephalocortical function. Unfortunately, most of the slowly advancing metabolic diseases of the second year may be so subtle in their effects that for a time the physician cannot be sure whether a regression of intellectual functions is taking place or mental retardation is becoming apparent for the first time. To distinguish the two is more difficult if the parents have been unobservant. Repeated examination and testing will usually settle the matter. Suspicion of a progressive encephalopathy is heightened by the presence of certain ocular, visceral, and skeletal abnormalities, as described below.

Once a neurologic syndrome is clearly established, there is an advantage in determining whether its main characteristics reflect a disorder of the cerebral white matter (oligodendrocytes and myelin) or of gray matter (neurons). Indicative of white matter (*leukodystrophies* or leukoencephalopathies) are early onset of spastic paralysis of the limbs, with or without ataxia; loss of tendon reflexes; and visual impairment with optic atrophy but normal retinae. Seizures and intellectual deterioration are late events. Indicative of gray matter disease (*poliodystrophies* or polioencephalopathies) are early onset of seizures, myoclonus, blindness with retinal changes, mental regression, choreoathetosis and ataxia; spastic paralysis and signs of sensory-motor tract involvement occur later. Neuronal storage diseases, such as the ones described in the previous section, as well as neuroaxonal dystrophy and the lipofuscinoses conform to the pattern of gray matter diseases (Table 38-4). Metachromatic, globoid-body, and sudanophilic leukodystrophy exemplify white matter diseases (Table 38-5). This mode of categorization of the inherited metabolic diseases, though introduced in this section, is appropriate at all age periods and is also a useful device in the categorization of developmental, heredodegenerative, and other types of nervous system disease.

The following are inherited metabolic diseases that occur most frequently in late infancy and early childhood:

1. Many of the milder disorders of amino acid metabolism

2. Metachromatic leukodystrophy

3. Late infantile G_{M1} gangliosidosis

4. Late infantile Gaucher disease and Niemann-Pick disease

5. Neuroaxonal dystrophy

6. The mucopolysaccharidoses

7. The mucolipidoses

8. Fucosidosis

9. The mannosidoses

10. Aspartylglycosaminuria

11. Jansky-Bielschowsky ceroid lipofuscinosis

12. Cockayne syndrome

THE AMINOACIDURIAS

As was pointed out in the first part of this chapter, only a few of the many aminoacidurias declare their existence in the neonatal and early infantile period of life. More often the only clinical manifestation is simply a lag in psychomotor development which, if mild, does not become evident until the second and third years, or later. Like other inherited metabolic disorders, the aminoacidurias do not derange growth, development, and maturation in utero or interfere with parturition. No physical sign betrays their presence in the early months of life. The only possibility of detection is by screening all newborns. The relative frequency of these diseases is indicated in Table 38-1, and the practical tests for their identification are summarized in Table 38-2.

The aminoacidurias of the late infantile and early childhood period—phenylketonuria (PKU) and Hartnup disease—will be described here because of their clinical importance, and because they exemplify different types of biochemical defect. Reference will also be made to other aminoacidurias, described in the first part of this chapter, which, like Hartnup disease, cause intermittent ataxia. Only passing reference will be made to the other aminoacidurias, which are exceedingly rare or have only an uncertain effect upon the nervous system. A detailed and current account of these disorders can be found in the monograph of Scriver et al.

The Phenylketonurias (PKU) Apart from being the most frequent of the aminoacidurias, this entity has a unique historical significance. In the nearly 55 years that have elapsed since its discovery by Følling, it has become a classic example of a disorder that illustrates three principles of medical genetics. First, it is inherited as an autosomal recessive trait in accordance with Mendel's law of segregation. Second, PKU exemplifies Garrod's cardinal principle of gene action in which genetic factors specify chemical reactions and biochemical individuality. Third, PKU is a disease, and hyperphenylalinemia is a phenotype only when the allele is expressed in an environment that contains an abundance of L-phenylalanine. Thus, as recognized by Galton, the ultimate phenotype is a product of "nature and nurture" (Scriver and Clow).

One must refer to the phenylketonurias in the plural, for there are (1) the usual type and several mild and and severe variants thereof, in which phenylalanine (PA) tolerance is reduced and mental retardation is invariable if the disease is not treated early in life, and (2) other types, in which there is hyperphenylalininemia without phenylketonuria and without effect on the nervous system. Also there are a small number of patients (3 percent in our series) in whom a lowering of the hyperphenylalininemia does not prevent the progression of the neurologic lesion. At birth, the typical PKU infant has a normal nervous system. The disease appears later, only after long exposure of the nervous system to PA. The homozygous infant lacks the means of protecting the nervous system. However, if the mother is homozygous with high PA levels in the blood (and the infant is heterozygous), the CNS is damaged in utero and the infant is born mentally retarded.

Table 38-4
Differential diagnosis of poliodystrophies of infancy

	Tay-Sachs	Niemann-Pick	Gaucher	Alpers	Subacute necrotizing encephalopathy
Age of onset	4–6 months	Under 6 months	Under 6 months	Under 1 year	Under 1 year, rarely late childhood
Rate of progression	Rapid Death 2–3 years	Rapid Death before 3 years	Very rapid Death before 2 years	Rapid Death before 3 years	Usually rapid Death before 3 years
Ethnic group	Almost all Jewish	50% Jewish			
Genetic	Recessive	Recessive	Recessive		Recessive
Head size	Enlarges late	Normal	Normal	Reduces late	Normal
Skin and/or systemic lesions	Normal	Hepatosplenomegaly Xanthoma of skin, rare	Hepato-splenomegaly	Normal	Normal
Eye	Cherry-red macula Optic atrophy	Cherry-red macula Optic atrophy	Normal	Normal	Optic atrophy
Seizures	Frequent, but late	Rare	Rare	Onset with seizures Myoclonus and other types	Seizures late and rare
Neurologic signs	Early: flaccid paresis Late: spastic paresis Dementia: early Hyperacusis	Spastic paresis Early: dementia	Early: retroflexion of head, dementia Strabismus Bulbar palsy Spastic paralysis	Spastic paresis Dementia Cortical blindness and deafness	Bulbar palsy Weak, infrequent cry Flaccid paresis with immobility
Blood	Absent fructose-1-phosphate-aldolase ↑ SGOT ↑ Vacuolated lymphocytes	↑ Serum lipids ↑ SGOT ↑ Vacuolated lymphocytes	↑ Acid phosphatase	Normal	Normal
Urine	Normal	Normal	Normal	Normal	Normal
CSF	Normal	Normal		Normal	Normal
Biopsy	Rectal	"Foam cells" in bone marrow	Gaucher cells in bone marrow		
X-ray		Diffuse pulmonary infiltrates Demineralization of bone			

Electroretinogram Normal
Diagnostic biochemical abnormality See text

Source: Adapted from AL Drew, Jr, in S Carter, AP Gold (eds), *Neurology of Infancy and Childhood,* New York, Appleton-Century-Crofts, 1974.

In the classic form of PKU, the lag in *psychomotor development* can usually be recognized in the latter part of the first year; by 5 to 6 years, when the IQ can be estimated, it is usually under 20, occasionally 20 to 50, and excep-tionally above 50. *Hyperactivity,* aggressivity, clumsy gait, fine tremor of the hands, poor coordination, odd posturings, *repetitive digital mannerisms,* rhythmias, and slight cor-ticospinal tract signs are the usual clinical manifestations.

Table 38-5
Differential diagnosis of leukodystrophies of infancy

	Krabbe	Metachromatic leukodystrophy	Spongy degeneration	Palizaeus-Merzbacher	Schilder
Age of onset	3–6 months	1–2 years, rarely late childhood	0–4 months	6–24 months	5–10 years
Rate of progression	Rapid Death by 2 years	Slow Death by 3–5 years	Rapid Death by 3 years	Slow May survive to adult life	Abrupt onset Death in months to years
Sex or ethnic group			Most Jewish	Predominantly males	
Genetic	Recessive	Recessive	Recessive	Sex-linked recessive	Adrenoleuko-dystrophy form—X-linked recessive
Head size	Normal	Enlarges late	Enlarges early	Normal	Normal
Skin or systemic	Normal	Normal	Normal	Normal	Bronzing with adrenal atrophy
Eye	Late: optic atrophy	Late: optic atrophy	Optic atrophy, blindness	Slow optic atrophy	Optic neuritis or optic atrophy
Seizures	Tonic spasms	Rare	Uncommon	Late	Rare, late
Neurologic signs	Spastic paresis Nystagmus Head retraction Bulbar palsy Dementia	Changes in gait Ataxia Combined upper and lower motor neuron signs Bulbar palsy ⎫ Blindness ⎬ late Deafness ⎪ Dementia ⎭	Hypotonia→ spastic diplegia→ decerebrate rigidity	Pendular nystagmus Titubation of head and other cerebellar signs in early childhood Spastic diplegia, late childhood Slow dementia	Early spastic paralysis Dementia Late: cortical blindness, deafness, aphasia, pseudobulbar palsy
Miscellaneous		Reduced nerve conduction			EEG diffuse delta waves
Blood	Normal	Normal	Normal	Normal	Normal or ↓ cortisol
Urine	Normal	Metachromatic bodies	Normal	Normal	Normal
CSF	↑ Protein (150–300 mg/dL)	Normal or ↑ protein up to 200 mg/dL	↑ Pressure Normal or ↑ protein up to 200 mg/dL	Normal	Normal or ↑ gamma globulin
Biopsy	Brain	Sural nerve	Brain		
X-ray		Nonfilling of gallbladder	Suture separation		
Diagnostic biochemical abnormality	See text				

Source: Adapted from AL Drew, Jr, in S Carter, AP Gold (eds), *Neurology of Infancy and Childhood*, New York, Appleton-Century-Crofts, 1974.

Athetosis, dystonia, and frank cerebellar ataxia occur, but are relatively rare. Seizures occur in 25 percent of severely retarded patients and take the form of flexor spasms and later, petit mal and grand mal. The majority of patients are blue-eyed and fair in color. A musty body odor (due to phenylacetic acid excretion) is noted frequently. Two-thirds are slightly microcephalic. The fundi are normal, and there is no visceral enlargement or skeletal abnormality.

The finding of *high levels of serum phenylalanine* (above 15 mg/dL) and of *phenylpyruvic acid in the urine* is diagnostic of PKU. The addition of 3 to 5 drops of 10 percent ferric chloride to 1 mL of urine yields an emerald green color that reaches a peak intensity in 3 to 4 min and fades in 20 to 40 min. In contrast, the green-brown color in the urine of patients with histidinemia is permanent. In maple syrup urine disease, addition of ferric chloride gives a navy-blue color; ketones or salicylates in the urine yield a purple color.

The fundamental biochemical abnormality is a deficiency of the hepatic enzyme phenylalanine hydroxylase; the failure of conversion of phenylalanine to tyrosine results in the excretion of phenylpyruvic acid by affected individuals. The precise step that is faulty in the complex phenylalanine hydroxylating reaction is still unknown. The mutant allelic gene has been localized on chromosome 12. Pathologic examination shows poor staining of myelin in the cerebral hemispheres. Reduction in size of cortical neurons and their dendritic arborizations are demonstrable in some cases.

Low phenylalanine diets, if instituted in infancy, improve intellectual development. Once the neurologic picture unfolds, diet has no effect on the mental status, but may improve behavior. Prolonged dietary treatment has many untoward effects and should be supervised by physicians experienced in its use. This is particularly important since it has been shown that intellectual impairment is greatest among children who were the earliest to abandon their diets (as indicated by a phenylalanine concentration of 715 mg/dL) and least for children who maintained dietary control the longest (Holtzman et al). In children with the enzyme defect leading to hyperalininemia, but without phenylketonuria, dietary treatment is not indicated.

The late form of maple syrup urine disease, histidinemia, and hydroxyprolinemia evolve in much the same fashion as PKU, and raise similar problems in diagnosis and therapy.

A small number of infants have a variant of PKU in which a restricted phenylalanine diet does not prevent neurologic involvement. They have normal levels of phenylalanine hydroxylase in the liver. The defect is a failure to synthesize the active cofactor tetrahydrobiopterin, either because of an insufficiency of dihydropteridine reductase or an inability to synthesize biopterin. The urinary metabolites of catecholamines and serotonin are reduced. There is some evidence that the underlying neurotransmitter fault can be corrected by L-dopa and 5-hydroxytryptophan (Scriver and Clow).

Homocystinuria   This aminoaciduria, which simulates Marfan disease but is associated with mental retardation, is described further on in this chapter (page 809).

Hartnup Disease   This disease, named after the family in which it was first observed, is probably transmitted by an autosomal recessive gene. The onset of symptoms is in late infancy or early childhood. The clinical features consist of an *intermittent red, scaly rash over the face, neck, hands, and legs*, resembling that of pellagra; episodic personality disorder in the form of *emotional lability*, uncontrolled temper, and confusional-hallucinatory psychosis; *episodic cerebellar ataxia* (unsteady gait, intention tremor, and dysarthria); and occasionally spasticity, vertigo, nystagmus, ptosis, and diplopia. Episodes of disease are triggered by exposure to sunlight, emotional stress, and sulfonamide drugs. Attacks last for about 2 weeks, followed by variable periods of relative normalcy. The frequency of attacks diminishes with maturation.

The metabolic faults are a *transport error of neutral amino acids, with excretion of greatly increased amounts of these amino acids in the urine* and feces; the *excretion of large amounts of indicans*, mainly indoxyl sulfate, particularly after oral L-tryptophan loading; and an abnormally high excretion of nonhydroxylated indole metabolites. The pathologic basis of the disease is undetermined. Differential diagnosis includes a large number of intermittent and progressive cerebellar ataxias of childhood, described below.

Treatment consists of avoidance of sunlight and of sulfonamide drugs. Because of the similarities between pellagra and Hartnup disease, the usual practice is to give nicotinic acid, 25 mg daily, but the value of this measure has not been established.

Other Intermittent Metabolic Ataxias   In addition to Hartnup disease, a number of other metabolic diseases give rise to episodic ataxias during *early childhood*. These are (1) mild forms of maple syrup urine disease and the congenital hyperammonemias (type II hyperammonemia, citrullinemia, argininosuccinic aciduria, hyperornithinemia), described in an earlier part of the chapter; (2) necrotizing encephalomyelopathy (Leigh) and hyperalininemia, also described earlier; and (3) hyperalininemia and hyperpyruvic acidemia (Lonsdale et al, Blass et al).

In all these conditions the ataxia is highly variable from time to time and may follow a burst of seizures (as in argininosuccinic aciduria). The seizures are treated always with anticonvulsant drugs that may at first be held responsible for the ataxia. In time, however, it becomes apparent that the ataxia lasts a week or two, and bears no relationship to the medicine. Indeed, seizures and ataxia are both due to the common biochemical abnormality. Between attacks, in all the intermittent ataxias, the patient's movements are relatively normal, but most of the affected children are slow in learning and remain backward mentally to a varying degree.

PROGRESSIVE CEREBELLAR ATAXIAS OF EARLY CHILDHOOD

The problems in diagnosis of the *persistent early-childhood ataxias* are first, to make certain that ataxia exists; and second, to differentiate cerebellar ataxia from the sensory ataxia of peripheral nerve disease. Since cerebellar ataxia is more a disorder of voluntary than of postural movements, the presence of ataxia can usually not be determined with certainty until intentional (projected) movements become part of the child's repertoire of motor activity. As indicated in Chap. 28, the earliest signs become manifest in the arms when the infant reaches for an object and brings it to the mouth, or transfers it from hand to hand. A jerky, wavering, tremulous movement then appears; in sitting, a titubation of the head and a tremor of the trunk may be apparent. Once walking begins, apart from the usual clumsiness of the toddler, there is a similar incoordination of movement. Sensory ataxia is always difficult to distinguish, but is rare at this age and nearly always accompanied by weakness and absence of tendon reflexes. By the fourth or fifth year, when more detailed sensory testing becomes possible, the presence or absence of a proprioceptive disturbance can be demonstrated.

The group of persistent and progressive cerebellar ataxias is heterogeneous and of varied etiology, and some of them merge with Friedreich ataxia, Lévy-Roussy syndrome, and other adolescent-adult hereditary ataxias. These disorders are discussed in the chapter on degenerative diseases since neither their cause nor pathogenesis is known. There are many other childhood ataxias that probably belong in the category of degenerative disease—some in which cerebellar ataxia is the most prominent abnormality, and some in which other neurologic abnormalities are more prominent. To describe each one in detail would be inappropriate in a book on principles of neurology, and they will only be tabulated here. A more complete list of these disorders and appropriate references to each of them will be found in Ford's monograph. The following are noteworthy:

1. A disequilibrium and dyssynergia syndrome of Hagberg and Janner: early-life onset of relatively pure cerebellar ataxia, with psychomotor retardation.

2. Cerebellar ataxia with diplegia, hypotonia, and mental retardation (also called *atonic diplegia* of Foerster); this is either a fetal disease or birth injury, and the neuropathology is uncertain.

3. Agenesis of the cerebellum: early cerebellar ataxia (with or without mental retardation) and episodic hyperventilation (Norman's family with granule-cell degeneration falls into this category).

4. Cerebellar ataxia with cataracts and oligophrenia: onset from childhood to as late as adult years (Marinesco-Sjögren disease).

5. Cerebellar ataxia and retinal degeneration.

6. Cerebellar ataxia with cataracts and ophthalmoplegia, or with cataracts and mental as well as physical retardation.

7. Familial cerebellar ataxia with mydriasis.

8. Familial cerebellar ataxia with deafness and blindness, and a similar combination called retinocochleodentate degeneration, referring to loss of neurons in these three structures.

9. Familial cerebellar ataxia with choreoathetosis, corticospinal tract signs, and mental and motor retardation (Gökay and Tukel).

In none of the above-mentioned syndromes has a biochemical abnormality been established, so their metabolic nature can only be inferred. The persistent cerebellar ataxias of childhood in which a metabolic fault has been demonstrated are (1) Refsum disease, (2) abetalipoproteinemia (Bassen-Kornzweig syndrome), (3) ataxia-telangiectasia, and (4) possibly Friedreich ataxia (Chap. 43). Refsum disease is discussed with the hereditary polyneuropathies (page 1058). The Bassen-Kornzweig syndrome more often has its onset in late than in early childhood, and is more appropriately described in the following section of this chapter.

Ataxia-Telangiectasia This is a relatively frequent childhood ataxia, inherited as an autosomal recessive trait. The onset of the disease coincides, more or less, with the acquisition of walking, which is awkward and unsteady. Later, by the age of 4 to 5 years, the limbs become ataxic, and choreoathetosis, grimacing, and dysarthric speech are added. The eye movements become jerky, and there is also apraxia for voluntary gaze (the patient turns the head and not the eyes on attempting to look to the side). By the age of 9 to 10 years some intellectual decline appears, and signs of mild polyneuropathy are evident. The characteristic telangiectatic lesions appear at 3 to 5 years of age or later, and are most apparent in the outer parts of the bulbar conjunctivae, over the ears, on exposed parts of the neck, on the bridge of the nose and cheeks in a butterfly pattern, and in the flexor creases of the forearms. The disease is progressive, and death occurs usually in the second decade from intercurrent bronchopulmonary infection or neoplasia (usually lymphoma, less often glioma).

The significant abnormalities in the CNS are severe degeneration in the cerebellar cortex; loss of myelinated fibers in the posterior columns, spinocerebellar tracts, and peripheral nerves; degenerative changes in the posterior roots and cells of the sympathetic ganglia; and loss of anterior horn cells at all levels of the spinal cord. In a few cases, vascular abnormalities, like the mucocutaneous ones, have been found scattered diffusely in the white matter of the brain and spinal cord. Also, there may be a loss of pigmented cells in the substantia nigra and locus ceruleus, and cytoplasmic inclusions (Lewy bodies) in the remaining cells (Agamanolis and Greenstein).

An absence or decrease in immunoglobulin (IgA) has been found in practically every patient. This deficiency, shown by McFarlin and his associates to be due to decreased synthesis, is associated with hypoplasia of the thymus, failure of delayed hypersensitivity reactions, lymphopenia, and slow response to the formation of circulating antibodies. Probably this immunodeficient state accounts for the striking susceptibility of these patients to recurrent pulmonary infections and bronchiectasis.

METACHROMATIC LEUKODYSTROPHY

This is one of the sphingolipid storage diseases (Table 38-3). The basic abnormality, localized in chromosome 22, is the absence of the enzyme aryl sulfatase A, a deficiency of which prevents the conversion of sulfatide to cerebroside and results in an accumulation of the former. The disease is transmitted as an autosomal recessive trait, and usually becomes manifest between the first and fourth years of life (variants have their onset in late childhood and even in adult life). It is characterized clinically by *progressive impairment of motor function* in combination with *mental regression*. At first the tendon reflexes are usually brisk, but later, as the peripheral nerves become involved, the *reflexes are decreased and eventually lost*. Instead, there may be hypotonia and areflexia from the beginning, or spasticity throughout the illness with hyporeflexia and slowed conduction velocities. Signs of mental regression may be apparent from the onset or appear after the motor disorder has become established. Later there is impairment of vision, sometimes with squint and nystagmus; intention tremor in the arms and dysarthria; dysphagia and drooling; and optic atrophy (one-third of patients), sometimes with grayish degeneration around the macula. Seizures are rare. Head size is usually normal, but rarely there is macrocephaly. Progression to a bedridden quadriplegic state

without speech or comprehension occurs over a 1- to 3-year period, somewhat more slowly in late-onset types.

There is widespread degeneration of myelinated fibers in the cerebrum, cerebellum, spinal cord, and peripheral nerves. The presence of metachromatic granules in glial cells and engorged macrophages is characteristic, and enables the diagnosis to be made from a biopsy of a peripheral nerve. The stored material, sulfatide, stains brown-orange rather than purple with aniline dyes. Sulfatides are also PAS-positive in frozen sections.

The diagnostic laboratory findings, in addition to the histologic changes, are an elevated CSF protein (75 to 250 mg/dL) and a marked *decrease or absence of aryl sulfatase A* in the urine; methods are also available for detecting this abnormality in white blood cells, in serum, and in cultured fibroblasts. Assaying the aryl sulfatase A activity in cultured fibroblasts and amniocytes permits the identification of carriers and prenatal diagnosis of the disease.

The differential diagnosis is from neuroaxonal dystrophy (see below), early cases of Déjerine-Sottas polyneuropathy, late-onset Krabbe disease, and childhood forms of Gaucher disease and Niemann-Pick disease.

Forms of metachromatic leukodystrophy developing in adult years have been identified and are discussed further on.

NEUROAXONAL DYSTROPHY (DEGENERATION)

This is a rare disease, with an autosomal recessive pattern of inheritance. The onset is usually in the second year of life (rarely after the third or fourth year), with *progressive difficulty in walking*, weakness, and diminished or absent tendon reflexes. Later there are corticospinal and pseudobulbar signs, with hyperactive reflexes and Babinski signs, loss of sight and optic atrophy, and *diminished sensitivity to pain* over the limbs and trunk. *Mental deterioration* coincides with motor impairment. Effective communicative speech is never achieved; head circumference is normal or slightly reduced; seizures are infrequent. The course is relentlessly progressive with fatal issue in 3 to 8 years, in a decorticate state.

In the largest group of cases (77 collected by Aicardi and Castelein), the onset was near the beginning of the second year in 50 patients and before the third year in all instances. The clinical constellation comprised psychomotor deterioration (loss of ability to walk, stand, sit and speak), marked hypotonia but brisk reflexes and Babinski signs, and progressive blindness with optic atrophy but normal retinas. Seizures, myoclonus, and extrapyramidal signs were rare. Loss of sensation was found later in some cases. Terminally, bulbar signs, spasticity, and decerebrate rigidity often supervened.

Pathologic examination reveals eosinophilic spheroids of swollen axoplasm in the posterior columns and nuclei of Goll and Burdach and in Clarke's column of cells, substantia nigra, subthalamic nuclei, central nuclei of brainstem, and cerebral cortex. There is cerebellar atrophy, affecting the granule cell layer predominantly, and increased iron-containing pigment in the basal ganglia (like that observed in Hallervorden-Spatz disease).

The CT scans and CSF are normal. After the age of 2 years, the EEG shows characteristic high amplitude fast rhythms (16 to 22 Hz). Evoked responses may be abnormal. Nerve conduction velocities are normal despite the presence of denervation in the EMG. There are no biochemical or blood cell abnormalities. The diagnosis can be reliably and easily established during life by electron microscopic examination of skin and conjunctival nerves, which show the characteristic spheroids within axons.

There is a later-onset form of the disease in which the course is more protracted and the neurologic manifestations (rigidity and spasticity, cerebellar ataxia, and myoclonus) are more pronounced. In these cases the mental regression is slow. Vision may be retained and tapetoretinal degeneration has been documented. Some of the late onset cases are indistinguishable from Hallervorden-Spatz disease (see page 804).

LATE INFANTILE AND EARLY CHILDHOOD GAUCHER DISEASE AND NIEMANN-PICK DISEASE

As stated above, Gaucher disease usually develops in early infancy, but some cases—Gaucher disease, type III—may begin in childhood. The onset is between 3 and 8 years of age. The clinical picture is variable and combines features of infantile Gaucher disease, such as abducens palsies, dysphagia, trismus, rigidity of the limbs and dementia, with features of the late childhood-early adult form, such as supranuclear gaze palsies, diffuse myoclonus, generalized seizures, and a chronic course (Winkelman et al). Diagnosis is established by the finding of splenomegaly, Gaucher cells, glucocerebroside storage, and deficient activity of glucocerebrosidase in leukocytes or cultured fibroblasts.

Late infantile or childhood Niemann-Pick disease causes *mental retardation*, seizures, *dysarthria, ataxia,* and *paralysis of vertical eye movements;* horizontal gaze becomes involved eventually. A special syndrome called *juvenile dystonic lipidosis* is characterized by extrapyramidal symptoms and paralysis of vertical eye movements. The syndrome of "the sea-blue histiocyte" (liver, spleen, and bone marrow contain histiocytes with sea-blue granules) in which there is retardation in mental and motor development, grayish macular degeneration, and, in one of our cases, posterior column and pyramidal degeneration, may be another variant. In the latter, several types of glycolipids were found in the liver and spleen, and the urinary level of mucopolysaccharides was increased. In the classic form of Niemann-Pick disease, sphingomyelin is increased in the viscera and sphingomyelinase is reduced in leukocytes and cultured fibroblasts.

LATE INFANTILE-CHILDHOOD G_{M1} GANGLIOSIDOSIS

In so-called type 2, or "juvenile," G_{M1} gangliosidosis the onset is between 12 and 24 months, with survival for 3 to 10 years. The first sign is usually *difficulty in walking* (awkward gait, frequent falls), followed by awkwardness of arm movements, loss of speech, severe *mental regression,* gradual development of *spastic quadriparesis* and pseudobulbar palsy (dysarthria, dysphagia, drooling), and seizures. Retinal changes are variable—usually they are absent, but macular red spots may be seen at the age of 10 to 12 years; vision is usually retained, but squints (comitant) are common. There is a facial dysmorphism resembling that of the Hurler syndrome and the liver and spleen are enlarged. Important laboratory findings are hypoplasia of the thoracolumbar vertebral bodies, mild hypoplasia of the acetabula, and the presence in the marrow of histiocytes with clear vacuoles or wrinkled cytoplasm. Leukocytes and cultured skin fibroblasts show a *deficiency* or absence *of β-galactosidase* activity. G_{M1} ganglioside accumulates in the cerebral neurons.

JANSKY-BIELSCHOWSKY DISEASE

Designated by these names is a rare form of lipid storage disease that is inherited as an autosomal recessive trait. The onset of symptoms is between 2 and 4 years, after normal or slightly retarded earlier development, with survival to 4 to 8 years of age. In some cases the onset is even later (page 809). Usually the first neurologic manifestations are *seizures* (petit mal or grand mal) *and myoclonic jerks* evoked by proprioceptive and other sensory stimuli, including voluntary movement and emotional excitement. *Incoordination,* tremor, ataxia, and spastic weakness with lively tendon reflexes and Babinski signs, *deterioration of mental faculties,* and dysarthria proceed to dementia and eventually to mutism. In patients with relatively late onset, dementia is the cardinal manifestation. Visual failure may occur early in some cases because of *retinal degeneration* and pigmentation (degeneration of rods and cones), but in others vision is normal. The electroretinogram is isoelectric if vision is affected. Abnormal inclusions (translucent vacuoles) are seen in 10 to 30 percent of circulating lymphocytes, and azurophilic granules occur in neutrophils; EEG spikes are induced by photic stimuli. In early-onset cases there may be microcephaly.

Pathologic examination shows neuronal loss in the cerebral and cerebellar cortices (granule and Purkinje cells), and curvilinear storage particles and osmiophilic granules in the neurons. Inclusions are also observed in cutaneous nerve twigs and endothelial cells, which permits diagnosis during life (electron microscopy of skin or conjunctival biopsies). In the differential diagnosis, one needs to consider late infantile G_{M1} gangliosidosis, idiopathic epilepsy, Alpers disease, and other forms of neuronal ceroid-lipofuscinoses (page 809).

MUCOPOLYSACCHARIDOSES

This is a group of diseases in which a storage of lipid in neurons and of polysaccharides in connective tissues are combined. As a consequence there is a conjunction of neurologic and skeletal abnormalities that is virtually unique. The nervous system may also be involved secondarily as a result of skeletal deformities and thickening and hyperplasia of connective tissue at the base of the brain, leading to obliteration of the subarachnoid space and obstructive hydrocephalus. Depending on the degree of visceral-skeletal and neurologic changes, at least seven different subtypes are recognized (see Table 38-3).

Hurler Disease (MPS I, MPS IH)   This, the classic form, is inherited as an autosomal recessive trait. The onset is toward the end of the first year. *Mental retardation* is severe, and *skeletal abnormalities* are prominent (dwarfism; gargoyle facies; large head with synostosis of longitudinal suture; kyphosis; broad hands with short, stubby fingers; flexion contractures at knees and elbows). Conductive deafness and corticospinal signs are usually present. Protuberent abdomen, hernias, *enlarged liver and spleen,* valvular heart disease, chronic rhinitis, respiratory infections, and *corneal opacities* are the common medical findings. The biochemical abnormalities consist of the accumulation of *dermatan* and *heparan sulfate* in the tissues and their *excretion in the urine,* due probably to *absence of activity* of α-iduronidase. Also, there is an increase in the ganglioside content in the brains of these patients.

Hunter Disease (MPS II)   Unlike the Hurler and other types, the Hunter form is transmitted as an X-linked trait. The clinical syndromes are alike, except that the Hunter

form is milder: mental retardation is less severe than in the Hurler type, deafness is less common, and *corneal clouding is usually absent.* Probably there are two forms of the syndrome—a more severe form in which the patients do not survive beyond the midteens, and a less severe form, with relatively normal intelligence and survival to middle age. Excessive amounts of dermatan and heparan sulfate are excreted in the urine. The basic abnormality is a *deficiency of iduronate sulfatase activity.*

Sanfilippo Disease (MPS III)   This form is inherited as an autosomal recessive trait. The onset is between 2 and 3 years of age, with progressive intellectual deterioration. The patients are of short stature, but in other respects the physical changes are fewer and less severe than in the Hunter and Hurler syndromes. Three types of Sanfilippo disease, designated A, B, and C, are distinguished on the basis of different enzymatic defects (see Table 38-3); patients of all three types excrete excessive amounts of heparan sulfate in the urine.

Morquio Disease (MPS IV)   This form of the disease is characterized by marked *dwarfism* and *osteoporosis.* Skeletal deformity may cause compression of the spinal cord and medulla in some cases. Also, because of hypoplasia of the odontoid process, there may be atlantoaxial dislocation. The dura around the cervical cord and inferior surface of the cerebellum may be thickened. Intelligence is affected only slightly or not at all. *Corneal opacities may be present.* The mode of inheritance is autosomal recessive. Patients excrete large amounts of keratan sulfate in the urine; two types of enzymatic deficiency have been identified (Table 38-3).

Scheie Disease (MPS V, MPS IS)   This form of the disease is also inherited as an autosomal recessive trait. It differs from the Hurler type in that the patients are of normal intelligence and height. Some have a carpal tunnel syndrome. *Corneal clouding* is the main abnormality. Other skeletal and visceral abnormalities are the same as in the Hurler form, as are the pathologic biochemical defects. There is no plausible explanation for the phenotypic differences between the Hurler and Scheie forms.

Maroteaux-Lamy Disease (MPS VI)   This syndrome also is inherited as an autosomal recessive trait. Intelligence is normal, but there are severe skeletal deformities. Several of our cases have had a pachymeninx cervicalis with spinal cord compression and hydrocephalus during adult life.

Spinal cord function improved with cervical decompression and ventriculoatrial shunting (Young et al). Hepatosplenomegaly is often present. Large amounts of dermatan sulfate are excreted in the urine, as a result of an *aryl sulfatase B deficiency.*

β-Glucuronidase Deficiency (MPS VII, Sly Disease)

This is a rare and more recently described type of mucopolysaccharidosis. The clinical features still have to be sharply delineated. Short stature, progressive thoracolumbar gibbus, hepatosplenomegaly, and the bony changes of dysostosis multiplex (as in the Hurler type) are the main clinical features. There is excessive excretion of dermatan and heparan sulfate, the result of a deficiency of β-glucuronidase.

MUCOLIPIDOSES AND OTHER DISEASES OF COMPLEX CARBOHYDRATES (SIALIDOSES)

In recent years several new diseases have been described, in which there is an abnormal accumulation of mucopolysaccharides, sphingolipids, and glycolipids in visceral, mesenchymal, and neural tissues, due to an α-N-acetylneuraminidase defect. In some types there is an additional deficiency of β-galactosidase. They are autosomal recessive diseases that manifest many of the clinical features of Hurler disease, but in contrast to the mucopolysaccharidoses, normal amounts of mucopolysaccharides are excreted in the urine. Frequently, G_{M1} gangliosidosis, described above, is also classified with the mucolipidoses. The other members of this category are synopsized below.

Mucolipidoses   At least three and possibly four closely related forms have been described. In *mucolipidosis I (lipomucopolysaccharidosis)* the morphologic features are those of gargoylism, with slowly progressive mental retardation. Cherry-red spots in the maculae, corneal opacities, and ataxia have been noted in some patients. Vacuolation of lymphocytes, marrow cells, hepatocytes, and Kupffer cells in the liver, and metachromatic changes in the sural nerve have been described.

In *mucolipidosis II ("I-cell" disease),* the most common of the four forms, there is an early onset of psychomotor retardation, which is usually severe by the second year but may not appear until the second or third decade. *Abnormal facies and periosteal thickening (dysostosis multiplex,* like that of G_{M1} gangliosidosis and Hurler disease) are evident. *Gingival hyperplasia* is prominent, and the *liver* and *spleen are enlarged;* but deafness is not

found and corneal opacities are slower to develop. Tonic-clonic seizures are frequent in older patients. In most cases, death occurs by the third to eighth year, of heart failure. There is a typical vacuolation of lymphocytes, Kupffer cells, and cells of the renal glomeruli. Bone-marrow cells are also vacuolated and contain refractile cytoplasmic granules (hence the term *inclusion-,* or *I-cell, disease*). A deficiency of several lysosomal enzymes required for the catabolism of mucopolysaccharides, glycolipids, and glycoproteins has been described.

In *mucolipidosis III (pseudo-Hurler polydystrophy)* the biochemical abnormalities are like those of I-cell disease, but there are clinical differences. In the former, symptoms do not appear until 2 years of age or later, and are relatively mild. Retardation of growth, fine corneal opacities, and valvular heart disease are the major manifestations.

In recent years, yet another variant, so-called mucolipidosis IV, has been described (see Tellez-Nagel et al). Clouding of the corneas is noticed soon after birth, and profound retardation is evident by one year of age. Skeletal deformities, enlargement of liver and spleen, seizures, or other neurologic abnormalities are notably lacking. Ultrastructural examination of conjunctival and skin fibroblasts has demonstrated lysosomal inclusions of material similar to lipids and mucopolysaccharides, which remain to be characterized.

Mannosidosis   This is another rare hereditary disorder with poorly differentiated symptomatology. The onset is in the first 2 years, with *Hurler-like facial* and *skeletal deformities, mental retardation* and slight motor disability. Corticospinal signs, loss of hearing, variable degrees of gingival hyperplasia, and spoke-like opacities of the lens (but no corneal clouding) may be present. The liver and spleen are enlarged in some cases. Radiographs show beaking of the vertebral bodies and poor trabeculation of long bones. Vacuolated lymphocytes and granulated leukocytes are characteristic. The urinary mucopolysaccharides are normal. *Mannosiduria is diagnostic,* caused by a defect in α-mannosidase. Mannose-containing oligosaccharides accumulate in nerve cells, spleen, liver, and leukocytes (Kistler et al).

Fucosidosis   This also is a rare autosomal recessive disorder, with neurologic deterioration beginning usually at 12 to 15 months and progressing to spastic quadriplegia, decerebrate rigidity, absence of mental activity, and death within 4 to 6 years. *Hepatomegaly, splenomegaly, enlarged salivary glands,* thickened skin, excessive sweating, normal or typical gargoyle facies, *beaking of the vertebral bodies,* and vacuolated lymphocytes are the main features. A variant of this disease has been described with slower progression and survival into late childhood and adolescence, and even into adult life (Ikeda et al).The latter type is characterized by mental and motor retardation, along with the corneal opacities, coarse facial features and skeletal deformities of gargoylism and the dermatologic changes of Fabry disease (angiokeratoma corporis diffusum), but no hepatosplenomegaly. The basic abnormality in both types is a lack of lysosomal-L-fucosidase, resulting in accumulation of fucose-rich sphingolipids, glycoproteins, and oligosaccharides in cells of the skin, conjunctivae, and rectal mucosa.

Aspartylglycosaminuria This disease is characterized by the early onset of psychomotor regression; delayed, inadequate speech; severe behavioral abnormalities (*bouts of hyperactivity* mixed with apathy and hypoactivity or psychotic manifestations); *progressive dementia;* clumsy movements; corticospinal signs; corneal clouding (rare); retinal abnormalities and cataracts; coarse facies, low bridge of the nose, epicanthi, thickening of the lips and skin; enlarged liver; and abdominal hernias in some. Radiographs show minimal *beaking of the vertebral bodies*, and vacuolated lymphocytes are seen in the blood.

Autosomal recessive inheritance is probably operative in this entire group of diseases. Diagnostic methods applicable to amniotic fluid and cells are being developed so that prenatal diagnosis will be possible, prompted by the occurrence of the disease in an earlier child. Neurons are vacuolated rather than stuffed with granules, much like the lymphocytes and liver cells. The specific biochemical abnormalities, as far as they are known, are indicated in Table 38-3.

LATE INFANTILE AND CHILDHOOD FORMS OF NIEMANN-PICK DISEASE

A number of cases of subacute or chronic neurovisceral storage disease with early signs of hepatosplenomegaly and late signs (2 to 4 years) of neurologic involvement have been described. Crocker and Farber have classified them as types III and IV Niemann-Pick disease. The neurologic disorder consists of progressive dementia, dysarthria, ataxia, rarely extrapyramidal signs (choreoathetosis), and paralysis of vertical and lateral gaze. On looking to the side, some of the patients make head-thrusting movements of the same type that one observes in ataxia-telangiectasia and Cogan's oculomotor apraxia. Lateral eye movements are full on passive movement of the head (doll's head eye phenomenon). Convergence is also deficient. The diagnosis is reached by bone marrow biopsy which reveals vacuolated macrophages and sea-blue histiocytes. Sphingomyelinase activities are normal.

Probably this variant of Niemann-Pick disease is the same as the syndrome of sea-blue histiocytes and the juvenile dystonic lipidosis described by Elfenbein.

COCKAYNE SYNDROME

This disorder is probably inherited as an autosomal recessive trait. The onset is in late infancy after apparently normal early development. The main clinical findings are evident *stunting of growth* by the second and third years; *photosensitivity of the skin;* microcephaly; *retinitis pigmentosa, cataracts,* blindness and pendular nystagmus; nerve deafness; *delayed psychomotor* and speech development; *spastic weakness* and *ataxia of limbs* and gait; occasionally athetosis; amyotrophy with abolished reflexes and reduced nerve conduction velocities; wizened face, sunken eyes, prominent nose, prognathism, anhydrosis, and poor lacrimation (resembling progeria and bird-headed dwarf). Some cases show calcification of the basal ganglia. The CSF is normal, and there are no diagnostic biochemical findings.

Pathologic examination reveals a small brain, striatocerebellar calcifications, leukodystrophy like that of Pelizaeus-Merzbacher disease, and a severe cerebellar cortical atrophy. The peripheral nerve changes are those of a primary segmental demyelination. The pathogenesis is unknown. The variability in clinical and pathologic manifestations of reported cases suggests that not all of them are representative of the same disease.

OTHER DISEASES

Globoid cell leukodystrophy (Krabbe), subacute necrotizing encephalomyelopathy (Leigh), and Gaucher disease may also begin in late infancy or early childhood. They have been described in the preceding section of this chapter. Familial striatocerebellar calcification (Fahr disease) and Lesch-Nyhan disease may also become manifest in this age period, but usually they have a later onset and are therefore described with the diseases of later childhood, in the section that follows.

DIAGNOSIS

The metabolic disorders of late infancy and early childhood present many of the same problems in diagnosis as those of early infancy. Some symptoms—psychomotor regression, unsteady gait, seizures, progressive quadriplegia—are common to most of the diseases in this group and are therefore of little specific diagnostic value. On the other hand, certain neurologic, skeletal, dermal, ophthalmic, and laboratory findings, or groups of findings, are highly distinctive and often diagnostic. These signs are listed below:

1. Evidence of involvement of peripheral nerves (weak-

ness, hypotonia, areflexia, sensory loss, reduced conduction velocities) in conjunction with lesions of the central nervous system—metachromatic leukodystrophy, Krabbe leukodystrophy, neuroaxonal dystrophy, and Leigh disease (rare)

2. Ophthalmic signs

   a. Corneal clouding—several of the mucopolysaccharidoses (Hurler, Scheie, Morquio, Maroteaux-Lamy), mucolipidoses, aspartylglycosaminuria (rare)

   b. Cherry-red macular spot—G_{M2} gangliosidosis, G_{M1} gangliosidosis (rare), lipomucopolysaccharidosis, occasionally Niemann-Pick disease

   c. Retinal degeneration with pigmentary deposits—Jansky-Bielschowsky lipid storage disease, G_{M2} gangliosidosis, syndrome of sea-blue histiocytes

   d. Optic atrophy and blindness—metachromatic leukodystrophy, neuroaxonal dystrophy

   e. Cataracts—Marinesco-Sjögren syndrome, Fabry disease, mannosidosis

   f. Telangiectasia and optic apraxia—ataxia-telangiectasia

   g. Impairment of vertical eye movements—late infantile Niemann-Pick disease, juvenile dystonic lipidosis, sea-blue histiocyte syndrome

   h. Jerky eye movements, limited abduction—late infantile Gaucher disease

3. Extrapyramidal signs—late-onset Niemann-Pick disease (rigidity, abnormal postures), juvenile dystonic lipidosis (dystonia, choreoathetosis), ataxia-telangiectasia (athetosis), Sanfilippo mucopolysaccharidosis

4. Facial dysmorphism—Hurler, Scheie, Morquio, and Maroteaux-Lamy forms of mucopolysaccharidosis, aspartylglycosaminuria, mucolipidoses, G_{M1} gangliosidosis, mannosidosis, fucosidosis (some cases)

5. Dwarfism, spine deformities, arthropathies—Hurler and Morquio mucopolysaccharidoses, Cockayne syndrome

6. Enlarged liver and spleen—Niemann-Pick disease, Gaucher disease, all mucopolysaccharidoses, fucosidosis, mucolipidoses, G_{M1} gangliosidosis

7. Alterations of skin—photosensitivity (Cockayne syndrome and one form of porphyria); papular nevi (Fabry disease); telangiectasia of ears, conjunctiva, chest (ataxia-telangiectasia); ichthyosis (Sjögren-Larsen disease)

8. Beaked thoracolumbar vertebras—all mucopolysaccharidoses, mucolipidoses, mannosidosis, fucosidosis; aspartylglycosaminuria

9. Deafness—mucopolysaccharidoses, Cockayne syndrome

10. Hypertrophied gums—mucolipidoses, mannosidosis

11. Vacuolated lymphocytes—all mucopolysaccharidoses, mucolipidoses, mannosidosis, fucosidosis

12. Granules in neutrophils—all mucopolysaccharidoses, mucolipidoses, mannosidosis, fucosidosis

In our experience the most difficult diagnostic problems in this age period are raised by neuroaxonal dystrophy, metachromatic leukodystrophy, subacute necrotizing encephalomyelopathy (SNE), and the late form of G_{M1} gangliosidosis. In none of these diseases is the clinical picture entirely stereotyped. Most helpful in the clinical diagnosis of neuroaxonal dystrophy is the onset at 1 to 2 years of severe hypotonia with retained reflexes and Babinski signs, early visual involvement without retinal changes, lack of seizures, normal CSF, physiologic evidence of denervation of muscles, fast-frequency EEG, and normal CT scan. Metachromatic leukodystrophy can be excluded in the differential diagnosis if the CSF protein is normal and if nerve conduction velocities and enzymatic studies of leukocytes and fibroblasts are normal. Similar criteria enable one to rule out G_{M1} gangliosidosis. SNE may begin at the same age with hypotonia and optic atrophy but abnormalities of ocular movement and respiration appear early, and in many cases the lactic acidosis and pyruvate decarboxylase defect will corroborate the diagnosis. Also in SNE, CT scanning may disclose hypodense lesions in the basal ganglia and brainstem, in contrast to the normal CT scan in neuroaxonal dystrophy. In metachromatic leukodystrophy, the cerebral white matter shows a decreased attenuation diffusely.

INHERITED METABOLIC ENCEPHALOPATHIES OF LATE CHILDHOOD AND ADOLESCENCE

Unavoidably one must refer here to certain inherited metabolic diseases, already described, that permit survival to late childhood and adolescence and may even begin in adolescence or adult life, after a normal childhood. There is a tendency for them to be less severe and less rapidly progressive, an attribute shared by many diseases with a dominant mode of inheritance. Nonetheless, there are diseases, such as the Wilson-Westphal-Strümpell hepatocerebral degeneration, in which the onset of neurologic symptoms is always after the tenth year and even after the thirtieth year in rare instances, and the mode of inheritance is recessive in type. However, in the latter instance, manifestations of the disease have existed since early childhood in the form of a ceruloplasmin deficiency with early cirrhosis and splenomegaly; only the neurologic disorder is of late onset. This brings us to another principle—that the pathogenesis of the cerebral lesion may involve a factor or factors once removed from the basic abnormality, in this case cirrhosis of the liver.

Genetic heterogeneity poses another problem with respect to both the clinical and biochemical findings. It has been pointed out that a single clinical phenotype such as the one seen in Hurler disease can be the expression of a number of different alleles of a given gene mutation. Or a number of different clinical phenotypes may appear to be based on different degrees of the same enzyme deficiency. One must, therefore, not rely solely on clinical appearances for diagnosis but always turn to biochemical tests for confirmation.

The diseases in this category are probably of greater interest to neurologists than the preceding ones, for they evince familiar neurologic abnormalities such as epilepsy, polymyoclonia, dementia, cerebellar ataxia, choreoathetosis, dystonia, tremor, spastic-ataxic paraparesis, blindness, deafness, and stroke. These manifestations appear much the same in late childhood and adolescence as they do in adult life, and the neurologist whose experience has been mainly with adult patients feels quite comfortable with them.

Diseases in this age period have a diversity of manifestations, yet each disease has certain characteristic patterns of neurologic expression, as though the pathogenetic mechanism were acting selectively on particular systems of neurons. Such affinities between the disease process and certain anatomic structures raise the question of *pathoclisis,* i.e., specific vulnerability of particular neuron systems to certain morbid agents. Stated in another way, for each disease there is a common and stereotyped clinical syndrome and a small number of variants; conversely, certain other symptoms and syndromes are rarely observed with a given disease. At the same time, however, it is clear that more than one disease may cause the same syndrome.

In deference to these principles, *the diseases in this section are grouped according to their most common mode of clinical expression,* as follows:

1. The progressive cerebellar ataxias of childhood and adolescence

2. The parkinsonian syndrome, with other extrapyramidal symptoms

3. The syndrome of dystonia and generalized choreoathetosis

4. The familial polymyoclonias

5. The syndrome of bilateral hemiplegia, cerebral blindness and deafness, and other manifestations of focal cerebral disorder

6. Strokes in association with inherited metabolic diseases

7. Metabolic polyneuropathies

8. Personality changes and behavioral disturbances as manifestations of inherited metabolic diseases

It is of advantage to memorize these groupings, for a knowledge of them, like the age of onset and gray and white matter distinctions in earlier diseases, facilitates clinical diagnosis. Variants seen personally by the authors will be mentioned in the descriptions of the diseases themselves. One word of caution—it is a mistake to assume that the diseases in the aforementioned categories affect one and only one particular part of the nervous system, or to assume that they are exclusively neurologic. Once the biochemical abnormality is discovered, it is usually found to implicate cells of certain other organs and tissues; whether or not the effects of such involvement become symptomatic is often a quantitative matter.

THE PROGRESSIVE CEREBELLAR ATAXIAS OF CHILDHOOD AND ADOLESCENCE

It has already been pointed out that there is a large group of diseases, some with (but most without) a known metabolic basis, in which an acute, episodic, or chronic disorder of coordination begins early in life. Apparently the anatomic peculiarities of the cerebellar cortex render it particularly susceptible to a number of morbid processes. The acute forms are essentially nonmetabolic and are observed in postinfectious encephalomyelitis, in postanoxic, postmeningitic, and posthyperthermic states, and with certain drug intoxications. The hereditary metabolic ataxias are often episodic (see above), as well as chronic. The episodic ones are the hyperammonemias, Hartnup disease, late-onset maple syrup disease, and diamox-responsive episodic ataxia. The chronic progressive ones are the late-onset lipid storage diseases. Most of these begin in infancy and childhood. In the later age periods the number of ataxias of proven metabolic type diminishes markedly, and those that begin in adult life are rare. Of the latter, Friedreich ataxia and its variants are the most frequent; although hereditary, there is only presumptive evidence of a metabolic defect (Chap. 43). Of the other cerebellar ataxias of late childhood and adolescence only the Bassen-Kornzweig acanthocytosis falls into the category of a truly metabolic disease—and one could perhaps add Refsum disease, ataxia-telangiectasia, and prolonged vitamin E deficiency. Refsum disease is so clearly a polyneuropathy (cerebellar features only in exceptional cases) that it is presented in Chap. 46. Ataxia-telangiectasia is usually encountered in late childhood, but the ataxia may begin as early as the second year of life; therefore it has been described in the preceding section with the ataxias of early childhood. The effect of vitamin E deficiency on the nervous system is described on page 836.

Bassen-Kornzweig Acanthocytosis (Abetalipoproteinemia)

The delineation of this disease excited great interest, for it promised to be a breakthrough into a hitherto obscure group of "degenerative" disorders. In the authors' experience, however, it is an extremely rare disease. Not more than two dozen cases are on record, and several reports are based on the study of the same case. Further, the resemblance to Friedreich ataxia is not so close that an experienced clinician would be likely to confuse the two.

The inheritance of this disease is autosomal recessive in type. The initial symptoms, occurring between 6 and 12 years (range 2 to 17 years) are *weakness of the limbs with areflexia* and an *ataxia of sensory (tabetic) type,* to which a *cerebellar component* is added later. *Steatorrhea* (raising suspicion of celiac disease) often precedes the weak, unsteady gait. Later, in more than half the patients, vision may fail because of *retinal degeneration* (similar to retinitis pigmentosa). Kyphoscoliosis, pes cavus, and Babinski signs are other elements in the clinical picture. The neurologic disorder is relatively slowly progressive—by the second to third decade the patient is usually bedridden.

The diagnostic laboratory findings are spiky or *thorny red blood cells (acanthocytes),* low sedimentation rate, and a marked reduction in the serum *of low-density lipoproteins* (cholesterol, phospholipid, and β-lipoprotein levels are all subnormal). Pathologic study has revealed the presence of foamy, vacuolated epithelial cells in the intestinal mucosa (causing absorption block), diminished numbers of myelinated nerve fibers in sural nerve biopsies, depletion of Purkinje and granule cells in all parts of the cerebellum, loss of fibers in the posterior columns and spinocerebellar tracts, loss of anterior horn and retinal ganglion cells, muscle fiber loss, and fibrosis of the myocardium. It has been proposed that the basic defect is an inability of the body to synthesize the proteins of cell membranes, because of the impaired absorption of fat from the small intestine through the mucosa. The administration of a low-fat diet and high doses of vitamin A and E may prevent progression of the neurologic disorder (Illingworth et al).

An adult form of acanthocytosis and hereditary chorea has also been recognized but lacking is evidence of lipid malabsorption. It will be described in Chap. 43.

There are doubtless many other conditions of metabolic type in which cerebellar ataxia figures importantly in the clinical picture. Some of these are associated with polymyoclonia and cherry-red macular spots (sialidosis or neuraminodosis; see below). Cerebellar ataxia is a prominent feature of Unverricht-Lundborg (Baltic) disease and Lafora body disease. The Cockayne syndrome and Marinesco-Sjögren disease, already described under the metabolic disorders of early childhood, persist into later childhood and adolescence, or may even have their onset in this later period. In cerebrotendinous xanthomatosis (see further on) spastic weakness and pseudobulbar palsy are combined with cerebellar ataxia. The Prader-Labhart-Willi children have a broad-based gait and are clumsy in addition to being obese, genitally deficient, and diabetic. One family of five males with a syndrome of hyperuricemia, spinocerebellar ataxia, and deafness has been reported by Rosenberg et al; the enzymatic defect of Lesch-Nyhan disease was not present, however. Marsden and coworkers have observed cerebellar ataxia beginning in late childhood, as an expression of adrenoleukodystrophy (see below). We have observed several cases of an hereditary paroxysmal cerebellar ataxia, each attack lasting a few hours. The attacks were prevented by diamox, 250 mg tid (Lonsdale et al).

THE PARKINSONIAN SYNDROME WITH OTHER EXTRAPYRAMIDAL SYMPTOMS

Reference here is to the distinctive motor disorder described in Chap. 4, in which strength remains relatively intact and corticospinal signs are absent, but in which effectiveness of movement is nonetheless impaired by the patient's disinclination to use the affected parts (hypo- or akinesia), by slowness (bradykinesia) and by rigidity and tremor. Dystonic postures and spasms of gaze may be conjoined.

When these symptoms have their onset in middle or late adult life, they indicate paralysis agitans (Parkinson disease) or striatonigral degeneration. The development of an extrapyramidal motor disorder in late childhood and adolescence should always suggest (1) Wilson-Westphal-Strümpell hepatocerebral degeneration and (2) Hallervorden-Spatz disease.

Hepatolenticular Degeneration (Wilson Disease, Westphal-Strümpell Pseudosclerosis)

Wilson's classic description of "progressive lenticular degeneration: a familial nervous disease associated with cirrhosis of the liver" appeared in 1912. A similar neurologic disorder had been described previously by Gowers (1906) under the title of "tetanoid chorea" and by Westphal (1883) and Strümpell (1898), as "pseudosclerosis"; these authors, however, had not recognized the association with cirrhosis. The clinical studies of Hall (1921) and the histopathologic studies of Spielmeyer (1920), who reexamined the liver and brain tissues of Westphal's and Strümpell's cases, clearly established that the pseudosclerosis described by the latter authors was the same disease as the one described by Wilson. Interestingly, none of these authors had recognized the golden-brown (Kayser-Fleischer) corneal ring, the one pathognomonic sign of the disease. The corneal abnormality was first recognized by Kayser in 1902, and in the following year Fleischer related it to pseudosclerosis. Rumpell (quoted by Sass-Kortsak and Bearn) had demonstrated the greatly increased copper content of the liver and brain as early as 1913, but this discovery was generally neglected until Mandelbrote (1948) found, quite by chance, that the urinary excretion of copper was elevated in Wilson disease, and that it was increased further by intramuscular administration of the chelating agent BAL (British antilewisite). In 1952, Scheinberg and Gitlin discovered that ceruloplasmin, the serum enzyme that binds copper, is consistently reduced in Wilson disease. They postulated that the inherited defect is an inability to synthesize ceruloplasmin, but how this leads to excessive tissue deposition of copper is not understood. Moreover, it has since been determined that the serum concentration of ceruloplasmin is normal in about 5 percent of patients with Wilson disease. An alternate hypothesis is that the impairment of ceruloplasmin synthesis is secondary to an intrahepatic defect in copper metabolism. (See reviews by Adams and by Scheinberg and Sternlieb for a full historical account and references.)

Clinical features   The disease is transmitted as an autosomal recessive trait, and the abnormal gene has been assigned, by linkage analysis, to the esterase D locus on chromosome 13 (Frydman et al). The prevalence is approximately one per 35,000 of the general population. The onset of neurologic symptoms is usually in the second and less often in the third decades, and rarely beyond that time.

In all instances the first expression of the disease is a deposition of copper in the liver, leading to an acute or chronic hepatitis and eventually to multilobular cirrhosis and splenomegaly (Scheinberg and Sternlieb). This may be asymptomatic (except for elevated serum transaminases) or give rise in childhood to attacks of jaundice, unexplained hepatosplenomegaly, or hypersplenism with thrombocytopenia and bleeding.

The first neurologic manifestations are *tremor* of a limb or of the head, slowness of movement, *dysarthria, dysphagia,* hoarseness, and occasionally choreic movements or dystonic postures of the limbs. Exceptionally an abnormality of behavior (argumentative; excessively emotional), or a gradual impairment of intellectual faculties precedes other neurologic signs. As the disease progresses, the "classic syndrome" evolves: dysphagia and drooling; *rigidity* and slowness of movements of the limbs; flexed postures; fixity of facial muscles with mouth constantly agape, giving an appearance of grinning or a "vacuous smile"; dysarthria; and a tremor in repose which increases

when the limbs are outstretched (coarse, "wing-beating" tremor). Usually an element of cerebellar ataxia and intention tremor of variable degree are added. In this and other ways the syndrome differs from classic parkinsonism.

With further progression of neurologic disease, the *Kayser-Fleischer rings* become more evident. They take the form of a rusty-brown discoloration of the deepest layer of the cornea (Descemet's membrane). In the purely hepatic stage of the disease, the rings may not be evident (in 25 percent of cases), but they are invariably present once neurologic signs are present. A slit-lamp examination may be necessary for their detection, particularly in brown-eyed patients. The disability increases because of increasing rigidity and tremor. The patient becomes mute, immobile, extremely rigid, dystonic, and slowed mentally (late and variable effect).

The diagnosis is virtually certain when there is a similar syndrome in a sibling, or when an extrapyramidal motor disorder of this type is conjoined with liver disease and the corneal rings. Variants of the above syndrome that the authors have seen are an early choreoathetosis (like Sydenham chorea); prominent dystonic postures; a cerebellar ataxia with minimal rigidity; a syndrome of coarse action or action and intention tremor, resembling a cerebellar degeneration; an immobile mute state with profound rigidity; and, as was remarked, a dementia, character change, or psychosis with relatively few extrapyramidal signs. Action myoclonus has also been described.

In these variants the finding of a *low serum ceruloplasmin* level (less than 20 mg/dL), low serum copper (less than 80 μg/dL), and *increased urinary copper excretion* (more than 100 μg Cu in 24 h) corroborate the diagnosis in most cases. Early in the course of the illness the most reliable diagnostic findings are a *high copper content in a biopsy of liver tissue* (more than 250 μg Cu per gram dried weight) and a failure to incorporate[64] Cu into ceruloplasmin. Persistent aminoaciduria is present in most but not all patients. Liver function tests are abnormal; some patients are jaundiced and other signs of liver failure may appear late in the illness. The cirrhosis may not always be evident in a liver biopsy (some regenerative nodules are large, and the biopsy may be taken from one of them).

In studies of large groups of patients it has been established that copper deposition in the liver is the initial disturbance and over time it leads to cirrhosis. The hepatic stage of the disease precedes neurologic involvement. Cranial CT scans are abnormal, even in the hepatic stage, and are invariably so when the neurologic disorder supervenes. The lateral ventricles and often the third ventricle are enlarged, the cerebral and cerebellar sulci are widened, the brainstem appears shrunken, and the lenticular nuclei become hypodense. With treatment these radiologic changes become less marked (Williams and Walshe). MRI is an even more sensitive means of visualizing the structural changes, particularly those in the subcortical white matter, midbrain, pons, and cerebellum (Starosta-Rubinstein et al).

Neuropathologic changes These vary with the rate of progress of the disease. Exceptionally, in the rapidly advancing and fatal form, there is frank cavitation in the lenticular (putaminal and pallidal) nuclei, as was observed in Wilson's original cases. In the more chronic form there is only shrinkage and a light-brown discoloration of these structures. Nerve cell loss and some degree of degeneration of myelinated fibers in lenticular nuclei, substantia nigra, and dentate nuclei are usually apparent. More striking, however, is a marked hyperplasia of protoplasmic astrocytes (Alzheimer type II cells) in the cerebral cortex, basal ganglia, brainstem nuclei, and cerebellum.

Treatment Ideally treatment should be started before the appearance of neurologic signs and if this can be effected, the latter can be prevented to a large extent. It consists of (1) reduction of dietary copper to less than 1 mg/day, which can usually be accomplished by avoidance of copper-rich foods (liver, mushrooms, cocoa, chocolate, nuts, and shellfish); and (2) administration of the copper chelating agent D-penicillamine (1 to 2 g/day) by mouth. If sensitivity to the latter develops (rash, arthralgia, fever, leukopenia), temporary reduction of dosage or a course of cortisone may bring the reaction under control. Reinstitution of drug therapy should be undertaken, using low dosages (250 mg daily) and small, widely spaced increases. If the patient is still sensitive to D-penicillamine or if severe reactions (lupus-like or nephrotic syndromes) occur, the drug should be discontinued and zinc acetate (50 mg elemental zinc five times daily) or the chelating agent triethylene tetramine (trientene) should be substituted. The appropriate drug needs to be continued for the patient's lifetime.

In most patients, neurologic signs improve under the influence of treatment. The Kayser-Fleischer rings disappear and liver function tests may return to normal, although the abnormalities of copper metabolism remain unchanged. In moderately severe and advanced cases, clinical improvement may not begin for several weeks or months despite full doses of D-penicillamine, and it is important not to discontinue the drug during this latent period. In still other patients

(10 to 50 percent in different series) the neurologic signs actually worsen in the month or two after institution of D-penicillamine therapy, and some of these patients remain in a worsened condition despite the persistent use of the drug. In one reported case, new lesions of Wilson disease (shown by MRI) developed while the patient was receiving full doses of D-penicillamine and excellent decoppering of the liver had occurred (Brewer et al).

Hallervorden-Spatz Disease This disease is also known as *pigmentary degeneration of the globus pallidus, substantia nigra, and red nucleus.* It is inherited as an autosomal recessive trait. Onset is in late childhood or early adolescence, and it progresses slowly over a period of 10 to 20 years. The early signs are motor, both *corticospinal (spasticity,* hyperreflexia, Babinski signs) and *extrapyramidal (rigidity, dystonia, and choreoathetosis).* General deterioration of intellect is conjoined. In individual cases, ataxia and myoclonus have been described at some phase of the illness. The spasticity and rigidity are predominantly paraplegic in distribution, but in some instances they begin in the bulbar muscles, interfering with speech and swallowing, as happens in Wilson disease. Eventually the patient becomes almost completely inarticulate and unable to walk or to use the arms. Optic atrophy has been mentioned in a few reports, but we have not observed it.

There is no known biochemical test by which the diagnosis can be corroborated. The deposits of iron in basal ganglia have not been associated with demonstrable abnormality of serum iron or of iron metabolism. It has, however, been reported that there is a high uptake of radioactive iron in the region of the basal ganglia following intravenous injection of labeled ferrous citrate (Vakili et al, Szanto and Gallyas). This technique may prove to be useful in diagnosis. CT scans reveal hypodense zones in the lenticular nuclei, resembling those of Wilson disease and SNE (Leigh), although recently, high-density lesions have been described in an autopsy-proven case of this disease (Tennison et al).

The neuropathology proves to be the most distinctive attribute of the disease. There is an intense brown pigmentation of the globus pallidus, substantia nigra, (especially the anteromedial parts), and red nucleus. Granules and larger amorphous deposits of iron mixed with calcium stud the walls of small blood vessels; others lie free in the tissue. A loss of neurons and medullated fibers occurs in the most affected regions. Another unique feature is the presence of swollen axon fragments, that resemble those of neuroaxonal dystrophy; for this reason some authors regard Hallervorden-Spatz disease as a juvenile form of neuroaxonal dystrophy. However, iron deposits are not a conspicuous finding in the latter disease, leaving this interpretation in doubt.

No treatment is known to be effective. Some of our patients were temporarily improved by L-dopa, but the effect was slight. The use of chelating agents to reduce iron storage has not helped.

Differential Diagnosis   Disorders that need to be differentiated from Wilson and Hallervorden-Spatz disease are Chédiak-Higashi disease, juvenile paralysis agitans, early-onset Huntington chorea, status dysmyelinatus, and Lafora-body disease, Leigh disease and other rare, presumably biochemical, disorders of unknown type. Several of the latter have come to our attention, simulating the neurologic picture of Wilson disease but without evidence of liver involvement or copper abnormality.

In Chédiak-Higashi disease (which is characterized by massive granulation of leukocytes in blood and marrow, and by partial albinism) neurologic symptoms occur in approximately half the patients. Mental retardation, seizures, chronic polyneuropathy, cerebellar ataxia, and a parkinsonian syndrome have been mentioned. The polyneuropathy, however, is the main clinical problem.

In families known to have *Huntington chorea*, children may be afflicted. The age of onset may be as early as 1 to 4 years, but more often it is between 5 and 14 years. About 5 percent of all cases of Huntington chorea are of this juvenile type. Surprisingly, the slow decay in intellect is attended by slurred speech, rigidity of the limbs, short-stepped gait, and flexion hypertonia of the limbs and trunk, rather than a movement disorder. Nevertheless, choreoathetosis does occur in some cases, and not all juvenile cases are rigid. Ocular movements are full except for upward gaze. A less frequent abnormality is a decreased velocity of conjugate ocular movements, so that the eyes move as though floating in an oil bath. The tendon reflexes are not exaggerated and are later suppressed by the rigidity, but occasionally there are Babinski signs. Generalized seizures have occurred in some cases. Other neurologic abnormalities in the childhood syndrome are abnormal behavior, withdrawal and negativism, and catatonic posturing. Irritability and emotionality may raise the question of Sydenham chorea. Myoclonic jerks have also been reported, and cerebellar ataxia occurs in some families. The disease is inexorably progressive and eventually the patient becomes mute and rigidly immobile, with mouth agape, limbs flexed, and hands fisted in fixed, dystonic postures. See Chap. 43 for discussion of the neuropathology and treatment.

Juvenile paralysis agitans was described by Ramsay Hunt in 1917. From the descriptions the resemblance to adult Parkinson disease is close. The course was slowly progressive. Familial incidence (two brothers aged 10 and 19) was reported by van Bogaert, but most cases have been sporadic. Postmortem examination has allegedly shown a shrinkage of the lenticular nuclei and loss of large cells in the pallidum, but in an anatomic specimen from van Bogaert's laboratory (age of onset was 7 years), cell loss

was noted in both the substantia nigra and pallidum. There was no evidence of encephalitis lethargica, and the pathologic findings differed from those of paralysis agitans, Wilson disease, Hallervorden-Spatz disease, and Huntington chorea. The authors are puzzled about this entity and have had no personal experience with it upon which to rely.

The *status dysmyelinatus* of Vogt and Vogt represents another obscure disease in which all myelinated fibers and nerve cells in the lenticular nuclei (both striatofugal and pallidofugal) disappear. The principal clinical features are extrapyramidal rigidity and, later, athetosis. Eventually the child becomes helpless, with limbs in weird postures and contorted by spasms. At one phase it is said to resemble Parkinson disease.

In isolated late-life cases of *Lafora-body disease* (see further on in this chapter), there may be rigidity, akinesia, and tremor; but usually myoclonus, seizures, and dementia dominate the picture. Rarely *Leigh disease* gives rise to a slowly evolving extrapyramidal rigidity in late childhood or adolescence with cavitation of the putamens in CT scans.

The differential diagnosis of the above diseases presents certain difficulties. Hallervorden-Spatz disease cannot always be recognized for want of a satisfactory laboratory test; some cases presently included in this category may have some other disease. The similarities between the diseases included under the rubric of the Parkinson syndrome are in general smaller than the differences. Wilson disease, for example, shares certain signs with Parkinson disease, yet the appearance of each is quite distinctive. The special qualities of the facial expression in Wilson disease—as well as the dysarthria, severe ataxic tremor, and other signs of cerebellar ataxia—are not readily confused with Parkinson disease. Furthermore, in several of the diseases in this category there may be myoclonus and extrapyramidal signs such as choreoathetosis, dystonia, etc., which are essential parts of the syndromes described below. Hence one must not insist that each disease conform strictly to a unique clinical syndrome.

THE SYNDROME OF DYSTONIA AND GENERALIZED CHOREA AND ATHETOSIS

As indicated in Chap. 4, the authors find the differences between dystonia and athetosis recondite. If one examines many patients with these involuntary movements, every gradation between the two is seen, and not infrequently the quicker, unpatterned involuntary movements of chorea and ballismus as well. Even tremor and myoclonus may complicate the composite movement disorder. With reference to muscular tone in patients with athetosis and dystonia, there are unpredictable accessions of hypertonia and hypotonia.

A number of rare inherited metabolic diseases are characterized by the syndrome of chorea, athetosis, and dystonia.

The Lesch-Nyhan Syndrome and Hyperuricemia

This rare metabolic disease is inherited as an X-linked recessive trait. Although it carries the name of Lesch and Nyhan (1964) the occurrence of uricemia in association with spasticity and choreoathetosis in early childhood had been described earlier by Catel and Schmidt. Essentially it is a *hereditary choreoathetosis with self-mutilation and hyperuricemia.* The affected children appear normal at birth and usually develop on schedule up to 6 to 9 months of age. Maturational delay then sets in, initially with hypotonia that later gives way to hypertonia. Abnormal behavior also appears, with aggressiveness and compulsive actions. The compulsive self-mutilation, mainly of the lips, occurs early (during the second and third year), and spasticity, choreoathetosis, and tremor come later. Speech is delayed; once attained, it is dysarthric through life. Mental retardation is moderately severe. Most of the children learn to walk. In patients over 10 years of age, gouty tophi appear on the ears, and there is increasing risk from gouty nephropathy. The serum levels of uric acid are in the range of 7 to 10 mg/dL. Deficient activity of the enzyme hypoxanthine-guanine-phosphoribosyl transferase (HGPRT) has been found in all typical cases of this disease. As a result of this deficiency, hypoxanthine is either excreted or catabolized to xanthine and uric acid. The biochemical abnormality responsible for CNS dysfunction is unclear. Lloyd and colleagues measured dopamine in nerve terminals and found it reduced by 10 to 30 percent. Goldstein et al have ascribed self-mutilation to dopamine denervation.

In the differential diagnosis, one must consider nonspecific mental retardation with hand biting and mutilation, athetosis from *birth trauma,* and encephalopathies with chronic renal disease. *Hyperuricemia* has also been reported in a family with spinocerebellar ataxia and deafness, and in another with autism and mental retardation, neither of them with the enzymatic defect of Lesch-Nyhan disease.

Treatment with allopurinol, a xanthine oxidase inhibitor which blocks the last steps of uric acid synthesis, reduces the uric acid in the Lesch-Nyhan disease and prevents the uricosuric nephropathy, but has no effect on CNS symptoms. Guanosine 5'-monophosphate and inosine 5'-monophosphate, which are deficient, have been replaced without benefit to the patient. Transitory success has been achieved with the administration of 5-hydroxytryptophan in combination with L-dopa. Fluphenazine (Prolixin) is reported to have eliminated the self-mutilation after haloperidol had failed to do so. Behavior modification programs may be of some value.

Familial Calcification of Vessels in Basal Ganglia and Cerebellum (Hypoparathyroidism and Fahr Syndrome)

Ferruginization and calcification of vessels in the basal ganglia occur to a slight degree in many otherwise normal humans (and in other mammals). The widespread use of CT scans and MRI of the cranium have brought the condition to light with increasing frequency (Fig. 38-1). Usually it may be dismissed as an aging phenomenon of no clinical significance. When it occurs early in life and is of such degree as to be visible in plain films of the skull, it must always be regarded as abnormal. An adult case of this type was described by Fahr, so that his name is sometimes attached to this disorder, but it was known long before his publication appeared, and his account added little to our knowledge of the condition.

Many authors have called attention to a form of calcification of the basal ganglia and cerebellum, in which choreoathetosis and rigidity are prominent. The clinical state may take the form of a parkinsonian syndrome or double athetosis. In several of our patients there was a unilateral athetosis (arm and leg) which was replaced gradually by a parkinsonian syndrome. Some patients have been mentally retarded, others intellectually intact. We have observed a a familial form of calcification, inherited as an autosomal recessive trait. Its onset was in adolescence and early adult life and it presented as a complex neurologic syndrome that included choreoathetosis, tremor, ataxia, and dementia. The serum calcium levels in the aforementioned types of cases are usually normal, and there is no explanation of the calcification.

In hypoparathyroidism (idiopathic or acquired) and pseudohypoparathyroidism (a rare familial disease characterized by the symptoms and signs of hypoparathyroidism in association with distinctive skeletal and developmental abnormalities) not only does diminution in ionized serum calcium induce tetany and seizures, but choreoathetosis may be added. The latter symptom is presumably due to calcification of the basal ganglia, which occurs in about one-half of the patients. Also, in some instances there are signs of a cerebellar lesion.

Sly and his colleagues have described the familial occurrence (21 cases in 12 families) of calcification in the caudate and lenticular nuclei, thalami, and frontal lobe white matter, in association with osteopetrosis (''marble bones'') and renal tubular acidosis. Clinically there were multiple cranial nerve palsies, including optic atrophy,

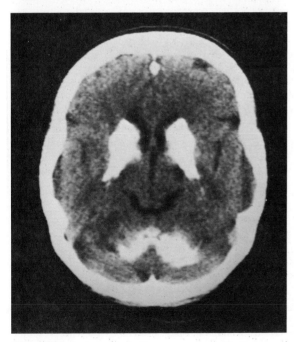

Figure 38-1

Above. Idiopathic basal ganglionic calcification in a 25-year-old woman who had no symptoms or signs of cerebral disease. Below. Idiopathic basal ganglionic and cerebellar calcification, discovered 5 years after the onset of a slowly progressive Parkinson syndrome in a 54-year-old woman.

psychomotor delay, and learning disabilities, but no extrapyramidal signs. The cranial nerve palsies, which are due to bony encroachment in neural foramina, were much less severe than in the lethal form of osteopetrosis. The pattern of inheritance of this disease is autosomal recessive, and the basic abnormality was found to be a deficiency in carbonic anhydrase II in red blood corpuscles and probably in kidney and brain.

Other Metabolic Disorders Associated with Choreoathetosis and Dystonia Exceptionally, ceroid-lipofuscinosis of the Kufs type, G_{M1} gangliosidosis, late-onset metachromatic leukodystrophy, Niemann-Pick disease, Hallervorden-Spatz disease, and Wilson disease may present with a syndrome of which dystonia or athetosis is an important component. Usually the other elements in the clinical picture are detectable, so that the correct diagnosis is seldom in doubt for long. Dal Canto et al have described a *variant* of *neuronal ceroid-lipofuscinosis* in which a boy and girl of unrelated non-Jewish parents developed severe choreoathetosis and dystonia at 6 to 7 years of age. Intellectual deterioration, gait abnormality, and seizures were the other clinical features. Cerebral biopsy showed intraneuronal inclusions consisting of *curvilinear bodies*. These observations support the notion of nosologic heterogeneity among the nonglycolipid neuronal storage disorders.

Finally, in regard to extrapyramidal motor disorders, it should be pointed out that those of acquired type are much more common than inherited ones. A prototype of athetosis is known to follow hypoxic encephalopathy of birth, leading to *état marbré* of the basal ganglia. This is the double athetosis syndrome that usually does not become manifest until after the first year of life and persists thereafter (page 993). The Rh and ABO blood incompatibilities that induce erythroblastosis fetalis and kernicterus may be the cause of a bilateral athetosis at about the same period of life, but are distinguished by deafness and paralysis of upward gaze (see page 994). The same is true of the Crigler-Najjar form of hereditary hyperbilirubinemia, wherein kernicterus (with ataxia or athetosis) may rarely appear as late as childhood or adolescence; the defect is one of glucuronide-bilirubin conjugation (Schmid and McDonagh).

A number of other rare diseases that can only be classified as heredofamilial degenerations, must also figure in the differential diagnosis of choreoathetotic or dystonic syndromes. *Torsion dystonia* is one of the best known examples (see page 64). A *nonprogressive familial choreoathetosis* with onset in early childhood has been described by Pincus and Chutorian; cerebellar signs are usually conjoined, but the intellect is spared. This syndrome is thought to be inherited as an autosomal recessive trait. The authors also have encountered families with hereditary choreoathetosis, uncomplicated, as an autosomal dominant trait. A paroxysmal form of *familial choreoathetosis* was recognized by Mount and Reback in 1940, and the subject has more recently been reviewed by Lance (see page 65). We have observed attacks of this kind in children with "cerebral palsy," as a manifestation of phenytoin toxicity; lowering the dose of phenytoin terminated the attacks. Clearly the metabolic effect of phenytoin on a damaged nervous system was capable of evoking this syndrome. Perhaps some unknown metabolite has a similar effect in other cases. Van Bogaert reported a syndrome of choreoathetosis and dystonia, the pathologic basis of which was an atrophy of the globus pallidus. Malamud and Demmy have placed on record two cases of choreoathetosis, mental deterioration, and hyperemotionality with spongy lesions in the subthalamic nuclei of Luys; these may be examples of the subacute necrotizing encephalomyelopathy of Leigh. No biochemical abnormalities or metabolic faults have been identified in any of the aforementioned diseases.

THE FAMILIAL POLYMYOCLONIAS

As was stated in Chap. 5, the term *myoclonus* is applied to many conditions, not at all alike, but sharing a single clinical feature—exceedingly brief, random, arrhythmic twitches of parts of muscles, muscles, and groups of muscles. Myoclonic jerks differ from choreoathetosis by virtue of their brevity (15 to 50 ms). Nevertheless, both phenomena are considered to be symptomatic of "gray matter" diseases.

Myoclonus may be mixed with any of the aforementioned syndromes of athetosis and dystonia, but more often it is associated with cerebellar ataxia. It may, in certain conditions, stand as a relatively pure syndrome. The many acquired forms of polymyoclonia, such as subacute sclerosing panencephalitis, have been mentioned in Chap. 5. Here we are concerned with those of known or presumed metabolic origin.

Myoclonic Encephalopathy of Infants Under this title Kinsbourne originally described a form of widespread, continuous myoclonus (except during deep sleep) affecting male and female infants, whose development had been normal until the onset of the disease (9 to 20 months). The myoclonus evolves over a week or less, affects all the muscles of the body, and interferes seriously with all the

natural muscular activities of the child. The eyes are notably affected by rapid (up to 8 per second) irregular conjugate movement ("dancing eyes"). The child is irritable and speech may cease. All laboratory tests are normal.

ACTH and dexamethasone, the latter in doses of 1.5 to 4.0 mg/day, suppress the myoclonus and permit developmental progress. Some patients have recovered from the myoclonus and have been mentally slow and mildly ataxic afterward. Others have required corticosteroid therapy for 5 to 10 years, with relapse whenever it is discontinued. Ordinary anticonvulsants have no effect.

A similar syndrome has been observed in conjunction with neuroblastoma, rarely with bronchogenic and other occult carcinomas, and as a transient illness of unknown cause (? viral) in young adults (Baringer et al).

Familial Progressive Myoclonus Four major categories of familial polymyoclonus of late childhood and adolescence have been delineated: (1) Lafora- or amyloid-body type, (2) juvenile cerebroretinal degeneration, (3) cherry-red spot-myoclonus (sialidosis or neuraminidosis), (4) mitochondrial encephalopathy, and (5) a more benign degenerative disease (dyssynergia cerebellaris myoclonica of Hunt). Familial myoclonus may also be a prominent feature of two other diseases—G_{M2} gangliosidosis and Gaucher disease—which occasionally have their onset in this age period.

Lafora-body polymyoclonus This disease, which is inherited as an autosomal recessive trait was first identified by Lafora, in 1911, on the basis of the postmortem finding of large basophilic cytoplasmic bodies in the dentate, brainstem, and thalamic neurons. They have been shown by Yokoi et al to be composed of a glucose polymer (polyglycosan), chemically but not structurally related to glycogen. Possibly some of the cases of familial myoclonus epilepsy reported by Unverricht and by Lundborg (see page 85) were of this type, but since they provided no pathologic data, one cannot be sure.

Beginning in late childhood and adolescence (11 to 18 years), in a previously normal individual, the disease announces itself by a seizure (petit mal or grand mal) or by many myoclonic jerks, or both. In about half the cases there are focal (occipital) seizures. The illness may at first be mistaken for ordinary epilepsy, but within a few months it becomes evident that it is far more serious. The myoclonus becomes widespread and can be initiated by noise, startle, excitement, or by certain sustained motor activities. An evoked train of myoclonic jerks may progress to a generalized seizure with loss of consciousness. As the disease advances, the myoclonus interferes increasingly with the patient's activities until function is seriously impaired. Close examination may also reveal an alteration in muscle tone and a slight degree of cerebellar ataxia. At this time, or even before the onset of myoclonus and seizures, the patient may experience visual hallucinations or exhibit irritability, odd traits of character, uninhibited or impulsive behavior, and, ultimately, progressive failure in all cognitive functions. Deafness has been an early sign in a few cases. Rigidity, hypotonia, impaired tendon reflexes, acrocyanosis, and rarely corticospinal tract signs are late findings. Finally the patient becomes cachectic and bedfast, and succumbs to intercurrent infection. Most do not survive beyond their twenty-fifth birthday. Nonetheless there are isolated reports of Lafora-body disease in which symptoms began as late as 40 years, with death at 50 years. These latter cases may constitute a separate genetic type.

No abnormalities of blood, urine, or CSF have been detected. The EEG shows diffuse slow waves and spikes as well as focal or multifocal discharges. Altered hepatocytes with homogeneous PAS-positive bodies that displace the nuclei have been observed in both the presymptomatic and symptomatic stages of the disease. Carpenter and Karpati have also observed these inclusions in duct cells of the eccrine sweat glands. These inclusions have been seen in skin and liver biopsies even though liver function tests were normal. Neuropathologic examinations have shown a slight loss of granule and Purkinje cells, and loss of neurons in the dentate nuclei, inner segment of globus pallidus, and cerebral cortex—in addition to the Lafora bodies. The latter may also be seen in the retina, myocardium, and striated muscles.

Anticonvulsant drugs help in the control of the seizures, but have no effect on the basic process.

Juvenile cerebroretinal degeneration (ceroid storage) This is one of the most variable forms of the lipidoses. The original observations were from Scandinavia, by Unverricht and Lundborg. Kolodny (1981), on the basis of a large experience with the neuronal ceroid-lipofuscinoses, has divided them into four subtypes, according to their age of onset: (1) *The infantile type* (Santavuori-Haltia), which presents with impaired vision and psychomotor delay in the first year or two of life; it is particularly common among Finnish children (Balkan disease). (2) *The late infantile type* (Jansky-Bielschowsky), which begins with seizures at the age of 2 to 4 years; it has been described on page 796. (3) *The juvenile type* (Spielmeyer-Vogt), which begins with visual symptoms between 3 and 8 years. Types (2) and (3) are often referred to as Batten or Batten-Mayou disease. (4) *The adult or Kufs type,* which begins in adolescent or adult years with alterations of personality, progressing to dementia.

The salient clinical features of types (1), (2), and (3) are severe myoclonus, seizures, and visual loss. The maculae are the site of the first lesions; they appear as yellow-gray

areas of degeneration, in contrast to the cherry-red spot and the encircling gray ring of Tay-Sachs disease. At first the particles of pigment are fine, and dust-like; later they agglomerate to resemble more the bone-corpuscular shapes in retinitis pigmentosa. The liver and spleen are not enlarged, and there are no osseous changes. The usual development of these and other manifestations of the disease has been outlined by Sjögren, who has studied a large number of the late infantile and juvenile types of cases in Sweden. He divides the illness into five stages:

1. Visual impairment, sometimes preceding retinal changes by months.

2. After approximately 2 years, the onset of generalized seizures and myoclonus, often with irritability, poor control of emotions, and stuttering, jerky speech.

3. Gradual intellectual deterioration (poor memory, reduced mental activity, inattentiveness). By this stage the movements have usually become slow, stiff, and tremulous, resembling somewhat those of Parkinson disease—to which are added elements of cerebellar ataxia and intention tremor, coming in this way to resemble Wilson disease.

4. Stage of severe dementia in which the patient needs assistance to get about, no longer speaks, and may scream when disturbed or forced to move. The muscles are wasted, though the tendon reflexes are lively and the plantar reflexes are extensor.

5. Finally the patient lies curled up in bed, blind and speechless, with strong extensor plantar reflexes, occasionally adopting dystonic postures. Mercifully the illness ends in 10 to 15 years.

In the early stages the EEG picture of random, high-voltage, triphasic waves is diagnostic; later, as the seizures and myoclonic jerks become less frequent and finally cease, only delta waves are seen. The electroretinographic waveforms are lost if the retina is affected. The lateral ventricles are slightly dilated. The CSF is normal. Diagnosis is best confirmed by electron microscopic study of biopsy material, particularly of the eccrine sweat glands of the skin. The enzymatic defect has not been demonstrated.

The Kufs type, which develops later (15 to 25 years), is often unattended by visual or retinal changes, and is even slower in its evolution. Personality change and seizures, usually with some degree of myoclonus, are the principal abnormalities. As the disease progresses, cerebellar ataxia, spasticity and rigidity, or athetosis, or mixtures thereof, are combined with dementia. Van Bogaert (personal communication) has noted that relatives of these patients may have retinal changes without neurologic accompaniments.

Of all the lipidoses, the cerebroretinal degenerations have defied biochemical definition. There is no deficiency in hexosaminidase activity in the serum nor increase in gangliosides in the brain. Zeman et al have shown that the cytoplasmic inclusions are autofluorescent and give a positive histochemical reaction for ceroid and lipofuscin, but accumulation of this latter substance is a nonspecific aging phenomenon. Williams and his colleagues find that there is a fusiform enlargement of proximal axon segments of pyramidal and polymorphic neurons. In addition to the presence of curvilinear bodies in the cytoplasm of neurons, some in a fingerprint pattern, there is a reduction in type II synapses in the dilated parts of the axon. All these changes precede nerve cell loss.

Childhood or juvenile G_{M2} gangliosidosis

Rarely, instances of the recessive type of G_{M2} gangliosidosis have their onset at this age period. Twenty-four such cases (from 20 kindreds) were found in the medical literature by Meek and his coworkers. Ataxia and dysarthria were frequently the presenting symptoms, followed by dementia, dysphagia, spasticity, dystonia, seizures, and myoclonus. Atypical cherry-red spots are observed in some patients. The biochemical abnormality, i.e., a deficiency of hexosaminidase A, is the same as in Tay-Sachs disease, but not as severe. Progression of the disease is slow, over a period of many years. Some of our patients are alive at 40 years, the disease having begun in adolescence.

Late Gaucher disease with polymyoclonia

A type of Gaucher disease is occasionally encountered in which seizures, severe diffuse myoclonus, supranuclear gaze disorders (slow saccades, saccadic palsy, saccadic and pursuit horizontal gaze palsies), and cerebellar ataxia begin in late childhood, adolescence, or adult life. The course is slowly progressive. The intellect is relatively spared. The spleen is enlarged. The pathologic and biochemical abnormalities are the same as those of Gaucher disease of early onset (Winkelman et al).

The cherry-red spot–myoclonus syndrome

This is a new and genetically distinct class of disease, characterized by the storage of sialidated glycopeptides in tissues and due to a neuraminidase deficiency. In some of the patients, the onset has been in late childhood or adolescence and in others even later. When Rapin et al described their patients, 24 similar cases had already been

reported in the medical literature and we had personally observed several at the EK Shriver Center.

In the cases of Rapin et al and in two of our own the first findings were the cherry-red macular spots, similar to those that are seen in Tay-Sachs disease, and less consistently in G_{M1} gangliosidosis, Niemann-Pick disease, and metachromatic leukodystrophy. In one case there was severe episodic pain in the hands and legs and feet during hot weather, reminiscent of Fabry disease. Polymyoclonia followed within a few years, and together with cerebellar ataxia, disabled the patients. Mental function remained relatively normal. Liver and spleen were not enlarged but storage material was found in Kupffer cells, neurons of the myenteric plexus, cerebral neurons, and presumably in cerebellar and retinal ones. In some of the reported cases a relative had clouded corneas, angiokeratomas of the skin, and burning pain in the hands and feet, suggesting an overlap with Fabry disease.

The cases of Thomas and colleagues were young adults, all members of one generation, who had developed dysarthria, intention myoclonus, cerebellar ataxia, and cherry-red macular lesions. Like the cases of Rapin et al, the heredity was autosomal recessive in type. There was urinary excretion of sialylated oligosaccharides and a sialidase deficiency in cultured fibroblasts. The two patients described by Tsuji et al are noteworthy, insofar as they were aged 50 and 30 years, respectively. In addition to the macular lesions, polymyoclonia, and cerebellar ataxia, there were gargoyle-like facial features, corneal opacities, and vertebral dysplasia. They too had a neuraminidase (partial β-galactosidase) deficiency.

Mitochondrial encephalomyopathy

In recent years this class of disease has undergone great expansion. A diversity of clinical syndromes has been grouped together on the basis of a shared morphologic change in skeletal muscle fibers—the "ragged-red fiber," as seen with modified Gomori stains.

One clinical phenotype, known as myoencephalopathy ragged-red fiber disease (MERRF), begins in the second decade or later with myoclonus and ataxia. Appearing later and advancing slowly are tonic-clonic seizures and decline in intellectual functions. Short stature, hearing loss, optic atrophy, and neuropathy are present in some cases. The lactate levels of the serum and CSF are elevated, indicating mitochondrial respiratory enzyme malfunction. In some families the disease has been transmitted by means of maternal mitochondrial DNA. Diagnosis of this and related syndromes is achieved by muscle biopsy and cytochrome oxidase tests of sarcoplasm (Berkovic et al).

Benign familial polymyoclonia

This, the fifth major polymyoclonus syndrome of childhood, adolescence, and early adult life, should probably be listed as a degenerative disease, for it has not been associated with any biochemical abnormalities. The inheritance is autosomal dominant in type, and in some families the disease has been traced through several generations.

The onset of the illness is with shock-like myoclonic contractions in the muscles of the shoulders and upper arms. As the years pass, all truncal and appendicular muscles are implicated, and finally the face, eyes, tongue, and palate. Parts of a muscle may be involved, resembling fasciculations, or whole muscles and groups of muscles. The frequency of the myoclonic jerks is highly variable. Some are rhythmic, but there are times when they are barely detectable, and others when they are so strong as to seriously interfere with all activities and even throw the patient out of a chair or bed. The myoclonus may begin at any age from infancy to adult life. Some of the most benign forms may virtually subside for a few years only to reappear later.

Mentation is usually preserved until late, when it may become slightly impaired. In a few patients, dementia has been a prominent feature. If any other neurologic abnormality develops, it is likely to be a cerebellar ataxia, which was the combination described by Hunt as *dyssynergia cerebellaris myoclonica* (page 951). A few have been combined with choreoathetosis. Some patients have seizures, but many do not. A form of polymyoclonia associated with nerve deafness has also been reported. The neuropathologic basis of this illness is unsettled.

BILATERAL HEMIPLEGIA, CEREBRAL BLINDNESS AND DEAFNESS, AND OTHER MANIFESTATIONS OF DECEREBRATION

This is the "white matter" syndrome by which most of the chronic familial leukodystrophies are expressed. There are several varieties, some of unquestionable metabolic origin and others of uncertain status. All differ from the preceding cerebral gray matter diseases (poliodystrophies), which have a slightly different mode of presentation—seizures, myoclonus, chorea, choreoathetosis, and tremor being prominent. Clinically, the diagnosis of the entire group of leukodystrophies is based on identification of symptoms and signs that are attributable to the interruption of tracts (corticospinal, corticobulbar, cerebellar peduncular, sensory, medial longitudinal fasciculi), and visual pathways (optic nerve, optic tract, geniculocalcarine), with infrequency or absence of seizures, myoclonus, and spike and wave abnormalities in the EEG.

The syndrome of progressive spasticity and rigidity with spastic dysarthria and pseudobulbar palsy poses a difficult problem. One's first impulse is to assume a corticospinal disorder, especially if tendon reflexes are brisk, but frequently the plantar reflexes are flexor and the facial reflexes not excessively brisk. Unsteadiness of gait and sudden breaks or interruptions of speech suggest a cerebellar defect; unusual postures and a more plastic type of rigidity are consonant with an extrapyramidal disorder. Such combinations, with mental backwardness and dementia, characterize the mild and late forms of *metachromatic leukodystrophy*—which may be taken as an example of a leukoencephalopathy with only a slight degree of neuronal storage. However, a similar syndrome may be observed in other less-well-characterized degenerative diseases, such as the one reported by Willvonseder and colleagues—in which a mild dementia, spastic dysarthria, paresis of vertical eye movements, gait disturbance, and splenomegaly came on during early adult life. Here abnormalities of copper metabolism were found (slightly decreased serum ceruloplasmin, copper turnover values in the range of those of heterozygous carriers of Wilson disease, but no increase in urinary copper excretion). The authors have seen several such patients.

Sudanophilic Leukodystrophy with Bronzing of Skin and Adrenal Atrophy (Adrenoleukodystrophy)

This combination of leukodystrophy and Addison disease, originally included under the rubric of Schilder disease, is now set apart as an independent metabolic encephalopathy.

The onset is usually betweeen 4 and 8 years, sometimes later, and, in the commonest form of this disorder, only males are affected (probably sex-linked recessive). The signs of either the adrenal insufficiency or the cerebral lesion may be the first to appear. In the case of Siemerling and Creutzfeldt, the first recorded example of this disorder, *bronzing of the skin* of the hands appeared at 4 years of age; *quadriparesis, with dysarthria and dysphagia* (pseudobulbar palsy) became evident at 7 years; a single seizure occurred at 8 years; and by 9 years, shortly before death, the patient was *decerebrate* and unresponsive. In personally observed cases, the first abnormalities appeared at 9 to 10 years and took the form of episodic vomiting, decline in scholastic performance, and change in personality, with silly, inappropriate giggling and crying. After a time, severe vomiting and even an episode of circulatory collapse occurred, following which the gait became unsteady and arms ataxic, with an action or intention tremor. Only then did increasing pigmentation of the oral mucosa and the skin around nipples and over elbows, knees, and scrotum become evident. *Cortical blindness* followed in some instances. In the late stages, bilateral hemiplegia (at first asymmetrical), pseudobulbar paralysis, blindness, deafness, and impairment of all higher cerebral functions occurred.

Griffin et al have described a spinal-neuropathic form of the disease (*adrenomyeloneuropathy*). In their patients evidence of adrenal insufficiency was present since early childhood, but only in the third decade did a progressive spastic paraparesis and a relatively mild polyneuropathy develop.

Moser and his colleagues, using clinical and biochemical criteria have identified the following subtypes: (1) familial instances of Addison disease without neurologic involvement in males but with a mild spastic paraparesis in females; (2) progressive degeneration of cerebral white matter in young males, often with cortical blindness; (3) an intermediate form of juvenile or young adult males with cerebral and spinal involvement; (4) a progressive spinal cord degeneration in adult males; (5) a chronic nonprogressive spinal cord disorder in heterozygous females; and (6) possibly a "connatal" form in male infants. Marsden and colleagues and, more recently, Kobayashi et al have described a familial spinocerebellar syndrome, and Ohno et al have reported a sporadic instance of adrenoleukodystrophy presenting as olivopontocerebellar atrophy—illustrating how variable the symptomatology of this disorder· can be.

The important laboratory findings are low sodium and chloride and elevated potassium levels—reflecting the atrophy of the adrenal glands. The latter results in reduced excretion of corticosteroids, low serum cortisol levels, and lack of rise in 17-hydroxyketosteroids after ACTH stimulation. The CSF protein may be elevated.

Massive degeneration of the myelin occurs, often asymmetrically in various parts of the cerebrum, brainstem, optic nerves, and sometimes spinal cord. Degradation products of myelin are visible in macrophages in recent lesions, viz., sudanophilic demyelination. Axis cylinders are damaged, but to a lesser degree. The cortex of the adrenal glands is atrophic, and the cells and invading histiocytes contain an abnormal lipid material. The testes show marked interstitial fibrosis and atrophy of the seminiferous tubules. Electron microscopically, the macrophages of the brain and adrenals and the Leydig cells of the testes show characteristic lamellar cytoplasmic inclusions.

Igarashi and his associates demonstrated that both the brain and adrenals of patients with adrenoleukodystrophy contain abnormally large amounts of very-long-chain fatty acids. Moreover, cultured fibroblasts from such patients contain abnormally high levels of the same fatty acids (Moser et al), a finding that permits accurate diagnosis and is helpful in genetic counseling.

Adrenal replacement therapy may prolong life, and occasionally effects a partial neurologic remission. Trials of dietary control with avoidance of long-chain fatty acids are underway.

Familial Orthochromic Leukodystrophy This is a diffuse, symmetrical cerebral, cerebellar, and spinal degeneration of white matter without visceral lesions. It is believed to be inherited as an autosomal recessive trait but the data are meager.

The age of onset has varied from 1 to 15 years. Some of the sporadic cases reported in the adult were probably examples of cerebral multiple sclerosis, but we have seen orthochromic or metachromatic leukodystrophy (MLD) begin as late as middle adult life, and Bosch and Hart have described dementia and polyneuropathy in a man with MLD whose illness began at 62 years. In all cases, the clinical picture is one of intellectual decline with spastic weakness, hyperreflexia, Babinski signs, and stiff, short-stepped gait. As the disease progresses over 3 to 5 years, there is a loss of vision and speech, then hearing, and finally a state of virtual decerebration. Variants not seen by us include cases wth sudanophilic dystrophy and striato-cerebellar calcification and those with microcephaly, large ears, hypertelorism, and epicanthal folds, who later developed quadriparesis, optic atrophy, and mild choreoathetosis.

In some of these cases it is impossible to distinguish the demyelinative disease from that of Pelizaeus-Merzbacher and of Cockayne, described in the preceding section.

Cerebral Sclerosis of Scholz This is a closely related white-matter disease that begins in childhood and is characterized by cerebral blindness, deafness, aphasia, and spastic quadriparesis. Choreoathetosis has been described in a few cases.

Polycystic White Matter Degeneration This disease of early or late childhood is probably transmitted as an autosomal recessive trait, and causes quadriparesis, blindness, deafness, and loss of speech and other higher cerebral functions. Seizures may be present but are infrequent.

Cerebrotendinous Xanthomatosis This rare disease is probably transmitted by an autosomal recessive gene. It usually begins in late childhood, with *cataracts* and *xanthomata of tendon sheaths and lungs*. As it progresses, mild mental retardation (the earliest neurologic manifestation) gives way to dementia, unsteady ataxic or *ataxic-spastic gait, dysarthria* and *dysphagia, and polyneuropathy*. In the late stages (after 5 to 15 years) the patient becomes bedfast and helpless; death occurs at 20 to 30 years of age. In other cases the clinical course is much more benign. The lesions are visible by CT and MR scanning. Neuropathologic examination shows masses of crystalline cholesterol deposits in the brainstem and cerebellum and sometimes in the spinal cord, with symmetrical destruction of myelin in the same areas.

The serum cholesterol levels were normal in five of seven cases and in the others were as high as 450 mg/dL. The tendon xanthomas contain cholesterol of which 4 to 9 percent is cholestanol (dihydrocholesterol). Cholestanol levels in the serum and red cells are increased.

Long-term treatment with chenodeoxycholic acid, 750 mg daily, cleared up the corticospinal and cerebellar signs and dementia in 10 of 17 patients followed by Berginer et al. This drug corrects the defective synthesis of bile acids and the absence of chenodeoxycholic acid.

This disease should not be confused with that described by Wolman, in which there is an hereditary malabsorption syndrome with hepatosplenomegaly, calcification of the adrenal glands, lymph node enlargement, and storage of cholesterol esters and triglycerides in the tissues (Crocker et al). Neurologic symptoms are usually limited to impaired intellectual development.

STROKES IN ASSOCIATION WITH INHERITED METABOLIC DISEASES

On page 661 it was remarked that strokes occur from time to time in children. Two metabolic diseases must always be considered in the diagnosis of such cases: homocystinuria and Fabry disease. Other less common ones are Tangier disease, familial hypercholesterolemia, and protein C deficiency.

Homocystinuria This aminoaciduria is inherited as an autosomal recessive trait and simulates Marfan disease. Tall, slender habitus, great length of limbs, sometimes scoliosis and arachnodactyly (long, spidery fingers and toes), thin and rather weak muscles, knock-knees, highly arched feet, and kyphosis are the main skeletal features. Sparse, blond, brittle hair and malar flush are often noted, and a *dislocation of one or both lenses* (usually downward) may occur, giving the iris a tremulous appearance. The only neurologic abnormality is *mental retardation,* setting this syndrome apart from Marfan disease, in which intellect is unimpaired.

The basis of the vascular lesions is uncertain. An abnormality of platelets, favoring clot formation and thromboses of cerebral arteries has been suggested. A number of reported cases have died of coronary occlusions during adolescence, and a myocardial lesion may be the source of emboli to cerebral arteries.

Homocystine is elevated in the blood, CSF, and urine. There is an inherited cystathionine synthase deficiency that results in an inadequacy of cystathionine formation, a substance essential to many tissues, including the brain. This may be the explanation of the mental retardation. The

infarcts in the brain are clearly related to thrombotic and embolic arterial occlusions. The administration of a low-methionine diet and large doses of pyridoxine (a cystathionine synthase coenzyme) reduces the excretion of homocystine, but is of uncertain clinical benefit.

Homocystinuria may also be an expression of 5, 10-methylenetetrahydrafolate reductase deficiency. The clinical manifestations consist of multiple cerebrovascular lesions, dementia, epilepsy, and polyneuropathy. The latter is believed to be due to a coincidental folic acid deficiency, but it may be incidental to dilantin toxicity (Nishimura et al).

Fabry Disease (Anderson-Fabry Disease, Hereditary Dystopic Lipidosis) This disease, also known as *angiokeratoma corporis diffusum,* is inherited as an X-linked recessive trait. It occurs in its complete form in men and incomplete form in female carriers. The primary deficit is in the enzyme α-galactosidase, the result of which is accumulation of ceramide trihexoside in endothelial, perithelial, and smooth muscle cells of the blood vessels, as well as in renal tubular and glomerular cells and other viscera and in nerve cells in many parts of the nervous system (hypothalamic and amygdaloid nuclei, substantia nigra, reticular and other nuclei of the brainstem, anterior and intermediolateral horns of the spinal cord, sympathetic and dorsal root ganglia). The disease becomes manifest clinically in childhood or adolescence, with intermittent lancinating pains and dysesthesias of the extremities. A notable feature of the latter is their evocation by fever, hot weather, and vigorous exercise. Usually there is no sensory loss, but autonomic disturbances have been recorded in a series of our cases. Later, the diffuse vascular involvement leads to hypertension, renal damage, cardiomegaly, and myocardial ischemia. Thrombotic infarctions occur in the brain during early adult years. Desnick and Sweeley have reviewed the neurologic, neuropathologic, and biochemical findings in this disease. Its painful neuropathic character is discussed on page 1059.

PERSONALITY CHANGES AND BEHAVIORAL DISTURBANCES AS MANIFESTATIONS OF INHERITED METABOLIC DISEASE

Although rare among the large numbers of maladjusted, neurotic, sociopathic, and psychotic adolescents, certain metabolic diseases may derange the mind and behavior; the management of these metabolic diseases is so special that one must take pains to identify them.

All the metabolic diseases of late childhood and

adolescence share the property of deranging behavior, thinking, feelings, and emotional reactions. The most obvious and easily detectable of these derangements are in the cognitive sphere, i.e., reduction in the capacity to learn and remember, to calculate, to solve problems, and to develop verbal skills. More pronounced forms of these impairments are recognized as neurologic deficits such as "the amnesic state," aphasia, dyscalculia, and visual-perceptual disorientation. Each of these phenomena has its own cerebral anatomy, as was pointed out in Chap. 21, and the state known as dementia comprises various degrees and combinations of these abnormalities.

In early childhood, when the composite of intellectual functions is but little developed, it is difficult to decide upon qualities of the mind. Slowness in learning, in acquiring language functions, etc., may be interpreted loosely as mental retardation. At this age these intellectual functions have not developed sufficiently to permit recognition of their regression. Only in late childhood do mental retardation and dementia become clearly distinguishable.

Far less tangible are subtle changes in personality and behavior, that must always be judged against the standards of the cultural group of which the patient is a member. The occurrence in adolescence of scholastic failure, withdrawal from the family circle, unwillingness to accept parental and societal standards, abuse of drugs, bizarre thinking, somatic delusions, hallucinations, and depressed mood, all raise difficult questions about adolescent maladjustment, sociopathy, schizophrenia, or manic-depressive disease.

The principle that most neuropsychiatrists follow in selecting from the large mass of maladjusted adolescents those with a metabolic brain disease is that the latter will sooner or later cause a regression in cognitive or intellectual functions. Schizophrenia and manic-depressive psychosis and the sociopathies and character disorders do so little or not at all. This is not to say that personality changes and emotional disturbances do not occur in the metabolic encephalopathies; of course they do. However, their recognition depends on the demonstration of failing memory, impaired thinking, inability to learn, and loss of verbal and arithmetic abilities, many of which are measured quantitatively by intelligence tests.

If one reviews all the diseases described in this chapter and selects the ones that demonstrate early regression of cognitive function in association with personality change and alteration of behavior, and that may for a time be unaccompanied by other neurologic abnormalities, the following merit special consideration:

1. Wilson disease

2. Hallervorden-Spatz pigmentary degeneration

3. Lafora-body myoclonic epilepsy

4. Late-onset neuronal ceroid-lipofuscinosis (Kufs form)

5. Juvenile Gaucher disease (type III)

6. Some of the mucopolysaccharidoses

7. Adolescent Schilder disease, without or with adrenal atrophy (sudanophilic leukodystrophy)

8. Metachromatic leukodystrophy

9. Adult G_{M2} gangliosidosis

10. Mucolipidosis I (type I sialidosis)

11. Non-wilsonian copper disorder with dementia, spasticity, and paralysis of vertical eye movements

12. Childhood Huntington chorea

In each of the above diseases, dementia and personality disorder may gradually develop and persist for many months, even a year or two, before other neurologic signs appear. Special problems in diagnosis are raised by each. Personality and behavioral change may so predominate that cognitive losses seem subordinate. The latter need to be sought in a carefully elicited history and review of mental status. One must look also for the earliest signs of movement disorders and other neurologic abnormalities which greatly clarify the diagnostic problem. Often a psychogenesis is incorrectly assumed and prolonged psychotherapy, completely fruitless, has been undertaken.

ADULT FORMS OF INHERITED METABOLIC DISEASES

The increasing range and precision of biochemical and cytologic tests have brought to light a number of inherited metabolic diseases that sometimes have their onset in adult life. Such disorders are uncommon but nevertheless important because they must be considered in the differential diagnosis of degenerative diseases and atrophies, for which explanations are beginning to be found.

In the last few years the authors have personally observed or have otherwise come to know of examples of the following diseases, the onset of which was in late adolescence or adult life.

1. Metachromatic leukoencephalopathy

2. Adrenoleukodystrophy

3. Kufs form of lipid storage disease

4. G_{M2} gangliosidosis

5. Wilson disease

6. Leigh disease

7. Gaucher disease

8. Niemann-Pick disease

9. Polysaccharide encephalopathy

10. Mucolipidosis: type I

11. Polyneuropathies (Andrade disease, porphyria, Refsum disease)

In the encephalopathic forms of these diseases the diagnosis was usually made only after symptoms had been present for months or years and the disease was in most instances mistaken for some other condition. One of our patients with metachromatic leukodystrophy, a 30-year-old man, began failing in college and was later unsuccessful in holding a job because of carelessness and mistakes in his work and indifference, irritability, and stubborness (clearly traceable to a mild dementia). Only when Babinski signs and loss of tendon reflexes in the legs were detected was the diagnosis entertained for the first time. By then he had been ill for nearly 10 years. Bosch and Hart (1978) described a patient with the onset of dementia at 62 years of age, and drew attention to 27 other cases of adult-onset metachromatic leukoencephalopathy. Overt signs of neuropathy are usually lacking in adult-onset cases, but EMG and sural nerve biopsy will disclose the characteristic abnormalities.

One of our adult patients with Wilson disease had been committed to a psychiatric hospital for paranoid tendencies and fighting with his family; the presence of a tremor and mild rigidity of the limbs had been attributed at first to phenothiazine drugs. In some of Griffin's cases of adrenomyeloneuropathy, a spastic weakness of the legs and sensory ataxia, progressing over several years, were the main clinical manifestations; a spinocerebellar degeneration was suspected. One of our patients with Kufs lipid storage disease began to deteriorate mentally in early adult life and later showed an increasing rigidity with athetotic posturing of limbs and difficulty in walking; he succumbed to his disease after more than 10 years. Cerebellar ataxia, polymyoclonus, and progressive blindness have been observed in several adolescents and adults with a variant of G_{M2} gangliosidosis; cherry-red macular spots provided the clue to diagnosis. Several such cases have been reported in the last decade, particularly among the Japanese (Miyatake). We have observed several adult patients with progressive spinal muscular atrophy who proved to have the hexosaminidase deficiency of Tay-Sachs disease.

Dementia, optic atrophy, mild cerebellar ataxia and corticospinal signs have been features of several personally observed patients with Leigh disease who survived in a relatively helpless state for nearly 20 years. Kalimo et al have reported a similar family.

One of our patients, an adolescent with severe diffuse

myoclonus and seizures and slight intellectual deterioration, was found after several years to have one of the rare variants of Gaucher disease. Another with dementia, rigidity, choreoathetosis, slight cerebellar ataxia, and Babinski signs had a variant of Niemann-Pick disease. We also have under observation a family with Gaucher disease, several members of which developed seizures, generalized myoclonus, supranuclear gaze palsies, and cerebellar ataxia in early adult life (Winkelman et al).

We have had the experience of finding laboratory evidence of adrenal insufficiency in several young men with white matter lesions of the frontal lobes and other parts of the cerebrum; there was no bronzing of the skin, and earlier a diagnosis of multiple sclerosis or Schilder disease had been made. Eldridge et al have described a large kindred with widespread noninflammatory degeneration of the cerebral and cerebellar white matter; individual members were thought to have multiple sclerosis before a pattern of autosomal dominant inheritance became evident. Adrenoleukodystrophy presenting in adult life as a spinocerebellar or olivopontocerebellar syndrome has already been mentioned.

These rare forms of inherited metabolic disease are notable for their chronicity and for the early prominence of a particular neurologic symptom or syndrome. Once the disease is established, however, there is nearly always evidence of involvement of multiple neuronal systems, reflected in a subtle or overt dementia, character disorder, or signs referable to cerebellar, pyramidal, extrapyramidal, visual, and peripheral nerve structures. This multiplicity of neuronal system involvement is much more a feature of heritable metabolic disease than of degenerative disease, and the finding of such involvement should always stimulate a search for an inherited metabolic disorder. The dictum that tract involvement (corticospinal, cerebellar, peduncular, sensory, optic nerve) indicates a leukodystrophy and that "gray matter" signs (seizures, myoclonus, dementia, retinal lesions) indicate a poliodystrophy is useful mainly in the early stages of a disease. Some of the lysosomal storage diseases affect both galactolipids (galactocerebrosides and sulfatides) as well as gangliosides; hence both white and gray matter are involved.

In concluding this last section, which classifies the inherited metabolic diseases in accordance with their salient clinical characteristics, the careful reader will appreciate its artificiality. Nearly every one of the diseases of each category may present some neurologic abnormality other than the ones we have emphasized, so that the potential number of variations is almost limitless. However, it is hoped that the plan adopted here—of thinking of these diseases in reference to age periods and syndromic relationships—will facilitate the development of a clinical approach to this relatively new and extremely difficult part of neurologic medicine.

REFERENCES

ADACHI M, TORII J, SCHNECK L, VOLK BW: Electron microscopic and enzyme histochemical studies of the cerebellum in spongy degeneration. *Acta Neuropathol* 20:22, 1972.

ADAMS RD: Hereditary hepatocerebral degeneration of Wilson-Westphal-Strümpell with reference to acquired hepatocerebral degeneration, in Bammer HG (ed): *Future of Neurology*. Stuttgart, Georg Thieme Verlag, 1967, pp 45–69.

ADAMS RD, LYON G: *Neurology of Hereditary Metabolic Diseases of Children*. New York, Hemisphere, 1982.

ADAMS RD, PROD'HOM LS, RABINOWICZ TH: Intrauterine brain death. *Acta Neuropathol* 40:41, 1977.

AGAMANOLIS DP, GREENSTEIN JI: Ataxia-telangiectasia. *J Neuropathol Exp Neurol* 38:475, 1979.

AICARDI J, CASTELEIN P: Infantile neuroaxonal dystrophy. *Brain* 102:727, 1979.

ALPERS BJ: Diffuse progressive degeneration of cerebral gray matter. *Arch Neurol Psychiatry* 25:469, 1931.

AUBORG P, SCOTTO J, RICHICIOLLI F: Neonatal adrenoleukodystrophy. *J Neurol Neurosurg Psychiatry* 49:77, 1986.

BANKER BQ, VICTOR M: Spongy degeneration of infancy, in Goodman RM, Motulsky AG (eds): *Genetic Diseases among Ashkenazi Jews*. New York, Raven Press, 1979, pp 210–216.

BARINGER JR, SWEENEY VP, WINKLER GF: An acute syndrome of ocular oscillations and truncal myoclonus. *Brain* 91:473, 1968.

BAUMANN RJ, KOCOSHIS SA, WILSON D: Lafora disease: Liver histopathology in presymptomatic children. *Ann Neurol* 14:86, 1983.

BERKOVIC SF, ANDERMANN F, CARPENTER S et al: Progressive myoclonus epilepsies and specific causes and diagnosis. *N Engl J Med* 315:296, 1986.

BERGINER VM, SALEN G, SHEFER S: Long-term treatment of cerebrotendinous xanthomatosis with chenodeoxycholic acid. *N Engl J Med* 311:1649, 1984.

BLASS JP, AVIGAN J, UHLENDORF BW: A defect in pyruvate decarboxylase in a child with intermittent movement disorder. *J Clin Invest* 49:423, 1970.

BOSCH EP, HART MN: Late adult onset metachromatic leukodystrophy. *Arch Neurol* 35:475, 1978.

BRADY RO: Sphingomyelin lipidoses: Niemann-Pick disease. In Stanbury JB, Wyngaarden JB, Fredrickson DS et al (eds): *The Metabolic Basis of Inherited Disease*. 5th ed. New York, McGraw-Hill, 1983, chap 41, pp 831–841.

BREWER GJ, TERRY CA, AISEN AM, HILL GM: Worsening of neurologic syndrome in patients with Wilson's disease with initial penicillamine therapy. *Arch Neurol* 44:490, 1987.

BRUSILOW SW, DANNEY M, WABER LJ et al: Treatment of episodic hyperammonemia in children with inborn errors of urea synthesis. *N Engl J Med* 310:1630, 1984.

BURTON BK, NADLER HL: Clinical diagnosis of the inborn errors of metabolism in the neonatal period. *Pediatrics* 61:398, 1978.

CARPENTER S, KARPATI G, ANDERMANN F et al: The ultrastructural characteristics of the abnormal cytosomes in Batten-Kufs' disease. *Brain* 100:137, 1977.

CARTER S, GOLD AP (eds): *Neurology of Infancy and Childhood*. New York, Appleton-Century-Crofts, 1974.

COWEN D, OLMSTEAD EV: Infantile neuroaxonal dystrophy. *J Neuropathol Exp Neurol* 22:175, 1963.

CROCKER AC, FARBER S: Niemann-Pick disease: A review of 18 patients. *Medicine* 37:1, 1958.

CROCKER AE, VAWTER GF, NEUHAUSER EBD, ROSOWSKY A: Wolman's disease: Three new patients with a recently described lipidosis. *Pediatrics* 35:627, 1965.

CROME L: A case of galactosaemia with the pathological and neuropathological findings. *Arch Dis Child* 37:415, 1962.

DAL CANTO MC, RAPIN I, SUZUKI K: Neuronal storage disorder with chorea and curvilinear bodies. *Neurology* 24:1026, 1974.

DANKS DM, CARTWRIGHT E, STEVENS BJ, TOWNLEY RRW: Menkes' kinky-hair disease: Further definition of the defect in copper transport. *Science* 179:1140, 1973.

DESNICK RJ, SWEELEY CC: Fabry's disease: galactosidase A deficiency, in Scriver CR, Beaudet AL, Sly WS, Valle D (eds): *The Metabolic Basis of Inherited Diseae*, 6th ed. New York, McGraw-Hill, 1989, pp 906–944.

DEVIVO DC, HAYMOND MW, OBERT KA, et al: Defective activation of the pyruvate dehydrogenase complex in subacute necrotizing encephalomyelopathy (Leigh disease). *Ann Neurol* 6:483, 1979.

DIMAGNO EP, LOWE JL, SNODGRASS PJ et al: Ornithine transcarbamalase deficiency—a cause of bizarre behavior in a man. *N Engl J Med* 315:744, 1986.

DREW AL JR: The degenerative and demyelinating diseases of the nervous system, in Carter S, Gold AP (eds): *Neurology of Infancy and Childhood*. New York, Appleton-Century-Crofts, 1974, chap 4, pp 57-89.

ELDRIDGE R, ANAYIOTOS CP, SCHLESINGER S et al: Hereditary adult-onset leukodystrophy simulating chronic progressive multiple sclerosis. *N Engl J Med* 311:948, 1984.

ELFENBEIN LB: Dystonic juvenile idiocy without amaurosis. *Johns Hopkins Med J* 123:205, 1968.

FAHR T: Idiopathische Verkalkung der Hirngefässe. *Zentralbl Allg Pathol* 50:129, 1930–1931.

FARRELL DF, SWEDBERG K: Clinical and biochemical heterogeneity of globoid cell leukodystrophy. *Ann Neurol* 10:364, 1981.

FØLLING A: Über Ausscheidung von Phenylbrenztraubensaure in den Harn als Stoffwechselanomalie in Verbindung mit Imbezilität. *Hoppe-Seyler's Z Physiol Chem* 227:169, 1934.

FORD FR: *Diseases of the Nervous System in Infancy, Childhood and Adolescence,* 6th ed. Springfield, IL, Charles C Thomas, 1973.

FRYDMAN M, BONNE-TAMIR B, FARBER LA et al: Assignment of the gene for Wilson disease to chromosome 13: Linkage to the esterase D locus. *Proc Natl Acad Sci USA* 82:1819, 1985.

GOLDFISCHER S, MOORE CL, JOHNSON AB et al: Peroxisomal and mitochondrial defects in the cerebro-hepato-renal syndrome. *Science* 182:62, 1973.

GOLDMAN JE, KATZ O, RAPUR I et al: Chronic G$_{M1}$ gangliosidosis presenting as dystonia. Clinical and pathological features. *Ann Neurol* 9:465, 1981.

GOLDSTEIN M, ANDERSEN LT, RUBEN R et al: Self-mutilation in Lesch-Nyhan disease caused by dopaminergic denervation. *Lancet* 1:338, 1985.

GRIFFIN JW, GOREN E, SCHAUMBURG H et al: Adrenomyeloneuropathy: A probable variant of adrenoleukodystrophy. *Neurology* 27:1107, 1977.

HARDING BN, EGGER J, PORTMANN B, ERDOHAZI M: Progressive neuronal degeneration of childhood with liver disease. *Brain* 109:181, 1986.

HERS HG: Inborn lysosomal diseases. *Gastroenterology* 48:625, 1965.

HOLMES LB, MOSER HW, HALLDORSSON S et al: *Mental Retardation: An Atlas of Diseases with Associated Physical Abnormalities.* New York, Macmillan, 1972.

HOLTZMAN NA, KRONMAL RA, VAN DOORNINCK W et al: Effect of age and loss of dietary control on intellectual performance and behavior of children with phenylketonuria. *N Engl J Med* 314:593, 1986.

HOMMES FA, POLMAN HA, REERINK JD: Leigh's encephalomyelopathy: An inborn error of gluconeogenesis. *Arch Dis Child* 43:423, 1968.

HUNT JR: Dyssynergia cerebellaris myoclonica. *Brain* 44:490, 1921.

IGARASHI M, SCHAUMBURG HH, POWERS J et al: Fatty acid abnormality in adrenoleukodystrophy. *J Neurochem* 26:851, 1976.

IKEDA S, KONDO K, OGUCHI K et al: Adult fucosidosis: Histochemical and ultrastructural studies of rectal mucosa biopsy. *Neurology* 34:451, 1984.

ILLINGWORTH DR, CONNOR WE, MILLER RG: Abetalipoproteinemia. Report of two cases and review of therapy. *Arch Neurol* 37:659, 1980.

JOHNSON RC, MCKEAN CM, SHAH SN: Fatty acid composition of lipids in cerebral myelin and synaptosomes in phenylketonuria and Down syndrome. *Arch Neurol* 34:288, 1977.

JOPPICH G, SCHULTE FJ: *Neurologie des Neugeborenen.* Berlin, Springer-Verlag, 1968.

KALIMO H, LUNDBERG PO, OLSSON Y: Familial subacute necrotizing encephalomyelopathy of the adult form (adult Leigh syndrome). *Ann Neurol* 6:200, 1979.

KENDALL BE, KINGSLEY DPE, LEONARD JV et al: Neurological features and computed tomography of the brain in children with ornithine carbamoyl transferase deficiency. *J Neurol Neurosurg Psychiatry* 46:28, 1983.

KERR DS, LAP HO, BERLIN CM et al: Systemic deficiency of the first component of the pyruvate dehydrogenase complex. *Pediatr Res* 22:312, 1987.

KINSBOURNE M: Myoclonic encephalopathy in infants. *J Neurol Neurosurg Psychiatry* 25:271, 1962.

KISTLER JP, LOTT IT, KOLODNY EH et al: Mannosidosis. *Arch Neurol* 34:45, 1977.

KOBAYASHI T, NODA S, UMEZAKI H et al: Familial spinocerebellar degeneration as an expression of adrenoleukodystrophy. *J Neurol Neurosurg Psychiatry* 49:1438, 1986.

KOIVISTO M, BLENCO-SEQUIROS M, KRAUSE U: Neonatal symptomatic hypoglycemia. A follow up of 151 children. *Dev Med Child Neurol* 14:603, 1972.

KOLODNY EH: Storage diseases of the reticuloendothelial system, in Nathan DG, Oski FA (eds): *Hematology of Infancy and Childhood,* 2nd ed. Philadelphia, Saunders, 1981, chap 33, pp 1104–1144.

KOLODNY EH, CABLE WJL: Inborn errors of metabolism. *Ann Neurol* 11:221, 1982.

KOLODNY EH, RAGHAVAN SS: G$_{M2}$ gangliosidosis hexosaminidase mutations not of the Tay-Sachs type produce unusual clinical variants. *Trends Neuro Sci* 6:16, 1983.

LANCE JW: Familial paroxysmal dystonic choreoathetosis and its differentiation from related syndromes. *Ann Neurol* 2:285, 1977.

LESCH M, NYHAN WL: A familial disorder of uric acid metabolism and central nervous system function. *Am J Med* 36:561, 1964.

LEVY HL: Newborn screening for metabolic disorders. *N Engl J Med* 288:1299, 1973.

LEVY HL, MADIGAN PM, SHIH V: Mass metabolic disorder screening program. *Pediatrics* 49:825, 1972.

LLOYD RG, HORNYKIEWICZ O, DAVIDSON L et al: Biochemical evidence of dysfunction of neurotransmitters in Lesch-Nyhan syndrome. *N Engl J Med* 305:1106, 1981.

LONSDALE D, FAULKNER WR, PRICE JW, SMEBY RR: Intermittent cerebellar ataxia associated with hyperpyruvic acidemia, hyperalininemia and hyperalininuria. *Pediatrics* 43:1025, 1969.

LOTT IT, COULOMBE T, DIPAOLO RV et al: Vitamin B$_6$-dependent seizures: Pathology and chemical findings in brain. *Neurology* 28:47, 1978.

LUNDBORG H: *Die progressive Myoklonus-epilepsie (Unverricht's Myoklonie).* Uppsala, Almqvist and Wiksell, 1903.

MALAMUD N, DEMMY N: Degenerative disease of the subthalamic bodies. *J Neuropathol Exp Neurol* 19:96, 1960.

MARSDEN CD, OGESO JA, LANG AE: Adrenoleukomyeloneuropathy presenting as spinocerebellar degeneration. *Neurology* 32:1031, 1982.

MCFARLIN DE, STROBER W, BARLOW M et al: The immunological deficiency state in ataxia-telangiectasia. *Res Publ Assoc Res Nerv Ment Dis* 49:275, 1971.

MCKUSICK VA: *Mendelian Inheritance in Man,* 8th ed. Baltimore, Johns Hopkins, 1988.

MEEK D, WOLFE LS, ANDERMANN E, ANDERMANN F: Juvenile progressive dystonia: A new phenotype of G$_{M2}$ gangliosidosis. *Ann Neurol* 15:348, 1984.

MELCHIOR JC, BENDA CE, YAKOVLEV PI: Familial idiopathic cerebral calcifications in childhood. *Am J Dis Child* 99:787, 1960.

MIYATAKE T, ATSUMI T, OBAYASHI T et al: Adult type neuronal storage disease with neuraminidase deficiency. *Ann Neurol* 6:232, 1979.

MOSER AE, SINGH I, BROWN FR III et al: The cerebrohepatorenal (Zellweger) syndrome. *N Engl J Med* 310:1141, 1984.

MOSER HW, MOSER AB, KAWAMURA N et al: Adrenoleukodystrophy: Studies of the phenotype, genetics and biochemistry. *Johns Hopkins Med J* 147:217, 1980.

MOSER HW, MOSER AB, KAWAMURA N et al: Adrenoleukodystrophy: Elevated C26 fatty acid in cultured skin fibroblasts. *Ann Neurol* 7:542, 1980.

MOSER AE, SINGH ABI, BROWN FR et al: The cerebrohepatorenal Zellweger syndrome. *N Engl J Med* 311:1141, 1984.

MOUNT LA, REBACK S: Familial paroxysmal choreoathetosis: Preliminary report on a hitherto undescribed clinical syndrome. *Arch Neurol Psychiatry* 44:841, 1940.

MSALL M, BATSHAW ML, SUSS R et al: Neurologic outcome in children with inborn errors of urea synthesis. *N Engl J Med* 310:1500, 1984.

NISHIMURA M, YOSHIMO K, TOMITA Y: Central and peripheral nervous system pathology due to methylenetetrahydrofolate reductase deficiency. *Pediatr Neurol* 1:375, 1985.

OHNO T, TSUCHIDA H, FUKUHARA N et al: Adrenoleukodystrophy: A clinical variant presenting as olivopontocerebellar atrophy. *J Neurol* 231:167, 1984.

O'NEILL BP, MOSER HW, SAXENA KM: Familial X-linked Addison's disease as an expression of adrenoleukodystrophy (ALD): Elevated C26 fatty acid in cultured skin fibroblasts. *Neurology* 32:543, 1982.

PAVLAKIS SG, PHILLIPS PC, DIMAURO S et al: Mitochondrial myopathy, encephalopathy, lactic acidosis, and stroke-like episodes: A distinctive clinical syndrome. *Ann Neurol* 16:481, 1984.

PINCUS JH: Subacute necrotizing encephalomyelopathy (Leigh's disease): A consideration of clinical features and etiology. *Dev Med Child Neurol* 14:87, 1972.

PINCUS JH, CHUTORIAN A: Familial benign chorea with intention tremor: A clinical entity. *J Pediatr* 70:724, 1967.

PRADER A, LABHART A, WILLI H: Ein Syndrom von Adipositas, Kleinwuchs, Kryptorchismus und Oligophrenie nach Myatonieartigem Zustand im Neugeborenenalter. *Schweiz Med Wochenschr* 86:1260, 1956.

PRECHTL H, BEINTEMA D: *The Neurological Examination of the Full-Term Newborn Infant.* London, Spastics Society, 1964.

PRENSKY AL, MOSER HW: Brain lipids, proteo-lipids and free amino acids in maple syrup urine disease. *J Neurochem* 13:863, 1966.

RAPIN I, GOLDFISCHER S, KATZMAN R et al: The cherry-red spot-myoclonus syndrome. *Ann Neurol* 3:134, 1978.

ROSENBERG AL, BERGSTROM L, TROOST BT, BARTHOLOMEW BA: Hyperuricemia and neurologic deficits: A family study. *N Engl J Med* 282:992, 1970.

ROWE PC, NEWMAN SL, BRUSILOW SW: Natural history of symptomatic partial ornithine transcarbamylase deficiency. *N Engl J Med* 314:541, 1986.

SALAM M: Metabolic ataxias, in Vinken PJ, Bruyn GW (eds): *Handbook of Clinical Neurology,* vol 21. Amsterdam, North-Holland, 1975, chap 32, pp 573–585.

SANDER J, PACKMAN S, BERG BO et al: Pyruvate carboxylase activity in subacute necrotizing encephalopathy (Leigh's disease). *Neurology* 34:515, 1984.

SANTAVUORI P, HALTIA M, RAPOLA J, RAITTA C: Infantile type of so-called neuronal ceroid-lipofuscinosis. Part 1: A clinical study of 15 patients. *J Neurol Sci* 18:257, 1973.

SASS-KORTSAK A, BEARN AG: Hereditary disorders of copper metabolism, in Scriver CR, Beaudet AL, Sly WS, Valle D (eds): *Metabolic Basis of Hereditary Disease,* 6th ed. New York, McGraw-Hill, 1989, chap 48, pp 1098–1126.

SCHEINBERG IH, GITLIN D: Deficiency of ceruloplasmin in patients with hepatolenticular degeneration (Wilson's disease). *Science* 116:484, 1952.

SCHEINBERG IH, STERNLIEB I: *Wilson's Disease. Major Problems in Internal Medicine,* vol 23. Philadelphia, Saunders, 1984.

SCHMID R, MCDONAGH AF: Hyperbilirubinemia, in Scriver CR, Beaudet AL, Sly WS (eds): *The Metabolic Basis of Inherited Diseases,* 6th ed. New York, McGraw-Hill, 1988, chap 51, pp 1238–1243.

SCRIVER CR, BEAUDET AL, SLY WS, VALLE D (eds): *The Metabolic Basis of Inherited Disease,* 6th ed. New York, McGraw-Hill, 1989.

SCRIVER CR, CLOW CL: Phenylketonuria: Epitome of human biochemical genetics. *N Engl J Med* 303:1335, 1980.

SHIH VE: *Laboratory Techniques for the Detection of Hereditary Metabolic Disorders,* Long JW (ed). Cleveland, OH, CRC Press, 1973.

SHIH VE, ABROMS IF, JOHNSON JL et al: Sulfite oxidase deficiency. *N Engl J Med* 297:1022, 1977.

SHUMAN RM, LEECH RW, SCOTT CR: The neuropathology of the nonketotic and ketotic hyperglycinemias: Three cases. *Neurology* 28:139, 1978.

SIEMERLING E, CREUTZFELDT HG: Bronzekrankheit und sklerosierende Encephalomyelitis (Diffuse Sklerose). *Arch Psychiatr Nervenkr* 68:217, 1923.

SJÖGREN T: Die juvenile amaurotische Idiotie: Klinische und erblichkeitsmedizinische Untersuchungen. *Hereditas* 14:197, 1931.

SLY WS, WHYTE MP, SUNDERAM V: Carbonic anhydrase II deficiency in 12 families with the autosomal recessive syndrome of osteopetrosis with renal tubular acidosis with cerebral calcification. *N Engl J Med* 313:139, 1985.

SMITH I, CLAYTON BE, WOLFF OH: New variant of phenylketonuria with progressive neurological illness unresponsive to phenylalanine restriction. *Lancet* 1:1108, 1975.

STAROSTA-RUBINSTEIN S, YOUNG AB, KLUIN K et al: Clinical assessment of 31 patients with Wilson's disease. *Arch Neurol* 44:365, 1987.

SZANTO J, GALLYAS F: A study of iron metabolism in neuropsychiatric patients: Hallervorden-Spatz disease. *Arch Neurol* 14:438, 1966.

TELLEZ-NAGEL I, RAPIN I, IWAMOTO T, et al: Mucolipidosis IV. *Arch Neurol* 33:828, 1976.

TENNISON MB, BOULDIN TW, WHALEY RA: Mineralization of the basal ganglia detected by CT in Hallervorden-Spatz syndrome. *Neurology* 38:155, 1988.

THOMAS PK, ABRAMS JD, SWALLOW D, STEWART G: Sialidosis type I: Cherry-red spot-myoclonus syndrome with sialidase deficiency and altered electrophoretic mobilities of some enzymes known to be glycoproteins. *J Neurol Neurosurg Psychiatry* 42:873, 1979.

TSUJI S, CHOUDARY PV, MARTIN BM et al: A mutation in the human glucocerebrosidase gene in neuropathic Gaucher's disease. *N Engl J Med* 311:570, 1987.

TSUJI S, YAMADA T, TSUTSUMI A, MIYATAKE T: Neuraminidase deficiency and accumulation of sialic acid in lymphocytes in adult type sialidosis with partial β-galactosidase deficiency. *Ann Neurol* 11:541, 1982.

UNVERRICHT H: *Die Myoclonie* Leipsig, Franz Denticke, 1891, pp 1-128.

VAKILI S, DREW AL, VON SCHUCHING S, et al: Hallervorden-Spatz syndrome. *Arch Neurol* 34:729, 1977.

VAN BOGAERT L: Contribution clinique et anatomique a l'étude de la paralysie agitante juvenile primitive. *Rev Neurol* 2:315, 1930.

VAN BOGAERT L: Le cadre des xanthomatoses et leurs differents types: Xanthomatoses secondaires. *Rev Med* 17:433, 1962.

VOGT C, VOGT O: Zur Lehre der Erkrankungen des striaren Systems. *J Psychol Neurol* 25:627, 1920.

WALSER M: Urea cycle disorders and other hereditary hyperammonemic syndromes, in Stanbury JB, Wyngaarden JB, Fredrickson DS, et al (eds): *The Metabolic Basis of Inherited Disease*, 5th ed. New York, McGraw-Hill, 1983, pp 402–438.

WALSH PJ: Adrenoleukodystrophy. *Arch Neurol* 37:448, 1980.

WALSHE JM: Wilson's disease (hepatolenticular degeneration), in Vinken PJ, Bruyn GW (eds): *Handbook of Clinical Neurology, Metabolic and Deficiency Diseases of the Nervous System, Part I*. Amsterdam, North-Holland, 1976, pp 379–414.

WILLIAMS FJB, WALSHE JM: Wilson's disease: An analysis of the cranial computerized tomographic experiences found in 60 patients and the changes in response to treatment with chelating agents. *Brain* 104:735, 1981.

WILLIAMS RS, LOTT IT, FERRANTE RJ, CAVINESS VS: The cellular pathology of neuronal ceroid-lipofuscinosis. *Arch Neurol* 34:298, 1977.

WILLIAMS RS, MARSHALL PC, LOTT IT et al: The cellular pathology of Menkes steely hair syndrome. *Neurology* 28:575, 1978.

WILLVONSEDER R, GOLDSTEIN NP, McCALL JT, et al: A hereditary disorder with dementia, spastic dysarthria, vertical eye movement paresis, gait disturbance, splenomegaly, and abnormal copper metabolism. *Neurology* 23:1039, 1973.

WILSON SAK: Progressive lenticular degeneration: A familial nervous disease associated with cirrhosis of the liver. *Brain* 34:295, 1912.

WINKELMAN MD, BANKER BQ, VICTOR M, MOSER HW: Non-infantile neuronopathic Gaucher's disease: A clinico-pathologic study. *Neurology* 33:994, 1983.

YOKOI S, NAKAYAMA H, NEGESHI T: Biochemical studies on tissues from a patient with Lafora disease. *Clin Chim Acta* 62:415, 1975.

YOUNG R, KLEINMAN G, OJEMANN RG et al: Compressive myelopathy in Maroteaux-Lamy syndrome: Clinical and pathological findings. *Ann Neurol* 8:336, 1980.

ZEMAN W, DONAHUE S, DYKEN P, GREEN J: The neuronal ceroid-lipofuscinoses (Batten-Vogt syndrome), in Vinken PJ, Bruyn GW (eds): *Handbook of Clinical Neurology*, vol 10. Amsterdam, North-Holland, 1970, chap 25, pp 588–679.

CHAPTER 39

DISEASES OF THE NERVOUS SYSTEM DUE TO NUTRITIONAL DEFICIENCY

Among nutritional disorders, those of the nervous system occupy a position of special interest and importance. The early studies of beriberi, at the turn of the century, were largely responsible for the discovery of thiamine, and, consequently, for the modern concept of deficiency disease. Despite the notable achievements in the science of nutrition that followed the discovery of vitamins, diseases due to nutritional deficiency—and particularly those of the nervous system—still represent a worldwide health problem of serious proportions. In Far Eastern communities, where the diet consists mainly of highly milled rice, there is still a significant incidence of beriberi. In other underdeveloped countries, deficiency diseases are endemic, the result of chronic dietary deprivation. It comes as a surprise to many physicians that deficiency diseases are also common in the United States and other parts of the western world. Mainly this is due to the prevalence of alcoholism. Dietary faddism and impaired absorption of dietary nutrients (which occurs in patients with sprue, pernicious anemia, or surgical exclusion of portions of the gastrointestinal tract, for treatment of obesity or other reasons) account for a relatively small number of cases. Occasionally, manifestations of nutritional deficiency may be induced by the use of vitamin antagonists or certain drugs, such as isonicotinic acid hydrazide, which is used in the treatment of tuberculosis and which interferes with the enzymatic function of pyridoxine.

GENERAL CONSIDERATIONS

The term *deficiency* will be used throughout this chapter in its strictest sense, to designate disorders that result from *the lack of an essential nutrient or nutrients in the diet, or from a conditioning factor that increases the need for these nutrients.*

The most important of these nutrients are the vitamins, and more specifically, certain members of the B group—

thiamine, nicotinic acid, pyridoxine, pantothenic acid, and cobalamin (vitamin B_{12}). Most deficiency diseases cannot be related to the lack of a single vitamin (pernicious anemia or vitamin B_{12} deficiency being a notable exception); usually the effects of deficiency of several vitamins can be recognized. This truism should neither obscure the fact that certain manifestations of deficiency disease (e.g., the ocular palsies of Wernicke disease) are indeed related to a deficiency of a specific nutrient, nor diminish the need to identify such relationships.

Nutritional diseases of the nervous system are, however, not simply a matter of vitamin deprivation. Practically always, these diseases are associated with the general signs of undernutrition, such as circulatory abnormalities and loss of subcutaneous fat and muscle bulk. Furthermore, a total lack of vitamins, as in starvation, is very rarely associated with the classic deficiency syndromes of beriberi or pellagra; a certain amount of food is necessary to produce them. An excessive intake of carbohydrate relative to the supply of thiamine favors the development of a thiamine deficiency state. Deficiency diseases in general, including those of the nervous system, are influenced by factors such as exercise, growth, pregnancy, and infection, and by disorders of the liver and the gastrointestinal tract, which might interfere with the synthesis and the absorption of essential nutrients.

As has been mentioned, alcoholism is an important factor in the causation of nutritional diseases of the nervous system, at least in the United States. Alcohol acts mainly by displacing food in the diet, but also by adding carbohydrate calories (alcohol is burned almost entirely as carbohydrate), thus increasing the need for thiamine. There is some evidence as well that alcohol impairs the absorption of thiamine and other vitamins from the gastrointestinal tract.

In infants and young children, a reduction of protein and caloric intake (so-called protein-calorie malnutrition, or PCM) has a devastating effect upon body growth; even those with relatively mild degrees of PCM may be permanently stunted. Whether or not PCM also hinders the growth of the brain, with consequent effects upon intellectual and behavioral development, cannot be answered as readily. The data bearing on this matter are discussed in the last part of the chapter.

Deficiency diseases of the nervous system may occur in pure form and will be so described, but usually they occur in various combinations. Stated in another way, the nutritional disorders are characterized by involvement of both the central and peripheral nervous systems, an attribute shared with certain hereditary metabolic disorders.

The following are the deficiency diseases to be discussed in this chapter:

1. Wernicke disease and Korsakoff psychosis

2. Nutritional polyneuropathy (neuropathic beriberi)

3. Deficiency amblyopia (nutritional optic neuropathy; "tobacco-alcohol" amblyopia)

4. Pellagra (with some remarks on spinal spastic ataxia and nicotinic acid deficiency encephalopathy)

5. The syndrome of amblyopia, painful neuropathy and orogenital dermatitis (Strachan syndrome)

6. Subacute combined degeneration of the spinal cord (vitamin B_{12} deficiency)

7. Neurologic disorders due to a deficiency of pyridoxine, of other B vitamins (pantothenic acid, riboflavin, folic acid), and of vitamin E

In addition, attention will be drawn to several distinctive neurologic disorders in which nutritional factors may be operative: (1) "alcoholic" cerebellar degeneration, (2) central pontine and extrapontine myelinolysis, and (3) primary degeneration of the corpus callosum (Marchiafava-Bignami disease).

Also, some comments will be made about protein-calorie malnutrition, the neurologic disorders consequent upon intestinal malabsorption, and the vitamin-responsive hereditary diseases.

Deficiencies of trace elements, because of their rarity, will not be discussed. Only iodine deficiency is of much importance in humans. Deficiencies of other elements have been reviewed by Fowden et al.

THE WERNICKE-KORSAKOFF SYNDROME

DEFINITION OF TERMS

Wernicke disease and Korsakoff psychosis are common neurologic disorders that have been recognized since the 1880s. *Wernicke disease* (polioencephalitis hemorrhagica superioris) is characterized by nystagmus, abducens and conjugate gaze palsies, ataxia of gait, and mental confusion. These symptoms usually have an abrupt onset and may occur singly or, more often, in various combinations. Wernicke disease is due to nutritional deficiency, more specifically to a deficiency of thiamine and is observed mainly though not exclusively in alcoholics.

Korsakoff psychosis (amnesic or amnestic-confabulatory psychosis; psychosis polyneuritica) refers to a unique mental disorder in which retentive memory is impaired out of all proportion to other cognitive functions, in an otherwise alert and responsive patient. This disorder, like Wernicke disease, is usually associated with alcoholism and malnutrition, but it may be a symptom of various other disorders that have their basis in lesions of the diencephalon or the temporal lobes. Thus, classic instances of Korsakoff psychosis may be observed in patients with third ventricular tumors, infarction (or surgical resection) of the inferomedial portions of the temporal lobes, or as a sequela of herpes simplex encephalitis. A transient impairment of retentive memory of the Korsakoff type may be the salient manifestation of temporal lobe epilepsy, concussive head injury, and so-called transient global amnesia; a permanent abnormality of this sort may be the most prominent feature of anoxic encephalopathy and Alzheimer disease.

In the alcoholic, nutritionally deficient patient, Korsakoff psychosis is usually associated with Wernicke disease. Stated in another way, Korsakoff psychosis is the psychic manifestation of Wernicke disease. For this reason, and others to be elaborated later, the term *Wernicke disease* should be applied to a symptom complex of ophthalmoparesis, nystagmus, ataxia, and an acute apathetic-confusional state. A symptom complex that comprises both the manifestations of Wernicke disease and a persistent or enduring defect in learning and memory is appropriately designated as the *Wernicke-Korsakoff syndrome*.

HISTORICAL NOTE

In 1881, Carl Wernicke first described an illness of sudden onset, characterized by paralysis of eye movements, ataxia of gait, and mental confusion. Swelling of the optic discs and retinal hemorrhages were also said to be present. His observations were made in three patients, of whom two were alcoholics and one was a young woman with persistent vomiting following the ingestion of sulfuric acid. In each of these patients there was progressive stupor and coma, culminating in death. The pathologic changes described by Wernicke consisted of punctate hemorrhages, primarily affecting the gray matter around the third and fourth ventricles and aqueduct of Sylvius; he considered these changes to be inflammatory in nature and confined to the gray matter, hence his designation "polioencephalitis hemorrhagica superioris."

In the belief that Gâyet had described an identical disorder in 1875, the term *Gâyet-Wernicke* is used frequently by French authors. Such a designation is hardly justified insofar as the lesion in Gâyet's patient consisted of a single hemorrhagic focus that occupied practically all of the pons (it was probably an instance of hemorrhagic leukoencephalitis); also the clinical features differed from those of Wernicke's patients in all essential details.

In a similar vein, a number of early writers, beginning with Magnus Huss in 1852, made casual reference to a disturbance of memory in the course of chronic alcoholism. However, the first comprehensive account of this disorder was given by the Russian psychiatrist S. S. Korsakoff, in a series of articles published between 1887 and 1891 (for English translation and commentary, see references). Korsakoff stressed the relationship between "neuritis" (a term used at that time for all types of peripheral nerve disease) and the disorder of memory (psychosis polyneuritica), which, he proposed, represented "two facets of the same disease." But he also made the point, generally disregarded by subsequent authors, that neuritis need not accompany the characteristic amnesic syndrome. Korsakoff's observations of the neuritic and mental aspects of the syndrome were made in both alcoholic and nonalcoholic patients. His clinical descriptions are remarkably complete and have hardly been surpassed to the present day.

It is of interest that the relationship between Wernicke disease and Korsakoff polyneuritic psychosis was appreciated neither by Wernicke nor by Korsakoff. Murawieff, in 1897, first postulated that a single cause was responsible for both. The intimate clinical relationship was established by Bonhoeffer in 1904, who stated that in all cases of Wernicke disease he found neuritis and an amnesic psychosis. Confirmation of this relationship on pathologic grounds came much later.

CLINICAL FEATURES

The incidence of the Wernicke-Korsakoff syndrome cannot be stated with precision, but it is a common disorder, judging from our experience. At the Cleveland Metropolitan General Hospital, for example, in a consecutive series of 3548 autopsies in adults, the pathognomonic lesions were found in 77 cases (2.2 percent). The disease affects males only slightly more frequently than females, and the age of onset is fairly evenly distributed, between 30 and 70 years.

The triad of clinical features described by Wernicke—ophthalmoplegia, ataxia, and disturbances of mentation and consciousness—is still diagnostically useful, provided the diagnosis is suspected and the signs carefully sought. Often the disease begins with ataxia, followed in a few days or weeks by mental confusion; or there may be the simultaneous onset of ataxia and ocular symptoms with or without confusion. A description of each of the major manifestations follows.

Ocular Abnormalities The diagnosis of Wernicke disease is made most readily on the basis of the ocular signs. These consist of (1) nystagmus that is both horizontal and vertical, (2) weakness or paralysis of the external rectus muscles, and (3) weakness or paralysis of conjugate gaze. Usually these abnormalities are combined.

The palsy of conjugate gaze varies from merely a nystagmus on extreme gaze to a complete loss of ocular movement in that direction. This applies to both horizontal and vertical movements, abnormalities of the former being somewhat more frequent. Paralysis of downward gaze is an unusual manifestation, but internuclear ophthalmoplegia is common. Next to nystagmus, the most frequent ocular abnormality is a lateral rectus weakness, which is always bilateral but not necessarily symmetrical, and which is accompanied by diplopia and internal strabismus. With complete paralysis of the lateral rectus muscles, nystagmus is initially absent in the abducting eyes, but it becomes evident as the weakness improves. In advanced stages of the disease there may be a complete loss of ocular movements, and the pupils, which are usually spared, may become miotic and nonreacting. Ptosis, small retinal hemorrhages, involvement of the near-far focusing mechanism, and evidence of optic neuropathy occur occasionally, but we have never observed papilledema in this disease.

Ataxia Essentially the ataxia is one of stance and gait, and in the acute stage of the disease it may be so severe that the patient cannot stand or walk without support. Lesser degrees of this disorder are characterized by a wide-based stance and by a slow, uncertain, short-stepped gait; in its mildest form the ataxia can be brought out only by tandem walking. In contrast to the gross disorder of locomotion is the relative infrequency of a clear-cut intention tremor. When present, it is more likely to be brought out by heel-to-knee than by finger-to-nose testing. Scanning speech is present only rarely.

Disturbances of Consciousness and Mentation These are present in all but 10 percent of patients. Four types of deranged mentation and consciousness can be recognized:

1. About 15 percent of patients show the signs of alcohol withdrawal, i.e., hallucinations and other disorders

of perception, confusion, agitation, tremor, and overactivity of autonomic nervous system function. These symptoms are evanescent in nature and usually mild in degree.

2. By far the commonest derangement of mental function is a *global confusional state*. Typically, the patient is apathetic, inattentive, and indifferent to the surroundings. Spontaneous speech is minimal and many questions are unanswered, or the patient may suspend the conversation in the middle of a sentence and drift off to sleep—although he can be aroused from this state without difficulty. The questions that are answered by the patient betray disorientation in time and place, misidentification of those around him, and an inability to grasp the meaning of the illness or immediate situation. Many of the patient's remarks are irrational and lack consistency from one moment to another. If the patient's interest and attention can be maintained long enough to ensure adequate testing, one finds that memory and learning ability are also impaired. Under the influence of thiamine or of an adequate diet, the patient rapidly becomes more alert and attentive and more capable of taking part in mental testing. Then the most prominent abnormality is one of retentive memory (Korsakoff psychosis).

3. Although drowsiness is common, stupor and coma are rare as *initial* manifestations of Wernicke disease. However, if the early signs are not recognized and the patient remains untreated, there occurs a progressive depression of the state of consciousness with stupor, coma, and death, in a matter of a week or two, as occurred in Wernicke's original cases. Autopsy series of Wernicke disease are heavily weighted with cases of this type (Torvik et al).

4. Some patients are alert and responsive from the time they are first seen, and already show the characteristic features of the Korsakoff amnesic state. In yet others Korsakoff psychosis is the only manifestation of the syndrome, and no ocular or ataxic signs can be discerned. The memory disorder, which constitutes the chronic and truly crippling feature of the Wernicke-Korsakoff syndrome, is described below.

The Amnesic State   The general features of the amnesic (Korsakoff) syndrome have been discussed in Chap. 20, and are entirely applicable to the amnesic state as it is observed in the alcoholic, nutritionally depleted patient.

Invariably there is a permanent gap in the patient's memory for the acute phase of the illness, attributable no doubt to the impairment of registration and general confusion that are so prominent during that period.

As indicated in Chap. 20, the core of the amnesic disorder is a defect in learning (anterograde amnesia) and loss of past memories (retrograde amnesia). The defect in learning or memorization is never complete but may be

very severe in degree. Immediate memory is intact as indicated by the patient's ability to repeat series of numbers. Short-term memory, in contrast, is markedly impaired. The patients may be incapable, for example, of committing to memory three simple facts (such as the examiner's name, the date, and the time of day) despite countless attempts; they can repeat each fact as it is presented, indicating that they understand what is wanted of them and that "registration" is intact, but by the time the third fact is repeated, the first may have been forgotten. Since the adaptation to new situations requires the formation of new memories and their integration with past experience, it is this learning defect that renders the patient helpless in society and capable of performing only the most habitual tasks.

The anterograde amnesia is always coupled with a *disturbance of past or remote memory*. As a rule, the latter disorder is also severe in degree, though rarely complete, and covers a period that antedates the onset of the illness by several years. Characteristically, isolated events and information from the past are retained, but these are related without regard for the intervals that separated them or for their proper temporal sequence. Usually the patient "telescopes" events, sometimes the opposite. This aspect of the memory disorder becomes prominent after the acute stage of the illness has passed and some improvement in memory function has occurred, and may account for certain instances of confabulation (see below).

It is probably true that memories of the recent past are more severely impaired than those of the remote past, but this is not to say that remote memories are intact. The latter are not as readily tested as more recent memories and the two are therefore difficult to compare. It is our impression that memories of the distant past are impaired in practically all cases of Korsakoff psychosis and seriously impaired in many of them.

It should be emphasized that all the manifestations of the Korsakoff syndrome cannot be explained in terms of memory loss alone, even though this is the most critical functional loss. Formal psychologic testing, using the Wechsler Adult Intelligence Scale, discloses a characteristic though nonspecific pattern of impairment of cognitive functions. The most consistent failure is with the digit symbol task, and to a lesser degree, with arithmetic and block design. However, patients have a relatively normal capacity to reason with data immediately before them—i.e., circumstances in which memory function is not the major factor.

Using a battery of tests of perceptual functions, Talland has demonstrated a number of defects in Korsakoff patients that could not be attributed to a primary abnormality in learning or memorizing. Whereas patients showed no deficit in immediate apprehension, they were greatly handicapped if the task was changed and a new "mental set" required, especially if the first task was continued. It seemed that patients were excessively dependent upon the immediate sensory input; their inability to detach themselves from it by imagery or to change their orientation toward it prevented them from assimilating a diversity of newly presented material. In addition, Korsakoff patients showed serious defects in the formation of concepts. Talland proposed that the inability to adopt new attitudes of orientation to a situation is the basic abnormality in both the perceptual and conceptual deficits.

Confabulation is generally considered to be an indispensable attribute of Korsakoff psychosis. The validity of this view depends largely on how one defines confabulation, and there is no uniformity of opinion on this point. Some patients simply do not confabulate, no matter how broadly one interprets this term. In our experience, confabulation is associated with two phases of the Wernicke-Korsakoff syndrome; the initial phase, in which profound general confusion dominates the disease; and the convalescent phase in which the patient recalls fragments of past experience in a distorted fashion. Events that were separated by long intervals are juxtaposed or related out of sequence, so that the narrative has an implausible or fictional aspect. Whether one designates this defect as confabulation or as a particular defect of retentive memory is academic. In the chronic, stable state of the disease, confabulation is usually absent.

The statement is often made that the Korsakoff patient fills the gaps in his or her memory with confabulation. In the sense that gaps in memory exist and that whatever the patient supplies in place of the correct answers fills these gaps, the statement is incontrovertible. It is hardly explanatory, however. The implication that confabulation is a deliberate attempt to hide the memory defect, out of embarrassment or for other reasons, is probably not correct. In fact, the opposite seems to pertain: as the patient improves and becomes more aware of a defect in memory, the tendency to confabulate becomes less.

Prognosis Once the Korsakoff amnesic state is established, complete or almost complete recovery occurs in only about 20 percent of patients. Of the remainder, some improve slightly, to the point where they can find their way to their room or dining hall; others improve somewhat more, so they are eventually able to carry out routine household or institutional tasks under supervision. Improvement may begin within a few weeks after the amnesic syndrome is recognized and treated, but in the majority of cases the onset of improvement is delayed for 1 to 3 months, and the maximum degree of recovery may not be attained for a year or longer.

Other Clinical Abnormalities Signs of *peripheral nerve disease* are found in more than 80 percent of patients with the Wernicke-Korsakoff syndrome. In the majority of patients the neuropathic affection is mild in degree and does not account for the disorder of gait, but it may be so severe that stance and gait cannot be tested. In a small number of patients, retrobulbar neuropathy is added. Despite the frequency of peripheral neuropathy overt signs of beriberi heart disease are rare. However, indications of *disordered cardiovascular function* such as tachycardia, exertional dyspnea, postural hypotension, and minor electrocardiographic abnormalities are frequent; occasionally, the patient dies suddenly, following only slight exertion. These patients may show an elevation of cardiac output disproportionate to oxygen consumption, associated with low peripheral vascular resistance—abnormalities that revert to normal after the administration of thiamine. *Postural hypotension* and syncope are common findings in Wernicke disease and are probably due to impaired function of the autonomic nervous system, more specifically to a defect in the sympathetic outflow (Birchfield). In the chronic stage of the disease, many patients demonstrate an *impaired capacity to discriminate between odors*. The studies of Mair et al suggest that this deficit is attributable not to a lesion of the peripheral olfactory system or to the rapid decay of memory stores, but to a lesion of the medial dorsal nucleus of the thalamus and its neocortical connections.

Ancillary Findings Vestibular function, as measured by the response to standard ice-water caloric tests, is universally impaired in the acute stage of Wernicke disease (Ghez). To this abnormality of function, which is bilateral and more or less symmetrical, the term *vestibular paresis* has been applied. It probably accounts for the severe disequilibrium in the initial stage of the illness. The *CSF* in uncomplicated cases of the Wernicke-Korsakoff syndrome is normal or shows only a modest elevation of the protein content. Protein values above 100 mg/dL or a pleocytosis should suggest the presence of a complicating illness—subdural hematoma and meningeal infection being the most common.

Blood pyruvate is consistently elevated in untreated cases of Wernicke disease. The usefulness of this estimation as an index of thiamine deficiency is limited, mainly because of its lack of specificity. This shortcoming has been overcome to a large extent by the introduction of the *blood transketolase assay* as an index of thiamine deficiency.

Transketolase, one of the enzymes of the hexose mono-phosphate shunt, requires thiamine pyrophosphate (TPP) as a cofactor. In normal adult subjects, transketolase values (expressed as sedoheptulose-7-phosphate produced per milliliter per hour) range from 90 to 140 μg and the TPP effect from 0 to 10 percent, depending upon the degree of vitamin supplementation. Before specific treatment with thiamine, patients with Wernicke disease show a marked reduction in their transketolase activity (as low as one-third of normal values) and a striking TPP effect (up to 50 percent). Restoration of these values toward normal occurs within a few hours of the administration of thiamine, and completely normal values are usually attained within 24 h.

An interesting abnormality of transketolase has been described by Blass and Gibson. They found that transketolase in fibroblasts from four alcoholics with Wernicke-Korsakoff disease bound TPP less avidly than did the transketolase from control lines. Presumably this defect in transketolase would be insignificant if the diet were adequate, but would be deleterious if the diet were low in thiamine. These findings implicate a hereditary factor in the genesis of Wernicke-Korsakoff disease and explain why only a small proportion of nutritionally deficient alcoholics develop this disease.

Only about half the patients with Wernicke-Korsakoff disease show EEG abnormalities, consisting of diffuse slow activity, mild to moderate in degree. Total cerebral blood flow and cerebral oxygen and glucose consumption may be greatly reduced in the acute stages of the disease, and these defects may still be present after several weeks of treatment (Shimojyo et al). These observations indicate that profound reductions in brain metabolism need not be reflected in EEG abnormalities or in depression of the state of consciousness, and that the latter is a function of the location of the lesion, not the overall degree of metabolic defect.

COURSE OF THE ILLNESS

The mortality rate in the acute phase of Wernicke disease was 17 percent in our series of patients. Most of the fatalities were attributable to infection (pneumonia, pulmonary tuberculosis, and septicemia being the most common) and decompensated liver disease due to cirrhosis. Some deaths undoubtedly were due to the effects of thiamine deficiency that had reached an irreversible stage.

Patients who recover respond to specific treatment (administration of thiamine) in a fairly predictable manner. The most dramatic improvement is in the *ocular manifestations*. Recovery often *begins* within hours after the administration of thiamine, and practically always within several days. This effect is so constant that a failure of the ocular palsies to respond to thiamine should raise doubts about the diagnosis of Wernicke disease. Sixth nerve palsies,

ptosis, and vertical gaze palsies recover completely, within a week or two in most cases, but vertical nystagmus may occasionally persist for several months. Horizontal gaze palsies recover completely as a rule, but in 60 percent of cases a fine horizontal nystagmus remains as a permanent sequela of the disease. In this respect, horizontal nystagmus is unique among the ocular signs.

In comparison to the ocular signs, improvement of *ataxia* is somewhat delayed. In most patients improvement is noted within a week, and in most of the remainder, within 1 to 3 weeks after treatment is begun. About 40 percent of patients recover completely from ataxia. The remainder recover incompletely or not at all, and are left with a slow, shuffling, wide-based gait and inability to walk tandem. The residual gait disturbances and horizontal nystagmus provide a means of identifying obscure and chronic cases of dementia as alcoholic-nutritional in origin.

Vestibular function, as disclosed by caloric testing, improves at about the same rate as the ataxia of stance and gait, i.e., over a period of weeks or months, and recovery is usually but not always complete.

The early symptoms of apathy, drowsiness, and global confusion invariably recede, and as they do so the defect in memory and learning (Korsakoff psychosis) stands out more clearly. The memory disorder, once it becomes established, recovers in only a small proportion of patients, as indicated above.

It is apparent, from the foregoing account, that Wernicke disease and Korsakoff psychosis do not comprise separate diseases; rather, the changing ocular and ataxic signs and the transformation of the global confusional state into an amnesic syndrome are successive stages in the recovery of a single disease process. Of 186 patients in our series who presented with Wernicke disease and survived the acute illness, 157 (84 percent) showed this sequence of clinical events. As a corollary, a survey of alcoholic patients with Korsakoff psychosis in a state mental hospital disclosed that in most of them the illness had begun with the symptoms of Wernicke disease, and that about 60 percent of them still showed the ocular or cerebellar stigmata, or both, of Wernicke disease, many years after the onset.

NEUROPATHOLOGIC FINDINGS AND CLINICAL-PATHOLOGIC CORRELATION

Patients who die in the acute stages of Wernicke disease show symmetrical lesions in the paraventricular regions of the thalamus and hypothalamus, in the mammillary bodies, the periaqueductal region of the midbrain, and floor of the fourth ventricle, particularly in the regions of the dorsal motor nuclei of the vagus and vestibular nuclei, and in the superior vermis. Lesions are consistently found in the mammillary bodies, less consistently in other areas. The microscopic changes are characterized by varying degrees of necrosis of parenchymal structures, though it is seldom complete. The tissue appears loose and vacuolated. Within the area of necrosis, nerve cells are lost, but usually some remain; some of these are damaged, but others are intact. These changes result in a prominence of the blood vessels, although in some cases there is a true endothelial proliferation. In the areas of parenchymal damage there is a density of cells, representing astrocytic and microglial proliferation. These alterations are most intense in the center of the lesion, shading off toward the periphery. Discrete hemorrhages were found in only 20 percent of our cases, and many of them appeared to be agonal in nature. The cerebellar changes consist of a degeneration of all layers of the cortex, particularly of the Purkinje cells; usually this lesion is confined to the superior parts of the vermis, but in advanced cases the cortex of the most anterior parts of the anterior lobes is involved as well.

Correlation of the clinical manifestations with the anatomic localization of lesions indicates that the ocular muscle and gaze palsies are attributable to lesions of the sixth and third nerve nuclei and adjacent tegmentum, and the nystagmus to lesions in the regions of the vestibular nuclei. The latter lesions are also responsible for the loss of caloric responses and probably for the gross disturbance of equilibrium that characterizes the initial stages of the disease. The lack of significant destruction of nerve cells in these lesions accounts for the rapid improvement and the high degree of recovery of oculomotor and vestibular function. The persistent ataxia of stance and gait is due to the lesion of the superior vermis of the cerebellum; ataxia of individual movements of the legs is attributable to an extension of the lesion into the anterior parts of the anterior lobes. Hypothermia occurs sometimes in the acute stages of Wernicke disease and is probably attributable to lesions in the posterior and posterolateral nuclei of the hypothalamus, since experimentally placed lesions in these parts have been shown to cause hypothermia in monkeys.

The neuropathologic changes in patients who die in the chronic stages of the disease, when the amnesic symptoms predominate, are much the same as the changes in the acute stages of Wernicke disease. Apart from the expected differences with respect to the age of the glial and vascular reactions, the only important difference has to do with the involvement or lack of involvement of the medial dorsal nucleus of the thalamus and the posterior nucleus as well. These structures were consistently involved in patients who had shown Korsakoff psychosis during life; they were not involved in patients who had had no symptoms of Korsakoff psychosis. The mammillary bodies were involved in all of the patients, both in those with the amnesic defect and in those without. These observations suggest that the lesions responsible for the memory disorder are those of the medial thalami, rather than of the mammillary bodies, as is frequently stated.

The lesion responsible for the olfactory deficit is uncertain. It may be in the mammillary nuclei, ventromedial nucleus of the hypothalamus, or dorsomedial nucleus of the thalamus, all of which are thought to function as relay nuclei in the central connections that mediate olfactory sensation (Mair et al).

McEntee and his colleagues have pointed out that the paraventricular lesions of the Wernicke-Korsakoff syndrome lie in the monoamine-containing pathways. In 25 such patients they found that levels of 3-methoxy-4-hydroxyphenylglycol (MHPG), the primary brain metabolite of norepinephrine, are decreased in the CSF of patients with Korsakoff psychosis. They found further that the administration of clonidine, a putative alpha-noradrenergic agonist, seemed to improve the disorder of memory in these patients. On the basis of these observations, these authors have theorized that damage to ascending norepinephrine-containing neurons in the brainstem and diencephalon may be the basis for the amnesia in Korsakoff psychosis.

THE NUTRITIONAL DEFECT IN WERNICKE DISEASE AND KORSAKOFF PSYCHOSIS

For many years it was believed that Wernicke disease was due to the toxic effects of alcohol. The first steps in its identification as a nutritional disorder were taken when it was recognized to be a complication of gastric carcinoma and other disturbances of the alimentary tract, and of hyperemesis gravidarum. Shortly thereafter, Alexander and his colleagues drew attention to the similarity of the pathologic changes in pigeons deprived of B vitamins and the changes observed in Wernicke disease; it then became evident that the lesions in many thiamine-deficient mammalian species also bore such a resemblance.

Thiamine is the specific nutritional factor responsible for most if not all the symptomatology of Wernicke disease. Ophthalmoplegia, nystagmus, and ataxia can be reversed by the administration of thiamine alone, although horizontal nystagmus and ataxia may persist in mild form for months or years after their onset. The marked sensitivity of the ophthalmoplegia to the administration of thiamine accounts for the rapid disappearance of this sign after a meal or two, and the quality of prompt reversibility indicates that the symptoms are due more to a biochemical abnormality than to structural change.

Many of the initial mental symptoms—apathy, drowsiness, listlessness, inattentiveness, and inability to concentrate and to sustain a conversation—clear rapidly under the influence of thiamine alone. With respect to memory defect and confabulation, the specific role of thiamine is less certain. The amnesic symptoms recover slowly and incompletely, and at much the same rate both in patients who are given a full diet and all vitamins from the outset, and in those who receive a deficient diet, supplemented only with thiamine. These observations suggest that the memory loss is due to a structural lesion rather than to a reversible biochemical process.

INFANTILE BERIBERI

This term designates an acute and frequently fatal disease of infants, which until recently was very common in rice-eating communities of the Far East. It affects only breast-fed infants, usually in the second to the fifth months of life. Acute cardiac symptoms dominate the clinical picture, but neurologic symptoms (aphonia, strabismus, nystagmus, spasmodic contraction of facial muscles, and convulsions) have been described in many cases. This syndrome can be reversed dramatically by the administration of thiamine, so that some authors prefer to call it *acute thiamine deficiency in infants*.

Infantile beriberi bears no consistent relationship to beriberi in the mother. Infants of mothers with overt signs of beriberi may be quite normal. Conversely, mothers of infants with beriberi are themselves frequently free of the disease. The levels of thiamine in the breast milk of such mothers have not been determined, however. The absence of beriberi in the mothers of affected infants suggested that infantile beriberi might be due to a toxic factor in breast milk, but such a factor, if it exists, has never been isolated.

In the few neuropathologic studies that have been made of this disorder, changes like those of Wernicke disease in the adult have been described.

Rarely, the clinical manifestations of beriberi in infancy represent an inherited (autosomal recessive) thiamine-dependent state, responding to the continued administration of massive doses of thiamine (Mandel et al; see also Table 39-3).

TREATMENT OF THE WERNICKE-KORSAKOFF SYNDROME

Wernicke disease constitutes a medical emergency, and its recognition demands the immediate administration of thiamine. The prompt use of thiamine prevents the progression of the disease and reverses those lesions that have not yet progressed to the point of fixed structural change. In patients

who show only ocular signs and ataxia, the administration of thiamine is crucial in preventing the development of an amnesic psychosis.

Although 2 to 3 mg of thiamine may be sufficient to modify the ocular signs, much larger doses are needed to sustain the improvement and to replenish the depleted thiamine stores—50 mg intravenously and 50 mg intramuscularly, the latter dose being repeated each day until the patient resumes a normal diet.

The further management of Wernicke disease involves the use of a balanced diet and all the B vitamins, since the patient is usually deficient in more than thiamine alone. It is also good practice to give B vitamins to all alcoholic patients, particularly those being treated with parenteral glucose. The alcoholic's reserve of thiamine may be exhausted after 7 or 8 weeks, at which time the administration of glucose often serves to precipitate Wernicke disease or cause an early form of the disease to progress rapidly.

A problem in management may arise once the patient has recovered from Wernicke disease and the amnesic psychosis becomes prominent. The onset of recovery of mental function may be delayed for several weeks or even months, and then it proceeds very slowly over a period of many months. The extent to which the amnesic symptoms will recover cannot be predicted accurately during the acute stages of the illness; one must guard against the premature commitment of the patient to a mental hospital. Interestingly, the alcoholic Korsakoff patient, once more or less recovered, seldom demands alcohol, but will drink it if it is offered.

NUTRITIONAL POLYNEUROPATHY (Neuropathic Beriberi)

Most physicians have a somewhat bemused notion about beriberi, which they recall as an ill-defined, predominantly cardiac disorder occurring among the rice-eating people of the Orient. In fact, beriberi is a rather distinct clinical entity that is not confined to any particular part of the world. Essentially it is a disease of the heart and of the peripheral nerves (which may be affected separately), with or without edema, the latter feature providing the basis for the classic division into wet and dry forms. The cardiac manifestations range from tachycardia and exertional dyspnea to acute and rapidly fatal heart failure. The latter is the most dramatic manifestation of beriberi, but is uncommon. Here we will be concerned with the affection of the peripheral nerves, or *neuropathic beriberi*, as it will be designated.

That beriberi is essentially a degenerative disorder of the peripheral nerves was established in the latter part of the nineteenth century by the classic studies of the Dutch investigators, Eijkman, Pekelharing and Winkler, and Grijns. Only after beriberi gained acceptance as a nutritional disease (this followed Funk's discovery of vitamins in 1911) was it suspected that the neuropathy of alcoholics was also nutritional in origin. The similarity between beriberi and alcoholic neuropathy was commented upon by several authors, but it was Shattuck, in 1928, who first seriously discussed the relationship of the two disorders. He suggested that "polyneuritis of chronic alcoholism was caused chiefly by failure to take or assimilate food containing a sufficient quantity of vitamin B . . . and might properly be regarded as true beriberi." Convincing evidence that "alcoholic neuritis" is not due to the neurotoxic effect of alcohol was supplied by Strauss. He allowed 10 patients to continue their daily consumption of whiskey while they consumed a well-balanced diet supplemented with yeast and vitamin B concentrates; improvement occurred in all the patients. Our own observations are supportive of Strauss' contention that all alcoholic polyneuropathy is nutritional.

The nutritional factor(s) responsible for the neuropathy of alcoholism and beriberi have not been defined precisely. Because of the difficulties in producing peripheral neuropathy in Mammalia by means of a thiamine-deficient diet, several authors have questioned whether thiamine is the antineuritic vitamin. Very few of the animal experiments undertaken to settle this point are satisfactory from a nutritional and pathologic point of view. Nevertheless, several studies in birds and in humans do indeed indicate that uncomplicated thiamine deficiency may result in peripheral nerve disease. The necessity of either accepting or rejecting the specific role of thiamine became less urgent when it was demonstrated, both in animals and in humans, that a deficiency of pyridoxine or of pantothenic acid could result in degeneration of the peripheral nerves.

PATHOLOGIC FEATURES

The essential pathologic change is axonal degeneration with destruction of both axon and myelin sheath. Segmental demyelination may also occur but affects only a small proportion of fibers. The latter change may be difficult to discern in myelin-stained sections of whole nerve trunks, but can be observed in teased nerve fibers stained with osmium. The most pronounced changes are observed in the distal parts of the longest and largest myelinated fibers in the crural and, to a lesser extent, in the brachial nerves. In advanced cases the degenerative changes involve the anterior and posterior nerve roots. The vagus and phrenic nerves and paravertebral sympathetic trunks may be implicated in advanced cases.

Anterior horn and dorsal root ganglion cells undergo chromatolysis, indicating axonal damage. Degenerative changes in the posterior columns are seen in some cases, and are probably secondary to the changes in the posterior roots.

CLINICAL FEATURES

The symptomatology of nutritional polyneuropathy is diverse. In fact, many patients are asymptomatic, and evidence of peripheral nerve affection is found only on examination. In the latter circumstance the neuropathic signs are mild in degree, consisting only of thinness and tenderness of the leg muscles, loss or depression of the Achilles reflexes and perhaps of the patellar reflexes as well, and at times a patchy blunting of pain and touch sensation over the feet and shins.

The majority of patients, however, are symptomatic—weakness, paresthesias, and pain being the usual complaints. The symptoms are insidious in onset and slowly progressive, although occasionally they seem to evolve or to worsen rapidly over a matter of days. The initial symptoms are often referred to the distal portion of the limbs and progress proximally if the illness remains untreated. The lower limbs are always affected earlier and more severely than the upper ones. Usually some aspect of motor disability constitutes the chief complaint, but in about one-quarter of the patients the main complaints are pain and paresthesias. The discomfort takes several forms: a dull constant ache in the feet or legs; sharp and lancinating pains, momentary in duration, like those of tabes dorsalis; cramping sensations in the muscles of the feet and calves; "tightness" of the calves; or band-like feelings around the legs. Coldness of the feet is a common complaint, but it is purely subjective. Far more distressing are feelings of heat or "burning"; these affect the soles mainly, less frequently the dorsal aspects of the feet. The dysesthesias fluctuate in severity; characteristically, they are worsened by contactual stimuli. In severe cases patients cannot bear to have the bedclothes touch their feet, nor can they bear to walk, despite the relative preservation of motor power. The term *burning feet* has been applied to this syndrome, but is not particularly apt, since the patient complains not only of "burning" but of other types of paresthesia and pain, and these symptoms may involve the hands as well as the feet.

Examination discloses varying degrees of motor, sensory, and reflex loss. As the symptoms suggest, the signs are symmetrical, usually more severe in distal than in proximal portions of the limbs, and often confined to the legs. The disproportionate affection of motor power may be striking, taking the form of a foot and wrist drop, but even in these patients the proximal muscles are usually affected. Involvement of thigh muscles is indicated by difficulty in arising from a squatting position. In other patients, all the leg muscles are affected more or less equally, and in still others the proximal muscles are disproportionately weakened. Absolute paralysis of the legs is observed only rarely; immobility due to contractures at the knees and ankles is a more common occurrence. Tenderness of muscles on pressure is a highly characteristic finding. This is elicited most readily in the muscles of the feet and calves, but all muscles of the limbs may be painful on pressure—even if they show only minimal weakness. Deep tendon reflexes in the legs are almost always lost, even when weakness is slight in degree. In the arms, tendon reflexes are sometimes retained, despite a loss of strength in the hands. In a small number of patients, particularly those in whom pain and dysesthesias are prominent and motor loss is slight, the reflexes may be of greater than average briskness.

Excessive sweating of the soles and dorsal aspects of the feet, and of the volar surfaces of the hands and fingers, is a common manifestation of alcohol-induced nutritional neuropathy. Postural hypotension is sometimes associated. The latter symptoms are indicative of involvement of the peripheral sympathetic nerve fibers.

Sensory loss or impairment may involve all the modalities, although one modality may be affected out of proportion to the others. One cannot predict from the patient's symptoms which mode of sensation might be affected disproportionately. In cases with impairment of superficial sensation (i.e., of touch, pain, and temperature), the border between normal and impaired sensation is not sharp but shades off gradually over a considerable vertical extent of the limbs.

Patients in whom pain is the outstanding symptom do not constitute a distinct group in terms of their neurologic signs. Pain and dysesthesias may be prominent symptoms in cases with either severe or with slight degrees of motor, reflex, and sensory loss. The term *hyperesthetic* is used commonly to designate the exquisitely painful form of neuropathy but is not well chosen; as pointed out on page 128, the term implies a heightened receptiveness of the nervous system or an increased response of the receptors to tactile and painful stimuli. Actually, in patients with severe "hyperesthesia" one is usually able, by using finely graded stimuli, to demonstrate an elevated threshold to painful, thermal, and tactile stimuli in the "hyperesthetic" zone. Once the stimulus is perceived, however, it has a painful and diffuse, unpleasant quality (hyperpathia).

In most patients with nutritional polyneuropathy only the limbs are involved; the abdominal, thoracic, and bulbar

musculature is usually spared. In patients with severe neuropathy, hoarseness and weakness of the voice and dysphagia due to affection of the vagus nerves may be added to the clinical picture.

An idea of the incidence of the motor, reflex, and sensory abnormalities and the combinations in which they occur can be obtained from Table 39-1, which is based on our study of 189 nutritionally depleted alcoholic patients. The legs were affected in all cases and exclusively in 132 (70 percent) of the 189 cases. In the remaining 57 cases, both the arms and legs were involved; in these cases the neuropathic signs were severe in degree and almost always more severe in the legs than in the arms. In no case were the arms alone affected. Only 66 (35 percent) of the 189 patients showed the clinical picture of polyneuropathy in its entirety—i.e., a symmetrical impairment or loss of tendon reflexes, sensation, and motor power affecting legs more than the arms, and the distal more than the proximal segments of the limbs. In the remaining patients the motor-reflex-sensory signs occurred in various combinations, as indicated in Table 39-1. In about two-thirds of the patients with sensory abnormalities, both superficial and deep sensation were impaired more or less equally; 25 percent showed a predominant affection of superficial sensation (touch, pain, and temperature); and in the remaining 10 percent, deep sensation (deep pressure, vibratory and position sense) was seemingly impaired to a greater extent. Usually vibratory and position sense were involved together, but in some cases one or the other was selectively affected.

Stasis edema and pigmentation, glossiness, and thinness of the skin of the lower legs and feet are common findings in patients with severe forms of neuropathy. Major

Table 39-1

Neuropathic abnormality	Legs (189 cases)	Arms (57 cases)
Loss of reflexes alone	45 (24)*	6 (10)†
Loss of sensation alone	10 (5)	10 (18)
Weakness alone	—	5 (9)
Weakness and sensory loss	2 (1)	10 (18)
Reflex and sensory loss	40 (21)	2 (3)
Sensory, motor, and reflex loss	66 (35)	17 (30)
Data incomplete	26 (14)	7 (12)

* Figures in parentheses indicate percent of 189 cases.
† Figures in parentheses indicate percent of 57 cases.

dystrophic changes, in the form of perforating plantar ulcers and painless destruction of the bones and joints of the feet (ulcero-osteolytic neuropathy; "Charcot forefeet"), are less frequent. Repeated trauma to insensitive parts with super-imposed infection is thought to be responsible for the neuropathic arthropathy.

In the alcoholic patient, skin changes (dryness and scaliness, pigmentation over the forehead and malar em-inences, acne vulgaris, rhinophyma, or frank lesions of pellagra), folic acid–deficiency anemia, liver disease, and stigmata of the Wernicke-Korsakoff syndrome are frequently associated. The CSF is usually normal, although a modest elevation of protein content is found in a small number of cases. The usual electromyographic findings include mild to moderate degrees of slowing of motor and sensory conduction and a marked reduction of the amplitudes of sensory action potentials; moreover, the conduction veloc-ities in distal segments of the nerves may be reduced, while conduction in proximal segments is normal. There are fibrillation potentials in the denervated muscles.

TREATMENT AND PROGNOSIS

The first consideration in treatment is to supply adequate nutrition in the form of a balanced diet, supplemented with B vitamins. It is equally important to make certain that the patient follows the prescribed diet. If persistent vomiting or other gastrointestinal complications prevent the patient from eating, then parenteral feeding becomes necessary; the vitamins may be given intramuscularly or added to intravenous fluids. A suitable parenteral preparation is Berroca-C, one injection daily.

Where pain and sensitivity of the feet are the major complaints, the pressure of bedclothes may be avoided by placing a cradle support over the legs. Aching of the limbs may be related to their immobility, in which case they should be moved passively on frequent occasions. Acetyl-salicylic acid, in a dosage of 0.3 to 1.0 g (5 to 15 grains) or acetaminophen (Tylenol) every 4 h, usually is sufficient to control hyperpathia; occasionally codeine in doses of 15 to 30 mg has to be added. Opiates and the addicting synthetic analgesics should be avoided, particularly if the pain is chronic in nature. Some of our patients with severe burning pain (similar to causalgia) in the feet have been helped by blocking the lumbar sympathetic ganglia. How-ever adrenergic blocking medication has been of little value.

The regeneration of peripheral nerves, which may take many months, will be of no avail if the muscles have been allowed to undergo contracture and the joints to become fixed. During the day, the patient's legs should be positioned so that the soles rest firmly against a footboard, in order to prevent shortening of the heel cords. In cases of severe paralysis, molded splints should be applied to the arms, hands, legs, and feet during periods of rest. Pressure on the heels and elbows can be avoided by padding the splints and by turning the patient frequently or by asking the patient to turn. As soon as the patient's general condition permits, the limbs must be passively moved through a full range of movement several times daily. Gentle massage is also useful. As function returns, more vigorous physio-therapeutic measures can be undertaken.

Recovery from nutritional polyneuropathy is a slow process. In the mildest cases there may be a considerable restoration of motor function in a few weeks. In severe forms of the disease, several months may pass before the patient is able to walk unaided. The slowness of recovery creates a special problem for the alcoholic patient in whom the great danger to continued recovery is the resumption of drinking. Suitable arrangements must therefore be made for close supervision during the long and tedious convalescence.

DEFICIENCY AMBLYOPIA (Nutritional Optic Neuropathy, "Tobacco-Alcohol Amblyopia")

These terms refer to a characteristic form of visual impair-ment that results from nutritional deficiency. The defect in vision is due not to an abnormality of the cornea or other parts of the refractive mechanism, but to a lesion of the optic nerve, more or less confined to the region of the papillomacular bundle.

Typically, the patient complains of dimness or blur-ring of vision for near and distant objects, evolving gradually over a period of several days or weeks. Examination discloses a reduction in visual acuity due to the presence of central or centrocecal scotomata, which are larger for colored than for white test objects. Pallor of the temporal portion of the optic disc is observed in some cases. These abnormalities are practically always bilateral and roughly symmetrical. Untreated, they may progress to irreversible optic atrophy. With nutritious diet and vitamin supplements, improvement occurs in all but the most chronic cases, the degree of recovery depending upon the severity of the amblyopia and particularly upon its duration before therapy is instituted.

The nutritional basis of this visual disorder was established beyond doubt during World War II and the Korean War, when innumerable instances were observed in prisoners-of-war who had been confined for prolonged periods under conditions of severe dietary deprivation. Fisher has described the optic nerve lesions in four such patients who died of unrelated causes between 8 and 10 years after the onset. The optic nerves in each case showed a distinct loss of myelin and axis cylinders, restricted to the region of the papillomacular fibers. Three of the four cases also showed demyelination of the posterior columns of the spinal cord, no doubt an expression of the associated sensory polyneuropathy.

In the Western world, a visual disorder indistinguishable clinically and pathologically from that observed in prisoners of war is observed sporadically, mainly among undernourished alcoholics. This was, for many years, referred to as *tobacco-alcohol amblyopia*—the implication being that the visual loss is due to the toxic effects of alcohol or tobacco, or both. Actually, the evidence is overwhelming that so-called tobacco-alcohol amblyopia is due to nutritional deficiency. A specific nutrient has not been established, however. There is evidence in humans and in animals that under certain conditions a deficiency of one or more of the B vitamins—thiamine, vitamin B_{12}, and perhaps riboflavin—may cause degenerative changes in the optic nerves—a situation that pertains in the peripheral nerves as well.

In the 1960s, a popular theory held that the combined effects of vitamin B_{12} deficiency and chronic poisoning by cyanide (generated in tobacco smoke) were responsible for "tobacco amblyopia." Vitamin B_{12} deficiency is a rare but undoubted cause of optic neuropathy, but the notion that cyanide or other substances in tobacco smoke have a damaging effect upon the optic nerves is supported neither by logic nor by experimental data. The arguments leading to this conclusion have been fully marshaled in two reviews, one by Potts and another by Victor, to which the reader is referred for a more detailed account than can be presented here.

PELLAGRA

In the early 1900s, pellagra attained epidemic proportions in the southern part of the United States and in the alcoholic population of large urban centers. Since 1940, the prevalence of pellagra has diminished greatly because of the general practice of enriching bread with niacin. Nevertheless, among the vegetarian, maize-eating people of underdeveloped countries and among the black population of South Africa, pellagra is still a common disease (Bomb et al, Shah et al, Ronthal and Adler). In the developed countries, pellagra is practically confined to the alcoholic population (Ishii and Nishihara, Spivak and Jackson, Serdaru et al).

In its fully developed form, pellagra affects the skin, alimentary tract, and hematopoietic and nervous systems. Only the effects upon the nervous system will concern us here.

The most clearly defined neurologic manifestations are the *cerebral* ones. In the early stages the symptoms may be mistaken for those of psychoneurosis. Insomnia, fatigue, nervousness, irritability, and feelings of depression are common complaints; examination may disclose mental dullness, apathy, and an impairment of memory. Sometimes an acute confusional psychosis dominates the clinical picture. Pellagra may not only produce insanity but occasionally may result from it, by virtue of anorexia and the refusal of food that accompanies certain mental illnesses. The manifestations of *spinal cord involvement* have not been clearly delineated, perhaps because the patient's mental state often precludes accurate testing; in general, the signs are referable to both the posterior and lateral columns, predominantly the former. Signs of *peripheral nerve affection* are relatively less common and are indistinguishable from those of neuropathic beriberi.

Spinal Spastic Syndrome This syndrome is observed occasionally in nutritionally depleted alcoholics. The main clinical signs are spastic weakness of the legs, with absent abdominal and increased tendon reflexes, clonus, extensor plantar responses, and a loss of position and vibratory senses. In our experience this syndrome is usually associated with other nutritional disorders, such as Wernicke disease and peripheral and optic neuropathy. In prisoner-of-war camps, the "spastic syndrome" was observed in association with mental and emotional changes, dimness of vision, and at times with widespread muscular rigidity, delirium, coma, and death. Unfortunately, this latter syndrome was never studied pathologically so that it is impossible to state whether the lesions are the same as or different from those of pellagra.

The syndrome of spastic paraparesis is far more common in tropical climates than in temperate ones (*tropical spastic paraparesis*). Probably more than one disease has been included under this rubric. The spastic weakness of the legs, which is the main feature of the illness, may be acute or chronic in nature and may occur sporadically or in large outbreaks. The acute form begins with painful paresthesias of the legs, followed within hours or days by weakness, often accompanied by dysarthria and visual complaints; in such cases, recovery is the rule, but it may be incomplete. The abrupt onset and epidemic nature of the spastic paraparesis suggests an infectious etiology (Carton et al). Many but not all of the patients test positively for antibodies to HTLV-1. Some cases of chronic spastic paraparesis in tropical climates have been attributed to chronic cyanide intoxication (due to ingestion of insufficiently detoxified cassava). Lathyrism, another form of spastic paraplegia that is common in India and certain parts of Africa, was for many years suspected of being nutritional in origin, but is now thought to be due to a toxin—β, *N*-oxalylaminoalanine—in chick-peas (*Lathyrus sativus*). These types of tropical spastic paraplegia are discussed in greater detail with the spinal cord diseases (page 747). A chronic tropical disease of the *peripheral nerves*, designated as "ataxic neuropathy of Nigeria," has also been attributed to the ingestion of inadequately detoxified cassava (Osun-tokun).

Nicotinic Acid Deficiency Encephalopathy   Under this title, Jolliffe et al in 1940 described an acute cerebral syndrome in alcoholic patients, consisting of clouding of consciousness progressing to coma, extrapyramidal rigidity and tremors ("cogwheel" rigidity) of the extremities, and uncontrollable grasping and sucking reflexes. Most of their patients showed overt manifestations of nutritional deficiency, such as Wernicke disease, pellagra, scurvy, and polyneuropathy. These authors concluded that the encephalopathy represented an acute form of nicotinic acid deficiency, since most of their patients recovered when treated with a diet of low vitamin B content supplemented by intravenous glucose and saline and large doses of nicotinic acid. Sydenstricker and his colleagues (1938) had previously reported the salutary effects of nicotinic acid on the unresponsive state of elderly undernourished patients, and Spillane (1947) described a similar syndrome and response to nicotinic acid in the indigent Arab population of the Middle East.

The status of this syndrome and its relation to pellagra are uncertain. The clinical and nutritional features were never delineated precisely and the pathologic basis never determined. Serdaru et al have reported 22 presumed examples of this syndrome in the alcoholic population of the Saltpetriere, all reviewed retrospectively after finding chromatolysis of nerve cells in postmortem material. Prominent were confusional states, oppositional rigidity (gegenhalten), ataxia, and polymyoclonia—a picture unlike that described by Joliffe et al (above). Skin lesions were absent. We have rarely encountered such cases among the undernourished patients in the alcoholic populations of Boston and Cleveland.

PATHOLOGIC CHANGES AND PATHOGENESIS

These are most readily discerned in the large cells of the motor cortex, the cells of Betz—although the same changes are seen to a lesser extent in the smaller pyramidal cells of the cortex, the large cells of the basal ganglia, the cells of the cranial motor and dentate nuclei, and the anterior horn cells of the spinal cord. The affected cells appear swollen and rounded, with eccentric nuclei and loss of the Nissl particles. These changes were originally designated by Adolf Meyer as "central neuritis" and are frequently referred to as "axonal reaction" because of their similarity to the changes that occur in anterior horn cells whose axons are severed. It has never been decided whether or not the central neuritis of pellagra is the same as the axonal reaction and whether it is, in fact, dependent on injury to the axons of the Betz cells. One argument against this possibility is the frequency with which the motor tracts are interrupted in the brain and spinal cord without an axonal reaction appearing in their cells of origin. Furthermore, in pellagra the cortical nerve cell changes are not always associated with corticospinal tract lesions; this may mean that the cytoplasmic alterations reflect a purely biochemical abnormality in the axon that only reaches the stage of visible myelin degeneration in certain of the more severe cases. In the pathologic material of Hauw et al, the chromatolytic changes were most pronounced in the brainstem nuclei (upper reticular and pontine) and not in the Betz cells. They, too, concluded that these changes were not due to a retrograde axonal lesion, but did not comment on the status of the spinal cord.

The spinal cord lesions in pellagra take the form of a symmetrical degeneration of the dorsal columns, especially of Goll, and to a lesser extent of the corticospinal tracts. Such a posterior column degeneration, affecting a specific system of fibers, is likely to be secondary to degeneration of the posterior roots or ganglion cells. The reason for the corticospinal tract degeneration is not clear, as has already been indicated.

The few studies that have been made of the peripheral nerves in pellagra have disclosed changes like those in alcoholics and other patients with nutritional deficiency.

ETIOLOGY

It has been known since 1937, when Elvehjem and his coworkers showed that nicotinic acid cured black tongue, a pellagra-like disease in dogs, that this vitamin is effective in the treatment of pellagra. Many years before, Goldberger had demonstrated the curative effects of dietary protein and proposed that pellagra was caused by a lack of specific amino acids. Now it is known that pellagra may result from a deficiency of either nicotinic acid or of tryptophan, the amino acid precursor of nicotinic acid. This explains the frequent occurrence of pellagra in persons who subsist mainly on corn, which contains only small amounts of tryptophan and of niacin—some of the niacin being in bound form and unavailable to the organism.

It should be pointed out that in experimental subjects only the cutaneous-gastrointestinal-neurasthenic manifestations of pellagra have been produced by the feeding of tryptophan- or niacin-deficient diets; neurologic symptoms were not produced by these diets (Goldsmith). As a corollary, only the dermal, gastrointestinal, and neurasthenic manifestations respond to treatment with niacin and tryptophan; neurologic disturbances in pellagrins have proved to be recalcitrant to prolonged treatment with nicotinic acid, although the peripheral nerve disorder may subsequently respond to treatment with thiamine. In monkeys, degeneration of peripheral nerves as well as the unique cerebral cortical changes of pellagra were induced by a deficiency of pyridoxine (Victor and Adams), and Vilter and his colleagues have produced polyneuropathy in human subjects rendered pyridoxine-deficient; these subjects also showed seborrheic dermatitis and glossitis (indistinguishable from that of niacin deficiency), and the cheilosis and angular stomatitis that are usually attributed to riboflavin deficiency. The foregoing observations indicate that certain lingual and cutaneous manifestations that are characteristic of pellagra may be produced by a deficiency of pyridoxine or other B vitamins, and that the neurologic manifestations of pellagra are most likely due not to niacin deficiency but to pyridoxine deficiency.

THE SYNDROME OF AMBLYOPIA, PAINFUL NEUROPATHY, AND OROGENITAL DERMATITIS (Strachan Syndrome)

There remains to be considered a neurologic syndrome that almost certainly is nutritional in origin but does not conform clinically to the classic deficiency diseases, beriberi and pellagra. This syndrome was originally described by Strachan (1897), a medical officer in Jamaica. The main symptoms in his patients were pain, numbness, and paresthesias of the extremities; objectively there was ataxia of gait, weakness, wasting, and loss of deep tendon reflexes and sensation in the limbs. Dimness of vision and impairment of hearing were common findings as were soreness and excoriation of the mucocutaneous junctions of the mouth. This disorder, originally known as "Jamaican neuritis," was quickly recognized in other parts of the world, particularly in the undernourished populations of tropical countries. Subsequently, many cases of this syndrome were observed in the besieged population of Madrid during the Spanish Civil War, and during World War II among prisoners of war in the Middle and Far East.

The clinical descriptions from these varied sources are not entirely uniform, but certain features are common to all of them, and others occur with sufficient frequency to allow the delineation of a neurologic syndrome and its identification with the one described by Strachan. Essentially, the disorder is one of the peripheral and optic nerves. The former is characterized mainly by sensory symptoms

and signs and the latter by failing vision which may go on to complete blindness and pallor of the optic discs. Deafness and vertigo are in general rare complications, but in some outbreaks among prisoners of war these symptoms were common enough to earn the epithet "camp dizziness." In all these respects the syndrome differs from beriberi. Along with the neurologic signs there may be varying degrees of stomatoglossitis, corneal degeneration, and genital dermatitis (the orogenital syndrome). These mucocutaneous lesions are distinct from those of pellagra—at least from the classic form of the disease.

There have been only a few neuropathologic studies of this syndrome. Aside from the changes in the papillomacular bundle of the optic nerve, the most consistent abnormality has been a loss of medullated fibers in each column of Goll adjacent to the midline. Fisher has interpreted this change to indicate a systemized degeneration of the central processes of the bipolar sensory neurons of the dorsal root ganglions. The fact that the primary sensory neuron is the chief site of this disease is consistent with the predominantly sensory symptomatology. The authors find it difficult to see the line that separates nutritional peripheral (and optic) neuropathy from the Strachan syndrome.

THE NEUROLOGIC MANIFESTATIONS OF VITAMIN B$_{12}$ DEFICIENCY

The spinal cord, brain, optic nerves, and peripheral nerves may all be involved in pernicious anemia. The spinal cord is usually affected first and often exclusively. The term *subacute combined degeneration* (SCD) is used customarily to designate the spinal cord lesion in pernicious anemia and to distinguish it from other forms of so-called combined system disease, in which the posterior and lateral columns are affected. Pernicious anemia and its neurologic manifestations are distinctive insofar as they result not from a dietary lack of vitamin B$_{12}$, but from the inability to transfer minute amounts of this nutrient across the intestinal mucosa—"starvation in the midst of plenty," as Castle has aptly put it. This is referred to as a *conditioned deficiency,* insofar as it is conditional upon a lack of intrinsic factor in the gastric secretion.

CLINICAL MANIFESTATIONS

Symptoms of nervous system disease occur in the majority of patients with pernicious anemia. The patient first notices general weakness and paresthesias, consisting of tingling, "pins and needles" feelings, or other vaguely described sensations. The paresthesias tend to be constant, to progress steadily, and to be the source of much distress. They are localized to the distal parts of all four limbs in a symmetrical pattern; occasionally the lower extremities are involved before the upper ones. As the illness progresses, the gait becomes unsteady and stiffness and weakness of the limbs, especially of the legs, develop. If the disease remains untreated, an ataxic paraplegia with variable degrees of spasticity and contracture may develop.

Early in the course of the illness, when only paresthesias are present, there may be no objective signs. Later, examination discloses a disorder of the posterior and lateral columns of the spinal cord, predominantly of the former. Loss of vibration sense is by far the most consistent sign; it is more pronounced in the legs than in the arms, and frequently it extends over the trunk. Position sense is usually impaired as well. The motor signs include loss of strength, spasticity, changes in tendon reflexes, clonus, and extensor plantar responses. These signs are usually limited to the legs. At first the patellar and Achilles reflexes are found to be diminished as frequently as they are increased, and they may even be absent. With treatment the reflexes may return to normal or become hyperactive. The gait at first is predominantly ataxic, later ataxic and spastic.

Loss of superficial sensation below a segmental level on the trunk may occur in isolated instances, implicating the spinothalamic tracts, but such a finding should always suggest the possibility of some other disease of the spinal cord. The defect of cutaneous sensation may take the form of impaired tactile sensation, pain, and thermal perception over the limbs in a distal distribution, implicating the *peripheral nerves*, but such findings are also relatively uncommon.

The nervous system involvement in subacute combined degeneration is roughly symmetrical and a definite asymmetry of motor or sensory findings maintained over a period of weeks or months should always cast doubt on the diagnosis.

Mental signs are frequent, ranging from irritability, apathy, somnolence, suspiciousness, and emotional instability to a marked confusional or depressive psychosis, or intellectual deterioration. *Visual impairment* may occasionally be the earliest or sole manifestation of pernicious anemia; examination discloses roughly symmetrical centrocecal scotomata and optic atrophy in the most advanced cases. The fact that visual-evoked potentials may be abnormal in vitamin B_{12}-deficient patients without clinical signs of visual impairment suggests that the visual pathways may be affected more often than is evident from the neurologic examination alone (Troncoso et al, Krumholz et al).

The CSF is usually normal; in some cases there is a moderate increase of the protein.

NEUROPATHOLOGIC CHANGES AND PATHOGENESIS

The pathologic process takes the form of a diffuse though uneven degeneration of white matter of the spinal cord and occasionally of the brain. The earliest histologic event is a swelling of myelin sheaths, characterized by separation of myelin lamellae and formation of intramyelinic vacuoles. This is followed by a coalescence of small foci of tissue destruction into larger ones, imparting a vacuolated, sieve-like appearance to the tissue. The myelin sheaths and axis cylinders are both involved in the degenerative process, the former more obviously and perhaps earlier than the latter. There is relatively little fibrous gliosis in the early lesions, but in more chronic ones, particularly those in which considerable tissue is destroyed, the gliosis is pronounced. The changes begin in the posterior columns of the lower cervical and upper thoracic segments of the cord and spread from this region up and down the cord, as well as forward into the lateral and anterior columns. The lesions are not limited to specific systems of fibers within the posterior and lateral funiculi but are scattered irregularly through the white matter. For this reason, the term *combined system disease,* which is used frequently to designate the myelopathy of pernicious anemia, is less appropriate than subacute combined degeneration.

In rare instances, foci of spongy degeneration are found in the optic nerves and chiasm and in the central white matter of the brain. The peripheral nerves may show a loss of myelin, but there is no unequivocal evidence that axis cylinders are significantly affected.

It has been shown that monkeys who are sustained on a vitamin B_{12}-deficient diet for a prolonged period develop neuropathologic changes indistinguishable from those of subacute combined degeneration in humans (Agamanolis et al). The time required for the production of CNS changes in monkeys—33 to 45 months—is comparable to the time required to deplete the vitamin B_{12} stores of humans. It is noteworthy that the vitamin B_{12}-deprived monkeys do not become anemic, despite the prolonged period of B_{12} deficiency. Also, in distinction to the human condition, involvement of the optic nerves is particularly severe in the monkeys and probably precedes the degeneration of the spinal cord. The optic nerve lesion appears first in the papillomacular bundles, in the retrobulbar portions of the nerves, and subsequently spreads caudally and beyond the confines of this bundle. These changes are much the same as those of "tobacco-alcohol amblyopia" (see above). The peripheral nerves were not affected in the experimentally produced vitamin B_{12} deficiency.

Clinical-Pathologic Correlation The paresthesias, impairment of deep sensation, and ataxia are due to lesions in the posterior columns, and these may also account for the loss of tendon reflexes. Weakness, spasticity, increased tendon reflexes, and Babinski signs depend on involvement of the corticospinal tracts. The spinothalamic tract may be involved in the pathologic process, which explains the occasional finding of a sensory level on the trunk. The distal and symmetrical impairment of superficial sensation and loss of tendon reflexes that occur in some cases is best explained by involvement of peripheral nerves.

Pathogenesis Little is known about the role of cobalamin in normal nervous system function or the mechanism of damage to nervous tissue in the case of cobalamin deficiency. It has been proposed that impairment of DNA synthesis in vitamin B_{12} deficiency accounts for the hematologic abnormalities and particularly for the production of megaloblasts; however, since neurons do not divide, this factor does not appear to be operative in regard to the CNS. One of the better-understood functions of vitamin B_{12} is its role as a coenzyme in the methylmalonyl CoA–mutase reaction. In this reaction, which is a key step in propionate metabolism, methylmalonyl CoA is transformed to succinyl CoA, which subsequently enters the Krebs cycle. A lack or failure of the cobalamin-dependent enzyme, methylmalonyl CoA mutase, leads to the accumulation of propionyl CoA (Cardinale et al). The latter displaces succinyl CoA, which is the usual primer for the synthesis of even-chain fatty acids, and results in the anomalous insertion of odd-chain fatty acids into membrane lipids, such as myelin sheaths. Conceivably this biochemical abnormality underlies the lesions of myelinated fibers that characterize this disease. However, Carmel et al have described a hereditary form of cobalamin deficiency, in which the methylmalonyl CoA mutase activity was normal, despite the presence of typical neurologic abnormalities. These authors attributed the neurologic abnormalities to an impairment of methionine synthase activity. These and other hypotheses are discussed by Agamanolis et al, Carmel et al, and Beck.

The role of folate deficiency in the genesis of SCD is even less certain. Nevertheless, cerebral and spinal cord lesions, indistinguishable from those due to vitamin B_{12} deficiency have been described occasionally in patients with defective folate metabolism—both in adults with acquired deficiency (Pincus) and in children with an inborn metabolic error (Clayton et al).

DIAGNOSIS AND TREATMENT

The chief obstacle to *early diagnosis* is a lack of parallelism between the hematologic and neurologic signs. This occurs particularly in patients who have taken dietary or medicinal folate, which serves to maintain a hematologic remission for an indefinite period while the neurologic signs worsen, often to an irreversible stage. But anemia may be absent, sometimes for many months, in a signifi cant number of patients who have not taken folate. In a retrospective study of 141 patients with neuropsychiatric abnormalities due to cobalamin deficiency, there were 19 patients in whom both the hematocrit and mean cell volume were normal (Lindenbaum et al). In such patients, subtle morphologic abnormalities—hypersegmented polymorphonuclear leukocytes, megaloblastosis in bone marrow smears—must be carefully sought. In these circumstances the most reliable diagnostic procedures are the measurement of the serum vitamin B_{12} level (the *Euglena gracilis* assay is the most reliable method), assays for serum antibodies to intrinsic factor, and the two-stage Schilling test. In rare instances, even these tests may be inconclusive, in which case the finding of high serum concentrations of cobalamin metabolites—methylmalonic acid and homocysteine—may be diagnostically useful (Lindenbaum et al).

The diagnosis of subacute combined degeneration demands the immediate administration of vitamin B_{12} and the continuation of treatment for the rest of the patient's lifetime. Initially the patient should be given 1000 μg of cyanocobalamin or hydroxycobalamin intramuscularly each day during hospitalization. Thereafter this dose is repeated weekly for a month, and then monthly for the remainder of the patient's life. Although most of this injected cobalamin is excreted, these patients must be flooded with the vitamin because the degree of repletion of cobalamin stores is a direct function of the dose.

The most important factor influencing the response to treatment is the duration of symptoms before treatment is begun; other factors such as age, sex, presence of arteriosclerosis and hypertension, and the degree of anemia are relatively unimportant. The greatest improvement occurs in those patients whose disturbance of gait has been less than 3 months in duration, and recovery may be complete if therapy is instituted within a few weeks after the onset of symptoms. In practically all instances at least partial improvement is effected, although in the long-standing cases often the best that can be accomplished is arrest of progression. All neurologic symptoms and signs may improve, mostly during the first 3 to 6 months of therapy, and then, at a slower tempo, during the ensuing year or even longer.

NEUROPATHY DUE TO DISORDERED PYRIDOXINE METABOLISM

A special type of nutritional neuropathy is encountered in tuberculous and hypertensive patients who are being given isonicotinic acid hydrazide (INH; isoniazid) and hydralazine, respectively.

The occurrence of a neuropathy due to INH was recognized in the early 1950s, soon after the introduction of this drug for the treatment of tuberculosis. The neuropathy was characterized by paresthesias and burning pain of the feet and legs, followed by weakness of these parts and loss of ankle reflexes. Rarely, with continued use of the drug, the hands were affected as well. The nature of INH-induced neuropathy was clarified by Biehl and Vilter. They found that the administration of isoniazid results in a marked excretion of pyridoxine, and that the administration of pyridoxine in conjunction with INH prevents the development of neuropathy. As a result of this simple expedient, very few examples of this disorder are now observed.

The same mechanism that is operative in INH-induced neuropathy is probably responsible for the neuropathy that complicates antihypertensive treatment with hydralazine (Apresoline). The latter drug is closely related to isoniazid and the clinical features of the neuropathy induced by these drugs are very much the same. Hydralazine causes the formation of pyridoxal-isoniazid complexes (hydrazones), thus making pyridoxal (the main form of vitamin B_6) unavailable to the tissues. Hydralazine-induced neuropathy responds favorably to discontinuation of the drug and the administration of pyridoxine.

Paradoxically, pyridoxine may cause a peripheral neuropathy, if it is consumed in large amounts for a prolonged period of time (Schaumburg et al; Albin et al). There is no weakness; the symptoms are purely sensory and can be quite disabling. Improvement is the rule when the drug is withdrawn. This disorder is probably due to the direct toxic effect of pyridoxine on dorsal root ganglion cells.

A predominantly sensory neuropathy has also been induced in humans by a deficiency of *pantothenic acid* (a constituent of coenzyme A), as reported by Bean et al. In some patients the administration of pantothenic acid reverses the painful dysesthesias of the ''burning foot'' syndrome.

In summary, polyneuropathy may be caused by a deficiency of at least four B vitamins—thiamine, pyridoxine, pantothenic acid, and vitamin B_{12}. There is no certain evidence that a deficiency of riboflavin or nicotinic acid causes lesions of the central or peripheral nervous system.

Despite the commonality of folic acid deficiency and its hematologic effects, its role in the pathogenesis of nervous system disease has not been established beyond doubt (see the review by Reynolds). The polyneuropathy that occasionally complicates the chronic administration of phenytoin has been attributed, on uncertain grounds, to folate deficiency. Botez and colleagues have described a group of 10 patients with motor-sensory polyneuropathy (four also had spinal cord disease), presumably due to intestinal malabsorption, all of whom improved over several months, while receiving large doses of folic acid. This experience is unique, however. The possible role of folate deficiency in the pathogenesis of spinal cord disease has been mentioned above, in relation to vitamin B_{12} deficiency.

Vitamin E Deficiency A rare neurologic disorder of childhood, consisting essentially of a spinocerebellar degeneration in association with a polyneuropathy and pigmentary retinopathy, has been related to a deficiency of vitamin E, consequent upon prolonged intestinal malabsorption (Muller et al; Satya-Murti et al). The same mechanism has been proposed to explain the neurologic disorders that sometimes complicate abetalipoproteinemia, fibrocystic disease, and extensive intestinal resections (Harding et al). Vitamin E deficiency has also been observed in young children with chronic cholestatic hepatobiliary disease. Ataxia, loss of tendon reflexes, ophthalmoparesis, proximal muscle weakness with elevated serum CK, and decreased sensation are the usual manifestations. These symptoms are referable to parts of the nervous system and musculature that are found to be diseased in animals deprived of vitamin E—degeneration of Clark's columns, spinocerebellar tracts, posterior columns, nuclei of Goll and Burdach, and sensory roots (Nelson et al). In affected children, neurologic function improves after the long-term correction of vitamin E deficiency.

One postulated mechanism of vitamin E deficiency is the peroxidation of membrane phospholipids rich in polyunsaturated fatty acids. Vitamin E serves as an antioxidant for free-radical scavenging of various toxic elements. Local differences in the vitamin E content of various parts of the nervous system and musculature may account for the localization of the lesions.

DISEASES OF THE NERVOUS SYSTEM OF PROBABLE NUTRITIONAL ORIGIN

The disorders comprising this category will be discussed only briefly because their nutritional etiology has not yet been proved. They are found mainly in alcoholics, but their relationship to alcohol is probably not fundamental, since each of them has been observed in nonalcoholic patients as well. The belief that these disorders are nutritional in origin is based on certain indirect evidence: (1) Usually a prolonged period of undernutrition, associated with a significant loss of weight, precedes the neurologic illness. In some of these cases the amount of alcohol consumed need not be large, but the dietary deprivation is always severe. (2) Examination, at the onset of the illness, frequently discloses physical evidence of undernutrition as well as the presence of neurologic disorders of known nutritional etiology. (3) Certain attributes of the neuropathologic changes, namely their symmetry and constancy of localization, are precisely the features that characterize neurologic disorders of known nutritional etiology.

"ALCOHOLIC" CEREBELLAR DEGENERATION

This term refers to a common and uniform type of cerebellar degeneration in alcoholics. This disorder is about twice as frequent as Wernicke disease, but unlike the latter, is considerably more frequent in men than in women. It is characterized clinically by a wide-based stance and gait, varying degrees of instability of the trunk, and ataxia of the legs, the arms being affected to a lesser extent and often not at all. Nystagmus and dysarthria are infrequent signs. In addition to an ataxic (intention) tremor, there may be a tremor of the fingers or hands resembling a parkinsonian tremor but appearing only when the limbs are placed in certain sustained postures. Mauritz et al have demonstrated that the instability of the trunk in these cases consists of a specific 3-Hz rhythmic swaying in the anteroposterior direction; by contrast patients with lesions of the cerebellar hemispheres show only slight postural instability without directional preponderance.

In most cases, the cerebellar syndrome evolves subacutely, over a period of several weeks or months, after which it remains unchanged for many years. In some instances, it evolves more rapidly or more slowly, but in these cases also the disease stabilizes eventually. Occasionally, the cerebellar disorder progresses in a saltatory manner, the symptoms worsening in relation to a severe infectious illness or an attack of delirium tremens.

The *pathologic changes* consist of a degeneration of all the neurocellular elements of the cerebellar cortex, but particularly of the Purkinje cells, and are restricted to the anterior and superior aspects of the vermis and, in advanced cases, to the anterior parts of the anterior lobes. The cerebellar atrophy is readily visualized by CT scan (Fig. 39-1).

Two particular forms of this syndrome have not been emphasized sufficiently. In one, an instability of station and gait are the main symptoms, individual movements of the limbs being unaffected; the pathologic changes in such cases are restricted to the anterior-superior portions of the vermis. A second type is acute and transient in nature; the cerebellar symptoms, except for their reversibility, are identical to the ones that characterize the chronic, fixed form of the disease. In this transient type, the derangement is only one of function (''biochemical lesion'') and has probably not progressed to the point of fixed structural changes.

These forms of cerebellar disease, and particularly the restricted and reversible varieties, cannot be distinguished from the cerebellar manifestations of Wernicke disease either on pathologic or on clinical grounds. As a general rule, the cerebellar lesions in Wernicke disease tend to be more abrupt in onset, less severe, and more likely to improve than those occurring apart from Wernicke disease—but these distinctions are hardly fundamental. The cerebellar lesions in Wernicke disease may be very severe, comparable to the most advanced instances of so-called alcoholic cerebellar degeneration.

It is our opinion that the cerebellar ataxia of Wernicke disease and that referred to as *alcoholic cerebellar degeneration* represent the same disease process, the former term being used when the cerebellar abnormalities are associated with ocular and mental signs, and the latter when the cerebellar syndrome occurs alone. Alcoholic cerebellar degeneration is in all likelihood due to nutritional deficiency and not to the toxic effects of alcohol or other causes, for reasons that have already been indicated. Insofar as the cerebellar ataxia may improve to some extent under the influence of thiamine alone (see above, under Wernicke disease) it is likely that a deficiency of this vitamin is responsible for the cerebellar lesion.

CENTRAL PONTINE MYELINOLYSIS

This unique lesion was long thought to be of alcoholic-nutritional origin, but is probably due neither to nutritional deficiency nor to the toxic effects of alcohol. Most likely central pontine myelinolysis is related in some way to a profound electrolytic disturbance, perhaps to the rapid correction of hyponatremia or to hyperosmolality. For this reason it is more appropriately considered with other acquired metabolic disorders of the nervous system (Chap. 40).

MARCHIAFAVA-BIGNAMI DISEASE (PRIMARY DEGENERATION OF THE CORPUS CALLOSUM)

In 1903, the Italian pathologists Marchiafava and Bignami described a unique alteration of the corpus callosum, in

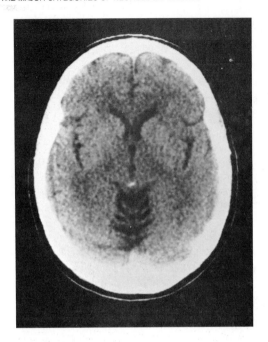

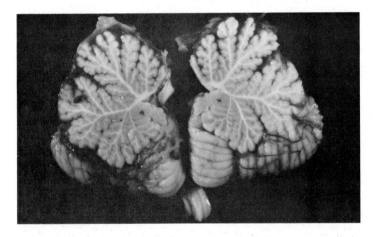

Figure 39-1

CT scan from a 60-year-old alcoholic showing prominence of midline cerebellar sulci. A broad-based gait and ataxia of the legs had been present for many years. Death was from myocardial infarction. The cerebellum, cut in the midsagittal plane (below), shows folial atrophy of the anterior-superior vermis, characteristic of alcoholic cerebellar degeneration.

three alcoholic patients. In each case, coronal sectioning of the fixed brain disclosed a pink-gray discoloration of the central portion of the corpus callosum, throughout the longitudinal extent of this structure. Microscopically, the lesion proved to be confined to the middle lamina (which makes up about two-thirds of the thickness of the corpus callosum), in which there was a loss of myelin with relative preservation of the axis cylinders; macrophages were abundant in the altered zone. The clinical observations in these patients were few and incomplete; in two of them, a chronic, ill-defined psychosis had been present and in all three, seizures and coma had occurred terminally. Bignami, in 1907, described a case in which the corpus callosum lesion was accompanied by a similar lesion in the central portion of the anterior commissure.

These early reports were followed by a spate of articles which confirmed and amplified the original clinical and pathologic findings. By 1931 about 40 cases of this disorder had been described in the Italian literature (Mingazzini). With one exception, all the reported cases were in males and all of them were insatiable drinkers. They drank red wine for the most part, but other forms of liquor also. Beginning with King and Meehan, in 1936, the disease has been described in patients native to France, Germany, Switzerland, England, and North and South America, and the notion that it has a special racial predisposition or geographic restriction has had to be abandoned.

Pathologic Features Marchiafava-Bignami disease is more readily defined by its pathologic than its clinical features. The principal alteration, as has repeatedly been emphasized, is in the middle portion of the corpus callosum, which on gross examination appears somewhat rarefied and sunken and reddish or gray-yellow in color, depending on its age. In the anterior portion of the corpus callosum, the lesion tends to be more severe in the midline than in its lateral parts but in the splenium, the opposite may pertain. The most chronic lesion takes the form of a centrally placed gray cleft or cavity, with collapse of the surrounding tissue and reduction in thickness of the corpus callosum. Microscopically, corresponding to the gross lesions, one observes clearly demarcated zones of demyelination, with relative sparing of the axis cylinders and an abundance of fatty macrophages. Inflammatory changes are absent.

Less consistently, lesions of a similar nature are found in the central portions of the anterior and posterior commissures and the brachia pontis. These zones of myelin destruction are always surrounded by a rim of intact white matter. The predilection of this disease process for commissural fiber systems has been stressed, but it certainly is not confined to these fibers. Symmetrically placed lesions have been observed in the columns of Goll, superior cerebellar peduncles, and cerebral hemispheres, involving the centrum semiovale and extending, in some cases, into the convolutional white matter. As a rule, the internal capsule and corona radiata, subcortical arcuate fibers, and cerebellum are spared. In several cases, the lesions of deficiency amblyopia (see above) have been observed and in others, the lesions of Wernicke disease.

Many of the reported cases of Marchiafava-Bignami disease, as first pointed out by Jequier and Wildi, have had cortical lesions of a special type: the neurons in the third layer of the frontal and temporal lobe cortices had disappeared and were replaced by a fibrous gliosis. Morel, who first described this *cortical laminar sclerosis*, did not observe an association with Marchiafava-Bignami disease. However, in subsequent reports, comprising 14 cases of cortical laminar sclerosis, the cortical lesion, which is easily seen, has consistently been associated with a corpus callosum lesion (see the review of Delay et al).

Clinical Features The disease affects persons in middle and late adult life. With few exceptions, all the patients have been males and severe chronic alcoholics. The clinical features of the illness are otherwise quite variable, and a clear-cut syndrome of uniform type has not emerged. Many patients have presented in a state of terminal stupor or coma, precluding a detailed neurologic assessment. In others, the clinical picture was dominated by the manifestations of chronic inebriation and alcohol withdrawal—tremor, seizures, hallucinosis, and delirium tremens. In some of these patients, following the subsidence of the withdrawal symptoms, no signs of neurologic disease could be elicited, even in the end stage of the disease which lasted for several days to weeks. In yet another group, a progressive dementia has been described, evolving slowly over a 3- to 6-year period before death. Emotional disorders leading to acts of violence, marked apathy, moral perversions, and sexual misdemeanors have been noted in these patients; dysarthria, slowing and unsteadiness of movement, transient sphincteric incontinence, hemiparesis, and apractic or aphasic disorders were superimposed. The last stage of the disease is characterized by physical decline, seizures, stupor, and coma. An impressive feature of these varied neurologic deficits has been their tendency toward remission.

In two cases that have come to our attention, the clinical manifestations were essentially those of bilateral frontal lobe disease: motor and mental slowness; apathy; prominent grasping and sucking reflexes; gegenhalten; incontinence; and a slow, hesitant, wide-based gait. In both of these cases, the neurologic abnormalities evolved over a period of about 2 months, and both patients recovered from these symptoms within a few weeks of hospitalization. Death occurred several years later as a result of liver disease and subdural hematoma, respectively. In each case, autopsy disclosed an old lesion typical of Marchiafava-Bignami disease, confined to the central portion of the corpus callosum.

In view of the great variability of the clinical picture, and the obscuration in many patients of subtle mental and neurologic abnormalities by the effects of chronic inebriation and other alcoholic neurologic disorders, the *diagnosis* of Marchiafava-Bignami disease is understandably difficult. In fact, the diagnosis is rarely made during life. The occurrence, in a chronic alcoholic, of a frontal lobe syndrome or a symptom complex that points to a diagnosis of frontal or corpus callosum tumor, but in whom the symptoms remit, should suggest the diagnosis of Marchiafava-Bignami disease. The CT scan and MRI have disclosed some unsuspected instances of this disease (Fig. 39-2; see also Kawamura et al).

Pathogenesis and Etiology   Originally, Marchiafava-Bignami disease was attributed to the toxic effects of alcohol, but this is an unlikely explanation in view of the prevalence of alcoholism and the rarity of corpus callosum degeneration. Further, the distinctive callosal lesions have not been observed with other neurotoxins. More importantly, undoubted examples of Marchiafava-Bignami disease have occurred in abstainers, so that alcohol cannot be an indis-pensable factor. A nutritional etiology has been invoked, for reasons given in the introduction to this section (see pages 836–837), but the deficient factor has not been defined. The mechanisms involved in the selective necrosis of particular areas of white matter remain to be elucidated. Enzymatic failure by virtue of vitamin deficiency, "edema damage," and a "vasocirculatory" defect have all been suggested, but these notions are purely speculative. Perhaps, when its mechanism becomes known, Marchiafava-Bignami disease, like central pontine myelinolysis (which it resem-bles histologically), will need to be considered in a chapter other than one on nutritional disease.

PROTEIN-CALORIE MALNUTRITION (PCM) AND MENTAL RETARDATION

The reader might gather from the foregoing descriptions that the nervous system is rarely affected by nutritional deficiency except when subjected to the influence of chronic alcoholism, and then the essential problem is an unbalanced diet with an inadequacy of B vitamins in the face of an adequate or near-adequate caloric intake. It is true that the CNS resists the effects of starvation better than other organs. Nonetheless there is increasing evidence that severe dietary deprivation during critical phases of brain development may result in permanent impairment of cerebral function and mental retardation. Inasmuch as there are an estimated 100 million children in the world who are undernourished and suffer from varying degrees of protein, calorie, and other dietary inadequacies, this is one of the most pressing problems in medicine and society.

Two overlapping syndromes have been defined in malnourished infants and children: kwashiorkor and mar-asmus. *Kwashiorkor* is a syndrome of weanling children due to protein deficiency and consisting of edema (and sometimes ascites), hair changes (sparsity and depigmen-tation), and stunting of growth. The edema is due to hypoalbuminemia, and there is in addition an abnormal pattern of blood amino acids as well as a fatty liver. Sometimes there are skin changes suggestive of pellagra or riboflavin deficiency. *Marasmus* consists of an extreme degree of cachexia and growth failure in early infancy. Infants with marasmus usually have been weaned early or were never breast-fed. Common to both groups of children is an apathy and indifference to the environment, combined with irritability when handled or moved. The children are underactive, and even after an adequate diet has been instituted, their tendency is to follow with the eyes rather than to move. At one stage of early convalescence some kwashiorkor children pass through a phase of rigidity and tremor for which there is no explanation.

As a rule, the clinical signs of polyneuropathy or subacute combined degeneration of the cord are lacking in

Figure 39-2

CT scan from a 43-year-old man with Wernicke disease. Although the ophthalmoparesis and disequilibrium improved rapidly under the influence of thiamine, he remained very apathetic, with prominent grasping and sucking reflexes, apraxias, and palilalia. The scan showed an area of de-creased attenuation between the anterior horns of the lateral ventricles, in the genu of the corpus callosum, suggesting a diagnosis of Marchiafava-Bignami disease. Also, the quad-rigeminal cistern is enlarged, suggesting atrophy of the superior vermis.

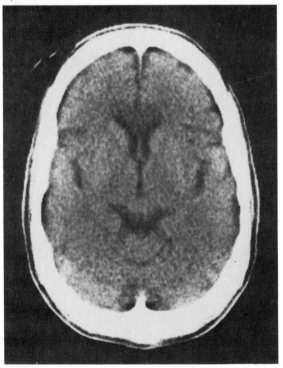

Table 39-2
Mechanisms whereby malabsorption may be related to neurological disease

Gastrointestinal defect	Substance malabsorbed	Associated neurological disorder
Localized gastric lesions:		
Pernicious anemia	Vitamin B_{12}	Myelopathy, neuropathy, etc.
Congenital lack of intrinsic factor	Vitamin B_{12}	Myelopathy, neuropathy, etc.
Partial gastrectomy	Vitamin B_{12}	Myelopathy, neuropathy, etc.
	Vitamin D	Osteomalacic myopathy
Localized lesions of small intestine:		
Predominantly proximal	? Water-soluble vitamins	? Hypovitaminosis B
	Vitamin D	? Osteomalacic myopathy
	Folic acid	Probably none
Predominantly distal	Vitamin B_{12}	Neuropathy, myelopathy, etc.
Bacterial contamination of small bowel (jejunal diverticulosis, blind-loop syndrome, strictures	Vitamin B_{12}	Neuropathy, myelopathy, etc.
Congenital absorptive defect	"Neutral" amino acids	Hartnup disease
	Tryptophan	"Blue diaper" syndrome
	Methionine	"Oast-house" urine disease
	Folic acid	Mental retardation, seizures, ataxia, choreoathetosis
	Vitamin B_{12}	Neuropathy, myelopathy
Transmucosal transport disorders associated with steatorrhoea:	Fat-soluble vitamins	Xerophthalmia
Endocrine causes		Keratomalacia
Postirradiation		? Osteomalacic myopathy
Drug-induced		
Defective synthesis of chylomicrons with prolonged intestinal malabsorption	Vitamin E (carrier lipoprotein not synthesized in liver)	Bassen-Kornzweig disease; spinocerebellar degeneration with polyneuropathy
Infiltration of villous cores	Fats (defective chylomicron release)	Encephalopathy of Whipple disease
Competition for essential nutrients (e.g. fish tapeworm)	Vitamin B_{12}	Neuropathy, myelopathy, etc.

Source: Pallis and Lewis.

children with PCM. However, electrophysiologic testing may disclose a reduction of motor nerve conduction velocity and abnormalities of sensory conduction (Chopra et al). And in children with severe degrees of PCM there may be evidence, in sural nerve biopsies, of retarded myelination (persistence of small myelinated fibers) and segmental demyelination.

Of great interest is whether the children who are rescued from these states of undernutrition by proper feeding are left with an underdeveloped or damaged brain. This subject has been studied extensively in many species of animals, as well as in humans, by clinical, biochemical, and neuropathologic methods. The literature is too large to review here, but excellent critiques have been provided by Winick, Birch et al, Latham, and Dodge et al.

In contrast to the devastating effect of PCM upon body growth, brain weight is only slightly reduced. Nevertheless, on the basis of experiments in dogs, pigs, and rats, it is evident that early (prenatal and early postnatal) malnutrition retards cellular proliferation in the brain. All cells are affected, including oligodendroglia, with a proportional reduction in myelin. Also, the process of dendritic branching may be retarded by early malnutrition. A limited number of studies in humans suggest that PCM has a similar effect upon the brain during the first 8 months of life. In animals, varying degrees of recovery from the effects of early malnutrition are possible if normal nutrition is reestablished during the vulnerable periods. Presumably this is true for humans as well, although it remains to be proved. In every series of severely undernourished infants and young children

Table 39-3
Vitamin-responsive inherited disorders affecting the nervous system

Vitamin	Disorder	Therapeutic dose	Enzymatic defect	Neurologic manifestations
Thiamine (B$_1$)	Branched-chain ketoaci-duria	5–20 mg	Branched-chain keto acid decarboxylase	Lethargy, coma
	Lactic acidosis	5–20 mg	Pyruvate carboxylase	Mental retardation
	Pyruvic acidemia	5–20 mg	Pyruvate dehydrogenase	Cerebellar ataxia
	Anemia	50 mg	—	Same as thiamine-deficient beriberi of infancy and childhood
Pyridoxine (B$_6$)	Homocystinuria	>25 mg	Cystathionine synthase	Mental retardation, cerebrovascular accidents, psychoses
	Infantile convulsions	10–50 mg	Glutamic acid decarboxylase	Seizures
	Xanthurenic aciduria	5–10 mg	Kynureninase	Mental retardation
Cobalamin (B$_{12}$)	Methylmalonic aciduria	1000 μg	Methylmalonyl CoA mutase apoenzyme	Lethargy, coma
	Methylmalonic aciduria and homocystinuria	> 500 μg	Defects in synthesis of adenosylcobalamin and methylcobalamin	Developmental arrest, cerebellar ataxia
Folic acid	Megaloblastic anemia	<0.05 mg	Intestinal malabsorption	Mental retardation
	Formiminotransferase deficiency	>5 mg	Formiminotransferase	Mental retardation
	Homocystinuria and hy-pomethioninemia	>10 mg	N^5, N^{10}-Methylene-tetrahydrofolate reductase	Schizophrenic syndrome
Biotin	β-Methylcrotonylglycin-uria	↑ 5–10 mg	β-Methylcrotonyl CoA carboxylase	Mental retardation
	Propionic acidemia	↑ 5–10 mg	Propionyl CoA carboxylase	Lethargy, coma
Nicotinamide	Hartnup disease	>400 mg	Intestinal malabsorption of tryptophan	Cerebellar ataxia

Source: Adapted from Rosenberg and from Matsui et al.

who have been observed for a period of many years, a variable proportion has been left mentally backward to a modest degree; the majority recover, however. Unfortunately, the neurologic and intellectual consequences of PCM have defied accurate assessment because of the difficulty of isolating the effects of malnutrition from those of infection, social deprivation, and other factors. The relative importance of these various factors is still under study.

NUTRITIONAL DEFICIENCIES SECONDARY TO DISEASES OF THE GASTROINTESTINAL TRACT

The vitamins that are known to be essential to the normal functioning of the central and peripheral nervous systems cannot be synthesized by the human organism. Each is ingested as an essential part of the normal diet and absorbed at certain points in the gastrointestinal tract. Impairment or failure of absorption due to diseases of the gastrointestinal tract gives rise to several malabsorption syndromes. In these diseases, the site of the block in transport from the intestinal lumen varies; it may be at the surface of the enterocytes or at their interface with the lymphatic channels and portal capillaries.

Table 39-2, which is modified from Pallis and Lewis, lists the malabsorptive diseases and their relationships to the intestinal abnormalities. From personal experience we have found the most frequent neurologic complication of intestinal malabsorption, e.g., sprue (idiopathic steatorrhea), to be a symmetrical sensorimotor polyneuropathy, similar to that of beriberi. Polyneuropathy and subacute combined degeneration of the cord, manifesting themselves many years after gastrectomy, are encountered only rarely.

An important effect of malabsorption is a deficiency of vitamin E, which in turn may give rise to neurologic symptoms, particularly in young children. This topic has been discussed in an earlier part of this chapter (page 836).

VITAMIN-RESPONSIVE NEUROLOGIC DISEASES

While humans lack the capacity to synthesize essential vitamin molecules, they are able nonetheless to use them in a series of complex chemical reactions involved in intestinal absorption, transport in the plasma, entry into the organelles of many organs, activation of the vitamin into coenzyme, and finally in their interaction with certain specific apoenzyme proteins. This compels consideration of another aspect of nutrition wherein one or more of these steps in vitamin utilization may be defective as a result of a genetic abnormality. Under these circumstances, the signs of vitamin deficiency result not from vitamin deficiency in the diet but from a genetically deranged control mechanism. In some instances the defect is only quantitative, and by loading the organism with a great excess of the vitamin in question, the biochemical abnormality can be overcome. Rosenberg has listed these hereditary vitamin-responsive diseases, which we have simplified for the reader who is interested in this subject (Table 39-3). The diseases of this category, being of hereditary type, have already been described in Chap. 38, "The Inherited Metabolic Diseases of the Nervous System."

REFERENCES

AGAMANOLIS DP, CHESTER EM, VICTOR M et al: Neuropathology of experimental vitamin B$_{12}$ deficiency in monkeys. *Neurology* 26:905, 1976.

AGAMANOLIS DP, VICTOR M, HARRIS JW et al: An ultrastructural study of subacute combined degeneration of the spinal cord in vitamin B$_{12}$ deficient rhesus monkeys. *J Neuropathol Exp Neurol* 37:273, 1978.

AGAMANOLIS DP, GREEN R, HARRIS JW: The neuropathology of cobalamin deficiency, in Dreosti IE, Smith RM (eds): *Trace Element Neurobiology and Deficiencies*, vol 1. Clifton, NJ, Humana Press, 1983, chap 9, pp 293–336.

ALBIN RL, ALBERS JW, GREENBERG HS et al: Acute sensory neuropathy-neuronopathy from pyridoxine overdosage. *Neurology* 37:1729, 1987.

ALEXANDER L, PIGOAN M, MYERSON A: Beriberi and scurvy. *Trans Am Neurol Assoc.* 64:135, 1938.

BEAN WB, HODGES RE, DAUM KE: Pantothenic acid deficiency induced in human subjects. *J Clin Invest* 34:1073, 1955.

BECK WS: Cobalamin and the nervous system. *N Engl J Med* 318:1752, 1988.

BIEHL JP, VILTER RW: The effect of isoniazid on vitamin B$_6$ metabolism and its possible significance in producing isoniazid neuritis. *Proc Soc Exper Biol Med* 85:389, 1954.

BIGNAMI A: Sulle alterazione del corpo calloso e della commissura anteriore ritrovate in un alcoolista. *Policlinico* (sez prat) 14:460, 1907.

BIRCH HG, PINEIRO C, ALCADE E et al: Relation of kwashiorkor in early childhood and intelligence at school age. *Pediatr Res* 5:579, 1971.

BIRCHFIELD RE: Postural hypotension in Wernicke's disease: A manifestation of autonomic nervous system involvement. *Am J Med* 36:404, 1964.

BLASS JP, GIBSON GE: Abnormality of a thiamine-requiring enzyme in patients with Wernicke-Korsakoff syndrome. *N Engl J Med* 297:1367, 1977.

BOMB BS, BEDI HK, BHATNAGAR LK: Post-ischaemic paresthesiae in pellagrins. *J Neurol Neurosurg Psychiatry* 40:265, 1977.

BOTEZ MI, PEYRONNARD JM, CHARRON L: Polyneuropathies responsive to folic acid therapy, in Botez MI, Reynolds EH (eds): *Folic Acid in Neurology, Psychiatry, and Internal Medicine.* New York, Raven Press, 1979, pp 401–412.

CARDINALE GJ, CARTY TJ, ABELES RH: Effect of methylmalonyl coenzyme A, a metabolite which accumulates in B$_{12}$ deficiency, on fatty acid synthesis. *J Biol Chem* 245:3771, 1970.

CARMEL R, WATKINS D, GOODMAN SI, ROSENBLATT DS: Hereditary defect of cobalamin metabolism (*cb1G* mutation) presenting as a neurologic disorder in adulthood. *N Engl J Med* 318:1738, 1988.

CARTON H, KAYENBE K, KABEYA et al: Epidemic spastic paraparesis in Bandundu (Zaire). *J Neurol Neurosurg Psychiatry* 49:620, 1986.

CHOPRA JS, DHAND UK, MEHTA S et al: Effect of protein calorie malnutrition on peripheral nerves. *Brain* 109:307, 1986.

CLAYTON PT, SMITH I, HARDING B et al: Subacute combined degeneration of the cord, dementia, and parkinsonism due to an inborn error of metabolism. *J Neurol Neurosurg Psychiatry* 49:920, 1986.

DELAY J, BRION S, ESCOUROLLE R, SANCHEZ A: Rapports entre la degenerescence du corps calleux de Marchiafava-Bignami et la sclerose laminaire corticale de Morel. *L'encephale* 49:281, 1959.

DODGE PR, PRENSKY AL, FEIGIN R: *Nutrition and the Developing Nervous System.* St Louis, Mosby, 1975.

DREYFUS PM, MONIZ R: The quantitative histochemical estimation of transketolase in the nervous system of the rat. *Biochim Biophys Acta* 65:181, 1962.

FISHER CM: Residual neuropathological changes in Canadians held prisoners of war by the Japanese. *Can Serv Med J* 11:157, 1955.

FOWDEN L, GARLON GA, MILLS CF: Metabolic and physiological consequences of trace element deficiencies in animals and man. *Physiol Trans Royal Soc London* 294:1, 1981.

GHEZ C: Vestibular paresis: A clinical feature of Wernicke's disease. *J Neurol Neurosurg Psychiatry* 32:134, 1969.

GOLDSMITH GA: Niacin-tryptophan relationships in man and niacin requirement. *Am J Clin Nutr* 6:479, 1958.

HARDING AE, MATHEWS S, JONES S, ELLIS CJK et al: Spinocerebellar degeneration associated with a selective defect of vitamin E absorption. *N Engl J Med* 313:32, 1985.

HAUW J-J, DE BAECQUE C, HAUSSER-HAUW C, SERDARU M: Chromatolysis in alcoholic encephalopathies: Pellagra-like changes in 22 cases. *Brain* 111:843, 1988.

JEQUIER M AND WILDI E: Le syndrome de Marchiafava-Bignami. *Schweiz Arch Neurol Psychiat* 77:393, 1956.

ISHII N, NISHIHARA Y: Pellagra among chronic alcoholics: Clinical and pathological study of 20 necropsy cases. *J Neurol Neurosurg Psychiatry* 44:209, 1981.

JOLLIFFE N, BOWMAN KM, ROSENBLUM LA, FEIN HD: Nicotinic acid deficiency encephalopathy. *JAMA* 114:307, 1940.

KAWAMURA M, SHIOTA J, YAGISHITA T, HIRAYAMA K: Marchiafava-Bignami disease: Computed tomographic scan and magnetic resonance imaging. *Ann Neurol* 18:103, 1985.

KING LS, MEEHAN MC: Primary degeneration of the corpus callosum (Marchiafava's disease). *Arch Neurol Psychiatry* 36:547, 1936.

KRUMHOLZ A, WEISS HD, GOLDSTEIN PJ, HARRIS KC: Evoked responses in vitamin B_{12} deficiency. *Ann Neurol* 9:407, 1981.

LATHAM MC: Protein-calorie malnutrition in children and its relation to psychological development and behavior. *Physiol Rev* 54:541, 1974.

LEVENTHAL CM, BARINGER JR, ARNASON BG et al: A case of Marchiafava-Bignami disease with clinical recovery. *Trans Am Neurol Assoc* 90:87, 1965.

LINDENBAUM J, HEALTON EB, SAVAGE DG et al: Neuropsychiatric disorders caused by cobalamin deficiency in the absence of anemia or macrocytosis. *N Engl J Med* 318:1720, 1988.

MAIR RG, CAPRA C, MCENTEE WJ, ENGEN T: Odor discrimination and memory in Korsakoff's psychosis. *J Exp Psychology* 6:445, 1980.

MANDEL H, BERANT M, HAZANI A, NAVEH Y: Thiamine-dependent beriberi in the ''thiamine-responsive anemia syndrome.'' *N Engl J Med* 311:836, 1984.

MARCHIAFAVA E, BIGNAMI A: Sopra un alterazione del corpo calloso osservata in soggetti alcoolisti. *Riv Patol Nerv* 8:544, 1903.

MATSUI SM, MAHONEY MJ, ROSENBERG LE: The natural history of inherited methylmalonic acidemias. *N Engl J Med* 308:857, 1983.

MAURITZ KH, DICHGANS J, HUFSCHMIDT A: Quantitative analysis of stance in late cortical cerebellar atrophy of the anterior lobe and other forms of cerebellar ataxia. *Brain* 102:461, 1979.

MCENTEE WJ, MAIR RG: Memory enhancement in Korsakoff's psychosis by clonidine: Further evidence for a noradrenergic deficit. *Ann Neurol* 7:466, 1980.

MCENTEE WJ, MAIR RG, LANGLAIS PJ: Neurochemical pathology in Korsakoff's psychosis: Implications for other cognitive disorders. *Neurology* 34:648, 1984.

MINGAZZINI G: *Der Balken*. Berlin, Springer, 1922.

MOREL F: Une forme anatamo-clinique particuliere de l'alcollisme chronique. Sclerose corticale laminaire alcoolique. *Rev Neurol* 71:280, 1939.

MULLER DPR, LLOYD JK, WOLFF OH: Vitamin E and neurological function. *Lancet* 1:225, 1983.

NELSON JS, FITCH CD, FISHER VW et al: Progressive neuropathologic lesions in vitamin E deficient rhesus monkey. *J Neuropathol Exp Neurol* 40:166, 1981.

OSUNTOKUN BO: Cassava diet, chronic cyanide intoxication and neuropathy in the Nigerian Africans. *World Rev Nutr Diet* 36:141, 1981.

PALLIS CA, LEWIS PD: *The Neurology of Gastrointestinal Disease*. Philadelphia, Saunders, 1974.

PINCUS JH: Folic acid deficiency. A cause of subacute combined system degeneration, in Botez MI, Reynolds EH (eds): *Folic Acid in Neurology, Psychiatry, and Internal Medicine*. New York, Raven Press, 1979, pp 427–433.

POTTS AM: Tobacco amblyopia. *Surv Ophthalmol* 17:313, 1973.

REYNOLDS EH: Folic acid, vitamin B_{12}, and the nervous system: Historical aspects, in Botez MI, Reynolds EH (eds): *Folic Acid in Neurology, Psychiatry and Internal Medicine*. New York, Raven Press, 1979, pp 1–5.

RONTHAL M, ADLER H: Motor nerve conduction velocity and the electromyograph in pellagra. *S Afr Med J* 43:642, 1969.

ROSENBERG LE: Vitamin-responsive inherited diseases affecting the nervous system, in Plum F (ed): *Brain Dysfunction in Metabolic Disorders*, vol 53. New York, Raven Press, 1974, pp 263–270.

SATYA-MURTI S, HOWARD L, KROHEL G, WOLF B: The spectrum of neurologic disorder from vitamin E deficiency. *Neurology* 36:917, 1986.

SERDARU M, HAUSSER-HAUW C, LAPLANE D, et al: The clinical spectrum of alcoholic pellagra encephalopathy. *Brain* 111:829, 1988.

SCHAUMBURG H, KAPLAN J, WINDEBANK A, et al: Sensory neuropathy from pyridoxine abuse. A new megavitamin syndrome. *N Engl J Med* 309:445, 1983.

SHAH DR, SINGH SV, JAIN IL: Neurological manifestations in pellagra. *J Assoc Phys India* 19:443, 1971.

SHATTUCK GC: Relation of beriberi to polyneuritis from other causes. *Am J Trop Med Hyg* 8:539, 1928.

SHIMOJYO S, SCHEINBERG P, REINMUTH OM: Cerebral blood flow and metabolism in the Wernicke-Korsakoff syndrome. *J Clin Invest* 46:849, 1967.

SPILLANE JD: *Nutritional Disorders of the Nervous System*. Baltimore, Williams & Wilkins, 1947.

SPIVAK JL, JACKSON DL: Pellagra: An analysis of 18 patients and a review of the literature. *Johns Hopkins Med J* 140:295, 1977.

STRACHAN H: On a form of multiple neuritis prevalent in the West Indies. *Practitioner* 59:477, 1897.

STRAUSS MB: Etiology of ''alcoholic'' polyneuritis. *Am J Med Sci* 189:378, 1935.

SYDENSTRICKER VP, SCHMIDT HL JR, FULTON MC et al: Treatment of pellagra with nicotinic acid: Observations in 45 cases. *South Med J* 31:1155, 1938.

TALLAND GA: *Deranged Memory*. New York, Academic Press, 1965.

TORVIK A, LINDBOE CF, ROGDE S: Brain lesions in alcoholics. *J Neurol Sci* 56:233, 1982.

TRONCOSO J, MANCALL EL, SCHATZ NJ: Visual evoked responses in pernicious anemia. *Arch Neurol* 36:168, 1979.

VICTOR M: Tobacco amblyopia, cyanide poisoning and vitamin B_{12} deficiency: A critique of current concepts, in Smith JL (ed): *Miami Neuroophthalmology Symposium,* vol 5. Hallandale, FL, Huffman, 1970, chap 3, pp 33–48.

VICTOR M: Polyneuropathy due to nutritional deficiency and alcoholism, in Dyck PJ, Thomas PK, Lambert EH, Bunge R (eds): *Peripheral Neuropathy,* 2nd ed. Philadelphia, Saunders, 1984, pp 1899–1940.

VICTOR M, ADAMS RD: Neuropathology of experimental vitamin B_6 deficiency in monkeys. *Am J Clin Nutr* 4:346, 1956.

VICTOR M, ADAMS RD: On the etiology of the alcoholic neurologic diseases: With special reference to the role of nutrition. *Am J Clin Nutr* 9:379, 1961.

VICTOR M, ADAMS RD, COLLINS GH: *The Wernicke-Korsakoff Syndrome: And Related Neurologic Disorders Due to Alcoholism and Malnutrition.* Philadelphia, Davis, 1989.

VICTOR M, ADAMS RD, MANCALL EL: A restricted form of cerebellar degeneration occurring in alcoholic patients. *Arch Neurol* 1:577, 1959.

VICTOR M, LAURENO R: Neurologic complications of alcohol abuse: Epidemiologic aspects, in Schoenberg BS (ed): *Advances in Neurology,* vol 19. New York, Raven Press, 1978, pp 603–617.

VICTOR M, MANCALL EL, DREYFUS PM: Deficiency amblyopia in the alcoholic patient: A clinicopathologic study. *Arch Ophthalmol* 64:1, 1960.

VICTOR M, YAKOVLEV PI: SS Korsakoff's psychic disorder in conjunction with peripheral neuritis: A translation of Korsakoff's original article with brief comments on the author and his contribution to clinical medicine. *Neurology* 5:394, 1955.

VILTER RW, MUELLER JF, GLAZER HS et al: The effect of vitamin B_6 deficiency induced by desoxypyridoxine in human beings. *J Lab Clin Med* 42:335, 1953.

WINICK M: *Malnutrition and Brain Development.* New York, Oxford University Press, 1976.

CHAPTER 40

THE ACQUIRED METABOLIC DISORDERS OF THE NERVOUS SYSTEM

An important segment of neurologic medicine, and one that is seen with great frequency in general hospitals, consists of a number of diverse disorders, in which a disturbance of cerebral function is consequent upon a failure in some other organ system—heart (and circulation), lungs (and respiration), kidneys, liver, pancreas, and the endocrine glands. Unlike the diseases that were considered in Chap. 38, in which a genetic abnormality affects many organs and tissues, including the brain, the cerebral disorders being discussed in this chapter are strictly secondary to derangements of the visceral organs themselves.

Relationships of this type, between a primary acquired disease of some thoracic or abdominal organ and the brain, have rather interesting implications. In the first place, recognition of the neurologic syndrome may guide one to the diagnosis of the visceral disease; indeed, the neurologic symptoms may be more informative and significant than the symptoms referable to the organ primarily involved. Then too, neurologists must have an understanding of the underlying medical disorder, for this may provide the means of controlling the neurologic part of the disease. In other words, the therapy for what appears to be a neurologic disease lies squarely in the field of internal medicine—a clear reason why every neurologist should be well trained in internal medicine. Lastly, and more of theoretical importance, the investigation of the acquired metabolic diseases promises new insights into the chemistry and pathology of the brain. To select a single example, the discovery of the episodic encephalopathy that is associated with portocaval shunt (Eck fistula) has opened a new and still unclear area in brain chemistry, pertaining to the effect of ammonium ions on glutamic acid and glutamine metabolism; and it has brought to light a curious histopathologic change—a relatively pure hyperplasia of protoplasmic astrocytes. Each visceral disease affects the brain in a somewhat different way, and since the pathogenic mechanism is not completely understood in any one of them, the study of these metabolic diseases promises rich rewards to the neurologic scientist.

In Table 40-1 the acquired metabolic diseases are classified according to their most common modes of clinical expression.

METABOLIC DISEASES PRESENTING AS A SYNDROME OF EPISODIC CONFUSION, STUPOR, OR COMA

The *syndrome of impaired consciousness,* its general features, the terms used in describing it, and the mechanisms involved in its genesis have been discussed in Chap. 16, which should be reread as an introduction to this section. There it was pointed out that metabolic disturbances are frequent causes of impaired consciousness, and that their presence has always to be considered when there are no focal or lateralizing signs of cerebral disease and the CSF is clear. Intoxication with alcohol and other drugs figures prominently in the differential diagnosis.

Laboratory examinations provide reliable clues to the cause(s) of the syndromes described below. In every patient who may fall into these categories, the following determinations should be made: serum Na, K, Ca, glucose, BUN, NH_3, pH, Pco_2, Po_2 (if there is evidence of hypoxia), and osmolality. Serum osmolality can be calculated from the values of Na, glucose, and BUN, using the following formula:

$$Osmolality = Na\,(1.86) + \frac{glucose}{18} + \frac{BUN}{2.8} + 9$$

EEG and measurements of evoked sensory, auditory, and visual potentials may be helpful in the assessment of different causes of impaired consciousness. If an exogenous toxin is suspected, a "toxin screen," using the newer methods of gas liquid or high performance chromatography, should be done. A point to be remembered is that the brain may suffer damage, even to an irreparable degree, by a disturbance of blood chemistry (e.g., hypoglycemia) that is no longer present when the patient is first seen.

HYPOXIC-HYPOTENSIVE ENCEPHALOPATHY

Here the basic disorder is a lack of oxygen to the brain, the result of failure of the heart and circulation or of the lungs and respiration. Often both are responsible and one cannot say which predominates, hence the ambiguous allusion in clinical records to "cardiorespiratory failure."

Hypoxic encephalopathy in various forms and degrees of severity is one of the most frequent and disastrous cerebral accidents encountered in the emergency and recovery rooms of every general hospital. The medical conditions that most often lead to it are (1) suffocation (from drowning, strangulation, aspiration of vomitus or blood, compression of the trachea by a surgical pack or hemorrhage or foreign body in the trachea); (2) carbon monoxide (CO) poisoning, in which respiration fails first and then the cardiovascular system (Fig. 40-1); (3) diseases that paralyze the respiratory apparatus (Guillain-Barré syndrome and poliomyelitis) or damage the CNS diffusely (trauma and vascular disease of the brain, certain encephalopathies of children, and epilepsy), again with respiratory failure being the initial factor, preceding cardiac failure; and (4) myocardial infarction or hemorrhage with shock and circulatory collapse; cardiac arrest during inhalation or spinal anesthesia; and infective and traumatic shock, in all of which cardiac action is paralyzed before respiration.

The terms *anoxic, anemic,* and *stagnant,* introduced by Barcroft to designate the various forms of anoxia, still appear in medical writings but have limited clinical value, since the ultimate effect of all three is the same, namely to deprive the brain and other organs of their critical oxygen supply. *Anoxic anoxia* implies a reduced arterial pressure

Table 40-1
Classification of the acquired metabolic disorders of the nervous system

I. Metabolic diseases presenting as a syndrome of episodic confusion, stupor, or coma
   A. Hypoxic-hypotensive encephalopathy
   B. Hypercapnia
   C. Hypoglycemia
   D. Hyperglycemia
   E. Hepatic failure and Eck fistula
   F. Reye syndrome
   G. Uremia
   H. Other metabolic encephalopathies: acidosis due to diabetes mellitus or renal failure (see also inherited forms of acidosis in Chap. 38); Addison disease; bismuth subgallate intoxication

II. Disturbances of sodium and potassium: changes in osmolality

III. Metabolic diseases presenting as a progressive extrapyramidal syndrome
   A. Acquired hepatocerebral degeneration
   B. Hyperbilirubinemia and kernicterus
   C. Hypoparathyroidism

IV. Metabolic diseases presenting as cerebellar ataxia
   A. Hypothyroidism
   B. Hyperthermia and hypothermia
   C. Hyperthyroidism

V. Metabolic diseases causing psychosis or dementia
   A. Cushing disease and steroid encephalopathy
   B. Thyroid psychoses
   C. Hyperparathyroidism
   D. Pancreatic encephalopathy (?)
   E. Whipple disease

Figure 40-1

Unenhanced CT scan of brain of a 30-year-old woman who attempted suicide by carbon monoxide inhalation. The only neurologic residua were a mild defect in retentive memory and areas of decreased attenuation in the pallidum bilaterally (arrows).

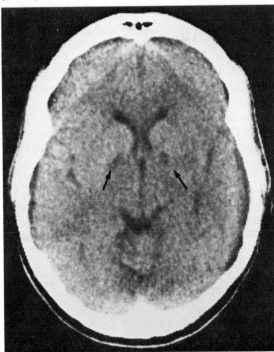

of oxygen, as might occur at high altitudes or with pulmonary disease, in which sufficient oxygen cannot cross the alveolar capillary membrane. In *anemic anoxia* there is insufficient hemoglobin to bind and transport the oxygen (CO poisoning, profound anemia). *Stagnant anoxia* is more appropriately designated *ischemic anoxia,* since circulatory failure, the underlying cause, never results in hypoxia alone; here the blood may contain sufficient oxygen, but cerebral blood flow (CBF) is insufficient to supply the cerebral tissues. Seldom is there a need to use the term *histotoxic anoxia,* which refers to chemical interference with the cellular utilization of oxygen, as occurs when cyanide blocks the cytochrome system.

Reduced to the simplest formulation, a deficient supply of oxygen to the brain is caused by a decrease in either the rate of blood flow (ischemia) or the content of arterial oxygen, secondary to a lowered oxygen saturation or a reduction in hemoglobin content.

Physiologic mechanisms of a homeostatic nature protect the brain under conditions of both ischemia and hypoxia. When the cerebral perfusion pressure is reduced, there is a compensatory dilatation of resistance vessels that maintains blood flow at a constant rate. When the perfusion pressure falls below 60 to 70 mmHg, increased oxygen extraction still allows normal energy metabolism to continue. When it falls below 40 mmHg, ischemic injury occurs within a few minutes in certain sites of predilection (border zones between major arteries of supply, parts of the hippocampus, and deep folia of cerebellum). This is explained by the fact that the brain is not a homogeneous organ; different parts have variable rates of metabolism (Sokoloff). Acidosis and hypercapnia are factors that interfere with constancy of blood flow. In total ischemia the tissue is depleted of its sources of energy in about 5 min, but longer periods are tolerated under conditions of barbiturate coma and hypothermia.

Energy failure due to hypoxia is counteracted by an increase in cerebral blood flow; at a Po_2 of 25 mmHg the increase is approximately 400 percent. A similar increase occurs with a decrease in hemoglobin to 20 percent or less, but here the decrease in viscosity facilitates the circulatory response.

In most of the clinical situations in which the brain is deprived of adequate oxygen there is a combination of ischemia and hypoxia (Seisjö et al). The pathophysiology of neuronal and tissue damage in cerebral and cerebellar cortices and pallidum under conditions of ischemia is discussed fully in Chap. 34 (page 622). Essentially, the *mechanism* in hypoxic-ischemic injury is an arrest of all aerobic metabolic processes necessary to sustain the Krebs (tricarboxylic acid) cycle and the electron-transport system. There is some evidence that synaptic transmission (neurotransmitters) fails before cell death occurs. The neurons, if completely deprived of their source of energy, proceed to catabolize themselves in an attempt to maintain their activity, and in so doing are damaged to a degree that does not permit their survival. The accumulation of catabolic products (particularly lactic acid) in the interstitial tissue contributes to the parenchymal damage.

There is also a phenomenon of delayed neurologic deterioration after anoxia that is not understood but may be due to the blockage or exhaustion of some enzymatic process during the period when brain metabolism is restored or even increased (as in hyperthermia or possibly with seizures or increased motor activity).

Clinical Features   Mild degrees of hypoxia induce only inattentiveness, poor judgment, and motor incoordination; there are no lasting effects. With severe hypoxia or anoxia, as occurs with cardiac arrest, consciousness is lost within seconds, but recovery will be complete if breathing, oxygenation of blood, and cardiac action are restored within 3 to 5 min. Beyond 5 min there is usually permanent injury. As shown by Ames and his colleagues, one of the reasons for the irreversibility of the lesion is swelling of the endothelium and blockage of circulation into the ischemic cerebral tissues (no-reflow phenomenon). Clinically, however, it is difficult to judge the precise degree of hypoxia since slight heart action or an imperceptible blood pressure may have served to maintain the circulation to some extent. Hence some individuals have made an excellent recovery after cerebral hypoxia that allegedly lasted 8 to 10 min or longer. Subnormal body temperatures, as might occur when the body is immersed in ice water, greatly prolong the tolerated period of hypoxia. *An important clinical rule is that degrees of hypoxia that at no time abolish consciousness rarely if ever cause permanent damage to the nervous system.* Also, generally speaking, anoxic patients who demonstrate intact brainstem function (as indicated by normal pupillary light and ciliospinal responses, intact doll's-head eye movements, and oculovestibular reflexes) have a good outlook for recovery of consciousness and perhaps all of their faculties. Conversely, absence of these reflex activities, particularly a fixity of the pupils to light, implies a hopeless outlook.

The most severe degrees of oxygen lack, most often caused by circulatory collapse (ischemic anoxia), are manifested by a state of complete unawareness and unresponsiveness with abolition of all brainstem reflexes. Natural respiration cannot be sustained; only the *cardiac action and blood pressure are maintained.* No electrical activity is seen in the EEG (it is isoelectric). This is the *brain death syndrome* (Chap. 16). When caused by hypoxia-hypotension it is always irreversible. At autopsy one finds that most if not all the cerebral, cerebellar, and brainstem tissues, and in some instances even the spinal cord, have been destroyed.

When the syndrome of brain death occurs, one must consider the advisability of discontinuing all supportive measures (respiratory aid, vasopressor agents, etc.). Such victims often become donors of vital organs. One must exercise extreme caution in concluding that the patient has irreversible brain damage, because anesthesia, drug intoxication, and hypothermia may also cause deep coma and an isoelectric EEG, but permit recovery. Such cases have been brought increasingly to public attention because of ethical and moral issues that surround the question of discontinuing medical therapy. In the authors' experience, the vital functions of patients with the brain death syndrome usually cannot be sustained for more than several days; in other words, the problem settles itself and is not nearly so difficult as the one described below.

Patients who have suffered severe but lesser degrees of hypoxia will have stabilized their breathing and heart action when first seen; yet they may be profoundly comatose, with eyes slightly divergent and motionless but with reactive pupils, the limbs inert and flaccid or intensely rigid, and the tendon reflexes diminished. Within a few minutes after cardiac action and breathing have been restored, generalized convulsions and also isolated or grouped twitches of muscles (myoclonus) may supervene. The seizures, if severe and recurrent, double or treble the oxygen need of the cerebral tissues, a deficiency that can only be corrected by neurogenic hypertension and metabolic cerebral vasodilatation (Plum and Posner). If the damage is severe, coma persists and decerebrate postures may be present or occur upon pinching the limbs, and bilateral Babinski signs can be evoked. In the first 24 to 48 h, death may terminate this state in a setting of rising temperature, deepening coma, and circulatory collapse. Tragically, however, the individual may survive for an indefinite period in a state that is variously referred to as *cortical death, irreversible coma, or persistent vegetative state* (see Chap. 16).

In this lesser degree of injury, the cerebral and cerebellar cortices are partly or completely destroyed, but brainstem-spinal structures survive. Some patients remain mute, unresponsive, and unaware of their environment for weeks, months, or years. Long survival is usually attended by some degree of improvement, but the patient appears to have lost all knowledge of the present situation, past memories, power of reasoning, capacity for meaningful social interaction and independent existence. One has only to observe such patients and their families to appreciate the gravity of the problem, the heartache, the waste of hospital facilities, and the tremendous expense of medical care. The only person who does not suffer is the patient. The medical

profession is searching for criteria that will accurately predict this hopeless state early in the comatose period, but the data are as yet insecure. If intoxication can be excluded, the presence of fixed dilated pupils and paralysis of eye movement for 24 to 48 h, along with absence of motor responses to painful stimuli and marked slowing of the EEG, usually signifies irreversible cerebral damage. We have not observed deep coma of this type, lasting 5 days or more, to be attended by full recovery. The question of what to do with such cases of protracted coma is a societal and not a medical problem. The most that can be expected of the neurologist is to state the level and degree of brain damage, its cause, and the prognosis. Of course one prudently avoids heroic, lifesaving therapeutic measures once the state is established.

With still lesser degrees of injury the patients improve after a period of coma. Consciousness is regained and then various degrees of confusion, visual agnosia, or any one of several types of abnormal movement (action or intention myoclonus, extrapyramidal rigidity, choreoathetosis) becomes manifest. Some of these patients quickly pass through this acute posthypoxic phase and proceed to make a full recovery; others are left with a permanent degree of disability. The permanent neurologic sequelae or *posthypoxic syndromes* that we have observed most frequently are (1) *persistent coma or stupor* and, with lesser degrees of cerebral injury, (2) dementia with or without extrapyramidal signs, (3) *visual agnosia*, (4) *extrapyramidal (parkinsonian) syndrome with mental enfeeblement*, (5) *choreoathetosis*, (6) *cerebellar ataxia*, (7) *intention or action myoclonus*, and (8) *a Korsakoff amnesic state. Seizures* may or may not continue to be a problem. These sequelae rarely occur in pure form; they overlap in various combinations although any one of them may predominate.

A relatively uncommon and unexplained phenomenon is *delayed postanoxic encephalopathy*. Initial improvement, which appears to be complete, is followed after a variable period of time (1 to 4 weeks in most instances) by a relapse, characterized by apathy, confusion, irritability, and occasionally by agitation or mania. Most patients recover from this second episode but some of them remain with serious mental and motor disturbances (Choi). In many cases there is progression of the neurologic syndrome, with weakness, shuffling gait, diffuse rigidity and spasticity, sphincteric incontinence, coma, and death after 1 to 2 weeks. Postmortem examination of these cases has shown the major abnormality to be a widespread cerebral demyelination. Exceptionally, there is yet another delayed syndrome in which an episode of hypoxia is followed by a slow, deteriorative state that progresses for weeks to months until the patient is mute, rigid, and helpless. In such cases the basal ganglia are affected more than the cerebral cortex and white matter (Dooling and Richardson). Some children affected in this way are found at autopsy to have a polio-encephalopathy, of the type described by Alpers (page 786).

Diagnosis depends on (1) the history of an hypoxic event and evidence of reduced oxygenation of arterial blood (in general, a P_{O_2} of less than 50 mmHg causes confusion and less than 25 mmHg, coma) or carbon monoxide intoxication (the latter is indicated by a cherry-red color of the skin or a characteristic spectroscopic band that lasts only a few minutes to hours after the episode), blood pressures below 70 systolic, or cardiac arrest; (2) the typical clinical sequence of events outlined above after a possible hypoxic episode has terminated. Renal damage (anuria) and myocardial ischemia may also have occurred, and provide corroborative evidence of hypoxia.

Treatment is directed mainly to the prevention of a critical degree of hypoxic injury. After a clear airway is secured, cardiopulmonary resuscitation, the use of a cardiac defibrillator or pacemaker, and open-chest surgery all have their place, and every second counts in their prompt utilization. Once cardiac and pulmonary function are restored, there is some evidence that reducing cerebral metabolic requirements by continuous hypothermia for 48 to 72 h and by barbiturate medication may prevent the delayed worsening referred to above. Oxygen may be of value during the first hours, but it is probably of little use after the blood becomes well-oxygenated. Dexamethasone intravenously in doses of 6 to 12 mg every 6 h helps combat brain (cellular?) swelling. Seizures should be controlled by the methods indicated in Chap. 15. If the seizures are severe, continuous, and unresponsive to drugs, controlled respiration and curare may need to be used. Often the seizures cease after a few days. If they persist, they are often myoclonic, in which case mephobarbital (Mebaral), in divided doses up to 500 mg/day, phenobarbital, 300 mg/day, clonazepam, 8 to 12 mg daily in divided doses, or 5-hydroxytryptophane, 100 to 400 mg daily, may be useful in their control. Keeping the patient at bed rest for 10 days, even if consciousness has been regained in 24 to 48 h, may help to prevent the delayed form of postanoxic encephalopathy.

In cases of carbon monoxide poisoning, the use of hyperbaric oxygen has been recommended as a means of restoring consciousness more rapidly and perhaps more completely than with normobaric oxygen (Myers et al). Certainly such treatment should be utilized if it is available.

HIGH-ALTITUDE SICKNESS

Acute mountain sickness is a particular form of cerebral hypoxia (anoxic anoxia) that occurs when a sea-level inhabitant is abruptly transported to a high altitude. Headache, anorexia, nausea and vomiting, weakness, and insomnia appear at altitudes above 8000 ft; even modest physical exertion causes dyspnea. At somewhat higher altitudes, cerebral edema may declare itself by ataxia, abnormal behavior, drowsiness, and hallucinations. At 16,000 ft, according to Griggs and Sutton, 50 percent of patients are found to have retinal hemorrhages, and it is suggested that they may also occur in the cerebral white matter. Mental impairment develops and may progress to coma. Hypoxemia is intensified during sleep, as ventilation diminishes. The most effective preventive measure is acclimatization by a 2- to 4-day stay at intermediate altitudes of 6000 to 8000 ft.

Chronic mountain sickness, sometimes called Monge disease, is observed in long-term inhabitants of high-altitude mountainous regions. Pulmonary hypertension, cor pulmonale, and secondary polycythemia are the main features. There is usually hypercarbia as well, with the expected mental dullness, slowness, fatigue, nocturnal headache, and sometimes papilledema (see below).

Sedatives, alcohol, and slightly elevated P_{CO_2} in the blood all reduce one's tolerance to high altitude. Dexamethasone and acetazolamide prevent and counteract mountain sickness to some extent.

HYPERCAPNIA (AND HYPOXIA) IN PULMONARY DISEASE (HYPERCARBIA)

Chronic emphysema, chronic fibrosing lung disease, and in some instances a seeming inadequacy of the respiratory centers lead to chronic respiratory acidosis, with an elevation of P_{CO_2} and a reduction in arterial P_{O_2}. Secondary polycythemia, cor pulmonale, and heart failure often accompany these diseases of the lungs, and pulmonary infection may be superimposed.

The clinical syndrome comprises *headache, papilledema, mental dullness, drowsiness, confusion, and coma, asterixis,* and a kind of *action tremor and coarse twitching* of muscles that are in a state of sustained contraction. The headache tends to be generalized or frontal or occipital in location, and intense, persistent, steady, and aching in type; nocturnal occurrence is a feature in some cases. The papilledema is bilateral, but may be slightly more in one eye than the other, and hemorrhages may encircle the choked disc. The visual acuity is undiminished and the visual fields are full. The tremor is best seen in the outstretched fingers and has all the characteristics of a fast-frequency, slightly arhythmic action tremor. It continues all through voluntary movement and increases slightly with effort, sometimes being misinterpreted as an intention tremor. In addition there is inability to maintain a fixed posture or a voluntary movement because of brief interruptions of muscle-action potentials (asterixis).

Intermittent drowsiness, indifference to the environment, inattentiveness, reduction of psychomotor activity, imperception of sequences of events, and forgetfulness constitute the more subtle manifestations of this syndrome and may prompt the family to seek medical help. Such symptoms may last only a few minutes or hours and one cannot count on their presence at the time of a particular examination.

In fully developed cases, the CSF is under increased pressure. Pco_2 may exceed 75 mmHg, and the O_2 saturation of arterial blood ranges from 85 percent to as low as 40 percent. The EEG reveals slow activity, in the delta or theta range, sometimes bilaterally synchronous. The mechanism of the cerebral disorder is said to be CO_2 narcosis, but all the biochemical details are not known. Normally the CSF is slightly acidic in comparison to the blood; the Pco_2 of CSF is about 10 mmHg higher than that of the blood. With respiratory acidosis the pH of the CSF falls (in the range of 7.15 to 7.25) and cerebral blood flow increases because of cerebral vasodilatation. However, the brain rapidly adapts to respiratory acidosis through the generation and secretion of bicarbonate by the choroid plexuses. Brain water also increases, mainly in the white matter. In animal models of hypercarbia, NH_3 is elevated, which may explain the similarity of the syndrome to that of hyperammonemia (Herrera and Kazemi).

Forced ventilation with an intermittent positive-pressure device, using room air or oxygen if hypoxia is severe, the treatment of heart failure with digitalis and diuretics, venesection to reduce the viscosity of the blood, and antibiotics to combat pulmonary infection have been the most effective therapeutic measures; often they result in a surprising degree of improvement that may be maintained for months or years. The danger of administering morphine, which depresses the respiratory center (now insensitive to CO_2), and the danger of oxygen inhalation, which removes the sole stimulus to the respiratory center, are now widely recognized; patients treated in this way have lapsed into coma and some have died.

Unlike pure hypoxic encephalopathy, prolonged coma due to hypercapnia is exceptional, and in our experience has not led to irreversible brain damage. Papilledema and jerky, intermittent lapses of posture (asterixis) are features of diagnostic import. The syndrome is apt to be mistaken for a brain tumor, confusional psychosis of other type, or a disease causing chorea or myoclonus. The latter must be distinguished from other metabolic diseases presenting as chronic extrapyramidal syndromes, as described later in this chapter.

HYPOGLYCEMIC ENCEPHALOPATHY

This condition is a relatively infrequent but important cause of confusion, convulsions, stupor, and coma, and it merits separate consideration as a metabolic disorder of the brain. The essential biochemical abnormality is a critical lowering of the blood glucose. At a level of about 30 mg/dL, the cerebral disorder takes the form of a confusional state, and one or more seizures may occur; at a level of 10 mg/dL, there is profound coma that may result in irreparable injury to the brain if not corrected by the administration of glucose.

The normal brain has a glucose reserve of 1 to 2 g (30 μmol per 100 g of tissue), mostly in the form of glycogen. Since glucose is utilized by the brain at a rate of 60 to 80 mg/min, the glucose reserve will sustain cerebral activity for only about 90 min, once blood glucose is no longer available. Glucose is transported from the blood to the brain by a carrier system. When glucose enters the brain, it either undergoes glycolysis or is stored as glycogen. Of the glucose taken up by the brain, 85 to 90 percent is oxidized; the remainder goes into an amino acid pool and is utilized in the formation of proteins and other substances (notably neurotransmitters, GABA in particular).

The brain is the only organ, besides the heart, that suffers severe functional and structural disorder under conditions of hypoglycemia. The pathophysiology of the cerebral disorder has not been fully elucidated (see Ferrendelli; also, Wilkinson and Prockop). It is known that hypoglycemia reduces O_2 uptake and increases cerebral blood flow. Blood NH_3 rises and glutamine and glutamate levels in the brain fall. The levels of several brain phospholipid fractions decrease when animals are given large doses of insulin. However, the suggestion that hypoglycemia results in a rapid depletion and inadequate production of high-energy phosphate compounds has not been corroborated; some other glucose-dependent biochemical process must be involved.

When blood glucose falls, the central nervous system may utilize nonglucose substrates to a variable extent for its metabolic needs, especially keto acids and intermediates of glucose metabolism, such as lactate, pyruvate, fructose, and other hexoses. In the neonatal brain, which has a higher glycogen reserve, keto acids account for a considerable proportion of cerebral energy requirements, and this also happens after prolonged starvation. Hypoglycemia also activates the adrenal glands and the autonomic nervous system to induce a corrective gluconeogenesis. However, in the face of severe and sustained hypoglycemia these nonglucose substrates are not adequate to preserve the structural integrity of cerebral neurons. If convulsions occur, they do so during a period of confusion; the convulsions have been attributed to an altered integrity of neuronal membranes, and, on a gradient, to an elevated NH_3 and depressed GABA and lactate levels (Wilkinson and Prockop).

Etiology The most common causes of hypoglycemic encephalopathy are (1) accidental or deliberate overdose of insulin or an oral diabetic agent, (2) islet cell, insulin-secreting tumor of the pancreas, (3) depletion of liver glycogen that occasionally follows a prolonged alcoholic debauch, starvation, or some form of acute liver disease such as acute nonicteric hepatoencephalopathy of childhood (Reye syndrome), (4) glycogen storage disease of infancy, and (5) an idiopathic state in the neonatal period. Moderate degrees of hypoglycemia ($\leq$49 mg/dL) may be observed with chronic renal insufficiency (Fischer et al). In the past, hypoglycemic encephalopathy was a rather frequent complication of "insulin shock" therapy for schizophrenia. In functional hyperinsulinism the hypoglycemia is rarely of sufficient severity or duration to damage the central nervous system.

Clinical Features As the level of blood glucose descends, to about 30 mg/dL, the initial symptoms appear—nervousness, hunger, flushed facies, sweating, headache, palpitation, trembling, and anxiety, and these gradually give way to confusion, drowsiness, and occasionally excitement or overactivity. Many of these early and mild symptoms relate to adrenal overactivity. In the next stage, forced sucking, grasping, motor restlessness, muscular spasms, and decerebrate rigidity occur, in that sequence. Myoclonic twitching and convulsions may develop in some patients, but are by no means the rule. Blood levels of approximately 10 mg/dL are associated with deep coma, dilatation of pupils, pale skin, shallow respiration, slow pulse, and hypotonicity of limb musculature—the so-called medullary phase of hypoglycemia. If glucose is administered before the medullary phase appears, the patient can be restored to normalcy, retracing the aforementioned steps in reverse order. However, once the medullary phase has been reached, and particularly if it persists for a time before the hypoglycemia is corrected by intravenous glucose or spontaneously, as a result of the gluconeogenic activities of the adrenal glands and liver, recovery is delayed for a period of days or weeks and may be incomplete.

The EEG is altered as the blood glucose falls, but the correlations are inexact. There is a decrease in the frequency of brain waves diffusely, in the theta or delta range. During recovery sharp waves may appear and coincide in some cases with seizures.

A large dose of insulin, which produces intense hypoglycemia, even of relatively brief duration (30 to 60 min), is more dangerous than a series of less severe hypoglycemic episodes from smaller doses of insulin, possibly because the former impairs or exhausts essential enzymes—a condition that cannot then be overcome by large quantities of glucose intravenously.

The major clinical differences between hypoglycemic and hypoxic encephalopathy lie in the setting and the mode of evolution of the neurologic disorder. The effects of hypoglycemia usually unfold more slowly, over a period of 30 to 60 min, rather than in a few seconds or minutes. The recovery phase and sequelae of the two conditions are quite similar. A severe and prolonged episode of hypoglycemia may result in permanent impairment of intellectual function as well as other neurologic residua, like the ones that follow severe anoxia. We have also observed states of protracted coma and relatively pure Korsakoff amnesia. However, one should not be hasty in *prognosis,* for slow improvement may continue for 1 to 2 years. *Recurrent hypoglycemia,* as with an islet cell tumor, may masquerade for some time as an episodic confusional psychosis or convulsive illness, and diagnosis then awaits the demonstration of low blood glucose or hyperinsulinism in association with the neurologic symptoms.

Lesser degrees and more chronic forms of low blood glucose may produce two other distinct but not mutually exclusive syndromes, according to Marks and Rose, who have written an authoritative monograph on the subject. One of these syndromes, termed *subacute hypoglycemia,* is characterized by drowsiness and lethargy, diminution in psychomotor activity, deterioration of social behavior, and confusion. Oral or intravenous glucose will immediately alleviate the symptoms. In the other syndrome, termed *chronic hypoglycemia,* there is a gradual deterioration of intellectual functions, raising the question of dementia; and in some reported instances tremor, chorea, rigidity, cerebellar ataxia, and rarely signs of lower motor neuron involvement (*hypoglycemic amyotrophy*) are added. The latter feature has not been seen by the authors, who can only refer the reader to the report by Tom and Richardson.

These subacute and chronic forms of hypoglycemia have been observed in conjunction with islet cell hypertrophy and islet cell tumors of the pancreas, carcinoma of the stomach, fibrous mesothelioma, carcinoma of the cecum, and hepatoma. Supposedly an insulin-like substance is elaborated by these nonpancreatic tumors.

Functional or reactive hypoglycemia is the most ambiguous of all syndromes related to low blood glucose. This condition may precede diabetes mellitus or accompany peptic ulcer. The rise of insulin in response to a carbohydrate meal is delayed, but then causes an excessive fall in blood glucose, to 30 to 40 mg/dL. The symptoms are malaise, fatigue, nervousness, headache, tremor, etc., which may be difficult to distinguish from anxious depression. This syndrome is proved by finding an excessive reaction to insulin, a low blood glucose during the symptomatic period, and a salutary response to oral glucose. Treatment, which consists of a high protein–low carbohydrate diet, should be reserved for patients whose symptom complex correlates with hypoglycemia as documented by a 5-h glucose tolerance test.

Pathologically, in all forms of hypoglycemic encephalopathy, the major damage is to the cerebral cortex. Cortical nerve cells degenerate and are replaced by microgliacytes and astrocytes. The distribution of lesions is similar though not identical to that in hypoxic encephalopathy. (It appears that the cerebellar cortex is less vulnerable to hypoglycemia than to hypoxia.)

Treatment of all forms of hypoglycemia obviously consists of correction of the hypoglycemia at the earliest possible moment. It is not known whether hypothermia or other measures will increase the safety period in hypoglycemia or alter the outcome.

HYPERGLYCEMIA

Two syndromes have been defined, mainly in diabetics: (1) hyperglycemia with ketoacidosis and (2) hyperosmolar nonketotic hyperglycemia.

In diabetic acidosis the familiar picture is one of dehydration, fatigue, weakness, headache, abdominal pain, stupor or coma, and Kussmaul type of breathing. Usually the condition has developed over a period of days in a known diabetic. Insulin has often been omitted. The blood glucose level is found to be more than 400 mg/dL, the pH of the blood is less than 7.20, the P_{CO_2} is 10 meq/L or less, and the bicarbonate is less than 10 meq/L. Ketone bodies and β-hydroxybutyric acid are elevated in the blood and urine, and there is a marked glycosuria. The prompt administration of insulin, correction of the acidosis by molar lactate, and repletion of body fluids restore cerebral function over a period of hours.

Of considerable interest is a small proportion of patients, such as those reported by Young and Bradley, in whom deepening coma and cerebral edema develop as the blood level of glucose falls. The basis of this condition, which is indicated by rising CSF pressure, is ascribed by Prockop to an accumulation of fructose and sorbitol in the brain. The latter substance is a polyol that is formed during hyperglycemia, crosses membranes slowly, and causes a shift of water into the brain and an intracellular edema. According to Fishman, the increased polyols in the brain in hyperglycemia are not present in sufficient concentration

to be important osmotically; they may have other metabolic effects related to the encephalopathy. Attempts at therapy by the administration of urea, mannitol, salt-poor albumin, and dexamethasone are usually unsuccessful though recoveries are reported.

In *hyperosmolar nonketotic hyperglycemia* the blood glucose is extremely high, over 1000 mg/dL, but ketoacidosis does not develop. The effects on the brain are like those of hypernatremia (see further on). Modern appreciation of the neurologic syndrome is generally credited to Wegierko, who published descriptions of it in 1956 and 1957. Most of the patients are elderly diabetics, but some were not previously known to have been diabetic. An infection, enteritis, pancreatitis, or drugs known to upset diabetic control (thiazides, prednisone, phenytoin) lead to severe polyuria, fatigue, confusion, stupor, and coma. If testable when first seen, seizures and focal signs such as a hemiparesis, a hemisensory defect, or a homonymous visual field defect suggest the possibility of a stroke. Osmolality is usually around 350 mosmol per kilogram of serum water. There is also hemoconcentration and prerenal azotemia. Many of the patients are in shock when first seen, and the mortality rate has been as high as 40 percent. Fluids should be replaced cautiously, using isotonic saline and probably parenteral potassium. Correction of the markedly elevated blood glucose requires relatively small amounts of insulin since these patients often do not have insulin resistance.

HEPATIC STUPOR AND COMA (HEPATIC OR PORTAL-SYSTEMIC ENCEPHALOPATHY)

Chronic hepatic insufficiency with portocaval shunting of blood is often punctuated by episodes of stupor, coma, and other neurologic symptoms—a state that is often referred to as hepatic stupor or coma. This state complicates all varieties of liver disease. Less widely known is the fact that a portal-systemic shunt or shunts (Eck fistula) may be attended by the same clinical picture, in which case the liver itself may be normal. Also, there are a number of hereditary hyperammonemic syndromes of childhood, outlined in Chap. 38, that may lead to episodic coma, with or without seizures. Reye syndrome, a special type of acute nonicteric hepatic encephalopathy of children, is also associated with very high levels of ammonia in the blood (see further on in this chapter).

Clinical Features The clinical picture of acute or subacute hepatic encephalopathy consists essentially of a derangement of consciousness, presenting first as mental confusion with increased or decreased psychomotor activity, followed by progressive drowsiness, stupor, and coma. The confusional state, before coma intervenes, is frequently combined with a characteristic intermittency of sustained muscle contraction, imparting an irregular "flapping" movement to the outstretched hands. The latter phenomenon, which was originally described in patients with hepatic stupor by Adams and Foley and called *asterixis* (from the Greek *sterein*, "to fasten" or "to support"), is now recognized as a sign of various metabolic encephalopathies. The EEG is a sensitive and reliable indicator of impending coma, becoming abnormal during the earliest phases of the disordered mental state. The usual EEG abnormality consists of paroxysms of bilaterally synchronous slow waves, in the delta range, which at first are interspersed with alpha activity and later, as the coma deepens, displace all normal activity. A small number of patients show only random high-voltage asynchronous slow waves. A variable, fluctuating rigidity of the trunk and limbs, grimacing, suck and grasp reflexes, exaggeration or asymmetry of tendon reflexes, Babinski signs, and focal or generalized seizures round out the clinical picture.

The foregoing syndrome of hepatic encephalopathy, or hepatic coma, evolves over a period of days to weeks and often terminates fatally. In other patients, the syndrome does not advance beyond the stage of mild mental dullness and confusion, with asterixis and EEG changes. This relatively mild form must be differentiated from other acute confusional psychoses and deliria. In yet other patients, a disorder of mood, personality, and intellect may be protracted over a period of many months or even years; these symptoms tend to fluctuate in severity or may be intermittent, but are still reversible if proper therapeutic measures are instituted. Finally there is a group of patients (many of whom have experienced repeated attacks of hepatic coma) in whom an irreversible mild dementia and a disorder of posture and movement (grimacing, tremor, dysarthria, ataxia of gait, choreoathetosis) gradually appear; the condition must then be distinguished from other dementing and extrapyramidal syndromes (see below).

The concentrations of blood ammonia NH_3, particularly if measured repeatedly in arterial blood samples, usually exceed 200 μg/dL, and the severity of the neurologic and EEG disorders is roughly parallel to the ammonium levels. With treatment, the fall in the NH_3 levels precedes clinical improvement. Once recovery occurs, an intolerance to ammonium can be demonstrated by an oral dose of 6.0 g NH_3Cl, which raises the blood NH_3 and sometimes produces mild symptoms. In a normal person, this dosage does not alter the blood NH_3 levels.

Neuropathologic Changes The striking finding in patients who die in a state of hepatic coma is a diffuse increase in the number and size of the protoplasmic astrocytes in the deep layers of the cerebral cortex, lenticular nuclei, thalamus, substantia nigra, cerebellar cortex, and red, dentate, and pontine nuclei, with little or no visible alteration in the nerve cells or other parenchymal elements. These abnormal glial cells are generally referred to as Alzheimer type II astrocytes, having been described originally by von Hösslin and Alzheimer, in 1912, in a patient with Westphal-Strümpell pseudosclerosis (familial hepatolenticular degeneration). Cavanagh has studied the development of these astrocytes in rats subjected to portacaval shunts. He observed swelling of the end feet, cytoplasmic vacuolation (distended sacs of rough endoplasmic reticulum), formation of folds in the basement membrane around capillaries, and diminution in glycogen. Under the electron microscope some degeneration in myelinated nerve fibers in the neuropil and increase in the cytoplasm of oligodendrocytes were also seen. The authors, in their chronic cases, found neuronal loss in the deep layers of the cerebral and cerebellar cortex and in the lenticular nuclei and a vacuolization of tissue (? astrocyte vacuolation) resembling the lesions of Wilson disease.

These astrocytic alterations occur to some degree in all patients who die of progressive liver failure, and the degree of this glial abnormality is roughly parallel to the intensity and duration of the neurologic disorder. The clinical and EEG features, as well as the astrocytic hyperplasia, though highly characteristic of hepatic coma, are not specific features of this metabolic disorder. Nevertheless, taken together in a setting of liver failure, these manifestations constitute a distinctive clinicopathologic entity.

Pathogenesis of Hepatic Encephalopathy The most plausible hypothesis relates hepatic coma to an abnormality of nitrogen metabolism, wherein ammonia (NH_3), which is formed in the bowel by the action of urease-containing organisms on dietary protein is carried to the liver in the portal circulation, but fails to be converted into urea, either because of hepatocellular disease or portal-systemic shunting of blood, or both. As a result, excess amounts of NH_3 reach the systemic circulation, where they interfere with cerebral metabolism in a way that is not yet fully understood (see reviews of Zieve and of Cooper and Plum). Bessman and Bessman originally proposed that the effect of hyperammonemia is to deplete the brain of α-ketoglutarate (by reductive amination of α-ketoglutarate to glutamate, and amidation of the latter to glutamine), leading eventually to a depletion of high-energy phosphate compounds and to a decrease in cerebral metabolism and oxygen utilization. This hypothesis became improbable, however when it was shown that the brain's oxygen and glucose utilization were normal during the first 24 h of coma (Maiolo et al). An alternate theory is that CNS function in cirrhotic patients is impaired by short-chain fatty acids (from the diet or from bacterial metabolism of carbohydrate). Another suggestion (Fischer and Baldessarini) is that biogenic amines (e.g., octopamine), which arise in the gut and bypass the liver, act as false neurotransmitters, displacing the putative transmitters norepinephrine and dopamine. However, it has been shown in rats that the intraventricular infusion of large amounts of octopamine, causing up to 90 percent reduction of brain dopamine and norepinephrine concentrations, fails to alter the animals' alertness and activity (Zieve and Olsen). Zieve has presented evidence that mercaptans (methanethiol, methionine), which are also generated in the gastrointestinal tract and removed by the liver, act in conjunction with NH_3 to produce hepatic encephalopathy.

Hypoxia, hypokalemia, metabolic alkalosis, electrolyte depletion, excessive diuresis, and the use of sedative-hypnotic drugs predispose the cirrhotic patient to hepatic encephalopathy. Excessive dietary intake of protein, gastrointestinal hemorrhage, and constipation are the most important precipitating events.

Despite the incompleteness of our understanding of the role of disordered ammonium metabolism in the genesis of hepatic coma, an awareness of this relationship has provided the few effective means of treating this disorder: restriction of dietary protein; mechanical cleansing of the colon; oral administration of neomycin or kanamycin, which suppresses the urease-producing organisms in the bowel; and the use of lactulose, an inert sugar that acidifies the colonic contents. Should these measures not control the protein intolerance, surgical exclusion of the bowel may be undertaken, but this operation carries a prohibitively high risk of mortality. The salutary effects of these therapeutic measures, the common attribute of which is the lowering of the blood NH_3, lend strong support to the theory of *ammonia intoxication.* Convincing evidence for this concept was first provided by Gabuzda and his colleagues who produced a state of hepatic encephalopathy in cirrhotic patients by giving them ammonium cation-exchange resins, various ammonium salts and a diet high in protein.

More recent methods of treatment, the practicality of which remains to be established, include the use of bromocriptine and of keto analogues of essential amino acids. Theoretically, the keto analogues should provide a nitrogen-free source of essential amino acids (Maddrey et al), and bromocriptine, a dopamine agonist, should enhance dopaminergic transmission. Morgan and her associates have described clinical improvement as well as an increase in cerebral blood flow and oxygen consumption in patients with chronic hepatic encephalopathy who were treated with bromocriptine.

In *acute hepatitis,* delirious, confusional, and comatose states also occur, but their mechanisms are still unknown. Blood NH_3 may be elevated, but usually not to a degree that would be expected to affect central nervous system function.

In children with chronic cholestatic liver disease, Rosenblum and his colleagues reported a progressive neurological syndrome, characterized by ataxia, diminished vibratory and position sense, and paresis of gaze. The lesions, consisting of a degeneration of the posterior columns and large myelinated fibers of the peripheral nerves, are similar to those of experimentally induced vitamin E deficiency—leading to the speculation that the neurologic disorder is the result of vitamin E malabsorption (see also page 836).

Reye Syndrome (Reye-Johnson Syndrome) As indicated above, this is a special type of nonicteric hepatic encephalopathy, occurring in children and adolescents, and characterized by acute brain swelling in association with fatty infiltration of the viscera, particularly of the liver. Although individual cases of this disorder had been described for many years, its recognition as a clinical-pathologic entity dates from 1963, when a large series was reported from Australia by Reye and his colleagues and from the United States by Johnson et al. The disorder is not uncommon and tends to occur in outbreaks (286 cases were reported to the Centers for Disease Control during a 4-month period in 1974). Outbreaks of Reye syndrome have been observed with influenza B virus and varicella infections, but the disease has been described in association with a wide variety of other viral infections (influenza A, echovirus, reovirus, rubella, rubeola, herpes simplex, Epstein-Barr virus), and the toxic effects of aspirin.

Most cases occur in childhood, boys and girls being equally affected, but rare instances have been observed in infants (Huttenlocher and Trauner) and in young adults. In most cases the encephalopathy is preceded for several days to a week by fever, symptoms of upper respiratory infection, and protracted vomiting. These are followed by the rapid evolution of stupor and coma, associated in many cases with focal and generalized seizures, signs of sympathetic overactivity (tachypnea, tachycardia, mydriasis), decorticate and decerebrate rigidity, and loss of pupillary, corneal, and vestibulo-ocular reflexes. In infants, respiratory distress, tachypnea, and apnea are the most prominent features. Initially there is a metabolic acidosis, followed by a respiratory alkalosis (rising arterial pH and falling P_{CO_2}). The CSF is usually under increased pressure and is acellular; glucose values may be low, reflecting the hypoglycemia. SGOT and blood ammonia levels are increased, sometimes to an extreme degree. The EEG is characterized by diffuse arrhythmic delta activity, progressing to electrocerebral silence in patients who fail to survive.

Lesser degrees of cerebral involvement are also observed from time to time. The authors have seen children who became acutely confused, frightened, or mute; the liver was not enlarged and only the high levels of SGOT and modest elevation of serum ammonia provided clues to the nature of the illness. Recovery was complete within a few days. Such cases usually are found among more severe cases during epidemics of influenza.

The major *pathologic findings* are cerebral edema, often with cerebellar herniation, and infiltration of hepatocytes with fine droplets of fat (mainly triglycerides); the renal tubules, myocardium, skeletal muscle, pancreas, and spleen are infiltrated to a lesser extent. There are no inflammatory lesions in the brain, liver, or other organs. The pathogenesis of this disorder remains obscure.

Prognosis and Treatment   In a series of children with blood ammonia levels greater than 500 μg/dL, treated during the years 1967 to 1974, Shaywitz et al reported a mortality of 60 percent. Once the child became comatose, death was almost inevitable. In recent years, early diagnosis (elevations of SGOT, prothrombin time, and serum NH_3) and initiation of treatment before the onset of coma has reduced the fatality rate to 5 to 10 percent. Treatment is aimed at correcting the metabolic abnormalities and reducing intracranial hypertension and consists of the following measures: temperature control with a cooling blanket; nasotracheal intubation and controlled ventilation, to maintain Pco_2 above 20 mmHg; intravenous glucose covered by insulin, to maintain blood glucose at 150 to 200 mg/dL; neomycin enemas; control of intracranial pressure by means of continual monitoring and the use of hypertonic solutions (see Chap. 30), maintaining serum osmolality below 320 mosmol and intracranial pressure below 200 mmH$_2$O; and the maintenance of fluid and electrolyte balance (Trauner). Upon recovery, cerebral function has been normal unless there was deep and prolonged coma. Of 40 children followed for over 4 years by Brunner et al there was a strong correlation between impaired psychologic function and the severity of neurologic dysfunction when treatment was instituted.

UREMIC ENCEPHALOPATHY

Episodic confusion and stupor and other neurologic symptoms may accompany any form of severe renal disease—acute or chronic. In addition, a number of neurologic

syndromes complicate chronic hemodialysis and kidney transplantation. Chronic polyneuropathy, the most common neurologic complication of renal failure, is discussed on page 1052.

The cerebral symptoms attributable to the uremic state (first described by Addison in 1832) are best discerned in normotensive individuals in whom renal failure develops rapidly. Toxic nitrogenous and other products accumulate in the blood, rising day by day to high levels. Apathy, fatigue, inattentiveness, and irritability are usually the initial symptoms; later, confusion, disturbances of sensory perception, hallucinations, and stupor supervene. Sometimes this takes the form of a toxic psychosis, with hallucinations, delusions, and catatonia (Marshall). Characteristically these symptoms fluctuate from day to day, or even from hour to hour. In some patients, especially in those who become anuric, these symptoms may come on rather abruptly and progress rapidly to a state of coma. In others, mild visual hallucinations and a disorder of attention may persist for several weeks in relatively pure form. The EEG becomes diffusely slow. The CSF pressure is normal and the protein is not elevated. In several reports a low-grade mononuclear pleocytosis is mentioned, but we have not confirmed this.

In acute renal failure, clouding of the sensorium is practically always associated with a variety of motor phenomena, which usually occur early in the course of the encephalopathy, sometimes when the patient is still mentally clear. The patient begins to twitch and jerk, and may convulse. The twitches involve parts of muscles, whole muscles, or limbs, are lightning quick, arrhythmic, asynchronous on the two sides of the body, and incessant during wakefulness and sleep. At various times the term fasciculation, arrhythmic tremor, myoclonus, chorea, asterixis, or convulsion is applicable to a particular involuntary movement. At other times the motor phenomena are difficult to classify. The authors prefer to speak of the condition as the *uremic twitch-convulsive syndrome.*

Because of the similarity of this syndrome to tetany, one is prompted to measure serum calcium and magnesium, and of course hypocalcemia and hypomagnesemia do occur in uremia. But often the values for these ions are normal, and the administration of calcium and magnesium salts has little effect. The resemblance of uremic encephalopathy to hepatic and other metabolic encephalopathies has been stressed by Raskin and Fishman, yet the authors are more impressed with differences than similarities. We have observed the twitch-convulsive syndrome in association with a variety of diseases such as widespread neoplasia, delirium tremens, diabetes with necrotizing pyelonephritis, and lupus erythematosus, in which the blood urea nitrogen was only modestly elevated, but always the factor of renal failure was ultimately discovered. Glaser and his colleagues produced a state of twitching and convulsions in rats by the injection of urea alone.

As the uremia worsens, the patient lapses into a quiet coma. Unless the accompanying metabolic acidosis is corrected, Kussmaul breathing appears and gives way, before death, to Cheyne-Stokes breathing.

Since uremia is so frequently associated with hypertension, a major problem arises in distinguishing the cerebral effects of uremia per se from those of severe hypertension. Volhard was the first to make this distinction; he introduced the term *pseudouremia* to designate the cerebral effects of malignant hypertension and to separate them from *true uremia*. The name *hypertensive encephalopathy*, by which pseudouremia is now generally known, was first used by Oppenheimer and Fishberg. The clinical picture of the latter disorder and its pathophysiology are discussed on page 676.

Opinions vary as to the cause of uremic encephalopathy and the twitch-convulsive syndrome. It would appear that every level of the central nervous system is affected from spinal cord to cerebrum. The authors have been unable to detect a lesion in the brain or spinal cord other than a mild hyperplasia of protoplasmic astrocytes in some cases, but this astrocytic alteration is never of the degree observed in hepatic encephalopathy. Cerebral edema is notably absent. In fact, CT scans and MRI regularly show an element of cerebral shrinkage (enlarged lateral ventricles and widened sulci) in chronic renal failure. Restoration of renal function completely corrects the neurologic syndrome, attesting to a functional disorder of subcellular type. Whether caused by the retention of organic acids, elevation of phosphate in CSF (claimed by Harrison et al), or by the action of other toxins, has never been settled.

In the *treatment* of uremic encephalopathy the nature of the renal disease assumes paramount importance, for if it is irreversible and progressive the prognosis is poor without dialysis or renal transplantation. Convulsions, which occur in about 35 percent of cases, often preterminally, respond to relatively low plasma concentrations of anticonvulsants, the reason being that serum albumin is depressed in uremia, reducing the amount of bound phenytoin and increasing the unbound, therapeutically active portion. Phenobarbital is also useful in the treatment of uremic convulsions, but care must be taken to avoid sedation. One must be cautious in prescribing drugs in the face of renal failure, for inordinately high, toxic blood levels may result. Examples are gentamicin (vestibular damage), kanamycin (cochlear damage), nitrofurantoin, isoniazid, and hydralazine (peripheral nerve damage).

The "Disequilibrium Syndrome" This term refers to a group of symptoms that may occur during and following hemodialysis or peritoneal dialysis. The symptoms include headaches, nausea, muscular cramps, nervous irritability,

agitation, drowsiness, and convulsions. The headache, which may be bilateral and throbbing or resemble common migraine, develops in approximately 70 percent of patients, while all the other symptoms are observed in 5 to 10 percent, usually in those undergoing rapid dialysis or in the early stages of a dialysis program. The symptoms tend to occur in the third or fourth hour of dialysis and last for several hours. Sometimes the symptoms appear 8 to 48 h after completing dialysis. Originally these symptoms were attributed to the rapid lowering of serum urea, leaving the brain with a higher concentration of urea than the serum, and resulting in a shift of water into the brain to equalize the osmotic gradient (*reverse urea syndrome*). Now the condition is attributed to a shift of water into the brain which is akin to water intoxication, and to the inappropriate secretion of antidiuretic hormone.

The symptoms of subdural hematoma, which occurs in 3.3 percent of patients undergoing dialysis, may be mistakenly attributed to the dysequilibrium syndrome.

Dialysis Encephalopathy (Dialysis Dementia) This is another subacutely progressive syndrome that complicates chronic hemodialysis. Characteristically the condition begins with a hesitant, stuttering dysarthria, dysphasia, and sometimes apraxia of speech, to which are added facial and then generalized myoclonus, focal and generalized seizures, personality and behavioral changes, and intellectual decline. The EEG is invariably abnormal, taking the form of paroxysmal and sometimes periodic sharp wave or polyspike and wave activity (up to 500 μV and lasting 1 to 20 s) intermixed with abundant theta and delta activity. The CSF is normal, except for increased protein in a few cases.

At first the myoclonus and speech disorders are intermittent, occurring during or immediately after dialysis and lasting for only a few hours, but gradually they become more persistent and eventually permanent. Once established, the syndrome usually is steadily progressive over a 1- to 15-month period (average survival of 6 months in the 42 cases analyzed by Lederman and Henry). However, there is some variability in the clinical picture. Some patients have a waxing and waning course and survive for several years; in others the symptoms are transient. We have observed two patients in whom a syndrome, indistinguishable from the one described above, occurred between 1 and 2 weeks after successful renal transplantation, at a time when they were not being dialyzed and were receiving only small doses of immunosuppressant drugs. Both these patients recovered spontaneously. Nadel and Wilson, and others, have observed a dramatic reversal of the clinical symptoms and EEG abnormalities in patients with dialysis encephalopathy who were given diazepam, suggesting that some of the symptoms and EEG changes in dialysis dementia represent a form of seizure disorder.

The neuropathologic changes are subtle and consist of a mild degree of microcavitation of the superficial layers of the cerebral cortex. Although the changes are diffuse, they have been found, in one study, to be more severe in the left (dominant) hemisphere than the right, and more severe in the left frontotemporal operculum than in the surrounding cortex (Winkelman). The disproportionate affection of the frontotemporal opercular cortex would explain the distinctive disorder of speech and language.

The current view of the pathogenesis of dialysis encephalopathy is that it represents a form of aluminum intoxication. Alfrey and his associates found that the cerebral gray matter of patients who died with dialysis encephalopathy contained a much greater amount of aluminum than tissue from dialysis patients without encephalopathy. The aluminum may be derived from the dialysate or from orally administered aluminum gels. Moreover, interrupting aluminum intake may reverse the symptoms of encephalopathy (Poisson et al, Rozas and Port). In recent years this disorder has practically disappeared, the result no doubt of the universal practice of purifying the water used in dialysis and the effective removal of aluminum from the dialysate. The subject has been reviewed by Parkinson et al.

Complications of Kidney Transplantation The risk in immunosuppressed persons of developing a primary lymphoma of the brain has already been mentioned (page 529). Systemic fungal infections are found at autopsy in about 45 percent of patients who have had renal transplants and long periods of immunosuppressive treatment, and in about one-third of these patients the CNS is involved. *Cryptococcus, Listeria, Aspergillus, Candida, Nocardia,* and *Histoplasma* are the usual organisms (page 581). Other CNS infections that have complicated transplantation are toxoplasmosis and cytomegalic inclusion disease.

In some nutritionally depleted uremic patients who are subjected to treatment that involves major shifts of plasma water and electrolytes, diseases unrelated to uremia may develop. In our necropsy material we have found examples of Wernicke-Korsakoff disease and central pontine myelinolysis. A bleeding diathesis may result in subdural or cerebral hemorrhage. Two of our patients developed a typical Guillain-Barré syndrome, from which they recovered.

Uremic Polyneuropathy Peripheral neuropathy, which is probably the most frequent neurologic complication of chronic renal failure, is discussed in Chap. 46 (page 1052).

OTHER METABOLIC ENCEPHALOPATHIES

Limitation of space permits only brief reference to other important metabolic disturbances that present as episodic confusion, stupor, or coma. *Metabolic acidosis* due to diabetes mellitus or renal failure produces a typical syndrome of drowsiness, stupor, and coma with dry skin and Kussmaul breathing (page 281). This happens when the pH of the CSF falls below 7.24. The CNS depression does not correlate with the concentration of ketones. Probably there are associated effects on neurotransmitters, consequent upon the increase in osmolality and intracellular calcium.

In infants and children acidosis may occur in the course of hyperammonemia, isovaleric acidemia, maple syrup urine disease, hyperglycinemia, etc. (Chap. 38). High-voltage, slow activity predominates in the EEG, and correction of the acidosis restores nervous function to normal, provided that coma has not persisted for too long a time and has not become complicated by hypoxia or hypotension. There is no recognizable neuropathologic change in uncomplicated acidotic coma.

Extreme degrees of *hyperosmolality* of the blood may develop in the course of diabetes mellitus (blood glucose greater than 400 mg) resulting in alterations of the state of consciousness, ranging from lethargy and stupor to deep coma. Delirium, muscle twitches or jerks, and seizures may occur. In some cases the movement disorder resembles chorea and myoclonic twitching, like that of uremia.

Encephalopathy due to *Addison disease* (adrenal insufficiency) may be attended by episodic confusion, stupor, or coma without special identifying features; its basis remains unclear. Hypotension and diminished cerebral circulation and hypoglycemia are the most readily recognized metabolic abnormalities, and measures that correct these conditions appear to have been beneficial in some instances.

Intoxication with bismuth gives rise to a stereotyped encephalopathy, which is considered in Chap. 42, with other intoxications due to heavy metals.

In children more than adults, cholera being an exception, extremely *severe diarrhea* may be attended by an encephalopathy. Irritability, weakness, headache, seizures, stupor, and coma may develop over a period of 2 to 3 days and carry a grave prognosis unless promptly relieved. Presumably this is a metabolic encephalopathy due to loss of fluids and electrolytes and can be corrected by their replacement. In the more protracted illness of *typhoid fever,* approximately half the patients are delirious and a small number will exhibit meningism and become comatose with twitching and seizures, or spasticity and hyperactive reflexes in the legs—all of which are transitory. In none of the infective diarrheas has there been a definite lesion in the brain at autopsy, and the nature of such encephalopathic disorders is poorly understood.

DISORDERS OF ELECTROLYTE AND FLUID BALANCE

Drowsiness, confusion, stupor, and coma, in conjunction with seizures and sometimes with other neurologic deficits, may have as their basis a more or less pure abnormality of electrolyte or water balance. Some of these, such as hypocalcemia, hypercalcemia, hypophosphatemia, and hypomagnesemia, are considered in other parts of the text. Hypo- and hypernatremia, hypo- and hyperkalemia, and changes in osmolality may have similar effects.

Among the many causes of *hyponatremia,* the *syndrome of inappropriate antidiuretic hormone secretion (SIADH)* is of special importance, since it commonly complicates neurologic diseases of many types—head trauma, bacterial meningitis and encephalitis, cerebral infarction and subarachnoid hemorrhage, neoplasm, and sometimes Gullain-Barre disease. The diagnosis of SIADH should be suspected in any critically ill neurologic or neurosurgical patient who excretes urine that is hypertonic relative to the plasma. As the hyponatremia develops there is a decrease in alertness, which progresses through stages of confusion to coma, often with convulsions ("acute toxic encephalopathy"). Lack of recognition of this state may allow the serum Na to fall to dangerously low levels, 100 meq/L or lower. One's first impulse is to administer NaCl intravenously, but this must be done cautiously, especially in sick children who have suffered a head injury or have been given hypotonic fluids postoperatively. Kliman recommends restriction of water intake to 500 mL per 24 h if the serum Na is less than 120 meq and to 1000 mL per 24 h, if less than 130 meq. Even when the Na reaches 130 meq the fluid intake should not exceed 1500 mL per 24 h. Hypertonic saline is rarely needed unless the patient has extremely low levels of Na or is comatose or convulsing. Then it is best to reduce blood volume with intravenous furosamide, beginning with a dose of 1 mg/kg and increasing the dosage until a diuresis is obtained. Small amounts of hypertonic saline (3%) with KCl are given to raise the serum Na and osmolality to safe levels. While the syndrome of SIADH is self-limiting, it may continue for weeks or months, depending on the type of brain disease.

Arieff has emphasized the hazards of *severe hyponatremia.* He has reported a series of 15 patients, all of them women, in whom severe hyponatremia followed elective surgery. About 48 h after recovering from anesthesia, the serum Na fell to an average level of 108 meq/ L; the urinary sodium was 68 mmol/L, and the osmolality was 501 mosmol/kg. At this time, generalized seizures occurred, followed by respiratory arrest, requiring intubation. Five patients died, but there were no diagnostic pathologic findings and no lesions of central pontine myelinolysis (see below). Seven patients, whose serum Na was corrected slowly, improved over a period of several days, but then developed a rapidly progressive diminution in alertness and increasing nausea, headache, and obtundation, followed by a recurrence of seizures and coma. These patients survived in a persistent vegetative state.

The entire sequence of events is difficult to interpret. The initial hyponatremia was probably the result of inappropriate secretion of antidiuretic hormone. What happened later could have been the consequence of immediate and delayed hypoxia.

Therapy with osmotic agents, when combined with fluid restriction to counteract brain swelling, will usually induce a mild to moderate degree of *hypernatremia* (150 to 155 meq/L), easily corrected by giving hypotonic solutions. Severe hypernatremic dehydration (Na > 155 meq/ L) is observed in diabetes insipidus, in nonketotic diabetic coma, or in the stuporous patient who is not receiving fluids. The latter condition is usually associated with a brain lesion that impairs consciousness, so that the patient is unaware of thirst. Exceptionally, in patients with chronic hydrocephalus, the thirst center is rendered inactive, and severe hypernatremia, stupor, and coma may follow. The brain volume is manifestly reduced in CT scans. Retraction of the cerebral cortex from the dura may rupture a bridging vein and cause a subdural hematoma.

The main clinical effect of hypokalemia (K, 2.0 meq/ L or less), is generalized muscular weakness (see Chap. 51); a confusional state may be added. Both conditions are readily corrected by adding 40 meq of K to each liter of intravenous fluid, at a rate of 100 mL/h. *Hyperkalemia* (above 7 meq/L) also may be manifested by generalized muscle weakness (Chap. 51), although the main effect is cardiac arrest.

It is to be noted that hyponatremia is usually accompanied by hypo-osmolality of the serum and hypernatremia by hyperosmolality. However, there is no absolute correlation between hypo- or hyperosmolality and neurologic dysfunction (Katzman and Pappius; Fishman). The rate of change is more important than the level. In hyponatremia-hypo-osmolality, Fishman finds an increase in intracellular water and a diminution in intracellular K—but the dehydration is critical and coincides with the neuronal derangement. In hypernatremia-hyperosmolality, the neurons do not lose water as much as do other cells, a compensatory reaction that Fishman attributes to the presence of idiogenic osmoles—probably glucose, glucose metabolites, and amino acids. The impairment of neuronal function in this state is not understood. Theoretically one would expect neuronal shrinkage and possibly alteration of the synaptic surface of the cell.

The degree of CNS disturbance is generally related to the rate at which the serum Na rises. Slowly rising values, to levels as high as 170 meq/L or even higher, are usually asymptomatic. Rapid rises shrink the brain and may cause subdural hematomas, especially in infants. Extremely high levels cause impairment of consciousness, asterixis, myoclonus, seizures, and choreiform movements. In addition, muscular weakness, rhabdomyolysis, and myoglobinuria have been reported.

In recent years, the correction of severe hyponatremia has come to be viewed from a new aspect—that of its relationship to central pontine myelinolysis (CPM) and related brainstem, cerebellar, and cerebral lesions (extrapontine myelinolysis). These disorders are described below.

CENTRAL PONTINE MYELINOLYSIS

In 1950, the authors observed a rapidly evolving quadriplegia and pseudobulbar palsy in a young alcoholic man who entered the hospital 10 days earlier with symptoms of alcohol withdrawal. Postmortem examination several weeks later disclosed a large, essentially demyelinative lesion occupying the central part of the basis pontis. Over the next 5 years, one of us (R.D.A.) had the opportunity to study three other cases pathologically, and in 1959 these four cases became the subject of a communication by Adams, Victor, and Mancall, titled *Central Pontine Myelinolysis*. The term was chosen because it denotes both the specific anatomic localization of the disease and its essential pathologic attribute: the remarkable unsystematic dissolution of the sheaths of medullated fibers. Once attention was focused on this distinctive lesion, many other reports appeared. The exact incidence of this disease is not known, but in a series of 3548 consecutive autopsies in adults, the typical lesion was found in nine cases, or 0.25 percent (see review of Wright et al).

Pathologic Features of Central Pontine Myelinolysis (CPM) One is compelled to define this disease in terms of its pathologic anatomy because the latter stands as its most certain feature. Transverse sectioning of the fixed brainstem discloses a grayish discoloration and fine granularity in the center of the basis pontis. The lesion may be only a few millimeters in diameter, or it may occupy almost the entire basis pontis. There is always a rim of intact myelin between the lesion and the surface of the pons. Posteriorly it may reach and involve the medial lemnisci and, in the most advanced cases, other tegmental structures as well. Very rarely the lesion encroaches on the midbrain, but inferiorly it has never been seen to extend as far as the medulla. Particularly extensive pontine lesions may be associated with identical myelinolytic foci symmetrically distributed in the thalamus, subthalamic nucleus, striatum, internal capsule, amygdaloid nuclei, lateral geniculate body, white matter of the cerebellar foliae, and deep layers of the cerebral cortex and subjacent white matter. We have studied one such case (Wright et al, 1979), and at that time were aware of 11 similar cases in the medical literature.

Microscopic examination discloses the fundamental abnormality—destruction of the medullated sheaths throughout the lesion with relative sparing of the axis cylinders and intactness of the nerve cells of the pontine nuclei. These changes always begin and are most severe in the geometric center of the lesion, where they may proceed to frank necrosis of tissue. Reactive phagocytes and glial cells are in evidence throughout the demyelinative focus, but no oligodendrocytes are seen. Signs of inflammation are conspicuously absent.

This constellation of pathologic findings provides easy differentiation of the lesion from infarction and the inflammatory demyelinations of multiple sclerosis and postinfectious encephalomyelitis. Microscopically, the lesion resembles that of Marchiafava-Bignami disease (Chap. 39), with which it is rarely associated. Wernicke disease is not infrequently associated with CPM, but the topography and character of the lesions bear no resemblance to the latter condition.

Clinical Features CPM occurs only sporadically, with no hint of a genetic factor. The two sexes are affected equally and do not fall into any one age period. Whereas the cases first reported had occurred in adults, there are now many reports of the disease in children, particularly in those with severe burns (McKee et al).

The outstanding clinical characteristic of CPM is its invariable association with some other serious, often lifethreatening disease. In more than half the cases it has appeared in the late stages of chronic alcoholism, often in association with Wernicke disease and polyneuropathy. The other medical conditions and diseases with which CPM has been conjoined are chronic renal failure and dialysis treatment; hepatic failure; advanced lymphoma, carcinoma, and cachexia from a variety of other causes; severe bacterial infections, dehydration, and electrolyte disturbances; acute hemorrhagic pancreatitis; and pellagra.

In the majority of cases of CPM there are no symptoms or signs that betray the pontine lesion, presumably because it is so small, extending only 2 to 3 mm on either side of the median raphe and involving only a few corticopontine or pontocerebellar fibers. In others, the presence of CPM is obscured by coma from a metabolic or other associated disease. In only a small proportion of cases, exemplified by the first patient whom we observed, can CPM be recognized during life. In this patient, a serious alcoholic with delirium tremens and pneumonia, there evolved, over a period of several days, a flaccid paralysis of all four limbs and an inability to chew, talk, or swallow. Pupillary reflexes, movements of the eyes and lids, corneal reflexes, and facial sensation were spared. In some instances, however, conjugate eye movements have been limited, and there may be nystagmus. With survival for several days, reflexes may return; in several patients, spasticity and extensor posturing of the limbs on painful stimulation have been reported. Mutism and paralysis with relative intactness of sensation and comprehension, i.e., the "locked-in syndrome," or pseudocoma, has been described.

To summarize, whenever a patient gravely ill with a general medical disease develops a quadriplegia, pseudobulbar palsy, and pseudocoma over a period of several days, one is justified in making a clinical diagnosis of CPM. However, from the available data this will be possible in less than a third of the cases in which the disease is demonstrated in postmortem material. The capacity of CT scanning and MRI to visualize the pontine lesion and of brainstem auditory evoked responses to disclose lesions that encroach upon the pontine tegmentum have increased the possibility of making a premortem diagnosis.

Variants of this syndrome are being encountered with increasing frequency. In two of our elderly patients, confusion and stupor without signs of corticospinal or pseudobulbar palsy recovered, and for many months they were left with a severe dysarthria and cerebellar ataxis. By CT and MRI, lesions were observed in the tegmentum of the brainstem and cerebellum. After 6 or more months their nervous functions were essentially normal; originally both had serum Na levels of 99 meq/L.

Brainstem infarction due to basilar artery occlusion may be a source of confusion to the clinician. Sudden onset or step-like progression of the clinical state and more extensive involvement of tegmental structures of the pons as well as midbrain and thalamus are the distinguishing characteristics of vertebral-basilar disease. Massive pontine demyelination in acute or chronic relapsing multiple sclerosis rarely produces a pure basis pontis syndrome. Other features of this disease provide the clues to correct diagnosis.

Etiology and Pathogenesis. Nutritional deficiency is a commonly invoked cause of CPM, because it is observed so frequently in chronic wasting diseases and particularly in malnourished alcoholics, often in association with Wernicke disease. Nevertheless there are cases in which it is difficult to incriminate a nutritional factor. In recent years, attention has been drawn to the possible role of hyponatremia in the genesis of CPM, and more particularly to the rapid correction of the serum sodium to normal or higher than normal levels. Severe hyponatremia ($\leqslant 130$ meq/L) has been present in all our patients and in all 15 patients in the series of Burcar et al. That a derangement of serum sodium is important in the pathogenesis of this disease has been demonstrated by Laureno. Dogs were made severely hyponatremic (100 to 115 meq/L) by repeated injections of vasopressin and intraperitoneal infusions of water. The hyponatremia and profound weakness were corrected by infusion of hypertonic (3%) saline, following which the dogs developed a rigid quadriparesis and showed, at autopsy, pontine and extrapontine lesions that were indistinguishable in their distribution and histologic features from those of the human disease. Hyponatremia alone or slowly corrected hyponatremia did not produce the disease.

These observations indicate that in addition to the adverse effects of hyponatremia itself (seizures, stupor and coma, respiratory arrest), the very rapid and vigorous correction of hyponatremia carries a risk of producing CPM. Therapeutic guidelines for the correction of hyponatremia are still being elaborated. Sterns and coworkers have suggested that the hyponatremia be corrected by no more than 12 mmol/L per day; others have suggested that rapid correction, in itself, is not dangerous, provided that the uppermost level of serum sodium does not exceed 126 mmol/L during the first 48 h of therapy (Ayus et al). More prospective studies are needed to determine the most appropriate therapeutic regimen.

Recently, McKee and colleagues have adduced evidence that extreme serum hyperosmolality, rather than the rapid correction or overcorrection of hyponatremia, is the important factor in the pathogenesis of CPM. They found the characteristic pontine and extrapontine lesions in 10 of 139 severely burned patients who were examined after death. Each of the "burn patients" with CPM had suffered a prolonged, nonterminal episode of severe hyperosmolality, which coincided temporally with the onset of the lesion, as judged by its histologic features. Hyponatremia was not present in any of the burn patients with CPM; moreover, no particular independent factor, such as hypernatremia, hyperglycemia, or azotemia correlated with the development of CPM.

To summarize, the cause and pathogenesis of central pontine myelinolysis are only beginning to be understood. All that one can say at the present time is that specific regions or zones of the brain, most often the center of the basis pontis, have a special susceptibility to some acute metabolic fault (? rapid correction or overcorrection of hyponatremia, ? hyperosmolality), analogous perhaps to the selective vulnerability of the corpus callosum and anterior commisure in Marchiafava-Bignami disease (Chap. 39).

METABOLIC DISEASES PRESENTING AS PROGRESSIVE EXTRAPYRAMIDAL SYNDROMES

These syndromes are usually of mixed type, i.e., they include a number of basal ganglionic and cerebellar symptoms in various combinations, and may emerge as part of an acquired chronic hepatocerebral degeneration or chronic hypoparathyroidism, or as a sequela of kernicterus, or of hypoxic or hypoglycemic encephalopathy. The basal ganglionic-cerebellar symptoms that result from severe *anoxia* and *hypoglycemia* have been described in the preceding section and in Chap. 4. *Kernicterus* is considered on page 994, with the special neurologic diseases of infancy and childhood, and calcification of the basal ganglia and cerebellum (chronic parathyroid deficiency) on page 806, with the inherited metabolic disorders as well as further on in this chapter. It must be realized, however, that acquired hypoparathyroidism may lead to calcification of the basal ganglia (see below under diseases presenting as cerebellar ataxia). We have observed choreiform movements in patients with severe hyperthyroidism, ascribed by Weiner and Klawans to a disturbance of dopamine metabolism. Jejunoileal bypass operations for obesity, in addition to causing a chronic arthropathy and vasculitic skin lesions, may give rise to an episodic confusion and cerebellar ataxia, associated with a D-lactic acidosis and abnormalities of pyruvate metabolism. Overfeeding and fasting are provocative factors (Dahlquist et al). The acquired form of hepatocerebral degeneration remains to be discussed here.

ACQUIRED (NON-WILSONIAN) HEPATOCEREBRAL DEGENERATION

Patients who survive an episode or several episodes of hepatic coma are sometimes left with residual neurologic abnormalities, such as tremor of the head or arms, asterixis, grimacing, choreic movements and twitching of the limbs, dysarthria, ataxia of gait, or impairment of intellectual function; and these symptoms may worsen with repeated attacks of stupor and coma. In other patients with chronic liver disease, permanent neurologic abnormalities become manifest in the absence of discrete episodes of hepatic coma. In either event, patients thus afflicted deteriorate neurologically over a period of years. Examination of the brain of such patients discloses foci of destruction of nerve cells and other parenchymal elements in addition to a widespread transformation of astrocytes, changes that are very much the same as those of Wilson disease.

Probably the first to describe this acquired type of hepatocerebral degeneration was van Woerkom (1914), whose report appeared only two years after Wilson's classic description of the familial form. Since then, there have been sporadic reports of the acquired disease. A full account of these as well as of our own extensive experience with this disorder is contained in the article by Victor, Adams, and Cole, listed in the references.

Clinical Features   The first symptom may be a tremor of the outstretched limbs, fleeting arrhythmic twitches of the face and limbs (resembling either myoclonus or chorea), or a mild unsteadiness of gait with action tremor. As the condition evolves over months or years a rather characteristic dysarthria, ataxia, wide-based, unsteady gait, and choreoathetosis, mainly of the face, neck, and shoulders, are joined in a common syndrome. Mental function is slowly altered, taking the form of a simple dementia with lack of concern and indifference to the illness. A coarse rhythmic tremor of the arms, appearing with certain sustained postures, mild corticospinal tract signs, and diffuse EEG abnormalities complete the clinical picture. Other less-frequent signs are muscular rigidity, grasp reflexes, tremor in repose, nystagmus, asterixis, and action or intention myoclonus. In essence, each of the neurologic abnormalities that characterizes chronic hepatocerebral degeneration may also be observed in patients with hepatic coma, the only difference being that the abnormalities are evanescent in the latter and irreversible in the former.

As a rule, all measurable hepatic functions are altered, but the neurologic disorder correlates best with an elevation of serum ammonia (usually greater than 200 µg/dL). Unlike Wilson disease, where the cirrhosis usually remains occult for a long time, there is no question about its presence in the acquired syndrome; jaundice, ascites, and esophageal varices are manifest in most of the acquired cases. Wilson disease, which enters into the differential diagnosis, is usually not difficult to differentiate on clinical grounds, although the distinction in some cases requires the critical evidence of familial occurrence, Kayser-Fleischer rings (never found in the acquired type), and certain biochemical determinations (serum ceruloplasmin and copper levels, urinary copper excretion—see page 802).

Pathologic Findings   The chronic cerebral symptoms, like the transient ones, may occur with all varieties of chronic liver disease. Portal-systemic shunts are always present. Occasionally the liver is normal and an Eck fistula has formed as a result of a thrombosis or surgical ligation of the portal vein.

The cerebral lesion is localized more regularly in the cortex than is the case in Wilson disease. In some specimens an irregular gray line of necrosis or gliosis can be observed throughout both hemispheres, with a predilection for the parietal and occipital regions, and the lenticular nuclei may appear shrunken and discolored. These lesions resemble hypoxic ones, but tend to spare the hippocampus, globus pallidus, and deep folia of the cerebellar cortex—the sites of predilection in anoxic encephalopathy. Microscopically, a widespread hyperplasia of protoplasmic astrocytes is visible in the deep layers of the cerebral cortex, in the cerebellar cortex, as well as in thalamic and lenticular nuclei and many other nuclear structures of the brainstem. In the necrotic lesions the medullated fibers and nerve cells are destroyed, with marginal fibrous gliosis; at the corticomedullary junction, in the striatum (particularly in the superior pole of the putamen), and in the cerebellar white matter, polymicrocavitation may be prominent. Protoplasmic astrocytic nuclei contain periodic acid–Schiff (PAS) positive glycogen granules. Nerve cells may appear swollen and chromatolyzed, taking the form, we believe, of the so-called Opalski cells. The similarity of the neuropathologic lesion in the familial (Wilson) and acquired forms of hepatocerebral disease suggests a common hepatogenesis.

Pathogenesis It is evident that a close relationship exists between the acute transient form of hepatic encephalopathy (hepatic coma) and the chronic, largely irreversible hepatocerebral syndrome. As stated above, the latter syndrome frequently develops on a background of repeated episodes of hepatic coma; in these patients it is often impossible to identify the point at which the reversible illness ends and the permanent one begins, so imperceptibly does one blend into the other. This intimate relationship is reflected in the pathologic findings as well; the astrocytic hyperplasia and PAS-positive inclusions are identical in both forms of the disease, and the distribution of the destructive lesions follows closely the distribution of the astrocytic change. Also, both disorders are characterized by hyperammonemia, episodic in one and persistent in the other. Reducing the serum ammonia by the measures that are effective in acute hepatic encephalopathy will cause a recession of many of the chronic neurologic abnormalities, not completely but to an extent that the patient is able to function better.

All these considerations allow one to theorize about the genesis of the acquired form of hepatocerebral degeneration and its relation to hepatic coma. As has been postulated above, episodic stupor or coma, reflected pathologically by a diffuse astrocytic hyperplasia, is a metabolic disorder secondary to the rapid accumulation of ammonia in the blood. A prolongation of this effect would lead to a chronic and largely irreversible neurologic syndrome based on parenchymal lesions. One may theorize further that the symptoms in both forms of the disease have their basis in a parenchymal lesion of similar mechanism, being transitory and invisible (at least by light microscopy) in one and permanent and microscopically evident in the other. Stated in another way, the damage to parenchymal elements might simply represent the most severe degree of a pathologic process that in its mildest form is reflected in an astrocytic hyperplasia alone.

KERNICTERUS

Kernicterus, formerly a common cause of congenital choreoathetosis, has now been virtually eliminated. It is discussed on page 994.

HYPOPARATHYROIDISM

This condition and pseudohypoparathyroidism (page 806) were mentioned in relation to the hereditary metabolic disorders. In the past, the usual cause of hypoparathyroidism was surgical removal of the parathyroid glands during subtotal thyroidectomy, although there were always idiopathic cases as well. With the more widespread use of radiation and drug therapy for thyroid disease, the surgical group has become small in proportion to the idiopathic one. The latter occurs in pure form, presumably as an agenesis of parathyroid glands with unmeasurable levels of parathormone in the blood, or as part of the DiGeorge syndrome of agenesis of thymus and parathyroids, organs embryologically derived from the third and fourth branchial clefts. Hypoparathyroidism is also part of a familial disorder in which there is a deficiency of thyroid, ovarian, and adrenal function, pernicious anemia, and other defects, based presumably on a derangement of autoimmune mechanisms. Other causes are intestinal malabsorption, pancreatic insufficiency, and vitamin D deficiency. In all instances the low levels of parathormone and normal responses to injected hormone permit the recognition of a primary defect of the parathyroid glands and distinguish it from all other conditions in which there is hypocalcemia and hyperphosphatemia.

The clinical manifestations, mainly attributable to the effects of hypocalcemia, are tetany, paresthesias, muscle cramps, laryngeal spasm, and convulsions. Children with this disease state may be irritable and show personality changes. In adults with chronic hypocalcemia, calcium deposits occur in the basal ganglia, dentate nuclei, and cerebellar cortex. In such patients we have observed unilateral tremor, a restless choreoathetotic hand, bilateral rigidity, slowness of movement and flexed posture resembling Parkinson syndrome, and ataxia of the limbs and gait—in various combinations. Interestingly, the multiple skeletal and developmental abnormalities that characterize both pseudo- and pseudo-pseudohypoparathyroidism (short stature, round face, short neck, stocky body build, shortening of metacarpal and metatarsal bones and phalanges from premature epiphyseal closure) are rarely seen in pure hypoparathyroidism.

A similar deposition of ferrocalc in the walls of small blood vessels of the lenticular and dentate nuclei and to a lesser extent in other parts of the brain is a common finding in normal older individuals. It also occurs in animals. Occasionally it reaches a degree of severity that destroys striatal or dentate neurons. In such cases, films of the skull and particularly CT scans will reveal the deposits. Cases of this type have been reported for years (page 806). The cause of the deposits is unknown. Apparently some protein in the capillary walls has an avidity for all mineral elements. Other diseases in which the basal ganglia calcify as part of an inherited metabolic disease are described on page 806.

METABOLIC DISEASES PRESENTING AS CEREBELLAR ATAXIA

CEREBELLAR ATAXIA ASSOCIATED WITH MYXEDEMA

The association of myxedema and cerebellar ataxia has been mentioned sporadically in medical writings since the latter part of the nineteenth century. Interest in this problem was revived in recent years by Jellinek and Kelly, who described six such cases. All of them showed an ataxia of gait; in addition, some degree of ataxia of the arms and dysarthria were present in four instances, and nystagmus in two. Cremer et al have reported a similar clinical experience, based on a study of 24 patients with either primary or secondary hypothyroidism.

There have been only a few reports of the pathologic changes, and these are far from satisfactory. The myxedematous patient described by Price and Netsky had also been a serious alcoholic, and the clinical signs (ataxia of gait and of the legs) and pathologic changes (loss of Purkinje cells and gliosis of the molecular layer, most pronounced

in the vermis) cannot be distinguished from those due to alcoholism and malnutrition. Scattered throughout the nervous system of their case were unusual glycogen-containing bodies, similar but not identical to corpora amylacea. These structures, designated *myxedema bodies* by Price and Netsky were also observed in the cerebellar white matter of a second case of myxedema; there were no other neuropathologic changes, however, and this patient had shown no ataxia during life.

It is difficult to know whether these peculiar bodies have anything to do with myxedema. If they do, it should be possible to demonstrate them in more than two cases. We have not seen them in one carefully studied case of myxedema, nor have they been described by others. Thyroid medication corrects the defect in motor coordination, raising doubt as to whether it could be based on a visible structural lesion.

The authors have had no experience with this condition, but wonder whether the attribution of the faulty gait and ataxia of movement to a cerebellar change might not be in error. Theoretically, the slowness of muscle relaxation (a characteristic of hypothyroidism) might interfere with the timing of muscle actions during a coordinated movement, thus simulating ataxia.

THE EFFECTS OF HYPERTHERMIA AND HYPOTHERMIA ON THE CEREBELLUM

The damaging effects of hyperthermia, like those of anoxia, involve the brain diffusely. In the case of hyperthermia, however, the changes are disproportionately severe in the cerebellum. The acute manifestations of profound hyperthermia are coma and convulsions, frequently complicated by shock and renal failure. Patients who survive the initial stage of the illness frequently show signs of widespread cerebral affection, such as confusion, dementia, and pseudobulbar and spastic paralysis. These abnormalities tend to resolve gradually, leaving the patient with a more or less pure disorder of cerebellar function.

The most extensive account of the pathologic effects of hyperthermia is that of Malamud and colleagues. These authors studied 125 fatal cases of heat stroke, but their observations are equally applicable to hyperthermia of other types. In patients who survived less than 24 h, the changes consisted mainly of a loss of some of the Purkinje cells and swelling, pyknosis, and disintegration of those that remained. In cases surviving longer, there was almost complete degeneration of the Purkinje cells, with gliosis throughout the cerebellar cortex, as well as degeneration of the dentate nuclei. The changes in the cerebellar cortex were equally pronounced in the hemispheres and vermis. It is of interest that we have not seen this syndrome in patients with malignant hyperthermia or the malignant neuroleptic syndrome—either the neuropathologic syndrome or a clinical cerebellar syndrome in survivors.

Hypothermia is much better tolerated than hyperthermia. Usually hypothermia is due to alcoholic or other forms of drug intoxication and exposure to cold, and rarely to hypoglycemia, adrenal insufficiency, hypothyroidism, phenothiazine intoxication, or diencephalic lesions, such as occur in Wernicke encephalopathy. Hypothermia in healthy persons may be due to cold water immersion and prolonged exposure. At core temperatures below 32°C the patient may appear clinically dead—unresponsive with dilated, fixed pupils, rigid extremities, and undetectable pulse and respiration. Rewarming is best done slowly, in an intensive care unit with complete monitoring. Recovery may be complete with correction of cardiac arrhythmias, dehydration, and lactic acidosis, the main complications of the hypothermic state.

METABOLIC DISEASE PRESENTING AS PSYCHOSIS AND DEMENTIA

The point has been made that milder forms of diseases that cause episodic stupor and coma, if persistent, may present as states of protracted confusion, impossible to distinguish from dementia. Chronic portal-systemic encephalopathy, the syndromes of chronic hypoglycemia, chronic hypercalcemia, and dialysis encephalopathy all fall within this category. Unlike the common types of dementia, described in Chap. 20, the acquired metabolic diseases are nearly always accompanied by a disorder of attentiveness, alertness, and vigilance; i.e., they cause a clouding of the sensorium and inaccurate perceptions and interpretations—attributes that usually allow a confusional state to be distinguished from a dementia. If the onset is rapid rather than gradual (over weeks and months) and if therapy reverses the condition, restoring full mental clarity, the conclusion is justified that one is dealing with a confusional state; but on strict clinical analysis at any one time in the active phase of the disease the distinction may be impossible.

In general hospitals, an episodic confusional state lasting days and weeks in the course of a medical illness or following an operation should always raise the suspicion of one of the aforementioned metabolic states. Usually, however, all of them can be excluded, and one falls back on a rather unsatisfactory interpretation—that a combination of drugs, fever, toxemia, and unspecifiable metabolic disorders is responsible.

In the *endocrine encephalopathies,* which are described below, the clinical phenomena are even more abstruse. Confusional states may be combined with agitation, hallucinations, delusions, anxiety, and depression, and the time span of the illness may be in terms of weeks

and months, rather than days. Certain aspects of the endocrine psychoses are discussed further on pages 1233 and 1234.

CUSHING DISEASE AND CORTICOSTEROID PSYCHOSES

Derangement of higher nervous function by the administration of ACTH or corticosteroid agents has become the prototype of all iatrogenic psychoses. The same symptoms have been reported in Cushing disease (page 542).

Our experience with this neurologic condition comes mainly from observations of patients receiving ACTH or prednisone for a variety of neurologic and medical diseases. At low dose levels there is usually no psychic effect other than a sense of well being and decreased fatigability. At higher dose levels (80 units per day of ACTH and 60 to 100 mg/day of prednisone) approximately 10 to 15 percent of patients become overly active, emotionally labile, and unable to sleep. Unless the dose is promptly reduced, there follows a progressive shift in mood, usually toward euphoria and hypomania—but sometimes toward depression, and then inattentiveness, distractibility, and mild confusion. The EEG becomes less well-modulated and slower frequencies begin to appear. Frank hallucinations and delusions are expressed by a minority of patients, giving the illness a truly psychotic stamp, and raising suspicions of schizophrenia or manic-depressive disease. In nearly all instances, however, this mixture of confusion and mood change in association with disordered cognitive function distinguishes the iatrogenic corticosteroid psychosis. Withdrawal of medication relieves the symptoms, but full recovery may take several days to a few weeks. Later, as with all confusional states and deliria, the patient's recollection of events during the illness is fragmentary.

The neurologic basis of this condition is poorly understood. The ascription of it to premorbid personality traits or a disposition to psychiatric illness is plausible, but lacks convincing documentation. Part of the difficulty is the lack of knowledge of the role of these endocrine agents in normal cerebral metabolism. We have no information as to how they act to reduce the volume of the edematous cerebral tissue around a tumor or the volume of the tumor itself. Critical studies of cellular or subcellular metabolism and morphologic changes are lacking. "Cerebral atrophy" (ventricular enlargement) has been shown radiologically in patients with Cushing disease and after a prolonged period (years) of corticosteroid therapy, but its basis also is unexplained (Momose et al). In some cases treatment has led to reversal of symptoms and reduction in ventricular size, documented by repeated CT scans.

THYROID ENCEPHALOPATHIES: THYROTOXIC AND MYXEDEMATOUS PSYCHOSES AND CRETINISM

Hyperthyroidism The neurology of thyrotoxicosis has proved to be particularly elusive. Allusions to psychosis are widely recorded in the medical literature and some thyrotoxic patients have been observed with mental confusion, seizures, manic or depressive attacks, and delusions. Tremor is almost universal and chorea occurs occasionally in various combinations with muscular weakness and atrophy, periodic paralysis, and myasthenia. In descriptions of the chorea it is often not clear whether chorea or myoclonus was observed. A myoclonic twitch has a duration of 15 to 50 msec and chorea, 200 to 300 msec. Treatment of the hyperthyroidism gradually restores the mental state to normal, leaving one with no explanation of what had happened to the CNS.

Hypothyroidism The myxedematous patient as a rule is slow to react, and psychomotor activity is reduced; but only in exceptional cases have we noted a significant change in cerebral function. When we have observed such a change, drowsiness, inattentiveness, and apathy have predominated. In two personally observed cases the somnolence was so extreme that the patients could not stay awake long enough to be fed or examined. They were in a state of hypothermic stupor, but exhibited no other neurologic abnormality. The extreme somnolence can be reversed within a few weeks by thyroid medication.

Hypothyroidism is associated with a number of distinctive myopathic disburbances, which are discussed in Chap. 51. The ataxia and peripheral neuropathy that are sometimes observed in patients with myxedema are described in this chapter (above) and Chap. 46, respectively.

Cretinism This form of severe hypothyroidism, occurring during intrauterine life (hypothyroidism in mother and fetus) or postnatally as an hereditary or acquired thyroid disease, is one of the correctable forms of metabolic cerebral disease. Although frequent in goitrous regions in which there is a lack of iodine, there are also a number of genetically determined defects in thyroxin synthesis that have come to light in recent years (Scriver et al). The thyroid gland in sporadic cretinism is either absent or represented by cysts, indicating a failure of development or a destructive lesion.

As a rule, the symptoms and signs of congenital thyroid deficiency are not recognizable at birth, but only become apparent after a few weeks; and more often the diagnosis is first made between the sixth and twelfth months of life. Physiologic jaundice tends to be severe and prolonged (up to 3 months), and this, along with widening of the posterior fontanelle and mottling of the skin, should raise suspicion of the disease. In typical cases the face is pale and puffy; the skin dry; the hair coarse, scanty, and dry; the eyelids thickened; the heavy lips parted by the enlarged tongue; the forehead low; and the base of the nose broad. There are fat pads above the clavicles and in the axillae. The abdomen is protuberant, often with an umbilical hernia, and the head is small—a physical appearance that prompted William Boyd to remark: "What was intended to be created in the image of God has turned out to be the pariah of nature, all for the want of a little thyroid."

In the latter part of the first year, *stunting of growth and delay in psychomotor development* become evident. Untreated, the child is severely retarded but placid and good natured; such children sleep contentedly for longer periods than normal children. Sitting, standing, and walking are delayed. Movements are slow, and if tendon reflexes can be obtained, their relaxation time is clearly delayed. The body temperature is low, and the extremities are cold and cyanotic. Although the head is small, the fontanelles may not close until the sixth or seventh year, and there is delayed ossification. If the hypothyroidism in the mother was present in the first trimester of pregnancy, cochlear development is imperfect, and there is *congenital deafness*. The gait is slow and the movements are stiff and awkward, manifestations of a *spastic paraparesis*.

The electrocardiogram is of low voltage; the EEG is slower than normal with less alpha activity; the CSF contains an excess of protein (50 to 150 mg/dL) and the serum T_3 and T_4, protein-bound iodine, and radioactive iodine uptake are all subnormal. Serum cholesterol is increased (300 to 600 mg/dL).

At autopsy the brain, though small, is normally formed. A reduction in number of nerve cells was described by Marinesco, especially in the fifth cortical layer, but others have not confirmed this finding. The use of Golgi and other silver techniques has shown decreased interneuronal distances (packing density increased as in the immature cortex) and a deficiency of neuropil. The latter change is due to a poverty of dendritic branchings and crossings, and presumably there is a decrease of the synaptic surfaces of cells (Eayrs). Thyroid hormone appears to be essential, not for neuronal formation and migration, but for dendritic-axonic development and organization.

If the condition is recognized early and treated consistently with potent thyroid hormones, statural and mental development can be stimulated to normal or near-normal levels. Extent of recovery depends on the severity of the hypothyroidism, its duration before treatment was begun, and the adequacy of therapy. In most patients, some degree of mental backwardness persists throughout life.

Hyperparathyroidism We have not been much impressed with the effects of this endocrine disorder upon the nervous system. The neuromuscular effects are the most definite, and consist of weakness and reversible electrophysiologic disturbances of nerve and muscle (see page 1135). When serum calcium levels reach 15 mg/dL or higher, the patient sinks into a quiet state of inattentiveness, drowsiness, lethargy, and confusion. Stupor, coma, and death may be caused by extreme degrees of hypercalcemia such as occur occasionally in cases of excessive vitamin D administration and metastatic carcinoma of bone.

PANCREATIC ENCEPHALOPATHY

This term was introduced by Rothermich and Von Haam in 1941 to describe a relatively uniform clinical state observed in patients with acute abdominal symptoms referable to pancreatic disease. As to the latter, there is usually a sudden development of midabdominal pain (on a background of biliary tract disease or alcoholism), associated with vomiting, upper abdominal tenderness, and rigidity. An elevation of serum amylase occurs later and may last for a few days. The encephalopathy consists of an agitated, confused state, sometimes with hallucinations and clouding of consciousness, dysarthria, and changing rigidity of the limbs—all of which fluctuate over a period of hours or days. Coma and quadriplegia have been reported. At autopsy, a variety of lesions have been described; two cases have had central pontine myelinolysis, and others have had small foci of necrosis and edema, petechial hemorrhages, and "demyelination" scattered through the cerebrum, brainstem, and cerebellum. These have been uncritically attributed to the action of released lipases and proteolases from the action of pancreatic enzymes (see review of this subject by Sharf and Levy).

The status of this entity, in the authors' opinion, is uncertain. Pallis and Lewis also express reservations and suggest that before such a diagnosis can be seriously entertained in a patient with acute pancreatitis, one should exclude delirium tremens, cerebral circulatory insufficiency from shock, renal failure, hypoglycemia, diabetic acidosis, hyperosmolality syndrome, hypokalemia, and hypocalcemia or hypercalcemia—any one of which may complicate the underlying disease(s).

WHIPPLE DISEASE

This is a rare disorder, predominantly of middle-aged men; even more rarely, it is associated with a number of neurologic syndromes. Weight loss, fever, anemia, steatorrhea, abdominal pain and distension, arthralgias, lymphadenopathy, and hyperpigmentation are the usual systemic manifestations. Biopsy of the jejunal mucosa, which discloses macrophages filled with PAS-positive material, is diagnostic. PAS-positive histiocytes have also been identified in the CNS, either in periventricular, hypothalamic, and tuberal foci, or diffusely scattered in the brain. Electron microscopic examination of involved tissue demonstrates distinctive bacilliform bodies ("Whipple's bacilli"), but serologic definition and culture of these so-called bacilli have never been accomplished. The neurologic manifestations most often take the form of a slowly progressive memory loss or dementia, like that of Alzheimer disease; hypersomnia, supranuclear ophthalmoplegia, ataxia, and myoclonus have been noted less often (Schochet and Lampert, Adams et al).

REFERENCES

ADAMS RD, FOLEY JM: The neurological disorder associated with liver disease. *Res Publ Assoc Res Nerv Ment Dis* 32:198, 1953.

ADAMS M, RHYNER PA, DAY J et al: Whipple's disease confined to the central nervous system. *Ann Neurol* 21:104, 1987.

ALFREY AC, LEGENDRE GR, KAEHNY WD: The dialysis encephalopathy syndrome: Possible aluminum intoxication. *N Engl J Med* 294:184, 1976.

AMES A, WRIGHT RL, KOWADA M et al: Cerebral ischemia. II: The no-reflow phenomenon. *Am J Pathol* 52:437, 1968.

ARIEFF AI: Hyponatremia, convulsions, respiratory arrest, and permanent brain damage after elective surgery in healthy women. *N Engl J Med* 314:1529, 1986.

AYUS JC, KROTHAPALLI RK, ARIEFF AI: Treatment of symptomatic hyponatremia and its relation to brain damage. A prospective study. *N Engl J Med* 317:1190, 1987.

BARCROFT R: *The Respiratory Function of the Blood.* London, Cambridge, 1925.

BESSMAN SP, BESSMAN AN: The cerebral and peripheral uptake of ammonia in liver disease with an hypothesis for the mechanism of hepatic coma. *J Clin Invest* 34:622, 1955.

BRUNNER RL, O'GRADY DJ, PARTIN, JC et al: Neuropsychologic consequences of Reye syndrome. *J Pediatr* 95:706, 1979.

BURCAR PJ, NORENBERG MD, YARNELL PR: Hyponatremia and central pontine myelinosis. *Neurology* 27:223, 1977.

CAVANAGH JB: Liver bypass and the glia, in Plum F (ed): *Brain Dysfunction in Metabolic Disorders,* vol 53. New York, Raven Press, 1974, pp 13–38.

CHOI IS: Delayed neurologic sequelae in carbon monoxide intoxication. *Arch Neurol* 40:433, 1983.

CLAYTON PT, SMITH L, HARDING B et al: Subacute combined degeneration of the cord, dementia and parkinsonism due to an inborn error of metabolism. *J. Neurol Neurosurg Psychiatry* 49:920, 1986.

CREMER GM, GOLDSTINE NP, PARIS J: Myxedema and ataxia. *Neurology* 19:37, 1969.

COOPER AJL, PLUM F: Biochemistry and physiology of brain ammonia. *Physiol Rev* 67:440, 1987.

DAHLQUIST NR, PERRAULT J, CALLAWAY CW: D-Lactic acidosis and encephalopathy after jejunoileostomy: response to overfeeding and to fasting in humans. *Mayo Clin Proc* 59:141, 1984.

DEVIVO DC, KEATING JP: Reye's syndrome. *Adv Pediatr* 22:175, 1976.

DOOLING EC, RICHARDSON EP JR: Delayed encephalopathy after strangling. *Arch Neurol* 33:196, 1976.

EAYRS JT: Influence of the thyroid on the central nervous system. *Br Med Bull* 16:122, 1960.

FERRENDELLI JA: Cerebral utilization of nonglucose substrates and their effect on hypoglycemia, in Plum F (ed): *Brain Dysfunction in Metabolic Disorders*, vol 53. New York, Raven Press, 1974, pp 113–120.

FISHER KF, LEES JA, NEWMAN JH: Hypoglycemia in hospitalized patients. *N Engl J Med* 315:1245, 1986.

FISCHER JE, BALDESSARINI RJ: Pathogenesis and therapy of hepatic coma, in Popper H, Schaffner F (eds): *Progress in Liver Disease*. New York, Grune & Stratton, 1976, chap 23, pp 363–397.

FISHMAN RA: Cell volume, pumps and neurologic function: Brain's adaptation to osmotic stress, in Plum F (ed): *Brain Dysfunction in Metabolic Disorders*, vol 53. New York, Raven Press, 1974, pp 159–171.

FISHMAN RA: *Cerebrospinal Fluid in Diseases of the Nervous System*. Philadelphia, Saunders, 1980, p 95.

GABUZDA GJ, PHILLIPS GB, DAVIDSON CS: Reversible toxic manifestations in patients with cirrhosis of the liver given cation exchange resins. *N Engl J Med* 246:124, 1952.

GLASER GH: Brain dysfunction in uremia, in Plum F (ed): *Brain Dysfunction in Metabolic Disorders*, vol 53. New York, Raven Press, 1974, pp 173–201.

GRIGGS RC, SUTTON JR: Neurologic manifestations of respiratory diseases, in Asbury AK, McKhann GM, McDonald WI (eds): *Diseases of the Nervous System*. Philadelphia, Saunders, chap 120, 1986.

HARRISON TR, MASON MF, RESNICK H: Observations on the mechanism of muscular twitchings in uremia. *J Clin Invest* 15:463, 1936.

HERRERA L, KAZEMI H: CSF bicarbonate regulation in metabolic acidosis: Role of HCO_3 formation in CSF. *J Appl Physiol* 49:778, 1980.

HOYUMPA AM JR, DESMOND PV, AVANT GR et al: Hepatic encephalopathy. *Gastroenterology* 76:184, 1979.

HUTTENLOCHER P, TRAUNER D: Reye's syndrome in infancy. *Pediatrics* 62:84, 1978.

JELLINEK EH, KELLY RE: Cerebellar syndrome in myxedema. *Lancet* 2:225, 1960.

JOHNSON GM, SCURLETIS TD, CARROLL NB: A study of sixteen fatal cases of encephalitis-like disease in North Carolina children. *NC Med J* 24:464, 1963.

KATZMAN B, PAPPIUS HM: *Brain Electrolytes and Fluid Metabolism*. Baltimore, Williams & Wilkins, 1973.

KLIMAN B: Metabolic derangements, in Ropper AH, Kennedy SK, Zervas NT (eds): *Neurological and Neurosurgical Intensive Care*. Baltimore, University Park Press, 1983, pp 119–131.

LAURENO R: Central pontine myelinolysis following rapid correction of hyponatremia. *Ann Neurol* 13:232, 1983.

LEDERMAN RS, HENRY CE: Progressive dialysis encephalopathy. *Ann Neurol* 4:199, 1978.

MCKEE AC, WINKELMAN MD, BANKER BQ: Central pontine myelinolysis in severely burned patients: relationship to serum hyperosmolality. *Neurology* 38:1211, 1988.

MADDREY WC, WEBER FL JR, COULTER AW et al: Effects of keto analogues of essential amino acids in portal-systemic encephalopathy. *Gastroenterology* 71:190, 1976.

MAIOLO AT, PORRO GB, GALLI C et al: Brain energy metabolism in hepatic coma. *Exp Biol Med* 4:52, 1971.

MALAMUD N, HAYMAKER W, CUSTER RP: Heat stroke: A clinicopathologic study of 125 fatal cases. *Mil Surg* 99:397, 1946.

MARINESCO G: Lésions en myxoedème congénitale avec idiotie. *L'Encéphale* 19:265, 1924.

MARKS R, ROSE FC: *Hypoglycemia*. Oxford, Blackwell, 1965.

MARSHALL JR: Neuropsychiatric aspects of renal failure. *J Clin Psychiatry* 40:181, 1979.

MORGAN MY, JAKOBOVITS AW, JAMES IM, SHERLOCK S: Successful use of bromocriptine in the treatment of chronic hepatic encephalopathy. *Gastroenterology* 78:663, 1980.

MOMOSE KJ, KJELLBERG RN, KLIMAN B: High incidence of cortical atrophy of the cerebral and cerebellar hemisphere in Cushing's disease. *Radiology* 99:341, 1971.

MYERS RAM, SNYDER SK, EMHOFF TA: Subacute sequelae of carbon monoxide poisoning. *Ann Emerg Med* 14:1163 1985.

NADEL AM, WILSON WP: Dialysis encephalopathy: A possible seizure disorder. *Neurology* 26:1130, 1976.

NAVILLE F: Diplegia and thyroid disturbance in defective children. *Schweiz Arch Neurol Psychiatr* 13:559, 1923.

OPPENHEIMER BS, FISHBERG AM: Hypertensive encephalopathy. *Arch Intern Med* 41:264, 1928.

PALLIS CA, LEWIS PD: *The Neurology of Gastrointestinal Disease*. London, Saunders, 1974.

PARKINSON IS, WARD MK, KERR DNS: Dialysis encephalopathy, bone disease and anemia: The aluminum intoxication syndrome during regular hemodialysis. *J Clin Pathol* 34:1285, 1981.

PLUM F, POSNER JB: *Diagnosis of Stupor and Coma*, 3rd ed. Philadelphia, Davis, 1980.

PLUM F, POSNER JB, HAIN RF: Delayed neurological deterioration after anoxia. *Arch Int Med* 110:18, 1962.

POISSON M, MASHALY R, LAFFORGUE B: Progressive dialysis encephalopathy. *Ann Neurol* 6:88, 1979.

PRICE TR, NETSKY MG: Myxedema and ataxia: Cerebellar alterations and "neural myxedema bodies." *Neurology* 16:957, 1966.

PROCKOP LD: Hyperglycemia: Effects on the nervous system, in Vinken PJ, Bruyn BW (eds): *Handbook of Clinical Neurology*, vol 27: *Metabolic and Deficiency Diseases of the Nervous System*, pt I. Amsterdam, North-Holland, 1976, pp 79–99.

RASKIN NH, FISHMAN RA: Neurologic disorders in renal failure. *N Engl J Med* 294:143, 204, 1976.

REYE RDK, MORGAN G, BARAL J: Encephalopathy and fatty degeneration of the viscera: A disease entity in childhood. *Lancet* 2:749, 1963.

ROSENBLUM JL, KEATING JP, PRENSKY AL, NELSON JS: A progressive neurologic syndrome in children with chronic liver disease. *N Engl J Med* 304:503, 1981.

ROTHERMICH NO, VON HAAM E: Pancreatic encephalopathy. *J Clin Endocrinol* 1:872, 1941.

ROZAS VV, PORT FK: Progressive dialysis encephalopathy: Prevention through control of aluminum levels in water. *Ann Neurol* 6:88, 1979.

SALAM-ADAMS MZ, ADAMS RD: Acquired hepatocerebral syndromes, in Vinken PJ, Bruyn GW, Klawans HL (eds): *Handbook of Clinical Neurology*, vol 5(49):*Extrapyramidal Disorders*. Amsterdam, North-Holland, chap 11, 1986.

SCHOCHET SS JR, LAMPERT PW: Granulomatous encephalitis in Whipple's disease. Electron microscopic observations. *Acta Neuropathologica* 13:1, 1969.

SCRIVER CR, BEAUDET AL, SLY WS, VALLE D (eds): *The Metabolic Bases of Inherited Diseases* 6th ed. New York, McGraw-Hill, 1989.

SHARF B, LEVY N: Pancreatic encephalopathy, in Vinken PJ, Bruyn GW, Klawans H (eds): *Handbook of Clinical Neurology*, vol 27: *Metabolic and Deficiency Diseases of the Nervous System*, pt I. Amsterdam, North-Holland, 1976, pp. 449–458.

SEISJÖ BK, JOHANNSSON H, LJUNGGREN B, NORBERG K: Brain dysfunction in cerebral hypoxia and ischemia, in Plum F (ed): *Brain Dysfunction in Metabolic Disorders*, vol 53. New York, Raven Press, 1974, pp 75–112.

SHAYWITZ BA, ROTHSTEIN P, VENES JL: Monitoring and management of increased intracranial pressure in Reye syndrome: Results in 29 children. *Pediatrics* 66:198, 1980.

SOKOLOFF L: Metabolism of the central nervous system in vivo, in Field J, Magoun HW, Hall VE (eds): *Handbook of Physiology, Section 1: Neurophysiology*, vol 3. Washington, Physiologic Society, 1960, pp 1843–1864.

STERNS RH, RIGGS JE, SCHOCHET SS: Osmotic demyelination syndromes following correction of hyponatremia. *N Engl J Med* 314:1555, 1986.

TOM MI, RICHARDSON JC: Hypoglycaemia from islet cell tumor of pancreas with amyotrophy and cerebrospinal nerve cell changes. *J Neuropathol Exp Neurol* 10:57, 1951.

TRAUNER DA: Treatment of Reye syndrome. *Ann Neurol* 7:2, 1980.

TYLER HR: Neurological disorders seen in renal failure, in Vinken PJ, Bruyn BW (eds): *Handbook of Clinical Neurology*, vol 27: *Metabolic and Deficiency Diseases of the Nervous System*, pt I. Amsterdam, North-Holland, 1976, pp 321–348.

VAN WOERKOM W: La cirrhose hépatique avec alterations dans les centres nerveux evoluant chez des sujets d'age moyen. *Nouvelle Iconographie de la Salpêtrière* 27:41, 1914.

VICTOR M, ADAMS RD, COLE M: The acquired (non-Wilsonian) type of chronic hepatocerebral degeneration. *Medicine* 44:345, 1965.

VICTOR M, LAURENO R: Neurologic complications of alcohol abuse; Epidemiologic aspects, in Schoenberg BS (ed): *Advances in Neurology*, vol 19, New York, Raven Press, 1978.

VOLHARD F: Clinical aspects of Bright's disease, in Berglund H et al (eds): *The Kidney in Health and Disease*. Philadelphia, Lea & Febiger, 1935, chap 29, pp 665–673.

VON HÖSSLIN C, ALZHEIMER A: Ein Beitrag zur Klinik und pathologischen Anatomie der Westphal-Strümpellschen Pseudosklerose. *Z Gesamte Neurol Psychiatr* 8:183, 1912.

WEGIERKO J: Typical syndrome of clinical manifestations in diabetes mellitus with fatal termination in coma without ketotic acidemia: So-called third coma. *Pol Tyg Lek* 11:2020, 1956.

WEINER WJ, KLAWANS HL: Hyperthyroid chorea, in Vinken PJ, Bruyn BW (eds): *Handbook of Clinical Neurology*, vol 27: *Metabolic and Deficiency Diseases of the Nervous System*, pt I. Amsterdam, North-Holland, 1976, pp 279–281.

WILKINSON DS, PROCKOP LD: Hypoglycemia: Effects on the nervous system, in Vinken PJ, Bruyn BW (eds): *Handbook of Clinical Neurology*, vol 27: *Metabolic and Deficiency Diseases of the Nervous System*, pt I. Amsterdam, North-Holland, 1976, chap 4, pp 53–78.

WILSON SAK: Progressive lenticular degeneration: A familial nervous disease associated with cirrhosis of the liver. *Brain* 34:295, 1912.

WINKELMAN MD, RICANATI ES: Dialysis encephalopathy: Neuropathologic aspects. *Hum Pathol* 17:823, 1986.

WRIGHT DG, LAURENO R, VICTOR M: Pontine and extrapontine myelinolysis. *Brain* 102:361, 1979.

YOUNG E, BRADLEY RF: Cerebral edema with irreversible coma in severe diabetic ketoacidosis. *N Engl J Med* 276:665, 1967.

ZIEVE L: Pathogenesis of hepatic encephalopathy. *Metab Brain Dis* 2:147, 1987.

ZIEVE L, OLSEN RL: Can hepatic coma be caused by a reduction of brain noradrenaline or dopamine? *Gut* 18:688, 1977.

CHAPTER 41

ALCOHOL AND ALCOHOLISM

Intemperance in the use of alcohol creates many problems in modern society, the importance of which can be judged by the repeated emphasis they receive in contemporary writings, both literary and scientific. These problems may be divided into three categories: psychologic, medical, and sociologic. The main psychologic problem is why a person drinks excessively, often with full knowledge that such action will result in personal physical injury and irreparable harm to the family. The medical problem embraces all aspects of alcoholic habituation as well as the diseases that result from the abuse of alcohol. The sociologic problem consists of the effects of sustained drinking on the patient's work, family, and community.

These several problems engendered by excessive drinking cannot be separated from one another, and the physician must therefore be conversant with all aspects of the subject. The physician may be asked to help the patient overcome his or her drinking problem or to diagnose and treat the numerous diseases to which such a patient is subject; often the physician must admit or commit the patient to a general or mental hospital, according to the nature of the presenting clinical disorder; and lastly, the physician may be required to enlist the aid of available social agencies when their services are needed by either the patient or the patient's family.

Primary alcoholism has been defined as both a chronic disease and a disorder of behavior, characterized in either context by chronic, repetitive, excessive drinking to an extent that interferes with the drinker's health, interpersonal relations, or means of livelihood. Reduced to pharmacologic terms, it is addiction to alcohol. *Secondary alcoholism* refers to excessive drinking in the context of another major psychiatric illness. The term *alcoholism,* unqualified, refers to the primary variety.

The causation of alcoholism remains obscure, although environmental, cultural, and genetic factors are clearly implicated in certain groups of patients. No single personality type has been shown to predict reliably who will become addicted to alcohol and who will not. Similarly, no particular aspect of alcohol metabolism has been found to account for the development of addiction in some individuals and not in others, with the possible exception of aldehyde dehydrogenase (see below). Some persons drink excessively and become alcoholics in response to severe life stress, but many do not. Depression may precede the development of alcoholism, more so in women than in men, but far more often depression is a consequence of drinking. Social and cultural influences are undoubtedly important in the genesis of alcoholism, as evidenced, for example, by the remarkably high incidence of alcoholism and drinking problems in the American Indian and Eskimo populations and by the disparity in the prevalence of alcoholism, within a single community, between the Irish and Jews. However, no ethnic or racial group and no social or economic class is immune to alcoholism. Moreover, no particular pattern of child rearing or cultural attitude is universally effective in facilitating or protecting against the development of alcoholism (Bacon). The writings of Roebuck and Kessler, of Schuckit, and of Mello, listed in the references, provide critical overviews of the many etiologic theories.

The importance of genetic factors in the causation of alcoholism is being increasingly recognized. Goodwin et al studied 55 Danish men whose biologic parents were alcoholic and 55 control subjects whose biologic parents were not alcoholics. All of the subjects had been adopted before the age of 5 weeks and had no knowledge of their biologic parentage. Twenty percent of the offspring of biologic alcoholic parents, but only 5 percent of the control subjects, had become alcoholics by the age of 25 to 29 years. A Swedish adoption study (Bohman), and one in the United States (Cadoret et al), have corroborated these findings. Family studies have disclosed a three- to fourfold increased risk for alcoholism in sons and daughters of alcoholics, and twin studies have shown a twofold higher concordance rate for alcoholism in monozygotic than in dizygotic pairs.

Details of these studies can be found in the comprehensive reviews of the genetics of alcoholism, by Grove and Cadoret, and by Schukit. The search goes on for a biologic trait, or marker, that would identify those who are genetically vulnerable to the development of alcoholism, but to date, none has proved to be sufficiently practical or sensitive to identify all such persons (Reich).

The incidence of alcoholism in the United States cannot be stated precisely. In 1985, the National Institute on Alcohol Abuse and Alcoholism estimated that there were 10.6 million adults in the United States (about 10 percent of the work force) who were addicted to alcohol. In addition, there were approximately 4.6 million problem drinkers among adolescents (about 20 percent of the persons in this age group). Schuckit has estimated that the lifetime risk for alcoholism is at least 10 percent for men and 3 to 5 percent for women. It requires little imagination to conceive the havoc wrought by alcohol in terms of decreased productivity, increased incidence of suicide, accidents, crime, mental and physical disease, and disruption of family life.

PHARMACOLOGY AND METABOLISM OF ALCOHOL

Ethyl alcohol, or ethanol, is the active ingredient in beer, wine, whiskey, gin, brandy, and other less common alcoholic beverages. In addition, the stronger spirits contain enanthic ethers, which provide the flavor but have no important pharmacologic properties, and impurities such as amyl alcohol (fusel oil) and acetaldehyde, which act like alcohol but are more toxic. Contrary to popular opinion, the content of B vitamins in American beer and other liquors is so low as to have little nutritional value (Davidson).

Absorption, Distribution, and Excretion Alcohol is absorbed unaltered from the gastrointestinal tract, about 25 percent from the stomach and the rest from the upper small intestine. Its presence may be detected in the blood within 5 min after ingestion, and the maximum concentration is reached in 30 to 90 min. The ingestion of milk and fatty foods impedes and water facilitates its absorption. The rate of absorption increases after Billroth I and II gastrectomies; in these cases maximum blood alcohol concentrations are higher and are attained faster than in subjects with intact stomachs. In habituated persons the blood alcohol concentration rises somewhat faster and reaches a higher maximum than in abstainers.

Alcohol is carried chiefly in the plasma and enters the various organs of the body—as well as the CSF, urine, and pulmonary alveolar air—in concentrations that bear a constant relationship to the concentration in the blood. It

is metabolized chiefly by oxidation, less than 10 percent being excreted chemically unchanged in the urine, perspiration, and breath. The energy liberated by the oxidation of alcohol (7 kcal/g) can be utilized as completely as that of fats, sugars, and proteins, which it replaces isodynamically. It should be emphasized that alcohol cannot be stored in the body or used in the replacement of destroyed tissue. Therefore, unless the chronic drinker takes an adequate amount of protein (which the alcoholic frequently fails to do), muscle bulk is lost and other tissues are damaged.

Metabolism of Alcohol and Acetaldehyde This is accomplished mainly in the liver, where several enzyme systems (located in different subcellular compartments of the hepatocyte) can independently oxidize alcohol to acetaldehyde. The most important of these systems, accounting for 80 to 90 percent of ethanol oxidation in vivo, are alcohol dehydrogenase (ADH) and its isoenzymes; they are found in the cell sap or soluble fraction of the hepatocyte and utilize nicotinamide adenine dinucleotide (NAD) as the cofactor. This reaction leads to the formation of acetaldehyde and the reduction of NAD to NADH. A second pathway involves catalase, which is located in the peroxisomes and mitochondria; a third utilizes the "microsomal ethanol oxidizing system" (MEOS), located mainly in the microsomes of the endoplasmic reticulum. The MEOS, which is dependent upon reduced nicotinamide adenine dinucleotide phosphate (NADPH), does not account for much of the alcohol metabolized in normal circumstances, but it may be responsible for the increased rate of alcohol metabolism observed in chronic alcoholics.

The exact steps in the *metabolism of acetaldehyde* are still not settled. Most likely it is converted by aldehyde dehydrogenase to acetate. This reaction, which is accomplished mainly in the mitochondria, also requires NAD as a cofactor. Alternatively, it is possible that alcohol is converted to acetyl CoA, which in turn could yield acetate. In either event, acetyl CoA and acetate (the end products of alcohol metabolism in the liver) are metabolized further through well-established normal pathways, with the eventual release of carbon dioxide and water.

Acetaldehyde has a number of unique biochemical effects that are not produced by alcohol alone, and this has led to speculation that acetaldehyde might be responsible for the manifestations of alcoholic intoxication and addiction. Persons who flush easily after ingestion of alcohol (Chinese and other orientals) differ from "nonflushers" with respect to the metabolism of acetaldehyde, rather than alcohol. The flushing reaction has been traced to a lack of one of the isoenzymes of aldehyde dehydrogenase. The low rate of alcoholism among the Chinese has been related to the flushing reaction (which is in effect a modified alcohol-disulfiram reaction—see further on), but this can hardly be the case, since North American Indians, a group with an extremely high prevalence of alcoholism, show the same reaction.

Also it has been observed that aldehydes combine with certain amines (norepinephrine, epinephrine, and serotonin) to form alkaloids, the molecular structure of which is similar to a number of highly addictive plant alkaloids, such as morphine. Because of this similarity, it has been suggested that the addictive properties of ethanol are related to the formation of alkaloids from acetaldehyde, generated during the metabolism of ethanol. Although the notion that addiction to alcohol and to opiates depends upon a common biochemical pathway is an attractive one, it is not consistent with either clinical observations or pharmacologic data (Seevers).

There are important reasons for believing that acetaldehyde does not play a significant role in alcoholic intoxication and that ethanol itself, rather than its initial metabolite, is the major addicting agent in alcoholism. The rate of acetaldehyde metabolism is very rapid and greatly exceeds the rate of oxidation of ethanol to acetaldehyde, and for this reason, acetaldehyde concentrations in the blood remain low even in the face of high blood alcohol levels. Moreover, the acetaldehyde levels remain stable as the behavioral signs of intoxication (and the blood alcohol levels) increase and later recede. It is unlikely that these low blood acetaldehyde concentrations have serious toxic effects, considering the high doses of acetaldehyde required to produce such effects in animals.

For all practical purposes it may be accepted that once absorption is ended and an equilibrium established with the tissues, ethyl alcohol is oxidized at a constant rate, independent of its concentration in the blood (about 150 mg alcohol per kilogram of body weight per hour, or about 1 oz 90-proof whiskey per hour). Actually, slightly more alcohol is burned per hour when the initial concentrations are very high, but this increment is of little clinical significance. On the other hand, the rate of oxidation of acetaldehyde does depend on its concentration in the tissues. This fact is of importance in connection with the drug disulfiram (Antabuse) that acts by raising the tissue concentration necessary for the metabolism of a certain amount of acetaldehyde per unit of time. The patient taking both Antabuse and alcohol will accumulate an inordinate amount of acetaldehyde, resulting in nausea, vomiting, and hypo-

tension, sometimes pronounced in degree and even fatal. This pharmacologic principle underlies the treatment of alcoholism with Antabuse. Certain other drugs, notably the sulfonylureas, metronidazole, and furazolidone, have effects like those of disulfiram, but are less potent.

Very few factors are capable of increasing the rate of alcohol metabolism. There is some evidence that repeated ingestion of alcohol facilitates its metabolism in both normal and alcoholic subjects. Insulin, amino acids, and fructose enhance ethanol metabolism, but none has proved to be of practical value in the treatment of alcohol intoxication. Starvation slows the rate of alcohol metabolism in the liver, although this varies greatly in degree from one person to another.

ACUTE EFFECTS OF ALCOHOL ON NONNEUROLOGIC ORGAN SYSTEMS

The acute pharmacologic actions of alcohol are diverse and complicated and involve virtually every organ in the body. Although our primary concern is with the nervous system, rarely are the effects of alcohol confined to this system. For this reason, the actions of alcohol on the nonneurologic organ systems will be reviewed briefly.

Heart and Circulation   There appears to be a direct action of alcohol on the excitability and contractility of heart muscle. With intoxicating doses there is usually a cutaneous dilatation and an increase in heart rate or stroke volume. In other normal individuals, administration of alcohol depresses myocardial function (see review by Segel et al). Peripheral vasodilatation, increased heart rate, and decreased blood pressure in response to acute ingestion of alcohol are much more prominent in orientals than whites (Ewing et al), possibly providing a physiologic explanation for the purportedly low rate of alcoholism among the former (see above). Some investigators have suggested that prolonged intoxication may have a damaging effect on cardiac and skeletal muscle—a degeneration of fibers supposedly due to the suppression of myophosphorylase activity (page 1115). Increased sweating and vasodilatation cause a loss of body heat and a fall in temperature. Finally, it now seems clear that chronic excessive drinking is an important risk factor for hypertension (Saunders).

Gastrointestinal System   In low concentrations, by whatever the route of administration, alcohol stimulates the gastric glands to produce acid, apparently by releasing gastrin from the antral region and possibly by causing the mucosa to form or release histamine. With the ingestion of alcohol, in concentrations of more than 10 to 15 percent, the secretion of mucus is increased, the stomach mucosa becomes congested and hyperemic, and the secretion of acid then becomes depressed. Clinically these changes account for the state known as *acute gastritis*. The increase in appetite following ingestion of alcohol is due to the stimulation of the end organs of taste and to a general sense of well-being. Similarly, the reviving effect of alcohol in fatigue states is a cerebral one and is not the result of a direct stimulating effect on muscle or other organs.

Liver As indicated above, the oxidation of alcohol in the liver involves the reduction of NAD to NADH. This shift in the NADH/NAD ratio results in a number of metabolic derangements in carbohydrate and lipid metabolism. The synthesis of glucose declines, since the smaller carbon compounds that are required for gluconeogenesis enter this pathway via NAD-linked oxidation. The conversion of lactic to pyruvic acid, described above, is one such entry reaction. A significant lowering of blood glucose will occur only if the hepatic glycogen stores are depleted—as a result of fasting, for example. Also, the levels of serum lactate will be increased occasionally, to the point of lactic acidosis. In certain circumstances alcohol can also interfere with the peripheral utilization of glucose, resulting in hyperglycemia.

Also, as a result of the changed NADH/NAD ratio, there occurs a depression in the oxidation of fatty acids, the excess of which is converted to triglycerides, which leads in turn to a fatty liver.

Renal and Endocrine Effects The inhibitory action of lactic acid on the renal excretion of uric acid may result in a secondary hyperuricemia. Other renal effects are low serum levels of phosphate and magnesium, presumably because of the increased tubular excretion of these ions. There is also an increased urinary excretion of ammonium and titratable acidity following alcohol ingestion, owing to a mild degree of both metabolic and respiratory acidosis. The former is presumably the result of an accumulation of acid metabolites and the latter, the effect of the direct action of alcohol on the respiratory center.

Alcohol has a well-known effect on the renal excretion of water. The ingestion of 4 oz of 100-proof bourbon whiskey results in a diuresis qualitatively indistinguishable from the diuresis that follows the drinking of large amounts of water. This is most likely the result of transient suppression of release of antidiuretic hormone (ADH) from the supraopticohypophysial system, since a relatively small amount of alcohol injected directly into a carotid artery evokes a prompt diuresis without a detectable rise in the concentration of alcohol in the systemic blood. Alcohol does not alter the sensitivity of the kidney tubules to endogenous or exogenous ADH (Pitressin) and has no discernible effect on renal hemodynamic function in normal persons. The degree of diuresis seems to be more closely related to the duration of the rising blood alcohol level than

to the rate of increase or the absolute level attained, if the period of alcohol intoxication is sustained. Diuresis occurs only during the initial phase of alcohol administration and does not persist during prolonged drinking.

It has been demonstrated that the administration of alcohol to normal young men for periods up to 4 weeks decreases the rate of production and the plasma concentration of testosterone (Gordon et al). These abnormalities of testosterone metabolism have been traced to both a central (hypothalamus-pituitary) and gonadal effect of alcohol and are independent of nutritional deficiency and liver disease. Considerably less is known about the effects of chronic alcoholism on other endocrine systems (see review by Cicero).

Hematopoietic Effects Alcohol has a direct effect upon cells of the bone marrow. Human volunteers who were given alcohol in doses equaling half their caloric intake for several weeks manifested an increase in vacuolation of red and white cell precursors, particularly of the former. In addition, there was a depression of the platelet count. Serum iron fell, but only during the withdrawal period. All these hematologic defects occurred despite excellent nutrition and concomitant administration of folic acid (Lindenbaum and Lieber).

PHARMACOLOGIC AND BEHAVIORAL EFFECTS ON THE NERVOUS SYSTEM

Behaviorally, the effects of acute nonlethal doses of alcohol are those of alcohol intoxication. Pharmacologically, alcohol acts directly on neuronal membranes in a manner akin to the general anesthetics. These agents, as well as barbiturates, are lipid-soluble and are thought to produce their effects by dissolving in the membranes (in direct relation to the degree of their lipid solubility), and perhaps by interacting with the membrane lipoproteins. It is now generally accepted that alcohol is not a stimulant of the central nervous system, but a depressant. Some of the early effects of alcohol, manifested by garrulousness, aggressiveness, excessive activity, and increased electrical excitability of the cerebral cortex—all of which suggest stimulation—are due to the inhibition of certain subcortical structures (high brainstem reticular formation?) that ordinarily modulate cerebral cortical activity. Similarly, the initial hyperactivity of tendon reflexes may represent a transitory escape of spinal motor neurons from higher inhibitory centers. With increasing amounts of alcohol, however, the depressant action spreads to involve the cortical as well as other brainstem and spinal neurons.

All manner of motor performance—whether the simple maintenance of a standing posture, the control of speech and eye movements, or highly organized and complex motor skills—is adversely affected by alcohol. The movements involved in these acts are not only slower than normal but also more inaccurate and random in character and therefore less well adapted to the accomplishment of specific ends.

Alcohol also impairs the efficiency of mental function by interfering with the speed of and persistence in mental processing. The learning process is slowed and rendered less effective. The facility of forming associations, whether of words or of figures, tends to be hampered and the ability to focus and sustain attention and to concentrate is reduced. The subject is not as versatile as usual in directing thought along new lines appropriate to the problems at hand. Finally, alcohol impairs the faculties of judgment and discrimination and, all in all, the ability to think and reason clearly.

A scale relating various degrees of clinical intoxication to blood alcohol levels in *nonhabituated* persons was constructed by Miles. At a blood alcohol level of 30 mg/dL, a mild euphoria was detectable, and at 50 mg/dL, a mild incoordination. At 100 mg/dL, ataxia was obvious; at 200 mg/dL, there was confusion and a reduced level of mental activity; at 300 mg/dL, the subjects were stuporous; and a level of 400 mg/dL was accompanied by deep anesthesia and could prove fatal. These figures are valid, provided the alcohol content in the blood rises steadily over a 2-h period.

Tolerance   It should be emphasized that a scale such as the one above has virtually no value in the chronic alcoholic patient, for it does not take into account the adaptation of the organism to alcohol, i.e., the phenomenon of tolerance. It is common knowledge that a habituated person can drink more and show fewer effects than the moderate drinker or abstainer. This phenomenon accounts for the surprisingly large amounts of alcohol that can be consumed by the chronic drinker without significant signs of drunkenness. Sober-appearing alcoholics may have blood alcohol levels of 400 to 500 mg/dL. In such individuals, there is a narrow margin between the doses associated with low blood alcohol levels and sobriety and the doses associated with high blood levels and drunkenness. One must question the validity, therefore, of a single estimation of the blood alcohol concentration as a reliable index of drunkenness.

The organism is capable of adapting to alcohol after a very short exposure. Thus, if the alcohol concentration in the blood is raised very slowly, few symptoms appear, even at quite high levels. Contrariwise, the degree of intoxication is more severe when the blood alcohol level peaks rapidly. As mentioned earlier, the important factor in this rapid adaptability is not so much the height of the blood alcohol level, but the length of time the alcohol has been present in the body. If the dosage of alcohol that just causes blood levels to be high is held constant, the blood alcohol concentration falls gradually and clinical evidence of intoxication disappears. The cause of this fall in alcohol concentration is not clear.

The biochemical mechanisms that underlie tolerance are not known. There is little evidence that an enhanced rate of alcohol metabolism can adequately account for the degree of tolerance observed in alcoholics. An increased degree of neuronal adaptation to alcohol is a more likely explanation. As indicated above, alcohol has an important physicochemical effect on the cell membrane. Alcohol has been shown to increase the "fluidity" of membrane lipids; with the development of tolerance, neuronal membranes become resistant to the fluidizing effect of alcohol (Chin and Goldstein; Harris et al). Probably a more important effect of alcohol is on membrane receptor systems, which regulate ion channels, particularly the chloride and calcium channels. Alcohol reduces depolarization-induced calcium entry into neurons. An adaptation to this effect is to increase the number of calcium channels in the cell membrane. Hudspith and colleagues have adduced evidence that such an increase in the calcium channels initiates a stage of hyperexcitability, which would be exposed upon the withdrawal of alcohol. The effect of alcohol at a cellular level is now the subject of intense research activity (see Rubin).

Removal of alcohol from the habituated nervous system results in another disturbance in neuronal function, presumably an overactivity. The need to drink in order to suppress the discomfort engendered by alcohol withdrawal is spoken of as *physical dependence*. Clinically these effects are recognized as the alcohol *withdrawal or abstinence syndrome* (see further on).

CLINICAL EFFECTS OF ALCOHOL ON THE NERVOUS SYSTEM

A large number of neurologic disorders are associated with alcoholism. The factor common to all of them, of course, is the abuse of alcohol, but the mechanism by which alcohol produces its effects varies widely from one group of disorders to another. The classification that follows is based for the most part on known mechanisms.

I. Alcohol intoxication—drunkenness, coma, excitement ("pathological intoxication"), "blackouts"

II. The abstinence or withdrawal syndrome—tremulousness, hallucinosis, seizures, delirium tremens

III. Nutritional diseases of the nervous system secondary to alcoholism
   A. Wernicke-Korsakoff syndrome
   B. Polyneuropathy
   C. Optic neuropathy ("tobacco-alcohol amblyopia")
   D. Pellagra

IV. Diseases of uncertain pathogenesis, associated with alcoholism
   A. Cerebellar degeneration
   B. Marchiafava-Bignami disease
   C. Central pontine myelinolysis
   D. "Alcoholic" cardiomyopathy and myopathy
   E. Alcoholic dementia
   F. Cerebral atrophy

V. Fetal alcohol syndrome

VI. Neurologic disorders consequent upon Laennec cirrhosis and portal-systemic shunts
   A. Hepatic stupor and coma
   B. Chronic hepatocerebral degeneration

ALCOHOL INTOXICATION

The manifestations of alcohol intoxication are so commonplace that they require no elaboration. They consist of varying degrees of exhilaration and excitement, loss of restraint, irregularity of behavior, loquacity and slurred speech, incoordination of movement and gait, irritability, drowsiness, and, in advanced cases, stupor and coma.

Pathological Intoxication On rare occasions alcohol has an excitatory rather than a sedative effect. This reaction has been referred to as *pathological,* or *complicated, intoxication* and as *acute alcoholic paranoid state.* Since all forms of intoxication are pathologic, "atypical intoxication" would be a more appropriate designation. Nevertheless, *pathological intoxication* is the term that has survived. The boundaries of this syndrome have never been clearly drawn. In the past, variant forms of delirium tremens and epileptic phenomena as well as psychopathic and criminal behavior were indiscriminately included. Now the term is generally used to designate an outburst of blind fury with assaultive and destructive behavior. Often the patient is subdued only with difficulty. The attack terminates with deep sleep, which occurs spontaneously or in response to sedation, and on awakening the patient has no memory of the episode. Lesser degrees are also known wherein the patient, after several drinks, repeatedly commits gross social indiscretions. Allegedly this reaction may follow the ingestion of a small amount of alcohol, but in our experience the amount has always been substantial. Unlike the usual forms of alcohol intoxication and withdrawal, this atypical form has not been produced in experimental subjects, and the diagnosis depends upon these rather arbitrary anecdotal criteria.

Pathological intoxication has been ascribed to many factors, the common ones being constitutional differences in the susceptibility to alcohol (idiosyncratic reaction to alcohol), pre-existent craniocerebral trauma or other brain disease, an underlying "hysterical or epileptoid temperament or sociopathy." There are no meaningful data to support any of these beliefs. However, an analogy may be drawn between pathological intoxication and the paradoxic reaction that occasionally follows the administration of barbiturates.

The diagnosis of pathological intoxication may have important legal implications. A person suffering from alcoholism or the usual forms of drunkenness is considered responsible for any harmful actions, whereas a person with pathological intoxication is considered insane at the time and therefore not responsible. The main disorders to be distinguished from pathological intoxication are temporal lobe seizures that occasionally take the form of outbursts of rage and violence, and the explosive episodes of violence that characterize the behavior of certain sociopaths. The diagnosis in these cases may be difficult and depends on eliciting the other manifestations of temporal lobe epilepsy or sociopathy.

"Blackouts" In the language of the alcoholic, the term "blackout" refers to a transient circumscribed episode that occurs during a period of severe intoxication, for which the patient, when sober, has no memory—even though the state of consciousness, as observed by others, was not grossly altered during that time. However, a systematic assessment of mental function during the amnesic period has not been made. A few observations indicate that it is short-term (retentive) memory, rather than immediate or long-term memory, that is impaired; this feature and the subsequent amnesia for the episode are somewhat reminiscent of the disorder known as *transient global amnesia* (page 343).

The nature and significance of such episodes are unclear. Some psychiatrists deny that a loss of memory has occurred and view the blackout as a form of malingering; others speak of "repression," which prevents conscious awareness of painful memories. These views are purely speculative. It is widely held that the occurrence of blackouts is an early and serious indicator of the development of alcohol addiction. In our experience, blackouts may occur at any time in the course of alcoholism, even in the first drinking experience, and they may occur also in persons who never become alcoholics. The salient facts are that a degree of intoxication has occurred that prevented the formation of memories during the period of intoxication, and rarely will the amount of alcohol consumed in moderate social drinking produce this effect.

Alcoholic Stupor and Coma As has been indicated, the symptoms of alcoholic intoxication are the result of the depressant action of alcohol on cerebral and spinal neurons. In this respect alcohol acts on nerve cells in a manner akin to the general anesthetics. Unlike the latter, however, the margin between the dose of alcohol that produces surgical anesthesia and that which dangerously depresses respiration is a narrow one, a fact that adds an element of urgency to the diagnosis and treatment of alcoholic narcosis. One must also be alert to the possibility that barbiturates or other sedative-hypnotic drugs have potentiated the depressant effects of alcohol.

The signs of alcohol intoxication are distinctive and most forms present no problem in diagnosis or management. On the other hand, coma due to alcohol may present difficulties in differential diagnosis. It should be stressed that the diagnosis of alcoholic coma is made not merely on the basis of a flushed face, stupor, and the odor of alcohol, but only after the careful exclusion of all other causes of coma (see Table 16-3).

Treatment of Alcohol Intoxication Mild to moderate degrees of intoxication require no special treatment. Certain time-honored remedies such as a cold shower, strong coffee, forced activity, or induction of vomiting may be helpful, but there is no evidence that any of them influences the rate of disappearance of alcohol from the blood. Alcoholic stupor is also a relatively brief, self-limited state, and if the vital signs are normal, no special therapeutic measures are necessary. *Pathological intoxication* may require the use of restraints and the parenteral administration of phenobarbital sodium (200 mg), or amobarbital sodium (500 mg), or haldol (5 to 10 mg), repeated once in 30 to 40 min if necessary.

Coma due to alcohol intoxication represents a medical emergency. The main object of treatment is to prevent respiratory depression and the complications it engenders. The management of the comatose patient is described on page 286. One would like to lower the blood alcohol level as rapidly as possible, but the administration of fructose or of insulin and glucose for this purpose is of little practical value. Analeptic drugs such as amphetamine, and various mixtures of caffeine and picrotoxin are antagonistic to alcohol only insofar as they are powerful cerebral cortical stimulants and overall nervous system excitants; they do not hasten the oxidation of alcohol. The use of hemodialysis

should be considered in comatose patients with extremely high blood alcohol concentrations (> 500 mg/dL), particularly if accompanied by acidosis, and in those who have concurrently ingested methanol or ethylene glycol or some other dialyzable drug.

Methyl, Amyl, and Isopropyl Alcohols and Ethylene Glycol Poisoning with alcohols other than ethyl alcohol is a relatively rare occurrence. *Amyl alcohol* (fusel oil) and *isopropyl alcohol* are used as industrial solvents and in the manufacture of varnishes, lacquers, and pharmaceuticals; in addition isopropyl alcohol is readily available as a rubbing alcohol. Intoxication may follow the ingestion of these alcohols or inhalation of their vapors. The effects of both are much like those of ethyl alcohol, but much more toxic.

Methyl alcohol (methanol, wood alcohol) is a component of antifreeze and many combustibles and is used in the manufacture of formaldehyde, as an industrial solvent, and as an adulterant of alcoholic beverages, the latter being the most common source of methyl alcohol intoxication. The oxidation of methyl alcohol to formaldehyde and formic acid proceeds relatively slowly; thus, signs of intoxication do not appear for several hours or may be delayed for a day or longer. Many of the toxic effects are like those of ethyl alcohol, but in addition methyl alcohol poisoning may produce serious degrees of acidosis and damage to the retinal ganglion cells, giving rise to scotomata and varying degrees of blindness, dilated unreactive pupils, and retinal edema. The most important aspect of treatment is the intravenous administration of large amounts of sodium bicarbonate. Hemodialysis may be a useful adjunct because of the slow rate of oxidation of methanol.

Ethylene glycol, an aliphatic alcohol, is a commonly used industrial solvent and the major constituent of antifreeze. In the latter form it is sometimes consumed by skid-row alcoholics, with disastrous results. At first the patient merely appears drunk, but severe confusion, convulsions, and coma follow in rapid succession. Acidosis and CSF lymphocytosis are other characteristic features. The metabolic acidosis is due to the conversion of ethylene glycol by alcohol dehydrogenase into glycolic acid. The cause of the renal toxicity is less clear—probably it is due to the formation of oxalate from glycolate. The current treatment of ethylene glycol poisoning, which is not altogether satisfactory, consists of hemodialysis and the intravenous infusion of ethanol, which competes for alcohol dehydrogenase. Recently, Baud and his colleagues have described the salutary effects of intravenous 4-methylpyrazole, an inhibitor of alcohol dehydrogenase; this drug is administered in an initial dose of 10 mg/kg and, reduced as ethylene glycol, is cleared from the bloodstream. The acidosis of salicylism and methanol intoxication need to be distinguished.

THE ABSTINENCE OR WITHDRAWAL SYNDROME

Included under this title is the symptom complex of tremulousness, hallucinations, seizures, confusion, and psychomotor and autonomic overactivity. Although a sustained period of chronic inebriation is the most obvious factor in the causation of these symptoms, they become manifest only *after a period of relative or absolute abstinence* from alcohol—hence the designation *abstinence, or withdrawal, syndrome.* This concept is illustrated in Fig. 41-1. Each of the major manifestations of the withdrawal syndrome may occur in more or less pure form and will be so described, but usually they occur in various combinations. Major withdrawal symptoms are observed mainly in the spree, or periodic, drinker, although the steady drinker is not immune if, for some reason, he stops drinking.

Tremulousness The most common manifestation of the abstinence syndrome is tremulousness, often referred to as "the shakes" or "the jitters," combined with general irritability and gastrointestinal symptoms, particularly nausea and vomiting. These symptoms first appear after several days of drinking, in the morning, after a night's abstinence. The patient states that he "quiets his nerves" with a few drinks and then is able to drink for the rest of the day without undue distress. The symptoms return on successive mornings with increasing severity. The usual spree lasts about 2 weeks, but the duration varies greatly. Usually it is terminated because of increasing severity of recurrent

Figure 41-1

Relation of acute neurologic disturbances to cessation of drinking. The shaded drinking period is greatly foreshortened and not intended to be quantitative. The periodic notching in the baseline represents the tremulousness, nausea, etc., that occur following a night's sleep. The time relations of the various groups of symptoms to withdrawal are explained in the text. The unlabeled peak, conforming closely to that of "fits," represents the relationship of acute auditory hallucinosis to cessation of drinking. (From Victor and Adams, 1953.)

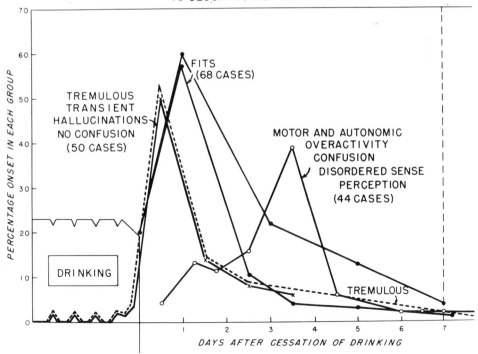

tremor and vomiting, but for other reasons as well, such as a lack of funds, weakness, self-disgust, injury, illness, or collapse. The symptoms then become greatly augmented, reaching their peak intensity 24 to 36 h after the complete cessation of drinking.

At this stage, the patient presents a distinctive clinical picture. The face is deeply flushed, the conjunctivas are injected, and there is usually tachycardia, anorexia, nausea, and retching. The patient is fully awake, startles easily, and complains of insomnia. He is inattentive and disinclined to answer questions, and may respond in a rude or perfunctory manner. The patient may be mildly disoriented in time and have a poor memory for events of the last few days of the drinking spree, but shows no serious confusion, being generally aware of his immediate surroundings and the nature of his or her illness.

Generalized tremor is the most obvious feature of this illness. It is of fast frequency (6 to 8 Hz), slightly irregular, and variable in severity, tending to diminish when the patient is in quiet surroundings and to increase with motor activity or emotional stress. The tremor may be so violent that the patient cannot stand without help, speak clearly, or eat without assistance. Sometimes there is little objective evidence of tremor, and the patient complains only of being "shaky inside."

The flushed facies, anorexia, tachycardia, and tremor subside to a large extent within a few days, but the overalertness, tendency to startle easily, and jerkiness of movement may persist for a week or longer and the feeling of uneasiness may not leave the patient completely for 10 to 14 days. These features are suggestive of adrenal hyperactivity, an idea that has received some support from the finding of elevated levels of norepinephrine and its metabolites in both the blood and CSF (Carlsson and Haggendal; Hawley et al). According to Porjesz and Begleiter, certain electrophysiologic abnormalities (diminished amplitudes of sensory-evoked potentials and prolonged latencies and conduction velocities of auditory brainstem potentials) remain altered long after the clinical abnormalities have subsided.

Hallucinosis Symptoms of disordered perception occur in about one-quarter of the tremulous patients. The patient may complain of "bad dreams"—nightmarish episodes associated with disturbed sleep, which he finds difficult to separate from real experience. Sounds and shadows may be misinterpreted, or familiar objects may be distorted and assume unreal forms. Although these are not hallucinations in the strict sense of the term, they represent the most common forms of disordered sense perception in the alcoholic.

Hallucinations may be purely visual in type, mixed visual and auditory, tactile, or olfactory, in that order of frequency. There is little evidence to support the popular belief that certain visual hallucinations (bugs, pink elephants) are specific to alcoholism. Actually, the hallucinations comprise the full range of visual experiences. They are more often animate than inanimate; persons or animals may appear singly or in panoramas, shrunken or enlarged, natural and pleasant, or distorted, hideous, and frightening.

Acute and Chronic Auditory Hallucinosis A special type of alcoholic psychosis, consisting essentially of a purely auditory hallucinosis, has been recognized for many years. Kraepelin referred to this as the *hallucinatory insanity of drunkards, or alcoholic mania*. The central feature of the illness, in the beginning, is the occurrence of auditory hallucinations despite an otherwise clear sensorium; i.e., the patients are not confused, disoriented, or obtunded, and they have an intact memory. The hallucinations may take the form of unstructured sounds such as buzzing, ringing, shots, and clicking (the elementary hallucinations of Bleuler), or they may have a musical quality, like a low-pitched hum or chant. The most common hallucinations, however, are human voices. When the voices can be identified, they are attributed often to the patient's family, friends, or neighbors—and rarely to God, radio, or radar. The voices may be addressed directly to the patient, but more frequently they discuss the patient in the third person. In the majority of cases the voices are maligning, reproachful, or threatening in nature and are disturbing to the patient; a significant proportion, however, are not unpleasant and leave the patient undisturbed. The voices are clearly audible and intensely real, and they tend to be exteriorized; i.e., they come from behind the door, from the corridor, or through the floor. Another quality of the formed auditory hallucinations (and the visual ones of delirium tremens) is the appropriateness of the patient's response to the hallucinatory content. The patient may call on the police for protection or put up a barricade against invaders; such a patient may even attempt suicide to avoid what the voices threaten. The hallucinations are most prominent during the night, and their duration varies greatly: they may be momentary, or they may recur intermittently for days on end and, in exceptional instances, for weeks or months.

Most patients, while hallucinating, have no appreciation of the unreality of their hallucinations. As improvement occurs, the patient begins to question their reality or is reluctant to talk about them, and may even question his own sanity. Full recovery is characterized by the realization that the voices were imaginary and by the ability to recall, sometimes with remarkable clarity, some of the abnormal thought content of the psychotic episode.

A unique feature of this psychosis is its evolution to a *chronic auditory hallucinosis* in a small proportion of the patients. The chronic disorder begins like the acute one, but after a short period, perhaps a week or two, the symptomatology begins to change. The patient becomes quiet and resigned, even though the hallucinations remain threatening and derogatory. Ideas of reference and influence and other poorly systematized paranoid delusions become prominent. At this stage the illness may be mistaken for paranoid schizophrenia, and indeed has been so identified by Bleuler. There are, however, important differences between the two disorders: the alcoholic illness develops in close relationship to a drinking bout and the past history rarely reveals schizoid personality traits. Alcoholic patients with hallucinosis are not distinguished by a high incidence of schizophrenia within their families (Schuckit and Winokur, Scott) and a large number of such patients, whom we evaluated long after their acute attacks, did not show an increased incidence of schizophrenia. There is some evidence that repeated attacks of acute auditory hallucinosis render the patient more susceptible to the chronic state.

Withdrawal Seizures ("Rum Fits") In this particular setting (i.e., where relative or absolute abstinence follows a period of chronic inebriation) there is a marked tendency to develop convulsive seizures. Over 90 percent of withdrawal seizures occur during the 7- to 48-h period following the cessation of drinking, with a peak incidence between 13 and 24 h. During the period of seizure activity the EEG may be abnormal, but it reverts to normal in a matter of days, even though the patient may go on to develop delirium tremens. Also during the period of seizure activity the patient is unusually sensitive to stroboscopic stimulation; almost half the patients respond with generalized myoclonus or a convulsive seizure (photomyogenic or photoparoxysmal response). By contrast, this type of response to photic stimulation is observed only rarely in nonalcoholic epileptics, and then usually in those with tonic-clonic seizures on awakening.

Seizures occurring in the abstinence period have a number of other distinctive features. There may be only a single seizure, but in the majority of cases the seizures occur in bursts of two to six, occasionally even more; two percent of our patients developed status epilepticus. The seizures are grand mal in type, i.e., generalized "tonic-clonic" convulsions with loss of consciousness. A focal seizure or seizures should always suggest the presence of a focal lesion (most often traumatic) in addition to the effects of alcohol. Almost 30 percent of our patients with generalized seizure activity developed delirium tremens, in which case the seizures invariably preceded the delirium.

The postictal confusional state may blend imperceptibly with the onset of the delirium, or there may be clearing of the postictal state over several hours or even a day or two, before the delirium sets in. Seizures of this type occur in patients who have been drinking for many years, and must be distinguished from other forms of epilepsy beginning in adult life.

It is suggested that the term *rum fits*, or *whiskey fits*—i.e., the names used by alcoholics themselves—be reserved for seizures with the attributes described above. This serves to distinguish this form of seizure activity, which occurs only in the immediate abstinence period, from seizures that occur in the interdrinking period, long after withdrawal has been accomplished.

It is important to note that the "idiopathic" or posttraumatic forms of epilepsy are also influenced by alcohol. In patients with the latter types of epilepsy, a seizure or seizures may be precipitated by only a short period of drinking (e.g., a weekend, or even one evening of heavy social drinking); interestingly, in these circumstances, the seizures occur not when the patient is intoxicated, but usually the morning after, in the "sobering-up" period.

The EEG findings in alcoholic subjects with rum fits do not support the notion that the seizures merely represent latent epilepsy made manifest by alcohol. Instead, the EEG reflects a sequence of changes induced by alcohol itself: a decrease in the frequency of brain waves during the period of chronic intoxication; a rapid return of the EEG to normal immediately after cessation of drinking; the occurrence of a brief period of dysrhythmia (sharp waves and paroxysmal discharges) that coincides with the flurry of convulsive activity; and again, a rapid return of the EEG to normal. Except for the transient dysrhythmia in the withdrawal period, the incidence of EEG abnormalities in patients who have had rum fits is no greater than in normal persons, in sharp contrast to patients who are indeed subject to seizures (see page 260).

Delirium Tremens This is the most dramatic and grave of all the alcoholic complications. It is characterized by profound confusion, delusions, vivid hallucinations, tremor, agitation, and sleeplessness—as well as by the signs of increased autonomic nervous system overactivity, i.e., dilated pupils, fever, tachycardia, and profuse perspiration. The clinical features of delirium have been presented in detail in Chap. 19.

Delirium tremens develops in one of several settings. The patient, an excessive and steady drinker of many years' duration, may have been admitted to the hospital for an unrelated illness, accident, or operation, and 2 to 4 days later becomes delirious. Or, following a prolonged spree, the patient may have already experienced several days of tremulousness and hallucinosis, or one or more seizures, and may even be recovering from these symptoms, when delirium tremens develops, rather abruptly as a rule.

In the majority of cases delirium tremens is benign and short-lived, ending as abruptly as it begins. Consumed by the relentless activity and wakefulness of several days' duration, the patient falls into a deep sleep and then awakens lucid, quiet, and exhausted, with virtually no memory of the events of the delirious period. Somewhat less commonly, the delirious state subsides gradually. In either case, when the delirium occurs as a single episode, the duration is 72 h or less in over 80 percent of the cases. Less frequently still, there may be one or more relapses, several episodes of delirium of varying severity being separated by intervals of relative or complete lucidity—the entire process lasting for only several days or as long as 4 to 5 weeks.

Between 5 and 15 percent of cases of delirium tremens, as defined above, end fatally. In many of the fatal cases there is an associated infectious illness or injury, but in a few no complicating illness is discernible. Other patients die in a state of hyperthermia or peripheral circulatory collapse; in some, death comes so suddenly that the nature of the terminal events cannot be determined. Reports of a negligible mortality in delirium tremens can usually be attributed to a failure to distinguish between delirium tremens and the minor forms of the withdrawal syndrome, which are far more common and almost invariably benign.

Closely related to typical delirium tremens and about as frequent are the *atypical delirious-hallucinatory* or *confusional states,* in which one facet of the delirium tremens complex assumes prominence to the practical exclusion of the other symptoms. The patient may simply exhibit a transient state of quiet confusion, agitation, or peculiar behavior lasting several days or weeks. Or there may be a vivid hallucinatory-delusional state and abnormal behavior, consistent with the various false beliefs. Unlike typical delirium tremens, the atypical states usually present as a single circumscribed episode without recurrences, are only rarely preceded by seizures, and do not end fatally. This may be another way of saying that they are a partial or less severe form of the disease.

Pathologic examination is singularly unrevealing in patients with delirium tremens. Edema and brain swelling have been absent in the authors' pathologic material except when shock or hypoxia had occurred terminally. There have

been no significant light-microscopic changes in the brain, which is what one would expect in an essentially reversible disease. Abnormalities of the CSF occur unpredictably, as do CT changes, and indicate the presence of some medical or surgical complication. The EEG findings have been discussed in relation to withdrawal seizures.

Rarely, blood glucose is seriously depressed in the alcohol withdrawal states, for the reasons given above, under "Pharmacology of Alcohol." Ketoacidosis with normal blood glucose is another infrequent laboratory finding. Disturbances of electrolytes are of varying frequency and significance. Serum sodium levels are altered infrequently, and are more often increased than decreased. The same is true for chlorides and phosphate. Serum calcium and potassium were found to be lowered in about a quarter of our patients. Most patients show a hypomagnesemia, low P_{CO_2} and high arterial pH, abnormalities that are probably important in the pathogenesis of withdrawal symptoms (see below).

Pathogenesis of the Tremulous-Hallucinatory-Delirious Disorders For many years, prior to 1950, it was generally held that these symptoms represented the most severe forms of alcohol intoxication—an idea that fails to satisfy the simplest clinical logic. The symptoms of toxicity—consisting of slurred speech, uninhibited behavior, staggering gait, stupor, and coma—are in themselves distinctive and quite different from the symptom complex of tremor, fits, and delirium. The former symptoms are associated with an elevated blood alcohol level, whereas the latter become evident only when the blood alcohol is reduced. Finally, the toxic symptoms increase in severity as more alcohol is consumed, whereas tremor and hallucinosis and even full-blown delirium tremens may be nullified by the administration of alcohol.

Although much discussed in the past, there is no evidence that an endocrine abnormality (other than the aforementioned increase in norepinephrine) or nutritional deficiency plays a role in the genesis of delirium tremens and related symptoms. Instead, the illness and its symptoms are of neural origin: the parts of the nervous system (including the autonomic nervous system) that become habituated to alcohol appear to overact when it is withdrawn. The duration of the illness seems to correspond to the time required for neuronal excitability to return to normal. The lesion is a biochemical one, of obscure nature still.

It is evident, from observations in both man and experimental animals, that the most important and the one indispensable factor in the genesis of delirium tremens and related disorders is the withdrawal of alcohol, following a period of sustained chronic intoxication. Further, these observations indicate that the emergence of withdrawal symptoms depends upon a *decline* in the blood alcohol level from a previously higher level and not necessarily upon the complete disappearance of alcohol from the blood.

The mechanism(s) by which the withdrawal of alcohol produces symptoms are only beginning to be understood. In all but the mildest cases, the early phase of alcohol withdrawal (beginning 7 to 8 h after cessation of drinking) is attended by a drop in serum magnesium concentration and a rise in arterial pH—the latter on the basis of respiratory alkalosis (Wolfe and Victor). Possibly the compounded effect of these two factors, both of which are associated with hyperexcitability of the nervous system, are responsible for seizures and for other symptoms that characterize the early phase of withdrawal. As an explanation of delirium tremens, however, hypomagnesemia is probably not important, since the serum magnesium level has frequently been restored to normal before the onset of the delirium. The respiratory alkalosis can be explained by the fact that with chronic alcohol intoxication the neurons of the "respiratory center" are rendered insensitive to circulating CO_2; in the "rebound" phase these cells become more sensitive than normal to CO_2, with resultant hyperventilation and a rise in arterial pH.

Treatment of Delirium Tremens and Minor Withdrawal Symptoms

The general aspects of management of the delirious and confused patient have been described on page 332.

More specifically, the treatment of delirium tremens begins with a careful search for associated injuries (particularly head injury with cerebral lacerations or subdural hematoma), infections (pneumonia or meningitis), pancreatitis, and liver disease. Because of the frequency and seriousness of these complications, skull and chest films and a CT scan should be obtained and lumbar puncture should be performed routinely. In severe forms of delirium tremens, the temperature, pulse, and blood pressure should be recorded at 30-min intervals in anticipation of peripheral circulatory collapse and hyperthermia, which, added to the effects of injury and infection, are the usual causes of death in this disease. In the case of shock, one must act quickly, utilizing whole-blood transfusions, fluids, and vasopressor drugs. The occurrence of hyperthermia demands the use of a cooling mattress in addition to specific treatment for any infection that may be present.

An important element in treatment is the correction of fluid and electrolyte imbalance. Severe degrees of agitation and perspiration may require the administration of 6000 to 8000 mL of fluid daily, of which 1500 to 2000 mL should be normal saline solution. The specific electrolytes and the amounts in which they are added are governed by the laboratory values for these electrolytes. If the serum sodium is extremely low one must be cautious in raising the level lest a central pontine myelinolysis be induced (see

page 860). In the rare case of hypoglycemia, the administration of glucose is an urgent matter. Patients who present with severe ketoacidosis and normal or only slightly elevated blood glucose concentrations usually recover promptly, without the use of insulin.

A special danger attends the use of glucose solutions in alcoholic patients. Typically these persons have subsisted on a diet disproportionately high in carbohydrate (alcohol is metabolized almost entirely as carbohydrate) and low in thiamine, and their reserves of B vitamins may have been further reduced by gastroenteritis and diarrhea. The administration of intravenous glucose may serve to consume the last available stores of thiamine and precipitate Wernicke disease. For this reason it is good practice to add B vitamins in all cases requiring parenterally administered glucose, even though the alcoholic disorder under treatment, e.g., delirium tremens, is not primarily due to vitamin deficiency.

With respect to the use of drugs, it is important to distinguish between mild withdrawal symptoms, which are essentially benign and responsive to practically all sedative drugs, and delirium tremens, which has a serious mortality and is relatively unresponsive to drugs. In the case of minor withdrawal symptoms, the purpose of medication is to ensure rest and sleep. In delirium tremens, the object of drug therapy is to blunt the psychomotor overactivity and prevent exhaustion and to facilitate the administration of parenteral fluid and nursing care; one should not attempt to suppress agitation at all costs, since to accomplish this would require an amount of drug that might seriously depress respiration.

A wide variety of drugs is effective in controlling withdrawal symptoms. Some of the ones that have been commonly used in recent years are prochlorperazine (Compazine), chlorpromazine (Thorazine), promazine (Sparine), meprobamate, hydroxyzine (Vistaril), chlordiazepoxide (Librium), and diazepam (Valium). There is little difference in the therapeutic efficacy of these drugs. More importantly, there are very few data to indicate that any one of them can prevent hallucinosis or delirium tremens, or shorten the duration or alter the mortality rate of the latter disorder. In general, phenothiazine drugs should be avoided because they reduce the threshold to seizures. At the moment, chlordiazepoxide and diazepam are the most popular drugs for the treatment of withdrawal symptoms, although the advantages of *oral* administration of these drugs over paraldehyde have not been proved by controlled studies (see review of Gessner). Paraldehyde has the advantage of being extremely safe, provided it is dispensed in ampoules, to prevent deterioration to acetic acid. If the patient can take medication orally, doses of 8 to 12 mL in orange juice should be given. Paraldehyde is also effective when given rectally, but intramuscular and intravenous administration should be avoided. If parenteral medication is necessary, sodium phenobarbital or sodium amytal in doses of 120 mg, or haloperidol (10 mg) repeated at 3- to 4-h intervals, may be given intramuscularly (provided there is no serious liver disease); or 10 mg diazepam may be given intravenously and repeated once or twice at 20- to 30-min intervals, until the patient is calm but awake. Beta blocking agents, such as propranolol and atenolol, are helpful in reducing heart rate and blood pressure, and the tremor to some extent. Lofexidine, an alpha$_2$ agonist that blocks autonomic outflow centrally, is similarly effective. Adrenal corticotropic hormone (ACTH) and cortisone have no place in the treatment of the withdrawal syndrome. These hormones do not significantly modify the course of the abstinence syndrome. In addition, they have many serious disadvantages: the masking of infection, a deleterious effect on tuberculosis and peptic ulcer, and a tendency to produce a negative nitrogen balance and excessive excretion of potassium. All these complications are of more than theoretical interest in the alcoholic patient.

Treatment of "Rum Fits" Most cases do not require the use of anticonvulsant drugs, since there may be only a single seizure or a brief flurry of seizures that have either ceased before the patient is seen by a physician or by the time certain medicines, such as phenytoin, become effective. The parenteral administration of sodium phenobarbital early in the withdrawal period could conceivably prevent "rum fits" in patients with a previous history of this disorder or in those who might be expected to develop seizures on withdrawal of alcohol. Also, the long-term administration of anticonvulsants is not practical: if such patients remain abstinent, they will be free of seizures; if they resume drinking, they usually abandon their medicines. The rare instances of status epilepticus should be managed like status of any other type (see page 270). Alcoholics with a history of idiopathic or posttraumatic epilepsy should drink only in moderation or not at all, because of the tendency of even short periods of drinking to precipitate seizures; such patients must be maintained on anticonvulsant drugs.

NUTRITIONAL DISEASES OF THE NERVOUS SYSTEM

Alcoholism provides the ideal setting for the development of nutritional diseases of the human nervous system. While the overall incidence of alcohol-induced nutritional diseases is relatively small, these diseases assume significance because of the frequency of alcoholism. From the medical standpoint their importance relates to the fact that they are preventable and that neglect of nutrition may lead to permanent disability. These illnesses are discussed in Chap. 39, "Diseases of the Nervous System Due to Nutritional Deficiency."

DISORDERS OF UNCERTAIN PATHOGENESIS, ASSOCIATED WITH ALCOHOLISM

Also discussed in Chap. 39 are several diseases (*alcoholic cerebellar degeneration, Marchiafava-Bignami disease*) in which a nutritional-metabolic etiology seems likely but has not been established. Central pontine myelinolysis, though frequently observed in alcoholics, is more appropriately considered with the acquired metabolic disorders (Chap. 40). Certain disorders of skeletal and cardiac muscle associated with alcoholism (*alcoholic myopathy and cardiomyopathy*) are described in Chap. 49, under the acute and subacute myopathic paralyses. There remain to be discussed several diverse disorders that have been attributed to alcoholism, but whose causal relationship to alcohol abuse or to nutritional deficiency or to some other factor is not clear.

Alcoholic Dementia (Alcoholic Deteriorated State)
These terms are used by some authors to designate a supposedly distinctive form of dementia that is attributable to the chronic, direct effects of alcohol on the brain. An immediate problem with this category of alcoholic disease is definitional. The syndrome subsumed under the title of *alcoholic dementia* or its many synonyms (*alcoholic deteriorated state, chronic alcoholic psychosis, chronic brain syndrome due to alcohol*) has never been delineated satisfactorily, either clinically or pathologically. In the *Comprehensive Textbook of Psychiatry* it is defined as "a gradual disintegration of personality structure, with emotional lability, loss of control, and dementia." To other psychiatrists (Strecker et al) the alcoholic deteriorated state denotes "the common end reaction of all chronic alcoholics who do not recover from their alcoholism or do not die of some accident or intercurrent episode." Purported examples of this state show a remarkably diverse group of symptoms, including jealousy and suspiciousness; coarsening of moral fiber and other personality and behavioral disorders; deterioration of work performance, personal care and living habits; disorientation, impaired judgment, and defects of intellectual function, particularly of memory; and even certain physical manifestations, such as dilatation of facial capillaries, a "bloated look," flabby muscles, chronic gastritis, tremors, and recurrent seizures. Some early authors were apparently

impressed with similarities between the alcoholic deteriorated state and general paresis, hence the term *alcoholic pseudoparesis*. Mercifully the latter term no longer appears in medical writings.

In recent years, there have been attempts to sharpen the diagnosis of alcoholic dementia. According to Seltzer and Sherwin, patients with alcoholic dementia, in distinction to those with the Korsakoff amnesic state, have difficulty with constructional tasks and prominent behavioral disturbances. Cutting has expressed the view that the term *Korsakoff psychosis* be limited to patients with a fairly pure disorder of memory of acute onset and that patients with more global symptoms of gradual evolution be considered to have alcoholic dementia. These are rather fragile diagnostic criteria. As pointed out in Chap. 39, Korsakoff psychosis may have an insidious onset and gradual progression, and patients with this disorder, in addition to an amnesic defect, characteristically show disturbances of cognitive functions that depend little or not at all on memory. More importantly, in none of the patients designated by these authors as having alcoholic dementia was there a pathologic examination, without which the clinical assessment must remain arbitrary and imprecise.

Courville described a series of cerebral cortical changes that he attributed to the toxic effects of alcohol and considered to be the basis of the alcoholic deteriorated state and alcoholic pseudoparesis: progressive atrophy of the cortex of the frontal lobes, associated with opacity and thickening of the overlying meninges and enlargement of the lateral ventricles; swelling, pyknosis, and "pigmentary atrophy" of nerve cells; irregular loss of the smaller pyramidal cells of the superficial and intermediate laminae; and secondary degeneration and loss of nerve fibers. Some of these changes such as neuronal pyknosis are insignificant artifacts, and many of the other changes are quite nonspecific. Opacity of the meninges and moderate dilatation of the lateral ventricles, for example, are observed both in alcoholics and nonalcoholics as well as in persons who had exhibited no neurologic or psychiatric abnormalities during life. Some of the cellular changes noted by Courville may have reflected a state of hepatic failure or terminal anoxia, and others reflect nothing more than the effects of aging or artifacts of tissue fixation and staining.

In our experience, the majority of cases that come to autopsy with the label of *alcoholic dementia* or *deteriorated state* prove to have the lesions of the Wernicke-Korsakoff syndrome. Traumatic lesions of varying degrees of severity are commonly added. Other cases show the lesions of anoxic or hepatic encephalopathy, communicating hydrocephalus, Alzheimer disease, ischemic necrosis, or some other disease quite unrelated to alcoholism. Practically always, in our material, the clinical state can be accounted for by one or a combination of these disease processes, and

there has been no need to invoke a hypothetical toxic effect of alcohol on the brain. This has also been the experience of Torvik et al. With a few exceptions, such as coincidental Alzheimer disease, all their cases that had been labeled *alcoholic dementia* turned out, on neuropathologic examination, to have the lesions of chronic Wernicke disease.

We have the impression, nevertheless, that one cannot dismiss altogether the possibility of there being another disease process linked to alcoholism. What is needed to settle this matter is a more sophisticated quantitative analysis of the neuropathology of such cases.

The subjects of alcoholic dementia and so-called alcoholic cerebral atrophy (see below) are discussed in greater detail by the authors (M.V. and R.D.A.) in the *Handbook of Clinical Neurology* and in our recently published monograph on the Wernicke-Korsakoff syndrome.

"Cerebral Atrophy" in Chronic Alcoholics This disorder, like the "alcoholic deteriorated state," does not constitute a clinical-pathologic entity. To some authors (e.g., Courville, see above) the concept of alcoholic cerebral atrophy is a pathologic one, but usually this diagnosis is made on the basis of radiologic findings. The concept was derived originally from pneumoencephalographic studies. Relatively young alcoholics, some with and some without symptoms of cerebral disease, showed enlarged cerebral ventricles and widened sulci, mainly of the frontal lobes (Brewer and Perrett, Haug). Similar findings have been reported in chronic alcoholics examined by CT scanning (see review of Carlen et al).

The clinical correlates of these radiologic findings are quite unclear. In some patients, so-called cerebral atrophy is associated with an overt complication of alcoholism; we found, for example, that about one-quarter of our autopsied patients with the Wernicke-Korsakoff syndrome showed enlargement of the lateral and third ventricles and convolutional atrophy of the frontal lobes. In other patients there is a history of recurrent seizures, or evidence of liver disease, cerebral trauma, or some other event that might have resulted in ventricular enlargement. In some alcoholic individuals, however, the finding of large ventricles comes as a surprise, no symptoms or signs of neuropsychiatric disease being found in the course of the usual neurologic and mental status testing.

The term *alcoholic cerebral atrophy* implies that chronic ingestion of alcohol causes an irreversible loss of cerebral tissue, a concept to which there is serious objection. One cannot assume that dilated ventricles and sulci, observed in a single CT scan, necessarily represent an irreversible tissue loss. Such CT changes may in fact be reversible to a varying extent, as has been observed in patients with the Cushing syndrome, anorexia nervosa, Lennox-Gastaut syndrome (treated with ACTH), as well as in alcoholic patients (Carlen et al, Lishman). This reversibility would suggest that a shift of fluids had occurred in the brain (over many months), rather than loss of tissue. Until this matter has been studied further, it would be preferable to refer to the asymptomatic ventricular enlargement and sulcal widening in alcoholics as such, rather than as cerebral atrophy.

Alcoholic Paranoia and Jealousy These are outmoded terms that were used in the past to designate what was thought to be a special type of paranoid reaction in chronic alcoholics, in which the patient, usually a male, developed ideas of infidelity on the part of his wife. The delusions of jealousy that might occur acutely in the course of alcoholic intoxication or withdrawal, or chronically, as part of the "alcoholic deteriorated state," were generally not included under this rubric. The notion that pathologic jealousy merits classification as a distinctive complication of alcoholism is not warranted, since the morbid jealousy that develops in alcoholics differs in no essential way from that in nonalcoholics. Nevertheless, among individuals with the syndrome of morbid jealousy, chronic alcoholism may be an important associated factor (11 of 66 cases reported by Langfeldt). Among the alcoholic patients, the delusions of jealousy may at first be evident only in relation to episodes of acute intoxication, but later they evolve, through a stage of constant suspicion and efforts to detect infidelity, into definite morbid beliefs that persist during periods of sobriety as well.

FETAL ALCOHOL SYNDROME

That parental alcoholism may have an adverse effect on the offspring has been a recurrent theme in medical lore. The documented occurrence of such a relationship was lacking, however, until the turn of the century, when Sullivan reported that the mortality among the children of drunken mothers was more than two times greater than among children of nondrinking women of "similar stock." The increased mortality was attributed by Sullivan and later by Haggard and Jellinek to postnatal influences such as poor nutrition and chaotic home environment rather than to the intrauterine effects of alcohol. Following Sullivan's studies there appeared isolated clinical reports in which damage to the fetus was ascribed to alcoholism in the mother, but in

general this idea was rejected and relegated to the category of superstitions about alcoholism.

In recent years, the effects of alcohol abuse on the fetus have been rediscovered, so to speak. Lemoine et al, in France, and Ulleland, and Jones and Smith, in the United States, described a distinctive pattern of abnormalities in infants born of severely alcoholic mothers. The affected infants are small in length in comparison to weight, and most of them fall below the third percentile for head circumference. They are distinguished also by the presence of short palpebral fissures (probably a reflection of microphthalmia) and epicanthal folds; maxillary hypoplasia, micrognathia, and cleft palate; dislocations of the hips, flexion deformities of the fingers, and a limited range of motion of other joints; cardiac anomalies (usually spontaneously closing septal defects); anomalous external genitalia; and capillary hemangiomata. The newborn infants suck and sleep poorly, and many of them are irritable, hyperactive, and tremulous; the latter symptoms resemble those of alcohol withdrawal, except that they persist. In one series of 23 infants born to alcoholic mothers there was a neonatal mortality of 17 percent (Jones et al), and among the infants who survived the neonatal period, almost half failed to achieve normal weight, length, and head circumference or remained backward mentally to a varying degree, even under optimal environmental conditions.

The pathologic changes that underlie the fetal alcohol syndrome have been studied in a small number of cases. Clarren et al found extensive leptomeningeal neuroglial heterotopias and an obstructive hydrocephalus, probably secondary to the dense heterotopias around the brainstem. Neuronal ectopias in the cerebral white matter and agenesis of the corpus callosum were also present. Peiffer et al described a broader spectrum of malformations, including cerebellar malformations similar to those of the Dandy-Walker syndrome, schizencephaly, agenesis of the corpus callosum, and signs of arrhinencephaly.

Although the relationship of this syndrome to severe maternal alcoholism seems undoubted, the mechanism by which alcohol produces its effects is not fully understood. It is noteworthy that infants born to nonalcoholic mothers who had been subjected to severe dietary deprivation during pregnancy (during World War II) were small and often premature, but these infants did not show the pattern of malformations that characterizes the fetal alcohol syndrome. Alcohol readily crosses the placenta in humans and animals, and in the mouse, rat, chick, miniature swine, and beagle dogs, alcohol has been shown to have both embryotoxic and teratogenic effects. Thus, the evidence to date favors a toxic effect of alcohol, rather than a nutritional or genetic factor.

The critical degree of maternal alcoholism that is necessary to produce the fetal alcohol syndrome and the critical stage(s) in gestation during which it occurs are not known. The various teratogenic effects described above were estimated to have occurred between the fourth week and the sixth month of gestation, a reflection perhaps of the varying periods during gestation when the fetus was exposed to particularly high alcohol levels. Cases observed to date have occurred only in infants born to severely alcoholic mothers (many of them with delirium tremens and liver disease), who continued to drink heavily throughout their pregnancy. Data derived from the collaborative study sponsored by the National Institutes of Health indicate that about one-third of the offspring of such women have the fetal alcohol syndrome. Abel and Sokol have estimated that the worldwide incidence of the fetal alcohol syndrome is 1.9 per 1000 live births and have pronounced it to be the leading known cause of mental retardation in the western world. In addition, components of the syndrome may occur in association with heavy maternal drinking, in the absence of the fully developed fetal alcohol syndrome; these have been termed *fetal alcohol effects*, and their incidence is more difficult to determine. A current account of this subject is contained in the Sixth Special Report to the U.S. Congress on Alcohol and Health (see References).

NEUROLOGIC DISORDERS CONSEQUENT UPON ALCOHOLIC CIRRHOSIS AND PORTAL-SYSTEMIC SHUNTS

This category of alcoholic disease is discussed in Chap. 40, in connection with the acquired metabolic disorders of the nervous system.

TREATMENT OF ALCOHOL ADDICTION

Following recovery from the acute medical and neurologic complications of alcoholism, the underlying problem of alcohol dependence remains. To treat only the medical complications and to leave the management of the drinking problem to the patient alone is shortsighted. Almost always, drinking is resumed, with a predictable recurrence of medical illness. For this reason the physician must be prepared to deal with the addiction or at least to initiate treatment.

The problem of excessive drinking is formidable, but not necessarily as hopeless as it is generally made out to be. A common misconception among physicians is that specialized training in psychiatry and an inordinately large amount of time are required to deal with the addictive drinker. Actually, a successful program of treatment can be initiated by any interested physician, using the standard techniques of history taking, establishing rapport with the patient, and setting up a schedule of frequent visits, though not necessarily for prolonged periods. Useful points at

which to undertake this task are during convalescence from a serious medical or neurologic complication of alcoholism, or in relation to loss of employment, arrest, or threatened divorce. Such a crisis may help convince the patient, more than any argument presented by family or physician, that the drinking problem has reached serious proportions.

The requisite for successful treatment is total abstinence from alcohol; for all practical purposes, this represents the only permanent solution. It is generally agreed that any attempts to curb the drinking habit will fail if the patient continues to drink. There are said to be alcohol addicts who have been able to reduce their intake of alcohol and eventually to drink in moderation, but they must represent only a small proportion of the addict population. Also, it is frequently stated that alcoholics must recognize that they are alcoholics—i.e., that their drinking is beyond their control—and must express willingness to be helped. Undoubtedly there is truth in both these statements, but they should not be interpreted to mean that alcoholic patients must gain this recognition and willingness entirely on their own initiative and that they will be helped only after they do so. The physician can do a great deal to help such patients understand the nature of their problem and thus to motivate them to accept treatment. The help of family, employer, courts, and clergy should be enlisted in an attempt to convince these patients that abstinence is preferable to chronic inebriety. Alcoholic patients must be made fully aware of the medical and social consequences of continued drinking and must also be made to understand that because of some constitutional peculiarity (like that of the diabetic, who cannot handle sugar) they are incapable of drinking in moderation. These facts should be presented in much the same way as one would explain the essential features of any other disease; there is nothing to be gained from adopting a punitive or moralizing attitude. Yet patients should not be given the idea that they are in no way to blame for their illness; there appears to be an advantage in making patients feel that they are responsible for doing something about their drinking.

The prevalent belief that an alcoholic will not stop drinking under duress also requires qualification. In fact, one of the few careful studies of this matter disclosed that relatively few patients would have sought help unless pressure had been exerted by family or employer; furthermore, patients who came to the clinic under duress of this sort did just as well as those who came voluntarily.

If an earnest and sustained effort by the physician fails to convince the patient that alcohol offers a problem, it is usually impossible to modify the alcoholic tendency.

The only way to make such individuals discontinue drinking is to commit them to a psychiatric hospital or special institution for the management of alcoholism, in the hope that with forced abstinence and improvement in their physical state they will gain insight and later accept psychiatric or other forms of therapy. This type of control is most often imposed by the courts and correctional system, although not for therapeutic purposes.

On the other hand, if patients come to realize that their drinking is beyond control and that they need to do something about it, their chances of being helped are raised considerably. Indeed, under these circumstances, many persons stop drinking on their own volition for several months or years. Some of these patients, despite the best of intentions, will relapse. This should not serve as an excuse to abandon treatment; many patients have attained a state of prolonged sobriety after several false starts.

A number of methods have proved valuable in the long-term management of patients. The more important of these are rehabilitative therapy, aversion treatment, the use of Antabuse, and the participation in self-help organizations for recovery from alcoholism.

Special clinics and hospital units for the treatment of alcoholism are now widely available. The physician should be fully aware of all the community resources that are available for the management of this problem and should be prepared to take advantage of them in appropriate cases. Most inpatient programs include individual and group counseling, didactics about the illness and recovery, and family intervention. Outpatient treatment (of individuals or groups) is widely available, either from specialized facilities or from specialized therapists in general mental health facilities; family counseling is usually offered as well, and is often beneficial. Most professional alcoholism treatment in the United States includes an introduction to the methods and utilization of Alcoholics Anonymous.

The aversion treatment consists of the simultaneous administration of a drink of alcohol and an injection of emetin. The violent nausea and vomiting that ensue are intended to create in the patient a strong revulsion for alcohol. This form of treatment, as well as other types of conditioned-reflex treatment, have been employed successfully in special clinics. Most of the facilities that offer aversion treatment also incorporate the features of conventional rehabilitation therapy and support involvement with Alcoholics Anonymous as well.

Antabuse (tetraethylthiuram disulfide, disulfiram) interferes with the metabolism of alcohol, so that a patient who takes both alcohol and Antabuse accumulates an inordinate amount of acetaldehyde in the tissues, resulting in nausea, vomiting, and hypotension, sometimes pronounced in degree. It is no longer considered necessary to demonstrate these effects to patients; it is sufficient to warn them of the severe reactions that may result if they drink while they have the drug in their bodies. Treatment with Antabuse is instituted only after the patient has been sober for several days, preferably longer. It should never be given to patients with cardiac or advanced liver disease. The drug is taken each morning, or at another suitable time daily, in a dosage of 0.25 g, preferably under supervision. This form of treatment may be of particular value in the spree or periodic drinker, in whom relapse from abstinence usually represents an impulsive rather than a carefully planned or premeditated act. The patient taking Antabuse, aware of the dangers of mixing liquor and the drug, is "protected" against the impulse to drink, and this protection may be renewed every 24 h by the simple expedient of taking a pill. The willingness with which such patients accept this form of treatment also serves as a rough test of their willingness to stop drinking. Should the patient drink while taking Antabuse, the ensuing reaction is usually severe enough to require medical attention, and a protracted spree can thus be prevented. Antabuse may cause a polyneuropathy if continued over a period of months or years, but this is a rare complication.

Alcoholics Anonymous (AA), an informal fellowship of recovering alcoholics, has proved to be the single most effective force in the rehabilitation of alcoholic patients. The philosophy of this organization is embodied in their "12 steps," a series of principles for sober living that guide the patient to recovery. These steps have been adopted by analogous fellowships for recovery from other addictive states, such as compulsive overeating and gambling and dependence on narcotics. The AA philosophy stresses in particular the practice of making restitution, the necessity to help other alcoholics, trust in a higher power, the group confessional, and the belief that the alcoholic is powerless over alcohol. AA philosophy also embodies the 24-h plan, in which the alcoholic strives to be abstinent for just 1 day at a time (a concept inspired by the Sermon on the Mount), as a means of facilitating the maintenance of sobriety. Although accurate statistics are lacking, it is stated that about one-third of the members who express more than a passing interest in the program attain a state of long-sustained or permanent sobriety (Baekeland et al). While the methods used by AA are not preferred by every patient, most who persist can benefit; in particular, the physician should not accept a patient's initial negative reaction as reason to abandon AA as a mode of treatment.

Finally, it should be noted that alcoholism is frequently associated with psychiatric disease of other type, particularly sociopathy (antisocial or psychopathic personality) and affective illness. In the latter case, the prevailing mood is far more often one of depression than of mania and is more often encountered in women, who are more apt to drink under these conditions than are men. In these circumstances expert psychiatric help should be sought, preferably from someone who is also familiar with addictive diseases.

REFERENCES

ABEL EL, SOKOL RJ: Incidence of fetal alcohol syndrome and economic impact of FAS-related anomalies. *Drug Alcohol Depend* 19:51, 1987.

BACON MK: Cross-cultural studies of drinking, in Bourne PG, Fox R (eds): *Alcoholism: Progress in Research and Treatment.* New York, Academic Press, 1973, pp 171–174.

BAEKELAND F, LUNDWALL LK, KISSIN B: Methods for the treatment of chronic alcoholism: A critical appraisal, in Israel Y (ed): *Research Advances in Alcohol and Drug Problems,* vol 2. New York, Wiley, 1975, pp 247–328.

BAUD FJ, GALLIOT M, ASTIER A et al: Treatment of ethylene glycol poisoning with intravenous 4-methylpyrazole. *N Engl J Med* 319:97, 1988.

BLEULER E [Brill AA (trans)]: *Textbook of Psychiatry.* New York, Macmillan, 1930, pp 163, 342–345.

BOHMAN M: Some genetic aspects of alcoholism and criminality. *Arch Gen Psychiatry* 35:269, 1978.

BREWER C, PERRETT L: Brain damage due to alcohol consumption: An air-encephalographic, psychometric and electroencephalographic study. *Br J Addict* 66(3):170, 1971.

CADORET RJ, CAIN C, GROVE WM: Development of alcoholism in adoptees raised apart from alcoholic biologic relatives. *Arch Gen Psychiatry* 37:561, 1980.

CARLEN PL, WORTZMAN G, HOLGATE RC et al: Reversible cerebral atrophy in recently abstinent chronic alcoholics measured by computed tomography scans. *Science* 200:1076, 1978.

CARLSSON C, HAGGENDAL J: Arterial noradrenaline levels after ethanol withdrawal. *Lancet* 2:889, 1967.

CHIN JH, GOLDSTEIN DB: Drug tolerance in biomembranes: A spin label study of the effects of ethanol. *Science* 196:684, 1977.

CICERO TJ: Endocrine mechanisms in tolerance to and dependence on alcohol, in Kissin B, Begleiter H (eds): *The Biology of Alcoholism,* vol 7: *The Pathogenesis of Alcoholism.* New York, Plenum Press, 1983, pp 285–357.

CLARREN SK, ALVORD EC JR, SUMI SM et al: Brain malformations related to prenatal exposure to ethanol. *J Pediatr* 92:64, 1978.

COURVILLE CB: *Effects of Alcohol on the Nervous System of Man.* Los Angeles, San Lucas Press, 1955.

CUSHMAN P JR, FORBES R, LERNER WD, STEWART M: Alcohol withdrawal syndrome: Clinical management with lofexidine. *Alcoholism* 9:103, 1985.

CUTTING J: The relationship between Korsakov's syndrome and "alcoholic" dementia. *Br J Psychiatry* 132:240, 1978.

DAVIDSON CS: Nutrient content of beers and ales. *N Engl J Med* 264:185, 1961.

EWING JA, ROUSE BA, PELLIZZARI ED: Alcohol sensitivity and ethnic background. *Am J Psychiatry* 131:206, 1974.

GESSNER PK: Drug therapy of the alcohol withdrawal syndrome, in Majchrowicz E, Noble EP (eds): *Biochemistry and Pharmacology of Ethanol,* vol II. New York, Plenum Press, 1979, pp 375–435.

GOLDSTEIN DB: *Pharmacology of Alcohol.* New York, Oxford University Press, 1983.

GOODWIN DW, SCHULSINGER F, MOLLER N et al: Drinking problems in adopted and nonadopted sons of alcoholics. *Arch Gen Psychiatry* 31:164, 1974.

GORDON GG, ALTMAN K, SOUTHREN AL et al: Effect of alcohol (ethanol) administration on sex-hormone metabolism in normal men. *N Engl J Med* 295:793, 1976.

GROVE WM, CADORET RJ: Genetic factors in alcoholism, in Kissin B, Begleiter H (eds): *The Biology of Alcoholism,* vol 7:*The Pathogenesis of Alcoholism.* New York, Plenum Press, 1983, pp 31–56.

HAGGARD HW, JELLINEK EM: *Alcohol Explored.* Garden City, New York, Doubleday Doran, 1942.

HARRIS RA, BAXTER DM, MITCHELL MA et al: Physical properties and lipid composition of brain membranes from ethanol tolerant-dependent mice. *Mol Pharmacol* 25:401, 1984.

HAUG JO: Pneumoencephalographic evidence of brain damage in chronic alcoholics: A preliminary report. *Acta Psychiatr Scand* 203(suppl):135, 1968.

HAWLEY RJ, MAJOR JF, SCHULMAN EA et al: CSF levels of norepinephrine during alcohol withdrawal. *Arch Neurol* 38:289, 1981.

HUDSPITH MJ, BRENNAN CH, CHARLES S, LITTLETON JM: Dihydropyridine-sensitive Ca^{2+} channels and inositol phospholipid metabolism in ethanol physical dependence, in Rubin E (ed): *Alcohol and the Cell.* Annals of the New York Academy of Sciences, vol. 492. New York, 1987, p. 156.

ISBELL H, FRASER HF, WIKLER A et al: An experimental study of the etiology of "rum fits" and delirium tremens. *Q J Stud Alcohol* 16:1, 1955.

JONES KL, SMITH DW: Recognition of the fetal alcohol syndrome in early infancy. *Lancet* 2:999, 1973.

JONES KL, SMITH DW, STREISSGUTH AP, MYRIANTHOPOULOS NC: Outcome in offspring of chronic alcoholic women. *Lancet* 1:1076, 1974.

LANGFELDT G: The erotic jealousy syndrome: A clinical study. *Acta Psychiatr Neurol Scand* 36(suppl 151):7, 1961.

LEMOINE P, HAROUSSEAU H, BORTEYRU JP, MENUET JC: Les enfants de parents alcooliques: Anomalies observées à propos de 127 cas. *Ouest-Med* 25:477, 1968.

LINDENBAUM J, LIEBER CS: Hematologic effects of alcohol in man in the absence of nutritional deficiency. *N Engl J Med* 281:333, 1969.

LISHMAN WA: Cerebral disorder in alcoholism: Syndromes of impairment. *Brain* 104:1, 1981.

MELLO NK: Etiological theories of alcoholism, in Mello NK (ed): *Behavioral and Biological Research,* vol III: *Advances in*

Substance Abuse. Greenwich, CN, JAI Press, 1983, pp 271–312.

MENDELSON JH, MELLO NK: Medical progress: Biologic concomitants of alcoholism. *N Engl J Med* 301:912, 1979.

MILES WR: The comparative concentrations of alcohol in human blood and urine at intervals after ingestion. *J Pharmacol Exp Ther* 20:265, 1922.

PEIFFER J, MAJEWSKI F, FISCHBACH H et al: Alcohol embryo- and fetopathy: Neuropathology of 3 children and 3 fetuses. *J Neurol Sci* 41:125, 1979.

PORJESZ B, BEGLEITER H: Brain dysfunction and alcohol, in Kissin B, Begleiter H (eds): *The Biology of Alcoholism,* vol 7: *The Pathogenesis of Alcoholism.* New York, Plenum Press, 1983, pp 415–483.

REICH T: Biologic-marker studies in alcoholism. *N Engl J Med* 318:180, 1988.

ROEBUCK JB, KESSLER RG: *The Etiology of Alcoholism: Constitutional, Psychological, and Sociological Approaches.* Springfield, Illinois, Charles C Thomas, 1972.

ROSETT HL: A clinical perspective of the fetal alcohol syndrome. *Alcoholism Clin Exp Res* 4:119, 1980.

ROSETT HL, OUELLETTE EM, WEINER L: A pilot prospective study of the fetal alcohol syndrome at the Boston City Hospital. Part I: Maternal drinking. *Ann NY Acad Sci* 273:118, 1976.

RUBIN E (ed): *Alcohol and the Cell.* Annals of the New York Academy of Sciences, vol. 492. New York, 1987.

SAUNDERS JB: Alcohol: An important cause of hypertension. *Br Med J* 294:1045, 1987.

SCHUCKIT MA: Genetic aspects of alcoholism. *Ann Emerg Med* 15:991, 1986.

SCHUCKIT MA, WINOKUR G: Alcoholic hallucinosis and schizophrenia: A negative study. *Br J Psychiatry* 119:549, 1971.

SCOTT DF: Alcoholic hallucinosis—an aetiological study. *Br J Addict* 62:113, 1967.

SEEVERS MH: Morphine and ethanol physical dependence: A critique of a hypothesis. *Science* 170:1113, 1970.

SEGEL LD, KLAUSNER SC, GNADT JTH, AMSTERDAM EA: Alcohol and the heart. *Med Clin North Am* 68:147, 1984.

SELTZER B, SHERWIN I: Organic brain syndromes: An empirical study and critical review. *Am J Psychiatry* 135:13, 1978.

SIXTH SPECIAL REPORT TO THE U.S. CONGRESS ON ALCOHOL AND HEALTH. U.S. Department of Health and Human Services. Publication ADN 87–1519. Rockville, Maryland, 1987.

STRECKER EA, EBAUGH FG, EWALT JR: *Practical Clinical Psychiatry.* New York, McGraw-Hill, 1951, pp 150–170.

SULLIVAN WC: A note on the influence of maternal inebriety on the offspring. *J Mental Sci* 45:489, 1899.

TORVIK A, LINDBOE CF, ROGDE S: Brain lesions in alcoholics. *J Neurol Sci* 56:233, 1982.

ULLELAND C: The offspring of alcoholic mothers. *Ann NY Acad Sci* 197:167, 1972.

VICTOR M: Treatment of alcoholic intoxication and the withdrawal syndrome: A critical analysis of the use of drugs and other forms of therapy. *Psychosom Med* 28(no 4, pt 2):636, 1966.

VICTOR M: The pathophysiology of alcoholic epilepsy. *Res Publ Assoc Res Nerv Ment Dis* 46:431, 1968.

VICTOR M: The alcohol withdrawal syndrome. *Ann NY Acad Med* 215:210, 1973.

VICTOR M, ADAMS RD: The effect of alcohol on the nervous system. *Res Publ Assoc Res Nerv Ment Dis* 32:526, 1953.

VICTOR M, ADAMS RD: The alcoholic dementias, in Vinken PJ et al (eds): *Handbook of Clinical Neurology,* vol 2: *Neurobehavioral Disorders,* 2nd ed. Amsterdam, North-Holland, 1985.

VICTOR M, ADAMS RD, COLLINS GH: *The Wernicke-Korsakoff Syndrome and Other Disorders Due to Alcoholism and Malnutrition.* Philadelphia, Davis, 1989.

VICTOR M, HOPE J: The phenomenon of auditory hallucinations in chronic alcoholism. *J Nerv Ment Dis* 126:451, 1958.

WOLFE SM, VICTOR M: The relationship of hypomagnesemia and alkalosis to alcohol withdrawal symptoms. *Ann NY Acad Sci* 162:973, 1969.

WOLFE SM, MENDELSON J, OGATA M et al: Respiratory alkalosis and alcohol withdrawal. *Trans Assoc Am Physicians* 82:344, 1969.

CHAPTER 42

DISORDERS OF THE NERVOUS SYSTEM DUE TO DRUGS AND OTHER CHEMICAL AGENTS

Subsumed under this title is a diverse group of disorders of the nervous system that result from the introduction into the body of injurious or poisonous substances. In textbooks of neurology, these disorders are customarily designated as *toxic,* and the offending agents are termed *exogenous* if they are introduced from outside the body, and *endogenous* if they are generated from within—a division that cannot always be sharply drawn, as in the case of toxins of certain bacteria that have invaded the body.

The so-called endogenous bacterial toxins (e.g., those of tetanus and botulism) rank among the most powerful nervous system poisons. While few in number and relatively uncommon, they assume importance because their effects are always serious and frequently fatal. By contrast, exogenous poisons that impair nervous system function are so numerous that it would hardly be possible to mention them all, let alone to describe their actions in detail. Falling into this latter category are the myriad of household products, insecticides, industrial solvents, proprietary medicines, water and air pollutants, and other poisons with which we are surrounded in modern life. The primary effect of most of these agents is on organs and systems other than the nervous system, but practically all of them, in large enough amounts, can give rise to neurologic symptoms such as headache, drowsiness, insomnia, confusion, delirium, seizures, and coma. An important principle derives from this fact—that the sudden development of such neurologic symptoms should always raise the suspicion of poisoning.

A full understanding of neurotoxicology would involve a knowledge of the special biochemical affinities that exist between each of the many neurotoxins and the neurons and interstitial tissues of the brain, spinal cord, and nerves. These affinities are varied with respect to both their topography within the nervous system and their mechanism. Arsenic, for example, forms bonds with sulfhydryl (SH) radicals, which are abundant in the axons of peripheral nerves and the endothelial cells of capillaries in the cerebral white matter. This explains the occurrence of polyneurop-

athy and hemorrhagic leukoencephalopathy in arsenic poisoning, but the molecular pathobiology is unknown. Diphtheria toxin, which causes a delayed polyneuropathy, proves to be a polypeptide chain composed of two fragments. The so-called fragment B binds with specific surface receptors on sensitive cell membranes, whereas fragment A crosses the plasma membrane of the cell and inhibits protein synthesis by inactivating the eukaryotic translocating enzyme ("elongation factor 2"); a cofactor, nicotinamide adenine dinucleotide, must be present if the toxin is to be active. How impaired protein synthesis damages the medullated sheaths of Schwann cells in the most vascular parts of the peripheral nerve is unknown. In the myocardium the toxin decreases the rate of oxidation of long-chain fatty acids by interfering with the metabolism of carnitine.

These few examples provide a glimpse of the complexity of the mechanisms of interaction of toxins and the cells of the nervous system. The elucidation of the mode of action of the several hundred known neurotoxins promises to yield important information about the biochemical physiology of neurons and opens for study one of the most inviting fields of experimental neuropathology.

It would hardly be possible, in the confines of this chapter, to recount the clinical aspects of the many neurotoxins in any degree of completeness. A number of comprehensive references which identify their symptoms, signs, and active ingredients are listed under "General References" at the end of this chapter. An up-to-date handbook of toxicology should be part of the library of every physician.

The scope of this chapter on neurotoxicology will be somewhat limited for other reasons. The toxic effects of ethyl, methyl, amyl, and isopropyl alcohol as well as ethylene glycol are considered in Chap. 41 on alcohol, and the adverse effects of antibiotics on cochlear and vestibular function in Chap. 14. The deleterious effects of the common drugs used in the treatment of extrapyramidal motor symptoms (e.g., atropine and related belladonna alkaloids), pain and headache (salicylates), convulsive seizures, sleep disorders, psychiatric illnesses, and so forth are considered in the chapters dealing with each of these disorders. Cyanide and carbon monoxide poisoning are discussed in relation to anoxic encephalopathy (Chap. 40). The chronic administration of various therapeutic agents (e.g., disulfiram, lithium, dapsone, etc.) often damages the peripheral nerves; these drugs are considered in Chap. 46. Rarely used drugs do not justify detailed description. The following discussion will be centered on the more common categories of drugs and chemical agents that affect the nervous system selectively or predominantly. The references at the end of the chapter are listed in relation to each of these categories.

1. The addicting drugs: opiates and synthetic analgesics.
2. Sedative-hypnotic drugs
3. Antipsychotic drugs
4. Antidepression drugs
5. Stimulants
6. Psychoactive drugs
7. Bacterial toxins
8. Plant poisons, venoms, bites, and stings
9. Heavy metals
10. Industrial toxins
11. Antineoplastic agents

OPIATES AND OTHER SYNTHETIC ANALGESIC DRUGS

The opiates, strictly speaking, include all the naturally occurring alkaloids in *opium,* which is prepared from the sap of the poppy, *Papaver somniferum.* For clinical purposes, opiates refer only to the alkaloids that have a high degree of analgesic activity, i.e., morphine and codeine. Thebaine, another opium alkaloid which, like morphine, possesses a phenanthrene nucleus, has few or no analgesic properties and is therefore not ordinarily considered an opiate. The terms *opioid* and *narcotic-analgesic* designate drugs with actions similar to those of morphine. Compounds that are chemical modifications of morphine include diacetylmorphine, or heroin (now the most commonly abused opioid), hydromorphone (Dilaudid), codeine, hydrocodone (Hycodan), oxymorphone (Numorphan), and oxycodone (Percodan). A second class of opioids comprises the purely synthetic analgesics meperidine (Demerol), the meperidine derivatives anileridine (Leritine) and alphaprodine (Nisen-

til), methadone (Dolophine or Amidone), racemorphan (Dromoran), levorphanol (*l*-Dromoran), *d*-propoxyphene (Darvon), pentazocine (Talwin), diphenoxylate (the main component of Lomotil), and phenazocine (Prinadol). These synthetic analgesics are similar to the opiates, both in their pharmacologic effects and patterns of abuse, the differences being mainly quantitative. Pentazocine was originally thought to have such low addictive liabilities that it was not controlled by the federal narcotic laws. It is now a controlled substance, in the same category as the barbiturates and diazepam, and although its addictive quality is relatively low, prolonged use undoubtedly causes physical dependence. Butorphanol and the related drugs nalbuphine and buprenorphine are more recently introduced synthetic analgesics, which, like pentazocine, combine the properties of an opioid and an opioid antagonist. They have about the same analgesic effectiveness (and the same shortcomings) as pentazocine.

The clinical effects of the opioids will be considered from two points of view: (1) acute poisoning and (2) addiction.

OPIOID POISONING

Because of the high incidence of addiction, which leads to the irregular and nonmedical use of opioids, poisonings may occur. This happens as a result of ingestion or injection with suicidal intent, errors in the calculation of dosage, the use of a substitute or contaminated street product, or unusual sensitivity. Children exhibit an increased susceptibility to opioids, so that relatively small doses may prove toxic. This is true also of adults with myxedema, Addison disease, chronic liver disease, or pneumonia. Acute poisoning may also occur in addicts who are unaware that available opioids vary greatly in potency and that tolerance for opioids declines quickly after the withdrawal of the drug; upon resuming the habit, a formerly well-tolerated dose can be fatal.

Varying degrees of unresponsiveness, shallow respirations, slow respiratory rate (e.g., two to four per minute) or periodic breathing, pinpoint pupils, bradycardia, and hypothermia are the well-recognized clinical manifestations of acute opioid poisoning. In the most advanced stage the pupils dilate, the skin and mucous membranes become cyanotic, and the circulation fails. The immediate cause of death is usually respiratory depression, with consequent asphyxia. Patients who suffer a cardiorespiratory arrest are sometimes left with all the known residua of anoxic encephalopathy. Others who recover from coma may occasionally reveal a hemiplegia, presumably due to vascular occlusion. Mild degrees of intoxication are betrayed by anorexia, nausea, vomiting, constipation, and loss of sexual interest.

Treatment consists of gastric lavage if the drug was taken orally. This procedure may be efficacious many hours after ingestion, since one of the toxic effects of opioids is severe pylorospasm, which may cause much of the drug to be retained in the stomach. Other measures must be directed toward the maintenance of an adequate airway (a cuffed endotracheal tube should be inserted if the patient is comatose) and oxygenation, as described in the following section on barbiturate intoxication. If the patient does not respond rapidly to these measures, *naloxone* (Narcan) should be administered. This is a specific antidote to the opiates and also to the synthetic analgesics. It is now preferred to *N*-allylnormorphine (Nalline) because naloxone has no agonist action; hence, naloxone will not depress respiration further if the diagnosis of opiate poisoning is mistaken. The dose of naloxone is 0.7 mg per 70 kg *intravenously,* repeated if necessary once or twice at 5-min intervals. In cases of opioid poisoning the improvement in circulation and respiration is usually dramatic. In fact, failure of naloxone to produce such a response should cast doubt on the diagnosis of opioid intoxication. If an adequate respiratory response to naloxone is obtained, the patient should be observed carefully for 24 h and further doses of naloxone (50 percent higher than previously found effective) should be given *intramuscularly* as often as necessary. Naloxone has little direct effect on consciousness, however, and the patient may remain drowsy for many hours. This is not harmful, provided respiration is well maintained.

Once the patient regains consciousness, usually in about 8 h, other complaints such as pruritus, sneezing, persistent obstipation, and urinary retention may necessitate symptomatic treatment. Nausea and severe abdominal pain, due presumably to pancreatitis (from spasm of the sphincter of Oddi), are other troublesome symptoms. Antidote must be used with great caution in an addict who has taken an overdose of opioid, because in this circumstance it may precipitate withdrawal phenomena.

In addition to the toxic effects of the opioid itself, the addict is exposed to a variety of neurologic and infectious complications, resulting from the injection of contaminated adulterants (quinine, talc, lactose, powdered milk, and fruit sugars) and of various infectious agents (injections administered by unsterile methods). Amblyopia, due probably to the toxic effects of quinine in the heroin mixtures, has been reported, as well as transverse myelopathy and several types of peripheral neuropathy. The spinal cord disorder expresses itself clinically by the abrupt onset of paraplegia with a level on the trunk below which all forms of sensation are lost or impaired. Pathologically, there is an acute necrotizing lesion involving both gray and white matter over a considerable vertical extent of the thoracic and occasionally the cervical cord. In some cases a myelopathy follows the first intravenous injection of heroin after a prolonged period of abstinence. Damage to single peripheral nerves at the injection site and from compression are relatively common

occurrences. Bilateral compression of the sciatic nerves, caused by sitting for a prolonged period in the lotus position while "stoned," has been observed several times. More difficult to understand is the involvement of individual nerves, particularly of the radial nerve, and painful affection of the brachial plexus, presumably unrelated to compression and remote from the site of injections.

An acute generalized myonecrosis with myoglobinuria and renal failure has been ascribed to the intravenous injection of adulterated heroin. Brawny edema and fibrosing myopathy (the Volkmann contracture) are the sequelae of venous thrombosis resulting from the administration of heroin and its adulterants by the intramuscular and subcutaneous routes. Occasionally there may be an inexplicable and sometimes massive swelling of an extremity into which heroin had been injected subcutaneously or intramuscularly. Infection and venous thrombosis appear to be involved in its causation.

The diagnosis of drug addiction or the suspicion of this diagnosis should always encourage surveillance for infectious complications, particularly abscesses and cellulitis at injection sites, septic thrombophlebitis, hepatitis, and periarteritis. Tetanus, endocarditis (due mainly to *Staphylococcus aureus*), spinal epidural abscess, meningitis, brain abscess, and tuberculosis are found less frequently.

OPIOID ADDICTION

Just 20 years ago there were about 60,000 persons addicted to narcotic drugs in the United States, not including those who were receiving drugs because of incurable painful diseases. This represented a relatively small public health problem in comparison with the abuse of barbiturates and alcohol. Moreover opioid addiction was of serious proportions in only a few cities—New York, Chicago, Los Angeles, Washington, and Detroit. Since the late 1960s a remarkable increase in opioid (mainly heroin) addiction has taken place. The precise number of opioid addicts is not known, but was estimated by the Drug Enforcement Administration, in 1970, to be more than 600,000 (half of this number in New York City). The peak incidence of heroin dependence occurred in 1972. The incidence declined between 1972 and 1974, then increased again, and has fluctuated at peak or near peak levels since then. The prevalence and patterns of opioid abuse have been reviewed recently by Brust.

Etiology and Pathogenesis A number of factors, socioeconomic, psychologic, and pharmacologic, contribute to the genesis of opioid addiction. In our culture, the most susceptible subjects are young men or delinquent youths living in the economically depressed areas of large cities, but significant numbers are now found in the suburbs and in small cities. The onset of opioid use is usually in adolescence, with a peak at 17 to 18 years. Fully two-thirds of addicts start using the drugs before the age of 21. A disproportionately large number are American blacks and persons of Puerto Rican or Mexican descent. Almost 90 percent of addicts engage in criminal activity, often to obtain their daily ration of drugs, but most of them have a history of arrests or convictions antedating their addiction. Also many of them have psychiatric disturbances, character disorder and sociopathy being the most common. Monroe et al examined a group of 837 opioid addicts, using the Lexington Personality Inventory, and found evidence of antisocial personality in 42 percent, emotional disturbance in 29 percent, and thinking disorder in 22 percent; only 7 percent were asymptomatic. Nevertheless, the precise "personality factor" that renders one vulnerable to addiction has not been defined.

Association with addicts is the apparent explanation for beginning addiction. One addict recruits another person into addiction, and the new recruit does likewise. In this sense opioid addiction is contagious, and as a result of this pattern, heroin addiction has attained epidemic proportions. A small, almost insignificant, proportion of addicts are introduced to drugs by physicians in the course of an illness.

Opioid addiction consists of three recognizable phases: (1) episodic intoxication, or "euphoria," (2) pharmacogenic (physical) dependence, or addiction, and (3) the propensity to relapse after a period of abstinence.

Some of the symptoms of opioid intoxication have already been considered. In patients with severe pain or pain-anticipatory anxiety, the administration of opioids produces a sense of unusual well-being, a state that has traditionally been referred to as *morphine euphoria*. It should be emphasized that only a negligible proportion of such persons continue to use opioids habitually after their pain has subsided. The vast majority of potential addicts are not suffering from painful illnesses at the time they initiate opioid use, and the term *euphoria* is not an apt description of the initial effects. These persons, as indicated above, are mainly teenagers who self-administer opioids under the tutelage of their peers. They learn, after several repetitions, to recognize what they refer to as a "high," despite the subsequent recurrence of unpleasant, or *dysphoric*, symptoms (nausea, vomiting, faintness). The repeated self-administration of the drug ("reinforcement" in

the language of operant psychology) is the most important factor in the genesis of addiction. Regardless of how one characterizes the state of mind that is produced by episodic injection of the drug, the individual quickly discovers the need to increase the dose in order to obtain the original effects. Although the initial effects may not be fully recaptured, the progressively increasing dose of the drug does abate the discomfort that arises as the effects of each injection wear off. In this way a new *pharmacogenically induced need* is developed, and the use of opioids becomes self-perpetuating. At the same time a marked degree of tolerance is produced, so that enormous amounts of drugs, e.g., 5000 mg morphine daily, have eventually been administered without the development of toxic symptoms.

The classic pharmacologic criteria of addiction, as indicated in the preceding chapter on alcoholism, are tolerance and physical dependence. The latter refers to the symptoms and signs that become manifest when the drug is withdrawn, following a period of continued use. These symptoms and signs constitute a specific clinical state, termed the *abstinence syndrome*. The mechanisms that underlie the development of tolerance and physical dependence are not fully understood, although they are the subject of much interest and speculation. A large and complex literature describing agonist and antagonist receptors in specific parts of the nervous system and the isolation of endogenous opioid substances, the enkephalins and endorphins, offers new explanations of pain, tolerance, and dependence (see reviews of Wikler and of Fields).

The intensity of the opioid abstinence syndrome depends on the doses of the drug and the duration of addiction. With morphine, the majority of individuals receiving 240 mg daily for 30 days or more will show moderately severe abstinence symptoms following withdrawal. Mild signs of opiate abstinence can be precipitated by narcotic antagonists in persons who have taken as little as 15 mg morphine or an equivalent dose of methadone or heroin, three times daily for 3 days.

The abstinence syndrome that occurs in the morphine addict may be taken as the prototype of the opioid group. The first 8 to 16 h of abstinence usually pass asymptomatically. At the end of this period, yawning, rhinorrhea, sweating, and lacrimation become manifest. Mild at first, these symptoms increase in severity over a period of several hours and then remain constant for several days. The patient may be able to sleep during the early abstinence period but is restless, and thereafter insomnia remains a prominent feature. Dilatation of the pupils, recurring waves of gooseflesh, and twitchings of the muscles appear. The patient complains of severe aching in the back, abdomen, and legs and of "hot and cold flashes"; requests for blankets are frequent. By the end of about 36 h the restlessness becomes more severe, and nausea, vomiting, and diarrhea usually develop. Temperature, respiratory rate, and blood pressure are slightly elevated. All these symptoms reach their peak intensity 48 to 72 h after withdrawal, and then gradually decline. The opioid abstinence syndrome is rarely fatal (it is life-threatening only in infants). After 7 to 10 days, the clinical signs of abstinence are no longer evident, although the patient may complain of insomnia, nervousness, weakness, and muscle aches for several more weeks, and small deviations of a number of physiologic variables can be detected with refined techniques for up to 10 months (protracted abstinence).

Two types of abstinence changes are recognized—*nonpurposive* and *purposive*. The former comprise the various autonomic and neuromuscular signs already described and are relatively transient in nature. That these symptoms represent an altered physiologic state and are not psychic in origin has been clearly demonstrated experimentally. Signs of physical dependence on morphine and other opioid drugs can be induced in the lower limbs of dogs whose spinal cords have been transected; the flexor and crossed extensor spinal reflexes that are depressed or abolished by the opioid become remarkably exaggerated when the drug is withdrawn. The purposive changes refer to the patient's craving for the drug and the manipulative activity directed toward obtaining it. These symptoms may persist indefinitely and are important in relation to that characteristic of addiction referred to as *habituation, emotional dependence,* or *psychologic dependence.* These terms are used interchangeably and refer to the substitution of drug-seeking activities for all other aims and objectives in life.

Habituation, or psychologic dependence, is regarded as the most important quality of addiction, since it is this feature that fosters relapse to the use of the drug long after the nonpurposive abstinence changes seem to have disappeared. The cause for relapse is imperfectly understood. It has been theorized that fragments of the abstinence syndrome may remain as a conditioned response, and that these abstinence signs may be evoked by the appropriate environmental stimuli. Thus, when a "cured" addict is in a situation where narcotic drugs are readily available, or in a setting that was associated with the initial use of drugs, the incompletely extinguished drug-seeking behavior may reassert itself.

The characteristics of addiction and of abstinence are qualitatively similar with all drugs of the opiate group as well as the related synthetic analgesics. The differences are mainly quantitative and are related to the differences in dosage, potency, and length of action. Heroin is two to three times more potent than morphine, but the heroin withdrawal syndrome encountered in hospital practice is usually mild in degree because of the low dosage of the drug in the street product. Dilaudid and metopon are more potent than morphine and have a shorter duration of action; hence the addict requires more doses per day, and the abstinence syndrome comes on and subsides more rapidly. The length of action of racemorphan is somewhat longer than that of morphine, but withdrawal phenomena are similar. Abstinence symptoms from codeine, while definite, are less severe than those from morphine. The addiction liabilities of *d*-propoxyphene are negligible. Abstinence symptoms from methadone are less intense than those from morphine and do not become evident until 3 or 4 days after withdrawal. For these reasons methadone is used in the treatment of morphine addiction. Meperidine addiction is of particular importance because of the high incidence among physicians and nurses and because there is still a widespread belief that this drug is nonaddicting. Tolerance to the toxic effects of this drug is not complete, so that the addict may show tremors, twitching of the muscles, confusion, hallucinations, and at times convulsions. Signs of abstinence appear 3 to 4 h after the last dose and reach their maximum intensity in 8 to 12 h, at which time they may be worse than those of morphine abstinence.

Diagnosis of Addiction Diagnosis is usually made when the patient admits to using and needing drugs. Should the patient decide to conceal this fact, one must rely on collateral evidence such as miosis, needle marks, emaciation, abscess scars or chemical analyses. Meperidine addicts are likely to have dilated pupils and muscles that twitch. Several methods for testing the urine for opiates are now generally available. The finding of morphine or opiate derivatives (heroin is excreted as morphine) in the urine is confirmatory evidence that the patient has taken or has been given a dose of such drugs within 24 h of the test.

Formerly it was necessary to isolate questionable cases and to observe the patient over a period of at least 2 days for signs of abstinence. Through use of the specific morphine antagonist naloxone (Narcan), a diagnosis of addiction to opiates and related analgesic drugs can be made within an hour. The drug is given intravenously, slowly, using a syringe containing one ampul (0.4 mg). The injection is stopped when the pupils dilate and the respiratory rate increases. If, after 5 to 10 min, these or other signs of abstinence do not appear, a second injection may be given in the same way. If again the patient shows no abstinence signs, one may assume that there is no physical dependence upon opiates. Naloxone may be injected subcutaneously in the same dosage as intravenously, in which case the abstinence signs become evident within 5 min, reach their peak intensity in 20 min, begin to decline in 60 min, and disappear after 3 h. Naloxone does not precipitate abstinence symptoms in meperidine addicts unless the patient has been taking more than 1600 mg daily.

Management and Avoidance of Addiction The ambulatory treatment of addiction never succeeds and should therefore not be undertaken, except in special settings, such as a carefully supervised methadone treatment program (see below). Addicts who are refused opiates may ask for methadone, meperidine, or racemorphan on the grounds that these drugs are synthetic and nonaddicting. However, these are addicting drugs and have been legally defined as such. The physician should also be aware that to prescribe narcotics for an addict merely for the purpose of preventing abstinence symptoms is to break both the letter and the spirit of the law. Occasional exceptions may be made in cases of seriously ill addicts who are awaiting treatment in a hospital or methadone program, or of patients who are suffering from incurable, painful disease.

The method that is now used almost exclusively is to substitute methadone for opioid, in the ratio of 1 mg methadone for 3 mg morphine, 1 mg heroin, or 20 mg meperidine. Since methadone is long-acting and effective orally, it need be given only twice daily by mouth—10 to 20 mg per dose being sufficient to suppress abstinence symptoms. After a stabilization period of 3 to 5 days on this dosage of methadone alone, the dosage is reduced and the drug withdrawn over a similar period of time. An alternate method is to use clonidine, a drug that counteracts most of the noradrenergic withdrawal symptoms. Gold et al practically eliminated abstinence symptoms with doses of 5 mg/kg twice a day for a week. Hypotension may be a problem, however, and others have not found this drug to be completely effective (Jasinski et al). Regardless of the method employed, withdrawal is best carried out in an institution with proper facilities for postwithdrawal rehabilitation. Such institutions, private or municipal, are available in most large communities.

The physician must be constantly alert to the dangers of addiction, particularly in susceptible individuals, i.e., in those with unstable and antisocial personalities or alcoholism. The use of opioids should be limited to patients in whom pain is the chief problem. These drugs should not be used primarily as sedatives, for the relief of asthma, or even in patients with chronic pain until all other measures have been exhausted. It follows that it is most important to make a precise diagnosis of the cause of pain, since in some cases measures other than opioids will suffice, while in others, such as hysteria and depression, narcotics are contraindicated.

If narcotics have to be used for the relief of pain, consideration should be given to the choice of the appropriate drug and to the mode of administration. Morphine is still the drug of choice for most patients requiring relief of severe pain for short periods. Meperidine may be useful in patients who cannot tolerate morphine. Patients with chronic pain should be managed with the least potent effective drug, given in the smallest effective dosage; doses should be spaced as far apart as possible and discontinued as soon as the need for pain relief has passed. In general, opioids should be administered orally whenever possible; should parenteral administration become necessary, one must be aware of the ratio of oral to parenteral dosage required to produce equivalent analgesia. In general, also, the intravenous route should be avoided, since this method produces maximum "euphoria" and, hence, the greatest danger of addiction. The oral administration of codeine and aspirin is a useful way to begin treatment of the patient with chronic pain, since the analgesic effects of these drugs are additive. On the other hand, the analgesic effects of a narcotic in combination with diazepam or phenothiazine are not additive. If these drugs fail to control the pain, the parenteral administration of codeine should be tried. If the more potent opioids are needed, methadone and levorphanol should be used because of their effectiveness by the oral route and the relatively slow development of tolerance. Should long-continued injections of morphine or meperidine become necessary, maximum analgesic effect is obtained with 10 mg morphine rather than with 15 mg, as is often prescribed, and with 60 to 70 mg meperidine rather than with 100 mg. In such cases, the use of pentazocine (Talwin) might be considered, administered parenterally in doses of 40 to 60 mg. The respiratory depression produced by pentazocine, like that due to opioids, can be counteracted by naloxone.

Ambulatory Treatment of Opiate Addiction The most significant development in the treatment of opiate (almost exclusively heroin) addiction has been the establishment and growth of ambulatory methadone maintenance clinics. The scope of this activity, like the incidence of addiction, cannot be stated precisely, but can be judged by the fact that in 1988 nearly 100,000 former heroin addicts are participating in methadone clinics approved by the Food and Drug Administration.

The method of treatment consists of the oral administration of methadone beginning with 40 mg or less once daily and then increasing the dose to an amount sufficient to suppress the craving for heroin and to abolish the euphoria-producing effects of that drug given intravenously (heroin blockade). The daily dosage of methadone required to achieve these effects varies between 60 and 100 mg; some patients can be maintained on as little as 40 mg/day, and with higher dosage they need take the drug only once in 48 h. A longer-acting form of methadone—*l*-acetylmethadol—can be taken three or even two times weekly. In principle, these effects could be achieved by multiple daily injections of heroin or morphine, but the effectiveness of methadone orally, its prolonged duration of action, and the fact that it precludes the desire and need for taking other opioids make methadone far more practical.

Methadone is no longer dispensed in tablet form; it is given only as a liquid (dissolved in fruit juice) which is taken under supervision. The collection of urine samples is also supervised, and these are analyzed for opiates and other drugs, to monitor the patient's adherence to the program. Once this has been established, the patient is allowed to take home a 1- to 3-day supply. These measures are designed to prevent the diversion of methadone into illicit channels. Various forms of individual psychotherapy, group psychotherapy, social service counseling, and vocational guidance are included in most programs and are of great importance. The use of former heroin addicts (who are themselves in methadone treatment) as counselors is considered to be a particularly important adjunct to methadone treatment.

The results of methadone treatment are difficult to assess and vary considerably from one program to another. Even the most successful programs suffer an attrition rate of about 25 percent after several years. Of the patients who remain, between 75 and 85 percent achieve a high degree of social rehabilitation, i.e., they are gainfully employed and no longer engage in criminal behavior or prostitution. Another notable achievement of the methadone maintenance programs has been to offer an alternative mode of treatment to chronic intravenous drug abusers—one-quarter of whom are seropositive for the AIDS virus and represent the chief source of transmission of the disease to newborns and to the heterosexual nonaddicted population.

Although the effectiveness of methadone treatment in the social rehabilitation of many addicts cannot be doubted, a number of questions about this method remain. The usual practice of methadone programs is to accept only addicts over the age of 16 years, with a history of heroin addiction for at least 1 year. This leaves untreated many adolescent addicts. The number of addicts who can withdraw from methadone and maintain a drug-free existence is very small. This means that the large majority of addicts now enrolled in methadone programs are committed to an indefinite period of methadone maintenance, and the effects of such a regimen are uncertain.

An alternate method of ambulatory treatment of the opiate addict involves the use of narcotic antagonists. Cyclazocine is the best-known of these. After withdrawal of the opiate, cyclazocine is administered orally, in increasing amounts over a period of 2 to 6 weeks, until a dosage of 2 mg per 70 kg is taken twice daily. The cyclazocine-stabilized individual is highly refractory to the euphoria-producing and pharmacologic effects of opiates. The idea of treatment is to continue the administration of cyclazocine until all drug-seeking behavior is extinguished, after which it is withdrawn. Good results have been achieved with this drug, but only in small numbers of highly motivated patients. The search for improved methods of using opioid antagonists continues.

SEDATIVE-HYPNOTIC DRUGS

This class of drugs, also referred to as *depressants*, may be divided into two main groups. The first includes the barbiturates, the bromides, chloral hydrate, and paraldehyde. In the past two decades, these drugs have been largely replaced by a second group, comprising *meprobamate* and other glycerol derivatives and the *benzodiazepines*, the most important of which are chlordiazepoxide (Librium) and diazepam (Valium). The advantages of the latter sedative-hypnotic drugs are their *relatively* low toxicity and addictive potential and their minimal interactions with other drugs.

BARBITURATES

Despite the marked reduction in the medical use of barbiturates during the past 20 years, the improper use of these drugs—particularly their nonmedical and illicit use—is still an important source of suicide, accidental death, and addiction. In the past, about 50 barbiturates were marketed for clinical use, but only the following are encountered with any regularity: pentobarbital (Nembutal), secobarbital (Seconal), amobarbital (Amytal), aprobarbital (Alurate), thiopental (Pentothal), barbital (Veronal), and phenobarbital (Luminal). The first three are the ones most commonly abused. All the barbiturates are similar pharmacologically and differ only in their speed of onset and duration of action. The clinical problems posed by the barbiturates are different, however, depending on whether the intoxication is acute or chronic.

Acute Barbiturate Intoxication   This results from the ingestion of large amounts of the drug either accidentally or with suicidal intent. The latter is most frequently the act of a depressed person. The hysteric or sociopath may take an overdose as a suicidal gesture and become seriously intoxicated because of a miscalculation or ignorance of the toxic dosage. Often the drug is taken while the individual is inebriated—a dangerous situation since alcohol and barbiturate have an additive effect.

Symptoms and signs   The symptoms and signs of acute barbiturate intoxication vary with the type and the amount of drug, as well as with the length of time that has elapsed since it was ingested. Pentobarbital and secobarbital produce their effects quickly, and recovery is relatively rapid. Phenobarbital induces coma more slowly, and its effects tend to be prolonged. The duration of action of these drugs can be judged by the hypnotic effect of an average oral dose. In the case of long-acting barbiturates, such as phenobarbital, barbital, and diallylbarbituric acid, it lasts 6 h or more; with the intermediate-acting drugs, amobarbital and aprobarbital, 3 to 6 h; and with the short-acting drugs, secobarbital and pentobarbital, less than 3 h. Most fatalities follow the ingestion of secobarbital, amobarbital, or pentobarbital. The ingestion by adults of more than 3.0 g of these drugs at one time will prove fatal unless intensive and skilled treatment is applied promptly.

In regard to prognosis and treatment, it is useful to recognize three grades of severity of acute barbiturate intoxication. *Mild intoxication* follows the ingestion of approximately 0.6 g pentobarbital or its equivalent. The patient is drowsy or asleep, although readily roused if called or shaken. The symptoms resemble those of alcohol intoxication. The patient thinks slowly, and there may be mild disorientation, lability of mood, impairment of judgment, slurred speech, drunken gait, and nystagmus. Reflex activity and vital signs are not affected.

Moderate intoxication follows the ingestion of 5 to 10 times the oral hypnotic dose. Here the state of consciousness is more severely depressed and is usually accompanied by depressed or absent deep reflexes, and slow but not shallow respiration. Corneal reflexes are retained, with occasional exceptions. At times the patient can be roused by vigorous manual stimulation. When awakened, the patient is confused and dysarthric and after a few moments drifts back into stupor. At other times the patient is comatose and cannot be roused by any means. In the latter case the depth of coma and seriousness of respiratory depression may be roughly estimated by the response of respiration to the inhalation of 10% carbon dioxide or to painful stimulation such as the application of firm pressure to the sternum or supraorbital ridge. If these stimuli cause an increase in the depth and rate of respiration, the outlook for recovery is good, and only symptomatic treatment is indicated.

Severe intoxication occurs with the ingestion of 15 to 20 times the oral hypnotic dose. The patient cannot be roused by any means. Respiration is slow and shallow or irregular, and pulmonary edema and cyanosis may be present. The deep tendon reflexes are usually but not invariably absent. Most patients show no response to plantar stimulation, but in those who do, the plantar responses are extensor. In the most advanced cases the corneal and gag reflexes may also be abolished. Ordinarily the pupillary light reflex is retained in severe intoxication and is lost only if the patient is asphyxiated. In the early hours of coma, there may be a phase of rigidity of the limbs, hyperactive reflexes, ankle clonus, extensor plantar signs, and decerebrate posturing; persistence of these signs indicates a severe degree of anoxic damage. The temperature may be subnormal, the pulse thready and rapid, and the blood pressure at shock levels.

Diagnosis If a reasonable suspicion of the diagnosis exists, then a careful search for drugs or their containers may be rewarding. One should also examine the mouth and gastric contents for any characteristically colored capsules. Acute barbiturate intoxication that presents as a state of coma must be distinguished from other forms of coma by methods outlined on pages 289 and 290. Actually there are few conditions other than barbiturate intoxication that cause a flaccid coma with reactive pupils, hypothermia, and hypotension. Glutethimide poisoning may produce an identical clinical picture, except that the pupils are fixed (a parasympathomimetic action). Laryngeal spasm and sudden apnea also characterize glutethimide intoxication. In the differential diagnosis, an hysterical trance presents the main problem.

The use of gas and high pressure liquid chromatography provides a reliable means of identifying the type and amount of barbiturate in the blood. A patient who has also ingested alcohol may be comatose with relatively low blood barbiturate concentrations. Contrariwise the addicted (tolerant) patient may show only mild signs of intoxication with very high blood barbiturate concentrations.

The *EEG* may also be useful in diagnosis. In mild intoxication, the normal activity is replaced by fast activity, in the range of 20 to 30 cycles per second, and is most prominent in the frontal regions. In more severe intoxication, the fast waves become less regular and interspersed with 3- to 4-per-second slow activity. In still more advanced cases, there are short periods of suppression of all activity, separated by bursts of slow (delta) waves of variable frequency. In extreme overdosage, all electrical activity ceases. This is one instance in which a "flat" EEG cannot be equated with brain death, and the effects are fully reversible unless anoxic damage has supervened.

Management In mild or moderate intoxication, recovery is the rule, and vigorous treatment is not required. If the patient is unresponsive, special attention should be given to maintaining respiration and to the prevention of infection. It is most important to maintain a patent airway, at first by the insertion of an endotracheal tube; suctioning should be used when necessary, and the patient should be turned frequently. Tracheostomy and bronchoscopic suctioning usually become necessary if atelectasis becomes manifest, or if intubation must be maintained for longer than 72 to 96 h. If there is any risk of respiratory depression or underventilation, it is advisable to support respiration by machine. Also, early on, an intravenous fluid line should be established to promote the renal clearance of barbiturate and permit rapid administration of drugs and electrolytes.

Cases of severe respiratory depression, with cyanosis and pupillary dilatation, represent a serious medical emergency. A clear airway should be secured immediately and assisted respiration begun with a positive-pressure respirator. If the patient is in shock, the foot of the bed should be elevated, and norepinephrine and whole blood or plasma administered. Catheterization is required to determine the adequacy of urinary output, to obtain samples for laboratory examination, and to prevent distention of the bladder. Since the amount of barbiturate cleared by the kidney is directly proportional to the amount of urine formed, 8 to 10 L of 5% glucose in saline solution should be given daily. Forced diuresis is also important because toxic amounts of barbiturate have an antidiuretic effect. Coma of any significant duration requires the administration of other electrolytes as well, the amounts being governed by their serum and urinary concentrations. The occurrence of pulmonary and urinary infections calls for the use of appropriate antibiotic treatment.

Hemodialysis has proved to be an effective form of therapy and should be used in all patients with profound coma who fail to respond to the measures outlined above. It is particularly useful in cases of coma due to long-acting barbiturates and is mandatory if anuria or uremia has developed.

The treatment of severe barbiturate intoxication with analeptic drugs (Metrazol, picrotoxin, Megimide), which enjoyed a brief period of popularity, has been generally abandoned since they do not affect the rate of metabolism or the excretion of barbiturate. Alkalinization of the blood, by the use of large amounts of bicarbonate solution, as a means of mobilizing the barbiturate and increasing its rate of excretion, seems to be a useful measure, but only when phenobarbital is the responsible agent.

Occasionally, in the case of a barbiturate addict who has taken an overdose of the drug, recovery from coma is followed by the development of abstinence symptoms which have to be managed by the methods outlined below.

Chronic Barbiturate Intoxication (Barbiturate Addiction)
Chronic barbiturate intoxication, like other drug addictions, tends to develop on a background of some psychiatric disorder, most commonly depression or psychoneurosis with symptoms of anxiety and insomnia, or

so-called character disorder. Individuals with character disorders are usually introduced to the drug by associates; since the drug is taken for its intoxicating effect, the dose tends to be increased rapidly. Addiction to alcohol or to opiates may predispose such individuals to barbiturate addiction. Alcoholics find that barbiturates effectively relieve their nervousness and tremor. They may then continue to take both alcohol and barbiturate, or the barbiturate may replace the alcohol. Heroin and morphine addicts may turn to barbiturates when they are unable to obtain opiates. As with other addicting drugs, the incidence of barbiturism is particularly high in individuals with ready access to drugs, such as physicians, pharmacists, and nurses.

The toxic manifestations of chronic barbiturism are much the same as those of alcohol intoxication. The barbiturate addict thinks slowly, exhibits increased emotional lability, and becomes untidy in dress and personal habits. The neurologic signs are quite characteristic and include dysarthria, nystagmus, and cerebellar incoordination. Both the mental and neurologic signs fluctuate greatly, being more severe if the drug is taken in the fasting state and tending to increase during the day as more of the drug is ingested. If the dosage is elevated rapidly, the signs of moderate or severe intoxication become manifest.

A characteristic feature of chronic barbiturate intoxication is the development of tolerance, sometimes striking in degree. The average addict will ingest about 1.5 g of a potent barbiturate daily and will not develop signs of severe intoxication unless this amount is exceeded. Tolerance to barbiturates does not develop as rapidly as to opiates. Most persons can ingest 0.4 g daily for as long as 3 months without developing major withdrawal signs (seizures or delirium). With a dosage of 0.8 g daily for a period of 2 months, abrupt withdrawal will result in serious symptoms in the majority of patients. Even after 2 weeks at this dosage, some patients will show mild withdrawal symptoms, including anxiety, insomnia, paroxysmal EEG changes in response to photic stimulation, and rebound increase in REM sleep. Individuals taking 0.4 to 0.7 g daily fall into an intermediate category; practically all show some mental dulling and episodes of forgetfulness, and occasionally severe withdrawal symptoms may occur.

Abstinence or withdrawal syndrome Immediately following withdrawal the patient seemingly improves over a period of 8 to 12 h, as the symptoms of intoxication diminish. After this short period a new group of symptoms develops, consisting of nervousness, tremor, insomnia, postural hypotension, and weakness. With chronic phenobarbital or barbital intoxication, withdrawal symptoms may not become apparent until 48 to 72 h after the final dose. Generalized seizures with loss of consciousness may occur, usually between the second and fourth days of abstinence, occasionally as long as 6 or 7 days after withdrawal. There may be a single seizure, several seizures, or rarely, status epilepticus. The convulsive phase may be followed directly by a delusional-hallucinatory state or a full-blown delirium, indistinguishable from delirium tremens, or a varying degree of improvement may follow the seizures before the delirium becomes manifest. Death has been reported under these circumstances. The abstinence syndrome may occur in varying degrees of completeness; some patients have seizures and recover without developing delirium and others have a delirium without preceding seizures. The abrupt onset of seizures or an acute psychosis in adult life should always raise the suspicion of addiction to barbiturates or other sedative-hypnotic drugs.

The EEG shows a number of changes during chronic barbiturate intoxication and withdrawal. During chronic intoxication, the predominant pattern is one of fast activity of moderate voltage, interspersed with some 6- to 8-Hz activity chiefly in the frontal and parietal regions. On withdrawal, the fast activity diminishes and paroxysmal bursts of mixed spike and slow waves or 4-Hz "spike and dome" paroxysmal discharges appear; these may or may not be associated with seizures. Characteristically, in the withdrawal period, there is a greatly heightened sensitivity to photic stimulation, to which the patient responds with myoclonus or a seizure, accompanied by paroxysmal changes in the EEG. Most of these abnormalities disappear after 4 or 5 days and the EEG pattern is usually completely normal in 2 weeks.

Treatment of chronic barbiturate intoxication

This should always be carried out in the hospital. If the diagnosis of addiction is made before signs of abstinence have appeared, the first step should be the determination of the "stabilization dosage." This is the amount of short-acting barbiturate required to produce mild symptoms of intoxication (nystagmus, slight ataxia, and dysarthria). Usually 0.2 g of pentobarbital given orally every 6 h is sufficient for this purpose. The patient is examined 1 h after each dose. If the signs of intoxication are severe, the next scheduled dose is reduced or omitted. If, instead, tremulousness and postural tachycardia appear, an additional 0.1 g of pentobarbital is given, and the next scheduled dose is increased. This method is preferable to a blind reduction of dosage, since patients frequently underestimate the amount of drug taken. An alternate method is to stabilize the patient with phenobarbital rather than pentobarbital. The longer-acting barbiturate is safer than the shorter-acting one and permits a withdrawal that is characterized by fewer fluctuations in blood concentrations (Wesson and Smith). Then a gradual withdrawal of the drug is undertaken, 0.1 g daily, the reduction being stopped for several days if abstinence symptoms appear.

With either of these methods, a severely addicted person can be withdrawn in 14 to 21 days. Patients undergoing withdrawal treatment require careful observation for symptoms of abstinence, and special precautions have to be taken to prevent the smuggling or concealment of drugs.

The patient presenting with severe withdrawal symptoms, such as seizures, is given 0.3 to 0.5 g phenobarbital intramuscularly and then enough to maintain a state of mild intoxication. Most other anticonvulsant medicines are ineffective against barbiturate withdrawal convulsions. Withdrawal should then be carried out as indicated above. If the abstinence symptoms are not severe, it is not necessary to reintoxicate the patient, but treatment can proceed along the lines laid down for the delirious and confused patient (pages 332 and 881).

After recovery has taken place, whether from symptoms of acute or chronic intoxication, the psychiatric problem requires evaluation and an appropriate plan of therapy. Many of the considerations in the management of alcoholism are equally applicable to the patient addicted to barbiturate and to nonbarbiturate hypnotic drugs.

Barbiturate Provocation of Other Diseases At times the administration of one of the barbiturates may induce an attack of another disease. The most striking example of this is in hereditary porphyria where a severe and sometimes fatal attack of abdominal pain, psychosis, and polyneuropathy may follow the ingestion of a few capsules of secobarbital. With severe liver disease, detoxification of barbiturates may be impaired.

BROMIDES

These drugs are no longer prescribed by physicians, but are contained in certain "nerve tonics" and proprietary remedies (Nervine, Neurosine), so that cases of bromide intoxication are still encountered occasionally. Acute bromide poisoning is rare because large doses of the drug are irritating to the gastric mucosa and vomiting prevents the attainment of significant blood concentrations. Taken in smaller doses, however, bromide tends to accumulate in the body because of its slow excretion by the kidney, and toxic symptoms may appear in a matter of weeks. These symptoms are due to the bromide ion and not simply to a displacement of the chloride by the bromide ion.

The symptoms of chronic bromide intoxication range from dizziness, drowsiness, irritability, and emotional lability to a quiet confusional state, with impairment of thinking and memory and, in severe cases, to delirium and stupor and coma. Skin manifestations are often associated, taking the form usually of an acne-like eruption and less frequently of proliferative nodular lesions, resembling those of tertiary syphilis. Headache, mild conjunctivitis, gastric distress, anorexia, and constipation may be associated as well. The blood bromide concentrations and the severity of toxic symptoms do not necessarily correspond. Values of 75 mg/dL (9 meq/L) or more are considered abnormal and diagnostic of bromism, if the clinical picture suggests it. However, higher levels are sometimes well tolerated, and symptoms of bromism may persist for some days after the blood concentrations have been reduced to normal or near-normal.

Treatment consists of administering sodium chloride (at least 6 g daily, in divided doses). Ammonium chloride may be substituted if an accumulation of sodium is to be avoided and if there is no danger of an uncompensated acidosis or hepatic failure. The administration of a mercurial or thiazide diuretic serves to promote a bromide diuresis. Hemodialysis should be utilized in the most severe cases of intoxication.

CHLORAL HYDRATE

This is the oldest and one of the safest, most effective, and inexpensive of the sedative-hypnotic drugs. After oral administration, chloral hydrate is reduced rapidly to trichloroethanol, which is responsible for the depressant effects on the central nervous system. A significant portion of the trichloroethanol is excreted in the urine as the glucuronide, which may give a false-positive test for glucose.

Tolerance and addiction to chloral hydrate develop only rarely, and for these reasons it is an appropriate medication for the management of insomnia, particularly the type that is associated with depression. Poisoning with chloral hydrate is a rare occurrence and resembles acute barbiturate intoxication, except for the finding of miosis, which is said to characterize the former. Treatment follows along the same lines as for barbiturate poisoning. Death from poisoning is due to respiratory depression and hypotension; patients who survive may show signs of liver and kidney disease.

PARALDEHYDE

This is also an effective and safe hypnotic, providing that certain precautions are taken in its preparation and administration (page 881). It is particularly effective in suppressing the tremulousness, restlessness, and insomnia that characterize the early phase (6 to 60 h) of the alcohol withdrawal period and is also an effective anticonvulsant. Its uses are discussed in the chapters on epilepsy and alcoholism (pages 881 and 270.

BENZODIAZEPINES

As remarked above, the foregoing drugs have been replaced to a large extent by drugs of the *benzodiazepine group*, particularly chlordiazepoxide (Librium) and diazepam (Valium). Indeed, the benzodiazepines are the most commonly prescribed drugs in the world today. According to Hollister, 15 percent of all adults in the United States use a benzodiazepine at least once yearly and about half this number use the drug for one month or longer. The use of these agents more than doubled from 1964 to 1972, then remained stable for several years, and since the late 1970s has declined by about 20 percent.

The benzodiazepines have been used extensively for the treatment of anxiety and insomnia, and they are especially effective when the anxiety symptoms are severe. Also, they have been used to control overactivity and destructive behavior in children and the symptoms of alcohol withdrawal. Diazepam is particularly useful in the treatment of delirious patients who require parenteral medication. The benzodiazepines possess anticonvulsant properties, and the intravenous use of diazepam is an effective means of controlling status epilepticus, as described on page 270. Alprazolam may be useful in the management of mild and moderate depression, and diazepam has been used with considerable success in the management of muscle spasm in tetanus and in "stiff man" syndrome. Diazepam has been far less successful in the treatment of extrapyramidal movement disorders and dystonic spasms.

Other important benzodiazepine drugs are flurazepam, triazolam, and temazepam, which are widely used in the treatment of insomnia (see page 310) and clonazepam, which is useful in the treatment of certain types of seizures and tremor (pages 269 and 80). Lorazepam, oxazepam, and many other benzodiazepine compounds have appeared in recent years, but a clear advantage over the original ones remains to be demonstrated (Greenblatt et al).

The benzodiazepine drugs, while quite safe in the recommended and even in excessive dosages, are far from ideal. They frequently cause unsteadiness of gait and drowsiness and at times hypotension and syncope, confusion, and impairment of memory, especially in the elderly. Triazolam in particular, but also lorazepam, are the most likely to disturb memory function. Signs of physical dependence and true addiction, though relatively rare, undoubtedly occur in chronic benzodiazepine users, even in those taking therapeutic doses. The withdrawal symptoms are much the same as the ones that follow the chronic use of other sedative drugs; they may not appear until the third day after the cessation of the drug, and may not reach their peak of severity until the fifth day (Hollister). The gradual tapering of dosage, over a period of 1 to 2 weeks, in chronic benzodiazepine users minimizes the withdrawal effects (Greenblatt et al).

CARBONIC ACID DERIVATIVES

These drugs are capable of modest depressant action and are effective in relieving mild degrees of nervousness, anxiety, and muscle tension. Meprobamate (Equanil, Miltown) is the best-known member of this group. It was the first of the new antianxiety drugs, a chemical variant of the weak and ineffective muscle relaxant, mephenesin. With average doses (400 mg three or four times a day) the paient is able to function quite effectively; larger doses cause ataxia, drowsiness, stupor, coma, and vasomotor collapse.

In recent years there has been a resurgence of misuse of meprobamate, including deaths from overdosage. Also, it should be emphasized that addiction to meprobamate may occur, and if four or more times the daily recommended dose is administered over a period of weeks to months, withdrawal symptoms (including convulsions) may appear, resembling those that follow withdrawal of barbiturate in a chronically intoxicated patient. Because of this tendency to develop physical dependence and other disadvantages (serious toxic reactions and high degree of sedation), meprobamate and meprobamate-like drugs are now seldom prescribed.

OTHER SEDATIVE-HYPNOTIC DRUGS

Several other nonbarbiturate sedative drugs have the same intoxicating and addicting effects as barbiturates: glutethimide (Doriden), ethinamate (Valmid), ethchlorvynol (Placidyl), methyprylon (Noludar), methaqualone (Quaalude), and perhaps oxazepam (Serax). The toxic effects of these drugs consist of slurred speech, nystagmus, ataxic gait, drowsiness, confusion, and coma. Furthermore, if the daily dose exceeds a minimal safe range, a state of physical dependence develops and withdrawal of them precipitates symptoms—hallucinations, seizures, and delirium—indistinguishable from those of the barbiturate and alcohol withdrawal syndromes. The seriousness of the abstinence syndrome in these cases is emphasized by reports of death following withdrawal of meprobamate, methyprylon, and diazepam (Essig). In view of these observations, physicians must exercise caution in prescribing new sedative drugs which are continually being introduced and are said to possess no addicting or habit-forming properties.

The treatment of addiction to these sedatives follows the same principles that apply to the treatment of barbiturate addiction. Thus if the drug and its dosage can be determined, it should be withdrawn at the rate of one therapeutic dose per day. Should abstinence symptoms appear, the reduction in dosage is stopped for several days. If the offending drug cannot be identified, a barbiturate such as secobarbital should be administered to the point of mild intoxication and then withdrawn at a rate not to exceed 0.1 g daily. Phenytoin and phenothiazine derivatives are not effective against abstinence convulsions.

ANTIPSYCHOTIC DRUGS

In the mid-1950s, a large new series of pharmacologic agents, loosely referred to as tranquilizers, came into prominent use—mainly for the control of schizophrenia, psychotic states associated with ''organic brain syndromes,'' and certain instances of manic-depressive disease. The mechanisms by which these drugs ameliorate disturbances of thought and affect in psychotic states are poorly understood, but have been attributed to inhibition or partial blocking of postsynaptic dopamine receptors in the brain; probably the parkinsonian side effects can be attributed to this mechanism also.

There are a large number of antipsychotic drugs on the market, and no attempt will be made here to describe or even list all of them. Some have had only an evanescent popularity, and others have yet to prove their value. Chemically these compounds form a heterogeneous group; six categories are of particular clinical importance: (1) the phenothiazines, (2) the thioxanthines, (3) the butyrophenones, (4) the rauwolfia alkaloids, (5) an indole derivative, molindone (Moban), and (6) a dibenzoxazepine derivative, loxapine (Loxitane). The last two drugs, introduced more recently than the others, are about as effective as the phenothiazines in the management of schizophrenia, and their side effects are also the same; their main use is in patients who are not responsive to the older drugs or who suffer intolerable side effects from them. The antipsychotic agent, clozapine (a dibenzodiazepine derivative), attracted great interest since it appeared to be uniquely free of extrapyramidal side effects, but a marked tendency to produce hypotension and agranulocytosis has largely precluded its clinical use.

PHENOTHIAZINES

This group comprises some of the most widely used tranquilizers, such as chlorpromazine (Thorazine, Largactil), promazine (Sparine), triflupromazine (Vesprin), prochlorperazine (Compazine), perphenazine (Trilafon), fluphenazine (Permitil, Prolixin), thioridazine (Mellaril), mesoridazine (Serentil), and trifluoperazine (Stelazine). In addition to their psychotherapeutic effects, these drugs have a number of other actions, so that certain members of this group are used as antiemetics (prochlorperazine) and antihistaminics (promethazine).

The phenothiazines have had their widest application in the treatment of the psychoses (schizophrenia and to a lesser extent manic-depressive psychosis). Their use outside of psychiatry should be discouraged. Under the influence of these drugs, many patients who would otherwise be hospitalized are able to live at home and even work productively. In the hospital, the use of these drugs has greatly facilitated the care of hyperactive and combative patients.

Side effects of the phenothiazines are frequent and often serious. All of them may cause a cholestatic type of jaundice, agranulocytosis, convulsive seizures, orthostatic hypotension, skin sensitivity reactions, mental depression, and disorders of the extrapyramidal motor system. Several types of extrapyramidal symptoms have been noted in association with all of the *phenothiazine* drugs [as well as with the *butyrophenones* and, to a lesser exent, the neuroleptics *metoclopramide* (Raglen, Maxofon) and *pimozide,* which have the ability to block dopaminergic receptors]:

1. A *parkinsonian syndrome*—masked facies, tremor, generalized rigidity, shuffling gait, and slowness of movement. These symptoms appear after several weeks of drug therapy.

2. Muscle spasms and dystonia, taking the form of involuntary movements of facial muscles and protrusion of the tongue (*buccolingual* or *oral-masticatory syndrome*), dysphagia, torticollis and retrocollis, oculogyric crises, and tonic spasms of a limb (dyskinesias). These complications usually occur early in the course of administration of the drug, sometimes after the initial dose, in which case they can be improved dramatically by discontinuation of the drug and the intravenous administration of diphenhydramine hydrochloride (Benadryl).

3. An inner restlessness, a persistent shifting of the body and feet, and an inability to sit still, so that the patient paces the floor constantly (*akathisia*). This disorder often responds to oral propranolol.

4. Lingual-facial-buccal-cervical dyskinesias as well as choreoathetotic and dystonic movements of the trunk and limbs may occur as late and persistent complications of long-term therapy with phenothiazines or haloperidol (*tardive dyskinesia*). Snyder has postulated that the movements are due to hypersensitivity of dopamine receptors in the basal ganglia, secondary to prolonged blockade of the receptors by antipsychotic medication. Baldessarini and Tarsy estimate that 40 percent of patients receiving long-term antipsychotic medication develop tardive dyskinesia.

5. The *neuroleptic malignant syndrome* of catatonic rigidity, stupor, unstable blood pressure, diaphoresis and other signs of autonomic dysfunction, high serum CK values, and hyperthermia. This complication proves fatal in 20 percent of cases. Fluphenazine and haloperidol are the neuroleptics most often associated with this syndrome and are thought to act through blockade of dopamine receptors in the basal ganglia and hypothalamus.

Neuroleptic medication must be discontinued as soon as these reactions are recognized. The purely parkinsonian syndrome and acute dystonic spasms will usually improve, but the tardive dyskinesias may persist for months or years, and may be permanent. Administration of antiparkinsonian drugs of the anticholinergic type (trihexyphenidyl, procyclidine, and benztropine) may hasten the recovery from some of the symptoms. Oral, lingual, and laryngeal dyskinesias are affected relatively little by any antiparkinsonian drugs. Amantadine (Symmetrel) in doses of 50 to 100 mg thrice daily has been useful in some cases of postphenothiazine dyskinesia, and reserpine in others. Many other drugs, including deanol, baclofen, pyridoxine, choline and lecithin, have been tried in the treatment of tardive dyskinesia with uncertain results. No treatment has been uniformly successful in the authors' experience. Nevertheless, we have noted a tendency for most of the obstinate forms of tardive dyskinesia to subside slowly even after several years of unsuccessful therapy. The use of low doses of these drugs in psychotic patients and frequent use of drug holidays, especially in the more susceptible older patients, helps to prevent the development of tardive dyskinesia.

In the case of the neuroleptic malignant syndrome, dantrolene and the dopamine agonist bromocriptine (5 mg orally three times daily) have been administered with some success (see also Chap.57).

BUTYROPHENONES

These drugs (haloperidol, trifluperidol) have much the same antipsychotic effects as the phenothiazines, as well as the same side effects. Unlike the phenothiazines, they have little or no adrenergic blocking action. The butyrophenones are effective substitutes for the phenothiazines in patients who are intolerant of the latter drugs, particularly of their autonomic effects.

RESERPINE

This is the prototype of the *rauwolfia alkaloids*. It was in relation to the sedative effects of these drugs that the term *tranquilization* was used for the first time. These drugs, so effective in controlling hypertension and vasospasm, are no longer recommended for the treatment of mental disorders, except perhaps in patients who cannot tolerate phenothiazines. When given in therapeutic doses, the rauwolfia alkaloids often provoke a parkinsonian syndrome or a serious depression of mood, which may prove more troublesome than the disorder for which they were prescribed.

Meprobamate, chlordiazepoxide, and diazepam are often referred to as "minor tranquilizers," the implication being that these drugs share the antipsychotic properties of the phenothiazines. This is not the case. In fact, the minor tranquilizers resemble the barbiturates in their pharmacologic (depressant) effects, including the ability to produce tolerance and physical dependence, and are more appropriately referred to clinically as *anti-anxiety* drugs.

It hardly needs to be pointed out that the tranquilizing drugs have been much abused. This would be suspected just from the frequency with which they are being prescribed. It is stated that in the decade 1955 to 1965, 50 million patients in the United States received chlorpromazine alone. These powerful medications have specific indications, noted above, and the physician should be certain of the diagnosis before using them. The fact the tranquilizing drugs can produce tardive dyskinesia in nonpsychotic patients is reason enough not to use them for nervousness, apprehension, anxiety, mild depression, and the many normal psychologic reactions to trying environmental circumstances. These drugs are not curative, but only suppress or partially alleviate symptoms, and they should not serve as a substitute for, or divert the physician from, the use of other measures for the relief of the abnormal mental state.

ANTIDEPRESSANT DRUGS

Two classes of drugs—the monoamine oxidase (MAO) inhibitors and dibenzazepine derivatives—are particularly useful in the treatment of depression. The adjective *antidepressant,* to describe these drugs, refers to their therapeutic effect, and is used here in deference to common clinical practice. *Antidepressive* or *antidepression* drugs would be preferable, since the term *depressant* still has a pharmacologic connotation that does not necessarily equate with the therapeutic effect. For example, barbiturates and chloral hydrate are depressants in the pharmacologic sense and mood elevators or antidepressants in the clinical sense. These commonly used terms must not be confused—the one referring to a drug that reduces nervous system excitability and the other to the capacity of the drug to ameliorate the symptoms of mental depression.

MONOAMINE OXIDASE INHIBITORS

The observation that iproniazid, an inhibitor of monoamine oxidase (MAO), had a mood-elevating effect in tuberculous patients initiated a great deal of interest in compounds of this type, and led quickly to their exploitation in the treatment of depression. Iproniazid (Marsilid) proved exceedingly toxic and was soon taken off the market, as were several subsequently developed MAO inhibitors; but other drugs, much better tolerated, have become available. These include isocarboxizide (Marplan), nialamide (Niamid), phenelzine (Nardil), and tranylcypromine (Parnate), the latter two being the most frequently used. Tranylcypromine, which bears a close chemical resemblance to dextroamphetamine, has proved to be the most potent therapeutically, but it has also produced the most serious toxic effects.

The exact mode of action of the MAO inhibitors has not been determined. They have in common the ability to block the oxidative deamination of naturally occurring amines (norepinephrine, epinephrine, and serotonin), and it has been suggested that the accumulation of these neurohormonal substances is responsible for the antidepressant effect. However, many enzymes other than monoamine oxidases are inhibited by MAO inhibitors, and the latter drugs have numerous actions unrelated to enzyme inhibition. Furthermore, many agents with antidepressant effects like those of the MAO inhibitors do not inhibit monoamine oxidase. At the present time, one cannot assume that the therapeutic effect of these drugs has a direct relation to the property of MAO inhibition.

The MAO inhibitors must be dispensed with great caution and constant awareness of their potentially serious side effects. They may at times cause excitement, restlessness, agitation, insomnia, and anxiety; occasionally, with the usual dose and more often with an overdose, mania and convulsions may occur (especially in epileptic patients). Other side effects are muscle twitching and involuntary movement of an extremity, urinary retention, skin rashes, tachycardia, jaundice, visual impairment, enhancement of glaucoma, impotence, sweating, muscle spasms, paresthesias, and a serious degree of orthostatic hypotension may develop.

Patients taking MAO inhibitors must be warned

against the use of phenothiazines, CNS stimulants, dibenzazepine derivatives (see below), and also sympathomimetic amines and tyramine, since the combination of an MAO inhibitor and any of these drugs may induce severe hypertension, atrial and ventricular arrhythmia, pulmonary edema, stroke, and even death. Sympathomimetic amines are contained in some of the commonly used nasal sprays, nose drops, and in so-called coryza tablets and in tyramine-containing cheeses, yogurt, beer, and wine. Exaggerated responses to the usual dose of meperidine (Demerol) and other narcotic drugs have also been observed; respiratory function may be depressed to a serious degree, and hyperpyrexia, agitation, and pronounced hypotension may occur as well, sometimes with fatal issue. Unpredictable side effects may also accompany the simultaneous administration of barbiturates and MAO inhibitors.

DIBENZAZEPINE DERIVATIVES (TRICYCLIC ANTIDEPRESSANTS)

Soon after the first successes with MAO inhibitors, a new class of tricyclic compounds appeared. The first was imipramine (Tofranil), which was soon followed by amitriptyline (Elavil), and then by desipramine (Norpramin) and nortriptyline (Aventyl). The first two members of this group have proved to be the most popular. Another important dibenzazepine derivative is carbamazepine (Tegretol), which is widely used in the treatment of lancinating pains (page 150), seizures (page 268), and depression. In recent years a number of new antidepression drugs has been introduced. Included are variants of the conventional tricyclic drugs (amoxapine), tetracyclics (maprotiline), bicyclics (zimelidine) and others (trazodone, buproprion, nomifensine). An account of these drugs, which cannot be attempted here, will be found in Hollister's monograph. Of importance is that none of these so-called second generation drugs has established a clear advantage over the conventional ones.

The exact mode of action of these agents is not established, but there is evidence that they block the reuptake of amine neurotransmitters. Blocking this amine pump mechanism (which ordinarily terminates synaptic transmission) permits the persistence of neurotransmitter substances in the synaptic cleft. Such a mechanism supports the hypothesis that endogenous depression is due to a deficiency of noradrenergic or serotonergic transmission.

The so-called tricyclic antidepressants are presently the most effective drugs for the treatment of patients with depressive illnesses, particularly those with retarded depressions, associated with hyposomnia, early morning awakening, and decreased appetite and libido. After the drug is stopped, the pharmacologic effects persist for only a short time, in comparison with the MAO inhibitors, and their side effects are far less frequent and serious.

The tricyclic or dibenzazepine compounds are potent anticholinergic agents, accounting for their most prominent and serious side effects—orthostatic hypotension and urinary bladder weakness. They may also produce CNS excitement, leading to insomnia, agitation, and restlessness, but usually these effects are controlled readily by the use of phenothiazines or chlordiazepoxide given concurrently or in the evenings. Occasionally they may cause ataxia and blood dyscrasias. The dibenzazepine drugs should never be given with an MAO inhibitor, as indicated above; serious reactions have allegedly occurred when small doses of imipramine were given to patients who had discontinued the MAO inhibitor one week previously. It is common for the intoxicated patient to have taken several drugs, in which case chemical analyses are particularly helpful in determining the drugs involved and in sorting out therapeutic and toxic concentrations. Finally it needs to be repeated that both the MAO inhibitors and the tricyclic antidepressants are extremely dangerous drugs when taken in excess. They are a frequent cause of accidental poisoning and a favorite instrument of depressed patients for committing suicide.

LITHIUM

The discovery of the therapeutic effects of lithium salts in mania has led to its widespread use in the treatment of manic-depressive disease (Chap. 56). The drug has proved relatively safe and blood levels are easily monitored. Its value is much more certain for the treatment and prevention of mania and hypomania than for anxiety and depression.

With blood levels of lithium in the upper therapeutic range, it is not uncommon to observe a fast-frequency action tremor or asterixis. Above a level of 1.5 meq/L serious intoxication becomes manifest—clouding of consciousness, confusion, delirium, dizziness, nystagmus, ataxia, stammering, and diffuse myoclonic twitching. The clinical state may at times resemble that of Creutzfeldt-Jakob disease, but there is no probem in diagnosis if the time frame of the disease and the administration of lithium are known. At a level of 3.5 meq/L, these symptoms are replaced by stupor and coma, sometimes with convulsions, and may end fatally.

Discontinuing the administration of lithium in the intoxicated patient, which is the initial step in therapy, does not result in the immediate recession of symptoms. This may be delayed by a week or two. Fluids, sodium chloride, aminophylline, and acetazolamide promote its excretion.

Lithium coma may require hemodialysis, which has proved to be the most rapid means of reducing the blood lithium concentration.

STIMULANTS

Drugs that act primarily as CNS stimulants have a relatively limited therapeutic use but assume clinical importance for other reasons. Some members of this group, e.g., the amphetamines, are much abused, and others are not infrequent causes of poisoning.

AMPHETAMINE (BENZEDRINE)

This drug and its *d* isomer, dextroamphetamine, are powerful analeptics and in addition have significant hypertensive, respiratory-stimulant, and appetite-depressant effects. They are useful in the management of narcolepsy, but have been much more widely and indiscriminately used for the control of obesity and the abolition of fatigue. Undoubtedly, they are able to reverse fatigue, postpone the need for sleep, and elevate mood, but these effects are not entirely predictable and certainly not indefinite, and the user must pay for the period of wakefulness with even greater fatigue and often with depression. The intravenous use of a high dose of amphetamine produces an immediate ecstasy, "the flash."

Because of the popularity of the amphetamines and ease with which they can be procured, instances of acute and chronic intoxication are observed frequently. The toxic signs are essentially an exaggeration of the analeptic effects—restlessness, excessive speech and motor activity, tremor, and insomnia. In severe cases, hallucinations, delusions, and changes in affect and thought processes may occur, a state that may be indistinguishable from paranoid schizophrenia. Other complications of chronic intoxication—amphetamine vasculitis and intracerebral and subarachnoid hemorrhage—have been the subject of numerous articles (Harrington et al). The pathogenesis of the vascular lesion is unknown.

Chronic use of amphetamines can lead to a high degree of tolerance and psychologic dependence. Withdrawal of the drug, after sustained oral or intravenous use, is regularly followed by a period of prolonged sleep (a disproportionate amount of which is REM sleep), from which the patient awakens with a ravenous appetite, muscle pains, and profound fatigue and depression.

Treatment consists of discontinuing the use of amphetamine and administering antipsychotic drugs. Nitrites may be useful if the blood pressure is markedly elevated.

METHYLPHENIDATE (RITALIN)

This drug has much the same type of action as dextroamphetamine and is useful in the treatment of narcolepsy. Paradoxically, like amphetamine, it is useful in the management of hyperactive children.

CAFFEINE

The therapeutic value of caffeine and other xanthine derivatives stems from their diuretic effect and their ability to stimulate the heart and nervous system. The major use of these agents is to abolish fatigue and maintain wakefulness, and the usual mode of administration is in coffee, a cup of which contains 100 to 150 mg of caffeine. Overdosage leads to insomnia, mild delirium, tinnitus, tachycardia, prominent diuresis, and cardiac arrhythmias. Caffeine and theophylline are frequently used in premature neonates to combat apnea, presumably through their stimulant effects on the respiratory center. These drugs are reasonably safe if used in small dosage; the excitatory, diuretic, and hyperglycemic effects are easily controlled and fatalities due to caffeine poisoning are extremely rare.

OTHER STIMULANTS

A number of nervous system excitants, much used in the past, are now of little interest, either as therapeutic agents or as causes of accidental poisoning. The use of *picrotoxin* in patients with coma due to barbiturates and other sedatives was abandoned long ago, because of its tendency to produce seizures. The use of *pentylenetetrazol* (*Metrazol*) which once served as the convulsive agent in the "shock treatment" of depression and schizophrenia, has been discontinued, even for experimental purposes. The same is true for bemegride and nikethamide (Coramine), which were used as cardiorespiratory stimulants. The incidence of *strychnine* poisoning, of some significance in past years, is now negligible; strychnine never had any therapeutic value.

Camphor (camphorated oil), formerly a popular stimulant, is now rarely used therapeutically; however, occasional cases of poisoning are still seen as a result of ingestion of liniment or moth flakes. The manifestations of poisoning are headache, sensation of warmth, confusion, clonic convulsions, and terminal respiratory depression; the characteristic odor of camphor facilitates the diagnosis. Treatment consists of supportive care and the cautious use of barbiturates to control convulsions.

PSYCHOACTIVE DRUGS

Included in this category is a heterogeneous group of drugs, the primary effect of which is to alter perception, mood, and thinking out of proportion to other aspects of cognitive function and consciousness. This group of drugs comprises *lysergic acid derivatives* [e.g., lysergic acid diethylamide (LSD)], *phenylethylamine derivatives* (mescaline or peyote), *psilocybin,* certain *indolic derivatives, cannabis* (marijuana), *phencyclidine* (PCP) and a number of less important compounds. They are also referred to as *psychotomimetic* or *psychotogenic drugs,* hallucinogens, illusogens, and psychedelics—but none of these names is entirely suitable. The problem of the nontherapeutic use of these drugs, which is less than before but still of serious proportions, has been reviewed by Nicholi.

Tolerance to LSD, mescaline, and psilocybin develops rapidly, even on a once-daily dosage. Furthermore, subjects tolerant to any one of these three drugs are cross-tolerant to the other two. Tolerance is lost rapidly when the drugs are discontinued abruptly, but no characteristic signs of physical dependence (abstinence syndrome) ensue. In this sense, addiction does not develop, although users may become dependent upon them for emotional support (psychologic dependence or habituation).

MARIJUANA

The effects of *marijuana,* when taken by inhaling the smoke from cigarettes, are prompt in onset and evanescent. In low doses the symptoms are like those of mild intoxication wth alcohol (drowsiness, euphoria, dulling of the senses, and perceptual distortions). With increasing amounts, the effects are similar to those of LSD, mescaline, and psilocybin (see below), and they may be quite disabling for many hours. With even larger doses, severe depression and stupor may occur, but death is unusual.

In the case of marijuana, *reverse tolerance* (i.e., increasing sensitization) may be observed initially, but on continued use, tolerance to the *euphoriant* effects of the drug has been observed. In one of the few chronic experimental studies that have been made, the subjects reported "jitteriness" during the first 24 h after abrupt cessation of marijuana cigarette smoking, although no objective withdrawal signs could be detected.

COCAINE

The conventional use of cocaine as a local anesthetic has for many years been overshadowed by its illicit and widespread use as a stimulant and mood elevator. Originally, cocaine was sold as a white lactose-adulterated powder that was usually administered intranasally ("snorting"); less often it was smoked or injected intravenously or intramuscularly. Since 1985 there has been an alarming escalation in the use of cocaine, mainly because a relatively pure and inexpensive form of the drug ("free-base" or "crack") became readily available at that time. This form of cocaine is heat-stable and therefore suitable for smoking. In 1985, it was estimated that about 5 million persons in the United States used cocaine regularly and that with each passing day an additional 5000 persons used it for the first time (Cregler and Mark).

A sense of well-being, euphoria, loquacity, and restlessness are the familiar effects. Pharmacologically, cocaine is thought to act like the tricyclic antidepressants; i.e., it blocks the presynaptic reuptake of biogenic amines, thus producing vasoconstriction, hypertension, and tachycardia, and predisposing to generalized tremor, myoclonus, seizures, and psychotic behavior. These actions as well as its mood-elevating and euphoric effects are similar to, but briefer than, those of dextroamphetamine (page 904). As with marijuana, the cocaine abuser readily develops psychologic dependence or habituation, i.e., an inability to abstain from frequent compulsive use ("craving"). The manifestations of physical dependence are more subtle and difficult to recognize. Nevertheless, abstinence from cocaine, following a period of chronic abuse, is regularly attended by insomnia, restlessness, anorexia, depression, hyperprolactinemia, and signs of dopaminergic hypersensitivity—a symptom complex that constitutes an identifiable withdrawal syndrome.

With the increasingly widespread use of cocaine, a variety of new complications continue to emerge. The symptoms of severe intoxication, noted above, may lead to coma and death and require emergency treatment in an intensive care unit, along the lines indicated for the management of barbiturate coma. Seizures in this setting are treated more effectively with benzodiazepines than with standard anticonvulsant drugs. Several instances of myocardial infarction, spontaneous subarachnoid hemorrhage, and cerebral infarction have followed the intranasal use and smoking of cocaine; these complications are presumably the result of vasospasm, induced by the sympathomimetic actions of cocaine. Roth and his colleagues have described 39 patients who developed acute rhabdomyolysis after cocaine use; 13 of these patients had acute renal failure, severe liver dysfunction, and disseminated intravascular coagulation, and 6 of them died. Some recent reports indicate that cocaine use during pregnancy may cause fetal damage or abortion, or persistent signs of toxicity in the newborn infant.

Paranoia and other manifestations of cocaine psychosis are best treated with haloperidol.

MESCALINE, LSD, AND PSILOCYBIN

These drugs produce much the same clinical effects if given in comparable amounts. The perceptual changes are the most dramatic: the user describes vivid visual hallucinations, alterations in the shape and color of objects, unusual dreams, and feelings of depersonalization. An increase in auditory acuity has been described, but auditory hallucinations are rare. Cognitive functions are difficult to assess because of inattention, drowsiness, and inability to cooperate in mental testing. The somatic symptoms consist of dizziness, nausea, paresthesias, and blurring of vision. Sympathomimetic effects—pupillary dilation, piloerection, hyperthermia, and tachycardia—are prominent, and the user may also show hyperreflexia, incoordination of the limbs, and ataxia.

LSD is not an approved drug, and the use of marijuana is governed by the federal narcotic laws. Nevertheless, these drugs are very widely used. They are taken by narcotic addicts as a temporary substitute for more potent drugs; by "drug heads," i.e., individuals who use practically any agent that alters consciousness; and by many troubled, unhappy college and high school students, often for reasons that they cannot ascertain. The unsupervised use of these drugs is attended by a number of serious adverse reactions taking the form of acute panic attacks; long-lasting psychotic states resembling paranoid schizophrenia; *flashbacks* (spontaneous recurrences of the original LSD experience, often precipitated by smoking marijuana and accompanied by panic attacks); or by serious physical injury, consequent upon impairment of the user's critical faculties. Whether prolonged usage leads to permanent damage to the nervous system is not certain; there are some data suggesting that this may happen. The reports claiming that LSD may cause chromosomal damage remain to be validated.

PHENCYCLIDINE (PCP, "ANGEL DUST")

During the past decade the abuse of phencyclidine or its many analogues has become a significant problem, since these drugs are relatively cheap, easily available, and quite powerful. PCP is used legally as an animal immobilizing agent and illicitly as a granular powder, frequently mixed with other drugs, that is smoked or snorted. PCP is usually classified as a hallucinogen, although it also has stimulant and depressant properties. The effects of intoxication are like those of LSD and other hallucinogens and resemble those of an acute schizophrenic episode, which may last several days to a week or more. PCP will be present in the blood and urine after ingestion of a large amount (10 mg or more) for only a few hours. Its manufacture was stopped in 1979.

The fact that small quantities of these drugs can produce gross mental aberrations has stimulated the search for similar endogenous substances that may be responsible for schizophrenia and other psychoses. The mechanisms involved in producing and antagonizing the *psychotomimetic* effects are also being studied intensively, in the hope of elucidating the mechanisms of the psychoses and finding improved psychotherapeutic agents. Numerous claims have been made that LSD and related drugs are effective in the treatment of mental disease and a wide variety of social ills and that they have the capacity to increase one's intellectual performance, creativity, and self-understanding. At this time, there are no acceptable studies that validate any of these claims.

A discussion of the legal implications of the illicit use of the aforementioned drugs and their social impact is beyond the scope of this chapter, but can be found in the appended references.

DISORDERS DUE TO BACTERIAL TOXINS

The most important diseases in this category are tetanus, botulism, and diphtheria. Each is caused by an extraordinarily powerful bacterial toxin that acts primarily upon the nervous system. Other bacterial toxins, e.g., ammonium and other amines, which are produced in the colon by the action of urease-splitting organisms and are thought to be responsible for hepatic encephalopathy, are more appropriately considered with the metabolic disorders.

TETANUS

The cause of this disease is the anaerobic, spore-forming rod, *Clostridium tetani*. The organisms are found in the feces of some humans and many animals, particularly horses, whence they readily contaminate the soil. The spores may remain dormant for many months or years, but when they are introduced into a wound, especially if a foreign body or suppurative bacteria are present, they are converted into their vegetative forms, which produce the exotoxin *tetanospasmin*. In underdeveloped countries, tetanus is still a common disease, particularly in newborns in whom the spores are introduced via the umbilical cord (*tetanus neonatorum*). In the United States, injection of contaminated heroin is a significant cause of tetanus. About two-thirds of all injuries leading to tetanus occur in the home and about 20 percent in gardens and on farms. In the

United States, the incidence rate of tetanus is about one case per million of population per year.

Since 1903, when Morax and Marie proposed their theory of centripetal migration of the tetanus toxin, it has been taught that spread to the nervous system occurs via the peripheral nerves, the toxin ascending in the axis cylinders or the perineural sheaths. Modern studies, utilizing fluorescein-labeled tetanus antitoxin, have disclosed that the toxin is also widely disseminated via blood or lymphatics, probably accounting for the generalized form of the disease. However, in local tetanus, direct neural spread seems probable.

Mode of Action of Tetanus Toxin This is not fully understood, but is analogous to that of strychnine. The toxin interferes with the function of the reflex arc by suppressing spinal and brainstem inhibitory neurons. In tetanus, the elicitation of the jaw jerk, for example, is not followed by the usual abrupt suppression of motor neuron activity, which is manifested in the electromyogram as a "silent period." There appears to be a failure of this normal inhibitory mechanism, with a resulting increase in activation of the neurons that innervate the masseter muscles (*trismus*). Of all neuromuscular systems the masseter innervation seems to be the most sensitive to the toxin, and in the monkey it is the only muscle to be affected. Not only do afferent stimuli produce an exaggerated effect, but they also abolish reciprocal innervation; both agonists and antagonists contract, giving rise to the characteristic muscular spasm. In addition to its generalized effects on the motor neurons of the spinal cord and brainstem, there is evidence that the toxin acts directly on skeletal muscle at the point of injection or entrance into the organism, accounting perhaps for the localization of signs of tetanus intoxication. The toxin is also thought to act at the cerebral cortical level and upon the sympathetic nervous system, in the hypothalamus.

The incubation period varies greatly, from a day or two to a month or even longer. Long incubation periods are associated with mild and localized types of tetanus.

Clinical Features There are several clinical types of tetanus, generally designated as local, cephalic, and generalized.

Local tetanus This is the most benign form. The initial symptoms are stiffness, tightness, and pain in the muscles in the neighborhood of a wound, followed by twitchings and brief spasms of the affected muscles. Local tetanus occurs most often in relation to a wound of the hand or forearm, or in the abdominal or paravertebral muscles after an operation. Gradually, some degree of continuous involuntary spasm becomes evident. This is referred to as *rigidity, hypertonic contractions,* or *tetanic*

spasticity, terms that denote the sustained tautness of the affected muscles and the resistance to passive movement. Superimposed on this background of more or less continuous motor activity are brief intense spasms, lasting from a few seconds to minutes, and occurring "spontaneously" or in response to all variety of stimulation. Early in the course of the illness there may be periods when the affected muscles are palpably soft and appear to be relaxed. A useful diagnostic maneuver at this stage is to have the patient perform some repetitive voluntary movements, such as opening and closing the hand, in response to which there occurs a gradual increase in the tonic contraction and spasms of the affected muscles, followed by spread of the spasms to neighboring muscle groups (*recruitment spasm*). The phenomenon resembles paradoxical myotonia (see page 1163). Even with mild localized tetanus there may be a slight trismus, a useful diagnostic sign.

Symptoms may persist in localized form for several weeks or months. Gradually the spasms become less frequent and more difficult to evoke, and they finally disappear without residue. Complete recovery is to be expected, since there are no pathologic changes in muscles, nerves, spinal cord, or brain, even in the most severe generalized forms of tetanus.

Cephalic tetanus This form of tetanus follows wounds of the face and head. The incubation period is short, 1 or 2 days as a rule. The affected muscles (most often the ocular and facial) are weak or paralyzed. Nevertheless, during accessions of tetanic spasm, the palsied muscles are seen to contract. Apparently the disturbance in the facial motoneurons is sufficient to prevent voluntary movement but insufficient to prevent the strong reflex impulses that elicit facial spasm. The spasms may involve the tongue and throat, with persistent dysarthria, dysphonia, and dysphagia. In a strict sense these cephalic forms of tetanus are examples of local tetanus that frequently become generalized. Many cases prove fatal.

Generalized tetanus This is the most common form. It may begin as local tetanus which after a few days becomes generalized, or it may be diffuse from the beginning. Trismus is frequently the first manifestation. In some cases this is preceded by a feeling of stiffness in the jaw or neck, slight fever, and other general symptoms of infection. The localized muscle stiffness and spasms spread quickly to involve other bulbar musculature, as well as muscles of the neck, trunk, and limbs. A state of unremitting rigidity develops in all the involved muscles: the abdomen is board-like, the legs are rigidly extended, and the lips are pursed or retracted (risus sardonicus); the eyes are partially closed by contraction of the orbicularis oculi or the eyebrows are elevated by spasm of the frontalis. Superimposed on this persistent state of enhanced muscle activity are paroxysms of tonic contraction or spasm of muscles (tetanic seizures or convulsions), which occur spontaneously or in response to the slightest external stimulus. They are agonizingly painful. Consciousness is not lost during these paroxysms. The tonic contraction of groups of muscles results in opisthotonus or in forward arching of the back, flexion and adduction of the arms, clenching of the fists, and extension of the legs. Spasms of the pharyngeal, laryngeal, or respiratory muscles carry the constant threat of apnea or suffocation. Fever and pneumonia are common complications. Death is usually attributable to asphyxia or heart failure, the result of constantly recurring spasms, or to circulatory collapse, the result of action of the toxin on the sympathetic nervous system.

Diagnosis This is made from the clinical features and a history of preceding injury. The latter is sometimes disclosed only after careful questioning, the injury having been trivial and forgotten. The organisms may or may not be recovered from the wound by the time the patient is seen by the physician, and other laboratory tests are of little value. Tetany, the spasms of strychnine poisoning (identical to tetanic spasms), trismus due to painful conditions in and around the jaw, the dysphagia of rabies, hysterical spasms, rigidity and dystonic spasms caused by neuroleptic drugs, and the spasms of the "stiff man" syndrome—all resemble the spasms of tetanus but should not be difficult to distinguish when all aspects of these disorders are considered.

The death rate from tetanus is about 50 percent overall; it is highest in newborns, heroin addicts, and in patients with the cephalic form of the disease. The patient usually recovers if there are no severe convulsions during the course of the illness or if the muscle spasms remain localized.

Treatment This needs to be directed along several lines. At the outset, a single dose of antitoxin (3000 to 6000 units of tetanus-immune human globulin) should be given, and a 10-day course of penicillin (1.2 million units of procaine penicillin daily) or tetracycline (2 g daily) is begun. Both of these drugs are effective against the vegetative forms of C. tetani. Immediate surgical treatment of the wound (excision or debridement) is imperative, and the tissue around the wound should be infiltrated with antitoxin.

Tracheostomy is a requisite in all patients with recurrent tonic convulsions, and should not be delayed until apnea or cyanosis has occurred. The patient must be kept as quiet as possible. This requires a darkened, isolated room, the judicious use of sedation, and expert and constant nursing care. Short-acting barbiturates (secobarbital or pentobarbital) in combination with chlorpromazine are the most useful drugs. Paraldehyde is an excellent medication, if it can be taken by mouth. The aim of drug therapy is to suppress muscle spasms and to keep the patient drowsy but rousable. All treatments and manipulations should be kept to a minimum; they should be carefully planned and coordinated, and the patient should be sedated beforehand.

Failure of these measures to control the tetanic paroxysms demands that all muscle activity be abolished by the use of d-tubocurarine, given intramuscularly in doses of 15 mg hourly, for as long as necessary, breathing being maintained entirely by a positive-pressure respirator.

From all that has been said, the importance of prevention of tetanus is evident. All persons should be immunized and receive a booster dose of toxoid every 10 years. Injuries that carry a threat of tetanus should be treated by an injection of toxoid if the patient has not received a booster injection in the preceding year, and a second dose of toxoid should be given 6 weeks later. If the injured person has not received a booster injection since the original immunization, he or she should receive an injection of both toxoid and human antitoxin; the same applies to the injured person who has never been immunized. An attack of tetanus does not confer permanent immunity, and all persons who recover should be actively immunized.

DIPHTHERIA

Diphtheria, an acute infectious disease caused by *Corynebacterium diphtheriae,* is now quite rare in the United States and western Europe. The faucial form of the disease, which is the most common clinical type, is characterized by the formation of an inflammatory exudate of the throat and trachea, and from this site the bacteria elaborate an exotoxin, which affects the heart and nervous system in about 20 percent of cases.

The involvement of the nervous system follows a predictable pattern. It begins locally, with *palatal paralysis* (nasal voice, regurgitation, and dysphagia) between the fifth and twelfth days of illness. At this time, or shortly afterward, other cranial nerves (trigeminal, facial, vagus, and hypoglossal) may also be affected. *Ciliary paralysis* with loss of accommodation and blurring of vision appears usually in the second or third week. Very rarely the extraocular muscles are involved. The cranial nerve signs may clear without further involvement of the nervous system, or a sensorimotor polyneuropathy may develop between the fifth and eighth weeks of the disease. The latter varies in severity, from a mild, predominantly distal affection of the limbs to a rapidly evolving, ascending paralysis of the Guillain-Barré type. The neuropathic symptoms progress for a week or two, and if the patient does not succumb to respiratory paralysis or cardiac failure (cardiomyopathy), they stabilize and then improve slowly and completely.

The early bulbar symptoms, the unique ciliary paralysis, and the subacute evolution of a delayed symmetrical sensorimotor peripheral neuropathy distinguish diphtheritic from all other forms of polyneuropathy. The long latency between the initial infection and the involvement of the nervous system has no clear explanation. Experimentally it has been shown that the toxin reaches the Schwann cells in the most vascular parts of the peripheral nervous system within 24 to 48 h of infection, but its metabolic effect on cell membranes extends over a period of weeks.

The source of diphtheritic infection may be extrafaucial—a penetrating wound, skin ulcer, or umbilicus. All the systemic and neurologic complications of faucial diphtheria may be observed in the extrafaucial form of the disease, after a similar latent period. It is probable, therefore, that the toxin reaches its neural site via the bloodstream; but in addition some action is exerted locally, as evidenced by palatal paralysis in faucial cases and by initial weakness and sensory impairment in the neighborhood of the infected wound.

There is no specific treatment for any of the neurologic complications of diphtheria. It is generally agreed that the administration of antitoxin within 48 h of the earliest symptoms of the primary diphtheritic infection lessens the incidence and severity of complications.

The polyneuropathy of diphtheria is discussed further in Chap. 46.

BOTULISM

Botulism is a rare form of food-borne illness, caused by the exotoxin of *Clostridium botulinum*. Outbreaks of poisoning are more often due to home-preserved than to commercially canned products, and vegetables are incriminated more commonly than any other food product. Although the disease is ubiquitous, five western states (California, Washington, Colorado, New Mexico, and Oregon) account for more than half of all reported outbreaks in the United States.

It is now well established, on the basis of observations both in animals and man, that the primary site of action of botulinus toxin is at the neuromuscular junction, more specifically on the presynaptic endings. The toxin interferes with the release of acetylcholine quanta, by a mechanism that is not fully understood. The defect is similar to the one that characterizes the myasthenic syndrome of Lambert-Eaton (page 1159), but different from that of myasthenia gravis.

Symptoms usually appear within 12 to 36 h of ingestion of the tainted food. Anorexia, nausea, and vomiting occur in some patients, not in others. As a rule, blurred vision and diplopia are the initial neural symptoms; their association with ptosis, strabismus, and extraocular muscle palsies may suggest a diagnosis of myasthenia gravis early in the illness. In many cases of botulism, however, the pupils are dilated and unreactive. Other symptoms of bulbar involvement—vertigo, deafness, nasality of the voice and hoarseness, dysarthria, and dysphagia—follow in quick succession, and these in turn are followed by progressive weakness of muscles of the neck, trunk, and limbs. Tendon reflexes are lost in cases of severe weakness. These symptoms and signs evolve rapidly, over 2 to 4 days as a rule, and may be mistaken for those of polyneuritis of the Guillain-Barré type. Sensation remains intact, however, and the spinal fluid shows no abnormalities. Severe constipation is characteristic of botulism, due perhaps to paresis of smooth muscle of the intestine. Consciousness is retained throughout the illness, unless severe degrees of anoxia develop. Until 1950, the death-to-case ratio was consistently above 60 percent, but it has declined since then, due probably to improvements in the intensive care of acute respiratory failure and the effectiveness of *C. botulinum* antitoxins.

The clinical diagnosis can be confirmed by electrophysiologic studies. Improvement, in patients who recover, begins within a few weeks, first in ocular movement, then in other cranial nerve function. Complete recovery of paralyzed limb and trunk musculature may take many months. Outbreaks of a neonatal and infantile form of the disease have been reported.

The three types of botulinus toxin, A, B, and E, cannot be distinguished by their clinical effects alone, so that the patient should receive the trivalent antiserum as soon as the clinical diagnosis is made. This antitoxin can be obtained from the Centers for Disease Control, in Atlanta. An initial dose of 10,000 units is given intravenously after intradermal testing for sensitivity to horse serum, followed by daily doses of 50,000 units intramuscularly, until improvement begins.

Guanidine hydrochloride (50 mg/kg) has reportedly been useful in reversing the weakness of limb and extraocular muscles. Actually, antitoxin and guanidine have changed the course of the illness relatively little: recovery, in the final analysis, depends upon the effectiveness of respiratory care, maintenance of fluid and electrolyte balance, prevention of infection, etc.

POISONING DUE TO PLANTS, VENOMS, BITES, AND STINGS

ERGOTISM

Ergotism is the name applied to poisoning with ergot, a drug derived from the rye fungus, *Claviceps purpurea*. Ergot is used therapeutically to control postpartum hemorrhage due to uterine atony; one of its alkaloids, ergotamine, is the drug of choice in the treatment of migraine. Chronic overdosage of the drug is the usual cause of ergotism; in the past, ingestion of bread made from contaminated flour was a common source of chronic poisoning. Acute overdosage in the postpartum state may cause an alarming rise in blood pressure.

Two types of ergotism are recognized: *gangrenous*, due to a vasospastic, occlusive process in the small arteries of the extremities, and *convulsive,* or *neurogenic*. The latter is characterized by fasciculations, myoclonus, and spasms of muscles, followed by seizures. In nonfatal cases, a tabes-like neurologic syndrome may develop, with loss of knee and ankle jerks, ataxia, and loss of deep and superficial sensation. The pathologic changes are said to consist of degeneration of the posterior columns, the dorsal roots, and peripheral nerves, but they are poorly described. The relation of these changes to ergot poisoning is also not clear, since most of the cases have occurred in areas in which malnutrition was endemic.

LATHYRISM

Lathyrism is a neurologic syndrome characterized by the relatively acute onset of pain, paresthesias, and weakness in the lower extremities, progressing to a permanent spastic paraplegia. It is a serious medical problem only in India and in some North African countries, and is probably due to a toxin contained in the chickling pea, *Lathyrus sativus,* a legume that is consumed in excess during periods of famine. This disorder is discussed more fully with the spinal cord diseases (page 747).

MUSHROOM POISONING

The gathering of wild mushrooms, a popular pastime in late summer and early fall, always carries with it the danger of poisoning. As many as one hundred species of mushrooms are poisonous. Most of them cause only transient gastrointestinal symptoms, but certain ones elaborate toxins that can be fatal. The most important of these toxins are the cyclopeptides, which are contained in several species of *Amanita phalloides* and account for more than 90 percent of fatal mushroom poisonings. These toxins disrupt RNA metabolism, causing hepatic and renal necrosis. Symptoms of poisoning with *Amanita* usually appear between 10 and 14 hours after ingestion, and consist of nausea, vomiting, colicky pain and diarrhea. On the second to fourth day there may be temporary recovery, which is followed by renal shutdown, convulsions and coma.

Other important toxins are methylhydrazine (contained in the *gyromitra* species) and muscarine (*inocybe* and *clitocybe* species). The former gives rise to a clinical picture much like that caused by the cyclopeptides. The symptoms of muscarine poisoning, which appear within minutes or an hour or two, are essentially those of parasympathetic stimulation—miosis, lacrimation, salivation, nausea, vomiting, diarrhea, perspiration, bradycardia, and hypotension. Tremor, seizures, and delirium occur in cases of severe poisoning.

The mushroom toxins have no effective antidotes. If vomiting has not occurred, it should be induced with ipecac, following which activated charcoal should be administered orally, in order to bind what toxin remains in the gastrointestinal tract. A local poison control center may help identify the poisonous mushroom and its toxin.

VENOMS, BITES, AND STINGS

These are relatively rare but nonetheless important causes of mortality in the United States. The venoms of certain species of snakes, lizards, spiders, and scorpions contain neurotoxins that may cause a fatal depression of respiration and curare-like failure of neuromuscular transmission. Ticks, while engorging, may inject a neurotoxin that has similar effects. The serious effects of *Hymenoptera* stings (bees, wasps, hornets, and fire ants) are due mainly to hypersensitivity and anaphylaxis. These are discussed in detail in *Harrison's Principles of Internal Medicine.*

From a neurologic point of view the most notable disorder that follows tick bite is what has come to be known as *Lyme disease*—so named for the Connecticut community in which it was discovered. The causative agent is a spirochetal organism, *Borrelia burgdorferi,* which is transmitted by the tick *Ixodes dammini*. The disorder is discussed fully with other infectious diseases in Chap. 32 (page 580).

HEAVY METALS

LEAD

Lead Poisoning in Children The causes and clinical manifestations of lead poisoning are quite different in children and adults.

In the United States, the disease occurs most often in 1- to 3-year-old children who inhabit the urban slum areas where old, deteriorated housing prevails. (Lead paint was used in most houses built before 1940 and in many built before 1960). The chewing of leaded paint, the most common sources of which are window sills and painted plaster walls, and the compulsive ingestion of these nonfood items (pica) are the important factors in the causation of lead poisoning. The development of an acute encephalopathy is the most serious complication, leading to death in 5 to 20 percent of cases and to neurologic and mental disturbances in more than 25 percent of survivors.

Clinical Manifestations These develop over a period of 3 to 6 weeks. The child becomes anorectic, less playful and alert, and more irritable. These symptoms may be misinterpreted as a behavior disorder or mental retardation. Intermittent vomiting, vague abdominal pain, clumsiness, and ataxia may be added. If these early signs of intoxication are not recognized and the child continues to ingest lead, more flagrant signs of acute encephalopathy may develop—most frequently in the summer months, for reasons that are not understood. Vomiting becomes more persistent, apathy progresses to drowsiness and stupor, interspersed with periods of hyperirritability, and finally coma and seizures supervene. This syndrome evolves in a period of a week or less, and most rapidly in children under 2 years of age; in older children, recurrent and less severe episodes are more likely to occur. This clinical syndrome must be distinguished from tuberculous meningitis, viral meningoencephalitis, and other causes of acute increased intracranial pressure. It follows that lumbar puncture should be done only if it is essential for diagnosis and with the utmost caution. Usually, in lead encephalopathy, the CSF pressure is increased and there is an increase of lymphocytes and protein but glucose values are normal.

The brains of children who die of acute lead encephalopathy show massive swelling and herniation of the temporal lobes and cerebellum, multiple ischemic foci in the cerebrum and cerebellum, and endothelial damage and deposition of proteinaceous material and mononuclear inflammatory cells around many of the small blood vessels.

Diagnosis Since the symptoms of plumbism are nonspecific, the diagnosis depends upon an appreciation of the causative factors, a high index of suspicion, and certain laboratory tests. The presence of *lead lines* at the metaphyses of long bones and basophilic stippling of red cells are too inconstant to be relied upon, but basophilic stippling of bone marrow normoblasts is uniformly increased. Impairment of heme synthesis, which is exquisitely sensitive to the toxic effects of lead, results in the increased excretion of urinary coproporphyrin (UCP) and of δ-aminolevulinic acid (ALA).

These urinary indexes and the blood lead concentrations bear only an imperfect relationship to the clinical manifestations. In the test for UCP, which is readily performed in the clinic and emergency room, a few milliliters of urine are acidified with acetic acid and shaken with an equal volume of ether. If coproporphyrin is present, the ether layer will reveal a reddish fluorescence under a Wood's lamp. This test is strongly positive when the whole blood concentration of lead exceeds 80 μg/dL. The diagnosis can be confirmed by promoting the lead excretion with calcium disodium edetate (CaNa$_2$ EDTA), three doses (25 mg/kg) at 8-h intervals. Excretion of over 500 μg in 24 h is indicative of plumbism. The measurement of zinc protoporphyrin (ZPP) in the blood is another reliable means of determining the presence and degree of lead exposure. The binding of erythrocyte protoporphyrin to zinc occurs when lead impairs the normal binding of erythrocyte protoporphyrin to iron. Elevated ZPP can also occur when access to iron is limited by other conditions such as iron deficiency anemia.

At blood lead concentrations of 70 μg/dL, symptoms may be minimal, but acute encephalopathy may occur abruptly and unpredictably, and the child should be hospitalized for chelation therapy. Some children with a blood lead level of 50 μg/dL may have symptoms of severe encephalopathy, whereas others may be asymptomatic. In the latter case, an attempt should be made to discover and remove the source of lead intoxication and the child should be reexamined at frequent intervals. The seriousness of lead encephalopathy in children is indicated by the fact that of those who become stuporous or comatose most remain mentally retarded despite treatment. The physician's aim, therefore, is to institute treatment before the severe symptoms of encephalopathy have become manifest.

The plan of therapy includes the following:

1. Establishment of urinary flow, following which intravenous fluid therapy is restricted to basal water and electrolyte requirements.

2. Combined chelation therapy with 2,3-dimercaptopropanol (BAL) and CaNa$_2$ EDTA for 5 to 7 days in cases of acute encephalopathy. This is followed by a course of oral penicillamine. Once the absorption of lead has stopped, chelating agents remove lead only from soft tissues and not from bone, where most of the lead is stored. Any intercurrent illness that causes demineralization results in a mobilization of lead into the soft tissues and an exacerbation of symptoms of lead intoxication.

3. Repeated doses of mannitol for relief of cerebral edema.

4. Microcytic hypochromic anemia is treated with iron, once the chelating agents have been discontinued.

5. Seizures are best controlled with intravenous diazepam.

Prevention   The prevention of reintoxication demands that the child be removed from the source of lead. While this is axiomatic, it is often difficult to accomplish, despite the best efforts of local health departments and hospital and city social workers. Nevertheless, an attempt to correct the environmental factor must be made in each case. Such attempts, among many other factors, have resulted in a marked decrease in the incidence of acute lead encephalopathy in the past decade. Although florid examples of this encephalopathy are now uncommon, undue exposure to lead (blood levels > 30 μg/dL) remains inordinately prevalent and a continuing source of concern to public health authorities. Mass screening has disclosed elevated blood levels in 2 percent of the general population, higher in children than in adults, and much higher (12.2 percent) in black children and in urban children from low income families, both black and white (Mahaffey et al). The clinical significance of these elevated levels remains uncertain. Rutter has presented evidence that persistent blood levels above 40 μg/dL may cause slight cognitive impairment and, less certainly, may increase the risk of developing behavioral difficulties.

Lead Intoxication in Adults   This is much less common than in children. The hazards to adults are exposure to dust of inorganic lead salts and to fumes resulting from the burning of lead or processes that require the remelting of lead. Painting, printing, pottery glazing, lead smelting, and storage battery manufacturing are the industries in which these hazards are likeliest to occur. Miners and brass foundry and garage workers (during automobile radiator repair, when soldered joints are heated) are the ones most at risk.

Intoxication with tetraethyl and tetramethyl lead, used as additives in gasoline, presents a special problem. It is caused by inhalation of gasoline fumes and has occurred most often in workers who clean gasoline storage tanks. Insomnia, irritability, delusions, and hallucinations are the usual clinical manifestations, and a maniacal state may develop. The hematologic abnormalities of inorganic lead poisoning are not found and chelating agents are of no value in treatment. Organic lead poisoning is usually reversible, but fatalities have been reported. The pathologic changes have not been well described.

The usual manifestations of lead poisoning in adults are colic, anemia, and peripheral neuropathy. Encephalopathy is decidedly rare; usually it results from consumption of illicit liquor contaminated by lead solder in the pipes of stills. Lead colic, frequently precipitated by an intercurrent infection or by alcohol intoxication, is characterized by severe, poorly localized abdominal pain, often with rigidity of abdominal muscles. There is no fever or leukocytosis. The pain responds to the intravenous injection of calcium salts, at least temporarily, but very little to morphine. Mild anemia is common. A black line of lead sulfide may develop along the gingival margins. Peripheral neuropathy, usually a bilateral wrist drop, is a rare manifestation and is discussed in Chap. 46.

The diagnostic tests for plumbism in children are generally applicable to adults, with the exception of bone films, which are of no value in adults. Also the treatment of adults with chelating agents follows the same principles as in children.

ARSENIC

In the past, medications such as Fowler's solution (potassium arsenite) and the arsphenamines, used in the treatment of syphilis, were frequent causes of intoxication, but now it is most commonly the result of the suicidal or accidental ingestion of herbicides, insecticides or rodenticides containing copper acetoarsenate (Paris green) or calcium or lead arsenate. In rural areas, arsenic-containing insecticide sprays are a common source of poisoning. Arsenic is used also in the manufacture of paints, enamels, and metals, and as a disinfectant for skins and furs and also in galvanizing, soldering, etching and lead plating. Occasional cases of poisoning are reported in relation to these occupational hazards.

Arsenic exerts its toxic effects by reacting with the sulfhydryl radicals of certain enzymes necessary for cellular metabolism. The effects on the nervous system are those of an encephalopathy or peripheral neuropathy. The latter may be the product of chronic poisoning, or may become manifest between 1 and 2 weeks after recovery from the acute effects. It takes the form of a distal axonopathy and is described in Chap. 46.

The symptoms of encephalopathy (headache, drowsiness, mental confusion, delirium, and convulsive seizures) may also occur as part of acute or chronic intoxication. In the latter case, they are accompanied by weakness and muscular aching, hemolysis, chills and fever (in patients exposed to arsine gas), mucosal irritation, a diffuse scaly desquamation, and transverse white (Mees) lines, 1 to 2 mm in width, above the lunula of each fingernail. Acute poisoning by the oral route is associated with severe gastrointestinal symptoms, with circulatory collapse and death in a large proportion of patients. The CSF is normal.

Examination of the brain in such cases discloses numerous punctate hemorrhages in the white matter. Microscopically the lesions consist of pericapillary zones of degeneration, which in turn are ringed by red cells (*brain purpura* or *encephalorrhagia*, incorrectly referred to as hemorrhagic encephalitis). These neuropathologic changes are not specific for arsenical poisoning, but have been observed in such diverse conditions as pneumonia, gram-negative bacillary septicemia from urinary tract infections, sulfonamide and phosgene poisoning, dysentery, disseminated intravascular coagulation, and others.

The diagnosis of arsenical poisoning depends upon the demonstration of increased levels of arsenic in the hair and urine. Arsenic is deposited in the hair within two weeks of exposure and may remain fixed there for years. Concentrations of more than 0.1 mg arsenic per 100 mg hair are indicative of poisoning. Arsenic also remains within bones for long periods and is slowly excreted in the urine and feces. Excretion of more than 0.1 mg arsenic per liter of urine is considered abnormal; levels greater than 1 mg/L may occur soon after acute exposure. The CSF protein level may be raised (50 to 100 mg/dL).

Acute poisoning is treated by gastric lavage, vasopressor agents, BAL, maintenance of renal perfusion, and exchange transfusions if massive hemoglobinuria occurs. Once polyneuropathy has occurred, it is little affected by treatment with BAL, but other manifestations of chronic arsenical poisoning respond favorably. There is gradual recovery from the polyneuropathy.

MANGANESE

Manganese poisoning results from the chronic inhalation and ingestion of manganese particles and occurs in miners of manganese ore and in workers who separate manganese from other ore. Several clinical syndromes have been observed. The initial stages of intoxication may be marked by a prolonged confusional-hallucinatory state. Later, the symptoms are predominantly of extrapyramidal type, resembling those of postencephalitic parkinsonism: impassive facies; drooling; faint, monotonous, dysarthric speech; stiffness and awkwardness of the limbs, often with tremor of the hands; "cogwheel" phenomenon and gross rhythmic movements of the trunk and head; and retropulsive and propulsive gait. Corticospinal and corticobulbar signs may be added. Progressive weakness, fatigability, and sleepiness are other prominent clinical features. Rarely, severe axial rigidity and dystonia, like those of Wilson disease, are the outstanding manifestations.

Neuronal loss and gliosis, affecting mainly the pallidum and striatum, but also the frontoparietal and cerebellar cortex and hypothalamus, have been described, but the pathologic changes have not been carefully studied.

The neurologic abnormalities have not responded to treatment with chelating agents. In the chronic "dystonic form" of manganese intoxication, dramatic and sustained improvement has been reported with the administration of L-dopa; patients with the more common "parkinsonian type" of manganese intoxication have shown only slight improvement with L-dopa.

MERCURY

Chronic mercury poisoning, particularly with methyl mercury compounds, gives rise to a wide array of serious neurologic symptoms, including tremors of the extremities, tongue, and lips; mental confusion; and a progressive cerebellar syndrome, with ataxia of gait and of the arms, intention tremor, and dysarthria. Choreoathetosis and parkinsonian facies have also been described. Changes in mood and behavior are prominent, consisting at first of weakness and fatigability and later of extreme depression and lethargy alternating with irritability. The pathologic changes are characterized by neuronal loss and gliosis of the calcarine cortex and to a lesser extent of other parts of the cortex and a striking degeneration of the granular layer of the cerebellar cortex, with relative sparing of the Purkinje cells.

This form of poisoning occurs in persons exposed to large amounts of the metal used in the manufacture of thermometers, mirrors, incandescent lights, x-ray machines, and vacuum pumps. Since mercury volatizes at room temperature, it readily contaminates the air and then condenses on the skin and respiratory mucous membranes. Nitrate of mercury, used in the manufacture of felt hats, and phenyl mercury, used in the paper, pulp, and electrochemical industries, are other sources of intoxication.

The presence of mercury in industrial waste has contaminated many sources of water supply and fish, which are ingested by humans and cause mercurial poisoning. So-called Minamata disease is a case in point. Between 1953 and 1956, a large number of villagers living near Minamata Bay in Kyushu Island, Japan, were afflicted with a syndrome of chronic mercurialism, probably due to the ingestion of fish that had been contaminated with industrial wastes containing methyl mercury. Concentric constriction of the visual fields, hearing loss, cerebellar ataxia, postural and action tremors and sensory impairment of the legs and arms, and sometimes of the tongue and lips, were the usual clinical manifestations. Pathologically there was diffuse neuronal loss in both cerebral and cerebellar cortices, most marked in the anterior parts of the calcarine cortex and granule cell layer of the cerebellum. CT scans in survivors, years after the mass poisoning, disclosed bilaterally symmetric areas of decreased attenuation in the visual cortex and diffuse atrophy of the cerebellar hemispheres and vermis, especially the inferior vermis (Tokuomi et al).

In the treatment of chronic mercury poisoning, *N*-acetyl-*dl*-penicillamine is probably the drug of choice, since it can be administered orally and appears to chelate mercury selectively, with less effect on copper, which is an essential element in many metabolic processes.

ORGANOPHOSPHATES

Nervous system function may be deranged as part of acute and usually fatal poisoning with inorganic phosphorous compounds (found in rat poisons, roach powders, and matchheads). More important clinically is poisoning with organophosphorous compounds, the best known of which is triorthocresyl phosphate (TOCP).

Organophosphates are widely used as insecticides. Since 1945, approximately 15,000 individual compounds have come into use. Certain ones, such as tetraethylpyrophosphate, have been the cause of major outbreaks of neurologic disorder, especially in children. These substances have an acute anticholinesterase effect but no delayed action. Chlorophos, which is a 1-hydroxy-2,2,2-trichlorethylphosphonate, has in addition a delayed action, as does TOCP.

The immediate anticholinesterase effect is manifested by headache, vomiting, sweating, abdominal cramps, salivation, wheezing secondary to bronchial spasm, miosis, and muscular weakness and twitching. Most of these symptoms can be reversed by atropine and pralidoxine. Some of the patients suffer a delayed effect, 2 to 5 weeks following acute organophosphorus insecticide poisoning. This takes the form of a distal symmetric sensorimotor (predominantly motor) neuropathy, progressing to atrophy. Recovery occurs to a variable degree and then, in patients poisoned with TOCP, signs of corticospinal damage become detectable. The severity of paralysis and its permanence vary with the dosage of TOCP.

In addition to the acute and delayed neurotoxic effects of organophosphorus, an intermediate syndrome has been described (Senanayake and Karalliedde). Symptoms come on 24 to 96 h after the acute cholinergic phase and consist of weakness or paralysis of proximal limb muscles, neck flexors, motor cranial nerves, and respiratory muscles. Respiratory paralysis may prove fatal. In patients who survive, the paralytic symptoms last for 2 to 3 weeks, and then subside. The intermediate and delayed symptoms do not respond to atropine or other drugs.

Several striking outbreaks of TOCP poisoning have been reported. During the latter part of the prohibition era and to a lesser extent thereafter, outbreaks of so-called jake paralysis were traced to the drinking of an extract of Jamaica ginger that had been contaminated with TOCP. Another was in Morocco, in 1959, when lubricating oil containing TOCP was used deliberately to dilute olive oil. Other outbreaks have been caused by the ingestion of grain and cooking oil that had been stored in inadequately cleansed containers previously used for TOCP.

The experimental studies of Cavanagh and Patangia in the cat revealed a dying back from the terminal ends of the largest and longest medullated motor nerve fibers, including those from the muscle spindles (annulospiral endings). The long fiber tracts of the spinal cord showed a similar dying-back phenomenon. Abnormal membrane bound vesicles and tubules were observed by Prineas to accumulate in axoplasm before degeneration. These effects have been traced to the inhibitory action of TOCP on esterases. Johnson found that one of three enzymes that hydrolyzed phenylphenacetate was always inhibited by TOCP. There is still uncertainty as to the details of these reactions, and no treatment for the prevention or control of the neurotoxic effects has been devised.

THALLIUM

In the late nineteenth century, thallium was used medicinally in the treatment of venereal disease, ringworm, and tuberculosis and in rodenticides and insecticides. Poisoning was fairly common. Sporadic instances of poisoning still occur, usually as a result of accidental or suicidal ingestion of thallium-containing rodenticides, rarely, from overuse of depilatory agents. Patients who survive the effects of acute poisoning develop a rapidly progressive and painful sensorimotor polyneuropathy, optic atrophy, and occasionally ophthalmoplegia—followed, 15 to 30 days after ingestion, by diffuse alopecia. The latter feature should always suggest the diagnosis of thallium poisoning, which can be confirmed by finding the drug in the urine. The use of potassium chloride by mouth may hasten thallium excretion.

OTHER METALS

Iron, antimony, zinc, barium, bismuth, copper, silver, gold, platinum and lithium may all produce serious degrees of intoxication. The major manifestations in each case are gastrointestinal or renal, but certain neurologic symptoms—notably headache, irritability, confusional psychosis, stupor, coma, and convulsions—may be observed in cases of profound poisoning, often as terminal events.

Gold preparations, which are still used occasionally in the treatment of arthritis, may, after several months of treatment, give rise to focal or generalized myokymia and a rapidly progressive, symmetrical polyneuropathy (Katrak et al). The adverse effects of *platinum* are discussed below, with the antineoplastic agents. *Lithium* has been discussed above (page 903).

Attention has already been drawn to the possible causative role of *aluminum intoxication* in so-called dialysis dementia or encephalopathy (page 857) and in Alzheimer disease (page 927). Removal of aluminum from the water used in renal dialysis has practically eliminated dialysis dementia. Also the deionization of the dialysate has had a salutary effect on the special types of osteomalacia and anemia that complicate renal dialysis and are thought to be due to aluminum intoxication. However, the neuropathology of experimental aluminum intoxication (see below) is not that of dialysis dementia. The causative role of aluminum toxicity in Alzheimer disease is less convincing. Neurofibrillary tangles have been produced in animals by the intrathecal injection of aluminum, but these tangles differ ultrastructurally from those of Alzheimer disease. Whether there is an increase of aluminum in the brains of patients with Alzheimer disease is still a matter of disagreement. Perl and his colleagues have reported the accumulation of aluminum in tangle-bearing neurons of patients with Alzheimer disease and guamanian Parkinson-dementia-ALS complex; the significance of these findings remains to be determined.

Organic compounds of *tin* may seriously damage the nervous system. Diffuse edema of the white matter of the brain and spinal cord has been produced experimentally with *triethyltin*. Presumably this was the basis of the mass poisoning produced by a triethyltin-contaminated drug called Stalinon. The illness was characterized by greatly elevated intracranial pressure and by a spinal cord lesion in some cases (Alajouanine et al). *Trimethyltin* intoxication is much rarer; the few pathologic studies have shown neuronal loss in the hippocampus, largely *sparing* the Sommer sector (see review by Le Quesne).

A highly stereotyped episodic encephalopathy has been associated with *bismuth intoxication,* usually taken orally as bismuth subgallate. Large outbreaks have been reported in Australia and France (Burns et al; Buge et al). The onset of the neurologic disturbance is usually subacute, with a mild and fluctuating confusion, somnolence, difficulty in concentration, tremulousness, and sometimes hallucinations and delusions. With continued ingestion of bismuth, there occurs a rapid (24 to 48 hours) worsening of the confusion and tremulousness, along with diffuse myoclonic jerks, seizures, ataxia and inability to stand or walk. These symptoms regress over a period of a few days to weeks when the bismuth is withdrawn, but some patients have died of acute intoxication. High concentrations of bismuth were found in the cerebral and cerebellar cortices and in

the nuclear masses throughout the brain. These concentrations can be recognized as hyperdensities in the CT scan (Buge et al).

CLIOQUINOL

This compound, sold as Entero-Vioform, has been used in many parts of the world to prevent traveller's diarrhea and as a treatment for chronic gastroenteritis. In 1971 clinical observations began to appear in medical journals of a subacute myelo-opticoneuropathy (SMON). During the 1960s more than 10,000 cases of this neurotoxic disease were collected in Japan by Tsubaki et al. The usual symptoms are gastrointestinal disturbance followed by ascending numbness and weakness of the legs, paralysis of sphincters, and autonomic disorder. Later, vision is affected. In about two-thirds of the cases the onset is acute, and in the remainder, subacute. The occurrence of these neurologic complications was found to be related to the prolonged use of clioquinol, though there is still not full agreement on this point. In Japan the drug was withdrawn from the market, and the incidence of SMON immediately fell, supporting the theory that it was caused by clioquinol.

Recovery is usually incomplete. Two patients seen by the authors several years after onset of the disease had been left with optic atrophy and a spastic-ataxic paraparesis.

INDUSTRIAL TOXINS

Some of these, the heavy metals, have already been considered. In addition, a large number of synthetic organic compounds are widely used in industry and are frequent sources of toxicity, and the list is constantly being expanded. The reader is referred to the references at the end of the chapter for details concerning these compounds; here we can do little more than enumerate them: chlorinated diphenyls (e.g., DDT) or chlorinated polycyclic compounds (Kepone), used as insecticides; diethylene dioxide (Dioxane); carbon disulfide; the halogenated hydrocarbons (methyl chloride, tetrachloroethane, carbon tetrachloride, trichloroethylene, and methyl bromide); naphthalene (used in moth repellants); benzine (gasoline); benzene and its derivatives [toluene, xylene, nitrobenzene, phenol, and amyl acetate (banana oil)] and the hexacarbon solvents (*n*-hexane and methyl *n*-butyl ketone).

The toxic effects of these substances, which are not exerted primarily on the nervous system, are much the same from one compound to another. Neural symptoms are also not specific. They consist of varying combinations of headache, restlessness, drowsiness, confusion, delirium, coma, and convulsions, which, as a rule occur late in the illness or preterminally. Some of these industrial toxins (carbon disulfide, carbon tetrachloride and tetrachloroethane, *n*-hexane) may cause polyneuropathy, which becomes evident with recovery from acute toxicity. Extrapyramidal symptoms may result from chronic exposure to carbon disulfide.

Of the aforementioned industrial toxins, the ones most likely to cause neurologic disease are *toluene* (methyl benzene) and the *hexacarbons*. The chronic inhalation of products containing toluene (usually glue or certain brands of spray paint) may lead to severe and irreversible tremor and cerebellar ataxia, affecting movements of the eyes (opsoclonus, ocular dysmetria) and limbs as well as stance and gait. Cognitive impairment is usually associated; corticospinal tract signs, progressive optic neuropathy, sensorineural hearing loss, and hyposmia occur in some patients. Generalized cerebral atrophy and particularly cerebellar atrophy are evident in CT scans (Fornazzari et al, Hormez et al). Also, it has become apparent that acute toluene intoxication is an important cause of seizures, hallucinations and coma in children (King et al).

The prolonged exposure to high concentrations of *n*-hexane or methyl *n*-butyl ketone may cause a sensorimotor neuropathy. These solvents are metabolized to 2.5-hexanedione which is the agent that damages the peripheral nerves. The neuropathy may result from exposure in certain industrial settings (mainly the manufacture of vinyl products) or, more often, from the deliberate inhalation of vapors from solvents, lacquers, glue, or glue thinners containing *n*-hexane (see also Chap. 46).

ANTINEOPLASTIC AGENTS

The increasing use of potent antineoplastic agents has given rise to a diverse group of neurologic complications, the most important of which are summarized below.

VINCRISTINE

This drug is used in the treatment of acute lymphoblastic leukemia, lymphomas, and some solid tumors. Its most important toxic effect, and the one that limits its use as a chemotherapeutic agent, is on the peripheral nerves. Paresthesias of the feet or hands, or both, may occur within a few weeks of the beginning of treatment; with continued use of the drug, a progressive symmetrical motor-sensory and reflex loss occurs. Cranial nerves are affected less

frequently; ptosis, lateral rectus and facial palsies, and vocal cord paresis are the usual manifestations. Autonomic nervous system function may also be affected: constipation and impotence are frequent complications; orthostatic hypotension, atonicity of the bladder, and adynamic ileus are less frequent. Inappropriate antidiuretic hormone secretion and seizures have been reported, but are relatively uncommon.

The neural complications of vinblastine are similar to those of vincristine, but are usually avoided because bone marrow suppression is the dose-limiting factor.

PROCARBAZINE

This drug, originally synthesized as an MAO inhibitor, is now an important oral agent in the treatment of Hodgkin disease and other lymphomas, bronchogenic carcinoma, and malignant gliomas. Neural complications are infrequent and usually take the form of somnolence, confusion, agitation, and depression. Diffuse aching pain in proximal muscles of the limbs and mild symptoms and signs of polyneuropathy occur in 10 to 15 percent of patients treated with relatively high doses. A reversible ataxia has also been described. Procarbazine, given in conjunction with phenothiazines, barbiturates, narcotics, and alcohol, may produce serious degrees of oversedation. Other toxic reactions, such as orthostatic hypotension, are related to the MAO inhibitory action of procarbazine.

L-ASPARAGINASE

L-Asparaginase is an enzymatic inhibitor of protein synthesis and is used in the treatment of acute lymphoblastic leukemia. Drowsiness, confusion, delirium, stupor and coma, and diffuse slowing of the electroencephalogram are the common neurologic effects and are dose related and cumulative. They may occur within a day of onset of treatment and clear quickly when the drug is withdrawn, or they may be delayed in onset, in which case they may persist for several weeks. These abnormalities are at least in part attributable to the systemic metabolic derangements induced by L-asparaginase, including liver dysfunction.

In recent years, increasing attention has been drawn to cerebrovascular complications of L-asparaginase therapy, including ischemic and hemorrhagic infarction and cerebral venous and dural sinus thrombosis. Fineberg and Swenson have analyzed the clinical features of 38 such cases. These cerebrovascular complications are attributable to transient deficiencies in plasma proteins that are important in coagulation and fibrinolysis.

5-FLUOROURACIL

This is a pyrimidine analogue, used mainly in treatment of cancer of the breast, ovary, and gastrointestinal tract. A small proportion of patients receiving this drug develops dizziness, cerebellar ataxia of the trunk and the extremities, dysarthria, and nystagmus. These abnormalities must be distinguished from metastatic involvement of the cerebellum and paraneoplastic cerebellar degeneration. The drug effects are usually mild and subside within 1 to 6 weeks after discontinuation of therapy. The anatomic basis of this cerebellar syndrome is not known.

METHOTREXATE

Administered in conventional oral or intravenous doses, methotrexate (MTX) is not neurotoxic. However, given intrathecally to treat meningeal leukemia or carcinomatosis, MTX commonly causes aseptic meningitis, with headache, nausea and vomiting, stiff neck, fever, and cells in the spinal fluid. Very rarely, probably as an idiosyncratic response to the drug, intrathecal administration results in acute, permanent paraplegia. The pathology of this condition has not been studied. The most vexing of all the neurologic problems associated with chemotherapy is the necrotizing leukoencephalopathy or leukomyelopathy caused by MTX in combination with cranial or neuraxis radiation therapy. This develops several months after repeated intrathecal or high systemic doses of MTX. The full-blown syndrome consists of the insidious evolution of dementia, pseudobulbar palsy, ataxia, focal cerebral cortical deficits or paraplegia. The brain shows disseminated foci of coagulation necrosis of white matter, usually periventricular. Yet unsettled is the role of MTX in the development of asymptomatic CT scan abnormalities or of mild neurologic abnormalities in children with acute lymphoblastic leukemia given intrathecal MTX and cranial irradiation as prophylaxis.

CISPLATIN

Cisplatin (*cis*-diamminedichloroplatinum) is a heavy metal effective in the treatment of gonadal and head and neck tumors as well as carcinoma of the bladder, prostate, and breast. The dose-limiting factor in its use is nephrotoxicity and vomiting. In addition, certain neurologic complications have been reported. Approximately one-third of patients receiving this drug experience tinnitus or high-frequency hearing loss (4000 to 8000 Hz) or both. These toxicities are dose-related, cumulative, and only occasionally reversible. Retrobulbar neuritis occurs rarely. Seizures associated with drug-induced hyponatremia and hypomagnesemia have been reported. Peripheral neuropathy manifested primarily by numbness and tingling in fingers and toes is being observed with increasing frequency; this toxic manifestation appears to be related to the total amount administered, and it usually improves after the drug has been discontinued. Biopsies of peripheral nerve have shown primary axonal degeneration.

CARMUSTINE (BCNU)

BCNU, a nitrosourea used to treat malignant cerebral gliomas, is not neurotoxic when given in conventional intravenous doses. Intracarotid injection of the drug, however, causes orbital, eye, and neck pain, focal seizures, and transient confusion. It is not yet known whether this relatively new mode of administration of the drug causes permanent cerebral damage.

CYTOSINE ARABINOSIDE (ARA-C)

This drug, long used in the treatment of acute nonlymphocytic leukemia, has not been neurotoxic when given in systemic daily doses of 100 to 200 mg/m². The administration of very high doses of Ara-C (up to 30 times the usual dose) has been shown to induce remissions in patients refractory to conventional treatment; it also produces a severe degree of cerebellar degeneration in a considerable proportion of cases (4 of 24 patients reported by Winkelman and Hines). Ataxia of gait and limbs, dysarthria, and nystagmus develop as early as 5 to 7 days after the beginning of high-dose treatment and worsen rapidly. Postmortem examination has disclosed a diffuse degeneration of Purkinje cells, most marked in the depths of the folia, as well as a patchy necrosis of the cerebellar cortex, affecting all the cellular elements. Other patients receiving high-dose Ara-C develop a mild, reversible cerebellar syndrome, with the same clinical features as the irreversible one.

REFERENCES

GENERAL

ARENA JM: *Poisoning: Toxicology-Symptoms-Treatments,* 5th ed. Springfield, IL, Charles C Thomas, 1986.

DREISBACH RH: *Handbook of Poisoning: Prevention, Diagnosis and Treatment,* 12th ed. Los Altos, CA, Lange, 1987.

FELDMAN RG, RICKS NL, BAKER EL: Neuropsychological effects of industrial toxins: A review. *Am J Ind Med* 1:211, 1980.

GILMAN AG, GOODMAN LS, GILMAN A, MURAD F (eds): *The Pharmacological Basis of Therapeutics,* 7th ed. New York, Macmillan, 1985.

GOLDFRANK LR (ed): *Toxicologic Emergencies,* 3rd ed. New York, Appleton-Century-Crofts, 1986.

HADDAD LM, WINCHESTER JF: *Clinical Management of Poisoning and Drug Overdose.* Philadelphia, Saunders, 1983.

Hamilton and Hardy's Industrial Toxicology, 4th ed, revised by J Finkel. Littleton, MA, John Wright/PSG, 1982.

LEVY BS, WEGMAN DH: *Occupational Health: Recognizing and Preventing Work-Related Disease,* 2nd ed. Boston, Little Brown, 1988.

PROCTOR N, HUGHES JP: *Chemical Hazards of the Workplace,* 2nd ed. Philadelphia, Lippincott, 1988.

ROM WN (ed): *Environmental and Occupational Medicine.* Boston, Little Brown, 1983.

SPENCER PS, SCHAUMBERG HH (eds): *Experimental and Clinical Neurotoxicology.* Baltimore, Williams & Wilkins, 1980.

TEMPLE AR (ed): *Clinical Toxicology.* Emerg Med Clin North Am 2(1):1–202, 1984.

VINKEN PJ, BRUYN GW (eds): *Handbook of Clinical Neurology,* vols 36 and 37: *Intoxications of the Nervous System,* pts 1 and 2. Amsterdam, Elsevier North-Holland, 1979.

OPIATES AND SYNTHETIC ANALGESICS

BRUST JCM: Drug dependence, in Baker AB, Joynt RJ (eds): *Clinical Neurology,* vol 2. Hagerstown MD, Harper and Row, 1986, chap 21.

BRUST JCM: The nonimpact of opiate research on opiate abuse. *Neurology* 33:1327, 1983.

DOLE VP, NYSWANDER ME: Methadone maintenance and its implication for theories of narcotic addiction. *Res Publ Assoc Res Nerv Ment Dis* 46:359, 1968.

FIELDS HL: *Pain.* New York, McGraw-Hill, 1987.

GOLD MS, REDMOND DE, KLEBER HD: Clonidine blocks acute opiate-withdrawal symptoms. *Lancet* 2:599, 1978.

HOLLISTER LE: Effective use of analgesic drugs. *Annu Rev Med* 27:431, 1976.

JASINSKI DR, JOHNSON RE, KOCHER TR: Clonidine in morphine withdrawal. *Arch Gen Psychiatry* 42:1063, 1985.

MARTIN WR: Realistic goals for antagonist therapy. *Am J Drug Alcohol Abuse* 2:353, 1975.

MONROE JJ, ROSS WF, BERZINS JI: The decline of the addict as "psychopath": Implications for community care. *Int J Addictions* 6:601, 1971.

NEWMAN RG: Methadone treatment. Defining and evaluating success. *N Engl J Med* 317:447, 1987.

PEARSON J, RICHTER RW: Addiction to opiates: Neurological aspects, in Vinken PJ, Bruyn GW (eds): *Handbook of Clinical Neurology,* vol 37: *Intoxication of the Nervous System,* pt 2. Amsterdam, Elsevier North-Holland, 1979, pp 365–400.

WIKLER A: Theories related to physical dependence, in Mule SJ, Brill H (eds): *The Chemical and Biological Aspects of Drug Dependence.* Cleveland, CRC Press, 1972, pp 359–377.

WIKLER A: Characteristics of opioid addiction, in Jarvik ME (ed): *Psychopharmacology in the Practice of Medicine.* New York, Appleton-Century-Crofts, 1977, p 417.

WIKLER A: *Opioid Dependence: Mechanisms and Treatment.* New York, Plenum Press, 1980.

BARBITURATES AND OTHER SEDATIVE-HYPNOTIC DRUGS

BLOOMER HA, MADDOCK RK JR: An assessment of diuresis and dialysis for treating acute barbiturate poisoning, in Mathew H (ed): *Acute Barbiturate Poisoning.* Amsterdam, Excerpta Medica, 1971, chap 15.

CLEMMESEN C, NILSSON E: Therapeutic trends in the treatment of barbiturate poisoning: The Scandinavian method. *Clin Pharmacol Ther* 2:220, 1961.

ESSIG C: Chronic abuse of sedative-hypnotic drugs, in Zarafonetis CJD (ed): *Drug Abuse.* Philadelphia, Lea & Febiger, 1972, pp 205–215.

GREENBLATT DJ, SHADER RI, ABERNATHY DR: Current status of benzodiazepines. *N Engl J Med* 309:354, 410, 1983.

HARVEY SC: Hypnotics and sedatives, in Gilman AG, Goodman LS, Gilman A, Murad F (eds): *The Pharmacological Basis of Therapeutics,* 7th ed. New York, Macmillan, 1985, pp 339–371.

ISBELL H, ALTSCHUL S, KORNETSKY CH et al: Chronic barbiturate intoxication: An experimental study. *Arch Neurol Psychiatry* 64:1, 1950.

PLUM F, SWANSON AC: Barbiturate poisoning treated by physiological methods. *JAMA* 163:827, 1957.

WESSON DR, SMITH DE: *Barbiturates: Their Use, Misuse, and Abuse.* New York, Human Sciences Press, 1977.

STIMULANTS (INCLUDING COCAINE AND AMPHETAMINES) AND PSYCHOTOGENIC DRUGS

ALTURA BT, ALTURA BM: Phencyclidine, lysergic acid diethylamide and mescaline: Cerebral artery spasms and hallucinogenic activity. *Science* 212:1051, 1981.

BALDESSARINI RJ: Drugs and the treatment of psychiatric disorders, in Gilman AG, Goodman LS, Gilman A, Murad F (eds): *The Pharmacological Basis of Therapeutics,* 7th ed. New York, Macmillan, 1985, pp 387–445.

BALDESSARINI RJ, TARSY D: Tardive dyskinesia, in Lipton MA et al (eds): *Psychopharmacology: A Generation of Progress.* New York, Raven Press, 1978, pp 993–1004.

CREGLER LL, MARK H: Medical complications of cocaine abuse. *N Engl J Med* 315:1495, 1986.

GAWIN FH, ELLINWOOD FH: Cocaine and other stimulants. Actions, abuse, and treatment. *N Engl J Med* 318:1173, 1988.

GREENBLATT DJ, HARMATZ JS, ZINNY MA, SHADER RI: Effect of gradual withdrawal on the rebound sleep disorder after discontinuation of triazolam. *N Engl J Med* 317:722, 1987.

HARRINGTON H, HELLER A, DAWSON D: Intracerebral hemorrhage and oral amphetamine. *Arch Neurol* 40:503, 1983.

HOLLISTER LE: Drug-induced psychiatric disorders and their management. *Med Toxicol* 1:428, 1986.

HOLLISTER LE: *Clinical Pharmacology of Psychotherapeutic Drugs,* 2nd ed. New York, Churchill Livingstone, 1983.

IVERSEN SD, IVERSEN LL: *Behavioral Pharmacology.* New York, Oxford University Press, 1975.

MARKS J: *The Benzodiazepines: Use, Overuse, Misuse, Abuse.* Baltimore, University Park Press, 1978.

NICHOLI AM: The nontherapeutic use of psychoactive drugs. *N Engl J Med* 308:925, 1983.

PETERSON RC, STILLMAN RC: Phencyclidine: An overview, in Peterson RC, Stillman RC (eds): *Phencyclidine (PCP) Abuse,* Research Monograph Series 21. Washington, National Institute on Drug Abuse, 1978, chap 1.

ROTH D, ALARCON FJ, FERNANDEZ JA et al: Acute rhabdomyolysis associated with cocaine intoxication. *N Engl J Med* 319:673, 1988.

SNYDER SH: Receptors, neurotransmitters and drug responses. *N Engl J Med* 300:465, 1979.

TETANUS

ABEL JJ, FIROR SM, CHALIAN W: Researches on tetanus. IX: Further evidence to show that tetanus toxin is not carried to central neurons by way of axis cylinders of motor nerves. *Bull Johns Hopkins Hosp* 63:373, 1938.

STRUPPLER A, STRUPPLER E, ADAMS RD: Local tetanus in man. *Arch Neurol* 8:162, 1963.

WEINSTEIN L: Current concepts: Tetanus. *N Engl J Med* 289:1293, 1973.

ZACKS SI, SHEFF MF: Studies on tetanus. V: In vivo localization of purified tetanus neurotoxin in mice with fluorescein-labelled tetanus antitoxin. *J Neuropathol Exp Neurol* 25:422, 1966.

DIPHTHERIA

FISHER CM, ADAMS RD: Diphtheritic polyneuritis: A pathological study. *J Neuropathol Exp Neurol* 15:243, 1956.

McDONALD WI, KOCEN RS: Diphtheritic neuropathy, in Dyck PJ, Thomas PK, Lambert EH (eds): *Peripheral Neuropathy,* 2nd ed. Philadelphia, Saunders, 1984, pp 2010–2017.

PAPPENHEIMER AM: Diphtheria toxin. *Annu Rev Biochem* 46:69, 1977.

BOTULISM

CHERINGTON M: Botulism: Ten-year experience. *Arch Neurol* 30:432, 1974.

GANGAROSA EJ: Botulism in the United States, 1899–1967. *J Infect Dis* 119:308, 1969.

KOENIG MG, DRUTZ DJ, MUSHLIN AI et al: Type B botulism in man. *Am J Med* 42:208, 1967.

LAMBERT EH: Defects of neuromuscular transmission in syndromes other than myasthenia gravis. *Ann NY Acad Sci* 135:367, 1966.

MAYER RF: The neuromuscular defect in human botulism, in Locke S (ed): *Modern Neurology.* Boston, Little Brown, 1969, pp 169–186.

PETTY CS: Botulism: The disease and toxin. *Am J Med Sci* 249:345, 1965.

ZACKS SJ, METZGER JF, SMITH CW, BLUMBERG JM: Localization of ferritin-labelled botulinus toxin in the neuromuscular junction of the mouse. *J Neuropathol Exp Neurol* 21:610, 1962.

MUSHROOM POISONING

Mushroom poisoning. *The Medical Letter* 26:67 (July 20), 1984.

VENOMS, BITES, AND STINGS

FINKEL M: Lyme disease and its neurologic complications. *Arch Neurol* 45:99, 1988.

LEAD

ALBERT JJ, BREAULT HJ, FRIEND WK et al: Prevention, diagnosis, and treatment of lead poisoning in childhood. *Pediatrics* 44:291, 1969.

BAKER EL, LANDRIGAN PJ, BARBOUR AG et al: Occupational lead poisoning in the United States. *Br J Ind Med* 36:314, 1979.

CHISHOLM JJ JR: Management of increased lead absorption and lead poisoning in children. *N Engl J Med* 289:1016, 1973.

GOLDMAN RH, BAKER EL, HANNAN M, KAMEROW DB: Lead poisoning in automobile radiator mechanics. *N Engl J Med* 317:214, 1987.

LIN-FU JS: Children and lead. *N Engl J Med* 307:615, 1982.

MAHAFFEY KR, ANNEST JL, ROBERTS J, MURPHY RS: National estimates of blood lead levels: United States, 1976–1980. *N Engl J Med* 307:573, 1982.

PERLSTEIN MA, ATTALA R: Neurologic sequelae of plumbism in children. *Clin Pediatr* 5:292, 1966.

RUTTER M: Raised lead levels and impaired cognitive/behavioural functioning: A review of the evidence. *Dev Med Child Neurol* 22 (suppl 42):1–26, 1980.

ARSENIC

HEYMAN A, PFEIFFER JB JR, WILLETT RW, TAYLOR HM: Peripheral neuropathy caused by arsenical intoxication. *N Engl J Med* 254:401, 1956.

JENKINS RB: Inorganic arsenic and the nervous system. *Brain* 89:479, 1966.

MANGANESE

MENA I, MARIN O, FUENZALIDA S, COTZIAS GC: Chronic manganese poisoning: Clinical picture and manganese turnover. *Neurology* 17:128, 1967.

MERCURY

KARK RAP, POSKANZER DC, BULLOCK JD, BOYLEN G: Mercury poisoning and its treatment with *N*-acetyl-*dl*-penicillamine. *N Engl J Med* 285:10, 1971.

KURLAND LT, FARO SN, SIEDLER H: Minamata disease. *World Neurol* 1:370, 1960.

RUSTAM H, VON BURG R, AMIN-ZAKI L, EL HASSANI S: Evidence for neuromuscular disorder in methyl mercury poisoning. *Arch Environ Health* 30:190, 1975.

TAKEUCHI T: Neuropathology of Minamata disease in Kumamoto, especially at the chronic stage, in Roizin L, Shiraki H, Grcevic

N (eds): *Neurotoxicology.* New York, Raven Press, 1977, pp 235–260.

Tokuomi H, Uchino M, Imamura S et al: Minamata disease (organic mercury poisoning): Neuroradiologic and electrophysiologic studies. *Neurology* 32:1369, 1982.

ORGANOPHOSPHATES

Cavanagh JB, Patangia GN: Changes in the central nervous system of the cat as the result of tri-*o*-cresyl phosphate poisoning. *Brain* 88:165, 1965.

Johnson MK: A phosphorylation site in brain and the delayed neurotoxic effect of organophosphorus compounds. *Biochem J* 111:487, 1969.

Namba IT, Nolte CT, Jackrel J, Grob D: Poisoning due to organophosphate insecticides: Acute and chronic manifestations. *Am J Med* 50:475, 1971.

Prineas J: The pathogenesis of the dying-back polyneuropathies. *J Neuropathol Exp Neurol* 28:571, 1969.

Senanayake N, Karalliedde L: Neurotoxic effects of organophosphate insecticide. *N Engl J Med* 316:761, 1987.

THALLIUM

Bank WJ, Pleasure DE, Suzuki D et al: Thallium poisoning. *Arch Neurol* 26:456, 1972.

GOLD

Katrak SM, Pollock M, O'Brien CP et al: Clinical and morphological features of gold neuropathy. *Brain* 103:671, 1980.

ALUMINUM

Le Quesne PM: Toxic substances and the nervous system: The role of clinical observation. *J Neurol Neurosurg Psychiatry* 44:1, 1981.

Perl DP, Brody AR: Alzheimer's disease: X-ray spectrometric evidence of aluminum accumulation in neurofibrillary tangle-bearing neurons. *Science* 208:297, 1980.

Perl DP, Gajdusek DC, Garruto RM et al: Intraneuronal aluminum accumulation in amyotrophic lateral sclerosis and parkinsonism-dementia of Guam. *Science* 217:1053, 1982.

BISMUTH

Buge A, Supino-Viterbo V, Rancurel G, Pontes C: Epileptic phenomena in bismuth toxic encephalopathy. *J Neurol Neurosurg Psychiatry* 44:62, 1981.

Burns R, Thomas DQ, Barron VJ: Reversible encephalopathy possibly associated with bismuth subgallate ingestion. *Br Med J* 1:220, 1974.

CLIOQUINOL

Tsubaki T, Honmay Y, Hoshl M: Neurological syndrome associated with clioquinol. *Lancet* 1:696, 1971.

INDUSTRIAL TOXINS AND SOLVENTS

Alajouanine TH, Derobert L, Thieffry S: Etude clinique d'ensemble de 210 cas d'intoxication par les sels organiques d'étain. *Rev Neurol (Paris)* 98:85, 1958.

Editorial: Hexacarbon neuropathy. *Lancet* 2:942, 1979.

Elofsson SA, Gamberale F, Hindmarsh T et al: Exposure to organic solvents. *Scand J Work Environ Health* 6:239, 1980.

Fornazzari L, Wilkinson DA, Kapur BM, Carlen PL: Cerebellar, cortical and functional impairment in toluene abusers. *Acta Neurol Scand* 67:319, 1983.

Hormes JT, Filley CM, Rosenberg NL: Neurologic sequelae of chronic solvent vapor abuse. *Neurology* 36:698, 1986.

King MD, Day RE, Oliver JS et al: Solvent encephalopathy. *Br Med J* 283:663, 1981.

ANTINEOPLASTIC AGENTS

Allen JC: The effects of cancer therapy on the nervous system. *Pediatrics* 93:903, 1978.

Fineberg WM, Swenson MR: Cerebrovascular complications of l-asparaginase therapy. *Neurology* 38:127, 1988.

Kaplan RS, Wiernik PH: Neurotoxicity of antineoplastic drugs. *Semin Oncol* 9:103, 1982.

Ostrow S, Hahn D, Wiernik PH, Richards RD: Ophthalmologic toxicity after *cis*-dichloro-diammineplatinum therapy. *Cancer Treat Rep* 62:1591, 1978.

Shapiro WR, Chernik NL, Posner JB: Necrotizing encephalopathy following intraventricular instillation of methotrexate. *Arch Neurol* 28:96, 1973.

Winkelman MD, Hines JD: Cerebellar degeneration caused by high-dose cytosine arabinoside: A clinicopathological study. *Ann Neurol* 14:520, 1983.

Young DF: Neurologic complications of cancer chemotherapy, in Silverstein A (ed): *Neurological Complications of Therapy: Selected Topics.* Mt Kisco, NY, Futura, 1982, pp 57–113.

CHAPTER 43

DEGENERATIVE DISEASES OF THE NERVOUS SYSTEM

The adjectival term *degenerative* has no great appeal to the modern neurologist. For one thing, it has an unpleasant literary connotation, referring, as it does, to a state of moral degradation or deviant sexual behavior, as the consequence of a sociopathic tendency. More important, it is not a satisfactory term medically, since it implies an inexplicable decline from a previous level of normalcy to a lower level of function—an ambiguous conceptualization of disease that satisfies neither theoretician nor scientist. Unquestionably some of the diseases included in this category depend on genetic factors, or at least they appear in more than one member of the same family and are, therefore, more properly designated as *heredodegenerative*. An even larger number of diseases, not differing in any fundamental way from the heredofamilial ones, occurs only sporadically, i.e., as isolated instances in given families. Gowers in 1902 suggested the term *abiotrophy* for diseases of this type, by which he meant a lack of "vital endurance" of the affected neurons, resulting in their premature death. This concept embodies an untested, unproven hypothesis—that aging and degenerative disease of cells are based on the same process, and contemporary neuropathologists are understandably reluctant to attribute to simple aging the diverse processes of cellular disease that are constantly being revealed by ultrastructural techniques.

There are, within recent memory, several examples of disease that were formerly classed as degenerative but are now known to have a metabolic, toxic, or nutritional basis or to be caused by a "slow virus." It seems reasonable to expect that with increasing knowledge, more and more diseases whose causes are now unknown will find their way into these categories. Until such time as the causation of all neurologic diseases is known, there has to be a name and a place for a group of diseases that have no known cause and are united only by the common attribute of gradually progressive disintegration of part or parts of the nervous system. In deference to traditional practice, they are collected here under the rubric of degenerative diseases.

The reader may be perplexed by the inconsistent use of the terms *atrophy* and *degeneration,* both of which are applied to diseases of this category. Spatz argued that on purely histopathologic grounds they are different. Atrophy specifies a gradual decay and loss of neurons, leaving in their wake no degradative products and only a sparsely cellular, fibrous gliosis. Degeneration refers to a more rapid process of neuronal, myelin, or tissue breakdown, with resulting degradative products that evoke a more vigorous reaction of phagocytosis and cellular gliosis. The difference is both in the speed and type of breakdown. It is of some interest that many of the diseases that are characterized by degeneration, in Spatz's sense of the term, are now known to be of established metabolic origin, but very few of the purely atrophic ones have been shown to have a metabolic basis.

GENERAL CLINICAL CHARACTERISTICS

The diseases included in the degenerative category *begin insidiously, after a long period of normal nervous system function, and pursue a gradually progressive course that may continue for many years, often a decade or longer.* In this respect they differ from most of the metabolic diseases. Frequently it is impossible to assign a date of onset. Sometimes, the patient or the patient's family gives a history of abrupt appearance of disability, particularly if some injury, infection, or other memorable event coincided with the initial symptoms. In such instances a skillfully taken history will elicit the fact that the patient or family suddenly became aware of a condition that had, in fact, been present for some time, but had attracted little attention. Whether trauma or other stress can actually evoke or aggravate a degenerative disease is a question that cannot be answered with certainty, but it seems highly improbable that this could occur. Anyone who states otherwise must offer evidence that at present is nonexistent. Instead, these disease processes by their very nature appear to develop de novo, without relation to known antecedent events, and their symptomatic expressions become possible only when the degree of neuronal loss reaches or exceeds the "safety factor" for a particular neuronal system. In other words, the degree of correspondence between the clinical state and its pathologic basis is only relative.

The *familial occurrence* of disease is of great importance, but it must be emphasized that such information is often difficult to obtain on first contact with the patient. The family may be small and widely scattered, so that the patient is unaware of the health of other members. The patient or the patient's relatives may be ashamed to admit that a neurologic disease has "tainted" the family. Furthermore, it may not be realized that an illness is hereditary if other members of the family have a much more or much less severe form of the disorder than the patient. Sometimes, in the latter case, only the careful examination of other family members will disclose the presence of an hereditary disease. It should be remembered, however, that familial occurrence of a disease does not prove heredity, but may indicate instead that more than one member of a family has been exposed to the same infectious or toxic agent.

In general, the degenerative diseases of the nervous system run a *ceaselessly progressive course*, uninfluenced by all medical and surgical measures, so that dealing with a patient with this type of illness may be an anguishing experience for all concerned. However, some of these diseases are characterized by long periods of stability; moreover, some symptoms can be alleviated by wise and skillful management, and the physician's interest may be of great help even though curative measures cannot be offered.

The bilateral symmetry of the clinical manifestations and lesions is another noteworthy feature of the degenerative diseases, and it alone may distinguish members of this group from many other diseases of the nervous system. Again, this principle requires qualification, for in the earliest stages of some degenerative diseases (e.g., paralysis agitans, amyotrophic lateral sclerosis) there may be greater involvement of one limb or one side of the body. Sooner or later, however, despite the asymmetric beginning, the inherently symmetric nature of the process asserts itself.

Many of the degenerative diseases are characterized by the *selective involvement of anatomically and physiologically related systems of neurons*. This feature is exemplified by amyotrophic lateral sclerosis, in which the pathologic process is limited to motor neurons of the cerebral cortex, brainstem, and spinal cord, and by certain forms of

progressive ataxia in which only the Purkinje cells of the cerebellum are affected. Many other examples could be cited (e.g., Friedreich ataxia) in which certain neuronal systems disintegrate, leaving others unscathed. These degenerative diseases have therefore been called *system atrophies* or *systemic neuronal atrophies,* and many of them turn out to be strongly hereditary. The selective vulnerability of certain systems of neurons is not an exclusive property of the degenerative diseases, however: several disease processes of known cause have similarly circumscribed effects on the nervous system. Diphtheria toxin, for instance, selectively affects the myelin of the peripheral nerves near the spinal ganglia, and triorthocresyl phosphate affects both the corticospinal tracts of the spinal cord and the spinal motor neurons. Other examples are the special vulnerability of the Purkinje cells to hyperthermia and cerebellar granule cells to methyl mercury compound. Conversely, in Alzheimer disease and similar degenerative diseases (according to the criteria of Spatz) the pathologic changes are quite diffuse and seemingly unselective.

As one would expect of any pathologic process that is based on the slow disintegration of neurons, not only do the cell bodies disappear but also their dendrites, axons, and myelin sheaths—unaccompanied by an intense tissue reaction or cellular response. The CSF, therefore, shows little if any change—at most a slight increase in protein content. Moreover, since these diseases invariably result in tissue loss (rather than in new tissue formation, as occurs with neoplasms or inflammations), radiologic examination shows either no change or a volumetric reduction with enlargement of the CSF compartments. The blood-brain barrier tends not to be altered. These negative laboratory findings help distinguish the neuronal atrophies from other large classes of progressive disease of the nervous system, viz., tumors, infections, and other processes of inflammatory type.

CLASSIFICATION

Since grouping of the degenerative diseases in terms of etiology is impossible (save that in many a hereditary, or genetic, factor can be recognized) we resort, for practical reasons, to dividing them according to the presenting clinical syndromes and their pathologic anatomy. Although this approach is a reversion to the most elementary mode of classification of naturally occurring phenomena, it is a necessary prelude to diagnosis and scientific study, and preferable to a haphazard listing of diseases by the names of the neurologists or neuropathologists who first described them.

  I. Syndrome of progressive dementia, other neurologic signs being absent or inconspicuous

A. Diffuse cerebral atrophy
   1. Alzheimer disease and senile dementia
   2. Nonspecific types
B. Circumscribed cerebral atrophy (lobar sclerosis)—Pick disease
C. Other types of dementia
   1. Arteriosclerotic (multi-infarct)
   2. Posttraumatic
   3. Postencephalitic
   4. Hydrocephalic
   5. Mitochondrial
II. Syndrome of progressive dementia in combination with other neurologic abnormalities
   A. Huntington chorea
   B. Cortical-striatal-spinal degeneration (Jakob) and the dementia–Parkinson–amyotrophic lateral sclerosis complex (guamanian and others)
   C. Cerebrocerebellar degeneration (Greenfield)
   D. Familial dementia with spastic paraparesis
   E. Cortical-basal ganglionic degeneration
   F. Familial myoclonic dementia
III. Syndrome of disordered posture and movement
   A. Paralysis agitans (Parkinson disease)
   B. Striatonigral degeneration with or without Shy-Drager syndrome and olivopontocerebellar atrophy
   C. Progressive supranuclear palsy (Steele-Richardson-Olszewski)
   D. Dystonia musculorum deformans (torsion spasm)
   E. Hallervorden-Spatz disease
   F. Spasmodic torticollis and other restricted dyskinesias
   G. Familial tremor
   H. Multiple tic disease (Gilles de la Tourette)
IV. Syndrome of progressive ataxia
   A. Predominantly spinal forms of hereditary ataxia
      1. Friedreich
      2. Strümpell-Lorrain
   B. Predominantly cerebellar forms of hereditary ataxia
      1. Holmes familial cortical cerebellar atrophy
      2. Late cerebellar cortical atrophy of Marie-Foix-Alajouanine
   C. Cerebellar-brainstem atrophies
      1. Olivopontocerebellar
      2. Dentatorubral
      3. Azorean disease
   D. Carcinomatous and other cerebellar degenerations
V. Syndrome of slowly developing muscular weakness and atrophy (nuclear amyotrophy)
   A. *Without sensory changes:* motor system disease
      1. Amyotrophic lateral sclerosis
      2. Progressive spinal muscular atrophy
      3. Progressive bulbar palsy
      4. Primary lateral sclerosis
      5. Hereditary forms of progressive muscular atrophy and spastic paraplegia
   B. *With sensory changes* (see Chap. 46)
      1. Hereditary sensory neuropathies
      2. Hereditary sensorimotor neuropathies [peroneal muscular atrophy (Charcot-Marie-Tooth); hypertrophic interstitial polyneuropathy (Déjerine-Sottas); heredopathia atactica polyneuritiformis (Refsum); etc.]
VI. Syndrome of progressive blindness
   A. Hereditary optic neuropathy (Leber)
   B. Pigmentary degeneration of retina (retinitis pigmentosa)
   C. Stargardt disease
VII. Syndromes characterized by neurosensory deafness
   A. Pure neurosensory deafness
   B. Hereditary hearing loss with retinal diseases
   C. Hereditary hearing loss with system diseases of the nervous system

DISEASES CHARACTERIZED MAINLY BY PROGRESSIVE DEMENTIA

ALZHEIMER DISEASE

This is the most common and important degenerative disease of the brain. Some clinical aspects of the intellectual deterioration that characterize this disease have already been described in Chap. 20, under the neurology of dementia, and the relationship of this disease to the aging process has been fully discussed in Chap. 29. There it was pointed out that some degree of shrinkage in size and weight of the brain, i.e., "atrophy," is an inevitable accompaniment of advancing age, but that these changes alone are of slight clinical significance. By contrast, severe degrees of diffuse cerebral atrophy that evolve over a few years are invariably associated with dementia, and the underlying pathologic changes in these cases most often prove to be those of Alzheimer disease (see below). When these changes occur in old age (and the definition of old age and just when it begins are hardly precise), it is usual to speak of senile dementia; when a pathologically identical progressive dementia appears *before* the senile period, the term *Alzheimer disease* is frequently used. This practice of giving Alzheimer disease and senile dementia the status of separate diseases is probably attributable to the relatively young age (51 years) of the patient originally studied by Alzheimer. The illogicality of such a division is at once apparent, since the two conditions, except for their age of onset, are clinically and pathologically indistinguishable.

Clinical Features   Although Alzheimer disease has been described at every period of adult life, the majority of our patients have been in their late fifties or early sixties or older. It is one of the most frequent mental illnesses, making up some 20 percent of all patients in psychiatric hospitals. In the United States, in 17 series comprising 15,000 persons over the age of 60 years, the mean incidence of moderate to severe dementia was calculated to be 4.8 percent (Wang). According to Terry and Katzman, there were in the United States in 1983, about 1.3 million patients with severe dementia, and an additional 2.8 million with mild to moderate intellectual impairment; in the majority of these patients the dementia was due to Alzheimer disease. The most careful epidemiologic study to date has been conducted in the community of Rochester, Minnesota, by Schoenberg and his colleagues. The incidence rate for dementia in general was 187 new cases per 100,000 population per year, and for Alzheimer disease, 123 cases per 100,000 annually.

The familial occurrence of Alzheimer disease has been well documented, the pedigrees being consistent with an autosomal dominant mode of inheritance (Nee et al; Fitch et al; Goudsmit et al). However, the concordance rate of Alzheimer disease is the same in monozygotic and dizygotic twin pairs (about 40 percent), supporting the belief that the disease cannot be accounted for by a single autosomal dominant gene (Nee et al). Reports of a substantial familial aggregation of dementia, without a specific pattern of inheritance, also suggest the operation of a genetic factor (see Heyman et al). Nearly all our own cases have been sporadic, and males and females have been about equally affected. Genetic studies are difficult because the disease does not appear at the same age in a given proband. Even in identical twins it may develop at the age of 60 years in one of the pair and at 80 years in the other. Death from other diseases may prevent its detection. In one-third of the cases reported by Fitch et al, the abnormal gene was not expressed until after the age of 70 years.

The onset of mental changes is usually so insidious that neither the family nor the patient can date the time of its beginning. Occasionally, however, it is brought to attention by an unusual degree of confusion in relation to a febrile illness, an operation, mild head injury, or the taking of medication.

The gradual development of forgetfulness is the major symptom. Small day-to-day happenings are not remembered. Seldom-used names are particularly elusive. Little-used words from an earlier period of life also tend to be lost. Appointments are forgotten and possessions misplaced. Questions are repeated again and again, the patient having forgotten what was just discussed. It is said that remote memories are preserved and recent ones lost (Ribot's law of memory), but this is only relatively true; it is difficult to check the accuracy of ancient memories. Warrington and her associates, who tested the patient's recognition of dated political events and pictures of prominent people, past and present, found the memory loss to extend to all decades of life.

Once the memory disorder has become pronounced, other failures in cerebral function become increasingly apparent. The patient's speech is halting because of failure to recall the needed word. The same difficulty interrupts writing. Comprehension of spoken words seems at first to be preserved, until it is observed that the patient does not carry out a complicated request; even then it is uncertain whether the request was not understood or was forgotten. Almost imperceptible at first, all these disturbances of language become more apparent as the disease progresses. Finally, there is a failure to speak in full sentences; to find words requires a continuous search; and little that is said or written is fully comprehended. Occasionally there is a rather dramatic repetition of every spoken phrase (echolalia). The deterioration of verbal skills has by then progressed beyond a groping for names and common nouns to an obvious dysphasia.

Skill in arithmetic suffers a similar deterioration. Faults in balancing the checkbook, mistakes in figuring the price of items and in making the correct change—all these and others progress to a point where the patient can no longer carry out the simplest calculations. This type of conceptual loss is called *acalculia,* or *dyscalculia.*

Visuospatial orientation becomes defective. The car cannot be parked; the arms do not find the correct sleeves of the dressing gown; the corners of the tablecloth cannot be oriented with the corners of the table; the patient turns in the wrong direction on the way home or becomes lost. The route from one place to another cannot be described nor can given directions be understood. As this state worsens, the simplest of geometric forms and patterns cannot be copied.

Eventually the patient forgets how to use common objects and tools while retaining the necessary motor power and coordination for these activities. The razor is no longer correctly applied to the face; the latch of the door cannot be unfastened; and eating utensils are no longer used properly. Finally, only the most habitual and virtually automatic actions are preserved. Tests of commanded and demonstrated actions cannot be executed or imitated. *Ideational* and *ideomotor apraxia* are the terms applied to the advanced forms of this motor incapacity (pages 46 and 47).

As these many amnesic, aphasic, agnosic, and apraxic deficits declare themselves, the patient at first seems unchanged in overall motility, behavior, temperament, and conduct. Social graces, whatever they were, are retained in the initial phase of the illness, but, gradually, troublesome alterations in these spheres appear. Restlessness and agitation or their opposites—hypokinesia and placidity—become evident. Dressing, shaving, and bathing are neglected.

A poorly organized paranoid delusional state, sometimes with hallucinations, may become manifest. The patient may suspect his elderly wife of having an illicit relationship or his children of stealing his possessions. Imprudent business deals may be made. A stable marriage may be disrupted by an infatuation with a younger person. Sexual indiscretions may astonish the community. The affect coarsens; the patient is more egocentric and indifferent to the feelings and reactions of others. A gluttonous appetite sometimes develops, but more often eating is neglected, with gradual weight loss. Later, grasping and sucking reflexes can be readily elicited, sphincteric continence fails, and the patient sinks into a state of relative akinesia and mutism, as described in Chap. 20. Difficulty in locomotion, a kind of unsteadiness with shortened steps but with only slight motor weakness and rigidity, frequently supervenes. Later, elements of parkinsonian akinesia and rigidity, and tremor can be perceived in the motor disability. Ultimately the patient loses the ability to stand and walk, being forced to lie inert in bed, having to be fed and bathed. The legs may curl into a *paraplegia in flexion*, in this instance of cerebral–basal ganglionic origin (see page 99).

The course of this tragic illness usually extends over a period of 5 or more years; surprisingly, throughout this period, corticospinal and corticosensory functions, visual acuity, and visual fields remain relatively intact. If there are hemiplegia, homonymous hemianopia, etc., either the diagnosis of Alzheimer disease is incorrect or the disease has been complicated by a stroke, tumor, or subdural hematoma. The tendon reflexes are little altered and the plantar reflexes almost always remain flexor. There is no true sensory or cerebellar ataxia. Convulsions are rare. Occasionally, widespread myoclonic jerks or mild choreoathetotic movements are observed. Eventually, in a bedfast state, an intercurrent infection such as aspiration pneumonia or some other disease mercifully terminates life.

The sequence of neurologic disabilities may not follow this described order, and one or another deficit may take precedence, presumably because the disease process affects one particular part of the brain earlier or later in one patient than in another. This allows for a relatively restricted deficit to become the source of early medical complaint, long before the full syndrome of dementia has declared itself. We have observed five limited deficits of this type, as follows:

1. *Korsakoff amnesic state.* The early stages of Alzheimer disease may be dominated by a disproportionate failure of retentive memory, with integrity of other cognitive abilities. In such patients, immediate memory, tested by the capacity to repeat a series of numbers or words, is essentially intact. It is the longer-term (retentive) memory that fails. Such a restricted disability constitutes the *senile*

amnesic state, or *presbyophrenia*. Retentive memory may become impaired to the point where the patient can recall nothing of what he had learned a minute or two previously. Yet as a business executive, for example, he may continue to make acceptable decisions if the work utilizes long-established habit patterns. In such cases, the temporal horns tend to be enlarged more than the rest of the ventricular system.

2. *Dysnomia.* Forgetting words, especially proper names, may first bring the patient to a neurologist. Later the difficulty involves common nouns and progresses to the point where fluency of speech is seriously impaired. Every sentence is broken by a pause and search for the wanted word. If not found, a circumlocution is substituted or the sentence is left unfinished. Repetition of the spoken words of others, at first flawless, later brings out a lesser degree of the same difficulty. A useful test for the failure to find names (dysnomia), which is probably the most common abnormality of language in this disease, is the category-fluency test. The patient is given 1 min to name as many items as possible in each of four categories: vegetables, vehicles, tools, and clothing. All Alzheimer patients fall below a score of 50 items. Other components of language may be relatively intact, but before long it is evident that the patient does not understand all that he hears or reads. In contrast, nonverbal memory and the ability to calculate and make simple judgments, may still be preserved. Mesulam and Chawluk and their colleagues have described a number of such patients, in whom an aphasic disorder began with anomia and eventually affected reading, writing, and comprehension, without the additional intellectual and behavioral disturbances of dementia. Two of the patients developed a more generalized dementia, but only after 7 years of progressive aphasia. These authors regard this syndrome as a focal degenerative disorder distinct from Alzheimer disease, but the pathologic data that would permit this conclusion are not yet available. Usually the EEG is normal or shows only a mild degree of slowing, and the lateral ventricles are either of normal size or slightly enlarged (especially the temporal lobes).

3. *Spatial disorientation.* Parietal lobe function, commonly deranged in the course of Alzheimer disease, may fail while other functions are relatively preserved. As remarked above, losing one's way in familiar surroundings, inability to interpret a road map, distinguish right from left, park or garage a car, or moor a boat, and difficulty in setting the table or dressing are all manifestations of a

special failure to orient the schema of one's body with that of surrounding space.

4. *Paranoia and other personality changes.* Not uncommonly, the most prominent event in the development of senile dementia is the occurrence of paranoia or bizarre behavior. The patient becomes convinced that relatives are stealing his or her possessions or that an elderly and even infirm husband or wife is guilty of infidelity. He may hide his belongings, even relatively worthless ones, and go about spying on family members. Hostilities arise, and wills may be altered irrationally. Many of these patients are constantly worried, tense, and agitated.

Of course, paranoid delusions may be part of a depressive psychosis and of other dementias, but the senile patients in whom paranoia is the presenting problem seem not to be depressed, and their cognitive functions are for a time well preserved. It is tempting to think that a very early senile change has exposed a lifelong trait of suspiciousness, but this is purely hypothetical.

Sometimes other oddities of behavior will announce the oncoming dementia. Social indiscretions, rejection of an old friend, embarking on an imprudent financial venture, or an amorous pursuit that is out of character are examples of these types of behavioral change.

5. *Gait disorder.* While it is true that most patients with Alzheimer disease walk normally until relatively late in their illness, not infrequently, in the older patients, a short-stepped gait and poor balance may call attention to the disease (see page 98).

Some clinicians attempt to subdivide the Alzheimer–senile dementia syndrome into subtypes. Amnesic defect without lexical-semantic abnormalities represents more than 50 percent of cases. Chin et al observed more prevalent and severe language disorder in early-onset familial cases. Whether such distinctions reveal any important facet of the disease process is questionable.

It has been our impression that each of the restricted cerebral disorders described above is only relatively pure. Careful testing of mental function, and this is of diagnostic importance, frequently discloses subtle abnormalities in several cognitive spheres. Initially, most patients have a disproportionate affection of the temporal-parietal parts of the cerebrum, hence the impairment on the performance parts of the Wechsler Adult Intelligence Scale. Within several months to a year or two, the more generalized aspects of mental deterioration become apparent, and the aphasic-agnosic-apraxic aspects of the syndrome become increasingly prominent. If one of the foregoing restricted deficits remains uncomplicated over a period of years, one is justified in suspecting some cause other than the Alzheimer disease, such as embolic infarction of one part of the temporal or parietal lobe; or perhaps an unrecognized herpes simplex encephalitis involving the temporal lobes. Also, as stated earlier, a visual field defect, cortical sensory loss, or hemiparesis is seldom if ever due to Alzheimer disease alone. More psychologic studies of a large group of Alzheimer cases are needed to confirm the various patterns of dementia that we are seeing clinically.

Pathology The brain presents a diffusely atrophied appearance. Cerebral convolutions are narrowed and sulci are widened. The third and lateral ventricles are symmetrically enlarged to a varying degree. Usually the atrophic process involves the frontal, temporal, and parietal lobes more or less evenly, but cases vary considerably. Microscopically, there is widespread loss of nerve cells (40 percent or more of cells over 90 μm in diameter), most marked in the cerebral cortex. The neurons of the nucleus basalis of Meynert (the substantia innominata) and locus ceruleus are are also reduced in number, a finding that has aroused great interest because of its possible role in the pathogenesis of the disease (see below). Residual neurons are said to lose dendrites and crowd upon one another due to loss of neuropil. Astrocytic proliferation follows as a compensatory or reparative process. In addition, three microscopic changes give this disease its distinctive character: (1) deposits of amorphous material, scattered throughout the cerebral cortex and most easily seen with silver-staining methods (so-called *senile* or "*neuritic*" *plaques*), (2) the presence within the nerve cell cytoplasm of thick, fiber-like strands of silver-staining material, often in the form of loops, coils, or tangled masses (*Alzheimer neurofibrillary change*), and (3) *granulovacuolar degeneration* of neurons, most evident in the pyramidal cell layer of the hippocampus. Electron-microscopic studies have shown the neurofibrillary tangle to be composed of clusters of twisted tubules that are different from the normal microtubules of nerve cells. The senile plaques contain a core of amyloid, surrounded by products of degenerated nerve terminals, mainly dendritic, containing lysosomes, abnormal mitochondria, and often twisted tubules. Also, amyloid can be found in the walls of small blood vessels near the plaques, the so-called dyshoric, or congophilic, angiopathy. Hinton and colleagues have described yet another feature—degeneration of retinal ganglion cells and optic nerves in a high proportion of patients with Alzheimer disease.

Neuritic plaques and neurofibrillary changes are uniformly distributed in all the association areas of the cerebral cortex. If any part is more affected, it is the hippocampus, particularly the CA1 zone (of Lorente de No) and the parahippocampal gyrus. The parietal lobes are another favored site. A few tangles and plaques are found in the hypothalamus, thalamus, lenticular nuclei, pontine tegmentum, and granule-cell layer of the cerebellum.

Experienced neuropathologists recognize a form of Alzheimer disease, particularly in older patients (>75 years), in which there are senile plaques but no neuronal tangles (20 percent of 150 cases reported by Joachim et al). Another problem for the neuropathologist is to distinguish between the normal aged brain and that of Alzheimer disease. It is not unusual to find a few senile plaques in normal individuals. Henderson and Hubbard have addressed themselves to this problem. They studied 27 demented individuals, aged 64 to 92 years, and 20 age-matched controls. In the former, 3 to 38 percent of the hippocampal neurons contained neurofibrillary tangles; in all but two of the controls, the number of hippocampal neurons with tangles fell below 2.5 percent.

Of interest also is the observation of Joachim et al that 18 percent of their Alzheimer cases had sufficient neuronal loss and Lewy bodies in the substantia nigra to justify a diagnosis of Parkinson disease. Leverenz and Sumi found that 25 percent of their Alzheimer patients showed the pathologic (and clinical) changes of Parkinson disease—a much higher incidence than can be attributed to chance. This subject is discussed further in the section on Parkinson disease.

It is of passing historical interest that Alzheimer was not the first to describe senile plaques, the hallmark of this pathologic state. These miliary lesions ("Herdchen") had been observed in senile brains by Blocq and Marinesco in 1892, and were named "senile plaques" by Simchowicz, in 1910. In 1907, Alzheimer described the case of a 51-year-old woman who died after a 5-year illness characterized by progressive dementia. Throughout the cerebral cortex he found the miliary lesions, but he also noted—thanks to the use of Bielschowsky's silver impregnation method—a clumping and distortion of fibrils in the neuronal cytoplasm, the change which now, appropriately, carries Alzheimer's name.

Pathogenesis The pathogenesis of the aforementioned changes is unknown. Interest in recent years has centered about the marked reduction in choline acetyltransferase (ChAT) and acetylcholine in the hippocampus and neocortex of patients with Alzheimer disease. This loss of cholinergic synthetic capacity has been attributed to the loss of cells in the basal forebrain nuclei, from which the major portion of neocortical cholinergic terminals originate (Whitehouse et al). Also, the reduction in ChAT activity has been correlated with the severity of the dementia and the increase in senile plaque formation (Perry et al), though there is no uniform agreement on this point, especially with reference to the number of plaques. It should be noted, however, that 50

percent reductions in ChAT activity have also been found in regions such as the caudate nucleus, which show neither plaques nor tangles (see review of Selkoe). Increasing skepticism is being voiced about the specificity of the nucleus basalis-cholinergic-cortical changes. A carefully tested group of patients with traumatic lesions localized to the basal forebrain did not show the syndrome of dementia (Salazar et al). Also, the Alzheimer brain shows a loss of monoaminergic neurons other than cholinergic ones, and a diminution of noradrenergic and serotonergic functions in the affected neocortex. The concentration of amino acid transmitters, particularly of glutamate, is also reduced in cortical and subcortical areas (Sasaki et al). Moreover, the Alzheimer cortex shows a markedly decreased concentration of putative neuropeptide transmitters, notable substance P and somatostatin (Beal and Martin). Most importantly, it has not been determined whether any of the aforementioned biochemical abnormalities, including the cholinergic ones, are primary or are secondary to neuronal loss. And finally, the administration of cholinomimetics—whether they be acetylcholine precursors (e.g., choline or lecithin), or degradation inhibitors (e.g., physostigmine), or muscarinic agonists that act directly on postsynaptic receptors—does not have a meaningful or sustained therapeutic effect.

The initial reports of transmissibility of Alzheimer disease have not been corroborated (Goudsmit et al). The significance of a presumed scrapie-like infective agent ("prion"), described by Prusiner, remains to be determined. The prions are structurally related to amyloid, the presence of which suggests a disordered immune process. Chase et al have demonstrated a 30 percent reduction in cerebral glucose metabolism in Alzheimer disease, greatest in the parietal lobes, but the significance of this finding, whether due to loss or to hypofunction of neurons, remains to be decided. The presence of increased amounts of aluminum (and calcium) in tangle-bearing neurons is also unexplained.

The role of vascular changes in the pathogenesis is controversial. It is definite that Alzheimer disease is not related to any of the usual types of arteriosclerosis. There are, however, small-vessel changes, accounting for the reduced cerebral blood flow reported by many investigators, e.g., by Yamaguchi et al. This small-vessel change is probably secondary to the cerebral atrophy since a lesser degree of reduction in blood flow is found in the brains of mentally intact, old individuals.

A recent advance of great interest and potential importance has been the discovery, in patients with the clearly inherited form of Alzheimer disease, of the locus of the defective gene (St. George-Hyslop et al). Using genetic linkage analysis, these workers have localized the gene to chromosome 21, thus providing an explanation for the Alzheimer changes that characterize practically all patients with the trisomy 21 defect (Down syndrome). The localization of the defective gene constitutes the first step in identifying the biochemical defect of the hereditary and perhaps the "sporadic" cases of Alzheimer disease—an approach that is being used successfully in the study of Duchenne muscular dystrophy, cystic fibrosis, and Huntington chorea.

Associated pathologic states The histologic changes of Alzheimer disease have a number of rather interesting associations. These changes are far more common in the brains of patients with Parkinson disease than in the brains of age-matched controls (Hakim and Mathieson). As a corollary, large numbers of Lewy bodies (a characteristic feature of Parkinson disease) have been found in 10 percent of 96 patients with Alzheimer disease (Woodard). These findings undoubtedly explain the high incidence of dementia in patients with Parkinson disease (see further on, under paralysis agitans), yet not more than 20 to 30 percent of patients with Parkinson disease have plaques and tangles. Another association between the two diseases is apparent in the guamanian Parkinson-dementia complex, which is also discussed below. In this latter entity, the symptoms of dementia and parkinsonism are related to neurofibrillary changes in the cerebral cortex and substantia nigra, respectively; senile plaques and Lewy bodies are unusual findings.

There are instances, such as those reported by Malamud and Lowenberg and by Löken and Cyvin, in which dementia begins in late childhood, with the finding at postmortem examination of the typical Alzheimer lesions in the cerebral cortex and basal ganglia. The clinical picture in these juvenile and early adult cases has been more varied than in the older ones. In some, paucity of speech, mutism, tremor, stooped posture, marked grasp and suck reflexes, and pyramidal and cerebellar signs leading to inability to stand or walk, have appeared at various stages of the disease.

The finding of fibrillary changes, like those of Alzheimer disease, in boxers ("punch-drunk" syndrome, or "dementia pugilistica") is another interesting ramification of this disease process (page 707). Hydrocephalus is present also, but there is insufficient information to determine whether it is a normal-pressure tension hydrocephalus from multiple subarachnoid hemorrhages or a hydrocephalus ex vacuo from cerebral atrophy.

Alzheimer disease in relation to mongolism, first emphasized by Jervis, is now widely recognized. The characteristic plaques and neurofibrillary tangles appear in the third decade and increase with age, and are present in practically all patients with the Down syndrome after 40 years of age. Relatively few of these patients, however, manifest a deterioration of behavior from their previously subnormal level (recognizable deterioration occurred in only 3 of the 20 cases of Ropper and Williams).

Lobar sclerosis (Pick) has, on occasion, been associated with the histologic alterations of Alzheimer disease, as was pointed out originally by Moyano and later by Berlin. The latter referred to this combination as the *double disease*. A close relationship between Pick, Alzheimer, and Parkinson diseases has been demonstrated in a large family with dysphasic dementia (Morris et al). Other isolated combinations have been reported wherein Alzheimer disease and hypopituitarism or neurosyphilis were conjoined, but these are probably a matter of chance and prove nothing. However, where the association is more frequent, as in mongolism and dementia pugilistica, one must consider both endogenous and exogenous factors in causation. From time to time other atypical examples come to light, such as the cases of familial dementia with spastic paraplegia reported by Worster-Drought and by van Bogaert and their associates (see further on in this chapter).

Diagnostic Studies There is no available biologic marker of Alzheimer disease. The most important diagnostic measure is the CT scan. In patients with advanced Alzheimer disease the lateral and third ventricles are enlarged to about twice normal size, and the cerebral sulci are widened. Early in the disease, however, the changes do not exceed those found in many mentally intact old persons. For this reason, one cannot rely on the CT scan alone for the diagnosis of Alzheimer disease. It is most valuable in excluding brain tumor, subdural hematoma, multi-infarct dementia, and obstructive hydrocephalus. The EEG undergoes a diffuse slowing, to the theta and delta range, but only late in the course of the illness. The CSF is normal, though occasionally the total protein is slightly elevated. Using the constellation of clinical data, CT, and MRI, along with the age of the patient and time-course of the disease, the diagosis of senile dementia of Alzheimer-type is being made correctly in 85 to 90 percent of cases.

Differential Diagnosis Formerly, when virtually all forms of presenile and senile dementia were untreatable, there was little advantage to either the patient or the family in ascertaining the cause of the cerebral disease. Such patients were customarily left at home or committed to an institution for care of the psychiatrically or chronically ill. Now that a few treatable dementing diseases have been discovered, a great premium attaches to correct diagnosis. The physician is compelled to exercise care in their detection even though they may be relatively infrequent.

The treatable forms of dementia are those due to general paresis, normal-pressure hydrocephalus, chronic subdural hematoma, nutritional deficiencies (Wernicke-Korsakoff syndrome, Marchiafava-Bignami disease, pellagra, vitamin B_{12} deficiency with subacute degeneration of the spinal cord and brain), chronic drug intoxication (e.g., barbiturates, bromides, and alcohol), certain endocrine-metabolic disorders (myxedema, Cushing disease, chronic hepatic encephalopathy), certain forms of frontal and temporal lobe tumors, and the pseudodementia of depression. To exclude these several diseases requires admission to a hospital where examinations of blood and CSF, EEGs, and special radiologic studies of the cerebrum (CT scan, MRI, scintigraphic cisternography) can be undertaken.

The most difficult problem in differential diagnosis, in the authors' experience, has been the distinction between a late-life depression and senile dementia, especially when some degree of both are present. Multi-infarct dementia may be difficult to separate from senile dementia, for patients with the latter illness may have had one or more clinically inevident infarcts. Normal-pressure hydrocephalus may be confused with senile dementia. The differential diagnosis of these several conditions is discussed in Chaps. 30, 34, and 56.

Treatment   There is no evidence that any of the proposed forms of therapy for the Alzheimer–senile dementia complex—cerebral vasodilators, stimulants, L-dopa, massive doses of vitamins B, C, and E, and many others—has any salutary effect whatsoever. There is no harm in using vitamins, however, for they keep the neurologic problem on a medical plane and provide repeated medical surveillance that proves helpful in counseling the family. Trials of oral physostigmine, choline, and lecithin have yielded mostly negative or uninterpretable results (Little et al). The use of chlorpromazine and related drugs may suppress some of the aberrant behavior, when this is a problem, and make life more comfortable for the patient and the family.

The general management of the demented patient should proceed along the lines outlined in Chap. 20.

LOBAR ATROPHY (PICK)

As the name implies, this is a special form of cerebral degeneration in which the atrophy is circumscribed (most often in the frontal and/or temporal lobes), with involvement of both gray and white matter—hence the term *lobar* rather than cortical. Arnold Pick of Prague first described its gross characteristics but gave no microscopic details; he was interested particularly in disproving a tenet advanced by

Wernicke that the manifestations of senile brain atrophy were always diffuse and nonfocal. In a series of publications Pick elaborated upon the aphasic symptoms of this condition. Alzheimer in 1911 presented the first careful study of the microscopic changes. The most complete analyses of the pathologic changes are those of Spatz, van Mansvelt, Morris et al, and Tissot et al, and since the recognition of Pick disease rests on these pathologic rather than on clinical criteria, they will be described first.

In contrast to Alzheimer disease, in which the atrophy is relatively mild and diffuse, the pathologic change in Pick disease is more circumscribed, as indicated above. The atrophy may extend to the island of Reil and the amygdaloid-hippocampal structures. The parietal lobes are involved less frequently. The affected gyri become paper-thin; the brain resembles the kernel of a dried walnut. The cut surface reveals not only a markedly thinned cortical ribbon but a grayish appearance and reduced volume of the white matter. The corpus callosum and anterior commissure share in the atrophy. The overlying pia-arachnoid is thickened, and the ventricles are enlarged. The pre- and postcentral, superior temporal, and occipital convolutions are relatively unaffected and stand out in striking contrast to the wasted parts. Pick insisted that the disease involves essentially the association areas of Flechsig. In some instances, atrophy of the caudate nuclei has been pronounced, almost to the degree seen in Huntington chorea. The thalamus, subthalamic nucleus, substantia nigra, and globus pallidus may also be affected.

The salient histologic feature is a loss of neurons most marked in the first three cortical layers. Surviving neurons are often swollen and contain argentophilic (Pick) bodies within the cytoplasm. Ultrastructurally, the Pick bodies are made up of straight fibrils, thus differing from the paired helical filaments that characterize Alzheimer disease. These bodies predominate in the medial parts of the temporal lobes, especially in the atrophic hippocampi. "Ballooning" of cortical neurons is found mainly in the frontal cortex; in such cases, atrophy of the basal ganglia and substantia nigra is especially frequent, according to Tissot et al. In some cases, however, these neuronal alterations are not demonstrable. There is a loss of medullated fibers in the white matter beneath the atrophic cortex. A heavy astrocytic gliosis is seen in both the cortex and subcortical white matter. Most neuropathologists consider the loss of myelinated fibers to be consequent to neuronal loss; Spatz believed that the site of primary damage was in the axon near the cell body and that swelling of the latter represented an "axonal reaction." Senile plaques and

Alzheimer neurofibrillary changes are frequently seen in the atrophic zones, and there is granulovacuolar degeneration of neurons in the hippocampus, but not to the degree seen in Alzheimer disease.

Symptomatology Whether the diagnosis is possible during life is doubtful; our clinical predictions as to the existence of the pathologic changes have been erratic, but they should improve with the use of CT scanning and MRI. In our opinion, the gradual onset of forgetfulness and confusion with respect to place and time, slowness of comprehension, inability to cope with unaccustomed problems, depreciation of social and work habits, and impairments in personality and behavior do not in any way distinguish between Pick and Alzheimer diseases. Focal disturbances are said to be early and prominent in Pick disease, pointing to a lesion in the frontal, temporal, or parietal lobes. Apathy, abulia, impairment of gait and upright stance, with prominent grasp and suck reflexes, indicate predominant affection of the frontal lobes. Language disorder has been reported in two-thirds of all patients with temporal lobe atrophy. At first the patient speaks less but language is intact; later he or she may forget and misuse words and fail to understand much of what is heard or read. Speech becomes a "medley of disconnected words and phrases" and eventually is reduced to an incomprehensible jargon. Finally, the patient is altogether mute, seemingly without impulse to speak or ability to form words. Verbal perseveration, palilalia, and echolalia have been described. Bulimia and alterations in sexual behavior occur to a distressing degree in some patients (Tissot et al).

Wilson distinguished two patterns of abnormal behavior: in one, the patient is talkative, lighthearted, and gay or anxious and uneasy, constantly on the move, occupied with trifles, and attentive to every passing incident; in the other, the patient is taciturn, inert, emotionally dull, and lacking in initiative and impulse. Probably these two patterns represent the temporal and frontal types, respectively. Those who have tried to distinguish Alzheimer and Pick diseases clinically have chosen the frontal type of Pick disease as the prototype. According to Tissot et al, the frontal, temporal, and parietal lobes are all affected in 75 percent of patients by the time the disease terminates.

Exceptionally, cerebellar ataxia or shuffling gait, weakness, rigidity, and pseudocontractures of the limbs may be prominent features. Van Mansvelt remarks upon seven or eight cases in which there was an associated amyotrophic lateral sclerosis, a relationship that we have been unable to corroborate in a pathologic study of several cases of Pick disease.

The cause of Pick disease is unknown. Sjögren et al concluded from a genetic survey of the cases in Stockholm that it was probably transmitted as a dominant trait with polygenic modification. Women seem to be affected more often than men. No chemical, vascular, traumatic, or other factor of possible causal importance has been identified.

The course of the illness is usually 2 to 5 years, occasionally longer, and nothing can be done therapeutically except to postpone the end by careful nursing.

"SUBCORTICAL" DEMENTIA

Of late there has been considerable interest in differentiating cortical and subcortical dementias. Senile dementia of the Alzheimer type is held to be the classic example of a cortical dementia. Huntington chorea, Parkinson disease, progressive supranuclear palsy, Wilson disease, Hallervorden-Spatz disease, and multiple infarct disease represent types of subcortical dementia. On the basis of psychometric analyses, the cortical dementias are featured by amnesia, aphasia, agnosia, and apraxia, whereas the subcortical ones are characterized by lesser degrees of dementia and amnesia and a lack of aphasia, agnosia, and apraxia. Movement disorder is often conjoined (Brandt et al).

Anatomically, no form of dementia is strictly cortical or subcortical, not even Alzheimer disease, in which the changes extend far beyond the confines of the cerebral cortex, involving the striatum, thalamus, and even the cerebellum. Also, it should be pointed out that severe degrees of dementia and impairment of memory and language function may be caused by lesions in subcortical structures (e.g., thalamus). There is no cogent evidence that a distinctive pattern of psychologic impairment can be related to diseases with a predominantly subcortical pathology. The proposed qualitative differences between cortical and subcortical dementia are probably attributable to differences in severity of the dementing processes, an argument that has been made convincingly by Mayeux, by Stern, and by Tierney and his colleagues.

Thus, the authors agree with Whitaker that a categorical distinction between these two forms of dementia cannot presently be validated on clinical, pathologic, or biochemical grounds. Yet there is no doubt that each of these cerebral diseases exhibits certain recognizable clinical peculiarities based on its distinctive pathology and anatomy. To cover all their mental and behavioral abnormalities by the generic term dementia obscures rather than clarifies the main issues.

There are other forms of progressive, diffuse brain atrophy leading to dementia that show none of the pathologic features of either Alzheimer or Pick disease, or any of the other diseases associated with dementia (Wilson disease, Creutzfeldt-Jakob disease, amyotrophic lateral sclerosis, etc.).

In Sweden, for example, Sjögren has found familial cases of this type, as have Schaumburg and Suzuki in this country, and we have seen occasional sporadic examples. The clinical picture in these cases has been indistinguishable from that of Alzheimer disease, and autopsy has disclosed widespread cerebral atrophy, most pronounced in the frontal and temporal lobes. Microscopically these cases were characterized by a diffuse neuronal loss, slight glial proliferation, and secondary demyelination of the white matter, but no other histologic changes of note. Other instances of sporadic and familial presenile dementia have shown subcortical gliosis or nonspecific cellular changes (atrophy of nerve cells and nuclei, loss of Nissl substance). Some examples of the latter type have in the past been described under the rubric of "Kraepelin disease." Another dementing syndrome clinically indistinguishable from Alzheimer disease is that in which the cortical neurons contain Lewy bodies and in which no neurofibrillary changes or senile plaques can be observed.

"Thalamic Dementia" A relatively pure degeneration of thalamic neurons has also been found in relation to a progressive dementia (Stern; Schulman). The dementia in these cases evolved relatively rapidly (several months) and was associated with choreoathetosis. Garcin and his colleagues described three cases of subacutely developing dementia, which they considered to be examples of Creutzfeldt-Jakob disease; in each of them the pathologic changes consisted primarily of neuronal loss and gliosis of the thalamus. A large kindred of such cases, characterized by subacute dementia and myoclonus and inherited as an autosomal trait, has been reported by Little and his coworkers. The clinical presentation in members of this kindred was very similar to Creutzfeldt-Jakob disease; however, the pathologic changes were confined to the thalami, particularly to the medial-dorsal and medial nuclei, and transmission of the disease to primates was unsuccessful.

In addition to these poorly classified forms of dementia, there are other somewhat better characterized dementing diseases, such as the following:

1. *Arteriosclerotic dementia* refers to an impairment of intellectual function due to multiple infarcts. As would be expected, vascular lesions in particular regions such as the medial temporal lobes, the medial frontal lobes, the corpus callosum, and the nondominant parietal lobe induce special types of mental abnormality, already described in Chaps. 21 and 34. In all such instances the history of one or more strokes can usually be elicited, and the focal deficit will have had the characteristic temporal profile of such an event. The degree of focal neurologic deficit may be small in comparison to the cognitive impairment, especially if many "silent areas" had been involved. Slow progression of dementia unpunctuated by strokes or only by some minor cerebrovascular incident is usually indicative of the Alzheimer–senile dementia complex, even in the face of hypertension and atherosclerotic occlusion of coronary and other arteries. Multiple lacunar infarcts produce a picture of pseudobulbar palsy with its typical labile emotionality, slurred speech, dysphagia, lively facial and mandibular reflexes, etc., but again this rarely happens without at least one incident of stroke. It is now generally agreed that the so-called progressive subcortical encephalitis of Binswanger is a form of arteriosclerosis with multiple infarcts (lacunar and larger infarcts) that tend to be localized to the cerebral white matter and to be associated with dementia.

A special problem relates to the interpretation of CT scans in Alzheimer disease and multi-infarct dementia. Often in both groups of diseases there are periventricular zones of white matter rarefaction, to be distinguished from infarcts. These lucencies were observed in one-third of the cases of Alzheimer disease reported by Steingart and his colleagues.

2. *Severe trauma* may also leave in its wake certain lasting cerebral deficits, usually under circumstances in which prolonged coma and stupor followed the injury. Enduring mental enfeeblement is exceptional, however, except in association with severe neurologic disability of other type (page 703). McMenemey quotes a number of cases in which a relatively minor cranial injury had marked the beginning of a dementia in which the histologic changes of Alzheimer disease were eventually demonstrated. The authors can only assume that trauma had called attention to an unrelated, ongoing Alzheimer disease.

3. In exceptional instances, *hypoxic encephalopathy and acute inclusion-body (herpes simplex) encephalitis* have left the individual relatively intact, except for impairment of memory and difficulty in learning and assimilating new information. In several such cases, examined pathologically many years later, we have observed destructive lesions limited to the inferomedial portions of both temporal lobes. Unless one knew about the initial event and had accurate

information concerning the long-term stability of the intellectual deficit, it would be impossible to differentiate such states clinically from a progressive cerebral degenerative disease.

DISEASES IN WHICH DEMENTIA IS ASSOCIATED WITH OTHER NEUROLOGIC ABNORMALITIES

HUNTINGTON CHOREA

This disease, distinguished by the triad of dominant inheritance, choreoathetosis, and dementia, commemorates the name of George Huntington, a medical practitioner of Pomeroy, Ohio. In 1872, in a paper read before the Meigs and Mason Academy of Medicine and published later that year in the *Medical and Surgical Reporter* of Philadelphia, Huntington gave a succinct and graphic account of the disease, based on observations of patients that his father and grandfather had gathered in the course of their practice in East Hampton, Long Island. Reports of this disease had appeared previously (see reference to DeJong for historical background), but lacked the accuracy and completeness of Huntington's description. Vessie, in 1932, was able to show that practically all the patients with this disease in the eastern United States could be traced to about six individuals who had emigrated in 1630 from the tiny East Anglian village of Bures, in Suffolk, England. One remarkable family was traced for 300 years through 12 generations, in each of which the disease had expressed itself.

To quote Huntington, the rule has been that "When either or both of the parents have shown manifestations of the disease . . . one or more of the offspring invariably suffer of the disease, if they live to adult life. But if by any chance these children go through life without it, the thread is broken and the grandchildren and great-grandchildren of the original shakers may rest assured that they are free from disease." Davenport, in a review of 962 patients with Huntington chorea, found only five who had descended from unaffected parents. Possibly, in these latter patients, a parent had the trait, but in very mild form. More likely, they represented rare sporadic instances of Huntington chorea, i.e., ones in whom a mutation had occurred from a normal gene to the mutant, disease-producing form.

In university hospital centers this is one of the most frequently observed types of hereditary nervous disease. Seldom does a month pass without one coming to our

notice. Its frequency is estimated at 4 to 5 per million. Males are said to be affected more often, but we have been unable to substantiate this point. The usual age of onset is in the fourth and fifth decades, but 3 to 5 percent begin before the fifteenth year, and some even in childhood. Twenty-eight percent begin after 50 years. The progression of the disease is slower in older patients. Once begun, the disease progresses relentlessly, until only a restricted existence in a nursing home or psychiatric hospital is possible, and some other disease terminates life.

Exhaustive genealogic documentation has established the cause to be a monohybrid autosomal gene of dominant type with complete penetrance. Martin has made the observation that young patients usually inherit the disease from their father and older patients from their mother. It has been observed in four sets of identical twins beginning at almost the same age.

Until recently, it had not been possible to foretell which of the children of a patient will be stricken with the disease. Based on the hypothesis that the disease is related to an enhanced sensitivity of striatal neurons to dopamine, the claim has been made that a "challenge" with 3.0 g L-dopa daily (which tends to induce choreoathetosis in parkinsonian patients) for a period of a month will cause chorea in prospective victims. The predictive value of this test has not been established (Klawans et al), and, until it is, L-dopa should not be administered to patients at risk of developing the disease. Also, caudate glucose metabolism, measured by positron emission tomographic scanning, is not a useful means of detecting persons at risk for Huntington disease, since it has proved to be normal in such persons (Young et al).

The most promising achievement in respect to the presymptomatic detection of Huntington disease has been the discovery, by Gusella and his colleagues, of a marker that is linked to the Huntington gene and is localized to the short arm of chromosome 4. This discovery has made possible the development of a test for the detection of carriers of the defective gene. Since the test does not identify the gene itself but depends upon linkage analysis, it requires that all available members of the affected family be tested; also certain ethical considerations need to be resolved before widespread testing can be realized (Martin).

Symptomatology   The mental disorder assumes several subtle forms long before the deterioration of cognitive function becomes evident. In approximately half the cases, slight alterations of character are often a source of annoyance to others. Patients begin to find fault and complain about everything and to nag other members of the family; they may be suspicious, irritable, impulsive, eccentric, or excessively religious, or they may exhibit a false sense of superiority. Poor self-control may be reflected in outbursts of temper, fits of despondency, alcoholism, or sexual promiscuity. These emotional disturbances and changes in character may reach such proportions as to constitute a virtual psychosis. Disturbances of mood, particularly depression, are common and may constitute the most prominent symptoms early in the disease. Invariably, intellect begins to fail. Diminished work performance and inability to manage household responsibilities may prompt medical consultation. Memory and attentiveness are the first faculties to be reduced. The gradual dilapidation of intellect resembles that of certain other types of dementia; elements of aphasia, agnosia, and apraxia are observed rarely. Often the process is so slow that even though the patient is mentally impaired, some degree of functional capacity is retained for many years.

The abnormality of movement is at first slight, involving the hands and face; the patient is merely considered to be fidgety or restless and "nervous." Slowly it becomes more pronounced until the entire musculature is implicated. Seldom in the advanced stage of the disease is the patient still for more than a few seconds. The movements are slower than the brusque jerks and postural lapses of Sydenham chorea, and they involve many more muscles. They tend to recur in stereotyped patterns yet not so stereotyped as tics. In more advanced cases they acquire an athetoid or dystonic quality, as pointed out by Denny-Brown. The disorder of movement is described more fully in Chap. 4. There is no weakness and no real ataxia. Voluntary movements are initiated and executed more slowly than normal. Muscle tone is variable. The speech becomes dysarthric and explosive. Ocular motor function is impaired in most patients (Leigh et al; Lasker et al). Particularly characteristic are impaired initiation and slowness of saccadic movements, inability to make a volitional saccade without movement of the head, and excessive distractibility during attempted fixation. The patient feels compelled to glance at extraneous stimuli even when specifically instructed to ignore them. Denny-Brown has pointed out that when the Huntington patient is suspended, the upper limbs assume a flexed posture and the legs an extended one, a posture that he consideres to be expressive of the striatal syndrome.

As Wilson stated, the relation of the choreic to mental symptoms "abides by no general rule." Most often the emotional and mental symptoms accompany the chorea, but they may follow or precede the onset of chorea, sometimes by several years. Either the chorea or the mental changes may be present for a long time without the other. A recurrent theme in older medical writings, unproven in our opinion, is that Huntington families have an inordinately high incidence of other neuropathic or psychopathic tendencies—mental retardation, constitutional psychopathy (sociopathy), neuroses, and the like. Of undoubted neuro-

psychiatric importance is the high suicide rate in huntingtonians (Schoenfeld et al). Also there is a high incidence of trauma; nearly half the patients with Huntington chorea dying at the Massachusetts General Hospital have had chronic subdural hematomas.

The first signs of the disease may appear in childhood, before puberty (even under the age of 4), and several series of such cases have been described (Farrer and Conneally; van Dijk et al). Mental deterioration at this early age is more often accompanied by seizures, bradykinesia, rigidity, and dystonia than by chorea. However, a rigid form of the disease is known also to occur in adults (Westphal variant). The functional decline in children is much faster than in adults (Young et al).

Earlier onset in successive generations (*anticipation*) has been reported in the past, but has not been confirmed by the study of Chandler et al. The latter authors have shown that the disease is generally more severe in cases of early onset (15 to 40 years) than in those of later onset (55 to 60 years). Furthermore, in adult patients with early onset of the disease, the emotional disturbance tends to be initially prominent and precedes the chorea and intellectual loss by many years; with older age of onset, choreiform movements and progressive dementia are more often the initial components and have their onset at nearly the same age.

Pathology Gross wasting of the head of the caudate nucleus and putamen bilaterally is the characteristic abnormality, usually accompanied by a moderate degree of gyral atrophy in the frontal and temporal regions. The caudatal atrophy alters the configuration of the frontal horns of the lateral ventricles; the inferolateral borders do not show the usual bulge created by the head of the caudate nucleus, and in addition the ventricles are diffusely enlarged (Fig. 43-1). In CT scans the bicaudate-cranial index is increased in the majority of patients. This finding corroborates the clinical diagnosis in the moderately advanced case.

The early articles of Alzheimer, Ramsay Hunt, and Dunlap, and the more recent one of Von Sattel et al contain the most authoritative descriptions of the microscopic changes. The latter authors have graded the disease into early, moderately advanced, and far advanced. In five early cases no striatal lesion was found, which suggests that the first clinical manifestations are based on a biochemical disorder without visible structural change, at least by light microscopy. This view is supported by the observation that Huntington patients studied with positron emission computed tomography (PET) show a characteristic decrease in glucose utilization, which appears early in the disease and

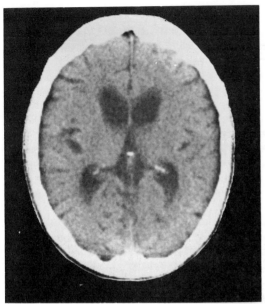

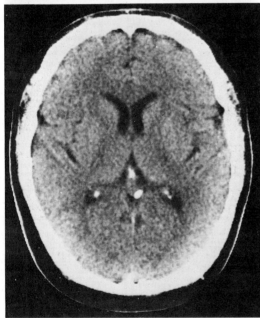

Figure 43-1

The upper CT scan is from a 54-year-old mildly demented woman with a 10-year history of Huntington chorea. The bulge in the inferolateal border of the lateral ventricle, normally created by the head of the caudate nucleus (lower scan), has been obliterated. There is also a diffuse enlargement of the lateral ventricles.

precedes the loss of tissue (Kuhl et al; Hayden et al). The striatal degeneration begins in the medial part of the caudate nucleus and spreads, tending to spare the nucleus accumbens. Of the six cell types in the striatum (differentiation based on size, dendritic arborizations, spines, and axon trajectories), it is not known if certain ones are more susceptible. In general the smaller cells are affected before the larger ones and are replaced by fibrous astrocytes; the large cells are relatively preserved and exhibit no special alterations. The anterior parts of the putamen and caudatum are more affected than the posterior parts. With the neuronal loss the myelinated fibers also disappear. In our own cases we have not been impressed with changes in the globus pallidus, subthalamic nucleus, red nucleus, or cerebellum; others have observed slight changes in these parts and in the substantia nigra. In the atrophic parts of the cerebral cortex, there is said to be slight neuronal loss in layers 3, 5, and 6, with replacement gliosis. Cases are reported with typical striatal lesions but normal cortices, in which only senile chorea had been present during life. In our early to moderately advanced cases even quantitative analyses of the cortex have not disclosed a significant loss of neurons. Several neuropathologists have observed marked cell loss and gliosis in the subthalamic nuclei in children or young adults with chorea and behavior disorders.

The biochemical defects in Huntington chorea are only beginning to be undertstood. The decreased glucose utilization by caudate cells, preceding visible atrophy, has already been mentioned. Since at least a partial explanation for L-dopa induced involuntary movements is an excess of dopamine (in contrast to Parkinson disease, in which there is a decrease), it has been postulated that the abnormal movements of Huntington chorea represent a heightened sensitivity of striatal dopamine receptors. The induction of *tardive dyskinesias* by the chronic administration of phenothiazines in patients without striatal lesions would support such a concept. There is a disturbance in the metabolism of other putative neurotransmitters as well. Spokes has reported that noradrenaline is increased in the striatum and lateral pallidum. Bird and Iversen found that glutamic acid decarboxylase and choline acetyltransferase were reduced in these areas. γ-Aminobutyric acid (GABA) and acetylcholine are also reduced since they are dependent on the activity of these two enzymes. Enna has shown that the GABA-binding sites on striatal neurons are not depleted beyond what would be expected from loss of nerve cells. Therefore one would expect that the strategy of facilitating GABA-ergic transmission would be effective. So far, however, the treatment of Huntington chorea with GABA-mimetic drugs has met with only limited success (Shoulson et al). Beal and Martin have found an increase in somatostatin in the striatum. In contrast, in Alzheimer disease, where there is little or no striatal neuron loss, the level of somatostatin is reduced. The significance of this biochemical finding is unknown.

Diagnostic Problems Once the disease has been observed in its fully developed form, it requires no great clinical acumen to recognize it. The main difficulty arises in patients who lack a family history but in whom the progressive chorea, emotional disturbance, and dementia beginning in adult life are typical. Sometimes it is learned later that the family history was incomplete or falsified, or that an illness in a parent had been misinterpreted. Chorea that begins in late life, with only mild or questionable intellectual impairment and without a family history of similar disease, is another source of difficulty; referring to it as *senile chorea* does not solve the problem. Indeed, senile chorea may have more than one cause. We have seen it appear with infections and drug therapy, only to disappear after a few weeks. *Recurrent chorea* in early adult life always raises the question of a late form of Sydenham chorea, an illness in which neither family history nor mental deterioration are seen. Other progressive neurologic disorders that are inherited in an autosomal dominant pattern and begin in adolescence or adult life (polymyoclonus with or without ataxia, double athetosis) always raise questions of atypical Huntington chorea; these matters are impossible to resolve clinically. Even the pathologic picture may not settle the matter, for the typical striatal lesions of Huntington chorea are seen in striatonigral degeneration and in other diseases.

Other problems in differential diagnosis include acanthocytosis with progressive chorea, a rare familial disease that is described below, bilateral thalamic degeneration with dementia and chorea, paroxysmal choreoathetosis of Mount and Reback (page 65), acquired hepatocerebral degeneration (page 862), and most often schizophrenia or manic-depressive psychosis with tardive dyskinesia (page 901).

Therapy The authors have not been impressed with any of the currently available drugs. Levodopa makes the chorea worse and, in the rigid form of the disease, evokes chorea. Drugs that block dopamine receptors, such as reserpine and tetrabenazine, suppress the chorea to some degree, but their side effects (drowsiness, akathisia, and tardive dyskinesia) outweigh their desired effects. Haloperidol, in daily doses of 2 to 10 mg, is probably the most effective agent in suppressing the chorea. Because of the danger of superimposing tardive dyskinesia on the chronic disorder, the chorea should be treated only if it is functionally disabling, using the smallest possible dosages of haloperidol and providing numerous drug holidays. Haloperidol may also help alleviate abnormalities of behavior or emotional lability, but it does not alter the progress of the disease. Drugs that facilitate GABA and acetylcholine synthesis have been

unsuccessful. The juvenile form of the disease is probably best treated with antiparkinsonian drugs. The disease pursues a steady progressive course and death occurs, on an average, 15 to 16 years after onset, sometimes much earlier or later. The psychologic and social consequences of the disease require supportive therapy, and genetic counseling is essential.

ACANTHOCYTOSIS WITH CHOREA

In recent years a few reports of a slowly progressive familial chorea in association with an abnormality of erythrocytes have appeared in English, American, and Japanese journals. The disease has the following characteristics: (1) onset in adolescence or early adult life of generalized involuntary movements (described as chorea), usually beginning as an orofacial dyskinesia and spreading to other parts of the body; (2) mild to moderate mental deterioration in some but not all of the cases; (3) decreased or absent tendon reflexes and evidence of denervation atrophy of muscles; (4) erythrocyte acanthocytosis; (5) atrophy and gliosis of the caudate nuclei and putamens but no neuronal loss in the cerebral cortex or other parts of the brain. The pattern of inheritance has been autosomal recessive, but was dominant in one New England family. The glutamic acid decarboxylase levels were not decreased as they are in Huntington chorea. The spinal cord is reported to be normal. The disorder differs, therefore, from Huntington chorea and from Bassen-Kornzweig, Wilson, and Hallervorden-Spatz diseases.

CORTICOSTRIATOSPINAL DEGENERATION [PARKINSON-DEMENTIA (PD) AND AMYOTROPHIC LATERAL SCLEROSIS (ALS) COMPLEX]

Under the title "spastic pseudosclerosis," Jakob, in 1921, described a chronic disease of middle to late adult life, characterized clinically by abnormalities of behavior and intellect; weakness, ataxia, and spasticity of the limbs (chiefly the legs); extrapyramidal symptoms such as rigidity, slowness of movement, tremors, athetotic postures, and hesitant, dysarthric speech; and normal spinal fluid. The lesions were diffuse and consisted mainly of an outfall of neurons in the frontal, temporal, and central motor gyri, corpus striatum, ventromedial thalamus, and bulbar motor nuclei. In one of Jakob's cases, there were prominent changes in the anterior horns and corticospinal tracts in the spinal cord, like those of amyotrophic lateral sclerosis

(ALS). The latter finding probably gave rise to Wilson's concept of the disease as a *corticostriatospinal degeneration*. A degenerative and probably familial disorder that had been described earlier by Creutzfeldt was considered by Spielmeyer to be sufficiently similar to the one of Jakob to warrant the designation Creutzfeldt-Jakob disease.

The disorder described by Creutzfeldt and Jakob has been a source of endless controversy because of its indeterminate character. On the one hand, it has been confused with the subacutely evolving myoclonic dementia, sometimes called Heidenhain disease (when visual disorder is prominent) or "subacute spongiform encephalopathy" and that now is known to be an infection akin to kuru, due to a transmissible agent. The authors believe that this latter disease, which is described on page 609, bears at best only a superficial resemblance to the one described by Creutzfeldt and Jakob, and that the two disorders should be clearly separated. Unfortunately, the eponym is so entrenched in medical usage that any attempt to remove it stands little chance of success.

On the other side, the disease described by Creutzfeldt and Jakob merges with a rather heterogeneous but overlapping group of degenerative disorders, including progressive dementia and spastic paraplegia, progressive dementia and ALS, the Parkinson-dementia-ALS complex of Guam, and the corticopallidospinal degeneration of Davison. One is tempted to conclude that the spastic pseudosclerosis of Jakob should not be reckoned with as a disease type, and certainly everyone agrees that the term *pseudosclerosis* (also used for the Westphal-Strümpell form of hepatolenticular degeneration) is worthless. Wilson's arguments for retaining the entity described by Jakob are rational, but we doubt that it refers to a disease *sui generis*.

The authors have observed several patients in whom extreme rigidity, pyramidal signs, and evidences of amyotrophic lateral sclerosis have developed over a period of several years. In the later stages of the disease the patient, while alert, is totally helpless, unable to speak, swallow, or move the limbs. Only eye movements are retained. Intellectual functioning is better preserved than movement but is difficult to assess. Other bodily functions are intact. The course is slowly progressive and ends fatally in 5 to 10 years. There is no family history, and there are no clues as to causation.

CORTICAL-BASAL GANGLIONIC SYNDROMES

Over the years the authors have observed several elderly patients, both men and women, in whom the essential abnormality was a progressive extrapyramidal rigidity and/ or tremor (suggestive in some respects of Parkinson disease) combined with signs of corticospinal disease. The relation of such cases to corticostriatospinal degeneration is indeterminate. The patients, though able to exert considerable muscle power, cannot voluntarily direct their efforts. Attempts to move a limb to accomplish some purposeful act might result in a totally inappropriate movement, always with great enhancement of the rigidity in the limb and in other affected parts. Other attempts might result in a persistent elevation of an arm or leg, sometimes without the patient being aware of it—a kind of involuntary catalepsy. With progression of the disease the limbs on both sides of the body and the cranial muscles are involved; and a variable combination of apraxia, rigidity, sensory ataxia, and action tremor finally renders the patient helpless, unable to sit, stand, speak, or take care of his basic needs. Mental deterioration of nonspecific type occurs late, but only in some cases. In a few of the cases there is some involvement of lower motor neurons. The condition progresses for 5 years or more before some medical complication overtakes the patient.

Postmortem examination has disclosed a combination of findings that stamps the disease process as unique. Cortical atrophy [mainly in the frontal (motor-premotor) and parietal lobes] is associated with degeneration of the substantia nigra and, in one instance, of the dentatorubrothalamic fibers. The loss of nerve cells is fairly marked, but there is no gross lobar atrophy, as occurs in Pick disease. The neuronal degeneration may be more on one side than the other. There is moderate gliosis in the cortex and underlying white matter. Many of the residual nerve cells are swollen and chromatolyzed with eccentric nuclei, a state to which Rebeiz and his colleagues have given the name *achromasia;* it resembles the central chromatolysis of axonal reaction. No Pick bodies, Alzheimer fibrillary changes, senile plaques, granulovacuolar changes, amyloid deposits, or Lewy bodies are seen.

We have searched unsuccessfully for clues as to the cause and pathogenesis of these diseases. There is no family history. No other organ is affected. The progression is relentless. None of the drugs in common use for spasticity, rigidity, and tremor have been helpful. We know of no attempt to transfer the disease to primates.

Marinescu has described a rather different state resembling more a severe form of Alzheimer disease, but with signs of both pyramidal and extrapyramidal disease (rigidity, tremor, nystagmus, incoordination, confusion, disorientation, and loss of memory). There was amyloidosis of blood vessels (so-called Scholz's perivascular plaques) in the cerebral white matter as well as in the liver and kidney. The disease bears some resemblance to the corticostriatospinal degeneration ("spastic pseudosclerosis") of Jakob.

GERSTMANN-STRAUSSLER DISEASE (ALSO GERSTMANN-STRAUSSLER-SCHEINKER DISEASE)

These terms denote an entity, usually familial (sometimes sporadic), that was first observed in an Austrian family by Gerstmann in 1936; other cases have since appeared in the United States and Japan. Seitelberger has provided an informative study of the neuropathologic changes.

The usual clinical picture is that of an adult who slowly develops dysarthria and cerebellar ataxia, raising the question of an hereditary ataxia. As time passes elements of bradykinesia and pyramidal signs begin to appear and finally, after some years, a form of dementia. The tendon reflexes in the legs diminish and are eventually lost, but there is no clear cut evidence of a sensorimotor polyneuropathy. Nystagmus is present in some cases. The span of the disease is 1 to 3 or 4 years. Light microscopy of the somewhat atrophied brain reveals: (1) massive multiform plaques (like so-called kuru bodies) mainly in the cerebellar cortex; (2) degeneration of fiber systems (spinocerebellar and corticospinal tracts and posterior columns of spinal cord) and gray matter (Purkinje cells, granule cells, neurons of cerebral cortex and caudate nuclei); (3) spongy change in the cerebral cortex and caudate nuclei in some cases but not in others. There are no senile plaques or neurofibrillary changes. The cores of the kuru-like plaques consist of radially arranged amyloid fibrils. Some of the anterior horn cells show chromatolysis. Some cases of this disease have been successfully transmitted to monkeys.

This relationship of Gerstmann-Straussler disease to kuru and to Creutzfeldt-Jakob disease received confirmation in the study of two bothers by Tateichi et al. Although in one case there was no spongiform change, immunostaining with antikuru plaque core protein and anti-B-protein peptide revealed many kuru plaques, and the disease was successfully transmitted to mice. It appears likely that Gerstmann-Straussler disease represents a familial form of Creutzfeldt-Jakob spongiform encephalopathy.

FAMILIAL DEMENTIA WITH SPASTIC PARAPARESIS

From time to time the authors have encountered families in which several members during middle adult years developed a spastic paraparesis and a gradual failure of intellect. The mental horizon of the patient narrowed gradually, and the capacity for high-level thinking diminished; in addition the examination showed appropriately exaggerated tendon reflexes, clonus, and Babinski signs. In one such family this illness had occurred in two generations; in another, three brothers in a single generation were afflicted. Skre described two recessive types of hereditary spastic paraplegia in Norway, one with onset in childhood,

the other in adult life. In contrast to the dominant form (see below) the recessive types displayed evidence of more widespread involvement of the nervous system, incuding dementia, cerebellar ataxia, and epilepsy. Also, Cross and McKusick have observed a recessive type of paraplegia, accompanied by dementia, that began in adolescence. They named it the Mast syndrome, after the afflicted family.

Worster-Drought et al have reported the pathologic findings in two cases of this type. In addition to senile plaques and neurofibrillary changes, there was demyelination of the subcortical white matter and corpus callosum and a "patchy but gross swelling of the arterioles" which gave the staining reactions for amyloid ("Scholz's perivascular plaques"). Van Bogaert et al have published an account of similar cases which showed the characteristic pathologic features of Alzheimer disease.

Adult forms of metachromatic leukoencephalopathy, as in the families described by Austin et al, may present with a similar clinical picture. Another interesting association of familial spastic paraplegia is with progressive cerebellar ataxia. Fully a third of the cases that we have seen with such a spastic weakness were also ataxic and would fall in the category of spinocerebellar degenerations.

DISEASES CHARACTERIZED BY ABNORMALITIES OF POSTURE AND MOVEMENT

PARALYSIS AGITANS (PARKINSON DISEASE)

This rather common disease, known since ancient times, was first cogently described by James Parkinson, in 1817. In his words, it is characterized by "involuntary tremulous motion, with lessened muscular power, in parts not in action and even when supported; with a propensity to bend the trunk forward, and to pass from a walking to a running pace, the senses and intellect being uninjured." Strangely, his essay contains no reference to rigidity or to slowness of movement, and, in the authors' opinion, it stresses unduly the reduction in muscular power. The same criticism can be leveled against the term *paralysis agitans,* which appeared for the first time in Marshall Hall's textbook *Diseases and Derangements of the Nervous System,* in 1841.

Certain biometric data are of interest. As a rule, the disease begins between 40 and 70 years of age with the peak age of onset in the sixth decade. It is infrequent before 30 years of age (only 4 of 380 cases in one series) and although some observers comment on a higher incidence in men, we have not been impressed with such a difference. Trauma, emotional upset, overwork, exposure to cold, etc., have been suggested as predisposing or exciting factors, but there is no convincing evidence to support any such claim. The malady is observed in all countries, all ethnic groups, and all socioeconomic classes. Familial cases are on record, but the evidence is rather unsubstantial, especially when one allows the possibility that some of these cases may have been examples of postencephalitic parkinsonism or striatonigral degeneration.

The disease is frequent. In the United States there are approximately a half-million patients; about 1 percent of the population over the age of 50 years is affected. The incidence in all countries where vital statistics are kept is the same. Considering its frequency, coincidence in a family on the basis of chance occurrence might be as high as 5 percent.

Symptomatology   The core syndrome of expressionless face, poverty and slowness of voluntary movement, "resting" tremor, stooped posture, rigidity, and festinating gait has been fully described in Chap. 4, and only certain diagnostic problems and variants in the clinical picture will be considered here. The early symptoms may be difficult to perceive and are often overlooked. Advancing years have a way of rendering the spine and limbs less pliable and elastic; and in the senium the gait may become short-stepped and then reduced to a shuffle, and the voice tends to become soft and monotonous. Hence it is all too easy to attribute the early symptoms to the effects of aging. The patient may for a long time not be conscious of the inroads of the disease; at first the only complaints will be of aching, fatigue, and malaise. A slight stiffness and slowness are ignored until one day it occurs to the physician or to a member of the family that the patient has Parkinson disease. Infrequency of blinking, as pointed out originally by Pierre Marie, is often a helpful early sign. The usual rate (about 20 blinks per minute) is reduced in the parkinsonian patient to 5 to 10. And with it there is a slight widening of the palpebral fissures (Stellwag sign). When seated, the patient makes fewer little shifts and adjustments of position than the normal person, and the fingers straighten and assume a flexed and adducted posture at the metacarpal-phalangeal joints.

The characteristic tremor, which usually involves a hand, is often listed as the initial sign; but in at least half the cases, observant family members will have remarked earlier on the relative immobility and the poverty of movement. Other warning symptoms are aching in the neck, shoulders, back, and hips which may be passed off as osteoarthritis, a surmise that may be correct except that parkinsonian rigidity may have aggravated the pain.

The tremor of the fully developed case takes several forms, as was remarked in Chap. 5. The 4-per-second "pill-rolling" tremor of the thumb and fingers is typically present when the hand is motionless, i.e., not used in voluntary movement (hence the term *resting tremor*). Complete rest, however, abolishes or reduces the tremor, and a volitional movement usually but not always dampens it momentarily. The rhythmic beat coincides with an alternating burst of activity in agonists and antagonists in the EMG. Arm, jaw, tongue, eyelids, and foot are less often involved. The least degree of tremor is felt during passive movement of a rigid part (cogwheel phenomenon or Negro's sign). The tremor shows surprising fluctuations from moment to moment and is aggravated by excitement.

Lance et al have called attention to another type of tremor in paralysis agitans—a fine, 7- to 8-per-second, slightly irregular action tremor of the outstretched fingers and hands. Unlike the slower tremor, this one persists throughout voluntary movement and is more easily suppressed by relaxation. Electromyographically, it lacks the alternating bursts of action potentials seen in the more typical tremor. The patient may have either type of tremor or both.

We have been less impressed with rigidity and hypertonus as important early findings. They tend to appear in the more advanced stages of the disease. Once rigidity develops, it is constantly present, and can be felt by the palpating finger and seen as a salience of muscle groups, even when the patient relaxes. When the examiner passively moves the limb, a mild resistance appears from the start (without the short free interval that characterizes spasticity), and it continues evenly throughout the movement, being altered only by the cogwheel phenomenon.

The basic postural hypertonus predominates in the flexor muscles of trunk and limbs and confers upon the patient the characteristic flexed posture. Particulars of the parkinsonian disorders of muscle tone and of stance and gait are discussed in Chaps. 4 and 6.

As regards the quality of volitional and postural movements, a few additional points may be made. The patient is slow and ineffective in attempts to deliver a quick hard blow. According to Hallett and Khoshbin, the parkinsonian patient cannot complete a quick movement by a single burst of agonist-antagonist-agonist sequence of energizing activity, like the normal person (see also page 58). Alternating movements, at first successful, become progressively impeded and finally are blocked completely or adopt the rhythm of the patient's tremor. Originally it was thought that rigidity interferes with facility of movement, but the observation that appropriately placed surgical lesions can abolish rigidity without affecting the disorder of movement refutes this interpretation. Thus the difficulty is not one of rigidity but of *bradykinesia* (slowness of movement) and of *akinesia* or *hypokinesia*. The latter deficits underlie the characteristic poverty of movement, shown by infrequency of swallowing, slowness of chewing, a limited capacity to make postural adjustments of the body and limbs in response to displacement of these parts, a lack of small "movements of cooperation" as in arising from a chair without first adjusting the feet, absence of arm swing in walking, etc. As was stated, the patient is able to generate normal or near-normal power, especially in the large muscles, but in the small ones strength is somewhat diminished.

As the disorder of movement worsens, all customary activities show the effects. Handwriting becomes small (micrographia), tremulous, and cramped, as was first noted by Charcot. The voice softens and the speech seems hurried and monotonous; the voice becomes less audible and finally the patient only whispers. Exceptionally "mumbling" is an early complaint. The consumption of a meal takes an hour. Each morsel of food must be swallowed before the next bite is taken. Walking becomes reduced to a shuffle; the patient frequently loses his balance, and in walking forward or backward must "chase the body's center of gravity" in order to avoid falling (festination). Defense and righting reactions are faulty. Persistent extension or clawing of the toes and other dystonic postures may enter the picture.

These various motor impediments and tremor often begin in one limb and spread to one side (monoplegic and hemiplegic pattern) and later to both sides until the patient is quite helpless. Yet in the excitement of some unusual circumstance (a fire, for example) the patient is capable of brief but remarkably effective movement (*kinesis paradoxica*).

The tendon reflexes vary as they do in normal individuals, from being barely elicitable to brisk. Even when parkinsonian symptoms are confined to one side of the body, the reflexes are usually equal on the two sides, and the plantar responses are flexor. Exceptionally the reflexes on the affected side are slightly more brisk, which raises the question of corticospinal involvement, but the plantar reflex remains flexor. In these respects, the clinical picture differs from that of cortical-basal ganglionic achromasia, in which rigidity, hyperactive tendon reflexes, and Babinski signs are combined (see above). There is an inability to inhibit blinking in response to a tap over the bridge of the nose (Meyerson sign). Commonly there is an impairment of upward gaze and convergence. The bradykinesia may extend to eye movements, in that the patients may show a delay in the initiation of gaze to one side and slowing of conjugate movements (decreased maximal saccadic velocity). There are no sensory changes. Drooling is troublesome; an excess flow of saliva has been assumed, but actually the problem is one of failure to swallow with normal frequency. Seborrhea and excessive sweating are also secondary, the former to failure to wash the face often enough, the latter to the effects of the constant motor activity. There is a tendency to syncope in some cases; this was found by Rajput and Rozdilsky to be related to cell loss in the sympathetic ganglia. However, it is never as prominent as in striatonigral degeneration.

As indicated earlier in this chapter, dementia is commonly associated with Parkinson disease. In the series reported by Lieberman et al, 168 of 520 patients (32 percent) with Parkinson disease had moderate to severe dementia—an incidence that was tenfold higher than that in their age-matched spouses. In this series, the demented patients, in addition to being somewhat older than nondemented ones, were also more severely involved in a shorter time and responded less well to L-dopa.

Taylor and colleagues have questioned these figures. In 100 successive cases (with a mean age of 65), they found only 8 percent to be demented, another 7 percent to be either questionably demented or confused, and another 8 percent to be depressed. MRI in Parkinson patients with dementia reveals lesions in the cerebral white matter (in T1-weighted images) not seen in parkinsonians without dementia.

Diagnosis As pointed out on page 604, the epidemic of encephalitis lethargica (von Economo encephalitis) that spread over western Europe and the United States after the First World War left great numbers of parkinsonian cases in its wake. The interval between the encephalitis and the development of extrapyramidal signs varied from months to years. The early age of onset, the rapid progression of symptoms and signs followed by stabilization, and the presence of a variety of other neurologic disorders (sociopathic behavior, tics, spasms, oculogyric crises and other restricted motor disorders, breathing arrhythmias, hyperphagia, and bizarre movements, postures, and gaits) distinguished this disease from the one described by Parkinson. Strangely, no definite instances of this form of encephalitis were recorded before the period 1914–1918, and virtually none has been seen since 1930; hence postencephalitic parkinsonism has nearly disappeared. Rarely, a Parkinson-like syndrome has been described with other forms of encephalitis (Coxsackie B, Japanese B, and St. Louis viral infections).

In England and Europe an "arteriopathic" or "arteriosclerotic" form of Parkinson disease is much diagnosed, but the authors have never been convinced of its reality. Pseudobulbar palsy from a series of lacunar infarcts (see page 643) can create a clinical picture simulating Parkinson disease, but unilateral and bilateral corticospinal tract signs, hyperactive facial reflexes, spasmodic crying and laughing, and other characteristic features distinguish spastic bulbar palsy from Parkinson disease. Rigidity, the hallmark of the arteriosclerotic form, is in reality a combination of spasticity and rigidity. Of course, the parkinsonian patient in advancing years is not impervious to cerebrovascular disease, and the two conditions then overlap.

Senile (familial or essential) tremor is distinguished by its fine, quick quality, by its tendency to become manifest during volitional movement and to disappear when the limb is in a position of repose, and by the lack of associated slowness of movement, flexed postures, etc. The head is more often involved in senile tremor than in Parkinson disease. Some of the slower, alternating beat forms of essential tremor are difficult to distinguish from the tremor of Parkinson disease and one can only wait to see whether it was the first manifestation of that disease.

Progressive supranuclear palsy (see further on in this section) is characterized by rigidity and dystonic postures of the neck and shoulders, a staring and immobile facies, and a tendency to topple when walking—all of which are suggestive of Parkinson disease. Paralysis of vertical gaze and eventually of lateral gaze with retention of certain reflex eye movements establish the diagnosis.

Paucity of movement, unchanging attitudes and postural sets, and a slightly stiff and unbalanced gait may be observed in patients with a retarded depression or normal-pressure hydrocephalus. Since as many as 25 to 30 percent of parkinsonian patients are depressed, the separation of these two conditions may be difficult. The authors have seen patients, called parkinsonian by competent neurologists, whose movements became normal when antidepressant drugs or electroconvulsive therapy were given.

The rapid onset of the Parkinson syndrome, especially in conjunction with other medical diseases, should always raise the suspicion of phenothiazine effects; reserpine, haloperidol, and the neuroleptics pimozide and metoclopramide, all cause a slight masking of the face, stiffness of the trunk and limbs, lack of arm swing, fine tremor of the hands, and mumbling speech. Also they may evoke an inner restlessness, a "muscular impatience," an inability to sit still, and a compulsion to move about, much like that which occurs at times in the parkinsonian patient (akathisia, see page 901). Spasms of the neck, facial, and jaw muscles (open mouth, protruded tongue, retrocollis or torticollis,

grimacing) may also be provoked by such drugs. A mild, localized rigidity of an arm, due to local tetanus, was studied by one of the authors (R.D.A.) in a patient who had been referred as a case of acute parkinsonism.

Early in the course of paralysis agitans, when only a slight asymmetry of stride or an ineptitude of one hand is present, and tremor has yet to appear and impart the unmistakable stamp of the disease, a number of small signs may be helpful in diagnosis. Lack of a Babinski sign or increased tendon reflexes in the affected limbs eliminates a corticospinal lesion, and lack of a grasp reflex helps to exclude a premotor cerebral disorder. Blepharoclonus, a Meyerson sign, digital impedance (a tendency for rapid alternating movements to block or to assume a tremor rhythm), and a lack of arm swing are all indicative of early Parkinson disease.

Pathology and Pathogenesis It is now accepted, by all modern neuropathologists, that a loss of pigmented cells in the substantia nigra and other pigmented nuclei (locus ceruleus, dorsal motor nucleus of the vagus) is the most constant finding in both paralysis agitans and postencephalitic Parkinson disease. The substantia nigra is visibly pale in gross specimens; microscopically, the pigmented nuclei show a marked depletion of cells and replacement gliosis, findings that enable one to state with confidence that the patient must have suffered from Parkinson disease. Also, many of the remaining cells of the pigmented nuclei contain eosinophilic cytoplasmic inclusions, called *Lewy bodies.* These are seen in practically all cases of paralysis agitans. They may be present in postencephalitic cases as well, but in the latter neurofibrillary tangles are more usual. Both of these cellular abnormalities appear occasionally in the substantia nigra of aging, nonparkinsonian individuals, however. Possibly these individuals would have developed paralysis agitans if they had lived a few more years. Noteworthy is the fact that nigral cells diminish with age, from 425,000 to 200,000 at age 80 (McGeer et al). The number in most cases of Parkinson disease is less than 100,000. Tyrosine β-hydroxylase, the rate limiting enzyme for dopamine, also diminishes with age suggesting that aging may increase the vulnerability to Parkinson disease.

Other depletions of cells are widespread, but they have not been quantitatively evaluated, and their significance is less clear. There is neuronal loss in the mesencephalic reticular formation, near the substantia nigra. These cells project to the thalamus and limbic lobes. In the sympathetic ganglia there is slight neuronal loss and Lewy bodies, and this is also true of several of the lower brainstem nuclei as well as of the putamen, caudatum, pallidum, and substantia innominata. In most patients, a rigorous search will disclose a few Lewy bodies in cortical neurons. The lack of a consistent lesion in either the striatum or pallidum is noteworthy, in view of the reciprocal connections between the striatum and nigra and the depletion of striatal dopamine that characterizes the parkinsonian state.

The statistical data relating Parkinson and Alzheimer diseases are difficult to assess because of different methods of examination from one reported series to another (Quinn et al). Nevertheless, the overlap of the two diseases is more than fortuitous, as was indicated in an earlier part of this chapter (page 927). In our own pathologic material the majority of the demented Parkinson patients showed the Alzheimer changes, but there were several in whom no plaques or neurofibrillary changes could be found. In two of the latter, the cortical neuronal loss was accompanied by a widespread distribution of Lewy bodies (Lewy-body dementia).

Of great interest in recent years has been the observation, both in human opiate addicts and in monkeys, that a neurotoxin (known as MPTP) can produce irreversible signs of parkinsonism and selective destruction of cells in the substantia nigra. This toxin was discovered in persons who self-administered an analogue of meperidine and has been shown to bind with high affinity to an extraneural enzyme, monoamine oxidase, which transforms it to a toxic metabolite, pyridinium MPP+. The latter is bound by the melanin in the dopaminergic nigral neurons in sufficient concentration to destroy the cells. It is postulated that a similar toxin may cause parkinsonism (Uhl et al; see also the review by Snyder and D'Amato).

Treatment Although there is no known treatment that will halt or reverse the neuronal degeneration that presumably underlies Parkinson disease, methods are now available that afford considerable relief from symptoms. Treatment can be medical or surgical, although the latter is rarely necessary, and reliance is placed almost exclusively on drugs, particularly on L-dopa and to a lesser extent on anticholinergic and other agents.

At present, *L-dihydroxyphenylalanine* (*L-dopa*) is unquestionably the most effective agent for the treatment of Parkinson disease, and the therapeutic results, even in those with far-advanced disease, are far better than have ever been obtained with other drugs. Some degree of response is so nearly universal that some neurologists use it as a diagnostic criterion (Young). The theoretic basis for the use of this compound rests on the observation that striatal dopamine is depleted in patients with Parkinson disease. Initially, 500 mg of L-dopa should be given daily, in several divided doses. The daily dose should be increased by 500 mg each week until 4.0 to 5.0 g/day are being given. The combination of L-dopa with a decarboxylase inhibitor (Sinemet) prevents its rapid destruction in the blood and permits the control of symptoms more quickly and with a much lower dose (10 to 25 mg inhibitor with 100 to 250 mg L-dopa, three or four times a day).

L-Dopa is not without serious toxic effects, so that it is not universally applicable. Approximately two-thirds of patients tolerate the drug initially and experience few serious side effects; and one-third will show dramatic improvement, especially in hypokinesia. Many patients are at first troubled by nausea, especially if the medication is not taken with meals, and a few have hypotensive episodes. Nausea can be allayed by antiemetic medication, but usually it disappears with continued use. Psychiatric symptoms may also present problems, and they are to be expected in 15 to 25 percent of patients. Depression is the main problem, even to the point of suicide; delusional thinking may occur in these circumstances. This combination of disorders is extremely difficult to treat, and one must turn to a medical antidepressant regimen, as described in Chap. 56. In most patients, however, the mood improves and activity increases, with the danger in frail elderly patients of accidental fractures and heart failure or myocardial infarction. Excitement and aggressiveness appear in a few. An increase in or a return of libido may lead to sexual assertiveness.

The most common and troublesome effect of L-dopa, and the limiting factor in its use, is the induction of involuntary movements—restlessness, head wagging, grimacing, lingual-labial dyskinesia, and choreoathetosis and dystonia of the limbs, neck, and trunk. Above a certain daily dose, which varies from patient to patient (usually 3 to 5 g), very few patients escape these effects, forcing a reduction in dosage. Often some degree of dyskinesia must be accepted as the price to be paid for the therapeutic effect.

If involuntary movements are induced by relatively small doses of L-dopa, the therapeutic effect may be enhanced to some extent by the addition of other dopaminergic agents such as amantadine or bromocriptine. *Amantadine,* an antiviral agent, is thought to act by releasing dopamine from striatal neurons; also it has an anticholinergic property. It is given in doses of 50 to 100 mg three times daily. Its benefit appears almost immediately; both hypokinesia and rigidity are reduced and tremor also, to a lesser degree. The side effects are similar to L-dopa but much milder. Edema of the legs has been troublesome in some patients. Amantadine is effective in combination with L-dopa and anticholinergic drugs. Given alone or in combination with the latter, it offers an alternative treatment for patients with early Parkinson disease or those who do not tolerate standard doses of L-dopa.

Bromocriptine is an ergot derivative, whose action in Parkinson disease is explained by its stimulating effect on dopamine receptors. The drug should be introduced cautiously, 7.5 to 10 mg daily in three to four divided doses, and the dosage increased very slowly to an optimal level of 40 to 60 mg daily. L-Dopa or Sinemet should be reduced concomitantly by 50 percent. It has a longer action than L-dopa and causes nausea and vomiting less often, but otherwise the action and side effects of the two drugs are much the same.

Lisuride and *pergoline* are newer dopaminergic ergoline derivatives that have much the same clinical utility as bromocriptine, i.e., an adjuvant in patients who are not responding satisfactorily to L-dopa alone. The side effects are also much the same as those of bromocriptine, but the newer drugs are less expensive, a feature that will probably determine their use.

Anticholinergic agents related to atropine have long been in use and favored by some neurologists as the initial therapy. They can be given in conjunction with L-dopa or to patients who cannot tolerate the latter drug. Several synthetic preparations are available, the most widely used being trihexyphenidyl (Artane) and benztropine mesylate (Cogentin). In order to obtain maximum benefit from the use of these drugs, they should be given in gradually increasing dosage to the point where toxic effects begin to appear: dryness of the mouth (which can be beneficial when drooling of saliva is a problem), blurring of vision from pupillary mydriasis (for which corrective spectacles may be indicated), constipation, and sometimes urinary retention (especially with prostatism). Unfortunately, mental slowing, confusional states, hallucinations, and impairment of memory—especially in patients with already impaired mental function—are frequent side effects of these drugs and sharply limit their usefulness. The optimum dosage level is the point at which the greatest relief from tremor is achieved within the limits of tolerable side effects. Occasionally further benefit may accrue from the addition of one of the antihistaminic drugs, such as diphenhydramine or phenindamine. In some patients, particularly in those in whom tremor is prominent, ethopropazine (Parsidol) 30 to 60 mg daily in divided doses, is useful. An important note of warning: anticholinergic agents should never be stopped suddenly. If this is done, the patient is likely to become totally immobilized and incapacitated by an abrupt and severe increase of tremor and rigidity.

Long-term treatment with L-dopa has not prevented the slow advance of the disease. Late complications appear in approximately 80 percent of treated patients. In some instances the patient becomes so sensitive to L-dopa that as slight an excess as 50 to 100 mg will precipitate violent choreoathetosis, and if the dose is lowered by the same

amount, the patient develops disabling rigidity. Frequently and unpredictably, in a matter of minutes or from one hour to the next, the patient may change from a state of relative mobility to one of complete or nearly complete immobility—the so-called *on-off phenomenon*. In such cases, close study shows wide fluctuations in blood levels of L-dopa. Attempts are being made to stabilize the blood levels by using a sustained release form of the drug (Juncos et al). Some patients function quite well in the morning and much less well in the afternoon, or vice versa. In such cases, one must literally titrate the dose of L-dopa and space the doses during the 24-h day; combining it with anticholinergic medicines and amantadine is helpful. Sometimes temporarily withdrawing L-dopa and at the same time substituting other medications will control the on-off phenomenon and the severe choreoathetosis.

Based on the hypothesis that alimentary-derived amino acids antagonize the clinical effects of L-dopa, Pincus and Barry have recommended the use of a low-protein diet to control the motor fluctuations described above. In 11 such patients, they reduced these symptoms by the simple expedient of eliminating dietary protein from breakfast and lunch. Moreover, this dietary regimen permits the patient to reduce the total daily dose of L-dopa. Such dietary manipulation is worth trying in appropriate patients; it is not harmful, and most of our patients who have persisted with this diet have reported improvement in their symptoms.

Because of the serious side effects with chronic levodopa treatment, some neurologists avoid all types of pharmacotherapy if the parkinsonian symptoms are not troublesome. When they do become more annoying, initial therapy with either amantadine 100 mg bid or an anticholinergic medication such as Artane 2 to 4 mg three to four times per day is advised. If tremor is the main problem, Parsidol 50 mg qid is often effective. Recently, Koller and Herbster have reported that long-acting propranolol (160 mg daily) is useful in suppressing the tremor. Only when the symptoms begin to interfere with social life or occupation is Sinemet introduced and then at the lowest possible dose—10 and 100 mg tid. The latter is slowly increased until maximal benefit is achieved. Small doses are believed to delay the appearance of clinical fluctuations and loss of drug effectiveness.

From what has been said, it is clear that the best combination of drugs and their dosages will vary from patient to patient. The patients who can be expected to benefit the most from treatment with anti-Parkinson drugs are those with relatively mild disease in whom relief from the symptoms is sufficient to warrant toleration of some side effects. In those more severely affected, the relief is partial, and eventually a degree of incapacity is reached which is not significantly responsive to the most carefully planned regimen of medications. With the advent of L-dopa therapy the authors have the impression that a much larger proportion of patients can be kept in a stable state for many years. This has been borne out by a recent multicenter study, in which patients who were started early on L-dopa survived longer with less disability than those starting late (Diamond et al). Some cases are remarkably benign, but, in general, the disease is progressive and eventually disabling. Approximately two-thirds of the patients are disabled within 5 years and 80 percent after 10 years.

Success with L-dopa has practically obviated the need for surgical therapy. The latter involves the stereotactic placement of lesions in the central nuclei of the brain, either in the globus pallidus or ventrolateral thalamus, contralateral to the side of the body chiefly affected. The best results occur in patients who are relatively young and in good health with sound mentality, in whom unilateral tremor or rigidity, rather than akinesia, are the predominant symptoms. The cerebral implantation of adrenal medullary tissue is purely experimental and of no proven value.

Finally, in the management of the patient with Parkinson disease, one must not neglect the maintenance of optimum general health and neuromuscular efficiency by a planned program of exercise, activity, and rest; and expert physical therapy may be of great help in achieving these ends. In addition, the patient often needs much emotional support in meeting the stress of the illness, in comprehending its nature, and in carrying on courageously in spite of it.

STRIATONIGRAL DEGENERATION

Closely related to paralysis agitans clinically but with a different pathologic basis is a state termed by Adams, van Bogaert, and Vander Eecken *striatonigral degeneration.* We found this lesion by chance in four middle-aged patients, all without a family history of similar disease, in three of whom a clinical picture of Parkinson syndrome had been described. In one of the three, examined by the authors, the typical rigidity, stiffness, and akinesia had begun on one side of the body, then spread to the other, and progressed over a 5-year period. A flexed posture of the trunk and limbs, slowness of all movements, poor balance, mumbling speech, and a tendency to faint were other elements in the clinical picture. Mental function was intact, and there were no reflex changes, no suck and grasp reflexes, and no cerebellar signs, tremor, or involuntary movements. The other two patients had been seen by competent neurologists who had made a diagnosis of Parkinson disease. Some of the symptoms had been partially relieved by anticholinergic drugs.

In each case the postmortem examination disclosed extensive loss of neurons in the zona compacta of the substantia nigra, but there were no Lewy bodies or neurofibrillary tangles in the remaining cells. More striking, however, were the degenerative changes in the putamens and to a lesser extent in the caudate nuclei. These structures were greatly reduced in size and had lost most of their neurons—more of the small than the large ones, and more on the side opposite the first clinical symptoms. The findings were suggestive of the striatal lesion of Huntington chorea, except that the cell loss was greater in the putamen than caudatum. Secondary pallidal atrophy (mainly a loss of striatopallidal fibers) was present. In the fourth patient there was in addition a widespread olivopontocerebellar degeneration.

In the past 25 years, we have seen many other patients in whom the changes of olivopontocerebellar and striatonigral degeneration were combined, and in whom the symptoms and signs of cerebellar ataxia had been prominent and had preceded the parkinsonian manifestations. Also, nearly half of the patients are handicapped by orthostatic hypotension, which proves at autopsy to be associated with loss of intermediolateral horn cells and pigmented nuclei of the brainstem (Shy-Drager syndrome), and many of them have disturbances of continence of micturition. The latter abnormalities are of several types (Kirby et al)—involuntary detrusor contractions, perhaps the result of a loss of striatonigral inhibitory influences; inability to initiate voluntary micturition, which may reflect the degeneration of neurons in pontine and medullary nuclei and in the sacral intermediolateral columns; and impaired sphincteric function, perhaps the result of degeneration of sacral anterior horn cells (Onuf's nucleus).

The combination of striatonigral degeneration and olivopontocerebellar degeneration has been reviewed by Gosset et al. They found 35 recorded cases of which 18 had the Shy-Drager autonomic syndrome. These authors and others speak of this combination of disorders as "multiple system atrophy." In several of the cases there were Babinski signs, slight muscular atrophy with denervation by EMG, polymyoclonia of intention type, impotence in males, upward gaze palsy, and sometimes sleep and respiratory disorders. One should suspect this type of striatal degeneration in patients with the Parkinson syndrome who have elements of ataxia, vertical gaze palsy, Babinski signs, and autonomic failure. The autonomic disorder involves not only preganglionic neurons but postganglionic ones as well, as demonstrated in a series of 36 cases by Cohen et al. MRI should be useful in showing the loss of tissue in the putamens.

Interestingly, except in a few early cases, levodopa has had no effect or has made the patient worse. This may be attributed to the loss of striatal dopamine receptors.

PROGRESSIVE SUPRANUCLEAR PALSY (PSP)

In 1963 Richardson, Steele, and Olszewski crystallized medical thought about a clinicopathologic entity to which there had been only ambiguous reference in the past. The condition is no longer unusual. In 1972, when Steele reviewed the subject, 73 cases (22 with postmortem examinations) had been described in the medical literature, and several examples are to be found in every large neurologic center. No toxic, encephalitic, racial, or geographic factor has been incriminated as a possible cause.

Clinical Features Characteristically the disease has its onset in the sixth decade (range 45 to 73 years) with some combination of difficulty in balance, abrupt falls, visual and ocular disturbances, slurred speech, dysphagia, and vague changes in personality, often with an apprehensiveness and fretfulness suggestive of an agitated depression. At first the neurologic and ophthalmologic examinations may be rather unrevealing, and it may take a year or longer for the characteristic syndrome—comprising supranuclear ophthalmoplegia, pseudobulbar palsy, and axial dystonia—to develop fully. Difficulty in voluntary movement of the eyes, usually downward, is a relatively early development, and so is impairment or loss of the fast component of optokinetic and caloric-induced nystagmus. Later, all vertical motions of the eyes are lost, and then the lateral ones as well. However, if the eyes are fixated on a target and the head is turned, full movements can be obtained, proving the supranuclear, nonparalytic character of the gaze disorder. Bell's phenomenon (reflexive up-turning of eyes on forced closure of eyelids) and ability to converge are also lost, and the pupils then become small. The upper eyelids may be retracted, imparting an expression of perpetual surprise. In the late stages the eyes may be fixed centrally, and all oculocephalic and vestibular reflexes may be lost.

Along with the oculomotor disorder, there is a gradual stiffening and extension of the neck (in one of our cases it was sharply flexed), but this is not an invariable finding. The limbs may be slightly stiff, with Babinski signs in a few cases. The signs of pseudobulbar palsy are always prominent. The face becomes "masked" and less expressive, speech is slurred, the mouth hangs open, and swallowing is difficult. The gait disturbance has proved difficult to analyze. Walking becomes more and more awkward and tentative, with a tendency to totter and fall repeatedly, but with only mild ataxia of the limbs. Some patients tend to lean and fall backward. One of our patients, a large man, fell repeatedly, wrecking household furniture as he went

down, yet an analysis of his stance and gait provided no clue as to the basic defect. In some ways this "toppling phenomenon" is similar to that seen in lower brainstem lesions such as occurs in lateral medullary infarction. Recent reports have emphasized a number of atypical features, such as palilalia, disturbances of vestibular function, and minimal or lack of ocular abnormalities, all of which the authors have observed in occasional cases. Finally the patient becomes anarthric, immobile, and quite helpless. Dementia of some degree is probably present in all the cases, but is mild in most of them. The CSF remains normal.

Postmortem examinations have disclosed a bilateral loss of neurons and gliosis in the periaqueductal gray matter, the superior colliculus, subthalamic nucleus of Luys, red nucleus, pallidum, dentate nucleus, pretectal and vestibular nuclei, and to some extent in the oculomotor nucleus. The cerebral and cerebellar cortices are usually spared. Loss of the medullated fiber bundles arising from these nuclear structures has been observed. A remarkable finding has been the neurofibrillary degeneration of many of the residual neurons.

The cause and nature of this disease are quite obscure. Attempts to transmit it to primates by the inoculation of fresh brain tissue from 10 patients have failed. By positron-emission tomography, Leenders et al have demonstrated, in mildly demented patients, a decrease in blood flow—most marked in the frontal lobes—and a lesser extent of oxygen utilization. Striatal dopamine formation and storage was significantly decreased when compared to control values. The disease should be suspected whenever an older adult develops extrapyramidal symptoms, particularly dystonia of the neck, ocular palsies, a picture of pseudobulbar palsy, or inexplicable imbalance and falling. Some patients whom we have seen had earlier been thought to have Parkinson disease or ocular myasthenia (there may be a partial response to tensilon), but the resemblances are superficial. However, there is a small group of parkinsonians with gaze palsies, especially of upward gaze, which must be distinguished (see above).

L-Dopa has been slightly beneficial in some of our patients and combinations of L-dopa and anticholinergic drugs in others. Unfortunately, these medications were of help for only short periods of time.

DYSTONIA MUSCULORUM DEFORMANS (TORSION SPASM)

Dystonia as a symptom has been discussed on page 64. Here we are concerned with a disease or diseases of which dystonia is the major manifestation. Schwalbe's account, in 1908, of three siblings of a Jewish family who were afflicted with progressive involuntary movements of trunk and limbs, probably represents the first description of the disease. In 1911, Oppenheim contributed other cases and coined the term *dystonia musculorum deformans,* in the belief that the disorder was primarily one of muscle and always associated with deformity. Flatau and Sterling, in the same year, first suggested that the disease might have a hereditary basis, and gave it the more accurate name *torsion dystonia of childhood.* At first thought to be a manifestation of hysteria, it gradually came to be established as a morbid entity with a preference for Russian and Polish Jews. Wider experience has defined a primary form of dystonia that affects non-Jews, and also symptomatic forms of dystonia due to vascular lesions, encephalitis lethargica, Wilson disease, Hallervorden-Spatz disease, and Huntington chorea, among many other disorders (see classification of Eldridge and Fahn).

The interesting epidemiologic study of Eldridge, who analyzed all reported cases up to 1970, revealed two patterns of inheritance, one autosomal recessive, the other dominant. The recessive form begins in early childhood, is progressive over a few years and restricted to Jewish patients, often with superior intelligence. The dominant form begins later, usually in late childhood and adolescence, progresses more slowly, and is not limited to any ethnic group. Our own clinical experience with the dominant form of the disease reveals a later age of onset and a milder, more slowly progressive course. Only the paravertebral or cranial muscles may be involved with little change from year to year. In one of our cases a dystonia of the foot appeared during adolescence and later disappeared.

Symptomatology The first manifestations of the disease may be rather subtle. The patient (usually a child between 6 and 14 years, less often an adolescent), begins intermittently to invert one foot, or to extend one leg and foot in an unnatural way, or to hunch one shoulder, raising the question of a nervous tic. As time passes, however, the motor peculiarity becomes more persistent and interferes increasingly with the patient's activities. Soon the muscles of the spine and shoulder or pelvic girdles become implicated in involuntary spasmodic twisting movements. The spasms are intermittent at first, and in free intervals muscular tone and volitional movements are normal. Indeed, in some instances the muscles are hypotonic. Gradually the spasms become more frequent; finally they are continuous, and the body is grotesquely contorted. For a time recumbency relieves the spasms; but later, position has no influence. The hands are seldom involved, though at times they may be fisted. Cranial muscles do not escape, and in a number of instances a slurring staccato-type speech has even been the initial manifestation. In two of our patients, severe dysarthria and dysphagia were the first signs of the disease, caused by dystonia of the tongue, pharyngeal, and laryngeal

muscles; in another it was blepharospasm. Other manifestations of the movement disorder include torticollis, tortipelvis, dromedary gait, propulsive gait, action tremor, myoclonic jerks during voluntary movement, and mild choreoathetosis of the limbs. Excitement worsens the condition, and sleep abolishes it; but as the years pass the postural distortion may become fixed to the point where it does not disappear even in sleep. Tendon reflexes are at all times normal; corticospinal signs are absent; there is no ataxia, sensory abnormality, convulsive disorder, or dementia.

Pathology No agreement has been reached concerning the pathologic substratum of the disease. In several reported cases the ferrocalcinosis of Hallervorden-Spatz disease, the lesions of Wilson disease or of kernicterus, the *état marbré* of hypoxia, or the CT lucencies of familial striatal necrosis were observed in the basal ganglia. Obviously in these cases the dystonia was symptomatic of another disease. However, in the particular hereditary form, which is the subject of this section, one cannot be certain of any specific lesions that would account for the clinical manifestations. The brain is grossly normal, and the ventricular size is not increased. According to Zeman and Dyken, who reviewed all the reported autopsy studies, there are no significant changes in the striatum or pallidum, or elsewhere. This does not mean that there are no lesions, only that the techniques being used (qualitative analysis of random sections by light microscopy) are inadequate for their demonstration. Dopamine β-hydroxylase is elevated in the plasma of patients with the autosomal dominant form of the disease and also the plasma norepinephrine levels are raised (Ziegler et al) but the meaning of these findings is not clear.

Treatment Early in the course of the illness, several drugs, including L-dopa, bromocriptine, carbamazepine, diazepam, and tetrabenazine, seem to be helpful, but only in a few patients, and the benefit is not lasting. The hereditary form of dystonia-parkinsonism (described below) responds well to L-dopa and dopamine agonists and is exceptional in this respect. Burke and coworkers advocate the use of very high doses (30 mg daily, or more) of trihexyphenidyl (Artane). Apparently dystonic children can tolerate these high doses, if they are attained gradually—by 5-mg increments weekly. In adults, high-dose anticholinergic treatment is less successful, but worthy of a trial, nevertheless. The most spectacular results have been obtained by Cooper, using stereotactic techniques (cryo- or chemothalamectomy) to make lesions that are centered in the ventrolateral nuclei of the thalamus. Some frightfully deformed children, unable to sit or stand, have been restored to near normalcy. Approximately 70 percent were moderately to markedly improved by unilateral or bilateral operations. The improvement was usually sustained, according to Cooper's 20-year follow-up.

OTHER FORMS OF HEREDITARY DYSTONIA

Other degenerative diseases have been described which combine hereditary dystonia with neural deafness and intellectual impairment (Scribanu and Kennedy) and with amyotrophy in a paraplegic distribution (Gilman and Romanul). In recent years, attention has been drawn to yet another form of hereditary dystonia (Allen and Knopp; Nygaard and Duvoisin). The pattern of inheritance is probably autosomal dominant, and again there is no ethnic predilection. The dystonic manifestations become evident in childhood, usually between 4 and 8 years of age. Sometimes parkinsonian features can be detected early in the course of the illness, but characteristically they are added to the clinical picture many years later. The unique feature of this *juvenile dystonia–parkinsonism syndrome,* as it is called, is the dramatic response of both the dystonic and parkinsonian symptoms to treatment with L-dopa and dopamine agonists.

Another sizable group of dystonic patients are adults *without* a family history. We have observed the dystonia to be relatively restricted in these patients and to overlap with spasmodic torticollis, as pointed out by Marsden.

HALLERVORDEN-SPATZ DISEASE

See Chap. 38 (page 804).

CALCIFICATION OF THE BASAL GANGLIA

See Chap. 38 (page 806).

SPASMODIC TORTICOLLIS AND OTHER RESTRICTED DYSKINESIAS

With advancing age, a large variety of degenerative *movement disorders* come to light. Supposedly there is loss of neurons in certain parts of the basal ganglia, but their pathologic basis has never been divulged. Groups of muscles begin to manifest arrhythmic involuntary spasms. The patient's inability to suppress them and the recognition that they are beyond voluntary control distinguish them from the common tics, habit spasms, and mannerisms described in Chap. 5. If the muscle contraction is frequent and prolonged, it is accompanied by an aching pain that may mistakenly be blamed for the spasm. Worsening under conditions of excitement and stress and improvement during quiet and relaxation are typical of this group of disorders.

The most frequent and familiar type is *torticollis,* wherein an adult, more often a woman, becomes aware of turning of the head to one side as she walks. Usually it worsens gradually to a point where it may be more or less continuous, but in some patients the condition remains mild for years on end. When followed over the years, the condition is observed to remain limited to the same muscles (mainly the scalene, sternocleidomastoid, and upper trapezius). Occasionally torticollis is combined with dystonia of the arm and trunk, or with tremor, facial spasms, or dystonic writer's cramp.

Other restricted dyskinesias involve the neck in combination with facial muscles, the orbicularis oculi (*blepharospasm* and *blepharoclonus*), the throat and respiratory muscles (*"spastic dysphonia,"* orofacial dyskinesia, and *respiratory and phonatory spasms*). All these conditions and their treatment are discussed fully in Chap. 5 (pages 87 to 89).

SYNDROME OF PROGRESSIVE ATAXIA

The cerebellum and its major connections are subject to a number of diseases that are more or less confined to these parts of the nervous system. Many of these diseases are so chronic that one would expect a close correspondence between their symptomatology and anatomic pathology, yet attempts to determine these relationships have been singularly disappointing. Traditionally, the classic examples of chronic progressive cerebellar disease are subsumed under the system atrophies, but all efforts to give some semblance of order to the anatomy and pathology of the various reported types have been unsuccessful. Wilson wrote that "The group of degenerative conditions strung together by the common feature of ataxia is one for which no very suitable classification has yet been devised,"—a statement that is as appropriate today as when it was written 50 years ago.

The difficulties in nosologic classification and clinical-anatomic correlation stem from several obvious and some inapparent sources. *First,* many of the clinical and anatomic studies have been incomplete, especially on the anatomic side. Rarely have all parts of the cerebellum been examined in quantitative fashion, and often myelin-stained sections of the spinal cord were either not made or marred by uninterpretable artifacts; axis cylinder and glial stains were either omitted or inadequate. Equally incomplete in most cases has been the examination of noncerebellar parts of the nervous system. *Second,* the established and "classic" types of disease seem to be infrequent in comparison to aberrant and transitional types. Hence, one is never certain that the patient under study is a typical example. At times it seems to the authors that every new patient deviates from known types in some way. *Third,* a large part of the neocerebellum has no assigned functions. It plays no recognizable role in motor function, and much of what it contributes to auditory and visual reflexes is obscure. Thus, an undeveloped cerebellar hemisphere may be discovered at postmortem examination in an individual who has had no symptoms of cerebellar deficit during life. Also, cerebellar symptoms from acute lesions have a way of disappearing, a phenomenon attributed to compensation by other parts of the nervous system. Finally, it is well known that lesions of the brainstem, spinal cord, and parietal lobe may cause a cerebellar type of ataxia with no visible abnormality being noted in the cerebellum itself—a situation exemplified by the cases described by Marie as hereditary cerebellar ataxia (see below). This is possible because of the manifold links between the cerebellum and the cerebrum, brainstem, and spinal cord.

Greenfield has reviewed the many early clinical and pathologic reports of heredofamilial spinocerebellar diseases. Becker has drawn attention to at least 60 different diseases and syndromes. He points out that in many of the reported conditions it is not possible to decide if one is dealing with a variant of a known genetic entity or a new and separate disease caused by a pathogenic gene. The monograph edited by Kark et al reviews the subject of the inherited ataxias and considers the role of metabolic, viral, and immunologic factors in their causation. The monograph of Harding is certainly the most thorough and scholarly effort to give order to the hereditary ataxias. Setting aside those of congenital type and those with an identifiable metabolic disorder, she has grouped them by age of onset, pattern of heredity, and associated features. A modification of Greenfield's classification is presented below, but it must be admitted that many of the fresh cases being published today are difficult to place for reasons that have just been given.

I. *Predominantly* spinal forms of hereditary ataxia
   A. Friedreich ataxia
   B. Non-Friedreich, predominantly spinal ataxias
II. *Predominantly* cerebellar forms of hereditary ataxia
   A. Cortical cerebellar atrophies
      1. Holmes type of cerebello-olivary atrophy
      2. Late cortical cerebellar atrophy of Marie-Foix-Alajouanine
   B. Cerebellar-brainstem atrophies
      1. Olivopontocerebellar atrophy of Menzel and of Déjerine and André-Thomas (cerebellopetal)
      2. Other types of olivopontocerebellar atrophy (Konigsmark and Weiner) including cases with striatonigral degeneration, retinal degeneration, and dementia
      3. Dentatorubral atrophy (Ramsay Hunt; Woods and Schaumburg; and others) (cerebellofugal)
III. Idiopathic late-onset cerebellar ataxias

PREDOMINANTLY SPINAL ATAXIAS

Friedreich Ataxia   This is the prototype of all forms of progressive ataxia and accounts for about half of all cases of hereditary ataxia in Sweden (86 of 171 cases in Sjögren's series). Friedreich, of Heidelberg, began in 1861 to report on a form of familial progressive ataxia that he had observed among nearby villagers. Already it was known through the writings of Duchenne in Paris that locomotor ataxia was the prominent feature of spinal cord syphilis, i.e., tabes dorsalis, and it was Friedreich who proved that a nonsyphilitic hereditary type also existed. This concept was greeted with some skepticism, but soon Duchenne himself affirmed the existence of the new disease and other case reports appeared in England, France, and the United States. In 1882, in a thesis on this subject by Brousse of Montpelier, the name of Friedreich was attached to the new entity.

As new cases appeared, it was noted that in about half of them the disease had its onset before the tenth year and sometimes as early as the third or fourth; Mollaret could find no examples with onset after the age of 25 years. Bell and Carmichael identified two inheritance patterns, the common one being autosomal recessive with an average age of onset at 11.75 years, and the other dominant, with an average age of onset at 20.4 years. The disease is invariably and steadily progressive, and within 5 years of the onset walking is no longer possible in many cases. The median age at death is 26.5 years in patients with the recessive type of the disease and 39.5 years in those with the dominant type. Genetic linkage studies of 22 families with 3 or more affected siblings have led to the assignment of the gene mutation to chromosome 9 (Chamberlain et al). Despite the variability of the clinical picture of Friedreich ataxia, current evidence favors a single gene locus for the disease.

Symptomatology   Ataxia of gait is nearly always the initial symptom. Occasionally it begins rather abruptly after a febrile illness, and one leg may become clumsy before the other. A "hemiplegic" pattern, the arm and leg on one side becoming ataxic before the other, has been remarked upon but is exceptional; usually both legs are affected simultaneously. Difficulty in standing steadily and in running are early symptoms, and Wilson has commented on fatigability, leg pains, and postexertional cramps—symptoms that we have seldom elicited. The hands usually become clumsy months or years after the gait disorder, and dysarthric speech appears after the arms are involved (rarely is it an early symptom).

In some patients pes cavus and kyphoscoliosis precede the neurologic symptoms, and in others they follow by several years. The characteristic foot deformity takes the form of a high plantar arch with retraction of the toes at the metatarsal-phalangeal joints and flexion at the interphalangeal joints (hammer toes).

In the fully developed state the abnormality of gait is of mixed sensory and cerebellar type, aptly called tabetocerebellar by Charcot. According to Mollaret, the author of an authoritative monograph on this disease, the cerebellar component predominates, but in our relatively small series we have been impressed as much with the sensory (tabetic) aspect. The patient stands with feet wide apart, constantly shifting position to maintain balance. Friedreich referred to the constant teetering and swaying as *static ataxia*. In walking, as with all sensory ataxias, the movements of the legs tend to be brusque, with sudden lurches, the feet resounding irregularly as they strike the floor. Closure of the eyes causes the patient to fall (Romberg sign), and attempts to correct the imbalance may result in abrupt, wild movements. Often there is a rhythmic tremor of the head. The arms become grossly ataxic, and both action and intention tremors are manifest. Speech is slow, slurred, explosive, and finally almost incomprehensible. Breathing, speaking, swallowing, and laughing may be so incoordinate that the patient nearly chokes while speaking. Holmes remarked upon an ataxia of respiration that causes "curious short inspiratory whoops." Facial, buccal, and arm muscles may display tremulous and sometimes choreiform movements.

Mentation has been preserved in all of our patients. However, emotional lability has been sufficiently prominent to provoke comment. Horizontal nystagmus may be present in the primary position, and is increased on lateral gaze. Rotatory and vertical nystagmus are rare. Deafness has been recorded along with vertigo and, more rarely, with inexcitability of the labyrinths and blindness with optic atrophy. Ocular movements usually remain full, and pupillary reflexes are normal. The facial muscles may seem slightly weak, and deglutition may become impaired. Amy-

otrophy occurs late in the illness and is usually slight, but it may be extreme in patients with an associated neuropathy (see below). The tendon reflexes are abolished in nearly every case; rarely they may be obtainable when the patient is examined early in the illness. Plantar reflexes are extensor, and flexor spasms may occur even with complete absence of tendon reflexes. The abdominal reflexes are usually retained until late in the illness. Loss of vibratory and position sense are invariable from the beginning, and later there may be some diminution of tactile, pain, and temperature sensation as well. Sphincter control is usually preserved.

Abortive and atypical forms are numerous. Peroneal muscular atrophy is sometimes associated with Friedreich ataxia, as is true of the hereditary areflexic dystasia of Roussy and Levy. These disorders are discussed with the hereditary neuropathies, on pages 1056 and 1058. Hereditary forms of optic atrophy, retinitis pigmentosa, and deafness are occasionally combined with Friedreich ataxia as well, but we agree with Skre that they probably represent genetically independent entities.

A cardiopathy is demonstrable in about half of the patients. Many of them die as a result of cardiac arrhythmia or congestive failure. Russell has described a degeneration of cardiac muscle fibers, and presumably the conducting system is similarly affected. Kyphoscoliosis and restricted respiratory function are important contributary causes of death. Harding remarks that about 10 percent have diabetes mellitus.

Pathology The spinal cord is small. The posterior columns and the corticospinal and spinocerebellar tracts are all depleted of medullated fibers, and there is a fibrous gliosis that does not replace the bulk of the lost fibers. The nerve cells in Clarke's column and the large neurons of the dorsal root ganglia, especially lumbosacral ones, are reduced in number—but seldom to a degree that would explain the tract degeneration. Betz cells are also diminished in some cases, but the corticospinal tracts are relatively intact down to the medullary-cervical junction. The nuclei of cranial nerves VIII, X, and XII all exhibit a reduction of cells. Slight to moderate neuronal loss is seen also in the dentate nuclei, and the superior cerebellar peduncles are thin. Depletion of Purkinje cells in the superior vermis and neurons in corresponding parts of the inferior olivary nuclei has been described in some cases.

As stated above, the myocardial muscle fibers are degenerated, and replaced by myophages and fibroblasts.

Blass and Kark and their colleagues have found reduced levels of pyruvate dehydrogenase and lipoamide dehydrogenase (LAD) in platelets and cultured skin fibroblasts in the majority of their patients with Friedreich ataxia. Barbeau (1980a) was unable to duplicate these findings, although he consistently found a decrease in serum LAD activity which he did not consider to be a primary abnormality. Some of the reported patients also had Kearns-Sayre myopathy and retinitis pigmentosa; hence, the clinical classification of the patients with these chemical abnormalities is unclear.

Clinical-pathologic correlations   The pes cavus is not greatly different from that seen in diseases with mild hypertonus of the long extensors and flexors of the feet, and in diseases (polyneuropathies) that cause amyotrophy of intrinsic feet muscles, occurring at a time when the bones of the feet are malleable. The kyphoscoliosis is probably due to spinal muscular imbalance. The tabetic aspects of the disease are explained by the degeneration of the columns of Goll and Burdach, and the cerebellar ataxia is attributable to a degeneration of the spinocerebellar tracts, the superior vermis and the dentatorubral pathways in various combinations. Loss of large neurons in the sensory ganglia causes abolition of tendon reflexes and contributes to the sensory impairment. Corticospinal lesions account for the weakness and Babinski signs.

Diagnosis   Friedreich disease and its variants must be distinguished from "hereditary cerebellar ataxia of Marie," familial spastic paraparesis with ataxia, and the Strümpell-Lorrain syndrome (these are discussed further on in this chapter); and peroneal muscular atrophy and the Lévy-Roussy syndrome, which are discussed in Chap. 46.

Treatment   Rodriguez-Budelli et al reported improvement of the ataxia with parenteral and oral doses of physostigmine (60-mg tablets). Kark and colleagues have claimed that a diet high in fat and low in carbohydrate is helpful. Sobue, in Japan, has attributed salutary effects upon ataxia to the administration of thyrotropin-releasing hormone (TRH) and its synthetic analogue DN-1417. None of these claims has been confirmed. Therapeutic trials, using choline chloride, lecithin, 5-hydroxytryptophan, and benserazide, have not yielded any benefit.

Non-Friedreich, Predominantly Spinal Ataxias   In the large literature on cerebellar ataxias, there are a respectable number of cases that resemble Friedreich ataxia except that the limbs are spastic and the tendon reflexes hyperactive. The unanswered question is whether they represent a variant of Friedreich ataxia or a different disease. The distinction between Friedreich ataxia and ataxia with retained tendon reflexes is an important one clinically, insofar as kyphoscoliosis and heart disease do not occur in the latter group and the prognosis is better. Usually cited in this regard are the cases of Sanger Brown, and also some of the cases of the Strümpell-Lorrain form of familial spastic

paraplegia and of optic atrophy with spasticity (Behr)—in both the latter groups there is sometimes a prominent ataxic component. Cerebellar atrophy has not been a prominent feature, and we would adopt the position that they are forms of spinocerebellar degeneration that are transitional between Friedreich ataxia and some of the other heredoataxias with cerebellar atrophy. In the few autopsied cases, the main abnormality has been in the spinal cord and the spinocerebellar (cerebellopetal) tracts.

PREDOMINANTLY CEREBELLAR FORMS OF HEREDITARY ATAXIA

Soon after the publication of Friedreich's descriptions of a spinal type of hereditary ataxia, reports began to appear of somewhat different diseases in which the ataxia was related to degenerative changes in the cerebellum and brainstem rather than the spinal cord. Claims of their independence from the spinal type were based largely on a later age of onset, a more definite hereditary transmission, the persistence or hyperactivity of tendon reflexes, and the more frequent concurrence of ophthalmoplegia and optic atrophy. Several of these clinical features, particularly briskness of tendon reflexes, are obviously alien to Friedreich ataxia.

By 1893 Pierre Marie thought it desirable to create a new category of hereditary ataxia that would embrace all of the non-Friedreich cases. He collated the familial cases of progressive ataxia that had been described by Fraser, Nonne, Sanger Brown, and Klippel and Durante (see Greenfield and Harding for references), and proposed that all of them were examples of an entity to which he applied the name *heredoataxie cerebelleuse*. Marie's proposition was based almost entirely on clinical observations—not his own, but those made by the aforementioned authors. Later, as more members of these families died, postmortem examinations disclosed that Marie's hereditary cerebellar ataxia included not one but several disease entities. Indeed, as pointed out by Holmes (1907*b*) and later by Greenfield, in three of the four families the cerebellum showed no significant lesions at all. Yet there was by then no doubt of a separate class of predominantly cerebellar atrophies, some purely cortical and others associated with a variety of noncerebellar lesions. The trouble is, however, that the clinical pictures and underlying pathologic lesions of the subtypes became less rather than more distinct as new cases were found. We can do no more than put all the cases with major cerebellar lesions together and tentatively subdivide them according to the type of lesion and its noncerebellar linkages.

CEREBELLAR ATROPHY WITH PROMINENT BRAINSTEM LESIONS

Familial Cortical Cerebellar Atrophy Holmes in 1907 described a family of eight siblings of whom three brothers and one sister were affected by a progressive ataxia, beginning with a reeling gait and followed by clumsiness of the hands, dysarthria, tremor of the head, and a variable nystagmus. The ataxia began insidiously in the fourth decade and progressed slowly over many years.

The late cortical cerebellar atrophy of Marie, Foix, and Alajouanine, reported in 1922, is probably the same disease. In their patients also, the onset was in later life (average age 57 years). The onset was rather abrupt in some, though usually insidious, and the progress was extremely slow (survival 15 to 20 years). Ataxia of gait, instability of the trunk, tremor of the hands and head, and slightly slowed, hesitant speech conformed to the usual clinical picture of a progressive cerebellar ataxia. Nystagmus was rare. Intelligence was usually preserved. The patellar reflexes were increased in many cases, the ankle jerks were often absent, and the plantar reflexes were said to be of extensor type in some cases. (It should be noted that this latter finding, in the absence of hyperreflexia and spasticity, is difficult to accept at face value, for withdrawal responses are often mistaken for extensor reflexes.)

Postmortem examination disclosed a symmetrical atrophy of the cerebellum most obvious on the upper surface (anterior lobe), the vermis being more affected than the hemispheres. The Purkinje cells were absent in the lingula, centralis, and pyramis of the superior vermis, and reduced in number in the quadrangularis, flocculus, biventral, and pyramidal lobes. The granule cells were affected, but less than the Purkinje cells. The white matter was slightly pale in myelin stains. The roof nuclei and pontine nuclei were normal. There was cell loss in the dorsal and medial parts of the inferior olivary nuclei. A questionable pallor was noted in the corticospinal and spinocerebellar tracts in myelin stains of the spinal cord.

The pathologic findings in Holmes' cases were essentially the same. Both familial and sporadic cases of this type have since been reported. The similarity of the pathology to that of *alcoholic cerebellar degeneration* always raises the question of a nutritional cause of single cases (Chap. 39).

Striatonigral degeneration (described above) has rarely been combined with a cortical cerebellar atrophy. As with olivopontocerebellar atrophy, cerebellar ataxia is then superseded by a parkinsonian syndrome.

Familial Olivopontocerebellar and Spinocerebellar Degeneration Menzel in 1891 described a male patient whose illness began at 28 years of age with ataxia of gait and of the limbs, dysarthria, and dysphagia—tendon reflexes being retained. When the patient died 18 years later, there was a conspicuous atrophy of the cerebellum involving mainly the middle cerebellar peduncles, pontine and olivary nuclei, and to a lesser extent the dentate nuclei and superior cerebellar peduncles. Some loss of Purkinje cells and thinning of the granule cells was noted, but these changes were less conspicuous than the loss of fibers in the pontine and cerebellar white matter. The dorsal columns and spinocerebellar and corticospinal tracts were also degenerated, along with a slight loss of cells in the anterior horns of the spinal cord and motor nuclei of the brainstem. Greenfield concluded that this was an example of olivopontocerebellar degeneration, but with "additional and anomalous" features. The latter (presumably spinal) features are of considerable interest, since they relate the Menzel type of hereditary ataxia to the Friedreich type.

Many other families with roughly similar lesions have since been reported (see review by Konigsmark and Weiner). Most of them were middle-aged at the time of death; the pattern of inheritance was usually autosomal dominant but occasionally recessive; and a variety of other clinical findings were present in single cases (hemiballismus, athetosis, contractures of the legs, fixed pupils, ophthalmoplegia, ptosis, gaze palsy, retinal degeneration, mental retardation and epilepsy, claw foot and scoliosis, incontinence, parkinsonian symptoms and signs, dementia).

Olivopontocerebellar Atrophy A sporadically occurring form of a closely related disorder was described by Déjerine and André-Thomas, who named it *olivopontocerebellar atrophy*. Here there were the same brainstem lesions as in the Menzel form, but the spinal cord was not affected. Hence it could hardly be designated as "spinocerebellar." The onset was in the fifth decade of life, and the main manifestations were ataxia—first in the legs, then the arms and hands and bulbar musculature—a symptomatology common to all the cerebellar atrophies. As more and more cases of this type were collected (by 1943, Rosenhagen had collected 45 from the literature, to which he added 11 of his own), a hereditary pattern (dominant) was evident in some, and degeneration of one or more long tracts in the spinal cord was found in several. About half the cases later developed the symptoms of Parkinson disease with degeneration of nigral cells and, in a few, of striatal cells as well.

Thus there was an overlap with the Menzel type of disease on one side and with Parkinson disease on the other.

Of considerable interest in both the Menzel and Déjerine–André-Thomas types is the extensive degeneration of the middle cerebellar peduncles, the cerebellar white matter, and the pontine, olivary, and arcuate nuclei; loss of Purkinje cells has been variable. Opinion is divided as to whether this is a degeneration of myelin with relative sparing of pontine neurons and their axons, or a terminal "dying-back" of axons of these nuclei with secondary myelin degeneration. Greenfield favors the latter idea, which seems to us the most plausible.

The boundaries of the entity of olivopontocerebellar atrophy have gradually been extended; Konigsmark and Weiner subdivided them into the following types: (1) hereditary (dominant) type of Menzel; (2) hereditary (recessive) type of Fickler-Winkler; (3) hereditary (dominant) type with retinal degeneration; (4) hereditary (dominant) type of Shut-Haymaker, with spastic paraplegia and areflexia; (5) hereditary (dominant) type with dementia, ophthalmoplegia, and extrapyramidal signs.

A decrease in glutamate dehydrogenase (GDH) activity has been reported in leukocyte and fibroblast homogenates of some patients with sporadic and dominantly inherited olivopontocerebellar atrophy (Finocchiaro et al). A similar deficiency of GDH activity has been found in the platelets of patients with both dominant and nondominant forms of the disease. The significance of these findings is not clear.

Dentatorubral Degeneration In 1921, Ramsay Hunt published an account of six cases (two in twin brothers) in which myoclonus was combined with progressive cerebellar ataxia. The age of onset in the four nonfamilial cases was between 7 and 17 years, and the cerebellar ataxia followed the myoclonus by an interval of 1 to 20 years. Hunt named this disorder *dyssynergia cerebellaris myoclonica.* In the twin brothers there were signs of Friedreich ataxia; postmortem examination of one of them showed a degeneration of the posterior columns and spinocerebellar tracts, but not of the corticospinal tracts. The only lesion in the cerebellum was an atrophy and sclerosis of the dentate nuclei with degeneration of the superior cerebellar peduncles. Louis-Bar and van Bogaert in 1947 reported a similar case, and they noted, in addition to the above findings, degeneration of the corticospinal tracts and loss of fibers in the posterior roots. Thus the pathology was identical to that of Friedreich ataxia except for the more severe atrophy of dentate and other roof nuclei.

Earlier (1914), under the title of *dyssynergia cerebellaris progressiva,* Hunt had drawn attention to a progressive disease in young adults manifested by what he

considered to be a pure cerebellar syndrome. One of the three patients described in this paper died 13 years after the onset of her illness, and necropsy disclosed cavitary lesions in the lenticular nuclei, cerebellum, and pons, and a diffuse increase of Alzheimer (type 2) glia cells, associated with nodular cirrhosis of the liver—i.e., findings typical of progressive lenticular degeneration (Wilson). Hunt's reports emphasize the hazard of classifying cerebellar ataxias on the basis of clinical findings alone, a point made effectively by Holmes in relation to the hereditary cerebellar ataxia of Marie (see above).

Dentatorubropallidoluysian Atrophy This is a rare familial disorder in which symptoms of cerebellar ataxia are coupled with those of choreoathetosis and dystonia. Pathologically there is degeneration of the dentatorubral and pallidoluysian systems (Smith; Iizuka et al).

Azorean Disease of the Nervous System (Machado-Joseph Disease) In recent years a special form of hereditary ataxia, aside from the Andrade type of amyloid polyneuropathy, has been described in patients of Portuguese-Azorean origin. One such case was described by Woods and Schaumburg in 1972 under the name *nigrospinodentatal degeneration with nuclear ophthalmoplegia.* The disorder was characterized by an autosomal dominant pattern of inheritance and by a slowly progressive ataxia beginning in adolescence or early adult life, in association with hyperreflexia, extrapyramidal (parkinsonian) rigidity, dystonia, bulbar signs, distal motor weakness, and ophthalmoplegia. The conjunction of the Parkinson syndrome with cerebellar ataxia was reminiscent of the cases of olivopontocerebellar degeneration, but the onset is earlier and there is a higher incidence of dystonia and amyotrophy. Postmortem examination disclosed a degeneration of the dentate nuclei and spinocerebellar tracts, and a loss of anterior horn cells and neurons of the pons, substantia nigra, and oculomotor nuclei. The heredoataxia was unaccompanied by signs of polyneuropathy, which was an important feature of the disease in Portuguese emigrants, described earlier by Nakano and colleagues as Machado disease, this being the name of the progenitor of the afflicted family.

A similarly affected Azorean family named Joseph was described by Rosenberg et al (1976), under the name of *autosomal dominant striatonigral degeneration.* The disease had its onset in early adult life and was characterized by progressive ataxia of gait, followed by dysarthria, nystagmus, slowness of eye movements, reduced facial mobility, slow lingual movements, fasciculations of face and tongue, dystonic postures, rigidity of the limbs, cerebellar tremor, hyperreflexia, and Babinski signs. Rosenberg et al considered the disorder to be a striatonigral degeneration, on the basis of their findings in one autopsied case. The choice of this designation was unfortunate, as the clinical and pathologic picture was quite unlike that of the striatonigral degeneration reported by Adams et al. The diagnosis of striatonigral degeneration was disputed also by Nielsen and by Romanul who were able to study the brain of the patient reported by Rosenberg et al.

Under the name *Azorean disease of the nervous system,* Romanul et al described yet another family of Portuguese-Azorean descent, the members of which suffered a progressive ataxia of gait, parkinsonian features, limitation of conjugate gaze, fasciculations, areflexia, nystagmus, cerebellar tremor, and extensor plantar responses; the pathologic changes closely resembled those described by Woods and Schaumburg. Romanul et al compared the genetic, clinical, and pathologic features of their cases with those of the three other Portuguese disorders and proposed that all of them represent a single genetic entity with variable expression. This concept of the disease has been corroborated by the observations of Rosenberg and of Fowler, who studied 20 patients with the Machado-Joseph-Azorean disease over a 10-year period.

This disease is not limited to Azoreans. Cases conforming to the above descriptions have now been observed among black, Indian, and Japanese families (Sakai et al; Yuasa et al; Bharucha et al).

There is no treatment. Early diagnosis of patients at risk is possible by the examination of ocular movements. Hotson et al found dysmetric horizontal and vertical saccades, similar to those of symptomatic patients.

OTHER CHRONIC CEREBELLAR ATAXIAS OF DEGENERATIVE TYPE

To be briefly mentioned here are the hereditary ataxias with optic atrophy described by van Leeuwen and van Bogaert; an autosomal recessive syndrome of cerebellar ataxia with pigmentary retinal degeneration and congenital deafness of Hallgren; an autosomal dominant hereditary ataxia with muscular atrophy, retinal degeneration and diabetes mellitus; Friedreich ataxia with juvenile parkinsonism of Biemond and Sinnige; an autosomal recessive ataxia with total albinism of Skre and Berg; and an autosomal recessive ataxia with cataracts, oligophrenia, pyramidal signs, and stunting of growth of Marinesco and Sjögren (see Kark et al for references). Probably these disorders are genetically distinct. No metabolic abnormalities have been detected in any of them. There is however a rare variant of Tay-Sachs disease (G_{M2} gangliosidosis) that presents as a childhood form of progressive and disabling spinocerebellar degeneration (Kolodny and Raghavan). Moreover, familial incidence in itself does not establish a genetic causation, for it is now known that diseases caused by transmissible agents, such as subacute spongiform encephalopathy, may begin with cerebellar ataxia. Also an immunologic defect, like the one underlying ataxia-telangiectasia, may cause cerebellar degeneration.

There is a form of *hereditary paroxysmal cerebellar ataxia,* the episodes occurring without explanation and lasting several hours; between episodes the patient is normal or exhibits only minimal ataxia of the limbs and nystagmus. The attacks can be prevented by acetazolamide (Griggs et al).

The metabolic ataxias are discussed further in Chap. 38 and the ataxias caused by transmissible agents in Chap. 33.

HEREDITARY POLYMYOCLONIA

The syndrome of quick, arrhythmic, involuntary single or repetitive twitches of a muscle or group of muscles was described in Chap. 5, and it was pointed out that the condition has many causes. Familial forms are known, one of which, associated with cerebellar ataxia, was described above (dyssynergia cerebellaris myoclonica of Ramsay Hunt). But there is another form, known as *hereditary essential benign myoclonus,* that occurs in relatively pure form unaccompanied by ataxia. In the latter condition, it may at times be difficult to evaluate coordination because willed movement is marred by the myoclonus, which may be mistaken for intention tremor. This hereditary myoclonus usually begins early in life and is inherited as an autosomal dominant trait. Once established it persists with little or no change in severity throughout life, often with rather little disability. It can by its natural course be differentiated from some of the hereditary metabolic diseases such as the Unverricht and Lafora types of myoclonic epilepsy, the lipidoses, tuberous sclerosis, and certain viral infections that are described in Chap. 33.

Of particular interest is the response of this form of movement disorder to new pharmacologic agents, notably clonazepam, valproic acid, and 5-hydroxytryptophan, the amino acid precursor of serotonin.

SYNDROME OF MUSCULAR WEAKNESS AND WASTING WITHOUT SENSORY CHANGES

MOTOR SYSTEM DISEASE

This general term is used to designate a progressive degenerative disorder of motor neurons in the spinal cord, brainstem, and motor cortex, manifested clinically by muscular weakness, atrophy, and corticospinal tract signs in varying combinations. It is a disease of middle life, for the most part, and progresses to death in a matter of 2 to 6 years, or longer in exceptional cases.

Customarily, motor system disease is subdivided into several types, on the basis of the particular grouping of symptoms and signs. The most frequent form, in which amyotrophy and hyperreflexia are combined, is called *amyotrophic lateral sclerosis* (amyotrophy is the term applied to denervative atrophy and weakness of muscles). Less frequent are cases in which weakness and atrophy occur alone, without evidence of corticospinal tract dysfunction. For these the term *progressive spinal muscular atrophy* is used. When the weakness and wasting predominate in muscles innervated by the motor nuclei of the lower brainstem, i.e., in muscles of the jaw, face, tongue, pharynx, and larynx, it is customary to speak of *progressive bulbar palsy* ("bulb" being the old name for medulla oblongata). In a small proportion of patients the clinical state is dominated for a time by spastic weakness, hyperreflexia, and Babinski signs, lower motor neuron affection becoming apparent at a later stage of the illness. *Primary lateral sclerosis* designates a rare form of motor system disease in which the degenerative process remains confined to the corticospinal pathways (Beal and Richardson). The authors believe that the pure spastic paraplegias without amyotrophy represent a special class of disease, to be described separately.

Special types of familial, progressive muscular atrophy also occur in infancy and childhood. The best known is the Werdnig-Hoffmann type or *infantile muscular atrophy;* but there are other familial forms beginning in later childhood, adolescence, or adult life. In some of these a spastic weakness is a prominent feature; others are characterized by a slowly progressive amyotrophy. In respect to the nonfamilial forms there is no reason to believe that the subgroups are anything other than variants of a single pathologic process—a motor neuron degeneration or atrophy.

History Credit for the original delineation of amyotrophic lateral sclerosis is appropriately given to Charcot. With Joffroy in 1869 and with Gombault in 1871 he studied the pathologic aspects of the disease, and in a series of lectures given from 1872 to 1874 he gave a lucid account of the clinical and pathologic findings. Although called Charcot disease in France, amyotrophic lateral sclerosis (the term recommended by Charcot) has been preferred in the English-speaking world. Duchenne had earlier (1858) described "labioglossolaryngeal paralysis," a term that Wachsmuth in 1864 changed to "progressive bulbar palsy." In 1869 Charcot called attention to the nuclear origin of progressive bulbar palsy, and in 1882 Dejerine established its relationship to amyotrophic lateral sclerosis. Most authors credit Aran and Duchenne with the earliest descriptions of progressive spinal muscular atrophy, which, they believed, was of myogenic origin. This interpretation was of course incorrect; Cruveilhier, a few years later, noted the slender anterior roots and soon thereafter the disease was brought into line with amyotrophic lateral sclerosis as a myelopathic or spinal muscular atrophy.

Amyotrophic Lateral Sclerosis (ALS)   This is a common disease, with an annual incidence rate of 0.4 to 1.76 per 100,000 population. Men are affected somewhat more frequently than women. Most patients are more than 50 years old at the onset of symptoms and the incidence increases with each decade of life (Mulder). The disease occurs in a random pattern throughout the world except for a dramatic clustering of patients among inhabitants of the Kii peninsula in Japan, and in Guam, where ALS is often combined with dementia and parkinsonism. In about 5 percent of cases the disease is familial, being inherited as an autosomal dominant trait. The familial cases do not differ in their symptoms and clinical course from nonfamilial ones, although as a group the former have a somewhat earlier age of onset, an equal distribution in men and women, a slightly shorter survival, and a greater tendency for the weakness to begin in the legs.

In its most typical form, uselessness of a hand, awkwardness in tasks requiring fine finger movements, stiffness of the fingers, and slight weakness or wasting of the hand muscles are the first indications of the disease. Cramping beyond what seems natural and fasciculations of the muscles of the forearm, upper arm, and shoulder girdle muscles also appear. As the weeks and months pass, the other hand and arm may be similarly affected. Before long, the triad of atrophic weakness of the hands and forearms, slight spasticity of the legs, and generalized hyperreflexia—all in the absence of sensory change—leaves little doubt as to the diagnosis. Muscle strength and bulk diminish in parallel; yet despite the amyotrophy, the tendon reflexes are notable for their liveliness. Abductors, adductors, and extensors of fingers and thumb tend to become weak before the long flexors, on which the handgrip depends, and the dorsal interosseous spaces become hollowed, giving rise to the "cadaveric" or "skeleton hand." The muscles of the upper arm and shoulder girdles are involved later. All the while the thigh and leg muscles seem relatively normal, and there may come a time when the patient walks about with useless, dangling arms. Later the atrophic weakness spreads to the neck, tongue, pharyngeal and laryngeal muscles, and eventually those in the trunk and lower extremities yield to the onslaught of the disease.

The affected parts may ache and feel cold, but true paresthesias, except from poor positioning and nerve pressure, do not occur. Sphincteric control is usually well maintained even after both legs have become weak and spastic, and the abdominal reflexes may be elicitable even when the plantar reflexes are extensor. Extreme spasticity is rarely seen. Coarse fasciculations are usually evident in the weakened muscles but may not be noticed by the patient until the physician calls attention to them.

Variants There are many patterns of neuromuscular involvement other than those just described. The leg may be affected before the hand. A foot drop with weakness and wasting of the pretibial muscles may be incorrectly attributed to a peroneal nerve compression until weakness of the gastrocnemius and other muscles betrays a more widespread involvement of lumbosacral neurons. In our experience this crural amyotrophy is nearly as frequent as the brachial-manual type. Another variant is the early involvement of thoracic, abdominal, or posterior neck muscles. The pattern of proximal or shoulder girdle amyotrophy, as in Wohlfart-Kugelberg-Welander disease (see further on), is also well known and simulates muscular dystrophy. On several occasions we have observed a pattern of involvement of arm and leg on the same side—sometimes called the *hemiplegic*, or *Mills, variant*. Again the first manifestations may be a spastic weakness of the legs; a diagnosis of primary lateral sclerosis may be made, and only after a year or two do the hand and arm muscles weaken, waste, and fasciculate. It is cases of this type that led to the inclusion of spastic paraparesis as a variant of ALS. Exceptionally, cramps or fasciculations of the limb muscles may precede recognizable weakness and wasting by a month or two. ALS has been observed in conjunction with presenile and senile dementia, and with Parkinson disease, a complex similar to that observed among the natives of Guam.

The course of this illness, irrespective of its particular mode of onset and pattern of evolution, is inexorably progressive. Half the patients succumb within 3 years and 90 percent within 6 years (Mulder and Espinosa).

Progressive Muscular Atrophy (PMA) This type of motor system disease is more common in men than in women, in a ratio of 3.6:1 (Chio et al). In about half the patients, PMA takes the form of a symmetrical (sometimes asymmetrical) wasting of intrinsic hand muscles, slowly advancing to the more proximal parts of the arms; less often the legs and thighs are the sites of onset of atrophic weakness, and less often still the proximal parts of the limbs are affected before the distal parts. These purely nuclear amyotrophies tend to progress at a slower pace than the usual case of amyotrophic lateral sclerosis, some patients surviving for 15 years or longer. Chio and his colleagues, who analyzed the factors affecting life expectancy in 155 patients with PMA, found that younger patients had a more benign course—the 5-year survival was 72 percent in patients with onset of PMA before age 50, and 40 percent in patients with onset after age 50. Some of the most chronic varieties of PMA are familial. Otherwise they differ from ALS only in that the tendon reflexes are diminished or absent, and signs of corticospinal tract disease cannot be detected. Fascicular twitchings and cramping are variably present.

Progressive Bulbar Palsy Here reference is made to a condition in which the first and dominant symptoms relate to weakness of muscles innervated by the motor nuclei of the lower brainstem, i.e., muscles of the jaw, face, tongue, pharynx, and larynx. This weakness gives rise to an early defect in articulation, in which there is difficulty in the pronunciation of lingual (r, n, l), labial (b, m, p, f), dental (d, t), and palatal (k, g) consonants. As the condition worsens, syllables lose their clarity and run together until finally speech becomes unintelligible. In other patients, slurring is due to spasticity of the tongue, pharyngeal, and laryngeal muscles or to a combination of atrophic and spastic weakness, as indicated below. Defective modulation of the voice with variable degrees of rasping and nasality is another characteristic. The pharyngeal reflex is lost, and the palate and vocal cords move imperfectly or not at all during attempted phonation. Mastication and deglutition are impaired; the bolus of food cannot be manipulated and may lodge between the cheek and teeth; and the pharyngeal muscles do not force it properly into the esophagus. Liquids and small particles of food find their way into the trachea or reflux into the nose. The facial muscles, particularly of the lower face, weaken and sag. Fasciculations and focal loss of tissue of the tongue are usually early manifestations; eventually the tongue becomes shriveled, and lies useless in the floor of the mouth. The chin may also quiver from fascicular twitchings, but the disease should never be diagnosed on the basis of fasciculations alone, i.e., in the absence of weakness or atrophy. Fasciculations may be entirely benign or a part of the syndrome of myokymia or of "continuous muscular activity" (see page 1170).

The jaw jerk may be present at a time when the muscles of mastication are markedly weak. In fact, spasticity of the jaw muscles may be so pronounced that the slightest tap on the chin will evoke clonus, and, rarely, attempts to open the mouth elicit a "bulldog" reflex (jaws snap shut involuntarily). The signs of spastic weakness may at all times surpass those of atrophic weakness, and pathologic laughter and crying may infrequently reach extreme degrees. *This is the only common clinical situation in which spastic and atrophic bulbar palsy co-exist.* Strangely, the ocular muscles always escape; nor have we ever observed an instance of the sporadic disease with sensory loss. Such cases have been reported, but they are so rare that the diagnosis must remain in doubt.

There is little need for laboratory investigation once one is familiar with the clinical picture, but there are a few aids. The electromyogram, as expected, displays widespread fibrillations and fasciculations, and motor nerve conduction studies reveal only a slight slowing. If the atrophic paresis is restricted to an arm or hand, raising the question of cervical spondylosis, evidence of denervation over many segments favors the diagnosis of ALS. The CSF protein is normal or sometimes slightly elevated.

As with other forms of motor system disease, the course of bulbar palsy is inexorably progressive. Eventually the weakness spreads to the respiratory muscles, and deglutition fails entirely; the patient dies of inanition and aspiration pneumonia, usually within 2 to 3 years of onset. Strangely, decubitus ulcers are rarely seen in bedfast patients, a point remarked upon by Charcot. About 25 percent of cases of motor system disease begin with bulbar symptoms but rarely, if ever, does the sporadic form of progressive bulbar palsy run its course as an independent syndrome (pure heredofamilial forms of progressive bulbar palsy and progressive ocular palsy in the adult are known, but are rare). Practically always, after a few months, the other manifestations of ALS become evident. The earlier the onset of the bulbar involvement in the course of ALS, the shorter the course of the disease.

Pathology The principal finding is a loss of nerve cells in the anterior horns of the spinal cord and motor nuclei of the lower brainstem. Many of the surviving nerve cells are small, shrunken, and filled with lipofuscin. Lost cells are replaced by fibrous astrocytes. Large neurons tend to be affected before small ones. The anterior roots are thin, and there is a disproportionate loss of large myelinated fibers in motor nerves (Bradley et al). The muscles show typical denervation atrophy of different ages. Whitehouse et al found a depletion of muscarinic, cholinergic, glycinergic, and benzodiazepam receptors in regions of the spinal cord, where motor neurons had disappeared.

The corticospinal tract degeneration is most evident in the lower parts of the spinal cord, but it can be traced up through the brainstem to the posterior limb of the internal capsule and corona radiata by means of fat stains, which show the macrophages that accumulate in response to the myelin degeneration. There is a loss of Betz cells in the motor cortex. Other fibers in the ventral and lateral funiculi are depleted, imparting a characteristic pallor in myelin stains. McMenemey interprets this as evidence of involvement of nonmotor neurons and, hence, objects to the term *motor system disease*. However, we regard this as due to a loss of collaterals of motor neurons which contribute to the lamina propria. One observes the same effect in severe, long-standing poliomyelitis.

Neuropathologic studies of cases of ALS with dementia are few in number. In addition to the usual affection of motor neurons, these cases have shown an extensive neuronal loss and gliosis involving the premotor area, particularly the superior frontal gyri, and the inferolateral cortex of the temporal lobes. The histologic changes of Alzheimer or Pick disease have not been seen in our cases; neurofibrillary degeneration has been observed but is inconsequential in comparison to that seen in the guamanian Parkinson-dementia-ALS complex (Finlayson et al; Mitsuyama). Attempts to transmit this ALS-dementia syndrome (33 cases) to subhuman primates have been unsuccessful (Salazar et al). Rare families with amyotrophy, chorea, mental changes, acanthocytosis, and hypobetalipoproteinemia have been observed in Great Britain, the United States, and Japan. This represents a separate disease.

Diagnosis Motor system disease may be simulated by a central spondylotic bar or ruptured cervical disc, but usually, with these latter conditions, there are pain in the neck and shoulders, limitation of neck movements, and sensory changes, and the lower motor neuron affection is restricted to one or two spinal segments. A mild corticospinal hemiparesis or monoparesis due to multiple sclerosis may for a time be difficult to distinguish from early ALS.

Progressive spinal muscular atrophy may be differentiated from peroneal muscular atrophy (Charcot-Marie-Tooth neuropathy) by the lack of family history and the complete lack of sensory change. Motor system disease beginning in the proximal limb muscles may be misdiagnosed as a limb girdle type of muscular dystrophy. The spastic form of bulbar palsy may suggest the pseudobulbar palsy of lacunar disease. A crural form of progressive muscular atrophy may be confused with diabetic mononeuropathy multiplex or polymyositis. There is also a very rare form of subacute poliomyelitis (possibly viral) in patients with lymphoma or carcinoma; it leads to an amyotrophy that progresses to death over a period of several months.

Some patients who have recovered from paralytic poliomyelitis may develop progressive muscular weakness 30 or 40 years later; the nature of this relationship is quite obscure. We favor the explanation that atrophy of anterior horn cells with aging brings to light a critically depleted motor neuron population.

A recent observation of considerable interest is the finding of a form of progressive spinal muscular atrophy in patients with G_{M2} gangliosidosis, the storage disease that presents in infancy as Tay-Sachs disease (Kolodny and Raghavan). The onset is in late adolescence and early adult life and the atrophic paralysis is progressive, so that these patients are often mistaken for Kugelberg-Welander disease or ALS. A number of cases of this type have been uncovered in Ashkenazi Jews by the use of lysosomal enzyme analysis.

All these caveats notwithstanding, amyotrophic lateral sclerosis or the more discrete forms of motor system disease rarely offer any difficulty in diagnosis.

Causation and Treatment The cause and pathogenesis of motor system disease are not known. The progressive weakness of affected muscles, occurring in some patients 30 or 40 years after recovery from an attack of paralytic poliomyelitis, should not be confused with progressive muscular atrophy (PMA), as indicated above. Genuine PMA and ALS have been described in patients who had suffered a remote attack of poliomyelitis and probably represent chance occurrences. There is no evidence that such cases represent a reactivation of the poliomyelitis virus or the presence of some other slow or unconventional virus. Trauma, particularly traction injury of an arm, has been reported from time to time as an antecedent event in patients with ALS, but the nature of this relationship has not been settled. Shy et al have reported that the incidence of paraproteinemia in patients with motor system disease is higher than can be accounted for by chance; the significance

of this observation remains to be determined. It has never been proved that intoxication with heavy metals (lead, mercury, aluminum) can cause motor system disease. There is no specific treatment for this disease, and only supportive measures can be utilized. It has been our practice to give the patient some idea of the seriousness of the condition, but not to make a devastating statement that it is invariably fatal. Usually it is advisable to give medication of some type "to try to halt the disease," even though none is known to be effective. Guanidine hydrochloride and injections of cobra venom, gangliosides, interferons, high-dose intravenous cyclophosphamide, and thyrotropin-releasing hormone are but the latest in a long series of agents that have been said to arrest the process, but no convincing evidence has been forthcoming to support these claims.

Heredofamilial Forms of Progressive Muscular Atrophy and Spastic Paraplegia *Werdnig-Hoffmann disease (infantile progressive spinal muscular atrophy)* This is the classic form of a spinal muscular atrophy of hereditary type. It is described fully in Chap. 52, along with the early-life myopathies, since these are the disorders from which it always needs to be distinguished.

Chronic proximal spinal muscular atrophy (PSMA, Wohlfart-Kugelberg-Welander syndrome) This is a somewhat different form of heredofamilial spinal muscular atrophy which, as the name indicates, involves the proximal muscles of the limbs predominantly, and is only slowly progressive. It was first clearly separated from other forms of motor system disease and from muscular dystrophy by Wohlfart and by Kugelberg and Welander in the mid-1950s. In about a third of the cases, the onset is before 2 years of age and in 50 percent, between 3 and 18 years. Males are preponderantly affected, especially among patients with juvenile and adult onset. The usual form of transmission is by an autosomal recessive gene, but families with dominant and sex-linked inheritance have been described.

The disease begins insidiously, with weakness and atrophy of the pelvic girdle and proximal leg muscles, followed by involvement of the shoulder girdle and upper arm muscles. Unlike the sporadic form of spinal muscular atrophy, the Wohlfart-Kugelberg-Welander variety is bilaterally symmetric from the beginning, and fasciculations are observed in only half the cases. Ultimately the distal limb muscles are involved, and tendon reflexes are lost. Bulbar musculature and corticospinal tracts are spared, although Babinski signs and an associated ophthalmoplegia (presumably neural) have been reported in rare instances.

The presence of fasciculations and the EMG and muscle biopsy findings, all of which show the characteristic abnormalities of neural atrophy, permit distinction from muscular dystrophy. Only a few cases have been examined postmortem, and they have shown loss and degeneration of the anterior horn cells.

In addition to the characteristic changes of denervation, muscle biopsies from these cases have disclosed necrosis of single muscle fibers with phagocytosis and attempts at regeneration, changes that may account for elevated creatine levels (Mastaglia and Walton). The nature of these latter changes—whether a primary process in muscle or in some way secondary to denervation—remains to be settled.

The disease progresses very slowly, and some patients survive to old age without serious disability. In general, the earlier the onset, the less favorable the prognosis; however, even the most severely affected patients retain the ability to walk for at least 10 years after the onset. Admittedly, it is difficult to make a sharp distinction between these latter cases of Wohlfart-Kugelberg-Welander disease and certain instances of Werdnig-Hoffmann disease with onset in late infancy and early childhood and prolonged survival (Byers and Banker). Some of these cases of "nuclear amyotrophy," as Wilson called them, have been mistaken for limb-girdle dystrophy (see Chap. 50).

Hereditary spastic paraplegia or diplegia

This disease was described by Seeligmüller in 1874 and later by Strümpell in Germany and Lorrain in France, and has now been identified in nearly every part of the world. The pattern of inheritance is usually autosomal dominant, rarely recessive, and the onset may be in any age period from childhood to the senium. The clinical picture is that of a gradual development of spastic weakness of the legs with increasing difficulty in walking. The tendon reflexes are hyperactive and the plantar reflexes extensor, and, in the pure form of the disease, sensory and other nervous functions are entirely intact. If the onset is in childhood, the feet are usually arched and shortened and there is a pseudocontracture of calf muscles, forcing the child or adolescent to "toe-walk." Sometimes the knees are slightly flexed, or the legs are fully extended and adducted. Weakness is variable and is difficult to estimate. Sphincteric function is usually retained. The arms are involved in varying degree, sometimes not at all. In some, the hands are stiff, movements are clumsy, and speech is mildly dysarthric. Conjoined findings such as nystagmus, ocular palsies, optic atrophy, pigmentary macular degeneration, ataxia (both cerebellar and sensory), epilepsy, and dementia have all been described in isolated families (see further on).

The few available pathologic studies have shown that aside from the degeneration of the corticospinal tracts throughout the spinal cord, there is a thinning of the columns of Goll, mainly in the lumbosacral regions, and of the spinocerebellar tracts, even though no sensory abnormalities

had been detected during life. These were the pathologic findings described by Strümpell in his original (1880) report of two brothers with spastic paraplegia; one of them in addition had a cerebellar syndrome, but again there were no sensory abnormalities. A reduction in number of Betz and anterior horn cells has also been reported.

In the differential diagnosis of this disorder, one must always consider an indolent spinal cord or foramen magnum tumor, familial multiple sclerosis (this was the clinical diagnosis in Strümpell's original cases), Arnold-Chiari malformation, and compression of the cord by a variety of congenital bony malformations at the craniocervical junction (see Chap. 36).

Available medications to suppress spasticity have had only limited success in the authors' hands. Recently we have had some success in ameliorating the spasticity with oral threonine, which is an activator of spinal cord glycine (an inhibitory neurotransmitter).

Other Hereditary Forms of Motor System Disease As mentioned above, instances of *familial amyotrophic lateral sclerosis (ALS)* in adults have long been recognized. The authors have had several under their care, beginning in the third, fourth, or fifth decades of life and transmitted as an autosomal dominant trait. Less well known, however, were the familial types of spinal muscular atrophy that occurred between the infancy–early childhood period (the Werdnig-Hoffmann type) and adulthood—until Emery collected all the cases in northern England and Scotland and found examples that began at every age. Moreover, a number of forms of familial spinal muscular atrophy have been combined with spastic paraplegia; families with later age of onset have tended to have more definite signs of corticospinal tract disease.

A remarkable number of subtypes have been recognized, both of the spinal and brainstem muscular atrophies and of the familial spastic paraplegias. It is not possible to describe all of them, but the following are the major ones, beginning with the lower motor neuron variants.

Progressive bulbar paralysis of childhood (Fazio-Londe syndrome)

Fazio in 1892 and Londe in 1893 described children, adolescents, and young adults who developed progressive bulbar palsy. As subsequent cases were identified, the full picture of facial diplegia, dysarthria, dysphagia, and dysphonia was observed and noted to become increasingly pronounced until the time of death some years after onset. In some there was a late development of corticospinal signs. Also jaw and oculomotor weakness appeared occasionally, and in one case there was progressive deafness. Pathologic examination has shown a loss of motor neurons in the hypoglossal, ambiguus, facial, and trigeminal motor nuclei. In a few cases, the nerve cells in the oculomotor nuclei were also diminished. This disease, the few times we have encountered it, had to be differentiated from a pontomedullary glioma and brainstem multiple sclerosis.

Ophthalmoplegia with neural disease   Ocular motor or gaze disorders have been observed in cases of Friedreich ataxia and spastic paraplegia, and in some of the early cases of hereditary ataxia reported by Sanger Brown. Ferguson and Critchley have described a heredofamilial syndrome comprising gaze palsies, spastic paraparesis, cerebellar ataxia, and optic atrophy (see below). Drachman has discussed these and other cases of presumably neural origin under the term *ophthalmoplegia plus*. His chapter and that of Rowland in the *Handbook of Clinical Neurology* summarize the extensive literature on the heredodegenerative ocular palsies.

Variants of familial spastic paraplegia   The literature contains a number of reports of familial spastic paraplegia combined with other neurologic abnormalities. Some of the syndromes had developed early in life and in conjunction with moderate degrees of mental retardation. Nevertheless the rest of the neurologic picture appeared many years after birth and was progressive. Because of limitations of space, each syndrome cannot be described in detail. The following list includes the best-known entities.

1. *Hereditary spastic paraplegia with spinocerebellar and ocular symptoms (Ferguson-Critchley syndrome).* Instances of this syndrome, characterized by a disorder of gaze, have been remarked upon above. Far more impressive are the manifestations of spinocerebellar ataxia beginning during the fourth and fifth decades of life accompanied by weakness of the legs, alterations of mood, pathologic crying and laughing, dysarthria and diplopia, dysesthesias of limbs, and poor bladder control. The tendon reflexes are lively, with bilateral Babinski signs. Sensation is diminished distally in the limbs. The whole picture resembles multiple sclerosis. In other cases, running through several generations of a family, the extrapyramidal features were more striking; such cases overlap with the following syndromes.

2. *Hereditary spastic paraplegia with extrapyramidal symptoms.* Action and static tremors, parkinsonian rigidity, dystonic tongue movement, and athetosis of the limbs have all been found in combination with spastic paraplegia. Gilman and Romanul have reviewed the literature on this subject. The picture of parkinsonism with spastic weakness and corticospinal signs has been the most frequent combination, in the authors' experience.

3. *Hereditary spastic paraplegia with optic atrophy.* Known as the Behr syndrome, this will be described below in connection with the Leber form of hereditary optic atrophy. Some of the members of the large family reported by Bruyn and Went also had athetosis. The onset was in childhood.

4. *Hereditary spastic paraplegia with retinal degeneration (Kjellin syndrome).* Spastic paraplegia with amyotrophy, oligophrenia, and central retinal degeneration constitutes the syndrome described in 1959 by Kjellin. While the mental retardation is stationary, the spastic weakness and retinal changes are of late onset and progressive. When ophthalmoplegia is added, it is called the *Barnard-Scholz syndrome.*

5. *Hereditary spastic paraplegia with mental retardation or dementia.* Many of the children with progressive spastic paraplegia have either been mentally retarded since early life or have regressed mentally as other neurologic symptoms developed. Examples of this syndrome and its variants are too numerous to be considered here, but are contained in the review of Gilman and Romanul. The recessive syndrome of Sjögren-Larsson, with the onset in infancy of spastic weakness of the legs in association with mental retardation, stands somewhat apart because of the associated ichthyosis.

6. *Hereditary spastic paraplegia with polyneuropathy.* We have observed several patients in whom a fairly typical sensorimotor polyneuropathy was combined with unmistakable signs of corticospinal disease. The age of onset was in childhood or adolescence, and the disability progressed to the point where the patient was chair-bound by early adult life. In two of the cases a sural nerve biopsy revealed a typical hypertrophic polyneuropathy; in a third case there was only a depletion of large myelinated fibers.

If the term *hereditary spastic paraplegia* is to have any neurologic significance, it should only be applied to the relatively rare, pure form of the progressive syndrome. The more common "atypical" cases with amyotrophy, cerebellar ataxia, tremors, dystonia, athetosis, optic atrophy, retinal degeneration, amentia, and dementia should be put in separate categories and their identity retained for nosologic purposes until such time as some biochemical data related to pathogenesis are forthcoming. Separable also are all the congenital nonprogressive types of spastic diplegia and athetosis.

THE MITOCHONDRIAL CYTOPATHIES

Another group of multisystem, multiorgan diseases, as heterogeneous and confusing as the spastic paraplegias, is the mitochondrial cytopathies. Again, classification defies the best attempts of clinicians, pathologists, and biochemists, mainly because the only factor that so far unites these disorders is a nonspecific morphological finding. As more is learned of their nature, it may be necessary to group them with the hereditary metabolic disorders (see page 810).

This interesting class of diseases came to medical attention through the study of a group of children with ophthalmoplegia and retinal degeneration, heart block, and physical and mental retardation—a group of symptoms now known as Kearns-Sayre syndrome (page 1144). The identifying histologic feature was the ''ragged-red muscle fiber,'' so named because of the presence of many enlarged mitochondria in the modified Gomori stains. More recently the ragged-red fibers have also been found in patients with disease of the central nervous system with few or no retinal or ocular muscle changes.

In childhood, these CNS mitochondrial abnormalities have been associated with retarded mental development, short stature, seizures, myoclonus, and ataxia. In adults a great variety of clinical syndromes, including combinations of seizures, ataxia, progressive intellectual decline, deafness, blindness, and peripheral neuropathy, have been reported. *M*yopathy and *e*ncephalopathy have been combined with *l*actic *a*cidosis and *s*troke-like episodes (MELAS), and *m*yopathy and *e*ncephalopathy with *r*agged-*red f*ibers (MERRF). In some instances the blood and visceral organs (endocrine system, heart, liver) have been deranged. The diseases progress over several years.

Petty et al have described the encephalopathy in 18 cases. Ataxia was present in all, 13 had become demented, 7 were deaf, 11 had visual difficulties due to a retinopathy, and 11 had abnormal eye movements. The onset was gradual and the course progressive. Severe brain atrophy was noted in CT scans and the CSF protein was elevated.

The clinical syndromes are too heterogeneous to classify systematically, and the biochemical abnormalities (various cytochrome and carnitine abnormalities) are too diverse to link to specific mitochondrial defects. Impressive to the authors is how the observation of a single morphological finding—an excessive number and size of mitochondria in a muscle fiber—is opening a new field of obscure disease. Another major discovery has been that these mitochondrial diseases are transmitted via the mitochondrial DNA of the mother more often than that of the father, and not by the usual nuclear genetic systems (Egger et al).

SYNDROME OF PROGRESSIVE BLINDNESS

There are two main classes of progressive blindness in children, adolescents, and adults—progressive optic neuropathy and retinal (pigmentary or tapeto-) degeneration. Of course there are many congenital anomalies and retinal diseases beginning in infancy that result in blindness and microphthalmia. Some of them of neurologic interest were described briefly in Chap. 12.

HEREDITARY OPTIC ATROPHY OF LEBER

While familial amaurosis was known in the early eighteenth century, it was Leber in 1871 who gave the definitive description of this disease and traced it through many genealogies. The pattern of inheritance does not conform to conventional mendelian principles. Male preference is evident in most families, but this cannot be adequately explained on the basis of X-linked transmission, since females are also affected and transmit the carrier state to their daughters more frequently than would be expected. In most patients the visual loss begins between 18 and 25 years, but the range of age of onset is much greater. A few of the affected women have their first symptom at the menarche. In some families the disease has been followed for five and six generations (Carroll and Mastaglia).

Usually the visual loss has an insidious onset and a subacute or slow evolution, but it may begin so abruptly as to suggest a retrobulbar neuritis; moreover, in these latter instances aching in the eye or brow may accompany the visual loss. Subjective visual phenomena are reported by some. Usually both eyes are affected simultaneously— though in some one eye is affected first, followed by the other after an interval of several weeks or months. In practically all cases, the second eye is affected within a year of the first, very rarely after a longer period. In the unimpaired eye, abnormalities of visual evoked potentials may be found before impaired visual acuity is recognized (Carroll and Mastaglia).

Once started, the visual impairment progresses over a period of weeks to months. Usually central vision is impaired before peripheral, and there is a stage in which bilateral central scotomata are readily demonstrated. Disturbances of color vision are said to be characteristic; early on, perception of blue-yellow is deficient, while that of red and green is relatively preserved. In the more advanced stages, however, the patients are totally color-blind. Constriction of the fields may be added later. Usually there is no nystagmus. At first there may be only blurring of the disc margins, but soon they become atrophic. Peripapillary telangiectasia and tortuosity of the more peripheral vessels have also been noted in the early stages of the disease (Smith et al). As visual symptoms develop, fluorescein angiography shows shunting in the abnormal vascular bed, with reduced filling of capillaries of the papillomacular bundle. The vasculopathy seems to be the primary change and the nerve fiber atrophy is secondary (Nikoskelainen). Of some importance is the fact that the visual impairment is seldom complete; and although patients are declared legally blind because of the large central scotomata, they still can do certain types of work.

The optic nerve lesion has been examined on a number of occasions. The central parts of the nerves are degenerated from papillae to the lateral geniculate bodies, the papillomacular bundles being particularly affected. Presumably axis cylinders and myelin degenerate together, as would be expected from the loss of nerve cells in the superficial layer of the retina. Both astrocytic glial and endoneurial connective tissue are increased.

As so often happens in heredofamilial diseases, this type of optic atrophy may be combined with degeneration in many other parts of the nervous system. Behr in 1909 reported six cases in which corticospinal and cerebellar signs came on with optic atrophy in early life. In others, spastic paraplegia and neuropathy, striatal degeneration with dystonia, and tremor and mental retardation have been associated, and epilepsy and imbecility were found in some members of the family studied by Ferguson and Critchley; spastic ataxia was seen in another.

Important in differential diagnosis is the recognition of congenital optic atrophy (of which recessive and dominant forms are known) and of retrobulbar neuritis.

RETINITIS PIGMENTOSA

This remarkable retinal abiotrophy, known since Helmholtz first invented the ophthalmoscope in 1851, usually begins in childhood and adolescence. Unlike the Leber type which affects only the third neuron of the visual neuronal chain, retinitis pigmentosa affects all the retinal layers, both the neuroepithelium and pigment epithelium. For this combination Leber proposed the term *tapetoretinal degeneration*, thinking it preferable to retinitis pigmentosa, since there is no evidence of inflammation. The incidence of this disorder is two or three times greater in males than in females. Inheritance is more often recessive than dominant; in the former, consanguinity, which increases the likelihood of

disease by approximately 20 times, plays an important part. Sex-linked types are also known.

The first symptom is usually a failure of twilight vision (nyctalopia). Under dim light the visual fields tend to constrict, but slowly, as the disease progresses, there is permanent visual impairment in all degrees of illumination. The perimacular zones tend to be the first and most severely involved, giving rise to partial or complete ring scotomata. Peripheral loss sets in later. Usually both eyes are affected simultaneously, but rare cases are on record where one eye was affected first and more severely. Color vision is lost relatively late. The electrical activity of the eye (measured by the electroretinogram, which depends on the activity of all components of the retina) is extinguished, in contrast to the Leber type of optic atrophy, in which it is retained.

Ophthalmoscopic examination shows the characteristic triad of pigmentary deposits that assume the appearance of bone corpuscles, attenuated vessels, and pallor of the optic discs. The pigment is due to clumping of epithelial cells that migrate from the pigment layer to the degenerating, superficial parts of the retina. The pigmentary degeneration spares only the fovea, so that eventually the world is perceived by the patient as though he or she were looking through narrow tubes.

Syndromes to which retinitis pigmentosa may be linked are oligophrenia, obesity, syndactyly and hypogonadism (Bardet-Biedl syndrome); hypogenitalism, obesity and mental deficiency (Laurence-Moon syndrome); Friedreich and other types of spinocerebellar and cerebellar ataxia; spastic paraplegia and quadriplegia with Laurence-Moon syndrome; neurogenic amyotrophy, progressive external ophthalmoplegia with or without heart block (Kiloh-Nevin and Kearns-Sayre syndromes); deaf mutism; Leber optic atrophy; myopia and color blindness; and polyneuropathy and deafness (Refsum syndrome).

Differential diagnosis includes the Batten form of cerebroretinal degeneration, Pelizaeus-Merzbacher disease, and Gaucher disease, and retinal infections such as syphilis, toxoplasmosis, and cytomegalic inclusion disease.

Virtual blindness is the outcome in many cases, but in others the visual failure stops short of that. It is doubtful if any of many proposed modes of therapy (sympathectomy, steroids, vitamins A and E) have any effect in halting the progress of the disease.

STARGARDT DISEASE

This is a bilaterally symmetrical, slowly progressive macular degeneration, differentiated from retinitis pigmentosa by Stargardt in 1909. In essence it is a hereditary (usually recessive) tapetoretinal degeneration or dystrophy (the latter term preferred by Waardenburg), with onset between 6 and 20 years, rarely later, and leading to a loss of central vision. The region of the macula becomes gray or yellow-brown with pigmentary spots, and the visual fields show central scotomata. Later the periphery of the retina may become dystrophic. The lesion is well visualized by fluorescein angiography. Activity in the electroretinogram is diminished or abolished.

This disease is clearly different from retinitis pigmentosa. According to Cohan et al it may be associated with epilepsy, Refsum syndrome, Kearns-Sayre syndrome, Bassen-Kornzweig syndrome, Sjögren-Larsson syndrome, with spinocerebellar and other forms of cerebellar degeneration, familial paraplegia, and the syndrome of hyperkinesia with statokinetic trembling of Vancea and Tudor.

SYNDROME OF PROGRESSIVE DEAFNESS

There is an impressive group of hereditary, progressive cochleovestibular atrophies that are linked to atrophies and degenerations of the nervous system. These are the subject of an informative review by Konigsmark. Such neuro-otologic syndromes must be set alongside a group of five diseases that affect the auditory and vestibular nerves exclusively: dominant progressive nerve deafness; dominant, low-frequency hearing loss; dominant midfrequency hearing loss; sex-linked, early-onset neural deafness; and hereditary episodic vertigo and hearing loss. The last of these is of special interest to neurologists because both balance and hearing are affected.

HEREDITARY HEARING LOSS WITH RETINAL DISEASES

Konigsmark has separated this overall category into three subgroups: patients with typical retinitis pigmentosa, those with Leber optic atrophy, and those with other retinal changes.

With respect to retinitis pigmentosa, four syndromes are recognized. Retinitis pigmentosa in combination with congenital hearing loss is referred to as the Usher syndrome. Retinitis pigmentosa and hereditary hearing loss may also be combined with polyneuropathy (Refsum syndrome); with hypogonadism and obesity (Alstrom syndrome); and with dwarfism, mental retardation, premature senility, and photosensitive dermatitis (Cockayne syndrome).

Hereditary hearing loss with optic atrophy forms the core of four syndromes: dominant optic atrophy, ataxia, muscle wasting, and progressive hearing loss (Sylvester disease); recessive optic atrophy, polyneuropathy, and neural hearing loss (Rosenberg-Chutorian syndrome); optic atrophy, hearing loss, and juvenile diabetes mellitus (Tunbridge-Paley syndrome); opticocochleodentate degeneration with optic atrophy, hearing loss, quadriparesis, and mental retardation (Nyssen-van Bogaert syndrome).

Hearing loss has also been observed with other retinal changes, two of which might be mentioned: *Norrie disease* with retinal malformation, hearing loss, and mental retardation (oculoacousticocerebral degeneration); *Small disease* with recessive hearing loss, mental retardation, narrowing of retinal vessels, and muscle atrophy. In the former, the infant is born blind, with a white vascularized retinal mass behind a clear lens; later the lens and cornea become opaque. The eyes are small, and the iris is atrophied. In the latter the optic fundi show tortuosity of vessels, telangiectases, and retinal detachment. The nature of the progressive generalized muscular weakness has not been ascertained.

HEREDITARY HEARING LOSS WITH DISEASES OF THE NERVOUS SYSTEM

Several conditions are known in which hereditary deafness accompanies degenerative disease of the peripheral or central nervous system.

1. *Hereditary hearing loss with epilepsy.* The seizure disorder is mainly one of myoclonus. In one dominantly inherited form, photomyoclonus is associated with mental deterioration, hearing loss, and nephropathy (Hermann disease). In May-White disease, also dominant, myoclonus and ataxia accompany hearing loss. Congenital deafness and mild chronic epilepsy of recessive type have also been observed (Latham-Monro disease).

2. *Hereditary hearing loss and ataxia.* Here Konigsmark was able to delineate five syndromes, the first two of which show a dominant pattern of heredity, the last three a recessive pattern: piebaldism, ataxia, and neural hearing loss (Telfer syndrome); hearing loss, hyperuricemia, and ataxia (Rosenberg-Bergstrom syndrome); ataxia and progressive hearing loss (Lichtenstein-Knorr syndrome); ataxia, hypogonadism, mental deficiency, and hearing loss (Richards-Rundles syndrome); ataxia, mental retardation, hearing loss, and pigmentary changes in the skin (Jeune-Tommasi syndrome).

3. *Hereditary hearing loss and other neurologic syndromes.* These include dominant sensory radicular neuropathy (Denny-Brown); progressive polyneuropathy, kyphoscoliosis, skin atrophy, eye defects (myopia, cataracts, atypical retinitis pigmentosa), bone cysts and osteoporosis (Flynn-Aird syndrome); chronic polyneuropathy and nephritis (Lemieux-Neemeh syndrome); congenital pain asymbolia and auditory imperception (Osuntokun syndrome); and bulbopontine paralysis (facial weakness, dysarthria,

dysphagia, and atrophy of the tongue with fasciculations) with progressive neural hearing loss. The onset of the latter syndrome occurs at 10 to 35 years of age; the pattern of inheritance is recessive. The disease progresses to death. It resembles the progressive hereditary bulbar paralysis of Fazio-Londe, except for the progressive deafness and loss of vestibular responses.

References which describe the details of these many syndromes are contained in Konigsmark's review, listed below. The syndromes are summarized here in order to increase awareness of the large number of hereditary neurologic diseases for which the clue is provided by the detection of impaired hearing and labyrinthine functions.

REFERENCES

ADAMS RD, VAN BOGAERT L, VANDER EECKEN H: Striato-nigral degeneration. *J Neuropathol Exp Neurol* 23:584, 1964.

ALLEN N, KNOPP W: Hereditary parkinsonism-dystonia with sustained control by L-dopa and anticholinergic medication, in Eldridge R, Fahn S (eds): *Advances in Neurology*, vol 14: *Dystonia*. New York, Raven Press, 1976, pp 201–215.

ALZHEIMER A: Über eine eigenartige Erkankung der Hirnrinde. *Allg Z Psychiatr* 64:146, 1907.

ALZHEIMER A: Über eigenartige Krankheitsfälle des späteren Alters. *Z Gesamte Neurol Psychiatr* 4:356, 1911.

AUSTIN JG, ARMSTRONG D, FOUCH S et al: Metachromatic leukodystrophy. *Arch Neurol* 18:225, 1968.

BARBEAU A: Biochemistry of Friedreich's ataxia, in *Spinocerebellar Degenerations*. Tokyo, University of Tokyo Press, 1980*a*, pp 303–311.

BARBEAU A: High-level levodopa therapy in severely akinetic parkinsonian patients—12 years later, in Rinne U, Klingler M, Stamm S (eds): *Parkinson's Disease: Current Progress, Problems and Management*. Elsevier/North Holland, New York, 1980*b*, pp 229–239.

BEAL MF, MARTIN JB: Somatostatin: Normal and abnormal observations in the CNS, in Wurtman RJ, Corkin SH, Growdon JH (eds): *Alzheimer Disease: Advances in Basic Research and Therapies*. Cambridge, MA, Center for Brain Science and Metabolism Charitable Trust, 1984, pp 229–258.

BEAL MF, RICHARDSON EP Jr: Primary lateral sclerosis: A case report. *Arch Neurol* 38:630, 1981.

BECKER PE: Genetic approaches to the nosology of nervous system defects, in Bergsma D (ed): *Birth Defects: Original Article Series*, vol 7: *Nervous System*, pt VI. New York, Alan R Liss, 1971, pp 10–22.

BEHR C: Die komplizierte, hereditär-familiäre Optikusatrophie des Kindesalters. Ein bisher nicht beschriebener Symptomkomplex. *Klin Mbl Augenheilk* 47, pt 2: 138, 1909.

BELL J: On hereditary ataxia and spastic paraplegia, in Fisher RA (ed): *Treasury of Human Inheritance*, vol IV: *Nervous Diseases and Muscular Dystrophies*, pt III. London, Cambridge University Press, 1939, pp 141–281.

BERLIN L: Presenile sclerosis (Alzheimer's disease) with features resembling Pick's disease. *Arch Neurol Psychiatry* 61:369, 1949.

BHARUCHA NE, BHARUCHA EP, BHABHA SR: Machado-Joseph-Azorean disease in India. *Arch Neurol* 43:142, 1986.

BIRD TD, CEDERBAUM S, VALPEY RW, STAHL WL: Familial degeneration of the basal ganglia with acanthocytosis: A clinical, neuropathological, and biochemical study. *Ann Neurol* 3:253, 1978.

BIRD ED, IVERSEN LL: Huntington's chorea: Postmortem measurement of glutamic acid decarboxylase, choline acetyl-transferase and dopamine in basal ganglia. *Brain* 97:457, 1974.

BLASS JP, KARK RAP, MENON NK: Low activities of the pyruvate and oxoglutarate dehydrogenase complexes in five patients with Friedreich's ataxia. *N Engl J Med* 295:62, 1976.

BRADLEY WG, GOOD P, RASOOL CG et al: Morphometric and biochemical studies of peripheral nerves in amyotrophic lateral sclerosis. *Ann Neurol* 14:267, 1983.

BRANDT J, FOLSTEIN SE, FOLSTEIN ME: Differential cognitive impairment in Alzheimer's disease and Huntington's disease. *Ann Neurol* 13:555, 1988.

BRUYN GW, WENT LN: A sex-linked heredodegenerative neurological disorder associated with Leber's optic atrophy. I: Clinical studies. *J Neurol Sci* 159, 1964.

BURKE RE, FAHN S, MARSDEN CD: Torsion dystonia: A double-blind, prospective trial of high-dosage trihexyphenidyl. *Neurology* 36:160, 1986.

BYERS RK, BANKER BQ: Infantile muscular atrophy. *Arch Neurol* 5:140, 1961.

CARROLL WM, MASTAGLIA FL: Leber's optic neuropathy. *Brain* 102:559, 1979.

CHAMBERLAIN S, SHAW J, ROWLAND A et al: Mapping of mutation causing Friedreich's ataxia to human chromosome 9. *Nature* 334:248, 1988.

CHANDLER JH, REED TE, deJONG RN: Huntington's chorea in Michigan: III. Clinical observations. *Neurology* 10:148, 1960.

CHASE TN, FOSTER NL, MANSI L: Alzheimer's disease and the parietal lobe. *Lancet* 2:225, 1983.

CHAWLUK JB, MESULAM M-M, HURTIG H et al: Slowly progressive aphasia without generalized dementia: Studies with positron emission tomography. *Ann Neurol* 19:68, 1986.

CHIN HC, TENG EC, HENDERSON EL et al: Clinical subtypes of dementia of Alzheimer type. *Neurology* 35:1544, 1985.

CHIO A, BRIGNOLIO F, LEONE M et al: A survival analysis of 155 cases of progressive muscular atrophy. *Acta Neurol Scand* 72:407, 1985.

COHAN SL, KATTAH JC, LIMAYE SR: Familial tapetoretinal degeneration and epilepsy. *Arch Neurol* 36:544, 1979.

COHEN J, LOW P, FEELEY R: Somatic and autonomic function in progressive autonomic failure and multiple system atrophy. *Ann Neurol* 22:692, 1987.

COOPER IS: 20-year followup study of the neurosurgical treatment of dystonia musculorum deformans, in Eldridge R, Fahn S (eds): *Advances in Neurology*, vol 14. New York, Raven Press, 1976, pp 423–453.

CREUTZFELDT HG: Über eine eigenartige herdförmige Erkrankung des Zentralnervensystems. *Z Gesamte Neurol Psychiatr* 57:1, 1920.

CROSS HE, MCKUSICK VA: The Mast syndrome. *Arch Neurol* 16:1, 1967.

DAVENPORT CB: Huntington's chorea in relation to heredity and eugenics. *Proc Natl Acad Sci* 1:283, 1915.

DAVISON C: Spastic pseudosclerosis (cortico-pallido-spinal degeneration). *Brain* 55:247, 1932.

DEJONG RN: The history of Huntington's chorea in the United States of America, in Barbeau A et al (eds): *Advances in Neurology*, vol 1: *Huntington's Chorea, 1872–1972*. New York, Raven Press, 1973, pp 19–27.

DIAMOND SG, MARKHAM CH, HOEHN MM et al: Multi-center study of Parkinson mortality with early versus late dopa treatment. *Ann Neurol* 22:8, 1987.

DRACHMAN DA: Ophthalmoplegia plus: A classification of the disorders associated with progressive external ophthalmoplegia, in Vinken PJ, Bruyn GW (eds): *Handbook of Clinical Neurology*, vol 22. Amsterdam, North-Holland, 1975, chap 9, pp 203–216.

DUNLAP CB: Pathologic changes in Huntington's chorea, with special reference to corpus striatum. *Arch Neurol Psychiatry* 18:867, 1927.

EGGER J, LAKE BD, WILSON J: Mitochondrial cytopathy: A multisystem disorder with ragged-red fibers on muscle biopsy. *Arch Dis Child* 56:741, 1981.

ELDRIDGE R: The torsion dystonias: Literature review and genetic and clinical studies. *Neurology* 20:1, 1970.

ELDRIDGE R, FAHN S (eds): *Advances in Neurology*, vol 14: *Dystonia*. New York, Raven Press, 1976.

EMERY AEH: Review of the nosology of progressive muscular atrophy. *J Med Genet* 8:481, 1971.

ENNA SJ: Huntington's chorea: Changes in neurotransmitter receptors in the brain. *N Engl J Med* 294:1305, 1976.

FARRER LA, CONNEALLY M: Predictability of phenotype in Huntington's disease. *Arch Neurol* 44:109, 1987.

FERGUSON F, CRITCHLEY M: A clinical study of an heredofamilial disease resembling disseminated sclerosis. *Brain* 52:203, 1929.

FINLAYSON MH, GUBERMAN A, MARTIN JB: Cerebral lesions in familial amyotrophic lateral sclerosis and dementia. *Acta Neuropathol* 26:237, 1973.

FINOCCHIARO G, TARONI F, DIDONATO S: Glutamate dehydrogenase in olivopontocerebellar atrophies: Leukocytes, fibroblasts, and muscle mitochondria. *Neurology* 36:550, 1986.

FITCH N, BECKER R, HELLER A: The inheritance of Alzheimer's disease: A new interpretation. *Ann Neurol* 23:14, 1988.

FLATAU E, STERLING W: Progressiver Torsionsspasmus bei Kindern. *Z Gesamte Neurol Psychiatr* 7:586, 1911.

FOWLER HL: Machado-Joseph-Azorean Disease. A ten-year study. *Arch Neurol* 41:921, 1984.

GARCIN R, BRION S, KHOCHNEIVISS AA: Le syndrome de Creutzfeldt-Jakob et les syndromes cortico-stries du presenium (à l'occasion de 5 observations anatomiocliniques). *Rev Neurol* 109:419, 1963.

GILMAN S, ROMANUL FCA: Hereditary dystonic paraplegia with amyotrophy and mental deficiency: Clinical and neuropathological characteristics, in Vinken PJ, Bruyn GW (eds): *Handbook of Clinical Neurology*, vol 22. Amsterdam, North-Holland, 1975, chap 19, pp 445–465.

GOSSET A, PELISSIER JF, DELPEUCH F, KHALIL R: Striatonigral degeneration associated with olivopontocerebellar degeneration. *Rev Neurol* 139:125, 1983.

GOUDSMIT J, MORROW CH, ASHER DM et al: Evidence for and against the transmissibility of Alzheimer's disease. *Neurology* 30:945, 1980.

GOUDSMIT JAAP, WHITE BJ, WEITKAMP LR et al: Familial Alzheimer's disease in two kindreds of the same geographic and ethnic origin. *J Neurol Sci* 49:79, 1981.

GREENFIELD JG: *The Spino-Cerebellar Degenerations*. Springfield, IL, Charles C Thomas, 1954.

GRIGGS RC, MOXLEY RT, LAFRANCE RA et al: Hereditary paroxysmal ataxia; response to acetazolamide. *Neurol* 28:1259, 1978.

GUSELLA JF, WEXLER NS, CONNEALLY PM et al: A polymorphic DNA marker, genetically linked to Huntington's disease. *Nature* 306:234, 1983.

HAKIM AM MATHIESON G: Basis of dementia in Parkinson's disease. *Lancet* 2:729, 1978.

HALLETT M, KHOSHBIN S: A physiological mechanism of bradykinesia. *Brain* 103:301, 1980.

HARDING AE: *The Hereditary Ataxias and Related Disorders*. New York, Churchill Livingstone, 1984.

HAYDEN MR, MARTIN WRW, STOESSL AJ et al: Positron emission tomography in the early diagnosis of Huntington's disease. *Neurology* 36:888, 1986.

HENDERSON JM, HUBBARD BM: Definition of Alzheimer disease. *Lancet* 1:408, 1985.

HEYMAN A, WILKINSON WE, HURWITZ BJ et al: Alzheimer's disease: Genetic aspects and associated clinical disorders. *Ann Neurol* 14:507, 1983.

HINTON DR: Optic nerve degeneration in Alzheimer disease. *N Engl J Med* 315:485, 1986.

HIRANO A, KURLAND LT, KROOTH RS, LESSELL S: Parkinsonism-dementia complex, an endemic disease on the Island of Guam: I. Clinical features. *Brain* 84:642, 1961.

HIRANO A, MALAMUD M, KURLAND LT: Parkinsonism-dementia complex on the Island of Guam. II: Pathological features. *Brain* 84:662, 1961.

HOLMES GM: A form of familial degeneration of the cerebellum. *Brain* 30:466, 1907a.

HOLMES GM: An attempt to classify cerebellar disease with a note on Marie's hereditary cerebellar ataxia. *Brain* 30:545, 1907b.

HOTSON JR, LANGSTON EB, LOUIS AA: The search for a physiologic marker of Machado-Joseph disease. *Neurol* 37:112, 1987.

HUFF FJ, BOLLER F, LUCHELLI F: The neurologic examination in patients with probable Alzheimer disease. *Arch Neurol* 44:929, 1987.

HUNT JR: Dyssynergia cerebellaris progressiva—a chronic progressive form of cerebellar tremor. *Brain* 37:247, 1914.

HUNT JR: Progressive atrophy of the globus pallidus. *Brain* 40:58, 1917.

HUNT JR: Dyssynergia cerebellaris myoclonica—primary atrophy of the dentate system: A contribution to the pathology and symptomatology of the cerebellum. *Brain* 44:490, 1921.

HUNT JR: The striocerebellar tremor. *Arch Neurol Psychiatry* 8:664, 1922.

HUNTINGTON G: On chorea. *Med Surg Reporter* 26:317, 1872.

IIZUKA R, HIRAYAMA K, MAEHARA K: Dentato-rubro-pallido-luysian atrophy: A clinico-pathological study. *J Neurol Neurosurg Psychiatry* 47:1299, 1984.

JACKSON JA, JANKOVIC J, FORD J: Progressive supranuclear palsy: Clinical features and response to treatment in 16 patients. *Ann Neurol* 13:273, 1983.

JAKOB A: Über eigenartige Erkrankungen des Zentralnervensystems mit bemerkenswertem anatomischen Befunde (spastische Pseudosclerose-Encephalomyelopathie mit disseminierten Degenerationsherden). *Z Gesamte Neurol Psychiatr* 64:147, 1921.

JAKOB A: Über eine der multiplen Sklerose klinisch nahestehende Erkrankung des Zentralnervensystems (spastische Pseudosklerose) mit bemerkenswertem anatomischen Befunde. *Med Klin* 17:382, 1921.

JERVIS GA: Early senile dementia in mongoloid idiocy. *Am J Psychiatry* 105:102, 1948.

JOACHIM CL, MORRIS JH, SELKOE DJ: Clinically diagnosed Alzheimer disease: autopsy results in 150 cases. *Ann Neurol* 24:50, 1988.

JOHNSON WG, WIGGER J, KARP HR: Juvenile spinal muscular atrophy: A new hexosamine deficiency phenotype. *Ann Neurol* 11:11, 1982.

JUNCOS J, SERRATI C, FABBRINI G: Fluctuating levadopa concentrations and Parkinson's disease. *Lancet* II:440, 1985.

KANTER W, WOOTEN F, ELDRIDGE R: Dopamine-beta-hydroxylase and the torsion dystonias, in Eldridge R, Fahn S (eds): *Advances in Neurology,* vol 14: *Dystonia.* New York, Raven Press, 1976, pp 303–307.

KARK RAP, ROSENBERG RN, SCHUT LJ (EDS): *Advances in Neurology,* vol 21: *The Inherited Ataxias.* New York, Raven Press, 1978.

KIRBY R, FOWLER C, GOSLING J, BANNISTER R: Urethro-vesical dysfunction in progressive autonomic failure with multiple system atrophy. *J Neurol Neurosurg Psychiatry* 49:554, 1986.

KJELLIN KG: Hereditary spastic paraplegia and retinal degeneration (Kjellin syndrome and Barnard-Scholz syndrome), in Vinken PJ, Bruyn GW (eds): *Handbook of Clinical Neurology,* vol 22. Amsterdam, North-Holland, 1975, chap 20, pp 467–473.

KLAWANS HL, GOETZ CG, PAULSON GW, BARBEAU A: Levodopa and presymptomatic detection of Huntington's disease—eight year follow up. *N Engl J Med* 302:1090, 1980.

KOLLER WC, HERBSTER G: Adjuvant therapy of parkinsonian tremor. *Arch Neurol* 44:921, 1987.

KOLODNY EH, RAGHAVAN SS: G$_{M2}$-gangliosidosis hexosaminidase mutations not of the Tay-Sachs type produce unusual clinical variants. *Trends Neurosci* 6:16, 1983.

KONIGSMARK BW: Hereditary diseases of the nervous system with hearing loss, in Vinken PJ, Bruyn GW (eds): *Handbook of Clinical Neurology,* vol 22. Amsterdam, North-Holland, 1975, chap 23, pp 499–526.

KONIGSMARK BW, WEINER LP: The olivopontocerebellar atrophies: A review. *Medicine* 49:227, 1970.

KUGELBURG E: Chronic proximal (pseudomyopathic) spinal muscular atrophy: Kugelberg-Welander syndrome, in Vinken PJ, Bruyn GW (eds): *Handbook of Clinical Neurology,* vol 22. Amsterdam, North-Holland, 1975, chap 3, pp 67–80.

KUHL DE, PHELPS ME, MARKAM CH et al: Cerebral metabolism and atrophy in Huntington's disease determined by [18]FDG and computed tomographic scan. *Ann Neurol* 12:425, 1982.

LANCE JW, SCHWAB RS, PETERSON EA: Action tremor and the cogwheel phenomenon in Parkinson's disease. *Brain* 86:95, 1963.

LASKER AG, ZEE DS, HAIN TC et al: Saccades in Huntington's disease: Initiation defects and distractibility. *Neurology* 37:364, 1987.

LEBER T: Ueber hereditäre und congenital angelegte Sehnervenleiden. v. *Graefes Arch Ophthal* 17:249, 1871.

LEENDERS KL, FRACKOWIAK SJ, LEES AJ: Steele-Richardson-Olszewski syndrome. *Brain* 111:615, 1988.

LEIGH RJ, NEWMAN SA, FOLSTEIN SE et al: Abnormal ocular motor control in Huntington's disease. *Neurology* 33:1268, 1983.

LEVERENZ J, SUMI SM: Parkinson's disease in patients with Alzheimer's disease. *Arch Neurol* 43:662, 1986.

LIEBERMAN A, DZIATOLOWSKI M, KUPERSMITH M et al: Dementia in Parkinson disease. *Ann Neurol* 6:355, 1979.

LITTLE A, CHUAQUI-KIDD P, LEVU R et al: Early results of a double blind, placebo controlled trial of high-dose lecithin in Alzheimers disease, in Wurtman RJ, Corkin SH, Growdon JG (eds): *Alzheimer's Disease: Advances in Basic Research and Therapies.* Cambridge, MA, The Center for Brain Science and Metabolism Charitable Trust, 1984, pp 313–332.

LITTLE BW, BROWN PW, RODGERS-JOHNSON P et al: Familial myoclonic dementia masquerading as Creutzfeldt-Jakob disease. *Ann Neurol* 20:231, 1986.

LÖKEN H, CYVIN K: Case of clinical juvenile amaurotic idiocy with histological picture of Alzheimer's disease. *J Neurol Neurosurg Psychiatry* 17:211, 1954.

LOUIS-BAR D, VAN BOGAERT L: Sur la dyssynergie cérébelleuse myoclonique (Hunt). *Mschr Psychiatr Neurol* 113:215, 1947.

MALAMUD W, LOWENBERG K: Alzheimer's disease: Contribution to its etiology and classification. *Arch Neurol Psychiatry* 21:805, 1929.

MARIE P: Sur l'hérédo-ataxie cérébelleuse. *Sem Med* 13:444, 1893.

MARIE P, FOIX C, ALAJOUANINE T: De l'atrophie cérébelleuse tardive à prédominance corticale. *Rev Neurol* 38:849, 1082, 1922.

MARINESCU G: Sur une affection particulière simulant, au point de vue clinique, la sclérose en plaques et ayant pour substratum des plaques du type senile spécial. *Arch Roum Pathol Exp Microbiol* 4:41, March 1931 (*Rev Neurol* 2:453, October 1931).

MARSDEN CD: The problems of adult onset idiopathic torsion dystonia and other isolated dyskinesias of adult life, in Eldridge R, Fahn S (eds): *Advances in Neurology,* vol 14: *Dystonia.* New York, Raven Press, 1976, pp 259–277.

MARTIN JB: Genetic testing in Huntington's disease. *Ann Neurol* 16:511, 1984.

Martin JB: Huntington's disease: New approaches to an old problem. *Neurology* 34:1059, 1984.

Mastaglia FL, Walton JN: Histologic and histochemical changes in skeletal muscles from cases of chronic juvenile and early adult spinal muscular atrophy (the Kugelberg-Welander syndrome). *J Neurol Sci* 12:15, 1971.

Masters CL, Gajdusek DC, Gibbs CJ Jr: The Gerstmann-Straussler syndrome and the various forms of amyloid plaques which occur in the transmissible spongiform encephalopathies. *J Neuropathol Exp Neurol* 39:374, 1980.

Mayeux R, Stern Y: Subcortical dementia. *Arch Neurol* 44:129, 1987.

Mayeux R, Stern Y, Rosen J et al: Is subcortical dementia a recognizable clinical entity? *Ann Neurol* 14:278, 1983.

McGeer PL, McGeer EG, Suzuki J: Aging and the extrapyramidal system. *Arch Neurol* 34:33, 1977.

McGeer PL, McGeer EG, Suzuki J et al: Aging, Alzheimer disease and the cholinergic system of the basal forebrain. *Neurology* 34:741, 1984.

McMenemey WH: The dementias and progressive diseases of the basal ganglia, in Blackwood W et al (eds): *Greenfield's Neuropathology,* 2d ed. London, Arnold, 1963, chap 9, pp 520–580.

Mesulam M-M: Slowly progressive aphasia without generalized dementia. *Ann Neurol* 11:592, 1982.

Mitsuyama Y: Presenile dementia with motor neuron disease in Japan: Clinico-pathological review of 26 cases. *J Neurol Neurosurg Psychiatry* 47:953, 1984.

Mollaret P: La Maladie de Friedreich. Paris, Legrand, 1929.

Morris JC, Cole M, Banker BQ, Wright D: Hereditary dysphasic dementia and the Pick-Alzheimer spectrum. *Ann Neurol* 16:458, 1984.

Moyano BA: Coloración de la neuroglia por el metodo de Holzer. *Sem Med* 2:1919, 1930.

Mulder DW (ed): *The Diagnosis and Treatment of Amyotrophic Lateral Sclerosis.* Boston, Houghton-Mifflin, 1980, p 41.

Mulder DW, Espinosa RE: Amyotrophic lateral sclerosis: Comparison of the clinical syndrome in Guam and the United States, in Norris FH, Kurland LT (eds): *Motor Neuron Diseases.* New York, Grune & Stratton, 1969, pp 12–19.

Mulder DW, Kurland LT, Offord KP, Beard CM: Familial adult motor neuron disease: amyotrophic lateral sclerosis. *Neurology* 36:511, 1986.

Nakano, KK, Dawson DM, Spence A: Machado disease. A hereditary ataxia in Portuguese emigrants to Massachusetts. *Neurology* 22:49, 1972.

Nee LE, Eldridge R, Sunderland T et al: Dementia of the Alzheimer type: Clinical and family study of 22 twin pairs. *Neurology* 37:359, 1987.

Nee LE, Polinsky RJ, Eldridge R et al: A family with histologically confirmed Alzheimer's disease. *Arch Neurol* 40:203, 1983.

Nielsen SL: Striatonigral degeneration disputed in familial disorder. *Neurology* 27:306, 1977.

Nikoskelainen E: New aspects of the genetic, etiologic, and clinical puzzle of Leber's disease. *Neurology* 34:1482, 1984.

Nygaard TG, Duvoisin RC: Hereditary dystonia-parkinsonism syndrome of juvenile onset. *Neurology* 36:1424, 1986.

Perry EK, Tomlinson BE, Blessed G et al: Correlation of cholinergic abnormalities with senile plaques and mental test scores in senile dementia. *Br Med J* 2:1457, 1978.

Petty RKH, Harding AE, Morgan-Hughes JA: The clinical features of mitochondrial myopathy. *Brain* 109:915, 1986.

Pick A: Über die Beziehungen der senilen hirnatrophie zur Aphasie. *Prager Med Wochenschr* 17:165, 1892.

Pincus JH, Barry K: Influence of dietary protein on motor fluctuations in Parkinson's disease. *Arch Neurol* 44:270, 1987.

Prusiner SB: Some speculations about prions, amyloid, and Alzheimer's disease. *N Engl J Med* 310:661, 1984.

Quinn NP, Rossor MN, Marsden CD: Dementia and Parkinson's disease—pathological and neurochemical considerations. *Br Med Bull* 42:86, 1986.

Rajput AH, Rozdilsky B: Dysautonomia in Parkinsonism: A clinicopathologic study. *J Neurol Neurosurg Psychiatry* 39:1092, 1976.

Rebeiz JJ, Kolodny EH, Richardson EP: Corticodentatonigral degeneration with neuronal achromasia. *Arch Neurol* 18:20, 1968.

Richardson JC, Steele J, Olszewski J: Supranuclear ophthalmoplegia, pseudobulbar palsy, nuchal dystonia and dementia. *Trans Am Neurol Assoc* 88:25, 1963.

Rocca WA, Amaducci LA, Schoenberg BS: Epidemiology of clinically diagnosed Alzheimer's disease. *Ann Neurol* 19:415, 1986.

Rodriguez-Budelli M, Kark RAP, Blss JP: Action of physostigmine on inherited ataxias, in Kark RAP, Rosenberg RN, Schut LJ (eds): *Advances in Neurology,* vol 21: *The Inherited Ataxias.* New York, Raven Press, 1978, pp 195–203.

Romanul FCA: Azorean disease of the nervous system. *N Engl J Med* 297:729, 1977.

Romanul FCA, Fowler HL, Radvany J et al: Azorean disease of the nervous system. *N Engl J Med* 296:1505, 1977.

Ropper AH, Williams RS: Relationship between plaques, tangles and dementia in Down syndrome. *Neurology* 30:639, 1980.

Rosenberg RN: Joseph disease: An autosomal dominant motor system degeneration, in Duvoisin RC, Plaitakis A (eds): *The Olivopontocerebellar Atrophies.* New York, Raven Press, 1984, pp 179–183.

Rosenberg RN, Nyhan WL, Bay C, Shore P: Autosomal dominant striatonigral degeneration: A clinical, pathologic and biochemical study of a new genetic disorder. *Neurology* 26:703, 1976.

Rosenhagen H: Die primäre Atrophie des Brächenfusses und der unteren Oliven. *Arch Psychiatr Nervenkr* 116:163, 1943.

Roussy G, Levy G: Sept cas d'un maladie familiale particulaire. *Rev Neurol* 1:427, 1926.

Rowland LP: Progressive external ophthalmoplegia, in Vinken PJ, Bruyn GW (eds): *Handbook of Clinical Neurology,* vol 22. Amsterdam, North-Holland, 1975, chap 8, pp 177–202.

Russell DS: Myocarditis in Friedreich's ataxia. *J Path Bacteriol* 58:739, 1946.

Sakai T, Ohta M, Ishino H: Joseph disease in a non-Portuguese family. *Neurology* 33:74, 1983.

SALAZAR AM, GRAFMAN J, SCHLESSELMAN S et al: Penetrating war injuries of the basal forebrain: Neurology and cognition. *Neurology* 36:459, 1986.

SALAZAR AM, MASTERS CL, GAJDUSEK C, GIBBS CJ: Syndromes of amyotrophic lateral sclerosis and dementia: Relation to transmissible Creutzfeldt-Jakob disease. *Ann Neurol* 14:17, 1983.

SASAKI H, MURAMOTO A, KANAZAWA I et al: Regional distribution of amino acid transmitters in postmortem brains of presenile and senile dementia of Alzheimer type. *Ann Neurol* 19:263, 1986.

SCHAUMBURG HH, SUZUKI K: Non-specific familial presenile dementia. *J Neurol Neurosurg Psychiatry* 31:479, 1968.

SCHOENBERG BS, KOKMEN E, OKAZAKI H: Alzheimer's disease and other dementing illnesses in a defined United States population: Incidence rates and clinical features. *Ann Neurol* 22:724, 1987.

SCHOENFELD M, MYERS RH, CUPPLES LA et al: Increased rate of suicide among patients with Huntington's disease. *J Neurol Neurosurg Psychiatry* 47:1283, 1984.

SCHULMAN S: Bilateral symmetrical degeneration of the thalamus. A clinicopathological study. *J Neuropathol Exp Neurol* 16:446, 1957.

SCHWALBE MW: *Eine eigentümliche tonische Krampffor mit hysterischen Symptomen.* Berlin, G Schade, 1908, 35 pp.

SCRIBANU N, KENNEDY C: Familial syndrome with dystonia, neural deafness and possible intellectual impairment: Clinical course and pathologic features, in Eldridge R, Fahn S (eds): *Advances in Neurology,* vol 14: *Dystonia.* New York, Raven Press, 1976, pp 235–245.

SELKOE DJ: Recent advances in Alzheimer's disease, in Petersdorf RG et al (eds): *Update V: Harrison's Principles of Internal Medicine.* New York, McGraw-Hill, 1984, pp 15–33.

SHY ME, ROWLAND LP, SMITH T et al: Motor neuron disease and plasma cell dyscrasia. *Neurology* 36:1429, 1986.

SJÖGREN T: Klinische und erbbiologische Untersuchungen über die Heredoataxien. *Acta Psychiatr (Kbh)* Suppl 27, 1943.

SJÖGREN T, SJÖGREN H, LINDGREN AGH: Morbus Alzheimer and Morbus Pick: A genetic, clinical and pathoanatomical study. *Acta Psychiatr Neurol Scand,* suppl 82, 1952.

SKRE H: Hereditary spastic paraplegia in Western Norway. *Clin Genet* 6:165, 1974.

SMITH JK: Dentatorubropallidoluysian atrophy, in Vinken PJ, Bruyn GW (eds): *Handbook of Clinical Neurology,* vol. 21. Amsterdam, North-Holland, 1975, pp 519–534.

SMITH JL, HOYT WF, SUSAC JO: Ocular fundus in acute Leber optic neuropathy. *Arch Ophthalmol* 90:349, 1973.

SNYDER SH, D'AMATO RJ: MPTP: A neurotoxin relevant to the pathophysiology of Parkinson's disease. *Neurology* 36:250, 1986.

SOBUE I (ed): *TRH and Spinocerebellar Degeneration.* Amsterdam, Elsevier, 1986.

SPATZ H: Die Systematischen Atrophien. *Arch Psychiatry* 108:1, 1938.

SPIELMEYER W: *Histopathologie des Nervensystems.* Berlin, Springer-Verlag, 1922, pp 223–229.

SPOKES EGS: Neurochemical alterations in Huntington's chorea: A study of post-mortem brain tissue. *Brain* 103:179, 1980.

ST. GEORGE-HYSLOP PH, TANZI RE, POLINSKY RJ et al: The genetic defect causing familial Alzheimer's disease maps on chromosome 21. *Science* 235:885, 1987.

STARGARDT K: Über familiäre, progressive Degeneration in der Maculagegend. v. *Graefes Arch Ophthal* 71:534, 1909.

STEELE JC: Progressive supranuclear palsy. *Brain* 95:693, 1972.

STEINGART A, HACHINSKI VC, LAU C et al: Cognitive and neurologic findings in demented patients with diffuse white matter-lucencies on computed tomographic scans (leukoaraiosis) *Arch Neurol* 44:36, 1987.

STERN K: Severe dementia associated with bilateral symmetrical degeneration of the thalamus. *Brain* 61:339, 1938.

TATEICHI J, KITAMOTO T, HASHIGUCHI H et al: Gerstmann-Straussler-Scheinker disease. Immunohistological and experimental studies. *Ann Neurol* 24:35, 1988.

TAYLOR A, SAINT-CYR JA, LANG AE: Dementia prevalence in Parkinson's disease. *Lancet* 1:1087, 1985.

TERRY RD, KATZMAN R: Senile dementia of the Alzheimer type. *Ann Neurol* 14:497, 1983.

TIERNEY MC, SNOW WG, REID DW et al: Psychometric differentiation of dementia. *Arch Neurol* 44:720, 1987.

TISSOT R, CONSTANTINIDIS J, RICHARD J: *La Maladie de Pick.* Paris, Masson et Cie, 1975.

TOMLINSON BE, CORSELLIS JAN: Ageing and the dementias, in Adams JH et al (eds): *Greenfield's Neuropathology,* 4th ed. New York, Wiley, 1984, pp 951–1025.

UHL JA, JAVITCH JA, SNYDER SN: Normal MPTP binding in Parkinson substantia nigra. *Lancet* 1:956, 1985.

VAN BOGAERT L, VAN MAERE M, DESMEDT E: Sur les formes familiales précoces de la maladie d'Alzheimer. *Monatsschr Psychiatr Neurol* 102:249, 1940.

VAN DIJK JG, VAN DER VELDE EA, ROOS RAC et al: Juvenile Huntington's disease. *Hum Genet* 73:235, 1986.

VAN MANSVELT J: Pick's disease: A syndrome of lobar cerebral atrophy. Clinicoanatomical and histopathological types, Thesis, Utrecht, 1954.

VESSIE PR: On the transmission of Huntington chorea for 300 years—the Bures family group. *J Nerv Ment Dis* 76:553, 1932.

VICTOR M, ADAMS RD, MAMCALL EL: A restricted form of cerebellar degeneration occurring in alcoholic patients. *Arch Neurol* 1:577, 1959.

VONSATTEL JP, FERRANTE RJ, RICHARDSON EP: Neuropathologic classification of Huntington's disease. *J Neuropathol Exp Neurol* 42:345, 1983.

WAARDENBURG PJ: Über familiär-erbliche Fälle von seniler Maculadegeneration. *Genetica* 18:38, 1936.

WANG HS: Dementia in old age, in Smith LW, Kinsbourne M (eds): *Aging and Dementia.* New York, Spectrum, 1977, pp 1–4.

WHITAKER PJ: The concept of subcortical and cortical dementia. *Ann Neurol* 19:1, 1986.

WHITEHOUSE PJ, HEDREEN JC, WHITE CL et al: Basal forebrain neurons in the dementia of Parkinson disease. *Ann Neurol* 13:243, 1983.

WHITEHOUSE PJ, PRICE DL, CLARK AW et al: Alzheimer disease: Evidence for loss of cholinergic neurons in nucleus basalis. *Ann Neurol* 10:122, 1981.

WHITEHOUSE PJ, WAMSLEY JK, ZARBIN MA et al: Amyotrophic lateral sclerosis: Alterations in neurotransmitter receptors. *Ann Neurol* 14:8, 1983.

WILSON SAK: *Neurology.* Baltimore, Williams & Wilkins, 1940.

WOHLFART G, FEX J, ELIASSON S: Hereditary proximal spinal muscular atrophy: A clinical entity simulating progressive muscular dystrophy. *Acta Psychiatr Neurol Scand* 30:395, 1955.

WOODS BT, SCHAUMBURG HH: Nigrospinodentatal degeneration with nuclear ophthalmoplegia, in Vinken PJ, Bruyn GW (eds): *Handbook of Clinical Neurology,* vol 22. Amsterdam, North-Holland, 1975, chap 7, pp 157–176.

WOODARD JS: Concentric hyaline inclusion body formation in mental disease. Analysis of 27 cases. *J Neuropathol Exp Neurol* 21:442, 1962.

WORSTER-DROUGHT C, GREENFIELD JG, McMENEMEY WH: A form of familial progressive dementia with spastic paralysis. *Brain* 67:38, 1944.

YAMAGUCHI F, MEYER JS, YAMAMOTO M et al: Noninvasive regional cerebral blood flow measurements in dementia. *Arch Neurol* 37:410, 1980.

YOUNG AB, PENNEY JB, STAROSTA-RUBINSTEIN et al: Normal caudate glucose metabolism in persons at risk for Huntington's disease. *Arch Neurol* 44:254, 1987.

YOUNG AB, SHOULSON I, PENNEY JB et al: Huntington's disease in Venezuela: Neurologic features and functional decline. *Neurology* 36:244, 1986.

YOUNG RR: The differential diagnosis of Parkinson's disease. *Int J Neurol* 12:210, 1977.

YUASA T, OHAMA E, HARAYAMA H et al: Joseph's disease: Clinical and pathological studies in a Japanese family. *Ann Neurol* 19:152, 1986.

ZEMAN W: Pathology of the torsion dystonias (dystonia musculorum deformans). *Neurology* 20 (pt 2):79, 1970.

ZEMAN W, DYKEN P: Dystonia musculorum deformans. Clinical, genetic and pathoanatomical studies. *Psychiatr Neurol Neurochir* 70:77, 1967.

ZIEGLER MG et al: Plasma norepinephrine and dopamine-β-hydroxylase in dystonia, in Eldridge R, Fahn S (eds): *Advances in Neurology,* vol 14: *Dystonia.* New York, Raven Press, 1976, pp 307–318.

CHAPTER 44

DEVELOPMENTAL DISEASES OF THE NERVOUS SYSTEM

Under this broad heading are subsumed a diversity of developmental malformations and diseases acquired during the intrauterine period of life. They number in the hundreds, according to the tabulation of Dyken and Krawiecki, although many of them are very rare. Taxonomically they include many unrelated pathologic processes of different origins: some stem from germ plasm abnormalities; others are associated with triplication, deletion, and translocations of chromosomes; and still others are due to the effects of a variety of noxious agents acting at different times on the nervous system, i.e., during the embryonal, fetal, and paranatal periods of life.

It would be intellectually satisfying if all the morbid states that originate in the intrauterine period could be separated into genetic (hereditary) or nongenetic (congenital) forms, but in many instances the biologic information and the pathologic changes in the brain at this early age have not been characteristic of one group or another and do not allow such a division. For example, in the large group of diseases in which the neural tube fails to close (rachischisis), more than one member of a family may be affected, but it cannot be stated whether a genetic factor is operative or an exogenous factor has acted upon several members during a succession of pregnancies of one mother. Even what appears to be an outright malformation of the brain may be no more than a reflection of the timing of a pathologic process that has affected the nervous system and other organs early in the embryonal period, derailing later processes of development. Teratology, the scientific study of neurosomatic malformations, is replete with such examples.

The authors do not wish to imply that medical and biologic ideas about these conditions are completely unsettled, for there are diseases that are transmitted from one generation to another, affecting both of identical (monovular) twins and only one of fraternal (biovular) twins. In these, a genetic determinant cannot be questioned, for the unaffected fraternal twin shares the same intrauterine environment as the twin sibling. Then, too, a few diseases

destroy parts of the brain in utero in specific ways; others affect it in nonspecific ways but leave little doubt as to the action of an exogenous pathogen.

A perusal of the following pages makes it evident that there is a great variety of structural defects of the nervous system in early life; in fact, every part of the brain, spinal cord, nerves, and musculature may be affected. However, certain principles are applicable to the entire group. *First,* the abnormality of the nervous system is frequently accompanied by an abnormality of some other structure or organ (eye, nose, cranium, spine, ear, and heart), which implicates a certain period of embryogenesis. Unfortunately, this principle is far from absolute; in certain maldevelopments of the brain that must have originated in the embryonic period, all other organs are normal. One can only assume that the brain is more vulnerable than any other organ to prenatal as well as natal influences. *Second,* a maldevelopment of whatever cause should be present at birth and remain stable thereafter, i.e., be nonprogressive; but again, this principle requires qualification—the abnormality may have affected parts of the brain that are not functional at birth so that an interval of time must elapse postnatally before the manifestations of a defect can appear. *Third,* birth should have been nontraumatic. However, the occurrence of a traumatic birth is not proof of a causative relationship between the injury (or infection) and the abnormality, because a defective nervous system may interfere with the birth process or may be excessively vulnerable to an intoxication or infection. *Fourth,* if the birth abnormality has occurred in other members of the family of the same or previous generations, it is usually genetic—although, as noted above, this does not exclude the possible adverse effects of exogenous agents. *Fifth,* many of the teratologic conditions that cause birth defects also cause spontaneous abortions. For example, the incidence of chromosomal abnormalities associated with birth defects is about 0.6 percent of live births, but this incidence among spontaneous abortions at 5 to 12 weeks gestational

Table 44-1
Classification of congenital neurologic disorders

I. Neurologic disorders associated with craniospinal deformities
  A. Enlarged head
    1. Hydrocephalus
    2. Hydranencephaly
    3. Macrocephaly
  B. Craniostenoses
    1. Turricephaly
    2. Scaphocephaly
    3. Brachycephaly
  C. Microcephaly
    1. Primary (vera)
    2. Secondary to cerebral disease
  D. Combinations of cerebral, cranial, and other anomalies
    1. Syndactylic craniocerebral anomalies
    2. Other craniofacial anomalies
    3. Oculoencephalic defects
    4. Oculoauriculocephalic anomalies
    5. Dwarfism
    6. Dermatocephalic anomalies
  E. Rachischisis
    1. Anencephaly, cephalic and spinal meningocele, meningoencephalocele, Dandy-Walker syndrome, meningomyelocele
    2. Arnold-Chiari malformation
    3. Platybasia and cervical-spinal anomalies (Chap. 36)
  F. Chromosomal abnormalities

II. The phakomatoses
  A. Tuberous sclerosis
  B. Neurofibromatosis
  C. Cutaneous angiomatosis with CNS abnormalities

III. Restricted developmental abnormalities of the nervous system
  A. Möbius syndrome
  B. Congenital apraxia of gaze
  C. Other restricted congenital abnormalities (Horner syndrome, unilateral ptosis, anisocoria, etc.)

IV. Congenital abnormalities of motor function (*cerebral palsy*)
  A. Cerebral spastic diplegia
  B. Infantile hemiplegia, double hemiplegia, and quadriplegia
  C. Congenital extrapyramidal disorders (double athetosis; erythroblastosis fetalis and kernicterus)
  D. Congenital and acquired ataxias
  E. The flaccid paralyses

V. Prenatal and paranatal infections
  A. Rubella
  B. Cytomegalic inclusion disease
  C. Congenital neurosyphilis
  D. Toxoplasmosis
  E. Other viral and bacterial infections

VI. Epilepsies of infancy and childhood

VII. Mental retardation

age is over 5 percent. According to the data compiled by Kalter and Warkany, 3 percent of all live-born children have some type of malformation. *Sixth,* low birth weight and gestational age, indicative of premature birth, increase the risk of mental subnormality, seizures, cerebral palsy, and death. In Holland, newborns weighing less than 1500 g have a mortality rate of 233 per 1000, and the rate rises in relation to a diminishing birth rate.

Regarding *etiology,* which is really the crux of the problem of birth defects, some order and classification have emerged. In general, malformations may be subdivided into five groups: (1) a group in which a single mutant gene is responsible (2.25 per 1000 live births); (2) another, in which an hereditary tendency interacts with nongenetic, usually undefined factors; (3) a group associated with chromosomal aberrations; (4) a group attributable solely to exogenous factors (a virus or other infectious agent, x-irradiation, or toxin); (5) and a last group, the largest of all (60 percent of cases), in which no cause can be identified.

Unfortunately, most of the severe birth defects are associated with abnormalities of brain development. Why this occurs is speculative. Perhaps it is because the nervous system, of all organ systems, requires the longest time for its development and maturation, during which it is vulnerable to disease.

A textbook on principles of neurology is not the place to present a detailed account of all the hereditary and congenital developmental abnormalities that might affect the nervous system. Instead we shall only outline the major groups and discuss a few of the more common disease entities. The classification in Table 44-1 adheres to a *grouping in accordance with the main presenting abnormality or abnormalities.* Represented are all the common problems that cause families to seek consultation with the pediatric neurologist: (1) structural defects of the cranium, spine, and limbs, and of eyes, nose, ears, jaws, and skin; (2) disturbed motor function—retarded development or abnormal movements; (3) mental retardation; and (4) epilepsy. The following discussion will focus on each of these clinical states.

NEUROLOGIC DISORDERS ASSOCIATED WITH CRANIOSPINAL DEFORMITIES

The majority of cases in this group are due to a mutant gene, a chromosomal abnormality, or an unknown factor. One has only to walk through an institution for the mentally retarded to appreciate the remarkable number of physical disfigurements that attend abnormalities of the nervous system: heads small and large, encephaloceles with absence of a cranial bone, dwarfed bodies, and odd physiognomies—some of them appallingly grotesque. Indeed, a normal-appearing individual stands out in such a crowd, and will be found frequently to have an inherited metabolic defect or birth injury.

The intimate relationship between the cranium and the growth and development of the brain deserves comment. In embryonic life the most rapidly growing parts of the neural tube induce special changes in and at the same time are influenced by the overlying mesoderm (a process known as induction); hence abnormalities in the formation of skull, orbits, nose, and spine are regularly associated with anomalies of the brain and spinal cord. During early fetal life the cranial bones and vertebral arches enclose and protect the developing brain and spinal cord; throughout the period of rapid brain growth, as pressure is exerted on the inner table of the skull, the latter accommodates to the increasing size of the brain. This adaptation is facilitated by the membranous fontanels, which remain open until maximal brain growth has been attained; only then do they ossify (close).

In addition, stature is controlled by the nervous system, as shown by the fact that the majority of mental retardates are also stunted physically to a varying degree. Thus disorders of craniovertebral development assume importance not merely because of their unsightly appearance but also because they may reflect an abnormality of the underlying brain and spinal cord, i.e., they become diagnostic signs.

CRANIAL MALFORMATIONS AT BIRTH

Certain alterations in size and shape of the head in the infant, child, or even adult always signify a pathologic process that affected the brain before birth or in early infancy. The size of the cranium reflects the size of the brain, and the tape measure is the most useful tool in pediatric neurology. No examination is complete without a measurement of the circumference of the head. A newborn, whose head circumference is below the third percentile for age and sex and whose fontanels are closed, may be judged to have a developmental abnormality of the brain. A head that is normal in size at birth but fails to keep pace with body length reflects a later failure of growth and maturation

of the cerebral hemispheres (microcephaly and microencephaly).

ENLARGEMENT OF THE HEAD

This can be due to hydrocephalus, hydranencephalus, or excessive brain growth (macrocephaly and macroencephaly). The *hydrocephalic head* is distinguished by several features—frontal bossing, a tendency for the eyes to turn down so that sclera is visible between the upper eyelids and iris (sunset sign), prominence of scalp veins due to blockage of blood flow into the dural sinuses, separation of the cranial sutures, thinning of the scalp, and a "cracked-pot" sound on percussion of the skull.

The *hydranencephalic* head (hydrocephalus and destruction or failure of development of parts of the cerebrum) is often associated with enlargement of the skull. When it is transilluminated with a strong flashlight in a darkened room it glows like a jack-o'-lantern. Hydranencephaly is not a well-defined entity. It can be caused by intrauterine vascular occlusion or diseases such as toxoplasmosis and cytomegalic virus disease, in which parts of each cerebral hemisphere are destroyed. *Destruction* of the cerebral mantle in the embryonal period may lead to the formation of huge porencephalic defects (encephaloclastic porencephaly), with subsequent failure of development (evagination) of brain. In the marginal parts of the porencephaly the cortex is malformed, but this indicates only that the lesion preceded neuronal migration. Lack of resistance of the defective brain to ventricular pressure enlarges the head. In still other cases, there appears to be a *primary* failure of development, more specifically varying degrees of failure of evagination. Yakovlev and Wadsworth speak of these as *schizencephalies.*

The *macrocephalic head* (a large head with normal or only slightly enlarged ventricles) may be indicative of the syndrome of macrocephalic idiocy or an advancing metabolic disease that enlarges the brain, as in the later phases of *Tay-Sachs disease, Alexander disease,* and *spongy degeneration of infancy. Subdural hematomas* may also enlarge the head and cause bulging of the fontanelles and separation of the sutures. In the latter condition, the infant is usually irritable, listless, and takes nourishment poorly. MRI or CT scans disclose the subdural blood or fluid (hygroma) and small ventricles. Infants and children with neurofibromatosis, osteogenesis imperfecta, and achondroplasia also have enlarged heads; in the latter condition some degree of hydrocephalus appears to be responsible.

Apart from these pathologic states there is another group of patients with large heads and brains who are normal in all other respects. Many come from families with large heads; Schreier et al, who traced this condition through three generations of some families, declared it to be an autosomal dominant trait. This group comprised 20 percent of 557 children referred to a clinic because of cranial enlargement (Lorber and Priestley).

Patients with hydrocephalus usually come to medical attention because of a rapidly expanding cranium. These problems are discussed in Chap. 30.

Finally, agenesis of the corpus callosum may be associated with macrocephaly and varying degrees of mental impairment and seizures. CT scans reveal the ''bat-wing'' deformity of the ventricles, and there is asynchrony of electrical activity of the two cerebral hemispheres. In a few of the patients an autosomal dominant inheritance has been found (Lynn et al). Agenesis of the corpus callosum is also part of the Aicardi syndrome (see further on).

CRANIOSTENOSES

Some of the most arresting cranial deformities are caused by an obscure malady in which the cranial sutures (membranous junctions between bones of the skull) close prematurely. Such conditions are estimated to occur in 1 of every 1000 births, with a predominance in males (Lyon and Evrard). The growth of the cranium is inhibited in a direction perpendicular to the involved suture(s), with a compensatory enlargement in other dimensions allowed by the patent sutures. For example, when the lambdoid and coronal sutures are both affected, the thrust of the growing brain enlarges the head in a vertical direction (*tower skull,* or *oxycephaly,* also referred to as *turricephaly* and *acrocephaly*). The orbits are shallow, the eyes bulge, and skull films show islands of bone-thinning (Lückenschädel). When only the sagittal suture is involved, the head is long and narrow (*scaphocephalic*), and the closed suture projects, keel-like, in the midline. With premature closure of the coronal suture, the head is excessively wide and short (*brachycephalic*). The nervous system is usually normal in these restricted craniostenoses. If recognized in early infancy, the surgeon can make artificial sutures that may permit the shape of the head to become more normal. Once brain growth has been completed, nothing can be done. When several sutures (usually coronal and sagittal) are closed so as to diminish the cranial capacity, intracranial pressure may increase, impairing cerebral function and later causing headache, vomiting, and papilledema. Obviously an operation is then needed to increase the capacity of the skull. In craniostenoses that are combined with syndactyly, there are often added complications—mental retardation, deafness, convulsions, and loss of sight secondary to papilledema. The so-called clover-shaped skull is the most

severe and lethal of the craniostenoses, because of the associated developmental anomalies of the brain.

When, for any reason, an infant lies with the head turned constantly to one side (because of a shortened sternomastoid muscle, for example), the occiput on that side becomes flattened, as does the opposite frontal bone. The other occipital and frontal bones bulge, so that the maximum length of the skull is not in the sagittal but in the diagonal plane. This condition is called *plagiocephaly,* or *wry head.* Craniostenosis of one half of a coronal suture may also distort the skull in this way.

MICROCEPHALY

There is a form of hereditary microcephaly called *microcephaly vera* in which the head is extremely small (circumference less than 45 cm in adult life, i.e., 5 standard deviations below the mean). In contrast, the face is of normal size, the forehead is narrow and recedes sharply, and the occiput is flat. Stature is only moderately reduced. Such individuals can be recognized at birth by their anthropoid appearance and later by their lumbering gait, extremely low intelligence, and lack of communicative speech. Vision, hearing, and cutaneous sensation are spared. Tendon reflexes in the legs are brisk, and the plantar reflexes may be extensor. Skull films show that the cranial sutures are present, and there are convolutional markings on its inner table. There are two types of inheritance of microcephaly vera, autosomal recessive and sex-linked. The brain often weighs less than 300 g (normal adult range, 1100 to 1500 g) and shows only a few primary and secondary sulci. The cerebral cortex is thick and unlaminated and grossly deficient in neurons. In a few reported cases there has been an associated cerebellar hypoplasia or an infantile muscular atrophy. Lesser degrees of microcephaly have been associated with progressive motor neuron disease and degeneration of the substantia nigra (Halperin et al).

COMBINED CEREBRAL, CRANIAL, AND SOMATIC ABNORMALITIES

As has been remarked, many diseases that interfere with cerebral development also deform the cranial and facial bones, the eyes, the nose, and the ears. Such somatic stigmata therefore assume significance as indicators of altered cerebral structure and function. Moreover, they constitute irrefutable evidence that the associated neural abnormality is in the nature of a maldevelopment, either hereditary or the result of a disease acquired during the intrauterine period.

There are so many of these cerebrosomatic anomalies that one can hardly retain visual images of them, much less recall all the physicians' names by which they are known. Of necessity one turns to atlases, one of the best of which has been composed by our colleagues Holmes and Moser et al, and is based on clinical material drawn from the Massachusetts General Hospital, the Fernald School, and the Eunice K. Shriver Center. The reader should turn to this book or to the one by Gorlin and colleagues for specific information. Ford's monograph on *Diseases of the Nervous System in Infancy, Childhood, and Adolescence* and Jablonski's *Illustrated Dictionary of Eponymic Syndromes, and Diseases, and Their Synonyms* are other valuable references.

There is some advantage in grouping these anomalies according to whether the extremities, face, eyes, ears, and skin are associated with a cerebral defect. For the convenience of the reader and for the purpose of conveying some notion of the number and variety of these anomalies, many of the more common types are summarized below. Unfortunately, no very useful leads as to their origin have been forthcoming.

The Syndactylic-Craniocerebral Anomalies Commonly, fusion of two fingers or two toes or the presence of a tab of skin, representing an extra digit, is present from birth in an otherwise normal individual. However, as pointed out above, when syndactylism of variable degree is accompanied by premature closure of cranial sutures, the nervous system usually proves to be abnormal as well. The following are summaries of some of the better-known syndromes.

1. *Acrocephalosyndactyly types I and II (typical and atypical Apert syndrome).* Type I: turribrachycephalic skull, flat occiput, complete syndactyly of hands and feet ("mitten hands," "sock feet"), protuberant and widely spaced eyes, flat and underdeveloped maxilla and nasal bridge but well-developed chin (relative prognathism), moderate to severe mental retardation, dilated cerebral ventricles. Type II, or atypical form: less extensive syndactyly, probably a phenotypic variant of type I.

2. *Acrocephalosyndactyly III (Saethre-Chotzen syndrome).* Transmission as an autosomal dominant trait, various types of craniostenosis, low frontal hairline, beaked nose with deviated nasal septum, hypertelorism, ptosis, prognathism, cryptorchidism, sometimes low-set ears, proximally fused and shortened digits, moderate degree of mental retardation.

3. *Acrocephalosyndactyly IV (Pfeiffer syndrome).* Autosomal dominant heredity, turribrachycephaly, protruding, widely spaced eyes and divergent strabismus, antimongoloid obliquity of palpebral fissures, low-set ears, irregularly aligned teeth, broad enlarged thumbs and great toes, partially flexed elbows (radiohumeral or radioulnar synostoses), mild and variable mental retardation.

4. *Acrocephalopolysyndactyly (Carpenter syndrome).* Autosomal recessive heredity, premature fusion of all cranial sutures with acrocephaly, flat bridge of nose, medial canthi displaced laterally, epicanthal folds and micrognathia, microcorneas and corneal opacities, hypogenitalism in males, excess digits and syndactyly, obesity, cardiac abnormality in some, subnormal intelligence.

5. *Acrocephalosyndactyly with absent digits.* High, bitemporally flattened head, widely spaced, prominent eyes, small posteriorly rotated ears, high-arched palate, defect in parietal bones, flexed arms, absent toes and syndactylic fingers, moderate mental retardation.

6. *Acrocephaly with cleft lip and palate, radial aplasia, and absent digits.* Microbrachycephaly due to craniostenosis, hypertelorism, misshapen ears, curved mandible, cleft lip and palate, absent radial bones, severe mental retardation.

7. *Dyschondroplasia, facial anomalies, and polysyndactyly.* Probably inherited as an autosomal recessive trait with keel-shaped skull and ridge through center of forehead (metopic suture), macrostomia, micrognathia, upward slant of eyes, high palate, thick alveolar ridges, short neck, short arms and legs, postaxial polydactyly and short digits, genu recurvatum, redundancy of skin, rib anomalies and short sternum, overfolding of helices of ears, moderate mental retardation.

In all the foregoing types of syndactylism and cranial abnormality, which may be regarded as variants of a common syndrome, the diagnosis can be made at a glance, because of the deformed head, protuberant eyes, and abnormal hands and feet. The mental retardation proves to be variable, usually moderate to severe, but occasionally intelligence is normal or nearly so. The brain has been examined in only a few instances and not in a fashion to display fully a developmental abnormality.

Other Craniocephalic-Skeletal Anomalies In the following group of anomalies, the cranium, face, and other parts have special peculiarities, but craniostenosis is not a consistent feature.

1. *Craniofacial dysostosis (Crouzon syndrome).* Autosomal dominant inheritance, variable types and degrees of craniosynostosis, broad forehead with prominence in the anterior fontanel region, shallow orbits with proptosis,

midline facial hypoplasia and short upper lip, malformed auditory canals and ears, high narrow palate, crowded, malaligned upper teeth, moderate mental retardation.

2. *Median cleft facial syndrome (frontonasal dysplasia; hypertelorism of Greig).* Autosomal dominant type of heredity in some cases, widely spaced eyes, broad nasal root, cleft nose and premaxilla, V-shaped frontal hairline, sometimes median frontal lipomas, dermoids and teratomas, heterotypic anterior frontal fontanel (midline cranial defect), strabismus and epibulbar dermoids, sometimes absence of entire prolabium and premaxilla and midline cleft in upper lip, mild to severe mental retardation. Surgical repair possible.

3. *Chondrodystrophia calcificans congenita (chondrodysplasia punctata, Conradi-Hünerman syndrome).* Autosomal recessive or dominant transmission with prominent forehead; flat nose; widely separated eyes; cataracts (in 18 percent); short neck and trunk with kyphoscoliosis; dry, scaly, atrophic skin; cicatricial alopecia; punctate calcifications of epiphyses of long bones and vertebral column with irregularly deformed vertebral bodies; mental retardation infrequent. Severe shortening of limbs in some cases.

4. *Orofaciodigital syndrome.* All the patients are female. It has been suggested that this condition is inherited as a dominant trait which is lethal in males. There are pseudoclefts involving the mandible, tongue, maxilla, and palate; lateral displacement of medial canthi; broad root of nose; hypertrophied buccal frenuli; hamartomas of tongue; sparse scalp hair; subnormal intelligence in one-third to one-half of cases.

5. *Pyknodysostosis.* Autosomal recessive inheritance, large head and frontal-occipital bossing, underdeveloped facial bones, micrognathia, unerupted and deformed teeth, dense and defective long bones with shortened limbs, short and broad terminal digits of fingers and toes, kyphosis and scoliosis in some cases, mental retardation in 25 percent.

6. *Craniotubular bone dysplasias and hyperostoses.* Included under this title are several different genetic disorders of bone, characterized by modeling errors of tubular and cranial bones. Some are inherited as an autosomal recessive trait, and others as a dominant trait. Frontal and occipital hyperostosis, overgrowth of facial bones, and widening of long bones occur in various combinations. Hypertelorism, broad nasal root, nasal obstruction, seizures, visual failure, deafness, prognathism, and retardation of growth are the major features. The serum alkaline phosphatase may be elevated.

Oculoencephalic Defects In this category of anomalies there is simultaneous failure or imperfect development of eye and brain. One member of this group, the oculocerebrorenal syndrome of Lowe has already been mentioned

on page 788, and of course a number of the mucopolysaccharidoses cause corneal opacities, skeletal changes, and psychomotor regression. Also congenital syphilis, rubella, toxoplasmosis, and cytomegalic inclusion disease may affect retina and brain; hypoxia at birth requiring treatment with oxygen may injure the brain and lead to *retrolental fibrodysplasia.*

1. *Anophthalmia with mental retardation.* A sex-linked recessive disease, in which the child is born without eyes; the orbits and maxillae remain underdeveloped, but adnexal tissues of eyes (lids) are intact; occasional kyphoscoliosis and equinovarus deformities of feet; subnormal intelligence.

2. *Norrie disease.* Also inherited as a sex-linked recessive trait; some sight may be present at birth; retrolental opacities; later eyes become shrunken and recessed (phthisis bulbi); some patients have short digits; outbursts of anger; hallucinations; regression of psychomotor function (?).

3. *Oculocerebral syndrome with hypopigmentation.* Autosomal recessive type of heredity with absence of pigment of hair and skin; small, cloudy, vascularized corneas and small globes (microphthalmia); marked mental retardation; athetotic movements of limbs; flexion contractures of elbows; spasticity of legs; persistent grasp and sucking reflexes.

4. *Microphthalmia with corneal opacities, spasticity, and mental retardation.* Microcephaly, broad flat nose, small eyes, corneal opacities, eccentric pupils, stiff extended spastic legs, severe mental retardation.

5. *Aicardi syndrome* with *ocular abnormality* (chorioretinopathy, retinal lacunae, staphyloma, coloboma of optic nerve, microphthalmos), *mental retardation, infantile spasms* and other forms of epilepsy, *agenesis of corpus callosum,* and cortical heterotopias. The *"bat-wing"* deformity of the third and lateral ventricles and asynchronous burst-suppression discharges and sleep spindles are diagnostic. The condition is found only in females.

6. *Lissencephaly of the Walker type (syndrome of Warburg or of Harde).* Ocular lesions are constant but variable (retinal dysplasia, microphthalmia, coloboma, cataracts, corneal opacities). There may be a hydrocephalus. By CT scans or MRI, the lack of cerebral sulci, abnormal eyes and orbits, and absence of cerebellar vermis are diagnostic. Some of the reported cases are familial.

7. *Septo-optique dysplasia (de Morsier syndrome).* Diminished visual acuity, small optic disc, absence of septum pellucidum, and precocious puberty comprise the

syndrome. The neuroendocrine abnormality is discussed further in Chap. 27.

Oculoauriculocephalic Anomalies These are less important from the neurologic standpoint.

1. *Mandibulofacial dysostosis (Treacher Collins syndrome, Franceschetti-Zwahlen-Klein syndrome).* Autosomal dominant heredity with abnormalities of external ears, atresia of external auditory canals, middle and inner ear anomalies, downward palpebral slant, colobomas of lower eyelids, malar, mandibular, and zygomal hypoplasia, microphthalmia and colobomas of iris in a few, mental retardation rare.

2. *Oculoauriculovertebral dysplasia (Goldenhar syndrome).* Autosomal dominant or recessive type of heredity with preauricular appendages, auricular deformities, epibulbar dermoids (lipodermoids), small receding chin, hypoplasia of the soft and bony tissues of the mandible and face (hemifacial microsomia), and vertebral anomalies (hemivertebrae, cervical spine anomalies, spina bifida). Congenital ophthalmoplegia and mild mental retardation are present in some patients.

3. *Oculomandibulodyscephaly with hypotrichosis (Hallermann-Streiff syndrome).* Prominent brow and parietal bones, open fontanels, long, tapering, beaked nose, mandibular hypoplasia, congenital cataracts and microphthalmia, teeth may be present at birth (others missing), skin thin and tense, hair thin and sparse, short stature (25 percent of cases), slight mental retardation.

Dwarfism Midgets are abnormally small but perfectly formed people of normal intelligence; they differ from dwarfs who are not only very small but whose bodily proportions are markedly abnormal. The majority of oligophrenic patients fall below average for height and weight, but there is a small group whose height is well below 135 cm (4½ ft), and who stand apart by this quality alone.

1. *Nanocephalic dwarfism (Seckel bird-headed dwarfism).* The uncomplimentary term *bird head* has been applied to individuals with a small head, large-appearing eyeballs, beaked nose, and underdeveloped chin. Such a physiognomy is not unique to any disease, but when combined with dwarfism it includes a few more or less specific syndromes. Up to 1976 approximately 25 cases had been reported, some with other skeletal and urogenital abnormalities such as medial curvature of middle digits; occasional syndactyly of toes; dislocations of elbow, hip,

knee; premature closure of cranial sutures; and clubfoot deformity. They are short at birth and remain so, living until adolescence or adult years. Retardation is severe. A recessive autosomal type of inheritance is probable. At autopsy the brain is found to have a simplified convolutional pattern, and one of our patients had a type of myelin degeneration similar to that of Pelizaeus-Merzbacher disease.

2. *Russell-Silver syndrome.* Possibly an autosomal dominant pattern of inheritance with short stature of prenatal onset, craniofacial dysostosis, short arms, *congenital hemihypertrophy* (arm and leg on one side larger and longer), pseudohydrocephalic head (normal-sized cranium with small facial bones), abnormalities of genital development in one-third of cases, delay in closure of fontanels and in epiphyseal maturation, elevation of urinary gonadotropins.

3. *Smith-Lemli-Opitz syndrome.* Autosomal recessive inheritance with monocephaly (one cerebral ventricle), broad nasal tip and anteverted nares, wide-set eyes, epicanthal folds, ptosis, small chin, low-set ears, enlarged alveolar maxillary ridge, cutaneous syndactyly, hypospadius in boys, short stature, subnormal neonatal activity, normal amino acids and serum immunoglobulins.

4. *Rubinstein-Taybi syndrome.* Microcephaly but no craniostenosis, downward palpebral slant, heavy eyebrows, beaked nose with nasal septum extending below alae nasi, mild retrognathia, "grimacing smile," strabismus, cataracts, obstruction of nasolacrimal canals, broad thumbs and toes, clinodactyly, overlapping digits, excessive hair growth, hypotonia, lax ligaments, stiff gait, seizures, hyperactive tendon reflexes, absence of corpus callosum, and mental retardation.

5. *Pierre Robin syndrome.* Possible autosomal recessive pattern of inheritance with microcephaly but no craniostenosis, small and symmetrically receded chin ("Andy Gump" appearance), glossoptosis (tongue falls back into pharynx), cleft palate, flat bridge of nose, low-set ears, mental deficiency, and congenital heart disease in half the cases.

6. *DeLange syndrome.* The phenotype shows some degree of variability, but the essential diagnostic features are intrauterine growth retardation and stature falling below the third percentile at all ages, microbrachycephaly, generalized hirsutism and eyebrows that meet across the midline (synophrys), anteverted nostrils, long upper lip, and skeletal abnormalities (flexion of elbows, webbing of second and third toes, clinodactyly of fifth fingers, transverse palmar crease). All are severely retarded mentally, which, with craniofacial abnormalities, is diagnostic. There are no chromosomal abnormalities. A polygenic inheritance has been postulated, but most cases are sporadic.

Neurocutaneous Anomalies with Mental Retardation

It is not surprising that skin and nervous system should share in pathologic states that impair development, since both have a common ectodermal derivation. Nevertheless, it is difficult to find a common theme to the diseases that affect both organs. In some instances it is clear that ectoderm has been malformed from early intrauterine life; in others a number of acquired diseases of skin must be considered. For reasons to be elaborated later, neurofibromatosis, tuberous sclerosis, and Sturge-Weber encephalofacial angiomatosis need to be set apart as a different category of disease.

Hemangiomas of the skin are without doubt the most frequent cutaneous abnormalities that are present at birth, and usually they are entirely innocent. Many recede in the first months of life. On the other hand, an extensive vascular nevus, located in the territory of the trigeminal nerve and sometimes in other parts as well, causes permanent disfigurement and usually portends a cerebral lesion.

Other neurocutaneous diseases are summarized below. A more complete review of these diseases will be found in the article by Adams, and in the monograph edited by Gomez, listed in the references. The importance of recognizing the cutaneous abnormalities relates to the fact that the nervous system is usually abnormal, and often the skin lesion appears before the neurologic symptoms are detectable. Thus the skin lesion becomes a prognosticator of potential neurologic involvement.

1. *Basal-cell nevus syndrome.* This condition is transmitted as an autosomal dominant trait, and is characterized by superficial pits in the palms and soles; multiple solid or cystic tumors over the head, face, and neck appearing in infancy or early childhood; mental retardation in some cases; frontoparietal bossing; hypertelorism and kyphoscoliosis.

2. *Congenital ichthyosis, hypogonadism, and mental retardation.* This disorder is inherited as a sex-linked recessive trait. Aside from the characteristic triad of anomalies, there are no special features.

3. *Xeroderma pigmentosum.* An autosomal recessive pattern of inheritance. Skin lesions appear in infancy, taking the form of erythema, blistering, scaling, scarring, and pigmentation on exposure to sunlight; old lesions are telangiectatic and parchment-like, covered with fine scales; skin cancer later; loss of eyelashes, symblepharon, dry bulbar conjunctivae; microcephaly, hypogonadism, and mental retardation (50 percent of cases).

4. *Sjögren-Larssen syndrome.* Autosomal recessive with congenital ichthyosiform erythroderma; normal or thin scalp hair; sometimes defective dental enamel; and pigmentary degeneration of retinae, spastic legs, and mental retardation.

5. *Poikiloderma congenitale (Rothmund-Thompson syndrome).* Autosomal recessive heredity; appearance of skin changes from the third to sixth month of life; diffuse, pink coloration of cheeks spreading to ears and buttocks, later replaced by macular and reticular pattern of skin atrophy mixed with striae, telangiectasia, and pigmentation; skin changes appear from the third to sixth month of life; sparse hair in half of the cases; cataracts; small genitalia; abnormal hands and feet; short stature and mental retardation.

6. *Linear sebaceous nevus syndrome.* Genetics uncertain, linear organoid nevus of one side of face and trunk, lipodermoids on bulbar conjunctivae, vascularization of corneas, mental retardation, focal seizures, and spike and slow waves in EEG.

7. *Incontinentia pigmenti (Bloch-Sulzberger syndrome).* Only females affected; appearance of dermal lesions in first weeks of life; vesicles and bullae followed by hyperkeratoses and streaks of pigmentation, scarring of scalp, and alopecia; abnormalities of dentition; hemiparesis; quadriparesis; seizures; mental retardation; up to 50 percent eosinophils in blood. Status of this disease is uncertain.

8. *Focal dermal hypoplasia.* Also a disease limited to females, areas of dermal hypoplasia with protrusions of subcutaneous fat, hypo- and hyperpigmentation, scoliosis, syndactyly in a few, short stature, thinness, intelligence occasionally subnormal.

Other rare entities are neurocutaneous melanosis; neuroectodermal melanolysosomal disease with mental retardation; progeria; Cockayne syndrome; ataxia telangiectasia (Chap. 28; see also Gomez).

CEREBRAL ABNORMALITY IN MULTIPLE CONGENITAL ANOMALY SYNDROMES

Actually there is little information about the state of the cerebral tissues in the aforementioned neural-somatic syndromes, and in many of them the nervous system has never been examined. In some instances the brain is small with virtually no sulcation, a state known as *lissencephaly* (smooth brain) or agyria (Fig. 44-1). This abnormality, readily seen with MRI or CT scans, is combined with severe mental retardation, infantile spasms, small nares, and micrognathia. Anomalies of chromosome 17 have been found in some cases. In others only a few sulci are present, resulting in an admixture of microgyria and macrogyria (pachygyria). In all these major malformations, the cerebral cortex is thickened, and the architecture is abnormal in that the inner cortical layers (layers 4, 5, and 6) are superficial to a band of medullated fibers beneath which there is a layer of neurons that have failed to migrate to their normal superficial position. This type of cortex has been referred to as undifferentiated. Other types of cortical dysgenesis, as, for example, the type described by one of the authors (R. D. A.) as the "driftwood cortex," represent special examples of disturbances in cellular migration.

RACHISCHISIS (DYSRAPHISM)

Included under this heading are the disorders of fusion of dorsal midline structures of the primitive neural tube, a process that takes place during the first 3 weeks of postconceptual life. Exogenous factors are presumed to be operative. The entire cranium may be missing at birth, and the undeveloped brain lies in the base of the skull, a small vascular mass without recognizable nervous tissue. Such a state, called *anencephaly,* is the most frequent of the rachischises and has many associations with other conditions in which the vertebral laminae fail to fuse. Its incidence is 0.1 to 0.7 per 1000 births and females predominate in ratios

Figure 44-1

Lissencephaly. CT demonstrates an absence of gyri, prominence of the subarachnoid space in the opercular region, and moderate ventricular enlargement.

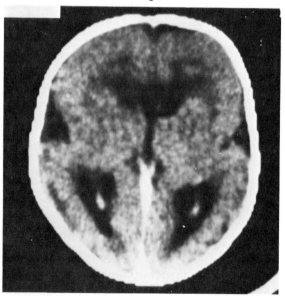

of 3:1 to 7:1. The concordance rate is low, being the same in identical and fraternal twins, but the incidence of the malformation is several times the expected rate if one child in the sibship has already been afflicted. Anencephaly is more frequent in certain geographic areas, e.g., Ireland. Most such fetuses are stillborn or live only a few hours. Lesser degrees of the defect are well known and are small or hidden, the infant presenting with a polypoid lesion of the forehead or of the nasal cavity, or as a *meningoencephalocele* connected with the rest of the brain through a small opening in the skull. Another common site is the occipital region, where parts of one or both occipital lobes or the cerebellum, or both, form a protruding mass, sometimes as large as the head itself. The small nasal encephaloceles may cause no neurologic signs, but if they are innocently snipped off, CSF rhinorrhea may result. The larger occipital ones are associated with blindness, ataxia, and mental retardation.

A failure of development of the midline portion of the cerebellum forms the basis of the *Dandy-Walker syndrome* (Fig. 44-2). A cyst-like structure, representing the greatly dilated fourth ventricle, expands in the midline, causing the occipital bone to bulge posteriorly and to displace the tentorium and torcula upward. In addition the corpus callosum may be deficient or absent, and there is dilatation of the aqueduct, third, and lateral ventricles.

Somewhat less frequent are abnormalities of closure of the vertebral arches. These take the form of a *spina bifida occulta, meningocele,* and *meningomyelocele* of the lumbosacral or other regions.

In *spina bifida occulta* the cord remains inside the canal, and there is no external sac, although a subcutaneous lipoma, or a dimple or wisp of hair on the overlying skin may mark the site of the lesion. In *meningocele* there is a protrusion of dura and arachnoid through the defect in the vertebral laminae, forming a cystic swelling; the cord remains in the canal, however. In *meningomyelocele,* which is 10 times as frequent as meningocele, the cord (more often the cauda equina) is extruded also and is closely applied to the fundus of the cystic swelling. Like anencephaly, the incidence of spinal rachischisis (myeloschisis) varies widely from one country to another, and the disorder is more likely to occur in a second child (if one child has already been affected, the incidence rises from 1 per 1000 to 40 to 50 per 1000). Exogenous factors (e.g., potato blight), have been suspected in the genesis of both myeloschisis and anencephaly. Vitamin A and folate, given before the twenty-eighth day of pregnancy, are said to be protective.

Typically the child is born with a large lumbosacral meningomyelocele covered by delicate, weeping skin. It may have ruptured in utero or during birth, but more often the covering is intact. Stroking the sac may elicit involuntary movements of the legs. As a rule the legs are motionless; urine dribbles, keeping the patient constantly wet; there is no response to pinprick over the lumbosacral zones; and the tendon reflexes are absent. In contrast, craniocervical structures are normal unless an Arnold-Chiari malformation is associated. The neurologic abnormalities of the legs prove that the sac contains elements of spinal cord or cauda equina. Differences are noted in the neurologic picture depending on the level of the lesion. If entirely sacral, bladder and bowel sphincters are affected, but legs escape; if lower lumbar and sacral, the buttocks, legs, and feet are more impaired than hip flexors and quadriceps; if upper lumbar, the feet and legs are sometimes spared and ankle reflexes retained, and there may be Babinski signs.

Pathology and Treatment The dreaded complications of these severe spinal defects are ascending meningitis and progressive hydrocephalus from an Arnold-Chiari malformation, which is often associated (see below). Transverse sections through the meningomyelocele show spinal roots and meninges matted together with connective tissue and incompletely covered by skin. The spinal cord is often included, and may appear incomplete with a defect in the posterior half, a widened central canal, and duplication of the central canal and parts of the central gray matter. The

Figure 44-2

Dandy-Walker syndrome. CT scan of a 14-year-old mildly retarded girl. A large midline cyst, representing the greatly dilated fourth ventricle, occupies the posterior fossa.

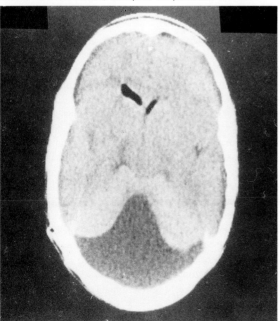

leg muscles are extremely small, owing to a lack of innervation.

Opinions as to the proper management are in a state of flux. Excision of the meningomyelocele in the first few days of life is advised if the objective is to prevent a fatal meningitis. Later (after a few weeks or months), as hydrocephalus reveals its presence by rapid increase in head size and enlargement of the ventricles in the CT scan, a ventriculoatrial or ventriculoperitoneal shunt is required if the hydrocephalus is to be controlled. In some centers such as the Massachusetts General Hospital, this mode of therapy has been routine for several years. Only patients with high spinal lesions and total paraplegia, hydrocephalus, and other congenital anomalies have been rejected for treatment. But the long-term results have not been encouraging. Lorber and others report that 80 to 90 percent of their surviving patients are mentally retarded to some degree and are paraplegic—thus totally dependent on others for their care. The decision to undertake these rather formidable surgical procedures is being questioned more and more frequently. In mothers suspected of having an affected child, the diagnosis can often be confirmed by the presence of α-fetoprotein in the amniotic fluid (removed at 15 to 16 weeks of pregnancy) and checked by ultrasound or plain films. Blood contamination is a source of error (Milunsky). Acetylcholinesterase immunoassay, done on amniotic fluid, is another highly reliable means of confirming neural tube defects. Some parents on receiving this information demand abortion.

Delayed Effects of Failure of Midline Fusion Meningomyelocele and its complications are so strictly pediatric and surgical that the neurologist seldom becomes involved except in the initial evaluation of the clinical problem, in the treatment of meningeal infection, or in the case of shunt failure with decompensation of hydrocephalus. Of greater interest to the neurologist are a series of closely related abnormalities that produce symptoms for the first time in late childhood, adolescence, or even in adult life. These include sinus tracts with meningeal infections, lumbosacral lipomas, and myeloschisis with low tethering of the spinal cord and a delayed radicular or spinal syndrome; diastematomyelia, cysts or tumors with spina bifida and a progressive myeloradiculopathy; and an adolescent or adult Arnold-Chiari malformation and syringomyelia. Yet another class of disorders is an occult lumbrosacral dysraphism that is not inherited but is due to faulty development of the caudal cell mass that lies caudal to the posterior neuropore (normally this undergoes canalization and regression). Occult spinal dysraphism of this type is also associated with meningoceles, lipomas, and sacrococcygeal teratomas.

Sinus tracts in the lumbosacral or occipital regions are of importance, for they may lead to bacterial meningitis at any age. They are often indicated by a small dimple in the skin or by a tuft of hair along the posterior surface of the body in the midline. (The pilonidal sinus, in the opinion of the authors, should not be included in this group.) They may be associated with dermoid cysts or fibrolipomas in the central part of the tract. Evidence of such tracts should be sought in every instance of meningitis, especially when the infection has recurred.

There are, in addition, other *congenital cysts* and *tumors,* particularly lipoma and dermoid, which may produce progressive symptoms and signs by stretching and tethering the spinal cord or by implicating nerve roots. Some of these children have bladder and leg weakness soon after birth. Others deteriorate neurologically at a later age (1.5 to 16 years). According to Chapman and Davis it is not the leptomyelolipoma (the most common form of occult spinal dysraphism) but the tethering of the cord that gives rise to symptoms. Removal of the tumor is of little benefit unless the cord is untethered at the same time. This may be difficult, for the lipoma may be fused with the dorsal surface of the spinal cord (Fig. 44-3).

Diastematomyelia is another unusual abnormality of the spinal cord often associated with spina bifida. Here a bony spicule or fibrous band protrudes into the spinal canal from the body of one of the thoracic or upper lumbar vertebras, splitting the spinal cord in two, each half being surrounded by a dural sac. This longitudinal fissuring and apparent doubleness of cord is spoken of as diplomyelia. With growth, this leads to a *traction myelopathy.*

Several clinical *syndromes of delayed progressive disease* (adolescents or adults) have been delineated:

1. *Progressive spastic weakness* in some of the weak muscles of the legs in a patient known to have had a meningocele or meningomyelocele. Presumably the spinal cord, which is securely attached to the lumbar vertebras, is stretched during the period of rapid lengthening of the vertebral column.

2. *An acute cauda equina syndrome* following some unusual activity or accident (e.g., rowing or a fall in a sitting position), in patients who have had an asymptomatic or symptomatic spina bifida or meningocele. The implicated sensory and motor roots are believed to be injured by sudden or repeated stretching. Weakness of bladder control, impotence (in the male), and numbness of the feet and legs

or foot drop comprise the clinical manifestations of the tethered cord syndrome (Pang and Wilberger).

3. *Progressive cauda equina syndrome* with lesions in the lumbosacral region.

4. *Syringomyelia* (page 748).

Also there are a variety of neurologic problems associated with spinal abnormalities in the high cervical region [fusion of atlas and occiput or of cervical vertebras (Klippel-Feil syndrome), congenital dislocation of the odontoid process and atlas, platybasia and basilar impression]. These spinal abnormalities are reviewed in Chap. 36, with diseases of the spinal cord.

Arnold-Chiari Malformation (ACM)   Encompassed by this term are a number of congenital anomalies at the base of the brain, the most consistent of which are (1) extension of a tongue of cerebellar tissue, posterior to the medulla and spinal cord, into the cervical canal, and (2) displacement of the medulla into the cervical canal, along with the inferior part of the fourth ventricle. These and associated anomalies were first clearly described by Chiari (1891, 1896), who divided them into four types. Arnold's contribution to our understanding of these malformations was relatively insignificant, but the double eponym is so widely accepted that a dispute over priorities at this late date will probably not alter its usage. In recent years the term Arnold-Chiari malformation has come to be restricted to Chiari's types I and II—i.e., to the cerebellomedullary malformation without and with a meningomyelocele, respectively. Type III is no more than a high cervical or occipitocervical meningomyelocele with cerebellar herniation, and type IV consists only of cerebellar hypoplasia.

Several other morphologic features are characteristic. The medulla and pons are elongated, and the aqueduct is narrowed. The displaced tissue (medulla and cerebellum) occludes the foramen magnum; and the remainder of the cerebellum, which is small, is also displaced so as to obliterate the cisterna magna. The foramens of Luschka and Magendie open into the cervical canal, and the arachnoidal tissue around the herniated brainstem and cerebellum is fibrotic. All these factors are probably operative in the production of hydrocephalus, which is always associated. Just below the herniated tail of cerebellar tissue there is a kink or spur in the spinal cord, pushed posteriorly by the lower end of the fourth ventricle. In this type of malformation, a meningomyelocele is nearly always found; hydromyelia of the cervical cord is also common.

Developmental abnormalities of the cerebrum (particularly polymicrogyria) may coexist, and the lower end of the spinal cord (i.e., filum terminale) may extend as low as the sacrum. There are usually bony abnormalities as well. The posterior fossa is small; the foramen magnum is enlarged and grooved posteriorly. Often the base of the skull is flattened or infolded by the cervical spine (basilar impression).

Clinical manifestations In type II Chiari malformation (with meningomyelocele) the problem is essentially one of progressive hydrocephalus. Cerebellar signs cannot be discerned in the first few months of life. However, lower cranial nerve abnormalities—laryngeal stridor, fasciculations of the tongue, sternomastoid paralysis (head lag), facial weakness, deafness, bilateral abducens palsies—may be present in varying combinations. If the patient survives to later childhood or adolescence, one of the syndromes that occurs with the type I malformation may become manifest.

In type I Chiari malformation (without meningocele or other signs of dysraphism), neurologic symptoms may not develop until adolescence or adult life. The symptoms may be those of (1) increased intracranial pressure, (2) progressive cerebellar ataxia, or (3) syringomyelia (segmental amyotrophy, and sensory disorders, with or without pain). Or the patient may show a combination of disorders of the lower cranial nerves, cerebellum, medulla and spinal cord (sensory and motor tract disorders), usually in conjunction with headache. Often the disease is mistaken for multiple sclerosis or a foramen magnum or high cervical cord tumor. The symptoms may have an acute onset after neck extension, chiropractic manipulation, or dental extraction. The physical habitus of such patients may be normal, but about 25 percent have signs of an arrested

Figure 44-3

MRI of a 5-month-old male infant with a lipomyelomeningocele (T1-weighted images). The sagittal view (left) *shows an intraspinal lipoma, continuous with the sacral fat; a tethered cord projects into the intraspinal lipoma (arrow). The extensive lumbrosacral dysraphism is evident in the coronal view* (right) *(From BR Friedman et al, Principles of MRI, New York, McGraw-Hill, 1988.)*

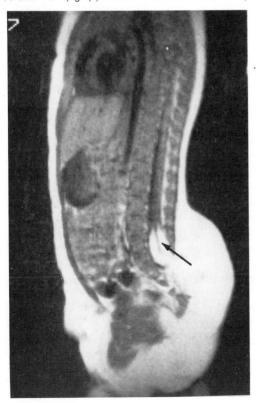
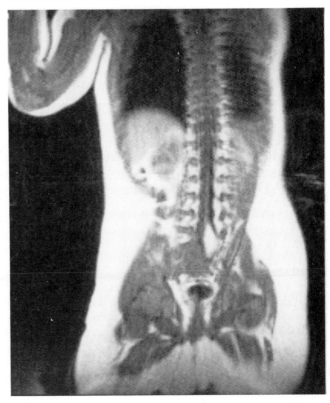

hydrocephalus or a short "bull neck." When basilar impression and ACM coexist, it is impossible to decide which of the two is responsible for the clinical findings.

Diagnosis and Treatment   Pantopaque or metrizamide myelography, performed with the patient supine, was until recently the most reliable means of corroborating the clinical diagnosis. The tongue of cerebellar tissue and the kinked cervical cord obstruct the upward flow of metrizamide and give a highly characteristic radiologic profile. This procedure and all others have been superceded by MRI, because of the clarity with which it exposes abnormalities of the craniocervical region (Figs. 2-2 and 36-5). CSF is usually normal, but may show an elevated pressure and protein level in some cases.

The treatment of basilar impression and Chiari malformation is far from satisfactory. If clinical progression is slight or uncertain, it is probably best to do nothing. If progression is certain and disability is increasing, upper cervical laminectomy and enlargement of the foramen magnum are indicated. Often this procedure halts the progress of the illness or results in some improvement. The surgical procedure must be done cautiously. Opening of the dura and extensive manipulation of the malformation or excision of tissue may aggravate the symptoms or even cause death. The treatment of Chiari malformations and other developmental abnormalities in this region is discussed further on page 750.

CHROMOSOMAL ABNORMALITIES (CHROMOSOMAL DYSGENESES)

A mid-twentieth century discovery of outstanding significance was the recognition of a group of developmental anomalies of the brain and other organs associated with a demonstrable abnormality of an autosomal or sex chromosome. Lejeune was the first to note a triplication of the twenty-first chromosome in the Down syndrome, and there followed the discovery of a number of other trisomies as well as deletions or translocations of certain of the autosomal chromosomes, and a lack or an excess of one of the sex chromosomes. Such an event must take place sometime after the formation of the oocyte, during the long period that it lies fallow in the aging ovary or during the process of conception or germination and first cell divisions. All the cells in the embryo may be affected or only part of them, the latter condition being called *mosaicism.*

The manner in which triplication or some other imperfection of a chromosome is able to derail the pathways of ontogenesis is a mystery. One can imagine that the sequential release of genes and their transcription of nuclear and messenger RNA to form certain basic proteins might affect the development of organs—especially of the brain, whose embryogenesis, growth, and maturation are the most complex and protracted of all organ systems.

Certain of the chromosomal abnormalities are incompatible with life, and it has been found that the cells of many unexplained abortuses and stillborns show abnormal karyotypes. On the other hand, the organism may survive and exhibit any one of the following syndromes: (1) Down syndrome (mongolism, trisomy 21); (2) one type of arrhinencephaly (trisomy 13, Patau syndrome); (3) trisomy 18 (Edwards syndrome); (4) cri-du-chat syndrome (deletion of short arm of chromosome 5); (5) monosomy 21 (antimongolism); (6) ring chromosomes; (7) Klinefelter syndrome (XXY); (8) Turner syndrome (XO); (9) others (XXXX, XXX, XYY, YY, XXYY). An account of these less-frequent chromosomal aberrations can be found in the article by Lemieux et al. The overall frequency of chromosomal abnormalities in live births is 0.6 percent (Kalter and Warkany).

Down Syndrome (Mongolism)   Described first in 1866, by Langdon Down, this is the best known of the chromosomal dysgeneses. The frequency is 1 in 700 births. Familiarity with the condition permits its recognition at birth, but it becomes more obvious with advancing age. The round head, open mouth, stubby hands, slanting palpebral fissures, and short stature create an unforgettable clinical picture. The ears are low-set and oval with small lobules. The palpebral fissures slant slightly upward and outward owing to the presence of medial epicanthal folds that partly cover the inner canthi. The bridge of the nose is poorly developed. The tongue is usually enlarged, heavily fissured, and protruding. Gray-white specks of depigmentation are seen in the irides (Brushfield spots). The little fingers are often short (hypoplastic middle phalanx) and incurved (clinodactyly). The hands are broad with a single transverse (simian) palmar crease and other characteristic dermal markings. Lenticular opacities and congenital heart lesions (septal defects) are frequent. The patient with Down syndrome is of average size at birth, but is characteristically short at later periods of life. The height attained in adult life seldom exceeds that of a 10-year-old child. Most affected children do not walk until 3 to 4 years of age; their acquisition of speech is delayed, but over 90 percent talk by 5 years. The intelligence quotient (IQ) is variable, and that of a large group follows a gaussian curve; the median IQ is 40 to 50, and the range is 20 to 70.

One cannot distinguish the Down syndrome with a triplication of chromosome 21 from that with a translocation. There is a strong correlation between the trisomy 21 type and age of the mother, whereas the less-frequent translocation is found equally in the offspring of young and old mothers. Mosaics have atypical forms of the syndrome, and some such individuals are of normal intelligence. Laboratory tests are not helpful in clarifying the mechanism of the disorder; abnormalities include decreased serotonin, increased alkaline phosphatase in the white cells, increased glucose diphosphate in red cells, and a 50 percent increase in superoxide dismutase. The latter enzyme derives from a gene located on the long arm of chromosome 21 and is a convenient marker of the trisomy, but is not believed to be responsible for the dysmorphism or mental retardation.

The pathologic findings have been difficult to define. The brain is approximately 10 percent lighter than average. The convolutional pattern is rather simple. The frontal lobes are smaller than normal, and the superior temporal gyri are thin. There are claims of delayed myelination of cerebral white matter, and also of immature and poorly differentiated cortical neurons. Alzheimer neurofibrillary changes and neuritic plaques are practically always found in Down cases beyond 40 years of age. There is a higher than expected incidence of leukemia, and the cardiac lesion may lead to heart failure.

It is possible to make the diagnosis by demonstrating the chromosomal abnormalities in cells of the amniotic fluid. About one-third of pregnant mothers (in the second trimester) also have abnormalities of serum α-fetoprotein. One could eliminate a considerable proportion of the population of mongoloids by doing amniocentesis on all pregnant women over 35 years of age and aborting those with positive tests.

The other chromosomal dysgeneses will only be synopsized.

1. *Trisomy 13 (Patau syndrome)*. Frequency 1:2000 live births, more female than male, average maternal age 30.8 years, microcephaly and sloping forehead, microphthalmus, coloboma of iris, corneal opacities, low-set ears, cleft lip and palate, capillary hemangiomata, polydactyly, flexed fingers, posterior prominence of heels, dextrocardia, umbilical hernia, impaired hearing, hypertonia, severe mental retardation, death in early childhood.

2. *Trisomy 18*. Frequency 1:4000, more in females, average maternal age 34.4 years, growth slow, occasional seizures, severe mental retardation, hypertonia, ptosis and lid abnormalities, low-set ears, small mouth, mottled skin, clenched fist with index finger over third, syndactyly, rocker-bottom feet, shortened big toe, ventricular septal defect, umbilical and inguinal hernias, short sternum, small pelvis, small mandible, death in early infancy.

3. *Cri-du-chat syndrome*. Abnormal cry like a kitten, severe mental retardation, hypertelorism, epicanthal folds, brachycephaly, moon face, antimongoloid slant of palpebral fissures, micrognathia, hypotonia, strabismus.

4. *Ring chromosomes*. Mental retardation with variable physical abnormalities.

5. *Klinefelter syndrome*. Only males. Eunuchoid appearance; wide arm-span, sparse facial and body hair; high-pitched voice; gynecomastia; small testicles; usually mentally retarded; high incidence of psychosis, asthma, and diabetes.

6. *Turner syndrome*. Only females. Triangular face, small chin, occasionally hypertelorism and epicanthal folds, widely spaced nipples, clinodactyly, cubitus valgus, hypoplastic nails, short stature, webbed neck, delayed sexual development, mild mental retardation.

7. *Colpocephaly*. This is a rare type of malformation of the brain consisting of marked dilatation of the occipital horns of the lateral ventricles, thickening of the overlying rim of cortical gray matter, and thinning of the white matter. The associated clinical picture comprises mental retardation, spasticity, seizures, and visual abnormalities (due to optic nerve hypoplasia). This disorder is probably of diverse causation but is being listed with the chromosomal abnormalities because some cases have been associated with the mosaicism for trisomy 8 (Herskowitz).

Several generalizations can be made about these chromosomal dysgeneses. First, the autosomal ones are often lethal, and they almost always have a devastating effect on cerebral growth and development, whether the infant survives or not. Somatic, nonnervous anomalies are regularly present, an association so constant that one may safely predict that a normally formed infant will not have a detectable chromosomal defect. Only in the Down syndrome and trisomy 13 (and possibly trisomy 18) are the physiognomy and bodily configuration of predictive value, however. Surprisingly, some of the most grotesque disfigurements, like anencephaly and multiple congenital anomalies, are rarely related to a morphologic abnormality in chromosomes. By contrast, an insufficiency of sex chromosomes exerts only the most subtle effects on the brain, intellect, and personality, and to some extent this is true of supernumerary sex chromosomes (XYY, for example).

The abnormality of the brain underlying the mental retardation in these several chromosomal dysgeneses has not been ascertained. The cerebra are slightly small, but only minor changes are seen in the convolutional pattern and cortical architecture. These brain anomalies are under active study.

ENVIRONMENTAL TERATOLOGIC FACTORS

A number of recent observations have led to a repudiation of the belief that the human embryo is shielded against exogenous causes of maldevelopment. Irradiation during the first trimester, rubella and cytomegalus virus infections of the mother during this same period, and the action of aminopterin, alcohol, and thalidomide all give rise to serious disorders of development. Concerning other teratogens there is much controversy. Claims and counterclaims have been made concerning the pathogenicity of the substances listed in Table 44-2. Usually the only data are from animals given amounts far in excess of any possible therapeutic doses in humans. The data are so meager that they will not be discussed here. The reader may refer to the article by Kalter and Warkany for further information.

THE PHAKOMATOSES (CONGENITAL ECTODERMOSES)

As was stated, there are two broad categories of neurocutaneous diseases. In one, the infant is born with a special

Table 44-2
Environmental substances suspected of causing congenital malformations in human beings

A. Contaminants and food additives	C. Habituating and addicting drugs
Cadminium	Alcohol
Cyclamates	Cigarettes
Dioxin	Coffee
Dichlorodiphenyl trichloroethane	Gasoline sniffing
Food coloring	Lysergic acid diethylamide
Hair dyes	Marijuana
Lead	Methadone
Love Canal pollutants	Phencyclidine
Mercury	Tea
Monosodium glutamate	Tobacco chewing
Nitrates	Toluene sniffing
Nitrites	D. Occupational exposure
Polyhalogenated biphenyls	Anesthetic gases
Saccharin	Fat solvents
Sodium fluoride	Hair-spray adhesives
B. Natural substances	Hexachlorophene
Blighted potatoes	Hydrocarbons
Cyanide in cassava	Organic solvents
Goitrogens in brassicae	Printing trades
	Smelter
	Chemical laboratories

Source: Kalter and Warkany. Of the substances listed here only mercury is a *proven* human teratogen.

type of skin disease or develops it in the first weeks of life; in the other, particular forms of cutaneous abnormality, though often present in minor degree at birth, later evolve as quasineoplastic disorders. The latter, to which van der Hoeve (1920) applied the term *phakomatoses* (from the Greek *phakos*, meaning "mother spot," "mole," or "freckle") includes tuberous sclerosis, neurofibromatosis, and cutaneous angiomatosis with CNS abnormalities. These diseases have many features in common—hereditary transmission, special involvement of organs of ectodermal origin (nervous system, eyeball, retina, and skin), slow evolution of lesions in childhood and adolescence, tendency to form hamartomas (benign tumorlike formations due to maldevelopment), and disposition to fatal malignant transformation. These disorders are discussed below.

TUBEROUS SCLEROSIS (BOURNEVILLE DISEASE, EPILOIA)

Tuberous sclerosis is a congenital disease of hereditary type in which a variety of lesions, due to a limited hyperplasia of ectodermal and mesodermal cells, arise in the skin, nervous system, heart, kidney, and other organs. It is characterized clinically by the triad of adenoma sebaceum, epilepsy, and mental retardation.

It is stated that Virchow had recognized scleromas of the cerebrum in the 1860s and that von Recklinghausen had reported a similar lesion combined with multiple myomata of the heart in 1862, but Bourneville's articles, appearing between 1880 and 1900, presented the first systematic account of the disease and related the cerebral lesions to those of the skin of the face. Vogt (1890) fully appreciated the significance of the neurocutaneous relationship and formally delineated the triad of adenoma sebaceum, epilepsy, and mental retardation. Epiloia, a term introduced by Sherlock in 1911, never gained general acceptance. These and other historical aspects are reviewed in Gomez's monograph on tuberous sclerosis.

Epidemiology The incidence of the disease is estimated to be from 5 to 7 per 100,000. It has been described in all parts of the world, and is equally frequent in all races and in both sexes. Heredity is evident in approximately one-third of reported cases (a dominant autosomal gene of variable penetrance). The remaining cases are attributed to a gene mutation, the frequency of which is calculated to be 1 in 20,000 to 1 in 50,000. The disease involves many organs in addition to the skin and brain and may assume a diversity of forms, the least severe of which, i.e., the *forme fruste*, is difficult to diagnose; hence, one cannot be certain of the true incidence of the disease. Among the feebleminded in institutions the frequency ranges from 0.1 to 0.7 percent. The medical literature contains a number of reports of patients whose mentality is preserved and who have never had convulsions. It is likely that data drawn from mental hospital populations exaggerate the overall frequency of mental retardation in this disorder (Gomez).

Etiology and Pathogenesis Tuberous sclerosis is a genetic disease but its pathogenesis remains unknown. The abnormal gene has been localized to chromosome 9. The lesions involve cells derived from ectoderm as well as mesoderm. The cellular elements within the lesions are abnormal both in number and size. The tumor-like growths in different organs may include cells of more than one type (e.g., fibroblast, cardiac myoblast and angioblast or glioblast and neuroblast), and their number is locally excessive. Something appears to have gone awry with the proliferative process in embryologic development, yet it is usually kept under control, and only rarely does the growth undergo malignant transformation. Highly specialized cells within the lesions may attain giant size; neurons three to four times normal size may be observed in the cerebral scleroses. These facts emphasize the blastomatous character of the process and suggest that some inhibitory growth factor is lacking at crucial moments in embryonic life and later, accounting for both the hyperplasia and hypertrophy of well-differentiated cells. How the underlying trait is transmitted remains a mystery. The focal character of the pathologic process seems to exclude a systemic metabolic abnormality.

Clinical Manifestations The disease may be present at the time of birth (the diagnosis has been made by CT scan in neonates), but more often the infant is judged at first to be normal. In approximately 75 percent of cases, attention is drawn to the disease initally by the occurrence of focal or generalized seizures or by retarded psychomotor development. As with any condition that leads to mental retardation, the first suspicion is raised by delay in reaching the milestones of natural maturation. Whatever the initial symptom, the convulsive disorder and mental retardation become more prominent within 2 to 3 years. The facial cutaneous abnormality, the so-called adenoma sebaceum, appears later in childhood, usually between the fourth and tenth years, and is progressive thereafter.

As the years pass, the seizures change pattern. In the first year or two they take the form of salaam spasms or flexion myoclonus with hypsarrhythmia (irregular dysrhythmic bursts of high-voltage spikes and slow waves in the EEG); later they change to more typical generalized motor and psychomotor attacks or atypical petit mal; any one of the seizure types may be brief, especially if the patient is receiving anticonvulsant medication. Seizures are always the most reliable index of the cerebral lesions, and focal neurologic abnormalities, which one might expect to

occur from the size and location of the cerebral lesions, are distinctly uncommon.

Mental function continues to deteriorate slowly. Exceptionally there may be a spastic weakness or mild choreoathetosis of the limbs; in a few cases there is obstructive hydrocephalus. As in any state of imbecility or idiocy, a variety of nonspecific motor peculiarities such as constant crying, muttering, rocking and swaying movements, and digital mannerisms may be observed. Behavioral and affective derangements may be added to the intellectual deficiency, resulting in what may be loosely classified as a primary type of psychosis.

The lack of parallelism of the epilepsy, mental deficit, and cutaneous abnormalities has been noted by all experienced clinicians. Some patients are subject to recurrent seizures while retaining relatively normal mental function; in others, trivial skin lesions or a retinal phakoma may suggest the diagnosis in a mentally normal person with few seizures. In such cases, recognition may elude competent neurologists and dermatologists. As a general rule, early onset of seizures is predictive of mental retardation. Whether the seizures damage the brain, as suggested by Gomez et al, or whether severe epilepsy and mental retardation are evidence of a more severe involvement of the brain by the lesions of tuberous sclerosis, is difficult to state.

Limitation of space does not allow more than a catalog of other visceral abnormalities. In about half the cases, gray or yellow plaques (in reality gliomatous tumors) may be found in the retina in or near the optic disc or at a distance from it. It is from this lesion, called phakoma, that van der Hoeve derived the term that is applied to all neurocutaneous diseases of this class. About half of all benign rhabdomyomas of the heart are associated with tuberous sclerosis, and if located in the wall of the atrium, they may cause a conduction defect. Other benign tumors of mixed cell type (angiomyolipomas) have been found in the kidneys, liver, lungs, thyroid, testes, and gastrointestinal tract. Cysts of the pleura or lungs, bone cysts in digits, and zones of marbling or densification in bones are some of the less-common abnormalities.

The well-developed facial lesions (adenomas of Pringle), pathognomonic of tuberous sclerosis, are present in 90 percent of patients over 4 years of age. Typically they are red to pink nodules with a smooth, glistening surface, and tend to be limited to the nasolabial folds, cheeks, and chin; sometimes they also involve the forehead and scalp. Although called "adenoma sebaceum," these nodules are actually angiofibromas; the sebaceous glands are only passively involved. The earliest manifestation of facial angiofibromatosis may be a mild erythema over the cheeks and forehead, intensified by crying. The occurrence of large plaques of connective tissue on the forehead is usually expressive of a severe form of the disease.

On the trunk the diagnostic lesion is the "shagreen patch" (in reality a plaque of subepidermal fibrosis) found most often in the lumbosacral region. It appears as a flat, slightly elevated, flesh-colored area of skin 1 to 10 cm in diameter, with a "pigskin," "elephant hide," or "orange peel" appearance. Another common site of fibromatous involvement is the nail bed; subungual fibromas usually appear at puberty and continue to develop with age. Other common skin changes, not in themselves diagnostic, include fibroepithelial tags (soft fibromas), café au lait spots, and port-wine hemangiomas.

In approximately 90 percent of patients with tuberous sclerosis, congenital hypomelanotic macules (formerly mistaken for "partial albinism" or "vitiligo") appear before any of the other skin lesions (Fitzpatrick et al). They are arranged in linear fashion over the trunk or limbs and range in size from a few millimeters to several centimeters; their configuration is oval, with one end round and the other pointed, in the shape of an ash leaf. A Wood's lamp, which transmits only ultraviolet rays, facilitates the demonstration of these lesions because of the absence of melanoblasts, which normally absorb light in the ultraviolet range (360-nm wavelength). They become pink when rubbed and contain sweat glands. Although not present on the face, there is occasionally a white tuft of hair. Electron microscopic examination shows a normal or reduced number of melanocytes, but their dopa reaction is reduced and melanosomes are small. This type of leukoderma had been recognized for many years, but only relatively recently have Gold and Freeman and Fitzpatrick et al emphasized their frequency and their value in the diagnosis of tuberous sclerosis during infancy, before the appearance of other cutaneous lesions.

Pathology The brain exhibits a number of anomalies that are at once diagnostic. Broadening, unnatural whiteness, and firmness of parts of some of the cerebral convolutions are simulated by no other disease. These are the *tubers,* after which the disease is named. On the surface of the brain, they range in width from 5 mm to 2 or 3 cm. Their cut surface reveals a lack of demarcation of cortex from white matter and the presence of white flecks of calcium; the latter, which are readily seen in CT scans and MRI, are called *brain stones.* The floors of the lateral ventricles may be encrusted with white or pink-white masses resembling candle gutterings. When calcified, they appear in radiographs as curvilinear opacities that follow the outline of the ventricle. Rarely, nodules of abnormal tissue are observed in the basal ganglia, thalamus, cerebellum, brainstem, and spinal cord.

Under the microscope the tubers are seen to be composed of interlacing rows of plump fibrous astrocytes (much like an astrocytoma though lacking in glial fibrillar protein). Elsewhere in the cerebral cortex, derangements of architecture result from the presence of abnormal-appearing glial cells. Monstrous neurons and glial cells, often difficult to distinguish, and displaced normal-sized neurons contribute to the chaotic histologic appearance of cerebral cortex and ganglionic structures. Gliomatous deposits may obstruct the foramina of Monro or the aqueduct or floor of the fourth ventricle, causing hydrocephalus. Neoplastic transformation of abnormal glial cells, a not infrequent occurrence, usually takes the form of a large-cell astrocytoma, less often of a glioblastoma; sometimes meningiomas are added.

The phakomas of the retina are composed mainly of neuronal and glial components, but occasionally there is an admixture of fibrous tissue.

Diagnosis When the full combination of mental, convulsive, and dermal abnormalities are conjoined, the diagnosis is self-evident. It is the early stage of the disease and the *forme fruste* that give trouble, and here the experienced dermatologist can be of great help. Epilepsy, i.e., flexion spasms in infancy, and delay in psychomotor development, are by no means diagnostic of tuberous sclerosis, since they occur in many diseases. It is in these cases and also in every sizable population of the epileptic or mentally retarded, especially when the family history is unrevealing, that a search for the dermal equivalents of the disease—the hypomelanotic nevus, adenoma sebaceum, collagenous patch, phakoma of the retina, or subungual or gingival fibromas—is so rewarding. The finding of any one of these lesions provides confirmation of the partial and atypical case. Adenoma sebaceum may occasionally occur alone and is easily confused with acne vulgaris in the adolescent. The history of epilepsy and/or the demonstration of a dull mentality is helpful but not necessary for the diagnosis of tuberous sclerosis (Gomez).

The most useful laboratory measures for corroborating the disease are CT scanning and MR scanning. The periventricular calcific lesions are particularly well shown on the CT scan, whereas MR is more sensitive in detecting cortical lesions. An increasing number of cortical lesions demonstrated with MRI appears to correlate with an increased impairment of neurologic function (Roach et al).

Treatment Nothing can be offered in the way of prevention other than to counsel affected individuals against childbearing. The slow march of the disease, once it has begun, cannot be halted. Anticonvulsant therapy of the standard type suppresses the convulsive tendency more or less effectively and should be applied assiduously. It is rather pointless to attempt the excision of tumors, especially in individuals who are severely affected. However, there are patients who are not mentally impaired and who can benefit from dermabrasion of their facial lesions, with the knowledge that they will slowly regrow; and neurosurgeons have partially excised brain tumors that were causing recalcitrant epilepsy or increased intracranial pressure.

Course and Prognosis   In general, the disease advances so slowly that years must elapse before one is sure of the progression. Of the severe cases, approximately 30 percent die before the fifth year, and 50 to 75 percent before attaining adult age. Worsening is mainly in the mental sphere. Status epilepticus accounted for many deaths in the past, but improved anticonvulsant therapy has reduced this hazard. Neoplasias take their toll, and the authors have had several such patients who died of malignant gliomas arising in striatothalamic zones.

NEUROFIBROMATOSIS OF VON RECKLINGHAUSEN

Neurofibromatosis is a comparatively common hereditary disease in which the skin, nervous system, bones, endocrine glands, and sometimes other organs are the sites of a variety of congenital abnormalities, often taking the form of benign tumors. The typical clinical picture, usually identifiable at a glance, consists of multiple circumscribed areas of increased skin pigmentation accompanied by dermal and neural tumors of various types.

History   The condition known as multiple idiopathic neuromas was the subject of a monograph by R. W. Smith in 1849, and even at that time he referred to examples recorded by other writers. It was von Recklinghausen, however, who in 1882 gave the definitive account of its clinical and pathologic features. The articles of Yakovlev and Guthrie, Lichtenstein, Riccardi, Martuza and Eldridge and the monographs of Crowe et al and Riccardi et al provide a complete analysis of the clinical, pathologic, and genetic data and include extensive bibliographies.

Incidence and Epidemiology   Crowe and his associates have calculated the prevalence of the disease to be 30 to 40 per 100,000 and expect one case in every 2500 to 3300 births. Approximately half of their cases had affected relatives, and in all instances the distribution of cases within a family was consistent with an autosomal dominant mode

of inheritance. They provided evidence that the remaining sporadic cases were due to a mutation of the dominant gene. The disease has been observed in all races in different parts of the world, and males and females are about equally affected.

Cause and Pathogenesis   The hereditary nature of neurofibromatosis has been appreciated for many years. Recently it has been established that neurofibromatosis is comprised of two distinct disorders, the genes for which are located on two separate chromosomes. The classic form of the disease, described below, has been shown by linkage analysis to be caused by a gene that is located near the centromere on chromosome 17 (Barker et al). Bilateral acoustic neurofibromatosis, described on page 538, has been linked to a DNA marker on chromosome 22 (Rouleau et al). These two forms of neurofibromatosis have been loosely referred to as peripheral and central, respectively, but the terms neurofibromatosis 1 and 2 are less confusing (Martuza and Eldridge).

The pathogenesis remains obscure. Cellular elements derived from the neural crest (i.e., Schwann cells, melanocytes, and possibly endoneurial fibroblasts, the natural components of skin and nerves) proliferate excessively in multiple foci, and the melanocytes function abnormally; but the hormones and growth factors that are involved in this proliferative process and the mechanism(s) by which it is accomplished are as unclear as in tuberous sclerosis.

Clinical Manifestations   In the majority of patients, spots of hyperpigmentation and cutaneous and subcutaneous tumors are the basis of clinical diagnosis. Pigmentary changes in the skin are nearly always present at birth, but neurofibromas are infrequent at that age. Both lesions increase in number during late childhood and adolescence. There may be a spurt of new lesions at puberty or during pregnancy. Exceptionally, a neurofibroma of a spinal or cranial nerve root, disclosed during neurosurgical intervention, may be the initial manifestation of the disease. In the study of a large series of patients with neurofibromatosis, approximately one-third were discovered to have the cutaneous manifestations while being examined for symptoms of some other disease; that is to say, the neurofibromatosis was asymptomatic and incidental. Usually these are the cases with the slightest degree of cutaneous abnormality. Of the remainder, many consulted a physician because of the disfigurement produced by the tumors or because some of the neurofibromas were producing symptoms.

Canale and colleagues noted that neurologic symptoms led to hospital admission in one-third of their series of 92 cases. Typical syndromes were traced most often to unilateral or bilateral tumors of the eighth cranial nerve (nerve deafness, dizziness, headache, and staggering), trigeminal neuromas (facial pain and numbness), optic nerve gliomas (progressive monocular blindness, optic atrophy, nystagmus, enlargement of optic foramen, abnormal contour of sella turcica, and failure to thrive, if the hypothalamus is invaded), other cranial nerve involvement, spinal-root tumors with or without compression of the spinal cord, and multiple cranial or spinal meningiomas. Seldom are the more peripheral tumors of nerve or skin painful or distressing.

In type 1 (peripheral) neurofibromatosis, patches of cutaneous pigmentation, appearing shortly after birth and occurring any place on the body, constitute the most striking clinical expression of the disease. They vary in size from a millimeter or two to many centimeters, and in color from a light to dark brown (café au lait), and are rarely associated with any other pathologic state. In a survey of pigmented spots in the skin, Crowe and his associates found that 10 percent of the normal population had one or more lesions of this type, but anyone with more than six spots, some exceeding 1.5 cm in diameter, nearly always proved to have von Recklinghausen disease. Of their 223 patients with neurofibromatosis, 95 percent had at least one spot, and 78 percent had more than six large ones. Freckle-like or diffuse pigmentation of the axillae and other intertriginous areas (groin, under breast), and small, round whitish spots are characteristic and almost pathognomonic of the syndrome (Crowe).

Multiple cutaneous and subcutaneous tumors appearing in late childhood or early adolescence are the other principal features of the disease. The cutaneous tumors are situated in the dermis and form discrete, soft or firm papules varying in size from a few millimeters to a centimeter or more (*molluscum fibrosum*). They assume many shapes—flattened, sessile, pedunculated, conical, lobulated, etc. They are flesh-colored or violaceous and often topped with a comedo. When pressed, the soft tumors tend to invaginate through a small opening in the skin, giving the feeling of a seedless raisin or a scrotum without a testicle. This phenomenon, spoken of as "buttonholeing," is useful in distinguishing the lesions of this disease from other tumors, e.g., multiple lipomas. A patient may have from a few of these dermal tumors to thousands.

The subcutaneous tumors, which are also multiple, take two forms: (1) firm, discrete nodules attached to a nerve or (2) an overgrowth of subcutaneous tissue, some-

times reaching enormous size. These latter, which are called *plexiform neuromas* (also pachydermatocele, elephantiasis neuromatosis, *la tumeur royale*), occur most often in the face, scalp, neck, and chest and may cause hideous disfigurement. When palpated, these growths feel like a bag of worms or strings; the bone underlying the tumor may enlarge. As a rule, congenital neurofibromas tend to be highly vascular and invasive and are especially prominent in the orbital, periorbital, and cervical regions. They are often accompanied by segmental hypertrophy. When the hyperpigmentation overlies a plexiform neurofibroma and extends to the midline one should suspect an intraspinal tumor at that level.

Other abnormalities associated with peripheral neurofibromatosis include bone cysts, pathologic fractures (pseudoarthrosis), cranial bone defects with pulsating exophthalmos, bone hypertrophy, precocious puberty, pheochromocytoma, scoliosis, syringomyelia, nodules of abnormal glial cells in brain and spinal cord, and macrocephaly, sometimes with obstructive hydrocephalus due to overgrowth of glial tissue around the sylvian aqueduct and fourth ventricle. Some degree of intellectual impairment is common (40 percent of Riccardi's series of 133 patients) but in our series the figure is nearer 5 percent and it is not profound, as a rule. Learning difficulty, developmental disorder, or hyperactivity have been more frequent abnormalities, occurring in almost 40 percent of patients. Rosman and Pearce have ascribed mental retardation to congenital malformation of the cerebral cortex (cortical dysgenesis). The incidence of seizures is about 20 times higher than that in the general population. Another unique finding is the Lisch nodule. This is a small whitish spot (hamartoma) in the iris, present in 94 percent of Riccardi's typical cases, but not found in patients with bilateral acoustic neuromas or in normal individuals.

Exceptionally neurofibromatosis has been associated with peroneal muscular atrophy, congenital deafness, and partial albinism (Bradley et al).

Pathology   The cutaneous tumors are characterized by a rather thin epidermis whose basal layer may or may not be pigmented. The collagen and elastin of the dermis is replaced by a loose arrangement of elongated connective tissue cells. It lacks the compactness of the normal dermal collagen, which accounts for the palpable opening in the skin.

The pigmented (café au lait) lesions contain only the normal numbers of melanocytes and the dark color of the skin is due instead to an excess of melanosomes in the malpighian cells; abnormally large melanosomes, measuring up to several microns in diameter, appear in some of the basal cells of the epidermis.

The nerve tumors are composed of a mixture of fibroblasts and Schwann cells, except the optic nerve tumors, which contain a combination of astrocytes and fibroblasts. Occasionally, along spinal roots or sympathetic chains, one may find a tumor made up of partially or completely differentiated nerve cells (a typical ganglioneuroma). Clusters of abnormal glial cells may be found in the brain and spinal cord, and, according to Bielschowsky, they form a link with tuberous sclerosis. Clinically, however, the two diseases are quite independent.

Malignant degeneration of the tumors is found in 2 to 5 percent of cases; peripherally they become sarcomas and centrally, astrocytomas or glioblastomas.

Diagnosis   If skin tumors and café au lait spots are numerous and Lisch nodules are present, the identification of the disease as type 1 neurofibromatosis offers no difficulty. A history of the illness in antecedent and collateral family members makes recognition even more certain. Uncertainty arises most frequently in patients with bilateral acoustic neuromas or other cranial or spinal neurofibromas or schwannomas with no skin lesions or only a few random ones. This tendency for these forms of neurofibromatosis to be accompanied by a paucity of skin lesions is well recognized. Plexiform neuromas with muscle weakness, due to nerve involvement, and abnormalities of underlying bone may be confused with other tumors, especially in young children who tend to have few café au lait spots and few cutaneous tumors. Enormous hypertrophy of a limb, which may also occur, requires differentiation from other developmental anomalies.

Crowe et al believe that 80 percent of patients with von Recklinghausen disease can be diagnosed by the presence of more than six café au lait spots. Of the remaining 20 percent, those over 21 years of age will be found to have multiple cutaneous tumors, axillary freckling, and a few pigmented spots; in those under 21, with no dermal tumors and only a few café au lait patches, a positive family history and radiographic demonstration of bone cysts will be helpful in some instances. Café au lait spots and cutaneous tumors should always be sought, for they may help the neurologist diagnose a progressive spinal syndrome, a cerebellopontine angle syndrome, bilateral deafness, progressive blindness, and an occasional case of precocious puberty, hydrocephalus, or mental retardation.

Because of the many conditions that accompany classic neurofibromatosis and because they are potentially dangerous, the initial clinical evaluation should be supplemented by a number of ancillary examinations: measurement of IQ, EEG, slit-lamp examination of irides, radiography of optic foramens and internal auditory meati, visual evoked responses, CT scans or MRI of cranium and sometimes of spine and mediastinum; if there is suspicion of a pheochromocytoma, a 24-h urine should be tested for metabolites of epinephrine. Each of these tests is not only an aid to diagnosis but is essential to the intelligent management of the illness.

Treatment   The skin tumors should not be excised unless they are cosmetically objectionable or show an increase in size, suggesting malignant change. The effects of radiotherapy are so insignificant that they do not justify the risk of heavy exposure. Plexiform neuromas about the face offer difficult problems. Here one must resort to plastic surgery, but the results are not always satisfactory because the growths may involve cranial nerves superficially (with risk of greater paralysis after surgical excision) or alter the underlying bone, the latter being either eroded from pressure or hypertrophied from increased blood supply. Cranial and spinal neurofibromas are amenable to excision, and the gliomas and meningiomas usually demand surgical measures. Here the differentiation of hamartomas from gliomas of structures such as the optic nerves, hypothalamus, or pons may be difficult. Peripheral nerve tumors that have undergone malignant (sarcomatous) degeneration pose special surgical problems. Affected individuals should be advised not to have children—a precaution that may not be necessary, because fertility, especially in males, seems to be reduced by the disease.

Prognosis varies with the grade of severity, being most favorable in those with ony a few lesions. But the disease is always progressive, and the patient should remain under continuous surveillance.

CUTANEOUS ANGIOMATOSIS WITH ABNORMALITIES OF THE CENTRAL NERVOUS SYSTEM

There are seven diseases in which a cutaneous vascular anomaly is associated with an abnormality of the nervous system: (1) encephalofacial (encephalotrigeminal) angiomatosis with cerebral calcification (Sturge-Weber syndrome); (2) dermatomal hemangiomas and spinal vascular malformations (sometimes with limb hypertrophy as in Klippel-Trenauney-Weber syndrome); (3) the epidermal nevus syndrome; (4) familial telangiectasia (Osler-Rendu-Weber disease); (5) hemangioblastoma of cerebellum and retina (Lindau and von Hippel disease); (6) ataxia-telangiectasia (Louis-Bar disease); and (7) angiokeratosis corporis diffusum (Fabry disease). The latter three disorders are considered elsewhere: ataxia-telangiectasia and Fabry disease on pages 794 and 813, respectively, and von Hippel-Lindau disease on page 535.

Meningofacial (Encephalofacial) Angiomatosis with Cerebral Calcification (Sturge-Weber Syndrome)

In this condition a vascular nevus is observed at birth to cover a large part of the face and cranium on one side (in the territory of the ophthalmic division of the trigeminal nerve). The lesion varies in extent, the most limited being an involvement of only the upper eyelid and forehead, and the most extensive being the entire head and even other parts of the body. The nevus is deep red (*port-wine nevus*), and its margins may be raised or flat; soft or firm papules, evidently composed of vessels, cause surface elevations and irregularities. The orbital tissue, especially the upper eyelid, is almost invariably involved, and congenital glaucoma (buphthalmos) may develop later in the eye on that side, causing blindness. The choroid is implicated in some cases. The increased cutaneous vascularity may result in an overgrowth of connective tissue and underlying bone, giving rise to a deformity like that of the Klippel-Trenauney-Weber syndrome (see below). Indications of cerebral affection appear as early as the first year of life or later in childhood; the most frequent clinical manifestations are unilateral seizures followed by increasing degrees of spastic hemiparesis with smallness of the arm and leg, hemisensory defect, and homonymous hemianopia, all on the side contralateral to the trigeminal nevus. Skull films (usually negative after birth) taken at the end of the second year reveal a characteristic *tramline calcification* which outlines the convolutions of the parieto-occipital cortex. CT scans and MRI at an earlier age show hyperdensity of the involved cortex.

This condition is generally referred to as the Sturge-Weber syndrome, since it was W. Allen Sturge, in 1879, who originally described a child with sensorimotor seizures contralateral to a facial "port-wine mark," and Parkes Weber (1922, 1929) who gave the first radiographic demonstration of the atrophy and calcification of the cerebral hemisphere homolateral to the skin lesion. This eponym overlooks the important intervening contributions of Kalischer (1897, 1901), who first described the meningeal angioma in conjunction with the facial one; of Volland (1913), who demonstrated the intracortical calcific deposits; and of Dimitri (1923), who described the characteristic double-contoured radiographic shadows. Krabbe (1932, 1934) showed conclusively that the calcification lay not in the blood vessels (as Dimitri and many others had concluded) but in the second and third layers of the cortex (see Wohlwill and Yakovlev for historical review and bibliography).

It must not be thought that all cranial hemangiomas affect the cerebrum; facial nevi, especially the flat midline ones and the elevated strawberry nevi, are of no neurologic significance. And a cerebral meningeal angiomatosis may be present without skin lesions. The involvement of the upper eyelid is of greatest importance; nearly all such cases are associated with cerebral lesions. There seems to be a close correlation between the maldevelopment of the embryonic vasculature of the eyelid and forehead and that of the occipitoparietal parts of the brain. When the nevus lies entirely below the upper eyelid and nose or high on the scalp (Gorbachev), a cerebral lesion is usually absent, although in a few instances such an angioma has been associated with a vascular malformation of the meninges overlying the brainstem and cerebellum. In angiograms, the abnormal meningeal vessels, which are largely veins, are not well seen; thus they can be distinguished from the arteriovenous malformations described in Chap. 34. Meningeal nevi are rarely the source of subarachnoid or cerebral hemorrhage, and they do not enlarge to form a "mass lesion." The cortical lesion is destructive in type; lost neurons are replaced by glial tissue that calcifies. Possibly diversion of blood to the meninges during seizures causes the progressive ischemia of the cerebral cortex. Barlow believes the seizures to be responsible for the progressive neurologic deficits and suggests that they be prevented by carefully regulated medical therapy or surgical excision of the discharging foci. The latter may not be feasible, in view of the magnitude of the cerebral lesion. Radiotherapy offers no hope of reducing the skin blemish; sensitive individuals usually try to hide it with cosmetics.

While of congenital origin, the cause and pathogenesis of the encephalotrigeminal syndrome are unknown. Familial coincidence has been observed but is exceptional. The chromosomes appear to be normal.

Dermatomal Hemangiomas with Spinal Vascular Malformations

Hemangiomas of the spinal cord may rarely be accompanied by vascular nevi in the corresponding dermatome of skin, as was first pointed out by Cobb. Like the encephalofacial nevi, they tend to conform to a dermatomal pattern. They are nearly always unilateral and are most frequent in the arm and trunk. When the cutaneous lesion involves an arm or leg, there may be enlargement of the entire limb or fingers in combination with underdevelopment of certain parts (Klippel-Trenauney-Weber syndrome). Some of these angiomatous syndromes, as well as the ones described by Wyburn-Mason, combine a spinal or retinodiencephalic arteriovenous malformation (AVM) with a trunkal or facial nevus. Such cases provide a link to the common AVMs described in Chap. 34.

The Epidermal Nevus Syndrome

This is a closely related congenital neurocutaneous disorder, in which a specific skin lesion (epidermal nevus or linear nevus sebaceus) is associated with a variety of hemicranial and neurologic abnormalities. The skull and brain abnormalities are ipsilateral to the nevus. One-sided thickening of the bones of the skull is characteristic. Mental retardation, seizures, and hemiparesis are the usual neurologic manifestations and have their basis in a wide variety of cerebral lesions—unilateral cerebral atrophy, porencephalic cyst, leptomeningeal hemangioma, arteriovenous malformation, and atresia of cerebral arteries and veins. The somatic and neurologic abnormalities have been comprehensively reviewed by Solomon and Esterley and by Baker and his associates.

Familial Telangiectasia (Osler-Rendu-Weber Disease) This, a vascular anomaly transmitted as an autosomal dominant trait, affects the skin, the mucous membranes, the gastrointestinal and genitourinary tracts, and occasionally the nervous system. The basic lesion is probably a defect in the vessel wall, and bleeding is thought to be due to the mechanical fragility of the vessel. The lesions range from the size of a pinhead to 3 mm or more; they are bright red or violaceous and blanch under pressure. Located sparsely in the skin of any part of the body, they first appear during childhood, enlarge during adolescence, and may assume spidery forms, resembling the cutaneous telangiectases of cirrhosis, in late adult life. The lesions cause trouble only because of their hemorrhagic tendency. During adult years they may give rise to severe and repeated epistaxis or gastric or intestinal or urinary tract hemorrhages, and result in an iron-deficiency anemia.

The angiomas of this disease may form in either the spinal cord or brain, where they can produce apoplectic syndromes; or an intermittently progressive focal cerebral syndrome may result from enlargement of the vascular lesions or from a succession of small hemorrhages. An unexplained gastrointestinal, genitourinary, intracranial, or intraspinal hemorrhage warrants a search for these small cutaneous lesions, which are easily overlooked. Pulmonary fistulae constitute another important feature of the generalized vascular dysplasia; patients with such lesions are peculiarly subject to brain abscesses. Cautery eradicates a bleeding lesion but satellite ones tend to form. Treatment may require the application of oxidized cellulose (Oxycel or Gelfoam).

RESTRICTED OR PARTIAL DEVELOPMENTAL ABNORMALITIES OF THE NERVOUS SYSTEM

In the course of clinical practice one encounters a remarkable number of restricted disorders of the nervous system, many of which are transmitted from generation to generation as

a mendelian dominant trait. Only a few of the more striking examples will be described here. The reader may turn to books on genetics for an account of such oddities as hereditary unilateral ptosis, hereditary Horner syndrome, pupillary inequalities, jaw winking, absence of a particular muscle, etc.

BIFACIAL AND ABDUCENS PALSIES (MÖBIUS SYNDROME)

The syndrome of congenital facial diplegia with convergent strabismus is generally referred to as Möbius syndrome, although it had been described earlier by von Graefe. Its presence at birth is disclosed by the lack of facial movements and full eye closure. The most complete review of the subject in the English literature is that of Henderson. In his analysis of 61 cases of the congenital facial diplegia syndrome, there were 45 instances of abducens palsy, 15 of complete external ophthalmoplegia, 18 of lingual palsy, 17 of clubfeet, 13 of brachial disorders, 6 of mental defect, and 8 of pectoral muscle defect. Thus the overlap with other neuromuscular and CNS abnormalities is evident. Early in life the mouth hangs open, the lower lip is everted, and there is difficulty in sucking. Usually it can be distinguished from the facial palsy of forceps or birth injury by its bilaterality and other associated weaknesses. Occasionally more than one family member is affected (usually autosomal dominant inheritance). The cause of this peculiar condition is not known. The few adequate pathologic studies have shown a lack of nerve cells in the motor nuclei of the brainstem. Rarely there may be an aplasia of facial muscles. This syndrome is also referred to on pages 1096 and 1141.

Partial paralysis of facial muscles, which dates from birth and cannot be attributed to obstetric trauma, is not infrequent. In a common type, the lower lip on the involved side remains immobile when the child smiles or cries; the lip on the unaffected side is drawn downward and outward, resulting in a prominent asymmetry of the lower face. Often it is not appreciated that the side that droops during crying is the normal side (Hoefnagel and Penry).

CONGENITAL LACK OF LATERAL GAZE (OCULOMOTOR APRAXIA OF COGAN)

Children with this congenital defect are unable to turn their eyes to either side volitionally or on command. Attempting to look to the right, the child turns the head to the right (there is no associated apraxia of head turning, as in the acquired condition), but the eyes lag and turn to the left.

As a result, the patient has to overshoot the mark with the head in order to attain fixation straight ahead. Once the eyes fixate, the head returns to the primary position. To compensate for the deficiency of eye movements the patient develops jerky thrusts of the head, which characterize all attempts at voluntary gaze. Caloric stimulation of the labyrinth causes tonic movement (cold to the side of stimulus, warm to the opposite side) but not nystagmus, as in the normal person. Also, optokinetic nystagmus cannot be induced. Vertical movements are normal, however. A similar ocular condition may occur in conjunction with ataxia-telangiectasia. These children are slow to walk, and Ford has observed one such child whose sibling had an absence of the vermis of the cerebellum. Aside from this observation, the anatomic basis of this condition has not been studied.

CONGENITAL ABNORMALITIES OF MOTOR FUNCTION

In this group of congenital disorders, a major disturbance of motor function, usually nonprogressive, has been present since infancy or early childhood. The popular term for these conditions is *cerebral palsy*. The name is not altogether appropriate, nor is it useful from the physician's viewpoint, collocating, as it does, diseases of widely differing etiologic and anatomic types; the hereditary and acquired, the intrauterine, natal, and postnatal diseases lose their identity. Nevertheless, the name has been adopted as a slogan for fund-raising societies and for a major rehabilitation movement throughout the United States, and it will not soon disappear from medical terminology.

Motor abnormalities that have had their onset early in life are numerous and diverse in their clinical manifestations. To ascertain the etiologic and pathogenic factor(s), it is helpful to categorize a given case according to the extent and nature of the motor abnormality. A careful history of possible prenatal, perinatal, or postnatal insults to the developing nervous system must always be sought; certain correlations of these factors with the resulting pattern of neurologic deficit are outlined below. Most patients with these motor abnormalities of infancy and childhood reach adult years. Many of them have some degree of mental retardation in addition to the motor abnormalities and there is an unavoidable overlapping in any consideration of the causes and mechanisms of the two clinical states.

Three major etiologic syndromes have been delineated—matrix hemorrhages in the immature infant, Little disease, and developmental abnormalities.

MATRIX (SUBEPENDYMAL) HEMORRHAGE IN PREMATURE INFANTS

In low-weight immature infants (20 to 35 weeks gestational age), there often occurs, within a few days after birth, a catastrophic decline in cerebral function. Respiratory distress (hyaline-membrane disease) with cyanosis and apneic spells usually precedes the reduced responsivity, failure of brainstem automatisms (sucking and swallowing), bulging of the fontanelles, and appearance of sanguineous CSF. Once the infant becomes completely unresponsive, death usually ensues within a few days. Autopsy discloses a small lake of blood in the highly cellular (subependymal) germinal matrix, near the caudate nucleus at the level of the foramen of Monro. This region is supplied by Heubner's recurrent, lenticulostriate, and choroidal arteries. In about 25 percent of cases the blood remains loculated in the matrix zone, while in the others it ruptures into the lateral ventricle. In a series of 914 consecutive autopsies in infants at the Cleveland Metropolitan General Hospital, subependymal hemorrhage was found in 284 (31 percent); practically all of these infants were immature (Banker and Bruce-Gregorios).

Lesser degrees of this complex of cerebral lesions are now being identified by CT scans, MRI, and ultrasound, and it is apparent that many infants with such lesions survive. Some rapidly develop a meningeal obstructive hydrocephalus and require a ventricular shunt. In others, the hydrocephalus stabilizes and there is clinical improvement. Several series of surviving cases have now been followed for many years. Those in whom the hemorrhage was severe are often left with motor and intellectual handicaps. In the series of 20 cases of posthemorrhagic hydrocephalus observed by Chaplin et al, 40 percent had significant motor deficits and over 60 percent had IQ scores of less than 85. In a personal experience with 12 less severe cases (mean birth weight 1.8 kg and gestational age of 32.3 weeks), only one had a residual motor deficit (a moderate spastic diplegia) and 9 of the 12 had IQs in the low normal or normal range. The average age of the children at the time of the last evaluation was 4.5 years.

The cause of this unique syndrome is unsettled. In all probability the hemorrhages are related to a greatly increased pressure in the thin-walled veins of the germinal matrix, coupled with a lack of adequate supporting tissue in these zones. The increased blood pressure or venous pressure is, in turn, manifestly related to the pulmonary disorders that occur in immature infants. These infants are also prone to the development of characteristic lesions of the cerebral white matter (*periventricular leukomalacia*), and the residual neurologic deficits are the result of these lesions, added to the hemorrhagic complications (mainly hydrocephalus). The zones of necrosis lie deep in the white matter, near the walls of the lateral ventricles, in a position to involve the occipital and sensorimotor radiations in the vascular border zones of the frontoparietal regions. These white matter lesions occur in about one-third of cases of subependymal hemorrhage, but they may develop separately and account for the visual, perceptive, and motor dysfunctions found in some of the older surviving patients (Banker and Larroche; Shuman and Selednik). Recently, claims have been made that the administration of ethamsylate, a drug that reduces capillary bleeding, and the intramuscular injection of vitamin E for the first 3 days after birth reduce the incidence of periventricular hemorrhage (Benson et al; Sinha et al).

CEREBRAL SPASTIC DIPLEGIA (LITTLE DISEASE)

Little's conception of the hypoxic-ischemic form of "birth injury" enunciated in 1862 has been subjected to searching study over the years. While it is evident that many newborns suffer some degree of perinatal asphyxia, few of them seem to manifest brain damage. One has the impression that the central nervous system of the newborn tolerates hypoxia and reduced blood flow better than at any other time in life. Indeed, animal experimentation supports this view. Not until the arterial O_2 tension is reduced to 10 to 15 percent of normal does brain damage occur, and even then the impaired function of other organs contributes to the damage; nearly always there are irregularities of the heart and hypotension from myocardial damage, as well as hepatic and renal failure. Thus it is more correct to think of the encephalopathy in terms of both hypoxia and ischemia, which usually occur in utero and are expressed postnatally by recognizable clinical syndromes.

These cerebral syndromes have been subdivided by Fenichel into three groups, according to their severity: (1) In patients with *mild hypoxic-ischemic encephalopathy*, the symptoms are maximum in the first 24 h and take the form of hyperalertness and tremulousness of limbs and jaw (the "jittery baby"), and a low threshold of the Moro reaction. The tone of the limbs is normal except for a mild increase in head lag during traction. The reflexes are brisk and there may be ankle clonus. The anterior fontanelle is soft. The EEG is normal. Recovery is complete and the risk of handicap is extremely low. (2) In newborns with *moderate hypoxic-ischemic encephalopathy*, the patient is lethargic, obtunded, and hypotonic, with normal movements. After 48 to 72 h the patient may improve, passing through a jittery hyperactive phase, or worsen, becoming less responsive in association with convulsions, cerebral edema, hyponatremia, and hyperammonemia from liver damage. The EEG is abnormal; Fenichel associates epileptiform activity and voltage suppression with an unfavorable outcome. Visual and auditory evoked potentials, if abnormal,

are other poor prognostic signs. (3) In patients with *severe hypoxic-ischemic encephalopathy,* stupor or coma are present from birth; respirations are irregular, requiring mechanical ventilation. There are usually convulsions within the first 12 h. The limbs are hypotonic and motionless even in attempts to elicit the Moro response. Sucking and swallowing are depressed, but chewing, sucking, pupillary reactions, and eye movements may at first be retained, only to be lost as the coma deepens.

It is from the second and third categories, i.e., the states of moderate to severe encephalopathy, in which correction of the respiratory insufficiency and the metabolic abnormalities permits survival, that a number of motor abnormalities (corticospinal and extrapyramidal) and mental retardation eventually emerge. According to Levene et al, the outcome was poor in 97 percent of such cases, because of developmental abnormalities or cerebral palsy or both, seizures, and sensorineural hearing loss. Of their 122 cases of perinatal asphyxia, 14 died within a few days to weeks, 6 had cerebral palsy, and 6 had developmental delay.

Included in the third category of severe hypoxic-ischemic encephalopathy are newborns with a variety of developmental anomalies of the brain and other organs. Some are born at term; others are premature, and the birth process may have been abnormal. But one must then consider the possibility, originally pointed out by Sigmund Freud, that the abnormality of the birth process, instead of being causal, was actually the consequence of prenatal pathology. The latter might include preterm intrauterine hypoxia-ischemia.

In a search for the antecedents of cerebral palsy, Nelson and Ellenberg found that maternal mental retardation, birth weight below 2000 g, and fetal malformation were among the leading predictors. Breech presentation was another factor, but a third of these cases also had a noncerebral malformation. Twenty-one percent of their 189 children with cerebral palsy had also suffered some degree of asphyxia. Other factors were maternal seizures, a motor deficit in an older sibling, two or more prior fetal deaths, hyperthyroidism in the mother, pre-eclampsia, and eclampsia.

The factors enumerated above operate to different degrees in the outcome of pregnancies but are informative because they bring to light the significant proportion of cases of cerebral palsy in which hypoxia-ischemia, matrix hemorrhages, and leukomalacia were *not* operative.

With reference to the types of motor disorder evolving from these three categories of cerebral disease, spastic paraparesis is the most frequent (motor disturbances in the upper extremities are mild). Two main groups can be recognized. In one, the spastic diplegia is associated with a relatively slight diminution in head size and intelligence. The neuropathology is unsettled; the condition is not related to matrix hemorrhages and periventricular leukomalacia. The frequency of this form of cerebral spastic diplegia, which is closely related to the degree of prematurity, has declined significantly since the introduction of neonatal intensive care facilities, and there is reason to believe that heredogenetic factors are of importance.

A second group, in which the major insult is intrapartum asphyxia and attendant fetal distress, is characterized by the development of severe spastic quadriplegia and mental retardation. Such infants will usually have required resuscitation and will have had low Apgar scores, which in this circumstance have important predictive value. The pathologic lesions of the brain in this second group consist of hypoxic-ischemic infarction in distal fields of arterial flow, primarily in the cortex and white matter of parietal and posterior frontal lobes.

The pattern of paralysis is actually more variable than the term spastic diplegia implies; several types may be distinguished: the paraplegic, diplegic, quadriplegic, pseudobulbar, and generalized. Pure paraplegic and pseudobulbar types are relatively rare. Usually all four extremities are involved, but the legs are much more affected than the arms, which is the real meaning of diplegia. As a rule, damage to the nervous system is suspected at birth or soon thereafter because of some abnormality of breathing, sucking, swallowing, or responsiveness. If the motor system is affected (corticospinal, extrapyramidal, or cerebellar), hypotonia with retained tendon reflexes and hypoactivity are usually present. Only after the first few months will evident weakness and spasticity appear, first in the adductors of the legs. The plantar reflexes are often ambiguous in the normal infant, but here the reflexes are clearly extensor, a finding that is pathologic at any age. Also, stiff, awkward movements of the legs, which are maintained in an extended, adducted posture when the infant is lifted by the axillae, often do not attract attention until several weeks or months have passed. Seizures occur in approximately a third of the cases, and it is not uncommon to observe a delay in all developmental sequences, especially those that depend on the motor system. Once walking is attempted, usually at a much later date than normal, the characteristic stance and gait become manifest. The legs are advanced stiffly in short steps, each describing part of an arc of a circle; adduction of the thighs is often so strong that the legs may actually cross (scissors gait); and the feet are flexed and turned in

with the heels not touching the ground. In the adolescent and adult, the legs tend to be short and small, but the muscles are not markedly atrophic, as in spinal muscular atrophy . Passive manipulation of the limbs reveals spasticity in the extensors and adductors and slight shortening of the calf muscles. The hands and arms may be affected only slightly, or not at all; there may be awkwardness and stiffness of the fingers, and, in a few, pronounced weakness and spasticity. In reaching for an object the hand may overpronate. Speech may be well articulated or noticeably slurred, and in some instances the face is set in a spastic smile. The deep tendon reflexes are exaggerated, those in the legs more than the arms; and the plantar reflexes are extensor in the majority of cases. Usually there is no disturbance of sphincteric function, though delay in acquiring voluntary control is usual. Athetotic postures and movements of the face, tongue, and hands are present in some patients and may actually conceal the spastic weakness; ataxic and hypotonic forms also exist (see further on).

These prenatal and parturitional types of spastic diplegia must be distinguished from the familial types of spastic paraparesis, which have already been discussed in Chap. 43.

In addition to diplegia, hypoxic-ischemic injury occurring in the term or preterm infant may take the form of a hemiplegia, double hemiplegia (quadriplegia), or a mixed pyramidal-extrapyramidal syndrome. Some of the latter are caused by other factors, such as kernicterus, as will be indicated below.

INFANTILE HEMIPLEGIA, DOUBLE HEMIPLEGIA, AND QUADRIPLEGIA

Hemiplegia is a common condition of infancy and early childhood. The functional difference between the two sides may be noticed soon after birth or not until after the first 4 to 6 months of life. In other cases, the child is in excellent health for a year or longer before the abrupt onset of hemiplegia (see below). In hemiplegia that dates from earliest infancy, the parents first notice that movements of prehension and exploration are carried out with only one arm. A manifest hand preference at an early age should always raise the suspicion of a unilateral motor defect. The affection of the leg is usually recognized later, i.e., during the first attempts to stand and walk. Mental defect may be associated with infantile hemiplegia but is less common than with cerebral diplegia and much less common than with bilateral hemiplegia. There may also be speech delay, regardless of the side of the lesion, but when present, one should look for mental retardation and bilaterality of the motor abnormality. Convulsions occur in 35 to 50 percent of children with congenital hemiplegia, and these may persist throughout life. They may be generalized, but are frequently unilateral and limited to the hemiplegic side. Often, after a series of seizures, the weakness on the affected side will be increased for several hours or longer (Todd's paralysis). Gastaut has described a hemiconvulsive-hemiplegic syndrome in which the progressive paralysis and cerebral atrophy are attributed to the convulsions. In our experience, however, the destruction of tissue, as shown by CT scan, suggests that a vascular or encephalitic lesion had occurred and resulted in both destruction of brain tissue and seizures.

A relatively frequent neurologic syndrome is that of *acquired hemiplegia.* A normal infant or young child, usually between the ages of 3 to 18 months, develops a massive hemiplegia, with or without aphasia, within hours. The disorder often begins with seizures, and the hemiplegia may not be recognized until the seizures have subsided. In Banker's autopsy series, arterial or venous thrombosis was found, but arteriography may be negative; some of the latter may be embolic (?cardiac). If this accident occurs at an early age, the recovery of speech may be complete though reduced scholastic capacity remains. The degree of recovery of motor function varies.

Double hemiplegia is a much less frequent condition. The bilateral weakness of the face, arms, and legs arises under conditions of severe acquired cerebral disease at any age. The arms are severely affected, in contrast to their minimal involvement in cerebral diplegia.

Encephaloclastic (destructive) lesions underlie most of the cases of infantile hemiplegia and of bilateral hemiplegias. The pathologic change is essentially that of ischemic necrosis. In many cases, the lesions must have been incurred in utero. The lesions reflect not only the effects of anoxia but also those of circulatory insufficiency (ischemia), the result of hypotension or circulatory failure. The ischemia of circulatory failure tends to affect the tissues lying in arterial border zones, and there may also be venous stasis with congestion and hemorrhage (occurring particularly in the deep central structures such as the basal ganglia and periventricular matrix zones). Myers has reproduced such lesions in the neonatal monkey by reducing the maternal circulation over a period of several hours. As the lesions heal, the monkeys develop the same ulegyric sclerotic changes in the cortex and white matter of the cerebrum (lobar sclerosis) and the ''marbling'' (*état marbré*) that characterize the brains of patients with spastic diplegia and double athetosis (see below).

The quadriplegic state differs from bilateral hemiplegias in that the bulbar musculature is often involved in the latter. The condition is relatively rare and is due usually to a bilateral cerebral lesion. However, one should also be alert to the possibility of a high cervical cord lesion. In the infant, this is usually the result of a fracture-dislocation of the cervical spine, incurred during a difficult breech delivery.

Similarly, in *paraplegia,* with weakness or paralysis limited to the legs, the lesion may be either a cerebral or a spinal one. Sphincteric disturbances and a loss of somatic sensation below a certain level on the trunk always point to a spinal localization. Congenital cysts, tumors, and diastematomyelia are more frequently causes of paraplegia than of quadriplegia. Another recognized cause of infantile paraplegia is spinal cord infarction from thrombotic complications of umbilical artery catheterization.

CONGENITAL EXTRAPYRAMIDAL SYNDROMES

The spastic cerebral diplegias discussed above shade almost imperceptibly into the congenital extrapyramidal syndromes. Patients with these latter syndromes are found in every cerebral palsy clinic, and ultimately they reach adult neurology clinics as well. Corticospinal tract signs may be completely absent, and the student, familiar only with the syndrome of pure spastic diplegia, is always puzzled as to their classification. Some cases of extrapyramidal type are undoubtedly attributable to severe perinatal hypoxia and others to diseases such as erythroblastosis fetalis with kernicterus. In order to state the probable pathologic basis and future course of these illnesses, it is desirable to separate the extrapyramidal syndromes due to prenatal and natal diseases, which usually become manifest during the first year of life, from the acquired or hereditary postnatal syndromes, such as familial athetosis, dystonia musculorum deformans, and hereditary cerebellar ataxia, which become manifest later. The latter have been discussed in Chaps. 38 and 43.

Congenital Choreoathetosis (Double Athetosis)
Double athetosis is probably the most frequent of the congenital extrapyramidal disorders. Like the spastic states, it may not be recognized at birth, but only after several months or a year have elapsed. In some cases the appearance of choreoathetosis is delayed for several years, and it may progress during adolescence and even early adult life. Chorea and athetosis dominate the clinical picture, but various combinations of these involuntary movements with hemiballismus, dystonia, and even myoclonus and ataxic tremor may be found in a single case. Furthermore, in all instances there is in addition a primary defect in voluntary movement.

Choreoathetosis in infants and children varies greatly in severity. In some the abnormal movements are so mild as to be misinterpreted as restlessness or ''the fidgets''; in others, every attempted voluntary act precipitates violent involuntary movements, leaving the patient nearly helpless. The clinical appearance of choreoathetosis and other involuntary movements has been discussed in Chap. 4.

An early hypotonia, followed by retardation of motor development, is the rule in these cases. Erect posture and walking may be delayed until the age of 3 to 5 years, and may never be attained in some patients. Tonic neck reflexes or fragments thereof tend to persist well beyond their usual time of disappearance. The plantar reflexes are characteristically flexor, though they may be difficult to interpret because of the continuous flexion and extension of the toes. Sensory abnormalities are not elicited. Because of the motor and speech impairment, patients are often erroneously classified as mentally defective. In some this conclusion is doubtless correct, but in others intellectual function is adequate, and a few can be educated to a high level.

With growth and development, new postures and motor capacities are acquired. The less severely affected patients can even make successful occupational adjustments. The more severely affected ones, even with all the help that can be provided by rehabilitation clinics, rarely achieve a degree of motor control that permits them to lead an independent life. One sees some of these unfortunate persons bobbing and twisting laboriously as they make their way in public places.

The most frequent pathologic finding in the brain has been a whitish, marble-like appearance of the putamen, thalamus, and border zones of the cerebral cortex. These whitish strands represent foci of nerve cell loss and gliosis with condensation of myelinated fibers—so-called *status marmoratus* (*état marbré*). This lesion does not develop after infancy, i.e., after the myelination glia have completed their developmental cycle.

Kernicterus This is now a rare cause of extrapyramidal motor disorder in children and adults. Such cases raise the broader question of the neurologic sequelae of erythroblastosis fetalis secondary to Rh and ABO incompatibilities.

The symptoms of kernicterus appear in the jaundiced neonate on the second or third postnatal day. The infant becomes listless, sucks poorly, develops respiratory difficulties, and becomes stuporous as jaundice intensifies. The serum bilirubin is usually greater than 25 mg/dL. In acidotic and hypoxic infants (e.g., those with prematurity and hyaline membrane disease) the kernicteric lesions develop with much lower levels of serum bilirubin.

The majority of infants with this disease die within the first week or two of life. Many of those who survive are mentally retarded, deaf, totally unable to sit, stand, or walk, and spend their lives in homes for the feebleminded. There are exceptional patients, however, obviously less damaged, who are mentally normal or at most only slightly backward. These are the ones who develop a variety of persistent neurologic sequelae—choreoathetosis, dystonia, and rigidity of the limbs—a picture not too different from that of cerebral spastic diplegia with involuntary movements. Kernicterus should always be suspected if an extrapyramidal syndrome is accompanied by bilateral deafness and palsy of upward gaze.

Neonates who die in the acute stage of kernicterus show a characteristic yellow staining of nuclear masses in the basal ganglia, brainstem, and cerebellum—a finding from which the disease takes its name. In surviving patients the pathologic changes consist of a symmetrically distributed nerve cell loss and gliosis in the subthalamic nucleus of Luys, the globus pallidus, thalamus, and oculomotor and cochlear nuclei; these lesions are the result of the hyperbilirubinemia. In the newborn, unconjugated bilirubin can pass through the poorly developed blood-brain barrier into these central and brainstem nuclei, where it is directly toxic. Acidosis and hypoxia exacerbate the effect. Also, in the newborn, the development of hyperbilirubinemia is enhanced by transient deficiency of the enzyme glucuronyl transferase, essential for the conjugation of bilirubin. *Hereditary hyperbilirubinemia,* due to lack of this enzyme (*Crigler-Najjar syndrome*), may have the same effect on the nervous system at a later period of infancy or childhood as hyperbilirubinemia due to the excessive hemolysis of Rh incompatibility.

Phototherapy and exchange transfusions with female blood, designed to prevent high levels of unconjugated serum bilirubin, have been shown to protect the nervous system. If the blood bilirubin level can be held to less than 20 mg/dL (10 mg/dL in prematures), the nervous system may escape damage. The effective use of these measures has greatly reduced the incidence of kernicterus.

CONGENITAL AND ACQUIRED ATAXIAS

The combination of cerebral diplegia with cerebellar ataxia has already been mentioned. In these patients difficulty in standing and walking cannot be attributed to spasticity or paralysis. Again, hypotonia is the initial motor abnormality, and the cerebellar defect becomes manifest at a later time, when the patient begins to sit, stand, and walk. The ataxia of the trunk is evident in sitting and that of the arms in reaching for a preferred toy. These defects may be of such severity that the individual is never able to sit or stand. Yet the muscles are of normal size, and voluntary movements, though weak, are possible in all the limbs. In less severe cases, sitting, standing, and walking are merely delayed, and, with maturation of the corticospinal systems, cerebellar ataxia and tremor become manifest. Relative improvement may occur in later years. The tendon reflexes are present, and the plantar reflexes are either flexor or extensor. Many of these patients suffer a degree of retardation of speech and mental development that results in their placement in homes for the feebleminded. In only a few cases have the pathologic changes been studied. Aplasia or hypoplasia of the cerebellum has been observed, but sclerotic lesions of the cerebellum are more common. The CT scan or MRI verifies the diagnosis.

As to causation, radiation of the maternal abdomen during the first trimester of pregnancy is said to have resulted in cerebellar hypoplasia. Mercury poisoning in utero is another cause of congenital ataxia. A cerebral and cerebellar lesion may coexist in patients with congenital ataxia, which is the reason for the term *cerebrocerebellar diplegia.*

Aside from the congenital ataxias (of which some are cerebellar and others probably cerebral in type), there are forms of childhood ataxia that have an acute onset and persist during adolescence and adult life. A few of these are familial. Also, the progressive hereditary ataxias are likely to begin at a later age than the congenital ones; some are intermittent or episodic, and others are persistent and progressive. They are discussed in Chap. 38.

THE FLACCID PARALYSES

The cerebral form, first described by Foerster and called *cerebral atonic diplegia,* has already been mentioned. It can usually be distinguished from spinal and peripheral nerve paralysis and muscular dystrophy by the retention of postural reflexes (flexion of the legs at the knees and hips when the infant is lifted by the axillae), the preservation of tendon reflexes, and the coincident failure of mental development.

The syndrome of *infantile spinal muscular atrophy* (*Werdnig-Hoffmann disease*) is the leading example of flaccid paralysis of lower motor neuron type. Perceptive mothers may be aware of a paucity of fetal movements in utero, and in most cases the motor defect becomes evident soon after birth. Several other types of familial progressive muscular atrophy have been described in which the onset is in early or late childhood, adolescence, or early adult life. Weakness, atrophy, and reflex loss without sensory change are the main features and are discussed in further detail in Chaps. 43 and 52. A few patients suspected of having infantile or childhood muscular atrophy prove, with the passage of time, to be merely inactive ''slack'' children, whose motor development has proceeded at a slower rate than normal. A few may remain weak throughout life, with thin musculature. These and several other myopathologic entities, e.g., *central core disease, rod-body myopathy, pleoconial, megaconial, and myotubular myopathies,* are

described in Chap. 52. Rarely polymyositis and acute idiopathic polyneuritis may manifest themselves as a syndrome of congenital hypotonia.

Infantile muscular dystrophy and *lipid and glycogen storage diseases* may also produce a clinical picture of progressive atrophy and weakness of muscles. The diagnosis of *glycogen storage* disease (usually the Pompe form) should be suspected when progressive muscular atrophy is associated with enlargement of the tongue, heart, liver, or spleen. The motor disturbance in this condition may be related in some way to the abnormal deposits of glycogen in skeletal muscles, though it is more likely due to degeneration of anterior horn cells that are also distended with glycogen and other substances.

Brachial plexus palsies, well-known complications of dystocia, usually result from forcible extraction of the fetus by traction on the shoulder in a breech presentation, or from traction and tipping of the head in a shoulder presentation. The effects of such injuries are sometimes lifelong. Their neonatal onset is later betrayed by the small size and inadequate osseous development of the affected limb. Either the upper brachial plexus and the fifth and sixth cervical roots or the lower brachial plexus and the seventh and eighth cervical and first thoracic roots suffer the brunt of the injury. Upper plexus injuries (*Erb*) are about 20 times more frequent than lower ones (*Klumpke*). Sometimes the entire plexus is involved (see page 1064).

Facial paralysis, due to forceps injury to the facial nerve immediately distal to its exit from the stylomastoid foramen, is another common peripheral nerve affection in the newborn. The failure of one eye to close and the difficulty in sucking make this condition easy to recognize. It must be distinguished from the congenital facial diplegia that is often associated with abducens palsy, i.e., the Möbius syndrome (page 989). In most cases of facial paralysis due to physical injury, function is recovered after a few weeks; in some, the paralysis is permanent and may account for facial asymmetry observed in later life.

INTRAUTERINE AND NEONATAL INFECTIONS

Throughout the intrauterine period the embryo and fetus are subject to particular types of infection. Since the infective agent must reach the fetus through the placenta, it is evident that the permeability of the latter at different stages of gestation and the immune status of the maternal organism are determinative.

Until the third to fourth month of gestation the large microbial organisms such as bacteria, spirochetes, protozoa, and fungi cannot invade the embryo, even though the mother harbors the infection. Viruses may do so, however—specifically rubella and cytomegalus viruses, and possibly others. The rubella virus enters embryonal tissues during the first trimester, *Treponema pallidum* in the fourth to fifth postconceptional month, and toxoplasma after that period. Bacterial meningitis (except for that due to *Listeria monocytogenes*, described below) is essentially a paranatal infection contracted during or immediately after parturition. Neonatal herpes simplex encephalitis, due to the type 2 (genital) virus, is also usually acquired during passage through an infected birth canal.

Embryonal and fetal infections are difficult to diagnose, for the mother may be entirely asymptomatic. Isolation of the organism from fetal and neonatal tissues is possible, but the demonstration of antibodies and other immune responses may be impossible because of the early stage of the infection or imperfections of the infant's immunity.

RUBELLA

Gregg, in 1941, first reported the association of maternal rubella and congenital cataracts in the neonate. His observations were quickly verified, and soon it became widely known that cataracts, deafness, congenital heart disease, and mental retardation constituted a kind of tetrad, diagnostic of this disease. That a virus could affect so many tissues, causing in essence a noninflammatory developmental disorder of multiple organs, was a novel concept, and it raised the exciting prospect that other viruses might have similar effects. Surprisingly, however, only the cytomegalovirus and possibly herpes simplex viruses have been incriminated in embryonal neuropathology. A large number of other viruses (e.g., influenza, Epstein-Barr, hepatitis) have been implicated in human teratogenesis, but in none is the relationship beyond doubt.

It is now well established that most instances of congenital rubella infection occur in the first 10 weeks of gestation, and that the earlier the occurrence of infection, the greater the risk to the fetus. However, there is considerable risk even beyond the first trimester (Hardy, 1973).

Following the massive rubella epidemic of 1964 and 1965, the congenital rubella syndrome has been expanded to include: low birth weight; bilateral deafness of neurocochlear type; microphthalmia, pigmentary degeneration of the retina (salt and pepper chorioretinitis), cloudy cornea, glaucoma and cataracts of special type; hepatosplenomegaly,

jaundice and thrombocytopenic purpura; patent ductus arteriosus or interventricular septal defect. One, a few, or many of these abnormalities may occur in various combinations. The mental retardation is severe and may be accompanied by seizures and motor defects such as hemiplegia or spastic diplegia.

Infection of the fetus after the first trimester results in a less impressive neonatal syndrome. The infant may seem lethargic and fail to thrive. The cranium is abnormally small. Only a cardiac abnormality, deafness, or chorioretinitis may provide clues to the diagnosis. The CSF shows an increase of mononuclear cells and an elevated protein. The infection may persist for a year or two.

The maternal infection may be inapparent but even when evident the fetus may be spared in 30 percent of cases. Diagnosis can be verified in the neonate by demonstrating IgM antibodies to the virus or by the isolation of the virus from the throat, urine, stool, or CSF. Also, the virus has been obtained from cells in the amniotic fluid.

The *neuropathology* is of considerable interest. In the nervous system of abortuses (the abortion performed because of proven maternal rubella in the first trimester), one of the authors (R.D.A.) found no visible lesions by light microscopy even though the virus had been isolated from the brain by Enders. At this period of development there is no inflammatory reaction because of the absence of polymorphonuclear leukocytes, lymphocytes, and other mononuclear cells in the fetus. At birth the brain is usually of normal size, and there may be no discernible lesions. In a few, a mild meningeal infiltration of lymphocytes, a few zones of necrosis, and calcification of vessels are seen. Smallness of the brain and delay in myelination have been observed in children dying at 1 to 2 years of age. None of the brains in our series have been malformed. Rubella virus continues to be recovered from the CSF for at least 18 months after birth. A delayed progressive rubella encephalitis in childhood has also been described (page 608).

The obvious approach to the problem of congenital rubella infection is to make sure that every woman has been vaccinated against rubella or has had the infection prior to pregnancy. The widespread use of rubella vaccine has reduced the chance of major epidemics, but sporadic infections continue to occur, and an outbreak of epidemic proportions is still possible because of laxity of vaccination programs. There is no effective treatment for the established infection.

CYTOMEGALIC INCLUSION DISEASE (CID)

For many years it was known that in the tissues of some infants who died in the first weeks and months of life there were swollen cells containing intranuclear and cyto-plasmic inclusions. This cytologic change seemed related to the fatalities. In 1956 and 1957, three different labora-tories isolated what have come to be called the human cytomegaloviruses (see Weller, 1970). They have proved to be the most frequent intrauterine viral infections (see below).

Infection of the fetus occurs in the first trimester of pregnancy, or later, by way of an inapparent maternal viremia and active infection of the placenta. The newborn can also be infected in the course of delivery or afterward by the mother's milk or by transfusions. However, only a small proportion of women known to harbor the cytomeg-alovirus give birth to infants with active infection. Early infection of the fetus may result in a malformation of the cerebrum; later, there is only inflammatory necrosis in parts of the normally formed brain. In the premature or in the full-term infant, the clinical picture is one of jaundice, petechiae, hematemesis, melena, direct hyperbilirubinemia, thrombopenia, hepatosplenomegaly, microcephaly, mental defect, and convulsions. Cells in the urine may show cytomegalic changes. There is a pleocytosis and an increased protein in the CSF. There are disseminated inflammatory foci in the cerebrum, brainstem, and retinas. In the centers of aggregates of lymphocytes, mononuclear cells, and plasma cells are microglial cells containing inclusion bodies; some astrocytes are similarly affected. The granulomas later calcify, particularly in the periventricular regions. Often there is hydrocephalus.

Several studies indicate that about 1 percent of infants born in the United States excrete virus in their urine and may continue to do so for as long as 4 years postnatally. Of the infected infants, about 17 percent have some degree of nervous system damage (Hanshaw, 1971). The latter consist of simple mental retardation, sensorineural deafness, delay in development, chorioretinitis, optic atrophy, sei-zures, and learning disability—occurring singly or in com-bination. Why one infected fetus develops normally and another develops CNS disease is not understood.

Congenital cytomegalovirus infections pose a much greater problem than rubella. There is no way of identifying the infected fetus prior to birth or to prevent inapparent infections in the pregnant woman. Moreover, some infected infants (with viruria) may appear normal at birth but develop neural deafness and mental retardation several years later (Reynolds et al). Virus replication in infected organs continues after the first year and health workers are at risk. A second child may be infected.

There is no known treatment. The difficulties in prenatal diagnosis of maternal infection preclude abortion. Routine serologic testing is of little value, since 2 percent of pregnant women, all of them asymptomatic, have a primary infection.

CONGENITAL NEUROSYPHILIS

The clinical syndromes and pathologic reactions of con-genital neurosyphilis are similar to those of the adult. Such differences as exist are determined principally by the immaturity of the nervous system at the time of spirochetal invasion.

The syphilitic infection may be transmitted to the fetus at any time from the fourth to the seventh months. The fetus may die, with resulting miscarriage or stillbirth, or may survive only to be born with florid manifestations of secondary syphilis. The dissemination of the spirochetes throughout the body, the time of appearance of the secondary manifestations, and the time of formation of syphilitic reagin in the blood are all governed by the same biologic principles that apply to adult syphilis.

At birth the spirochetemia may not have had time to cause syphilitic reagin to appear; hence a negative VDRL reaction in umbilical cord blood does not exclude syphilis. In unselected groups of syphilitic mothers, 25 to 80 percent of fetuses are infected, and in 20 to 40 percent of those infected the CNS is invaded, as judged by the finding of abnormal CSF. In general, the incidence of congenital neurosyphilis is approximately the same as adult neurosy-philis, and the types (asymptomatic and symptomatic men-ingitis, meningovascular disease, hydrocephalus, general paresis, and tabes dorsalis) are also the same except for the rarity of tabes dorsalis. The Hutchinson triad (dental de-formities, interstitial keratitis, and bilateral deafness) is infrequently observed in complete form; deafness is rare. The sequence of neurologic syndromes is the same as for the adult, all stemming basically from a chronic spirochetal meningitis. The latter may become symptomatic in the first weeks and months of postnatal life, meningovascular lesions and hydrocephalus reaching maximal frequency during the 9-month to 6-year period. Congenital paresis and tabes usually appear between the ninth to fifteenth years. The pathologic basis of each neurosyphilitic syndrome is, re-spectively, meningoarteritis (vascular syphilis), menin-goencephalitis (general paresis), and meningoradiculitis (tabes dorsalis).

The authors have observed fewer and fewer cases of congenital neurosyphilis as the years pass, but there may be a recent recrudescence of the disease. If the syphilitic mother is treated before the fourth month of pregnancy, the fetus will not be infected. The infant may be normal at birth or exhibit only mucocutaneous lesions, hepatosple-nomegaly, lymphadenopathy, and anemia. There are in the neonatal period no signs of meningeal invasion, or only an asymptomatic meningitis. If the latter is actively treated, until the CSF is normal, vascular lesions of brain and spinal cord, hydrocephalus, general paresis, and tabes dorsalis will not develop. If cases of meningovascular syphilis, general paresis, and tabes dorsalis are treated for 3 to 4 weeks with penicillin until the CSF is rendered acellular and the protein reduced to normal, the neurologic disorder will be arrested, and often there is a functional improvement.

The various neurosyphilitic syndromes are described fully in Chap. 32. Only those features pertinent to the congenital forms are mentioned below.

1. *Meningovascular syphilis* declares itself by a stroke with involvement of cerebrum, brainstem, or spinal cord in the first months or years of life. It enters the differential diagnosis of *infantile hemiplegia.* Several infarctive lesions may leave the patient mentally backward, and any one of them may become epileptogenic.

2. *Early hydrocephalus* and *retarded psychomotor development* should always raise the possibility of congenital syphilis though less than 1 percent of cases have a syphilitic basis. Such children may be permanently retarded.

3. *Congenital paretic neurosyphilis.* Approximately half the patients who decline mentally because of neurosyphilis during late childhood will have been defective physically and mentally since infancy. The other half will have developed normally. In 23 personally observed patients the initial symptom was either mental or physical. If already feebleminded, the patient becomes more deficient; or, if intelligence had been normal, behavior becomes eccentric and school performance declines. Silliness, forgetfulness, irascibility, and inattentiveness are noteworthy behavioral abnormalities. There may be outbursts of agitation and depression. Approximately half of the patients have seizures. Peculiar choreiform movements, twitches, and action tremors are frequent. The tendon reflexes are hyperactive, and plantar reflexes extensor. The pupils are fixed to light and sometimes to accommodation, and tend to be dilated rather than miotic. Optic atrophy and chorioretinitis may be conjoined.

4. *Congenital tabetic neurosyphilis.* Failing vision and urinary incontinence are the usual early symptoms. Sensory ataxia and lightning pains are rare. The legs are areflexic but not weak, and the bladder hypotonic and dilated. The pupils are unreactive to light and more frequently dilated than miotic; optic atrophy and strabismus are often present as well.

Congenital syphilis must be considered a potential albeit an increasingly rare cause of epilepsy and amentia. Once the syphilitic infection has been treated in early life and rendered inactive (acellular CSF, normal protein), the occurrence of a congenital luetic infection can only be substantiated by an accurate history, the finding of the syphilitic stigmata in the eyes, teeth, and ears, or a positive serologic reaction in the CSF.

Treatment of syphilis in the child follows the same lines as treatment of the syphilitic adult (page 579), with appropriate adjustment of dosage in accordance with weight.

TOXOPLASMOSIS

This tiny protozoan, *Toxoplasma gondii,* occurring freely or in pseudocyst form, was established by Cowan and his associates as a frequent cause of meningoencephalitis in utero or in the perinatal period of life. The disease exists in all parts of the United States, but is more frequent in western European countries. The mother is most often infected by handling uncooked infected mutton or other animal foods, but she is nearly always asymptomatic or has only a mild fever and lymphadenopathy.

The precise times of placental and fetal invasion are not known, but presumably they are late in the gestational period. The clinical syndrome usually becomes manifest in the first days and weeks of life when seizures, spastic paralysis of the extremities, progressive hydrocephalus, and chorioretinitis appear. The retinal lesions consist of large pale areas surrounded by deposits of pigment. If severe, the maculae are destroyed, and optic atrophy and microphthalmus follow. In older infants, we have several times observed hemiplegias, first on one side then on the other, followed by hydrocephalus. The latter is present in about one-third of the cases. The CSF contains a moderate number of white blood cells, mostly lymphocytes and mononuclear cells, and increased protein in the range of 100 to 400 mg/dL. The glucose values are normal. Less than 10 percent of infected children recover. In these latter cases the infection must have been mild and soon burned itself out.

Granulomatous masses and zones of inflammatory necrosis abut on the ependyma or meninges. The organisms, 6 to 7 μm in length and 2 to 4 μm in width, are visible in and near the lesions. Microcysts may be found also, lying free in the tissues without inflammatory reaction. The necrotic lesions calcify rapidly and after several weeks or months are readily visible in plain films of the skull. These appear as periventricular and multiple nodular densities.

We have observed the disease coming on later in life—in childhood, adolescence, and even late adult years. Many instances are now being observed in patients with AIDS. It gives rise to a rapidly evolving meningitis and multifocal encephalitis in conjunction with myocarditis, hepatitis, and polymyositis. The latter syndrome is described on page 611 as are the diagnostic tests and treatment. In the infant, infections such as rubella, syphilis, cytomegalic inclusion disease, and herpes simplex must be considered in the differential diagnosis.

In women who develop antibodies in the first 2 or 3 months of pregnancy, treatment with spiramycine (Rovamycine) prevents fetal infection. Once the fetus is infected, one must resort to pyrimethamine and sulfadiazine, as described on page 585.

OTHER VIRAL AND BACTERIAL INFECTIONS

Several other infections of late fetal life or the neonatal period will only be mentioned here, for to describe them all would be tedious and would elucidate no new neurologic principles. Meningitis due to a small gram-positive rod, *Listeria monocytogenes,* may be acquired in the usual way, at the time of passage through an infected birth canal, or in utero, as a complication of maternal and fetal septicemia due to this organism. In the latter case, it causes abortion or premature delivery. *Neonatal meningitis* is a particularly devastating and often fatal type of bacterial infection, not easily diagnosed unless the pediatrician is alert to the possibility of a silent meningitis in every case of neonatal infection (page 558).

Herpes simplex encephalitis may destroy large parts of the brain, particularly of the temporal lobes, and is frequently fatal. Coxsackie B, polioviruses, and arboviruses (western equine) seem to be able to cross the placental barrier late in pregnancy and cause encephalitis or encephalomyelitis in the fetus at term which is indistinguishable from the disease in the very young infant.

Infectious mononucleosis is another not infrequent cause of meningoencephalitis. In some instances it may present as an aseptic meningitis or a Guillain-Barré type of acute polyneuritis. This disease is more apt to affect the nervous system of children than of adults. It is estimated that approximately 2 percent of children and adolescents with this disease have some type of neurologic dysfunction and rarely this will be the only manifestation of the disease (Friedland and Yahr). Stupor, chorea and aseptic meningitis were the main neurologic findings in the case reported by Friedland and Yahr and acute cerebellar ataxia and deafness in the case of Erzurum et al (see also Chaps. 32 and 33).

EPILEPSIES OF INFANCY AND CHILDHOOD

In Chap. 15 the major types of seizures were discussed in some detail. In bringing up this subject here, attention is drawn to the fact that epilepsy is mainly a disease of infancy and childhood. Approximately 75 percent of epileptics fall into these age periods, and some of the most interesting and unique types of seizure are peculiar to these epochs of life.

One principle that emerges is that the form taken by seizures in early life is in part age-linked. Neonatal seizures are predominantly partial or focal; infantile seizures take the form of myoclonic flexor (sometimes extensor) spasms; and petit mal is essentially a disease of childhood (4 to 13 years). Further, certain epileptic states tend to occur during certain epochs of life—febrile seizures from 6 months to 6 years and generalized or temporal spike-wave activity with benign motor and complex partial seizures from 6 to 16 years. In general, idiopathic epilepsy, so-called because the cause cannot be determined, is predominantly a pediatric neurologic problem. This is not to say that seizures of unknown cause do not occur in adult life, but rather that the proportion of such seizures is much greater in childhood and steadily diminishes once adulthood is reached.

The characteristics of certain forms of infantile and childhood seizures that are not observed in adult life—neonatal seizures, infantile spasms, febrile seizures, typical and atypical petit mal, acquired aphasia with convulsive disorder, and so-called rolandic epilepsy—have been fully described in Chap. 15.

MENTAL RETARDATION

In reconsidering this subject (see also Chap. 28), it is important to emphasize that only a small proportion (about 10 percent) of cases of mental retardation—representing the most severely retarded—can be traced to the congenital anomalies of development and related disorders that have been reviewed in the preceding pages. When these patients are studied clinically, a reasonably accurate diagnosis of the brain disease can be made in almost half of them. According to Penrose, chromosome abnormalities account for 15 percent, single gene disorders for 7 percent, and environmental factors for 20 percent; no cause could be found for the remaining cases. Males outnumber females 3:1.

When the cerebra of the severely retarded are examined by conventional histopathologic methods, gross lesions are found in approximately 90 percent of cases and in fully three-quarters of them an etiologic diagnosis is possible. Interestingly, the destructive vascular and hypoxic-ischemic lesions and other diseases (chromosomal, metabolic, and genetic) that are found in this group, are much the same as would be found if the group had been selected on the basis of cerebral palsy rather than severe mental retardation (see Table 44-3). Noteworthy is the fact that the cerebra in the remaining 10 percent of the "pathologically retarded" are grossly and microscopically normal; it is a remarkable fact that current technology does not enable the neuropathologist to visualize a lesion which had caused a lifelong idiocy.

Here it is important to repeat a point made in Chap. 28, that the large majority of mentally retarded persons does not have recognizable cerebral pathology, or exhibit any of the familiar and conventional symptoms and signs of cerebral disease. For this reason, some physicians do not regard them as having disease of the brain, even though most informed individuals believe that the brain is the organ of the mind.

This less severely affected group of retarded persons represents the segment of the normal population that is the opposite of genius. On the gaussian curve of human intelligence they represent the lowest 3 percent (see Fig. 28-4), the group that lies between the second and third standard deviations from the mean. Lewis was one of the first to call attention to this large group of simple mental retardates, and he referred to them as *subcultural*. In many of the families other members of the same and previous generations are feebleminded or have other mental disorders

Table 44-3
Causes of severe and mild mental retardation in 1372 patients at the W. E. Fernald State School

| Disease category | Number of patients | | Percent of all patients |
	IQ<50	IQ>50	
Acquired destructive lesions	278	79	26.0
Chromosomal abnormalities	247	10	18.7
Multiple congenital anomalies	64	16	5.8
Developmental abnormality of brain	49	16	4.7
Metabolic and endocrine diseases	38	5	3.1
Progressive degenerative disease	5	7	0.9
Neurocutaneous diseases	4	0	0.3
Psychosis	7	6	1.0
Mentally retarded (cause unknown)	385	156	39.5

so that the term *familial* has been applied to the group. There are several types of hereditary mental retardation, but they have not been well-defined clinically or pathologically. Some of them are characterized by maldevelopment of the cerebral cortex. Again males, in general, tend to be affected more frequently than females, and there has arisen a recent interest in the "fragile X chromosome" which some geneticists hold accountable for at least part of this sex difference. Another probable mutation of one X chromosome results in the *Rett syndrome* of autism, dementia, ataxia, and loss of purposeful hand movements. None of the 35 cases reported by Hagberg et al were male. Presumably the abnormality is lethal to males. After normal general and psychomotor development up to the age of 7 to 18 months, deterioration begins and higher cerebral functions are lost. Epilepsy, a mild spastic paraparesis, and vasomotor disturbances in the legs are late findings. The cause is unknown. Some of the translocations and deletions of parts of chromosomes are also found in this group of familial retardates. Nevertheless, it appears that factors other than purely genetic ones are operative in this "subcultural" group. The majority come from families in the lowest social and economic strata. A high incidence of prematurity and complicated births, exposure to toxic substances such as lead, and undernutrition also characterize this group. Of course, these factors may affect only a single child in a family.

The factor of *malnutrition* as a worldwide cause of mental retardation has received considerable attention in recent years. Animal experiments (Winick) demonstrate that severe undernutrition in early life will lead to biochemical and morphologic changes in the brain and behavioral abnormalities, and these may be permanent (see Chap. 39). However, the data proving that human mental retardation is widely caused by malnutrition is far from convincing. Although there seems to be little doubt that severe protein-calorie deficiency in the first 8 months of life may retard mental development, the authors are more impressed with the ability of the nervous system to resist the effects of nutritional deficiency, perhaps better than any other organ. Examples abound of infantile cachexia, as in cystic fibrosis, where, after a lag in development, dietary supplementation has resulted in rapid improvement in functioning of the nervous system—"catching up" to normal—and a spurt of brain and head growth, even with temporary separation of sutures. In most of the groups of malnourished children who remain feebleminded it has not been possible to separate the effects of polygenic inheritance, impoverished environment, and infectious disease.

The action of exogenous toxins during pregnancy or early infancy is another factor to be considered. It has been suggested that low-grade lead intoxication in utero or during infancy, insufficient to cause flagrant lead encephalopathy, may be associated with a lowering of IQ, but so far much of the evidence is statistical (Bellinger et al). Kalter and Warkany, however, state that they know of no evidence linking lead exposure to the development of human congenital malformations. Severe maternal alcoholism has been linked to a dysgenetic syndrome (see Chap. 41, under fetal alcohol syndrome). Surprisingly, maternal addiction to opiates, while causing withdrawal symptoms in the infant for weeks or even months (Wilson et al), seems not to result in permanent injury to the nervous system. However, such children have been observed for an insufficient length of time to be sure of this. Trimethadione, when taken as an anticonvulsant during pregnancy, is said to cause a slight increase in the incidence of mental retardation; phenytoin is reported to have no effect on mental development but does result in a slight (two- to threefold) incidence of cleft-lip and palate and other selected congenital malformations (page 269).

In all the aforementioned conditions the neuropathology is essentially unknown. For the most part the cases fall into the category of mental retardation without morphologic changes, akin to the 10 percent of the severely retarded with normal brains and to practically all of the less severely retarded. As indicated in Chap. 28 (page 475), there is now an active interest in devising new cytopathologic methods for exposing the defect which must surely have a structural component.

As an aid to the pediatrician and neurologist who must assume responsibility for the diagnosis and management of backward children, the following descriptions may be of some value. The differentiation of the various classes of mental backwardness by clinical criteria is facilitated if they are subdivided into the dysmorphic, the neurologic, the systemic, and the simple, or uncomplicated (see Table 44-4 for a framework of reference).

Table 44-4
Types of mental retardation

I. Mental defect with associated developmental abnormalities in nonnervous structures
    A. Those affecting cranioskeletal structures
        1. Microcephaly
        2. Macrocephaly
        3. Hydrocephalus (including myelomeningocele with Arnold-Chiari malformation and associated cerebral anomalies)
        4. Down syndrome (mongolism)
        5. Cretinism (congenital hypothyroidism)
        6. Mucopolysaccharidoses (Hurler, Hunter, and Sanfilippo types)
        7. Acrocephalosyndactyly (craniostenosis)
        8. Arthrogryposis multiplex congenita (in certain cases)
        9. Rare specific syndromes: De Lange
        10. Dwarfism, short stature: Russell-Silver dwarf, Seckel bird-headed dwarf, Rubinstein-Taybi dwarf, Cockayne-Neel dwarf, etc.
        11. Hypertelorism, median cleft face syndromes, agenesis of corpus callosum
    B. Those affecting nonskeletal structures
        1. Neurocutaneous syndromes: tuberous sclerosis, Sturge-Weber, neurofibromatosis (uncommon)
        2. Congenital rubella syndrome (deafness, blindness, congenital heart disease, small stature)
        3. Chromosomal disorders: Down syndrome, some cases of Klinefelter syndrome (XXY), XYY, Turner (XO) syndrome (occasionally), and others.
        4. Laurence-Moon-Biedl syndrome (retinitis pigmentosa, obesity, polydactyly)
        5. Eye disorders: toxoplasmosis (chorioretinitis), galactosemia (cataract), congenital rubella
        6. Prader-Willi syndrome (obesity, hypogenitalism)
II. Mental defect without developmental anomalies in nonnervous structures, but with focal cerebral and other neurologic abnormalities.
    A. Cerebral spastic diplegia
    B. Cerebral hemiplegia, unilateral or bilateral
    C. Congenital choreoathetosis or ataxia
        1. Kernicterus
        2. Status marmoratus
    D. Congenital ataxia
    E. Congenital atonic diplegia
    F. Syndromes resulting from hypoglycemia, trauma, meningitis, and encephalitis
    G. Associated with other neuromuscular abnormalities (muscular dystrophy, Friedreich ataxia, etc.)
    H. Cerebral degenerative diseases (lipidoses)
    I. Lesch-Nyhan syndrome
    J. Rett syndrome
III. Mental defect without signs of other developmental abnormality or neurologic disorder (epilepsy may or may not be present)
    A. Simple mental retardation, familial mental retardation, subcultural mental retardation
    B. Some cases of encephaloclastic disease (hypoxia, hypoglycemia)
    C. Infantile autism
    D. Associated with inborn errors of metabolism (phenylketonuria, other aminoacidurias, organic acidurias)
    E. Congenital infections (some cases of congenital syphilis, cytomegalic inclusion disease)

CLINICAL CHARACTERISTICS

Some of the clinical aspects of mental retardation, particularly of the "subcultural" type, have been discussed in Chap. 28. There it was pointed out that mental retardation manifests itself most obviously in the spheres of motor, language, social, and intellectual development. The severely retarded infant with an IQ of less than 20 (idiot level in the older classifications) often does not sit up, walk, or stand; and if any one of these motor activities is acquired, it appears late and is imperfectly performed. Language never develops; at most a few words are understood and fewer are uttered, or the patient vocalizes in a meaningless way. Such a patient is continuously idle and interacts little with people and objects in his or her surroundings. There is no effort to make known bodily needs for water, food, excretion, etc. Only the most primitive emotional reactions are exhibited. Physical growth is usually retarded, nutrition may be poor, and susceptibility to respiratory infections is increased. Sphincteric control may never be accomplished. A variety of physical deformities, particularly microcephaly, is common in this group; affections of the nervous system which have their onset later in life are usually not attended by bodily disfigurement.

If the mental defect is less pronounced [IQ of 20 to 45 (i.e., imbecile), or 45 to 70 (i.e., moron)], and if specific motor defects do not coexist, then sitting, walking, and speech are acquired, but only after a delay in many cases. The existence of a cerebral defect may be noted for the first time when the child fails to speak normally during the second and third years of life, and seems not to be able to learn the usual household and play activities as well as other children. However, delay in speech development must not by itself be taken as a mark of mental retardation, for some children who can obviously comprehend what is said to them and communicate by gesture are slow in talking. Also the deaf child may be singled out by an indifference to noise and reduced vocalization—but otherwise normal development. Toilet training also may be difficult to accomplish in the retarded child; but, again, it may be delayed in an otherwise normal child.

Within the spectrum of mental retardation, even within a group of persons of similar IQs, there are vast differences in overall behavioral functioning. Some retardates are pleasant and amiable, and achieve a rather satisfactory social adjustment; this is especially true of the subcultural group. At the opposite extreme is the ill-understood syndrome of autism, associated with varying degrees of retardation, in which the child or older person fails to manifest any kind of interpersonal, social contact—including communicative language—and demonstrates a limited interest in inanimate objects (see page 481). It is impossible to list all variations of mental retardation here, but the point should be made that all aspects of intellectual life and personality are affected in differing degrees. Many retarded individuals are dull, apathetic, and underactive. Others display an incessant hyperactivity, characterized by a very short attention span, a restless inquisitive searching of the environment, and low frustration tolerance; they may be destructive or recklessly fearless, and may seem strangely impervious to injury. Some display a peculiar *anhedonia* and are indifferent to either punishment or reward. Strangely, as with the mentally normal but hyperactive, inattentive child, improvement in these children can often be achieved by using amphetamines, methylphenidate, and related drugs. Other aberrant types of behavior, such as violent aggressiveness and even self-mutilation, are not uncommon, being many times more frequent than in the normal or nonmentally disabled child. Rhythmic rocking, rolling, head-banging, and bouncing movements are features of the motor activities of retarded persons, and may be performed hour after hour without fatigue, often to the accompaniment of bleating sounds, squeals, and other ejaculations. The retarded person can often suppress them when asked to do so, and they cease during other volitional movement. Here the abnormality is not the appearance of rhythmic movements of the body—which are to be observed at one period in the development of many normal children—but their persistence. Music may encourage rhythmic movement, and it gives pleasure to many retarded children and adults.

The least severely retarded individual (IQ of 45 to 70) grows and develops in many ways not different from normal ones, and can be taught useful occupational skills. A few of these persons can work under careful supervision. All scholastic pursuits are relatively unsuccessful, and vocational training is of more value than other types of education.

It is apparent that the clinical and behavioral characteristics of retarded individuals cannot be adequately described by a single parameter, the IQ; many other factors determine the social success of the retarded child and should give direction to the education and training of such a child. These include recognition of specific sensory or motor handicaps, such as blindness and deafness as well as athetosis or hemiplegia; specific language or speech deficits; behavioral disturbances, such as lack of socialization and hyperactivity; and the presence of seizures. Measures can be taken which help the handicapped person to compensate for these deficiencies. This becomes a primary consideration in functional diagnosis and in guiding the parents or guardians.

Lesser degrees of cognitive impairment and more

specific defects such as autism, partial autism, dyslexia, dyscalculia, learning defects, and hyperactivity also are believed to be expressions of certain abnormalities of brain structure and function. Some are caused by the same pathologic states that underlie cerebral palsy, epilepsy, and mental retardation. They have already been discussed in Chap. 28.

CONCLUSIONS

Viewed in their entirety these many genetic and acquired anomalies of development pose a formidable problem to medicine and science. In the United States, significant fetal abnormalities occur at a rate of about 3 percent of live births and a large but imprecisely determined number of individuals are lost to spontaneous abortion or stillbirth.

As regards the disease processes themselves, once they have acted to prevent development or to destroy the immature brain, little or nothing can be done medically. The lesion is completed. If the pathologic process is encountered in a stage of evolution, further damage can sometimes be prevented by effective therapy. An objective of more fundamental importance is the identification of pathogenic factors and their control or elimination as ways of preventing cerebral maldevelopment or injury before they occur.

A number of maternal health factors have been recognized within recent years as having injurious effects on the fetal brain. Rubella is now being controlled by vaccination of all young women or girls before the child-bearing age. Congenital syphilis has been eliminated almost completely by widespread serologic testing and by treatment of all syphilitic women in the first half of pregnancy. Kernicterus has been greatly reduced by preventing high degrees of bilirubinemia. Although more than 50 medications are suspect as fetal pathogens, only thalidomide, folic acid antagonists, steroid hormones, and alcohol are convincingly dangerous. Evidence of others being harmful may be forthcoming, and until such time it seems advisable for the pregnant woman to take only those drugs that are absolutely essential to her health. The same must be said of street drugs, which may possess teratogenic effects. Smoking diminishes the birth weight of neonates by more than 150 g, but whether this predisposes to cerebral damage is uncertain. Nutritional deficiency is surely associated with an increase of associated disease and subnormal mentality and should be corrected at all costs.

In mothers of advanced age or with diseases that place the fetus at risk, amniocentesis before the twentieth week of fetal life is advisable. The information which it yields at least warns of the possibility of disease in the neonate and offers the option of abortion. This is but a glimpse of future prospects. Increasing knowledge of the specific defects that underlie the congenital and hereditary diseases and newer methods (e.g., fetoscopy) for the direct measurement of these defects promise to control and eliminate many congenital diseases.

REFERENCES

ADAMS RD: Neurocutaneous diseases, in Fitzpatrick TB et al (eds): *Dermatology in General Medicine*, 3rd ed. New York, McGraw-Hill, 1987, chap 172, pp 2022–2062.

AICARDI J, LEFEBVRE J, LERIQUE-KOECHLIN A: A new syndrome: Spasm in flexion, callosal agenesis, ocular abnormalities. *Electroencephalogr Clin Neurophysiol* 19:609, 1965.

ANNEGERS JF, HAUSER WA, ELVEBACK LP, KURLAND LT: The risk of epilepsy following febrile convulsions. *Neurology* 29:297, 1979.

BAKER RS, ROSS PA, BAUMAN RJ: Neurologic complications of the epidermal nevus syndrome. *Arch Neurol* 44:227, 1987.

BANKER BQ: Cerebral vascular disease in infancy and childhood. 1. Occlusive vascular disease. *J Neuropathol Exp Neurol* 20:127, 1961.

BANKER BQ, BRUCE-GREGORIOS J: Neuropathology, in Thompson GH et al (eds): *Comprehensive Management of Cerebral Palsy*. New York, Grune & Stratton, 1983, chap 4, pp 25–31.

BANKER BQ, LARROCHE J-C: Periventricular leukomalacia of infancy. *Arch Neurol* 7:386, 1962.

BARKER E, WRIGHT K, NGUYEN K et al: Gene for von Recklinghausen neurofibromatosis in the pericentromeric region of chromosome 17. *Science* 236: 1100, 1987.

BARLOW CF: *Mental Retardation and Related Disorders*. Philadelphia, Davis, 1978.

BELLINGER D, LEVITON A, WATERNAUX C et al: Longitudinal analyses of prenatal and postnatal lead exposure and early cognitive development. *N Engl J Med* 316:1037, 1987.

BENSON JWI, HAYWARD C, OSBORNE J et al: Multicentre trial of ethamsylate for prevention of periventricular hemorrhage in very low birth weight infants. *Lancet* 2:1297, 1986.

BIELSCHOWSKY M: Über tuberöse Sklerose und ihre Beziehungen zur Recklinghausenschen Krankheit. *Z Gesamte Neurol Psychiatr* 26:133, 1914.

BRADLEY WG, RICHARDSON J, FREW IJC: The familial association of neurofibromatosis, peroneal muscular atrophy, congenital deafness, partial albinism and Axenfeld's defect. *Brain* 97:521, 1974.

CANALE D, BEBIN J, KNIGHTON RS: Neurologic manifestations of von Recklinghausen's disease of the nervous system. *Confin Neurol* 24:359, 1964.

CHAPLIN ER, GOLDSTEIN GW, MYERBERG DZ et al: Posthemorrhagic hydrocephalus in the preterm infant. *Pediatrics* 65:901, 1980.

CHAPMAN PH, DAVIS KR: Surgical treatment of spinal lipomas in childhood, in Raimondi AJ (ed): *Concepts in Pediatric Neurosurgery.* Munich, S. Karger, 1983.

CHAPMAN PH: Congenital intraspinal lipomas. Anatomic considerations and surgical treatment. *Child's Brain* 9:37, 1982.

COBB S: Haemangioma of the spinal cord associated with skin naevi of the same metamere. *Ann Surg* 62:641, 1915.

COGAN DC: A type of congenital ocular motor apraxia presenting jerky head movements. *Trans Am Acad Ophthalmol* 56:853, 1952.

COWAN D, WOLF A, PAIGE BH: Toxoplasmic encephalomyelitis. VI: Clinical diagnosis of infantile or congenital toxoplasmosis; survival beyond infancy. *Arch Neurol Psychiatry* 48:689, 1942.

CROWE FW: Axillary freckling as a diagnostic aid in neurofibromatosis. *Ann Intern Med* 61:1142, 1964.

CROWE FW, SCHULL WJ, NEEL JV: *A Clinical, Pathological and Genetic Study of Multiple Neurofibromatosis.* Springfield, IL, Charles C Thomas, 1956.

DENNIS J: Neonatal convulsions: aetiology, late neonatal status and long-term outcome. *Dev Med Child Neurol* 20:143, 1978.

DYKEN P, KRAWIECKI N: Neurodegenerative diseases of infancy and childhood. *Ann Neurol* 13:351, 1983.

ELDRIDGE R: Central neurofibromatosis with bilateral acoustic neuroma, in Riccardi VM, Mulvihill JJ (eds): *Advances in Neurology,* vol 29, *Neurofibromatosis (Von Recklinghausen Disease).* New York, Raven Press, 1981, pp 57–65.

ERZURUM S, KALAVSKY SM, WATANAKUNAKORN C: Acute cerebellar ataxia and hearing loss as initial symptoms of infectious mononucleosis. *Arch Neurol* 40:760, 1983.

FENICHEL GM: Hypoxic-ischemic encephalopathy in the newborn. *Arch Neurol* 40:261, 1983.

FENICHEL GM: *Neonatal Neurology,* 2nd ed. New York, Churchill Livingstone, 1985.

FITZPATRICK TB, SZABO G, HORI Y et al: White leaf-shaped macules, earliest visible sign of tuberous sclerosis. *Arch Dermatol* 98:1, 1968.

FORD FR: *Diseases of the Nervous System in Infancy, Childhood and Adolescence,* 6th ed. Springfield, Illinois, Charles C Thomas, 1973.

FRIEDLAND R, YAHR MD: Meningoencephalopathy secondary to infectious mononucleosis: Unusual presentation with stupor and chorea. *Arch Neurol* 34:186, 1977.

GARCIA CA, DUNN D, TREVOR R: The lissencephaly (agyria) syndrome in siblings. *Arch Neurol* 35:608, 1978.

GASTAUT H, POIRIER F, PAYAN H et al: H.H.E. syndrome: Hemiconvulsion, hemiplegia, epilepsy. *Epilepsia* 1:418, 1960.

GOLD AP, FREEMAN JM: Depigmented nevi, the earliest sign of tuberous sclerosis. *Pediatrics* 35:1003, 1965.

GOMEZ MR: *Neurocutaneous Disease (a Practical Approach).* Boston, Butterworth, 1987.

GOMEZ MR: *Tuberous Sclerosis.* New York, Raven Press, 1979.

GOMEZ MR, KUNTZ NL, WESTMORELAND BF: Tuberous sclerosis, early onset of seizures, and mental subnormality: Study of discordant homozyous twins. *Neurology* 32:604, 1982.

GORLIN RS, PINDBORG JJ, COHEN MM JR: *Syndromes of the Head and Neck.* New York, McGraw-Hill, 1976.

GREGG NM: Congenital cataract following German measles in the mother. *Trans Ophthalmol Soc Australia* 3:35, 1941.

HAGBERG B, AICARDI J, DIAS K et al: A progressive syndrome of autism, dementia, ataxia and loss of purposeful hand movements in girls. Rett's syndrome. *Ann Neurol* 14:471, 1983.

HALPERIN JJ, WILLIAMS RS, KOLODNY EH: Microcephaly vera, progressive motor neuron disease and nigral degeneration. *Neurology* 32:317, 1982.

HANSHAW JB: Congenital cytomegalovirus infection: A fifteen year perspective. *J Infect Dis* 123:555, 1971.

HARDY JB: Clinical and developmental aspects of congenital rubella. *Arch Otolaryngol* 98:230, 1973.

HENDERSON JL: The congenital facial diplegia syndrome: Clinical features, pathology and etiology. *Brain* 62:381, 1939.

HERSKOWITZ J, ROSMAN P, WHEELER CB: Colpocephaly: Clinical, radiologic and pathogenetic aspects. *Neurology* 35:1594, 1985.

HOEFNAGEL D, PENRY JK: Partial facial paralysis in young children. *N Engl J Med* 262:1126, 1960.

HOLMES LB, MOSER HW, HALLDØRSSON S et al: *Mental Retardation: An Atlas of Diseases with Associated Physical Abnormalities.* New York, Macmillan, 1972.

JABLONSKI S: *Illustrated Dictionary of Eponymic Syndromes, and Diseases, and Their Synonyms.* Philadelphia, Saunders, 1969.

JOHNSON KP: Viral infections of the developing nervous system, in Thompson RA, Green JR (eds): *Advances in Neurology,* vol 6. New York, Raven Press, 1974, pp 53–67.

KALTER H, WARKANY J: Congenital malformations: Etiologic factors and their role in prevention. *N Engl J Med* 308:424, 1983.

KRISHNAMOORTHY KS, KUEHNLE KJ, TODRES ID, DELONG GR: Neurodevelopmental outcome of survivors with posthemorrhagic hydrocephalus following grade II neonatal intraventricular hemorrhage. *Ann Neurol* 15:201, 1984.

LEMIEUX BG, WRIGHT FS, SWAIMAN KF: Genetic and congenital structural defects of the brain and spinal cord, in Swaiman KF, Wright FS (eds): *The Practice of Pediatric Neurology,* 2nd ed. St Louis, Mosby, 1982, chap 24, pp 344–471.

LEVENE MI, GRINDULIS H, SANDS C, MOORE JR: Comparison of two methods of predicting outcome in perinatal asphyxia. *Lancet* I:67, 1986.

LEWIS EO: Types of mental deficiency and their social significance. *J Ment Sci* 79:298, 1933.

LICHTENSTEIN BW: Neurofibromatosis (Von Recklinghausen's disease of the nervous system). *Arch Neurol Psychiatry* 62:822, 1949.

LORBER J: Spina bifida cystica. Results of treatment of 270 cases with criteria for selection in the future. *Arch Dis Child* 47:854, 1972.

LORBER J, PRIESTLEY BL: Children with large heads: A practical approach to diagnosis in 557 children with special reference to 109 children with megalencephaly. *Dev Med Child Neurol* 23:494, 1981.

LYNN RB, BUCHANAN DC, FENICHEL GM, FREEMAN FR: Agenesis of the corpus callosum. *Arch Neurol* 37:444, 1980.

LYON G, EVRARD PH: *Neuropediatrie,* Masson, Paris, 1987.

Martuza RL, Eldridge R: Neurofibromatosis 2 (bilateral acoustic neurofibromatosis). *N Engl J Med* 318:684, 1988.

Milunsky A: Prenatal detection of neural tube defects. VI. Experience with 20,000 pregnancies. *JAMA* 244:2731, 1980.

Myers RE: Experimental models of perinatal brain damage: Relevance to human pathology, in Glueck L (ed): *Intrauterine Asphyxia and the Developing Fetal Brain.* Bethesda, MD, Year Book, 1977, pp 37–97.

Nelson KB, Ellenberg JH: Antecedents of cerebral palsy. *N Engl J Med* 315:81, 1986.

Pang D, Wilberger JE: Tethered cord syndrome in adults. *J Neurosurg* 57:32, 1982.

Penrose LS: *The Biology of Mental Defect.* New York, Grune & Stratton, 1949.

Purpura DP: Normal and aberrant neuronal development in the cerebral cortex of human fetus and young infant, in Buchwald NA, Brazier MA (eds): *Brain Mechanisms in Mental Retardation.* New York, Academic Press, 1975, pp 141–171.

Reynolds DW, Stango S, Stubbs KG et al: Inapparent congenital cytomegalovirus infection with elevated cord IgM levels: Causal relation with auditory and mental deficiency. *N Engl J Med* 290:291, 1974.

Riccardi VM: Von Recklinghausen neurofibromatosis. *N Engl J Med* 305:1617, 1981.

Riccardi VM, Mulvihill JJ (eds): *Advances in Neurology,* vol 29: *Neurofibromatosis (Von Recklinghausen Disease).* New York, Raven Press, 1981.

Roach ES, Williams OP, Laster DW: Magnetic resonance imaging in tuberous sclerosis. *Arch Neurol* 44:301, 1987.

Rosman NP, Pearce J: The brain in neurofibromatosis. *Brain* 90:829, 1967.

Rouleau GA, Wertelecki W, Haines JL et al: Genetic linkage of bilateral acoustic neurofibromatosis to a DNA marker on chromosome 22. *Nature* 329:246, 1987.

Schreier H, Rapin I, Davis J: Familial megalencephaly or hydrocephalus? *Neurology* 24:232, 1974.

Shuman RM, Selednik LJ: Periventricular leukomalacia. *Arch Neurol* 37:231, 1980.

Sinha S, Davies J, Toner N et al: Vitamin E supplementation reduces frequency of periventricular hemorrhage in very premature babies. *Lancet* 1:466, 1987.

Solomon LM, Esterley NB: Epidermal and other congenital organoid nevi. *Curr Prob Pediatr* 6:1, 1975.

van der Hoeve J: Eye symptoms of tuberous sclerosis of the brain. *Trans Ophthalmol Soc UK* 40:329, 1920.

Volpe JJ: *Neurology of the Newborn,* 2nd ed. Philadelphia, Saunders, 1986.

Weber F Parkes: Association of extensive haemangiomatous naevus of skin with cerebral (meningeal) haemangioma, especially cases of facial vascular naevus with contralateral hemiplegia. *Proc R Soc Med* 22:25, 1929.

Weller TH: Cytomegaloviruses: The difficult years. *J Infect Dis* 122:532, 1970.

Weller TH: The cytomegaloviruses: Ubiquitous agents with protean clinical manifestations. *N Engl J Med* 285:267, 1971.

Wilson GS, Desmond MM, Verniand W: Early development of infants of heroin-addicted mothers. *Am J Dis Child* 126:457, 1973.

Winick M: *Malnutrition and Brain Development.* New York, Oxford University Press, 1976.

Wohlwill FJ, Yakovlev PI: Histopathology of meningofacial angiomatosis (Sturge-Weber's disease). *J Neuropathol Exp Neurol* 16:341, 1957.

Wyburn-Mason R: *Vascular Abnormalities and Tumors of the Spinal Cord and Its Membranes.* St. Louis, Mosby, 1944.

Yakovlev PI, Guthrie RH: Congenital ectodermoses (neurocutaneous syndromes) in epileptic patients. *Arch Neurol Psychiatry* 26:1145, 1931.

Yakovlev PI, Wadsworth RC: Schizencephalies. A study of the congenital clefts in the cerebral mantle. *J Neuropathol Exp Neurol* 5:116, 169, 1946.

DISEASES OF PERIPHERAL NERVE AND MUSCLE

CHAPTER 45

LABORATORY AIDS IN THE DIAGNOSIS OF NEUROMUSCULAR DISEASE

The clinical suspicion of neuromuscular disease, evinced by the recognition of any one of the symptoms or syndromes that will be discussed in the succeeding chapters, now finds ready confirmation in the laboratory. The intelligent use of the laboratory requires some knowledge of the biochemistry and physiology of muscle fiber contraction, nerve action potentials, and neuromuscular conduction. These subjects will therefore be reviewed briefly, as an introduction to the descriptions of the laboratory methods and findings.

BIOCHEMISTRY AND PHYSIOLOGY OF NEUROMUSCULAR DISEASE

Biochemical tests in common use include the measurement of serum electrolytes and enzymes and the detection of myoglobin in the blood and urine. Also, in certain circumstances, measurements of urinary creatine and creatinine may be useful. The quantitative measurement of certain essential constituents of muscle (carnitine, carnitine palmityl transferase, phosphorylase, acid maltase, phosphofructokinase) is now possible by application of microchemical methods to small pieces of muscle taken at biopsy. Abnormalities of these constituents have proved to be specific for certain myopathies, and will be mentioned in the sections that deal with these particular diseases.

ELECTROLYTES AND NEUROMUSCULAR ACTIVITY

This is not the place to review all the biochemical and biophysical data that explain nerve impulse formation and conduction. Since the early studies of Hodgkin (1951) and of Hodgkin and Huxley (1952), tomes have been written on these subjects. Suffice it to say that the nerve and muscle fibers, like other bodily cells, maintain a fluid internal environment that is distinctly different from the external or interstitial medium. The main intracellular constituents are

potassium (K), magnesium (Mg), and phosphorus (P), whereas those outside the cell are sodium (Na), calcium (Ca), and chloride (Cl). In both nerve and muscle the intracellular concentrations of these ions are held within a narrow range by electrical and chemical forces, which maintain the membranes in electrochemical equilibrium (*"resting membrane potential"*). These forces are the result of selective permeability of the membranes to various ions and the continuous expulsion of intracellular Na by a pump mechanism ("the sodium pump"). The function of the pump mechanism is dependent on the enzyme Na-K ATPase, which is localized in the membranes. The resulting electrochemical equilibrium is such that the inside of the cell is kept negative in respect to the outside by a potential difference of 70 to 90 mV.

This resting membrane potential shows an interesting dependence on the concentrations of K and Na. The interior of the cell is some 30 times richer in K than the extracellular fluid, and the concentration of Na is 10 to 12 times greater in the extracellular fluid. In the resting state the chemical forces that promote diffusion of K ions out of the cell (down their concentration gradient) are counterbalanced by electrical forces (the external positivity opposes further diffusion of K to the outside). At the resting potential, the situation of Na ions is the opposite; they tend to diffuse into the cell, both because of their concentration gradient and because of the relative negativity inside the cell. Because the membrane is less permeable to Na than to K, the amount of K leaving the cell exceeds the amount of Na entering the cell, thus creating the difference in charge across the membrane (the outside of the cell is positive relative to the inside).

The permeability of the cell membrane to Na is controlled by the electrical potential of the membrane. As the latter is depolarized by slight electrical or chemical change, there is an increased permeability to Na. The subsequent movement of K outward repolarizes the membrane and thereby reduces its permeability to Na. These slight fluxes of ions in the resting state are known as *passive decay*. If a greater degree of depolarization occurs, a situation arises in which the outward movement of K is unable to stabilize the membrane. It then becomes even more depolarized and progressively more permeable to Na, and an "explosive" regenerative Na current develops; Na rushes down its chemical and electrical gradients into the cell. Eventually an equilibrium potential is reached where the interior of the cell becomes about 40 mV positive. This is the *action potential* and it lasts only a millisecond or less before the membrane loses its permeability to Na and becomes much more permeable to K. The resulting efflux of K repolarizes the membrane to a resting level. During this time the nerve and muscle fibers are refractory, at first absolutely then relatively, to another depolarizing stimulus. If the process of recovery is delayed, this *depolarization inactivation* prevents the development of further action potentials until the membrane regains its resting potential.

Action currents in the axon and muscle cell occur when one region of the membrane becomes depolarized. As the action currents flow into the depolarized zone, the contiguous membrane becomes depolarized; the depolarization may reach the threshold for development of an action potential, and a new zone of increased Na permeability then spreads in this way, in an all-or-none fashion, down the length of the nerve or muscle membrane. This is the *conducted action potential* (see Kuffler et al for further details).

As the motor nerve impulse passes centrifugally from the parent axon into its terminal branches, transmission "breaks down," especially if the repetition rate is excessive and impulses arrive too frequently at branch points. Impulses may then fail to be transmitted across the myoneural junction. This happens in certain peripheral neuropathies (Guillain-Barré syndrome) and in myasthenia gravis and may result in an EMG picture indistinguishable from that of a myopathy (see further on).

These events, the hallmarks of all excitable tissues, are clearly influenced by the concentration of K ions in the extracellular fluids.

THE NEUROMUSCULAR JUNCTION (MOTOR END PLATE)

This interface between the finely branched nerve fiber and the muscle fiber, where nervous activity is translated into muscle action, has special properties (Figs. 45-1 and 45-2). The nerve fiber, as it indents the muscle cell membrane, always leaves a *synaptic cleft* between the axolemma and

sarcolemma (Fig. 45-2). Relatively fixed numbers of molecules (quanta) of acetylcholine (ACh) in the nerve terminals, liberated by the arrival of action potentials, diffuse into the synaptic cleft and attach to the receptor sites on the sarcolemma. Calcium ions facilitate this release, whereas botulinus toxin and a high concentration of Mg ions interfere with it. ACh is the chemical transmitter. It is bound by the ACh receptor protein and acts on the postsynaptic part of the motor end plate by causing a local increase in the conductance of Na and K and other small ions. It produces a depolarization known as the *end-plate potential*. Small end-plate potentials are continuously formed and regenerated as the membranes repolarize, similar to the process of passive decay described above. If ACh release exceeds a certain threshold (if hundreds of quanta of ACh are released), an independent all-or-nothing muscle action potential spreads up and down the muscle membrane, much like the nerve action potential. The sarcolemma, once depolarized, is refractory to another action potential until repolarized. Molecules of ACh combine with cholinesterase at receptor sites and are hydrolyzed.

THE CHEMISTRY OF MUSCLE CONTRACTION

The plasmalemma (the plasma membrane of the sarcolemma), the transverse tubules, and the sarcoplasmic reticulum each play a role in the control of the activity of muscle fibers. The structural components involved in excitation, contraction and relaxation of muscle are illustrated in Fig. 45-3. Following nerve stimulation, an action potential is transmitted by the plasmalemma from the motor end-plate region to both ends of the muscle fiber. Depolarization spreads quickly to the interior of the fiber along the walls of the transverse tubules, probably by a conducted action potential. The transverse tubules and the terminal cisternae of the sarcoplasmic reticulum come into close proximity at points referred to as *triads*. Here, by a mechanism that is not understood, depolarization of the transverse tubules is transmitted to the sarcoplasmic reticulum, which releases Ca stored in its interior. Ca binds to the regulatory protein, *troponin*, thereby removing the inhibition exerted by the troponin-tropomyosin system upon the contractile protein, *actin*. This allows an interaction to take place between the actin molecules of the thin filaments and the cross bridges of the myosin molecules in the thick filaments and enables myosin adenosine triphosphatase (ATPase) to split adenosine triphosphate (ATP) at a rapid rate, thereby providing the energy for contraction. This chemical change produces a force that causes the filaments to slide past each other. Relaxation occurs as a result of active (energy-dependent) Ca reuptake by the sarcoplasmic reticulum.

The pyrophosphate bonds of ATP, which supply the energy for muscle contraction, must be replenished constantly by a reaction that involves interchanges with the muscle phosphagen, creatine diphosphate, where high-energy phosphate bonds are stored. These interactions, in both contraction and relaxation, require the action of creatine kinase (CK). Myoglobin, another important muscle protein, functions in the transfer of oxygen, and a series of oxidative enzymes are involved in this exchange. The intracellular Ca, as noted above, is released by the muscle action potential and must be reaccumulated within the cisternae before actin and myosin filaments can slide back past one another in relaxation. The reuptake of Ca requires the expenditure of considerable energy. When ATP is lacking, the muscle remains shortened, as in the *contracture* of phosphorylase deficiency (McArdle disease) or phospho-fructose kinase deficiency. The same sort of shortening occurs under normal conditions in some of the "catch muscles" of certain mollusks and is the basis of rigor mortis in mammals.

Many glycolytic and other enzymes (transaminases, aldolase, CK) are also implicated in the metabolic activity of muscle, particularly under relatively anaerobic conditions. Muscle fibers differ in their relative content of oxidative and glycolytic enzymes; the latter determine the capacity of the muscle fiber to sustain anaerobic metabolism

during periods of contraction with inadequate blood flow. Muscle cells rich in oxidative enzymes contain more mitochondria and larger amounts of myoglobin (appear red), have slower rates of contraction and relaxation, fire more tonically, and are less fatigable than muscle fibers poor in oxidative enzymes. The latter fire in bursts and are utilized in quick phasic rather than sustained postural reactions. The amount of myosin ATPase activity, which governs the speed of contraction, is low in oxidative-rich fibers and high in glycolytic-rich fibers. The Ca-activated myosin ATPase stain at pH 9.4 has been used to classify these two types of fibers in microscopic sections. Type I (oxidative-rich) fibers have a low content of myosin ATPase, and type II (phosphorylative-rich) fibers have a high content of this enzyme; hence type I fibers stain lightly and type II darkly (the reverse reaction occurs at pH 4.6). Other less well-differentiated histochemical types have also been identified. All the fibers within one motor unit are of the same type.

The chemical energy required to maintain the various activities of the muscle cell is derived mainly from the metabolism of carbohydrate (blood glucose, muscle glycogen) and fatty acids (plasma free fatty acids, esterified fatty acids, and ketone bodies). There is a lesser contribution from branched chain and other amino acids, but it may increase with prolonged exercise.

The most readily available source of energy is glycogen, which is synthesized and stored in muscle cells. It provides over 90 percent of the energy needs of muscle under conditions of high work intensity and during the early stages of submaximal exercise. Blood glucose and free fatty acids supplement intracellular glycogen as exercise proceeds. The free fatty acids are obtained from endogenous triglycerides (found mostly in type I fibers), from the triglycerides released by circulating lipoproteins, and from

Figure 45-1

Motor end plate showing relationship between various structures in nerve and muscle. Last segment of myelin, with Schwann nucleus (S), terminates abruptly, leaving axis cylinder covered by sheaths of Schwann and Henle. End-plate nuclei (EP) of muscle fiber lie embedded in sarcoplasm and have same staining reactions as sarcolemmal nuclei (M). Ramifications of axis cylinder (telodendria) lie in grooves or pouches in granular sarcoplasm, each lined by spiny "subneural apparatus" of Couteaux, which is continuous with membranous sarcolemma and also Schwann membrane. Nucleus (S) of sheath of Schwann commonly lies near point of branching of axon. Sheath of Henle has small nuclei (H) and fuses with endomysial sheath of muscle fiber. (Courtesy of D Denny-Brown.)

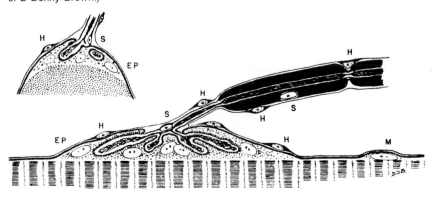

the lipolysis of adipose tissue. Most of the energy needs of resting muscle are provided by fatty acids.

The enzymatic reactions involved in the transport of these substrates into muscle cells and their intracellular synthesis and degradation during anaerobic and aerobic cell conditions have been thoroughly investigated and most of the enzymes identified. This subject is too complicated to present in a textbook of neurology. Detailed information can be found in the review by Morgan-Hughes. Enough is known about these matters to state confidently that a number of diseases can impair the contractile functions of muscle in different ways without destroying the fiber. Specific enzymatic defects under genetic control may affect carbohydrate utilization (myophosphorylase deficiencies, de-

Figure 45-2

Normal human end plate. The nerve terminal with its synaptic vesicles is seen in upper and central part of picture. The adjacent nucleus is that of a Schwann cell. Below the nerve terminal the postsynaptic region is composed of folds and clefts. The synaptic space contains homogeneous material. The line indicates 1 μm. × 30,000. (From Engel et al.)

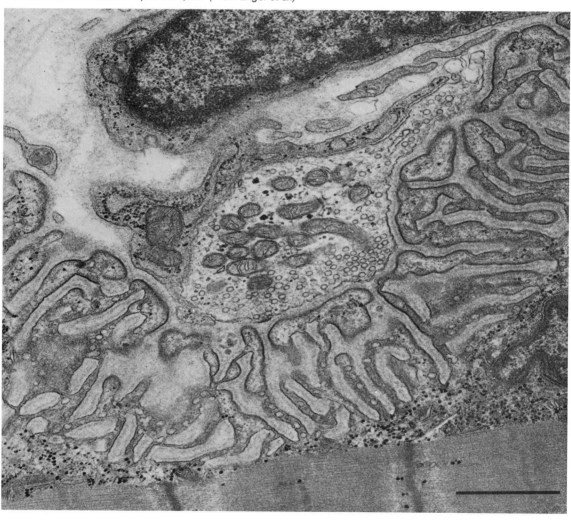

brancher enzyme deficiencies, phosphofructokinase deficiency, phosphoglyceromutase deficiency, and myoadenylate deaminase deficiency), fatty acid utilization (carnitine and carnitine palmityl transferase deficiencies), pyruvate metabolism, and cytochrome oxidase activity. These will be discussed in later chapters.

The mechanical events of muscle contraction (twitch) last much longer than the action potential and depend upon the following factors: (1) an end-plate potential of sufficient magnitude to produce a muscle action potential, (2) the availability and rate of release of Ca ions from the sarcoplasmic reticulum, (3) the rate of hydrolysis of ATP, (4)

the rate of sarcomere shortening, (5) the elasticity of the muscle fiber and surrounding connective tissues, and (6) the rate of reuptake of Ca ions by the sarcoplasmic reticulum. Factors (2) and (3) affect the latency of onset of the twitch (i.e., the interval between the action potential and beginning of contraction); (4) and (5) determine the velocity of rise to peak tension at a given length; and (6) determines the duration of the twitch (viz., the period of full tetanic tension

Figure 45-3

Schematic illustration of the major subcellular components of a myofibril. The transverse (T) system, which is an invagination of the plasma membrane of the cell, surrounds the myofibril midway between the Z lines and the center of the A bands; the T system is approximated to, but apparently not continuous with, dilated elements (terminal cisternae) of the sarcoplasmic reticulum on either side. Thus, each sarcomere (the repeating Z-line-to-Z-line unit) contains two "triads," each composed of a pair of terminal cisternae on each side of the T tubule. (From Peter.)

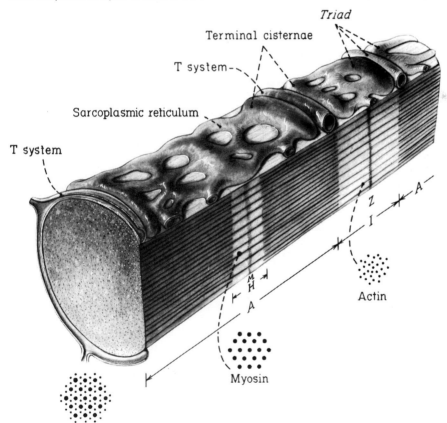

attained during the twitch). The total twitch time is the sum of all the above plus the time required for the twitch to be transmitted to the tendon.

If a second muscle action potential arrives after the refractory phase of the previous action potential but before the muscle has relaxed, the contraction will be prolonged. Thus, at frequencies of anterior horn cell firing of 40 to 50 per s, the twitches fuse into a sustained contraction or *tetanus*. In this fashion the mechanical phenomena are smoothed into a continuous process, even though the electrical potentials present as a series of depolarizations, separated by intervals during which the muscle membrane resumes its resting polarized state.

At the motor end plate, repolarization is possible only if ACh is inactivated. This is accomplished by acetylcholinesterase, which is located at the receptor site on the muscle fiber. If this chemical reaction does not occur, the end plate remains depolarized and therefore is unable to respond to further nerve impulses. Anticholinesterase drugs, such as neostigmine (Prostigmine), pyridostigmine (Mestinon), edrophonium (Tensilon), physostigmine (Eserine), succinylcholine, decamethonium, diisopropyl fluorophosphate (DFP), tetraethylpyrophosphate (TEPP), and several of the so-called nerve gases and pyrophosphate insecticides act in this way to paralyze muscle. These substances are called *depolarizing blocking agents* because they maintain the end-plate region in a depolarized state, refractory to activation by the arrival of successive action potentials (and quanta of ACh). The quaternary ammonium ions (such as curare) are called *competitive blocking agents* and paralyze muscles by occupying the receptor sites on the muscle fiber so that acetylcholine cannot reach them, thereby maintaining them in a nondepolarized state. Antibodies to the end-plate receptor protein (in myasthenia gravis) act in the same way.

Biochemical changes may cause not only an impairment of neuromuscular activity (paresis, paralysis) but also excessive irritability, tetany, spasm, and cramp. In the latter instances, spontaneous discharges may occur from an instability of axon polarization, hence a single nerve impulse may initiate a train of action potentials in nerve and muscle, as in the tetany of hypocalcemia and in idiopathic facial spasm. In tetany, there may also be paresthesias, on the basis of irritability of the neurilemma of sensory nerve fibers. The common cramps of calf and foot muscles (painful, sustained, contractions with motor unit discharges at frequencies up to 200 per second) may be due to increased excitability (or unstable polarization) of the motor axons. Quinine, procaine amide, diphenhydramine (Benadryl), and

warmth reduce the irritability of nerve and muscle fiber membranes.

To summarize, the muscle fiber, which is wholly dependent on the nerve for its stimulus to contract, may be physiologically paralyzed in a number of ways. The nerve may fail to conduct impulses; the neuromuscular junction may not release ACh, or once released, it may not be inactivated by cholinesterase; the receptor zone on the muscle cell may be blocked by a competing substance; the sarcolemma may not distribute the nerve impulse to all parts of the muscle fiber; and finally, the metabolic or contractile elements of the muscle may not react, or, once contracted, may not relax. Similarly, the mechanisms involved in fasciculations, cramps, and muscle spasms may be traced to a number of different loci in the neuromuscular apparatus. There may be an unstable polarization of the nerve fibers as in tetany and in dehydration with salt depletion, or unexplained hyperirritability of the motor fibers, as in amyotrophic lateral sclerosis. The threshold of mechanical activation or electrical reactivation of the sarcolemmal membrane may be reduced, as in myotonia; or, impairment of an energy mechanism within the fiber may slow the contractile process, as in hypothyroidism; or a deficiency of phosphorylase, which deprives muscle of its carbohydrate energy source, may prevent relaxation, as in the contracture of McArdle disease. By a mechanism not understood, lesions of the most peripheral branches of nerves may give rise to continuous activity of motor units. This is expressed clinically as a rippling of muscle known as *myokymia*.

In recent years, new technologies such as isolation of complementary DNA have made it possible to isolate each of the proteins involved in neuromuscular transmission and the excitation-contraction-relaxation of muscle fibers. And the amino acid composition of most of these proteins has been determined. This information is beginning to be applied to the analysis of gene products in the normal and diseased organism (see Fishbeck for a recent review of this subject). Other pertinent references will be found in the chapters that follow.

EFFECTS OF ABNORMALITIES OF SERUM ELECTROLYTES

Diffuse muscle weakness or the occurrence of muscle twitchings, spasms, and cramps, should always raise the question of a disorder of serum electrolytes. The latter reflect the concentrations of electrolytes in intra- and extracellular fluids. The ECG may reveal alterations of their intracellular levels in the heart. If the plasma level of *potassium falls below 2.5 meq/L or rises above 7 meq/L*, weakness of extremity and trunk muscles results. Below a level of 2 meq/L or above 9 meq/L, there is almost always flaccid paralysis of these muscles and later of the respiratory ones as well, only the extraocular and other cranial muscles being spared. In addition, the tendon reflexes are diminished or absent. The reaction of muscle to percussion is also reduced or abolished, suggesting impairment of transmission along the sarcolemmal membranes themselves. *Hypocalcemia* of 7 mg/dL or less (as in rickets or hypoparathyroidism) or relative reduction in the proportion of ionized calcium (as in hyperventilation) causes increased irritability and spontaneous discharge of sensory and motor nerve fibers, i.e., tetany, and sometimes convulsions from similar effects upon cerebral neurons; frequent repetitive and finally prolonged spontaneous discharges appear in the EMG, and convulsive effects are reflected in the EEG. *Hypercalcemia* above 12 mg/dL (as in vitamin D intoxication, hyperparathyroidism, and carcinomatosis) causes weakness and lethargy, perhaps on a central basis. *Reduction in the plasma concentration of magnesium* also results in tremor, muscle weakness, tetanic muscle spasms, and convulsions; a considerable *increase in magnesium levels* leads to muscle weakness and depression of central nervous function (confusion). The weakness of muscle may be due, in part at least, to reduced release of ACh at the motor end plate.

CHANGES IN SERUM LEVELS OF ENZYMES ORIGINATING IN MUSCLE CELLS

In all diseases causing extensive damage to striated muscle fibers, intracellular enzymes leak out of the fiber and enter the blood. Those being measured in most hospital laboratories are the transaminases, lactic acid dehydrogenase, aldolase, and creatine kinase (CK). Of these, the level of CK in serum has proved to be the most sensitive measure of muscle damage. Since high concentrations of this enzyme are found in heart muscle and brain, raised serum values may be due to myocardial or cerebral infarction as well as to the necrotizing diseases of striated muscle (polymyositis, muscle trauma, muscle infarction, paroxysmal myoglobinuria, and the more rapidly advancing muscular dystrophies). For serum CK levels to be interpretable, one has to be certain that heart or brain are undamaged. This can be determined by the quantitation of serum isoenzymes of CK. The isoenzymes are referred to as MB, MM, and BB (M—muscle, B—brain) and their measurement provides a more sensitive means for the detection of damage to myocardium, skeletal muscle, and nervous tissue, respectively.

The MM form of CK is found in highest concentration in striated muscle, but there is also 5 to 6 percent MB. Heart contains 17 to 59 percent MB; hence, in myocardial infarction, CK-MB is more than 6 percent. Embryonic and regenerating muscle contains more CK-MB. In patients with destructive lesions of striated muscle, serum values of CK often exceed 1000 units and may reach 40,000 units

or more (the upper limit of normal varies from 65 to 200 units, depending on the method). Even more interesting is its rise in some children with progressive muscular dystrophy before there is enough destruction of fibers for the disease to be clinically manifest, at least as judged by crude tests of muscle strength. Moreover, the unaffected female carrier of the Duchenne pseudohypertrophic form may often be identified by a slightly elevated serum level of CK. Alterations of serum enzyme levels are nonspecific for dystrophy since they occur in all types of disease that damage the muscle fiber. Moreover, in the more slowly evolving types of dystrophy, such as that of Landouzy-Déjerine, the serum levels of CK may be normal. It would be expected that the values would always be normal in denervation paralysis with muscular atrophy, but unfortunately they may be slightly elevated in some patients with progressive spinal muscular atrophy and amyotrophic lateral sclerosis. Even vigorous exercise may elevate CK in normal persons, and sometimes CK may be persistently elevated without evidence of muscle or other diseases. An unexplained alteration of the sarcolemma with high serum CK occurs in hypothyroidism and in alcoholism. An idiopathic creatinekinasemia is also seen in most large clinics.

ENDOCRINOPATHIES

In a number of disorders of endocrine glands, muscle weakness may be a prominent feature, and occasionally it may be the chief complaint. While these diseases are discussed in detail elsewhere (Chap. 51), it should be noted that such weakness, local or generalized, acute or chronic, may occur in the absence of changes in serum electrolytes or enzymes. Specific hormone assays are then necessary for diagnosis. This is particularly true of prolonged corticosteroid therapy and of thyrotoxicosis, in which severe muscle paresis may appear without the classic signs of Graves disease.

MYOGLOBINURIA

The red pigment, myoglobin, responsible for much of the color of muscle, is an iron-protein compound present in the sarcoplasm of striated skeletal and cardiac fibers. Of the total body hematin compounds, about 25 percent is in muscle, the remainder in red blood corpuscles and other cells. Destruction of striated muscle, regardless of the process—whether trauma, ischemia, or metabolic disease—liberates myoglobin, and because of its relatively small size, the molecule filters through the glomeruli and appears in the urine, imparting to it a burgundy red color. Lack of ATP is believed to injure the sarcolemma. Because of the low renal threshold, the excretion of myoglobin is so rapid that the serum remains uncolored. In contrast, because of the high renal threshold, the hemoglobin released by destruction of red blood corpuscles colors both the serum and urine. Myoglobinuria should thus be suspected when the urine is deep red and the serum normal in color. It is estimated that 200 g of muscle must be destroyed to visibly color the urine (Rowland). As in hemoglobinuria, the guaiac and benzidine tests are positive. The urine does not fluoresce, as it does in porphyria. On spectroscopic analysis, myoglobin shows an absorption band at 581 nm, but the most sensitive method for measuring myoglobin in the urine and serum is by radioimmunoassay techniques (Rosano and Kenny). Hyperkalemia, hyperphosphatemia, and hypercalcemia may complicate massive rhabdomyolysis. The conditions giving rise to myoglobinuria are listed on page 1112.

CREATINURIA

Creatine, an amino acid, is a prominent constituent of striated muscle. It may be ingested (exogenous creatine), but it is also synthesized in the liver from glycine, arginine, and methionine and then delivered to the skeletal muscles, which contain more of this compound than any other organ (150 mg per 100 g fresh-weight muscle tissue). Creatinine, the anhydride of creatine, is a degradation product that is excreted in the urine. The creatinine content of muscles is low (about 5 mg/dL), since it diffuses readily through the sarcolemma. The serum level of creatine in normal males varies from 0.2 to 0.6 mg/dL; in females from 0.4 to 0.9 mg/dL. Creatinine serum levels range from 0.8 to 1.4 mg/dL and are increased only in serious renal disease. Adult 24-h urine excretion of creatine averages from 60 to 150 mg in normal men and 100 to 300 mg in women. Creatinine excretion is remarkably constant at 1.0 to 1.6 g/day. In diseases such as progressive muscular dystrophy, the creatine content of the muscle fiber is diminished, and there is a decrease in creatinine excretion, increase in creatine excretion, and hypercreatinemia. The same alterations occur with reduction in muscle mass in neurogenic atrophy, polymyositis, hyperthyroidism, Addison disease, and male eunuchoidism. Ingestion of 1 to 3 g creatine will not significantly raise the level in blood or urine in a normal person, for the muscles are not saturated, but in an individual with a reduced muscle mass, creatinemia and creatinuria result. Thus, this type of creatine tolerance test merely indicates a reduction in functional muscle mass.

ELECTRODIAGNOSIS OF NEUROMUSCULAR DISEASE

Long ago it was discovered that muscle would contract when a pulse of electric current was applied to the skin, near the point of entrance of the muscular nerve (*motor point*). The effective electrical pulse is brief, less than a millisecond, and is induced by a rapidly alternating (faradic) current. After denervation, an electrical pulse of several milliseconds, induced by a constant (galvanic) stimulus, is required to produce the same response. This change, in which the galvanic stimulus remains effective after the faradic one has failed, was the basis of *Erb's reaction of degeneration,* and varying degrees of this change were plotted in the form of *strength-duration curves.* For decades, this was the standard electrical method for evaluating denervation of muscle. This method, though still valid, is outmoded. Now, reliance is placed on the demonstration of fibrillation potentials and characteristic changes in motor unit potentials (MUPs) by the insertion into muscle of needle electrodes. This type of study is based on the concept of the "motor unit," introduced by Sherrington (page 37), and is generally referred to as the "needle examination." The terms *electromyography* and *electromyogram* (EMG) were coined originally to describe only the needle examination, but are now commonly used to include the *nerve conduction studies* as well.

NEEDLE EXAMINATION OF MUSCLE

The needle examination of skeletal muscles is laborious. Usually a large number of muscles must be tested, one at a time, because of the varying topography of muscle and peripheral nerve diseases, which may involve some muscles and not others, or only parts of muscles. Normal findings in one or a few muscles do not exclude the possibility of pathologic phenomena elsewhere. External plate or surface electrodes, such as those used in electrocardiography or electroencephalography, can be used to record summated MUPs, but they do not delineate single MUPs. The latter requires the use of monopolar or concentric needle electrodes, which are inserted into the muscle to be studied. With concentric needle electrodes, the tip of the wire in the lumen of the needle will be in proximity to several muscle fibers, belonging to several motor units; this is the recording electrode. The shaft of the needle, in contact over most of its length with intercellular fluid and many other muscle fibers, is the indifferent reference electrode. With monopolar electrodes, the reference electrode may be another monopolar needle electrode or a surface plate electrode placed in subcutaneous tissue or on the skin overlying the muscle being tested.

The following is a summary of the electrical events

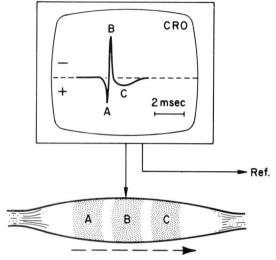

Figure 45-4

The shaded area represents the zone of the action potential which is negative to all other points on the fiber surface. It is shown at three points in its course (from left to right) along the fiber. At each point, the correspondingly lettered portion of the triphasic muscle-action potential displayed on the cathode ray oscilloscope (CRO) reflects the potential difference between the active (vertical arrow) and reference (Ref.) electrodes. Polarity in this and subsequent figures is negative upward as depicted. The time calibration is on the CRO screen.

that occur in relation to the recording electrode. When the electrical impulse travels along the surface of the muscle, current begins to flow through the normally polarized region under the recording electrode to the depolarized zone. As shown in Fig. 45-4, the recording electrode becomes positive (by convention) relative to the reference electrode, and the beam of the cathode ray oscilloscope (CRO) is deflected downward (at A). When the depolarized zone moves under the recording electrode, the latter rapidly becomes negative and the beam is deflected upward (at B). As the depolarized zone continues to move along the sarcolemma, away from the recording electrode and toward the reference electrode, the membrane under the latter slowly becomes repolarized. Current once again begins to flow outward through the membrane toward the distant depolarized region, and the recording electrode becomes relatively positive again (at C). It then returns to its resting isopotential position. The net result is a triphasic action potential recorded on the CRO, as in Fig. 45-4. This configuration is typical of fibrillation potentials that are recorded at a distance from the end-plate zone. Fibrillation potentials are seen only when single muscle fibers are functionally or structurally

denervated, and are so brief (<5 ms) that the inertia-free CRO must be used to record them; ink-writing apparatus does not have the necessary frequency response.

As indicated above, single muscle fibers do not discharge in normally innervated muscle but are activated in motor unit activity, which involves the almost simultaneous discharge or depolarization of all the muscle fibers innervated by a single anterior horn cell. The potential recorded from a motor unit necessarily has a greater duration and amplitude than a fibrillation potential. The typical configuration of a motor unit potential is also triphasic, as indicated in Fig. 45-9. Up to 10 percent of normal MUPs consist of four or more phases (*polyphasic potentials*).

Normally, resting muscle should be electrically silent; the small tension spoken of as muscle tone has no EMG equivalent. There are, however, two types of normal spontaneous activity. One is an irregularity in the baseline caused by 10- to 40-μV negative potentials of very brief duration. These are believed to represent single or synchronized miniature end-plate potentials (mepps), and are most in evidence when the recording needle electrode is accidentally placed near a motor end plate ("end-plate noise"). The other type of normal spontaneous activity is characterized by irregularly discharging (5- to 50-Hz) initially negative spike discharges of 100 to 200 μV in amplitude. These potentials have been termed end-plate spikes and are believed to represent discharges of single muscle fibers provoked by mechanical stimulation of intramuscular nerve terminals by the needle electrode. These potentials need to be distinguished from fibrillation potentials.

Insertion of the needle electrode into the muscle injures and mechanically stimulates many fibers, causing a burst of potentials of short duration (< 300 ms). This is referred to as *normal insertional activity*. When muscle is voluntarily contracted, the action potentials of motor units begin to appear on the CRO. One can observe the way force is built up by watching the progressive recruitment of MUPs, the initial ones firing at rates of 4 to 5 per second. As more and more MUPs are recruited, a great crowd of them appears on the CRO screen, firing simultaneously but asynchronously on vigorous contraction at much higher rates (40 to 50 per second; see Fig. 45-5A). Since individual MUPs can no longer be distinguished, this is referred to as a *complete interference pattern*. The largest normal MUPs are up to 5 mV in amplitude. As muscles relax, more and more units drop out. If a muscle is weakened by denervation, there will obviously be fewer MUPs, firing at a moderately rapid to rapid rate (*decreased interference pattern*). In contrast, with poor voluntary effort, the decreased MUPs fire at slower rates and often in an irregular pattern.

THE ABNORMAL ELECTROMYOGRAM

Clinically important deviations from the normal EMG include (1) increased or decreased insertional activity, (2) the occurrence of abnormal "spontaneous" activity during relaxation (fibrillation potentials, positive sharp waves, fasciculation potentials, cramps, myotonia, myokymia, etc.), (3) abnormalities in the amplitude, duration, and shape of single MUPs, (4) a decrease in the number of MUPs and changes in their firing pattern, (5) variation in amplitude of MUPs during voluntary contraction of muscle, and (6) the demonstration of special phenomena, such as electrical silence during obvious shortening of the muscle (contracture).

Insertional Activity   At the moment the needle is inserted into muscle, there is usually a brief burst of action potentials that cease once the needle is stable, providing it is not in a position to irritate an intramuscular nerve fiber. Increased

insertional activity is seen in all forms of denervation, as well as in polymyositis, Duchenne dystrophy, myotonia, and disorders that dispose to muscle cramps. In cases of advanced denervation or myopathy, in which muscle fibers have been largely replaced by connective tissue and fat, insertional activity may be decreased and there may be increased mechanical resistance to insertion of the needle electrode.

Abnormal "Spontaneous" Activity   Spontaneous activity of single muscle fibers and of motor units, known respectively as *fibrillation* potentials and *fasciculation* potentials, is abnormal. The two phenomena are often confused. Fibrillation is the spontaneous contraction of a *single muscle fiber* and appears when the muscle fiber has lost its nerve supply. Fasciculation represents a spontaneous contraction of a motor unit. (Each is discussed below.)

Fibrillation potentials   When a motor neuron is destroyed by disease, or when its axon is interrupted, the distal part of the axon degenerates, a process that takes several days. The muscle fibers formerly innervated by the branches of the dead axon, viz., the motor unit, are disconnected from the nervous system. For reasons that are still obscure, the chemosensitive region of the sarcolemma at the motor end plate "spreads" after denervation to

Figure 45-5

Patterns of motor unit recruitment. A. Normal. With each increment of voluntary effort, more and larger units are brought into play until, with full effort at the extreme right, a complete "interference pattern" is seen in which single units are no longer recognizable. B. After denervation, only a single motor unit is recorded despite maximal effort. It is seen to fire repetitively. C. With myopathic diseases, a normal number of units is recruited on minimal effort, though the amplitude of the pattern is reduced. Calibrations: 50 ms (horizontal) and 1 mV in A and B; 200 µV in C (vertical).

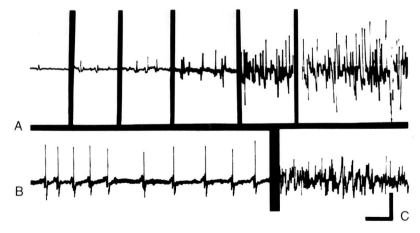

involve the entire surface of the muscle fiber. Then, 10 to 25 days after death of the axon, the denervated fibers develop spontaneous activity; i.e., even while no effort is being made by the patient to contract the muscle, each fiber contracts at its own rate and without relation to the activity of neighboring fibers. There results a totally random conglomeration of brief, di- or triphasic fibrillation potentials (Fig. 45-6A), having a duration of 1 to 5 ms and rarely exceeding 300 μV in amplitude. When brief spontaneous potentials of this sort are observed firing regularly at two or three different locations outside the end-plate zone of a resting muscle, one may conclude that some of the fibers are denervated. Closer analysis reveals that about half of the fibrillation potentials discharge at a constant rate and the rest in irregular sequence. The latter appear to originate from discharges in the end-plate zone and the former from potential oscillations in the sarcolemma. Fibrillation potentials may be seen, in considerable numbers, in certain primary diseases of muscle, such as polymyositis, or in Duchenne dystrophy. Diseases such as poliomyelitis, which damage spinal motor neurons, or injuries of peripheral nerves or anterior spinal roots, frequently produce only partial denervation of the involved muscles. In such muscles, one electrode placement may record fibrillation potentials at rest from denervated fibers and normal potentials during voluntary contraction from nearby healthy fibers. Fibrillation potentials continue until the muscle fiber is reinnervated by

the outgrowth of new axons from nearby healthy nerve fibers, or until the muscle fiber degenerates and is replaced by connective tissue, a process that may take many years. In addition, fibrillation potentials may take the form of *positive sharp waves*, i.e., spontaneous, initially positive diphasic potentials, of longer duration and slightly greater amplitude than the biphasic or triphasic spikes of fibrillation potentials (Fig. 45-6A). The latter configuration reflects the position of the recording needle near the denervated fiber, whereas positive sharp waves probably arise from fibers that have been damaged by the recording needle electrode.

Fasciculation potentials Fasciculation is the spontaneous or involuntary contraction of a motor unit or part of a motor unit. Such contractions may cause a visible dimpling or twitching of the skin, though ordinarily they are of insufficient force to move a joint. The form of the accompanying EMG potential, like that of an ordinary MUP, is relatively constant for any one fasciculation potential. Commonly, it will have three to five phases, a duration of 5 to 15 ms (somewhat less in the facial muscles), and an amplitude of several millivolts (Fig. 45-6B). Fasciculation potentials usually fire irregularly. They are evidence of motor nerve fiber irritability and not necessarily of nerve fiber destruction and motor unit denervation. Occasional fasciculation potentials, particularly in the calves and hands, occur in many normal persons and constantly in some of them, and need not be taken as evidence of disease at all (benign fasciculation). Shivering induced by low temperature and twitchings associated with low serum calcium levels are also forms of fasciculatory activity. Whether or not fasciculations are related to denervation in any particular case cannot be decided on the basis of their configuration, firing rate, or rhythm, but only by the presence or absence of associated fibrillation potentials and certain changes in MUPs (see below).

Fasciculation potentials occur in chronic, slowly advancing, destructive diseases of the anterior horn cells, such as amyotrophic lateral sclerosis and progressive spinal muscular atrophy. In these diseases, fasciculation potentials are numerous and may exceed 15 ms in duration. They are seen often in the early stages of poliomyelitis but only occasionally in the chronic phase of the disease, perhaps because the affected cells die rapidly. Occasionally, they are also seen with compressive anterior root lesions, such as those caused by a protruded intervertebral disc; large numbers of axons may be affected, with the result that the fasciculations (or even cramps) may be more prominent than with disease of anterior horn cells. Fasciculation

Figure 45-6

A. *Fibrillations and positive sharp waves. This spontaneous activity was recorded from a totally denervated muscle—no motor unit potentials were produced by attempts at voluntary contraction. The fibrillations (above arrow) are 1 to 2 ms in duration, 100 to 300 μV in amplitude, and largely negative (upward) in polarity following an initial positive deflection. A typical positive sharp wave is seen above the star.* B. *Fasciculation. This spontaneous motor unit potential was recorded from a patient with amyotrophic lateral sclerosis. It has a serrated configuration and it fired once every second or two. Calibrations: 5 ms (horizontal) and 200 μV in A; 1 mV in B (vertical).*

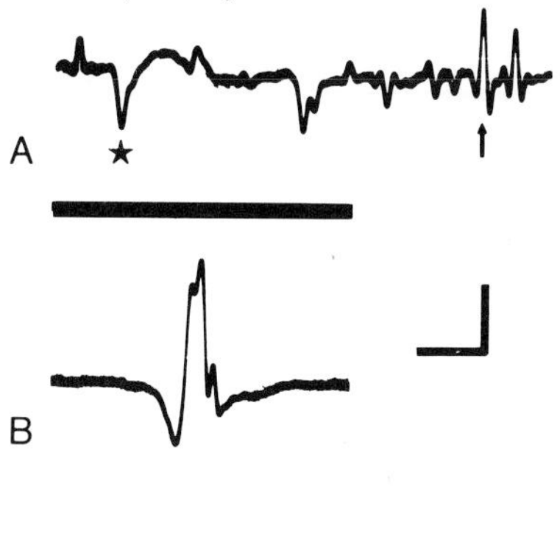

potentials have also been observed early in the course of acute idiopathic polyneuritis and other peripheral nerve lesions, giving way to fibrillation potentials upon death of the axon. In all these cases, the damaged neuron or its axon seems to be "irritated" by the disease process and fires repetitively, and, in doing so, produces activity in all the muscle fibers that it innervates.

Less common types of spontaneous activity In *myokymia*, a term introduced by Schultze to refer to a persistent quivering and rippling of muscles at rest, the EMG picture is distinctive. The spontaneously firing MUPs are often smaller but more numerous than fasciculation potentials and fire at rates up to 50 per second. This activity may be blocked by xylocaine infusion of peripheral nerve and may be diminished by carbamazepine.

In the *syndrome of continuous muscle fiber activity,* EMG discloses high frequency (up to 300 Hz) repetitive discharges of varying wave forms that show decrements in the amplitude of successive discharges. The origin of these discharges (*neuromyotonia*) is probably in the distal peripheral nerve, where activity of afferent fibers, possibly via ephaptic transmission, excites distal motor terminals. This activity persists during sleep and general anesthesia.

The phenomenon of myotonia (see pages 1095 and 1172) is characterized by high-frequency repetitive discharges that wax and wane in amplitude and frequency, producing a "dive-bomber" sound on the audio monitor. It is elicited mechanically by percussion or movement of the needle electrode. This electrical picture is also seen following voluntary contraction or electrical stimulation of the muscle via its motor nerve (after-discharge). With myotonia congenita, the MUPs may appear normal during voluntary contraction but they are not followed by the silence that normally occurs on relaxation; instead there is a burst of potentials that may take as long as several minutes to subside (Fig. 45-7A). These EMG findings correspond to the clinical failure of voluntary relaxation of muscle following a forceful contraction. Some of the potentials of this prolonged discharge have the duration, amplitude, and form of single muscle fiber potentials, while others appear to have the characteristics of motor unit potentials. If the muscle is activated repeatedly at short intervals, the late discharge becomes briefer and briefer and eventually disappears (Fig. 45-7B), as the patient becomes able to relax the exercised muscle at will ("warm-up" effect). In the paradoxical myotonia observed in some cases with the paramyotonia of von Eulenberg, Nielsen and colleagues have found a decreasing recruitment pattern and increasing

activity after each of a succession of voluntary contractions. This is the converse of what happens in congenital myotonia. Cold abolishes the myotonic discharges in paramyotonia congenita and induces an electrically silent contracture.

Complex repetitive discharges without waxing and waning, formerly referred to as bizarre high-frequency discharges and *pseudomyotonia,* are seen in some myopathies and in certain types of denervation and reinnervation. High-frequency coupling of action potentials into doublets, triplets, or higher multiples of single units, indicating instability in repolarization of the nerve fiber, occurs in tetany and in the early stages of myokymia.

The *contracture* of McArdle disease is associated with relative electrical silence of muscle. This feature is important in the definition of this syndrome.

Abnormalities in Amplitude, Duration, and Shape of Motor Unit Potentials *Motor unit potentials in denervation* Figure 45-8 depicts, schematically, ways in which disease processes affect the motor unit and the appearance, in each case, of the MUP in the EMG. Early in the course of denervation, many motor units with functional connections to the spinal cord are unaffected, and though the number of MUPs appearing during contrac-

Figure 45-7

A. Myotonia congenita (Thomsen disease). The five lines are a continuous record of activity in the biceps brachii following a tap on the tendon. The initial response is within normal limits, but it is followed by a prolonged burst of rapid activity, gradually subsiding over a period of many seconds or minutes. B. Same electrode placement as in A. Response to the fifth of a series of tendon taps. "Warm-up" has occurred, and the characteristic prolonged myotonic activity is no longer evident.

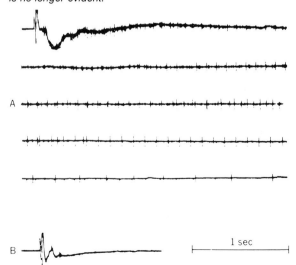

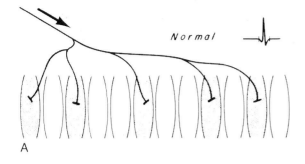

Normal

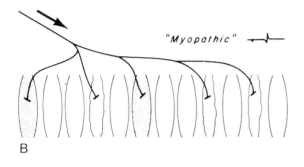

"Myopathic"

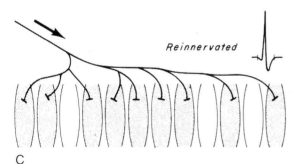

Reinnervated

C

Figure 45-8

The shaded muscle fibers are functional members of one motor unit, whose axon enters from the upper left and branches terminally to innervate the appropriate muscle fibers. The action potential produced by each motor unit is seen in the upper right: its duration is measured between the two vertical lines. The normal-appearing but unshaded fibers belong to other motor units. A. Hypothetical situation, with five muscle fibers in the active unit. B. In this myopathic unit, only two fibers remain active, the other three (shrunken) have been affected by one of the primary muscle diseases. C. Four fibers which originally belonged to other motor units and had been denervated have now been reinnervated by terminal sprouting from an undamaged axon. Both the motor unit and its action potential are now larger than normal. Note that only under these abnormal circumstances do fibers in the same unit lie next to one another.

tion is reduced, the configurations of the remaining ones are quite normal. In time, the remaining MUPs often increase in amplitude, perhaps two to three times normal, and become longer in duration and sometimes *polyphasic* (more than four phases). Such large and sometimes *giant potentials* (Fig. 45-9C) are believed to arise from motor units containing more than the usual number of muscle fibers that are spread out over a greatly enlarged territory within the muscle (Fig. 45-8C). Presumably, new nerve twigs have sprouted from undamaged axons and have reinnervated previously denervated fibers, thus adding them to their own motor units. Some of these units may become low in amplitude, extremely prolonged and polyphasic, findings pathognomonic of reinnervation (Fig. 45-9B). These units are to be differentiated from (1) polyphasic potentials of normal duration, which, as was said, make up as much as 10 percent of the total number of MUPs in normal muscle, and (2) polyphasic MUPs of short duration and low amplitude, which are characteristic of myopathies and myasthenia gravis and other disorders of neuromuscular transmission.

The motor unit potential in myopathy
Diseases such as polymyositis, the muscular dystrophies, and other myopathies that randomly destroy muscle fibers or render them nonfunctional obviously reduce the popu-

Figure 45-9

Single voluntary motor unit potentials. A. Normal. B. Prolonged polyphasic potential seen with reinnervation. C. "Giant unit"—normally shaped but of much greater amplitude than normal. D. Brief, low-amplitude "myopathic" units. Calibrations: 5 ms (horizontal) and 1 mV in A and B; 5 mV in C; 100 μV in D (vertical).

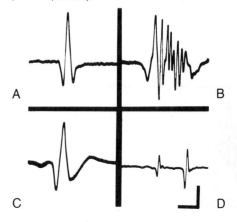

lation of fibers per motor unit, as in Fig. 45-8*B*. Therefore, when such a unit is activated, its potential is of lower voltage and shorter duration than normal (Fig. 45-9*D*), and it may also appear polyphasic, as the compound motor unit potential becomes fragmented into its constituent single fiber potentials. Slowing of the propagated muscle fiber action potential in affected muscle fibers is also believed to contribute to the changes in the myopathic MUP. When most of the muscle fibers are affected, the MUPs are very small and of short duration and are recruited out of proportion to the tension generated—so-called increased recruitment. Both types of alterations produce a characteristic high-pitched crackling sound from the audio monitor. They occur in all forms of progressive muscular dystrophy and, unfortunately, are indistinguishable from those of polymyositis, dermatomyositis, and other chronic myopathies. Fibrillation potentials are often seen in the myositides and in the rapidly progressive muscular dystrophies, perhaps because of segmental necrosis of muscle fibers, which may isolate a segment of the fiber from its nerve supply. In myasthenia gravis, where transmission of impulse fails at the neuromuscular junction, a single MUP may vary in amplitude during sustained weak contraction. EMG recordings of single muscle fibers belonging to the same motor unit disclose varying interpotential intervals on successive discharges; this phenomenon is called ''jitter'' and increases with deficits in neuromuscular transmission.

Abnormalities of the interference pattern

Diseases that reduce the population of functional motor neurons or axons within the peripheral nerve obviously decrease the number of motor units that can be recruited in the affected muscles. The decreased number of motor units available for activation now produce an incomplete interference pattern, which is manifested by a decreased number of units firing at a moderate to rapid rate. A severe reduction in the interference pattern may result in a single unit pattern (Fig. 45-5*B*).

If muscle power is reduced in diseases such as polymyositis or muscular dystrophy, in which individual muscle fibers are affected, there will be little or no reduction in the number of motor units available for recruitment, though each unit will consist of fewer muscle fibers than normal. A modest effort produces a full interference pattern despite marked weakness (increased recruitment). Because fewer muscle fibers are firing, the amplitude of the pattern will be reduced from normal. A full highly complex interference pattern of less than usual amplitude, in the face of dramatic weakness, is the hallmark of myopathy (Fig. 45-5*C*).

SINGLE FIBER ELECTROMYOGRAPHY (SF-EMG)

This is a special technique for the recording of single muscle fiber action potentials, and is used to measure fiber density and jitter. Fiber density is an index of the number and distribution of muscle fibers within a motor unit. Jitter is the variability of the interpotential interval of successive discharges of two single muscle fiber action potentials belonging to the same motor unit. Jitter is due largely to the variability of synaptic delay at the neuromuscular junction. For this reason, SF-EMG is particularly useful in the detection of disorders of neuromuscular transmission, especially myasthenia gravis. Fiber density and jitter are often increased markedly in neuropathic disorders causing denervation with reinnervation. They are usually normal or only slightly increased in myopathic disorders. The details of this technique and its clinical applications are discussed fully by Stålberg and Trontelj.

CONDUCTION STUDIES OF NERVE

Techniques are available for the percutaneous stimulation of peripheral nerve fibers and recording of the muscle and sensory action potentials. The results of these *motor and sensory nerve conduction studies*, expressed as amplitudes, conduction velocities, and distal latencies, yield certain information unavailable from needle examination studies.

Hodes et al in 1948 were the first to perform nerve conduction studies in patients. An accessible nerve is stimulated through the skin by surface electrodes, and the resulting compound action potential is recorded by electrodes on the skin (1) over the nerve more proximally using orthodromic techniques for sensory fibers stimulated in the digital nerves, (2) over the nerve more distally, using antidromic techniques for sensory nerve conduction studies (this has many technical advantages over orthodromic techniques and is widely used for routine sensory nerve conduction studies), and (3) over the muscle more distally in the case of motor fibers stimulated in a mixed nerve (Fig. 45-10). The conduction times from the most distal stimulating electrode, measured in milliseconds, from the stimulus artifact to the onset and to the peak of the response are termed the distal and peak latencies, respectively. If a second stimulus can be applied to a mixed nerve more proximally (or if recording or stimulating electrodes can be placed more proximally in the case of sensory fibers), a new and longer conduction time can be measured. When the distance (in millimeters) between the two sites of stimulation of motor fibers or recording of sensory fibers is divided by the difference in conduction times (in milliseconds), one obtains a *maximal conduction velocity* (in meters per second), which describes the velocity of propagation of the action potentials in the largest and fastest

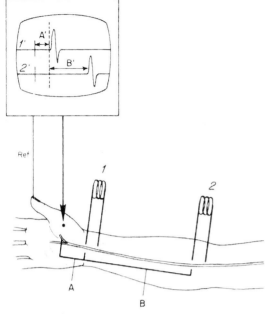

Figure 45-10

*The median nerve is stimulated percutaneously (1) at the
wrist and (2) in the antecubital fossa with the resultant
compound muscle action potential recorded as the potential
difference between a surface electrode over the thenar
eminence (arrow) and a reference electrode (Ref.) more
distally. Sweep 1' on the CRO depicts the stimulus artifact
followed by the compound muscle action potential. The distal
latency, A', is the time from the stimulus artifact to the take-
off phase of the compound muscle action potential and
corresponds to conduction over distance A. The same is
true for sweep 2', where stimulation is at 2 and the time from
the artifact to the response is A' + B'. The maximum motor
conduction velocity over segment B is calculated by dividing
distance B by the time B'.*

nerve fibers. These velocities in normal subjects vary from
a minimum of 40 or 45 m/s, to a maximum of 75 to 80 m/s,
depending upon which nerve is studied. Values are lower
in infants, reaching the adult range by the age of 2 to 4
years. Values decrease again with advancing age (also with
exposure to cold). Normal values have also been established
for distal latencies from the distalmost site of stimulation
on various mixed nerves to the appropriate muscles; when
one stimulates the median nerve at the wrist, for example
(Fig. 45-10A), the latency for motor conduction through
the carpal tunnel to the median-innervated thenar muscles
is always less than 4.5 ms in normal adults. Similar tables
of normal values have been compiled for orthodromic and
antidromic sensory conduction velocities and distal latencies.

In addition to the study of distal latency and conduction velocity, the amplitudes of the evoked muscle action
potential and the sensory nerve action potential can yield
valuable information about peripheral nerve function. These
amplitudes can be used as an index of the number of nerve
fibers that respond to a given stimulus and conduct to the
various recording points, hence allowing for the detection
of conduction blocks and axonal loss. In addition, segmental
demyelinative lesions or axonal loss affecting the large and
fast conducting fibers may be detected by finding evidence
of differential slowing causing a dispersal of the response.
Motor and sensory amplitudes are often more sensitive than
conduction velocity or distal latencies in detecting disorders
that cause axonal loss. Conversely, prolonged distal latencies, slowed motor conduction velocities, and conduction
blocks are the hallmarks of segmental demyelinative lesions.

When motor fibers in a mixed nerve are stimulated,
the compound action potential of many hundreds of microvolts can easily be recorded from electrodes on the skin
over the muscle. However, when one attempts to measure
sensory potentials, activity must be recorded from nerve
fibers themselves; one then lacks the "amplification"
provided by all the muscle fibers in one motor unit, as
noted above, and much greater electronic amplification is
required. Abnormal sensory potentials are sometimes very
small or absent even when powerful computer-averaging
techniques are used, and sensory conduction measurements
are often difficult or impossible to record. By contrast, it
is always possible to obtain a reliable motor conduction
velocity as long as some functioning nerve fibers remain.
These conduction velocities reflect the status of surviving
fibers and, if the latter are unaffected by the disease process,
may be normal despite widespread axonal degeneration.
Thus, following incomplete transection of a nerve, the
maximal motor conduction velocity may be normal in the
few remaining fibers, although the muscle involved is
almost paralyzed and its compound muscle potential very
low.

Disease processes that preferentially injure the fastest
conducting, large-diameter fibers in peripheral nerves should
reduce the maximal conduction velocity slightly because
the remaining fibers with smaller diameters conduct more
slowly. Such a reduction in velocity can be determined by
comparing values recorded from the patient with those from
a control group of the same age and sex.

In most neuropathies, only a part of the axons are
affected (either by the "dying-back" phenomenon or wallerian degeneration), and nerve conduction velocities are
then relatively uninformative. This is true for typical

alcoholic, nutritional, carcinomatous, uremic, other meta-bolic, and some diabetic neuropathies, in which conduction velocities range from low in the normal range to 35 or 40 m/s. On the other hand, the motor and particularly the sensory amplitudes are usually diminished, and there may be fibrillations and changes in motor unit potentials on needle examination. In contrast, neuropathies of the acute Guillain-Barré type and those associated with diphtheria, infantile metachromatic leukodystrophy, Krabbe disease, and Charcot-Marie-Tooth disease (as it is seen in most kinships) affect Schwann cells primarily and produce seg-mental demyelination, with markedly slow conduction velocities or conduction block.

Focal compression of nerve, as in entrapment syn-dromes, may produce localized slowing or blocks in con-duction, perhaps because of segmental demyelination at the site of compression. The demonstration of such localized changes of conduction affords ready confirmation of nerve entrapment; for example, if the distal latency of the median nerve (Fig. 45-10A) exceeds 5.0 ms while that of the ulnar nerve remains normal, compression of the median nerve in the carpal tunnel is likely. Similar focal slowing of con-duction may be recorded from the ulnar nerve at the elbow.

Repetitive Stimulation Studies Skeletal muscle may be activated by the application of brief electrical pulses to the skin overlying a motor nerve. By adjusting the strength of the stimulus to supramaximal range, a maximal compound muscle action potential may be obtained for each stimulus; the form of the response will depend on the number of motor units activated and the number of muscle fibers sampled by the recording apparatus. If repeated stimuli are given, each response will have the same form and amplitude until fatigue supervenes. A normal response will follow each stimulus even with rates of stimulation up to 25 per second for periods of 60 s or more, before a decrement of the compound muscle action potential appears. The latter is due to the failure of some muscle fibers to respond, presumably because of failure of the nerve impulse to be transmitted through certain branching points of the terminal axon.

In certain disorders, notably myasthenia gravis, the initial compound muscle action potential produced by electrical stimulation is normal. After a few stimuli at rates of 1 to 10 per second (optimal rate 2 to 3 per second) the amplitude of the potentials decreases, though not to zero, and then, after four or five stimuli, may increase somewhat (Fig. 45-11A). This partial block of neuromuscular trans-mission in myasthenics is similar to the one produced by

curare and can be partially corrected with neostigmine. Similar decremental responses may occur in poliomyelitis and certain other diseases of the motor unit, but the pattern described for myasthenia is not present.

The myasthenic syndrome of Lambert-Eaton, often associated with oat-cell carcinoma of the lung, is charac-terized by a different type of defect of neuromuscular transmission. Following rapid (up to 50 per second) repet-itive stimulation of nerve, the muscle action potentials, which are small or practically absent with the first stimulus, increase in voltage with each successive response until a more nearly normal amplitude is attained (Fig. 45-11B). Exercising the muscle for 10 s will also cause the amplitude to increase dramatically (>100 percent). Neostigmine has no effect on this phenomenon, but it may be reversible with guanidine and 3,4-diaminopyridine, which stimulate the release of ACh. The effects of the myasthenic syndrome are similar to those produced by botulinus toxin or by neomycin and other antibiotics (pages 909 and 1160).

ELECTRODIAGNOSTIC STUDIES OF SPINAL REFLEXES

Information about the conduction of impulses through the proximal segments of a nerve, not obtainable by routine nerve conduction techniques, may be provided by the study

Figure 45-11

Compound action potentials evoked in hypothenar muscles by electrical stimulation of the ulnar nerve at the wrist. A. Patient with myasthenia gravis—typical pattern of decrement in first four responses followed by slight increment. At this rate of stimulation (4 per second) the decrement in response does not continue to zero. B. Patient with Lambert-Eaton syndrome and oat-cell carcinoma—typical marked increase toward normal amplitude with rapid repetitive stimulation (20 per second). Horizontal calibration: 250 ms.

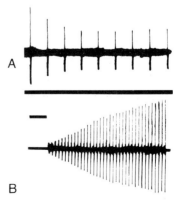

of the H reflex and the F wave. In 1918, Hoffmann, after whom the H reflex was later named, showed that submaximal stimulation of mixed motor-sensory nerves, insufficient to produce a direct motor response, produces a muscle contraction (H wave) after a latency that is much longer than that of the direct motor response (M wave). This reflex is based on activation of fusimotor afferent fibers, and the long delay in muscular response reflects the time required for the sensory impulses to reach the spinal cord, synapse with anterior horn cells, and then be transmitted along motor fibers to the muscle (Fig. 3-1). The H reflex is particularly useful in the diagnosis of S1 radiculopathy, certain predominantly proximal polyneuropathies, and predominantly sensory polyneuropathies. With more intense stimulation of the nerve, the response is blocked by antidromic conduction along motor fibers. Stimuli of increasing frequency, but low intensity, cause a progressive depression and finally obliteration of H waves. The latter phenomenon has been used to study spasticity, rigidity, and cerebellar ataxia in which there are differences in the frequency-depression curves of H waves.

The F response, so named because it was initially elicited in the feet, was first described by Magladery and McDougal in 1950. It is evoked by a supramaximal stimulus of a motor-sensory nerve. Again, after a latency longer than that for the direct motor response, a second small muscle action potential is recorded (F wave). The F wave is produced by the stimulation of motor fibers that travel antidromically to the anterior horn cells; a certain number of anterior horn cells may be activated and produce an orthodromic response.

When conduction studies of the distal segments of peripheral nerves are normal, prolonged latencies of the H and F waves can be taken as evidence of disease in the most proximal segments of the nerves or spinal roots. Normal F responses and absent H reflexes indicate proximal disease of sensory nerves and roots.

BIOPSY MYOPATHOLOGY

Muscle biopsy can be of great diagnostic value, but both surgical and microscopic techniques must be exacting. The muscle chosen for study should be accessible; there should be evidence that it has been affected but not totally destroyed by the disease in question, and it should not have been the site of a recent injection or electromyographic study, since the trauma of the needles produces focal necrotizing and inflammatory lesions. Muscle biopsy is helpful in distinguishing several basic disorders in patients with neuromuscular disease.

1. *Denervation atrophy.* Reduction in the size of muscle fibers with enlargement of intact motor units (due to collateral reinnervation) and delayed degenerative changes in some fibers are the main changes of denervation atrophy. This change typifies all peripheral nerve and many spinal cord diseases and is particularly well shown in histochemical stains for ATPase, phosphorylase, and oxidases, where the normal mosaic pattern of fiber types is altered (i.e., muscle fibers of similar histochemical types form groups of 15 or more fibers).

2. *Segmental necrosis of muscle fibers with myophagia and various manifestations of regeneration.* These are the typical changes in idiopathic polymyositis (in combination with infiltrates of inflammatory cells), infective polymyositis (in the presence of trichina, toxoplasma, etc., as well as inflammation), and paroxysmal myoglobinuria, and may be observed also in Duchenne and other rapidly progressive muscular dystrophies.

3. *Unusual changes of muscle fibers.* Included here are sarcoplasmic masses and ringbinden in myotonic dystrophy, glycogen masses in glycogen storage diseases, rods (nemaline), central cores, aggregates of lipid bodies, and other cytoplasmic changes (such as aggregation and other abnormalities of mitochondria) in certain congenital myopathies. Histochemical stains for fiber typing and electron microscopy are the important techniques in the diagnosis of these disorders.

4. *Alterations in number and size of fibers as a reflection of abnormalities of growth, maturation, and aging.* Many states of dwarfism and congenital myopathies of myotubular type present principally with numerical or volumetric changes, which must be distinguished from denervation, disuse effects, cachexia, and work hypertrophy.

5. *Disorders of the conduction apparatus (neuromuscular junctions) in which nerve fibers and muscle fibers appear to be intact.* Here the abnormality can be revealed only by performing motor point biopsy (to include the motor end plate) and using electron microscopy and special staining techniques for nerve terminals, acetylcholinesterase, and the outlining of acetylcholine receptors. Myasthenia gravis, botulism, Lambert-Eaton syndrome, and myasthenic syndrome with motor end-plate acetylcholinesterase deficiency fall into this category.

Further details of pathology will be presented with the descriptions of specific muscle diseases.

As a rule, the biopsy procedure requires no more than a cleanly excised block of muscle, 1.0 to 2.0 cm, which is prevented from contracting by a clamp or by tying at full length to a stick, and is then fixed in 10% neutral formalin, embedded in paraffin, sectioned in a cross and longitudinal fashion, and stained by hematoxylin and eosin and Gomori trichrome methods. Special techniques should be applied if it is desirable to visualize particular qualities of a disease. Various histochemical stains for enzyme content of muscle fibers are required to establish the diagnosis of many of the unusual myopathies. The latter require rapid freezing (cryostat) rather than formalin fixation. Electron microscopy, performed on carefully selected blocks of muscle and nerve fixed in glutaraldehyde, is useful in confirming abnormalities detected by histochemical staining and provides a refined means of studying other myopathies.

Sural nerve biopsies, processed by the fixation, staining, and embedding techniques of electron microscopy, can provide very valuable histopathologic data, even when examined by ordinary microscopy. These biopsies can also be studied physiologically in vitro, where fibers of all sizes can be stimulated and their activity recorded—in contrast to routine nerve conduction studies where only the largest fibers can be sampled. All these special techniques are of interest to research workers and are available in centers where nerve and muscle diseases are under investigation.

USE OF LABORATORY TESTS IN THE STUDY OF MUSCLE DISEASE

None of the results of the diagnostic laboratory procedures described above may be taken as an infallible index of a specific disease of muscle. Each procedure is subject to technical error and the findings to misinterpretation. A biopsy specimen may be excised from an unaffected muscle or portion of a muscle and, because of this sampling error, be negative in the face of clinical evidence of obvious disease; rough excision and improper fixation and staining may produce artifacts that may be misinterpreted as marks of disease when, in fact, the muscle is microscopically normal. Similarly, EMG study may fail to record fibrillations in obviously denervated muscle, particularly in slowly progressive disorders. Also, in some of the muscles of the feet, fibrillations and fasciculations may be found in normal asymptomatic older individuals (Falck and Alaranta). As in the study of all disease, laboratory data have significance only if evaluated in the light of the clinical findings.

REFERENCES

ADAMS RD, KAKULAS BA: *Diseases of Muscle: Pathological Foundations of Clinical Myology,* 4th ed. New York, Harper & Row, 1985.

AMINOFF MJ: *Electromyography in Clinical Practice,* 2nd ed. New York, Churchill Livingstone, 1987.

BUCHTHAL F, KAMIENIECKA Z: Diagnostic yield of quantified electromyography and quantified muscle biopsy in neuromuscular disorders. *Muscle & Nerve* 5:265, 1982.

BUCHTHAL F, ROSENFALCK A: Evoked action potentials and conduction velocity in human sensory nerves. *Brain Res* 3:1, 1966.

ELMQUIST D, LAMBERT EH: Detailed analysis of neuromuscular transmission in a patient with the myasthenic syndrome associated with bronchogenic carcinoma. *Mayo Clin Proc* 43:689, 1968.

ENGEL AG, BANKER BQ: *Myology: Basic and Clinical.* New York, McGraw-Hill, 1986.

ENGEL AG, JERUSALEM M, TSUJIHATA M, GOMEZ MR: The neuromuscular junction in myopathies. A quantitative ultrastructural study, in Bradley WG, Gardner-Medwin D, Walton JN (eds): *Recent Advances in Myology.* New York, Elsevier, 1975, pp 132–143.

FALCK B, ALARANTA H: Fibrillation potentials, positive sharp waves and fasciculations in the intrinsic muscles of the foot in healthy subjects. *J Neurol Neurosurg Psychiatry* 46:681, 1983.

FISHBECK K: Structure and function of striated muscle, in Asbury AK, McKhann GM, McDonald W (eds): *Diseases of the Nervous System.* Philadelphia, Saunders, 1986, chap 15.

FRANZINI-ARMSTRONG C: Membrane particles and transmission at the triad. *Fed Proc* 34:1382, 1975.

GOODGOLD J, EBERSTEIN A: *Electrodiagnosis of Neuromuscular Diseases,* 3rd ed. Baltimore, Williams & Wilkins, 1983.

HODES R, LARRABEE MG, GERMAN W: The human electromyogram in response to nerve stimulation and conduction velocity of motor axons: Studies on normal and on injured peripheral nerves. *Arch Neurol Psychiatry* 60:340, 1948.

HODGKIN AL: Ionic basis of electrical activity in nerve and muscle. *Biol Rev* 26:339, 1951.

HODGKIN AL, HUXLEY AF: Currents carried by sodium and potassium ions through the membranes of the giant axon of *Loligo. J Physiol* 116:449, 1952.

HUXLEY HE: Molecular basis of contraction in cross-striated muscles, in Bourne GH (ed): *The Structure and Function of Muscle,* 2nd ed, vol 1: *Structure.* New York, Academic Press, 1972, pt 1, chap 7, pp 301–387.

KATZ B: *Nerve, Muscle and Synapse.* New York, McGraw-Hill, 1966.

KIMURA J: *Electrodiagnosis in Diseases of Nerve of Muscle: Principles and Practice,* 2nd ed. Philadelphia, Davis, 1989.

KUFFLER SW, NICHOLLS JG, MARTIN AR: *From Neuron to Brain,* 2nd ed. Sunderland, MA, Sinauer Associates, 1984.

MAGLADERY JW, McDOUGAL DB: Electrophysiological studies of nerve and reflex activity in normal man. *Johns Hopkins Med J* 86:265, 1950.

MORGAN-HUGHES JA: Defects of the energy pathways of skeletal muscle, in Mathews WB, Glaser GH (eds): *Recent Advances in*

Clinical Neurology. London, Churchill Livingstone, 1982, chap 1, pp 1–46.

NEWHAM DJ, JONES DA, EDWARDS RHT: Large delayed CK changes after stepping exercise. *Muscle & Nerve* 6:380, 1983.

NIELSEN VK, FRIIS ML, JOHNSEN T: Electromyographic distinction between paramyotonia congenita and myotonia congenita: effect of cold. *Neurology* 32:827, 1982.

PETER JB: Skeletal muscle: Diversity and mutability of its histochemical, electron-microscopic, biochemical and physiologic properties, in Pearson CM, Mostofi FK (eds): *The Striated Muscle.* Baltimore, Williams & Wilkins, 1973, chap 1, pp 1–18.

ROSANO TG, KENNY MD: A radioimmunoassay for human serum myoglobin. Method development and normal values. *Clin Chem* 23:69, 1977.

ROWLAND LP: Myoglobinuria. *Canad J Neurol Sci* 11:1, 1984.

STÅLBERG E, TRONTELJ JV: *Single Fiber Electromyography.* Old Woking, Surrey, UK, The Miraville Press, 1979.

SUMNER AJ (ed): *The Physiology of Peripheral Nerve Disease.* Philadelphia, Saunders, 1980.

WILBOURN AJ: The value and limitations of electromyographic examination in the diagnosis of lumbosacral radiculopathy, in Hardy RW (ed): *Lumbar Disc Disease.* New York, Raven Press, 1982, pp 65–109.

CHAPTER 46

DISEASES OF THE PERIPHERAL NERVES

Disease of the peripheral nervous system stands as one of the most difficult subjects in neurology. Since the structure and function of this system are relatively simple, one might suppose that our knowledge of its diseases would be complete. Such is not the case. For example, in patients with chronic polyneuropathy who were investigated intensively in a highly specialized center for the study of peripheral nerve diseases, a suitable explanation for the neuropathy could not be found in 24 percent of the cases (Dyck, Oviatt, and Lambert). The pathologic changes have not been fully determined in any one of the neuropathies. Moreover, the physiologic basis of many of the neural symptoms continues to elude experts in the field.

In recent years there has been a surge of interest in disease of the peripheral nervous system which promises to change this rather discouraging state of affairs. Electron-microscopic studies, new quantitative histometric methods, and refined physiologic techniques are rapidly expanding our knowledge of the structure and function of peripheral nerves under conditions of disease. These methods permit more precise correlations between structural and functional changes than has been possible until now, and biochemical advances hold promise of providing a better understanding of disease processes as well.

GENERAL CONSIDERATIONS

It is important to have a clear concept of the extent of the peripheral nervous system and of the possible mechanisms whereby it can be affected by disease.

The peripheral nervous system (PNS) includes all neural structures lying outside the pial membrane of the spinal cord and brainstem. The optic nerves and olfactory bulbs are not included, for they are special extensions of the brain. The parts of the PNS within the spinal canal and attached to the ventral and dorsal surfaces of the cord are called the *spinal nerve roots;* those attached to the ventro-lateral surface of the brainstem are the *cranial roots.* The dorsal (afferent or sensory) roots consist of central axonal processes of the dorsal root and cranial ganglion cells; on reaching the spinal cord and brainstem they extend for a variable distance into the posterior columns (funiculi) and spinal trigeminal and other tracts in the medulla and pons. The peripheral axons of the dorsal root ganglion cells are the sensory nerve fibers. They terminate as freely branching endings or in specialized corpuscular endings in the skin, joints, and other tissues. The ventral (efferent, or motor) roots are composed of the emerging axons of anterior and lateral horn cells; they terminate on muscle fibers, or in sympathetic or parasympathetic ganglia. Traversing the subarachnoid space, and lacking epineurial sheaths (Fig. 46-1), the cranial and spinal roots (both sensory and motor) are bathed in and susceptible to substances in the cerebrospinal fluid (CSF), the lumbosacral roots having the longest exposure.

The vast extent of the peripheral ramifications of cranial and spinal nerves is noteworthy, as are their thick protective and supporting sheaths of perineurium and epineurium, and their unique vascular supply through longitudinal arrays of richly anastomosing nutrient arterial branches that run in the epineurium and perineurium (see Fig. 46-4). The nerves traverse narrow foramina (intervertebral and cranial) and a number pass through tight channels peripherally (e.g., median nerve between the carpal ligament and tendon sheaths of flexor forearm muscles; the ulnar nerve in the cubital tunnel). These anatomic features explain the susceptibility of certain nerves to compression and entrapment.

Sympathetic and parasympathetic motor fibers from the spinal cord end in ganglia whose cells in turn send axons (unmedullated) to peripheral nerves and thence to blood vessels, sweat glands, and viscera. The medullated nerves are coated with short segments of myelin of variable length (250 to 1000 μm), each of which is enveloped by a Schwann cell plasma membrane. This latter characteristic is noteworthy because some anatomists define the PNS as the part of the nervous system that is invested by Schwann cells. Each myelin segment has a symbiotic relationship to the axon but is always morphologically independent.

These anatomic features enable one to conceptualize the possible mechanisms by which disease may affect the peripheral nerves. Pathologic processes may be directed at any one of several groups of nerve cells whose axons compose the nerves, e.g., those of the anterior or lateral horns of the spinal cord, the dorsal root ganglia, or sympathetic ganglia. Each cell type exhibits specific vulnerabilities to disease processes, and if destroyed—as are the motor nerve cells in poliomyelitis—there results a secondary degeneration of the axons and myelin sheaths of the peripheral fibers of these cells. On the other hand, the function and structure of the peripheral nerves might be affected by disease processes that involve the ventral and dorsal columns (funiculi) of the spinal cord, which contain the fibers of exit and entry of anterior horn and dorsal root

Figure 46-1

Diagram showing the relationships of the peripheral nerve sheaths to the meningeal coverings of the spinal cord. The epineurium (EP) is in direct continuity with the dura mater (DM). The endoneurium (EN) remains unchanged from the peripheral nerve and spinal root to the junction with the spinal cord. At the subarachnoid angle (SA) the greater portion of the perineurium (P) passes outward between the dura mater and the arachnoid (A), but a few layers appear to continue over the nerve root as part of the root sheath (RS). At the subarachnoid angle, the arachnoid is reflected over the roots and becomes continuous with the outer layers of the root sheath. At the junction with the spinal cord, the outer layers of the root sheath become continuous with the pia mater (PM). (From FR Haller, FM Low, Am J Anat 131:1, 1971.)

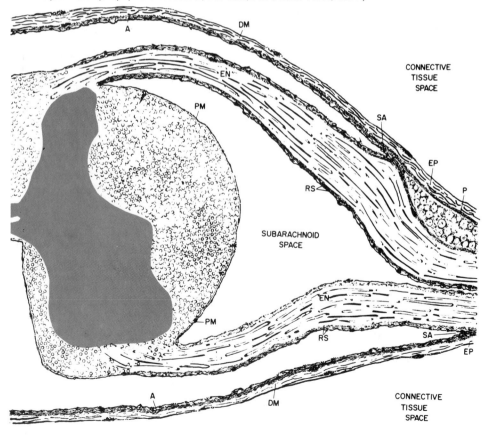

ganglion cells, respectively. The myelin of these centrally located fibers is constituted differently than that of the peripheral nerves, being enveloped by oligodendrocytes rather than Schwann cells, and the fibers are supported by fibrous astrocytes rather than fibroblasts. Because of the intimate relation of the roots to the CSF and to specialized arachnoidal cells (villi), a pathologic process in the CSF or leptomeninges may damage the exposed spinal roots. Destruction of anterior roots results in wallerian degeneration of the motor axons in peripheral nerves; destruction of posterior roots results in wallerian degeneration of the posterior columns of the spinal cord, but not of peripheral nerves. Disease of the connective tissues may affect the peripheral nerves that lie within their sheaths. Diffuse or localized arterial diseases may injure nerves by occluding their nutrient arteries. Noxious agents that selectively damage the Schwann cells or their membranes, which compose the myelin sheaths, cause demyelination of peripheral nerves, leaving axons relatively intact. Finally, one might suppose that axons of the motor or sensory nerves, or sympathetic fibers of varying diameter and length, or the end organs to which they are attached, might each have a particular liability to disease.

Much of this is theoretical and somewhat speculative. At present we can cite examples of diseases that are based on only a few of these potential disease pathways, e.g., diphtheria, in which the bacterial toxin acts directly on the membranes of the Schwann cells near the dorsal root ganglia and adjacent parts of motor and sensory nerves (the most vascular parts of the peripheral nerve); polyarteritis nodosa, which causes widespread occlusion of vasa nervorum; tabes dorsalis, in which there is a treponemal meningoradiculitis of the posterior roots (mainly of the lumbosacral segments) that lie next to the arachnoidal villi (for resorption of CSF); and poisoning with arsenic, which combines with the axoplasm of the largest sensory and motor nerves, via sulfhydryl bonds. Analogous anatomic pathways are probably implicated in other diseases whose mechanisms remain to be divulged.

Pathologically, several distinct processes are recognized, although they are not disease-specific and may be present in varying combinations in any given patient. The major ones are wallerian degeneration, segmental demyelination, and axonal degeneration (diagrammatically illustrated in Fig. 46-2). The myelin sheath is the most susceptible element of the nerve fiber, for it may break down as part of a primary process involving the Schwann cells (or some component thereof) or secondarily, consequent to disease affecting its axon. Focal degeneration of the myelin

sheath with sparing of the axon is called *segmental demyelination*. Degeneration of myelin secondary to axonal disease has been called medullary-axonic and may occur either distal to the most proximal site of axonal interruption *(wallerian degeneration)* or as a "dying-back" phenomenon in more generalized, metabolically determined polyneuropathies *(axonal degeneration)*. The latter form of degeneration affects the terminal parts of the central axons in the posterior columns of the spinal cord as well as the distal axons in peripheral nerves. Wallerian degeneration of axons causes a breakdown of the myelin into blocks or ovoids in which lie fragments of axons (the digestion chambers of Cajal). Degeneration of myelin secondary to neuronal disease has been called neuronolytic (Adams and Richardson) and here also the myelin breaks up into fragments. When the myelin sheath degenerates (the axon being left intact), the highly structured lipoprotein disintegrates into fine particles that are then converted, through the action of macrophages, into neutral fats and cholesterol esters, and carried by these cells to the bloodstream.

In segmental demyelination, recovery of function may be rapid because the intact but denuded axon needs only to become remyelinated. The newly formed internodal segments are of variable length. By contrast, with wallerian or axonal degeneration, recovery is slower, often requiring months to a year or more, because the axon must first regenerate and reconnect to muscle, sensory organ, blood vessel, etc., before function returns. When the axon becomes myelinated, the internodal segments are of uniform length, a point of value to the neuropathologist in the interpretation of teased fiber preparations. When a nerve is severed and continuity is not re-established, regenerating axonic filaments and connective tissue at the end of the central portion of the interrupted nerve form a pseudoneuroma. When nerve cells are destroyed, no recovery of their function is possible except by collateral regeneration from axons of intact nerve cells.

These few pathologic reactions cannot in themselves differentiate the 40 or more diseases of the peripheral nerves, but when considered in relation to the selective effects of pathologic processes on various types and sizes of fibers, the topography of the lesions, and the time course of the process, a set of criteria is provided whereby many diseases can be differentiated. Then, too, there are particular pathologic changes that characterize certain diseases of the peripheral nervous system. In acute idiopathic polyneuritis and infectious mononucleosis there are infiltrations of lymphocytes, plasma cells, and other mononuclear cells in the roots, sensory and sympathetic ganglia and nerves; and frequently the destruction of myelin has a perivenous distribution. In polyarteritis nodosa, a characteristic *necrotizing panarteritis* with occlusion of vessels and focal infarction of peripheral nerves and, less often, with rupture of vessels and hemorrhage into nerves, are the dominant findings. Deposition of amyloid in the endoneurial connective tissue and walls of vessels, affecting the nerve fibers secondarily by compression or ischemia, are the distinctive features of amyloid polyneuropathy. In one of the inherited polyneuropathies of childhood the axons are enlarged by tightly packed masses of neurofilaments. Diphtheritic polyneuropathy is typified by the predominantly demyelinative character of the nerve fiber change, the location of this change in and around the roots and sensory ganglia, the subacute course, and the lack of inflammatory reaction. Other polyneuropathies (paraneoplastic, nutritional, porphyric, arsenical, and uremic) are topographically symmetric but are not presently distinguishable from one another by histopathologic means. The least is known about the familial types of polyneuropathy; although genetic factors are clearly involved, their biochemical mechanisms and pathology are just beginning to be understood.

Concerning the pathogenesis of the mononeuropathies, our knowledge is also incomplete. Compression producing local or segmental ischemia, violent stretch, and laceration of nerves are understandable mechanisms, and the pathologic changes they cause have been reproduced in animals. Vascular disease with ischemic infarction of nerve accounts for some cases. Of infections localized to single nerves, only leprosy, sarcoid, and herpes zoster represent identifiable disease states. For most of the acute mononeuropathies the pathologic changes have yet to be defined, since they are usually benign, reversible states that provide no opportunity for complete pathologic examination.

SYMPTOMATOLOGY

There are a number of motor, sensory, reflex, autonomic, and trophic symptoms and signs that are more or less typical of peripheral nerve disease and provide the criteria for diagnosis.

Figure 46-2

Diagram of the basic pathologic processes affecting peripheral nerves. In wallerian degeneration, *there is degeneration of the axis cylinder and myelin distal to the site of axonal interruption (arrow), and central chromatolysis. In* segmental demyelination *the axon is spared. In* axonal degeneration *there is a distal degeneration of myelin and axis cylinder as a result of neuronal disease. Both wallerian and axonal degeneration cause muscle atrophy. Further details in text. (Courtesy of A Asbury.)*

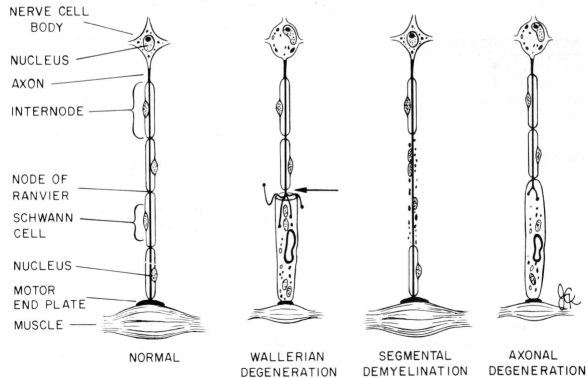

NERVE CELL BODY
NUCLEUS
AXON
INTERNODE
NODE OF RANVIER
SCHWANN CELL
NUCLEUS
MOTOR END PLATE
MUSCLE

NORMAL WALLERIAN DEGENERATION SEGMENTAL DEMYELINATION AXONAL DEGENERATION

IMPAIRMENT OF MOTOR FUNCTION

Whereas anesthetic agents, nerve toxins, cooling, and ischemia may temporarily cause weakness or paralysis, persistent impairment of motor function over days, weeks, or months always signifies segmental demyelination, axonal interruption, or destruction of motor neurons. The degree of weakness is proportional to the number of alpha motor neurons affected, although kinesthetic loss adds to the functional disorder.

Most polyneuropathies are marked by a characteristic distribution of the weakness and paralysis. Usually the muscles of the feet and legs are affected first and most severely, and those of the hands and forearms later and less severely. In milder form, only the lower legs are involved. Most of the nutritional, metabolic, and toxic neuropathies assume this pattern. The pathologic changes in such cases begin in the distal parts of the largest and longest nerves and advance along the affected fibers toward their nerve cell bodies ("dying-back neuropathy," "distal axonopathy"). One explanation for this process is that the primary damage is to the neuronal perikaryon, which fails in its function to synthesize proteins and to deliver them to the distal parts of the axon. Spencer and Schaumburg have theorized that neurotoxic compounds inhibit axonal enzymes required for energy synthesis and that the neuronal soma fails to meet the increased demand for enzyme replacement in the axon, causing the latter to degenerate in the distal regions. Another plausible hypothesis would be that the functional impairment is proportional to the number of affected Schwann cells and myelin segments, there being more of them in long nerves.

Another characteristic pattern of paralysis is one in which all the muscles of the limbs, trunk, and neck are involved, leading often to respiratory paralysis. The vast majority of neuropathies requiring respiratory support are of the acute idiopathic variety, most often referred to as the Guillain-Barré syndrome or GBS. This disease may at times affect proximal limb muscles more than the distal ones. Porphyric, diphtheritic, and certain toxic polyneuropathies are far less common causes of such a pattern of paralysis, but fatalities, when they do occur, are usually due to respiratory paralysis.

A predominantly bibrachial paralysis is rare but may occur in porphyric, lead, and amyloid polyneuropathy, and Tangier disease; occasionally Guillain-Barré disease begins in the cranial nerves and upper extremities. Bifacial and other cranial nerve paralyses are also most likely to occur in the latter syndrome, and less frequently with polyarteritic

or some of the rare metabolic neuropathies (Refsum, Bassen-Kornzweig, Tangier, and Riley-Day).

Atrophy of affected muscles proceeds slowly over several months and its degree is proportional to the number of damaged nerve fibers. The atrophy is a product of disuse, especially in demyelinative neuropathies, and of disuse and denervation in diseases that interrupt axons or destroy motor neurons. Atrophy, therefore, does not coincide with or correspond to acute paralysis and is least prominent in the demyelinative neuropathies such as diphtheritic and some cases of acute idiopathic polyneuritis. In chronic neuropathies, the degrees of paralysis and atrophy correspond. Finally there is degeneration and loss of the denervated muscle fibers. This process begins in 6 to 12 months; in 3 to 4 years most of the denervated fibers will have degenerated. If reinnervation takes place within a year, motor function and muscle volume may be completely restored.

TENDON REFLEXES

The rule is that diminution or loss of tendon reflexes is an invariable sign of peripheral nerve disease. Moreover, reflexes can be diminished out of proportion to weakness because of involvement of the afferent and efferent fibers that innervate the muscle spindles. Another hypothesis is that slowing of conduction velocities in sensory and motor fibers may prevent the reflex by dispersing the volley of impulses initiated by the tendon tap. Early in an acute polyneuropathy the reflexes may be diminished, but not absent, and may be perceptibly more reduced from day to day. In the newly recognized class of small fiber neuropathies, however, tendon reflexes may sometimes be retained, even with marked loss of perception of painful and thermal stimuli and loss of autonomic function.

FASCICULATIONS AND CRAMPS

In most polyneuropathies, fasciculations and cramps are not important findings. Occasionally one observes a state of mild motor polyneuropathy that, upon recovery, leaves the muscles in a state that has been variably referred to as *myokymia, continuous muscular activity* and *neuromyotonia* (see Chap. 54). All the affected muscles ripple and quiver and occasionally cramp. Use of the muscles increases this activity, and there is a reduction in their efficiency which the patient senses as a stiffness and heaviness. Stimulation of a motor nerve, instead of causing a brief burst of action potentials in the muscle, results in a prolonged or dispersed series of potentials lasting several hundred milliseconds. Also the distal latencies are prolonged. Evidently, branched axons involved in collateral innervation have an unstable polarization that may last for years. Another closely related phenomenon results in spasms (e.g., hemifacial spasm) or

neuropathy limits the etiologic possibilities. The *time-course* of the disease is also informative. An acute onset (i.e., rapid evolution) is nearly always diagnostic of an inflammatory, immunologic, or vascular etiology. A polyneuropathy evolving slowly over years is indicative of a hereditary or metabolic disease. Most of the toxic, nutritional, and systemic diseases of nerve develop subacutely over weeks and months.

Also, the diagnosis of both polyneuropathy and mononeuropathy multiplex is facilitated by determining whether the myelin sheath or the axon is primarily involved (*demyelinative disease* or *axonopathy*). This requires that one resort to nerve conduction studies and needle examination of muscles (EMG). The latter also helps to distinguish primary disorders of muscle (myopathies) from disorders that are secondary to denervation and neuromuscular block. The electrical examinations of nerve and muscle are described fully in Chap. 45. Other useful laboratory tests are (1) biochemical tests to identify the metabolic, nutritional, or toxic states that produce neuropathy, (2) CSF examination (increase in protein and sometimes in cells with radicular and meningeal involvement), and (3) nerve (usually sural) and muscle biopsy.

Having established that the patient has a disease of the peripheral nerves and having ascertained its pattern and time-course, one must attempt to determine its nature. This is accomplished most readily by allocating the case in question to one of the categories in Table 46-1, in which the peripheral nerve diseases are classified syndromically, according to their mode of evolution and clinical presentation. Having characterized the neuropathic syndrome in this way, one then seeks to identify the case in question with a particular disease within that category.

Diseases of the peripheral nerves are considered in the most comprehensive fashion in the two-volume monograph *Peripheral Neuropathy,* edited by Dyck, Thomas, Lambert and Bunge, and in the two volumes (7 and 8) on diseases of the nerves in the *Handbook of Clinical Neurology,* edited by Vinken and Bruyn. Also available are more concise monographs on this subject by Schaumburg, Spencer, and Thomas, and by Asbury and Gilliat.

SYNDROME OF ACUTE ASCENDING MOTOR PARALYSIS WITH VARIABLE DISTURBANCE OF SENSORY FUNCTION

Only minor semiologic differences separate the polyneuropathies of (1) acute inflammatory demyelinating type (Landry-Guillain-Barré), (2) acute infectious mononucleosis, (3) viral hepatitis, (4) diphtheria, (5) porphyria, (6) certain intoxications, and (7) acute axonal polyneuropathy. The first of these is by far the most common.

ACUTE IDIOPATHIC POLYNEURITIS [LANDRY-GUILLAIN-BARRÉ DISEASE, GUILLAIN-BARRÉ SYNDROME (GBS), ACUTE INFLAMMATORY DEMYELINATING POLYRADICULONEUROPATHY, ACUTE IMMUNE-MEDIATED POLYNEURITIS (AIMP)]

This inflammatory disease occurs in all parts of the world and in all seasons; it affects children and adults of all ages and both sexes. Its cause is unknown. A mild respiratory or gastrointestinal infection precedes the neuritic symptoms by 1 to 3 weeks in 60 to 70 percent of the patients. Other preceding events include surgical procedures, viral exanthems and other viral illnesses (including AIDS), mycoplasma infections, the spirochetal infection of Lyme disease, and lymphomatous (particularly Hodgkin) disease. The administration of outmoded antirabies vaccines and the A/New Jersey (swine) influenza vaccine, given in late 1976, were associated with a severalfold increase in the incidence of GBS.

Historical It has been difficult to find the earliest description of this syndrome. The important landmarks are Landry's report of an acute, ascending, predominantly motor paralysis with respiratory failure and death; Osler's febrile polyneuritis; the account by Guillain, Barré, and Strohl of a benign childhood polyneuritis with albuminocytologic dissociation in the CSF (increase in protein without cells); and the elaboration of the clinical picture by many British and American investigators (for details of the historical and other aspects of this disease see reference to Asbury, Arnason, and Adams).

Incidence Our experience with this disease at the Massachusetts General and Cleveland Metropolitan General Hospitals has shown it to be nonseasonal and nonepidemic. Year after year between 15 and 25 patients have been admitted to each institution. Males and females are equally susceptible. The age range of 160 consecutive patients was 8 months to 81 years, with attack rates highest in persons 50 to 74 years of age. The incidence rate worldwide is from 1 to 1.5 cases per 100,000 persons per year, and slightly higher in the United States.

Symptomatology The major clinical manifestation is weakness, which evolves, more or less symmetrically, over a period of several days or a week or two. Proximal as well as distal muscles of the limbs are involved, usually the lower extremities before the upper; the trunk, intercostal and neck muscles, and the cranial muscles are affected later. The weakness can progress to total motor paralysis

Table 46-1
Principal neuropathic syndromes

I. Syndrome of acute ascending motor paralysis with variable disturbance of sensory function
   A. Acute idiopathic polyneuritis (inflammatory polyradiculoneuropathy), Landry-Guillain-Barré syndrome (GBS), acute immune-mediated polyneuritis (AIMP)
   B. Infectious mononucleosis and polyneuritis
   C. Hepatitis and polyneuritis
   D. Diphtheritic polyneuropathy
   E. Porphyric polyneuropathy
   F. Certain toxic polyneuropathies (triorthocresyl phosphate, thallium)
   G. Acute axonal polyneuropathy
   H. Rarely, paraneoplastic, vaccinogenic (smallpox, rabies), serogenic, polyarteritic, or lupus polyneuropathy
   I. Acute panautonomic neuropathy

II. Syndrome of subacute sensorimotor paralysis
   A. Symmetric polyneuropathies
      1. Deficiency states: alcoholism (beriberi), pellagra, vitamin B_{12} deficiency, chronic gastrointestinal disease
      2. Poisoning with heavy metals and industrial solvents: arsenic, lead, mercury, thallium, methyl *n*-butyl ketone, *n*-hexane, methyl bromide, organophosphates (TOCP, etc.), acrylamide.
      3. Drug intoxications: isoniazid, ethionamide, hydralazine, nitrofurantoin and related nitrofurazones, disulfiram, carbon disulfide, vincristine, chloramphenicol, phenytoin, amitriptyline, dapsone, stilbamidine, trichlorethylene, thalidomide, Clioquinol, etc.
      4. Uremic polyneuropathy
   B. Asymmetric neuropathies (mononeuropathy multiplex)
      1. Diabetes
      2. Polyarteritis nodosa and other inflammatory angiopathic neuropathies
      3. Subacute idiopathic polyneuropathies
      4. Sarcoidosis
      5. Ischemic neuropathy with peripheral vascular disease.

III. Syndrome of chronic sensorimotor polyneuropathy, acquired forms
   A. Carcinoma, myeloma, and other malignancies
   B. Paraproteinemias
   C. Uremia (occasionally subacute)
   D. Beriberi (usually subacute)
   E. Diabetes
   F. Hypothyroidism
   G. Connective tissue diseases
   H. Amyloidosis
   I. Leprosy
   J. Benign form in the elderly
   K. Sepsis and chronic illness

IV. Syndrome of chronic polyneuropathy, genetically determined forms
   A. Inherited polyneuropathies of predominantly sensory type
      1. Dominant mutilating sensory neuropathy in adults
      2. Recessive mutilating sensory neuropathy of childhood
      3. Congenital insensitivity to pain
      4. Other inherited sensory neuropathies, including those associated with spinocerebellar degenerations and Riley-Day syndrome and the universal anesthesia syndrome
   B. Inherited polyneuropathies of mixed sensorimotorautonomic types
      1. Idiopathic group
         a. Dominant peroneal muscular atrophy (Charcot-Marie-Tooth)
         b. Dominant hypertrophic polyneuropathy of Déjerine-Sottas, adult and childhood forms
         c. Roussy-Lévy polyneuropathy
         d. Polyneuropathy with optic atrophy, with spastic paraglegia, with spinocerebellar degeneration, with mental retardation, and with dementia
      2. Inherited polyneuropathies with a recognized metabolic disorder (see also Chap. 38)
         a. Refsum disease
         b. Metachromatic leukodystrophy
         c. Globoid-body leukodystrophy (Krabbe disease)
         d. Adrenoleukodystrophy
         e. Amyloid polyneuropathy of Andrade
         f. Porphyric polyneuropathy
         g. Anderson-Fabry disease
         h. Abetalipoproteinemia and Tangier disease

V. Syndrome of recurrent or relapsing polyneuropathy
   A. Idiopathic polyneuritis (GBS)
   B. Porphyria
   C. Chronic inflammatory polyradiculoneuropathy
   D. Certain forms of mononeuritis multiplex
   E. Beriberi or intoxications
   F. Refsum disease, Tangier disease

VI. Syndrome of mononeuropathy or multiple neuropathies
   A. Pressure palsies
   B. Traumatic neuropathies (including irradiation and electrical injuries)
   C. Idiopathic brachial and sciatic neuropathy
   D. Serum and vaccinogenic (smallpox, rabies) neuropathy
   E. Herpes zoster
   F. Neoplastic infiltration of roots and nerves
   G. Leprosy
   H. Diphtheritic wound infections with local neuropathy
   I. Migrant sensory neuropathy

with death from respiratory failure within a few days. Pain and aching in the muscles are frequent complaints. Paresthesias (tingling and numbness) are frequent but tend to be evanescent; occasionally they are absent throughout the illness. Objective sensory loss occurs to a variable degree and in a few is barely detectable; when present, deep sensibility tends to be more affected than superficial.

The weakness develops so rapidly that muscle atrophy does not occur. Hypotonia and reduced and then absent reflexes are consistent findings. There is in many cases tenderness on deep pressure of muscles. At an early stage the arm muscles may be less weak than the leg muscles or are spared entirely. Facial diplegia, occurring in about half of all cases, and other cranial palsies usually come later, after the arms are affected. Disturbances of autonomic function (sinus tachycardia and less often bradycardia, facial flushing, fluctuating hypertension and hypotension, loss of sweating or episodic profuse diaphoresis) are common, but rarely do these abnormalities persist for more than a week or two. Retention of urine occurs rarely, and catheterization is seldom required for more than a few days.

Variants of this clinical picture are frequent. Whereas in most patients the paralysis ascends from legs to trunk, arms, and cranial muscles (Landry's ascending paralysis) and reaches a peak of severity within 10 to 14 days (90 percent of our cases), occasionally cranial and arm muscles are affected first, or simultaneously with those of the legs. A syndrome comprising complete ophthalmoplegia with ataxia and areflexia, and thought to represent a variety of acute idiopathic polyneuritis, has been described by Fisher. Cases with stepwise progression over several weeks, some of which show asymmetries of involvement, probably represent a different disease. A relapsing form of the latter is also known (see further on).

The body temperature is usually normal, and lymphadenopathy and splenomegaly do not occur. T-wave and other electrocardiographic changes of minor degree have been reported frequently but are evanescent. The CSF is under normal pressure and is acellular in all but 10 percent of patients; in the latter, 10 to 50 cells (rarely more) per cubic millimeter, predominantly lymphocytes, is found. About a week after the onset of symptoms the protein level begins to rise, reaching a peak in 4 to 6 weeks. The increase in CSF protein is probably a reflection of the widespread inflammatory disease of the nerve roots. In the peripheral blood, there is a moderate leukocytosis and shift to immature forms early in the illness, but the blood picture soon returns to normal. Nerve conduction velocities are slowed soon after the paralysis develops, sometimes more in proximal parts of the nerves (abnormal H and F responses) than distal. Denervation potentials (fibrillations), if they are to appear at all, come later. Transient diabetes insipidus is a rare complication for unexplained reasons.

Pathologic Findings These have had a consistent pattern and form. Even when the disease is fatal within a few days, perivascular lymphocytic infiltrates have been found. Later the characteristic inflammatory cell infiltrates and perivenous demyelination are combined with segmental demyelination and a variable degree of wallerian degeneration. Infiltrates are scattered throughout the cranial nerves, ventral and dorsal roots, dorsal root ganglia, and along the entire length of the peripheral nerves. Infiltrates of inflammatory cells (lymphocytes and other mononuclear cells) are also found in lymph nodes, liver, spleen, heart, and other organs, and reflect the systemic nature of the disease.

Pathogenesis and Etiology Most of the evidence suggests that the clinical manifestations of this disorder are the result of a cell-mediated immunologic reaction directed at peripheral nerve. Waksman and Adams demonstrated that a peripheral nerve disease, clinically and pathologically indistinguishable from acute idiopathic polyneuritis, develops in animals about 2 weeks after immunization with peripheral nerve homogenate (experimental allergic neuritis or EAN). Brostoff and his colleagues determined that the antigen in this reaction is a basic protein, designated as P_2 protein, found only in peripheral nerve myelin. Subsequent investigations by these authors indicated that the neuritogenic factor was a specific peptide in the P_2 protein. The pathologic steps in this proposed reaction are diagramatically illustrated in Fig. 46-3. All attempts to isolate a virus or microbial agent have failed. However, the occurrence of a similar polyneuritis in patients with AIDS and with a preceding Epstein-Barr or cytomegalus virus infection, opens again the possibility of a viral etiology.

Differential Diagnosis Acute idiopathic polyneuritis (GBS) is not only one of the most frequent forms of polyneuropathy seen in a general hospital but also the most rapidly evolving and potentially fatal form. Any polyneuropathy that brings the patient to the brink of death within a few days will usually be of this type. The predominantly motor paralysis is its other major characteristic. Because of the latter feature, one must include poliomyelitis (distinguished by an epidemic occurrence, meningeal symptoms, fever, purely motor and usually asymmetric areflexic paralysis) and acute myelopathy (marked by sensorimotor paralysis below a given spinal level and sphincteric paralysis) in the differential diagnosis. Other forms of acute polyneuropathy described below must also be differentiated from this syndrome.

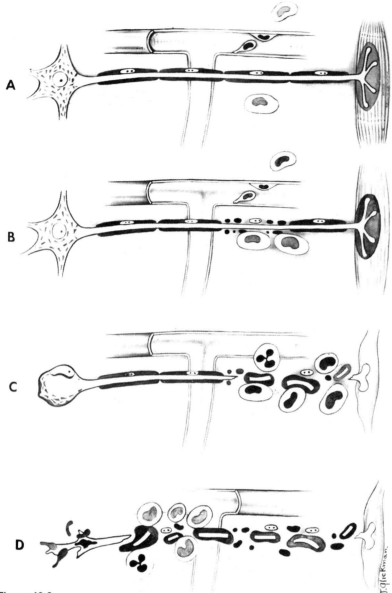

Figure 46-3

Diagram of probable cellular events in idiopathic polyneuritis. A. Lymphocytes attach to the walls of endoneurial vessels, migrate through the vessel wall, enlarging and transforming as they do so. At this stage no nerve damage has occurred. B. More lymphocytes have migrated into the surrounding tissue. The first effect upon the nerve is breakdown of myelin, the axon being spared (segmental demyelination). This change appears to be mediated by the mononuclear exudate, but the mechanism is uncertain. C. The lesion is more intense, polymorphonuclear leukocytes being present as well as lymphocytes. The axon is interrupted in addition to myelin sheath damage; as a result, the muscle undergoes denervation atrophy and the nerve cell body shows central chromatolysis. If the axonal damage is distal, the nerve cell body will survive, and regeneration and clinical recovery is likely. If, as in D, axonal interruption has occurred proximally because of a particularly intense root or proximal nerve lesion, the nerve cell body may die and undergo dissolution. In this situation, there is no regeneration, only the possibility of collateral reinnervation of muscle from surviving motor fibers. (From Asbury et al, 1969.)

Treatment The essence of therapy is respiratory assistance and careful nursing, for the disease remits naturally and recovery is complete in the majority of cases. Not every patient needs respiratory assistance, but since the patient's condition may deteriorate rapidly, he or she should be in a hospital where such aid is available. Respiratory assistance should be instituted at the first sign of dyspnea (expiratory vital capacity below 12 to 15 mL/kg) or decrease in oxygen saturation of the blood (arterial Po_2 below 70 mmHg). Tracheostomy may become necessary at this time, especially if the patient has difficulty in clearing secretions from the pharynx and tracheobronchial tree, but may be postponed and an endotracheal tube used for a few days if the physician is uncertain. Once tracheostomy is performed, careful tracheal toilet and control of infections by the use of appropriate antibiotics are required. Support of the blood pressure in the face of hypotension by vasopressor agents is another essential part of the therapeutic regimen. The best results are obtained by admitting the patient to an efficient respiratory care unit, skilled in maintaining adequacy of ventilation and circulation, preferably before respiratory failure occurs. Under these conditions the mortality from the disease can be reduced to 3 percent or less (Ropper and Kehne).

A controlled trial of the use of *plasmapheresis*, involving 245 cases of GBS in several hospital centers, has indicated that it is a useful therapeutic measure in the rapidly evolving phase of GBS (Guillain-Barré Study Group). A controlled study by the French Cooperative Group has reinforced this conclusion. In patients who were treated within 2 weeks of onset, there was a distinct reduction in the period of hospitalization, in the length of time that the patient required mechanical ventilation, and in the time required for the patient to resume walking. However, if plasmapheresis was instituted 3 weeks or longer after the onset of the disease, the procedure had little value. The most important predictors of early responsiveness to plasmapheresis treatment were the patient's age (responders were younger), and the preservation of amplitudes of compound muscle action potentials prior to instituting plasmapheresis (McKhann et al; Gruener et al).

Our practice, as advocated by McKhann and Griffin, is to observe the patient closely, even if mildly affected; if the patient reaches or appears to be reaching an inability to walk unaided, or shows a significant reduction in vital capacity (see above) or bulbar weakness, pheresis is instituted promptly. This procedure, like the management of respiratory failure, should be carried out in centers with special competence in the technique and complications of plasmapheresis. Patients who fail to meet these criteria should not undergo plasmapheresis. There is some evidence (Osterman et al) that patients who are exchanged very early may suffer a relapse when plasmapheresis is discontinued.

Corticosteroids are said to have no therapeutic value, yet we have observed high doses to reverse a progressive course in individual cases.

Physiotherapy (passive movement and positioning of limbs to prevent pressure palsies and, later, mild resistance exercises) should begin once the condition of the patient has stabilized. The decision to discontinue respiratory aid and to close the tracheostomy are based on the degree of recovery of the patient's respiratory function.

Prognosis As indicated above, about 3 percent of patients do not survive the illness, even in the best-equipped hospital. In the early stages, death is most often due to the accidental disconnection of the patient from the respirator, or some other type of machine failure. Occasionally death occurs suddenly, without adequate explanation. Later in the illness, pulmonary embolism and complications of prolonged tracheostomy (usually bacterial) are the main causes.

The majority of patients recover spontaneously and completely. In the multicenter study of GBS, referred to above, 10 to 23 percent required mechanical ventilatory assistance, and 7 to 22 percent were left with some degree of disability—usually mild motor or reflex deficits in the feet and legs. In about 10 percent of patients, however, the residual disability was severe; this occurred in the patients with the most severe and rapidly evolving form of the disease and the ones requiring early and prolonged mechanical ventilatory assistance (Ropper). In patients with respiratory failure, the average period of machine-assisted respiration has been 50 days and the period of hospitalization, 108 days. As indicated above, these periods can be reduced significantly by the early use of plasmapheresis.

The speed of recovery varies. Often it occurs within a few weeks or months; but if axons have degenerated, their regeneration may require 6 to 18 months or longer. Little or no improvement can be expected after 2 years. In general, elderly patients recover more slowly than younger ones and are more likely to be left with residual weakness.

About 3 percent of patients suffer one or more recurrences of acute polyneuropathy, and in the latter cases the nerves may gradually become palpably enlarged. An illness that in the beginning appears to be an acute inflammatory polyradiculoneuropathy may fail to stabilize and continue to progress steadily; or, there may be an incomplete remission followed by a chronic, fluctuating slowly progressive neuropathy. These chronic forms of neuropathy need to be distinguished from acute GBS and are described in a later section of this chapter.

INFECTIOUS MONONUCLEOSIS WITH POLYNEURITIS

Three neurologic syndromes have been described with infectious mononucleosis: (1) a rapidly evolving ascending sensorimotor paralysis, identical to that of the Guillain-Barré syndrome described above, (2) aseptic meningitis, and (3) meningoencephalitis. All three appear during the midphase of the infection. The polyneuritis varies in severity and has rarely been fatal. The few autopsied cases have shown heavy infiltrations of lymphocytes, monocytes, and sometimes plasma cells in the nerves, roots, and meninges. The CSF may contain only a few or as many as several hundred mononuclear cells, and the protein level is raised. The diagnosis is suggested by the other typical physical and laboratory findings in this disease.

VIRAL HEPATITIS WITH ACUTE POLYNEURITIS

An acute polyneuritis, indistinguishable clinically and pathologically from the GBS type, may be associated with viral hepatitis. The polyneuritis usually follows the jaundice by several days or weeks and probably has the same relation to it as to preceding respiratory or intestinal infections. Usually the type of hepatitis has remained unclear. Recovery from the hepatitis and polyneuritis has been the rule, but is not invariable.

Neuropathy may be associated with liver disease under two other conditions: (1) A mild and usually asymptomatic (nutritional?) polyneuropathy has been described with chronic liver disease of diverse types. (2) A mild subacute to chronic sensory neuropathy, due to xanthomatous involvement of the connective tissue sheaths of cutaneous nerves, is occasionally encountered in patients with biliary cirrhosis (Thomas and Walker). These *hepatic polyneuropathies,* in which the nerve lesions appear to be a consequence of the liver disease, should not be confused with conditions in which the polyneuropathy and liver disease are both complications of a systemic disease such as alcoholism and malnutrition, infectious mononucleosis, polyarteritis nodosa, amyloidosis, and certain intoxications.

DIPHTHERITIC POLYNEUROPATHY

Some of the neurotoxic effects of *C. diphtheriae* and mode of action of the exotoxin elaborated by the bacillus are described in Chap. 42. Local action of the exotoxin may paralyze pharyngeal and laryngeal muscles (dysphagia, nasal voice) within 1 or 2 weeks after the onset of the infection, and shortly thereafter may also cause blurring of vision due to loss of accommodation, but these and other cranial nerve symptoms may be overlooked. The polyneuropathy, coming 5 to 8 weeks later, takes the form of an acute to subacute limb weakness with paresthesias and distal loss of vibratory and position sense. The weakness characteristically involves all four extremities at the same time or may descend from arms to legs. After a few days to a week or more, the patient may be unable to stand or walk, and occasionally the paralysis is so severe and extensive as to impair respiration. The CSF protein level is usually elevated (50 to 200 mg/dL). Diphtheritic deaths that occur after the pharyngeal infection has been controlled are due usually to cardiomyopathy or to polyneuropathy with respiratory paralysis.

As indicated earlier, the important pathologic change is a demyelination without inflammatory reaction of spinal roots, sensory ganglia, and adjacent spinal nerves. Axons, anterior horn cells, peripheral nerves distally, and muscle fibers remain normal.

Diphtheria antitoxin, given within 48 h of the onset of the infection, reduces the incidence and severity of neuropathic complications. Antitoxin is of no value once the polyneuropathy begins. Otherwise, treatment is purely symptomatic, along the lines indicated for acute idiopathic polyneuritis. The prognosis for full recovery is excellent, once respiratory paralysis is circumvented.

PORPHYRIC POLYNEUROPATHY

A severe, rapidly advancing, more or less symmetric polyneuropathy, often with abdominal pain, psychosis (delirium or confusion), and convulsions mark the disease known as *acute intermittent porphyria* (pyrroloporphyria, or Swedish type). This type of porphyria is inherited as an autosomal dominant trait and is not associated with cutaneous sensitivity to sunlight. The metabolic defect is in the liver and is marked by increased production and urinary excretion of porphobilinogen and of the porphyrin precursor, δ-aminolevulinic acid. The peripheral and central nervous systems may also be affected in *variegate (South African) porphyria.* In this latter type, the skin is markedly sensitive to light and trauma, and porphyrins are at all times found in the stools. Both of these *hepatic* forms of porphyria are to be distinguished from the rare *erythropoietic (congenital photosensitive)* porphyria, in which the nervous system is not affected.

The most extensive study of acute intermittent porphyria was reported by Waldenstrom in 1937. The initial and often the most prominent symptom is moderate to severe colicky pain. It may be generalized or localized and is unattended by rigidity of the abdominal wall or tenderness. Radiographs show intestinal distention and spasm. Constipation is frequent. Attacks last for days to weeks and repeated vomiting may lead to inanition. In latent forms, the patient may be asymptomatic or complain only of slight dyspepsia.

The neurologic manifestations are usually those of a polyneuropathy, involving principally the motor nerves, less often both sensory and motor nerves, and sometimes autonomic nerves. It may begin in the feet and legs and ascend, or it may begin in the hands and arms (sometimes asymmetrically) and spread in a few days to the trunk and legs. Occasionally the weakness predominates in the proximal muscles of the limbs and limb girdles. Sensory loss, often involving the trunk, is present in half the cases. Facial paralysis, dysphagia, and ocular palsies are features of the most severe affections, simulating acute polyneuritis of the GBS type. The CSF protein content is normal or slightly elevated. The course of the polyneuropathy is variable. In mild cases the symptoms may regress in a few weeks. If severe, it may progress to a fatal respiratory or cardiac paralysis in a few days; or it may progress in a saltatory fashion over a period of several weeks, resulting in a severe sensorimotor paralysis that requires months to regress.

A disturbance of cerebral function (confusion, delirium, visual field defects, and convulsions) is more likely to precede the severe than the mild forms of polyneuropathy, but it may not appear at all. The cerebral manifestations usually subside in a few days to weeks though one of our patients was left with a homonymous hemianopia.

Tachycardia and hypertension are frequent in the acute phase of the disease, and fever and leukocytosis also may occur; these are said to reflect the activity of the pathologic process. The disease is characterized by recurrent attacks, often precipitated by drugs such as sulfonamides, griseofulvin, estrogens, barbiturates, phenytoin, and the succinimide anticonvulsants. The possibility of sensitivity to these drugs must always be kept in mind when treating convulsions in the porphyric patient. The first attack rarely occurs before puberty, and the disease is most likely to threaten life during adolescence and early adulthood. Death may result from respiratory paralysis or cardiac arrest and sometimes from uremia and cachexia.

In sum, the most characteristic clinical features are acute onset, initial abdominal pain and psychotic symptoms, predominantly motor neuropathy, often an early bibrachial distribution of weakness, truncal sensory loss, and tachycardia.

The pathologic findings in the peripheral nervous system vary according to the stage of the illness at which death occurs. If the patient dies in the first few days, the myelinated fibers may appear entirely normal, despite an almost complete paralysis. If symptoms had been present for weeks, degeneration of both axons and myelin sheaths will be found in most of the peripheral nerves. No inflammatory reaction, vascular lesion, or other change distin-

guishes this form of polyneuropathy. The relation between the abnormality of porphyrin biosynthesis in the liver and nervous dysfunction has never been explained satisfactorily.

Diagnosis is confirmed by the demonstration of large amounts of porphobilinogen and δ-aminolevulinic acid in the urine. The urine turns dark when standing due to the formation of porphobilin, an oxidation product of porphobilinogen.

In general, the *prognosis* for ultimate recovery is excellent, though relapse of the porphyria may result in further involvement of the peripheral nervous system (see *relapsing polyneuropathy,* further on).

Treatment consists of respiratory support, use of beta blockers (propranolol) if tachycardia and hypertension are severe, intravenous glucose to suppress the heme biosynthetic pathway, and pyridoxine (100 mg twice a day) on the supposition that vitamin B_6 depletion has occurred. The use of intravenous levulose and intravenous hematin (4 mg/kg once or twice a day) has been recommended (see review by Ridley).

Prevention is of the utmost importance, since attacks can be precipitated by porphyrinogenic drugs, the most common of which are the barbiturates (see above).

CERTAIN TOXIC POLYNEUROPATHIES

As indicated in Chap. 42 the peripheral nerves may be affected by a wide variety of toxins, including heavy metals, drugs and industrial solvents. The neuropathies induced by these agents are chronic in nature, as a general rule. Certain drugs, however, notably triorthocresylphosphate *(TOCP)* and other organophosphates (page 914) and *thallium* produce a polyneuropathy that may be fatal in a matter of days. *TOCP* causes severe and permanent motor paralysis that ultimately proves to be due to involvement of both upper and lower motor neurons.

Thallium salts, when taken in sufficient amount, may also produce a clinicial picture that resembles that of GBS. If taken orally there is first abdominal pain, vomiting, and diarrhea followed within a few days by pain and tingling in the toes and fingertips and then rapid weakening of muscles of the legs, hands, and arms. Initially the weakness is always distal. As it progresses, the tendon reflexes diminish. Pain sensation is reduced more than touch, vibratory, and position sense. All cranial nerves except the first and eighth may be affected; facial palsies, ophthalmoplegia, nystagmus, optic neuritis with visual impairment, and vocal cord palsies are the most prominent abnormalities. The CSF protein rises to over 100 mg. Death may occur in the first 10 days, due to cardiac arrest. The early onset of painful paresthesias, pain localized to joints, back, and chest, and rapid loss of hair (within a week or two) help differentiate this neuropathy from GBS, porphyria and other acute polyneuropathies. Relative preservation of reflexes is also noteworthy. From lesser degrees of intoxication there may be recovery. Thallium salts act like potassium and a high intake of KCl hastens the excretion of thallium; chelating agents are of unproven value.

ACUTE AXONAL FORM OF GBS

Most of the acute polyneuropathies are autoimmune and demyelinative in type. Acute axonal polyneuropathies are rare and usually they are due to toxins. Recently, however, Feasby and his colleagues have drawn attention to a nontoxic form. They described five patients with the clinical syndrome of GBS, each with a particularly rapid evolution and poor recovery. Unlike the usual form of the disease, all of their patients had inexcitable motor nerves and signs of severe muscle denervation, and lacked the characteristic decrease in conduction velocities and conduction block. Postmortem examination in one patient showed severe axonal degeneration affecting nerves and roots, without inflammation and with only minimal demyelination.

OTHER ACUTE POLYNEUROPATHIES

Occasionally, the *polyneuropathy associated with lupus erythematosus* or *polyarteritis nodosa* develops as rapidly as acute idiopathic polyneuritis, and muscle biopsy may be needed to distinguish these disorders. However, most cases of neuropathy due to polyarteritis evolve more slowly and the syndrome assumes a symmetric or asymmetric distribution. For this reason it will be described in the next section.

 We have observed a few patients with alcoholism, occult carcinoma, Hodgkin disease, and renal transplantation who developed an acute polyneuropathy, as rapid in its evolution as GBS, and acute episodes of this type have also been described in patients with Refsum disease. Formerly, the use of smallpox and rabies vaccines and injections of antitoxin in foreign serum were sometimes followed by a sensorimotor polyneuritis. The usual picture, however, is a brachial plexitis and these conditions are more appropriately discussed with the brachial plexus neuropathies (see further on in this chapter.)

PURE AUTONOMIC POLYNEUROPATHIES

Since the first description of such a case by Young and his colleagues, a number of similar cases has been recorded (Low et al). The condition is described in detail in Chap. 26.

SYNDROME OF SUBACUTE SENSORIMOTOR PARALYSIS

SUBACUTE SYMMETRIC POLYNEUROPATHIES

The neuropathic conditions in this category evolve over a period of a few weeks, and, after reaching their peak of severity, tend to persist for a variable period. In contrast to the acute polyneuropathies, most subacute ones are of axonal type; subacute demyelinative types occur but are rare (buckthorn berry and gold thioglucose poisoning). Some instances of diphtheritic (demyelinative) neuropathy evolve subacutely, but others evolve rapidly, like GBS. Pain, dysesthesias and paresthesias, "hyperesthesia," and tenderness of muscles are often prominent features, in addition to weakness and atrophy of muscles, and loss of sensation and tendon reflexes. A symmetric syndrome of this type usually proves to be due to alcoholism and nutritional deficiency, or to poisoning with arsenic, lead, nitrofurantoin, hydralazine, disulfiram (Antabuse), perhexiline, or isoniazid. Occasionally other drugs, heavy metals, and industrial solvents can be incriminated; these are discussed in Chap. 42.

Deficiency States In the western world, nutritional polyneuropathy is usually associated with alcoholism. As pointed out in Chap. 39, all data point to the identity of alcoholic neuropathy and neuropathic beriberi. A common nutritional factor is responsible for both, though in any given case it often remains unclear whether the deficiency is one of thiamine, pyridoxine, pantothenic acid, folic acid, or a combination of the B vitamins. We have not been able to define a form of polyneuropathy that is attributable to the direct toxic effect of alcohol. Neuropathic beriberi and other forms of deficiency neuropathy (Strachan syndrome, pellagra, vitamin B_{12} deficiency, and malabsorption syndromes) are described fully in Chap. 39.

Arsenical Polyneuropathy Of the neuropathies caused by metallic poisoning, that due to arsenic is particularly well known. In cases of chronic poisoning, the symptoms develop rather slowly, over a period of several weeks or months, and have the same sensory and motor distribution as the nutritional polyneuropathies. Gastrointestinal symptoms, the result of ingestion of arsenic, may precede the polyneuropathy which is nearly always associated with anemia, jaundice, brownish cutaneous pigmentation, hyperkeratosis of palms and soles, white transverse banding of the nails (Mees lines), and an excess of arsenic in the urine and hair. Pathologically, this form of arsenical neuropathy is of the ''dying-back'' (axonal degeneration) type.

In patients who survive the ingestion of a single massive dose of arsenic, a more rapidly evolving polyneuropathy may appear after a period of 8 to 21 days. The neuropathy may be preceded by severe gastrointestinal symptoms, renal and hepatic failure, and mental disturbances, convulsions, confusion, and coma, i.e., arsenical encephalopathy (brain purpura). Initially, the neuropathy that develops in this setting may resemble GBS, both clinically and electromyographically (partial conduction block, prolonged F responses).

Diagnosis and treatment of arsenical poisoning are discussed further in Chap. 42.

Lead Neuropathy Lead neuropathy is an uncommon disorder. It occurs following chronic exposure to lead, and its most characteristic clinical feature is the predominantly motor affection involving mainly the upper extremities. The radial nerves are most frequently involved, producing wrist and finger drop with few or no sensory manifestations. Less commonly, there is foot drop and weakness of the proximal arm muscles and the shoulder girdle. As pointed out in Chap. 42, lead neuropathy is a disease of adults; it seldom occurs in children, in whom lead poisoning usually results in an encephalopathy.

The diagnosis is established by the history of lead exposure, the characteristic motor involvement, the associated medical findings (anemia, basophilic stippling of red cell precursors in the bone marrow, a ''lead line'' along the gingival margins, colicky abdominal pain, and constipation), and the urinary excretion of lead and coproporphyrins. Blood lead levels of more than 70 μg/dL are always abnormal. In patients with lower levels, doubling of the 24-h urinary lead excretion following an infusion of the chelating agent CaNa$_2$ EDTA indicates a significant degree of lead intoxication. Coproporphyrin in the urine is abnormal in any amount, but it may be found in porphyria, alcoholism, iron deficiency, and other disorders, as well as in lead intoxication. Treatment consists of terminating the exposure to lead and eliminating lead from the blood stream and the bones by the measures described in Chap. 42. For this purpose, penicillamine, which is safe and can be administered orally, is preferable to BAL or edetate.

Other Metals and Industrial Solvents Poisoning with *mercury, thallium* (more chronic form of intoxication), and sometimes with *lithium, gold,* and *platinum* (in the antineoplastic agent cisplatin) may produce a sensorimotor polyneuropathy similar to arsenical polyneuropathy; these

intoxications are discussed in Chap. 42. Exposure to manganese, bismuth, antimony, zinc, and copper may give rise to systemic signs of poisoning; some of them affect the central nervous system, but one cannot be certain that any of them specifically involves the peripheral nerves. A distal, symmetric sensorimotor (predominantly sensory) neuropathy may follow exposure to certain hexacarbon industrial solvents, such as *n-hexane* (found in contact cements) and *methyl n-butyl ketone* (used in the production of plastic-coated and color-printed fabrics); to dimethylaminopropionitrile (DMAPN), used in the manufacture of polyurethane foam); to the fumigant *methyl bromide;* and to the gas sterilant *ethylene oxide.*

Detailed accounts of the clinical and experimental neurotoxicology of these agents can be found in the monograph edited by Spencer and Schaumburg.

Isonicotinic Acid Hydrazide (Isoniazid, INH) Neuropathy As mentioned in Chap. 39, isoniazid-induced polyneuropathy was a common occurrence in the early 1950s, when this drug was first used for the treatment of tuberculosis. Symptoms of neuropathy appeared in about 10 percent of patients receiving therapeutic doses of the drug (10 mg/kg daily), between 3 and 35 weeks after treatment was begun.

The initial symptoms are a symmetric numbness and tingling of the toes and feet, spreading, if the drug is continued, to the knees, and occasionally to the hands. Aching and burning pain in these parts then become prominent. In addition to sensory loss, examination discloses a loss of tendon reflexes and weakness in the distal parts of the limbs, almost exclusively of the legs. Severe degrees of weakness and loss of deep sensation are observed only rarely.

INH produces its effects on the peripheral nerves by interfering with pyridoxine metabolism, perhaps by inhibiting the phosphorylation of pyridoxine (the collective name for the B$_6$ group of vitamins), and decreasing the tissue levels of its active form, pyridoxal phosphate. The administration of 150 to 450 mg of pyridoxine daily, in conjunction with isoniazid, completely prevents the neuropathic disorder. The same mechanism is probably operative in the neuropathies that occasionally complicate the administration of the INH-related substances *ethionamide,* used in the treatment of tuberculosis, and the antihypertensive agent *hydralazine.* Paradoxically, the prolonged administration of extremely high doses of pyridoxine may actually cause a disabling, predominantly sensory neuropathy (Schaumburg et al).

Nitrofurantoin Neuropathy The introduction in 1952 of nitrofurantoin for the treatment of bladder infections was soon followed by reports of neurotoxicity attributable to this drug. The earliest symptoms are pain and tingling paresthesias of the toes and feet, followed shortly by similar sensations in the fingers. If the drug is not discontinued, this disorder may progress to a severe, symmetric, sensorimotor polyneuropathy. Neuropathic symptoms appear after the drug has been administered in high dosage for several weeks or months, but a few patients have experienced paresthesias after briefer periods. Patients with chronic renal failure and azotemia are particularly prone to neurotoxicity from nitrofurantoin, presumably because diminished excretion results in high tissue levels of the drug. To make matters more difficult, the uremic state itself may be responsible for a clinically similar polyneuropathy, so that the distinction between uremic and nitrofurantoin neuropathy in the presence of chronic renal failure may be impossible. The neuropathologic studies of Lhermitte et al reveal an axonal degeneration in peripheral nerves and sensory roots.

Other Drug-Induced Neuropathies The development of a sensorimotor neuropathy, similar to that produced by isoniazid, is sometimes associated with the chronic use of *disulfiram* (Antabuse). Its neurotoxic effects have been attributed to the action of *carbon disulfide*, which is produced during the metabolism of disulfiram and is known to produce polyneuropathy among workers in the viscose rayon industry. Pathologic data, though scant, tend to discredit this notion, insofar as disulfiram produced a wallerian-type axonal degeneration, whereas carbon disulfide neuropathy is characterized by swollen (giant) axons that are filled with neurofilaments (Bouldin et al).

Peripheral neuropathy commonly complicates the use of *vincristine,* an antineoplastic agent widely used in treatment of the reticuloses and leukemia (see page 916). Loss of ankle jerks is an early manifestation, along with paresthesias, mild sensory loss, and weakness of the fingers and toes, in that order. Weakness is observed first in the extensor muscles of the fingers and wrists, later in the dorsiflexors of the toes and feet, and if the dosage of vincristine is not reduced, weakness may spread rapidly to involve the proximal muscles of the limbs. The neuropathy is strictly dose-related and reduction in dosage is followed by rapid improvement of neuropathic symptoms; many patients are then able to continue the use of vincristine in low dosage, such as 1 mg every 2 weeks, for many months. Also, among chemotherapeutic agents, *cisplatin* is

known to evoke a predominantly sensory polyneuropathy, which begins several weeks after completion of therapy. Proprioception and vibratory sensation are most severely affected, and there may be degeneration in the posterior columns—the basis for Lhermitte's sign.

A relatively mild sensory neuropathy associated with optic neuropathy occasionally complicates *chloramphenicol* therapy. Patients who have taken *phenytoin* for many years may show absence of ankle and patellar reflexes, a mild, distal symmetric impairment of sensation, a reduced conduction velocity in the peripheral nerves of the legs, and, rarely, weakness of the distal musculature. The chronic administration of *metronidazole* (used in the treatment of Crohn disease) and of *amitriptyline* may occasionally have the same effect. A predominantly motor neuropathy may be induced by the chronic administration of *dapsone,* a sulfone used to treat leprosy and certain dermatologic conditions. *Stilbamidine,* used in the treatment of kala azar, may produce a purely sensory neuropathy, mainly in the distribution of the trigeminal nerves. The anesthetic agent *trichloroethylene* also has a predilection for cranial nerves, particularly the fifth. The neurotoxicity is apparently due to dichloroacetylene, formed in the course of decomposition of trichloroethylene. *Amiodarone,* a drug that is commonly used in Europe for treating angina pectoris and ventricular tachyarrhythmias, induces a motor-sensory neuropathy in about 5 percent of patients after several months of treatment. *Perhexiline maleate,* another drug for the treatment of angina pectoris, also may induce a generalized, predominantly sensory polyneuropathy in a small proportion of treated patients. Affected persons show a striking neuronal lipidosis, which has been attributed to an inherited metabolic impairment of oxidation of debrisoquine (Shah et al). *Triorthocresyl phosphate* and *acrylamide* are potent peripheral nerve poisons. Both of these drugs cause a ''dying-back'' polyneuropathy (axonal degeneration) and have been used experimentally to produce this effect.

Clioquinol (discussed in Chap. 42) and *thalidomide,* each of which can produce severe polyneuropathy, have been withdrawn from the market, but patients are still seen with the residual neurotoxic effects of these drugs.

A subacute symmetric polyneuropathy of varying severity is not an infrequent development in critically ill and septic patients who require prolonged intubation for cardiac or pulmonary disease (Zochodne et al). It may pose a major difficulty in weaning the patient from the ventilator as the critical illness comes under control. The EMG findings of a primary axonal degeneration and a normal CSF distinguish the neuropathy from GBS, and autopsies have disclosed no inflammatory changes in the peripheral nerves. The toxic effects of drugs and antibiotics and nutritional deficiency are always considered in causation, but rarely can these factors be established.

The most notable examples of this syndrome accompany diabetes, polyarteritis nodosa and other vasculitides, and uncommon forms of idiopathic polyneuritis. Rarely, sarcoidosis presents in this fashion.

Diabetic Neuropathy   About 15 percent of patients with diabetes mellitus have both symptoms and signs of neuropathy, but nearly 50 percent have either neuropathic symptoms or slowing of nerve conduction velocity. Neuropathy is most common in diabetics over 50 years of age, is uncommon in those under 30 years of age, and is rare in childhood.

Several clinical syndromes have been delineated: (1) diabetic ophthalmoplegia, (2) acute mononeuropathy, (3) a rapidly evolving, painful, asymmetric, predominantly motor, multiple neuropathy (so-called *mononeuropathy multiplex)*, which usually undergoes remission, (4) a symmetric, proximal motor weakness and wasting without pain and with variable sensory loss, which pursues a subacute or chronic course, (5) a distal, symmetric, primarily sensory polyneuropathy affecting feet and legs more than hands in a chronic, slowly progressive manner, (6) an autonomic neuropathy involving bowel, bladder, and circulatory reflexes, and (7) a painful thoracoabdominal radiculopathy. These forms of neuropathy often coexist, particularly the autonomic and the distal symmetric types.

Diabetic ophthalmoplegia is usually due to an isolated third nerve lesion; much less commonly the sixth nerve is involved. This disorder is described on page 216. Isolated affection of practically all the major peripheral nerves has been described in diabetes, but the ones most commonly involved are the femoral and sciatic. The acute mononeuropathies, cranial and peripheral, are presumably due to ischemic infarction of the nerve. The outlook for recovery is good.

Painful, asymmetric multiple neuropathy tends to occur in older patients with relatively mild or even unrecognized diabetes. Occasionally it may complicate longstanding diabetes. Pain often begins in the low back or hip and spreads to the thigh and knee on one side. It usually has a deep, aching character with superimposed lancinating jabs, and there is a propensity for the discomfort to be most severe at night. Muscle weakness and atrophy are most evident in the pelvic girdle and thigh, although the distal muscles may also be affected. The upper extremities are only rarely affected. Deep and superficial sensation may be intact or mildly impaired, conforming to either a multiple nerve or root distribution, or to both. The vesical and anal sphincters may be involved, and the knee jerk is often lost on the affected side. Recovery from this type of neuropathy

is the rule, although months and even years may elapse before it is complete. There is a tendency for the same syndrome to recur after a lapse of months or years in the opposite lower limb. This form of neuropathy is often referred to as *diabetic amyotrophy*, a term that draws attention to one facet of the syndrome but is otherwise uninformative.

There is a second type of proximal diabetic neuropathy, characterized by a symmetric weakness and wasting of insidious onset and gradual evolution over several months. The proximal muscles of the lower limbs, particularly the iliopsoas, quadriceps, and hamstrings, are involved in varying degrees. The muscles of the scapulae and upper limbs, especially the deltoid and triceps, are affected less frequently. Pain is not a consistent feature as it is in the acute asymmetric type, and sensory changes, if present, are distal, symmetric, and usually mild in degree.

The *distal, symmetric, primarily sensory form* is the most common type of diabetic neuropathy. Persistent and often distressing numbness and tingling, usually confined to the feet and lower legs and becoming worse at night, are the main symptoms. The ankle jerks are rarely preserved. As a rule the sensory signs are confined to the distal parts of the lower extremities, but in severe cases the hands may be involved and the sensory loss may spread to involve the anterior aspect of the lower abdomen, giving rise to confusion in diagnosis (Said et al). Trophic changes in the form of deep ulcerations and neuropathic joints are occasionally encountered, presumably due to severe sensory denervation of skin and joints. Muscle weakness is usually mild, but in some patients a distal sensory neuropathy is combined with a proximal weakness and wasting of the types described above.

The clinical picture may be dominated by deep sensory loss, ataxia, and atony of the bladder, with only slight weakness of the limbs, in which case it resembles tabes dorsalis (hence the term *diabetic pseudotabes*). The similarity is even closer if lancinating pains in the legs, unreactive pupils, and neuropathic arthropathy are present.

Symptoms of *autonomic involvement* include pupillary and lacrimal dysfunction, impairment of sweating and vascular reflexes, nocturnal diarrhea, atonicity of the gastrointestinal tract and bladder, sexual impotence, and postural hypotension. The basis of this type of involvement is not well understood. Duchen has studied the sympathetic ganglia in five diabetics with autonomic symptoms and has described vacuolated and granular neurons, cell necrosis, loss of myelinated nerve fibers in the vagus and splanchnic nerves, and loss of neurons in the intermediolateral columns of the spinal cord.

Attention has been drawn to the occurrence of a syndrome of severe thoracoabdominal pain and dysesthesia in long-standing diabetics (Kikta et al). The pain is distributed over segments of the chest or abdomen; it may be unilateral or bilateral, and is usually associated with marked weight loss. Superficial sensory loss can be detected over the involved area in most patients. The pathology of this state is not known but is presumed to be a widespread radiculopathy on the basis of the EMG changes, which characteristically consist of fibrillations of the paraspinal and abdominal wall muscles in multiple myotomes, corresponding to the painful area. Recovery may be protracted, but the prognosis for recovery is good.

In all these forms of diabetic neuropathy, the CSF protein may be elevated, 50 to 200 mg/dL, and rarely, even higher. The usual explanation for this phenomenon is involvement of spinal roots and ganglia.

Thomas and Lascelles have reviewed the neuropathology. Loss of myelinated nerve fibers is the most prominent finding in the distal symmetric type of polyneuropathy. In addition, segmental demyelination and remyelination of remaining axons are apparent in teased nerve fiber preparations. The latter findings are believed to be secondary to changes in the axon. Unmyelinated fibers are also reduced in number in some specimens. Similar lesions are found in the posterior roots and posterior columns of the spinal cord, and in the rami communicantes and sympathetic ganglia. Under the electron microscope the basement membranes of intraneural capillaries are seen to be thickened and duplicated.

Many uncertainties persist about the pathogenesis of the diabetic neuropathies. Both the cranial (diabetic ophthalmoplegia) and peripheral mononeuropathies, as well as the painful, asymmetric, predominantly proximal neuropathy of sudden onset, are thought to be ischemic in origin, secondary to disease of the vasa nervorum; obliterative vascular lesions were well illustrated by Raff et al (Fig. 46-4). In the other forms of diabetic neuropathy a metabolic basis, as yet undefined, has long been favored, but recent observations by Dyck and by Johnson and their associates suggest that these too might be vascular. They have described multiple foci of fiber loss throughout the length of the peripheral nerves, beginning high in the proximal segments and becoming more frequent and severe in the distal segments. This pattern of change was different from that observed in diffuse metabolic disease of Schwann cells and in dying-back neuropathy and suggested an ischemic etiology. Fascicular capillaries and epineural arterioles were noted to be thickened and their lumens narrowed. However, similar changes are observed in diabetics without neuropathy and in nondiabetics as well. Occlusion of vessels and frank infarction of nerve was not observed, so that a vascular pathogenesis remains to be established.

The several biochemical findings and their interpretations have been reviewed by Thomas and Eliasson. After reading their article, one can only conclude that a convincing biochemical pathogenesis has yet to be educed.

The only meaningful *treatment* is regulation of the diabetes and the maintenance of the blood glucose level in a normal range, since the prevailing view is that there is some relationship between peripheral nerve damage and inadequate diabetic control. There is evidence that tight glucose control, by means of an intravenous insulin infusion system, can significantly reduce painful neuropathic symptoms (Samanta and Burden). Culebras et al have reported therapeutic success with an aldose reductase inhibitor called *albrestatin*. The drug was given intravenously over a period of 5 days, after which 7 of 10 patients declared their weakness, sensory loss, and pains to have diminished; also there was improvement in nerve conduction velocities. Others have made similar but uncontrolled observations (see Thomas and Eliasson). Recent interest has centered around the use of gangliosides, which are normal components of neuronal membranes and can be administered exogenously. The authors have had no experience with either of these agents. *Prognosis* in the distal, symmetric, sensory neuropathy is uncertain, but in the other types improvement and eventual recovery may be expected over a period of months. During that time the management of the painful forms of neuropathy may be a trying experience because analgesic medication is required, raising the danger of drug addiction.

Ischemic Neuropathy One-half to two-thirds of patients with atherosclerotic ischemic disease of the legs will be found to have localized sensory changes or impairment of reflexes. Usually the other effects of ischemia—claudication and pain at rest, absence of distal pulses, and trophic skin changes—are so prominent that the neurologic changes are overlooked. The literature on this subject is to be found in the articles of Hutchinson and of Daube and Dyck, listed in the references.

Angiopathic Neuropathies A number of mononeuropathies are known to be caused by small vessel arteritis. Approximately one-third of all cases of chronic mononeuropathy multiplex can be traced to *a systemic vasculitis of the vasa nervorum*. Included in this category are polyarteritis nodosa, rheumatoid arthritis, lupus erythematosus, systemic sclerosis, cranial arteritis, and Wegener granulomatosis (see reviews of Conn and Dyck, and of Dyck, Benstead, et al). A small vessel arteritis is also the putative mechanism in the multiple mononeuropathies that complicate Lyme disease and AIDS.

Polyarteritis nodosa with polyneuropathy Perhaps 75 percent of cases of polyarteritis nodosa show involvement of the nutrient arteries of peripheral nerves (autopsy figures), but a symptomatic form of neuropathy develops in only about half this number. Yet involvement of the peripheral nerves may be the principal clue to the diagnosis of the underlying disease when, up to that time, the main components of the clinical picture—abdominal pain, hematuria, fever, eosinophilia, hypertension, vague limb pains, and possibly asthma—have not fully declared themselves or have been misinterpreted.

The polyneuropathy associated with polyarteritis nodosa may be diffuse and more or less symmetric in distribution, but more often it takes the form of a *mononeuropathy multiplex*, i.e., a random affection of two or more individual nerves. The onset in this latter form is usually abrupt, with symptoms of pain or numbness in the distribution of an affected nerve, followed in hours or days by motor or sensory loss in the distribution of that nerve, and then by involvement, in a saltatory fashion, of other peripheral nerves. Both spinal and cranial nerves may be affected. No two cases are identical. The CSF protein level is usually normal. Muscle biopsy, taken near the motor point so as to include nerve twigs, is useful in corroborating the clinical impression in the majority of cases.

Mononeuropathy multiplex due to polyarteritis calls for treatment with corticosteroids. Spontaneous remission and therapeutic arrest are known, but most cases have a fatal outcome.

Rheumatoid arthritis One to 5 percent of patients with rheumatoid arthritis will have involvement of one or more nerves at some time in the course of their disease. Apart from pressure neuropathies, there is a form of rheumatoid arteritis that may result in acute ischemic necrosis and demyelination of single or multiple nerves. The arteritis is of fibrinoid type and immune globulins are demonstrable in the walls of the vessel. Most of the affected patients have had arthritis for more than 10 years, and the disease is severe. They often have, in addition to the neuropathy, rheumatoid nodules, skin vasculitis, weight loss, fever, a high titer of rheumatoid factor and low serum complement.

Most polyneuropathies that complicate rheumatoid arthritis are chronic in nature and are described further on,

Figure 46-4

Three-dimensional drawing reconstructed from serial cross sections of left obturator nerve, taken from an elderly diabetic with mononeuropathy multiplex. Note organized thrombus in the interfascicular artery. Arteriolar branches from occluded segments supply three infarcted fascicles. The tendency for infarcts to occur in bridging interfascicular bundles is shown. (From Raff et al.)

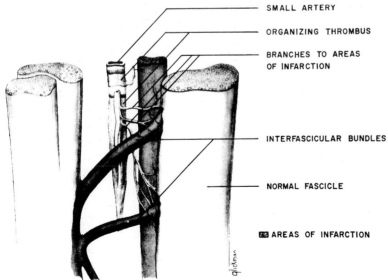

SMALL ARTERY

ORGANIZING THROMBUS

BRANCHES TO AREAS
OF INFARCTION

INTERFASCICULAR BUNDLES

NORMAL FASCICLE

▓ AREAS OF INFARCTION

under the chronic polyneuropathies associated with the connective tissue diseases.

Lupus erythematosus Approximately 10 percent of patients with this disease will exhibit symptoms and signs of peripheral nerve involvement. It usually appears in the established and more advanced stages of the disease but rarely has been the initial presentation. In several of our cases the polyneuropathy has taken the form of a symmetric, progressive sensorimotor paralysis, beginning in the feet and legs and extending to the arms, sometimes over a period of several days, mimicking GBS. In some, the weakness and areflexia were more prominent than the sensory loss; the latter involved mainly vibratory and position senses. Multiple mononeuropathy has also been seen, and the autonomic nervous system has been involved in some cases. An elevation of CSF protein in some cases suggests root involvement. The neuropathy may be due to occlusion of the nutrient arteries. More often in biopsies there is vasculitis (endothelial thickening and perivascular cuffing). McCombe et al demonstrated class II (Ia) antigen within nerve fascicles, perineurium, and endothelial cells in six cases. Vascular injury from deposition of immune complexes is a suspected mechanism.

Wegener granulomatosis (necrotizing granulomatous vasculitis of upper and lower respiratory tract, glomerulonephritis, and systemic vasculitis) This disorder has given rise to two neuropathic syndromes—one a symmetric or asymmetric polyneuropathy indistinguishable from the other angiopathic neuropathies described above, the other a direct involvement of lower cranial nerves as they issue from the skull and pass through the retropharyngeal tissues. The latter needs to be differentiated from carcinoma, chordoma, sarcoidosis, and zoster. This vasculitis is discussed further on page 679.

Nonsystemic Vasculitic Neuropathy
In contrast to the aforementioned disorders, which characteristically involve several tissues in addition to the peripheral nerves, a necrotizing vasculitis may rarely affect the peripheral nerves selectively. This affection takes the form of a multiple mononeuropathy and, less often, of a symmetric or asymmetric polyneuropathy and tends to be much more indolent and less life-threatening than the systemic forms of vasculitic neuropathy.

Subacute Asymmetric Idiopathic Polyneuropathy
This disorder, which accounts for about one-third of cases of mononeuritis multiplex, takes several forms. It usually develops over a period of weeks and continues to worsen in the following months, either gradually or in a stepwise manner. As time passes, some symptoms improve as others appear, resulting in a markedly asymmetric neuropathy. After a year or two, the nerves may become palpably enlarged, and the level of protein in the CSF extremely high (600 to 1500 mg/dL), with a virtual Froin syndrome (xanthochromia and spontaneous clotting). The high concentration of protein may induce headache, papilledema, and high CSF pressure (without hydrocephalus), possibly because of an increased CSF volume resulting from the osmotic effect of the protein. The pathology of this particular form of neuropathy has not been defined; infiltrates of inflammatory cells are found in some biopsies. Its relation to the acute or chronic relapsing variety of idiopathic polyneuritis is unknown.

Ultimately most patients recover to some extent, though late fatality is known to occur. Corticosteroids in full doses have proved to be beneficial in the majority of cases but may have to be continued over a period of months. Plasmapheresis has benefitted some patients after steroids have failed.

In another group of patients, an asymmetric sensorimotor neuropathy is evident from the onset. At first, only one or two nerves may be affected, usually the median or ulnar, but as the disease progresses, other nerves are involved, always more in the arms than in the legs. Tendon reflexes are lost in the arms and may be preserved in the legs. Pain is prominent in the distribution of the involved nerves, and the nerves themselves may be tender. Optic neuropathy is sometimes conjoined. The CSF in this group of patients is normal or slightly elevated. Electrophysiologically the involved nerves show a persistent focal conduction block. Sural nerve biopsies have shown demyelinating-remyelinating changes and varying degrees of fiber loss. Lewis and his colleagues have described this form of asymmetric sensorimotor neuropathy under the title of *multifocal demyelinating neuropathy with persistent conduction block*. This type of neuropathy also responds to treatment with corticosteroids.

A special variety of possibly the same disease, *hypertrophic mononeuropathy,* presents as an enlargement and tenderness of two or three nerves (back of neck and head or supraclavicular region) and raises suspicion of a nerve tumor (neurofibroma). A biopsy reveals the *onion bulb* type of enlargement of hypertrophic polyneuritis. There may be inflammatory cells in the interstitial tissue. Several patients whom we have followed responded well to corticosteroids only to relapse sometime later, after the treatment was terminated.

Sarcoidosis Sarcoidosis is a rare cause of subacute or chronic polyneuropathy of asymmetric type. It may be associated with lesions in muscles (polymyositis), or with signs of CNS involvement (stalk of the pituitary with diabetes insipidus, and cerebellum with ataxia).

Single nerve involvement with sarcoid most often takes the form of a facial palsy; in other cases, multiple cranial nerves are affected successively (see pages 1083 and 1089). Weakness and reflex and sensory loss in the distribution of one or more spinal nerves or roots may be added. The occurrence of large, irregular zones of sensory loss over the trunk is said to distinguish the neuropathy of sarcoidosis from other forms of mononeuropathy multiplex. This type of sensory loss, particularly when accompanied by pain, should also suggest a diagnosis of diabetic radiculopathy (see above).

Sicca Syndrome   Yet another type of asymmetric polyneuropathy may occur in association with keratoconjunctivitis sicca and xerostomia (Kennett and Harding). The latter features may be combined with rheumatoid arthritis (in which case it is called Sjögren syndrome) or with a wide range of other abnormalities, notably lymphoma, vasculitis, and renal tubular defects. An asymmetric loss of sensation, mostly of position sense and involving mainly the upper limbs, in association with tonic pupils and trigeminal anesthesia, are the common clinical features. The pathologic basis is unknown.

SYNDROME OF CHRONIC SENSORIMOTOR POLYNEUROPATHY

In this syndrome, impairment of sensation, weakness, and muscular atrophy progress over a period of many months or years. The time of onset is often uncertain. In infants the condition may be mistaken for muscular dystrophy or infantile muscular atrophy until sensory testing becomes possible. In the developing child, whose musculature naturally increases in power and volume, it may be difficult to decide whether the disease is progressive. Ataxia of the limbs may be pronounced at a stage when sensory loss exceeds paresis. The atrophy of muscle and trophic changes in the skin are more marked than in the acute and subacute forms of polyneuropathy; for this reason the chronic syndrome must be differentiated from the other forms of severe muscular atrophy, i.e., motor system disease, distal type of muscular dystrophy, and syringomyelia. The feet and hands may be extremely wasted, deformed (talipes equinus, claw hand), and subject to painless injuries, loss of tissue, and Charcot joints, while proximal structures are sound. Symmetry of distribution is the rule (tuberculoid leprosy is an exception), and in some of the familial sensory neuropathies only the nerves of the legs may be involved. The CSF protein content may remain elevated over a period of years.

There are two main categories of chronic polyneuropathy, one acquired and the other familial. These will be discussed separately.

ACQUIRED FORMS OF CHRONIC POLYNEUROPATHY

Carcinomatous and Myelomatous Polyneuropathy

A predominantly distal, symmetric sensory or sensorimotor polyneuropathy, evolving over a period of months, may occur as a remote effect of carcinoma or multiple myeloma, and less frequently, lymphoma. Severe weakness and atrophy, ataxia, and sensory loss of the limbs may advance to the point where the patient is confined to a wheelchair or bed; usually the CSF protein content is moderately elevated. All these symptoms may occur months or even a year or more before a small malignant tumor is found.

A mixed sensorimotor polyneuropathy is four to five times more frequent than a purely sensory one. It may spread slowly from the lower to the upper extremities, reaching its peak in a few months. Usually the condition remains unchanged until death, but on occasion it runs a remitting and relapsing course. The sensory polyneuropathy described originally by Denny-Brown is characterized by severe ataxia with retention of strength. All modalities of sensation are impaired over the limbs and even the face, and the reflexes disappear. Occasionally the evolution of the sensorimotor variety is subacute (weeks) and in a few instances the development seems to have been as rapid as that of the Guillain-Barré syndrome.

These forms of polyneuropathy are manifest clinically in 2 to 5 percent of all patients with malignant disease. The figures are much higher if one includes the mild neuropathies that occur in the terminal stages of cancer and those identified by EMG in asymptomatic patients (Henson and Urich). Carcinoma of the lung accounts for about 50 percent of the cases of sensorimotor polyneuropathy and 75 percent of the cases of pure sensory neuropathy (Croft and Wilkinson). These neuropathies have been joined to neoplasms of all types, however. They may also accompany a solitary plasmacytoma of bone or multiple myeloma. Thus polyneuropathy must be added to polymyositis or dermatomyositis, with which it is sometimes conjoined, as a paraneoplastic neurologic complication. The other remote neurologic effects of neoplasia may coexist: a type of myasthenic weakness (Lambert-Eaton syndrome; page 1159), spinocerebellar degeneration, limbic encephalits, and multifocal leukoencephalopathy (page 608).

The *pathology* of the neuropathy has not been completely defined. In the purely sensory type, there is a loss of nerve cells in the dorsal root ganglia, with secondary degeneration of the dorsal nerve roots and posterior columns of the spinal cord. In the sensorimotor type the pathologic picture is indistinguishable from that of a nutritional or metabolic disease of nerves (axonal degeneration). The degeneration is greater in the distal than in the proximal segments of the peripheral nerves, but extends into the roots in advanced cases. Dorsal root ganglion cells may be lost in small numbers. If the histologic examination is performed early in the course of the neuropathy, there are sparse infiltrates of lymphocytes distributed in foci around blood vessels. Their relation to both segmental demyelination and axonal degeneration of myelinated fibers is unclear. No tumor cells are seen in the nerves or spinal ganglia, unlike carcinomatous and lymphomatous mononeuropathy multiplex, in which tumor cells infiltrate nerves. Degeneration of the dorsal columns and chromatolysis of anterior horn cells are probably secondary to changes in the peripheral nerves and roots.

The *prognosis* is poor. Even though the polyneuropathy may stabilize and not progress or even remit to some extent with therapy, most of the patients succumb to the tumor within a year.

The *cause* of paraneoplastic polyneuropathy is not known. The occasional finding of infiltrates of inflammatory cells in the sensory ganglia, nerves, spinal roots, and spinal cord and the occasional association with multifocal leukoencephalopathy suggest a viral infection. Croft et al found circulating antibodies to nerve in four cases of sensory neuropathy but not in the more common sensorimotor neuropathy. This raises the question of an immunologic mechanism. A vitamin deficiency has also been proposed, but the administration of vitamins has been of no value.

Therapy consists of removing or controlling the tumor growth, which has resulted at times in improvement of neuropathic signs. Corticosteroid therapy has helped some patients. In cases of myelomatous polyneuropathy, particularly if the myeloma is "solitary," radiotherapy may result in prolonged remission of both the myeloma and neuropathy.

Chronic Inflammatory Polyradiculoneuropathy (CIP)

Only in recent years has this form of polyneuropathy been clearly separated from acute inflammatory polyradiculopathy, or the Guillain-Barré syndrome (GBS). Undoubtedly, similarities between these disorders can be discerned: clinically, both are symmetric polyradiculoneuropathies, usually but not invariably with cytoalbuminologic

dissociation of the CSF; both exhibit the nerve conduction abnormalities of a demyelinating neuropathy; and pathologically, both show inflammatory changes. But there are also important differences, the most striking of which are their modes of evolution and prognosis. GBS is an acute, monophasic disorder that evolves over a period of days or a week or two, after which it remains stationary for several weeks, and then recovers slowly. CIP is a considerably less common disorder. As a rule it begins insidiously and evolves slowly, either in a steadily progressive or stepwise manner, attaining its maximum severity after many months or even a year or longer. In only a small proportion of patients (16 percent in the series of McCombe et al) did the disease evolve at a tempo that mimicked GBS. Then it runs a persistent relapsing or fluctuating course, or it may simply worsen slowly and progressively.

Most cases of CIP respond favorably to the administration of prednisone; the response in GBS is less certain. Antecedent infections occur far less frequently in patients with CIP than those with GBS. Finally, CIP may be distinct immunologically, insofar as certain HLA antigens (A1, B8, DRw3, Dw3), reportedly occur with greater frequency in patients with this disorder than in the normal population and in patients with GBS (Adams et al).

Several large series of CIP have been reported. Dyck and his colleagues (1975) studied 53 such patients. All age groups were represented. The clinical course was monophasic and slowly progressive in about one-third of their patients, stepwise and progressive in another one-third, and relapsing in the remaining one-third. The periods of worsening or improvement were measured in weeks or months. In this series, infections and inoculations in the 3 months preceding the onset of CIP were no more frequent than in the population at large. Weakness of the limbs, particularly of the proximal leg muscles, or numbness, paresthesias, and dysesthesias of the hands and feet were the initial symptoms. In 45 of the 53 patients, the signs were those of a mixed sensorimotor polyneuropathy with weakness of the shoulder, upper arm, and thigh muscles, in addition to motor and sensory loss in the distal part of the limbs. In five patients the neuropathy was purely motor, and in three, purely sensory. Papilledema was observed in four patients, but other cranial nerve abnormalities were distinctly rare. Enlarged, firm nerves were found in six patients; thus CIP has to be distinguished from other chronic and recurrent hypertrophic neuropathies, particularly the hereditary ones.

More recently, McCombe and her colleagues have described the clinical and electromyographic findings in a group of 92 patients with CIP. Males outnumbered females, 57:35. These authors chose to classify their patients into two major subgroups—*relapsing* (corresponding to the relapsing and stepwise progressive groups of Dyck et al) and *nonrelapsing* (corresponding to Dyck's monophasic and gradually progressive groups). Again, all age groups were affected, although the age of onset was significantly earlier in patients with the relapsing disease (mean, 26.8 years) than in the nonrelapsing group (mean, 51.4 years). In other respects the clinical features of this series of patients did not differ substantially from those described by Dyck et al.

As first pointed out by Wartenberg, and more recently by Forrester and Lascelles, and by Thomas and his colleagues, chronic relapsing polyneuritis may rarely be associated with multiple sclerosis. We have seen two such cases as well.

The CSF protein is elevated in 90 percent of patients with CIP. Elevation of the CSF gamma globulin and a mild lymphocytic pleocytosis occur in some 10 percent of cases. Usually, the motor conduction velocities are distinctly reduced as are the amplitudes of muscle action potentials.

Pathologically, the peripheral nerves and roots, throughout their length, and the spinal ganglia are infiltrated by small clusters of mononuclear inflammatory cells, often perivenous in distribution. Myelinated fibers are lost to a varying degree, and many of the remaining ones are seen to be undergoing degeneration or show the changes of segmental demyelination or demyelination-remyelination. So-called onion-bulb formations (see above) are conspicuous in the recurrent and relapsing cases.

Prednisone is the *treatment* of choice and should be reserved for patients with moderately severe and severe disease. Dyck and Arnason recommend that 120 mg and 7.5 mg be given on alternate days for a period of a month, followed by a gradual reduction of the larger dosage at 4-week intervals. Should worsening occur with reduction of prednisone, it needs to be increased again. Should a sustained trial of prednisone therapy prove unsuccessful, a course (at least 3 months) of azathioprine, 3 mg/kg in a single daily dose, is recommended (Dalakas and Engel).

Some patients, but not all, have responded well to plasmapheresis. In a prospective, double-blind trial, Dyck and his colleagues found that plasma exchange, administered twice weekly for 3 weeks, had a beneficial effect on both the neurologic disability and nerve conduction. The type of patient who responded best could not be determined. Moreover, in those who did respond, the beneficial effects began to fade in 10 to 14 days. Just how plasma exchange should be used in practice remains to be established, therefore. Probably it should be tried in patients whose condition is worsening seriously, and who do not respond to prednisone or azathioprine.

Neuropathies Associated with Paraproteinemias and Dysproteinemias The occurrence of a relatively mild chronic sensorimotor polyneuropathy in association with an abnormality of gamma globulin or immunoglobulin

is being recognized with increasing frequency. In general, the immunoglobulin abnormalities are of two types—*dysproteinemias,* in which there is a purely quantitative change, usually an increase in the normal components of gamma globulin (so-called polyclonal gammopathy) and the *paraproteinemias,* in which a clone of abnormal plasma cells produces a homogenous immunoglobulin with restricted electrophoretic mobility. The paraproteinemias that give rise to polyneuropathy are multiple myeloma, macroglobulinemia, cryoglobulinemia and benign monoclonal gammopathy. To these can be added the neuropathy of ataxia-telangiectasia, a disease that is characterized by an absence or marked decrease in IgA.

The neuropathy that is associated with *multiple myeloma* has already been described (see above, under "Carcinomatous Neuropathy"). Polyneuropathy complicates 13 to 14 percent of cases of multiple myeloma, and has a disproportionately high association with the osteosclerotic form (McLeod et al). In a number of patients the neuropathy was associated with diffuse cutaneous hyperpigmentation, edema, enlargement of liver and spleen, and endocrinopathy (Tang et al). An abnormal gamma globulin (M component) is found in the serum of 80 percent of patients with myelomatous neuropathy; in the remainder, a monoclonal Bence-Jones protein is found in the urine. The neuropathy that complicates solitary plasmacytomas may improve markedly, following irradiation of the bone lesion.

Macroglobulinemia is the term applied by Waldenstrom to a systemic condition occurring mainly in elderly persons and characterized by fatigue, weakness, and a bleeding diathesis and by a marked increase in the 19S IgM plasma fraction, on immunoelectrophoresis. A significant proportion of cases with hyperproteinemia are complicated by a diffuse slowing of retinal and cerebral circulation *(Bing-Neel syndrome),* giving rise to episodic confusion, coma, and sometimes to strokes, as well as by a peripheral neuropathy. The latter may be subacute but is more often chronic in nature, sometimes markedly so, and either asymmetric, in a multiple nerve trunk pattern (particularly at the onset of the neuropathy), or symmetric and distal in distribution. In several of our cases the polyneuropathy was symmetric and sensorimotor in type, and limited to the feet and legs, with mild ataxia and loss of knee and ankle jerks. The CSF protein is usually elevated and the globulin fraction increased. In a case recorded by Rowland et al the polyneuropathy was purely motor and the clinical diagnosis had been motor neuron disease. Only the elevated CSF protein provided a clue as the nature of the disease.

Cryoglobulinemia is characterized by a serum protein

that precipitates on cooling. The cryoglobulins are usually IgG or IgM. Cryoglobulinemia may occur without any apparent associated condition (essential cryoglobulinemia) or, more frequently, with a wide variety of disorders such as myeloma, lymphoma, connective tissue disease, and chronic infection. Peripheral neuropathy occurs in a small proportion of both types of cases. It develops insidiously, on a background of the Raynaud phenomenon and purpuric eruptions of the skin. Originally, the neuropathic symptoms consist only of pain and paresthesias which are often precipitated by exposure to cold. Later, weakness and wasting gradually develop, often asymmetrically, more in the legs than in the arms and more or less in the distribution of the vascular changes.

The pathology of the neuropathies associated with macroglobulinemia and cryoglobulinemia has been incompletely studied, and the mechanisms by which these disorders cause neuropathy are quite obscure. In one of our most completely autopsied cases there was widespread distal axonal degeneration of nondescript type without amyloid deposition or inflammatory cells, yet in other reported cases amyloid has been found. Immune deposits were observed by Ongerboer de Visser et al; IgM had impregnated the inner layers of the perineurium. Dalakas and Engel have made similar observations. Paraproteins may also appear in the CSF. Their role in pathogenesis is uncertain. Possibly the neuropathy of cryoglobulinemia is ischemic in nature, the result of vasoconstriction, increased blood viscosity and thrombosis of small vessels, all of which occur in this disease.

The use of prednisone or the alkylating agent chlorambucil have at times led to improvement in the general and neuropathic symptoms, although recovery has been incomplete.

Benign monoclonal gammopathy refers to a paraproteinemia in which there is no evidence of macro- or cryoglobulinemia, multiple myeloma, or other malignant disease. Insofar as such diseases may become manifest many years after the ''benign'' gammopathy has been recognized, both the benign and malignant gammopathies are often subsumed under the rubric of *plasma cell dyscrasias*. Such disorders are common; Kelly et al reported that 6 percent of patients referred to the Mayo Clinic with peripheral neuropathy of unknown cause proved to have a monoclonal paraproteinemia (usually IgM, less often IgG, and rarely IgA).

The neuropathy affects males mainly, in the sixth and seventh decades of life. The onset is insidious, with numbness and paresthesias of the feet, then of the hands, followed by a symmetric weakness of the extremities. The course is usually slowly progressive, rarely remitting and relapsing. The Raynaud phenomenon is often associated; action tremor and ataxia may be present as well. Sural nerve biopsies have consistently shown an extensive loss of myelinated fibers of all sizes; unmyelinated fibers are spared; hypertrophic changes are seen in about half of the cases (Smith et al). The latter authors have demonstrated the presence of monoclonal IgM antibody on the surviving myelin sheaths, and Latov and his associates have shown that the serum IgM fraction displays antimyelin activity, indicating that the neuropathy is caused directly by the antimyelin antibody.

In *ataxia-telangiectasia*, in which there is a diminution in gamma globulin, specifically in IgA, a peripheral nerve dysfunction is manifested at first by hyporeflexia and decreased nerve conduction velocities, and then by the slow evolution of a symmetric and predominantly distal atrophic paralysis and sensory loss, the legs being affected more than the arms (see page 794).

Uremic Polyneuropathy Polyneuropathy is probably the most common complication of chronic renal failure. It has been stated by Robson to be present to some degree in two-thirds of all patients about to begin dialysis therapy. Bolton's figures are very much the same; 70 percent of patients being dialyzed regularly had uremic polyneuropathy, and in 30 percent the neuropathy was of moderate or severe degree. Usually the neuropathy takes the form of a painless, progressive, symmetric sensorimotor paralysis of the legs and then of the arms. In some patients, the neuropathy begins with burning dysesthesias of the feet or with sensations of creeping, crawling, and itching of the legs and thighs, which tend to be worse at night and are relieved by movement (restless legs syndrome of Ekbom; see page 308).

The combination of muscle weakness and atrophy, areflexia, sensory loss, and the graded distribution of the neurologic deficit in the limbs leave little doubt about the neuropathic nature of the disorder. Usually the neuropathy evolves slowly over many months, at times in subacute fashion. Rare instances of acute noninflammatory sensorimotor polyneuropathy have been reported as well (Asbury et al). Also, a uremic polymyositis with hypophosphatemia has been described (Layzer). The neuropathy has been observed with all types of chronic kidney disease. More important to the development of neuropathy than the nature of the renal lesion is the duration and severity of the renal failure and symptomatic uremia (not merely azotemia).

With long-term hemodialysis, the symptoms and signs of polyneuropathy stabilize, but they improve in relatively few patients. In fact, rapid hemodialysis may occasionally worsen the polyneuropathy temporarily. Peritoneal dialysis has been more successful than hemodialysis in improving the neuropathy. Complete recovery, occurring over a period of 6 to 12 months, usually follows successful renal transplantation, for the reason given below.

The pathologic findings are those of a nonspecific axonal degeneration. The changes are most intense in the distal segments of the nerves, with the expected chromatolysis of their cell bodies. Amyloid deposits in the nerves have not been found; there is no evidence of vitamin deficiency or of diabetes during life, although the latter diagnosis may be difficult to establish in the uremic patient. There are no signs of polyarteritis nodosa at autopsy.

The cause of uremic polyneuropathy is unknown. The "middle molecule" theory is currently the most plausible. The end stage of renal failure is associated with the accumulation of toxic substances in the 300- to 2000-molecular-weight range. Furthermore, the concentration of these substances, which include methylguanidine and myoinositol, has been shown to correlate with the degree of neurotoxicity (Funck-Brentano et al). These toxins (and the clinical signs of neuropathy) are not greatly reduced by chronic hemodialysis. On the other hand, the transplanted kidney deals effectively with substances of wide-ranging molecular weights, which would account for the invariable improvement of neuropathy after transplantation.

Alcoholic and Diabetic Neuropathy

In all patients with alcoholic-nutritional polyneuropathy who remain untreated for some reason, the weakness and atrophy of the legs, and to a lesser extent the arms, may reach an extreme degree. Thus this disease, though subacute in its evolution, becomes a frequent cause of chronic polyneuropathy. Certain cases of diabetic neuropathy behave similarly.

Chronic Polyneuropathy with Connective Tissue Diseases

In clinics devoted to connective tissue diseases, occasional examples of either subacute or chronic polyneuropathy or mononeuropathy are observed. The latter are usually related to rheumatoid arthritis, and are difficult to distinguish from pressure palsies. A small proportion of patients with rheumatoid arthritis develop a symmetric, predominantly sensory, and variably painful polyneuropathy. Some of the most painful polyneuropathies we have seen, extending over long periods of time, have had only minimal sensory loss, weakness, or reflex changes in the limbs, and the diagnosis has been difficult. An unexpected rise in the CSF protein level or electromyographic evidence of denervation may be an important lead.

Pallis and Scott have made an extensive study of the patterns of nerve involvement with rheumatoid arthritis. They divide the neuropathies into five groups, according to whether the upper or lower limbs are involved and whether the involvement takes the form of multiple pressure palsies

or a distal sensory loss in the digits. They allude also to a rare symmetric sensorimotor polyneuropathy. All these complications occur late, after the rheumatoid arthritis has been present for years. Of course, the carpal tunnel syndrome is frequent with rheumatoid arthritis.

Little is known of the mechanism or pathology of the neuropathies associated with rheumatoid arthritis. Several types of arterial lesions have been described in the nerves of these patients, particularly in a rare, subacutely evolving mononeuropathy multiplex that occurs in the setting of long-standing, severe, destructive joint changes and a high titer of rheumatoid factor (Dyck et al). The angiopathic neuropathy of rheumatoid arthritis and that of lupus erythematosus and polyarteritis have been discussed in a preceding section of this chapter.

Amyloid Neuropathy

Amyloid, defined as an amorphous extracellular substance with specific functional properties and fine fibrillar ultrastructure, has wide medical ramifications. Small amounts of it are often found in the small meningeal and cerebral vessels of older individuals, in which case it must be regarded as a product of aging. It is a major constituent of the so-called senile plaque of Alzheimer disease. Also, amyloid deposition is a consequence of many chronic infections and is often associated with multiple myeloma, medullary carcinoma of the thyroid and other malignancies. Then there are hereditary forms, in which no antecedent or associated disease can be discerned. Finally there are sporadic instances in which a peripheral neuropathy is associated with amyloid deposition in the heart, kidneys, and gastrointestinal tract (primary systemic amyloidosis). The peripheral nervous system is regularly affected in the familial and primary systemic forms but not in those secondary to infection.

The following forms of amyloid neuropathy have been identified: (1) chronic familial polyneuropathy, (2) familial amyloidosis with carpal tunnel syndrome, (3) polyneuropathy or carpal tunnel syndrome associated with multiple myeloma, and (4) peripheral neuropathy in primary systemic amyloidosis.

Insofar as the sporadic form of amyloid neuropathy does not differ clinically or pathologically from the familial form, they will be discussed together, under the genetically determined neuropathies (see further on).

Leprous Polyneuritis

This is the classic example of an infectious neuritis, being due to the direct invasion of nerves by the acid-fast *Mycobacterium leprae*, and is probably the most common disease of peripheral nerves in the world today. The disease is particularly frequent in India and Central Africa, but there are many lesser endemic foci, including parts of Florida, Texas, and Louisiana that border on the Gulf of Mexico.

The initial lesion in leprosy is an innocuous-appearing skin macule or papule, which is often hypopigmented and lacking in sensation and which is due to the invasion of cutaneous nerves by *M. leprae*. The disease may progress no further than this stage, which is spoken of as *indeterminate leprosy,* or it may evolve in several ways depending mainly upon the resistance of the host. The bacilli may be locally invasive, producing a circumscribed epithelioid granuloma that implicates cutaneous and subcutaneous nerves and results in a characteristic patch of superficial sensory loss (*tuberculoid leprosy*). The subcutaneous sensory nerves may be palpably enlarged. If a larger nerve in the vicinity of the granuloma is invaded (the ulnar, median, peroneal, and facial nerves are most frequently affected in this way), a sensorimotor deficit in the distribution of that nerve is added to the patch of cutaneous anesthesia.

Lack of resistance permits the proliferation and hematogenous spread of bacilli and the diffuse infiltration of skin, ciliary bodies, testes, lymph nodes, and nerves (*lepromatous leprosy*). Widespread invasion of the cutaneous nerves produces a symmetric pattern of pain and temperature loss, involving the pinnae of the ears, dorsal surfaces of hands, forearms and feet, and anterolateral aspects of the legs—a distribution that is apparently determined by the relative coolness of these parts of the skin. Eventually the anesthesia spreads to involve most of the cutaneous surface. Extensive sensory loss is followed by loss of motor function owing to invasion of muscular nerves where they lie closest to the skin (ulnar nerve is the most vulnerable). There is a loss of sweating in areas of sensory loss, but otherwise the autonomic nervous system is unaffected. In distinction to other polyneuropathies, tendon reflexes are usually preserved in leprosy, despite widespread sensory loss. Probably this depends upon sparing of the muscular nerves. Because of widespread anesthesia, injuries may be unrecognized, with resultant infections, trophic changes, and loss of tissue. Variations in host immunity result in patterns of disease having both tuberculoid and lepromatous characteristics (*dimorphous leprosy*).

All forms of leprosy require long-term treatment with sulfones, (dapsone being the most commonly used), rifampin, and clofazimine. The skin lesions of lepromatous leprosy are responsive to thalidomide (Barnhill and McDougall).

Polyneuropathy with Hypothyroidism   While characteristic disturbances of skeletal muscle are known to complicate hypothyroidism (see Chap. 49), the demonstration of a polyneuropathy has been infrequent. However, a number of elderly myxedematous patients complain of weakness and numbness of feet, legs, and, to a lesser extent, the hands for which no other explanation can be found. Loss of reflexes, diminution in vibratory, joint-position, and touch-pressure sensations, and weakness in the distal parts of the limbs are the usual findings. The neuropathic manifestations are seldom severe. Nerve conduction velocities are significantly diminished, and the protein content of the CSF is usually increased, to more than 100 mg/dL in some patients; probably this is a reflection of the increased protein content of the serum. Convincing evidence of a hypothyroid etiology is the subjective improvement and complete or near-complete reversibility of neuropathic signs following treatment with thyroid hormones. In biopsies of nerve, an edematous protein infiltration of the endoneurium and perineurium, a kind of metachromatic mucoid material, has been seen. Dyck and Lambert noted segmental demyelination in teased fiber preparations. In electron-microscopic sections, a slight increase in glycogen, acid mucopolysaccharides, and aggregates of glycogen and cytoplasmic laminar bodies in Schwann cells have been observed.

Polyneuropathy of sensorimotor type has also been observed in association with chronic lymphocytic thyroiditis and alopecia (Hart et al).

Chronic Benign Polyneuropathy of the Elderly   The authors have observed numerous cases of a benign, relatively nonprogressive sensory polyneuropathy in elderly patients. Tingling paresthesias of feet and legs, sensory loss, and absent ankle reflexes are the usual findings. The hands may be mildly affected. Laboratory studies confirm the neuropathy but do not disclose the cause. It has been our practice to prescribe B vitamins and to reassure the patient that there will be no serious disability.

GENETICALLY DETERMINED NEUROPATHIES

There has been much difficulty in classifying the chronic familial polyneuropathies. Dyck has proposed a scheme that divides them into three large groups, according to their main clinical features: (1) a *pure motor type,* which includes all the progressive spinal muscular atrophies, hitherto called myelopathic motor neuron diseases, (2) a *predominantly sensory type,* often with mutilating trophic lesions, and (3) a *mixed sensorimotor and autonomic* type. The second and third types each include four or five subgroups. All these diseases, which he designates as *system atrophies,* are notable for their hereditary nature, chronicity, fiber loss with few or no products of degeneration, progressivity, and symmetry of involvement.

We are reluctant to group motor system diseases with the neuropathies but would accept the other two categories, the predominantly sensory and sensorimotor groups. We would agree also that the distinction drawn between system atrophies and degenerations in the hereditary neuropathies probably has no validity. Special neuropathologic features such as pseudohypertrophy of nerves are also not acceptable as the basis of classification. Far better in our view is a division of hereditary polyneuropathies into those with an established gene-controlled biochemical mechanism and those in which the biochemical mechanism is unknown. These considerations have influenced us to propose the classification given in Table 46-1. It is evident from this classification that the major proportion of the familial polyneuropathies is of "degenerative" type. Some are associated with certain abnormalities of the CNS, whereas others are relatively pure. For convenience of exposition several of the hereditary metabolic polyneuropathies have already been discussed in Chap. 38, with the metabolic diseases of the nervous system. Here we will consider the other inherited neuropathies.

INHERITED POLYNEUROPATHIES OF PREDOMINANTLY SENSORY TYPE

Common to the several diseases comprising this group are lancinating pains, ulcers of the feet and hands, and osteomyelitis, leading to osteolysis, stress fractures, recurrent episodes of cellulitis and lymphangitis, and insensitivity to pain. Since similar symptoms and signs occur in syringomyelia, leprosy, and tabes dorsalis there has been uncertainty in many writings, especially those cited for historical interest, as to whether the reported clinical cases were examples of one or another of these diseases.

According to Dyck and Ohta, Leplat in 1846 described plantar ulcers (*mal perforant du pied*) as did Nélaton in 1852. Morvan in 1883 reported his observations of adult patients who had developed suppuration of the pulps of insensitive fingers (whitlows). It is now generally agreed that Morvan's cases were examples of syringomyelia, whereas the family described by Nélaton was probably an example of a recessive form of childhood sensory polyneuropathy, since familial syringomyelia in children is a rarity. Other examples of foot ulceration were later ascribed to lumbar syringomyelia or dysraphism, again an interpretation that has not been supported by postmortem studies. We would agree with Dyck and Ohta that most such cases are examples of sensory polyneuropathy.

Dominant Mutilating Sensory Polyneuropathy in Adults The characteristics of this group of polyneuropathies include autosomal dominant mode of inheritance; onset of symptoms in the second decade or later; normal life expectancy; involvement mainly of feet with calluses of soles and later episodes of blistering, ulceration, and lymphangitis, followed by osteomyelitis and osteolysis; analgesia or shooting pains; distal sensory loss with greater affection of pain and thermal sensation than of touch and pressure; loss of sweating; diminution or absence of tendon reflexes; and only slight loss of muscle power.

The plantar ulcer overlying the head of a metatarsal bone is the most dreaded complication and may develop into an osteomyelitis. Infection of the pulp of the fingers and paronychias are uncommon. Some patients have a mild pes cavus and weakness of the peroneal and pretibial muscles with foot drop and steppage gait. Lancinating pains may occur in the legs, thighs, and shoulders, and, exceptionally, the pain may last for days and be as disabling as in tabes dorsalis; however, in the majority of patients there is no pain whatsoever. Neural deafness was present in one of Denny-Brown's patients. In the latter case, which was studied post mortem, there was a loss of small nerve cells in the lumbosacral dorsal root ganglia. The spinal roots were thin, and the fibers in the posterior columns of the spinal cord and peripheral nerves were diminished in number. Myelinated fibers and unmyelinated ones were both affected. Both axonal degeneration and segmental demyelination have been demonstrated in teased nerve preparations. Sensory nerve conduction is usually untestable.

Recessive Mutilating Sensory Polyneuropathy of Childhood Here the pattern of inheritance is autosomal recessive. There are reports of several sibships in which multiple members had a sensory neuropathy manifested by an apparent insensitivity to pain. Onset is in infancy and early childhood and walking is delayed; there is pes cavus deformity and the first movements are ataxic. Ulcerations of the tips of toes and fingers and repeated infections of acral parts result in the formation of paronychias and whitlows. The tendon reflexes are absent, but muscular power is well-preserved. All sensory modalities are impaired (touch-pressure somewhat more than pain-temperature) mainly in the distal parts of the limbs, but also over the trunk. Light-touch, pain, thermal, vibratory, and position senses are all impaired in the distal parts of the extremities and trunk. The lesions and electrical findings are similar to those in the dominantly inherited sensory neuropathy.

In both types of sensory neuropathy measures must be taken to prevent stress fractures, acral mutilation, and infection. This is more difficult in the small child who does not fully understand the problem.

Congenital Insensitivity to Pain In *congenital indifference* to pain, a syndrome in which the patient throughout life seems totally unreactive to the pain of injury, there is no loss of the ability to distinguish pinprick and other painful stimuli from nonpainful ones. Furthermore, the nervous system of such individuals seems to be normal. There is, however, another variety characterized by universal analgesia. In 1963 Swanson et al described two brothers and about the same time Biemond reported two siblings in whom, in addition to complete *insensitivity* to pain, there was anhidrosis and mild mental retardation. During childhood, one of the patients of Swanson et al had high fever when the environmental temperature was raised, and the other possibly had orthostatic hypotension. One of the patients died in his twelfth year and was found to have an absence of small neurons in the dorsal root ganglia, an absence of Lissauer's tracts, and a decrease in the size of the descending spinal tracts of the trigeminal nerves. Sweat glands were present in the skin but were not innervated. Biemond observed similar neuropathologic changes in an autopsied case. Nothing was said about the anatomic basis of the low IQ (70) or the autonomic disorder.

Other Forms of Inherited Sensory Neuropathy Included here are the neuropathy of Friedreich ataxia, which has been discussed in Chap. 43, and the Riley-Day syndrome, which is discussed further on in this chapter, as well as the neuropathies in which there are recognized metabolic abnormalities. However, we have seen other unclassifiable examples of an almost pure sensory or sensorimotor type. Some years ago a young man and woman with universal anesthesia affecting head, neck, trunk, and limbs came to our attention (Adams et al). All forms of sensation were affected. The patients were areflexic but retained full motor power; the movements were ataxic. Autonomic functions were impaired but not abolished. In a sural nerve biopsy, nearly all fibers—large and small, myelinated and unmyelinated—had disappeared. Surprisingly there were no trophic changes of any kind. Another of our families with ulcers and loss of digits had a symmetric sensory and motor polyneuropathy of the extremities with areflexia. The inheritance was of dominant type, with onset in adolescence. Donaghy and others have described a unique variant of the recessively inherited form of sensory neuro-

pathy, in which there is an associated neurotrophic keratitis and a selective loss of small myelinated fibers in sural nerve biopsies.

We continue to observe variant and unclassifiable cases such as these every year. In general the mutilating effects are the result of injury to analgesic parts.

INHERITED POLYNEUROPATHIES OF MIXED SENSORIMOTOR-AUTONOMIC TYPES (IDIOPATHIC)

Peroneal Muscular Atrophy (Charcot-Marie-Tooth Disease) This disease is inherited as an autosomal dominant (occasionally recessive) trait, with onset during late childhood or adolescence. Described in 1886 almost simultaneously by Tooth in England and by Charcot and Marie in France, all their names were attached to it, even though similar cases had been recorded earlier by Eulenberg (1856), Friedreich (1873), Ormerod (1884), and Osler (1880). Because of changes in the spinal cord and its occasional overlap with Friedreich ataxia, the early observers considered it to be an hereditary myelopathy and did not class it with the neuropathies; but the evidence that supports this latter nosologic grouping is now unassailable.

Essentially this is a chronic degeneration of peripheral nerves and roots, resulting in distal muscle atrophy, beginning in the feet and legs and later involving the hands. The extensor hallucis and digitorum longus, the peronei, and the intrinsic muscles of the feet are affected early and produce an equinovarus deformity and *pied en griffe* (see page 1034). Later, all muscles of the legs and sometimes the lower third of the thigh become weak and atrophic. The thin legs have been likened to those of a stork or, if the lower thigh muscles are affected, to an "inverted champagne bottle." Eventually the nerves to the calf muscles degenerate and the ability to plantar flex the feet is lost. After a period of years, atrophy of the hand and forearm muscles develops. The hands become clawed (*main en griffe*). The wasting seldom extends above the elbows or above the middle third of the thighs. Paresthesias and cramps are invariably present to some degree and there is always some impairment, usually slight, of deep and superficial sensation in the feet and hands, shading off proximally. Rarely, the sensory loss is severe, and perforating ulcers may be associated. The tendon reflexes are absent in the involved limbs. The illness progresses very slowly, and it seems to stabilize for long periods.

The walking difficulty, which is the main disability, is due to a combination of sensory ataxia and weakness. Foot drop and instability of the ankles are additional handicaps. The feet and legs may ache after use and cramps may be troublesome, but otherwise pain is exceptional; the feet are often cold, swollen, and blue, secondary to inactivity of the muscles of the feet and legs and their dependent position. There is usually no disturbance of autonomic function. Fixed pupils, optic atrophy, nystagmus and endocrinopathies, epilepsy, and spina bifida, which have been reported occasionally in association with peroneal muscular atrophy, probably represent coincidental congenital disorders.

The age of onset varies, but we have not seen cases beginning in early childhood. An onset in middle adult life is not unknown, especially in mild forms. When combined with tremor, it may be difficult to draw a line between this disease and the Roussy-Lévy syndrome. One of our patients had a long family history of benign action tremor and peroneal muscular atrophy; but we discovered, in analyzing this genealogy, that some family members had tremor, some had peroneal muscular atrophy, and some had both. Restricted forms are known to affect only the peroneal and pectoral or scapular muscles (scapuloperoneal form of Dawidenkow). Other variants are (1) a rare type that begins in the proximal muscles of the arms and (2) the *"familial claw foot with absent tendon jerks"* of Symonds and Shaw.

Laboratory data are of little help. The CSF is usually normal. Nerve conduction velocities are diminished, and giant polyphasic units are seen in the EMG, with few fibrillation potentials.

Pathologic findings Degenerative changes in the nerves result in depletion of the population of large sensory and motor fibers leaving only the condensed endoneurial connective tissue. As best as one can tell, axons and myelin sheaths are both affected, the distal parts of the nerve more than the proximal. Anterior horn cells are slightly diminished in number and some are chromatolyzed. Dorsal root ganglion cells suffer a similar fate. The disease involves sensory posterior root fibers with degeneration of the posterior columns of Goll more than of Burdach. The autonomic nervous system remains intact. The muscles contain large fields of atrophic fibers (group atrophy). Some of the larger fibers have a target appearance and may show degenerative changes, a finding that has led some workers to postulate a myopathic effect. There is some physiologic evidence to support this idea, but the muscle lesion is of the denervative type, similar to that following poliomyelitis, a disease exclusively of motor neurons. Claims of a coincidental myelopathy and degeneration of spinocerebellar and corticospinal tracts probably indicate that the associated disease was really Friedreich ataxia.

Treatment No treatment is known. Stabilizing the ankles by arthrodeses is indicated if foot drop is severe and the disease has reached the point where it is not progressing. Fitting the legs with light braces and the shoes with springs, to overcome foot drop, can be helpful.

Differential diagnosis and nosologic differentiation involve the distal dystrophies (Chap. 50), late forms of familial motor system disease, Friedreich ataxia (Chap. 43), Roussy-Lévy syndrome (see below), and other familial polyneuropathies.

Progressive Hypertrophic Neuropathy (Déjerine-Sottas Disease) This type of neuropathy is usually inherited as a recessive trait and occasionally as a dominant one. It begins in childhood or in infancy, earlier than peroneal muscular atrophy, and is slowly progressive. Pain and paresthesias in the feet are early symptoms, followed by the development of symmetric weakness and wasting of the distal portions of the limbs. Talipes equinovarus postures with claw feet as well as claw hands are common. Sensation is impaired in a distal distribution, and the tendon reflexes are absent. Miotic, unreactive pupils, nystagmus, and kyphoscoliosis have been observed in some cases. There are no important changes in autonomic functions. Trunk and cranial parts of the body are spared. The ulnar, median, radial, posterior neck, and peroneal nerves stand out like tendons and are easily followed with the gently roving finger. The enlarged nerves are not tender. Patients are usually much more disabled than with peroneal muscular atrophy and are confined to a wheelchair at an early age.

It is important to emphasize that the occurrence of hypertrophic neuropathy is not confined to the particular inherited disease described above. If one groups all patients in whom the nerves are diffusely enlarged (incorrectly called "hypertrophic"), several different diseases, both genetic and acquired, are included. Enlarged nerves have been described in some cases of recurrent idiopathic polyneuritis, familial amyloidosis, Refsum disease, peroneal muscular atrophy, and other diseases. Basically any pathologic process that causes recurrent segmental demyelination and subsequent repair and remyelination may have this effect. In some patients with a history of early childhood hereditary polyneuropathy, the nerves are not palpably enlarged, yet the diagnosis can be established by biopsy of a cutaneous nerve. In Déjerine-Sottas disease the CSF protein is persistently elevated for the reason that the spinal roots are affected. Indeed they may enlarge to the point of blocking the subarachnoid space and compressing the spinal cord. Nerve conduction velocities are markedly reduced in this disease even when there is little or no functional impairment. The treatment is purely symptomatic.

Under the microscope the enlargement of nerves is seen to be due to a great increase in connective tissue (perineurial more than epineurial) and the fields of collagen often appear impregnated with an amorphous eosinophilic protein precipitate resembling mucus. However, the identifying lesion is the ''onion bulb,'' which consists of a whorl of overlapping, intertwined, attenuated Schwann cell processes that encircle naked or finely medullated axons. The so-called onion bulbs are also seen in the several other ''hypertrophic'' neuropathies listed above.

Hereditary Areflexic Dystasia (Roussy-Lévy Syndrome)

In 1926 Roussy and Lévy reported seven cases of a familial malady that had not previously been described. Its close relation to Friedreich ataxia and the amyotrophy of Charcot-Marie was recognized. For many years thereafter—in fact until the present day—the existence of this entity was disputed by reason of these latter relationships, and the original authors felt called upon to defend their thesis twice more in the medical literature.

The condition in question is a sensory ataxia (dystasia) with pes cavus and areflexia, affecting mainly the lower legs and later progressing to involve the hands. Some degree of sensory loss, mainly of vibratory and position sense, has been described in all cases. Atrophy of the muscles of the legs, with the electrical reactions of denervation, are prominent. None of the patients has had evidence of cerebellar ataxia. Kyphoscoliosis is described in several. The abdominal reflexes are preserved, but in some an uncertain extensor plantar reflex has been obtained on one or the other side. Although the feet may be cold or slightly discolored, no autonomic defects are documented. The nerves are not palpably enlarged. Electrocardiographic abnormalities similar to those of Friedreich ataxia have been noted in one family. Action tremor is variable.

The onset in many patients is during infancy, possibly dating from birth; the course is benign. Lapresle was able to find and reexamine four of the original seven patients of Lévy and Roussy, 30 years later, and found that the condition had changed little if at all in its general format. There are no complete postmortem studies.

The authors are faced repeatedly with the problem of diagnosis of this syndrome when a patient presents with either an ataxic gait or pes cavus and leg atrophy but without the usual signs of Friedreich ataxia or of peroneal muscular atrophy. The pattern of inheritance, slow course, lack of cerebellar, brainstem, and corticospinal tract signs, and prominence of atrophy serve to exclude Friedreich ataxia. The very early onset, the presence of a ''tabetic'' picture with sensory ataxia in association with definite atrophy, and the kyphoscoliosis, differentiate it from peroneal muscular atrophy. Our position is that it represents a type of chronic familial neural atrophy of different onset and course than peroneal muscular atrophy, but until the specific biochemical defects of these diseases have been discovered, final differentiation is impossible. We are not impressed with the recorded evidence of a myelopathy with pyramidal involvement in either peroneal muscular atrophy or the dystasia of Roussy-Lévy, based as it is on the interpretation of a wavering plantar reflex in a deformed foot with contracture of long extensor muscles of the great toes.

Chronic Polyneuropathy with Hereditary Spastic Paraplegia

From time to time we have observed children and young adults with unmistakable progressive spastic paraplegia superimposed on which was a sensorimotor polyneuropathy of extremely chronic evolution. Sural nerve biopsy in two of our cases disclosed a typical hypertrophic polyneuropathy. In another case only loss of nerve fibers was found. Cavanaugh et al and Harding and Thomas have reported similar patients. Our patients were severely disabled, being barely able to stand on their atrophic legs. The disease is slowly progressive. The cases described by Cavanaugh et al had mainly sensory deficits and were not disabled.

INHERITED POLYNEUROPATHIES WITH A RECOGNIZED METABOLIC DISORDER

Heredopathia Atactica Polyneuritiformis (Refsum Disease)

This rare disorder is inherited as an autosomal recessive trait and has its onset in late childhood, adolescence, or early adult life. Diagnosis is based on a combination of clinical manifestations—retinitis pigmentosa, cerebellar ataxia, and chronic polyneuropathy, coupled with an increase in blood phytanic acid. Cardiomyopathy and neurogenic deafness are present in most patients and pupillary abnormalities, cataracts, and ichthyotic skin changes are present in some. Also, anosmia and night blindness with constriction of the visual fields may precede the neuropathy by many years. Usually the latter develops gradually, sometimes rapidly. The polyneuropathy is sensorimotor, distal, and symmetric in distribution, affecting the legs more than arms. All forms of sensation are reduced and tendon reflexes are lost. The CSF protein is moderately increased.

Although the nerves may not be palpably enlarged, ''hypertrophic'' changes with onion-bulb formation are invariable pathologic features. The metabolic defect is in the utilization of dietary phytol; a failure of oxidation of phytanic acid, a tetramethylated 16-carbon fatty acid, allows its accumulation. The relation between the increased phytanic acid and the polyneuropathy is uncertain. Clinical diagnosis is confirmed by the finding of increased phytanic acid in the blood; the normal level is less than 0.3 mg/dL, but in patients with this disease it constitutes 5 to 30 percent of the total fatty acids of the serum lipids. Diets low in phytol may be beneficial, but this is difficult to judge, for after an acute attack there may be a natural remission. In other patients there is a very slow and gradual progression of the disease, and in still others a more rapid progression with death from cardiac complications.

Ataxia, Retinitis Pigmentosa, and Peripheral Neuropathy without Increase in Phytanic Acid Like Tuck and McLeod, we have observed several cases over a period of years in which there was a clinical syndrome almost identical to Refsum disease, but without demonstrable change in phytanic acid. A mild ichthyosis, sensorineural deafness, an ataxia of mixed tabetic-cerebellar type, areflexia, and retinitis pigmentosa were found. None of our cases had a positive family history. Sural nerve biopsy showed loss of large fibers. We have been unable to detect any biochemical abnormalities in the blood or cultured fibroblasts. The course has been slowly progressive with onset of the disease during adolescence.

Abetalipoproteinemia (Bassen-Kornzweig Syndrome, Acanthocytosis) This rare, autosomal recessive disorder is characterized by (1) near absence of β-lipoprotein and a low level of cholesterol in the serum, (2) retinal (macular) degeneration, (3) acanthocytosis (a thorny or spiky appearance of the red cells, best seen in wet preparations of fresh blood), and (4) a chronic, progressive neurologic deficit, usually beginning in childhood.

Patients with this disorder first come to medical attention as infants because of steatorrhea and retarded growth. The brunt of the neurologic disorder falls upon the cerebellum and peripheral nervous system. The first neurologic finding is diminution or absence of tendon reflexes, detected as early as the second year of life. Later, when the patient is able to cooperate in sensory testing, a loss of vibratory and position sense is found in the legs. Cerebellar signs (ataxia of gait, trunk and extremities, titubation of the head and dysarthria), muscle weakness, ophthalmoparesis, Babinski signs, and loss of pain and temperature sense are the other neurologic abnormalities, in more or less this order of frequency. Mental backwardness occurs in some patients. There are no signs of autonomic disorder. Irregular progression occurs over a few years and many patients are no longer able to stand and walk by the time they reach adolescence.

Skeletal abnormalities include pes cavus and kyphoscoliosis, which are secondary to the neuropathy. Constriction of the visual fields and ring scotomata are manifestations of the macular degeneration and retinitis pigmentosa. Cardiac enlargement and failure are serious and late complications.

Neuropathologic findings consist of *demyelination of peripheral nerves* and degeneration of nerve cells in the spinal gray matter and cerebellar cortex. Diagnosis is confirmed by the finding of acanthocytes, low serum cholesterol, and β (low-density)-lipoproteins. What is known about the pathogenesis and treatment is discussed in Chap. 38 (page 802).

A closely related disease, also with familial hypobetalipoproteinemia, has been described by van Buchem et al. It is associated with a malabsorption syndrome, an ill-defined weakness, ataxia, and dysesthesia of the legs, and Babinksi signs, but no sensory loss.

Tangier Disease This is an exceedingly rare familial disorder which also is inherited as a recessive trait. It is marked by a deficiency of high-density lipoprotein, low cholesterol, diminution of phospholipids, and high triglyceride levels in the serum. The presence of enlarged, yellow-orange (cholesterol-laden) tonsils is said to be a constant manifestation. About half of the reported cases have had neuropathic symptoms, taking the form of an asymmetric sensorimotor neuropathy, which fluctuates in severity. The polyneuropathy may come in attacks, viz., is recurrent, as in the two sisters reported by Engel et al.; onset of symptoms was in childhood and in infancy, respectively. The sensory loss is predominantly for pain and temperature and extends over the entire body; at times it is limited to the face and upper extremities. Tactile and proprioceptive sensory modalities tend to be preserved.

The muscular weakness affects either the lower or upper extremities, or both, and particularly the hand muscles, which may undergo atrophy and show denervation potentials by EMG. In one of our patients, only a facial diplegia was present. Nerve conduction is slowed. Tendon reflexes are lost or diminished. Facial muscles may be involved. Transient ptosis and diplopia have been reported.

Fat-laden macrophages are present in the bone marrow and elsewhere. No complete pathologic studies are available. There is no known treatment.

Anderson-Fabry Disease (Fabry Disease) The genetic and metabolic aspects of this sex-linked disorder have already been considered (page 813). Here, some additional remarks will be made about the painful neuropathic component.

The pain, which is usually the initial symptom in childhood and adolescence, often has a burning quality or occurs in brief lancinating jabs, mostly in the fingers and toes, and may be accompanied by paresthesias of the palms and soles. Changes in environmental temperature and exercise may induce pain. These abnormalities are due to the accumulation of glycolipid (ceramide trihexoside) in peripheral nerves, both perineurally and intraneurally, as well as in cells of the spinal ganglia and the anterior and intermediolateral horns of the spinal cord. Ohnishi and Dyck have demonstrated a preferential loss of small myelinated and unmyelinated fibers and small neurons of dorsal root ganglia. Involvement of the latter cells and the associated degenerative changes in the afferent fibers are thought to be the likely cause of the painful sensory phenomena (Kahn).

Later in the illness there occur progressive impairment of renal function (relatively mild in degree) and cerebral and myocardial infarction, but the most characteristic feature is an eruption of dark red macules and papules, up to 2 mm in diameter, over the trunk and limbs, most closely clustered over the thighs and lower trunk (*angiokeratoma corporis diffusum*).

Phenytoin or carbamazepine (Tegretol) may be helpful in alleviating the pain and dysesthesias, but there is no specific therapy for the disease.

Metachromatic Leukodystrophy (see also Chap. 38) Massive sulfatide accumulation throughout the central and peripheral nervous systems, and to a lesser extent in other organs, occurs in this disorder, because of congenital absence of the degradative enzyme, sulfatase. The abnormality is transmitted as an autosomal recessive trait. Progressive cerebral deterioration is the most obvious clinical aspect, but hyporeflexia, muscular atrophy, and diminished nerve conduction velocity reflect the presence of a neuropathy. Early in the course of the illness, the weakness, hypotonia, and areflexia may suggest Werdnig-Hoffmann disease; in older children there may be a complaint of paresthesias and demonstrable sensory loss. Bifacial weakness has been reported. Sensory and motor conduction velocities are slowed. Metachromatically staining granules accumulate in the cytoplasm of Schwann cells in all peripheral nerves, as well as in the central white matter. Sural biopsy may be used to establish the diagnosis, even early in the course of the illness.

Familial Dysautonomia (Riley-Day Disease) This is a recessively inherited disorder that affects Jewish children predominantly. The condition is manifest at birth (poor sucking, failure to thrive, unexplained fever, episodes of pneumonia). Hyporeflexia and impairment or loss of pain and temperature sensation, with relative preservation of

pressure and tactile sense, are the main neuropathic manifestations. Motor fibers are probably involved as well, but only to a slight degree, shown less by weakness than reduced conduction velocity in peripheral nerves. At a later age the neuropathy continues to be overshadowed by other manifestations of the disease, notably the repeated infections and abnormalities of the autonomic nervous system—lack of tears, corneal ulceration, blotchiness of the skin, defective temperature control, cold hands and feet, excessive sweating, lability of blood pressure, postural hypotension, difficulty in swallowing, esophageal and intestinal dilatation, emotional instability, recurrent vomiting, and stunted growth. The tongue shows an absence of fungiform papillae.

Nerve biopsy reveals a diminution of small myelinated and unmyelinated fibers, which explains the impairment of pain and temperature sensation. In autopsy material, sympathetic and parasympathetic ganglion cells and, to a lesser extent, nerve cells in the sensory ganglia are diminished in number. Patients excrete increased amounts of homovanillic acid and decreased amounts of vanillylmandelic acid and methoxyhydroxyphenylglycol. Weinshilboum and Axelrod have shown a significant decrease in serum dopamine β-hydroxylase, the enzyme that converts dopamine to norepinephrine. There is no treatment for the disease.

Other examples of congenital polyneuropathy with absence of autonomic function, probably different from the Riley-Day dysautonomia, have been reported. A congenital failure of development of neural elements derived from the neural crest is postulated.

The Amyloid Neuropathies Peripheral neuropathy is a common and often the most prominent manifestation of amyloidosis. The polyneuropathies associated with amyloidosis are of two main types—those associated with hereditary amyloidosis, and those associated with primary (nonfamilial) systemic amyloidosis.

The *familial amyloid polyneuropathies* comprise several distinct clinical groups. The pattern of inheritance in all types is autosomal dominant; males and females are affected with equal frequency.

(1) The Portuguese (Andrade) type Andrade, in 1939, first recognized that a chronic familial illness, known as "foot disease" among the inhabitants of Oporto, Portugal, was a special type of amyloid polyneuropathy. He was not the first to have seen amyloid in degenerating nerve but deserves credit for identifying the disease as one of the heredofamilial polyneuropathies. By 1969 he had studied 148 sibships including 623 individuals among whom there were 249 with polyneuropathy. Descendants of this family have been traced to Africa, France, and Brazil.

Other foci of the disease have been reported in Japan (Araki et al; Ikeda et al), in the United States (Kantarjian and deJong), in Germany (Delank et al), in Poland, Greece, and Sweden, and, most recently, in northwest Ireland (Staunton and others). As far as one can tell, these are separate unrelated probands in different ethnic groups.

Cohen and Rubinow, whose review contains the important references to this subject, are impressed with the degree to which the lower extremities are affected initially, and they distinguish this group from the one in which the legs and arms are seemingly affected together, as occurs in the large group of cases in Iowa, recorded by van Allen et al. The authors question the validity of this division, for in all of our patients the lower extremities were affected first and more severely, and the disease extended to the hands and arms much later. Thus, the patients would fall at first into one category or another, depending on the stage of the disease in which they were seen. We suggest that these two apparent categories are but different phases of one disorder. The fact that renal disease tends to occur later in the course of the Portuguese cases is also insufficient reason to separate them from the Iowa cases. The type affecting the hands alone (carpal tunnel syndrome) and the predominantly cranial nerve affection with corneal lattice dystrophy (Meretoja) are special problems.

The age of onset of this form of familial amyloid polyneuropathy is between 25 and 35 years. The disease progresses slowly and terminates fatally in 10 to 15 or more years. The initial symptoms are usually numbness, paresthesias, and sometimes pain in the feet and lower legs. Weakness is minimal, and the tendon reflexes, while diminished, may not be lost early in the course of the illness. Unlike most other polyneuropathies, pain and temperature sensation are reduced more than touch, vibration, and position (pseudosyringomyelia). Autonomic involvement is another important characteristic—loss of pupillary light reflexes and miosis, anhidrosis, vasomotor paralysis with orthostatic hypotension, alternating diarrhea and constipation, and impotence. These autonomic changes tend to be more extensive than the sensory ones. Difficulty in walking also develops and has its basis in a combination of faulty position sense and mild muscle weakness. Later, tendon reflexes are abolished and the legs become thin. The nerves are not enlarged. Cranial nerve involvement (facial weakness and numbness, loss of taste) are late manifestations and occur in only a few cases.

Cases vary somewhat. Irregularities in cardiac rhythm due to bundle branch or AV block and cardiac enlargement occur early in some and late in others. A few patients have had severe amyloid heart disease from the onset (Ikeda et al). Weight loss may be pronounced, owing to anorexia and disordered bowel function and the later development of a malabsorption syndrome, and the liver may become enlarged. Vitreous opacities (veils, specks, and strands) may progress to blindness, but this has been rare, and in a few there has been an impairment of hearing. CNS involvement, manifested as behavioral abnormalities, cerebellar ataxia, and bilateral corticospinal signs, has been reported in a few cases of familial amyloid polyneuropathy, but its pathologic basis is controversial (Ikeda et al). Albuminuria, the nephrotic syndrome, and uremia terminate life in a few of the patients. The CSF may be normal or the protein content may be increased (50 to 200 mg/dL); the blood is normal except for anemia in cases of amyloidosis of the bone marrow.

(2) Familial amyloidosis with carpal tunnel syndrome Falls et al in 1955 and later Rukavina et al described a large group of patients of Swiss stock living in Indiana who developed, in the fourth and fifth decades, a characteristic syndrome of acroparesthesias due to deposition of amyloid in the connective tissues in and deep to the carpal ligaments. There was sensory loss and atrophic muscle weakness in the distribution of the median nerves, which were compressed. Section of the carpal ligaments relieved the symptoms. In some of the patients other nerves of the arms were said to have become involved subsequently. Vitreous deposits were observed frequently in this form of the disease.

(3) Cranial neuropathy with corneal lattice dystrophy This unusual form of amyloid neuropathy was first described in three Finnish families by Meretoja—hence ''Finnish type.'' Subsequently, it has been reported from several different parts of the world, in families of other than Finnish heritage.

The disease usually begins in the third decade, with lattice corneal dystrophy. Vitreous opacities are not observed, and visual acuity is little affected. Peripheral neuropathy may not be evident until the fifth decade, at which time the facial nerves, and particularly their upper branches, become affected. The nerves of the limbs are involved even later, and to a much lesser extent than in other amyloid neuropathies. At postmortem examination, deposits of amyloid are found in virtually every organ, mainly in the kidneys and blood vessels, and in the perineurium of affected nerves.

The neuropathic picture in patients with *primary (nonfamilial) systemic amyloidosis* is much the same as that of hereditary amyloid polyneuropathy. The former type is more frequent in men (27 of 31 cases reported by Kelly et al) and, as a rule, has a considerably later age of onset (mean age 63 years) than the familial type. About one-half of the sporadic cases present with neuropathic symptoms and signs and the other half with renal, cardiac, hematologic, or gastrointestinal complications; the latter are usually responsible for the patient's death.

Multiple myeloma with amyloid neuropathy

Although multiple myeloma is frequently associated with amyloidosis or with a paraneoplastic neuropathy, amyloid neuropathy as a complication of myeloma has proved to be extremely rare. In the few such cases that have been seen, the clinical and pathologic manifestations did not differ from amyloid neuropathy of other type. Bilateral median nerve compression due to amyloid deposition in the carpal ligaments is a relatively frequent complication of myeloma, however.

Other unclassifiable syndromes

We have observed two cases of amyloid neuropathy in elderly persons with diabetes mellitus. Severe, chronic, sensorimotor, areflexive polyneuropathy with slightly enlarged nerves and elevated CSF protein were the identifying features. The diabetes was moderately severe and difficult to control and ended fatally, due presumably to Kimmelstiel-Wilson lesions in the kidney.

In the syndrome of urticaria, deafness, and amyloid nephropathy, in the syndrome of progressive amyloid cardiopathy, and in that of amyloid nephropathy, the peripheral nerves may also be affected, but only late in the course of the disease. Localized trigeminal neuropathy due to amyloid deposition in the gasserian ganglion has been reported (Daly et al).

Pathologic findings

In familial amyloid polyneuropathy, amyloid deposits are demonstrable in the blood vessels, in the interstitial (endoneurial) tissues of the peripheral somatic and autonomic nerves, and in the spinal and autonomic ganglia and roots. There is a loss of nerve fibers, the unmyelinated and small myelinated fibers being more depleted than the large myelinated ones. The anterior horn and sympathetic ganglion cells are swollen and chromatolysed due to involvement of their axons, and the posterior columns of the spinal cord degenerate.

The pathogenesis of the fiber loss is not fully understood. On the basis of their findings in a sporadic case of amyloid polyneuropathy, Kernohan and Woltman suggested that amyloid deposits in the walls of the small arteries and arterioles interfered with the circulation in the nerves and that amyloid neuropathy was essentially an ischemic neuropathy. In other cases, however, the vascular changes are relatively slight and the degeneration of the nerve fibers appears to be related to their compression and distortion by the endoneurial deposits of amyloid. Amyloid is also seen in the tongue, gums, heart, gastrointestinal tract, kidneys, and many other organs.

In all the amyloid polyneuropathies, the only specific diagnostic test is skin, muscle, gingival, or rectal mucosa biopsy, in which amyloid can be demonstrated by appropriate stains and electron microscopy. In familial amyloidotic polyneuropathy of the autosomal dominant (Portuguese) type, Saraiva et al have identified a biochemical marker in the form of a variant transthyretin (a protein formerly referred to as prealbumin)—thus making it possible to detect carriers of the mutant gene.

In personally observed cases we have been impressed with the prominence of autonomic effects, the pseudosyringomyelia, the relative sparing of motor nerves, and the retention of reflexes, at least early in the disease. The constellation of these clinical features should always raise suspicion of the disease. Diagnosis is affirmed by the demonstration of amyloid in the vitreous and nerve biopsy, the abnormal ECG, and renal abnormalities.

Unfortunately, there is no specific therapy. Life is prolonged by medical measures to maintain renal and cardiac function, the use of fludrocortisone acetate (Florinef) to prevent orthostatic syncope, and nutritional supplements to counteract weight loss.

SYNDROME OF RECURRENT AND RELAPSING POLYNEUROPATHY

Two types of neuropathy are particularly prone to recurrence: porphyria, in which the attacks recur spontaneously or because of the administration of barbiturates or other drugs (see above), or the Guillain-Barré syndrome (GBS). Approximately 3 percent of patients with the latter disorder have one or more sudden relapses, in which the clinical and pathologic changes differ in no essential way from those of the acute monophasic form of the disease. And, of course, chronic inflammatory polyneuropathy and some instances of mononeuritis multiplex are characterized by remission and relapse, although the remissions are incomplete. Enlargement of nerves may occur with repeated attacks, and it is probable that some patients classed originally as Déjerine-Sottas disease fall into this category. Rare neuropathies in which relapses may occur are Refsum disease and Tangier disease. Also it is obvious that patients who have recovered from an episode of alcoholic-nutritional or toxic polyneuropathy may develop a recurrence of their disease if they are subjected again to intoxication or nutritional deficiency.

This is the group that has given the authors the most difficulty. The cause of most of the acute and many of the subacute and relapsing forms can usually be established by the clinical and laboratory methods presently available in teaching centers. It is the chronic ones that continue to baffle the neurologist despite the respectable advances that have been made in this field of medicine.

Many of the chronic polyneuropathies prove to be heredofamilial. The observations of Dyck et al, referred to in the introduction to this chapter, are of interest in this respect. In a series of 205 patients who were referred to the Mayo Clinic with neuropathies of unknown cause, 86 were found to have an inherited form of the disease. With apporprite genealogic data, the diagnosis of the hypertrophic polyneuropathy of Déjerine-Sottas and the peroneal muscular atrophy of Charcot-Marie-Tooth, the two major types, can usually be made on clinical grounds alone. Sporadic cases become more difficult. Dyck et al found that direct examinations of the patients' kin, using all available clinical data, electromyography, nerve conduction studies, CSF examination, and nerve and muscle biopsy, was particularly helpful in revealing an hereditary basis of the neuropathy.

The several rare chronic hereditary diseases of nerve express themselves mainly by three syndromes: (1) progressive pseudosyringomyelic syndrome with autonomic paralysis, (2) progressive sensorimotor paralysis, and (3) chronic sensory polyneuropathy with ataxia.

One should always suspect familial amyloidosis and Riley-Day dysautonomia when impairment of autonomic function and of pain and thermal sensation is prominent and disproportionate to other sensory and motor symptoms. The diagnosis of both these diseases can usually be affirmed by proper laboratory tests; occasionally, however, we have seen patients with this syndrome when tests for amyloid and disordered catecholamine metabolism were normal. Bassen-Kornzweig, Tangier, and Refsum disease are being entertained as diagnostic possibilities now that the methods for confirming the diagnosis have become more widely available. They are so rare, however, that such a search is seldom rewarding.

The syndrome of chronic sensorimotor paralysis involving legs more than arms and distal parts more than proximal parts should, in an adult, always lead to a search for occult neoplasia (carcinoma, multiple myeloma, or plasmacytoma) or macroglobulinemia. In exceptional cases, the tumor remains hidden for as long as 2 or 3 years after the onset of neuropathy. In our experience, a toxic, endocrine, or nutritional cause is seldom found. Unusual causes of nutritional deficiency, such as celiac disease and other malabsorption syndromes (Whipple disease, chronic hepatic disease), have usually been obvious enough when present, so that the experienced clinician rarely overlooks them. A difficult type of case is the older person with a mild nonprogressive sensorimotor polyneuropathy who has mild hypothyroidism, marginally low vitamin B_{12} levels in the blood, a somewhat unbalanced diet, and an abnormal glucose tolerance curve. It is easy to imagine but hard to prove that any one of these abnormalities is relevant. Other patients develop a polyneuropathy for no discernible reason other than that they are chronically septic and critically ill (Zochodne et al).

In the chronic sensory polyneuropathies—some painful, some not, some with marked ataxia—the association with occult carcinoma is the primary consideration. Milder degrees may be seen with biliary cirrhosis (xanthomatous polyneuropathy of Thomas and Walker). When confined to the feet and legs, a sporadic example of hereditary sensory neuropathy must be considered. However, from year to year the authors regularly observe a few patients in whom the cause is not disclosed by any of the available tests. We have watched helplessly as some of these patients become reduced to a bed and wheelchair existence and others suffer from pain until they become addicted to opiates in spite of our admonitions.

Other peripheral nerve syndromes, whose anatomical bases are not well established, include (1) pure panautonomic polyneuritis (Chap. 26) and (2) possibly myokymia and continuous muscular activity (Chap. 54). Of course, tetany is essentially a peripheral nerve phenomenon—an unstable polarization of the axolemma due to diminished ionized serum calcium.

DIAGNOSIS OF MONONEUROPATHY AND MULTIPLE NEUROPATHY

The distinguishing feature of this group of neuropathies is that one or several individual peripheral nerves are involved by the disease process. The diagnosis rests on the finding of motor, reflex, or sensory changes confined to the territory of a single nerve or several individual nerves affected in a random manner *(mononeuritis or mononeuropathy multiplex)*, and the presence of other data pointing to its causation. A plexus of nerves or part of a plexus may be involved. Certain neuropathies of this type are due to leprosy, sarcoid, diabetes, and polyarteritis nodosa, and have already been discussed. A chronic inflammatory neuropathy should also be considered; in addition to mononeuritis multiplex, pain, erythema, and elevated CSF protein with pleocytosis are the main features (Bannwarth syndrome or Lyme disease). A zone of erythema on a limb or the chest, due to a tick bite, may be diagnostic. Cranial nerves can be affected at a distance from the bite (page 580).

COMMON BRACHIAL PLEXUS NEUROPATHIES

Brachial plexus neuropathies, usually unilateral, comprise an interesting group of neurologic disorders. Some may develop without apparent cause and manifest themselves by sensorimotor derangements ascribable to cords of the plexus. Others result from trauma in which the arm is hyperabducted or the shoulder violently separated from the neck. Difficult births are an important source of traction injuries. Rarely, the brachial plexus or other peripheral nerves may be damaged at the time of electrical injury, either from lightning or from household or industrial sources. Direct compression of parts of the plexus by adjacent skeletal anomalies (cervical rib, fascial bands) or by apical lung tumors represents another category of plexus injury. A subcutaneous or intramuscular injection of vaccine or foreign serum may be followed by a brachial plexopathy, usually partial. *Neuralgic amyotrophy* of obscure origin, also called *paralytic brachial neuritis*, stands as a special clinical entity, often difficult to distinguish from other types of brachial pain. Some of these latter are, surprisingly, familial; others occur in epidemic form. There are plexus lesions of presumed toxic nature, as in those following heroin injection. Finally, there may be impairment of function of the brachial plexus or portions thereof many months or years after radiation therapy.

These introductory remarks are intended to convey the idea that most brachial plexus disorders are due to trauma, tumors, compression, injections of serum, vaccine, or drugs, obscure (viral?) infections, and the delayed effects of radiotherapy.

For the anatomic plan of the brachial plexus and its relation to blood vessels and bony structures, one of the more detailed monographs on the peripheral nerves should be consulted. The one by Haymaker and Woodhall is recommended (see references). For quick orientation it is enough to remember that the brachial plexus is formed from the anterior and posterior divisions of cervical roots 5, 6, 7, and 8, and the first thoracic nerve roots (see Fig. 46-5). The fifth and sixth cervical roots merge into the upper trunk, the seventh root forms the middle trunk, and the eighth cervical and first thoracic roots form the lower trunk. Each trunk divides into an anterior and posterior division.

The posterior divisions of each trunk unite to form the posterior cord of the plexus. The anterior divisions of the upper and middle trunks unite to form the lateral cord. The anterior division of the lower trunk forms the medial cord. Two important nerves emerge from the upper trunk (dorsal scapular nerve to the rhomboid and levator scapulae muscles, and long thoracic nerve to the anterior serratus). The posterior cord gives rise mainly to the radial nerve. The medial cord gives rise to the ulnar nerve, medial cutaneous nerve to the forearm, and medial cutaneous nerve to the upper arm. This cord lies in close relation to the subclavian artery and apex of the lung and is the part of the plexus most susceptible to traction injuries and to compression by tumors that invade the costoclavicular space. The median nerve is formed by the union of parts of the medial and lateral cords.

Lesions of the Whole Plexus The entire arm is paralyzed and hangs uselessly at the side; the sensory loss is complete below a line extending from the shoulder diagonally downward and medially to the middle third of the upper arm. Biceps, triceps, radial periosteal, and finger reflexes are abolished. The usual cause is vehicular trauma.

Upper Brachial Plexus Paralysis This is due to injury to the fifth and sixth cervical nerves and roots, the most common causes of which are forceful separation of the head and shoulder during difficult delivery, pressure on the supraclavicular region during anesthesia, injections of foreign serum or vaccines, and idiopathic neuralgic amyotrophy. The muscles affected are the biceps, deltoid, brachialis anticus, supinator longus, supraspinatus and infraspinatus, and rhomboids. The arm hangs at the side, internally rotated and extended at the elbow. Hand motion is unaffected. The prognosis for spontaneous recovery is generally good though it may be incomplete; injuries of the upper brachial plexus and spinal roots which are incurred at birth (Erb-Duchenne palsy) may persist throughout life.

Lower Brachial Plexus Paralysis This is usually the result of traction on the abducted arm in falls or during operations on the axilla, or of infiltration or compression by tumors arising from the apex of the lung (superior sulcus or Pancoast syndrome or by cervical ribs or bands). Injury may occur during birth, particularly with breech deliveries (Déjerine-Klumpke paralysis). There is weakness and wasting of the small muscles of the hand and a characteristic claw-hand deformity. Sensory loss is limited to the ulnar border of the hand and the inner forearm; and if the first thoracic motor root is involved, there may be an associated paralysis of the cervical sympathetic nerves with a Horner syndrome. Invasion of the lower plexus by tumors is usually painful; postradiation lesions usually cause paresthesias without pain (Lederman and Wilbourn).

Lesions of the Cords of the Brachial Plexus (see Fig. 46-5) A lesion of the *lateral cord* causes weakness of the muscles supplied by the musculocutaneous nerve and the lateral root of the median nerve; it manifests itself mainly as a weakness of flexion and pronation of the forearm. The intrinsic muscles of the hand innervated by the medial root of the median nerve are spared. A lesion of the *medial cord* causes weakness of muscles supplied by the medial root of the median nerve and the ulnar nerve. The effect is that of a combined median and ulnar nerve palsy. A lesion of the *posterior cord* results in weakness of the deltoid muscle, extensors of the elbow, wrist, and

Figure 46-5

Diagram of the brachial plexus: the components of the plexus have been separated and drawn out of scale. Note that peripheral nerves arise from various components of the plexus: roots [indicated by (C) 5, 6, 7, 8, and (T) 1]; trunks (upper, middle, lower); divisions (anterior and posterior); and cords (lateral, posterior, and medial). The median nerve arises from the heads of the lateral and medial cords. (From Haymaker and Woodhall.)

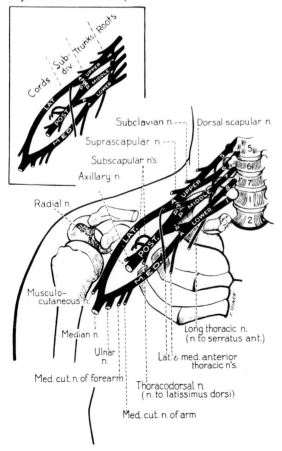

fingers, and sensory loss on the outer surface of the upper arm.

The most frequent causes of injury to the cords are dislocation of the head of the humerus, direct axillary trauma (stab wounds), pressure of a cervical rib, or band, and supraclavicular compression during anesthesia. All cords of the plexus may be injured, or they may be injured in various combinations.

Costoclavicular Syndrome This is discussed in Chap. 10 (pages 173 and 174).

Brachial Plexus Neuropathy (Neuralgic Amyotrophy, Brachial Neuritis) This illness, of obscure nature, may develop abruptly in an otherwise healthy individual, or it may complicate an infection, or an injection of serum, vaccine, antibiotic, or heroin. Magee and deJong in 1960, and Tsairis et al in 1972, reported large series of cases and amplified a well-known clinical picture that the authors have observed repeatedly. Our patients have nearly all been adults ranging from 25 to 65 years of age. Males are slightly more susceptible (2.4:1.0). Beginning as an ache in and around the shoulder, at the root of the neck or base of the skull, and suspected at first of being only a ''wry neck,'' the pain rapidly becomes more severe; it is followed after a period of 3 to 10 days by the rapid development of muscular weakness and sensory and reflex impairment. The pain is made worse by movements that involve the muscles in the region. In a few cases, the neurologic disorder occurs without antecedent pain. Unlike radicular lesions, which almost never cause complete paralysis of a muscle, here a muscle such as the serratus anterior, deltoid, biceps, or triceps may be totally or almost totally paralyzed. Rarely all the muscles of the arm are involved (4 of 99 of Tsairis' cases). Motor nerve conduction becomes slowed in 7 to 10 days. In a small proportion of cases both shoulders and arms are affected. Most of the neurologic deficits in our cases have been localized around the shoulder and upper arm; sometimes the hand has been affected. Either the biceps or triceps reflex may be abolished. Recurrence of brachial plexus neuropathy has been reported. In rare cases the symptoms are bilateral.

The term *neuralgic amyotrophy* was given to this symptom complex by Parsonage and Turner and is not inappropriate, since the clinical and EMG findings may suggest a lesion of the peripheral nerves rather than the cords of the plexus, and the exact site and nature of the pathologic changes have never been established. Such patients usually have no fever, leukocytosis, or increased sedimentation rate. Occasionally there is a mild pleocytosis (10 to 50 white blood cells per cubic millimeter) and slightly increased CSF protein. Duchowny et al have described a patient in whom a typical brachial neuritis occurred as part of a febrile illness that proved to be due to cytomegalic virus infection. A few outbreaks have been recorded and have prompted the suggestion that the Coxsackie virus is the cause.

As a rule, the pain subsides with the onset of weakness, but in some cases it lasts for weeks. Recovery of paralysis and restoration of sensation are usually complete in a matter of 6 to 12 weeks, but sometimes not for a year or longer. One must differentiate this disorder from the following conditions: (1) spondylosis or ruptured disc with root involvement; particularly C7 root with involvement of the serratus anterior and winging of the scapula; (2) brachialgia from bursitis or "rotator cuff syndrome"; (3) polymyalgia rheumatica; (4) serogenic and vaccinogenic plexitis; (5) local entrapment neuropathies.

Brachial Neuropathy Following Radiotherapy

This is usually a complication of irradiation of the axilla for carcinoma of the breast. Stoll and Andrews studied a group of 117 such patients who were treated with high-voltage, small-field therapy, using either 6300 or 5775 rads in divided doses. Of those receiving the larger dose, 73 percent developed weakness and sensory loss in the hand and fingers between 4 and 30 months after treatment, most of them after 12 months. In one autopsied case, the brachial plexus was ensheathed in dense fibrous tissue; below this zone, both myelin and axons had degenerated (wallerian degeneration), presumably as a result of *entrapment* of nerves in fibrous tissue; possibly a vascular factor was also operative.

Kori et al, who analyzed the brachial plexus lesions in 100 patients with cancer, also found that doses exceeding 6000 rads were associated with radiation damage. Usually the upper plexus was involved and was associated with a painless lymphedema. In patients who received lower doses, the development of brachial plexopathy usually indicated tumor infiltration; these lesions affected the lower plexus more than the upper, and were often painful and accompanied by a Horner syndrome (see also Lederman and Wilbourn).

Herpes Zoster Plexitis, Neuritis, and Ganglionitis

See Chap. 33.

Serum- and Vaccine-Induced Brachial Neuropathy

Formerly, when animal antisera were in common use, this entity was rather frequent, but now it is a great rarity. Three to 10 days after the administration of horse tetanus antitoxin, for example, there is the acute onset of severe pain in one or both shoulders and upper arms, coinciding with or following, within a day or two, the development of other systemic manifestations of serum sickness. Several days after the onset of pain, as with brachial neuritis of other types, weakness about the shoulder is noted, usually in the distribution of the upper (lateral) trunk of the brachial plexus. Or there may be only an isolated mononeuropathy (most often of the axillary, suprascapular, musculocutaneous, or long thoracic nerve). The most common isolated palsy is that of the serratus anterior.

Plexitis following vaccines is similar. It has been seen after injection of tetanus toxoid, typhoid-paratyphoid vaccine, triple vaccine (pertussis, diphtheria, and tetanus), and rarely after vaccination for smallpox.

No pathologic data are available. The disease has not been reproduced in the experimental animal. Therapy is purely symptomatic. Recovery may occur within a few weeks or may take up to 2 years, or even longer. In 10 to 20 percent of cases there is residual weakness and wasting of the affected muscles.

Heredofamilial Brachial Plexus Neuropathy

This term designates an acute brachial neuropathy that occurs in families. The pattern of inheritance is autosomal dominant, and the attacks occur most commonly in the second and third decades. Some of the affected individuals have had multiple attacks with recovery in between. Lower cranial nerve involvement and mononeuropathies in other limbs were conjoined in some instances (see Taylor). Again the clinical course is benign.

Madrid and Bradley have examined the sural nerves from two patients with familial recurrent brachial neuropathy. In teased, single nerve fibers they found sausage-like areas of thickened myelin and redundant loops of myelin with secondary constriction of the axon. In addition, nerve fibers showed a considerable degree of segmental demyelination and remyelination. To this aberration of myelin formation they applied the term "tomaculous neuropathy" (from the Latin *tomaculum*, "sausage"). These changes were not observed in the sural nerve of a sporadic case of recurrent acute brachial plexus neuropathy.

The genetic vulnerability to brachial neuropathy is comparable to the *familial occurrence of multiple pressure palsies* reported by Earl et al. Indeed, sausagelike swellings of the myelin sheaths have also been found in the nerves of patients with hereditary pressure-sensitive neuropathy (Behse et al). This would suggest that the nerves of patients with familial brachial plexus neuropathy may also be unduly sensitive to pressure or ischemia. Why the sensitivity should be largely restricted to the brachial plexus is not clear, however.

Brachial Mononeuropathies *Long thoracic nerve (of Bell)* This nerve is derived from the fifth, sixth, and seventh cervical nerves and supplies the serratus anterior muscle, which fixates the lateral scapula to the chest wall. Paralysis of this muscle results in winging of the medial border of the scapula when the outstretched arm is pushed forward against resistance, and inability to raise the arm over the head. It is injured most commonly by carrying heavy weights on the shoulder or by strapping the shoulder on the operating table. It sometimes follows immunization and is also involved at times in serum neuritis and neuralgic amyotrophy (brachial neuritis); it has been described as the sole manifestation of inherited brachial plexus neuropathy (Phillips). Occasionally it arises de novo.

Suprascapular nerve This nerve is derived from the fifth (mainly) and sixth cervical nerves and supplies the supraspinatus and infraspinatus muscles. Lesions may be recognized by the presence of atrophy of these muscles and weakness of the first 15° of abduction of the arm (supraspinatus) and of external rotation of the arm at the shoulder joint (infraspinatus). The latter is tested by having the patient flex the forearm and then, pinning the elbow to the side, asking the patient to swing the forearm backward against resistance. This nerve is often involved together with other nerves of the plexus in cases of brachial neuritis. Lesions of this nerve have also been reported in gymnasts and during infectious illnesses. An entrapment syndrome has been reported where pain and weakness on external rotation of the shoulder joint are the characteristic features. The infraspinatus muscle becomes atrophic. Decompression of the nerve where it enters the spinoglenoid notch relieves the condition.

Axillary nerve This nerve arises from the posterior cord of the brachial plexus (mainly from C5 root with a smaller contribution from C6) and supplies the teres minor and deltoid muscles. It may be involved in dislocations of the shoulder joint, fractures of the neck of the humerus, serum- and vaccine-induced neuropathies, brachial neuritis, or no cause may be apparent. The anatomic diagnosis depends on recognition of paralysis of abduction of the arm (in testing this function the angle between the side of the chest and the arm must be greater than 15° and less than 90°), wasting of the deltoid muscle, and slight impairment of sensation over the outer aspect of the shoulder.

Musculocutaneous nerve The origin of this nerve is from the fifth and sixth cervical roots. It is a branch of the lateral cord of the brachial plexus and innervates the biceps brachii, brachialis, and coracobrachialis muscles. Lesions of the nerve result in wasting of these muscles and weakness of flexion of the supinated forearm. Sensation may be impaired along the radial and volar aspects of the forearm (lateral cutaneous nerve). Isolated lesions of this nerve are usually the result of fracture of the humerus.

Radial nerve This nerve is derived from the sixth to eighth (mainly the seventh) cervical roots and, as was stated, is the termination of the posterior cord of the brachial plexus. It innervates the triceps, brachioradialis, and supinator muscles, the extensor muscles of the wrist and fingers, and the abductor of the thumb. A complete radial nerve lesion results in paralysis of extension of the elbow, flexion of the elbow with the forearm midway between pronation and supination (due to paralysis of the brachioradialis muscle), supination of the forearm, extension of the wrist and fingers, and extension and abduction of the thumb. Sensation is impaired over the posterior aspects of the forearm and a small area over the radial aspect of the dorsum of the hand. The nerve may be compressed in the axilla, for example in "crutch" palsy, but more frequently at a lower point, where the nerve winds around the humerus; pressure palsies incurred during sleep and fractures commonly injure the nerve at the latter site. It is susceptible to lead intoxication and is frequently involved as part of a neuralgic amyotrophy.

Median nerve This nerve originates from the fifth cervical to the first thoracic roots, but mainly from the sixth cervical root, and is formed by the union of the medial and lateral cords of the brachial plexus. It innervates the pronators of the forearm, long finger flexors, and abductor and opponens muscles of the thumb, and is a sensory nerve to the palmar aspect of the hand. Complete interruption of the median nerve results in inability to pronate the forearm or flex the hand in a radial direction, paralysis of flexion of the index finger and terminal phalanx of the thumb, weakness of flexion of the remaining fingers, weakness of abduction and opposition of the thumb, and sensory impairment over the radial two-thirds of the palmar aspect of the hand and the dorsum of the distal phalanges of the index and third fingers. The nerve may be injured in the axilla by dislocation of the shoulder and in any part of its course by stab, gunshot, or other types of wounds. Incomplete lesions of the median nerve between the axilla and wrist may result in causalgia (see below).

Compression of the nerve at the wrist (*carpal tunnel syndrome*) is the most common disorder affecting the median nerve. This is most often due to excessive use of the hands and occupational exposure to repeated trauma. Infiltration of the transverse carpal ligament with amyloid (as occurs in multiple myeloma); or thickening of connective tissue in rheumatoid arthritis, acromegaly, mucopolysaccharidosis, and hypothyroidism are less commonly identified causes. Often, the cause of the carpal tunnel syndrome is not apparent. apparent.

Dysesthesias and pain in the hand, referred to for many years as "idiopathic acroparesthesias," came to be recognized as a syndrome of median nerve compression only in the 1950s. The paresthesias are characteristically worse during the night. As pointed out in Chap. 10, the pain in carpal tunnel syndrome often radiates into the forearm, and even into the upper arm and shoulder. The syndrome is essentially a sensory one; the loss or impairment of superficial sensation affects the thumb, index, and middle fingers (especially the index finger) and may or may not split the ring finger (splitting does not occur with a plexus or root lesion). Weakness and atrophy of the abductor pollicis brevis and other median-innervated muscles occur in only the most advanced cases of compression. As indicated in Chap. 45, electrophysiologic testing confirms the diagnosis and explains cases in which operation has failed (see also the review by Stevens).

Surgical division of the carpal tunnel with decompression of the nerve is curative. Splinting of the wrist, to avoid flexion, almost always relieves the discomfort, but denies the patient the use of the hand. It is a useful temporizing measure, however, as is the injection of hydrocortisone into the carpal tunnel. The administration of pyridoxine has not been useful, in our experience, and in large doses it may be dangerous.

Ulnar nerve This nerve is derived from the eighth cervical and first thoracic roots. It innervates the ulnar flexor of the wrist, the ulnar half of the deep finger flexors, the adductors and abductors of the fingers, the adductor of the thumb, the third and fourth lumbricals, and muscles of the hypothenar eminence. Complete ulnar paralysis is manifested by a characteristic claw-hand deformity; this is the result of wasting of the small hand muscles, permitting hyperextension of the fingers at the metacarpophalangeal joints and flexion at the interphalangeal joints. The flexion deformity is most pronounced in the fourth and fifth fingers, since the lumbrical muscles of the second and third fingers, supplied by the median nerve, counteract the deformity. Sensory loss occurs over the fifth finger, the ulnar aspect of the fourth finger, and the ulnar border of the palm.

The ulnar nerve is most commonly injured at the elbow, by fracture or dislocation involving the joint. *Delayed ulnar palsy* may occur many years after an injury to the elbow which has resulted in a cubitus valgus deformity of the joint. Because of the deformity, the nerve is stretched in its groove over the ulnar condyle, and its more superficial location renders it vulnerable to compression. A shallow ulnar groove, quite apart from abnormalities of the elbow joint, may expose the nerve to compressive injury. Anterior transposition of the ulnar nerve is a simple and effective form of treatment for these types of ulnar palsy. Compression of the nerve may occur just distal to the medial epicondyle, where the ulnar nerve runs beneath the aponeurosis of the flexor carpi ulnaris (*cubital tunnel*). Flexion at the elbow causes a narrowing of the tunnel and constriction of the nerve. This type of ulnar palsy is treated by incising the aponeurotic arch between the olecranon and medial epicondyle. Yet another site of ulnar nerve compression is in the ulnar tunnel, at the wrist. Prolonged pressure on the ulnar part of the palm may result in damage to the deep palmar branch of the ulnar nerve, causing weakness of small hand muscles but no sensory loss. The site of the lesion is localizable by nerve conduction studies.

CAUSALGIA

This is the name applied by Weir Mitchell to a rare (except in time of war) type of peripheral neuralgia consequent upon trauma with partial interruption of the median or ulnar nerve, and occasionally the sciatic or peroneal nerve. It is characterized by persistent, severe pain in the hand or foot, most pronounced in the digits, palm of the hand, or sole. The pain has a burning quality and frequently it radiates beyond the territory of the injured nerve. The painful parts are exquisitely sensitive to contactual stimuli, so the patient cannot bear the contact of clothing or drafts of air; even ambient heat or cold or noise intensify the causalgic symptoms. The affected extremity is kept protected and immobile, often wrapped in a cloth moistened with cool water. Sudomotor and vasomotor and later, trophic abnormalities are usual accompaniments of the pain. The skin of the affected part is moist and warm or cool and soon becomes shiny and smooth, at times scaly and discolored. The most plausible explanation of causalgic pain is that it is due to a short-circuiting of impulses, the result of an artificial connection between efferent sympathetic and sensory somatic fibers at the point of the nerve injury. This theory would explain not only the vasomotor and sudomotor abnormalities, but the exacerbations of pain with all types of emotional stimuli. "True causalgia" of this type can be counted upon to respond favorably to procaine block of the appropriate sympathetic ganglia and, over the long run, to regional sympathectomy. Intravenous injection of guanethidine into the affected limb (with the venous return blocked for several minutes) may alleviate the pain for days or longer.

The term *causalgia* is best reserved for the syndrome described above—i.e., persistent burning pain and abnormalities of sympathetic innervation consequent upon trauma to a major nerve in an extremity. Others have applied the term to a wide range of conditions which are characterized by persistent burning (i.e., causalgic) pain, but which have only an inconsistent association with sudomotor, vasomotor, and trophic changes and an unpredictable response to sympathetic blockade. These latter states, which have been described under a plethora of titles (Sudeck atrophy, minor causalgia, shoulder-hand syndrome, reflex dystrophy, etc.), may follow nontraumatic lesions of the peripheral nerves or even lesions of the CNS. The role of the central and sympathetic nervous systems in causalgic pain is the subject of a critical review by Schott.

Under the title of *migrant sensory neuropathy,* Wartenberg described an ascending neuritis beginning in the foot or hand and involving sensory nerves. It can be extremely painful, even causalgic. The findings are predominantly sensory. The pathology and cause are unknown. After months, the condition remits, presumably with regeneration.

LUMBOSACRAL PLEXUS AND CRURAL NEUROPATHIES

The twelfth thoracic, first to fifth lumbar, and first, second, and third sacral spinal nerve roots compose the lumbosacral plexuses and innervate the muscles of the lower extremities (see Fig. 46-6). The following are the common plexus and crural nerve palsies.

Lumbosacral Plexus Lesions Extending as it does from the upper lumbar area to the lower sacrum and passing near several lower abdominal and pelvic organs, this plexus is subject to a number of injuries and diseases, most of them secondary. The cause of involvement may be difficult to ascertain, because the primary disease is often not within reach of the palpating fingers, either from the abdominal side or through the anus and vagina; even refined radiologic techniques may not reveal it. Differential diagnosis involves exclusion of spinal root (cauda equina) lesions by examination of CSF, myelography, and MRI. The clinical findings help to focus studies on the appropriate part of the lumbosacral plexus. Valuable diagnostic aids include the presence of autonomic disturbances (present with nerve but not

with root lesions), roentgenograms of spine, bone scans, CT body scans, aortic arteriography, intravenous pyelography, barium enema, and electromyography.

Characteristically, plexus lesions produce unilateral muscle weakness and sensory and reflex changes that are not confined to the territory of a single root or nerve. If pain is present, it may occasionally be accentuated by straight leg raising (Lasègue sign) or movement of the hip, but will be unaffected by increasing the intraspinal pressure by coughing, sneezing, and jugular compression. The main effects of upper plexus lesions are weakness of flexion and adduction of the thigh and extension of the leg, with sensory loss over the anterior thigh and leg; these effects must be distinguished from the symptoms of femoral neuropathy (see below). Lower plexus lesions weaken the posterior thigh, leg, and foot muscles and abolish sensation over the first and second sacral segments (sometimes the lower sacral segments also). Lesions of the entire plexus, which occur infrequently, cause a weakness or paralysis of all leg muscles, with atrophy, areflexia, anesthesia from toes to perianal region, and autonomic loss with warm, dry skin. Usually there is edema of the leg as well.

The types of lesions that involve the lumbosacral plexus are rather different than those affecting the brachial plexus. Trauma is a rarity except with massive pelvic, spine, and abdominal injuries, because the plexus is so well protected. Occasionally a pelvic fracture will damage the sciatic nerve as it issues from the plexus. In contrast, some part of the plexus may be damaged during surgical procedures on abdominal and pelvic organs, for reasons that may not be entirely clear. For example, hysterectomy has on a number of occasions led to neurologic consultation in our hospitals because of numbness and weakness of the anterior thigh. Either the cords of the upper part of the plexus were compressed by retraction against the psoas muscle or, in vaginal hysterectomy (when thighs are flexed, abducted, and externally rotated), the femoral nerve was compressed against the inguinal ligament. A similar type of injury may be associated with childbirth. Lumbar sympathectomy has also been associated with upper plexus lesions; the most disabling sequelae are burning pain and hypersensitivity of the anterior thigh. Appendectomy, pelvic explorations, and hernial repair may injure branches of the upper plexus (ilioinguinal, iliohypogastric, and genitofemoral nerves), with severe pain and slight sensory loss in the distribution of one of these nerves. The pain may last for months or a year or more.

The lumbar plexus may be compressed by an aortic, atherosclerotic aneurysm. Usually there is pain that radiates to the hip, anterior thigh, and occasionally to the flank. Slight weakness in hip flexion and altered sensation over the anterior thigh are the findings on examination. Plexus involvement with tumors is commonplace and at times presents special difficulties in diagnosis. Carcinoma of either the cervix or prostate may seed itself along the perineurial lymphatics and cause pain in the groin, thigh, knee, or back without much in the way of sensory, motor, or reflex loss. The pain may be bilateral. The CSF and spinal canal (by myelography) are normal. Testicular, uterine, and colonic tumors, or retroperitoneal lymphomas, by extending along the paravertebral gutter, implicate various parts of the lumbosacral plexus. The neurologic symptoms are projected at a distance in the leg, and may or may not be confined to the territory of any one nerve. Pelvic and rectal examinations may be negative and intravenous pyelography, visualization of the lymphatic system, CT, and MRI may be necessary to show such lesions. If

all these examinations are negative, exploratory laparotomy may be necessary.

Reference has already been made to femoral nerve injury during parturition, but other puerperal complications are also observed. Back pain in the latter part of pregnancy is common, but there are rare instances in which the patient complains of severe pain in the back of one or both thighs during labor, and after delivery has numbness and weakness of the leg muscles, with diminished ankle jerks. The attribution of these symptoms to pressure of the fetal head on the sacral portion of the plexus(es) is conjectural. Protrusion of an intervertebral disc may also occur during delivery.

A *neuralgic amyotrophy* or *lumbosacral plexitis*, analogous to the brachial variety, is observed from time to time. Bradley et al have recorded their observations of such cases. After causing widespread unilateral or bilateral sensory, motor, and reflex changes, lumbosacral plexitis may leave the patient with dysesthesias as troublesome as those that follow herpes zoster (which may also occur at this level). Some patients have had an exploration of the cauda equina (for ruptured disc) even though loss of sweating

Figure 46-6

Diagram of the lumbar plexus (left) *and the sacral plexus* (right). *The lumbosacral trunk is the liaison between the lumbar and the sacral plexuses. The three divisions of the sciatic nerve are indicated. (From Haymaker and Woodhall.)*

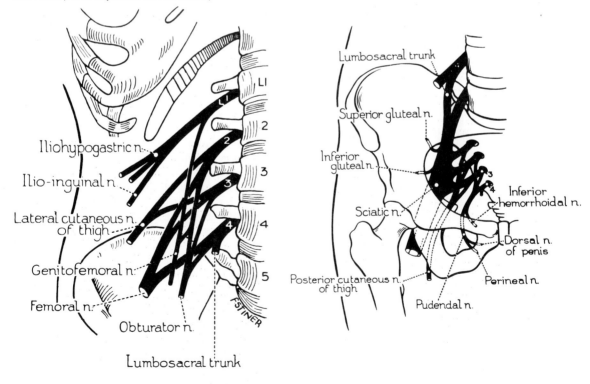

and warmth of the feet should have indicated interruption of autonomic fibers by lesions in peripheral nerves. Immunosuppressant drugs were beneficial in four of six cases (Bradley et al). *Diabetic amyotrophy*, due to involvement of the lumbar plexus(es), has a vascular origin, but probably there are also nondiabetic vascular lesions, which give rise to algesic paresis of proximal muscles. The plexus lesions of polyarteritis nodosa, unilateral or bilateral, may also be manifest as a mononeuropathy multiplex. The incidence of mononeuropathy multiplex in diabetics increases sharply if there is associated occlusive vascular disease of the lower extremities. Diabetic mononeuropathy multiplex is discussed in an earlier part of this chapter and protruded intervertebral disc syndromes are described in Chap. 10.

Lateral Cutaneous Nerve of the Thigh

This is a sensory nerve that originates from the second and third lumbar roots and supplies the anterolateral aspect of the thigh, from the level of the inguinal ligament almost to the knee. The nerve penetrates the psoas muscle, crosses the iliacus and passes into the thigh by coursing between the two prongs of attachment of the lateral part of the inguinal ligament to the anterior superior iliac spine. Compression (entrapment) may occur at the point where it passes between the two prongs of attachment of the inguinal ligament.

Compression of the nerve results in uncomfortable paresthesias and sensory impairment in its cutaneous distribution, a condition known as *meralgia paresthetica* (*meros*—thigh). Usually numbness and mild sensitivity of the skin to clothing are the only symptoms, but occasionally there is a persistent, distressing burning pain. Perception of touch and pinprick are reduced in the territory of the nerve; there is no weakness of the quadriceps or diminution of knee jerk. The symptoms are characteristically worsened in certain positions, usually with prolonged standing or walking. Occasionally, in an obese person, sitting is the most uncomfortable position. Obesity, pregnancy, and diabetes mellitus are contributory factors. Usually the neuropathy is unilateral; Ecker and Woltman found only 20 percent of their cases to be bilateral.

Most of our patients with meralgia paresthetica have requested no treatment once they learned of its benign character. A few with the most painful symptoms have demanded a neurectomy, but it is always wise to perform a xylocaine block first so that the patient can decide whether the persistent numbness is preferable. In one specimen of nerve obtained at operation we found a discrete traumatic neuroma. Hydrocortisone injections at the point of entrapment have helped in a few cases.

Obturator Nerve

This nerve arises from the third and fourth and to a lesser extent from the second lumbar roots. It supplies the adductors and to some extent the internal and external rotators of the thigh. The adductors have the added function of flexion at the hip. The nerve may be injured by the fetal head or forceps during the course of a difficult labor or compressed by an obturator hernia. Rarely, it is affected in diabetes, polyarteritis nodosa, and osteitis pubis; and rarely also by retroperitoneal spread of carcinoma of the cervix, uterus, and other tumors.

Femoral Nerve

This nerve is formed from the second, third, and fourth lumbar roots. Within the pelvis it passes along the lateral border of the psoas muscle and enters the thigh beneath Poupart's ligament, lateral to the femoral artery. Branches arising within the pelvis supply the iliacus and psoas muscles. Just below Poupart's ligament the nerve divides into anterior and posterior divisions. The former supplies the pectineus and sartorius muscles and carries sensation from the anteromedial surface of the thigh; the posterior division provides the motor innervation to the quadriceps and the cutaneous innervation to the medial side of the leg from the knee to the internal malleolus.

Following injury to the femoral nerve, there is weakness of extension of the leg and wasting of the quadriceps muscle; if the nerve is injured proximal to the origin of the branches to the iliacus and psoas muscles, there is weakness of hip flexion. The knee jerk is abolished.

The commonest cause of femoral neuropathy is diabetes. The nerve may be injured during pelvic operations (see above), and may be involved by pelvic tumors. Bleeding into the iliac muscle, observed in patients receiving anticoagulants and in hemophiliacs, is a relatively common cause of isolated femoral neuropathy (Goodfellow et al). The presenting symptom of iliacus hematoma is pain in the groin, spreading to the lumbar region or thigh, in response to which the patient assumes a characteristic posture of flexion and lateral rotation of the hip. A palpable mass in the iliac fossa and the signs of femoral nerve compression follow in a day or two. Infarction of the nerve may occur in the course of diabetes mellitus and polyarteritis nodosa. Not infrequently the nerve suffers acute damage of indeterminate cause. Biemond states this to be true of 60 percent of his cases; Calverley and Mulder found fewer occult cases, which is more in keeping with the authors' experience.

Sciatic Nerve

This nerve is derived from the fourth and fifth lumbar and first and second sacral roots. It supplies motor innervation to the hamstring muscles and all the muscles below the knee; it carries sensory impulses from the posterior aspect of the thigh, the posterior and lateral aspects of the leg, and the entire sole. In complete sciatic paralysis, the knee cannot be flexed and all muscles below the knee are paralyzed. Weakness of gluteal muscles and pain in the buttock and posterior thigh point to nerve involvement in the pelvis. Lesions beyond the sciatic notch spare the gluteal muscles but not the hamstrings.

The sciatic nerve is commonly injured by fractures of the pelvis or femur, gunshot wounds of the buttock and thigh, and the injection of toxic substances such as paraldehyde into the lower gluteal region. Tumors of the pelvis (sarcomas, lipomas) or gluteal region may compress the nerve. Sitting for a long period with legs flexed and abducted (lotus position) under the influence of narcotics or lying flat on a hard surface in coma may severely injure one or both sciatic nerves. The nerve may be involved by neurofibromas, infections, and ischemic necrosis in diabetes mellitus and polyarteritis nodosa. Cryptogenic forms also occur and are actually more frequent than those of identifiable cause. A ruptured lumbar disc often simulates sciatic neuropathy. Partial lesions of the sciatic nerve occasionally result in causalgia (see above).

Common Peroneal Nerve Just above the popliteal fossa the sciatic nerve divides into the *tibial nerve (medial, or internal, popliteal nerve)* and *the common peroneal nerve (lateral, or external, popliteal nerve).* The latter swings around the head of the fibula to the anterior aspect of the leg, giving off the musculocutaneous branch (to the peroneal muscles) and continuing as the *anterior tibial, or deep peroneal, nerve.* Branches of the latter supply the dorsiflexors of the foot and toes, and carry sensory fibers from the dorsum of the foot and lateral aspect of the lower half of the leg. Pressure or sleep palsy, or tight plaster casts, obstetrical stirrups, habitual and prolonged crossing of the legs while seated, and tight knee boots are the most frequent causes of injury to the common peroneal nerve, the compression being to that part of the nerve which passes over the head of the fibula. Emaciation greatly increases the incidence of these types of compressive injury. It may also be affected in diabetic neuropathy and injured by fractures of the upper end of the fibula.

Tibial Nerve This, the other of the two divisions of the sciatic nerve in the popliteal fossa, gives branches to all of the calf muscles, i.e., the plantar flexors of the foot and toes, after which it continues as the posterior tibial nerve. This nerve passes through the tarsal tunnel, an osseofibrous channel along the medial aspect of the calcaneus which is roofed by the flexor retinaculum. The canal also contains the tendons of the tibialis posterior, flexor digitorum longus,

and flexor hallucis longus muscles and the vessels to the foot. The posterior tibial nerve terminates under the flexor retinaculum by dividing into medial and lateral plantar nerves (supplying the small muscles of the foot).

Complete interruption of the tibial nerve results in a calcaneovalgus deformity of the foot, which can no longer be plantar-flexed and inverted. There is loss of sensation over the plantar aspect of the foot.

The posterior tibial nerve may be compressed in the tarsal tunnel (entrapment syndrome) by thickening of the tendon sheaths or the adjacent connective tissues or osteoarthritis. Tingling pain and burning over the sole of the foot develop after standing or walking for a long time. Usually there is no motor deficit. Relief is obtained by severing the flexor retinaculum.

ENTRAPMENT NEUROPATHIES

Reference has been made in several places in the preceding pages to entrapment neuropathies. A nerve, passing through a tight canal, is trapped and subjected to constant movement or pressure, forces not applicable to nerves elsewhere. The epineurium and perineurium become greatly thickened, strangling the nerve, with the additional possibility of demyelination. Function is gradually impaired, sensory more than motor, and the symptoms fluctuate with activity and rest. The two most frequently compressed nerves are the median and ulnar.

Listed in Table 46-2 are the more common entrapment neuropathies. A detailed account of these disorders is contained in the monograph of Dawson and his colleagues, listed in the references.

Table 46-2
Entrapment neuropathies

Nerve	Site of entrapment
Suprascapular	Spinoglenoid notch
Median	Carpal tunnel
Ulnar	
Elbow	Bicipital groove, cubital tunnel
Wrist	Palmar fascia-pisiform bone
Anterior interosseous (pronator syndrome)	Between heads of pronator muscle
Lateral femoral cutaneous (meralgia paresthetica)	Inguinal ligament
Obturator	Obturator canal
Posterior tibial	Tarsal tunnel, medial malleolus-flexor retinaculum
Plantar (Morton metatarsalgia)	Plantar fascia: heads of third and fourth metatarsals

REFERENCES

ADAMS D, FESTENSTEIN H, GIBSON JD et al: HLA antigens in chronic relapsing idiopathic inflammatory polyneuropathy. *J Neurol Neurosurg Psychiatry* 42:184, 1979.

ADAMS RD, RICHARDSON EP JR: The demyelinative diseases of the human nervous system: A classification; a review of salient neuropathological findings; comments on recent biochemical studies, in Folch-Pi J (ed): *Chemical Pathology of the Nervous System.* New York, Pergamon, 1961, pp 162–195.

ADAMS RD, SHAHANI BT, YOUNG RR: A severe pansensory familial neuropathy. *Trans Am Neurol Assoc* 98:67, 1973.

ANDRADE C, CANIJO M, KLEIN D, KAELIN A: The genetic aspect of the familial amyloidotic polyneuropathy. Portuguese type of peraamyloidosis. *Humangenetik* 7:163, 1969.

ARAKI S, MAWATARI S, OHTA M et al: Polyneurotic amyloidosis in a Japanese family. *Arch Neurol* 18:593, 1968.

ASBURY AK, ARNASON BGW, ADAMS RD: The inflammatory lesion in acute idiopathic polyneuritis. *Medicine* 48:173, 1969.

ASBURY AK, FIELDS HL: Pain due to peripheral nerve damage: An hypothesis. *Neurology* 34:1587, 1984.

ASBURY AK, GILLIAT RW (eds): *Peripheral Nerve Disorders.* London, Butterworth, 1984.

ASBURY AK, JOHNSON PC: *Pathology of Peripheral Nerve.* Philadelphia, Saunders, 1978.

ASBURY A, VICTOR M, ADAMS RD: Uremic polyneuropathy. *Arch Neurol* 8:113, 1963.

AUSTIN JH: Observations on the syndrome of hypertrophic neuritis (the hypertrophic interstitial radiculoneuropathies). *Medicine* 35:187, 1956.

BARNHILL RL, MCDOUGALL AC: Thalidomide: Use and possible mode of action in reactional lepromatous leprosy and in various other conditions. *J Am Acad Dermatol* 7:317, 1982.

BEHSE F, BUCHTHAL F, CARLSEN F, KNAPPEIS GG: Hereditary neuropathy with liability to pressure palsies. Electrophysiological and histopathological aspects. *Brain* 95:777, 1972.

BIEMOND A: Femoral neuropathy, in Vinken PJ, Bruyn GW (eds): *Handbook of Clinical Neurology,* vol 8. Amsterdam, North-Holland, 1970, chap 18, pp 303–310.

BOLTON CF: Peripheral neuropathies associated with chronic renal failure. *Can J Neurol Sci* 7(2):89, 1980.

BOULDIN TW, HALL CO, KRIGMAN MR: Pathology of disulfiram neuropathy. *Neuropathol Appl Neurobiol* 6:155, 1980.

BRADLEY WG, CHAD D, VERGBESE JP et al: Painful lumbosacral plexopathy, with elevated sedimentation rate: A treatable inflammatory syndrome. *Ann Neurol* 15:457, 1984.

BROSTOFF SW, LEVIT S, POWERS JM: Induction of experimental allergic neuritis with a peptide from myelin P_2 basic protein. *Nature* 268:752, 1977.

CALVERLEY JR, MULDER DW: Femoral neuropathy. *Neurology* 10:963, 1960.

CAVANAUGH NPC, EAMES RA, GALVIN RJ et al: Hereditary sensory neuropathy with spastic paraplegia. *Brain* 102:79, 1979.

COHEN AS, RUBINOW A: Amyloid neuropathy, in Dyck PJ, Thomas PK, Lambert EH, Bunge R (eds): *Peripheral Neuropathy,* 2nd ed. Philadelphia, Saunders, 1984, chap 81, pp 1866–1898.

CONN DL, DYCK PJ: Angiopathic neuropathy in connective tissue diseases, in Dyck PJ, Thomas PK, Lambert EH, Bunge R (eds):

Peripheral Neuropathy, 2nd ed. Philadelphia, Saunders, 1984, chap 88, pp 2027–2943.

CROFT PB, WILKINSON M: The incidence of carcinomatous neuromyopathy in patients with various types of carcinoma. *Brain* 88:427, 1965.

CROFT PB, HENSON RA, URICH H, WILKINSON PC: Sensory neuropathy with bronchial carcinoma: A study of four cases showing serological abnormalities. *Brain* 88:501, 1965.

CULEBRAS A, ALIO J, HERRERA J-L, LOPEZ-FRAILE IP: Effect of aldose reductase inhibitor on diabetic peripheral neuropathy. *Arch Neurol* 38:133, 1981.

DALAKAS MC, ENGEL WK: Chronic relapsing (dysimmune) polyneuropathy: Pathogenesis and treatment. *Ann Neurol* 9:134, 1981.

DALAKAS MC, ENGEL WK: Polyneuropathy with monoclonal gammopathy: Studies of 11 patients. *Ann Neurol* 10:45, 1981.

DAUBE JR, DYCK PJ: Neuropathy due to peripheral vascular diseases, in Dyck PJ et al (eds): *Peripheral Neuropathy,* 2nd ed. Philadelphia, Saunders, 1984, chap 63, pp 1458–1478.

DAWSON DM, HALLETT M, MILLENDER LH: *Entrapment Neuropathies.* Boston, Little Brown, 1983.

DELANK HW, KOCH G, KOHN G et al: Familiare amyloid Polyneuropathie typus Wohlwill-Corino Andrade. *Aerztl Forsch* 19:401, 1965.

DENNY-BROWN D: Hereditary sensory radicular neuropathy. *J Neurol Neurosurg Psychiatry* 14:237, 1951.

DONAGHY M, HAKIN RN, BAMFORD JM et al: Hereditary sensory neuropathy with neurotrophic keratitis. *Brain* 110:563, 1987.

DUCHEN LW: Neuropathology of the autonomic nervous system in diabetes, in Bannister R (ed): *Autonomic Failure,* Oxford, Oxford University Press, 1983, pp 437–452.

DUCHOWNY M, CAPLAN L, SIBER G: Cytomegalus virus infection of the adult nervous system. *Ann Neurol* 5:458, 1979.

DYCK PJ: Inherited neuronal degeneration and atrophy affecting peripheral motor, sensory and autonomic neurons, in Dyck PJ, Thomas PK, Lambert EH, Bunge R (eds): *Peripheral Neuropathy,* 2nd ed. Philadelphia, Saunders, 1984, pp 1600–1655.

DYCK PJ, ARNASON BGW: Chronic inflammatory demyelinating polyradiculoneuropathy, in Dyck PJ et al (eds): *Peripheral Neuropathy,* 2nd ed. Philadelphia, Saunders, 1984, chap 91, pp 2101–2114.

DYCK PJ, BENSTEAD TJ, CONN DL et al: Nonsystemic vasculitic neuropathy. *Brain* 110:843, 1987.

DYCK PJ, DAUBE J, O'BRIEN P et al: Plasma exchange in chronic inflammatory demyelinating polyneuropathy. *N Engl J Med* 314:461, 1986.

DYCK PJ, KARNES JL, O'BRIEN P et al: The spatial distribution of fiber loss in diabetic polyneuropathy suggests ischemia. *Ann Neurol* 19:440, 1986.

DYCK PJ, LAMBERT EH: Polyneuropathy associated with hypothyroidism. *J Neuropathol Exp Neurol* 29:631, 1970.

DYCK PJ, LAIS AC, OHTA M et al: Chronic inflammatory polyradiculoneuropathy. *Mayo Clin Proc* 50:621, 1975.

DYCK PJ, OHTA M: Neuronal atrophy and degeneration predominantly affecting peripheral sensory and autonomic neurons, in Dyck PJ, Thomas PK, Lambert EH, Bunge R (eds): *Peripheral Neuropathy*, 2nd ed. Philadelphia, Saunders, 1984, chap 68, pp 1557–1599.

DYCK PJ, OVIATT KF, LAMBERT EH: Intensive evaluation of referred unclassified neuropathies yields improved diagnosis. *Ann Neurol* 10:222, 1981.

EARL CJ, FULLERTON PM, WAKEFIELD GS, SCHUTTA HS: Hereditary neuropathy with liability to pressure palsies. *Q J Med* 33:481, 1964.

ECKER AD, WOLTMAN HW: Meralgia paresthetica: A report of one hundred and fifty cases. *JAMA* 110:1650, 1938.

EKBOM KA: Restless legs syndrome. *Neurology* 10:858, 1960.

ENGEL WK, DORMAN JD, LEVY RI, FREDRICKSON DS: Neuropathy in Tangier disease. *Arch Neurol* 17:1, 1967.

ENGLAND AC, DENNY-BROWN D: Severe sensory changes and trophic disorders in peroneal muscular atrophy (Charcot-Marie-Tooth type). *Arch Neurol Psychiatry* 67:1, 1952.

FALLS HF, JACKSON JH, CAREY JG et al: Ocular manifestations of hereditary primary systemic amyloidosis. *Arch Ophthalmol* 54:660, 1955.

FEASBY TE, GILBERT JJ, BROWN WF et al: An acute axonal form of Guillain-Barré polyneuropathy. *Brain* 109:1115, 1986.

FISHER CM: An unusual variant of acute idiopathic polyneuritis (syndrome of ophthalmoplegia, ataxia and areflexia). *N Engl J Med* 255:57, 1956.

FORRESTER C, LASCELLES RG: Association between polyneuritis and multiple sclerosis. *J Neurol Neurosurg Psychiatry* 42:864, 1979.

FRENCH COOPERATIVE GROUP: Efficiency of plasma exchange in Guillain-Barré syndrome. *Ann Neurol* 22:753, 1987.

FUNCK-BRENTANO JL, CUEILLE GF, MAN NK: A defense of the middle molecule hypothesis. *Kidney Int* 13(suppl 8):S31, 1978.

GOODFELLOW J, FEARN CB, MATTHEWS JM: Iliacus haematoma: A common complication of haemophilia. *J Bone Joint Surg* 49B:748, 1967.

GRUENER G, BOSCH P, STRAUSS R et al: Prediction of early beneficial response to plasma exchange in Guillain-Barré syndrome. *Arch Neurol* 44:295, 1987.

GUILLAIN-BARRÉ STUDY GROUP: Plasmapheresis and acute Guillain-Barré syndrome. *Neurology* 35:1096, 1985.

HARDING AE, THOMAS PK: Peroneal muscular atrophy with pyramidal features. *J Neurol Neurosurg Psychiatry* 47:168, 1984.

HART ZH, HOFFMAN W, WINBAUM E: Polyneuropathy, alopecia areata, and chronic lymphocytic thyroiditis. *Neurology* 29:106, 1979.

HAYMAKER W, WOODHALL B: *Peripheral Nerve Injuries*, 2nd ed. Philadelphia, Saunders, 1953.

HENSON RA, URICH H: *Cancer and the Nervous System*. Oxford, Blackwell, 1982, pp 368–405.

HUTCHINSON EC: Ischaemic neuropathy and peripheral vascular disease, in Vinken PJ, Bruyn GW (eds): *Handbook of Clinical Neurology*, vol 8. Amsterdam, North-Holland. 1970, chap 10, pp 149–153.

IKEDA S-I, HANYU N, HONGO M et al: Hereditary generalized amyloidosis with polyneuropathy. Clinicopathological study of 65 Japanese patients. *Brain* 110:315, 1987.

JOHNSON PC, DOLL SC, CROMEY DW: Pathogenesis of diabetic neuropathy. *Ann Neurol* 19:450, 1986.

KAHN P: Anderson-Fabry disease: A histopathological study of three cases with observations on the mechanism of production of pain. *J Neurol Neurosurg Psychiatry* 36:1053, 1973.

KANTARJIAN AD, DEJONG RN: Familial primary amyloidosis with nervous system envolvement. *Neurology* 3:399, 1953.

KELLY JJ, KYLE RA, O'BRIEN PC, DYCK PJ: The natural history of peripheral neuropathy in primary systemic amyloidosis. *Ann Neurol* 6:1, 1979.

KELLY JJ, KYLE RA, O'BRIEN PC, DYCK PJ: Prevalence of monoclonal protein in peripheral neuropathy. *Neurology* 31:1480, 1981.

KENNETT RP, HARDING AE: Peripheral neuropathy associated with the sicca syndrome. *J Neurol Neurosurg Psychiatry* 49:90, 1986.

KERNOHAN JW, WOLTMAN HW: Amyloid neuritis. *Arch Neurol Psychiatry* 47:132, 1942.

KIKTA DG, BREUER AC, WILBOURN AJ: Thoracic root pain in diabetes: The spectrum of clinical and electromyographic findings. *Ann Neurol* 11:80, 1982.

KORI SH, FOLEY KM, POSNER JB: Brachial plexus lesions in patients with cancer: 100 cases. *Neurology* 31:45, 1981.

LAPRESLE J, SALISACHS P: Roussy-Lévy syndrome, in Vinken PJ, Bruyn GW (eds): *Handbook of Clinical Neurology*, vol 21. Amsterdam, North-Holland, 1975, chap 9, pp 171–179.

LATOV N, GROSS RB, KASTELMAN J et al: Complement-fixing antiperipheral nerve myelin antibodies in patients with inflammatory polyneuritis and with polyneuropathy and paraproteinemias. *Neurology* 31:1530, 1981.

LAYZER RB: *Neuromuscular Manifestations of Systemic Disease*. Contemporary Neurology Series, vol 25. Philadelphia, Davis, 1984.

LEDERMAN RJ, WILBOURN AJ: Brachial plexopathy: Recurrent cancer or radiation? *Neurology* 34:1331, 1984.

LEWIS T, PICKERING GW: Circulatory changes in the fingers in some diseases of the nervous system with special reference to the digital atrophy of peripheral nerve lesions. *Clin Sci* 2:149, 1936.

LEWIS RA, SUMNER AJ, BROWN MJ, ASBURY AK: Multifocal demyelinating neuropathy with persistent conduction block. *Neurology* 32:958, 1982.

LHERMITTE F, FRITEL D, CAMBIER J et al: Polynévrites au cours de traitements par la nitrofurantoine. *Pressé Med* 71:767, 1963.

LOW PA, DYCK PJ, LAMBERT EH: Acute panautonomic neuropathy, *Ann Neurol* 13:412, 1983.

MADRID R, BRADLEY WG: The pathology of neuropathies with focal thickening of the myelin sheath (tomaculous neuropathy). *J Neurol Sci* 25:415, 1975.

MAGEE KR, DEJONG RN: Paralytic brachial neuritis. *JAMA* 174:1258, 1960.

McCOMBE PA, McLEOD JG, POLLARD JD et al: Peripheral sensorimotor and autonomic polyneuropathy associated with systemic lupus erythematosus. *Brain* 110:533, 1987.

McCOMBE PA, POLLARD JD, McLEOD JG: Chronic inflammatory demyelinating polyradiculoneuropathy. A clinical and electrophysiological study of 92 cases. *Brain* 111:1617, 1987.

McKHANN GM, GRIFFIN JW: Plasmapheresis and the Guillain-Barré syndrome. *Ann Neurol* 22:762, 1987.

McKHANN GM, GRIFFIN JW, CORNBLATH DR et al: Plasmapheresis and Guillain-Barré syndrome: Analysis of prognostic factors and the effect of plasmapheresis. *Ann Neurol* 23:347, 1988.

McLEOD JG, WALSH JC, POLLARD JD: Neuropathies associated with paraproteinemias and dysproteinemias, in Dyck PJ et al (eds): *Peripheral Neuropathy*. Philadelphia, Saunders, 1984, chap 80, pp 1847–1865.

MEDICAL RESEARCH COUNCIL: *Aids to the Examination of the Peripheral Nervous System*, Memorandum no 45 (superseding war memorandum no 7). London, HM Stationery Office, 1976.

MERETOJA J: Familial systemic paramyloidosis with lattice dystrophy of the cornea, progressive cranial neuropathy, skin changes and various internal symptoms: A previously unrecognized heritable syndrome. *Ann Clin Res* 1:314, 1969.

NATHAN PW: Painful legs and moving toes: Evidence on the site of the lesion. *J Neurol Neurosurg Psychiatry* 41:934, 1978.

OHNISHI A, DYCK PJ: Loss of small peripheral sensory neurons in Fabry disease. *Arch Neurol* 31:120, 1974.

ONGERBOER DE VISSER BW, FELTKAMP-VROOM TM, FELTKAMP CA: Sural nerve immune deposits in polyneuropathy as a remote effect of malignancy. *Ann Neurol* 14:261, 1983.

OSTERMAN PO, FAGIUS J, SAFWENBERG J et al: Early relapses after plasma exchange in acute inflammatory polyradiculoneuropathy. *Lancet* 2:1161, 1986.

PALLIS CA, SCOTT JT: Peripheral neuropathy in rheumatoid arthritis. *Br Med J* 1:1141, 1965.

PARSONAGE MJ, TURNER JWA: Neuralgic amyotrophy. The shoulder girdle syndrome. *Lancet* 1:973, 1948.

PHILLIPS LH: Familial long thoracic nerve palsy: A manifestation of brachial plexus neuropathy. *Neurology* 36:1251, 1986.

RAFF MC, SANGALANG V, ASBURY AK: Ischemic mononeuropathy multiplex associated with diabetes mellitus. *Arch Neurol* 18:487, 1968.

REFSUM S: Heredopathia atactica polyneuritiformis: Phytanic acid storage disease (Refsum's disease), in *Spinocerebellar Degenerations*, Japan Medical Research Foundation Publication no. 10. University of Tokyo Press, 1980, pp 313–338.

RIDLEY A: Porphyric neuropathy, in Dyck PJ, Thomas PK, Lambert EH, Bunge R (eds): *Peripheral Neuropathy*, 2nd ed. Philadelphia, Saunders, 1984, chap 72, pp 1704–1716.

ROBSON JS: Uraemic neuropathy, in Robertson RF (ed): *Some Aspects of Neurology*. Edinburgh, Royal College of Physicians, 1968, pp 74–84.

ROPPER AH: Severe acute Guillain-Barré syndrome. *Neurology* 36:429, 1986.

ROPPER AH, KEHNE SM: Guillain-Barré syndrome: Management of respiratory failure. *Neurology* 35:1662, 1985.

ROWLAND LP, DEFENDINI R, SHEMAN W et al: Macroglobulinemia with peripheral neuropathy simulating motor neuron diseases. *Ann Neurol* 11:532, 1982.

RUKAVINA JG, BLOCK WD, JACKSON CE et al: Primary systemic amyloidosis: A review and an experimental genetic and clinical study of 29 cases with particular emphasis on the familial form. *Medicine* 35:239, 1956.

SAID D, SLAMA G, SELVA J: Progressive centripetal degeneration of axons in small fiber type diabetic polyneuropathy: A clinical and pathological study. *Brain* 106:791, 1983.

SAID G: Perhexiline neuropathy: A clinicopathologic study. *Ann Neurol* 3:259, 1978.

SAMANTA A, BURDEN AC: Painful diabetic neuropathy. *Lancet* 1:348, 1985.

SARAIVA MJM, COSTA PP, GOODMAN DS: Genetic expression of a transthyretin mutation in typical and late-onset Portuguese families with familial amyloidotic polyneuropathy. *Neurology* 36:1413, 1986.

SCHAUMBURG HH, SPENCER PS, THOMS PK: *Disorders of Peripheral Nerves*. Philadelphia, Davis, 1983.

SCHAUMBURG HH, KAPLAN J, WINDEBANK A et al: Sensory neuropathy from pyridoxine abuse. *N Engl J Med* 309:445, 1983.

SCHOTT GD: Mechanisms of causalgia and related clinical conditions. *Brain* 109:717, 1986.

SHAH RR, OATES NS, IDLE JR et al: Impaired oxidation of debrisoquine in patients with perhexilene neuropathy. *Br Med J* 284:295, 1982.

SHAHANI BT, YOUNG RR, ADAMS RD: Neuropathic tremor: Evidence on the site of the lesion. *Electroencephalogr Clin Neurophysiol* 34:800, 1973.

SMITH IS, KAHN SN, LACEY BW et al: Chronic demyelinating neuropathy associated with benign IgM paraproteinemia. *Brain* 106:169, 1983.

SPENCER PS, SCHAUMBURG HH (eds): *Experimental and Clinical Neurotoxicology*. Baltimore, Williams & Wilkins, 1980.

STAUNTON H, DERVAN P, KALE R et al: Hereditary amyloid polyneuropathy in northwest Ireland. *Brain* 110:1231, 1987.

STEVENS JC: The electrodiagnosis of the carpal tunnel syndrome. *Muscle Nerve* 12:99, 1987.

SPILLANE JW, NATHAN PW, KELLY RE, MARSDEN CD: Painful legs and moving toes. *Brain* 94:541, 1971.

STOLL BA, ANDREWS JT: Radiation induced peripheral neuropathy. *Br Med J* 1:834, 1966.

SUN SF, STEIB EW: Diabetic thoracoabdominal neuropathy: Clinical and electrodiagnostic features. *Ann Neurol* 9:75, 1981.

SWANSON AG, BUCHAN GC, ALVORD EC JR: Anatomic changes in congenital insensitivity to pain: Absence of small primary sensory neurons in ganglia, roots and Lissauer's tract. *Arch Neurol* 12:12, 1965.

SYMONDS CP, SHAW ME: Familial clawfoot with absent tendon jerks: A "forme-fruste" of the Charcot-Marie-Tooth Disease. *Brain* 49:387, 1926.

TANG LM, HSI M, RYU S et al: Syndrome of polyneuropathy, skin hyperpigmentation, oedema, and hepatosplenomegaly. *J Neurol Neurosurg Psychiatry* 46:1108, 1983.

TAYLOR RA: Heredofamilial mononeuritis multiplex with brachial predilection. *Brain* 83:113, 1960.

THÉVENARD A: L'Acropathie ulcero-mutilante familiale. *Rev Neurol* 74:193, 1942.

THOMAS PK, ELIASSON SG: Diabetic neuropathy, in Dyck PJ, Thomas PK, Lambert EH, Bunge R (eds): *Peripheral Neuropathy*, 2nd ed. Philadelphia, Saunders, 1984, chap 76, pp 1773–1810.

THOMAS PK, LASCELLES RG: The pathology of diabetic neuropathy. *Q J Med* 35:489, 1966.

THOMAS PK, WALKER JG: Xanthomatous neuropathy in primary biliary cirrhosis. *Brain* 88:1079, 1965.

THOMAS PK, WALKER RWH, RUDGE P et al: Chronic demyelinating peripheral neuropathy associated with multifocal central nervous system demyelination. *Brain* 110:53, 1987.

TSAIRIS P, DYCK PJ, MULDER DW: Natural history of brachial plexus neuropathy: Report on 99 cases. *Arch Neurol* 27:109, 1972.

TUCK RR, MCLEOD JG: Retinitis pigmentosa, ataxia, and peripheral neuropathy. *J Neurol Neurosurg Psychiatry* 46:206, 1983.

VAN ALLEN MW, FROLICH JA, DAVIS JR: Inherited predisposition to generalized amyloidosis. *Neurology* 19:10, 1969.

VAN BUCHEM FSP, POL G, DE GIER J et al: Congenital β-lipoprotein deficiency. *Am J Med* 40:794, 1966.

VINKEN PJ, BRUYN GW (eds): *Handbook of Clinical Neurology,* vols 7 and 8: *Diseases of Nerves.* Amsterdam, North-Holland, 1970.

WAKSMAN BH, ADAMS RD: Allergic neuritis: An experimental disease of rabbits induced by the injection of peripheral nervous tissue and adjuvants. *J Exp Med* 102:213, 1955.

WALDENSTROM J: Studien über Porphyrie. *Acta Med Scand Suppl* 82: 1937.

WALDENSTROM J: The porphyrias as inborn errors of metabolism. *Am J Med* 22:758, 1957.

WARTENBERG R: *Neuritis, Sensory Neuritis, and Neuralgia.* New York, Oxford Press, 1959.

WATSON CJ, PIERACH CA, BOSSENMAIRET I et al: Use of hematin in the acute attack of the "inducible" hepatic porphyrias. *Adv Int Med* 23:265, 1978.

WEINSHILBOUM RM, AXELROD J: Reduced plasma dopamine-β-hydroxylase activity in familial dysautonomia. *N Engl J Med* 285:938, 1971.

WILLIAMS IR, MAYER RF: Subacute proximal diabetic neuropathy. *Neurology* 26:108, 1976.

WULFF CH, HANSEN K, STRANGE P, TROJABORG W: Multiple mononeuritis and radiculitis with erythema, pain, elevated CSF protein, and pleocytosis. Bannwarth's syndrome. *J Neurol Neurosurg Psychiatry* 46:485, 1983.

YOUNG RR, ASBURY AK, CORBETT JL et al: Pure panautonomia with recovery. *Brain* 98:613, 1975.

ZOCHODNE DW, BOLTON CF, WELLS GA: Critical illness polyneuropathy. A complication of sepsis and multiple organ failure. *Brain* 110:819, 1987.

CHAPTER 47

DISEASES OF THE CRANIAL NERVES

The cranial nerves are susceptible to many disorders that rarely if ever affect the spinal peripheral nerves; for this reason alone they deserve to be considered separately. Some of the cranial nerve disorders have already been discussed: viz., disorders of olfaction, in Chap. 11; of vision and extraocular muscles, in Chaps. 12 and 13; of cochlear and vestibular function, in Chap. 14; and craniofacial pain, referable to the trigeminal and glossopharyngeal nerves, in Chap. 9. There remain to be discussed the disorders of the seventh (facial) nerve and of the lower cranial nerves (IX to XII), as well as certain aspects of disordered trigeminal nerve function; these are considered below.

THE FIFTH, OR TRIGEMINAL, NERVE (See Fig. 47-1)

This is a mixed sensory and motor nerve. It conducts sensory impulses from the greater part of the face and head, from the mucous membranes of the nose and mouth, and from the cornea and conjunctiva. The cell bodies of the sensory part of the nerve lie in the gasserian, or semilunar, ganglion. The proximal axons of these cells form the sensory root. On entering the pons, they divide into short ascending and long descending branches. The former are concerned mainly with tactile and deep-pressure sense and terminate in the principal and mesencephalic nuclei, respectively. The long descending branches form the spinal trigeminal tract and mediate pain and temperature sensation (facial pain has been relieved after medullary trigeminal tractotomy). The spinal trigeminal tract, together with its nucleus, extends from the junction of the pons and medulla to the uppermost segments (C_2) of the spinal cord. From the nucleus, second-order fibers cross to the opposite side and ascend to the thalamus in the most medial part of the spinothalamic tract. This is called the *trigeminothalamic tract*.

The peripheral branches of the gasserian ganglion form the three sensory divisions of the nerve. The first (ophthalmic) division passes through the superior orbital fissure; the second (maxillary) division leaves the middle fossa through the foramen rotundum; and the third (mandibular), through the foramen ovale.

The motor portion of the fifth nerve, which supplies the masseter and pterygoid muscles, has its origin in the midpons; the fibers pass underneath the gasserian ganglion and become incorporated into the mandibular nerve. The masseter and pterygoid muscles are implicated in a number of brainstem reflexes, the best known of which is the jaw jerk. Tapping the chin with the jaw muscles relaxed stimulates proprioceptive afferents, which terminate in the mesencephalic nucleus of the midbrain. This nucleus sends collaterals to the motor trigeminal nucleus. The jaw jerk is enhanced in pseudobulbar palsy.

Because of their wide anatomic distribution, complete interruption of both the motor and sensory fibers of the trigeminal nerve is rarely observed. On the other hand, partial affection of the trigeminal nerve, particularly of the sensory part, is common. The various cranial nerve and brainstem syndromes in which the fifth nerve is involved are listed in Tables 47-1 and 47-2.

A variety of diseases may affect the peripheral branches of the trigeminal nerves, the gasserian (semilunar) ganglion, and the roots (sensory and motor). These have been ably described by Selby. The most frequent disorder, and the most elusive from the standpoint of its pathologic basis, is trigeminal neuralgia (in French, *tic douloureux*). Known since ancient times, it affects the elderly at a frequency of 155 cases per million with a female to male ratio of 3:2. The mean age of onset is 52 to 58 years for the idiopathic form and 30 to 35 years for the symptomatic form, the latter being caused by trauma or vascular, neoplastic, and demyelinative diseases. The nature of the pain, its unilaterality and tendency to involve the second and third divisions of the trigeminal nerve, an intensity that makes the patient grimace or wince (tic), the presence of an initiating or trigger point, the lack of sensory or motor deficit, and its response in approximately half or two-thirds of the cases to carbamazepine, phenytoin, baclofen, and clonazepam, have been presented on page 150. The surgical therapy in those not controlled by drugs was also discussed on page 150.

In rare instances trigeminal neuralgia is preceded or accompanied by hemifacial spasm, a combination that Cushing called *tic convulsif*. This usually is indicative of a tumor (cholesteatoma), an aneurysmal dilatation of the basilar artery, or an arteriovenous malformation that compresses the trigeminal and facial nerves. Trigeminal neuralgia and glossopharyngeal neuralgia (pain in the tonsillar region) may also be combined. Diagnosis of the idiopathic form and its differentiation from the symptomatic forms of facial neuralgia as well as from the atypical facial pain of younger women, cluster headache, dental neuralgia, and temporomandibular dysfunction, is not difficult, especially if there is a trigger point and no demonstrable signs of sensory or motor impairment.

Of the conditions that damage the branches of the trigeminal nerve, cranial injuries and skull fractures are the

Figure 47-1

Scheme of the trigeminal nuclei and some of the trigeminal reflex arcs. I, ophthalmic division; II, maxillary division; III, mandibular division. (From MB Carpenter and J Sutin, Human Neuroanatomy, 8th ed. Baltimore, Williams & Wilkins, 1982.)

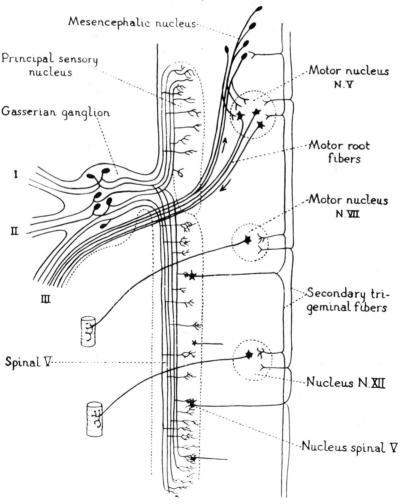

most common. The most superficial branches—the supra-trochlear, supraorbital, and infraorbital—are the ones usually involved. The sensory loss is present from the time of the injury, and partial regeneration may be attended by constant pain, often demanding nerve block and sectioning. Sinus tumors and metastatic disease may implicate the trigeminal nerve, causing pain and a gradually progressive sensory loss. The ophthalmic division of the fifth nerve may be implicated in the wall of the cavernous sinus in combination with the third, fourth, and sixth nerves. Stilbamidine and trichlorethylene are known to cause sensory loss, tingling, burning, and itching exclusively in the trigeminal sensory territory.

Of the various inflammatory diseases that affect the trigeminal nerves or ganglia, herpes zoster ranks first (see page 596). Herpes simplex virus has been isolated from the ganglion in as many as 50 percent of routine autopsies but, only with rare exceptions, is associated with skin lesions alone. Middle ear infections and petrositis may spread to the ganglion and root, also implicating the sixth cranial nerve (Gradenigo syndrome). Selby recounts cases of trigeminal neuropathy with systemic sclerosis, lupus erythematosus, and Sjögren syndrome. In the latter there is a sensory loss over the face as well as the usual keratocon-junctivitis and xerostomia (the sicca syndrome), parotitis, and some one of the connective tissue diseases.

The trigeminal root may be compressed or invaded by intracranial meningiomas, acoustic neuromas, trigeminal neuromas, cholesteatomas, and chordomas. Tumors in the sphenoid bone (myeloma, metastatic carcinoma) may compress branches of the trigeminal nerve at their foramens of exit. We have several times observed numbness of the chin and lower lip as the first sign of the primary disease. Massey et al have reported 19 such cases seen in their clinic.

Finally every neurologist from time to time encounters cases of idiopathic trigeminal neuropathy in which there is a purely sensory impairment in the territory of the trigeminal nerve on one or both sides of the face, sometimes associated with pain and paresthesias and disturbances of taste. Of 22 such cases described by Lecky and his colleagues, 9 had either systemic sclerosis (scleroderma) or mixed connective tissue disease, and a similar number had either organ or nonorgan specific serum autoantibodies. The condition may remain troublesome for years. Pathologic data are limited

Table 47-1
Cranial nerve syndromes

Site	Cranial nerves involved	Eponymic syndrome	Usual cause
Sphenoidal fissure	III, IV, ophthalmic, V, VI	Foix	Invasive tumors of sphenoid bone, aneurysms
Lateral wall of cavernous sinus	III, IV, ophthalmic (occasionally maxillary) V, VI	Tolosa-Hunt Foix	Aneurysms or thrombosis of cavernous sinus, invasive tumors from sinuses and sella turcica; sometimes recurrent, benign granulomatous reactions, responsive to steroids
Retrosphenoidal space	II, III, IV, V, VI	Jacod	Large tumors of middle cranial fossa
Apex of petrous bone	V, VI	Gradenigo	Petrositis, tumors of petrous bone
Internal auditory meatus	VII, VIII		Tumors of petrous bone (dermoids, etc.), acoustic neuroma
Pontocerebellar angle	V, VII, VIII, and sometimes IX		Acoustic neuromas, meningiomas
Jugular foramen	IX, X, XI	Vernet	Tumors and aneurysms
Posterior laterocondylar space	IX, X, XI, XII	Collet-Sicard	Tumors of parotid gland, carotid body, secondary and lymph node tumors, tuberculous adenitis
Posterior retroparotid space	IX, X, XI, XII, and Bernard-Horner syndrome	Villaret MacKenzie	Same as above, and granulomatous lesions (sarcoid, fungi)
Posterior retroparotid space	X and XII, with or without XI	Tapia	Parotid and other tumors of, or injuries to, the high neck

Table 47-2
Brainstem syndromes which involve cranial nerves

Eponym	Site	Cranial nerves involved	Tracts and nuclei involved	Signs	Usual cause
Weber syndrome	Base of midbrain	III	Corticospinal tract	Oculomotor palsy with crossed hemiplegia	Vascular occlusion; tumor; aneurysm
Claude syndrome	Tegmentum of midbrain	III	Red nucleus and brachium conjunctivum	Oculomotor palsy with contralateral cerebellar ataxia and tremor	Vascular occlusion; tumor; aneurysm
Benedikt syndrome	Tegmentum of midbrain	III	Red nucleus, corticospinal tract, and brachium conjunctivum	Oculomotor palsy with contralateral cerebellar ataxia, tremor and corticospinal signs	Softening; hemorrhage; tuberculoma; tumor
Nothnagel syndrome	Tectum of midbrain	Unilateral or bilateral III	Superior cerebellar peduncles	Ocular palsies, paralysis of gaze, and celebellar ataxia	Tumor
Parinaud syndrome	Dorsal midbrain		Supranuclear mechanism for upward gaze and other structures in periaqueductal gray matter	Paralysis of upward gaze and accommodation; fixed pupils.	Pinealoma, hydrocephalus and other lesions of dorsal midbrain
Millard-Gubler syndrome and Raymond-Foville syndrome	Base of pons	VII and often VI	Corticospinal tract	Facial and abducens palsy and contralateral hemiplegia; sometimes gaze palsy to side of lesion	Softening or tumor
Avellis syndrome	Tegmentum of medulla	X	Spinothalamic tract; sometimes descending pupillary fibers, with Bernard-Horner syndrome	Paralysis of soft palate and vocal cord and contralateral hemianesthesia	Softening or tumor
Jackson syndrome	Tegmentum of medulla	X, XII	Corticospinal tract	Avellis syndrome plus ipsilateral tongue paralysis	Softening or tumor
Wallenberg syndrome	Lateral tegmentum of medulla	Spinal V, IX, X, XI	Lateral spinothalamic tract Descending pupillodilator fibers Spinocerebellar and olivocerebellar tracts	Ipsilateral V, IX, X, XI palsy, Horner syndrome and cerebellar ataxia; contralateral loss of pain and temperature sense	Occlusion of vertebral or posterior-inferior cerebellar artery

but point to a lesion of the trigeminal ganglion or sensory root.

A less common form of idiopathic trigeminal sensory neuropathy has a more acute onset and a tendency to resolve completely or partially, in much the same manner as Bell's palsy (Blau et al).

A pure unilateral trigeminal motor neuropathy is a clinical rarity. Chia has described five patients in whom an aching pain in the cheek and unilateral weakness of mastication were the main features. EMG showed denervation changes in the ipsilateral masseter and temporalis muscles. The outcome was apparently benign.

THE SEVENTH, OR FACIAL, NERVE

The seventh cranial nerve is mainly a motor nerve supplying all the muscles concerned with facial expression on one side. The sensory component is small (the nervus intermedius of Wrisberg); it conveys taste sensation from the anterior two-thirds of the tongue and probably cutaneous sensation from the anterior wall of the external auditory canal. The taste fibers at first traverse the lingual nerve (a branch of the mandibular), and then join the chorda tympani. Secretomotor fibers innervate the lacrimal gland through the greater superficial petrosal nerve, and the sublingual and submaxillary glands through the chorda tympani (Fig. 47-2).

Several other anatomic facts are worth remembering. The motor nucleus of the seventh nerve lies anterior and lateral to the abducens nucleus, and the intrapontine fibers of the facial nerve hook around the abducens nucleus before emerging from the pons, just lateral to the corticospinal tract. The facial nerve enters the internal auditory meatus with the acoustic nerve and then bends sharply forward and downward around the anterior boundary of the vestibule of the inner ear. At this angle (*genu*) lies the sensory ganglion (named *geniculate* because of its proximity to the genu). The nerve continues its course in its own bony channel, the facial canal, and makes its exit from the skull at the stylomastoid foramen. It then passes through the parotid gland and subdivides into five branches to supply the facial muscles, the stylomastoid muscle, and the posterior belly of the digastric muscle. Within the facial canal, just distal to the geniculate ganglion, it gives off the branch to the pterygopalatine ganglion, i.e., the greater superficial petrosal nerve; somewhat more distally, it gives off a small branch to the stapedius and is joined by the chorda tympani.

A complete interruption of the facial nerve at the stylomastoid foramen paralyzes all muscles of facial expression. The corner of the mouth droops, the creases and skin folds are effaced, the forehead is unfurrowed, the palpebral fissure is widened, and the eyelids will not close. Upon attempted closure of the lids, the eye on the paralyzed side is seen to roll upward (Bell phenomenon). The lower lid sags also, and the punctum falls away from the conjunctiva, permitting tears to spill over the cheek. Food collects between the teeth and lips and saliva may dribble from the corner of the mouth. The patient complains of a heaviness or numbness in the face, but sensory loss can usually not be demonstrated. Taste is intact.

If the lesion is in the facial canal above the junction with the chorda tympani but below the geniculate ganglion, all the above symptoms occur; in addition, taste is lost over the anterior two-thirds of the tongue on the same side. If the nerve to the stapedius muscle is involved, there is hyperacusis (painful sensitivity to loud sounds), and the sound produced by moving the jaw and facial muscles is no longer present in the ear on the affected side. If the geniculate ganglion or the motor root proximal to it is involved, lacrimation may be reduced. Lesions at this point may also affect the adjacent eighth nerve, causing deafness, tinnitus, or dizziness. Intrapontine lesions that paralyze the face often affect the abducens nucleus and the corticospinal and sensory tracts.

If the peripheral facial paralysis has existed for some time and return of motor function has begun but is incomplete, a kind of contracture (in reality a continuous diffuse muscle contraction) may appear. The palpebral fissure becomes narrowed and the nasolabial fold deepens. Attempts to move one group of facial muscles result in contraction of all of them (associated movements, or synkinesis). Spasms of facial muscles develop and persist indefinitely, being initiated by every facial movement. This condition, called *hemifacial spasm*, occurs not infrequently in adults who have never had a facial palsy. Anomalous regeneration of the seventh nerve fibers may result in other curious disorders. If fibers originally connected with the orbicularis oculi become connected with the orbicularis oris, closure of the lids may cause a retraction of the corner of the mouth; or if visceromotor fibers originally innervating the salivary glands later come to innervate the lacrimal gland, anomalous tearing (crocodile tears) may occur whenever the patient salivates. With the passage of time, the corner of the mouth and even the tip of the nose become pulled to the unaffected side.

BELL'S PALSY (IDIOPATHIC FACIAL PARALYSIS)

The most common disease of the facial nerve is *Bell's palsy* (incidence rate of 23 per 100,000 annually, according to Hauser et al). This disorder, the cause of which is unknown, affects men and women more or less equally and occurs at all ages and at all times of the year. The incidence is not disproportionately high in pregnant women, contrary to popular belief, but is probably higher in diabetics than in the normal population. As one might expect, the opportunity of examining the facial nerve in the course of Bell's palsy happens very rarely. Only about a dozen such cases are on record, all showing varying degrees of degeneration of nerve fibers. Two cases were said to show inflammatory changes, but these were probably misinterpreted (see Karnes). A viral causation is suspected but unproved. There are no antibodies to the varicella-zoster or herpes simplex viruses.

The onset is acute; about one-half of the cases attain maximum paralysis in 48 h and practically all cases within 5 days. Pain behind the ear may precede the paralysis by a day or two. In a small proportion of patients a hypesthesia in one or more branches of the trigeminal nerve can be demonstrated. The explanation of this finding is not clear. Impairment of taste is present to some degree in almost all patients, but rarely persists beyond the second week of paralysis. It means that the lesion has extended to or above the point where the chorda tympani fibers join the facial nerve. Hyperacusis or distortion of sound in the ipsilateral ear indicates paralysis of the stapedius muscle. In some cases there is mild increase of lymphocytes and mononuclear cells in the CSF.

Fully 80 percent of patients recover within a few weeks or in a month or two. Recovery of taste precedes

Figure 47-2

Scheme of the seventh cranial (facial) nerve. The motor fibers are represented by the heavy black line. Parasympathetic fibers are represented by regular dashes; special visceral afferent (taste) fibers are represented by long dashes and dots. A, B, and C denote lesions of the facial nerve at the stylomastoid foramen, distal to the geniculate ganglion, and proximal to the geniculate ganglion. Disturbances resulting from lesions at each of these sites are described in the text. (From MB Carpenter and J Sutin, Human Neuroanatomy, 8th ed. Baltimore, Williams & Wilkins, 1982.)

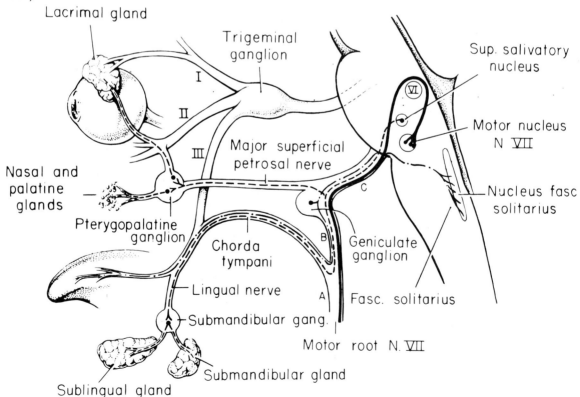

recovery of motor function, and if the former occurs in the first week, it is a good prognostic sign. Incomplete paralysis in the first 5 to 7 days is the most favorable prognostic sign. Electromyography may be of value in distinguishing temporary conduction defects from a pathologic interruption of nerve fibers; evidence of denervation after 10 days indicates a long delay in the onset of recovery (3 months, on the average). Recovery then proceeds by regeneration of nerve, a process that may take 2 years or longer and is often incomplete.

Protection of the eye during sleep, massage of the weakened muscles, and a splint to prevent drooping of the lower part of the face are the measures generally employed in the management of such cases. There is no evidence that surgical decompression of the facial nerve is effective, and it may be harmful. The administration of prednisone (40 to 60 mg/day) during the first week to 10 days after onset may be beneficial; it is thought to decrease the possibility of permanent paralysis from swelling of the nerve in the tight facial canal.

OTHER CAUSES OF FACIAL PALSY

Tumors that invade the temporal bone (carotid body, cholesteatoma, and dermoid) may produce a facial palsy; the onset is insidious and the course progressive. Fracture of the temporal bone (usually with damage to the middle or internal ear), otitis media, and middle ear surgery are relatively uncommon causes of facial palsy. The Ramsay Hunt syndrome, due presumably to herpes zoster of the geniculate ganglion, consists of severe facial palsy associated with a vesicular eruption in the external auditory canal, other parts of the cranial integument, and mucous membrane of the oropharynx. Often the eighth cranial nerve is affected as well (see Chap. 33). Acoustic neuromas, glomus jugulare tumors, and aneurysmal dilatations of the basilar artery may involve the facial nerve. Vascular lesions or tumors are the common forms of pontine disease that may cause facial palsy. Bilateral facial paralysis (facial diplegia) occurs in acute idiopathic polyneuritis and in a variety of sarcoidosis known as *uveoparotid fever (Heerfordt syndrome)*. *Melk-ersson-Rosenthal syndrome* comprises a triad of recurrent facial paralysis, facial (particularly labial) edema, and less constantly, plication of the tongue. The syndrome begins in childhood or adolescence and is quite rare; the cause is unknown. The facial nerve is frequently involved in leprosy.

Some of the muscles controlled by the facial nerve may be deranged in supranuclear disorders and in abnor-malities of brainstem reflexes. In a condition called "apraxia of the eyelids" the patients cannot close the eyes voluntarily but they will close reflexly. For example, stimulation of the supraorbital branch of the trigeminal nerve by a tap on the brow, which normally induces bilateral closure of the

eyes, or stimulation of the long ciliary branches of the trigeminal nerve by touching the cornea will still cause closure of the eyes. These are trigeminofacial reflexes. Actually the blink reflex is expressed by two responses, an early and a late one. The late response, which disappears in the Parkinson patient and is enhanced in pseudobulbar palsy, utilizes large fiber bundles in the supraorbital nerves and the corneal reflex, the small fiber bundles in the long ciliary nerves. Derangement of one of these reflexes or the jaw reflex may be found in 25 percent of multiple sclerotic patients. In pseudobulbar palsy, tapping the lips (orbicularis oris) elicits a buccal (trigeminofacial) reflex, and it may spread to cause closure of the eyes.

All forms of nuclear or peripheral facial palsy must be distinguished from the supranuclear type. In the latter the frontalis and orbicularis oculi muscles are involved less than those of the lower part of the face or not at all, since the upper facial muscles receive upper motor neuron in-nervation from both hemispheres, and the lower facial muscles, from the opposite hemisphere predominantly. In supranuclear lesions there may be a dissociation of emotional and voluntary facial movements, and often some degree of paralysis of the arm and leg or an aphasia (in dominant hemisphere lesions) is conjoined.

An obscure disorder is the *facial hemiatrophy of Romberg*. It occurs mainly in females and is characterized by a disappearance of fat in the dermal and subcutaneous tissues on one or both sides of the face. It usually begins in adolescence or early adult years and is slowly progressive. In its advanced form the affected side of the face is gaunt and the skin is thin, wrinkled, and rather dark; the hair may turn white and fall out, and the sebaceous glands become atrophic; the muscles and bones are not involved as a rule. The condition is a form of *lipodystrophy*, and the localization within a dermatome indicates the operation of some neural factor of unknown nature. Plastic surgery is the treatment of choice.

The facial muscles on one side may be involved in irregular clonic contractions of varying degree (*hemifacial spasm*). This condition develops in the fifth and sixth decades, affects women more than men, and is usually without known antecedent cause. It may prove to be due to an irritative lesion of the facial nerve [e.g., an aberrant artery, basilar artery aneurysm, or a tumor (acoustic neu-roma) pressing on the nerve], or it may represent a transient or permanent sequela of a Bell's palsy, as stated above. In the idiopathic variety the spasm usually begins in the orbicularis oculi muscle and gradually spreads to other muscles on that side of the face, including the platysma.

The spasm may be induced by all voluntary and other movements of the face.

Currently there is a controversy concerning its pathogenesis. Janetta attributes all ''idiopathic'' cases to a compression of the root of the facial nerve by an aberrant blood vessel. Microsurgical decompression of the root with the interposition of a nonabsorbable sponge between the vessel and the root has successfully relieved the facial spasm ''in most cases.'' Kaye and Adams, who performed posterior fossa surgery in 16 patients, could find a definite vascular abnormality in only 4 of them. However, wrapping of sponge around the nerve yielded a good or excellent result in 14 of the 16 patients, raising the possibility that operative manipulation of the nerve or circumferential fibrosis due to the sponge is responsible for the improvement. More recently, Auger and his colleagues reported that of 54 patients who underwent microvascular decompression, 70 percent obtained lasting benefit.

The pathophysiology of the spasm is believed to be nerve root compression and segmental demyelination, the latter permitting artificial synapses to form. A volley of impulses conducted centrifugally in one motor fiber results in the activation of neighboring fibers (ephaptic excitation). Also, the injured fibers are thought to be capable of ectopic excitation. Nielsen and Jannetta, who offer the same explanation for trigeminal neuralgia, have shown that ephaptic transmission disappears after the nerve is decompressed.

Many patients refuse surgical treatment, preferring to tolerate the abnormal movements. Alexander and Moses note that carbamazepine (Tegretol) in dosage of 600 to 1200 mg/day controls the spasm in two-thirds of the patients, but some patients cannot tolerate this high a dosage. Injections of botulinum A toxin into the orbicularis oculi relieves the major symptom—the spasms around the eye— for 3 to 5 months and can be repeated without danger. Two surgical procedures are in use: one in which the muscles most affected are denervated by crushing one or more of the branches of the facial nerve in the face itself; the other, mentioned above, involves a posterior fossa exploration with separation of the nerve from a compressing vessel and interposition of Gelfoam or muscle. The latter carries a higher risk and should be practiced only by neurosurgeons skilled in the procedure. One of the complications has been deafness due to injury of the adjacent eighth nerve. Also there is a significant risk of recurrence of the spasms within 2 years of the operation (Piatt and Wilkins).

Facial myokymia is a fine fibrillary activity of all the muscles of one side of the face which has usually developed in the course of multiple sclerosis or a brainstem glioma. It has also been seen in the Guillain-Barré-polyneuritis (Wasserstrom and Starr). The fibrillary nature of the involuntary movements and their arhythmicity distinguish them from the coarser intermittent facial spasms and contracture, tics, tardive dyskinesia, and clonus. The EMG pattern is one of spontaneous discharge of motor units, appearing singly or in doublets or triplets at a rate varying from 30 to 70 cycles per second. Irritation of the facial nucleus, demyelination of the intrapontine part of the facial nerve, and supranuclear disinhibition of the nucleus have been the postulated mechanisms. But the observation of facial myokymia in polyneuritis informs us that a lesion (? demyelinative) may occur at any point along the nerve.

A clonic or tonic contraction of one side of the face may be the sole manifestation of a cerebral cortical seizure. An involuntary recurrent spasm of both eyelids (*blepharospasm*) occurs in elderly persons as an isolated phenomenon, and there may be varying degrees of spasm of the other facial muscles (see also page 88). Relaxant and tranquilizing drugs are of little help in this disorder, but injections of botulinum toxin into the orbicularis oculi muscles give temporary or lasting relief. In many cases, blepharospasm subsides spontaneously. Rhythmic unilateral myoclonia, akin to palatal myoclonia, may be restricted to facial, lingual, or laryngeal muscles.

Hypersensitivity of the facial nerve occurs in tetany (Chvostek test of spasm of facial muscles on tapping in front of the ear).

THE NINTH, OR GLOSSOPHARYNGEAL, NERVE

This nerve arises from the lateral surface of the medulla by a series of small roots that lie just rostral to those of the vagus nerve. The glossopharyngeal, vagus, and accessory nerves leave the skull together through the jugular foramen and are then distributed peripherally. The ninth nerve has a sensory component with cell bodies in the inferior (petrosal) ganglion (the central processes of which end in the nucleus solitarius) and the small superior ganglion (the central fibers of which enter the spinal trigeminal tract and nucleus). It also receives the nerve of Hering from the carotid body. The somatic efferent fibers of the ninth nerve are derived from the nucleus ambiguus, and the visceral efferent (secretory) fibers, from the inferior salivatory nucleus. These fibers contribute to the motor innervation of the striated musculature of the pharynx (mainly of the stylopharyngeus, which elevates the pharynx) and the glands in the pharyngeal mucosa.

The sensory functions of the ninth nerve are not entirely clear. It is commonly stated that this nerve mediates sensory impulses from the faucial tonsils, posterior wall of the pharynx, and part of the soft palate, and taste sensation from the posterior third of the tongue. However, an isolated lesion of the ninth cranial nerve is a rarity, and the effects are not fully known. In one personally observed case of bilateral surgical interruption of the ninth nerves, verified at autopsy, there had been no demonstrable loss of taste or other sensory or motor impairment. This suggests that the tenth nerve may be responsible for these functions, at least in some individuals. There is some evidence that the ninth nerve, through its innervation of the carotid sinus, plays a part in the reflex control of circulation.

One may occasionally observe a glossopharyngeal palsy in conjunction with vagus and accessory nerve involvement due to a tumor in the posterior fossa or an aneurysm of the vertebral artery. The nerves are compressed as they pass through the jugular foramen. Hoarseness due to vocal cord paralysis, some difficulty in swallowing, deviation of the soft palate to the sound side, anesthesia of the posterior wall of the pharynx, and weakness of the upper trapezius and sternomastoid muscles comprise the clinical picture (see Table 47-1, jugular foramen syndrome).

Glossopharyngeal neuralgia is a syndrome that resembles trigeminal neuralgia in many respects. It is described on pages 295 and 1078. Rarely, herpes zoster may involve the glossopharyngeal nerve. Carotid sinus sensitivity with syncope was described on page 295.

THE TENTH, OR VAGUS, NERVE

This nerve has an extensive sensory and motor distribution. It has two ganglia: the *jugular*, which contains the cell bodies of the somatic sensory nerves (which innervate the skin in the concha of the ear); and the *nodose*, which contains the cell bodies of the afferent fibers from the pharynx, larynx, trachea, esophagus, and the thoracic and abdominal viscera. The central processes of these ganglia terminate in relation to the nucleus of the spinal trigeminal tract and the tractus solitarius, respectively. The motor fibers of the vagus are derived from two nuclei in the medulla, the nucleus ambiguus and the dorsal motor nucleus. The former supplies somatic motor fibers to the striated muscles of the larynx, pharynx, and palate; the latter supplies visceral motor fibers to the heart and other thoracic and abdominal organs. The distribution of vagal fibers is illustrated in Fig. 47-3.

Complete interruption of the intracranial portion of one vagus nerve results in a characteristic paralysis. The soft palate droops on the ipsilateral side and does not rise in phonation. Deviation of the uvula to the normal side on phonation is an inconstant sign. There is loss of the gag reflex on the affected side and of the *curtain movement* of

the lateral wall of the pharynx, whereby the faucial pillars move medially as the palate rises in saying "ah." The voice is hoarse, often nasal, and the vocal cord lies immobile in a "cadaveric" position, i.e., midway between abduction and adduction. With partial lesions, movements of abduction are affected more than those of adduction (Semon's law). There may also be a loss of sensation at the external auditory meatus and back of the pinna. Usually no change in visceral function can be demonstrated.

Complete bilateral paralysis is said to be incompatible with life, and this is probably true if the nuclei are completely destroyed in the medulla by poliomyelitis or some other disease. However, in the cervical region both vagi have been blocked with procaine (Novocain) for the treatment of intractable asthma, without mishap. Moreover, Johnson and Stern report a case of bilateral vocal cord paralysis in association with familial hypertrophic polyneuropathy, and Plott relates the history of three brothers with congenital laryngeal abductor paralysis with bilateral dysgenesis of the nucleus ambiguus. Bannister and Oppenheimer have called attention to defects of phonation and laryngeal stridor as a feature of orthostatic hypotension and multiple system atrophy. The posterior cricoarytenoid and interarytenoid muscles are denervated. The pharyngeal branches of both vagi may be affected, as in diphtheria; the voice has a nasal quality, and regurgitation of liquids through the nose occurs during the act of swallowing.

The vagus nerve may be implicated at the meningeal level by tumors and infectious processes and within the medulla by vascular lesions, e.g., the lateral medullary syndrome of Wallenberg, by motor system disease and occasionally by tumors. Dysphagia is then invariably present. Herpes zoster may attack this nerve. Polymyositis and dermatomyositis, which cause hoarseness and dysphagia owing to direct involvement of laryngeal and pharyngeal muscles, may be confused with disease of the vagus nerves.

Of importance is the fact that the left recurrent laryngeal nerve may be damaged as a result of thoracic disease. There is no dysphagia with lesions at this level, since the branches to the pharynx have already separated from the nerve. Aneurysm of the aortic arch, an enlarged left atrium, and a mediastinal or superior sulcus lung tumor are much more frequent causes of an isolated vocal cord palsy than are intracranial diseases.

Laryngeal neuralgia is a rare entity, in which paroxysms of pain are localized over the upper portion of the thyroid cartilage or hyoid bone on one or both sides. It is evoked by coughing, yawning, talking, or sneezing. In the case of Brownstone et al it was relieved by carbamazepine.

When confronted with a case of vocal cord palsy, the physician must attempt to determine the site of the lesion. If it is intramedullary, there are usually ipsilateral cerebellar signs, loss of pain and temperature sensation over the ipsilateral face and contralateral arm and leg, and an ipsilateral Bernard-Horner syndrome. If the lesion is extramedullary but intracranial, the glossopharyngeal and spinal accessory are frequently involved (jugular foramen syndrome, Table 47-1). If it is extracranial in the posterior laterocondylar or retroparotid space, there may be a combination of ninth, tenth, eleventh, and twelfth cranial nerve palsies and a Bernard-Horner syndrome. Combinations of

Figure 47-3

Anatomical features of the vagus nerve. Note the relationship to the spinal-accessory and glossopharyngeal nerves at the jugular foramen and the long course of the left recurrent laryngeal nerve.

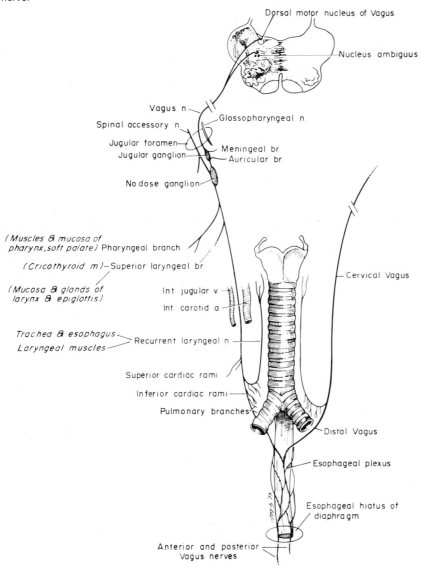

these lower cranial nerve palsies, which have a variety of eponymic designations (see Table 47-1), are caused by tumors of various types or chronic inflammations of lymph nodes. If there is no sensory loss of the palate and pharynx and no palatal weakness, the lesion is below the origin of the pharyngeal branches, which leave the vagus nerve high in the cervical region. The usual site of disease is then the mediastinum.

THE ELEVENTH, OR ACCESSORY, NERVE

This is a purely motor nerve. Its fibers arise from the anterior horn cells of the upper four or five cervical cord segments and enter the skull through the foramen magnum. Intracranially, the accessory nerve travels for a short distance with the part of the tenth nerve that is derived from the most caudal cells of the nucleus ambiguus (together, the two roots are referred to as the *vagal-accessory nerve* or the *cranial root of the accessory nerve*). The two roots leave the skull through the jugular foramen. The aberrant vagus fibers then rejoin the main trunk of the vagus, and the fibers derived from the cervical segments of the spinal cord form the external ramus and innervate the sternoclei-domastoid and trapezius muscles. Only the latter fibers constitute the accessory nerve in the strict sense. In patients with torticollis, however, division of the upper cervical motor roots or the spinal accessory nerve has often failed to ablate completely the contraction of the sternomastoid muscle. This suggests a wider innervation of the muscle, perhaps by fibers of apparent vagal origin that join the accessory nerve for passage through the jugular foramen.

A complete lesion of the accessory nerve results in weakness of the sternocleidomastoid muscle and upper part of the trapezius (the lower part of the trapezius is innervated by the third and fourth cervical roots through the cervical plexus). This can be demonstrated by asking the patient to shrug the shoulders; the affected trapezius will be found to be weaker, and there will often be evident atrophy of its upper part. With the arms at the sides, the shoulder on the affected side droops and the scapula is slightly winged; the latter defect is accentuated with lateral movement of the arm (with serratus anterior weakness, winging of the scapula occurs on forward elevation of the arm). When the patient turns the head forcibly against the examiner's hand, preferably from the deviated to the straight-ahead position, the sternomastoid of the opposite side does not contract firmly beneath the fingers. This muscle can be further tested by having the patient press the head forward against resistance or lift the head from the pillow.

Motor system disease, poliomyelitis, syringomyelia, and spinal cord tumors may involve the cells of origin of the spinal accessory nerve. In its intracranial portion, the

nerve is usually affected along with the ninth and tenth cranial nerves by lesions of the jugular foramen (glomus tumors, neurofibromas, metastatic carcinoma). In the posterior triangle of the neck, the eleventh nerve can be damaged during surgical operations and by external compression or injury.

A benign disorder of the eleventh nerve, akin to Bell's palsy, has been described by Eisen and Bertrand; it begins with pain that subsides in a few days, and is followed by weakness and atrophy in the distribution of the nerve. About one-quarter to one-third of eleventh nerve lesions are of this idiopathic type, and the majority of patients recover. Double sternomastoid and trapezius palsy, which occurs with primary disease of muscles, e.g., polymyositis and muscular dystrophy, may be difficult to distinguish from a lesion of both accessory nerves.

HYPOGLOSSAL NERVE

This also is a purely motor nerve, which supplies the somatic musculature of the tongue. It arises as a series of rootlets that issue from the medulla between the pyramid and inferior olivary complex. The nerve leaves the skull through the hypoglossal foramen and innervates the genioglossus muscle, which acts to protrude the tongue; the styloglossus, which retracts and elevates its root; and the hypoglossus, which causes the upper surface to become convex. Complete interruption of the nerve results in paralysis of one side of the tongue. The tongue curves slightly to the healthy side as it lies in the mouth, but on protrusion it deviates to the affected side owing to the unopposed thrust of the healthy genioglossus muscle. In the mouth the tongue cannot be moved with natural facility. The denervated side becomes wrinkled and atrophied, and fasciculations and fibrillations can be seen.

Lesions of the hypoglossal nerve roots are rare. Occasionally an intramedullary lesion damages the emerging fibers of the hypoglossal nerve, the corticospinal tract, and medial lemniscus. The result is paralysis and atrophy of one side of the tongue, together with spastic paralysis and loss of vibration and position sense in the opposite arm and leg. Poliomyelitis and motor system disease may destroy the hypoglossal nuclei. Lesions of the basal meninges and the occipital bones (platybasia, Paget disease) may involve the nerve in its extramedullary course, and it is sometimes damaged in operations on the neck. A dissecting aneurysm of the carotid artery was shown by Goodman et al to have compressed the hypoglossal nerve with resultant weakness and atrophy. Since the C_2 segment receives some of the sensory fibers from the tongue, lesions at this level may explain the numbness of the tongue in patients with bouts of pain on head turning—what Lance and Anthony have described as the *neck-tongue syndrome*.

SYNDROME OF BULBAR PALSY

This syndrome is the result of weakness or paralysis of muscles that are supplied by the motor nuclei of the lower brainstem, i.e., the motor nuclei of the fifth, seventh, and ninth to twelfth cranial nerves. (Strictly speaking, the motor nuclei of the fifth and seventh lie outside the "bulb," which is the old name for the medulla oblongata.) Involved are the muscles of jaw and face, the sternomastoids and upper parts of the trapezii, and the muscles of tongue, pharynx, and larynx. If weakness develops rapidly, as may happen in diphtheria or poliomyelitis, there is no time for muscle atrophy. The more chronic diseases, e.g., progressive bulbar palsy (a form of motor system disease and the childhood form of Fazio-Londe), result in marked wasting and fasciculation of the facial, tongue, sternomastoid, and trapezius muscles. These disorders need to be differentiated from pseudobulbar palsy (see pages 46 and 414).

MULTIPLE CRANIAL NERVE PALSIES

As one can readily understand, several cranial nerves may be affected by a single disease process. One of the clinical problems that arises is whether the lesion lies within or outside the brainstem. Lesions lying on the surface of the brainstem are characterized by involvement of adjacent cranial nerves (often occurring in succession) and late and rather slight involvement of the long sensory and motor pathways and segmental structures lying within the brainstem. The opposite is true of intramedullary, intrapontine, and intramesencephalic lesions. The extramedullary lesion is more likely to cause bone erosion or enlargement of the foramens of exit of the cranial nerves (seen radiographically). The intramedullary lesion involving cranial nerves often produces a crossed sensory or motor paralysis (cranial nerve signs on one side of the body and tract signs on the opposite side). In this way, a number of distinctive syndromes, to which eponyms have been attached, are produced. These are listed in Table 47-2.

Involvement of multiple cranial nerves outside the brainstem is frequently the result of trauma (sudden onset),

localized infections such as herpes zoster (less acute onset), granulomatous disease (subacute onset), or compression by tumors and saccular aneurysms (chronic development). Of the tumors, neurofibromas, schwannomas, meningiomas, cholesteatomas, carcinomas, and sarcomas have all been observed. Nasopharyngeal tumors may implicate several lower cranial nerves in succession, as do also platybasia and adult-onset Chiari malformation. Multiple or single cranial nerve palsies of abrupt onset may precede or accompany infectious mononucleosis. De Simone and Snyder have assembled a series of 20 cases; bilateral facial paralysis was the most common presentation, bilateral optic neuritis the next, and in three cases, three or four cranial nerves were involved. The prognosis is excellent. A purely motor disorder without atrophy always raises the question of myasthenia gravis (see Chap. 53). Owing to their anatomic relationships, the multiple cranial nerve palsies form a number of distinctive syndromes, listed in Table 47-1 and in the chapter on intracranial neoplasms (Table 31-3).

From time to time one observes an acute form of multiple cranial neuropathy of undetermined cause. Juncos and Beal have reported on 14 such patients from the files of the Massachusetts General Hospital, along with six well-documented cases of the Tolosa-Hunt orbitocavernous sinus syndrome with oculomotor palsies. In the former group, the onset was with facial pain and headache (temporofrontal) followed within days by abducens palsy (12 of 14), oculomotor palsy (6 of 14), trigeminal palsy (5 of 14) facial weakness (4 of 14) and less often by involvement of the eighth, ninth, and tenth cranial nerves (unilaterally in most instances). Increased protein of CSF and pleocytosis occurred in several. The prompt relief of pain upon receipt of steroids was similar to that obtained in the Tolosa-Hunt syndrome. The mode of recovery, which usually occurred within a few months, was also much the same in the two groups of patients. Juncos and Beal concluded that the clinical features of the two groups overlapped and that their separation into two syndromes was arbitrary.

The question of *viral infections of cranial nerves* is always raised by these acute palsies of the facial, trigeminal, and auditory nerves, especially when the affection is bilateral, involves several nerves in combination, or is associated with a CSF pleocytosis. Actually, the only proved virus etiology in this group of cases is that of herpes zoster; in every instance in which we have searched for this virus in cases of Bell's palsy or vestibular neuronitis, the results have been negative. Since perceptive deafness, vertigo, and other cranial nerve palsies have been observed in conjunction with the postinfectious encephalomyelitides of varicella, measles, rubella, mumps, and scarlet fever and also with the Guillain-Barré syndrome, an immune-mediated mechanism must be considered. Nothing is known of the pathology of the cranial nerve lesion nor has a virus been isolated in these latter diseases. In the Tolosa-Hunt cases, in which the orbital or cavernous sinus has been biopsied, a nonspecific granuloma has been found. Sarcoid and tuberculosis have been the causes of a few cases. In Wegener granulomatosis, multiple cranial nerve palsies, usually lower ones, have occurred. Treatment of postinfectious cases is symptomatic; fortunately the prognosis for recovery is excellent. In Wegener disease cyclophosphamide has led to remission.

There is also a benign form of cranial nerve affection, involving both sides of the face more or less symmetrically. Some of these cases probably represent a variant form of the Guillain-Barré syndrome, insofar as they may be preceded by a nonspecific infection and accompanied by areflexia, evanescent paresthesias and/or weakness of the extremities, and an elevated spinal fluid protein, without pleocytosis. In rare instances, none of these features are evident and the neuropathy is strictly confined to cranial structures—in which case the status of the cranial neuropathy remains uncertain. In either case, recovery is usually prompt, in a matter of several weeks, and quite complete.

REFERENCES

ALEXANDER GE, MOSES H: Carbamazepine for hemifacial spasm. *Neurology* 32:286, 1982.

AUGER RG, PIEPGRAS DG, LAWS ER JR: Hemifacial spasm: Results of microvascular decompression of the facial nerve in 54 patients. *Mayo Clin Proc* 61:640, 1986.

BANNISTER R, OPPENHEIMER DR: Degenerative diseases of the nervous system associated wth autonomic failure. *Brain* 95:457, 1972.

BLAU JN, HARRIS M, KENNET S: Trigeminal sensory neuropathy. *N Engl J Med* 281:873, 1969.

BRODAL A: *The Cranial Nerves.* Springfield, IL, Charles C Thomas, 1959.

BROWNSTONE PK, BALLENGER JJ, VICK NA: Bilateral superior laryngeal neuralgia. *Arch Neurol* 37:525, 1980.

CHIA L-G: Pure trigeminal motor neuropathy. *Br J Med* 296:609, 1988.

DESIMONE PA, SNYDER D: Hypoglossal nerve palsy in infectious mononucleosis. *Neurology* 28:844, 1978.

EISEN A, BERTRAND G: Isolated accessory nerve palsy of spontaneous origin. A clinical and electromyographic study. *Arch Neurol* 27:496, 1972.

ELSTON JS: Botulinum toxin treatment of hemifacial spasm. *J Neurol Neurosurg Psychiatry* 49:827, 1986.

GOODMAN JM, ZINK WL, COOPER DF: Hemilingual paralysis caused by spontaneous carotid artery dissection. *Arch Neurol* 40:653, 1983.

GROVES J: Bell's (idiopathic) facial palsy, in Hinchcliffe R, Harrison D (eds): *Scientific Foundations of Otolaryngology.* London, Heinemann, 1976, pp 446–459.

HAUSER WA, KARNES WE, ANNIS J, KURLAND LT: Incidence and prognosis of Bell's palsy in the population of Rochester, Minnesota. *Mayo Clin Proc* 46:258, 1971.

JOHNSON JA, STERN LZ: Bilateral vocal cord paralysis in a patient with familial hypertrophic neuropathy. *Arch Neurol* 38:532, 1981.

JANNETTA PJ: Hemifacial spasm caused by a venule: Case report. *Neurol Surg* 14(1):89–92, 1984.

JUNCOS JL, BEAL MF: Idiopathic cranial polyneuropathy. *Brain* 110:197, 1987.

KARNES WE: Diseases of the seventh cranial nerve, in Dyck PJ et al (eds): *Peripheral Neuropathy,* 2nd ed. Philadelphia, Saunders, 1984, chap 55, pp 1266–1299.

KAYE AH, ADAMS CBT: Hemifacial spasm: A long-term follow-up of patients treated by posterior fossa surgery and nerve wrapping. *J Neurol Neurosurg Psychiatry* 44:1100, 1981.

LANCE JW, ANTHONY M: Neck-tongue syndrome on sudden turning of the head. *J Neurol Neurosurg Psychiatry* 43:97, 1980.

LECKY BRF, HUGHES RAC, MURRAY NMF: Trigeminal sensory neuropathy. *Brain* 110:1463, 1987.

MASSEY EW, MOORE J, SCHOLD SC JR: Mental neuropathy from systemic cancer. *Neurology* 31:1277, 1981.

MAYO CLINIC AND MAYO FOUNDATION: *Clinical Examinations in Neurology,* 5th ed. Philadelphia, Saunders, 1981.

NIELSEN VK, JANNETTA PJ: Pathophysiology of hemifacial spasm: Effects of facial nerve decompression. *Neurology* 34:891, 1984.

PIATT JH, WILKINS RH: Treatment of tic douloureux and hemifacial spasm by posterior fossa exploration; therapeutic implications of various neurovascular relationships. *Neurosurgery* 14:462, 1984.

PLOTT D: Congenital laryngeal-abductor paralysis due to nucleus ambiguus dysgenesis in three brothers. *N Engl J Med* 271:593, 1964.

SELBY G: Diseases of the fifth cranial nerve, in Dyck PJ, Thomas PK, Lambert EH, Bunge R (eds): *Peripheral Neuropathy,* 2nd ed. Philadelphia, Saunders, 1984, chap 54, pp 1244–1265.

SWEET WH: The treatment of trigeminal neuralgia (tic douleureux). *N Engl J Med* 315:174, 1986.

WASSERSTROM WR, STARR A: Facial myokymia in the Guillain-Barré syndrome. *Arch Neurol* 34:578, 1977.

CHAPTER 48

PRINCIPLES OF CLINICAL MYOLOGY: DIAGNOSIS AND CLASSIFICATION OF MUSCLE DISEASES

GENERAL CONSIDERATIONS

Striated muscle constitutes the principal organ of locomotion as well as a vast metabolic reservoir. Disposed in more than 600 separate muscles, this tissue makes up as much as 40 percent of the weight of adult human beings. Intricacy of structure undoubtedly accounts for its diverse susceptibilities to disease, and for this reason the following anatomic considerations provide an appropriate introduction to this chapter.

A single muscle is composed of thousands of muscle fibers that course for variable distances along its longitudinal axis. Some fibers extend the entire length of the muscle; others are joined end to end by connective tissue. Each fiber is a relatively large and complex multinucleated cell varying in length from a few millimeters to several centimeters (34 cm in the human sartorius muscle) and in diameter from 10 to 100 μm. Although the muscle fiber represents an indivisible anatomic and physiologic unit, disease may affect only one part of it, leaving the remainder to atrophy, degenerate, or regenerate, depending on the nature and severity of the disease. The nuclei of each cell, which are oriented parallel to the longitudinal axis of the fiber and may number in the thousands, lie beneath the cytoplasmic membrane (true sarcolemma)—hence "sarcolemmal nuclei." The cytoplasm (sarcoplasm) of the cell is abundant and contains myofibrils, various organelles such as mitochondria and ribosomes, and endoplasmic (sarcoplasmic) reticulum. The myofibrils in turn are composed of longitudinally oriented interdigitating filaments (myofilaments) of contractile proteins (actin and myosin). Droplets of stored fat, glycogen, various proteins, many enzymes, and myoglobin, the latter imparting the red color to muscle, are contained within the sarcoplasm or its organelles.

The individual muscle fibers are enveloped by delicate strands of connective tissue (endomysium), which provide their support and permit unity of action. Capillaries, of which there may be several for each fiber, and nerve fibers lie within the endomysium. Muscle fibers are bound into groups or fascicles by similar reticular tissue and sheets of collagen (perimysium), which also bind together groups of fascicles and surround the entire muscle (epimysium). The latter connective tissue tunics are also richly and variably vascularized, different types of muscle having different arrangements of arteries and veins; and fat cells (lipocytes) are embedded within the interstices. The muscle fibers are attached at their ends to tendon fibers, which in turn connect with the skeleton. By this means muscle contraction maintains posture and effects movement.

Other notable characteristics of muscle are its natural mode of contraction, i.e., through innervation, and the necessity of intact innervation for the maintenance of its normal trophic state. Each muscle fiber receives a nerve twig from a motor nerve cell in the anterior horn of the spinal cord or nucleus of a cranial nerve; the nerve twig joins the muscle fiber at a point called the *neuromuscular junction* or *motor end plate*. As was pointed out on page 37, groups of muscle fibers with a common innervation from one anterior horn cell constitute the *motor unit*, which is the basic physiologic unit in all reflex, postural, and voluntary activity.

Acetylcholine (ACh), ACh receptors, and acetylcholinesterase (AChE), which play a special role in neuromuscular transmission, are concentrated at the neuromuscular junction. ACh is synthesized in the motor nerve terminal and stored in vesicles as packets or "quanta," each containing a relatively fixed number (about 10,000) molecules. Quanta of ACh are released at the nerve ending, diffuse into the narrow synaptic cleft, and combine with specialized receptors on the muscle cell. Small numbers of quanta of ACh are released spontaneously and produce miniature end-plate potentials (mepps) of about 0.5 μV. A nerve impulse triggers the release of many ACh quanta, producing a much larger end-plate potential (epp), which excites the muscle membrane and leads to muscle contraction. The process is terminated by the action of the enzyme AChE, which breaks down ACh (see Chap. 45).

In addition to the motor nerves, muscle has two types of sensory receptors (proprioceptors), the muscle spindles and Golgi tendon organs, which participate in reflex activity (see page 39). Also, there are free nerve endings that subserve the sensation of pain, and autonomic endings on blood vessels and possibly on muscle fibers.

All muscles are not equally susceptible to disease despite the apparent similarity of their structure. In fact, practically no disease affects all muscles in the body, and each disease has as one of its features a characteristic topography within the musculature. The topographic differences between diseases provide incontrovertible evidence of structural or physiologic differences between muscles, not presently disclosed by the light or electron microscope. The factors responsible for the selective vulnerability of certain muscles are not known. One factor may relate simply to fiber size; consider, for example, the large diameter and length of the fibers of the glutei and paravertebral muscles in comparison with the smallness of the ocular muscle fibers. The number of fibers composing a motor unit may be of significance; in the ocular muscles, a motor unit contains only 6 to 10 muscle fibers, but in the gastrocnemius, it contains as many as 1800 fibers. The eye muscles have a much higher metabolic rate than the large trunk muscles. Differences in patterns of vascular supply may permit some muscles to withstand the effects of hypoxia or vascular occlusion better than others. Subtle metabolic differences between fibers within any one muscle have been revealed by enzyme studies, certain fibers being richer in glycolytic and poorer in oxidative enzymes than others. Doubtless other differences will be discovered.

These anatomic and biochemical properties of muscle suggest some of the ways in which this tissue can be affected by disease. Thus, one may envisage causative agents that affect each of the different components of sarcoplasm, namely, an enzyme, an essential substrate, the filamentous proteins, the endoplasmic reticulum, or the sarcolemma itself. Again, the endomysial connective tissue could be the primary pathway in disease, since it so closely invests the muscle fiber. Inadequacy of blood supply in relation to the oxygen requirement of active muscle, or frank ischemia from vascular occlusion, could be another mechanism of disease. Finally, the nerve or its cell of origin in the spinal cord is known to bear the brunt of certain pathologic processes, paralyzing all the muscle fibers that it innervates and depriving them of the unique trophic influence that nerve normally has upon muscle.

Normal muscle possesses a limited capacity to regenerate, a point often forgotten. Acute destructive processes of the muscle fiber, e.g., inflammatory or metabolic,

are usually followed by fairly complete restoration of the muscle cells, providing some part of each fiber has survived and the endomysial sheaths of connective tissue have not been disturbed. Unfortunately, many pathologic processes of muscle are chronic and unrelenting and destroy the muscle fibers completely. Under such conditions any regenerative activity fails to keep pace with the disease, and the loss of muscle fibers is permanent.

APPROACH TO THE PATIENT WITH MUSCLE DISEASE

The number and diversity of diseases of striated muscle greatly exceed the number of symptoms and signs by which they express themselves clinically; thus, different diseases share certain common symptoms and even syndromes. To avoid excessive repetition in the description of individual diseases, we shall discuss in one place all their clinical manifestations, a subject that we call *clinical myology*.

The physician is put on the track of a myopathic disease by eliciting complaints of muscle weakness or fatigue, pain, limpness or stiffness, spasm, twitching, or a muscle mass or change in muscle volume. Of these, the symptom of weakness is by far the most frequent and, at the same time, the most elusive. As was remarked in Chap. 23, the patient, when speaking of weakness, often means excessive fatigability. Although fatigability is a feature of a few muscle diseases, such as myasthenia gravis, it is far more frequently a complaint of patients with anxiety, depression, and chronic systemic disease. To distinguish between fatigability and weakness, an assessment should be made of the patient's capacity to perform certain common activities such as walking, running, climbing stairs, and arising from a sitting, kneeling, squatting, or reclining position. Difficulty in performing these tasks signifies weakness rather than fatigue. The same is true of difficulty in working with the arms above shoulder level. Particular complaints may reveal a localized muscle weakness; e.g., drooping of the eyelids, diplopia and strabismus, change in facial expression and voice, difficulty in chewing, closing the mouth, pursing the lips, and swallowing indicate a paresis of the levator palpebrae, extraocular, facial, laryngeal, masseter, and pharyngeal muscles, respectively. Of course, the impairment of muscle function may be due to a neuropathic or a central nervous system disturbance rather than to a myopathic one, but usually these conditions can be separated by the methods indicated further on in this chapter and in Chaps. 3 and 23.

EVALUATION OF MUSCLE WEAKNESS AND PARALYSIS

Reduced strength of muscle contraction, manifested by diminished power of single contractions and resistance to opposition (peak power), and by endurance during the performance of demanded movements (i.e., work potential), is the indubitable sign of muscle disease. In such testing the physician may encounter difficulty in enlisting the patient's cooperation. The tentative, hesitant performance of the hysteric or malingerer poses difficulties that can be surmounted by the techniques described in Chap. 3. In infants and small children, who cannot follow commands, one assesses muscle power by their resistance to passive manipulation or observing their performance while they are engaged in certain activities. The patient may be reluctant to contract muscles fully in a painful limb, and indeed pain itself may reflexly diminish the power of contraction (algesic paresis). Estimating the strength of isometric contractions that do not require the painful part to be moved is a way around this difficulty. Sometimes the weakness of a group of muscles only becomes manifest after a period of activity; e.g., the feet and legs may "drag" only after walking a long distance. The physician, upon being told this by the patient, should conduct the examination under circumstances that duplicate the complaint(s).

Weakness of muscle contraction acquires added significance when associated with other abnormalities, such as tenderness or atrophy of muscle, change in tendon reflexes, twitching, and spasm. Also severe weakness of certain muscle groups may result in abnormalities of posture and gait. A waddling gait indicates affection of the medial glutei (or dysplasia of hip joints); excessive lumbar lordosis and protuberance of the abdomen indicate weakness of the iliopsoas and abdominal muscles; kyphoscoliosis points to an asymmetric weakness of the paravertebral muscles; and flaring of the shoulder blades is a sign of weakness of the lower trapezii, serratus magnus, and rhomboid muscles. Equinovarus deformities of the feet may be the result of pseudocontracture of the calf muscles.

The *physiologic mechanism of the weakness* varies in the many diseases of muscle. In the dystrophies the most obvious explanation is degeneration and loss of muscle fibers. The degree to which thin and altered fibers are a contributory factor is uncertain. In diseases like myasthenia gravis, Lambert-Eaton syndrome, aminoglycoside antibiotic paralysis, and botulism, weakness is clearly traceable to disorders of neuromuscular transmission. In the various metabolic polymyopathies the basis of weakness has not been fully elucidated; a failure of energy production has been postulated. In some diseases such as carnitine palmityl transferase deficiency, weakness is associated with storage of fat, muscle fiber destruction, and myoglobinuria, but it is not known whether intact fibers are capable of exerting full force. The same is true of fibers storing glycogen.

Ascertaining *the extent and severity of muscle weakness* requires a systematic examination of the main groups of muscles from forehead to feet. The patient is asked to contract each group quickly with as much force as possible, while the examiner opposes the movement and offers a graded resistance in accordance with the degree of residual power. Alternatively, the patient is asked to produce a maximal contraction, and the examiner estimates power by the force needed to "break" or overcome it. If the weakness is unilateral, one has the advantage of being able to compare it with the strength on the normal side. If it is bilateral, the physician must refer to a concept of what constitutes normalcy, based on experience in muscle testing. Ocular, facial, lingual, pharyngeal, laryngeal, cervical, shoulder, upper arm, lower arm and hand, truncal, pelvic, thigh, and lower leg and foot muscles are examined sequentially. The anatomic significance of each of the actions tested, i.e., what roots, nerves, and muscles are involved, can be determined by referring to Table 48-1. A practiced examiner can survey the strength of these muscle groups in 2 to 3 min. A word of caution: in opposing the patient's attempts to contract the large and powerful trunk and girdle muscles, one may fail to detect slight to moderate degrees of weakness. These muscle groups are best tested by asking the patient to squat and kneel and then to assume the erect posture; to step onto a chair without using the hands; to walk on toes and heels; and to lift a heavy object (textbook of medicine) over his head.

In order to quantitate the degree of weakness, which indicates the severity of affection, and to compare one examination with another, which is necessary to determine the course of the disease and the effects of therapy, a rating scale should be used. Most widely used is the one proposed by the Medical Research Council of Great Britain which recognizes five grades of muscle strength, as follows: 0, complete paralysis; 1, minimal contraction; 2, active movement, with gravity eliminated; 3, weak contraction, against gravity; 4, active movement against gravity and resistance; and 5, normal strength. Some physiatrists add further gradations, specified as 4+ for barely detectable weakness and 4− for easily detected weakness, etc. With practice, one can distinguish true weakness from unwillingness to cooperate, feigned weakness, and inhibition of movement by pain.

Table 48-1
Tests of muscle action

Action tested	Roots	Nerves	Muscles
CRANIAL			
Closure of eyes, pursing of lips, exposure of teeth	Cranial 7	Facial	Orbicularis oculi Orbicularis oris
Elevation of eyelids, movement of eyes	Cranial 3, 4, 6	Oculomotor, trochlear, abducens	Extraocular
Closing and opening of jaw	Cranial 5	Motor trigeminal	Masseters Pterygoids
Protrusion of tongue	Cranial 12	Hypoglossal	Lingual
Phonation and swallowing	Cranial 9, 10	Glossopharyngeal, vagus	Palatal, laryngeal, & pharyngeal
Elevation of shoulders, anteroflexion and turning of head	Cranial 11	Spinal accessory	Trapezius, sternomastoid
BRACHIAL			
Adduction of extended arm	*C5*, C6	Brachial plexus	Pectoralis major
Fixation of scapula	C5, 6, 7	Brachial plexus	Serratus anterior
Initiation of abduction of arm	*C5*, C6	Brachial plexus	Supraspinatus
External rotation of flexed arm	*C5*, C6	Brachial plexus	Infraspinatus
Abduction and elevation of arm up to 90°	*C5*, C6	Axillary nerve	Deltoid
Flexion of supinated forearm	C5, C6	Musculocutaneous	Biceps, brachialis
Extension of forearm	C6, *C7*, C8	Radial	Triceps
Extension (radial) of wrist	C6	Radial	Extensor carpi radialis longus
Flexion of semipronated arm	C5, *C6*	Radial	Brachioradialis
Adduction of flexed arm	C6, *C7*, C8	Brachial plexus	Latissimus dorsi
Supination of forearm	C6, C7	Posterior interosseous	Supinator
Extension of proximal phalanges	*C7*, C8	Posterior interosseous	Extensor digitorum
Extension of wrist (ulnar side)	*C7*, C8	Posterior interosseous	Extensor carpi ulnaris
Extension of proximal phalanx of index finger	*C7*, C8	Posterior interosseous	Extensor indicis
Abduction of thumb	*C7*, C8	Posterior interosseous	Abductor pollicis longus and brevis
Extension of thumb	*C7*, C8	Posterior interosseous	Extensor pollicis longus and brevis
Pronation of forearm	C6, C7	Median nerve	Pronator teres
Radial flexion of wrist	C6, C7	Median nerve	Flexor carpi radialis
Flexion of middle phalanges	C7, *C8*, T1	Median nerve	Flexor digitorum superficialis
Flexion of proximal phalanx of thumb	C8, *T1*	Median nerve	Flexor pollicis brevis
Opposition of thumb against fifth finger	C8, *T1*	Median nerve	Opponens pollicis
Extension of middle phalanges of index and middle fingers	C8, *T1*	Median nerve	First, second lumbricals
Flexion of terminal phalanx of thumb	*C8*, T1	Anterior interosseous nerve	Flexor pollicis longus

Table 48-1 (*continued*)
Tests of muscle action

Action tested	Roots	Nerves	Muscles
Flexion of terminal phalanx of second and third fingers	*C8*, T1	Anterior interosseous nerve	Flexor digitorum profundus
Flexion of distal phalanges of ring and little fingers	C7, *C8*	Ulnar	Flexor digitorum profundus
Adduction and opposition of fifth finger	C8, *T1*	Ulnar	Hypothenar
Extension of middle phalanges of ring and little fingers	C8, *T1*	Ulnar	Third, fourth lumbricals
Adduction of thumb against second finger	C8, *T1*	Ulnar	Adductor pollicis
Flexion of proximal phalanx of thumb	*C8*, T1	Ulnar	Flexor pollicis brevis
Abduction and adduction of fingers	C8, *T1*	Ulnar	Interossei
CRURAL			
Hip flexion from semiflexed position	*L1*, *L2*, L3	Femoral	Iliopsoas
Hip flexion from externally rotated position	L2, L3	Femoral	Sartorius
Extension of knee	L2, *L3*, *L4*	Femoral	Quadriceps femoris
Adduction of thigh	*L2*, *L3*, L4	Obturator	Adductor longus, magnus, brevis
Abduction and int. rotation of thigh	*L4*, *L5*, S1	Superior gluteal	Gluteus medius
Extension of thigh	L5, *S1*, S2	Inferior gluteal	Gluteus maximus
Flexion of knee	L5, *S1*, S2	Sciatic	Biceps femoris Semitendinosus Semimembranosus
Dorsiflexion of foot (medial)	*L4*, L5	Peroneal (deep)	Anterior tibial
Dorsiflexion of toes (proximal and distal phalanges)	*L5*, S1		Extensor digitorum longus and brevis
Dorsiflexion of great toe	*L5*, S1		Extensor hallucis longus
Eversion of foot	L5, S1	Peroneal (superficial)	Peroneus longus and brevis
Plantar flexion of foot	*S1*, S2	Tibial	Gastrocnemius, soleus
Inversion of foot	L4, *L5*	Tibial	Tibialis posterior
Flexion of toes (distal phalanges)	L5, *S1*, S2	Tibial	Flexor digitorum longus
Flexion of toes (middle phalanges)	*S1*, S2	Tibial	Flexor digitorum brevis
Flexion of great toe (proximal phalanx)	S1, S2	Tibial	Flexor hallucis brevis
Flexion of great toe (distal phalanx)	L5, *S1*, S2	Tibial	Flexor hallucis longus
Contraction of anal sphincter	S2, S3, S4	Pudendal	Perineal muscles

Modified from Walton. Italics indicate major nerve root involved.

In the *myasthenic states* there is a rapid failure of contraction in the most affected muscles during a sustained activity. For instance, after looking at the ceiling for a few minutes the eyelids progressively droop; and after closing the eyes and resting the levator palpebrae muscles, the ptosis lessens or disappears. Similarly, holding the eyes in a lateral position will induce diplopia and strabismus. This reaction, in combination with restoration of power by the administration of neostigmine or edrophonium (Tensilon), are the most valid criteria for the diagnosis of myasthenia gravis (see page 1156).

In addition to myasthenic weakness, there are other abnormalities that may be discovered by observing, during one or a series of maximal actions of a group of muscles, the speed and efficiency of contraction and relaxation. In myxedema, for example, slow waves of contraction in a muscle such as the quadriceps may be seen on change in posture (*contraction myoedema*); often it is associated with percussion myoedema and prolonged duration of the tendon reflexes. Slowness in relaxation of muscles is another feature of hypothyroidism, accounting for the complaint of uncomfortable tightness of proximal limb muscles.

A prolonged failure of relaxation with after-discharge is characteristic of the myotonic phenomenon, which characterizes certain diseases—congenital myotonia (of Thomsen), myotonic dystrophy (of Steinert), and the paramyotonia of von Eulenberg. True myotonia, with its prolonged discharges of action potentials, requires strong contraction for its elicitation, is more evident after a period of relaxation, and tends to disappear with repeated contractions (see page 1173). This persistence of contraction is demonstrable also by tapping a muscle (*percussion myotonia*), a phenomenon easily distinguished from the electrically silent local bulge (*myoedema*) induced by a sharp tap of a muscle in the myxedematous or cachetic patient and from the brief fascicular contraction that is induced by the tapping of normal or partially denervated muscle (idiomuscular contraction). (N.B., in patients with hyperactive tendon reflexes, striking the muscle rather than its tendon can elicit a stretch reflex.) *Paradoxical myotonia* refers to an increase in the degree of myotonia during a series of contractions (the reverse of what happens in the usual type of myotonia). It occurs in some cases of von Eulenberg paramyotonia.

Increase in power in a series of several voluntary contractions in the absence of myotonia is a feature of the *inverse myasthenic (Lambert-Eaton) syndrome,* which is associated in about 50 percent of cases with small-cell carcinoma of the lung. It, too, has its electromyographic equivalent—a rapid increase in the voltage of a series of action potentials with appropriate stimulation (page 1159).

The effect of cold on muscle contraction may also prove informative; either paresis or myotonia, lasting for a few minutes, may be evoked or enhanced by cold, as in the paramyotonia of von Eulenberg.

Myotonia and myoedema must also be distinguished from the recruitment and spread of involuntary spasm induced by strong and repeated contractions of limb muscles in patients with *mild or localized tetanus*. This is not a primary muscle phenomenon but is due to an abolition of inhibitory spinal mechanisms.

The repeated contraction of forearm or leg muscles, after the application of a tourniquet (exceeding arterial pressure) to the proximal part of a limb, will often elicit latent tetany. Its special mode of development, as well as its duration, its enhancement by hyperventilation, and the association of tingling, prickling paresthesias, separate tetany from ordinary cramp and also from true contracture.

In practice, the term *contracture* is applied to all states of fixed muscle shortening. Several distinct types can be recognized. In *true contracture* a group of muscles, after a series of strong contractions, may remain shortened for many minutes, because of failure of the metabolic mechanism necessary for relaxation; and the EMG, in this shortened state, remains relatively silent, in contrast to the high-voltage, rapid discharges observed with cramp, tetanus, and tetany. Such contracture occurs in McArdle disease (phosphorylase deficiency), in which it is aggravated by arterial occlusion, but it has been seen in phosphofructokinase deficiency and possibly in another disease, as yet undefined, where the tourniquet has no effect and phosphorylase seems to be present in adequate amounts, at least as judged by histochemical stains (page 1171). True contracture is to be distinguished from paradoxical myotonia (see above) and from cramp, which in certain conditions (dehydration, tetany, pathologic cramp syndrome, amyotrophic lateral sclerosis) may be initiated by one or a series of voluntary muscle contractions.

Pseudocontracture (myostatic contracture) is the common form of muscle shortening that inevitably follows prolonged fixation and complete inactivity of the normally innervated muscle. Here the shortened state of the muscle, which may persist for days or weeks, has no clearly established anatomic, physiologic, or chemical basis.

Far more frequent is a fibrosis of muscle, a state following fiber loss and immobility of muscle. Depending on the predominant position, certain muscles are both weakened and shortened (*fibrous contracture*). This accounts for the rigidity and kyphoscoliosis of the spine, so frequent in myopathic diseases. The latter state is distinguished from *ankylosis* by the springy nature of the resistance, coincident with increased tautness of muscle and tendon during passive motion, and from *Volkmann contracture,* where there is evident fibrosis of muscle and surrounding tissues due to ischemic injury, usually after a fracture of the elbow.

TOPOGRAPHY OR PATTERNS OF PARALYSIS

As was stated above, in almost all the diseases under consideration, some of the muscles are affected and others are spared. Each disease exhibits its own pattern. Moreover, the topography or distribution of involvement tends to follow a similar pattern in all patients with the same disease. Thus, topography or pattern of involvement becomes another valid diagnostic attribute of muscular disease, ranking next in importance after altered quantity, intensity, and quality of contraction.

The following patterns of muscle involvement constitute a core of essential clinical knowledge in this field:

1. *Ocular palsies presenting more or less exclusively as diplopia, ptosis, or strabismus,* sometimes in association with exophthalmos and pupillary change. As a rule, primary diseases of muscle do not involve the pupil, and in most instances their effects are bilateral. In lesions of the third, fourth, or sixth cranial nerves, the neural origin is disclosed by the pattern of ocular muscle palsies or abnormalities of the pupil, or both. When weakness of the orbicularis oculi (muscles of eye closure) is added to ocular palsies and ptosis, it nearly always signifies myopathic disease.

Myasthenia gravis (ocular form), progressive external ophthalmoplegia (ocular myopathy), oculopharyngeal muscular dystrophy, and exophthalmic ophthalmoplegia of thyroid disease are the most frequent causes of a relatively pure affection of eye muscles. There are several other myopathies in which external ophthalmoplegia is associated with involvement of other muscles or organs, namely, the Kearns-Sayre syndrome (retinitis pigmentosa, heart block, short stature, generalized weakness, and ovarian hypoplasia); congenital myotubular and mitochondrial myopathies; nuclear ophthalmoplegia with bifacial weakness (Möbius syndrome); and the myotonic dystrophy of Steinert. Eye muscle weakness may occur at a late stage in other dystrophies such as the facioscapulohumeral type. Conversely, most patients with oculopharyngeal dystrophy eventually develop weakness of limb and girdle muscles. Acute ophthalmoplegia may be an expression of botulism and the Fisher syndrome of ophthalmoplegia, arreflexia and ataxia (page 1037).

2. *Bifacial palsy presenting as an inability to smile, expose the teeth, and close the eyes.* Varying degrees of bifacial weakness are observed in myasthenia gravis, ptosis and ocular palsies being conjoined in about 90 percent of cases. The same is true of myotonic dystrophy. More severe or complete facial palsy occurs in facioscapulohumeral and related dystrophies, in congenital myopathies (centronuclear, nemaline, carnitine deficiency) in the Guillain-Barré syndrome (always with other signs of neuropathy), in polymyositis (rare), and in combination with abducens palsies in Moebius syndrome. Very rarely, Bell's palsy is bilateral. Sometimes bilateral facial paralysis occurs as a manifestation of sarcoid or as part of a cranial polyneuritis of unknown cause (page 1089).

3. *Bulbar palsy presenting as dysphonia, dysarthria, and dysphagia with or without weakness of jaw or facial muscles.* Myasthenia gravis is the most frequent cause of this syndrome and must also be considered whenever a hanging jaw or fatigue of the jaw while eating or talking presents as a solitary finding; usually, however, ptosis and ocular palsies are conjoined ($>$90 percent of cases). These combinations of palsies are also observed in myotonic dystrophy and botulism. Progressive bulbar palsy of lower motor neuron type may be the basis of this syndrome, and the diagnosis is most obvious when the tongue is withered and twitching. Basilar invagination of the skull and certain types of Chiari malformation may reproduce some of the findings of bulbar palsy by involving the lower cranial nerves; diphtheria and bulbar poliomyelitis are now rare diseases that may present in this way. The neurologic condition known as spastic bulbar paralysis, or pseudobulbar palsy, is readily distinguished by the presence of hyperactive facial and gag reflexes, lack of muscle atrophy, and the associated clinical findings (see pages 46 and 414). Dysphonia and dysphagia may rarely be the first manifestations of polymyositis.

4. *Cervical palsy presenting with inability to hold the head erect or to lift the head from the pillow.* The patient may be unable to hold up the head owing to weakness of the posterior neck muscles, or to lift it from a pillow because of weakness of the sternocleidomastoids and other anterior neck muscles. In advanced forms of this syndrome, the head may hang with chin on chest, unless it is held up by the patient's hands.

The hanging head with weakness of the posterior neck muscles occurs most often in idiopathic polymyositis, often combined with slight dysphagia, dysphonia, and weakness of girdle muscles. The major types of progressive muscular dystrophy, when advanced, usually affect the anterior neck muscles disproportionately. Rarely, syringomyelia, syphilitic meningoradiculitis, loss of anterior horn cells in conjunction with carcinomatosis, and motor system disease may differentially paralyze various neck muscles.

5. *Weakness of respiratory and trunk muscles.* Usually the chest and trunk muscles are affected in association with proximal limb muscles, but occasionally weakness of the former muscles is the initial or the dominant manifestation of disease. Involvement of the thoracic muscles and diaphragm, giving rise to dyspnea and diminished vital capacity, may first bring the patient to the pulmonary clinic. We have observed this to happen in patients with motor system disease, glycogen storage disease, and acute polymyositis. The paravertebral muscles may be severely affected in some types of muscular dystrophy but usually in conjunction with crural and shoulder muscle weakness. And of course, respiratory failure may terminate life in severe myasthenia gravis and Guillain-Barré syndrome. Chest expansion, speaking a consecutive series of numbers on one breath, and straightening up after touching the floor with unbent knees are ways of detecting these patterns of muscle weakness.

6. *Bibrachial palsy, sometimes presenting as a dangling-arm syndrome.* Weakness, atrophy, and fasciculations of the hands, arms, and shoulders characterize the common form of motor system disease, namely, amyotrophic lateral sclerosis. Primary diseases of muscle hardly ever weaken these parts disproportionately. Rarely, a diffuse weakness of both arms may occur in the early stages of acute idiopathic polyneuritis and porphyric and other polyneuropathies, but it soon becomes part of a more generalized paralysis.

7. *Bicrural palsy presenting as lower leg weakness with inability to walk on the heels and toes, or as paralysis of all leg and thigh muscles.* Symmetric weakness of the lower legs is usually due to polyneuropathy although peroneal and anterior tibial muscles are often weakened in dystrophy. Diabetic polyneuropathy may cause an asymmetric weakness of thigh and pelvic muscles, often with pain and little sensory change. In total leg and thigh weakness, one first thinks of a spinal cord disease, in which case there is often loss of control of the bladder and bowel sphincters, as well as loss of sensory function below a certain level on the trunk. Motor system disease may begin in the legs, asymmetrically as a rule, and affect them out of proportion to other parts. Thus the differential diagnosis of leg weakness involves more diseases than do the restricted paralyses of other parts of the body.

8. *Limb-girdle palsies presenting as inability to raise the arms or to arise from a squatting, kneeling, or sitting position.* Two groups of diseases—polymyositis and dermatomyositis and the progressive muscular dystrophies—most often manifest themselves in this fashion. The Duchenne and Leyden-Möbius types of dystrophy tend first to affect the muscles of the pelvic girdle, gluteal region, and thighs, resulting in a lumbar lordosis and protuberant abdomen, a waddling gait, and difficulty in arising from

the floor and climbing stairs without the assistance of the arms. The Landouzy-Déjerine type affects the muscles of the face and shoulder girdles foremost, and is manifested by incomplete eye closure, inability to whistle and to raise the arms above the head, winging of the scapulae, and thinness of the upper arms ("Popeye" appearance). In the milder forms of polymyositis, weakness may be limited to the neck muscles or those of the shoulder or pelvic girdles. In a similar vein, the early or mild forms of dystrophy may selectively involve only the peroneal and scapular muscles (scapuloperoneal dystrophy). A number of other diseases of muscle may express themselves by a disproportionate weakness of girdle and proximal limb musculature. A metabolic myopathy, such as the adult form of acid maltase deficiency and the familial (hypokalemic) type of periodic paralysis, may affect only the pelvic and thigh muscles. In a number of the congenital polymyopathies, cataloged by Bethlem, a relatively nonprogressive weakness affects girdle muscles more than distal ones. Proximal muscles are occasionally implicated in progressive spinal muscular atrophy, as in the syndrome first described by Wohlfart et al and by Kugelberg and Welander, which unfortunately adds to confusion in diagnosis.

Similarly, a *pure quadriceps femoris weakness* may be the expression of several diseases. If bilateral, it usually indicates a polymyositis or a restricted dystrophy. Thyrotoxic and steroid myopathies have major effects on the quadriceps muscles. If unilateral or bilateral, with loss of patellar reflex and sensory loss over the inner leg, it is due most often to a femoral neuropathy or to an upper lumbosacral plexus lesion. Injuries to the hip and knee cause rapid disuse atrophy of the quadriceps muscles.

9. *Distal limb palsies presenting usually as foot drop with steppage gait (and pes cavus), weakness of all lower leg muscles, and later wrist drop and weakness of hands (claw hand).* The principal cause of this neuromuscular syndrome is a familial polyneuropathy, such as the peroneal muscular atrophy of Charcot-Marie-Tooth, hypertrophic polyneuropathy of Déjerine and Sottas, and the hereditary polyneuropathy of Refsum. Rarely chronic nonfamilial polyneuropathies may also present such a picture, but once more, there are exceptions, such as some forms of familial progressive muscular atrophy and distal types of progressive muscular dystrophy (Gowers, Welander). In myotonic dystrophy there may be weakness of the leg muscles as well as those of the forearm, sternomastoid, face, and eyes. Despite these exceptions, the generalization that girdle weakness means myopathy and distal weakness neuropathy is clinically useful.

10. *Generalized or universal paralysis: limb (but usually not cranial) muscles, involved either in attacks or as part of a persistent, progressive deterioration.* When acute in onset and episodic, this syndrome is usually a manifestation of familial hypokalemic or hyperkalemic periodic paralysis. One variety of the former type is associated with hyperthyroidism, another with aldosteronism. Generalized paresis (rather than paralysis) that has an acute onset and lasts many weeks is a feature of a group of diseases called paroxysmal myoglobinuria of Meyer-Betz, and at times of a severe form of idiopathic or parasitic (trichinosis) polymyositis. Idiopathic polymyositis may involve all limb and trunk muscles but usually spares the facial and ocular muscles, whereas the weakness in trichinosis is mainly in the ocular and lingual muscles. In infants and young children, a chronic and persistent generalized weakness of all muscles except those of the eyes always raises the question of Werdnig-Hoffman spinal muscular atrophy or, if mild in degree and relatively nonprogressive, of congenital myopathy or polyneuropathy. In these diseases of infancy, paucity of movement, hypotonia, and retardation of motor development may be more obvious than weakness.

Universal ascending paralysis, developing over a few days, with involvement of cranial (including ocular) muscles, is usually due to acute idiopathic (Guillain-Barré) polyneuritis. Insidious onset and slow (months to years) progression of paralysis, atrophy, and fasciculation of limb and trunk muscles, without sensory loss, characterizes motor system disease. Here the eye muscles are nearly always spared. Mild degrees of generalized weakness are features of a number of metabolic myopathies, such as thyrotoxic myopathy, glycogen storage diseases, vitamin D deficiency, and rickets.

11. *Paralysis of single muscles or a group of muscles.* This is almost always neuropathic, rarely spinal. Muscle disease does not need to be considered except possibly in certain atypical forms of familial periodic paralysis (see page 1162).

From this exposition of the topographic aspects of weakness one can appreciate that each neuromuscular disease exhibits a predilection for particular groups of muscles. As a corollary, a given pattern of weakness should always suggest certain possibilities of disease and exclude others.

Diagnosis also depends on features of paralysis other than its topography, such as mode of onset and tempo of progression, the coexistence of medical disorders, and certain laboratory findings (serum enzymes, EMG, and biopsy findings). Other differentiating features, such as the age of onset, natural course of the disease, and its genetic determinants figure prominently in the delineation of muscle diseases.

MUSCLE FATIGUE AND EXERCISE INTOLERANCE

In the field of clinical myology a distinction is often drawn between weakness—an inability to generate force, and fatigue—an inability to maintain force (Edwards). In myopathic diseases, however, weakness and fatigability are usually conjoined. The term *exercise intolerance* may mean either a lack of endurance or discomfort (polymyalgia) and stiffness in the days following exercise. Exceptionally, muscle power appears to be normal in the performance of all the usual activities of daily life, yet the patient is unable to engage in activities that require repetitive muscle contractions. This is particularly true of some of the glycogen storage diseases of muscle and the mitochondrial myopathies. And as was stated above, fatigability, without weakness in tests of peak power or endurance, is most commonly nonmyologic. Surprisingly, fatigue is an infrequent complaint in patients who have polymyopathic diseases; usually the main symptom is weakness.

By contrast, one of the most frequently unsolved problems in "muscle clinics" is true exercise intolerance. This may be combined with weakness and fatigability. But often in the absence of demonstrable weakness, atrophy, or reflex change, every prolonged exertion leads to premature fatigue and myalgia, not unlike that experienced by a sedentary person after excessively vigorous exercise. Only the patient never can condition himself to the point of tolerating ordinary muscular activity. Sometimes this state appears to be familial. It is tempting to think of it in terms of an enzymatic defect causing inadequate availability of substrates needed for sustained muscle activity. Adenylate deaminase deficiency is postulated as one cause of exercise intolerance and Ca-ATPase deficiency another (Chap. 51). Since the symptoms are purely subjective and so variably described, one must not overlook a chronic anxiety neurosis, depression, or chronic postviral fatigue syndrome (Chap. 23). Many patients are destined to limp through life, hampered in this way, with no explanation or treatment.

MUSCLE TONE

All normal muscles display a slight resistance to stretch when fully relaxed. When stretched to their limit and released, they recoil, mainly because of the elasticity of the fibers and their connective tissue sheaths. In addition, the trunk and proximal limb musculature is intermittently or constantly activated in the maintenance of attitudes and postures. To relax, i.e., to completely disengage a muscle from all its natural activities, requires practice and seems increasingly difficult in the elderly (paratonic rigidity or "gegenhalten," page 62). Impairment of the innervation of muscle, atrophy, or loss of contracting fibers are causes of "hypotonia." In infants this state has been accepted as a mark of neuromuscular disease; the infant is said to be "floppy."

Muscle tone is used as a sign of disease in infants, a practice that stems mainly from the difficulty in testing strength at this age. Tone can be assessed by lifting the infant in a prone position; if hypotonic, the head and legs cannot be supported against gravity and dangle. Or when held under the arms the hypotonic infant slips through the examiner's hands. André-Thomas introduced the term "passivite" to refer to the amplitude of the flapping movement of the extremity when shaken and "extensibilite" to denote the resistance of a relaxed muscle to slow passive stretch. In our opinion these are but different ways of testing muscle tone. Diminution in tone is observed in infants suffering from Werdnig-Hoffman disease, benign hypotonia, the congenital myopathies, and also in sickly infants with a variety of systemic diseases. In adults hypotonia is a feature of many of the myopathies and neuropathies, all of which reduce the number of contracting motor units.

Excessive tone, apart from that observed as a consequence of extrapyramidal rigidity, is rare in infants. A purely myopathic form of hypertonia is difficult to substantiate. Various types of disease may lead to fibrous contracture and arthrogryposis. Myopathic weakness may lead to the "rigid spine syndrome," described by Dubowitz. Dudley and her colleagues have reported a "stiff-baby syndrome," resembling tetanus, which slowly disappeared after 2 years of age. For the most part, the muscle stiffness syndromes are due to continuous overactivity of motor units.

CHANGES IN MUSCLE VOLUME

Diminution or increase in muscle bulk stands as another feature of disease that can be observed in all except the most obese patients. There are, of course, innate differences in muscle development, a greater salience of muscle in the male than in the female, and differences due to use and disuse. Greatly increased size and strength of muscles (hypertrophia musculorum vera) is observed in cultists devoted to bodybuilding, in *congenital myotonia* (circus freaks with phenomenal muscular development often have this disease), in instances of a rare pathologic cramp syndrome, in the Bruck-DeLange syndrome of congenital hypertrophy of muscle, athetosis and feeblemindedness, and in some patients destined to develop muscular dystrophy. Far more often, muscle enlargement in progressive muscular dystrophy takes the form of *pseudohypertrophy*,

in which the increase in size is accompanied by weakness. Here large and small fibers are mixed with fat cells, which have replaced many of the degenerated muscle fibers; other muscles in the same patient are atrophied. Other diseases may also cause pseudohypertrophy. We have seen it in amyloidosis, sarcoidosis, eosinophilic monomyositis, and rarely in certain of the congenital myopathies. Hypothyroidism is often accompanied by an increase in volume of certain muscles, simulating hypertrophia musculorum vera and congenital myotonia (see page 1173).

Cachexia, malnutrition, and lipodystrophy tend to reduce muscle bulk without reducing the power of contraction proportionately (*pseudoatrophy*). Denervation is invariably attended by atrophy. Lesions of the peripheral nerve or anterior horn cells, if complete, lead to a loss of bulk up to 85 percent of the original volume within 3 months. The most severe degrees of atrophy are observed in the chronic neuropathies, motor system diseases, and the muscular dystrophies. The distribution of the atrophy corresponds to the paresis. Of interest is the fact that a number of diseases result in severe weakness with little or no atrophy; these are polymyositis, myasthenia gravis, periodic paralyses, steroid myopathy, hypothyroidism, and Addison disease.

TWITCHES, SPASMS, AND CRAMPS

Fascicular twitches at rest, if pronounced and combined with muscular weakness and atrophy, usually signify motor neuron disease (amyotrophic lateral sclerosis, progressive muscular atrophy, or progressive bulbar palsy); but they may be seen in other diseases that involve the gray matter of the spinal cord (e.g., syringomyelia or tumor), as well as in lesions of the anterior roots (e.g., protruded intervertebral disc), and in certain peripheral neuropathies. Widespread fasciculations may occur with severe dehydration, after an overdose of neostigmine, or with organophosphate poisoning. Slow and persistent fasciculations, spreading in a wave-like pattern along the entire length of a muscle and associated with slight reduction in the speed of contraction and relaxation, are part of the syndrome of continuous muscular activity (page 1170). The same sequence, evolving at a slightly slower pace, may occur in small fiber neuropathies. Fasciculations that occur with muscular contraction, in contrast to those at rest, indicate a state of heightened irritability of muscle; this may occur for no discernible reason or as a sequela of a disease (e.g., poliomyelitis) that leaves muscle with some paralyzed motor units, so that during contraction small and increasingly larger units are not enlisted smoothly. *Benign fasciculations,* a common finding in otherwise normal individuals, can be distinguished by the lack of muscular weakness and atrophy. *Myokymia* is a less common condition in which repeated twitchings impart a rippling appearance to the muscle. One type, associated with muscle cramping, is known as "myokymia with persistent spasm." These conditions and Isaac's continuous muscle activity are discussed in Chap. 54. The recurrent twitches of the eyelid or muscles of the thumb which are experienced by most normal persons are often referred to as myokymia but are probably more closely related to benign fasciculations.

Muscle cramps, despite their commonality, are a poorly understood phenomenon. They occur at rest or with movement (action cramps) and are frequently reported in motor system disease, tetany, dehydration after excessive sweating and salt loss and other metabolic diseases (uremia and hemodialysis, hypocalcemia, hypothyroidism, and hypomagnesemia) and in certain muscle diseases (e.g., some of the myoglobinurias, rare cases of Becker muscular dystrophy, and congenital myopathies). Far more frequent, however, is the benign form (*idiopathic cramp syndrome*), in which no other neuromuscular disturbance can be found. Most often the cramps occur at night and affect the muscles of the calf and foot, but they may occur at any time and involve any muscle group. Some patients state that cramps are more frequent when the legs are cold and daytime activity has been excessive. Cramps of this type are extremely common; they are provoked by the abrupt stretching of muscles, are very painful, and tend to wax and wane before they disappear. The electromyographic equivalent is a high-frequency discharge. Although of no pathologic significance, the cramps in extreme cases are so persistent and so readily provoked by innocuous movements as to be disabling.

In contrast to cramp is physiologic contracture, observed in McArdle disease and carnitine palmityl transferase deficiency, in which increasing muscle shortening and pain gradually develop during muscular activity. Unlike cramping, it does not occur at rest, the pain is less intense, and the EMG of the contractured muscle is relatively silent.

A particularly malignant and progressive form of painful spasm is known as the *stiff-man syndrome;* this appears to be a disease of the central nervous system, of unknown nature. Continuous spasm, intensified by the action of muscles, with no demonstrable disorder at a neuromuscular level, is a common manifestation of tetanus and also follows the bite of the black widow spider.

All of the foregoing conditions must be distinguished from sensations of cramp without muscle spasm. The latter is a dysesthetic phenomenon.

All the aforementioned phenomena are discussed in Chap. 54.

PALPABLE ABNORMALITIES OF MUSCLE

Altered structure and function of muscle are not accurately revealed by palpation. Of course, the difference between the firm hypertrophied muscle of a well-conditioned athlete and the slack muscle of a sedentary person is as apparent to the palpating fingers as to the eye; so also is the persistent contraction in tetanus, cramp, contracture, and extrapyramidal rigidity. The muscles in dystrophy are said to have a "doughy" or "elastic" feel, but we find this difficult to judge. In the Pompe type of glycogen storage disease, attention may be attracted to the musculature by an unnatural firmness and increase in bulk. For reasons not known, partial denervation and reinnervation may occasionally result in focal hypertrophy of muscle, as was first pointed out by Lhermitte (cf. Mielke et al). The swollen, edematous, weak muscles in acute paroxysmal myoglobinuria or severe polymyositis may feel taut and firm but are usually not tender. Areas of tenderness in muscles that otherwise function normally, a state called *myogelosis,* has been attributed to fibrositis or fibromyositis, but their nature has not been divulged by biopsy.

A mass may develop in part of a muscle, or throughout a muscle, and poses a series of special clinical problems that are discussed on pages 1176 and 1177.

TENDON (STRETCH) REFLEXES

The tendon reflexes are impaired in the majority of neuromuscular diseases, but particularly in those involving peripheral nerves. In muscular dystrophy and polymyositis they tend to be reduced in proportion to the reduction in muscular power. In the myopathy of hypothyroidism, in which contraction and relaxation of muscle is slowed, there is a characteristic prolongation of the tendon reflex; the opposite condition of quickening and brevity of the tendon reflex is less reliably demonstrated in hyperthyroidism.

MUSCLE PAIN

Notably, few of the primary muscle diseases are painful. When pain is prominent and continuous during rest and activity, there will usually be evidence of disease of the peripheral nerves or vasculature, as in polymyalgia rheumatica, alcoholic neuropathy, etc. Severe pain localized to a group of muscles occurs in wryneck, fibrositis and fibromyositis, acute brachial neuritis (neuralgic amyotrophy), radiculitis, and Bornholm disease, or pleurodynia, but little is known of the cause of the pain in any of them. Cramping also causes intense pain, and the latter is a prominent complaint in most of the muscle spasm and cramp syndromes mentioned above. Also, as was said above, contracted muscle is usually painful. Tenderness of muscle is a variable state normally. It tends to be more definite in polyneuritis, poliomyelitis, and polyarteritis nodosa than in polymyositis, the various forms of dystrophy, and other myopathies. In polymyositis, if pain is present, it usually indicates coincident involvement of connective tissues and joint structures. The myalgic states are considered further on pages 1175 and 1176.

The mechanism of muscle pain is probably multiple. Prolonged and continuous contraction gives rise to a deep aching sensation; allegedly this is the cause of "tension headache." Contraction under ischemic conditions, as when the circulation is occluded by tourniquet, induces pain. The pain of intermittent claudication is supposedly of this type and is not accompanied by cramp. It is postulated that lactic acid or some other metabolite accumulates in muscles and activates pain receptors, but this is unproven. Pain is not a feature of the mitochondrial myopathies, in which there is an increase in lactic acid. The pain, swelling, and tenderness after prolonged exercise of unconditioned muscles, which usually comes on the following day, is evidently due to fiber necrosis (Armstrong).

NONMUSCULAR ABNORMALITIES

Clinical studies have divulged the involvement of many organs in certain diseases formerly thought to be purely myopathic. Some of the nonmuscular abnormalities, such as congenital dislocation of the hips in several of the congenital myopathies, are probably secondary to the inadequate action of immature muscles. In other diseases, however, it is evident that the pathogenic agent has affected many systems and knowledge of these assumes diagnostic importance. For example, in congenital dystrophy of the Fukuyama type, in Duchenne dystrophy, and in myotonic dystrophy, cerebral development is blighted, with resulting mental retardation. The cardiac musculature or conducting system is often damaged in Duchenne dystrophy, myotonic dystrophy, Kearns-Sayre disease, and some other adult dystrophies. The retinas, eighth nerves, and ovaries are simultaneously involved in Kearns-Sayre disease, and the CNS in some of the mitochondrial myopathies.

DIAGNOSIS OF MUSCLE DISEASE

The aforementioned symptoms and signs attain significance only when considered in connection with the age of the patient at the time of onset, their mode of evolution and course, and the presence or absence of familial occurrence.

Since many diseases of muscle are hereditary, a careful family history is important. Stated differently, the familial occurrence of a muscle disease practically always indicates a genetic causation. The pattern of inheritance has diagnostic significance, as indicated below, and if genetic counselling or prenatal diagnosis is a consideration, the construction of a detailed genealogic tree becomes essential. Historical data may be insufficient, and it is necessary to examine siblings and parents of the proband.

The heritable muscle diseases are single-gene conditions, so that they often assume readily recognized mendelian patterns. The pattern of transmission in a particular kindred depends on whether the abnormal gene is X-linked or autosomal and whether the disease is inherited as a recessive or dominant trait.

X-linked disorders of muscle (Duchenne-Becker muscular dystrophies) are always inherited as recessive traits, i.e., they occur only in males, who transmit the gene on the X chromosome to all their daughters (carriers) but to none of their sons. Carrier women transmit the gene to their offspring (with a 50 percent risk that a son will have the disease and that a daughter will be a carrier). In suspected instances of this type of dystrophy, it is important to examine the status of the male relatives of the mother and also the possible female carriers.

Diseases that are inherited as *autosomal dominant* traits (e.g., myotonic dystrophy) affect males and females equally. The disease is transmitted from one affected (usually heterozygous) parent to an affected child. Each child has a 50 percent chance of inheriting the gene. In cases of dominant inheritance the expression of disease is often variable and mild degrees of it, undiagnosed, may be found in other members of the family.

In *autosomal recessive* muscle diseases, males and females also are affected equally but here the abnormal gene is inherited from *both* parents; the latter are heterozygous carriers who show no signs of the disease. For this reason, the history of a consanguineous marriage or a common ethnic or geographic background of the parents should be sought (see Thompson).

The clinical recognition of myopathic diseases is facilitated by a prior knowledge of a few syndromes. The ones listed in Table 48-2 occur with regularity. A description of these syndromes and the diseases of which they are a manifestation forms the content of the chapters that follow. Diagnostic accuracy is aided by the intelligent use of laboratory examinations, such as chemical analyses of serum and urine, electromyography, nerve conduction studies, and muscle biopsy. These procedures and the principles underlying them are discussed in Chap. 45.

Table 48-2
Syndromic classification of muscle diseases

I. Acute (evolving in days) or subacute (weeks)
paretic or paralytic disorders of muscle*
  A. Rarely fulminant myasthenia gravis
  or myathenic syndrome from a "mycin" antibiotic
  or hypokalemia
  B. Idiopathic polymyositis and dermatomyositis
  C. Viral polymyositis
  D. Acute paroxysmal myoglobinuria
  E. "Alcoholic" polymyopathy
  F. Familial (malignant) hyperpyrexia precipitated
  by anesthetic agents
  G. First attack of episodic weakness may enter
  into differential diagnosis (see below)
  H. Botulism
  I. Organophosphate poisoning

II. Chronic (i.e., months to years) weakness or paralysis
of muscle usually with severe atrophy
  A. Progressive muscular dystrophy
    1. Duchenne type
    2. Facioscapulohumeral type (Landouzy-Déjerine)
    3. Limb-girdle types
    4. Distal type (Gowers, Welander)
    5. Myotonic dystrophy
    6. Progressive ophthalmoplegic, oculopharyngeal,
    and Kearns-Sayre types
  B. Chronic idiopathic polymyositis (may be subacute)
  C. Chronic thyrotoxic and other endocrine myopathies
  D. Chronic, slowly progressive, or relatively
  stationary polymyopathies†
    1. Central core and multicore diseases
    2. Rod-body and related polymyopathies
    3. Mitochondrial and centronuclear polymyopathies
    4. Other congenital myopathies (reducing-body,
    fingerprint, zebra body, fiber-type atrophies and
    disproportions)
    5. Glycogen storage disease
    6. Lipid myopathies (carnitine deficiency
    myopathy, undefined lipid myopathies)

III. Episodic weakness of muscle
  A. Familial (hypokalemic) periodic paralysis
  B. Normokalemic or hyperkalemic familial periodic
  paralysis
  C. Paramyotonia congenita (von Eulenberg)
  D. Nonfamilial hyper- and hypokalemic periodic
  paralysis (including primary hyperaldosteronism)
  E. Acute thyrotoxic myopathy (also thyrotoxic
  periodic paralysis)
  F. Conditions in which weakness fluctuates
    1. Myasthenia gravis, immunologic type
    2. Myasthenia associated with:

      a. Lupus erythematosus disseminatus
      b. Polymyositis
      c. Rheumatoid arthritis
      d. Nonthymic carcinoma
    3. Familial and sporadic nonimmunologic types of
    myasthenia
    4. Myasthemia due to antibiotics and other drugs
    5. Lambert-Eaton syndrome

IV. Disorders of muscle presenting with myotonia,
stiffness, spasm, and cramp
  A. Congenital myotonia (Thomsen disease),
  paramyotonia congenita, myotonic dystrophy,
  and Schwartz-Jampel syndrome
  B. Hypothyroidism with pseudomyotonia (Debré-
  Semelaigne and Hoffmann syndromes)
  C. Tetany
  D. Tetanus
  E. Black widow spider bite
  F. Myopathy resulting from myophosphorylase defi-
  ciency (McArdle syndrome), phosphofructokinase
  deficiency, and other forms of contracture
  G. Contracture with Addison disease
  H. Idiopathic cramp syndromes
  I. Myokymia and syndromes of continuous muscle
  activity

V. Myalgic states‡
  A. Connective tissue diseases (rheumatoid arthritis,
  mixed connective tissue disease, Sjögren syndrome,
  lupus erythematosus, polyarteritis nodosa,
  scleroderma, polymyositis)
  B. Localized fibrositis or fibromyositis
  C. Trichinosis
  D. Myopathy of myoglobinuria and McArdle
  syndrome
  E. Myopathy with hypoglycemia
  F. Bornholm disease and other forms of viral
  polymyositis
  G. Anterior tibial syndrome
  H. Other
    1. Hypophosphatemia
    2. Hypothyroidism
    3. Psychiatric illness (hysteria, depression)

VI. Localized muscle mass(es)
  A. Rupture of a muscle
  B. Muscle hemorrhage
  C. Muscle tumor
    1. Rhabdomyosarcoma
    2. Desmoid
    3. Angioma
    4. Metastatic nodules

Table 48-2 (*continued*)
Syndromic classification of muscle diseases

D. Monomyositis multiplex
  1. Eosinophilic type
  2. Other
E. Localized and generalized myositis
  ossificans
F. Fibrositis (myogelosis)
	G. Granulomatous infections
	  1. Sarcoidosis
	  2. Tuberculosis
	  3. Wegener granulomatosis
	H. Pyogenic abscess
	I. Infarction of muscle in the diabetic

*The acute and subacute primary disorders of muscle need to be differentiated from acute spinal cord or peripheral nerve diseases, in which paralysis is often severe and widespread and atrophy may or may not be present (poliomyelitis, acute idiopathic polyneuritis, or other forms of polyneuropathy; see Chap. 46).

†The chronic myopathies need to be distinguished from the progressive muscular atrophies and other forms of motor system disease (amyotrophic lateral sclerosis, progressive bulbar palsy) and infantile spinal muscular atrophy (Werdnig-Hoffmann disease), as well as chronic neural muscular atrophies such as peroneal muscular atrophy (Charcot-Marie-Tooth), hypertrophic polyneuritis (Déjerine-Sottas), amyloid polyneuropathy, chronic nutritional, arsenical, leprous, and other polyneuropathies (see Chap. 46).

‡Pain and tenderness of muscle are characteristic also of many forms of polyneuropathy (see Chap. 46).

REFERENCES

ADAMS RD: Thayer lectures: I. Principles of myopathology. II. Principles of clinical myology. *Johns Hopkins Med J* 131:24, 1972.

ADAMS RD, KAKULAS BA: *Diseases of Muscle: Pathological Foundations of Clinical Myology,* 4th ed. Philadelphia, Harper and Row, 1985.

ANDRÉ-THOMAS, CHESNI Y, DARGASSIES ST. ANNE S: The neurological examination of the infant, in MacKeith RC, Polani PE, Clayton-Jones E (eds): *Little Club Clinics in Developmental Medicine,* No. 1. London, National Spastics Society, 1960.

ARMSTRONG RB: Mechanisms of exercise-induced, delayed onset muscular soreness. A brief review. *Med Sci Sports Exerc* 16:529, 1984.

BETHLEM J: *Myopathies.* Philadelphia, Lippincott, 1977.

BROOKE MH: *A Clinician's View of Neuromuscular Diseases,* 2nd ed. Baltimore, Williams & Wilkins, 1986.

DUBOWITZ V: *Muscle Disorders in Childhood.* Philadelphia, Saunders, 1978.

DUDLEY MA, DUDLEY AW, Bernstein LH et al: Biochemical aspects of a new familial myopathy. *J Neuropathol Exp Neurol* 37:609, 1979.

EDWARDS RHT: New techniques for studying human muscle function, metabolism and fatigue. *Muscle Nerve* 7:599, 1984.

ENGEL AG, BANKER BQ (eds): *Myology.* New York, McGraw-Hill, 1986.

GOWERS WR: A lecture on myopathy, a distal form. *Br Med J* 2:89, 1902.

KUGELBERG E, WELANDER L: Hereofamilial juvenile muscular atrophy simulating muscular dystrophy. *Arch Neurol Psychiatry* 75:500, 1956.

MIELKE U, RICKER K, EMSER W, BOXLER K: Unilateral calf enlargement following S1 radiculopathy. *Muscle Nerve* 5:434, 1982.

THOMPSON MW: The genetic transmission of muscle diseases. In Engel AG, Banker BQ (eds). *Myology.* New York, McGraw-Hill 1986, pp 1151–1179.

WALTON JN (ed): *Disorders of Voluntary Muscle,* 5th ed. Edinburgh, Churchill Livingstone, 1988.

WELANDER L: Myopathia distalis tarda hereditaria. *Acta Med Scand* 141(suppl 265):1, 1951.

WOHLFART G, FEX J, ELIASSON S: Hereditary proximal spinal muscle atrophy simulating progressive muscular dystrophy. *Acta Psychiatr Neurol* 30:395, 1955.

CHAPTER 49

POLYMYOSITIS AND OTHER ACUTE AND SUBACUTE MYOPATHIC PARALYSES

Of importance from a diagnostic standpoint is the principle that primary diseases of muscle seldom if ever are the cause of acute, widespread paralysis. Diffuse paralytic states of rapid evolution, i.e., over the period of a few days, are usually due to idiopathic polyneuritis (Guillain-Barré syndrome) and infrequently to poliomyelitis and other neuritides; one must also consider certain spinal cord diseases (Chaps. 36 and 46). Nevertheless, there are exceptions to this clinical rule, the most notable being disorders of neuromuscular transmission. For example, botulinum toxin can paralyze muscles within a few hours by blocking acetylcholine (ACh) release. Rarely, myasthenia gravis or a myasthenic syndrome related to aminoglycoside antibiotic therapy may develop over several days, or a week or two. In a thyroid "storm" there may be a widespread weakness of muscles, the defect evidently being in the contractile mechanism of the muscle fibers. Hypokalemic paralysis as in hyperaldosteronism and the initial attack of familial periodic paralysis due to either hypo- or hyperkalemia may come on within a few hours. Finally, a paroxysm of myoglobinuria, due to an infection or a metabolic myopathy, especially if there is unusually strenuous exertion, may be followed within hours by a rapidly developing paresis of limb muscles, usually in association with pain in the muscles.

Thus the occurrence of acute paralysis raises the consideration more of neurologic than of myologic disease. In the relatively rare instances of the latter, diagnostic suspicions are affirmed by measurements of electrolytes, muscle enzymes [creatine kinase (CK) and aldolase], and thyroid hormones in the serum, by nerve conduction studies and needle examination of muscles, and by urinary analysis for myoglobin.

Pareses of widespread distribution and subacute evolution (over the period of a few weeks) are attributable to a wider spectrum of diseases, some clearly myologic, such as infective and idiopathic polymyositis and dermatomyo-

sitis and several of the metabolic polymyopathies. These are the subject material of this chapter.

THE INFECTIVE (AND PRESUMABLY INFECTIVE) FORMS OF POLYMYOSITIS

TRICHINOSIS

The main features of this infection have been discussed in Chap. 32 (page 585). With respect to the myopathic aspect of the illness, the authors have been most impressed with the ocular muscle weakness which results in strabismus and diplopia; with weakness of the tongue, resulting in dysarthria; and weakness of the masseter and pharyngeal muscles, which interferes with chewing and swallowing. The involved muscles are slightly swollen and tender in the acute stage of the disease, and there is conjunctival, orbital and facial edema. As the trichinae become encysted, over a period of a few weeks, the symptoms subside, and recovery is complete. Many, perhaps the majority, of the infected patients are asymptomatic throughout the invasive period and as much as 1 to 3 percent of the population in certain regions of the country will be found at autopsy to have calcified cysts in the muscles, with no history of parasitic illness. Heavy infestations may end fatally, usually from cardiac and diaphragmatic involvement. In the more massive infections the brain may be involved, probably by emboli that arise in the heart, from an associated myocarditis (Chap. 32).

Clinically, one should always suspect the disease in a patient who presents with a puffy face and tender muscles. The diagnosis is always suggested by an eosinophilia (>700 per cubic millimeter), and there are many eosinophils in the muscle infiltrates. A skin test using trichina antigen is available, but it only turns positive in the third week of the disease. Precipitin, complement fixation, and bentonite flocculation tests are also available. Biopsy of almost any muscle (usually the deltoid or gastrocnemius), regardless of whether they are painful or tender, is the most reliable method of diagnosis. Both fiber types are invaded. The EMG may exhibit profuse fibrillations, probably because of the disconnection of segments of muscle fibers from their end plates (Gross and Ochoa).

No treatment is required in most cases. If the infestation is severe, thiabendazole 25 to 50 mg/kg daily in divided doses for 5 to 10 days and prednisone 40 to 60 mg/day, are recommended.

TOXOPLASMOSIS

An acute to subacute systemic illness due to the encephalitozoon toxoplasma, with some indication of retinal, myocardial, liver, and brain involvement, has occasionally been encountered in adults. In one such case we detected toxoplasma organisms and pseudocysts in skeletal muscle. Wherever the pseudocysts had ruptured, there was focal inflammation. Some muscle fibers had undergone segmental necrosis, but this was not prominent, accounting for the relative paucity of muscle symptoms. In fact, most infections with toxoplasma which occur in 10 to 30 percent of the population, are asymptomatic. The immunocompromised patient is particularly susceptible. Sulfadiazine, in combination with pyrimethamine or trisulfapyrimidine, which act synergistically against the toxoplasma trophozoites, are effective therapeutic agents. See Chap. 32 for further discussion.

OTHER PROTOZOAN AND FUNGAL INFECTIONS

Sarcosporoidosis, echinococcosis, cysticercosis, trypanosomiasis (Chagas disease), sparganosis, toxocariasis, actinomycosis, tuberculosis, and syphilis are all known to affect skeletal muscle on occasion, but the major symptoms relate more to involvement of other organs. Only cysticercosis may first claim the attention of the clinical myologist, because of a dramatic pseudohypertrophy of thigh and calf muscles. Hydatids infest paravertebral and lumbar girdle muscles in 5 percent of cases. Coenurosis and sparganosis are causes of moveable lumps in the rectus abdominis, thigh, calf, and pectoralis muscles. The reader who seeks more details may refer to the monograph on muscle diseases by Adams and Kakulas, and the chapter by Banker (see references).

VIRAL INFECTIONS

Most patients with pleurodynia (epidemic myalgia, Bornholm disease) have had negative muscle biopsies, and there is no clear explanation of the pain. However, group B Coxsackie virus has been isolated from striated muscle of patients with this disorder. In recent years a number of patients with viral influenza were found to have a necrotizing myositis, and virus was seen under the electron microscope in infected muscle fibers. Malaise, myalgia, slight weakness and stiffness were the reported clinical manifestations. From the descriptions it seems difficult to decide how much of the weakness was only apparent, because of the myalgia. Recovery was complete within a few weeks. In one patient with generalized myalgia and myoglobinuria, the influenza virus was isolated from muscle (Gamboa et al). These observations suggest that the intense muscle pain in certain viral illnesses might be due to a direct viral infection of muscle. However, there are many cases of influenzal myalgia, mainly of the calves and thighs, such as those reported by Lundberg and more recently by Antony et al, in which it was not possible to establish a cause of the muscular disorder. Also, in the disorder described as *epidemic neuromyasthenia* (benign myalgic encephalomyelitis, Icelandic disease)—in which influenza-like symptoms were combined with severe pain and weakness of muscles—a viral cause was postulated, but a virus has never been isolated (Johnson).

Viral myositis is an established entity in comparative myopathology. Echo 9, adenovirus 21, herpes simplex, the Epstein-Barr virus, and *Mycoplasma pneumoniae* are cited by Mastaglia and Ojeda as causes of myositis with rhabdomyolysis in humans. In our experience, other aspects of these infections are predominant, and the evidence of viral invasion of muscle has not been fully substantiated. In most instances the nonspecific Zenker degeneration could have explained the findings. Unsettled also is the existence of a postinfectious polymyositis.

SARCOIDOSIS

Patients with sarcoidosis may develop a polyneuritis or mononeuritis multiplex (Chap. 46) or, less frequently, a granulomatous meningoencephalitis or -myelitis (Chaps. 32 and 36). Much more puzzling to the authors, however, have been patients with an illness, the clinical features of which are virtually indistinguishable from those of idiopathic polymyositis, described further on; but the muscle biopsy reveals inflammation with Langhans giant cells or a noncaseating granulomatous lesion. Several of the reported cases have been middle-aged or elderly adults with no signs of sarcoidosis of the nervous system, lungs, bone, skin, or lymph nodes.

The question is whether such lesions in myositic

muscle are a sufficient basis for the diagnosis of sarcoidosis. We doubt that they are, but the matter cannot be settled until we have better laboratory tests than are now available. At present we prefer to designate these cases as granulomatous myositis and suspect that they have several clinical associations. In one syndrome, described by Namba et al, this type of myositis was combined with myasthenia gravis, myocarditis, and thyroiditis. It has on a few occasions been associated with Crohn disease. Electron microscopy in some instances has disclosed muscle fiber invasion by lymphocytes, suggesting a cell-mediated immune reaction (Matsubara).

IDIOPATHIC POLYMYOSITIS AND DERMATOMYOSITIS

DEFINITION

These are relatively common diseases that affect primarily the striated muscle and skin, and sometimes connective tissues as well. The term used varies according to the distribution of the pathologic process. If restricted clinically to the striated muscles, the disease is called polymyositis (PM); if the skin is involved, it is designated as dermatomyositis (DM); and if connective tissues also are implicated, the term of choice is PM or DM with rheumatoid arthritis, rheumatic fever, lupus erythematosus, scleroderma, or mixed connective tissue disease (also referred to as the ''overlap group'').

Polymyositis was first described by Wagner in 1863, and the dermatomyositic form was established as an entity by Wagner and by Unverricht in a series of articles written from 1887 to 1891. A survey of the literature since that time can be found in the monograph of Adams and Kakulas.

CLINICAL MANIFESTATIONS

Polymyositis and dermatomyositis tend to assume several clinical forms, as follows:

Polymyositis *A subacute symmetric weakness of proximal limb and trunk muscles without dermatitis.* The onset is usually insidious and the course progressive over a period of several weeks or months. The disease may develop at almost any age and in either sex. However, the majority of patients range from 30 to 60 years of age and a smaller group has a peak incidence at 15 years. Females outnumber males two to one. A febrile illness or benign infection may

precede the muscle weakness, but in most patients the first symptoms develop in the absence of these or other apparent initiating events.

The patient first becomes aware of a painless weakness of the proximal limb muscles, especially of the hips and thighs and to a lesser extent the shoulder girdles. Certain actions, such as arising from a deep chair or from a squatting or kneeling position, climbing or descending stairs, walking, putting an object on a high shelf, or combing the hair, become increasingly difficult. In restricted forms of the disease only the neck muscles or quadriceps may be involved. Pain of an aching variety in the buttocks, calves, or shoulders is experienced by only about 15 percent of patients and often indicates a combination of polymyositis and arthritis or other connective tissue disease.

When the patient is first seen, all the muscles of the trunk, shoulders, hips, upper arms, and thighs are usually involved. The facial, posterior and anterior neck muscles (the head may loll), the pharyngeal and laryngeal muscles (dysphagia and dysphonia) are usually involved as well. Ocular muscles are never affected except in the rare patient with both polymyositis and myasthenia gravis; and the forearm, hand, leg, and foot muscles are spared in all but 25 percent of cases. Occasionally the symptoms at first predominate in one limb, before becoming generalized. The muscles are usually not tender, and atrophy and reduction in tendon reflexes, though present, are not so pronounced as in cases of chronic denervation atrophy. When reflexes are disproportionately reduced, one must think of carcinomatosis with polymyositis and neuropathy or other more obscure forms of neuromyositis. The skin and mucous membranes and joints are unchanged.

In our cases of PM (and DM) a surprising number of cardiac abnormalities have been observed. Most of these were relatively minor ECG changes, but several patients have had arrhythmias of significance. Among the fatal cases about half showed clinical evidence of severe cardiac disease and had necrosis of myocardial fibers at autopsy, usually with only modest inflammatory changes. As a rule, evidence of systemic infection is absent. Exceptionally there is a low-grade fever, especially if joint pain coexists, and a patch or a few patches of dermatitis may be present at one stage of the illness.

Dermatomyositis The skin changes may precede, accompany, or follow the muscle syndrome and take the form of a localized or diffuse erythema, maculopapular eruption, scaling eczematoid dermatitis, or even an exfoliative dermatitis. Particularly characteristic is a lilac-colored (heliotrope) change in the skin over the bridge of the nose, cheeks, forehead, and around the fingernails. Itching may be troublesome in some cases. Periorbital and perioral edema are common findings particularly in more fulminating episodes. The skin lesions are observed frequently over the extensor surfaces of joints (elbows, knuckles and knees), particularly in childhood. The skin changes are quite transient in some cases, and in others they consist of only a patch or more of dermatitis. These evanescent and restricted manifestations are emphasized because they are frequently overlooked, and may provide the clues to diagnosis in otherwise difficult cases.

In the healing stage, the skin lesions become whitened and atrophic, with a flat, scaly base. Periarticular and subcutaneous calcification may occur but is not common except in the childhood form. Signs of other connective tissue diseases are more frequent than in examples of pure PM. The limb weakness is usually proximal but may be diffuse, i.e., distal and proximal, just as in PM. The Raynaud phenomenon is reported in nearly a third of the patients. Others will develop a mild form of scleroderma. Esophageal weakness may be demonstrated by fluoroscopy in approximately 30 percent of all patients. The superior constrictors of the pharynx are involved almost universally, but careful analysis by cinefluorography may be required to demonstrate the abnormality.

Connective Tissue Diseases with Polymyositis and Dermatomyositis

One-third to one-half of our cases of myositis, and particularly of DM, have occurred in patients who have or have had symptoms of rheumatoid arthritis, scleroderma, lupus erythematosus or mixtures of the aforementioned diseases (mixed connective tissue disease). The Sjögren syndrome (keratoconjunctivitis sicca, xerostomia, and rheumatoid arthritis) may also be associated. In these connective tissue diseases, the incidence of PM-DM is not high. A true necrotizing-inflammatory myopathy has been reported in only 8 percent of cases of lupus erythematosus, and an even smaller proportion of cases of systemic sclerosis, rheumatoid arthritis, and Sjögren syndrome. The treatment of rheumatoid arthritis with D-penicillamine is believed to increase the incidence of PM-DM.

In this so-called overlap group, there is greater muscular weakness and atrophy than can be accounted for by the original disease. Inasmuch as arthritis may limit motion because of pain, result in disuse atrophy, and cause mono- or polyneuritis, the interpretation of diminished strength in this disease is not easy. Sometimes diagnosis must depend on muscle biopsy, EMG findings, and measurements of muscle enzymes in the serum. Malaise, aches, and pains may be the only symptoms in the early stages of the disease. In these complicated cases the myositis may accompany the connective tissue disease or occur many years later.

Carcinoma with Polymyositis or Dermatomyositis

This syndrome is placed in a separate category, although the muscle and skin changes are indistinguishable from those described above. In different series, from 8 to 30 percent of all adults with DM (less often with PM), are found to have a carcinoma or some other tumor; if DM appears after the age of 40 years, the proportion of patients with carcinoma is higher. The neoplastic syndrome is slightly more frequent in men than in women and is linked most often with carcinomas of the breast and ovary in women and with lung and colon in men. The tumors, however, have arisen in nearly every organ of the body. The muscle and skin tissues show no tumor cells. In about half the cases, the PM-DM antedates the clinical manifestations of the malignancy, sometimes by 1 or 2 years. The relationship is not understood.

Dermatomyositis of Childhood

Idiopathic PM occurs in children, but much less frequently than in adults. Some of the myositic illnesses in children are relatively benign and do not differ from those in adults. Far more common in children is a distinctive syndrome, first described by Banker and Victor, which is generally designated as dermatomyositis, but which differs in many respects from the adult form of the disease. The childhood form of DM is equally distributed between the sexes. It begins as a rule with rather typical skin changes, accompanied by anorexia and fatigue. Erythematous discoloration of the upper eyelids, frequently with edema, is a particularly characteristic initial sign. The erythema spreads to involve the periorbital regions, nose, malar areas, and upper lip, as well as the skin over the knuckles, elbows, and knees. Symptoms of weakness, stiffness, and pain in the muscles usually follow but may precede the skin manifestations. The muscular weakness is generalized, but always more severe in the muscles of the shoulders and hips and proximal portions of the limbs. A tiptoe gait, the result of flexion contractures at the ankles, is a common abnormality. Tendon reflexes are depressed or abolished, commensurate with the degree of muscle weakness. Intermittent low-grade fever, substernal and abdominal pain (like that of peptic ulcer), melena, and hematemesis are common symptoms.

The mode of progression of DM of childhood, like that of the adult form, is variable. In some cases, the weakness advances rapidly, involving all the muscles—including those of chewing, swallowing, talking, and breathing—and leading to total incapacitation. Perforation of the gastrointestinal tract (with or without the contributing effects of steroids or gastric intubation) is usually the immediate cause of death. In other patients there is slow progression or arrest of the disease process, and in a small number there may be a remission of muscle weakness. Flexion contractures at the elbows, hips, knees, and ankles, and subcutaneous calcification and ulceration of the overlying skin, with extrusion of calcific debris, are common manifestations in chronic cases.

LABORATORY FINDINGS

In all forms of PM and DM, regardless of the clinical associations, the serum levels of the transaminases and other tissue enzymes such as CK and aldolase are elevated in the majority of cases. Serum alpha$_2$ and gamma globulin values may be increased. Tests for circulating rheumatoid factor (latex fixation and sensitized sheep cell procedure) and antinuclear antibody reactions (as in lupus erythematosus) are positive in fewer than half the cases. Myoglobinuria is found in the majority of patients with acute and severe muscle affection, providing a sensitive immunoassay procedure is used. The sedimentation rate may be normal or elevated. Lupus erythematosus preparations of blood smears are negative in 90 to 95 percent of cases. The EMG discloses a typical "myopathic pattern," i.e., many abnormally brief action potentials of low voltage and, in addition, numerous fibrillation potentials and salvos of pseudomyotonic activity (see Chap. 45). As stated, the ECG has been abnormal in many of our cases. The muscle biopsy, if taken from an affected muscle, usually demonstrates the typical pathologic changes of the disease.

PATHOLOGIC CHANGES

The principal changes in idiopathic PM consist of widespread destruction of segments of muscle fibers, with the expected cellular reaction thereto—phagocytosis (myophages) and infiltration with inflammatory cells (lymphocytes, mononuclear leukocytes, plasma cells, and rare neutrophilic leukocytes). Evidence of regenerative activity in the form of proliferating sarcolemmal nuclei, basophilic (ribonucleic acid–rich) sarcoplasm, and new myofibrils is almost invariable. Many of the residual muscle fibers are small, with increased numbers of sarcolemmal nuclei. Either the degeneration of muscle fibers or the infiltrations of inflammatory cells may predominate in any given biopsy specimen, though at autopsy both types of change are in evidence.

Probably because of sampling error, only part of the complex of pathologic changes may be divulged in any one biopsy specimen. There may be necrosis and phagocytosis of individual muscle fibers without infiltrates of inflam-

matory cells, or the reverse may be observed. Repeated attacks of a necrotizing myositis appear to exhaust the regenerative potential of the muscles so that fiber loss, fibrosis, and residual thin and large fibers in haphazard arrangement may eventually impart a dystrophic aspect to the lesions. For all these reasons the pathologic picture can be correctly interpreted only in relation to the clinical and other laboratory data.

In patients with skin lesions, i.e., dermatomyositis, there are several distinctive histopathologic changes. In contrast to the single fiber necrosis of PM, DM is characterized by perifascicular muscle fiber degeneration and atrophy of muscle fibers, and, electron microscopically, by the presence of tubular aggregates in the endothelial cells. Moreover, the inflammatory infiltrates in DM are primarily in the perimysial connective tissue, whereas in PM they are more prominent in relation to the muscle fiber membrane and to the endomysium.

The muscle lesions in dermatomyositis of childhood are similar to those of the adult form, only greatly accentuated. Perifascicular degeneration and atrophy of muscle fibers are particularly prominent. The fundamental changes are in the small intramuscular blood vessels. Vasculitis, endothelial alterations (tubular aggregates in the endothelial cytoplasm), and occlusion of vessels by fibrin thrombi are the main abnormalities. Occlusion of small vessels also involves the intrafascicular nerves, so that the affected muscle may show both zones of infarction and denervation atrophy. The same vascular changes underlie the lesions in the connective tissue of skin, subcutaneous tissue, and gastrointestinal tract.

ETIOLOGY AND PATHOGENESIS

The cause of idiopathic PM and DM, as the term indicates, is unknown. All attempts to isolate an infective agent have been unsuccessful. Several electron microscopists have observed particles in muscle fibers, resembling viruses, but their causative role has not been proved. Consistent rises of antibody titers have not been demonstrated, nor has a polymyositic illness been induced in animals by injections of affected muscle.

That an autoimmune mechanism might be operative in PM and DM was suggested by the association of these disorders with a number of other autoimmune diseases, such as myasthenia gravis, Hashimoto thyroiditis, scleroderma, Waldenstrom macroglobulinemia, monoclonal gammopathy, and agammaglobulinemia. Immunopathologic studies have substantiated this idea and have indicated further that PM and DM can be distinguished from one another on the basis of their autoimmune characteristics. In DM, immune complexes—IgG, IgM, and complement (C3)—and membrane-attack complexes are deposited in the walls of venules and arterioles, suggesting that the immune response is directed primarily against intramuscular blood vessels (Whitaker and Engel; Kissel et al); such a response is lacking in PM. Also, Engel and Arahata have demonstrated a difference between the two disorders on the basis of localization and quantitation of the subsets of lymphocytes that comprise the intramuscular inflammatory aggregates. In PM, the endomysial inflammatory exudate was found to contain a large number of T cells, T8 + cells, and activated T cells, whereas B cells were sparse; T cells, accompanied by macrophages, enclosed and invaded nonnecrotic muscle fibers. In DM, very few fibers were similarly affected, and the percentage of B cells at all sites was significantly higher than in PM. These observations, coupled with the morphologic differences described above, strongly suggest that in DM the effector response is predominantly humeral, whereas in PM the injury is mediated by T cells, clones of which had been sensitized to a muscle fiber–associated surface antigen.

The autoimmune basis of PM has been corroborated by animal experimental studies. When splenic cells, sensitized in vitro to syngeneic skeletal muscle, were injected into the syngeneic mouse, a myopathy, characterized by single muscle fiber necrosis and endomysial and perimysial inflammatory cells, was produced (Hart et al). These findings indicate a sensitized T-cell-mediated attack upon the muscle fiber, similar to that in human PM.

DIAGNOSIS

This is secure if there is rapidly evolving proximal weakness with dysphagia and dysphonia (with or without dermatitis), typical changes in the muscle biopsy, EMG abnormalities of myopathic type with fibrillations, and elevated serum levels of CK. All these criteria are satisfied in only 25 to 30 percent of our cases, even in those responsive to steroids. One must often accept the diagnosis, therefore, when only part of the criteria are met.

The following problems arise repeatedly in connection with the diagnosis of polymyositis:

1. *The patient with proximal muscle weakness incorrectly diagnosed as progressive muscular dystrophy.* Points in favor of polymyositis are (*a*) lack of family history, (*b*) older age at onset, (*c*) more rapid evolution of weakness, (*d*) evidence, past or present, of other connective tissue diseases, (*e*) high serum CK and aldolase values, (*f*) many fibrillation potentials in EMG, (*g*) marked degeneration and regeneration in muscle biopsy and finally, if there is still doubt, (*h*) unmistakable improvement with corticosteroid therapy.

2. *The patient with a connective tissue disease (rheumatoid arthritis, scleroderma, lupus erythematosus)* suspected of having polymyositis in addition. Pain in rheumatoid arthritis prevents strong exertion (algesic pseudoparesis). Points against the coexistence of polymyositis are (*a*) lack of weakness out of proportion to muscle atrophy, (*b*) normal EMG, (*c*) normal serum CK and aldolase, and (*d*) normal muscle biopsy, except possibly for infiltrations of chronic inflammatory cells in the endomysial and perimysial connective tissue (interstitial nodular myositis). Also, polymyalgia rheumatica must be differentiated. This syndrome is characterized by pain, stiffness, and tenderness in the muscles of the neck and shoulders and arms, and sometimes of the hips and thighs; biopsy of the temporal artery frequently discloses a giant-cell arteritis (see page 678). Rapid disappearance of pain with administration of prednisone is also diagnostic.

3. *The patient with restricted muscle weakness.* Weakness or paralysis of the posterior neck muscles, with inability to hold up the head, restricted bilateral quadriceps weakness, and other limited pelvicrural palsies are examples. Most often, the head-hanging or lolling syndrome proves to be due to polymyositis, and the other syndromes to restricted forms of dystrophy and neural atrophy. Muscle enzymes in the serum may be relatively normal. EMG and biopsy are helpful in diagnosis.

4. *The patient with diffuse myalgia and fatigability.* Features that exclude a polymyositis are (*a*) lack of reduced peak power of contraction and (*b*) normal EMG, serum enzymes, and muscle biopsy. Hypothyroidism, McArdle disease, hyperparathyroidism, steroid myopathy, adrenal insufficiency, hyperinsulinemia, and early rheumatoid arthritis must be ruled out by appropriate studies (see Chap. 51). Most of our patients with diffuse myalgia and fatigability have proved to be neurasthenic or depressed, rarely myopathic.

5. *The patient with a clinical picture of polymyositis,* in whom the muscle biopsy discloses a noncaseating granulomatous reaction consistent with sarcoid. More than 25 such cases have been reported.

TREATMENT

The following program is recommended:

1. *Prednisone,* 60 mg in three or four divided doses per day. Once recovery begins, as judged by careful tests of strength and serum enzyme levels, the dosage is reduced gradually, in steps of 5 mg every 2 to 3 weeks; when the dosage has been reduced to 20 mg daily, it is best to give

double this amount (i.e., 40 mg) on alternate days. After cautious reduction of prednisone over a period of 6 months to a year or longer, the patient can usually be maintained on doses of 7.5 to 20 mg daily. Corticosteroids should not be discontinued prematurely, for the relapse that may follow is often more difficult to treat than the original symptoms.

2. *Physiotherapy:* gentle massage, passive movement and stretching of affected muscles, followed by "resistance exercises" as strength returns and evidence of activity (elevated serum enzyme concentrations) subside.

All patients receiving corticosteroids and aspirin need to be protected by the liberal administration of potassium and antacids. Elderly patients in particular should be examined periodically for signs of malignancy.

Very few measures, other than the aforementioned, are of proven value in the treatment of polymyositis. Some patients who are refractory to prednisone may respond favorably to methotrexate (25 to 30 mg intravenously each week) or to oral azathioprine in doses of 150 to 300 mg/day, making certain to keep the WBC level above 3000 per cubic millimeter. Preferably the methotrexate or azathiaprine should be given along with relatively small daily doses (15 to 25 mg) of prednisone. Some clinicians favor, from the beginning, a combination of prednisone in low dosage and one of the immunosuppressant drugs. Cyclophosphamide is a useful drug in the treatment of Wegener granulomatosis, periarteritis, and perhaps other vasculitides, but is of little value in PM. Cyclosporin has also been used in recalcitrant cases, but its efficacy and safety are still under study. Vitamin E, or alpha tocopherol, which was used extensively in the past, is of no proven benefit.

PROGNOSIS

Only a small proportion of patients with PM succumb to the disease, and then usually from a pulmonary or cardiac complication. The majority improve with corticosteroid therapy. The period of activity of disease is usually around 2 years in both the childhood and adult groups, but many are left with varying degrees of weakness of the shoulders and hips. Approximately 20 percent of our patients have recovered completely, and long-term remissions have been achieved in about an equal number. The extent of recovery is roughly proportional to the acuteness and severity of the disease and the duration of symptoms prior to institution of therapy. Patients with acute or subacute PM, in whom treatment is begun soon after the onset of symptoms, have the best prognosis. In the series of deVere and Bradley, in

which patients were treated early, there was remission in over 50 percent of cases, whereas in the patients of Riddoch and Morgan-Hughes, treated more than 2 years after onset of the disease, the remission rate was considerably lower. Even in patients with a coexistent malignancy, muscle weakness may lessen and serum enzyme levels decline in response to corticosteroid therapy, but weakness returns after a few months, and may then be resistant to further treatment. If the tumor is successfully removed, the muscle symptoms remit.

The mortality after several years ranges about 15 percent, being higher in childhood DM, PM with connective tissue diseases, and, of course, with malignancy.

INCLUSION-BODY MYOSITIS

In 1965, one of the authors, with Kakulas and Samaha, described an example of inclusion-body myositis. Our patient was a 20-year-old man with a steadily progressive polymyopathy, involving mainly the pelvicrural muscles, but also the distal muscles of the legs. He was wheelchair-bound within 1 to 2 years and eventually required a cardiac pacemaker. Serum CK was only slightly elevated. He did not respond to large doses of steroids and succumbed to the disease after a protracted course. Several muscle biopsies during life disclosed intranuclear and intracytoplasmic inclusions, comprised of masses of filaments and subsarcolemmal whorls of membranes, combined with fiber necrosis, cellular infiltrates and regeneration. Since the original report, many cases, conforming to this clinical-pathologic picture, have been described (see Mikol for references). One of the larger series was recorded by Carpenter et al, who emphasized the greater frequency in males, the more generalized distribution of weakness in the upper and lower limbs (the upper limbs may be affected first), the muscle atrophy, and the rarity of dysphagia. Many of their patients were elderly. The filamentous inclusions have suggested a viral origin, but a virus has never been isolated and serologic studies have failed to substantiate a viral causation except for one patient in whom adenovirus type 2 was isolated from a biopsy specimen (Mikol). In inclusion-body myositis, as in PM, the injury to muscle appears to be T-cell-mediated. There is no effective treatment. Only a few have improved while receiving full doses of steroids.

OTHER FORMS OF IDIOPATHIC POLYMYOSITIS

Granulomatous myositis, giant-cell myositis with thymoma, and myositis with Wegener granulomatosis and with glomerulonephritis have all had isolated case documentation, but the data are too fragmentary to permit delineation of particular subgroups (see Banker). Exceptions are eosinophilic myositis and orbital myositis, which are described below.

EOSINOPHILIC MYOSITIS

This term has been applied to three separable but possibly overlapping clinical entities: (1) eosinophilic fasciitis, (2) eosinophilic monomyositis (sometimes multiplex), and (3) eosinophilic polymyositis.

Eosinophilic fasciitis is a rare entity in which an otherwise healthy individual develops a tenosynovitis manifested by local pain, stiffness, and eventual limitation of movement. One muscle after another is affected in a particular region of the body, such as the forearm and hand. Biopsy of the tendon sheath and fascia of the muscle reveals an intense inflammatory reaction with eosinophilic leukocytes predominating in the infiltrates. The muscle per se is not involved; the EMG is negative and the CK is normal. In the two cases we have seen there was no eosinophilia in the blood or evidence of involvement of other organs. No parasite or other microbe has been identified. The response to corticosteroids and salicylates is uncertain.

Painful swelling of a calf muscle, or less frequently some other muscle, has been the chief characteristic of *eosinophilic monomyositis*. A painful mass forms within the muscle. Biopsy reveals inflammatory necrosis and edema of the interstitial tissues; the infiltrates contain variable numbers of eosinophils. This disorder is typified by one of our cases—a young woman who developed such an inflammatory mass first in one calf and, 3 months later, in the other. The response to prednisone in this patient was dramatic; the swelling and pain subsided in 2 to 3 weeks, and power of contraction was then found to be normal. When the connective tissue and muscle are both damaged, a chaotic regeneration of fibroblasts and myoblasts may occur, forming a pseudotumor that persists indefinitely.

Layzer and his associates have described a third form of this disorder, which they classify as a true subacute *polymyositis*. Their patients were adults, in whom a predominantly proximal weakness of muscles had evolved over a period of several weeks. In each case the muscle disorder was part of a severe and widespread systemic illness, including cardiac involvement (conduction disturbances and congestive failure), vascular disorder (Raynaud phenomenon, subungual hemorrhages), pulmonary infiltrates, strokes, anemia, neuropathy, and hypergammaglobulinemia. The muscles were swollen and painful. The eosinophil counts in the blood were increased in some patients, but not in others. There was a favorable response to corticosteroids in two patients, but in a third patient the outcome was fatal within 9 months. Layzer et al related the syndrome to eosinophilic pulmonary disease. They felt that a lack of necrotizing arteritis distinguished it from polyarteritis nodosa. No infective agent could be isolated. An allergic mechanism seems a likely cause of the lesions, and in the authors' view one cannot exclude an angiitis as a cause of all of the lesions.

The last two of these syndromes have overlapping features as shown by Stark's cases, in which a monomyositis was accompanied by several of the systemic features described by Layzer et al.

Among the many cases of idiopathic orbital inflammatory disease (pseudotumor of the orbit), there is a small group in whom the inflammatory process appears to be localized to the extraocular muscles. To this latter group the term *acute orbital myositis* has been applied. The abrupt onset of orbital pain that is made worse by eye motion, redness of the conjunctiva adjacent to the muscle insertions, diplopia caused by restrictions of ocular movements, lid edema, and mild proptosis are the main clinical features. The erythrocyte sedimentation rate is usually elevated and the patient may feel generally unwell, but only rarely can the ocular disorder be related to a connective tissue disease or any other specific systemic disease. The enhanced CT scan has proved to be particularly useful in demonstrating the swollen ocular muscles and separating orbital myositis from the many other remitting inflammatory orbital and retro-orbital conditions (Keane). As a rule, acute orbital myositis resolves spontaneously in a matter of a few weeks or a month or two, although it may recur either in the same or opposite eye. Administration of corticosteroids appears to hasten recovery.

OTHER ACUTE AND SUBACUTE MYOPATHIES

NECROTIZING POLYMYOPATHY (RHABDOMYOLYSIS) WITH MYOGLOBINURIA

In any disease that results in rapid destruction of striated muscle fibers, myoglobin and other muscle proteins may enter the bloodstream and appear in the urine. The latter is burgundy red or brown in color, much like the urine in hemoglobinuria. In the latter case, however, the serum is initially pink because hemoglobin (but not myoglobin) is bound to haptoglobin, and this complex is not excreted in the urine as readily as myoglobin (also, the hemoglobin molecule is three times larger than the myoglobin molecule). The hemoglobin-haptoglobin complex is removed from the blood plasma over a period of hours, and if hemolysis continues, the haptoglobin may be depleted so that hemoglobinuria is present without grossly evident hemoglobinemia. Differentiation of the two pigments in urine is difficult. Both are guaiac-positive. Very small differences are seen on spectroscopic examination. Electrophoresis on starch gel or cellulose is preferred by many laboratories and ultrasensitive immunologic methods are now being used to an increasing degree.

Porphyrins are the other substances that color the urine. They change color on exposure to sunlight and are guaiac-negative. Moreover, the associated clinical findings are those of a neuropathy and not a myopathy.

Regardless of the cause of the rhabdomyolysis, the affected muscles become painful and tender within a few hours. Power of contraction is diminished. Sometimes the skin and subcutaneous tissues overlying the affected muscles (nearly always of the limbs and sometimes of the trunk) are swollen and congested. There may be a low-grade fever. Apart from the discoloration of the urine, albumin excretion rises, and there is a leukocytosis. If myoglobinuria is mild, recovery occurs within a few days, and there is only a residual albuminuria. When myoglobinuria is severe, renal damage may ensue and lead to anuria. The mechanism of the renal damage is not clear; probably it is not simply a mechanical obstruction of tubules by precipitated myoglobin. It is, however, more likely to occur with massive rhabdomyolysis and very high CK levels in the serum. Alkalinization of the urine by ingestion of sodium bicarbonate is said to protect the kidneys by preventing myoglobin casts, but in severe cases it is of doubtful value, and the sodium may actually be harmful if anuria has already developed. Therapy is the same as in the anuria which follows surgical shock (see *Harrison's Principles of Internal Medicine*).

The following conditions may give rise to rhabdomyolysis and myoglobinuria:

1. Crush injury.

2. Excessive use of muscles, especially the ones that are confined in the tight pretibial compartment (pretibial syndrome) or prolonged compression of muscle. There is then ischemic injury.

3. Extensive infarction of muscle, as in occlusion of the main artery of a limb or a subcutaneous infusion into the lower leg (with resultant swelling and probably ischemia).

4. Idiopathic PM and viral PM, when necrosis is exceptionally severe.

5. Protoplasmic toxins resulting from the bite of the Malayan Sea Snake or the eating of fish or eels poisoned by toxic resins [Haff disease, so-called because it was first reported in patients residing in the bay (*Haff*) area of Konigsberg, Germany].

6. Alcoholic polymyopathy (see below).

7. Disorders of muscle glycolysis (see below).

8. Familial recurrent, or paroxysmal, myoglobinuria (Meyer-Betz and related diseases) which occurs in families with or without a diffuse chronic myopathy or dystrophy (see below).

9. Malignant hyperthermia, especially with convulsions, following the use of succinyl choline, halothane, and other anesthetic agents (see below).

Probably common to all these conditions is an acute depletion of ATP, which is necessary for the maintenance of the sarcolemma.

PAROXYSMAL MYOGLOBINURIA

Recurrent paroxysmal myoglobinuria surely comprises a number of different diseases. Two clinical syndromes have been described. In the first an infection may be a precipitating factor, usually in conjunction with physical exertion; in the second, there is a period of excessive muscular activity, together with a period of fasting or a diet deficient in glucose or fatty acids. The first example was reported in 1911 by Meyer-Betz, and his name has often been attached to all types of paroxysmal myoglobinuria, even though at that time there was no way of identifying myoglobin.

A therapeutic role for dantrolene sodium has been suggested in the prevention of recurrent occupational rhabdomyolysis (Haverkort-Poels et al).

MYOGLOBINURIA FROM DISTURBANCES OF MUSCLE GLYCOLYSIS

In recent times myoglobinuria has been observed in conjunction with six hereditary metabolic diseases of muscle: myophosphorylase deficiency (McArdle disease), phosphofructokinase deficiency (Tarui disease), lipid storage polymyopathy, carnitine palmityl transferase deficiency, phosphoglycerate kinase deficiency, and malignant hyperthermia. The first two of these diseases will be described in Chap. 51; the others are described below. In each of these diseases, a period of intense physical activity is followed by aching stiffness of muscle and extremely high levels of CK. Only exceptionally do episodes of myoglobinuria result in nephrosis and anuria. Usually, the exact conditions of exercise that cause rhabdomyolysis cannot be defined; intensity and duration of muscle contraction are not the complete explanation. In most instances one presupposes one or another of the aforementioned enzyme deficiencies. Fasting at the time of exercise is another factor. The myoglobinuria in this and other metabolic myopathies probably results from a shortage of substrate due to a block at some point in the glycolytic pathway. Under conditions of vigorous exercise, glycogen (by way of glycolysis) is the main source of energy. Once the energy source is depleted, muscle cramps and myoglobinuria, resulting from muscle fiber necrosis, follows. The incidence of these types of exercise rhabdomyolysis is not known, since the diagnosis requires special laboratory facilities not available to most clinicians. One suspects the presence of this group of glycolytic derangements by the failure of serum lactic acid to rise after ischemic exercise. With the availability of dialysis none of our patients has died of myoglobinuria, and by limiting their level of physical activity they have been able to lead relatively normal lives. The possibility of warding off an attack of one of the glycogen diseases by frequent ingestion of fructose or glucose has not been sufficiently explored.

LIPID STORAGE POLYMYOPATHY

Lipid storage polymyopathy is another cause of exercise-related myoglobinuria.

Although it has long been known that lipids are an important source of energy in muscle metabolism (along with glucose) it was not until 1970 that WK Engel et al described the storage of lipid in muscle fibers of twin girls who complained of intermittent muscular discomfort and myoglobinuria. It was suggested that there must be a defect in the utilization of long-chain fatty acids. Bressler, in commenting on this observation, predicted three possible biochemical defects: (1) in carnitine, (2) in carnitine palmityl transferase I, or (3) in carnitine palmityl transferase II. His prediction was borne out by the discovery of two separate conditions, one in which the synthesis of carnitine by the liver appeared to be faulty, the other in which there was an enzymatic defect in muscle of carnitine palmityl transferase.

MUSCLE CARNITINE DEFICIENCY

(See Chap. 51.)

DEFECT IN CARNITINE PALMITYL TRANSFERASE (CPT)

Since 1973 when the first cases of this disorder were described by DiMauro and DiMauro many others have been reported. The following clinical picture emerges: Of the first 19 reported cases, 18 were males; the inheritance pattern is probably autosomal recessive with low penetrance in females. Sustained exertion leads to muscle aching and rapid fatigue. The attacks of myoglobinuria begin in the first or second decade. Cold and caloric deprivation (high-fat, low-carbohydrate diet), are provocative factors. CK rises to high levels not only during attacks of myoglobinuria

but also with vigorous exercise without myoglobinuria. Between attacks the patient's muscle function is normal. Lipid accumulates in vacuoles, mainly in type 1 muscle fibers, but this is variable and not marked. Serum triglycerides are elevated, and there is fat intolerance with reduced clearance of chylomicrons. The main defect is in CPT, which is necessary for the regulation of long-chain fatty acids. There is an associated deficiency of carnitine acetyltransferase, which regulates short-chain fatty acids.

The diagnosis of the disease is suggested by the occurrence of paroxysmal myoglobinuria in a patient with a normal rise in serum lactate following ischemic exercise. Myoglobinuria occurs only in CPT deficiency, not in carnitine deficiency, which is described in Chap. 51.

Treatment consists of a high-carbohydrate, low-fat diet, and the feeding of extra carbohydrate before vigorous exercise.

SYSTEMIC CARNITINE DEFICIENCY

(See Chap. 51.)

PHOSPHOGLYCERATE KINASE (PGK) DEFICIENCY

DiMauro and his associates identified this enzymatic deficiency as a cause of recurrent myoglobinuria. The defect is transmitted as an X-linked recessive trait. Clinically there is a severe hemolytic anemia that becomes evident soon after birth, in association with mental retardation, behavioral abnormalities, seizures, and tremor. The myopathy takes the form of recurrent episodes of muscle pain, weakness, and myoglobinuria, precipitated by vigorous activity and associated with extremely high serum CK values, often with renal failure. In some patients the disease takes a purely myopathic form, anemia and neurologic disturbances being absent.

MALIGNANT HYPERTHERMIA

This may also be a cause of myoglobinuria, but its clinical presentation is unusual, that of a hyperthermic anesthesia accident. As larger experience has been gained with this entity, since the original report by Denborough and Lovell in 1960, it has proved to be a metabolic polymyopathy inherited as a dominant trait, which renders the individual vulnerable to certain anesthetic agents, particularly halothane and succinylcholine and ether to a lesser extent.

The clinical picture is unforgettable. As halothane anesthesia is induced and suxamethonium is given for muscular relaxation, the jaw muscles unexpectedly become tense rather than relaxed, and soon the rigidity extends to all of the muscles. Thereafter the temperature rises to 42 or 43°C with coincidental tachypnea and tachycardia. Failure of brainstem reflexes, circulatory collapse, and death may ensue or the patient may survive with gradual recovery. In some cases there is the same sequence of events without muscular spasm. The CK rises to high levels.

The pathogenesis of this reaction has been the subject of a number of investigations. Muscle from affected individuals is abnormally sensitive to caffeine, which induces contracture. It has been postulated that halothane acts in a manner similar to caffeine, i.e., to release calcium from and prevent its reaccumulation in the sarcoplasmic reticulum, thus interfering with relaxation of the muscle. A breed of pigs (Landrace) has been found in which muscle spasm (true contracture) and hyperthermia follow the administration of anesthetic agents. The latter are found to increase O_2 consumption by 50 to 60 percent and to deplete the ATP of muscle fibers. A primary defect of phosphodiesterase, the enzyme involved in the degradation of cyclic AMP, has been suggested as a pathogenetic factor. The cause of the fever is not known; it is probably due to the muscle spasm, but an effect of the anesthetic on heat-regulating centers cannot be excluded.

Clues as to which patients are at risk for this condition come from several sources. Other members of the family may have collapsed or died during anesthesia. Some of the susceptible individuals exhibit certain myopathic and musculoskeletal abnormalities. As to the former, progressive congenital myopathy, high CK values, or hypertrophic muscular dystrophy going on to atrophic weakness has been noted in some families (King-Denborough Syndrome). Central core myopathy, in some instances, predisposes to malignant hyperthermia (see review of Frank et al). The most frequently observed musculoskeletal abnormalities are short stature, ptosis, strabismus, highly arched palate, dislocated patellae, and kyphoscoliosis.

The treatment consists of discontinuation of anesthesia at the first hint of masseter spasm or rise of temperature. The intravenous administration of dantrolene, which inhibits the release of calcium from the sarcoplasmic reticulum, may be lifesaving. Other measures should include body cooling, intravenous hydration, sodium bicarbonate infusions to correct acidosis, and mechanical hyperventilation to decrease respiratory acidosis. Halothane inhalation anesthesia and succinylcholine should be avoided in such individuals, and any surgical procedures, if necessary, should be done under local anesthesia (see Isaacs and Barlow for review of literature).

ALCOHOLIC MYOPATHY

Several forms of muscle weakness have been ascribed to alcoholism. In one type, a painless and predominantly proximal weakness develops over a period of several days or weeks in the course of a prolonged drinking bout, and is associated with severe degrees of *hypokalemia* (serum levels <2 meq/L). The urinary excretion of potassium is not significantly increased; depletion is probably the result of vomiting and diarrhea, which usually precede the onset of muscular weakness. In addition, serum levels of liver and muscle enzymes are markedly elevated. Biopsies from severely weakened muscles show single-fiber necrosis and vacuolation. Treatment consists of the administration of potassium chloride intravenously (about 120 meq daily for several days), after which oral administration suffices. Strength returns gradually in 7 to 14 days, and enzyme levels return to normal concomitantly.

Another type of myopathic syndrome, occurring acutely at the height of a prolonged drinking bout, is manifested by severe pain, tenderness, and edema of the muscles of the limbs and trunk, accompanied in severe cases by renal damage and hyperpotassemia (Hed et al). The muscle affection is generalized in some patients and remarkably focal in others. A swollen, painful, and tender limb or part of a limb may give the appearance of a deep phlebothrombosis or lymphatic obstruction. Myonecrosis is reflected by high serum levels of CK and aldolase and the appearance of myoglobin in the urine, leading in some cases to fatal myoglobinuric nephrosis. In fact, in a general hospital, alcoholism is by far the commonest cause of rhabdomyolysis and myoglobinuria. Some patients recover within a few weeks, but others require several months, and relapse during another drinking spree is commonplace. Restoration of motor power is attendant upon regeneration, but may be complicated by polyneuropathy and other syndromes of neuromuscular disability associated with alcoholism. Haller and Drachman have produced the main abnormalities of alcoholic rhabdomyolysis (myonecrosis, elevated CK, and myoglobinuria) in rats by subjecting the animals to a brief fast following a 2- to 4-week exposure to alcohol; these observations suggest that a period of fasting, after a prolonged drinking spree, may be the factor that precipitates myonecrosis in alcoholic individuals.

Perkoff and his associates have described yet another muscular disorder in alcoholics, characterized by severe muscular cramps and diffuse weakness, occurring in the course of a sustained drinking bout. They noted a number of biochemical abnormalities in these patients, as well as in asymptomatic alcoholics who had been drinking heavily for a sustained period before admission to the hospital. These abnormalities consisted of elevated serum levels of CK, evidence of myoglobin in the urine, and a diminished rise in blood lactic acid in response to ischemic exercise, as occurs in McArdle disease. In distinction to the latter, however, myophosphorylase levels were not consistently reduced in the alcoholic patients. How these biochemical abnormalities are related to muscle cramps and weakness is a matter of speculation.

From time to time one observes in alcoholics the subacute or chronic evolution of painless weakness and atrophy of the proximal muscles of the limbs, especially of the legs, with only minimal signs of neuropathy in the distal segments of the legs and feet. Cases such as these have been referred to as chronic alcoholic myopathy, but the data are insufficient to warrant this designation. Some of these cases have shown necrosis of muscle fibers with myoglobinuria and most cases, in the authors' experience, have proved to be neuropathic in nature. Treatment follows along the lines indicated for alcoholic neuropathy (page 826), and complete recovery can be expected if the patient abstains from alcohol and commences a regimen of good nutrition.

REFERENCES

ADAMS RD, KAKULAS BA: *Diseases of Muscle: Pathological Foundations of Clinical Myology,* 4th ed. Philadelphia, Harper & Row, 1985.

ADAMS RD, KAKULAS BA, SAMAHA FA: A myopathy with cellular inclusions. *Trans Am Neurol Assoc* 90:213, 1965.

ANGELINI G, GOVONI E, BRAGAGLIA MM, VERGANI L: Carnitine deficiency: Acute postpartum crisis. *Ann Neurol* 4:558, 1978.

ANTONY JH, PROCOPIS PG, OUVRIER RA: Benign acute childhood myositis. *Neurology* 29:1068, 1979.

BANKER BQ: Dermatomyositis of childhood. Ultrastructural alterations of muscle and intramuscular blood vessels. *J Neuropathol Exp Neurol* 34:46, 1975.

BANKER BQ: Parasitic myositis, in Engel AG, Banker BQ (eds): *Myology. New York, McGraw-Hill, 1986a,* Chap 49.

BANKER BQ: Other inflammatory myopathies, in Engel AG, Banker BQ (eds): *Myology.* New York, McGraw-Hill, *1986b,* Chap 50.

BANKER BQ, ENGEL AG: The polymyositis and dermatomyositis syndromes, in Engel AG, Banker BQ (eds): *Myology.* New York, McGraw-Hill, 1986, Chap 46, pp 1385–1422.

BANKER BQ, VICTOR M: Dermatomyositis (systemic angiopathy) of childhood. *Medicine* 45:261, 1966.

BRESSLER R: Carnitine and the twins. *N Engl J Med* 282:745, 1970.

CARPENTER S, KARPATI G, HELLER I ET AL: Inclusion body myositis. A distinct variety of idiopathic inflammatory myopathy. *Neurology* 28:8, 1978.

CURRIE S: Polymyositis and related disorders, in Walton JN (ed): *Disorders of Voluntary Muscle,* 5th ed. Edinburgh, Churchill Livingstone, 1988, chap 17, pp 588–610.

DEMOS MA, GITLIN EL, KAGAN LG: Exercise myoglobinuria and acute exertional rhabdomyolysis. *Arch Intern Med* 134:669, 1974.

DENBOROUGH MA, LOVELL RRH: Anaesthetic deaths in a family. *Lancet* 2:45, 1960.

DEVERE R, BRADLEY WG: Polymyositis, its presentation, morbidity and mortality. *Brain* 98:637, 1975.

DIMAURO S, HARTWIG GB, HAYS A et al: Debrancher deficiency. Neuromuscular disorder in 5 adults. *Ann Neurol* 5:422, 1979.

DIMAURO S, DALAKAS M, MIRANDA AF: Phosphoglycerate kinase deficiency: A new cause of recurrent myoglobinuria. *Ann Neurology* 10:90, 1981.

DIMAURO S, DIMAURO PMM: Muscle carnitine palmityl transferase deficiency and myoglobinuria. *Science* 182:929, 1973.

DIMAURO S, MIRANDA AF, OLERTE M et al: Muscle phosphoglycerate mutase deficiency. *Neurology* 32:584, 1982.

ENGEL AG: Metabolic and endocrine myopathies in Walton JN (ed): *Disorders of Voluntary Muscle,* 4th ed, Edinburgh, Churchill Livingstone, 1981, chap 18, pp 664–711.

ENGEL AG, ANGELINI C, NELSON RA: Identification of carnitine deficiency as a cause of human lipid storage myopathy, in Milhorat AT (ed): *Exploratory Concepts in Muscular Dystrophy,* vol 2. Amsterdam, Excerpta Medica, 1974, pp 601–618.

ENGEL AG, ARAHATA K: Mononuclear cells in myopathies: Quantitation of functionally distinct subsets, recognition of antigen-specific cell-mediated cytotoxicity in some diseases and implications for the pathogenesis of the different inflammatory myopathies. *Hum Pathol* 1986, 17:704.

ENGEL WK, VICK NA, GLUECK CJ: A skeletal muscle disorder associated with intermittent symptoms and a possible defect in lipid metabolism. *N Engl J Med* 282:697, 1970.

FRANK JP, HARATI Y, BUTLER JJ et al: Central core disease and malignant hyperthermia syndrome. *Ann Neurol* 7:11, 1980.

GAMBOA ET, EASTWOOD AB, HAYS AP et al: Isolation of influenza virus from muscle in myoglobinuric polymyositis. *Neurology* 29:556, 1979.

GROSS B, OCHOA J: Trichinosis: A clinical report and histochemistry of muscle. *Muscle Nerve* 2:394, 1979.

HALLER RG, DRACHMAN DB: Alcoholic rhabdomyolysis: An experimental model in the rat. *Science* 208:412, 1980.

HART MN, LINTHICUM DS, WALDSCHMIDT MM et al: Experimental autoimmune inflammatory myopathy. *J Neuropathol Exp Neurol* 46:511, 1987.

HAVERKORT-POELS PJE, JOOSTEN EMG, RUITENBEEK W: Prevention of recurrent exertional rhabdomyolysis by Dantrolens sodium. *Muscle Nerve* 10:45, 1987.

HED R, LUNDMARK C, FAHLGREN H, ORELL S: Acute muscular syndrome in chronic alcoholism. *Acta Med Scand* 171:585, 1962.

ISAACS H, BARLOW MB: Malignant hyperpyrexia. *J Neurol Neurosurg Psychiatry* 36:228, 1973.

JOHNSON RT: *Viral Infections of the Nervous System.* New York, Raven Press, 1982, p 120.

KEANE JR: Alternating proptosis: A case report of acute orbital myositis defined by the computerized tomographic scan. *Arch Neurol* 34:642, 1977.

KISSEL JT, MENDELL JR, RAMMOHEN KW: Microvascular deposition of complement membrane attack complex in dermatomyositis. *N Engl J Med* 314:329, 1986.

LAYZER RB, SHEARN MA, SATYA-MURTI S: Eosinophilic polymyositis. *Ann Neurol* 1:65, 1977.

LUNDBERG A: Myalgia cruris epidemica. *Acta Paediatr Scand* 46:18, 1957.

MASTAGLIA FL, OJEDA VJ: Inflammatory myopathies. *Ann Neurol* 17:278, 317, 1985.

MATSUBARA S: Ultrastructural changes in granulomatous myopathy. *Acta Neurolpathol* 50:91, 1980.

MEYER-BETZ F: Beobachtungen an einem eigenartigen mit muskellähmungen verbundenen Fall von Hämoglobinurie. *Dtsch Arch Klin Med* 85:85, 1911.

MIKOL J: Inclusion body myositis, in Engel AG, Banker BQ (eds): *Myology.* New York, McGraw-Hill, 1986, Chap 47.

NAMBA T, BRUNNER MG, GROG N: Idiopathic giant cell polymyositis. Report of a case and review of the syndrome. *Arch Neurol* 31:27, 1974.

PERKOFF GR, HARDY P, VELEZ-GARCIA E: Reversible acute muscular syndrome in chronic alcoholism. *N Engl J Med* 274:1277, 1966.

RIDDOCH D, MORGAN-HUGHES JA: Prognosis in adult polymyositis. *J Neurol Sci* 26:71, 1973.

STARK RJ: Eosinophilic polymyositis. *Arch Neurol* 36:721, 1979.

WHITAKER JN, ENGEL WK: Vascular deposits of immunoglobulin and complement in idiopathic inflammatory myopathy. *N Engl J Med* 286:333, 1972.

CHAPTER 50

THE MUSCULAR DYSTROPHIES

As indicated in the classification of the muscle disorders (Chap. 48), progressive muscular weakness and atrophy of chronic course may occur with four major groups of diseases: the *chronic polyneuropathies,* the various forms of *motor system disease* (also called progressive muscular atrophies), the *progressive muscular dystrophies* and certain *congenital* or *metabolic polymyopathies.* All are or may be of genetic origin.

As a rough clinical indicator, the pattern of muscle involvement is helpful in separating these four categories of disease. In most polyneuropathies, the distal muscles of the limbs, particularly of the legs, are predominantly involved; in the dystrophies and polymyopathies, the affection is mainly of the girdle, proximal limb, or oculopharyngeal muscles; and in the spinal muscular atrophies there is a variable, symmetric or asymmetric pattern of involvement. Concurrent sensory loss, reflex impairment out of proportion to weakness, decreased nerve conduction velocities, characteristic EMG changes, elevated CSF protein, and group atrophy in the muscle biopsy usually establish the existence of a disease of peripheral nerves; the various types are presented in Chap. 46. Variable patterns of weakness, fasciculations at rest in weak muscles, normal sensation, relatively normal nerve conduction velocities, the presence of fibrillation potentials in the EMG, and typical features of denervation atrophy in the muscle biopsy serve to identify the progressive muscular atrophies. The latter, considered to be degenerative diseases of the anterior horn cells, are more appropriately grouped with degenerative diseases of the nervous system (see Chap. 43). Only the progressive muscular dystrophies will be considered in the following pages.

THE MUSCULAR DYSTROPHIES

The muscular dystrophies are progressive, hereditary degenerative diseases of skeletal muscles. The innervation of the affected muscles, in contrast to that of the neuropathic and spinal atrophies, is sound. Indeed, final proof that the origin of these disorders is in muscle itself comes from the demonstration of intact spinal motor neurons, muscular nerves, and nerve endings, in the presence of severe degenerative changes in the muscle fibers. The symmetric distribution of muscular weakness and atrophy, intact sensibility, preservation of cutaneous reflexes, and liability to heredofamilial incidence are the characteristic features of this group of diseases and serve to set them apart on clinical grounds alone.

Some clinicians and researchers have suggested that the term *muscular dystrophy* be applied to other degenerative diseases of muscle, such as those in animals due to vitamin E deficiency and the Coxsackie viruses, and certain inherited metabolic diseases in humans; we would discourage this practice, as one leading to terminologic confusion. The intensity of the degenerative changes and cellular response and vigor of the regenerative changes distinguish the latter diseases historically and also imply a fundamental difference in pathogenesis. We therefore reserve the term *dystrophy* for the purely degenerative muscular disease of hereditary type and refer to the others as myopathies or polymyopathies. The more benign and relatively nonprogressive myopathies such as central core, nemaline, mitochondrial, and centronuclear diseases, present a greater difficulty in classification. Like the dystrophies, they are primarily diseases of muscle and are heredofamilial in nature, but again we prefer to place them in a separate category because of their nonprogressive or slowly progressive course and the special qualities of their morphology.

HISTORY

The differentiation of dystrophic diseases from those secondary to neuronal degeneration was an achievement of neurologists of the second half of the nineteenth century. As pointed out by Gowers, isolated cases of muscular dystrophy had been described earlier but no distinction was made between neuropathic and myopathic disease. Meryon in 1852 gave the first clear description of progressive weakness and atrophy of muscle in young boys, who at autopsy had an intact spinal cord and nerves, a fact that led him to postulate an "idiopathic disease of muscles, dependent perhaps on defective nutrition." In 1855, the French neurologist Duchenne, who had long devoted himself to the clinical analysis of muscle function, described the progressive muscular atrophy of childhood that now bears his name. However, it was not until the second edition of his famous monograph in 1861 that the "hypertrophic paraplegia of infancy" was recognized as a distinct syndrome of unknown pathology, but with speculation about the nature of hypertrophy of muscles. By 1868 he was able to write a comprehensive description of 13 cases and recognized the restriction of this disease to males. Gowers in 1879 gave a masterful account of 21 personally observed cases and called attention to the characteristic way in which such patients arose from the floor (Gowers sign).

Leyden in 1876 and Möbius 1879 reported a nonhypertrophic form of disease which began in the pelvic girdle muscles and could affect both sexes. Erb, in 1891, was the first to crystallize the clinical and histologic concept of a group of diseases due to primary degeneration of muscle, which he called muscular dystrophies. The first descriptions of facioscapulohumeral dystrophy were published by Landouzy and Déjerine in 1894; of progressive ocular myopathy, by Fuchs in 1890; of myotonic dystrophy, by Steinert and by Batten and Gibb in 1909; of distal dystrophy, by Gowers in 1888, by Milhorat and Wolff in 1943, and by Welander in 1951; and of oculopharyngeal dystrophy, by the authors with Hayes in 1962.

A number of variant syndromes have come to light in the last 50 years. Bramwell in 1922 described an hereditary quadriceps myopathy; Dreifuss in 1961 and Emery in 1966 placed on record a sex-linked humeroperoneal dystrophy; and Seitz in 1957 distinguished a form of scapuloperoneal dystrophy with cardiomyopathy from the larger group of scapuloperoneal syndromes. References to these and other writings of historical importance can be found in the monographs of Adams and Kakulas, of Walton, and of Engel and Banker (see References).

CLASSIFICATION OR CLINICAL PRESENTATION

The following classification of the muscular dystrophies is based largely on the foregoing clinical studies. Certain forms, namely myotonic dystrophy, and the ocular, oculopharyngeal, and distal dystrophies, are sufficiently distinctive to make their separation relatively easy. There is

still uncertainty about the classification of the childhood forms of proximal dystrophy with and without pseudohypertrophy and with and without facial involvement. Erb, in his comprehensive monograph, divided the dystrophies into those beginning in childhood and those beginning in adult life. The adult forms were again divided into two groups, those with and those without facial involvement; and the childhood forms into two subtypes, those with pseudohypertrophy and those with atrophy. A more strictly genetic approach was taken by Walton and his associates who put in one group the sex-linked childhood forms of Duchenne, Becker, and Emery-Dreifuss; in a second group, the autosomal dominant facioscapulohumeral form of Landouzy and Déjerine and scapuloperoneal form of Seitz; and in a third group with variable types of inheritance, the limb-girdle cases of Leyden-Möbius and of Erb.

The authors, while impressed with the relative purity of the first two of these hereditary groups, continue to find many examples that do not run true to form. As for the third ("limb-girdle") category, there undoubtedly are such forms of dystrophy, but they are relatively uncommon. Furthermore, many of the cases included in this group have proved to be instances of spinal muscular atrophy of familial type, as reported by Wohlfart et al and by Kugelberg and Welander, and of congenital myopathy and glycogen storage disease.

The most frequent types of muscular dystrophy are myotonic dystrophy and the pseudohypertrophic form of Duchenne. Nevertheless, for purposes of exposition, we shall consider all of the types of muscular dystrophy, i.e., progressive, hereditary diseases of muscle in which the pathologic changes consist of degeneration and loss of muscle fibers in a particular topographic pattern. (See Table 50-1.)

Duchenne Muscular Dystrophy (Severe Generalized Muscular Dystrophy of Childhood; Erb Childhood Type) This type of dystrophy usually begins in early childhood and runs a relatively rapid, progressive course. The incidence rate is in the range of 13 to 33 per 100,000 and the prevalence is about 3 per 100,000. It occurs in every part of the world. There is a strong familial liability; the disease occurs predominantly in males, and so-called pseudohypertrophy of certain muscles is a prominent feature. Approximately 40 percent of patients have a negative family history and are said to represent mutations. However, careful examinations of their mothers will show slight involvement in as many as half of the mutant cases, as pointed out by Roses et al. Instances of Duchenne muscular dystrophy occur in girls who have the Turner XO or other XX genotypes. However, most cases of female childhood dystrophy prove to be of autosomal recessive limb-girdle type (for discussion of hereditary features, see chapter by Engel listed in References).

Table 50-1
The progressive muscular dystrophies

Type of dystrophy	Age of onset	Pattern of muscular involvement	Special features	CK level	Inheritance
Duchenne	Infancey or early childhood	Pelvifemoral; later pectoral girdle	Hypertrophy-pseudohypertrophy; cardiac involvement; mental retardation	High	X-linked recessive
Becker	Childhood, adolescence, or early adult	Pelvifemoral, later pectoral girdle	Cardiac involvement, slight; mentation normal	Moderate	X-linked recessive
Emery-Dreifuss	Childhood, adolescence	Humeroperoneal	Contractures posterior neck and biceps muscles	Moderate	X-linked recessive
Landouzy-Déjerine	Late childhood, adolescence	Facioscapulo-humeral; pelvic girdle—late	Heart normal, mentation normal	Slight to moderate	Dominant
Scapulohumeral of Seitz	Childhood or adult	Spinati and humeral, later pelvic girdle	Cardiomyopathy	Slight to moderate	Dominant
Limb-girdle (Erb)	Childhood, adolescence, sometimes adult	Pectoral or pelvic or both	Heart usually normal, mentation normal	Slight to moderate	Variable, recessive, or dominant
von Graefe-Fuchs	Childhood, adolescence	Ocular (sparing pupils); later facial and other muscles (slight)	Kearns-Sayre group have retinitis pigmentosa, heart block, stunting of growth, and ovarian dysgenesis	Slight to moderate	Dominant; Kearns-Sayre recessive
Oculopharyngeal	Middle or late adult	Levators of lids; other ocular-pharyngeal muscles later		Slight to normal	Dominant
Myotonic (Steinert)	Infancy, childhood, adult	Ocular, facial, sternomastoid, forearm, peroneal	Cataracts, testicular atrophy	Slight to normal	Dominant
Congenital	Birth, infancy	Pectoral and pelvic girdles, or diffuse	Mental retardation, arthrogryposis	Slight to moderate	Dominant or recessive

The most frequent and best known of the childhood muscular dystrophies is the Duchenne pseudohypertrophic type, the name being taken from the unnatural enlargement of the calves and certain other muscles. The disease is usually recognized in the third year of life and nearly always before the sixth year, but nearly half of the patients show evidence of disease before beginning to walk. Many of them are backward in other ways (psychomotor retardation), and the muscle weakness may at first be overlooked. An elevated CK may be the first clue. In another group of young children, an indisposition to walk or run when they should do so brings them to medical attention; or, having achieved these motor milestones, they appear to be less sprightly than usual, and are prone to fall. Increasing difficulty in walking, running, and climbing stairs, sway-back, and waddling gait become ever-more obvious as time passes. The iliopsoas, quadriceps, and gluteal muscles are the first to be affected; then the pretibial muscles weaken (foot drop and toe walking). Muscles of the pectoral girdle and upper limbs are affected later than the pelvicrural ones; the serrati, lower parts of pectorals, latissimus dorsi, biceps, and brachioradialis are affected, more or less in this order.

Enlargement of the calves and certain other muscles is progressive in the early stages of the disease, but most of the muscles, even the ones that are originally enlarged, eventually decrease in size; only the gastrocnemii, and to a lesser extent the quadriceps and deltoids, are consistently large and this quality may be evident before weakness is noted. The enlarged muscles have a firm, resilient (rubbery) feel and as a rule are slightly less strong and more hypotonic than healthy ones of the same size. Rarely, all muscles are at first large and exceptionally strong, even the facial muscles, as in one of Duchenne's cases (a "Farnese Hercules"); this is a true hypertrophy.

Muscles of the pelvic girdle, lumbosacral spine, and shoulders become weak and wasted, accounting for certain clinical peculiarities. Weakness of abdominal and paravertebral muscles accounts for the lordotic posture and protuberant abdomen when standing and the rounded back, when sitting. Bilateral weakness of the extensors of the knees and hips interferes with equilibrium and with activities such as climbing stairs or rising from a chair or from a stooped posture. In standing and walking the patient places his feet wide apart in order to increase his base of support. To rise from a sitting position, he first flexes his trunk at the hips, puts his hands on his knees, and pushes the trunk upward by working the hands up the thighs (Gowers sign). In getting up from a recumbent position the patient turns his head and trunk and pushes himself sideways to a sitting

position. S. A. K. Wilson used an alliterative phrase to describe the characteristic abnormalities of stance and gait—the patient "straddles as he stands and waddles as he walks." According to Duchenne, the waddle is due to bilateral weakness of the gluteus medius (see page 97) Calf pain is a not infrequent complaint. Weakening of the muscles that fix the scapulae to the thorax (serratus anterior, lower trapezius, rhomboids) causes a winging of the scapulae, and the scapular angles can sometimes be seen when facing the patient.

Later, weakness and atrophy spread to the muscles of the legs and forearms. The muscles that are selectively affected include the neck flexors, wrist extensors, brachioradialis, the costal part of the pectoralis major, latissimus dorsi, biceps, triceps, anterior tibial, and peroneal muscles. The ocular, facial, bulbar, and hand muscles are usually spared although weakness of the facial and sternomastoid muscles and of the diaphragm have been reported as late events in the disease. As the trunk muscles atrophy the bones stand out like those of a skeleton. The space between the lower ribs and iliac crests diminishes with affection of the abdominal muscles.

The limbs are usually loose and flaccid, but as the disability progresses, fibrous contractures appear as a result of keeping the limbs in one position and the imbalance between agonists and antagonists. Early in the ambulatory phase of the disease the feet assume an equinovarus position, the result of contracture of the posterior calf muscles, which act without the normal opposition of the pretibal and peroneal muscles. Later, the hamstring muscles become permanently shortened because of a lack of counteraction of the weaker quadriceps muscles. Similarly, the strong hip flexors become contractured because of the relatively greater weakness of hip extensors and abdominal muscles. This leads to a pelvic tilt and compensatory lordosis to maintain standing equilibrium. The consequences of these contractures account for the habitual posture of the patient with Duchenne dystrophy: lumbar lordosis, hip flexion and abduction, knee flexion and ankle equinus. These contractures, as they become severe, contribute importantly to the eventual loss of ambulation. Scoliosis, due to unequal weakening of the paravertebral muscles, and flexion contractures of the forearms appear, usually after walking is no longer possible.

The tendon reflexes are lost as muscle fibers disappear, the ankle reflexes being the last to go. The bones are thin and demineralized and the appearance of ossification centers is delayed. Smooth muscles are spared, but the heart may be hypertrophied, and various types of arrhythmia may appear. The ECG shows prominent R waves in the right precordial leads and deep Q waves in the left precordial and limb leads, the result of cardiac fiber loss and replacement fibrosis of the basal part of the left ventricular wall (Perloff et al). Death is usually the result of respiratory weakness and pulmonary infections, and sometimes cardiac decompensation. Mild degrees of mental retardation, non-progressive, are observed in many cases. Death usually occurs during adolescence, and not more than 20 to 25 percent of patients survive beyond the twenty-fifth year. The last years of life are spent in a wheelchair; finally the patient becomes bedfast.

Roses et al have studied the female carriers of the disease and report a slight enlargement of calves, slight weakness, mildly elevated CK values, and slight abnormalities of EMG and muscle biopsy in over 80 percent, including families with affection of only one male patient.

Becker Type Muscular Dystrophy This is another well-characterized dystrophy, closely related to the Duchenne type. Its incidence rate is difficult to ascertain, perhaps 3 to 6 per 100,000 male births. Like the Duchenne form it is an X-linked disorder, affecting only males and transmitted by females. It causes weakness and hypertrophy in the same muscles as the Duchenne dystrophy, but the onset is much later (mean age, 11 years; range, 5 to 45 years). The course is more benign; the average age at which the patient becomes unable to walk is 25 to 30 years; death occurs usually in the fifth decade, but some patients live to an advanced age. If maternal uncles are affected by the disease and are still walking, the diagnosis is relatively easy. Cardiac involvement is less frequent than in Duchenne dystrophy and mentation is usually normal. Kuhn et al have added a genealogy in which early myocardial disease and cramping myalgia were prominent features.

The serum CK values are 25 to 200 times normal, which with the EMG and muscle biopsy findings, helps to exclude an hereditary spinal muscular atrophy. The EMG shows fibrillations, positive waves, low-amplitude and polyphasic motor unit potentials, and sometimes high-frequency discharges. The female carrier may occasionally display the same mild abnormalities as in Duchenne dystrophy.

Another benign X-linked muscular dystrophy has been described by Emery and Dreifuss and more recently by Hopkins and Merlini et al. The age of onset varies from childhood to late adolescence or adulthood. The weakness affects first the upper arm and pectoral girdle musculature, and later the pelvic girdle, the distal muscles being spared. Contractures appear in the flexors of the elbow, extensors of the neck, and posterior calf muscles. Facial muscles are affected occasionally. There is no hypertrophy or pseudo-hypertrophy and mentation is intact. A severe cardiomyopathy with dysrhythmias, conduction defects, and atrial paralysis is a common accompaniment. The course is generally benign like that of Becker dystrophy, but weakness and contractures are severe in some cases, and sudden death is a frequent occurrence. The X-linked *scapuloperoneal*

muscular atrophy with cardiopathy (Mawatari and Katayama) is probably a variant of this disease. The autosomal dominant, *adult-onset scapuloperoneal myopathy*, described by Thomas and his colleagues, and the humeroperoneal myopathy, described by Gilchrist and Leshner, though genetically different from the Emery-Dreifuss syndrome, are phenotypically much the same.

Etiology of Duchenne-Becker Dystrophy The most important development in our understanding of the Duchenne and Becker muscular dystrophies has been the recent discovery by Louis M. Kunkel and his associates of the abnormal gene that is shared by these disorders, and the gene product. "Dystrophin" is the name that has been applied by these investigators to the protein product of the affected gene (Hoffman et al). The biochemical assay of this protein has made possible the accurate diagnosis of the Duchenne and Becker phenotypes and has clarified the relationship between these two disorders. Whereas dystrophin is absent in patients with Duchenne phenotype, it is present but structurally abnormal in the Becker type. Moreover, the phenotype that falls between the classic Duchenne and Becker forms (intermediate or "outlier" types) is characterized by a lower than normal amount of dystrophin. The genetic research that led to the isolation of the Duchenne dystrophy locus and its protein product is described in the articles of Koenig and of Hoffman and their colleagues, and a readable account of these investigations has been given by Rowland (see references).

Facioscapulohumeral Dystrophy (Landouzy-Déjerine, Erb Adult Form with Facial Involvement, Relatively Mild Restricted Muscular Dystrophy This is a slowly progressive dystrophy involving primarily the musculature of the shoulders and face, often with long periods of nearly complete arrest. The pattern of inheritance is usually autosomal dominant. A subvariety is a slowly progressive form without facial weakness.

While less common than the Duchenne type, this form of dystrophy is not rare. The age of onset is usually between 6 and 20 years; cases with onset in early adult life are occasionally encountered. As a rule, the first manifestations are difficulty in raising the arms above the head and winging of the scapulae, although in some cases facial weakness may have attracted attention, even in early childhood. Weakness and atrophy of muscles are the major physical findings; pseudohypertrophy occurs only rarely and is slight. There is an inability to close the eyes firmly, to purse the lips, and to whistle; the lips have a peculiar looseness and tendency to protrude, likened by some to those of the tapir. The lower parts of the trapezius muscles and the sternal parts of the pectorals are almost invariably affected. By contrast the deltoids may seem to be unusually large and strong, an appearance that may be mistaken for pseudohypertrophy. The advancing atrophic process also involves the sternomastoid, serratus magnus, rhomboid, erector spinae, latissimus dorsi, and eventually the deltoid muscles. The bones of the shoulders become salient; the scapulae are winged and elevated, and the clavicles are prominent. The anterior axillary folds slope down and out as a result of wasting of the pectoral muscles. Usually the biceps waste less than the triceps, but both are affected, as are the brachioradialis muscles, so that the upper arm may be thinner than the forearm (Popeye effect). Pelvic muscles are involved later and to a milder degree, giving rise to a slight lordosis and pelvic instability. The pretibial muscles weaken, and foot drop is added to the waddling gait. At any one point the disease may become arrested and cease to progress.

An occasional feature of this group of diseases is the congenital absence of a muscle (one pectoral, brachioradialis, or biceps femoris), or part of a muscle, in patients who later develop the typical affection. Also, the external ocular muscles are known to become affected occasionally, late in the illness. Cardiac involvement is rare, but in a few of the cases tachycardia, cardiomegaly, and arrhythmias (ventricular and auricular extrasystoles) have occurred. Mental function is normal.

A probable variant is characterized by an early onset and relatively rapid progression, and an association with facial diplegia, sensorineural deafness, and sometimes with exudative retinal detachment (Coats' disease). Using fluorescein angiography, Fitzsimmons and others found a variety of other vascular abnormalities, comprising telangiectases, occlusion, leakage, and microaneurysms, in 56 of 75 persons with the usual form of facioscapulohumeral dystrophy—suggesting that these retinal abnormalities are an integral part of the disease.

Limb-Girdle Dystrophies (Scapulohumeral and Pelvifemoral Muscular Dystrophy)

Clearly there are many patients with muscular dystrophy who do not fit into the categories described above. Children of both sexes are affected and lack the hypertrophy of calves and other muscles; adults have either pelvic or shoulder girdle involvement, or both, and their facial muscles are spared. Insofar as Wilhelm Erb first called attention to these types of dystrophy, they have been grouped by Walton and his colleagues as the "limb-girdle dystrophies of Erb." The inheritance has been variable, but the recessive form is the most common. We believe that this group is separable but overlaps the Duchenne-Becker and the Landouzy-Déjerine types. In a review of 102 families with pelvifemoral dystrophy without calf hypertrophy, Lamy and deGrouchy found 9 out of 10 to have an X-linked inheritance and the remainder an autosomal recessive inheritance. The latter would fall into the Erb group. Sensorineural deafness and retinal telangiectases are added features in some probands.

Thus, in the limb-girdle group either the shoulders or hips may be first affected, and the weakness and atrophy may become evident either during childhood or in early adult life. The later the onset the more likely is the course to be benign; dominant inheritance and lack of family history are features favoring slow progression. In the latter group, while the EMG is myopathic, the CK values are often only moderately elevated and may even be normal in the most chronic forms. Cardiac involvement is infrequent and mental function is normal. Walton and Gardner-Medwin believe that the scapulohumeral cases, with the same pattern of muscle involvement (except for facial muscles) as the Landouzy-Déjerine form, are the ones to which the term *limb-girdle dystrophy* is the most applicable. They include also the late life muscular dystrophy of Nevin.

The problem with this group of limb-girdle dystrophy, as indicated in the introduction to this chapter, is that its status as a clinical-genetic entity is being steadily eroded. The delineation of the progressive spinal muscular atrophies and the congenital and metabolic myopathies have greatly narrowed the category of limb-girdle dystrophy as originally described. Nevertheless, there remains a small group of limb-girdle syndromes that are familial and progressive and possess the characteristic myopathologic features of muscular dystrophy.

Progressive External Ophthalmoplegia (Ocular Myopathy of von Graefe-Fuchs)

This is a slowly progressive myopathy, primarily involving and often limited to the extraocular muscles. Usually the levators of the eyelids are the first to be affected, causing ptosis, followed by progressive ophthalmoparesis. This disorder usually begins in childhood, sometimes in adolescence and rarely in adult life (as late as 50 years). Males and females are equally affected; the pattern of inheritance is autosomal dominant in some and recessive or uncertain in others. Once started, the disease progresses relentlessly until the eyes are motionless. Simultaneous involvement of all extraocular muscles permits the eyes to remain in a central position so that strabismus and diplopia are uncommon (in rare instances one eye is affected before the other). In an attempt to raise the eyelids and to see under them, the head is thrown back and the frontalis muscle is contracted, wrinkling the forehead (hutchinsonian facies). The eyelids are abnormally thin because of atrophy of the levator muscles.

The orbicularis oculi muscles are frequently involved, in addition to the extraocular muscles. Thus, in progressive external ophthalmoplegia, as in myasthenia gravis and myotonic dystrophy, there is a characteristic combination of weakness of eye closure and eye opening. As stated above, this is nearly always myopathic, for it would be unusual for all the oculomotor and facial nerves to be involved bilaterally from lesions of the third, fourth, sixth, and seventh cranial nerves or their nuclei. Other facial muscles, masseters, sternocleidomastoids, deltoids, or peronei are variably weak and wasted in about 25 percent of cases.

The absence of myotonia, cataracts, and endocrine disturbances distinguishes progressive external ophthalmoplegia from myotonic dystrophy, with which it might be confused because of the ptosis. The more extensive forms of the disease may resemble mild restricted muscular dystrophy, and indeed Landouzy and Déjerine described ocular palsy in one of their cases. The characteristic feature of progressive external ophthalmoplegia is that ptosis and ocular paralysis precede involvement of other muscles by many years. The relatively early age of onset and absence of dysphagia set it apart from the oculopharyngeal form of dystrophy, and the lack of retinal degeneration and the normality of growth, mentation, and CSF protein distinguish it from the Kearns-Sayre syndrome (see below).

Opinions vary as to whether all cases of progressive external ophthalmoplegia should be assigned a myopathic origin. In chronic diseases such as this, dystrophy and partial denervation are difficult to distinguish on the basis of the appearance of the biopsied eye muscle, as pointed out by Ringel et al. The categorization of progressive external ophthalmoplegia is complicated further by its frequent association with a variety of neurologic abnormalities and atypical pigmentary degeneration of the retina. Drachman has lumped all these complicated cases under the title of "ophthalmoplegia plus," in the belief that any further classification has little value. Nevertheless, the purely myopathic origin of some cases is proven by intactness of neurons in the brainstem nuclei and normality of the cranial nerves. Apart from myasthenia gravis, it has been possible to separate at least two distinctive syndromes from this group. One of these is the highly restricted oculopharyngeal dystrophy of late onset, which is described in the following section of this chapter. Another rather uniform syndrome comprises childhood ophthalmoplegia, pigmentary degeneration of the retina, varying degrees of heart block, short stature, and elevated CSF protein (Kearns and Sayre). Because of its special histopathologic features,

this latter syndrome will be discussed with the congenital mitochondrial myopathies (page 1144). (See review by Berenberg et al for further discussion of the progressive ophthalmoplegias and their classification.)

Oculopharyngeal Dystrophy This disease is inherited as an autosomal dominant trait and is unique with respect to its late onset (usually after the forty-fifth year) and the restricted muscular weakness, manifested mainly as a bilateral ptosis and dysphagia. E. W. Taylor first described the disease in 1915, and assumed that it was due to a nuclear atrophy (oculomotor-vagal complex); the authors, with Hayes in 1962, showed that the descendants of Taylor's cases had a late-life myopathy (myopathic EMG and biopsy). Subsequent studies by Barbeau traced the family that we had described through 10 generations, to an early French-Canadian immigrant who was the progenitor of several hundred descendants with the disease. Since then, other families showing a dominant pattern of inheritance and a number of sporadic cases have been described.

Associated with slowly progressive ptosis is a difficulty in swallowing and change in voice. Swallowing becomes so difficult that food intake is limited, resulting in cachexia. The latter is prevented at first by cutting the cricopharyngeus muscle, and, failing this measure, by a "feeding gastrostomy" or nasogastric intubation. In some families, the other external ocular muscles and shoulder and pelvic muscles become weakened and atrophic to a relatively slight extent. In the few autopsied cases, a loss of fibers of modest proportions was widespread in these and many other muscles. The brainstem nuclei and cranial nerves were normal. Like the other mild and restricted polymyopathies the serum CK and aldolase levels are normal, and the EMG is altered only in the affected muscles.

Dystrophia Myotonica (Myotonic Dystrophy) This form of dystrophy was described in 1909 by Steinert, who considered it to be a variant of congenital myotonia (Thomsen disease), and, in the same year, by Batten and Gibb, who recognized it as a separate clinical entity. It is distinguished by an autosomal dominant pattern of inheritance with a high level of penetrance, a unique topography of the muscle atrophy, an associated myotonia, and the occurrence of dystrophic changes in nonmuscular tissues (lens of eye, testicle and other endocrine glands, skin, and, in some cases, the cerebrum). Recently it has been shown, by genetic linkage analysis, that the gene for myotonic dystrophy lies in chromosome 19, within measurable distance of several genetic markers (Shaw et al). Its gene product has not yet been isolated. Certain muscles, namely the levator palpebrae, facial, masseter, sternomastoid, forearm, hand, and pretibial muscles, are consistently involved in the dystrophic process. In this sense, dystrophia myotonica is a distal type of myopathy. It is probable that Gowers' case of an 18-year-old youth with weakened and wasted anterior tibial and forearm muscles and sternomastoids, in conjunction with paresis of orbicularis and frontalis muscles, was an example of this disease, differing from the simple distal muscular dystrophy described by Welander (see below).

Usually the muscular wasting in myotonic dystrophy does not become manifest until the third decade of life, but we have seen a number of infants and young children with the typical facies. Moreover, in recent years a severe, often fatal, neonatal (congenital) form of the disease has been identified (see further on). The small muscles of the hands, along with the extensor muscles of the forearms, are often the first to become atrophied. In other cases, ptosis of the eyelids and thinness and slackness of the facial muscles may be the earliest signs, preceding other muscular involvement by many years. Atrophy of the masseters leads to narrowing of the lower half of the face, and the mandible is slender and malpositioned so that the teeth do not occlude properly. This, along with the ptosis, frontal baldness, and wrinkled forehead, imparts a distinctive physiognomy that, once seen, can be recognized at a glance. The sternomastoids are almost invariably implicated and are associated with a general thinness and an exaggerated forward curvature of the neck ("swan neck"). Atrophy of the anterior tibial muscle groups, leading to foot drop, is an early sign in other families.

Pharyngeal and laryngeal weakness results in a weak, monotonous nasal voice. The uterine muscle may be weakened, interfering with normal parturition, and the esophagus is often dilated because of loss of muscle fibers in the striated part. Megacolon occurs in some patients. Diaphragmatic weakness and alveolar hypoventilation, resulting in chronic bronchitis and bronchiectasis, are frequent. Cardiac abnormalities are also frequent. Most often, they are due to disease of the conducting apparatus, giving rise to bradycardia and a prolonged PR interval. Patients with extreme bradycardia may die suddenly, and for such subjects, insertion of a pacemaker has been recommended (Moorman et al). Mitral valve prolapse and left ventricular dysfunction (cardiomyopathy) are less frequent abnormalities.

The disease progresses slowly, with gradual involvement of the proximal muscles of the limbs and muscles of the trunk. Tendon reflexes are lost or much reduced. Contracture is rarely seen and the thin, flattened hands are consequently soft and pliable. Most patients are confined to a wheelchair or bed within 15 to 20 years, and death occurs before the normal age from pulmonary infection or heart failure.

The phenomenon of *myotonia*, which expresses itself in prolonged contraction of certain muscles following brief percussion or electrical stimulation and in delay of relaxation after strong voluntary contraction, is the third striking attribute of the disease. Not as widespread as in myotonia congenita (Thomsen disease), it is, nonetheless, easily elicited in the hands and tongue in over 95 percent of cases and in the proximal limb muscles in half of the cases. Gentle movements do not evoke it (eye blinks, movements of facial expression, and the like are not impeded), whereas strong closure of the lids and clenching of the fist are followed by a long delay in relaxation.

Myotonia may precede weakness by several years. Indeed, Maas and Paterson have claimed that many cases diagnosed originally as myotonia congenita eventually prove to be examples of myotonia dystrophica. Of interest is the fact that in congenital or infantile cases of myotonic dystrophy, the myotonic phenomenon is not elicited until after the second or third year of life. Moreover, the patient often becomes accustomed to the myotonia and no longer complains about it. The relation of myotonia to the dystrophy is not direct. Certain muscles that show the myotonia best (tongue, flexors of fingers) are seldom weak and atrophic. There may be little or no myotonia in certain families that show the other characteristic features of myotonic dystrophy.

The fourth major characteristic is the association of dystrophic changes in nonmuscular tissues. The most common of these are lenticular opacities, which are found by slit lamp examination in 90 percent of patients. At first dust-like, they then form small, regular opacities found in the posterior and anterior cortex of the lens just beneath the capsule; they are colored blue, blue-green, and yellow under the slit lamp and are highly refractile. Microscopically, the crystalline material, probably lipids and cholesterol (which cause the iridescence) lies in vacuoles and lacunae among the lens fibers. In older patients a stellate cataract slowly forms in the posterior cortex of the lens.

Feeblemindedness of mild to moderate degree is not infrequent, and the brain weight in several of our patients was 200 g less than normals of the same age. Late in adult life some patients become suspicious, argumentative, and forgetful. In some families, a hereditary, sensorimotor neuropathy may be associated with the muscle disease (Cros et al).

Other nonspecific abnormalities, such as hyperostosis of the frontal bones and calcification of the basal ganglia, both readily discerned by CT scanning, seem to be more common in patients with myotonic dystrophy than in normal persons.

Progressive frontal alopecia, beginning at an early age, is a characteristic feature in both men and women with this disease. Testicular atrophy with androgenic deficiency, reduced libido or impotence, and sterility are frequent manifestations. In some patients gynecomastia and elevated gonadotropin excretion are found. Testicular biopsy may show atrophy and hyalinization of tubular cells and hyperplasia of Leydig cells. Thus all the clinical characteristics of the Klinefelter syndrome may be present. However, the nuclei of skin or bone marrow cells only rarely show "sex chromatin mass." The majority of patients have the usual sex chromatin constitution. Ovarian deficiency occasionally develops in the female patient but is seldom severe enough to interfere with menstruation or fertility. The prevalence of clinical or chemical diabetes mellitus is only slightly increased in patients with myotonic dystrophy, but an increased insulin response to a glucose load has proved to be a common abnormality. Numerous surveys of other endocrine functions have yielded rather little of significance.

In an extensive clinical experience with this, the most frequent of all the dystrophies, we have been impressed with the variability of its clinical expression. In many patients intelligence has been unimpaired and the myotonia and muscle weakness have been so mild that they were unaware of any difficulty. Pryse-Philips et al emphasized these features in their description of a large Labrador kinship in which 27 of 133 patients had only a partial syndrome and only minor muscle symptoms at the time of examination.

Congenital Myotonic Dystrophy Brief mention was made above of this distinctive and potentially lethal form of myotonic dystrophy. That it occurs not infrequently is evident from Harper's (1975) study of 70 personally observed patients, and 56 others gathered from the medical literature. Profound hypotonia and facial diplegia at birth are the most prominent clinical features; myotonia is notable for its absence. The drooping of the eyelids, the tented upper lip ("carp mouth"), and open jaw impart a characteristic appearance, which allows immediate recognition of the disease in the newborn infant. Difficulty in sucking and swallowing, bronchial aspiration (due to palatal weakness), and respiratory distress (due to diaphragmatic and intercostal weakness and pulmonary immaturity) are present in varying degrees of severity, and the latter disorders are responsible for a previously unrecognized group of neonatal deaths (24 such deaths among sibs of affected families in Harper's study). In surviving infants, delayed motor and speech development, mild to moderately severe mental retardation, and talipes or generalized arthrogryposis are common. Once adolescence is attained, the disease follows the same course as the later form. As stated above, myotonia (clinical,

EMG) in the childhood form of the disease does not become evident before the second or third year, but is uniformly present after the tenth year. ECG changes occur in a third of the patients.

The affected parent, in the congenital form of this disease, is practically always the mother, in whom the disease need not be severe. Contrariwise, in cases of adult onset, transmission is predominantly paternal. These data suggest that in addition to inheriting the myotonic dystrophy gene, the congenital cases also receive some maternally transmitted factor, the nature of which is presently unknown. Genetic linkage studies, using apolipoprotein CII (apo CII) as a marker, have now made possible the prenatal diagnosis of myotonic dystrophy in informative (three affected generations) families. Bird et al have shown, in such families, that amniocentesis with apo CII haplotype determination can predict with great accuracy that the fetus has *not* inherited the myotonic dystrophy gene. Additional genetic markers, close to the myotonic dystrophy locus, should provide even more informative diagnostic possibilities.

Late-Onset Distal Muscular Dystrophy (Milhorat and Wolff: Welander) This is a slowly progressive distal myopathy with onset principally in middle adult life. Weakness and wasting of the muscles of the hands, forearms, and lower legs, especially the extensors, are the main clinical features. Although cases such as these had been reported by Gowers and others, their differentiation from myotonic dystrophy and peroneal muscular atrophy was unclear until relatively recent times.

Milhorat and Wolff, in 1943, presented the findings in 12 individuals of one family affected by "a progressive muscular dystrophy of atrophic distal type." The inheritance was autosomal dominant in type, and the onset was between 26 and 43 years; within 5 to 15 years the patients had become disabled. There was one autopsy, confirming the dystrophic nature of the disease.

Welander's account of this disorder, based on the study of 249 Swedish cases, appeared in 1951. In her series the mode of inheritance was autosomal dominant. The changes demonstrated in three autopsies and 22 biopsies were purely dystrophic. Fasciculations, cramps, pain, sensory disturbances, and myotonia were notably absent. Senile cataracts appeared after the age of 70 in three patients and surely can be discounted as having special significance. No endocrine disorders were detected. The central nervous system and peripheral nerves were normal. Progression of the disease was very slow; after 10 years or so some wasting of proximal muscles was seen in a few of the patients.

An apparently separate form of distal dystrophy with autosomal dominant inheritance and onset before 2 years of age was described by van der Does de Willebois et al. The condition is distinguished from spinal muscular atrophy and polyneuropathy by the high levels of CK in the serum, EMG, and biopsy.

Yet another type of distal dystrophy is characterized by an autosomal recessive pattern of inheritance and is particularly prevalent in Japan (Miyoshi et al). Onset of the disease is in early adult life, with weakness and atrophy of the leg muscles, especially of the gastrocnemius and soleus muscles, extending over many years to the thighs, gluteal muscles, and forearms. Serum CK concentrations are greatly increased in the early stages of the disease.

CONGENITAL MUSCULAR DYSTROPHY

From the beginning of the twentieth century there have been scattered reports of congenital myopathy, but the status of this condition was difficult to evaluate, mainly because of inadequacy of the pathologic studies. Some cases may have been examples of congenital myotonic dystrophy or one of the congenital myopathies described further on, in Chap. 52. In 1957 Banker and the authors described two patients (siblings), one dying at 1½ h after birth, the other at 10 months, of a congenital muscular dystrophy with arthrogryposis. The pathologic changes consisted of muscle fiber degeneration, variation in fiber size, fibrosis, and fat cell replacement. The central and peripheral nervous systems were intact. The severity of the degenerative changes was such that a developmental disorder of muscle could be excluded.

Pearson and Fowler, in 1963, reported a brother and sister with similar clinical and pathologic findings and Walton described still another patient, aged 4 years. By 1967 Vassella et al were able to collect 27 cases from the medical literature and add 8 cases of their own. The high incidence of sibling involvement suggests an autosomal recessive inheritance.

Defined as a muscle dystrophy already present at birth, often with contractures of proximal muscles and trunk, the severity of the weakness and degree of progressivity have varied widely. Of the eight cases reported by Rotthauwe et al, one had a benign course, but the others all had weakness and hypotonia at birth, and difficulty in sucking and swallowing had interfered with nutrition. Their oldest patients, aged 14 and 23 years, and several others had walked but at a late age. In the Finnish series of Donner

at al, congenital dystrophy accounted for 9 percent of the 160 cases of neuromuscular disease seen at their hospital over a decade. The weakness and hypotonia were generalized and three had ECG abnormalities. The CK values were elevated and the EMGs were myopathic.

More recently a series of papers have issued from Japan relating the details in over 100 patients with congenital dystrophy (Fukuyama et al). A feature of these cases was the coexistence of severe mental retardation and febrile convulsions. Lebenthal et al described a large Arab pedigree with congenital muscular dystrophy and patent ductus arteriosus. Some had contractures at birth; in others contractures developed at a later age. The EMG disclosed a myopathic pattern, and CK levels were moderately elevated.

At the moment it is still difficult to classify many of these cases, mainly because of the highly variable clinical course. In some cases there was improvement as the patient matured and the CK values returned toward normal. In our original report we cautioned against the too ready acceptance of the term dystrophy in categorizing all of these patients. The definite criterion of a dystrophy must be its progressivity.

Other Varieties   As remarked earlier, there are many patients with muscular dystrophy who do not conform to any one of the above types, and this calls into question the adequacy of our classification or of any nosologic system that is based on semiology alone.

Since the majority of early-life dystrophies are X-linked, it always comes as a surprise to observe a clinically manifest form of *progressive muscular dystrophy in young girls*. However, this happens occasionally and is the subject of several reports. Explanations easily come to mind: (1) As mentioned above, if the female has only one chromosome as in the Turner XO syndrome, she should have the same muscle affection as the male. (2) Some female carriers also have overt disease, probably through the operation of the Lyon principle of sex heredity. However, neither explanation accounts for several families in which only females have been subject to a proven muscular dystrophy, such as the one described by Henson et al. In the latter family, a proximal myopathy had its onset at the age of 5 to 20 years and led to severe disability by the age of 30 years. Waddling gait and lumbar lordosis were prominent, and the proximal limb and trunk muscles, especially the deltoids, glutei, hamstrings, and medial parts of the gastrocnemii were the most affected.

A familial hypertrophy of the quadriceps may be the first sign of a dystrophic disease that affects males in their third to fourth decades of life. It spreads slowly to other muscles, mainly of the pelvis and legs. A purely atrophic form of quadriceps or gastrocnemius dystrophy, with pain on exercise, has also been described. Mild forms of restricted scapuloperoneal dystrophy (see above) probably represent variants of Erb limb-girdle dystrophy.

A universal dystrophy, with affection of every skeletal muscle in the body, including the eye muscles, and occurring in three members of a family (two males and one female in two successive generations), has come under our observation. The onset was in adult life and progression to a state of severe weakness and atrophy occurred over a period of 10 years; there was no hypertrophy, pseudohypertrophy, cataracts, or myotonia.

We have also seen pure dysphagia with esophageal dilatation (upper striated part) as a probable dystrophic disease. This disorder has its onset in early adult life and is slowly progressive, without other signs of myotonic dystrophy.

From time to time, muscular dystrophy of either the classic or exceptional type occurs in conjunction with one or several more strictly neurologic disorders. Muscular dystrophy has been noted together with dementia, deafness, cerebellar ataxia, an extrapyramidal syndrome, and with spastic weakness of the legs. The association of progressive external ophthalmoplegia with mild peripheral neuropathy, cerebellar ataxia, and corticospinal tract disease and of myotonic dystrophy and peripheral neuropathy has already been mentioned. Wilson referred to these as "transitional states" implying that the disease process has extended from muscle to nervous tissue. Our view would be that these heredofamilial neurologic disorders have a closely related genetic mechanism. The sporadic claims that peroneal muscular atrophy is a combined polyneuropathy and polymyopathy must be examined critically, for there is often a tendency to misinterpret the degenerative muscle changes in the late stages of denervation.

LABORATORY FINDINGS IN MUSCULAR DYSTROPHY

Serum creatine kinase (the MM isoenzyme form) and other enzymes derived from muscles are often elevated. This is most marked in Duchenne dystrophy and least in the chronic benign forms. As the muscles are destroyed there is a tendency for the CK to fall. Myoglobin, when measured by sensitive immunologic techniques, is elevated in all the dystrophies. The EMG discloses the abnormally small action potentials during partial and full voluntary contractions and, of course, myotonic discharges in myotonic dystrophy. Some fibrillation potentials and other abnormalities, as described in Chap. 45, are also present. Biopsy provides the final corroboration.

PATHOLOGY

The histologic changes in the several forms of muscular dystrophy are plain to see, but elusive of interpretation.

The changes are loss of muscle fibers, residual fibers of larger and smaller size than normal in haphazard arrangement (no grouping), segmental necrosis (degeneration) of muscle fibers with phagocytosis and regenerative activity (abortive?), and increase in lipocytes and fibrosis. The basic problem revolves on the interpretation of these changes: Which are primary and which are secondary? Opinions on this subject vary.

The difficulty in resolving this problem can be appreciated if one considers the extreme chronicity of the pathologic process. While the Duchenne form may run its course in a 10- to 15-year period, the span of the disease in the Landouzy-Déjerine and limb-girdle types is reckoned in decades. The prospect of capturing an image of the fundamental defect at any one instant in a tiny fragment of one muscle is not encouraging. Further, a survey of end-stage pathologic changes at autopsy, when all the fibers in many muscles have disappeared, yields little information concerning the pathogenesis of the fiber loss.

That fibers disappear is undoubted. Undetermined is the manner in which they disappear. Two hypotheses merit consideration: (1) that recurrent segmental necrosis results in destruction of the entire fiber and (2) that progressive atrophy leads eventually to fiber death. Each is difficult to affirm. Segmental necrosis is demonstrated most readily in the Duchenne type of dystrophy. Often several closely approximated fibers are simultaneously affected, which has led to the suggestion, by analogy with the findings in experimental embolism of muscle, of a vascular pathogenesis of muscular dystrophy. Physiologic and pathologic studies of the vessels have shown this hypothesis to be untenable. In the chronic (i.e., benign) forms of dystrophy one often searches in vain for evidence of segmental necrosis. Whether this is a problem in sampling at the correct moment, there being much less likelihood of showing the necrotic change in a long-drawn-out process, or whether this is due to a different type of involvement, cannot be decided with certainty. One of the authors (R.D.A.) believes that segmental necrosis is a feature of all dystrophic muscle diseases and that its frequent recurrence exhausts the regenerative (restorative) potential of the fiber.

The smallness of residual fibers (atrophy?) is a prominent feature but may have a number of explanations. It could be, as some myopathologists argue, that the underlying disorder is one of gradual failure of metabolism with all sarcoplasmic constituents undergoing volumetric reduction. If studied in three dimensions by serial sections, however, one can see, in the Duchenne type of dystrophy, that regeneration of the muscle fiber, after segmental necrosis, results in forking or branching of the intact parts of a fiber and the formation of several new, thin fibers. This change raises the question of the regenerative capacity of dystrophic muscle. Walton and Adams and others have found that a single trauma to a relatively sound dystrophic muscle excites the same regenerative changes as trauma to a normal and myositic muscle. Yet in severely dystrophic muscle, where only a few thin fibers remained, it was impossible to evaluate their response to injury. The fibers do eventually degenerate and disappear, owing presumably to an exhaustion of regenerative capacity after repeated injuries, or more and more extensive necrosis.

Hypertrophy of muscle is believed by most pathologists to be a work hypertrophy of sound fibers in the face of fiber injury. But there are disturbing examples of true hypertrophy of entire muscles prior to the first sign of weakness, when only a few degenerating fibers are present. Erb contended that the hypertrophy was the first expression of the basic abnormality, which then progressed to segmental necrosis (atrophy?). Pseudohypertrophy is due to lipocytic replacement of degenerated muscle fibers, but in its earlier stages the presence of many enlarged fibers contributes importantly to the enlargement of muscle. It is a true hypertrophy that eventually gives way to pseudohypertrophy. The increase in lipocytes, fibrosis, and thickening of the walls of blood vessels are secondary changes.

In the early stages of Duchenne dystrophy the most distinctive features are prominent segmental degeneration and phagocytosis of single fibers or groups of fibers and evidence of regenerative activity (basophilia of sarcoplasm, hyperplasia and nucleolation of sarcolemmal nuclei, and the presence of myotubes and myocytes). Vitreous change of sarcoplasm in many fibers scattered throughout the muscle has also been emphasized as an early sign of degeneration and is found more often in Duchenne dystrophy than in other dystrophies. Mokri and Engel have postulated that degenerative foci in the plasma membrane, which allow calcium to enter the fibers, explain this change. This hypothesis is supported by the demonstration of an increase in intracellular calcium and a decrease in magnesium in Duchenne dystrophy (Bertorini et al). Also the cholesterol content of the sarcolemma is increased in this disease. Schotland, by the use of the freeze-fracture technique, has demonstrated ultrastructural alterations in the intramembranous architecture of the plasmalemma of muscle fibers of dystrophic patients. Thus, according to this hypothesis, plasmalemmal degeneration becomes the initial change leading to fiber necrosis. Nevertheless, the authors remain skeptical because such vitreous fibers do not progress to a state of necrosis and phagocytosis. Moreover, the fibers showing the vitreous change are nearly always in a state of contraction (contraction bands); hence it may be no more than a mark of irritability of dystrophic muscle. Also, some degree of this change occurs as a biopsy artifact in many muscle diseases.

Under the light microscope the end stages of all the types of dystrophy are essentially the same. Differences are mainly quantitative in the different muscles in any one patient and in the different diseases. Only myotonic dystrophy stands apart from the others by virtue of lack of hypertrophy (atrophy of type I fibers), spiral annulets (ringbinden), sarcoplasmic masses, and rowing of central nuclei.

In the late stages of the dystrophic process only a few scattered muscle fibers remain, almost lost in a sea of fat cells. It is of interest that the late or burned-out stage of chronic polymyositis resembles muscular dystrophy in that the fiber population is depleted, the residual fibers are of variable size but otherwise normal, and fat cells and endomysial fibrous tissue are increased; lacking only are the hypertrophied fibers of dystrophy. This resemblance informs us that many of the typical changes of muscular dystrophy are nonspecific, reflecting only the chronicity of the myopathic process.

All the dystrophies have been studied electronmicroscopically, but the results have been disappointing insofar as they have provided no information as to the initial or specific lesion. The same is true of histochemical studies.

Finally, it should be restated that in all forms of muscular dystrophy the spinal neurons and their axons in the roots and peripheral nerves are normal.

ETIOLOGY AND PATHOGENESIS

Known to be a hereditary disease, the central issue in dystrophy is how an abnormal gene induces a degeneration of muscle fibers. Probably it is not overly important whether the degeneration occurs as a consequence of repeated segmental necrosis or of progressive atrophy.

The search for essential data regarding pathogenesis began with a scrutiny of the normal-appearing hypertrophied and atrophied fibers. Under the light and electron microscopes they appear to be normal, although one occasionally observes focal degeneration of myofilaments, smudging and misalignment of Z bands, increased numbers of mitochondria, glycogen and lipofuscin granules, autophagic vacuoles, lipid droplets, crystalline inclusions, and filamentous and myelin-like bodies. None of these changes, nor any particular combination of them is specific. Residual fibers show no special histochemical features, and attempts at tissue culture have failed to demonstrate unique properties of the dystrophic fibers.

Biochemical studies have revealed the following abnormalities: decreased glycolytic enzymes and relative normality of mitochondrial oxidative enzymes; increase of cathepsins (lysosomal enzymes); decrease in isoenzyme 5 of lactic dehydrogenase; decrease in myoglobin; increased serum CK, aldolase, LDH, SGOT, and SGPT; decreased protein synthesis; creatinuria and short half-life of labeled creatine; increased serum alpha globulin and polysaccharides, and occasionally pentosuria and taurinuria. Most of these abnormalities are the result of degeneration or regeneration of the muscle fiber, and none has been shown to be the basic biochemical defect that leads to necrosis and/or atrophy under conditions of natural activity.

As indicated above, biochemical and biophysical studies in recent years have implicated an abnormality of the muscle surface membrane in the genesis of muscular dystrophy. Supporting evidence has come also from the study of the membranes of red blood cells. Abnormalities in the phosphorylation of membrane proteins have been reported, as have a variety of morphologic abnormalities (distortion and surface projections: ''echinocytes'' and ''stomatocytes''). Unfortunately, these abnormalities have been found only in patients with myotonic dystrophy. To date, morphologic abnormalities of red blood cells (or of lymphocytes or cultured fibroblasts) have failed to provide a reliable diagnostic test for dystrophy. (A more comprehensive account of the pathology and biochemistry of muscle dystrophy can be found in the chapter by A.G. Engel, listed in the references).

Certainly the most interesting developments, mentioned earlier, have been the localization of the defective gene in myotonic dystrophy and the isolation of the defective gene and its protein product (dystrophin) in Duchenne dystrophy. Already these discoveries have altered our clinical concepts of the X-linked dystrophies and have provided new insights into the dystrophic process. Several investigators have localized dystrophin to the plasma membrane of the muscle. By the technique of immunostaining with dystrophic antibody, Arahata and his colleagues have demonstrated that in Duchenne dystrophy the muscle surface membrane is completely devoid of this protein. In Becker dystrophy, which is allelically related to Duchenne dystrophy (they share the same gene), there is a sporadic staining pattern. These observations support the hypothesis that defects in the surface membrane may initiate the muscle degradation in Duchenne-Becker dystrophy (Mokri and Engel).

DIAGNOSIS

The following are some of the common problems that arise in the diagnosis of muscular dystrophy:

1. *The diagnosis of muscular dystrophy in a child who has not been walking for long, or whose locomotion is delayed.* Tests of peak power on command cannot be used with reliability in small children. The most helpful points are (*a*) unusual difficulty in climbing stairs, or arising from a crouch or from a recumbent position on the floor, showing greater weakness at the hips and knees than at the ankles; (*b*) unusually large, firm calves; (*c*) male sex; (*d*) high serum CK and aldolase values; (*e*) myopathic EMG; and (*f*) biopsy findings.

2. *The adult patient with diffuse or proximal muscle weakness of several months' duration, raising the question of polymyositis versus dystrophy.* Biopsy may be misleading in showing a few inflammatory foci in an otherwise dystrophic picture. The main points which help to distinguish polymyositis from dystrophy have been indicated in the preceding chapter. As a rule, polymyositis is associated with high CK and aldolase values (higher than any dystrophy except the Duchenne type, which does not begin in adults), and the EMG shows many fibrillation potentials (rare in adult forms of muscular dystrophy). With these points in mind, there may still be uncertainty, in which instance a trial of prednisone is indicated for a period of 6 months. Unmistakable improvement favors polymyositis; questionable improvement (physician's and patient's judgment not in accord) leaves the diagnosis unsettled.

3. *An adult with a slowly evolving proximal weakness.* Several of the congenital polymyopathies discussed in Chap. 52 may begin to cause symptoms or to worsen in adult years. These include central core and nemaline myopathy. Examples of a mild form of acid maltase or debrancher enzyme deficiency with glycogenosis, progressive hypokalemic polymyopathy, mitochondrial myopathy, and carnitine polymyopathy have been reported in the adult. Muscle biopsy and histochemical staining of the muscle usually provide the correct diagnosis.

4. *The occurrence of subacute or chronic symmetric proximal weakness in an adolescent or adult raises the question of spinal muscular atrophy (Kugelberg-Welander type) as well as of polymyositis and muscular dystrophy.* EMG and muscle biopsy usually settle the matter. Some of the same problems arise in an adult with distal dystrophy.

5. *Weakness of a shoulder or one leg of some weeks' standing with increasing atrophy.* Here one must differentiate between a mononeuritis, poliomyelitis, the beginning of motor system disease (progressive spinal muscular atrophy), and a muscle dystrophy. The first three may develop silently, in mild form, and only attract notice when wasting begins (the latter takes 2 to 3 months to reach its peak).

Points in favor of these acquired diseases are (a) confinement of the disease to muscles originally affected, (b) sparing of other muscles, and (c) EMG showing denervation effects. Biopsy is seldom performed under such circumstances, for by temporizing the problem eventually settles itself (stabilization or recovery with poliomyelitis, recovery with mononeuritis). Spinal muscular atrophy declares itself by the presence of fasciculations and relatively rapid progression of weakness.

6. The distinction, in the child or adolescent, between dystrophy and one of the congenital myopathies will be considered in relation to the latter disorders (Chap. 52).

TREATMENT

There is no specific treatment for any of the muscular dystrophies, and the physician is forced to stand by helplessly and witness the unrelenting progression of weakness and wasting. The various vitamins, steroids, amino acids and innumerable drugs, recommended in the past, have all proved to be ineffective.

Quinine has a mild curare-like action at the motor end plate and thus relieves myotonia. Although symptomatic relief of the myotonia is usually achieved, the drug has no effect on the progress of the muscle atrophy or other degenerative aspects of dystrophia myotonica. The usual dose is 0.3 to 0.6 g orally, repeated as needed about every 6 h. Mild toxic symptoms such as tinnitus may develop before enough quinine has been given to relieve the myotonia. Some patients find the side effects more distressing than the myotonia and prefer not to take quinine except on occasions when the myotonia is troublesome in a particular activity. Procainamide (0.5 to 1.0 g four times daily) phenytoin, ACTH, and corticosteroids are sometimes useful in alleviating myotonia.

Androgens may be administered in cases of myotonic dystrophy and provide symptomatic benefit when deficiency is apparent, but a relationship of the hormonal deficiency to the pathogenesis of the muscle disease is not established.

Needless to say, the common complications of muscular dystrophy, notably fractures, pulmonary infections, and cardiac decompensation can be treated symptomatically, with benefit to the patient. Surgical management of cataracts, when they are mature, is indicated.

Trials of new drugs will and should continue. Promising possibilities are agents that inhibit muscle proteases, such as the products of actinomycete fungi, and calcium blockers, which have been shown to interfere with cardiac muscle fiber necrosis. None has yet proven to be of therapeutic value. It is unlikely that a rational therapy will be discovered until more is known about the basic biochemical abnormalities in each of the dystrophies.

Until such time, physicians must rely on physical methods of rehabilitation. Vignos has reviewed studies that evaluate muscle strengthening exercises and has offered evidence that maximal resistance exercises, if begun early, can strengthen muscles in Duchenne, limb-girdle, and facioscapulohumeral dystrophies. None of the muscles were weaker at the end of a year than at the beginning. Cardiorespiratory function, after endurance exercise, was not significantly improved. Contractures were reduced by passive stretching of the muscles 20 to 30 times a day and by splinting at night. If contractures have already formed, fasciotomy and tendon-lengthening are indicated if the patient is still ambulatory. Preventive measures were more successful than restorative ones.

From such observations it is concluded that two factors are of importance in the management of patients with muscular dystrophy: avoiding prolonged bed rest and encouraging the patient to maintain as full and normal a life as possible. These help to prevent the rapid worsening associated with inactivity and to conserve a healthy attitude of mind. Obesity should be avoided; this requires careful attention to diet. Swimming is a useful exercise. Massage and electrical stimulation are worthless. The education of children with muscular dystrophy should continue with the purpose of preparing them for a sedentary occupation.

REFERENCES

ADAMS RD, KAKULAS BA: *Diseases of Muscle: Pathological Foundations of Clinical Myology,* 4th ed. Philadelphia, Harper & Row, 1985.

ARAHATA K, ISHIURA S, ISHIGURO T et al: Immunostaining of skeletal and cardiac muscle surface membrane with antibody against Duchenne muscular dystrophy peptide. *Nature* 333:861, 1988.

BAKKER E, HOFKER MH, GOOR N et al: Prenatal diagnosis and carrier detection of Duchenne muscular dystrophy with closely linked RFLPs. *Lancet* 1:655, 1985.

BANKER BQ, VICTOR M, ADAMS RD: Arthrogryposis multiplex due to congenital muscular dystrophy. *Brain* 80:319, 1957.

BARBEAU A: The syndrome of hereditary late onset ptosis and dysphagia in French Canada, in Kuhn EE (ed): *Progressive Muskeldystrophies, Myotonie, Myasthenie.* New York, Springer-Verlag, 1966.

BATTEN FE, GIBB HP: Myotonia atrophica. *Brain* 32:187, 1909.

BECKER PE: Two new families of benign sex-linked recessive muscular dystrophy. *Rev Can Biol* 21:551, 1962.

BERENBERG RA, PELLOCK JM, DiMAURO S et al: Lumping or splitting? ''Ophthalmoplegia plus'' or Kearns-Sayre syndrome? *Ann Neurol* 1:37, 1977.

BERTORINI TE, BHATTACHARYA SK, GENARO MA et al: Muscle

calcium and magnesium in Duchenne muscular dystrophy. *Neurology* 32:1088, 1982.

BIRD TD, BOEHNKE M, SCHELLENBERG DG et al: The use of apolipoprotein CII as a genetic marker for myotonic dystrophy. *Arch Neurol* 44:273, 1987.

BRAMWELL E: Observations on myopathy. *Proc Roy Soc Med* 16:1, 1922.

CHAKRABARTI A, PEARSE JMS: Scapuloperoneal syndrome with cardiomyopathy: Report of a family with autosomal dominant inheritance and unusual features. *J Neurol Neurosurg Psychiatry* 44:1146, 1981.

CROS D, HARNDEN P, POUGET J et al: Peripheral neuropathy in myotonic dystrophy: A nerve biopsy study. *Ann Neurol* 23:470, 1988.

DONNER M, RAPOLA J, SOMMER H: Congenital muscular dystrophy, a clinicopathological and follow-up study of 13 patients. *Neuropediatrie* 6:239, 1975.

DRACHMAN DA: Ophthalmoplegia plus: The neurodegenerative disorders associated with progressive external ophthalmoplegia. *Arch Neurol* 18:654, 1968.

EMERY AEH, DREIFUSS FE: Unusual type of benign X-linked muscular dystrophy. *J Neurol Neurosurg Psychiatry* 29:338, 1966.

ENGEL AG: Duchenne dystrophy, in Engel AG, Banker BQ (eds): *Myology*. New York, McGraw-Hill, 1986, chap 37, pp 1185–1240.

ENGEL AG, BANKER BQ (eds): *Myology*. New York, McGraw-Hill, 1986.

FITZSIMMONS RB, GURWIN EB, BIRD AC: Retinal vascular abnormalities in facioscapulohumeral muscular dystrophy. *Brain* 110:631, 1987.

FUKUYAMA Y, KAWAZURA M, HARUNA H: A peculiar form of congenital muscular dystrophy. Report of 15 cases. *Pediatrica Univ Tokyo*, No. 4, 5-8, 1960.

GARDNER-MEDWIN D: Clinical features and classification of the muscular dystrophies. *Br Med Bull* 36(2):109, 1980.

GILCHRIST JM, LESHNER RT: Autosomal dominant humeroperoneal myopathy. *Arch Neurol* 43:734, 1986.

GOWERS WR: *Pseudohypertrophic Muscular Paralysis*. London, Churchill Livingstone, 1879.

HARPER PS: Congenital myotonic dystrophy in Britain. *Arch Dis Child* 50:505, 514, 1975.

HARPER PS: *Myotonic Dystrophy*. Philadelphia, Saunders, 1979.

HAZAMA R, TSUJIHATA M, MORI M, MORI K: Muscular dystrophy in six young girls. *Neurology* 29:1486, 1979.

HENSON TE, MULLER J, DEMYER WE: Hereditary myopathy limited to females. *Arch Neurol* 17:238, 1967.

HOFFMAN EP, BROWN RH JR, KUNKEL LM: Dystrophin: The protein product of the Duchenne muscular dystrophy locus. *Cell* 51:919, 1987.

HOFFMAN EP, FISCHBECK KH, BROWN RH et al: Characterization of dystrophin in muscle-biopsy specimens from patients with Duchenne's or Becker's muscular dystrophy. *N Engl J Med* 318:1363, 1988.

HOPKINS LC, JACKSON JA, ELIAS LJ: Emery-Dreifuss humeroperoneal muscular dystrophy: an x-linked myopathy with unusual contractures and bradycardia. *Ann Neurol* 10:230, 1981.

KEARNS TP, SAYRE GP: Retinitis pigmentosa, external ophthalmoplegia and complete heart block. *Arch Ophthalmol* 60:280, 1958.

KOENIG M, HOFFMAN EP, BERTELSON CJ et al: Complete cloning of the Duchenne muscular dystrophy (DMD) cDNA and preliminary genomic organization of the DMD gene in normal and affected individuals. *Cell* 50:509, 1987.

KUGELBERG E, WELANDER L: Heredofamilial juvenile muscular atrophy simulating muscular dystrophy. *Arch Neurol Psychiatry* 75:500, 1956.

KUHN E, FIEHN W, SCHRÖDER JM et al: Early myocardial disease and cramping myalgia in Becker type muscular dystrophy: A kindred. *Neurology* 29:1144, 1979.

KUNKEL LM: Analysis of deletions in DNA from patients with Becker and Duchenne muscular dystrophy. *Nature* 322:73, 1986.

LAMY M, DEGROUCHY J: L'hérédité de la myopathie (formes basses). *J Génetique Humaine* 3:219, 1954.

LEBENTHAL E, SCHOCHET SR, ADAM A et al: Arthrogryposis multiplex congenita. 23 cases in an Arab kindred. *Pediatrics* 16:891, 1970.

MAAS O, PATERSON AS: Myotonia congenita, dystrophia myotonica, and paramyotonia. *Brain* 73:318, 1950.

MAWATARI S, KATAYAMA K: Scapuloperoneal muscular atrophy with cardiopathy. *Arch Neurol* 28:55, 1973.

MERLINI L, GRANATA C, DOMINICI P, BONFIGLIOLI S: Emery-Dreifuss muscular dystrophy: report of five cases in a family and review of the literature. *Muscle Nerve* 9(6):481–485, 1986.

MILHORAT AT, WOLFF HG: Studies in diseases of muscle. XIII. Progressive muscular dystrophy of atrophic distal type; report on a family; report of autopsy. *Arch Neurol Psychiatry* 49:655, 1943.

MIYOSHI K, KAWAI H, IWASA M et al: Autosomal recessive distal muscular dystrophy as a new type of progressive muscular dystrophy. *Brain* 109:31, 1986.

MÖBIUS PJ: Ueber die hereditaren Nervenkrankheiten. *Sammlung klinischer Vortage* 171:1505, 1879.

MOKRI B, ENGEL AG: Duchenne dystrophy: Electron microscopic findings pointing to a basic or early abnormality in the plasma membrane of the muscle fiber. *Neurology* 25:1111, 1975.

MOORMAN JR, COLEMAN RE, PACKER DL et al: Cardiac involvement in myotonic muscular dystrophy. *Medicine* 64:371, 1985.

NEVIN S: Two cases of muscular degeneration occurring in late adult life with a review of the recorded cases of late progressive muscular dystrophy (late progressive myopathy). *J Med* 5:51, 1936.

PEARSON CM, FOWLER WG: Hereditary nonprogressive muscular dystrophy inducing arthrogryposis syndrome. *Brain* 86:75, 1963.

PERLOFF JK, ROBERTS WC, DELEON AC et al: The distinctive electrocardiogram of Duchenne's muscular dystrophy. *Am J Med* 42:179, 1967.

PRYSE-PHILIPS W, JOHNSON GJ, LARSEN B: Incomplete manifestations of myotonic dystrophy in a large kinship in Labrador. *Ann Neurol* 11:582, 1982.

RINGEL SP, WILSON WB, BARDEN MT: Extraocular muscle biopsy

in chronic progressive ophthalmoplegia. *Ann Neurol* 6:326, 1979.

ROSES AD, HARPER PS, BOSSEN EH: Myotonic muscular dystrophy, in Vinken PJ, Bruyn GW (eds): *Handbook of Clinical Neurology*, vol. 40. Amsterdam, North-Holland, 1979, chap 13, p 485.

ROSES MS, NICHOLSON MT, KIRCHER CS, ROSES AD: Evaluation and detection of Duchenne's and Becker's muscular dystrophy carriers by manual muscle testing. *Neurology* 27:20, 1977.

ROTTHAUWE HW, MORTIER W, BEYER H: Neuer Typ einer recessiv X-chromosomal verebten Muskeldystrophie: Scapulo-humero-distale Muskeldystrophie mit fruhzeitigen Kontrakturen und Herzrhythmusstorungen. *Humangenetik* 16:181, 1972.

ROWLAND LP: Dystrophin. A triumph of reverse genetics and the end of the beginning. *N Engl J Med* 318:1392, 1988.

SCHOTLAND DL: Duchenne dystrophy—a freeze fracture study, in Rowland LP (ed): *Pathogenesis of Human Muscular Dystrophies*. Amsterdam, Excerpta Medica, 1977, pp 562–568.

SEITZ D: Zur nosologischen Stellung des sogenannten scapuloperonealen Syndroms. *Dtschr Z Nervenheilk* 175:547, 1957.

SHAW DV, BROOK JD, MEREDITH AL et al: Gene mapping and chromosome 19. *J Med Genet* 23:2, 1986.

STEINER TH: Uber das klinische und anatomische Bild des Muskelschwunds der Myotoniker. *Dtschr Z Nervenheilk* 37:58, 1909.

SWASH M, HEATHFIELD KWG: Quadriceps myopathy, a variant of the limb-girdle dystrophy syndrome. *J Neurol Neurosurg Psychiatry* 46:355, 1983.

THOMAS PK, SCHOTT GD, MORGAN-HUGHES JA: Adult onset scapuloperoneal myopathy. *J Neurol Neurosurg Psychiatry* 38:1008, 1975.

VAN DER DOES DE WILLEBOIS AEM, BETHLEM J, MEYER AEFH, SIMONS AJR: Distal myopathy with onset in early infancy. *Neurology* 18:383, 1968.

VASSELLA F, MUMENTHALER M, ROSSI E et al: Congenital muscular dystrophy. *Deutsche Z Nervenh* 190:349, 1967.

VICTOR M, HAYES R, ADAMS RD: Oculopharyngeal muscular dystrophy. A familial disease of late life characterized by dysphagia and progressive ptosis of the eyelids. *N Engl J Med* 267:1267, 1962.

VIGNOS PJ: Physical models of rehabilitation in neuromuscular disease. *Muscle Nerve* 6:323, 1983.

WALTON JN (ed): *Disorders of Voluntary Muscle*, 5th ed. Edinburgh, Churchill Livingstone, 1988.

WALTON JN, GARDNER-MEDWIN D: Muscular dystrophy and myotonias, in Walton JN, (ed): *Disorders of Voluntary Muscle*, 4th ed. Edinburgh, Churchill-Livingstone, 1981, chap 14, pp 481–524.

WALTON JN, NATTRASS FS: On the classification, natural history and treatment of myopathies. *Brain* 77:169, 1954.

WELANDER L: Myopathia distalis tarda hereditaria. *Acta Med Scand* 141 (suppl 265):1, 1951.

WOHLFART G, FEX J, ELIASSON S: Hereditary proximal spinal muscle atrophy simulating progressive muscular dystrophy. *Acta Psychiatr Neurol* 30:395, 1955.

CHAPTER 51

THE METABOLIC MYOPATHIES

Two classes of metabolic disease of muscle have been recognized—one in which a muscle disorder is the consequence of a disease of the thyroid, parathyroid, pituitary or adrenal gland, and another in which the myopathy is traceable to a hereditary metabolic abnormality. The first group is relatively common and of considerable interest to internists. Diseases of the second group, much less frequent, are of greater interest to the myologist, for they reveal certain aspects of the complex chemistry of muscle. Indeed, each year brings to light some new genetically determined enzymopathy. And a number of diseases, formerly classified as dystrophic or degenerative, have been added to the list of metabolic myopathies. Limitation of space precludes a detailed description of each entity; only the most representative forms will be presented on the following pages. Complete accounts of this subject can be found in the reviews by A. G. Engel and diMauro, and in the monograph of Engel and Banker, listed in the references.

Apropos the clinical manifestations of this group of diseases, the majority have shown few or no muscular abnormalities prior to a certain age. Then there gradually unfolds a progressive weakness over a period of months or years. The weakness may affect only the lower extremities (hip flexors and extensors and quadriceps) or both the lower and upper extremities. Ocular and facial muscles are affected in only a few cases. Sometimes the involvement is more diffuse. Clues to the myopathic nature of the weakness are the elevated CK and aldolase in the serum: brief, low voltage (myopathic) units in the EMG; and atrophy or degeneration of fibers in the muscle biopsy. The differential diagnosis includes chronic idiopathic polymyositis and some of the congenital myopathies, described in Chaps. 49 and 52, respectively.

THYROID MYOPATHIES

Several myopathic diseases are related to alterations in thyroid function: (1) chronic thyrotoxic myopathy, (2) exophthalmic ophthalmoplegia (infiltrative ophthalmopathy), (3) myasthenia gravis associated with toxic diffuse goiter or with hypothyroidism, (4) periodic paralysis associated with toxic goiter, and (5) muscle hypertrophy and slow muscle contraction and relaxation associated with myxedema and cretinism. Although not frequent, several examples of these diseases may be seen in a single year in a large general hospital.

Chronic thyrotoxic myopathy is characterized by progressive weakness and wasting of the skeletal musculature, occurring in conjunction with overt or covert (masked) hyperthyroidism. The thyroid disease is usually chronic, and the goiter is of the nodular rather than the diffuse type. The muscular disorder may reach such an advanced degree as to suggest progressive spinal muscular atrophy (motor system disease). This complication of hyperthyroidism is most frequent in middle age, and men are more susceptible than women. The onset is insidious and the weakness progresses over weeks and months. Exophthalmos and other classic signs of hyperthyroidism need not be present. Muscles of the pelvic girdle and thighs are weakened more than others (Basedow paraplegia), though all are affected to some extent, even the bulbar muscles and rarely the ocular ones. However, the shoulder and hand muscles show the most conspicuous atrophy. Tremor and twitching during contraction may occur, but we have not seen fasciculations at rest or fibrillations (in the EMG). The tendon reflexes are normal or lively. Creatine excretion in the urine is increased and tolerance to ingested creatine is diminished, but the degree of these impairments has not correlated with the degree of weakness. Serum levels of muscle enzymes are not elevated and may be reduced. Usually the EMG is normal, though occasionally the action potentials are abnormally brief or polyphasic. Biopsies of muscle, except for slight atrophy of both type I and II fibers, have been normal. Administration of neostigmine has no effect. Muscle power and bulk are gradually restored when thyroid activity is reduced to normal levels.

Exophthalmic ophthalmoplegia refers to weakness of the external ocular muscles conjoined with the exophthalmos of Graves disease (pupillary and ciliary muscles are always spared). The exophthalmos varies in degree, being absent sometimes at an early stage of the disease, and is not in itself responsible for the muscle weakness. Both the exophthalmos and the weakness of the extraocular muscles may precede the signs of hyperthyroidism or follow effective treatment of the disorder. The extraocular muscle palsies may occasionally be unilateral, especially in the beginning. Any of the external eye muscles may be affected, usually one more than others, accounting for strabismus and diplopia; the inferior and medial recti are the most frequently affected, and upward movements are usually limited to the greatest degree. Ultrasound studies of the orbit reveal thickening of the temporal wall and loss of retro-orbital fat. The muscles are swollen, a change visible in CT scans and MRI. Examination of the eye muscles from biopsies and autopsy material has shown many degenerated fibers and infiltrations of lymphocytes, mononuclear leukocytes, and lipocytes; hence the term *infiltrative ophthalmopathy*. These histopathologic findings are suggestive of a specific autoimmune disease—a hypothesis supported by the finding of serum antibodies that react with extracts of eye muscles (Kodama et al). The condition often runs a self-limited course as does the exophthalmos itself, and therapy is difficult to evaluate. Certainly the maintenance of a euthyroid state is desirable (Dresner and Kennerdell).

In patients with marked periorbital and conjunctival edema, high doses of corticosteroids (about 80 mg prednisone per day) may partially control the ophthalmic disorder, including the extraocular muscle weakness. Because of the hazards of corticosteroid therapy, it should be reserved for patients who would otherwise require surgical intervention. In a number of such cases it has been possible, with corticosteroids, to carry the patient over the crisis and to avoid the damaging effects of extreme exophthalmos and risks of surgery. If the exophthalmos reaches a degree that threatens to injure the cornea, tarsorrhaphy or decompression by removal of the roof of the bony orbit may save the patient's vision.

Thyrotoxic periodic paralysis resembles familial periodic paralysis (page 1163), and consists of attacks of mild to severe weakness of the muscles of the trunk and limbs; usually the cranial muscles are spared. The weakness develops over a period of a few minutes or hours and lasts for part of a day or longer. In some series of patients with periodic paralysis, as many as half have had hyperthyroidism and many of them have been males of Oriental extraction. Unlike the typical hypokalemic form, thyrotoxic periodic paralysis is not a familial disorder, and its onset is usually in early adult life. In most of the thyrotoxic cases, the serum potassium levels have been low during the attacks of weakness and the administration of several grams of KCl has terminated the attack. Propranolol in doses of 160 mg daily is helpful in suppressing the attacks. Treatment of the hyperthyroidism abolishes the symptomatic manifestations of the muscular disorder.

Myasthenia gravis, in its typical autoimmune, neostigmine-responsive form, may accompany hyper- or hypothyroidism. The latter are also believed to be autoimmune diseases. Approximately 5 percent of myasthenic patients have hyperthyroidism, and the frequency of myasthenia gravis in hyperthyroid patients is 20 to 30 times that of the general population. Either condition may appear first or they may coincide. In hyperthyroidism, weakness and atrophy of muscles, characteristic of the aforementioned chronic thyrotoxic myopathy, are added to the myasthenia, without appearing to affect the requirement for or response to neostigmine. By contrast, hypothyroidism, even of mild degree, seems to aggravate the myasthenia gravis, greatly increasing the need for neostigmine and at times inducing a myasthenic crisis. Thyroxine is beneficial and, with respect to myasthenia, restores the patient to the status that existed before the onset of the thyroid insufficiency. However, the myasthenia gravis is independent of the thyroid disease, and each must be treated separately.

Hypothyroidism, whether in the form of myxedema or of cretinism, is often accompanied by changes in skeletal muscle, consisting of diffuse myalgia and increased volume, stiffness, and slowness of contraction and relaxation. These changes probably account for the large tongue and dysarthria that one observes in myxedema. The presence of action myospasm (rare) and percussion myoedema, along with the slowness of tendon reflexes, assists the examiner in making a bedside diagnosis (see page 1171). Cretinism in association with these muscle symptoms is known as the *Kocher-Debré-Semelaigne syndrome,* and myxedema in childhood or later, with muscle hypertrophy, as the *Hoffmann syndrome.* The latter clinical syndrome simulates hypertrophia musculorum vera and myotonia congenita. In neither cretinism nor myxedema, however, is there evidence of true myotonia, either by clinical test or EMG, although muscle action potentials are myopathic. Muscle biopsies have disclosed only the presence of large fibers or an increase in small fibers (either type I or II) and slight distention of the sarcoplasmic reticulum and subsarcolemmal glycogen (probably all due to disuse atrophy).

Patients with the muscle disorder of hypothyroidism show a reduction in creatinine excretion and an increase in creatine tolerance. Transaminase values in the serum are normal, but the CK level is usually elevated. The administration of thyroxine corrects the muscle disturbance.

How thyroid secretion affects the muscle fiber in all these myopathies is still a matter of conjecture. Clinical data indicate that this hormone influences the contractile process in some manner, but does not interfere with the transmission of impulses in the peripheral nerve, across the myoneural junction, or along the sarcolemma. In hyperthyroidism this functional disorder enhances the speed of the contractile process and reduces its duration, the net effect being a weakening, an excess fatigability, and a loss of endurance of muscle action. In hypothyroidism, muscle contraction is slowed, as is relaxation, and its duration is prolonged.

The speed of the contractile process is thought to be related to the quantity of myosin ATPase, which is increased in hyperthyroid muscle and decreased in hypothyroid muscle. The speed of relaxation depends on the rate of release and reaccumulation of calcium in the endoplasmic reticulum. This is slowed in hypothyroidism and increased in hyperthyroidism (Ianuzzo et al).

A sensorimotor neuropathy has been reported in conjunction with hypothyroidism. It is described on page 1054.

CORTICOSTEROID POLYMYOPATHY

The widespread use of adrenal corticosteroids has created a new muscle disease, probably similar to the one that occurs in the Cushing syndrome (Müller and Kugelberg). The proximal limb and girdle musculature becomes weak, to the point where it is difficult to elevate the arms and to arise from a sitting, squatting, or kneeling position, and walking may be hampered. The EMG is either normal or mildly myopathic, with small and abundant action potentials but no fibrillations. Biopsies disclose a slight variation in fiber size, with atrophic fibers, mainly of type IIb, and little or no fiber necrosis and no inflammatory cells. Electron microscopically there are aggregates of mitochondria, accumulations of glycogen and lipid and slight myofibrillar loss (disuse atrophy). The serum CK and aldolase are usually normal, and there is creatinuria.

There is only a poor correlation between the total dose of corticosteroid and the severity of muscle weakness. Nevertheless, in patients who develop this type of myopathy, the corticosteroid dosage has usually been high and sustained over a period of months or years. All corticosteroids may produce the disorder although fluorinated ones are more culpable than others. Discontinuation or reduction of corticosteroid administration leads to improvement and recovery. The mechanism by which corticosteroids cause muscle weakness is not known.

PRIMARY ALDOSTERONISM

Adrenal adenomas producing an excess of aldosterone have been the subject of many articles, the most notable being that of Conn. Muscular weakness has been observed in three-quarters of the reported cases and nearly half of them had either episodic hypokalemic periodic paralysis or tetany. Chronic potassium deficiency may express itself either by periodic weakness or by a chronic myopathic weakness. An associated alkalosis causes the tetany.

Generalized weakness is a characteristic of *Addison disease*, related to the water and electrolyte disturbances and hypotension. Rarely, a contracture of hamstring muscles develops, preventing upright stance. Biopsy has not disclosed any abnormalities of muscle; the EMG is normal; and the tendon reflexes are retained.

Diseases of Parathyroid Glands and Osteomalacia

A small proportion of patients with parathyroid adenomas complain of weakness and fatigability. Vicale described the first example of this disorder and remarked on the atrophy and weakness and the pain on passive or active movement. The tendon reflexes were retained. A few scattered muscle fibers undergo degeneration. Claims for a denervative process are disputed. We have not been impressed with either a myopathy or neuropathy in this disease.

In hypoparathyroidism, muscle cramping is prominent but there are no other neuromuscular manifestations.

In osteomalacia, due to vitamin D deficiency and disorders of renal tubular absorption, muscle weakness and pain have been common complaints and also the source of lively discussion in the myologic literature (see Layzer for further comment).

More striking than any of the foregoing disturbances, in our view, has been a chronic proximal myopathy in conjunction with hypophosphatemia and solitary bone cysts, the removal of which restored serum phosphorus levels and cured the muscle weakness. The oral administration of phosphates, to raise the serum phosphorus, has been beneficial in nontumorous cases. Some of the latter are accompanied by pain and stiffness. Presumably the phosphorus depletion in these disorders had limited the phosphorylation reactions and the synthesis of ATP.

DISEASES OF THE PITUITARY GLAND

Proximal muscle weakness and atrophy are recorded as late developments in many acromegalic patients. Formerly thought to be the consequence of a polyneuropathy, these symptoms were convincingly shown by Mastaglia et al to be due to a chronic polymyopathy. The serum CK is slightly elevated in some cases, and myopathic potentials are observed in the EMG. Biopsy specimens have shown atrophy and reduced numbers of type II fibers, and necrosis of only a few fibers. Treatment of the pituitary adenoma and correction of the hormonal changes restores strength. A mild peripheral neuropathy of sensorimotor type has also been reported in a few acromegalic patients but is less frequent than the carpal tunnel syndrome.

The myopathic manifestations of Cushing disease have been mentioned above, and are also discussed on page 542.

POLYMYOPATHY WITH HYPOKALEMIC PERIODIC PARALYSIS

A rare complication of *familial periodic paralysis* (page 1161) takes the form of a subacute or chronic persistent weakness of the thigh and pelvic musculature. The onset may be in the middle adult years, long after a troublesome periodic paralysis during childhood or adolescence has ameliorated or ceased altogether. Biopsy reveals the characteristic vacuolization and hydropia of periodic paralysis, and the degeneration of some of the muscle fibers that may be consequent to it. Slightly elevated levels of muscle enzymes in the serum and a myopathic pattern in the EMG substantiates the diagnosis. The effective control of the acute attacks of paralysis by the administration of potassium appears to slow or halt the progress of the myopathy.

GLYCOGEN STORAGE MYOPATHIES

This relatively rare group of diseases has gradually enlarged as more has been learned about carbohydrate metabolism of muscle. Following the work of Illingworth, Larner, and the Coris (1952), several additional enzymatic steps have been discovered, and deficiencies in each of them have become the basis of the commonly accepted classification, which is presented in Table 51-1. These enzymatic deficiencies alter the metabolism of many cells but most strikingly those of the liver, heart, and skeletal muscle; in about half of the affected individuals a chronically progressive or intermittent myopathic syndrome is the major manifestation of the disease. The most impressive of these glycogen storage diseases, from the standpoint of the clinical myologist, are α-1,4-glucosidase (acid maltase) and myophosphorylase deficiencies.

Acid Maltase Deficiency This enzymopathy takes three clinical forms, each of which is inherited as an autosomal recessive trait. The first is the most malignant. It develops in infancy, between 2 and 6 months; dyspnea and cyanosis call attention to enlargement of the heart, and the skeletal muscles are found to be weak and hypotonic. The tongue may be enlarged, giving the infant a cretinoid appearance. Hepatomegaly, while often present, is not pronounced. Exceptionally, the heart is relatively normal in size, and the CNS and muscles bear the brunt of the disorder. The clinical picture then resembles infantile muscular atrophy (Werdnig-Hoffmann disease). The disease is rapidly progressive and ends fatally in a few months. The EMG is myopathic and there are fibrillations, heightened insertional activity, and pseudomyotonia. Large amounts of glycogen accumulate in muscle, heart, liver, and neurons of the spinal cord and brain. All tissues lack acid maltase. The abnormal gene is located on chromosome 17.

In the second (childhood) form, onset is during the second year, with delay in walking and slowly progressive weakness of shoulder and pelvic girdles and trunk muscles. The toe walking, waddling gait, enlargement of calf muscles, and lumbar lordosis resemble those in Duchenne dystrophy. Cardiomyopathy is exceptional. Hepatomegaly is less frequent than in the infantile form and mental retardation was present in only 2 of 18 cases reported by diMauro. Death occurred between 3 and 24 years of age.

In the third, or adult, form there is a more benign proximal and truncal myopathy. The weakness is slowly progressive over years, and death is usually the result of paralysis of respiratory muscles. At times the only severe weakness is of the diaphragm, as in the case of Sivak et al. The liver and heart are not enlarged. CK values are 2 to 12 times normal. The EMG reveals brief motor unit potentials, fibrillation potentials, positive waves, bizarre, high frequency discharges, and occasional myotonic discharges (without clinical evidence of myotonia). The disease must be differentiated from other chronic adult polymyopathies.

The diagnosis is readily confirmed by muscle biopsy. In routine preparations the sarcoplasm is vacuolated and alcohol fixation permits staining of the stored glycogen. The latter is increased 4 to 5 times above normal and the glycogen particles lie in aggregates, some surrounded by membranes and some free. Electron microscopy shows them to occupy lysosomal vesicles. The myofibrillae are disrupted. Some muscle fibers degenerate. The glycogen accumulation is more pronounced in type I fibers. In the more severe infantile form of acid maltase deficiency nerve cells and heart muscle may also accumulate glycogen and degenerate. The difference in severity between infant and adult forms may relate to the completeness of enzyme deficiency, but other factors may be at work. More than one of the three types may occur in the same family.

There is no effective treatment. Respiratory support (rocking bed) may prolong life.

Myophosphorylase Deficiency (Type V Glycogenosis; McArdle Disease) This disorder expresses itself by the syndrome of recurrent contracture, and the same is true of phosphofructokinase deficiency (type VII). Both are discussed in Chap. 54.

Of the other forms of glycogenosis only type III (*debranching enzyme deficiency*) affects muscle and then not consistently. A childhood form, less severe than that of acid maltase deficiency, sometimes weakens muscle and diminishes tone, and an adult form with chronic proximal and distal myopathy have been observed. In the series reported by diMauro and his colleagues several of the patients who developed weakness during adult life complained of rapid fatigue and aching of muscles, occurring with exertion, since an early age. Their CK values were elevated, and the EMG showed a myopathic picture, as well as increased insertional activity, pseudomyotonic discharges, and fibrillations. Rarely, in the adult form, glycogen accumulates in the peripheral nerves, giving rise to mild symptoms of polyneuropathy. The enzymatic defect is one of amylo-1,6-glucosidase deficiency.

CARNITINE DEFICIENCY

Carnitine, derived mainly from lysine and methionine, is synthesized in the liver and kidney and transported to muscle, where it facilitates the intramitochondrial oxidation of long-chain fatty acids. Three clinical syndromes have been associated with carnitine deficiency. One is a predominantly myopathic form, originally described by Engel et al. The main features are progressive muscle weakness with onset in childhood or in adult life, affection of the trunk and proximal limb muscles, lipid excess in muscle, and marked reduction of muscle carnitine. It is worsened by

Table 51-1
Glycogen storage diseases

Type	Clinical and laboratory findings	Enzyme defiency	Heredity	Proper name
I	Enlarged liver and kidneys, hyperlipidemia, hypoglycemia, ketoacidosis, hypotonia in infants	Glucose-6-phosphatase	Autosomal recessive	von Gierke
II	*Infantile form:* cardiomegaly, hypotonia and weakness, dysphagia, and respiratory difficulty; death in infancy *Childhood:* proximal weakness, enlarged calves, atonic anal sphincter, respiratory difficulties *Adult:* slowly progressive proximal myopathy; respiratory failure	α-1,4-Glucosidase (acid maltase)	Autosomal recessive	Pompe
III	Hepatomegaly, hypoglycemia, growth retardation, proximal and distal myopathy in some patients	Amylo-1,6-glucosidase (debranching)	—	Illingworth-Cori-Forbes
IV	Failure to thrive and growth failure, hepatosplenomegaly, cirrhosis, hypotonia with muscle atrophy in lower limbs in some patients	α-1,4-Glucan 6-glucosyltransferase (branching)	Autosomal recessive	Anderson
V	Cramp, pain, and weakness of muscles with exercise, sometimes myoglobinuria, lack of rise in blood lactate after ischemic exercise	Myophosphorylase	Probably autosomal recessive; autosomal dominant (rare)	McArdle
VI	Growth retardation, hepatosplenomegaly, hypoglycemia and mild ketosis	Hepatic phosphorylase	—	Hers
VII	Same as type V	Muscle phosphofructokinase	Same as type V	Tarui
Other		Phosphohexoisomerase Phosphorylase-*b*-kinase Phosphoglucomutase		

exercise and prolonged fasting. Cardiomyopathy may occur. Muscle enzymes in the serum are increased. Patients have responded favorably to prednisone, carnitine replacement (3 to 6 g DL carnitine per day orally), and a low-fat, high-carbohydrate diet, but interestingly, none has shown an increase in muscle carnitine.

A second syndrome, so-called systemic carnitine deficiency, was first described by Karpati et al. The dominant features of this condition are progressive, predominantly proximal muscle weakness, punctuated by attacks of vomiting, confusion, stupor, and coma, resembling the Reye syndrome. The age of onset has ranged in age from 11 months to 17 years. Lipid storage was more pronounced in type I than in type II fibers, as is the case also in the myopathic form. The administration of carnitine has a variable effect on the muscle weakness, and most patients succumb during an attack of acute encephalopathy. The nature of this disorder is not fully understood; recent studies suggest that it is due to a generalized defect of carnitine transport (see A. G. Engel).

The syndrome of *carnitine palmityl transferase deficiency* usually declares itself by attacks of myoglobinuria and has already been described in Chap. 50. All three of the carnitine deficiency syndromes are inherited as autosomal recessive traits.

Some carnitine deficiency syndromes are probably secondary to some other metabolic disorder, either one involving the mitochondrial respiratory chain, or an acquired state such as hemodialysis, cachexia, and cirrhosis.

MITOCHONDRIAL MYOPATHIES

As stated in Chap. 52, Shy and his colleagues, in their studies of hypotonic infants, were the first to recognize a number of morphologic abnormalities of muscle characterized mainly by abnormalities of mitochondria. The latter were either present in excessive number, a state that they called pleoconial, or were abnormal by virtue of their size or their inclusions, hence megaconial. In some obscure manner the mitochondrial changes had interfered with the normal maturation and development of the muscle fibers, and in some instances, the cells of other organs.

Much later, in connection with the Kearns-Sayre syndrome, it was found that muscle fibers with a great excess of mitochondria could be seen as ''ragged-red fibers'' in Gomori stains of muscle. These fibers also showed uniformly positive reactions with oxidative histochemical stains such as succinic dehydrogenase. Since many enzymes of the Krebs cycle reside in the mitochondria, where they remove high-energy electrons from acetyl CoA and convert them via nucleotide carriers into phosphate bonds and ATP synthetase, they are involved in a series of essential steps in the cycle. Cytochromes containing copper and particularly cytochrome C form the final link.

Further studies of deficiencies of mitochondrial enzymes in these diseases have brought to notice a new mode of inheritance, which differs from nuclear DNA inheritance and is called mitochondrial inheritance; the latter is contributed mainly by the maternal organism. Mutations of mitochondrial enzymes may block the oxidative phosphorylation pathway at any one of several points.

Most recently Morgan-Hughes and diMauro et al have written informatively about this group of diseases. Some of them present as muscle weakness and exercise intolerance in childhood or adult years. Others involve the retina, central nervous system (dementia and cerebellar ataxia, choreoathetosis), or peripheral nerves. Some cause stroke-like episodes. The latter aspects of the subject are discussed more completely in Chaps. 38 and 52.

ADENYLATE DEAMINASE DEFICIENCY

Since polymyalgia and exercise intolerance are the major symptoms, this condition is described in Chap. 54 (page 1175).

REFERENCES

ANGELINI G, GOVONI E, BRAGAGLIA MM, VERGANI L: Carnitine deficiency: Acute postpartum crisis. *Ann Neurol* 4:558, 1978.

CONN JW: Aldosteronism in man. Some clinical and climatological aspects. *JAMA* 183:871, 1963.

DIMAURO S: Metabolic myopathies, in Vinken PJ, Bruyn GW, (eds): *Handbook of Clinical Neurology, Diseases of Muscle,* vol 41. Amsterdam, North-Holland, 1979, chap 6, pp 175–234.

DIMAURO S, BONILLA E, ZEVIANI M et al: Mitochondrial myopathies. *Ann Neurol* 17:521, 1985.

DIMAURO S, MIRANDA AF, SAKODA S et al: Metabolic myopathies. *Am J Med Genet* 25:635, 1986.

DRESNER SC, KENNERDELL JS: Dysthyroid orbitopathy. *Neurology* 35:1628, 1985.

ENGEL AG: Metabolic and endocrine myopathies, in Walton JN (ed): *Disorders of Voluntary Muscle*, 5th ed. Edinburgh, Churchill Livingstone, 1988, pp 811–868.

ENGEL AG, ANGELINI C, NELSON RA: Identification of carnitine deficiency as a cause of human lipid storage myopathy, in Milhorat AT (ed): *Exploratory Concepts in Muscular Dystrophy II*. Amsterdam, Excerpta Medica, 1974, p 601.

ENGEL AG, BANKER BQ (eds): *Myology.* New York, McGraw-Hill, 1986.

IANUZZO D, PATEL P, CHEN V et al: Thyroidal trophic influence on skeletal muscle myosin. *Nature* 270:74, 1977.

ILLINGWORTH B, LARNER J, CORI GT: Structure of glucogens and amylopectins. I. Enzymatic determination of chain length. *J Biol Chem* 199:631, 1952.

ILLINGWORTH B, CORI GT: Structure of glycogens and amylopectins. III. Normal and abnormal human glycogen. *J Biol Chem* 199:653, 1952.

KARPATI G, CARPENTER S, ENGEL AG et al: The syndromes of carnitine deficiency. *Neurology* 25:16, 1975.

KODAMA K, SIKORSKA H, BANDY-DAFOE P et al: Demonstration of circulating autoantibody against a soluble eye-muscle antigen in Graves' ophthalmopathy. *Lancet* 2:1353, 1982.

LARNER J, ILLINGWORTH B, CORI GT, CORI CF: Structure of glycogens and amylopectins. II. Analysis by stepwise enzymatic degradation. *J Biol Chem* 199:641, 1952.

LAYZER RB: *Neuromuscular Manifestations of Systemic Disease.* New York, Davis, 1985.

MASTAGLIA FL, BARWICH DD, HALL R: Myopathy in acromegaly. *Lancet* 2:907, 1970.

MORGAN-HUGHES JA: Mitochondrial myopathies, in Engel AG, Banker BQ (eds): *Myology.* New York, McGraw-Hill, 1986, pp 1709–1743.

MÜLLER R, KUGELBERG E: Myopathy in Cushing's syndrome. *J Neurol Neurosurg Psychiatry* 22:314, 1959.

SIVAK ED, SALANGA VD, WILBOURN AJ et al: Adult onset acid maltase deficiency presenting as diaphragmatic paralysis. *Ann Neurol* 9:613, 1981.

SLONIM AE, WEISBERG MD, BENKE P: Reversal of debrancher deficiency myopathy by the use of high protein nutrition. *Ann Neurol* 11:420, 1982.

SPECTOR RH, CARLISLE JA: Minimal thyroid ophthalmopathy. *Neurology* 37:1803, 1987.

VICALE CT: The diagnostic features of a muscular syndrome resulting from hyperparathyroidism, osteomalacia owing to renal tubular acidosis, and perhaps to related disorders of calcium metabolism. *Trans Am Neurol Assoc* 74:143, 1949.

CHAPTER 52

THE CONGENITAL NEUROMUSCULAR DISORDERS

As skeletal muscle is subjected to increasingly careful study, more and more congenital, developmental, and aging abnormalities are being discovered. All are understandable in relation to the life cycle of the muscle fiber and are therefore presented together in this chapter. Such diseases are of particular importance in pediatric neurology, for most of them attract notice at an early age.

THE DEVELOPMENT AND AGING OF MUSCLE

The commonly accepted view of the embryogenesis of muscle is that muscle fibers form originally by fusion of myoblasts, soon after the latter differentiate from mesenchymal cells. The newly formed fibers are thin, centrally nucleated tubes (appropriately called *myotubes*) in which myofilaments begin to be produced from polyribosomes. As myofilaments become organized into myofibrils, the nuclei of the muscle fiber are displaced peripherally to a subsarcolemmal position. The intricacy of the steps whereby myoblasts seek one another, the manner in which each of a series of fused nuclei contribute to the myotube, the formation of actin and myosin fibrils, and the differentiation of a small residue of satellite cells are elaborated in the review by Allbrook.

The mechanisms that determine the number and arrangement of fibers in each muscle are not so well understood. Presumably the myoblasts themselves possess the genetic information that controls the program of development, but within any given species there are wide familial and individual variations, which account for obvious differences in the size of muscles and their power of contractility.

It is stated that the number of fibers which is assigned to each muscle is attained by birth, and growth of muscle thereafter depends mainly on the enlargement of fibers. Although the nervous system and musculature develop

independently, muscle fibers continue to grow after birth only when they are active and under the influence of nerve. Our observations are in accord with these principles, although one of the authors (R.D.A.) and deReuck found a twofold numerical increase in fibers in several muscles between birth and adult life. Probably this increase is related to the normal process of repeated injury and splitting of hypertrophied fibers (Schwartz et al).

Measurements of muscle fiber diameters from birth throughout life show the growth curve ascending rapidly in the early postnatal years and less rapidly in adolescence, reaching a peak during the third decade. After puberty, growth of muscle is less in females than in males; such differences are greater in the arm, shoulder, thigh, and pelvic muscles than in those of the leg, and growth in ocular muscles is about equal in the two sexes. At all ages, disuse decreases the fiber size by as much as 30 percent (at the expense of myofibrils), and overuse increases the size by about the same amount (work hypertrophy). Normally, type I (oxidative-enzyme-rich) fibers are slightly smaller than type II (phosphorylative-enzyme-rich) fibers.

During late adult life and the senium, the number of muscle fibers diminishes and variations in size increase. The variations are of two types, *group atrophy* (clusters of 20 to 30 fibers, all reduced in diameter to about the same extent) and *random atrophy*. Also, there is enlargement of other fibers. Exercising young animal muscle causes a hypertrophy of high-oxidative type I fibers and an increase in the proportion of low-oxidative type II fibers; aging muscle lacks this capacity [exercise produces only an increase in the proportion of type II fibers (Silbermann et al)]. No such data are available in humans, but clinical observation informs us of a diminished capacity in old age to respond to intense and prolonged exercise. Thus, it appears that muscle cells, like other cells of post-mitotic type, are subject to aging (lipofuscin accumulation, autophagic vacuolization, enzyme loss) and to death. Group atrophy, present in 90 percent of gastrocnemii in individuals past 60 years of age, represents denervation effect and corresponds to the 30 percent loss of lumbar motor neurons in old age (Tomlinson et al).

DERANGEMENTS OF THE LIFE CYCLE OF MUSCLE FIBERS

These have not been fully ascertained, but one can envision the following possibilities: (1) failure of muscle cells to differentiate in a given region (congenital absence of muscle); (2) congenital hypoplasia (local or universal); (3) congenital hyperplasia (local or universal); (4) faulty intrinsic development leading to certain disfigurations of fibers (improper arrangement of nuclei, myofilaments, and other organelles; this conceivably could reduce viability, i.e., cause abiotrophy); and (5) presenile abiotrophy or senescent polymyopathy.

Denervation from spinal or nerve disease at every age has roughly the same effect, viz., atrophy of muscle fibers (first in random distribution then in groups) and later dystrophic degeneration. Segmental necrosis at all ages excites a regenerative response from the intact parts of the fiber. As indicated on page 1128, if this occurs repeatedly, the regenerative potential presumably wanes, with ultimate death of the fiber. The latter leads to permanent depopulation of fibers and muscle weakness.

CONGENITAL ABSENCE OF MUSCLES

It is well known that some individuals are born without certain muscles. Not only is this true of certain inconstant and functionally unimportant ones, such as the palmaris longus, but of more constant and important ones as well. In the most authoritative writings on this subject (leDouble, Bing), the muscles found to be absent most frequently were the pectoralis, trapezius, serratus anticus, and quadratus femoris, but 27 others were missing in at least one case.

Congenital absence of a muscle is usually associated with congenital anomalies of other tissues. It would appear that an anomaly as crude as total failure of mesenchymal cells to differentiate into muscle fibers affects the anlage of neighboring nonmuscular tissues. For example, congenital absence of the pectoral muscle is accompanied by aplasia or hypoplasia of the mammary gland as well as syndactyly and microdactyly. Agenesis of the pectoral muscle may also be associated with scoliosis, webbed fingers, and underdevelopment of the ipsilateral arm and hand (Poland syndrome). Another unusual syndrome consists of congenital deficiency of the abdominal muscles in association with a defect of ureters, bladder, and genital organs.

There is another group of restricted palsies in which the essential abnormalities appear to lie in the nervous system (*nuclear amyotrophies*). One of the most frequent is *congenital ptosis,* due to an innervatory defect of the levator palpebrae muscles. Complete paralysis of all muscles supplied by the oculomotor nerve, due apparently to hypoplasia of the third nerve nuclei, has been observed in several members of one family, but has also been seen occasionally in only one member. A *congenital Horner syndrome* is another well-known phenomenon and may be familial. Bilateral abducens palsy is often associated with bifacial palsy in the newborn and is known as the *Möbius syndrome;* this usually nonfamilial anomaly, the cause of which is thought to be a nuclear hypoplasia or aplasia, is discussed with the developmental disorders (page 989). However, a primary muscle defect may also give rise to a bifacial weakness in Landouzy-Déjerine dystrophy.

In these familial nuclear amyotrophies the muscles develop independently of the nervous system but have no prospect of attaining their natural growth and function because of failure of innervation. It is a kind of congenital denervation hypotrophy.

CONGENITAL FIBROUS CONTRACTURES OF MUSCLES AND JOINT DEFORMITIES

Fibrous contracture refers to a fixation of limb posture due to a developmental lack or destruction of muscles, fibrosis of muscle and periarticular tissues, and shortening of ligaments. There are a surprising number of deformities in infants and children that appear to be due to shortening and fibrosis of muscles. The most common are congenital clubfoot (talipes), congenital torticollis, and congenital elevation of the scapula (Sprengel deformity). In all these conditions the postural distortion is produced and maintained either by a weakened, fibrotic muscle or by a normal one that is contracted and shortened because of the absence of a countervailing antagonist. Trauma to a muscle during intrauterine life or at birth leads to fibrosis and to fibrous contracture in some cases.

In congenital clubfoot the deformity may be one of plantar flexion of the foot and ankle (talipes equinus), inversion (talipes varus or clubfoot), eversion (talipes valgus or splayfoot), or dorsiflexion of foot and ankle (talipes calcaneus). About 75 percent are equinovarus. Usually both feet are affected. Multiple incidence in one family may occur. Several explanations of cause and pathogenesis have been offered: fetal malposition, an embryonic abnormality of tarsal and metatarsal bones, a primary defect in nerves or anterior horns of the spinal cord, or a congenital dystrophy of muscle. No one theory applies to all cases; available pathologic data exclude a single cause and pathogenesis. In some instances clubfoot is the only recognizable congenital abnormality, but more often it occurs as a manifestation of generalized arthrogryposis (see below) and as an indicator of widespread involvement of the CNS (see Adams and Kakulas and also Banker for pertinent literature on the subject).

Congenital wryneck, or torticollis, begins during the first months of life and is due to shortening of the sternomastoid muscle, which is firm and taut. The head is inclined to one side and the occiput slightly rotated to the side of the affected muscle. This disorder is nonfamilial and is usually ascribed to injury of the sternomastoid at birth. Whether the injury is purely mechanical in nature or ischemic, due to arterial or venous occlusion, is not entirely clear. It gives rise to a sternomastoid tumor (actually a pseudotumor) that appears, on exploration, as a white, spindle-shaped swelling of the muscle belly. The histologic findings are similar to those of Volkmann contracture, i.e., replacement of the muscle fibers by relatively acellular connective tissue, so that an ischemic mechanism appears most likely (page 1096).

Arthrogryposis Multiplex Congenita Multiple congenital contractures, multiple congenital articular rigidities, and amyoplasia congenita are some of the names that have been applied to congenital deformity and rigidity of the extremities. This disorder, now generally referred to as *arthrogryposis* (literal meaning—curved joints), has been shown to have at least two pathologic bases. By far the more common is the *myelopathic* type, in which there is a failure in development of anterior horn cells, resulting in uneven smallness and paresis of limb muscles. The unopposed contraction of normally innervated muscles causes the fixed deformities. Often this form is combined with multiple defects in the nervous system and somatic structures, i.e., some degree of mental retardation, webbed fingers, polydactyly, hydrocephalus, malformations of skull, small jaw, low-set ears, etc. In the less common or *myopathic* form, the nervous system is intact and the disease is that of a congenital muscular dystrophy (page 1126). In this form of arthrogryposis there is probably a hereditary factor. It is of interest that in the myopathic variety the limbs are fixed in a position of flexion at the hips and knees and adduction of the legs, in contrast to the variable postures of the myelopathic form. Also, the former type is less frequently conjoined with multiple anomalies than the latter.

It cannot be decided, from the available reports, whether there is a neuropathic form of arthrogryposis, in addition to these two well-recognized types.

RELATIVELY NONPROGRESSIVE CONGENITAL POLYMYOPATHIES

Beginning in 1956, with the account by Shy and Magee of a patient whose muscle fibers showed a peculiar central densification of sarcoplasm ("cores"), a series of new diseases of muscle has gradually been delineated. These include the central core, nemaline (rod-body), mitochondrial, centronuclear or myotubular myopathies, and myopathies with fiber-type disproportion. As the names imply, in each of these diseases there is a distinctive morphologic abnormality that expresses itself early in life by a retardation of motor development and hypotonia and weakness of the limbs.

Further study has revealed that the diseases of this group are not confined to infancy and early childhood. Each of the entities mentioned above has been observed at a later age, even in middle adult life; and if the disease is mild, there is often no way of deciding whether it has been present since birth. Lack of or extremely slow progression characterize most of the congenital myopathies, in contrast to the more rapid pace of muscular dystrophy, Werdnig-Hoffmann disease, and the other forms of hereditary motor system disease of childhood and adolescence. Yet exceptionally, examples of more rapid progression have been reported, and prior to muscle biopsy studies such patients were usually considered to have muscular dystrophy. Familial occurrence has also been established, so the clinical line of separation between this group of diseases and the muscular dystrophies remains ambiguous. There is no specific treatment for any of the congenital myopathies.

The lesions in the congenital myopathies are revealed most clearly by the systematic use of histochemical stains and phase and electron microscopy. Some of the abnormalities can also be disclosed by the conventional stains used in light microscopy. Thus, as a group, one might say that their discovery is a product of a new histologic technology.

A word of caution must be expressed about the specificity of some of the morphologic changes and the classifications of the congenital myopathies based upon them. It is treacherous to assume that a change in a single organelle or a subtle change in the sarcoplasm of a muscle fiber can be relied upon to characterize a pathologic process. Indeed, as more careful studies have been made of the following entities, the specificity of the lesions has been questioned. Central cores are sometimes found in the same muscle as nemaline bodies, etc., and each of the denotative lesions has been reported in other conditions or lesions, as pointed out by Bethlem and his associates. Therefore, the following subgroups must be regarded as only tentative.

Central Core Myopathy   In the original family of Shy and Magee, five members (four males) in three generations were affected, suggesting a dominant type of inheritance. The youngest was 2 years old; the oldest, 65 years old. In each, there was a general delay in motor development, particularly in walking, until the age of 4 to 5 years, and always the patient had had difficulty in arising from a chair, climbing stairs, and running. The weakness was more in proximal than distal muscles, though the latter did not escape, and shoulder girdle muscles were affected less than those of the pelvic girdle. Facial, bulbar, and ocular muscles were spared. The tendon reflexes were active and symmetric. Muscle atrophy was not a prominent feature, though poor muscular development was present in one patient and has since been reported in others. There were no fasciculations, cramps, or myotonia. The electrocardiograms were normal.

The disease is rare, but as additional cases were discovered, milder forms of the disease came to be recognized, with onset of symptoms in adult life. Originally some of these patients were thought to have limb-girdle dystrophy because of the disproportionate involvement of proximal muscles. In other families, such as the one reported by Patterson et al, the onset was in middle adult life with rapid progression of a proximal myopathy. These represent the two extremes of the clinical state. Dislocation of the hips and pes cavus has been found in a few children. In the majority of cases the progress of the disease is extremely slow, with slight worsening over many years. The EMG reveals only brief, small amplitude motor unit potentials with a normal interference pattern. Except for an increase in urinary creatine and decrease of urinary creatinine, no chemical abnormalities have been found in the blood or urine.

Pathologically, the majority of the fibers appear normal in size or enlarged, and no focal destruction or loss of fibers can be found. The unique feature of the disease is the presence in the central portion of each muscle fiber of a dense, amorphous, hyaline change in myofibrils. This altered zone characteristically lacks organelles and gives a positive periodic acid Schiff (PAS) reaction and an altered color with the Gomori trichrome stain, contrasting with the normal blue-green color of the peripheral fibrils. Most of the cores are in type I fibers, which predominate.

In other familial disorders of muscle, particularly in oculopharyngeal dystrophy but also in other forms of dystrophy, multiple cores or minicores have been seen within muscle fibers. These cores do not run the length of the muscle fiber, thus differing from the cores of central core disease.

Nemaline Myopathy   This disorder also expresses itself by hypotonia and impaired motility in infancy and early childhood, but unlike central core disease, the muscles of the trunk and limbs (proximal greater than distal) as well as the facial, lingual, and pharyngeal muscles are strikingly thin and hypoplastic. Tendon reflexes are diminished or absent. The young child with this disease usually suffers from inanition and frequent respiratory infections, which may shorten life. Strength slowly improves with growth, the latter process evidently exceeding the advance of the disease. Scoliosis becomes apparent in late childhood and adolescence. The milder cases reach adulthood and then worsen slowly over the years. A. G. Engel as well as W. K. Engel and Reznick have observed individuals who showed signs of the disease for the first time in middle age; the weakness was mainly in proximal muscles. The EMG is "myopathic" and serum enzymes are normal or only slightly elevated. The inheritance pattern has been both autosomal dominant and recessive.

A Gomori trichrome-stained section of frozen muscle discloses the characteristic lesion, which can be seen under the light microscope. Myriads of bacilli-like rods, singly and in small packets, are seen beneath the sarcolemma. They are composed of material that resembles that of Z bands under the electron microscope, and often actin filaments are attached just as they are to Z bands. The type I fibers, which usually predominate, are smaller than normal, as in central core disease. The cause of the disease is unknown but probably the weakness is related to a smallness and reduction in the number of muscle fibers and possibly to focal interruption of their cross striations. In one of the few autopsied cases, the anterior horn cells and their axons were present in normal number but were reduced in size (Robertson et al). These changes were interpreted as being secondary to the myopathic disorder.

Mitochondrial Myopathies   As stated in Chap. 57, a variety of myopathies have been associated with the presence of overly abundant and large mitochondria (often containing abnormal inclusions and cristae) in many muscle fibers. The terms *mitochondrial* and *lipid storage* have been used interchangeably to designate some of these myopathies, since the enzymes essential for intramuscular lipid metabolism are contained in the mitochondria, and a defect in the latter results in an abnormal accumulation of lipid bodies in muscle fibers.

One type of benign congenital myopathy was named *pleoconial* by Shy and his colleagues, because of the abundance of mitochandria that were seen in the muscle biopsy. The patient was an 8-year-old boy who had hypotonia and slow motor development since early life. It was reported that he craved salt and that there had been at least three prolonged episodes of flaccid quadriparesis, like periodic paralysis.

A closely related disorder was called *megaconial,* because of the presence, in the muscle biopsy, of giant mitochondria containing rectangular inclusions. This disorder also was detected in an 8-year-old child who had had hypotonia and weakness of muscles since birth. A sibling had died, probably of the same disease, though it had been called infantile muscular atrophy.

Over the years other cases have been reported. Dubowitz has summarized the findings in six patients, three of whom had ophthalmoplegia and generalized weakness, and fell into the waste basket of "ophthalmoplegia plus," a mixed neuromuscular group (page 1123). The other three had a severe weakness of shoulder and pelvic girdle muscles and neck flexors. Several had such severe weakness of respiratory muscles that pulmonary assistance was required; five of the six had ECG abnormalities, one an enlarged heart due to a cardiac myopathy. Unlike the Duchenne cases the respiratory center was unresponsive to CO_2 inhalation.

In all probability the increase in number of mitochondria, seen best in histochemical stains for oxidative enzymes, and as ragged-red fibers in Gomori stains, is a reaction to a number of different metabolic defects, the most serious being a defect of cytochrome b. Interestingly there is little or no destruction of fibers, and in a few instances the muscle strength improved with age.

Kearns-Sayre Syndrome This disorder, which was briefly referred to in relation to the adult forms of ocular myopathy (page 1123), is characterized by the clinical triad of progressive external ophthalmoplegia, atypical pigmentary degeneration of the retina, and heart block. The syndrome has its onset before the age of 20 years and appears to be sporadic rather than hereditary. Ptosis is usually the first manifestation, followed by ophthalmoplegia; retinitis and heart block come later, sometimes by many years. In practically all cases the CSF protein is increased (usually >100 mg/dL), and in the majority the gamma globulin is elevated as well. The defect in cardiac conduction is of varying degrees of severity; many patients have required pacemakers for AV block. The pigmentary degeneration of the retina takes the form of a fine stippling around the optic discs and rarely causes discrete field defects—hence, "atypical." Short stature, delayed sexual maturation, neurosensory hearing loss, and impaired cerebellar and vestibular

function are usually but not invariably associated. Some patients are retarded mentally. Postmortem examination in a few patients has disclosed a diffuse coarse vacuolation of cerebral tissue, particularly of the parts concerned with eye movements.

Patients with the Kearns-Sayre syndrome (as well as patients with adult type ocular myopathy) have shown striking mitochondrial abnormalities in skeletal as well as in eye muscles. Degenerating type I fibers appear red when stained by the modified Gomori trichrome method, owing to clusters of proliferating mitochondrial elements (hence "ragged-red fibers"). Electron microscopy discloses large numbers of abnormal mitochondria. In patients with progressive external ophthalmoplegia, accumulations of mitochondria in skeletal muscles have also been associated with excessive glycogen in muscle fibers. Similar accumulations of mitochondria have also been observed in the perinuclear zones of fibers in hypokalemic myopathy, in progressive muscular dystrophy, and in the sarcoplasmic masses of myotonic dystrophy.

Mitochondrial myopathy is a prominent feature of two additional familial syndromes. One of them, described by Pavlakis et al, is characterized by ragged-red fibers in skeletal muscle, short stature, seizures, lactic acidosis, and stroke-like episodes (see page 810). The other syndrome, also associated with ragged-red fibers, is characterized by myoclonus and ataxia, as well as atrophy of the optic nerves (Fukuhara et al). The acronym MELAS has been used to designate the first of these syndromes and MERRF, the second. Whether Kearns-Sayre, MELAS, and MERRF are distinctive syndromes or variants of a single syndrome must await definition of the inherited biochemical abnormality or abnormalities.

Congenital Myopathy with Fiber-Type Disproportion
Brooke first called attention to a congenital polymyopathy characterized by a disparity in size of type I and type II fibers, and since that time there have been several other reports. The infants are weak and floppy, and the condition appears to progress in some cases and improve in others. Histochemical stains (ATPase) reveal a smallness and increased proportion of type I fibers. Additional clinical features are: normal mental development, ophthalmoplegia, hip dislocations, and "contractures." A disproportionate increase in type II fibers has also been reported, sometimes with fatal outcome. In the report of Eisler and Wilson the onset of the weakness was in mid-childhood, and there were no nonmuscular abnormalities. The smallness of type I fibers without evidence of degeneration suggests a trophic defect related to one class of anterior horn cells. Unfortunately, quantitative studies of the spinal cord and motor nerve fibers have not been made. In this group, as well as the central core and rod-body myopathies, the small fibers in all probability account for the muscular weakness. An

autosomal recessive inheritance pattern is found in some of the reported families. Improvement with age may be explained by compensatory hypertrophy of type II fibers.

Centronuclear or Myotubular Myopathy In this familial disease, hypotonia and weakness become manifest soon after birth, or in infancy or early childhood. Rarely, in the mildest form, the diagnosis does not become evident until adult years. All the striated skeletal muscles are involved to some degree. Ptosis and ocular palsies are combined with weakness of facial, masticatory, lingual, pharyngeal, laryngeal, and cervical muscles in most of the infants with this disease, but not of the adults. In the limbs, distal weakness keeps pace with proximal weakness. The muscles remain thin and areflexic throughout life. Motor development is necessarily retarded, though some improvement with maturation can occur; later, however, motor functions that had been acquired may be lost as the disease slowly advances. Several patients have shown signs of cerebral abnormality, with seizures and an abnormal EEG, but this may not be part of the disease. Muscle enzyme levels in the serum have not been elevated. EMG shows myopathic potentials and fibrillations. The pattern of inheritance has not been constant; X-linked recessive, autosomal dominant, and autosomal recessive patterns have all been described. Heckmatt and his colleagues have classified this disorder into three types, based on their severity, mode of presentation, and genetic pattern: a severe neonatal X-linked recessive type, a less severe infantile or childhood autosomal recessive type, and a still milder autosomal dominant type.

The outstanding pathologic features of the disease are the smallness of muscles and their constituent fibers, and central nucleation. In one group of myotubular myopathies there is hypotrophy of type I fibers (Bethlem et al, Karpati et al). Surrounding most of the centrally placed nuclei is a clear zone, in which there is a lack of organization of contractile elements. Because of central nucleation, the disease has incorrectly been referred to as *myotubular myopathy,* implying an arrest in development of muscle at the myotubular stage. Actually, the nature of the pathologic process is quite obscure. The small, centrally nucleated fibers do not really resemble typical myotubes. Also, there is evidence, from electron-microscopic studies, of degenerative changes in the central parts of the fibers (in the clear zones surrounding the nuclei), leading in all probability to fiber loss. Such changes argue against a purely developmental abnormality.

OTHER CONGENITAL MYOPATHIES

In addition to the foregoing congenital myopathies, a number of other far less common types have been reported, each named according to a distinctive histochemical or electron-microscopic alteration. Each report is based on the study of only one or a few cases, insufficient to allow full categorization as a disease entity. A more complete account of these disorders than can be given here will be found in the review by Banker.

Reducing Body Myopathy First reported by Neville and Brooke, this is a progressive disorder beginning at or before birth and ending fatally between 1 and 2½ years. In a small number of fibers there were RNA-containing inclusions, surrounded by degenerating myofilaments. In the cases of Oh et al the weakness was nonprogressive throughout childhood.

Fingerprint Myopathy A. G. Engel et al reported a case in which subsarcolemmal inclusions assumed the appearance of fingerprints in electron microscopic examination. Their patient was a child, age 5 years, who was weak and hypotonic from birth and was mentally subnormal.

Zebra Body Myopathy This term was applied by Lake and Wilson to rod-shaped bodies which imparted a striped appearance in electron micrographs. The myopathy was congenital and nonprogressive. There was also variation in fiber size.

Sarcotubular Myopathy Jerusalem et al observed two brothers, aged 11 and 15 years, who suffered a congenital nonprogressive myopathy in which the endoplasmic reticulum was dilated.

In summary, it is not possible at present to decide whether these ultrastructural changes in the muscle fibers serve to differentiate the aforementioned congenital myopathies as clinical-pathologic entities. As indicated above, the weakness and hypotonia are probably not explained by the subtle disfigurations but are more likely due to the smallness of the fibers. Possibly a lack of trophic influence from anterior horn cells prevents the natural growth of type I fibers in motor units, at least in all of the nonprogressive congenital myopathies. There is no fiber destruction. It has been suggested that the nervous system may also be affected and in at least one case of centronuclear myopathy reported by Bormioli et al, the distribution of acetylcholine esterase (normally present in neuromuscular junctions, myomuscular junctions, and myotendinous junctions) was abnormal. This biochemical abnormality had been observed experimentally after denervation and reinnervation of muscle at birth. Unfortunately, mixed with this group are a number of metabolic myopathies in which there is a genetic enzyme defect. In the latter myopathies, there is definite progression of muscle weakness, sometimes leading to a fatal paralysis.

Much research is necessary to clarify the problematic features of the congenital myopathies, not only their genetic and biochemical nature but also their neuropathology.

THE SPINAL MUSCULAR ATROPHIES OF INFANCY AND CHILDHOOD

Of an entirely different nature, viz., nonmyopathic, is the group of diseases in which there is a progressive degeneration of the motor neurons of the spinal cord or brainstem or both. The muscular atrophy is secondary. In many respects these diseases resemble the motor system diseases described in Chap. 43 but differ with respect to their early age of onset and genetic determination. Conventionally, the spinal muscular atrophies of early life are classified with the other motor system diseases, but we are describing them here, because they must always be included in the differential diagnosis of the weak and limp infant or child.

HISTORY AND CLASSIFICATION

Werdnig in 1891 and 1894 and Hoffmann in 1893, and, at about the same time, Thomsen and Bruce, recorded instances of a hereditary progressive muscular atrophy of spinal origin. Soon thereafter, however, it became apparent that this disease was being confused with nonprogressive forms of weakness and hypotonia in infancy and childhood that Oppenheim was attempting to delineate under the name of myatonia congenita (later called amyotonia congenita, see below).

The cases that originally became known as Werdnig-Hoffmann disease were all infantile. Further clinical analyses indicated the inadequacy of this narrow grouping. Brandt, in his study of 112 Danish patients, found that in about one-third of them the weakness was already present at birth, and in 97 the onset was in the first year of life; in nine patients, the disease was not recognized until after the first year of life. Of the early-onset cases, 53 had died by the end of the first year, but 8 of the cases of later onset survived for 4 to 10 years. Wohlfart et al and Kugelberg and Welander identified a milder form of spinal muscular atrophy in which the onset was between 2 and 17 years, and walking was still possible in adult life. Byers and

Banker, in a study of 52 patients, subdivided them into three groups on the basis of age of onset; in one group the disease was recognized at birth or in the first month or two of life; in a second, between 6 and 12 months; and in a third, after the first year. In the last group, it was not unusual for the patient to survive into adolescence and adult life. Emery (1971), in a large Scottish survey, classified the progressive spinal muscular atrophies into five groups, on the basis of their clinical features and patterns of inheritance: (1) proximal spinal muscular atrophy, which included the three types of Werdnig-Hoffmann disease of Byers and Banker; (2) distal spinal muscular atrophy; (3) progressive juvenile bulbar palsy; (4) scapuloperoneal atrophy of spinal type; (5) facioscapulohumeral type. Thus it would seem, from a review of published accounts over the years, that inherited degeneration of lower motor neurons may develop at any age from birth to adult life; that most of the early life forms are severe, generalized, and rapidly fatal, and are transmitted as an autosomal recessive trait; and that later onset forms are more benign and likely to be inherited as an autosomal dominant or X-linked recessive trait. In a few of the late-onset type, signs of corticospinal tract involvement are conjoined. Bonduelle includes some patients with areflexic atrophy, pes cavus, Babinski signs, choreiform movements, and mental retardation. They resemble the cases of Grunnet and Donaldson, and their classification with the infantile muscular atrophies is seemingly justified by the presence of eosinophilic cytoplasmic inclusion bodies in anterior horn cells, similar to those seen in Werdnig-Hoffmann-disease.

Still a matter of uncertainty is the status of a pure hereditary motor neuropathy. Dyck includes a motor neuropathy as one of the three types of Charcot-Marie-Tooth peroneal muscular atrophy (see Chap. 46). The authors disagree and would classify the former as spinal muscular atrophy. In our autopsied cases of Charcot-Marie-Tooth disease there was no loss of anterior horn cells and many of them showed typical axonal reaction. The only cases of a relatively pure motor polyneuropathy with preserved anterior horn cells that we have found are the ones associated with macroglobulinemia (Rowland et al).

Finally, it should be mentioned that clinical disorders more or less similar to the spinal muscular atrophies may occur occasionally in certain hereditary metabolic diseases. For example, Johnson et al have described a patient who began experiencing weakness of legs, cramping, and fasciculations during adolescence in what proved to be a variant of hexosaminidase A deficiency, and biopsy of rectal mucosa showed nerve cells with the typical membranous cytoplasmic bodies of Tay-Sachs disease. Kaback et al had earlier presented a similar case. Progressive motor neuron or motor nerve disease has also been observed in glycogen storage disease affecting anterior horn cells. Motor nerve fibers suffer damage also in metachromatic and globoid body leukoencephalopathy, and in association with multiple myeloma (Rowland et al).

Clinical Manifestations In its most frequent form, an infant, usually born normally, is noted from birth to be unnaturally weak and limp. Some mothers report that fetal movement had been less than expected or lacking altogether. The muscle weakness in these children is generalized from the beginning, and death comes early, usually within the first year. Other infants seem to develop normally for several months before the weakness becomes apparent. In these, the trunk, pelvic, and shoulder girdle muscles are at first disproportionately affected, while the fingers and hands, toes and feet, and cranial muscles retain their mobility. Hypotonia attends the weakness, and since passive displacement of articulated parts is easier to judge than power of contraction at this early age, it may be singled out as the dominant clinical characteristic. As a rule the tendon reflexes are unobtainable. Volume of muscle diminishes but is difficult to evaluate because of the coverings of adipose tissue. Fasciculations are seldom visible except in the tongue. Perception of tactile and painful stimuli is undiminished, and emotional and social development measure up to age.

As the months pass, the weakness and hypotonia progress gradually and spread to all of the skeletal muscles except the ocular ones. Intercostal paralysis with severe collapse of the chest is the rule. Respiratory movements are paradoxical. The cry becomes feeble, and sucking and swallowing are less efficient. Such infants are unable to sit unless propped, and the head cannot be supported. They cannot roll over or support their weight when placed on their feet. The posture is characteristic: arms abducted and flexed at the elbow, legs in the "frog position," with external rotation and abduction at hips, and flexion at hips and knees. If the effects of gravity are removed, all muscles continue to contract; i.e., there is paresis, not paralysis. Until late in the illness these children appear bright-eyed, alert, and responsive.

The disease runs a steadily downhill course. Infants in whom the disease only becomes apparent after several months of life run a less precipitous course than those affected in utero or at birth. Some of the former become able to sit and creep and even to walk with support, and may survive for several years and even into adolescence or early adult life (see below).

The heredity of the disease is consistent with an autosomal recessive pattern.

Laboratory data of confirmatory value are few. Muscle enzymes in the serum are normal. The EMG shows fibrillations and/or fasciculations, proving the denervative basis of the weakness. Motor unit potentials are diminished in number and some are larger than normal (giant or polyphasic potentials). Motor nerve conduction velocities fall in the low normal range. Muscle biopsy reveals a typical picture of group atrophy, and many of the groups of normal fibers are hypertrophied. However, if the biopsy is obtained shortly after birth, the group atrophy may be unclear, and only slight variation in fiber size is seen.

INTERMEDIATE AND LATE-ONSET FORMS

In the intermediate and late-onset forms the child may be entirely normal for the first year or two, sometimes achieving walking at the usual time. Then a symmetrical weakness of proximal muscles, lower extremities more than upper, begins. The tendon reflexes may be obtainable or are absent. Intercostal muscles are affected late and there is usually no respiratory difficulty. Bulbar muscles are spared. The hands are tremulous in some cases. Progression of the disease is slow and may be masked by natural growth and development. Cardiac involvement does not occur.

In the Wohlfart-Kugelberg-Welander group with onset in childhood, the first difficulty may be in climbing stairs and arising from the floor (using Gowers maneuver) and there may be a waddling gait, a clinical picture suggestive of childhood dystrophy. The arms are involved to a lesser degree.

Serum enzymes are normal or slightly elevated. The EMG is typical of a neurogenic atrophy.

An unusual pattern of distal atrophy, sometimes with ocular palsies or bulbar signs, was first described by Kennedy. The time of onset has varied from childhood to adult age. Some cases have shown an X-linked pattern of inheritance and others, an autosomal dominant pattern. In the family described by Kaeser, in which 12 members in five generations were affected, the pattern of weakness was shoulder-shank, i.e., scapuloperoneal. In one autopsied case there was loss of motor neurons in the spinal cord and brainstem nuclei.

PROGRESSIVE BULBAR PALSY (FAZIO-LONDE SYNDROME)

This is a rare variant of lower motor neuron disease, described by Fazio and Londe almost simultaneously in Italy and France. The age of onset varies from childhood to late adolescence. There is progressive paralysis of the facial, lingual, pharyngeal, laryngeal, and sometimes ocular muscles. Death occurs in a few months to years. The skeletal muscle is spared. In one autopsied case (Gomez et al) with onset at 1 year and death at 3½ years, there was extensive neuronal degeneration in all of the motor nuclei of the brainstem.

Pathologic Findings Aside from the aforementioned multiple, successive motor unit atrophy of muscle, which is universal, the essential abnormalities are in the anterior horn cells in the spinal cord and the motor nuclei in the lower brainstem. Nerve cells are greatly reduced in number, and many of the remaining ones are in varying stages of degeneration; a few are chromatolytic and contain cytoplasmic inclusions. Occasionally neuronophagia has been observed. There is replacement gliosis and secondary degeneration in roots and nerves. Other systems of neurons, including the corticospinal and corticobulbar, remain intact.

Differential Diagnosis The major problem in diagnosis is to distinguish Werdnig-Hoffmann disease from an array of other diseases that cause hypotonia and delayed motor development in the neonate and infant. The congenital polymyopathies, as described in the preceding section, frequently present in this way. The preservation of tendon reflexes and relative lack of progression of muscle weakness distinguish these latter disorders. Of course, the muscle biopsy, if studied properly, usually yields the correct diagnosis.

Certain forms of muscular dystrophy, notably myotonic dystrophy, may become manifest in the neonatal period and interfere with sucking and motor development. As a rule, the weakness is not as severe or diffuse as that in Werdnig-Hoffmann disease. Also, a number of polyneuropathies may cause a serious degree of weakness in early childhood. Unfortunately, in respect to the latter, adequate sensory testing is not possible because of their age, but the CSF protein is often elevated; diagnosis is greatly facilitated by measurement of nerve conduction velocities (which are reduced) and nerve-muscle biopsy. Examination of parents and siblings may disclose a clinically inapparent neuropathy. Polymyositis of childhood may also simulate both muscular dystrophy and motor neuron disease (see Chap. 43).

Mental retardation with a flaccid rather than spastic weakness of the limbs is another major category of disease that must be distinguished. This may be difficult. Reliance must be placed on tests of psychosocial development, which are invariably delayed. Also, certain of the leukodystrophies may weaken muscles and abolish tendon reflexes, but usually there is evidence of cerebral involvement. The same may be said of mongolism, cretinism, achondrodysplasia, and certain forms of lipid and glycogen storage diseases. Finally,

very sick children with celiac disease, cystic fibrosis, and other chronic diseases may be hypotonic, to the point of simulating neuromuscular disease. Usually the tendon reflexes are not abolished in these purely medical states, and strength returns as the medical problem is corrected.

There remains, after the assiduous study of the "floppy infant," a group of cases of hypotonia and motor underdevelopment that are presently unclassifiable. The term *amyotonia congenita* (Oppenheim), once applied to all this group, is obsolete. Oppenheim provided no information about the clinical course of his patients and no pathologic data, so that the nature of the cases he described can never be settled with finality. Walton devised the term *benign congenital hypotonia* to designate patients who manifest limp and flabby limbs in infancy and delay in sitting up and walking and who improve gradually, some completely and others incompletely. Some of the cases of fiber-type disproportion and centronuclear myopathy fall into this category (see above). This hardly constitutes a homogeneous category of disease. The nature of the cases with complete recovery is quite obscure. One would suspect that among this group there are examples of congenital myopathy that await differentiation by application of modern histochemical and ultrastructural techniques. Neither amyotonia congenita nor benign congenital hypotonia is a categorization that serves the purpose of precise diagnosis, and should be retained only until other parameters of the pathologic process are discovered.

REFERENCES

Adams RD, Kakulas BA: *Diseases of Muscle: The Pathological Foundations of Clinical Myology,* 4th ed. Philadelphia, Harper & Row, 1985.

Allbrook D: Skeletal muscle regeneration. *Muscle Nerve* 4:234, 1981.

Banker BQ: Congenital muscular dystrophy, in Engel AG, Banker BQ (eds): *Myology.* New York, McGraw-Hill, 1986a, chap 45, pp 1367–1382.

Banker BQ: Congenital deformities, in Engel AG, Banker BQ (eds): *Myology.* New York, McGraw-Hill, 1986b, chap 73, pp 2109–2159.

Banker BQ, Victor M, Adams RD: Arthrogryposis multiplex due to congenital muscular dystrophy. *Brain* 80:319, 1957.

Bethlem J, Arts WF, Dingemans KP: Common origin of rods, cores, miniature cores, and focal loss of cross striations. *Arch Neurol* 35:555, 1978.

Bethlem J, Meyer AE, Schellons JP et al: Centronuclear myopathy. *Eur Neurol* 1:325, 1968.

Bing R: Uber angeborene Muskeldefecte. *Virchows Arch (Pathol Anat)* 170:175, 1902.

Bonduelle M: Amyotrophic lateral sclerosis, in Vinken RT, Bruyn GW (eds): *Handbook of Clinical Neurology,* vol 29. Amsterdam, North Holland, 1975, pp 281–338.

BORMIOLI SP, LUCKE S, ANGELINI C: Abnormal myomuscular junctions and AChE in congenital neuromuscular disease. *Muscle Nerve* 3:240, 1980.

BRANDT S: Werdnig-Hoffmann's infantile progressive muscular atrophy, in *Thesis*, vol 22. Copenhagen, Ejnar Munksgaard, 1950.

BROOKE MH: Congenital fiber type disproportion, in Kakulas BA (ed): *Clinical Studies in Myology*. New York, American Elsevier, 1973, pp 147–159.

BYERS RK, BANKER BQ: Infantile muscular atrophy. *Arch Neurol* 5:140, 1961.

DEREUCK J, ADAMS RD: The metrics of muscle, in Kakulas BA (ed): *Basic Research in Myology,* International Congress Series. Excerpta Medica Foundation, 1973, pp 1–11.

DUBOWITZ V: *Muscle Disorders in Childhood.* Philadelphia, Saunders, 1978.

EISLER T, WILSON JH: Muscle fiber type disproportion. *Arch Neurol* 35:823, 1978.

EMERY AEH: The nosology of the spinal muscular atrophies. *J Med Genet* 8:481, 1971.

ENGEL AG: Recent studies on neuromuscular disease. Late-onset rod myopathy (a new syndrome?). Light and electron microscopic observations in 2 cases. *Mayo Clin Proc* 41:713, 1966.

ENGEL AG, ANGELINI C, GOMEZ MR: Fingerprint body myopathy. *Mayo Clinic Proc* 47:377, 1972.

ENGEL WK, REZNICK JS: Late onset rod-myopathy: A newly recognized, acquired, and progressive disease. *Neurology* 16:308, 1966.

FAZIO F: Ereditarieta della paralisi bulbare progressiva. *Riforma Med* 4:327, 1892.

FUKUHARA N, TOKIGUCHI S, SHIRAKAWA K, TSUBAKI T: Myoclonus epilepsy associated with ragged-red fibers (mitochondrial abnormalities): Disease entity or a syndrome? *J Neurol Sci* 47:117, 1980.

GOMEZ MR, CLERMONT V, BERNSTEIN J: Progressive bulbar paralysis in childhood (Fazio-Londe's disease). Report of a case with pathologic evidence of nuclear atrophy. *Arch Neurol* 6:317, 1962.

GRUNNET ML, DONALDSON JO: Juvenile multisystem degeneration with motor neuron involvement and eosinophilic intracytoplasmic inclusions. *Arch Neurol* 42:144, 1985.

HECKMATT JZ, SEWRY CA, HODES D, DUBOWITZ V: Congenital centronuclear (myotubular) myopathy. *Brain* 108:941, 1985.

HENDERSON JL: The congenital facial diplegia syndrome; clinical features, pathology and aetiology. *Brain* 62:381, 1939.

JERUSALEM F, ENGEL AG, GOMEZ MR: Sarcotubular myopathy. *Neurology* 23:897, 1973.

JOHNSON WG, WIGGER J, KARP HR: Juvenile spinal muscular atrophy: a new hexosaminidase deficiency phenotype. *Ann Neurol* 11:11, 1982.

KAESER HE: Scapuloperoneal muscular dystrophy. *Brain* 88:407, 1965.

KABACK M, MILES J, YAFFE M et al: Hexosaminidase A deficiency: a new type of Gm₂ gangliosidosis. *Am J Human Genet* 30:31A, 1978.

KARPATI G, CARPENTER S, NELSON RF: Type I muscle fiber atrophy and central nuclei. *J Neurol Sci* 10:489, 1970.

KENNEDY WR, ALTER M, SUNG JH: Progressive proximal spinal and bulbar muscular atrophy of late onset. A sex-linked recessive trait. *Neurology* 18:617, 1968.

KUGELBERG E, WELANDER L: Heredofamilial juvenile muscular atrophy simulating muscular dystrophy. *Arch Neurol Psychiatry* 5:500, 1956.

LAKE BD, WILSON J: Zebra body myopathy. *J Neurol Sci* 24:437, 1975.

LEDOUBLE AF: *Traité des variations du système musculaire de l'homme.* Paris, Schliger Frères Editeurs, 1897.

LICHTENSTEIN BW: Congenital absence of the abdominal musculature: Associated changes in the genitourinary tract and the spinal cord. *Am J Dis Child* 58:339, 1939.

LONDE P: Paralysie bulbaire: progressive infantile et familiale. *Rev Med (Paris)* 13:1020, 1893.

NEVILLE HE, BROOKE MH: Central core fibers structured and unstructured, in *Proceedings of the Second International Congress of Muscle Diseases.* Amsterdam, Excerpta Medica, 1973, p 497.

OH SJ, MEYERS GJ, WILSON ER, ALEXANDER CB: A benign form of reducing body myopathy. *Muscle Nerve* 6:278, 1983.

OH SJ, DANON MJ: Nonprogressive congenital neuromuscular disease with uniform type I fiber. *Arch Neurol* 40:147, 1983.

OPPENHEIM H: Ueber allgemeine und localisierte Atonie der Muskulatur (Myatonie) in frühen Kindesalter. *Monatsschr Psychiatr Neurol* 8:232, 1900.

PAVLAKIS SG, PHILLIPS PC, DIMAURO et al: Mitochondrial myopathy, encephalopathy, lactic acidosis, and stroke-like episodes: A distinctive clinical syndrome. *Ann Neurol* 16:481, 1984.

PATTERSON VH, HILL TRG, FLETCHER PJH, HERON JR: Central core disease: Clinical and pathological progression within a family. *Brain* 102:581, 1979.

ROBERTSON WC, KAWAMURA Y, DYCK PJ: Morphometric study of motoneurons in congenital nemaline myopathy and Werdnig-Hoffmann disease. *Neurology* 28:1057, 1978.

ROWLAND LP, DEFENDINI R, SHERMAN W et al: Macroglobulinemia with peripheral neuropathy simulating motor neuron disease. *Ann Neurol* 11:532, 1982.

SCHWARTZ MS, SARGENT M, SWASH M: Longitudinal fiber splitting in neurogenic muscular disorders. Its relation to the pathogenesis of ''myopathic'' change. *Brain* 99:617, 1976.

SHY GM, GONATOS NK, PEREZ M: Two childhood myopathies with abnormal mitochondria. *Brain* 89:133, 1966.

SHY GM, MAGEE KR: A new congenital non-progressive myopathy. *Brain* 79:610, 1956.

SILBERMANN M, FINKELBRAND S, WEISS A et al: Morphometric analysis of aging skeletal muscle following endurance training. *Muscle Nerve* 6:136, 1983.

TOMLINSON BF, WALTON JN, REBEIZ JJ: The effects of aging and cachexia upon skeletal muscle: a histopathologic study. *J Neurol Sci* 8:201, 1969.

WOHLFART G, FEX J, ELIASSON S: Hereditary proximal spinal muscular atrophy. A clinical entity simulating progressive muscular dystrophy. *Acta Psychiatry Scand* 30:395, 1955.

CHAPTER 53

MYASTHENIA GRAVIS AND EPISODIC FORMS OF MUSCULAR WEAKNESS

The thread that connects the various types of muscle disease included in this chapter is the fluctuating or episodic nature of the weakness. This variability implicates important physiologic mechanisms rather than structural changes, located at the neuromuscular junction or in the transmitting mechanism of the distal ends of the motor nerve fibers, sarcolemma, transverse tubules, and endoplasmic reticulum (see Chap. 45). In *myasthenia gravis* and in a number of other myasthenic states related to abnormalities of the neuromuscular junction, there is usually some degree of weakness at all times, but it is made worse by activity. In the *periodic paralyses,* weakness occurs only in discrete attacks, associated with a derangement of serum electrolytes. These two categories of muscle disease form the subject matter of this chapter.

MYASTHENIA GRAVIS

This proves to be a group of maladies that exhibit several striking clinical features, the most important of which is a *fluctuant weakness* of certain voluntary muscles, particularly those innervated by motor nuclei of the brainstem, i.e., ocular, masticatory, facial, deglutitional, and lingual. Manifest weakening during continued activity, quick restoration of power with rest, and dramatic improvement in strength following the administration of anticholinesterase drugs such as neostigmine, are other notable features.

HISTORY

Several students of medical history affirm that Thomas Willis, in 1685, gave an account of a disease that could be none other than myasthenia gravis. Others give credit to Wilks (1877) for the first description, and for having noted that the medulla was free of disease, in distinction to other types of bulbar paralysis. The first reasonably complete accounts were those of Erb (1878), who designated the disease as a bulbar palsy without an anatomic lesion, and of Goldflam (1893). For many years thereafter the disorder was referred to as the Erb-Goldflam syndrome. Jolly (1895) was the first to use the name myasthenia gravis, to which he added the term *pseudoparalytica,* to indicate the lack of structural changes at autopsy. Also it was Jolly who originally demonstrated that myasthenic weakness of muscle could be reproduced by faradic stimulation of its motor nerve and that the "fatigued" muscle would still respond to galvanic stimulation. Interestingly, he suggested the use of physostigmine as a form of treatment, but there the matter rested until Remen, in 1932, and Walker, in 1934, demonstrated the therapeutic value of the drug.

Campbell and Bramwell (1900) and Oppenheim (1901) each analyzed over 60 cases and crystallized the clinical concept of the disease. The relationship between myasthenia gravis and the thymus gland was first noted by Laquer and Weigert in 1901, and in 1949 Castleman and Norris described in detail the pathologic changes in the gland.

In 1905 Buzzard published a detailed clinicopathologic analysis of the disease, commenting on both the thymic abnormalities and the infiltrations of lymphocytes (called lymphorrhages) in muscle. He postulated that an autotoxic agent caused the muscle weakness, the lymphorrhages, and the thymic lesions. He also commented on the close relation of myasthenia gravis to Graves disease and Addison disease, which also are now considered to have an autoimmune basis. In 1960, Simpson and, independently, Nastuk et al, theorized that an autoimmune mechanism must be operative in myasthenia gravis. Finally in 1973, and thereafter, the autoimmune nature of myasthenia gravis was established, through a series of investigations by Patrick and Lindstrom, Fambrough, Lennon, and Engel and their colleagues (see further on, under "Etiology and Pathogenesis").

These and other references to the early historical features of the disease are to be found in the reviews by Viets and by Adams and Kakulas; A. G. Engel's chapter in *Myology*, edited by Engel and Banker, is an excellent modern reference.

CLINICAL MANIFESTATIONS

Myasthenia gravis, as the name implies, is a muscular weakness having a grave prognosis. Repeated or persistent activity of a muscle group exhausts its contractile power, leading to a progressive paresis, and rest restores strength, at least partially. The demonstration of these two attributes, assuming the patient cooperates fully, is enough to establish the diagnosis.

The onset is usually insidious, but there are instances of fairly rapid development, sometimes initiated by an emotional upset or infection (usually respiratory). Symptoms may first appear during pregnancy or the puerperium, or in response to drugs used during anesthesia. Once started, a slow progression follows. Usually the muscles of the eyes, and somewhat less often of the face, jaws, throat, and neck, are the first to be affected, but in rare cases the initial complaint may be referable to the limbs. However, as the disease advances, it often spreads to other muscles.

The special vulnerability of certain muscles to myasthenia accounts for the mode of clinical presentation. In more than 90 percent of cases the levator palpebrae or extraocular muscles are involved. Ocular palsies and ptosis are usually accompanied by weakness of eye closure (orbicularis oculi), a combination observed regularly only in this disease and muscular dystrophy, viz., in purely myopathic states. The muscles of facial expression, mastication, swallowing, and speech are next most frequently affected (80 percent). The flexors and extensors of the neck, muscles of the shoulder girdle, and flexors of the hips are less often involved. Of the trunk muscles the erector spinae are the most frequently affected. In the most advanced cases, all muscles are weakened, including the diaphragm, abdominal, and intercostal muscles, and even the external sphincters of the bladder and bowel. The incidence of involvement of any group of muscles closely parallels the likelihood of their being initially affected by the disease. Clinically, myasthenia gravis is most accurately conceived as a fluctuating oculofaciobulbar palsy. In patients with affection of the trunk and limbs, the clinical rule holds firm, that in myopathy the proximal muscles are more vulnerable than distal ones.

To rephrase the topographic attributes of the illness in terms of symptoms, drooping of the eyelids and intermittent diplopia are the most common complaints. Bright sunlight aggravates the ptosis. Facial mobility and expression are altered. The natural smile becomes transformed

into a snarl. The jaw may hang so that it must be propped up by the patient's hand. Chewing tough food may be difficult, and the meal may have to be terminated because of inability to masticate and swallow. It may be more difficult to eat after talking, and the voice fades and becomes nasal after sustained conversation. Women may complain of inability to fix their hair because of fatigue of the shoulders, or of difficulty in applying lipstick because of inability to purse and roll the lips. Weakness of the neck muscles causes fatigue in holding up the head.

Weakness tends to increase as the day wears on, but patients seldom volunteer this information. And a few are worse on awakening, especially if they have not received medication during the night. A temporary increase in weakness has been attributed to vaccination, menstruation, and extremes of temperature.

A peculiarity of myasthenic muscle contraction is a sudden lapse of sustained posture, or interruption of movement by a kind of irregular tremor, similar to that of normal muscle nearing the point of exhaustion. A dynamometer or ergogram demonstrates the rapidly waning power of contraction, and repetitive stimulation of a motor nerve at slow rates, while recording muscle action potentials, reflects the same disorder in a more quantitative fashion (see page 1024; also, Fig. 45-11).

Weakened muscles in myasthenia gravis undergo atrophy in only a limited number of cases (about 10 percent of females and 20 percent of males); the atrophy is rarely marked in degree. Tendon reflexes are seldom altered. Even repeated tapping of a tendon does not usually tax muscles to the point where contraction fails. Smooth and cardiac muscles are not involved. Normal pupillary responses to light and accommodation in the face of weakness of extraocular muscles and orbicularis oculi are virtually diagnostic of myasthenia gravis, especially if strength is restored after a period of rest.

Other neural functions are preserved. The weakened muscles, especially those of the eyes and back of the neck, may ache, but pain is seldom an important complaint. Paresthesias of the face, hands, and thighs are sometimes reported but are not accompanied by demonstrable sensory loss. Anosmia and ageusia have been mentioned as rare findings, but whether they are coincidental has not been decided. The tongue may display one central and two lateral longitudinal furrows (trident tongue), as was pointed out by Buzzard.

Some statistical features of the disease are of clinical significance. Its prevalance is variously estimated to be from 43 to 84 per million of the population. The disease may begin at any age, but onset in the first decade is relatively rare (only 10 percent of cases occur under the age of 10 years). The peak age of onset in women is between 20 and 30 years, while the male incidence peaks in the sixth or seventh decade. Under the age of 40, females are affected two to three times as often as males, whereas in later life, the incidence in males is higher. Of patients with thymomas, the majority are older (50 to 60 years), and males predominate.

The course of the illness is extremely variable. Rapid spread from one muscle group to another occurs in some, but in others the disease remains unchanged for months before progressing. Remissions may take place without explanation, but these happen in less than half the cases and are seldom longer than a month or two. If the disease remits for a year or longer and then recurs, it tends to be progressive. Remission is more likely to occur in the early years of the disease than later. Relapse may follow remission and is occasioned by the same conditions as the initial attack. In Simpson's opinion, and this coincides with our observations, the danger of death from myasthenia gravis is greatest in the first year after the onset of the disease. A second period of danger in progressive cases is from 4 to 7 years after onset. After this time the disease tends to stabilize, and the risk of severe relapse diminishes. Fatalities then relate mainly to respiratory complications (infection, aspiration).

To facilitate clinical staging of therapy and prognosis the following classification, introduced by Osserman, has been adopted in many medical centers.

I. Ocular myasthenia
II. A. Mild generalized myasthenia with slow progression; no crises; drug-responsive
   B. Moderate generalized myasthenia; severe skeletal and bulbar involvement, but no crises; drug response less than satisfactory
III. Acute fulminating myasthenia; rapid progression of severe symptoms with respiratory crises and poor drug response; high incidence of thymoma; high mortality
IV. Late severe myasthenia, same as III but progression over two years from Class I to II

Prognosis and response to treatment varies with the pattern of muscle involvement and severity, though it remains difficult to predict the outcome in an individual case. According to Bever et al, an increasing duration of purely ocular myasthenia is associated with a decreasing risk of late generalization of weakness. These authors found, in a retrospective study of 108 such patients, that only 15 percent of the observed generalizations occurred after 2

years of solely ocular manifestations. Also they found that an increasing age at onset was associated with an increasing incidence of fatal respiratory crises; in general patients with a younger age of onset ran a more benign course.

Grob and his colleagues, who observed the course of 1036 patients for a mean duration of 12 years, found that the clinical manifestations remained confined to the extraocular muscles and orbiculares oculi in 168 (16 percent of the total). Their data indicate that if localized ocular myasthenia has been present for only one month, there is a 60 percent likelihood that the disease will become generalized. If the ocular myasthenia has been localized for a year, there is an 84 percent likelihood that it will remain localized indefinitely. These authors found that in two-thirds of 750 patients with generalized myasthenia gravis the disease attained its maximum severity within a year of onset, and in 83 percent of patients, within three years. In general, the progression of symptoms was more rapid in male than in female patients.

Associated Disorders *Thymic tumors* occur in some 10 percent of patients, predominantly in older males. Other differences in the myasthenic syndrome have been noted between older men and young women: (1) older men with thymomas react somewhat differently to anticholinesterase drugs than young women without thymomas; (2) weakness in young women tends to be more generalized than in older men, in whom the weakness tends to be restricted to ocular, pharyngeal, and respiratory muscles; (3) there are differences in HLA phenotype (early onset in women without thymoma has a strong association with HLA-B8 and -D/DR3, whereas the incidence of HLA-B5 is increased in older women). Another difference that may be significant is the finding of a higher incidence of antibody to receptor substance in the older male patients.

A biologic trait of interest is the coexistence of *thyrotoxicosis* in about 5 percent of myasthenic patients. Also, rheumatoid arthritis, lupus erythematosus, and polymyositis are associated more often than can be explained by chance. In the series of patients reported by Kerzin-Storrar et al, 30 percent had a maternal relative with one of these or other disorders of autoimmune nature, suggesting that myasthenia gravis patients inherit an autoimmune susceptibility. Aplastic anemia of autoimmune type has been reported, and in one of our cases was successfully treated by antilymphocyte serum. One or more nerves may also be affected.

Familial occurrence is known but rare and usually proves to be a nonimmunologic form of myasthenia (see below). We have seen the latter disease in father and daughter. There are reports of myasthenia in only one of identical twins, so that direct inheritance is probably not a factor in the autoimmune form. About 10 to 15 percent of babies born to myasthenic mothers show signs of myasthenia. This is a transitory phenomenon, lasting 1 to 12 weeks, and recovery is complete, without later relapse. Obviously, this *neonatal myasthenia* is due to some factor transmitted from the mother; anti-AChR antibodies that have passed through the placenta are found in affected newborns, and the antibodies disappear with clinical improvement.

CONGENITAL MYASTHENIA

Apart from neonatal myasthenics born of mothers with the disease, there have been several reports of a congenital myasthenia that persists throughout life. Several of the cases have been familial. The mother may have noticed weakness of fetal movements. Unlike the usual type of myasthenia gravis, the course is variable. In some there are no remissions or fluctuations of the weakness. Yet there are decremental responses on repetitive nerve stimulation. Considering the lack of response to anticholinesterase drugs and thymectomy, the condition is difficult to identify as myasthenia.

Engel and his colleagues have identified two of these types of congenital myasthenia, each different than the common variety of acquired myasthenia. In the first, with weakness of all muscles, there was a deficiency of end-plate acetylcholinesterase. In the second, in which there was selective amyotrophy of scapular and forearm muscles with variable involvement of oculofacial muscles, the myasthenic weakness was attributable to a prolonged open time of the acetylcholine (ACh)-induced ion channel (hence "slow-channel syndrome"). The unique electrophysiologic and ultrastructural characteristics of these disorders and two other types of congenital myasthenia—due, respectively, to a defect in ACh synthesis or mobilization (reduced quantal size) and to end-plate ACh receptor deficiency—are described in the review by A. G. Engel (1984).

PATHOLOGY

Reference has already been made to the involvement of the thymus gland in myasthenia gravis. True neoplasms of the gland are found in about 10 percent of patients (see below), and fully 80 percent of the remaining patients show a striking degree of hyperplasia of lymphoid follicles with active germinal centers, confined to the medulla of the thymus. The cells in the centers of the follicles are histiocytes; they are surrounded by helper T lymphocytes. B lymphocytes and plasma cell IgG protein are elaborated by germinal cells. The changes in the thymus gland resemble the reaction in the thyroid in Hashimoto thyroiditis. Since the latter has been reproduced in animals by injecting extracts of thyroid with Freund's adjuvants, it is probable

that the so-called thymitis of myasthenia gravis is of similar nature. Immunosuppression with steroids causes involution of the thymus.

Thymic tumors are localized growths, despite the potential malignancy of their cell type. Two forms have been described: one is composed of reticular (histiocytic) cells like those in the center of the follicles and the other is predominantly lymphocytic and specified as lymphosarcomatous. Some of the tumors are composed of spindle-shaped cells. Overlapping of the types is common in our material. Thymic tumors may be unattended by myasthenia, though in all of our cases myasthenia has eventually developed, sometimes 15 to 20 years after the tumor was first recognized and removed surgically. The relation of thymitis to thymoma is not understood, but one may speculate that the latter is a thymitis in which the removal of some restraining influence has permitted neoplastic transformation of local type, such as may happen in ataxia-telangiectasia, another disease with an immunologic defect.

As regards the nervous system, all current studies confirm Erb's original contention that it is a disease without a CNS lesion. The brain and spinal cord are normal unless damaged by hypoxia and hypotension from cardiorespiratory failure. The muscle fibers, except for slight reduction in volume (disuse effect?), are generally intact. In fatal cases with extensive paralysis, isolated fibers of esophageal, diaphragmatic, and eye muscles may undergo segmental necrosis with variable regeneration (Russell). Scattered aggregates of lymphocytes (lymphorrhages) are also observed, as originally noted by Buzzard, but none of these changes in muscle explain the widespread and severe weakness. The lymphorrhages, which are found more frequently in the tumor cases, are not located in the vicinity of the motor end plates.

Of major importance was the demonstration by Zacks et al and by Engel and associates of a reduction in the area of the nerve terminal, a simplification of the postsynaptic region (sparse, shallow, abnormally wide or absent secondary synaptic clefts), and a widening of the primary synaptic cleft (Fig. 53-1; compare with Fig. 45-2). The number and size of the presynaptic vesicles and their quanta of acetylcholine (ACh) were within the normal range. The observation of regenerating axons near the junction, the many simplified junctions, and the absence of nerve terminals supplying some postsynaptic regions, suggested to Engel et al that there was an active process of degeneration and repair of the neuromuscular junction in myasthenia gravis. Following these observations, Fambrough and his associates, by means of radioactive α-bungarotoxin binding,

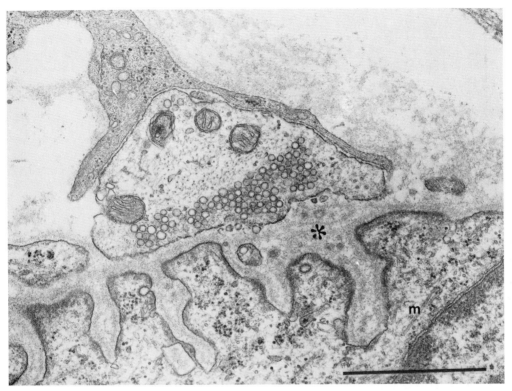

Figure 53-1

End plate from a patient with myasthenia gravis. The terminal axon contains abundant presynaptic vesicles, but the postsynaptic folds are wide and there are few secondary folds. The loose junctional sarcoplasm is filled with microtubules and ribosomes. The synaptic cleft (asterisk) is widened. The line indicates 1 μm (from Santa et al).

demonstrated a decrease in the number of ACh receptor sites on the postsynaptic part of the neuromuscular junction. Binding of IgG and C3 component of complement to receptors of end plates were demonstrated on the postsynaptic surface by Engel et al, indicating an immunologic block (Fig. 53-2).

ETIOLOGY AND PATHOGENESIS

The establishment of an immunologic mechanism, operative at the neuromuscular junction, is certainly one of the most significant developments in the field of myology in the last decade. Almost accidentally it was discovered by Patrick and Lindstrom that repeated immunization of rabbits with acetylcholine (ACh) receptor protein caused a muscular weakness, which Lennon and her colleagues recognized as being similar to myasthenia gravis. Soon thereafter it was

shown that in patients with myasthenia gravis there was a deficiency of ACh receptor at the neuromuscular junction (Fambrough et al). These observations were followed by the creation of an experimental model of the disease and the demonstration that the experimentally induced myasthenia had clinical, pharmacologic, and electrophysiologic properties identical with those of human myasthenia gravis [decreased miniature end-plate potentials (MEPPs) and decremental response on neuromuscular stimulation at 3 Hz] and that labeled antibodies were attached to the receptor site in proportion to the degree of decrease of the MEPPs (Engel et al). It was also shown that humoral antibodies to receptor protein could transfer the myasthenic weakness to normal animals and that the weakness, as well as the physiologic abnormalities, could be reversed by the administration of anticholinesterase drugs.

Antibodies to ACh receptor protein have been found

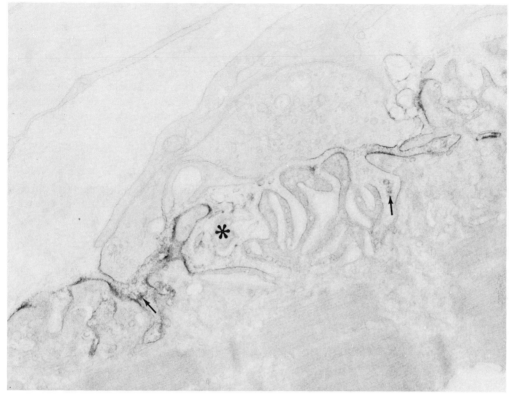

Figure 53-2

Localization of immune complexes (IgG) on segments of the postsynaptic membrane of a myasthenic end plate. IgG deposits are also seen on debris in the synaptic space (arrows). An asterisk marks a degenerated junctional fold. The IgG is directed against one or more of the antigenic determinants of AChR protein, resulting in destruction of the AChR-containing segments of the postsynaptic membrane. (Courtesy of Dr. A. G. Engel.)

to be present in approximately 85 percent of patients with generalized myasthenia and in 60 percent of those with ocular myasthenia (Newsom-Davies). Antibodies are also present in infants with neonatal myasthenia gravis and in animal species known to have a naturally occurring myasthenia. The presence of receptor antibodies has proved to be a sensitive and reliable test of the disease.

How the antibodies act at the receptor surface of the end plate has also been investigated, but the matter is not entirely settled. The nicotinic ACh receptors are located on the crests of the folds in the sarcolemma beneath the nerve fiber terminals, in a density of approximately 30,000 per square micrometer, and are also present in mammalian thymus gland. The receptor substance is a highly specialized glycoprotein, spanning the lipid layer of the postsynaptic membrane, with a molecular weight of 300,000 daltons.

Each receptor molecule, which controls an ion channel, has multiple binding sites for ACh. Attachment of the latter to the receptor molecule opens an ionic channel in the receptor membrane for the influx of Na and the efflux of K. The neurotoxin α-bungarotoxin, a small polypeptide, has a high affinity for the binding site, and like the receptor antibodies, it blocks the attachment of ACh or destroys in some manner the receptor membrane; C3 complement is also involved in the immunologic blockade. Hypotheses concerning the way in which ACh receptor antibodies might inhibit ACh binding are reviewed by Lennon.

The level of receptor antibodies in the blood stream does not correlate precisely with the severity of the myasthenia, which Lennon explains as a matter of heterogeneity of antigen specificities to ACh receptors. Also, the absence of measurable antibodies in 10 to 15 percent of patients with acquired myasthenia remains unexplained. It is of interest that Engel and Lambert and their associates have found several types of myasthenia that are only slightly responsive to anticholinesterase drugs and have a different mechanism from myasthenia gravis (see above, under "Congenital Myasthenia"); in these there are no receptor antibodies on the postsynaptic membrane. These new diseases are nonimmunologic forms of myasthenia, and it may be that other nonimmunologic forms of acquired myasthenia are being included in the overall collections of cases.

Thus the evidence that an autoimmune mechanism is responsible for the functional disorder of muscle in most cases of myasthenia gravis appears to be incontrovertible. What is not known is what stimulates the production of these antibodies and where they are formed. Lennon offers an attractive hypothesis. She proposes that the site of the disease is in the thymus, where there are known to be "myoid" cells (thymic cells resembling striated muscle) that elaborate the receptor antigen. One suggestion, unconfirmed, is that a virus with a tropism for thymic cells that have ACh nicotinic receptors might injure such cells and induce antibody formation. It might at the same time have a potential for oncogenesis, accounting for the 10 percent of myasthenic patients with thymic tumors. Scadding et al have suggested a somewhat different mode of thymic involvement. They have shown that thymic lymphocytes from patients with myasthenia gravis can synthesize anti-acetylcholine receptor antibody, both in culture and spontaneously. The loss of immune tolerance, basic to all autoimmune diseases, is not understood. This failure is postulated to be related to the activity of either suppressor lymphocytes or circulating blocking agents.

DIAGNOSIS

In patients who present with the typical myasthenic facies—unequally drooping eyelids, relatively immobile mouth turned down at the corners, a smile that looks more like a snarl, a hanging jaw supported by the hand—the diagnosis can hardly be overlooked. However, only a minority of patients present in this stage of the disease, and seldom is there a clear recognition—even by the patient—that the muscles tire during activity. Ptosis, diplopia, difficulty in speaking or swallowing, or weakness of the limbs are at first mild and inconstant. The finding that sustained activity of small cranial muscles results in weakness (e.g., increasing droop of eyelids while looking at the ceiling or diplopia when fixating in lateral or vertical gaze for 2 to 3 min) and that contraction improves after a brief rest is virtually

diagnostic, however, even in the early stages of the disease. Any other affected group of muscles may be critically tested in similar fashion. If the diagnosis remains in doubt, the measurement of specific antibody (anti-AChR), the EMG, and certain pharmacologic tests (see below) may be useful.

The rapid reduction in the amplitude of compound muscle action potentials evoked during repetitive stimulation of a peripheral nerve at a rate of 3 per second (*decrementing response*), and reversal of this response by neostigmine or edrophonium, has been a reliable confirmatory finding in the majority of cases, and it can be obtained from the facial, hand, or proximal limb muscles, which may or may not be clinically weak. Single-fiber EMG represents an even more sensitive method of detecting the defect in neuromuscular transmission by demonstrating increased variability of the interpotential interval ("jitter") or blocking of successive discharges from single muscle fibers belonging to the same motor unit. During a progressive phase of the disease or during steroid therapy, a *slight incrementing* response may be obtained (Mayer and Williams), not to be confused with the marked incrementing response after voluntary contraction that characterizes the Lambert-Eaton syndrome (see further on). Also characteristic of the myasthenic syndrome is the postactivation potentiation of single evoked action potentials, followed by exhaustion (see page 1024). Since the eye muscles exert a pull on the globe, which is reflected in intraocular tension, the increase of the latter in response to edrophonium can also be measured. Nerve conduction velocities and distal latencies are usually normal.

Equally valuable at this point are the edrophonium (Tensilon) and the neostigmine tests, which are performed in the following manner:

Edrophonium (Tensilon) Test After the strength of certain of the cranial muscles has been estimated (usually the levator palpebrae or an extraocular muscle), 10 mg (1 mL) of the drug is injected intravenously. Initially 2 mg (0.2 mL) is injected; if this dose is tolerated and no definite improvement in strength occurs after 45 s, another 3 mg is injected. If there is no response after another 45 s, the final 5 mg is given. Most patients who respond do so after 5 mg has been administered. The clinical effect lasts 4 to 5 min. A positive test consists of visible (objective) improvement in muscle contractility. The report of subjective improvement alone is not always dependable. Also one must be distrustful of equivocal test results, for they may occur with ocular palsies due to tumors or carotid aneurysms (pseudo-ocular myasthenia). Finally it should be noted that the electrical and pharmacologic tests are not specific for myasthenia gravis. The gaze palsies of progressive supranuclear palsy, for example, may improve in response to Tensilon. The drug carries a rare risk of ventricular fibrillation and cardiac arrest.

The Tensilon test is also helpful in determining whether or not increasing weakness is due to a *cholinergic crisis* (overdose of neostigmine). In this latter condition, there is no improvement with Tensilon; instead, weakness may actually increase, and there may be fasciculations about the eyes and face. The test is best done about 2 h after the last dose of neostigmine or pyridostigmine. The effect of the Tensilon is gauged by observing the respiratory and bulbar muscles, since weakness in these muscles may increase while there is no change in the ocular muscles.

Neostigmine Test Neostigmine methylsulfate is injected intramuscularly in a dose of 1.5 mg. Atropine sulfate (0.6 mg) should be available to counteract muscarinic effects (nausea, vomiting, sweating, salivation). The drug may be given intravenously in a dose of 0.5 mg but then should always be preceded by atropine sulfate to obviate the danger of ventricular fibrillation and cardiac arrest. Objective and subjective improvement occurs in 10 to 15 min and reaches its peak at 30 min, lasting 2 or 3 h. Oral prostigmine may also be given as a test dose. The effect is still slower in onset and lasts more than 2 to 3 h.

A negative test does not exclude myasthenia gravis but is a strong point against the diagnosis. A trial of oral prostigmine, 15 mg every 4 h during the day, is sometimes recommended in doubtful cases, but we have been misled more often than helped by it.

Measurement of Receptor Antibodies in Blood As was stated above, this is in general a sensitive and useful test, although the radioimmunoassay method has been the most accurate and widely used. Serum antibody against AChR can be found in 85 to 90 percent of patients with generalized myasthenia gravis and about 70 percent of patients whose symptoms are restricted to the ocular muscles (Vincent and Newsom-Davis). Adult myasthenics whose serum is persistently negative for AChR antibodies do not differ clinically or electromyographically from patients with serum antibodies. Mossman et al have adduced evidence that the former patients form an immunologically distinct group insofar as they possess an immunoglobulin antibody that binds to end-plate determinants other than AChR. The precise nature and site of action of this antibody remain to be defined. Antimyosin antibodies are found in the sera of some myasthenics, especially those with thymomas.

It is in milder myasthenic patients, who lack a decremental response in the EMG, that one most needs the help of laboratory diagnostic tests. Each of the commonly used tests proves to be about equally efficacious. Kelly et al obtained positive results with single muscle fiber recording in 79 percent, with the antireceptor antibody test in 71 percent, and with the edrophonium test in 81 percent.

Combined, they confirmed the diagnosis in 95 percent of clinically suspected cases.

SPECIAL DIAGNOSTIC PROBLEMS

We have sometimes been puzzled by the following clinical problems:

1. *The concurrence of myasthenia gravis and thyrotoxicosis.* As indicated on page 1133, thyrotoxicosis may produce its own type of myopathy. There is no certain evidence that thyrotoxicosis aggravates myasthenia gravis, and some have even observed a see-saw relationship, which we have not confirmed. The diagnosis of myasthenia must rest on objective clinical findings and be confirmed by the laboratory tests already described. The ophthalmoplegia of thyrotoxicosis can usually be distinguished by the presence of an associated exophthalmos (early in the disease exophthalmos may be absent) and the lack of response to neostigmine. Lupus erythematosus and polymyositis are distinguished by finding the signs of these diseases in combination with those of myasthenia (see Chap. 49).

2. *The neurasthenic patient who complains of weakness when actually referring to fatigability.* There is no ptosis, strabismus, or dysphagia, though a neurotic individual may complain of diplopia (usually of momentary duration, when drowsy) and also of tightness in the throat (globus hystericus). A number of such patients claim improvement with neostigmine, but objective weakness and reversal thereof can never be ascertained. Conversely, myasthenia may be mistaken for hysteria or other emotional illness, mainly because the physician is unfamiliar with myasthenia (or with hysteria) and has been overly impressed with the precipitation of the illness by an emotional crisis.

3. *Progressive external ophthalmoplegia and other restricted myopathies,* including the congenital myasthenic states, may be mistaken for myasthenia gravis. It should be emphasized that the ocular muscles may be permanently damaged by myasthenia and cease to respond to neostigmine. Another possibility is that restricted ocular myasthenia may not respond to anticholinesterase drugs from the beginning and the diagnosis of myasthenia is erroneously excluded. One must then turn to other muscles for clinical and electromyographic confirmation of the diagnosis.

4. *Illnesses with dysarthria and dysphagia, but without ptosis or obvious strabismus;* these may be mistaken for multiple sclerosis or some other neurologic disease.

5. Rarely, one encounters a typical syndrome of *myasthenic polymyopathy with hypersensitivity to neostig-*

mine. Here there is improvement on minute doses of neostigmine and worsening on the usual dose. The basis of this state has never been ascertained.

TREATMENT

The treatment of this disease involves the careful use of three groups of drugs—anticholinesterases, immunosuppressants, and corticosteroids—and of thymectomy and plasmapheresis.

Anticholinesterase Drugs The two drugs that have given the best results in counteracting myasthenic weakness are neostigmine (Prostigmin) and pyridostigmine (Mestinon). The oral dose of neostigmine ranges from 7.5 to 45.0 mg every 2 to 6 h. The dose of pyridostigmine is twice that of neostigmine. Delayed-action forms of both drugs are available. The average maintenance dose of neostigmine is approximately 150 mg (10 tablets) per day. The addition of potassium or ephedrine to fortify the anticholinesterase activity contributes little. For mild cases without thymic tumor, this should be the initial and only form of therapy.

If the response to anticholinesterase drugs is poor and large doses are not relieving symptoms, there is always the danger of a *cholinergic crisis.* This consists of an episode in which the muscarinic effects of neostigmine (nausea, vomiting, pallor, sweating, salivation, colic, diarrhea, miosis, bradycardia), occur and are coupled with increasing myasthenic weakness. An impending cholinergic effect is betrayed by constriction of pupils; (they should not be allowed to contract to less than 2 mm). If the blood pressure falls, 0.6 mg atropine sulfate should be given slowly by the intravenous route. If the muscarinic effects are not present and weakness from overdose of neostigmine is suspected, the Tensilon test should be done (see above). The weakness of a cholinergic crisis is unaffected by Tensilon. If the weakness does improve, the patient is not receiving enough anticholinesterase drug.

Thymectomy Removal of the thymus gland is indicated in practically all cases of *thymoma.* An exception would be an elderly person enfeebled by age and other diseases; radiation of the tumor could then be substituted. The operative approach is through the anterior thorax, with adequate exposure to remove all the tumor tissue. If the removal is incomplete, radiotherapy should be given.

Thymectomy is recommended in practically all patients with uncomplicated myasthenia gravis who are less than 45 to 50 years of age and who, after a period of treatment with anticholinesterase drugs, are responding poorly and requiring increasing doses of medication. A suprasternal approach has been developed and results in less postoperative pain and morbidity, but the transsternal approach is preferable because it assures a more complete removal of thymic tissue. In patients with myasthenia restricted to the ocular muscles for a year or longer, the prognosis is so good that operation is unnecessary. The remission rate in the nontumor patients is approximately 35 percent, providing the procedure is done in the first year or two after onset of the disease; the remission rate is progressively lower if operation is postponed beyond this time. Another 45 percent will improve to some extent. The response to thymectomy is maximal by 3 years. In favorably responding cases, levels of circulating receptor antibody are reduced or disappear entirely. As improvement occurs the dosage of neostigmine can be reduced.

The long-term outlook for myasthenic children is generally good, and their life expectancy is only slightly reduced. Rodriguez et al followed a group of 149 children for an average of 17 years; 85 of them had been thymectomized. Approximately 30 percent of the nonthymectomized and 40 percent of the thymectomized patients underwent remission and were free of symptoms. The remission occurred usually in the first 3 years. Those with bulbar symptoms and with no ocular or generalized weakness had the most favorable outcome. Similarly, Olanow et al reported complete remission in 9 of 11 late-onset myasthenics submitted as early as possible to thymectomy.

Corticosteroids For the moderately severe myasthenic, in whom a remission has not been induced by thymectomy and who is responding inadequately to anticholinesterase drugs, a trial of corticosteroids is worthwhile and, if beneficial, may be continued for years. Some physicians use corticosteroids from the beginning, in preference to anticholinesterase drugs, in the belief that high doses downregulate the receptor. Of course, one must contend with the side effects of long-term corticosteroid therapy and one would hesitate to undertake such a program in children. In neonatal myasthenia only neostigmine is required.

The usual form of corticosteroid therapy is prednisone in a dose of 40 to 45 mg/day, preferably given in twice this dose every other day. Since worsening in the first week or 10 days is expected, hospitalization and careful observation for respiratory difficulty is advisable. Improvement occurs in the next few weeks, and, once obtained, the dosage of prednisone can be reduced slowly to the lowest point at which it is still effective. Potassium supplements and antacids are prescribed liberally, as with any corticosteroid treatment regime. The anticholinesterase drugs are given simultaneously, and as the patient improves, their dosage may be adjusted downward.

Plasmapheresis and Immunosuppression For the severe myasthenic who does not respond adequately to anticholinesterase drugs, thymectomy, or prednisone, one must resort to other measures. Striking temporary remissions (4 to 6 weeks) may be obtained by the use of plasmapheresis (5 daily plasma exchanges every 5 weeks). This form of treatment may be lifesaving during a crisis. It is also useful before and after thymectomy and at the start of immunosuppressive drug therapy.

Immune suppression with azathioprine has been accompanied by clinical improvement and reduction in the levels of receptor antibodies (Reuther et al). Azathioprine is given in a dosage of 2.5 mL/kg daily, with prednisone in doses up to 1.5 mg/kg per day. Improvement may not be evident for several months after the onset of treatment (Witte et al). Similar improvement has been achieved with the immunosuppressant cyclophosphamide within the first month of treatment (Perez et al). Other cytotoxic drugs such as methotrexate, cyclosporin, with or without antilymphocyte serum, or total lymphoid radiation, are also being tried in patients who continue to do poorly after thymectomy. Eventually there may be a remission, hence the justification for using every possible measure to support the patient until this happens.

THE MYASTHENIC-MYOPATHIC SYNDROME OF LAMBERT-EATON

This special form of myasthenia, observed most often with oat-cell carcinoma of the lung, was first described by Eaton and Lambert, in 1957. Unlike myasthenia gravis, the muscles of the trunk and the pelvic and shoulder girdles are the ones that most frequently become weak and fatigable. Often the first symptoms are difficulty in arising from a chair, climbing stairs, and walking, and the shoulder muscles are affected later. While ptosis, diplopia, dysarthria, and dysphagia may occur, and may even be the presenting symptoms, this is less frequent. Increasing weakness after exertion stamps the condition as myasthenic, but as Eaton and Lambert originally pointed out, *there may be a temporary increase in muscle power during the first few contractions*. The tendon reflexes are often diminished but if abolished should raise the question of an associated carcinomatous polyneuropathy. Fasciculation is not seen. Other complaints are paresthesias, aching pain (suggesting arthritis), and a number of autonomic disturbances, such as dryness of the mouth, constipation, difficult micturition, and impotence. There may be other neurologic manifestations of neoplasia (polyneuropathy, polymyositis or dermatomyositis, multifocal leukoencephalopathy, cerebellar degeneration).

The onset is usually subacute and the course variably progressive. The myasthenia may precede discovery of the tumor by months or years. In addition to lung tumors, this syndrome has been associated with carcinoma of the breast, prostate, stomach, and rectum. Males are affected more often than females (5:1). In almost half of the patients no tumor is found. The condition may occur in children, usually without relation to tumor. In the tumor cases, death usually occurs in a few months to years from the effect of the tumor itself.

Also unlike myasthenia gravis, the response to neostigmine and pyridostigmine is variable. On the other hand, *d*-tubocurarine, suxamethonium chloride, gallamine, and other muscle relaxants have a deleterious effect and when given during anesthesia may dramatically increase the weakness and even result in fatality.

Electrodiagnostic studies have shown no abnormality in the peripheral nerves. A single stimulus of nerve may yield a low-amplitude muscle action potential (in contrast to myasthenia gravis, in which it is normal or nearly so), whereas at fast rates of stimulation (50 per second) and with strong voluntary contraction (for 15 s or longer) there is a marked increase in the amplitude of action potentials (incrementing response). Single fiber recordings show an increase in ''jitter'' (page 1022).

In patients with the Lambert-Eaton syndrome, there is an increased incidence of HLA-B8 and -DR3 haplotypes, as may occur in other autoimmune diseases. When injected into mice, IgG from patients with this syndrome transfers the physiologic abnormalities.

Elmquist and Lambert, from a series of studies of excised muscle, deduced that there is a defect in the release of acetylcholine quanta from the nerve terminals akin to that in paralysis due to botulinus toxin (see page 905). The presynaptic vesicles appear to be normal in electron micrographs. In contrast to myasthenia gravis the extent of the receptor surface in the myasthenic syndrome is actually increased, and no receptor antibody is present. Some factor(s) elaborated by oat-cell carcinoma appears to interfere with ACh release, according to Lindstrom and Lambert. How small-cell lung cancer evokes the physiologic changes is of interest. In tissue culture, the tumor cells, thought to be of neural crest origin, show a voltage-dependent Ca flux, which can be inhibited by known Ca channel blockers. This property is also blocked by the IgG of Lambert-Eaton cases. According to Roberts et al, these antibodies are responsible for the 40 percent reduction in the number of voltage-gated Ca channels at the motor nerve terminals.

Muscle biopsy has shown the same slight, nonspecific changes as in myasthenia gravis.

Elicitation of the Lambert-Eaton syndrome should lead to a search for occult tumor, especially of the lung. If found, it should of course be treated, and this alone may result in improvement in the neurologic syndrome. If none is found the search should be repeated at regular intervals. Guanidine hydrochloride (20 to 30 mg/kg/day in divided doses) has been more effective than neostigmine or pyridostigmine. More recently, this drug has been replaced by the less toxic 3,4-diaminopyridine, 20 mg orally five times daily, in conjunction with pyridostigmine (Lundh et al). Takamori et al recommend drugs which increase the content of cyclic AMP. Streib and Rothner were able to achieve long-term improvement with prednisone. Dau and Denys obtained the best results in nontumor cases with repeated courses of plasmapheresis in combination with prednisone and azathioprine. The dose of prednisone was 25 to 60 mg per day, and azathioprine, 2.3 to 2.9 mg/kg body weight daily. The response to treatment tends to be slow, over a period of months to a year. Some patients recover fully; in others, restoration of power is incomplete.

The only illnesses that might be confused with this myasthenic syndrome are hysterical paralysis, where the patient may do better with encouragement on successive voluntary contractions, and arthritis, where pain hampers the first movements more than successive ones. Then the electrodiagnostic tests are of value.

OTHER MYASTHENIC SYNDROMES

The phenomenon of decreasing power of muscle contraction with continued activity and restoration of strength with rest, along with the electrophysiologic demonstration of reduced "safety factor" of neuromuscular transmission, have been demonstrated in a number of other clinical settings. Walton et al observed a case of benign congenital myopathy with myasthenic features and we have already mentioned the various types of congenital myasthenia.

In Japan, a disorder referred to as "kubisagari" has been described, occurring as an outbreak of ptosis and bulbar weakness in nutritionally deprived children. The effect of Prostigmin on the weakness is not clear from the published reports; also, the question of a neurotoxin was raised. Similar cases had been observed among soldiers held prisoner by the Japanese. Denny-Brown stated that the parenteral administration of thiamine restored muscular power within a week.

A deficiency of pseudocholinesterase, either genetic or acquired, may cause prolonged weakness and apnea when succinylcholine or some other depolarizing relaxant is administered (usually during anesthesia). According to Lehmann and Liddell, the genetic form may be identified

by measuring the action of dibucaine or fluorine in serum. Phenelzine, several organophosphates, and liver disease are at times attended by a mysasthenic weakness of this type.

MYASTHENIC WEAKNESS WITH ANTIBIOTICS AND OTHER DRUGS

Many drugs may cause a worsening of myasthenia gravis by their action on pre- or postsynaptic structures. This is most likely to happen in patients who are already receiving some other drug(s) or suffering from hepatic or renal disease. Or the offending drug may induce an immunologic reaction. Again the drug may unmask a latent neuromuscular disease (Swift). Interestingly, the myasthenic state in all these conditions is acute and lasts hours or days, providing the patient does not succumb to respiratory failure; the ocular, facial, and bulbar muscles are involved as well as other muscles. The treatment in all instances is to provide respiratory support, discontinue the offending drug, and attempt to reverse the block by infusions of calcium gluconate, supplementation of potassium, and anticholinesterases, along the lines suggested by Argov and Mastaglia. The latter list more than 30 drugs in current clinical use (other than anesthetic agents) that may interfere with neuromuscular transmission. Of these, the most important are the aminoglycoside antibiotics. According to McQuillen et al and Pittinger et al, who have reviewed this subject, myasthenic weakness has been reported with 18 different antibiotics but particularly with neomycin, kanamycin, cholistin, streptomycin, polymyxin B, and certain tetracyclines. It has been shown that these drugs impair transmitter release (as does myasthenia gravis) by interfering with calcium-ion fluxes at nerve terminals. These drugs are especially dangerous when given to myasthenic patients. Also, several of the immunosuppressant drugs such as ACTH, prednisone, and azathioprine worsen myasthenia temporarily by depolarizing nerve terminals or impairing release of ACh.

Other drugs, such as anticholinesterase drugs, particularly insecticides and nerve gases, cause paralysis by binding to cholinesterase and blocking the hydrolysis of ACh. The end plate remains depolarized. The most notable of these drugs or toxins are *botulinum* toxin, which binds to cholinergic motor endings, blocking quantal release of ACh; black widow spider venom, which causes a massive release of ACh, resulting in muscular contraction and then paralysis from a lack of ACh; *d*-tubocurarine, which binds to ACh receptors; suxemethonium and decamethonium, which also bind to ACh receptors; organophosphates, which bind irreversibly to ACh esterases; malathione and parathione, which inhibit ACh esterase. The actions of all these agents are transitory except for the organophosphate "nerve gases."

The administration of D-penicillamine has also caused a type of myasthenia. The weakness is typical in that rest increases strength as do Prostigmin and Tensilon, and the electrophysiologic findings are also typical. In such cases, Vincent et al found anti-ACh receptor antibodies in the serum; hence, one must assume that this is a form of autoimmune myasthenia gravis. In these respects it differs from the weakness caused by aminoglycosides (see review of Swift). Rarely, typical autoimmune myasthenia gravis develops as part of a chronic graft-versus-host disease in long-term (2- to 3-year) survivors of allogenic marrow transplants.

EPISODIC (KALEMIC) PARALYSES

At least four hereditary syndromes of recurrent muscle weakness have now been identified:

1 Hypokalemic familial periodic paralysis

2. Hypokalemic periodic paralysis with hyperthroidism

3. Hyperkalemic periodic paralysis without myotonia (adynamica episodica hereditaria of Gamstorp)

4. Hyperkalemic, cold-evoked periodic paralysis with paradoxical myotonia (von Eulenberg)

In addition, transitory episodes of weakness are known to be associated with other derangements of potassium metabolism, mainly a hypokalemia, such as aldosteronism, 17α-hydroxylase deficiency (Yazaki et al), barium poisoning (Lewi et al), and abuse of thyroid hormone (Layzer). Other forms of secondary hypokalemic weakness have been observed in patients suffering from chronic renal and adrenal insufficiency or disorders due to a loss of potassium, such as occurs with excessive ingestion of thiazide or laxatives, etc. Renal failure with hyperkalemia can also induce paralysis.

In each of the periodic paralyses, the patient may, over a few hours, develop a disorder of trunk and limb muscles, varying from a diffuse weakness to total paralysis; the condition subsides after a few hours or days, leaving the musculature entirely normal. Clinical differences between these several syndromes are small, except in the von Eulenberg form, where evocation of the attacks by cold and a restricted or paradoxical myotonia are added features.

Periodic paralysis can be readily distinguished from cataplexy, which lasts only a few seconds or minutes, and is precipitated by emotion; from episodes of sleep paralysis, which also are very brief; and from presyncope, in which physical weakness is always combined with pallor and a disorder of consciousness. In textbooks, the differential diagnosis of episodic paralysis also includes ''drop attacks''

of the aged, myoclonic and akinetic epilepsy with falling attacks, and hydrocephalic attacks with limb weakness, but the resemblances to these states are remote.

FAMILIAL OR HYPOKALEMIC PERIODIC PARALYSIS (PAROXYSMAL MYOPLEGIA)

This is the best-known form of periodic paralysis. The history of the disease is difficult to trace. References to it can be found in writings of the early eighteenth century, but the first clear descriptions were given by Hartwig, in 1874, followed by Westphal (1885) and by Oppenheim (1891). Goldflam (in 1895) was the first to call attention to the remarkable vacuolization of the muscle fibers. In 1937, Aitken and his associates first described the occurrence of hypokalemia during attacks of paralysis and reversal of the paralysis by the administration of potassium, thus setting the stage for subsequent studies of the normo- and hyperkalemic forms of periodic paralysis. For English-speaking readers, Talbott's monograph serves as the best review of the subject and includes the historical references as well as all cases that had been reported prior to 1941; and the more recent articles of Grob et al, A. G. Engel, and Layzer bring the subject up to date.

A strong heredofamilial incidence characterizes fully three-quarters of all cases, as the name implies. The usual pattern of inheritance is autosomal dominant. Recessive inheritance is also known to occur. One suspects that in the sporadic cases an intensive exploration of family records might have divulged affected antecedents. Males are more susceptible, in a ratio of 3:1, but a sex-linked hereditary pattern has not been proved. Association with other neurologic or psychiatric conditions, e.g., migraine, is probably coincidental. The disease has been observed in all parts of the world.

Clinical Manifestations The onset of the disease is in late childhood or adolescence. In Talbott's review of 152 cases, there were 40 in which symptoms began before the tenth year of life and 92 before the sixteenth year. The typical attack comes on during sleep, after a day of unusually strenuous exercise; a meal rich in carbohydrates favors its development. Certain prodromata—a sense of well-being before retiring, or of weariness and fatigue—are reported but are difficult to evaluate. Excessive hunger or thirst, dry mouth, palpitation, sweating, diarrhea, and nervousness are also mentioned but do not necessarily precede an attack. Usually the patient awakens to discover a mild or severe weakness of the limbs. However, diurnal attacks also occur, especially after a nap following a large meal. The attack evolves over minutes to several hours, and at its peak may render the patient so helpless as to be unable to call for assistance. Once established, the weakness lasts a few hours, if mild, or several days, if severe.

The distribution of the paralysis varies. Limbs are affected earlier and often more severely than trunk muscles and proximal muscles are possibly more susceptible than distal ones. Legs are often weakened before the arms, but exceptionally the order is reversed. The muscles most likely to escape are those of the eyes, face, tongue, pharynx, larynx, diaphragm, and sphincters, but on occasion even these may be involved. At its peak, tendon reflexes are reduced or abolished and cutaneous reflexes may also disappear. Sensibility is preserved. As the attack subsides, strength generally returns first to the muscles that were last to be affected. Headache, exhaustion, diuresis, and occasionally diarrhea may follow the attack.

Attacks of paralysis tend to occur every few weeks and lessen in frequency with advancing age. Rarely, death may occur from respiratory paralysis or derangements of the conducting system of the heart.

Atypical forms include weakness of one limb or certain groups of muscles, bibrachial palsy (inability to lift arms or comb hair), and transient weakness during accustomed activities. Earlier descriptions of daily brief attacks, some associated with exposure to cold or coupled with muscular hypertrophy or exophthalmic goiter, preceded recognition of the other types of periodic paralysis and cannot be evaluated. A number of patients have developed a slowly progressive proximal myopathy, with vacuolated and degenerated fibers and myopathic action potentials, during middle adult life, long after attacks of periodic paralysis have ceased.

Laboratory Findings   The attacks are accompanied by reduction in serum K levels, as low as 1.8 meq/L, but usually at levels that would not be associated with paresis in normal subjects. The fall in serum K is associated with little or no increase in urinary K excretion; presumably the K enters the muscle fibers. The serum K levels return to normal during recovery. It has been calculated that as much as 100 meq K may move from the extracellular fluid compartment into muscle during an attack. Grob et al found the intramuscular K to increase after ingestion of carbohydrate, administration of glucose, and injection of insulin and possibly epinephrine. Although these shifts in K are of undoubted importance in the pathogenesis of muscle weak-

ness, the marked sensitivity to small reductions of serum K and to cold suggest that other factors, as yet undefined, are also of importance.

The muscular paralysis is associated with a decrease and eventual loss of muscle action potentials evoked by supramaximal stimulation of peripheral nerve and of voluntary motor unit potentials, recorded by needle examination. Decline in strength precedes loss of motor unit potentials and of propagation of the latter from the neuromuscular junction over the surface of the fiber. The polarization potentials of muscle fibers measured by intracellular recordings are normal, yet the muscle fiber does not propagate the action potential. The reason for the inexcitability of the muscle cell membrane is not yet known (Layzer). One would expect it to be hyperpolarized as K moves into the fiber, but actually it is hypopolarized. Rüdel et al attribute the latter to an increased Na conductance. ECG changes also begin at levels of K that are slightly below normal (about 3 meq/L); they consist of prolonged PR, QRS, and QT intervals and lowering of T waves.

Diagnosis at a time when the patient is normal may be facilitated by provocative tests. With the patient carefully monitored, the oral administration of 50 to 100 g of glucose or loading with 2 to 4 g of NaCl, followed by vigorous exercise, brings on an attack, which then responds to 2 to 4 g of oral KCl.

Pathologic Changes   The nervous system is entirely normal. The muscle fibers are relatively large and of similar size. The most striking change is vacuolization of sarcoplasm. The myofibrils are separated by round or oval vacuoles containing clear fluid, presumably water, and a few PAS-positive granules. Isolated muscle fibers may undergo segmental degeneration. Electron-microscopic studies have shown that the vacuoles arise by progressive dilatation of the sarcoplasmic reticulum.

Treatment   The daily administration of 5 to 10 g of KCl orally in aqueous solution prevents attacks in many patients, and apparently this program can be maintained indefinitely. When not successful, a low-carbohydrate, low-salt, high-K diet, combined with a slowly released K preparation, may be effective. A low-sodium diet (< 60 meq/day), avoidance of large meals and exposure to cold, acetozalamide 250 mg three times daily, and chlorthiazide 500 mg daily, may also be helpful in preventing attacks.

For an acute attack, 10 g of KCl should be given, or some other K salt if this is not tolerated. This dose may be insufficient, and if there is no improvement in 1 or 2 h, another 5 g may be required. Under exceptional conditions KCl may have to be given intravenously. Regular exercise (not too strenuous) to keep the patient fit is desirable.

THYROTOXICOSIS WITH PERIODIC PARALYSIS

This, too, is a form of hypokalemic periodic paralysis. It occurs mainly in young adult males, with a special predilection for those of Japanese and Chinese extraction. In Japan, Okinaka et al found that 8.9 percent of males with thyrotoxicosis had periodic paralysis but only 0.4 percent of females, and for the Chinese, the corresponding figures were 13.0 and 0.17 percent (McFadzean and Yeung). The paralytic disorder is unrelated to the severity of the hyperthyroidism. In the naturally occurring variety of familial periodic paralysis, the induction of hyperthyroidism is said not to increase the frequency or intensity of attacks. Therefore it seems likely that the thyrotoxicosis has unmasked another type of hereditary periodic paralysis, although a familial occurrence in the thyrotoxic cases is exceptional. Clinically, the attacks of paralysis are much the same as those of familial hypokalemic type, except for a greater liability to cardiac irregularity. As in the familial form, the paralyzed muscles are inexcitable, due possibly to overactivity of the Na-K pump, according to Layzer. KCl restores power in a paralytic attack, and treatment of the hyperthyroidism prevents their recurrence.

HYPERKALEMIC PERIODIC PARALYSIS WITHOUT MYOTONIA (ADYNAMIA EPISODICA HEREDITARIA)

Soon after the recognition of hypokalemia in familial periodic paralysis and its treatment with K replacement, another type of periodic paralysis was found in which the serum K was elevated and an attack would actually be induced by the administration of potassium salts. Tyler and colleagues (1951) studied such a family and concluded that it was an entity distinct from the usual type of familial periodic paralysis. Five years later, Gamstorp reported two families and named the newly defined state *adynamia episodica hereditaria*. As further examples were reported, it was noted that in many of them there were minor degrees of myotonia, which brought the condition into relationship with paramyotonia congenita described in 1886 by von Eulenberg (see below). Drager et al insist that the latter disease and that described by Tyler and Gamstorp are identical; Gamstorp does not agree. The dispute cannot be settled until the basic biochemical abnormality of each condition is elucidated.

Clinical Manifestations   Onset is usually in infancy and childhood. Characteristically, the attacks of weakness occur when the patient is resting in a chair, about 20 to 30 min after exercise. The paresis begins in the legs, thighs, and lower back and spreads to the hands, forearms, and shoulders. Only in the severest attacks are the neck and ocular

muscles involved. As the muscles become inexcitable, tendon reflexes are diminished or lost. Attacks are usually more frequent and briefer (30 to 60 min or somewhat longer) than in the hypokalemic variety, and recovery is hastened by exercise. If the patient continues to be active, further attacks may be averted, but then, with rest, they tend to recur. In young, active children the attacks may occur every day; others have them less frequently. During late adolescence and adult years, when the patient becomes more sedentary, the attacks may diminish and cease. In certain muscle groups, particularly the ocular muscles, it is difficult to separate the effects of paresis from those of myotonia. Indeed when an attack of paresis is prevented by continuous movement, firm painful lumps may form in the calf muscles. Some patients with repeated attacks may be left with a permanent weakness and wasting of the proximal limb muscles.

The *provocative test*, undertaken when the patient is functioning normally, consists of the oral administration of 2 g of KCl, repeated every 2 h for four doses. The patient needs to be carefully monitored by continuous ECG and serum K estimations, and the test should never be undertaken in the presence of an attack of weakness or reduced renal function.

The *treatment* of this syndrome is the same as that for paramyotonia congenita (see below).

PARAMYOTONIA CONGENITA OF VON EULENBERG

In this disease, attacks of periodic paralysis are associated with myotonia. In some patients the myotonia can be elicited even in a warm environment, but more characteristically, a widespread myotonia, often coupled with weakness, is induced by cold. The weakness may be diffuse, as in adynamia episodica hereditaria, or limited to the part of the body that is cooled. Once started the weakness persists for several hours, even after the body is rewarmed. Percussion myotonia can be evoked in the tongue and thenar eminence. Immersion of the arm and hand in ice water elicits both myotonia and weakness after a period of about 30 min. According to Haass et al, myotonia that is constantly present in a warm environment diminishes with repeated contraction, whereas myotonia induced by cold increases with repeated contraction (paradoxical myotonia).

Laboratory Findings   In the latter two diseases (adynamia and paramyotonia), which are similar, and in the view of some myologists, identical, the serum K is usually above normal range, but paralysis has been observed at levels of 5 meq/L or even lower. Each patient appears to have a critical level of serum K that if exceeded will be associated with weakness. The administration of KCl, raising serum K to above 7 meq/L, a level that has no effect on normal individuals, invariably induces an attack in the patient. There is evidence that during the attack intramuscular K falls and Na rises, and that between attacks they are normal. There may also be a hypocalcemia during attacks. The EMG of the weakened muscle shows a dropping out of some motor unit potentials and a reduced voltage and duration of others (as though some muscle fibers in each motor unit are no longer contracting). Other fibers show the typical hyperirritability and afterdischarge of myotonia.

The polarization of the resting muscle fiber is reduced between attacks and even more so during the attack. As temperature is reduced, the muscle membrane is progressively depolarized. Physiologic studies have shown that both the weakness and myotonia are due to a temperature-dependent abnormality of sodium conductance in the sarcolemma (Lehmann-Horn et al). In patients with paramyotonia—but not in those with hyperkalemic periodic paralysis—Subramony and his colleagues have observed a diminution of the compound muscle action potential in response to the cooling of muscle, suggesting that the two syndromes are indeed distinct.

There are either no histologic changes in the fibers or at most a few vacuoles. Aggregates of tubules are seen in electron microscopic preparations of muscle fibers in this and normokalemic periodic paralysis.

Treatment Many of the attacks are too brief and mild to require treatment. If severe, intravenous calcium gluconate (1 to 2 g) often restores power. If after a few minutes this treatment is unsuccessful, intravenous glucose or glucose and insulin and chlorothiazide should be tried.

The continuous use of diuretics such as chlorothiazide (about 0.5 g daily), keeping the serum K below 5 meq/L, prevents attacks. Acetazolamide or some longer-acting carbonic anhydrase inhibitors have also proved effective. When the myotonia is more troublesome than weakness, procainamide or the lidocaine derivative, tocainide, in doses of 400 to 1200 mg daily, is useful (Streib).

Some patients with paramyotonia, as with other forms of periodic paralysis, may slowly develop a mild polymyopathy that causes persistent weakness.

NORMOKALEMIC PERIODIC PARALYSIS

In this condition, described by Poskanzer and Kerr in 1961, the attacks tend to be more severe and prolonged than in the hyperkalemic form, and there is no myotonia or sensitivity to cold. Urinary K does not increase during paralysis. However, the paralysis is induced and made worse by the administration of K salts. Like other forms of periodic paralysis, the inheritance follows an autosomal dominant pattern. Acetazolamide, 250 mg tid, and appropriate daily doses of 9α-fluorohydrocortisone, prevented attacks in the patients reported by Poskanzer and Kerr, but these measures were unsuccessful in the family reported by Meyers et al. Also, in the affected members of the latter family, the attacks were shorter and were not provoked by large doses of K.

HYPOKALEMIC WEAKNESS IN PRIMARY ALDOSTERONISM

Hypokalemic weakness due to hypersecretion of the major adrenal mineralocorticoid aldosterone was first described by Conn, in 1955. In *primary aldosteronism,* the cause of the hypersecretion is in the adrenal itself—usually an adrenal cortical adenoma, less often adrenal cortical hyperplasia. The disorder is not common (occurring in about 1 percent of unselected hypertensive patients), but its recognition is essential since it can be treated effectively. Persistent aldosteronism is frequently associated with hypernatremia, polyuria, and alkalosis, which predisposes the patient to attacks of tetany as well as to hypokalemic weakness. Conn et al (1964), in an analysis of 103 patients with primary aldosteronism, found that persistent muscular weakness was a major complaint in 73 percent; intermittent attacks of paralysis occurred in 21 percent, and tetany in 21 percent. These manifestations were much more frequent in women than in men, in contrast to the preponderance of men among patients with hypokalemic periodic paralysis of familial type. Rarely, the typical syndrome of primary aldosteronism is produced by the chronic ingestion of licorice; this is due to its content of glycyrrhizic acid, a potent mineralocorticoid that causes sodium retention and potassium diuresis.

The muscle fibers of patients with primary aldosteronism show necrosis and vacuolation. Ultrastructurally, the necrotic areas are characterized by a dissolution of myofilaments with degenerative vacuoles; nonnecrotic fibers contain membrane-bound vacuoles and show dilatation of the sarcoplasmic reticulum and abnormalities of the T system, suggesting that a vulnerability of the latter structures may be responsible for the muscle fiber necrosis (Atsumi et al).

DIFFERENTIAL DIAGNOSIS
OF THE PERIODIC PARALYSES

The nocturnal occurrence of severe and prolonged attacks of periodic paralysis, with onset in early life, suggests the hypokalemic type. Infusions of carbohydrate after heavy exercise provokes attacks, which can be verified by measurements of serum K and electrodiagnostic testing. Such patients should be checked for hyperthyroidism, but this latter form of periodic paralysis is rare in North America, except in adult Oriental males. In our experience, hyperkalemic patients have all had some degree of sensitivity to cold and restricted myotonia. Moreover their attacks are brief and more frequent in early childhood. In the normokalemic type, the attacks are both severe and prolonged. The paralytic disorders due to renal disease and aldosteronism are not familial, and the serum electrolyte disorders are severe in degree, in distinction to the familial hypokalemic types.

REFERENCES

Adams RD, Kakulas BA: *Diseases of Muscle: Pathological Foundations of Clinical Myology,* 4th ed. Philadelphia, Harper & Row, 1985.

Almon RR, Andrew CG, Appel SH: Serum globulin in myasthenia gravis: Inhibition of α-bungarotoxin binding in acetylcholine receptors. *Science* 186:55, 1974.

Argov Z, Mastaglia FL: Disorders of neuromuscular transmission caused by drugs. *N Engl J Med* 301:409, 1979.

Atsumi T, Ishikawa S, Miyatake T, Yoshida M: Myopathy and primary aldosteronism: Electron microscopic study. *Neurology* 29:1348, 1979.

Bever CT Jr, Aquino AV, Penn AS et al: Prognosis of ocular myasthenia. *Ann Neurol* 14:516, 1983.

Buzzard EF: The clinical history and postmortem examination of 5 cases of myasthenia gravis. *Brain* 28:438, 1905.

Conn JW: Primary aldosteronism: A new clinical syndrome. *J Lab Clin Med* 45:6, 1955.

Conn JW, Knopf RF, Nesbit RM: Clinical characteristics of primary aldosteronism from an analysis of 145 cases. *Am J Surg* 107:159, 1964.

Conn JW, Rovner DR, Cohen EL: Licorice-induced pseudoaldosteronism. Hypertension, hypokalemia, aldosteronopenia and suppressed plasma renin activity. *JAMA* 205:492, 1968.

Dau PC, Denys EH: Plasmapheresis and immunosuppressive therapy in the Eaton-Lambert syndrome. *Ann Neurol* 11:570, 1982.

Denny-Brown D: Neurological conditions resulting from prolonged and severe dietary restriction. *Medicine* 26:41, 1947.

Drachman DB: Myasthenic antibodies cross-link acetylcholine receptors to accelerate degradation. *N Engl J Med* 298:136, 186, 1978.

Drager GA, Hammill JF, Shy GM: Paramyotonia congenita. *Arch Neurol Psychiatry* 30:1, 1958.

Eaton LM, Lambert EH: Electromyography and electric stimulation of nerves and diseases of motor unit: Observations on myasthenic syndrome associated with malignant tumors. *JAMA* 163:1117, 1957.

Elmquist D, Lambert EH: Detailed analysis of neuromuscular transmission in a patient with the myasthenic syndrome, sometimes associated with bronchial carcinoma. *Mayo Clin Proc* 43:689, 1968.

Engel AG: Evolution and content of vacuoles in primary hypokalemic periodic paralysis. *Mayo Clin Proc* 45:774, 1970.

Engel AG, Lambert EH, Howard FM: Immune complexes (IgG and C3) at motor end-plate in myasthenia gravis. *Mayo Clin Proc* 52:267, 1977.

Engel AG, Lambert EH, Santa T: Study of long-term anticholinesterase therapy. *Neurology* 23:1273, 1973.

Engel AG, Tsujihata M, Lambert EH, Lindstrom JM, Lennon VA: Experimental autoimmune myasthenia gravis: A sequential and quantitative study of the neuromuscular junction ultrastructure and electrophysiologic correlations. *J Neuropathol Exp Neurol* 35:569, 1976.

Engel AG, Tsujihata M, Lindstrom JM, Lennon VA: The motor end-plate in myasthenia gravis and in experimental autoimmune myasthenia gravis. *Ann NY Acad Sci* 274:60, 1976.

Fambrough DM, Drachman DB, Satyamurti S: Neuromuscular junction in myasthenia gravis: Decreased acetylcholine receptors. *Science* 182:293, 1973.

Gamstorp I: Adynamia periodica hereditaria. *Acta Paediatr Scand Suppl* 108:1, 1956.

Grob D, Brunner NG, Namba T: The natural course of myasthenia gravis and effect of therapeutic measures. *Ann NY Acad Sci* 377:652, 1981.

Haass A, Ricker K, Rüdel et al: Clinical study of paramyotonia congenita with and without myotonia in a warm environment. *Muscle Nerve* 4:388, 1981.

Kelly JJ, Daube JR, Lennon VA: The laboratory diagnosis of mild myasthenia gravis. *Ann Neurol* 12:238, 1982.

Kerzin-Storrar L, Metcalfe RA, Dyer PA: Genetic factors in myasthenia gravis: A family study. *Neurology* 38:38, 1988.

Lambert EH, Lindstrom JM, Lennon VA: End-plate potentials in experimental autoimmune myasthenia gravis in rats. *Ann NY Acad Med* 274:300, 1976.

Layzer RB: *Neuromuscular Manifestations of Systemic Disease.* Philadelphia, Davis, 1985.

Layzer RB: Periodic paralysis and the sodium pump. *Ann Neurol* 11:547, 1982.

Lehmann H, Liddell J: Human cholinesterase (pseudocholinesterase) genetic variants and their recognition. *Br J Anaesth* 41:235, 1968.

LEHMANN-HORN F, RÜDEL R, DENGLER R: Membrane defects in paramyotonia congenita with and without myotonia in a warm environment. *Muscle Nerve* 4:396, 1981.

LENNON VA: Immunologic mechanisms in myasthenia gravis—a model of a receptor disease, in Franklin E (ed): *Clinical Immunology Update—Reviews for Physicians.* New York, Elsevier/North-Holland, 1979, pp 259–289.

LENNON VA, LINDSTROM JM, SEYBOLD ME: Experimental autoimmune myasthenia gravis in rats and guinea pigs. *J Exp Med* 141:1365, 1975.

LEWI Z, BAR-KHAYIM Y: Food poisoning from barium carbonate. *Lancet* 2:342, 1964.

LINDSTROM JM, LAMBERT EH: Content of acetylcholine receptor and antibodies bound to receptor in myasthenia gravis, experimental autoimmune myasthenia gravis, and Eaton-Lambert syndrome. *Neurology* 28:130, 1978.

LUNDH H, NILSSON O, ROSEN I: Treatment of Lambert-Eaton syndrome: 3,4-Diaminopyridine and pyridostigmine. *Neurology* 34:1324, 1984.

MAYER RF, WILLIAMS IR: Incrementing responses in myasthenia gravis. *Arch Neurol* 31:24, 1974.

MEYERS KR, GILDEN DH, RINALDI CF, HANSEN JL: Periodic muscle weakness, normokalemia, and tubular aggregates. *Neurology* 22:269, 1972.

MCFADZEAN AJS, YEUNG R: Periodic paralysis complicating thyrotoxicosis in Chinese. *Br Med J* 1:451, 1967.

MCQUILLEN MP, CANTOR HE, O'ROURKE JR: Myasthenic syndrome associated with antibiotics. *Arch Neurol* 18:402, 1968.

MOSSMAN S, VINCENT A, NEWSOM-DAVIS J: Myasthenia gravis without acetylcholine receptor antibody: A distinct disease entity. *Lancet* 1:116, 1986.

NASTUK WL, PLESCIA OJ, OSSERMAN KE: Changes in serum complement activity in patients with myasthenia gravis. *Proc Soc Exp Biol Med* 105:177, 1960.

NEWSOM-DAVIS J: Diseases of the neuromuscular junction, in Asbury AK, McKhann GM, McDonald WI (eds): *Diseases of the Nervous System.* Philadelphia, Saunders, 1986.

OKINAKA S, SHIZUME K, IINO S et al: The association of periodic paralysis and hyperthyroidism in Japan. *J Clin Endocrinol Metab* 17:1454, 1957.

OLANOW CW, LANE RJM, ROSES AD: Thymectomy in late-onset myasthenia gravis. *Arch Neurol* 39:82, 1982.

OSSERMAN KE: *Myasthenia Gravis.* New York, Grune & Stratton, 1958.

PATRICK J, LINDSTROM JP: Autoimmune response to acetylcholine receptor. *Science* 180:871, 1973.

PATRICK J, LINDSTROM JP, CULP B, MCMILLAN J: Studies on purified eel acetylcholine receptor and antiacetylcholine receptor antibody. *Proc Natl Acad Sci USA* 70:3334, 1973.

PENN AS: Myoglobinuria, in Engel AG, Banker BQ (eds): *Myology.* New York, McGraw-Hill, 1986, Chap 62, pp 1785–1805.

PEREZ MC, BUOT WL, MERCADO-DONGUILAN C: Stable remissions in myasthenia gravis. *Neurology* 31:32, 1981.

PITTINGER CB, ERYASE Y, ADAMSON R: Antibiotic induced paralysis. *Anesth Analg* 49:487, 1970.

POSKANZER DC, KERR DNS: A third type of periodic paralysis with normokalemia and favorable response to NaCl. *Am J Med* 31:328, 1961.

REMAN L: Zur Pathogenese und Therapie der Myasthenia gravis pseudoparalytica. *Dtsch Z Nervenheilkd* 128:66, 1932.

REUTHER P, FULPIUS BW, MERTENS HB, HERTEL G: Antiacetylcholine receptor antibody under long-term azothiaprine treatment in myasthenia gravis, in Dau PC (ed): *Plasmapheresis and the Immunobiology of Myasthenia Gravis.* Boston, Houghton-Mifflin, 1979, pp 329–348.

ROBERTS A, PERERA S, LANG B et al: Paraneoplastic myasthenic syndrome IgG inhibits 45 Ca^{2+} flux in human small cell carcinoma lines. *Nature* 317:737, 1985.

RODRIGUEZ M, GOMEZ MR, HOWARD FM: Myasthenia gravis in children: long-term followup. *Ann Neurol* 13:504, 1983.

RÜDEL R, LEHMANN-HORN F, RICKER K et al: Hypokalemic periodic paralysis: In vitro investigation of muscle fiber membrane parameters. *Muscle Nerve* 7:110, 1984.

RUSSELL DS: Histological changes in myasthenia gravis. *J Pathol Bacteriol* 65:279, 1953.

SANTA T, ENGEL AG, LAMBERT EH: Histometric study of neuromuscular junction ultrastructure. I. Myasthenia gravis. *Neurology* 22:71, 1972.

SCADDING GK, VINCENT A, NEWSOM-DAVIS J, HENRY K: Acetylcholine receptor antibody synthesis by thymic lymphocytes: Correlation with thymic histology. *Neurology* 31:935, 1981.

SIMPSON JA: Myasthenia gravis: A new hypothesis. *Scot Med J* 5:419, 1960.

SIMPSON JA: Myasthenia gravis and myasthenic syndromes, in Walton JN (ed): *Diseases of Voluntary Muscle,* 5th ed. Edinburgh, Churchill Livingstone, 1988, chap 19, pp 628–665.

STREIB EW: Paramyotonia congenita: Successful treatment with tocainide. Clinical and electrophysiologic findings in seven patients. *Muscle Nerve* 10:155, 1987.

STREIB EW, ROTHNER D: Eaton-Lambert myasthenic syndrome: long-term treatment of 3 patients with prednisone. *Ann Neurol* 10:448, 1981.

SUBRAMONY SH, WEE AS, MISHRA SK: Lack of cold sensitivity in hyperkalemic periodic paralysis. *Muscle Nerve* 9:700, 1986.

SWIFT TR: Disorders of neuromuscular transmission other than myasthenia gravis. *Muscle Nerve* 4:334, 1981.

TAKAMORI M, ISHII N, MORI M: The role of c-AMP in neuromuscular transmission. *Arch Neurol* 29:420, 1973.

TALBOTT JH: Periodic paralysis: A clinical syndrome. *Medicine* 20:85, 1941.

TYLER FH, STEPHENS FE, GUNN FD, PERKOFF GT: Studies on disorders of muscle. VII. Clinical manifestations and inheritance of a type of periodic paralysis without hypopotassemia. *J Clin Invest* 30:492, 1951.

VIETS HR: A historical review of myasthenia gravis from 1672 to 1900. *JAMA* 153:1273, 1953.

VINCENT A, NEWSOM-DAVIS J: Acetylcholine receptor antibody as a diagnostic test for myasthenia gravis: Results in 153 validated cases and 2967 diagnostic assays. *J Neurol Neurosurg Psychiatry* 48:1246, 1985.

VINCENT A, NEWSOM-DAVIS J, MARTIN V: Antiacetylcholine

receptor antibodies in D-penicillamine associated myasthenia gravis. *Lancet* 1:1254, 1978.

WALKER MB: Treatment of myasthenia gravis with physostigmine. *Lancet* 1:1200, 1934.

WALTON JN, GESCHWIND N, SIMPSON JA: Benign congenital myopathy with myasthenic features. *J Neurol Neurosurg Psychiatry* 19:224, 1956.

WITTE AS, CORNBLATH DR, PARRY GJ et al: Azathioprine in the treatment of myasthenia gravis. *Ann Neurol* 15:602, 1984.

YAZAKI K, KURIBAYASHI T, YAMAMURA Y et al: Hypokalemic myopathy associated with a 17 α-hydroxylase deficiency: A case report. *Neurology* 32:94, 1982.

ZACKS SI, BAUER WC, BLUMBERG JM: The fine structure of the myasthenic neuromuscular apparatus. *J Neuropathol Exp Neurol* 21:335, 1962.

CHAPTER 54

DISORDERS OF MUSCLE CHARACTERIZED BY CRAMP, SPASM, PAIN, AND LOCALIZED MASSES

Quite apart from spasticity and rigidity, which are due to a disinhibition of spinal motor mechanisms (see pages 45 and 62), there are forms of muscular stiffness and spasm that can be traced to abnormalities of the lower motor neuron or the sarcolemma of the muscle fiber and its intrinsic conducting apparatus. Thus, muscles may go into spasm because of an unstable depolarization of motor axons, which sends volleys of impulses across neuromuscular junctions—as occurs in myokymia, hypocalcemic tetany, pseudohypoparathyroidism, and motor system disease. Or the innervation of muscle may be normal but contraction persists despite attempts at relaxation (myotonia); or, after one or a series of contractions the muscle may be slow in decontracting, as occurs in paradoxical myotonia and hypothyroidism; or, in the contracture of McArdle phosphorylase deficiency and phosphofructokinase deficiency, muscle, once contracted, may lack the energy to relax.

Each of these conditions evokes the complaint of cramp or spasm, which is variably painful and interferes with free and effective voluntary activity. Each condition has its own identifying clinical characteristics, registered also in the EMG, and most of them respond favorably to therapy. Premium attaches, therefore, to the clinical differentiation of these phenomena.

MUSCLE CRAMP

This subject has already been introduced in Chap. 48. There it was mentioned that everyone at some time or other has experienced muscle cramps. Usually they occur during the night, after a day of unusually strenuous activity; less often they occur during the day, either during a period of relaxation or occasionally after a strong voluntary or postural contraction. A random restless or stretching movement will induce a hard contraction of a single muscle (most frequently of the foot or leg) which cannot be voluntarily relaxed. The muscle is visibly and palpably taut and painful, and the

condition is readily distinguished from an illusory cramp, in which the patient experiences only a sensation of cramp but where little or no contraction of muscle occurs, as in intermittent claudication and in certain diseases of peripheral nerve. Massage and vigorous stretch of the cramped muscle will cause the spasm to yield, though for a time the muscle remains excitable and subject to recurrent cramps. Visible fasciculation may precede and follow the cramp, indicating an excessive excitability of the motor neurons supplying the muscle. Sometimes the cramp is so violent that the muscle appears to have been injured. It remains sore to touch and painful upon use for a day or longer. Particularly alarming are cramps of precordial chest muscles or diaphragm. Fear of heart or lung disease may be aroused. In the EMG the cramp is attended by bursts of high-frequency, high-voltage action potentials, and the precramp phase by runs of activity in motor units. Why cramps should be painful is not known; probably the demands of the overactive muscle exceed metabolic supply, causing a relative ischemia and accumulation of metabolites. Overwork of muscle with or without impairment of circulation is also painful. Between cramps the muscles are normal clinically and electromyographically.

Cramps are known to increase in frequency under certain conditions and with certain diseases. They are frequent during pregnancy for reasons not fully understood. Dehydration and sweating favor cramping, and athletes try to prevent this by ingestion of sodium chloride. Exertional cramps are frequent in motor system disease and hypothyroidism and less so in chronic polyneuropathies. Patients undergoing hemodialysis are subject to cramps, which can be suppressed by intravenous hypertonic saline or hypertonic glucose. Rapid rehydration after dehydration is another provocative factor.

The mechanism of muscle cramping is obscure. In a number of cases with exercise-induced stiffness and muscle pain, sometimes progressing to cramp, low levels of myoadenylate deaminase have been found. The significance of this observation is uncertain. This enzyme, which is present in high concentration in muscle, is said to remove cyclic AMP and to protect muscle against rapid fluctuations in ATP and ADP (see Morgan-Hughes for details). Others assert that low levels of this enzyme are not specific, occurring in such unrelated disorders as hypokalemic periodic paralysis and spinal muscular atrophy. Layzer has raised the possibility of some unknown metabolite(s) being released into the perineural spaces of intramuscular motor nerves; this could result in hyperactivity of the nerve and posttetanic repetitive activity.

Quinine sulfate (300 mg at bedtime and repeated in 4 h if necessary), or 300 mg tid for diurnal cramping, is the most useful medication; diphenhydramine hydrochloride (Benadryl) 50 mg or procainamide 0.5 to 1.0 g can be used if quinine cannot be tolerated. Phenytoin and carbamazepine may be helpful in alleviating repeated daytime cramping.

TETANY AND PATHOLOGIC CRAMP

As pointed out on page 1014, a reduction in ionizable calcium and magnesium are associated with involuntary cramplike spasms; in their mildest form they tend to be distal (carpopedal spasm), but they may involve any of the muscles, except the extraocular ones. Stimulation of a muscle through its nerve at certain frequencies (15 to 20 times per second) characteristically reproduces the spasms, and hyperventilation and ischemia increase the tendency. Indeed the Trousseau sign—carpal spasms with occlusion of the blood supply to the arm—takes advantage of the latter phenomenon. That hypocalcemic tetany is attributable to an unstable depolarization of the axonal membrane of the nerve fiber is shown by (1) the sensitivity of nerve to percussion (tapping over the facial nerve near its foramen of exit induces a facial twitch or Chvostek sign), (2) the appearance of fast-frequency doublets and triplets of motor unit potentials in the EMG, (3) evocation of spasm by application of a tourniquet to proximal parts of a limb (causing ischemia of segments of nerve beneath the tourniquet), (4) the regular association of tingling, prickling paresthesias from excitation of sensory nerve fibers. Hypocalcemia also causes a change of lesser importance in the muscle fibers themselves; hence nerve block does not completely eradicate tetany.

A condition resembling tetany, but without measurable hypocalcemia, is the aforementioned *benign cramp syndrome* (*pseudotetany*). In the most severe forms, all skeletal muscles are intermittently locked in spasm, and almost any strong postural or voluntary movement leads to cramp. When this phenomenon is repeated again and again, the overly active muscles begin to hypertrophy. In about half of the authors' cases, stimulation of nerve at 15 or more per second produced cramp discharges, as in tetany.

Muscle biopsies have been normal except for a few ring-binden. Calcium and diazepam were of no value, but some patients responded to phenytoin, quinine, procainamide, or chlorpromazine.

Satoyoshi has described a group of such patients who, in addition to the widespread severe cramping of muscle, also showed universal alopecia, amenorrhea, intestinal malabsorption, and sometimes epiphyseal destruction and retarded growth. The serum Ca in these patients was normal, and the EMG showed only high-frequency discharges. Jusic et al have described a familial (autosomal dominant) form of cramp of distal limb muscles beginning in childhood and persisting throughout life.

It is also to be noted that a tendency to cramp and pain are symptoms in a number of the congenital myopathies described in Chap. 51.

STATES OF PERSISTENT FASCICULATION, CONTINUOUS MUSCLE ACTIVITY, MYOKYMIA, NEUROMYOTONIA, AND "STIFF-MAN" SYNDROME

This is a confusing group of clinical states that are not fully differentiated from one another.

As is well known, a few random fasciculations in the muscles of the calf or elsewhere are to be seen in most normal individuals. They are of no significance but can be a source of worry to physicians and nurses who have heard or read that fasciculations are an early sign of amyotrophic lateral sclerosis. A simple clinical rule is that fasciculations in relaxed muscle are never indicative of motor system disease unless there is an associated weakness, atrophy, or reflex change.

Frequently a normal individual will experience intermittent twitching of a muscle (or even part of a muscle) such as one of the muscles of the thenar eminence or the orbicularis oculi. It may continue for days. Lay persons refer to it as "live flesh." Electromyographically this twitching, like that of the benign fasciculations described above, tends to be more constant in localization and more frequent and rhythmic than the malignant fasciculations of amyotrophic lateral sclerosis, but such distinctions are not entirely reliable.

There are in addition to the aforementioned benign states, three major syndromes of abnormal muscle activity: (1) *a state of almost continuous muscle activity* in association with slight weakness and fatigability that is not suppressed by nerve block but is by curare; (2) *myokymia*, a term that refers to a continuous rippling, more or less tonic contraction of muscles; and (3) *a state of continuous muscle spasm* that is arrested by spinal anesthesia and procaine nerve block. The latter has been called "stiff-man syndrome."

The syndrome of *widespread, continuous fasciculations* may last for months or even years, and is accompanied by slight weakness and fatigability. No reflex changes, sensory loss, nerve conduction, EMG abnormality (other than fasciculations), or increase in serum muscle enzymes are found. Low energy and fatigability may suggest an endogenous depressive illness, yet the fasciculations are indeed prominent. We suspect that this fasciculatory state reflects a disease of the terminal motor nerves, for several of our patients have shown slowing of distal latencies, and Cöers et al have found degeneration and regeneration of motor nerve terminals. Eventual recovery can be expected.

Myokymia, as defined above, may be generalized or limited to one part of the body such as the muscles of the shoulders or of the lower extremities. In some patients cramping is frequently associated, and indeed muscles about to cramp may twitch or show spontaneous rippling contractions; and the cramping may be associated with sweating. Other patients with the same condition never have cramps. Obviously myokymia, fasciculation, and cramping are closely related but not identical conditions. Some of the patients also complain of a slight weakness and inability to perform motor tasks in a normal fashion. We suspect that myokymia also represents a mild distal motor neuropathy for the reasons stated above. CK and aldolase levels are normal. This state is also called *neuromyotonia*, with the implication that a neuropathy has led to a pseudomyotonia. Possibly this represents a phase of nerve regeneration. In several of our cases the response to phenytoin (100 mg tid) has been dramatic. Usually the condition recedes after several years.

The relation of myokymia to states called *continuous muscular activity* and "stiff-man" syndrome is ambiguous. Gamstorp and Wohlfart and later Isaacs described patients whose muscles at some point begin to "work" continuously. Twitching and spasms are evident, as well as generalized muscle stiffness and reduced or abolished reflexes. Slight muscle atrophy is present in some cases. The muscle activity persists throughout sleep. General and spinal anesthesia do not always suppress the muscular activity, but curare does; nerve block may have no effect or may reduce it, as in the case of Lütschg et al. The EMG shows continuous normal motor unit discharges. The reported cases have varied. Some resemble the diffuse fasciculation-weakness syndrome and myokymia described above; others have continuous spasms and cramps that cause the muscles to be hard and

unavailable for voluntary movements. The stiffness and slowness of movement makes walking laborious ("armadillo syndrome"), and in some cases all voluntary movement is blocked.

Neuromyotonia is a condition, observed after lesions of the peripheral nerve, in which stiffness, delayed relaxation, fasciculatory activity, and myokymia interfere with voluntary contraction of muscle. Apparently regenerating motor neurons are hyperexcitable. Muscle hypertrophy may result. Lance et al observed myokymic discharges in the EMG, again unlike myotonic discharges. The condition is not well understood, and it overlaps with the aforementioned continuous muscle activity syndromes.

The condition in which the spasms are continuous, forcing the patient to lie helplessly in bed, the feet in equinus position, the legs extended, conforms to the one originally described by Moersch and Woltman in 1956 as *"stiff-man" syndrome*. Since then more than 100 isolated examples have been reported all over the world. The onset is usually in middle life, and men are affected more often than women. At first there is intermittent and then more or less continuous stiffness and spasms of limb and trunk muscles. Muscles of respiration, swallowing, and of the face may be involved in the more advanced cases, but trismus, a common feature of tetanus, does not occur. Any noise or attempted passive or voluntary movement precipitates severely painful spasms of all the involved musculature. In the case of Meinck et al, a variety of acoustic, vestibular, and somatosensory stimuli evoked muscular spasms; the myotatic reflexes were normal. Clomipramine, which is said to inhibit neuronal uptake of serotonin and norepinephrine, worsened the condition, whereas clonidine reduced the spasms. This suggested an imbalanced action of noradrenergic pathways in the brainstem and spinal cord.

Once started, the spasms continue for many years with little or no abatement. Unlike the syndrome of continuous muscular activity, spinal and general anesthesia usually abolish the spasms. However, this is not invariable, as pointed out by Wettstein. In patients in whom activity persists after nerve block the condition cannot be distinguished from the syndromes of continuous muscle activity and myokymia. The authors favor the view that all of these conditions (benign fasciculations, myokymia, continuous muscle activity, neuromyotonia, and stiff-man syndrome) represent states of neural degeneration and regeneration and, as Valli et al and Cöers et al point out, overlap one another. Distinctions based on the effect of nerve block, curare, and pharmacotherapeutic agents are probably not determinative.

In our experience one cannot predict the most efficacious therapy from the clinical state. While phenytoin in a dose of 100 mg tid or carbamazepine, 200 to 400 mg tid, usually have been beneficial in the benign fasciculation, myokymia, and continuous muscle activity syndromes, we have had patients who did not respond. Quinine sulfate gave better results. Similarly in the stiff-man syndrome, diazepam in doses of 10 to 50 mg/day is said to be most effective, though here also there are instances in which phenytoin is preferable. In general it seems that drugs which have a stabilizing effect on axonal membranes are most likely to reduce muscle activity and improve function.

These syndromes of continuous muscle activity, except perhaps the "stiff-man" syndromes, are readily distinguished clinically and electromyographically from extrapyramidal and corticospinal abnormalities such as dystonia, dyskinesia, rigidity, and spasticity.

CONGENITAL NEONATAL RIGIDITY

In four families of mixed heritage, Dudley et al observed a "stiff-infant" syndrome. The condition came to medical attention because of respiratory distress that was due to a generalized muscular rigidity beginning at about 2 months of age. The rigidity spread slowly from cervical muscles to those of the trunk and limbs, and, as it persisted, slight hypertrophy developed. The use of respiratory aid and a feeding gastrostomy enabled the infants to survive. The rigidity slowly diminished in the second year of life. The clinical course was unlike that of tetanus. In fatal cases there were zones of fiber loss with fibrosis in skeletal and cardiac muscles and a greater than normal variation in fiber size. Cytoplasmic crescents of reducing bodies and altered Z lines were observed in some fibers.

CONTRACTURE AND PSEUDOMYOTONIAS

Phosphorylase deficiency (McArdle) and phosphofructokinase deficiency (Tarui) provide examples of an entirely different type of painful shortening and hardness of muscle. In both these diseases an otherwise normal child, adolescent, or adult begins to complain of weakness and stiffness and sometimes pain on using the limbs. Muscle contraction and relaxation are normal when the patient is in repose, but strenuous activity, especially under conditions of ischemia, causes the muscles to shorten, unable to relax. With mild sustained exercise, the patient experiences progressive fatigue and weakness for several minutes, after which the symptoms diminish and then disappear ("second-wind" phenomenon). During the second wind phase, the patient copes with his symptoms by increasing cardiac output and substituting free fatty acids and blood-borne glucose for muscle glycogen (Braakhekke et al). The primary abnormality in McArdle disease is a defect in myophosphorylase (of autosomal recessive inheritance), which prevents the conversion of glycogen to glucose-6-phosphate. Phosphofructokinase deficiency interferes with the conversion of

glucose-6-phosphate to glucose-1-phosphate; the defect is also present in red blood cells (Layzer et al).

The contracted muscles in these disorders, unlike muscles in cramp and other involuntary spasms, no longer use energy, and they are more or less electrically silent; moreover, they do not produce lactic acid. This condition is spoken of as *pharmacologic contracture*. Ischemia contributes to this condition by denying glucose to the muscle, which cannot function adequately on fatty acids and non-glucose substrates. The diagnosis of either disease is confirmed by the failure of blood lactate to rise in the cubital vein after a 3-min period of ischemic exercise. Histochemical stains of biopsied muscle reveal an absence of phosphorylase activity (in McArdle disease) or of phosphofructokinase activity (in Tarui disease). The only known treatment is a planned reduction in activity. Fructose taken orally is said to be helpful in some cases. Improvement has been reported after the administration of glucagon (Kono et al) and after a high-protein diet (Slonim and Goans).

A kind of pseudomyotonia also accompanies *hypothyroidism*, where the muscle fibers contract and relax slowly. This response is readily demonstrated in eliciting tendon reflexes, particularly the Achilles reflex. The muscles are large and subject to myoedema, and when used may show waves of slow contraction. The basis of this disorder appears to be a slowness in the reaccumulation of calcium ions in the endoplasmic reticulum and in the disengagement of thin actin and thick myosin filaments. The EMG may reveal after-potentials following voluntary contraction; they do not resemble the waning, "dive-bomber" bursts of true myotonia.

TETANUS

In *tetanus*, the skeletal muscles are persistently contracted, owing to the effect of the tetanus toxin on spinal neurons (Renshaw cells) whose natural function is to inhibit the motor neurons (see also page 903). As the condition develops, activities that normally excite the neurons, i.e., voluntary contraction and startle from visual and auditory stimulation, all evoke involuntary spasms. Sleep tends to quiet them, and they are suppressed by spinal anesthesia and curare. The EMG shows the expected interference pattern of action potentials. Once the muscle is involved in persistent contraction, it is said that the shortened state is not abolished by procaine block or severance of nerve (in animals), but this so-called *myostatic contracture* has not been demonstrated in humans.

There is also an action of the toxin at the neuromuscular junction, which has been more difficult to evaluate in the face of its powerful central action. Injected locally in animals, Price et al have demonstrated its localization at motor end plates. It binds with ganglioside in the axon membrane and is transported by retrograde flow to the spinal cord where it induces local tetanus effects. Neurons that innervate slow-twitch type I muscle fibers are more sensitive than neurons that innervate fast-twitch type II fibers. Presynaptic vesicles increase, ACh is blocked, and terminal axon injury may paralyze muscle fibers. Fibrillation potentials and axonal sprouting follow.

BLACK WIDOW SPIDER BITE

The black widow spider (*Latrodectus* species) produces a toxin which, within a few minutes of the bite, leads to cramps and spasms, and then a painful rigidity of abdominal, trunk, and leg muscles. The spasms are followed by weakness. There is also vasoconstriction, hypertension, and autonomic hyperactivity. If death does not occur in 24 to 48 h, recovery is complete.

The spider venom has a presynaptic localization and rapidly releases quanta of ACh. The vesicles are depleted. There is some evidence that the venom prevents endocytosis of the vesicle membrane and by inserting itself into the membrane forms permanent ionic conductance channels (Swift).

Treatment, which is more or less empiric, consists of Ca gluconate infusions. Intravenous magnesium sulfate also helps to reduce the release of ACh and control convulsions that sometimes occur. There is a reconstituted antiserum that is available in regions where such envenomation is frequent.

MALIGNANT HYPERTHERMIA

This condition, described on page 1114, is also characterized by an acute onset of generalized muscular rigidity accompanied by rapid rise in body temperature, metabolic acidosis, and myoglobinuria. It is invariably induced by anesthetic agents and other drugs.

CONGENITAL MYOTONIA
(Thomsen Disease)

This is an uncommon hereditary disease of skeletal muscle that begins in early life and is characterized by myotonia and muscular hypertrophy.

HISTORY

This disease was first brought to the attention of the medical profession in 1876, by Julius Thomsen, a Danish physician who himself suffered from the disease as did 20 other members of his family over four generations. His designation *ataxia muscularis* was not apt, but he left no doubt as to the nature of the condition, which featured ''tonic cramps in voluntary muscles associated with an inherited psychical indisposition.'' The association of the latter condition was not borne out by subsequent studies and is now believed to be fortuitous.

Strümpell in 1881 assigned the name *myotonia congenita* to the disease, and Westphal in 1883 referred to it as *Thomsen's disease*. Erb provided the first description of its pathology and called attention to two additional unique features, muscular hyperexcitability and hypertrophy. In 1923, Thomsen's great-nephew, K. Nissen, extended the original genealogy to 35 cases in seven generations. In 1948, Thomasen updated the subject in a monograph that is still a useful reference.

GENETIC FEATURES

The cause of the disease is genetic. From the careful studies of Becker, two forms are now recognized. In one, the type described by Thomsen, the myotonia is inherited as an autosomal dominant trait. The myotonia usually has its onset early in infancy, sometimes later. In about half the patients in this group, the myotonia is worsened by exposure to cold, but episodes of paralysis do not occur. Hypertrophy of muscles is absent or slight. In the second type the inheritance is autosomal recessive, but males predominate in a ratio of 3:1. Here the myotonia begins later in childhood, and even as late as adult life, and tends to be more severe than in the dominant type. It appears first in the lower extremities and spreads to the trunk, arms, and face. Hypertrophy is invariably present. There may be an associated mild distal weakness and atrophy; this was found in the forearms in 28 percent of Becker's 148 patients, and in the sternomastoids in 19 percent. Dorsiflexion of the feet was limited and fibrous contractures were common. Weakness may also be present in the proximal leg and arm muscles. The most troublesome aspect of the disease is the transient weakness that follows initial muscle contraction after a period of inactivity. Progression of the disease continues to about 30 years of age, and then the course of the illness remains unchanged, according to Sun and Streib. The CK may be elevated. Thus, it would appear that the recessive form of myotonia shares certain features with myotonia dystrophica. However, testicular atrophy, cardiac abnormality, frontal baldness and cataracts are conspicuously absent.

The assertion that all cases of myotonia congenita eventually convert to myotonic dystrophy, long a point of dispute, has not been confirmed by deJong, who found, in a study of 100 cases, that the two diseases can be distinguished at all ages. Personal observations accord with this opinion. It is for this reason that we have not classified myotonia congenita with the dystrophies.

CLINICAL FEATURES

Tonic spasm of muscle after forceful voluntary contraction stands as the cardinal feature of the disease and is most pronounced after a period of inactivity. Repeated contractions "wear it out," so to speak, and later movements in a series become more swift and effective. Rarely the converse is observed—where the first movements of a series are less likely to induce myotonia than are later ones (*myotonia paradoxica*), but usually this is a feature of cold-induced paramyotonia. The spasm is painless, unlike cramp. Close observation reveals a softness of the muscles during rest, and the initial contraction appears not to be significantly slowed unless there is preexistent myotonia.

The congenital nature of the dominant form of the disease may be evident even in the crib, where the infant's eyes are noted to open slowly after crying or sneezing, and the legs are conspicuously stiff as the first steps are attempted. In the recessive form, myotonia may not become evident until adult years, which probably explains some cases of so-called *myotonia acquisita* or *tarda* (other cases are probably examples of myotonic dystrophy or the pseudomyotonia of hypothyroidism).

When severe, the myotonia tends to affect all skeletal muscles, being especially prominent in the lower limbs. Attempts to walk and run are sometimes impeded to the extent that the patient stumbles and falls. Other limb and trunk muscles are also thrown into spasm as are those of the face and upper limbs. Small, gentle movements such as blinking or elicitation of a tendon reflex do not initiate myotonia, whereas strong closure of the eyes, as in a sneeze, sets up a spasm that may prevent complete opening for many seconds. Spasms of extraocular muscles occur in some instances, leading to strabismus. Loosening of one set of muscles after a succession of contractions does not prevent the appearance of myotonia in another set, nor in the same ones if used in another pattern of movement. Smooth and cardiac muscles are never affected.

Myotonia can be induced in most cases by tapping a muscle belly with a percussion hammer. Unlike the lump or ridge produced in hypothyroid or cachectic muscle (myoedema), the myotonic contraction involves an entire fasciculus or a muscle and, unlike the phenomenon of idiomuscular irritability, it persists for several seconds. The tongue, if tapped, shows a similar reaction. The effect of an electrical (faradic) stimulus delivered to the motor point in a muscle also induces a prolonged contraction (Erb's myotonic reaction).

In severe cases of the recessive type, muscular hypertrophy may reach herculean proportions, and such adolescents and young adults may gain occupation as "strong men" in circuses. The hypertrophy affects particularly the muscles of the thighs, forearms, and shoulders. When relaxed, the large muscles have a natural consistency, but if the myotonia is severe and persistent, they feel firm and tense all the time. The power of large muscles may seem to be reduced, but this is related to difficulty in initiating movements, possibly owing to an inability to relax antagonists.

PATHOLOGIC FINDINGS

Biopsy reveals no abnormality other than enlargement of muscle fibers, and this change occurs only in hypertrophied muscles. As often happens in fibers of increased volume, central nucleation is somewhat more frequent than in normal muscle. However, central rowing of nuclei, so prominent in myotonic dystrophy, is not seen, nor are the sarcoplasmic masses and peripheral disorganization of myofibrils that occur in the latter disease. The large fibers contain increased numbers of normally structured myofibrils. Peripheral ring-binden or spiral annulets are visible in some fibers. In well-fixed biopsy material, examined under the electron microscope, Schroeder and Adams were unable to discern any significant morphologic changes. Tubular arrays, believed to be derived from the sarcoplasmic reticulum, have been seen in a few specimens, but this is not a consistent finding. There are no changes in the peripheral or central nervous system.

PATHOGENESIS

In view of the absence of morphologic changes and the prominence of the myotonic phenomenon in individual muscle fibers, one must assume the existence of a physiologic change in the sarcolemma or some other part of the conducting apparatus of the muscle fibers. The EMG shows that the tension in contracting muscle fibers is slow to diminish, due to persistence of very fine electrical potentials. Some of the latter are of the same size as fibrillation potentials, but others are larger (normal motor unit potentials). The small potentials indicate independent, incoordinate activity of single fibers. Their activity continues after the volley of nerve impulses that initiated the contraction has ceased. Denny-Brown and Foley, stimulating single muscle fibers directly, obtained this myotonic afterdischarge only by a volley of stimuli, never by a single stimulus, and the series of myotonic fibrillation potentials progressively diminished in size, as they do in natural myotonia. Percussion elicits myotonia because it, too, provides a brief but relatively intense repetitive excitation. Thus myotonia can be distinguished electrophysiologically from contracture of other types (e.g., that produced by perfusion of muscle with veratrum alkaloids). Myotonia probably has a biochemical basis. Denny-Brown considered it to be a byproduct of the preceding contraction. In addition Denny-Brown and Nevin noted that strong myotonia in one group of muscles may evoke reflex afterspasm in antagonist and synergist muscles, a reaction that depends on the operation of spinal mechanisms.

Reduction in chloride and, to a lesser degree, in potassium conductance has been found in myotonia congenita but not in myotonic dystrophy. In the latter there is an increased permeability to sodium (McComas and Johns). Substances such as the cholesterol-lowering agent diazacholesterol are capable of inducing myotonia in normal muscle (and cataracts as well), presumably by altering the membrane resistance of the fibers and decreasing chloride conductance. This suggests that myotonia depends on some basic alteration of the sarcolemma itself. Quinine, procainamide, and calcium lessen the duration of myotonic bursts; these substances are known also to act on the sarcolemma and endoplasmic reticulum.

DIAGNOSIS

In patients with very large muscles one must consider not only myotonia congenita but also familial hyperdevelopment, hypothyroid polymyopathy, hypertrophic polymyopathy (hypertrophia musculorum vera), and the Bruck-DeLange syndrome (congenital hypertrophy of muscles, mental retardation, and extrapyramidal movement disorder). The demonstration of myotonia by percussion and EMG study usually resolves the problem, although it should be noted that in exceptional cases of Thomsen disease the persistence of contraction may be difficult to demonstrate. In hypothyroidism, the EMG may show bizarre, high-frequency (pseudomyotonic) discharges (page 1020). However, true myotonia does not occur, myoedema is prominent, the contraction and relaxation of tendon reflexes is slowed, and there are other signs of thyroid deficiency.

In patients who complain of spasms, cramping, and stiffness, myotonia must be distinguished from myokymia,

"the syndrome of persistent muscle activity" of Gamstorp and Wolfahrt, the Schwartz-Jampel syndrome (see below), the pathologic cramp syndrome, the "stiff man" syndrome, and the contracture of phosphorylase or phosphofructose kinase deficiency. The distinguishing features of each of these states have been described in the preceding sections of this chapter. In none of them is there myotonia by percussion or by EMG. The only exception is the Schwartz-Jampel syndrome of hereditary stiffness combined with short stature and muscle hypertrophy. This is probably a form of myotonia and should be set apart from myokymia and the syndrome of continuous muscle activity.

Diagnostic uncertainty may arise in those patients who later prove to have myotonic dystrophy when only myotonia is noted in early life. The myotonia in these latter cases is usually mild and in several families that we have followed, some degree of weakness and a typical facies could be perceived even in early childhood. Also in paramyotonia congenita there is myotonia of early onset, but again it tends to be mild, involving mainly the orbicularis oculi, levator palpebrae, and tongue, and the diagnosis is seldom in doubt because of the cold-induced episodes of periodic paralysis.

TREATMENT

Quinine sulfate, 0.3 to 0.6 g, and procainamide, 250 to 500 mg tid, are clearly beneficial in myotonia congenita. Phenytoin, 100 mg tid, has also been useful in some cases. Recently, Streib has reported a diminution in myotonia and a generalized increase in muscle strength in a patient with the recessive form of congenital myotonia, treated with the cardiac antiarrhythmic drug, tocainide (1200 mg daily). It is reported that corticosteroids in moderate doses are capable of reducing myotonia, but the authors have had no experience with this treatment. The adverse effects of prolonged treatment with corticosteroids would probably outweigh their benefits.

SCHWARTZ-JAMPEL SYNDROME

Blepharospasm, dwarfism, pinched face with low-set ears, blepharophimosis, diffuse metaphyseal and epiphyseal bone dysplasia with flattened vertebrae, and a generalized myotonic muscular disorder were crystallized as a syndrome by Schwartz and Jampel in 1962. The syndrome has also been reported under the name of *myotonic chondrodystrophy*. The EMG displays typical myotonic discharges. Fariello et al, who have reviewed the 12 reported instances of this syndrome, do not believe that the reported cases constitute a homogeneous group. The only constant feature is the disturbed muscle function. The stiff muscles disturb gait. Pathologic studies of muscle have yielded inconsistent findings: group atrophy, dilated T system, Z-band streaming, and dilatation of mitochondria. The three latter changes are nonspecific and often artefactual. Treatment with procainamide, phenytoin, diazepam, or barbiturates is ineffective. Presently this should be regarded as the fourth myotonic syndrome, the other three being myotonia congenita (see above), myotonic dystrophy (pages 1123 to 1125), and the paramyotonia of von Eulenberg (page 1163). Aberfeld and his colleagues have described two siblings in whom myotonia was combined with dwarfism, diffuse bone disease, and unusual ocular and facial abnormalities; this appears to be a unique syndrome.

MYALGIC STATES

Many of the muscle diseases described in the preceding pages are associated with aching and discomfort. These are particularly prominent in conditions that are accompanied by cramp and biochemical contracture (phosphorylase and phosphofructokinase deficiency). Ischemia of muscle, viz., intermittent claudication, is also painful. Muscle weakness that imposes abnormal postures on the limbs may cause stretch injury of muscles and tendons. This is observed in a number of the congenital myopathies and dystrophies. In all these conditions clinical study will usually disclose the source(s) of the pain.

Diffuse muscle pain, which merges with malaise, is a frequent expression of a large variety of systemic infections, e.g., influenza, brucellosis, dengue, Colorado tick fever, glanders, measles, malaria, relapsing fever, rheumatic fever (cf. "growing pains"), salmonellosis, toxoplasmosis, trichinosis, tularemia, and Weil disease. When the pain is intense, and especially if it is localized to the lower chest and abdomen, the most likely diagnostic possibility is epidemic myalgia (also designated as pleurodynia, "devil's grip," and Bornholm disease). As indicated on page 1105, one of the group B Coxsackie viruses has been isolated from the striated muscles of patients with pleurodynia, and muscle biopsies of patients with viral influenza have been found to show both necrotizing myositis and virus particles. Poliomyelitis also may be accompanied by intense pain at the onset of neurologic involvement, and later the paralyzed muscles may ache. This is true also of the Guillain-Barré syndrome. Nothing is known about the pathologic basis of the muscular pains in these diseases. Herpes zoster is another well-known cause of segmental pain, and is related to inflammation in spinal nerves and dorsal root ganglia, which may precede the vesicular skin eruption by as long as 72 to 96 h.

Fibromyalgia and *myogelosis* would appear by definition to represent an inflammation of the fibrous tissues of the muscles, fascia, aponeuroses, and probably nerves

as well. Unfortunately, the pathologic changes remain obscure. Only some clinical facts are at hand. A muscle or group of muscles becomes painful and tender after exposure to cold, dampness, or minor trauma, or for no reason that can be discerned. The neck and shoulders are the most common sites. Firm, tender zones, sometimes several centimeters in diameter, can be palpated within the muscles (fibrositic nodules), and active contraction or passive stretching of the involved muscles increases the pain—points of diagnostic value. Usually the condition clears up in a few weeks, and local heat and massage and local injections of anesthetics or steroids, are found to give comfort while symptoms are present. The condition is a "favorite" with physiotherapists and osteopaths, who believe their physical measures and adjustments to be helpful, as they may be. Rarely a similar syndrome is the forerunner of what proves, after some days, with the onset of neurologic signs, to be a radiculitis, brachial neuritis, or an outbreak of herpes zoster.

Diffuse muscular soreness and aching may at times be the initial symptoms in rheumatoid arthritis, preceding the signs of joint involvement by a period of weeks or months. This may also be indicative of polymyalgia rheumatica, an acute illness in which every movement is stiff and painful. The muscles are tender, but since this may be found in otherwise normal individuals, particularly women, it is difficult to interpret. A 48-h trial of prednisone, by alleviating muscle pain, confirms the diagnosis of polymyalgia rheumatica.

Often the patient observes that aching pain occurs not at the time of activity but some hours or even a day or two later, resembling the discomfort following the excessive use of unconditioned muscles. However, a program of conditioning exercises does not alleviate the pain. An increased sedimentation rate, a positive latex-fixation test, or other laboratory aids may clarify the diagnosis. Muscle biopsy may reveal a nonspecific interstitial nodular myositis, or, in polymyalgia rheumatica, a vasculitis. These same symptoms most often occur without explanation, and one can only suspect an obscure infection or a subtle aberration of muscle metabolism, presently impossible to demonstrate. Reference was made above to the finding of a myoadenylate deaminase deficiency in some of these cases. The rapid rise of CK after strenuous exercise will sometimes provide a clue. Idiopathic leg pain during rest after activity occurs in some families and enforces a sedentary existence. The condition does not respond to analgesics. In two cases a deficiency of Ca-ATPase was found and reportedly alleviated by a calcium channel blocker (Walton). It must be distinguished from Fabry disease (page 809) and from the syndromes of painful legs and moving toes, and the restless legs of Ekbom (page 308).

Occasionally a localized weakness of muscle, a slightly reduced tendon reflex, or a zone of impaired cutaneous sensation within the territory of a nerve will indicate the existence of a disease of the peripheral nervous system—an interstitial mononeuritis or mononeuritis multiplex (see page 1045)—which can sometimes be confirmed by the finding of infiltrates of lymphocytes, mononuclear leukocytes, and plasma cells in a nerve or muscle biopsy.

In thin, asthenic adults who exhibit this rather vague symptomatology without other abnormalities, the authors have found it difficult to exclude hysteria or other neurosis and depression. However, before considering a psychiatric diagnosis, it is important in every such individual to search for evidence of a rheumatic state, brucellosis, as well as the myopathy which may accompany hypothyroidism, hyperparathyroidism and renal tubular acidosis, hypophosphatemia, hypoglycemia, the intrinsic phosphorylase or phosphofructokinase defect, and one of the paroxysmal myoglobinurias. Patients with these latter diseases often complain of soreness, stiffness, and lameness after strenuous muscular effort. Many of the patients with diffuse myalgic states referred to the authors with a questionable diagnosis of polymyositis have turned out to be suffering from an overlooked endogenous depression. Others probably have an obscure metabolic myopathy, presently undiagnosable.

LOCALIZED MUSCLE MASSES

Masses may be found in one or many muscles in a variety of clinical settings, and the clinical findings in each one have a different significance.

Muscle rupture is usually caused by a violent strain attended by an audible snap and then a bulge which appears when the muscle contracts. A weakening in contractile power and mild discomfort are usually noted by the patient. The biceps muscle is the one most often affected. Treatment is immediate surgical repair; if delayed, little can be done for the condition.

Hemorrhage into muscle may occur as a consequence of trauma, as a complication of the use of anticoagulants, in hematologic diseases, or after a minor trauma in a patient with Zenker degeneration who is convalescing from typhoid fever or some other infection.

Tumors include *desmoid tumor* (a benign massive growth of fibrous tissue in parturient women and after

surgery), *rhabdomyosarcoma* (a highly malignant tumor with strong liability to local recurrence and metastasis), and *angioma*. *Pseudotumorous* growths, sometimes massive, may follow injury of a muscle. Interlacing muscle fibers and fibroblasts compose the mass. Excision of the entire muscle has been undertaken in several cases in the belief that it was a rhabdomyosarcoma; the growth is a benign reaction.

Thrombosis of arteries or, more often, of *veins* causes congestion and infarction of muscle. A special type of *muscle infarction* occasionally involves the anterior thigh in patients with diabetes mellitus (Banker and Chester). The major symptoms are the sudden onset of pain and swelling of the thigh, with the formation of a tender, palpable mass. Recurrent infarction of the same or opposite thigh is characteristic. The stereotypical clinical picture obviates the need for diagnostic muscle biopsy. The extensive infarction of muscle is due to the occlusion of many medium-sized muscular arteries and arterioles, most likely the result of embolization of atheromatous material from eroded plaques in the aorta or iliac arteries. Recognition of this complication and immobilization of the limb are of prime practical importance, since muscle biopsy and early ambulation may cause serious hemorrhage into the infarcted tissue.

The *pretibial syndrome* is another well-recognized entity. After excessive activity (marching, exercising of unconditioned muscles) there is swelling of the extensor hallucis longus, extensor digitorum longus, and anterior tibial muscles. Being tightly enclosed by the bones and pretibial fascia, the swelling leads to ischemic necrosis and myoglobinuria. Permanent weakness of this group of muscles can be prevented by incising the pretibial fascia.

MYOSITIS OSSIFICANS

This refers to the deposit of bone within the substance of a muscle. Two types are recognized. One is a localized form which appears in a single muscle or group of muscles after trauma, and the other is a progressive, widespread ossifying process in many muscles of the body, entirely unrelated to trauma.

Localized (Traumatic) Myositis Ossificans After a muscle tear or a single blow to the muscle, or after repeated minor trauma, a painful area develops in the muscle. It is gradually replaced by a mass of cartilaginous consistency, and within 4 to 7 weeks' time, a solid mass of bone can be felt and seen in roentgenograms. As would be expected, this most frequently happens in vigorous adult men, and the thigh muscles (in those who ride horses) and to a lesser extent the pectoralis major and biceps brachii are the usual sites of the abnormality. The mass tends to subside after several months if the patient desists from the activity that produced the trauma.

Generalized Myositis Ossificans

This disease, also referred to as *myositis ossificans progressiva,* is rare, although Lutwak, in 1964, was able to collect 264 cases from the literature. The cause is unknown, but it is probably inherited as an autosomal dominant trait. It consists of widespread bone deposition along the fascial planes of muscles, and has its onset in infancy and childhood in 90 percent of cases.

Pathology The first stage is believed to be an interstitial myositis or fibrositis. Biopsies of early indurated swellings have revealed extensive proliferation of interstitial connective tissue in which little inflammatory cell reaction is found. Within a few weeks the connective tissue becomes less cellular and retracts, compressing the adjacent muscle fibers. Osteoid and cartilage formation occur at a later stage, developing in the connective tissue and enclosing relatively intact muscle fibers.

Clinical manifestations Nearly 75 percent of all reported cases have had congenital anomalies, the most frequent of which is a failure of development of the great toes or thumbs and less often other digits. Less frequently, there is hypogenitalism, deafness, and an absence of upper incisors. The first symptom is often a firm swelling and tenderness in a paravertebral or cervical muscle. There is, in addition, a mild discomfort during muscle contraction, and the overlying skin may be reddened and slightly swollen. A trauma may be recalled as the initiating factor, but as the months pass, other muscles not injured in any recognizable way become similarly involved. At first radiographs reveal no important changes, but within 6 to 12 months calcium deposits are observed and one can feel stony-hard masses within the muscles. As the disease advances, limitation of movement and deformities become increasingly evident. Calcified bridges between adjacent muscles and across joints lead to scoliosis; rigidity of spine, jaw, and limbs; and limited expansion of the thorax. Ultimately, the patient is virtually converted into "stone."

Diagnosis The principal problem in diagnosis is to differentiate this condition from *calcinosis universalis,* which usually occurs in relationship to scleroderma or polymyositis. In calcinosis universalis there is said to be calcinosis (calcium deposits) in the skin, subcutaneous tissues, and connective tissue sheaths around the muscles, whereas in myositis ossificans there is actual bone formation within the muscles. The pathologic data are too meager to justify this sharp distinction. The prolonged ingestion of large doses of vitamin D may also produce widespread deposition of masses of calcium around muscles, joints, and subcutaneous tissue. Calcific deposits, perhaps true ossification, may occur in the soft tissues around the hips and knees of paraplegics, and rarely following a hemiplegia ("paralytic myositis ossificans").

Prognosis The disease may undergo spontaneous remissions and may halt for many years at a stage where the patient is capable of adequate function. In other cases, progression leads to marked debilitation and respiratory embarrassment, the final illness often being a terminal pneumonia or other infection.

Treatment The administration of diphosphonate (10 to 20 mg/kg orally), a compound that inhibits the deposition of calcium phosphate, has been said to cause regression of new swellings and to prevent calcification (Russell et al). Some of the calcium deposits in calcinosis universalis have receded in response to prednisone, and because of the unclear relationship of this disease to generalized myositis ossificans, it is probably advisable to try this form of therapy as well. Excision of bony deposits may be undertaken if it is certain that they are the cause of particular disabilities.

REFERENCES

ABERFELD DC, HINTERBUCHNER LP, SCHNEIDER M: Myotonia, dwarfism, diffuse bone disease, and unusual ocular and facial abnormalities (a new syndrome). *Brain* 88:313, 1965.

ADAMS RD, KAKULAS BA: *Diseases of Muscle: Pathological Foundations of Clincial Myology,* 4th ed. Philadelphia, Harper & Row, 1985.

BANKER BQ, CHESTER CS: Infarction of thigh muscle in the diabetic patient. *Neurology* 23:667, 1973.

BECKER PE: Genetic approaches to the nosology of muscle disease: Myotonias and similar diseases, pt 7: Muscle, in Bergsma D (ed): *The Clinical Delineation of Birth Defects.* Baltimore, Williams & Wilkins, 1971.

BRAAKHEKKE JP, DE BRUIN MI, STEGEMAN DF et al: The second wind phenomenon in McArdle's disease. *Brain* 109:1087, 1986.

CÖERS, TELERMAN TN, DURDA J: Neurogenic benign fasciculations, pseudomyotonia, and pseudotetany. *Arch Neurol* 38:282, 1981.

CONNER JM, EVANS DA: Genetic aspects of fibrodysplasia ossificans progressiva. *J Med Genet* 19:35, 1982.

DEJONG JG: *Dystrophia Myotonica, Paramyotonica, and Myotonia Congenita.* Assen, Netherlands, Van Gorcum, 1955.

DENNY-BROWN D, FOLEY JM: Evidence of a chemical mediator in myotonia. *Trans Assoc Am Physicians* 62:187, 1949.

DENNY-BROWN D, NEVIN S: The phenomenon of myotonia. *Brain* 64:1, 1941.

DUDLEY MA, DUDLEY AW, BERNSTEIN LH et al: Biochemical aspects of a new familial myopathy. *J Neuropathol Exp Neurol* 37:609, 1979.

ERB W: *Die Thomsensche Krankheit (Myotonia Congenita)*. Leipsig, Vogen, 1886.

FARIELLO R, MELOFF K, MURPHY EG et al: A case of Schwartz-Jampel syndrome with unusual muscle biopsy findings. *Ann Neurol* 3:93, 1978.

GAMSTORP I, WOHLFART G: A syndrome characterized by myokymia, myotonia, muscular wasting and increased perspiration. *Acta Psychiatr Neurol Scand* 34:181, 1959.

HARPER PS: *Myotonic Dystrophy*. Philadelphia, Saunders, 1979.

ISAACS H: Continuous muscle fibre activity in an Indian male with additional evidence of terminal motor fibre abnormality. *J Neurol Neurosurg Psychiatry* 30:126, 1967.

JUSIC A, DOGAN S, STOJANOVIC V: Hereditary persistent distal cramps. *J Neurol Neurosurg Psychiatry* 35:379, 1972.

KONO N, MINEO I, SIMSUMI S et al: Metabolic basis of improved exercise tolerance: Muscle phosphorylase deficiency after glucagon administration. *Neurology* 34:1471, 1984.

LANCE JW, BURKE D, POLLARD J: Hyperexcitability of motor and sensory neurons in neuromyotonia. *Ann Neurol* 5:523, 1979.

LAYZER RB: Motor unit hyperactivity states, in Vinken PJ, Bruyn GW (eds): *Handbook of Clinical Neurology*, vol 41: *Diseases of Muscle II*. Amsterdam, North-Holland, 1979, chap 10, pp 295–316.

LAYZER RB, ROWLAND LP: Cramps. *N Engl J Med* 285:31, 1971.

LAYZER RB, ROWLAND LP, RANNEY HM: Muscle phosphofructokinase deficiency. *Arch Neurol* 17:512, 1967.

LÜTSCHG J, JERUSALEM F, LUDIN HP et al: The syndrome of "continuous muscle fiber activity." *Arch Neurol* 35:198, 1978.

LUTWAK L: Myositis ossificans progressiva: Mineral, metabolic and radioactive calcium studies of the effects of hormones. *Am J Med* 37:269, 1964.

McCOMAS AJ, JOHNS RJ: Potential changes in the normal and diseased muscle cell, in Walton JN (ed): *Disorders of Voluntary Muscle*, 4th ed. Edinburgh, Churchill Livingstone, 1981, pp 1008–1029.

MEINCK H-M, RICKER K, CONRAD B: The stiff-man syndrome: New pathophysiological aspects from abnormal exteroceptive reflexes and the response to clompramine, clonidine, and tizandine. *J Neurol Neurosurg Psychiatry* 47:280, 1984.

MOERSCH FP, WOLTMAN HW: Progressive fluctuating muscular rigidity ("stiff-man syndrome"): Report of a case and some observations in 13 other cases. *Mayo Clin Proc* 31:421, 1956.

MORGAN-HUGHES JA: Defects of the energy pathways of skeletal muscle, in Mathews WB, Glaser GH (eds): *Recent Advances in Clinical Neurology*. Edinburgh, Churchill Livingstone, 1982, pp 1–46.

NISSEN K: Beiträge zur Kenntnis der Thomsen'schen Krankheit (Myotonia congenita), mit besonderer Berücksichtigung des hereditären Momentes und seinen Beziehungen zu den Mendelschen Vererbungsregeln. *Z Klin Med* 97:58, 1923.

PRICE DL, GRIFFIN JW, PECK K: Tetanus toxin: Evidence for binding at presynaptic nerve endings. *Brain Res* 121:379, 1977.

RUSSELL RGG, SMITH R, BISHOP MC et al: Treatment of myositis ossificans progressiva with a diphosphonate. *Lancet* 1:10, 1972.

SATOYOSHI E: A syndrome of progressive muscle spasm, alopecia and diarrhea. *Neurology* 28:458, 1978.

SCHROEDER JM, ADAMS RD: The ultrastructural morphology of the muscle fiber in myotonic dystrophy. *Acta Neuropathol* 10:218, 1968.

SCHWARTZ O, JAMPEL R: Congenital blepharophimosis associated with a unique generalized myopathy. *Arch Ophthal* 68:52, 1962.

SLONIM AE, GOANS PJ: Myopathy in McArdle's syndrome. Improvement with a high protein diet. *N Engl J Med* 312:355, 1985.

STREIB EW: Successful treatment with tocainide of recessive generalized congenital myotonia. *Ann Neurol* 19:501, 1986.

SUN SF, STREIB EW: Autosomal recessive generalized myotonia. *Muscle Nerve* 6:143, 1983.

SWIFT TR: Disorders of neuromuscular transmission other than myasthenia gravis. *Muscle Nerve* 4:334, 1981.

THOMASEN E: *Myotonia, Thomsen's Disease, Paramyotonia, Dystrophia Myotonica*. Aarhus, Denmark, Universitetsforlaget i Aarhus, 1948.

THOMSEN J: Tonische Krämpfe in willkürlich beweglichen Muskeln in Folge von ererbter psychischer Disposition (ataxia muscularis?). *Arch Psychiatr Nervenkr* 6:706, 1876.

VALLI G, BARBIERI S, STEFANO C et al: Syndromes of abnormal muscular activity: Overlap between continuous muscle fiber activity and the stiff-man syndrome. *J Neurol Neurosurg Psychiatry* 46:241, 1983.

WALTON J: Diffuse exercise-induced pain of undetermined cause relieved by verapamil. *Lancet* 1:993, 1981.

WETTSTEIN A: The origin of fasciculations in motor neuron disease. *Ann Neurol* 5:295, 1979.

To understand mental disorders one must know something of how the brain functions, know something of human psychology, and at the same time be sensitive and responsive to other human beings and have a sincere desire to help them. The first two of these require special study; the third is more an innate quality, found in all good physicians.

Mental disorders pose a number of special problems not met in other fields of medicine. In the first place there are such wide variations in personality, character, and behavior that the point where normal ends and abnormal begins is often difficult to ascertain. Secondly, the methods of study of mental illness are quite subjective, depending mainly on the physician's almost intuitive perceptions of the "vital secrets" and occult purposes of the patient and on the powers of description and narration of the patient in revealing his or her symptoms; these latter capacities vary with intelligence, education, and status of cerebral function. Thirdly, the clinical entities to be presented in the following pages are wholly unverifiable; neither by laboratory test nor postmortem examination can one corroborate the clinical impression.

There is another, more abstruse and essentially theoretic problem of which one must be aware in attempting to study mental disorder. Physicians find that there are two different and seemingly antithetical approaches to disordered nervous function—one proceeding along strictly medical or neurologic lines, the other psychologic. They must learn to utilize two types of data, one drawn from their observations of the patient's behavior, the other from the introspections of the patient. It must be emphasized that the terms *neurologic* and *psychologic* in this context do not necessarily refer to the activities of neurologists and psychiatrists. They are merely convenient terms for two distinct modes of approach to mental disorders; both may be and frequently are used by the neurologist and the psychiatrist, as will be made clear.

The neurologic approach begins with the premise that all clinical manifestations of a nervous disorder are expressions of a pathologic process (disease) within the nervous system. This process may be obvious (such as a tumor or cerebral infarct), or may be impossible to detect with the light or even the electron microscope (such as the encephalopathy of delirium tremens). In all instances the pathologic process is traceable to some genetic, chemical, or physical factor acting on the brain and the visible lesion represents only the most advanced and irreversible stage of a dynamic morbid process. The particular clinical effect, qua symptom or sign, whether it be paralysis, sensory loss, visual or auditory perceptual failure, ataxia, aphasia, tremor, confusion, coma, convulsion, or hallucination, depends on the nature of the lesion and its locus within the nervous system. The clinical manifestations, therefore, are interpretable in terms of neurophysiology, neuroanatomy, and neuropsychology.

The symptoms and signs of the disease, i.e., the expressions of the pathologically altered nervous system, take two forms, either of overactivity or excitation (positive effects) or of loss of function (negative effects)—or first one, then the other. An example of an excitatory lesion would be a convulsive seizure. A destructive lesion abolishes the function of a certain part of the nervous system (negative effects), but at the same time there may be a disinhibition of intact parts, resulting in their overactivity. As pointed out in Chaps. 3 and 4, grasp and suck reflexes are explained in this way. In the delirious patient, as in the paralyzed one, one may speculate that something has been lost in the course of disease and something new in behavior has emerged, presumably because of the uninhibited activity of the undamaged parts of the nervous system. In many cerebral disorders, however, such distinctions between negative and positive effects cannot be made with certainty; in relation to processes such as perceiving, thinking, remembering, symbolization, etc., we lack the knowledge that would enable us to reduce them to this basic formulation.

This brings us face to face with other problems posed by the more complex diseases of the brain. Quite apart from differences in symptoms related to anatomic localization and nature of the pathologic process, the status of the nervous system at the time of onset of the disease makes a difference. Level of intelligence, degree of education, facility with language(s), peculiarities of personality and character, and stability of emotional control may all be reflected in the patient's symptoms. Thus in a syndrome like dementia or a partial aphasia, while the deficit symptoms may be much the same from patient to patient, the unbalanced behavior may differ widely even with the same disease in the same parts of the cerebrum. Only with some knowledge of the patient's natural endowment, education, premorbid personality, etc., can such differences be understood.

In assessing the symptoms of cerebral diseases the examiner must depend on two separate types of information—one subjective, the other objective. Subjective information is provided by the patients' awareness of their own deficits and their capacity to report and describe them; objective information is provided by behavioral changes that can be recognized by others. For example, information about hallucinations comes mainly from the patient's description of his or her abnormal sensory experience, and the objective side may not be evident or certain. In cerebral diseases causing complex disorders of perception, speech, and thinking, there is usually an impairment of both introspective ability (lack of insight) and a change in behavior. This dual loss provides the most certain proof that activities of the mind and behavior depend on the same physiologic processes in the brain. It leads inevitably to a psychophysical monism, the position on the mind-body problem most acceptable to thoughtful neurologists. One of the ideas most difficult to grasp and appreciate, though it follows clearly from the neurologic concept of disordered nervous function, is that there is no essential difference between diseases called *physical* or *organic* and others called *functional*. Every disorder of function must have a structural basis.

The methodology of neurologic analysis, already described in Chap. 1, is merely a series of techniques for eliciting in a systematic fashion the altered activities of the nervous system. The standard procedures of history taking and physical examination require supplementation by tests of the biochemical, physiologic, and psychologic type. Pathologic examination provides the final confirmation of diagnosis. The goals of the neurologic methodology and of neuropathology (the scientific study of nervous system disease) are to determine if a disease exists in the patient and, if so, to ascertain its cause and mechanism and the possibilities of prevention and therapy. A complete concept of a disease must incorporate all its essential elements—genetic, biochemical, physiologic, psychologic as well as pathologic.

A second mode of approach to disordered function of the nervous system, which one may term the psychologic approach, makes many of the same assumptions as the neurologic one. For example it assumes that in many patients the psychologic disorder is an expression of structural changes in the brain at the molecular, chemical, or tissue level. Again, the latter may be determined by a genetic abnormality, a developmental defect, or an acquired lesion of many types. The main premise, however, is that there is an additional category of disordered function, which, within broad limits, is understandable solely in terms of a reaction to previous or present life experiences. Certain abnormalities of personality, emotional immaturity, and inability to adjust to the challenges and opportunities of everyday life are thought to stem from an inadequate development of personality or hurtful experiences in early life, or both. Some of these experiences are remembered (i.e., "conscious"), others are said to be suppressed or forgotten (i.e., "subconscious or unconscious") and recalled only with difficulty or through the free association method of psychoanalysis. In either case the principal approach is to construct a type of psychologic autobiography of the individual and to search it for the roots of the present difficulty. Particular emphasis is placed on three lines of data, traced from early life: key events in the patient's life, their temporal association with medical illnesses, and their conjunction with psychiatric symptoms. The purpose of this approach is not only to determine causality, viz., psychogenesis, but to understand the patient's current behavior in the light of past experiences and to use this understanding to effect change. By frank discussion the physician endeavors to demonstrate the relationship of the patient's symptoms to abnormal behavior patterns and reactions, and by a kind of re-education, i.e., psychotherapy, to assist in bringing about an understanding of the problems and improved ways of coping with them.

Psychiatrists have formulated a number of psychologic mechanisms whereby symptoms are produced, and they speak of them in a language rather unfamiliar to most physicians—e.g., conflict, repression, projection, displacement of affect, conditioning, and arrest or fixation of libido. Some of the more narrowly trained psychoanalysts believe that all theories of mental disorder must be cast in psychologic terms and that anatomic, biochemical, and pathologic considerations have no place in such a formulation. Needless to say, most contemporary psychiatrists do not accept this restrictive psychologic concept of nervous disorders.

A HOLISTIC AND ECLECTIC POSITION

It seems to the authors that both the neurologic and the psychologic concepts and approach have their place in medicine. But the two methods operate at different levels and are of principal use in different types of nervous aberrations.

In the *diagnosis* of a disease of the nervous system one begins always with a careful recording of the symptoms and signs and their temporal aspects, obtained through a detailed history and physical and ancillary examinations. The interpretation of such data leads to diagnosis. Here the psychologic method is of little value, and the neurologic method stands as the only valid system of analysis. It permits one to approach the problem of nervous system disease as one does any other medical problem.

It must be acknowledged that special difficulties attend the diagnosis of psychiatric diseases. These illnesses are expressed mainly by symptoms—complaints about distressing thoughts or feelings or behavior disturbing to others. Seldom are there signs. Often patients are not consistent in what they say and their behavior may change with time. Symptoms are always more liable to varied interpretation than are signs. Nevertheless the physician must rely on the methodology of medicine, with due allowance for these added difficulties.

In *theorizing* about disease and investigating its causes, this broad neurologic or medical approach is essential, for it accepts data from all the medical sciences and is able to incorporate all biologic as well as psychologic facts. Here the psychologic method has limited application, and although yielding useful data concerning the evolution of particular symptoms and their form and content, will never provide a complete explanation of disease.

However, in the *diagnosis* and *management of disorders of character and social maladjustments,* which constitute such a large and important part of psychiatry, the psychologic approach takes precedence. Worry over loss of a job or the illness of a child, the death of a loved one, or domestic difficulty, with all their potential physiologic disturbances, would be acceptable to every thoughtful person as derangements consequent upon the social problem. Indeed, only when such worries and stresses are beyond the patient's control or the connection between the social problem and its physical effects is not perceived do they become medical problems. These are suitably looked upon as reactions to life's difficulties and dealt with entirely at a psychologic level. In the *management of all diseases,* knowledge of the patient's personality and general

reactions is quite indispensable. This is a province of medicine where the psychologic approach is of practical value, and the physician who knows the patient and how to deal with him or her as a troubled individual functions with great effectiveness.

This brings us to one of the crucial problems in neurology and psychiatry—that of defining a disease of the nervous system and in distinguishing it from a social or psychologic maladjustment. Failure to do this has resulted in much confusion as to the legitimate spheres of medical activity and has been an obstacle to research. The authors define a disease of the nervous system as *any condition in which there is a visible lesion in the nervous system or in which there is reasonable evidence of its existence on the basis of stereotypy of clinical expression and of genetic and collateral laboratory data.* Goodwin and Guze offer a slightly different definition of disease, one that is acceptable to many critical psychiatrists. For them *a disease is any cluster of symptoms and signs that occur with such consistency as to permit the prediction of their outcome. An abnormal psychologic reaction is defined as a disorder of psychic function and behavior caused by a maladjustment in social relations not based directly on a known disease process or lesion.*

Simple as this division might seem, it is not easily applied to every abnormal nervous state. How does one interpret disturbances of impulse control, hyperactivity, inability to learn at the accustomed pace, failure to read or master arithmetic at the usual age, criminality, and inadequacy in adjustment to school, work, marriage, and society? Some of these disturbances, as pointed out in Chap. 28, are surely due to *specific retardations in development;* others may be due to lack of proper training and education, unstable home environment, etc. Obviously in such a complex situation it may at times be impossible to separate cause and effect. An individual whose nervous system is affected by disease and who is unable to learn or to form stable social relationships may create an abnormal environment. Or a serious environmental stress may decompensate a patient with underlying nervous system disease.

Also, certain mental abnormalities have an uncertain status vis-à-vis this division and are currently subject to double interpretations, depending on one's premises. A persistent anxiety state without obvious cause in a previously healthy adult would be viewed by some psychiatrists as a reaction of fear to some unconscious threat. Others would consider it a genetic disease closely allied to endogenous depression, in which some biochemical disturbance, as mysterious as was hyperthyroidism a century ago, has developed de novo. Since the nature of the condition is unsettled, it is understandably treated by physicians using both psychologic methods and drugs. Anyone who proposes to investigate it, we would argue, should do so with a completely open mind and be prepared to review critically any reasonable hypothesis as to its cause.

There is also disagreement about the major psychiatric disorders—depression, mania, paranoia, and schizophrenia. Most psychiatrists and all neurologists regard them as genetically determined diseases of the nervous system, the mechanism, anatomy, and biochemistry of which are still obscure. Environmental stress at times seems important in their evocation and exacerbation, but is obviously not an essential or sufficient factor. Only a few psychiatrists insist, still, that such states represent deviate ways of living or abnormal psychologic reactions. It seems reasonable to assume that the more comprehensive methodology of the neurologic and medical sciences will eventually lead to their solution.

PSYCHOSOMATIC MEDICINE

In the recent past there has been great interest in a large category of disease called *psychosomatic*. Included here were peptic ulcer, mucous and ulcerative colitis, hay fever, bronchial asthma, urticaria, angioneurotic edema, essential hypertension, hyperthyroidism, rheumatoid arthritis, amenorrhea, and migraine—diseases in which a stressful life situation or emotional upset appeared to be associated with their development, exacerbation, or prolongation. Three lines of evidence were adduced, purportedly setting these diseases apart from others: (1) a series of observations, showing that the function of the offending organ had been excited and possibly deranged by strong emotions; (2) analyses of the biographies and personalities of patients with these diseases, which allegedly disclosed an inordinately high incidence of resentment, hostility, dependence, aggressiveness, suppressed emotionality, inability to communicate matters of emotional concern or to differentiate reality and subjective falsification—attributes that are difficult or impossible to define and quantitate; (3) longitudinal histories drawn from the memories of the patients, which were said to reveal a relationship between personal crises and outbreaks (relapses) of the chronic disease. Medical therapy was ineffective or failed, it was argued, when these psychologic phenomena were disregarded.

More than 50 years have passed since these ideas were first proclaimed, and an enormous literature followed, with the establishment of pathetically few unassailable facts. It became clear that these "psychosomatic" diseases are not neuroses in that (1) they have different symptoms and (2) the psychosomatic diseases have in most instances a known and easily demonstrable pathologic basis. No complete proof of psychic causation of the psychosomatic diseases has been adduced. Treatment has been concerned mainly with the relief of symptoms and has been directed for the most part by nonpsychiatric specialists. There is no evidence that the therapeutic results obtained by psychiatrists are better than those of a competent internist.

With the growth of the field of psychosomatic medicine, there was, on the part of many physicians, an overemphasis of the psychologic aspects of disease, out of all proportion to the somatic. As pointed out by Wolff in his scholarly exposition of the "mind-body" relationship, the fallacy of "psychogenic" or "psychosomatic" concepts is that they imply a mind acting in opposition to the body. Nevertheless, interest in the psychosomatic diseases contributed to the growing awareness of the diseased patient and not merely of the disease in isolation. First suggested by Claude Bernard and ably espoused and elaborated by Walter Cannon and Adolph Meyer is the view that the patient must always be regarded as a complex psychobiologic unit functioning in relationship to the immediate physical and social environment. Disease represents a faulty or inadequate adaptation of the organism to the environment. Sometimes the maladaptation can be traced to a single agent in the environment, such as an abnormal gene or the tubercle bacillus, without which the disease could not develop. Seldom, however, even in such a straightforward disease as tuberculosis, or, to take another example, the encephalopathy caused by phenylketonuria, can the problem be reduced to a single physical or psychic factor. Hence a rigid, narrowly physical or psychologic approach always proves to be inadequate and must be supplanted by a broader psychobiologic one, which attempts to weigh each of many factors in the equation of disease. At present this is difficult, especially with the so-called psychosomatic diseases, since not all the factors are known. Until such time as new facts are obtained, the physician must cope with a large population of patients, with inadequate methods of diagnosis and treatment. Fortunately most of these patients suffer from relatively minor ailments that time and reassurance alleviate.

The reader seeking further information as to the status of psychosomatic or "psychophysiologic" disorders, as they are called in the DSM III, is referred to the review by Sheehan and Hackett.

PLAN OF PSYCHIATRY SECTION

In the chapters that follow there will be a consideration of the neuroses, the affective disorders, the sociopathies, and the schizophrenias and paranoid states. The magnitude of these disorders and their clinical and social importance can hardly be overestimated. Some 10 to 15 percent of all individuals will at some period of their lives experience psychiatric symptoms and seek medical help for them. The headings that guide our exposition of neuropsychiatric illnesses might be questioned, but justification for their selection is that each can be diagnosed by a competent physician and each diagnosis, once made, has been validated by follow-up studies. If a given case does not lend itself to classification under this scheme, it is better left undiagnosed. All physicians should know something about these categories of psychiatric disease. Neurologists in particular need to be familiar with them, if only for the purpose of differentiating them from other neurologic diseases and initiating intelligent management.

Emphasis throughout these chapters will be on the biologic characteristics and the diagnosis of each state. This is in keeping with a significant trend in psychiatry, stimulated by the development of rigorous diagnostic criteria (the Feighner Research Diagnostic Criteria; see also writings of Rakoff et al, Goodwin and Guze, and McHugh). The prevention of suicide, the choice of appropriate therapy, communication with the patient's family and physician, predictions about the course of the illness (prognosis)—all begin with accurate diagnosis. Finally, strict diagnostic criteria are important in psychiatric research.

In adhering to the bias of neurologic medicine we do not wish to depreciate the importance of psychologic medicine. Our position on this matter has been fully stated in the preceding pages and needs no further elaboration. Theoretic aspects of personality and psychopathology and psychoanalytic concepts of symptom formation will be given little space, largely because the authors find themselves relatively unfamiliar with and unable to evaluate many of the tenets of these aspects of psychiatry. The reader will find them well presented in the references at the end of each chapter.

REFERENCES

Cobb S: *Emotions and Clinical Medicine.* New York, Norton, 1950.

Diagnostic and Statistical Manual of Mental Disorders (DSM III), 3rd ed. Washington, American Psychiatric Association, 1980.

Feighner JP, Robins E, Guze SB et al: Diagnostic criteria for use in psychiatric research. *Arch Gen Psychiatry* 26:57, 1972.

Goodwin DW, Guze SB: *Psychiatric Diagnosis,* 3rd ed. New York, Oxford University Press, 1984.

McHugh PR: William Osler and the new psychiatry. *Ann Intern Med* 107:914, 1987.

Rakoff V, Stancer HC, Kedward HB (eds): *Psychiatric Diagnosis.* New York, Brunner-Mazel, 1977.

Sheehan DV, Hackett TP: Psychosomatic disorders, in AM Nicholi (ed): *Harvard Guide to Modern Psychiatry.* Cambridge, MA, Harvard University Press, 1978, chap. 16, pp 319–353.

Wolf S, Wolff HG: *Human Gastric Function: An Experimental Study of Man and His Stomach.* New York, Oxford University Press, 1947.

Wolff HG: The mind-body relationship, in Bryson L (ed): *An Outline of Man's Knowledge of the Modern World.* New York, McGraw-Hill, 1960.

CHAPTER 55

THE NEUROSES AND PERSONALITY DISORDERS

From time immemorial, in every society, it has been realized that there are many mentally troubled individuals who are neither insane nor feebleminded. They differ from normal people in being plagued by feelings of inferiority, inexplicable fatigue, shyness, moodiness, sense of guilt, and unreasonable fears; or they behave in ways that are upsetting to those around them and to society at large. Yet these conditions seem not to preclude their partaking in many of the everyday affairs of life, such as attending school, working in the marketplace, and marrying and rearing a family. As these conditions were more carefully documented, the ones that caused an individual much personal suffering came to be called *neuroses,* and those that caused society to suffer were called *psychopathies,* and more recently, *sociopathies.*

The question of the purity and homogeneity of these mental states has excited a lively polemic in the psychiatric literature. The neuroses as a group appeared to be so diverse as to require subdivision into no less than eight different types: anxiety states, neurasthenia, phobic neurosis, obsessive-compulsive neurosis, hysteria, hypochondriasis, neurotic depression, and depersonalization. And the psychopathies, in older classifications, came to include conditions as disparate as criminality, sexual perversions, and drug and alcohol addictions.

Originally, Freud designated these disorders as *psychoneuroses,* and the subject became enmeshed in psychoanalytic theory. The assumption was that an undercurrent of anxiety arising in unconscious conflict was the explanation of all the different types of neurosis as well as the psychopathies. This substitution of an explanatory concept for a descriptive one was not acceptable to the more biologically oriented psychiatrists, with the result that the term psychoneurosis has been expunged from the Diagnostic and Statistical Manual of Mental Disorders (DSM III). The term neurosis has been replaced by *neurotic disorder,* which is applied to any mental disorder with the following characteristics: (1) symptoms that are distressing to the victim and regarded by him or her as unacceptable or alien; (2) reality testing that remains intact; (3) symptomatic behavior that does not seriously violate social norms, although personal functioning may be considerably impaired; (4) a disturbance that is enduring, not a transitory reaction to stress; and (5) absence of an organic cause.

The foregoing definition of neurotic disorder has the virtue of being descriptive without committing one to any hypothesis of causation. It retains the historical connotation of neurosis and provides a terminologic link between psychiatrists throughout the world, according to Bayer. Psychodynamic theorists may continue to imbue the term with their ideas of unconscious conflict.

The genesis of the neurotic disorders is a matter of great importance in psychiatry and not only to adherents of psychoanalysis. It is generally conceded that neurotic disorders do not arise de novo in otherwise normal individuals. Their natural antecedents are thought to be abnormalities in personality development, molded by stressful events in the life of the victim. Thus an informative discussion of neurotic disorders requires a brief digression into the origins of normal personality development and departures therefrom.

The concept of *personality* and its development were introduced in Chap. 28. There it was pointed out that the term embraces the totality of a person's observable behavior and reportable subjective experience—the sum of characteristics that distinguishes one individual from all others. Thus it includes elements of the individual's character, intelligence, instinctual drives, sentiments, motor control, and memories—in short, all forces from within the organism, as well as the prevailing influences of the environment that govern behavior. The term *character* is almost synonymous with personality but is less useful because of its more moralistic connotation.

The roots of personality are multiple. Certain personality traits, such as boldness and timidity, level of energy and activity, fearfulness and fearlessness, adaptability and rigidity or stubbornness, etc., are already evident in the first months of life. Monozygotic twins are alike (but not absolutely identical) in these respects, even when reared apart. Each of these personality characteristics is genetically determined, like intelligence; probably a multiplicity of genes set the general pattern of each person's constitution, viz., personality. In addition these patterns are subject to incessant modification through familial, educational, social, and other environmental influences. Personalities become as individualistic as fingerprints.

Pertinent to the subject matter of this chapter is the assumption that during maturation the development of certain portions of the personality lag or become dissociated from the personality synthesis, or they are repressed to the point of having no influence or a distorted influence on behavior. How this happens and why the deviations take such a variety of forms are not known. Psychoanalytic explanations abound but are difficult or impossible to validate. The extent to which the deviations reflect past experience or a genetically predetermined pattern is unsettled.

Another of the unsolved problems in psychiatry is whether each of the personality types listed in Table 55-1 (taken from the list of personality disorders accepted by the American Psychiatric Association) is predictive or determinative of a particular type of neurosis or psychosis. In this regard, two broad groups of personality disorders can be recognized. In one group, comprising the paranoid, schizoid, cyclothymic, and obsessive-compulsive personality types, there is a probable relationship to a major type of psychiatric illness. Thus, among patients who develop simple or paranoid schizophrenia, a considerable number will have had the attributes described under paranoid personality. Similarly, among patients who develop schizophrenia of other type, the history will frequently disclose a pre-existent schizoid personality. In fact, it may be difficult to judge where the personality disorder left off and the schizophrenic illness began. It seems clear from several family studies (reviewed by Winokur et al) that the cyclothymic personality is related to manic-depressive disease. Obsessive-compulsive personality is closely related to obsessive-compulsive neurosis, as one might expect, but it also appears to be related to depressive disease. A close relationship exists between sociopathy and the development of alcoholism.

In other personality disorders, such relationships are not evident. Care must be taken to distinguish between "hysterical personality" and the disease *hysteria* (Briquet disease); there are no data to support the idea that a

hysterical personality is a determinant in the development of the full-blown hysterical neurosis. Also, the evidence that the asthenic, inadequate, and passive-aggressive or -dependent personalities are related to a major psychiatric illness or neuroses is rather weak. In this sense they are "pure" personality disorders, which in themselves may be lifelong sources of personal distress and difficulties in functioning, but which do not, as a rule, lead to the development of any specific psychiatric illness.

It need hardly be stressed that many of the terms that specify the several well-recognized personality types (Table 55-1) are used indiscriminately by physicians and laity to judge the personalities and character of others, with no implication of neurosis. Nevertheless, an understanding of the nonneurotic personalities and the less obtrusive traits and peculiarities of patients may be of great help to the physician. Such knowledge makes it possible to distinguish disorders of personality from the neuroses and other mental disorders and to understand sources of family discord or a patient's reactions during a medical illness, which may result in his interference with diagnostic and therapeutic procedures.

Personality disorders are little influenced by the physician, although often the contacts between physician and patient over many years may in themselves serve as a stabilizing force; and, of course, one should never underestimate the power of maturation to tranquilize the passions of adolescence and to settle the mind. The use of sedatives to influence some aspect of personality should be avoided unless there is evidence that the peculiarity of personality has elaborated into a full-blown neurosis.

In the following pages, prototypes of the clinically recognized neuroses and psychopathies will be described along with current hypotheses of their causation and pathogenesis.

THE NEUROTIC DISORDERS

Though numbered as the most frequent mental illnesses, the neuroses are among the least understood. They were established as clinical entities in the late nineteenth century, but there are still major unresolved issues with respect to their nature, classification, and etiology. As stated earlier, when Freud made his original observations on hysteria and obsessional neuroses, he preferred to designate them as *psychoneuroses*, implying a psychogenesis; but even Freud was uncertain of their etiology and speculated that the underlying cause of anxiety neurosis would probably be traced to a biologic factor. We have therefore retained the terms *neurotic disorder* and *neurosis*, thinking them preferable to psychoneurosis. But of course this does not settle the great uncertainty about the neuroses—whether they have

Table 55-1
Personality disorders

Type*	Characteristics	Type*	Characteristics
Paranoid (16)	Chronic wariness, suspiciousness, litigiousness; hypersensitivity, jealousy, envy; lack of insight or humor; tendency to blame others; sense of self-importance and entitlement	Asthenic (1)	Chronic weakness, easy fatigability, sense of vulnerability, oversensitive to physically and emotionally taxing situations, little ambition or aggression; low energy level; anhedonia
Cyclothymic (3)	Recurring periods of depression (low energy, pessimism, hopelessness, despair) and elation (high energy, ambition, enthusiasm, optimism) not readily explained by circumstances	Passive-aggressive (78)	Obstructive behavior, stubborness, intentional errors or omissions; intolerance of authority with struggles over control often creating difficulties in medical settings; externalization of conflicts and blaming others for untoward events
Schizoid (30)	Isolation, seclusiveness, secretiveness; discomfort in relationships; often eccentric and lacking in energy; few friends; detachment; inability to express ideas and feelings, especially anger	Inadequate (17)	Chronic inability to meet ordinary life demands in the absence of mental retardation; severe dependency on others; tendency to become institutionalized or to become dependent on institutions
Explosive (4)	Outbursts of rage and aggression not in keeping with usual personality, often in response to minor provocation; sense of loss of control followed by regret	Antisocial (32)	Unsocialized or antisocial behavior in conflict with society; selfishness, callousness, impulsiveness, lack of loyalty, and little guilt; low frustration tolerance; tendency to blame others; long history of interpersonal and social difficulties and arrests
Obsessive-compulsive (anankastic) (21)	Chronic worries about standards; excessive concern about self-image; tension in relationships, leading to isolation; inability to relax and excessive inhibitions; overly meticulous, conscientious, and perfectionist; predisposition to depression and obsessive-compulsive neurosis	Passive-dependent (30)	Lack of self-confidence, indecisiveness, tendency to cling to and seek support from others
Hysterical (103)	Immaturity, histrionic behavior, excitability, emotional instability, sexualization of relationships, low frustration tolerance, and shallow interpersonal ties; dependency	Immature (12) Unspecified (14)	Ineffectual responses to social, psychologic, and physical demands; lack of stamina; poor adaptation to ordinary situations; a "loser"

* Figures in parentheses represent the number of diagnoses of each personality disorder out of a total of 361 patients with the diagnosis of personality disorder at the Psychiatric Service of the University of Iowa (Winokur and Crowe).

an organic basis or are social maladjustments due to faulty learning and leading to unnatural reactions to stress.

Descriptively, as already indicated, the neurotic disorders include the following syndromes: (1) anxiety neurosis, (2) neurasthenia, (3) phobic neurosis, which includes phobia of illness, social phobia, agoraphobia, etc., (4) obsessive-compulsive neurosis [(3) and (4) are also called *psychasthenia*], (5) hysteria, (6) hypochondriasis, and (7) neurotic depression. Former classifications included an additional type called "depersonalization neurosis" with which we have had little experience; most such cases would probably fall under (5).

Although each of these syndromes is clinically identifiable and separable when occurring in pure form, experience shows that most patients experience symptoms of more than one type and therefore are said to have "mixed neuroses." Tyrer refers to this state as "the general neurotic syndrome" and proposes as criteria for diagnosis at least three of the following features: (1) abnormal personality of passive-dependent type; (2) two or more of the following syndromes, past or present—social phobia, agarophobia, panic disorder, nonpsychotic depression, chronic anxiety, hypochondriasis; (3) a history of similar disorders in the family (first-degree relatives); (4) at least one episode of illness that appeared without relationship to stress. In DSM III, all of the neuroses have been replaced by two categories of disorders—(1) the *anxiety disorders* (which include panic states, and the phobic and obsessive-compulsive neuroses) and (2) the *somatiform disorders* (comprising hysteria, conversion symptoms, and hypochondriasis).

It is evident from these several attempts at definition that a single explanation—one that would satisfactorily cover the attributes of these seven (or eight) neuroses—is still forthcoming. Syndromes as different as neurasthenia and panic reaction do not lend themselves to a unitary explanation. If there is a central feature of the neuroses, it is thought to be *anxiety,* which runs as a kind of leitmotif through all of them. Even in hysterical neurosis, in which patients seem indifferent to their disabilities, there is often a strong undercurrent of anxiety. In psychoanalytic theory, anxiety is looked upon as the individual's response to a threat from within, in the form of a forbidden instinctual drive that is about to escape from the individual's control. The intensity of the anxiety is thought to be proportional to the intensity of the disguised threat, i.e., one of which the patient is unaware. The anxiety is seen as a signal to which the mind reacts by erecting psychologic defenses. Thus each neurotic syndrome is perceived as a particular defense mechanism for dealing with anxiety. These and other psychodynamic theories of the neuroses are discussed in detail by Nemiah in the *Comprehensive Textbook of Psychiatry* (see references at end of chapter).

INCIDENCE

There are few reliable data as to the incidence rate or prevalence of neurotic disorders or the relative incidence of the various types of neurosis. An analysis of 1045 consecutive psychiatric consultations at the New England Center Hospital, a tertiary referral hospital, during the years 1955 and 1956, disclosed that the dominant syndrome in about 20 percent was an anxiety state. In addition, symptoms of anxiety were present in some cases of depression, hysteria, and schizophrenia. In contrast, frank hysteria was diagnosed in only 6 percent of cases, and all the other neuroses together with schizophrenia, alcoholic psychoses, sociopathic states, and the dementias comprised only 10 percent. As indicated on page 1204, depression in one form or another was the most common psychiatric illness (50 percent); psychiatric disease was either absent or could not be diagnosed in the remaining 14 percent of this series.

Such information as is available suggests that the incidence of the neuroses is much the same in an urban population (midtown New York) and a rural one (Stirling County, Nova Scotia), indicating that socioeconomic, racial, and cultural factors are of relatively little importance. Further, in times of calamity, such as the bombing of London, the incidence of neurotic symptoms was said not to have increased. Thus one tends to dismiss as an oversimplification the notion that neuroses are merely a by-product of life in civilized society or reactions to environmental stress (see also Chap. 24). Neurosis of all types occurs in both sexes, except for hysteria which, with the qualifications to be indicated, is a disease of females. The onset is in late childhood, adolescence, and early adult life. Admittedly, neurotic symptoms may be recognized for the first time after this age, but a good clinical rule is to suspect any mental illness that appears for the first time after the age of 40 years to be either a depression or a dementia due to degenerative or other organic disease of the brain.

ANXIETY NEUROSIS
(Neurocirculatory Asthenia)

The term *anxiety neurosis* was introduced by Freud, in 1894, to describe a syndrome consisting of general irritability, anxious expectation, anxiety attacks, somatic equivalents of anxiety, and nightmares. In anxiety neurosis this symptom complex constitutes the entire illness. However, as indicated above and in Chap. 24, this syndrome may also occur in a number of other psychiatric diseases—manic-depressive psychosis, schizophrenia, hysteria, and phobic neurosis. Its closest link is with depression, which it resembles in another respect, viz., a strong hereditary factor. The term used in DSM III is *anxiety reaction,* of which phobias, acute and chronic anxiety states, and panic states are the important subdivisions. *Anxiety neurosis* is the term preferred by the authors.

CLINICAL PRESENTATION

Anxiety neurosis is a chronic disease, punctuated by recurrent attacks of acute anxiety or panic. The acute attacks are the hallmark of the disease, and many psychiatrists are reluctant to make a diagnosis of anxiety neurosis in their absence. Fully developed, they are nearly as dramatic as a seizure. They begin with distressing feelings of dread and foreboding. Patients are assailed by a feeling of strangeness, as though their body had changed or the surroundings were unreal (depersonalization; derealization). They are frightened, most often by the prospect of imminent death (angor animi), of losing their mind or self-control, or of smothering. "I am dying," "This is the end," "Oh, my God, I'm going," or "I can't breathe" are the characteristic expressions of alarm and panic. The heart races, breathing comes in rapid gasps, pupils are dilated, and the patient sweats and trembles. The palpitation and breathing difficulties are so prominent that a cardiologist is often called. The symptoms abate spontaneously after 15 to 30 min, leaving the patient shaken, tense, perplexed, and often embarrassed.

Hyperventilation is a special feature of the anxiety attack. Hyperventilation itself, by reducing the P_{CO_2} will cause giddiness, paresthesias of the fingers, tongue, and lips, and, at times, frank tetany. Some patients become frightened and cry during a period of forced overbreathing. A 3-min period of commanded deep breathing reproduces their symptoms and corroborates the diagnosis of hyperventilation syndrome.

Such attacks may occur at infrequent intervals or several times a day. They may occur in situations where there are no easily recognizable sources of fear, as when the patient is sitting quietly at home; or the attacks may awaken the patient from sleep. In other instances a trying or upsetting experience is followed by an anxiety attack, nonetheless excessive for the condition that provoked it. In some patients attacks are provoked by confinement to a closed space, an elevator for example, or by crowded surroundings, as in church or a movie house. An anxiety state not infrequently follows an accident and may, according to Modlin, be a source of disability. Symptoms of both anxiety and depression may be prominent features of the posttraumatic nervous instability syndrome.

Except in minor details all the attacks are alike in any one individual. Between attacks, some patients feel relatively well, but most complain of the symptoms of the panic attack in lesser but persistent fashion. Cohen and White listed the following symptoms in order of frequency: palpitation 97 percent, easy fatigue 93 percent, breathlessness 90 percent, nervousness 88 percent, chest pain 85 percent, sighing 79 percent, dizziness 78 percent, apprehensiveness 61 percent, headache 58 percent, paresthesias 58 percent, weakness 56 percent, insomnia 53 percent, unhappiness 50 percent.

Anxiety neurosis may begin with an acute panic attack, but more frequently the onset is insidious—feelings of tenseness, vague apprehension, fatigue, weakness, and giddiness having been present for weeks or months before the first panic attack. From the history alone, two patterns of chronic anxiety neurosis are discernible. In one, there is a nearly lifelong history of poor exercise tolerance, little stamina, inability to do heavy physical work or participate in vigorous sports, tenseness, nervousness, and intolerance of crowds. In the other, the patient is vigorous and symptom-free before the anxiety state begins. Most patients with chronic symptoms first consult a physician complaining of cardiorespiratory symptoms, but in a significant number gastrointestinal symptoms (dyspepsia, loss of appetite, or "irritable colon") are the initial symptoms. The former often come to light during military service and have been designated, since shortly after the American Civil War, as *neurocirculatory asthenia,* "irritable heart," or "soldier's heart."

The physical examination between acute attacks yields relatively little of diagnostic value. The common findings, disclosed by the study of Cohen et al, were slight tachycardia, sighing respirations, yawning, flushed face and neck, tremor of the outstretched hands, and brisk tendon jerks.

The onset of both acute and chronic anxiety neurosis is rare before 18 and after 35 to 40 years of age (average age of onset, 25 years). It is twice as frequent in women as men. There is a high familial incidence of this illness. In one study (Wheeler et al) there was a prevalence of 49 percent among the grown children of patients with anxiety neurosis, compared to a prevalence of about 5 percent in the general population. Among identical twins, there was a concordance rate of 40 percent, compared to 4 percent in dizygotic twins (Slater and Shields). Among the relatives of index cases, the mothers suffered from anxiety neurosis more often than the fathers; in the latter, alcoholism was more frequent than in the population at large (Modlin). The pattern of inheritance has not been established, but most closely approximates that of autosomal dominance.

The course of anxiety neurosis is variable. The symptoms fluctuate in severity, without apparent relation to environmental stress. A 20-year follow-up study by Wheeler and his associates showed that symptoms of anxiety neurosis were still present in 88 percent, but were moderately or severely disabling in only 15 percent. Most of the patients were able to work and to enjoy a reasonably normal family and social life. Their only liability to further psychiatric illness was to recurrent anxiety neurosis or anxious depression; so-called psychosomatic illnesses and other psychiatric illnesses did not occur more frequently than in the general population. The life span of patients with anxiety neurosis is not shortened. They rarely commit suicide.

ETIOLOGY AND PATHOGENESIS

Anxiety neurosis has been attributed to a genetic abnormality, to constitutional weakness of the nervous system, to social and psychologic factors, some of which have already been discussed, and more recently, to certain physiologic and biochemical derangements. None of these factors provides a completely satisfactory explanation of the primary disorder, however.

The symptoms of an anxiety attack resemble those of fear in many ways, though nearly always the former symptoms are longer in duration and less distinct. The most important difference, however, is that the cause of fear is known to the patient, whereas that of anxiety is not.

On the physiologic and biochemical side it has been observed that anger provokes an excessive secretion of norepinephrine, whereas fear is accompanied by increased secretion of epinephrine. Actually fear activates the whole autonomic nervous system, and the increase in epinephrine is more than counterbalanced by a parasympathetic discharge (see Chap. 24). The responsiveness of the autonomic nervous system remains heightened in patients with chronic anxiety. In such patients, a number of stimuli (cold, pain, muscular effort) produce abnormal responses in pulse, respiration, oxygen consumption, and work performance. Another interesting abnormality (first noted by Cohen et al) is that the blood lactic acid levels are higher than normal, especially after mild exercise, and infusions of lactic acid have been said to trigger anxiety symptoms in persons with anxiety neurosis. The presence of these derangements does not mean that they are causal; more likely they are secondary to the poor physical condition and apprehension associated with the syndrome.

DIFFERENTIAL DIAGNOSIS

Shorn of the psychologic components of apprehension and fear, the anxiety attack consists essentially of an autonomic discharge. Some of the autonomic symptoms are duplicated by chromaffin tumors, hyperthyroidism, and the menopause. The prominence of chest pain and respiratory distress during an acute anxiety attack may be mistaken for an episode of myocardial ischemia or angina pectoris, and the patient is subjected to a series of studies of cardiac function. Other medical diseases that simulate certain elements of an anxiety state are pulmonary embolism, cardiac arrhythmias, hypoglycemia, hypoparathyroidism, drug withdrawal, and complex partial seizures. Strict criteria for the clinical diagnosis of these disease states readily permit their differentiation from anxiety neurosis.

Of greater importance is the distinction between anxiety neurosis and other psychiatric illnesses, particularly depression. Symptoms of depression are frequently added to those of anxiety neurosis, and the majority of patients with depression have symptoms of anxiety. Indeed, some psychiatrists believe that anxiety neurosis is only a variant of depression. As has been mentioned, an anxiety state appearing for the first time after the fortieth year usually proves to be a depression. The uncovering of paranoid symptoms in a patient with an anxiety state should always raise the question of depression, as should the presence of symptoms such as self-depreciation and feelings of hopelessness. A number of patients with a condition diagnosed as anxiety neurosis by competent psychiatrists have been known to commit suicide.

Schizophrenia may begin with prominent anxiety symptoms. Here the diagnosis rests on finding the characteristic thought disorder of schizophrenia, which may emerge only after several interviews. Hysteria also includes anxiety symptoms, as do phobic and obsessive-compulsive neurosis, but each has other distinguishing attributes.

TREATMENT

Rather little information is available as to the efficacy of different methods of treatment. There is no evidence that sophisticated psychotherapy is of more value than an explanation of the nature of the illness and reassurance that the symptoms have no ominous significance. A cardiac consultation and some simple tests (ECG, chest films) may be needed to reinforce the diagnosis and to alleviate the patient's fear of heart disease. Brief admission to a hospital for this purpose is often justified. Propranolol, 10 to 20 mg tid, blocks many of the autonomic accompaniments, and diazepam, 5 mg tid, or chlordiazepoxide, 10 mg tid, may also suppress symptoms to some extent. A nonbenzodiazepine, buspirone, is equally as effective for the treatment of generalized anxiety disorder, although its long-term effects and safety remain to be determined. If depressive symptoms are in evidence, amitriptyline, 150 mg/day in divided doses, should be given. Tricyclic antidepressants or monoamine oxidase (MAO) inhibitors (particularly the latter) are said to be more effective than anxiolytic drugs in preventing panic attacks (Matuzas and Glass). These and other current concepts of the treatment of anxiety have been discussed by Rosenbaum and by Peroutka. In all types of neurosis, the physician must develop and maintain a psychotherapeutic program involving discussion of the patient's symptoms, reassurance, and explanation as to the nature of the illness.

With the use of these simple medical measures, the anxiety state remits within 3 months in about half the patients; the remission rate is not much higher with the most intense psychotherapy. Anxiety symptoms arising in relation to a threatening event carry a better prognosis. Patients whose anxiety state persists should always be suspected of having an endogenous depression.

NEURASTHENIA

Literally the word means "nervous weakness," and the closest equivalent as a medical symptom is chronic fatigability. The latter was discussed in Chap. 23, as one of the cardinal manifestations of disease. Once considered an important neurosis, the diagnosis of neurasthenia is now obsolete. The careful study of patients with the complaint of chronic fatigue usually reveals that they are suffering from anxiety neurosis or depression. When lifelong, it may resemble more a character disorder than a neurosis (the "asthenic psychopathy" of Kahn; see Table 55-1). In the authors' experience, most patients designated as chronic neurasthenics are depressed and most of them will recover under the influence of antidepressive therapy.

PHOBIC NEUROSIS

In this state, patients (women more than men) are overwhelmed by an intense and irrational fear of some animal, object, situation, or disease. Though acknowledging that there are no rational grounds for this fear (hence it is not a delusion), and that such provocative stimuli are innocuous, they are nonetheless powerless to suppress it. This disorder was known to Hippocrates who drew a distinction between normal and morbid fears. Westphal in 1871 was the first to give morbid fears the status of a disease.

Mild phobias of darkness, solitude, animals, and high places are commonplace in childhood; some persist into adult life and may be culturally acceptable, such as fear of snakes or mice. In phobic neurosis, an illness constituting only 1 to 2 percent of all psychiatric disorders, the patient is chronically fearful of a particular animal or situation and may be panic-stricken and incapacitated when placed in a situation that evokes the phobia. For example, it may be impossible for the patient to leave the house or neighborhood except when attended by a relative or friend, or to mingle in a crowd (ochlophobia). The patient may be unable to eat certain foods, ride in cars or planes, have sexual intercourse, eat in public, urinate in the presence of others, etc. Feelings of helplessness, pessimism, and de-

spondency may result. Often there are obsessive-compulsive tendencies as well, and some patients are hypochondriacal. The authors have observed a number of patients whose phobic (or obsessive-compulsive) neurosis decompensated as an endogenous depression developed. Recovery from the depression returned them to their earlier and milder phobic state. This suggests a linkage between these neuroses and depression.

OBSESSIVE-COMPULSIVE NEUROSIS

Like the pure phobic states, a neurosis dominated by obsessions and compulsions is rare, occurring in not more than 1 to 2 percent of patients seeking help in a psychiatric outpatient clinic. Minor compulsions (not stepping on cracks in the sidewalk, etc.), like minor phobias, are common in children, cause little or no distress, and tend to disappear in later life. Certain irrational habits and rigid obsessional ways of thinking are frequent and persistent but excite little attention medically until they interfere with some diagnostic procedure or the therapy of some disease.

Obsessive-compulsive or *obsessional neurosis,* as it is usually designated, begins, as do the other neuroses, in adolescence or early adult years, although treatment may not be sought until middle age is reached. The two sexes are equally affected. Onset is usually gradual and cannot be accurately dated, but in some cases it is precipitated by some event in the life of the patient, such as death of a relative, sexual conflict, etc. The family history will show a high incidence of obsessional personality. In most instances, the obsessive-compulsive neurosis is engrafted on a personality in which rigidity, inflexibility, and lack of adaptability are prominent. These traits are manifest in the individual's punctuality and in his dependability and reliability in the affairs of everyday life. There is always a prevailing undercurrent of insecurity.

Obsessions may be defined as imperative and distressing thoughts and impulses that persist in the patient's mind despite a desire to resist and to be rid of them. Obsessions take various forms. The most common are *intellectual obsessions,* in which phrases, rhymes, ideas, or vivid images (these are often absurd, blasphemous, obscene, and sometimes frightening) constantly intrude into consciousness; *impulsive obsessions,* in which the mind is dominated by an impulse to kill oneself, to stab one's children, or to perform some other objectionable act; and *inhibiting obsessions,* in which every act must be ruminated upon and analyzed before it is carried out—a state aptly called *doubting mania.* Every effort at distraction fails to rid the patient of the obsessive thought. It engulfs the mind, rendering the person miserable and inefficient. Probably the most disturbing obsessions are the impulsive ones, in which patients constantly struggle with the fear that they will put some terrible thought into action. Even as they tell of the obsession, they reveal their underlying anxiety and seek reassurance that they will not yield to it. Fortunately, such patients rarely obey their pathologic impulses. Phobias are essentially *obsessive fears* and should probably be included in this category of neurosis. The most common phobias are those of open, closed, or high places, dogs, cats, dirt, sprays and other contaminants, air travel, AIDS, cancer, insanity, and death.

Compulsions are acts that result from obsessions. These are single acts or a series of acts (rituals) which the patient must carry out in order to put the mind at ease. Examples are repeated checking of the gas jets or the locks on doors, adjusting articles of clothing, repeated hand washing, using a clean handkerchief to wipe objects that have been touched by others, tasting foods in specific ways, touching objects in a particular sequence, etc.

Certain motor disturbances, namely habit spasms or tics, are, in a sense, motor compulsions. They consist of repetitive movements of the shoulders, arms, hands, and certain of the facial muscles (see Chap. 5). The feature that separates tics from involuntary movements of extrapyramidal type is the feeling, on the part of the patient, that tics must be carried out to relieve tension (see page 89). Unlike compulsions, however, tics are not based on obsessive thoughts. It is of interest that in the Gilles de la Tourette syndrome, multiple tics are combined with compulsive utterances, often offensive ones.

In all these obsessions and compulsions, and in the phobias, patients recognize the irrationality of their ideas and behavior, yet are powerless to control them, much as they desire to do so. It is this insight into the obsessional experience and the struggle against it that distinguish obsessions from delusions.

The majority of patients with obsessive-compulsive neurosis are tense, irritable, and apprehensive. They suffer a curious feeling of insufficiency or incompetency in being unable to expel their troublesome thoughts. The most distraught emotional state, as mentioned above, is related to the fear that an idea may eventuate in reality. These patients may complain of typical anxiety attacks, and after the condition has persisted for a time they may become depressed. Fatigue, anorexia, and general lack of interest, which are often present, are probably related to the anxiety and depression.

MECHANISMS OF PHOBIC AND OBSESSIVE NEUROSES

Janet believed that individuals with phobias and obsessions differ from normal in their diminished capacity for mental inhibition and attention, for which reason distracting and irrelevant thoughts cannot be eliminated. Indecisiveness was thought to be another common manifestation of this state. For all these defects Janet suggested the term *psychasthenia;* by this he vaguely implied a genetic origin but offered no evidence on this point.

Psychoanalytic theory holds that psychasthenic behavior is the result of an overactive superego and imperfect repression of some disagreeable wish. This wish is conceived as having both an ideational and an emotional or affective content. If the disagreeable wish is completely repressed, the psychic energy may be converted into a physical symptom such as paralysis or anesthesia (conversion hysteria). If repression is imperfect or incomplete, so that only the ideational content is repressed, the psychic energy may be converted into fear (phobia), or into another idea which then becomes an obsession. To the analyst, obsessional symptoms have symbolic meanings.

To the neurologist, these are interesting but unverifiable speculations. There must be some more basic defect, as yet unexplained, that allows these irrational ideas or fears to dominate the mind.

DIAGNOSIS

Since the prevailing emotional state in patients with phobias and obsessions is one of anxiety and depression, it is necessary to distinguish between phobic and obsessional neuroses, anxiety neurosis, and depressive psychosis. In phobic and obsessive neuroses the depression tends to be inconstant and closely related to a sense of weariness and helplessness in overcoming the irrational fears and obsessive thinking. As the latter improve the depression lightens. In uncomplicated anxiety states, baseless fears are not uncommon, but are never so persistent or disabling as in psychasthenia; also the indecisiveness and compulsive tendencies are lacking. Schizophrenia must be considered when an adolescent or young adult begins to harbor peculiar ideas, but then a careful mental examination reveals the other characteristic disturbances of this disorder (Chap. 58).

TREATMENT OF PHOBIC AND OBSESSIONAL NEUROSES

This is best left to the psychiatrist. At least there should be a trial of therapy using behavioral modification techniques. In the case of phobic neurosis, the aim of such treatment is to reduce the patient's fear to the extent that exposure to the phobic situation can be tolerated. The most popular form of therapy in recent years has been so-called *systematic desensitization* (Wolpe), which consists of graded exposure of the patient to the object or the situation that arouses fear. Psychotherapy, if undertaken, need not be intensive, consisting instead of explanation, reassurance, and guidance in dealing with symptoms.

Cases of obsessional neurosis that are cyclic in nature, with exacerbations and remissions and with no apparent relationship to environmental factors, have the best prognosis. Some psychiatrists treat this cyclic form like cyclic depressions, with antidepressant drugs and electroconvulsive therapy (ECT). It is not certain that these measures accomplish more than can be attributed to the spontaneous changes in the disease. More often the course of obsessional neurosis is steady and severely disabling, and in these patients the outlook for recovery is poor. ECT has helped some patients, in whom there has been a strong element of depression. Tranquilizing drugs are being used, but their efficacy is uncertain.

Cingulotomy has reportedly produced symptomatic improvement in both phobic and obsessional neuroses. This measure, if it is to be used at all, should be considered only as a last resort in exceptionally severe cases, in which the patient has failed to respond to all other methods of treatment and is totally disabled.

Berg's long-term study of phobic neurosis showed that half the patients were improved after 5 years, a quarter unchanged, and the rest worse, whether treated or not. Pollitt, who observed a group of 150 obsessional patients for a period of 3½ years, found that nearly two-thirds of them had had previous attacks, from which they had recovered. Among a smaller group of 30 patients, followed for 4½ years, two-thirds had achieved a good social adjustment (see Insel for additional reading).

HYSTERIA (Hysterical Neurosis, Conversion Reaction, Briquet Disease)

Although hysteria has been known since ancient times, it was the French physician Briquet who in 1859 first described the disease as we know it today. Later, Charcot elaborated certain manifestations of the disease, and interested Freud and Janet in it. Charcot believed that the symptoms could be produced and relieved by hypnosis (mesmerism). Janet postulated *a dissociative state* of mind to account for certain features such as trance and fugue states. Freud and his students conceived of hysterical symptoms as a product of "ego defense mechanisms," in which psychic energy, generated by unconscious psychic conflicts, is converted into physical symptoms. This latter concept has been widely accepted, to the point that the term *conversion* has been incorporated into the nomenclature of the neurosis and the terms *conversion symptoms* and *conversion reaction* have come to be equated with the disease hysteria. In the authors' opinion, the term *conversion symptoms,* if it is used at all, should refer only to certain *unexplained symptoms,* such as amnesia, paralysis, blindness, aphonia, etc., which mimic neurologic disease. The term *hysteria* should be reserved for a *disease* that is practically confined to women and is characterized further by a distinctive age of onset, natural history, and many somatic symptoms and signs, which typically include "conversion symptoms" and dissociative reactions.

The term *hysteria* has a number of other connotations, most of them pejorative. Lay people refer to individuals with tantrums or loss of self-control in the face of an emotional crisis as "hysterical." Some psychiatrists dub any dramatic, histrionic, manipulative, or "seductive" behavior as hysterical (referring to the *hysterical personality*), or equate hysteria with hypersuggestibility and susceptibility to hypnosis. These are traditional ideas based on the incorrect belief that these qualities are typical of hysteria.

In clinical neurology one encounters two types of patients with hysteria: (1) young women with a chronic illness marked by multiple and often dramatically presented symptoms, the source of which they are unaware, and somatic abnormalities, for which no cause is evident; (2) men and women who develop physical symptoms or remain inexplicably disabled for the purpose of obtaining compensation, influencing litigation, avoiding military duty, imprisonment, etc. This latter state is called *compensation neurosis* or *compensation hysteria.*

CLASSIC, OR FEMALE, HYSTERIA (BRIQUET DISEASE)

This neurosis usually has its onset in the teens or early twenties. However, a few cases may begin before puberty. Once established, the symptoms continue to recur intermittently, though with lessening frequency, throughout adult years, even to an advanced age. There are, no doubt, cases of lesser severity in which symptoms occur only a few times or perhaps only once, just as there are mild forms of all diseases. The patient may be seen for the first time during middle life or later, and the earlier history may not at first be forthcoming. Careful probing, however, will almost invariably reveal that the earliest manifestations of the illness had appeared before the age of 25 years.

Other important data are also brought to light by a careful past history. During late childhood and adolescence, the normal activities of the patient, including education, have usually been interrupted by periods of illness. Rheumatic fever, tuberculosis, or some obscure disease may have been suspected. Later in life, problems in work adjustment and marriage are frequent. There is a notably high incidence of marital incompatibility, separation, and divorce. The patient's life history is punctuated by symptoms that do not conform to recognizable patterns of medical and surgical disease. For these, many forms of therapy, including surgical operations, will have been performed. Rarely has adult life been reached without at least one abdominal operation, usually done because of pain, persistent nausea and vomiting, or some vague gynecologic complaint. The indications for the surgical procedures have usually been unclear, and, further, the same symptoms or others recurred to complicate the convalescence. The biographies of these patients are also replete with disorders that center about menstrual, sexual, and procreative functions. Menstrual periods may be painfully prostrating, irregular, or excessive. Sexual intercourse may be painful, unpleasant, or unsatisfactory. Pregnancies may be difficult; the usual vomiting of the first trimester may persist all through the gestational period, with weight loss and prostration; labor may be unusually difficult and prolonged, and all manner of unpredictable complications are said to have occurred during and after parturition.

Hysteria is, then, a polysymptomatic disorder, involving almost every organ system. The most frequent symptoms, all statistically significant, which were elicited during a study of 50 unmistakable cases of female hysteria as compared with a control group of 50 healthy women, included the following: headache, blurred vision, lump in the throat, loss of voice, dyspnea, palpitation, anxiety attacks, anorexia, nausea and vomiting, abdominal pain, food dyscrasia, severe menstrual pain, urinary retention, sexual indifference, painful intercourse, paresthesias, dizzy spells, nervousness, and easy crying (Purtell et al).

The examination of the female hysteric demonstrates a number of useful findings, mostly in the sphere of mental status. Questions regarding the chief complaint usually elicit a vague reply or the narration of a series of incidents or problems, many of which prove to have little or no relevance to the question. However, unlike the situation in a psychotic illness, the patient's ideas about most aspects of her life are rational and coherent, and there is no evidence of hallucinations, delusions, disturbance in logical thinking, or loss of appreciation of the reality of the situation. The manner of the patient is often amiable and even ingratiating. The description of symptoms tends to be dramatic and exaggerated and does not accord with the facts as elicited

from other members of the family; yet at the same time a rather casual demeanor is manifested. The patient may insist that everything in her life is quite normal and controlled, when, in fact, her medical record is checkered with instances of dramatic behavior and unexplained illness. This calm attitude toward a turbulent illness and seemingly disabling physical signs is so common that it has been singled out as an important characteristic of hysteria, *la belle indifférence*. Other patients, however, are obviously tense and anxious, and frank anxiety attacks are reported by many of them; or the patient may be effusive in her enthusiasms, fickle and flighty, always putting on an act, and demanding constant attention. Her emotional reactions are superficial and she creates scenes that are disturbing to others, but are quickly forgotten. If physical disorders are present, attempts by the physician to disprove the somatic nature of the complaints usually meet with anxiety and vehement protest. Memory defects (amnesic gaps) are usually demonstrated while the history is being taken; the patient appears to have forgotten important segments of the history, some of which she had clearly described in the past and are part of the medical record. Antisocial behavior occurs in a minority of patients.

There are no characteristic physical findings. Although many writers have commented on the rather youthful, girlish appearance and coquettish manner of the patients, this by no means characterizes all of them. The so-called stigmata of hysteria, i.e., corneal anesthesia, absence of gag reflex, spots of pain and tenderness over the scalp, sternum, breasts, lower ribs, and ovaries, are often suggested by the examiner and are too inconsistent to be of much help in the diagnosis. The only limit to the variation and pleomorphism of the physical signs is the patient's ability to produce them by an effort of will. Accordingly, symptoms and signs that are beyond volitional control cannot be accepted as manifestations of hysteria. Some weight in diagnosis is attached to the development of physical signs similar to those of another member of the family or their evocation by a stressful event in the patient's personal life. However, this may not be disclosed at the time of the first examination.

SPECIAL HYSTERICAL SYNDROMES

A few hysterical syndromes recur with great regularity, and every physician may expect to encounter them. They constitute some of the most puzzling diagnostic problems in medicine.

Hysterical Pain This may involve any part of the body; generalized or localized headache, "atypical facial neuralgia," vague abdominal pain, back pain with camptocormia are the most frequent and most troublesome to the clinician. In many of these patients the response to analgesic drugs has been unusual, and some of them are addicted. They may respond to a placebo as though it were a potent drug, but it should be pointed out that this is a notoriously unreliable means of distinguishing hysterical pain from that of other diseases. The greatest error is to mistake the pain of osteomyelitis, metastatic carcinoma, or brain tumor, before other symptoms have developed, for a manifestation of hysteria. The most helpful diagnostic features of hysterical pain are the inability of the patient to give a clear, concise description of the type of pain; its location, which does not conform to the pattern of pain in the familiar medical syndromes; the dramatic elaborations of its intensity and effects; its persistence, either continuous or intermittent, for long periods of time; the absence of other diseases that could account for pain; the assumption of bizarre attitudes and postures; and, most important, the coexistence of other attacks of hysterical nature.

Hysterical Vomiting This is often combined with pain and tenderness in the lower abdomen and results in unnecessary appendectomies and removal of pelvic organs in adolescent girls and young women. The vomiting is somewhat unusual, in that it often occurs after a meal, leaving the patient hungry and ready to eat again; it may be induced by unpleasant circumstances. Some of these patients can vomit at will, regurgitating food from the stomach like a ruminant animal. Vomiting may persist for weeks with no cause being found. Weight loss may occur but seldom to the degree anticipated. As was remarked above, the usual first-trimester vomiting of pregnancy may continue throughout the entire 9 months, and occasionally pregnancy will be interrupted because of it. Anorexia may be another prominent symptom and must be differentiated from anorexia nervosa, another disease of young women (see page 1217).

Hysterical Seizures, Trances, and Fugues These conditions seem to be less frequent than in the days of Charcot, when *la grande attaque d'hystérie* was often exhibited before medical audiences. Nevertheless they do occur and must be distinguished from cerebral cortical seizures and catalepsy. To witness an attack is of great assistance in diagnosis. The lack of an aura, initiating cry, hurtful fall, and incontinence; the presence of peculiar movements such as grimacing, squirming, thrashing and flailing of the limbs, side-to-side motions of the head, and striking at or resisting those who offer assistance; the retention of consciousness during a motor seizure that involves both sides of the body; the long duration of the seizure, the abrupt termination by strong sensory stimulation, and lack of postictal confusion—are all typical of the hysterical attack. Sometimes hyperventilation will initiate an attack and is therefore a useful diagnostic maneuver. Both epilepsy and hysteria may be combined in the same

patient, in which instance the resulting illness invariably causes difficulty in diagnosis. Hysterical trances or fugues, in which the patient wanders about for hours or days and carries out complex acts, may also simulate temporal lobe epilepsy or any of the conditions that lead to confusional psychosis or stupor. Here the most reliable point of differentiation comes from observation of the patient, who, if hysterical, is likely to indicate a degree of alertness and promptness of response not seen in temporal lobe seizures or confusional states. Following the episode, an interview with the patient, under the influence of hypnosis, strong suggestion, or amobarbital, will often bring to light memories of what happened during the episode; this will exclude the possibility of an epileptic fugue.

Hysterical Paralyses and Tremors Hysterical palsies may involve an arm, a leg, one side of the body, or both legs. If the affected limb can be moved at all, muscle action is weak, and often the strength of voluntary movement is in proportion to the resistance offered by the examiner. Movements are characteristically slow, tentative, and poorly sustained. One can feel agonist and antagonist muscles contracting simultaneously. When the resistance is suddenly withdrawn, there is no follow-through or rebound, as is normally the case. The muscular tone in the affected limbs is usually normal, but rigidity may sometimes be found. Walking may be impossible, there may be a veritable astasia-abasia, or the gait may be bizarre (see page 98). This discrepancy between the inability to walk and to move the legs is, of course, not unique to hysteria; it also occurs in so-called frontal lobe apraxia and in ataxia from midline cerebellar lesions. If the limb has been held in a rigid posture for a long time, contractures may set in. The features of hysterical tremor have been described on page 81, and need not be repeated here. The tendon reflexes are always normal, but with hysterical hemianesthesia the abdominal and plantar reflexes may be suppressed on the affected side. Anesthesia or hypesthesia is almost always inadvertently suggested by the physician's examination. Seldom is sensory loss a spontaneous complaint of the patient, although complaints of "numbness" and paresthesias are not uncommon. The sensory loss may involve one or more limbs below a sharp line (stocking and glove distribution) or may involve one-half the body. Touch, pain, taste, smell, vision, and hearing may all be affected on that side, which is an anatomic impossibility from a single lesion.

Hysterical Amnesia Patients brought to a hospital in a state of amnesia, not knowing their own identity, are usually hysterical females or sociopathic males involved in a crime. Usually after a few hours or days, with encouragement, they divulge their life history. Epileptic patients or victims of a concussion or acute confusional psychosis do not come to a hospital asking for help in establishing their identity. Moreover, the complete loss of memory for all previous life experiences by a patient who is otherwise able to comport herself normally is not observed in any other conditions.

In the *Ganser syndrome* (amnesia, disturbance of consciousness, and hallucinations), patients pretend to have lost their minds or to have become insane. They act in an absurd manner, in the way they believe an insane or feebleminded person should act, and give senseless answers to every question asked of them.

Unexplained Hyperpyrexia Among patients with unexplained fever who turn up in every diagnostic clinic, there are always a few hysterics. One cannot help but be impressed with the number of student nurses, nurses, and nurses' aides among this group of patients. Some of them will be found to have no fever if the nurse or doctor checks the temperature. Others have oral temperatures of 37 to 38°C (99 to 100°F), which must be regarded as normal for some individuals. Finally, there are a few well-documented cases of hyperpyrexia that appear to be of psychogenic origin; in these the possibility of some obscure hypothalamic disorder cannot be excluded. Diagnosis is assisted by a longitudinal history and the elicitation of the other symptoms of hysteria.

Dermatitis Factitia (Hysterical Dermatoneurosis)
This condition is seen more often in the sociopath than in the hysterical patient. The skin eruptions induced by the patient are characterized by erythema, ulcerations, gangrene, and variable degrees of dermatitis. Usually a caustic or irritant chemical or a sharp instrument such as a nail file has been used. The lesions are most commonly observed on parts of the body accessible to the right hand, i.e., right side of the face, neck, anterior trunk, anterior surface of left arm. They are multiple, sharply outlined, appear at variable intervals of time, and do not conform to any of the standard dermatologic diseases. They resist all treatment until protected from the persistent manipulations of the patient, and then they heal promptly.

HYSTERIA IN MEN (COMPENSATION NEUROSIS IN MEN AND WOMEN)

As stated before, hysterical symptoms do occur in men, most often in those trying to avoid legal difficulties or

military service, or to obtain disability payments, veteran's pensions, or compensation following injury. Male sociopaths may also present with this type of illness. Unless such a factor is present, the diagnosis of hysteria in the male should be made with great caution. In compensation neurosis, as in the classic form of hysteria, multiple symptoms are often noted; in the majority of cases; furthermore, many of the symptoms are the same as those listed under female hysteria. Or, the patient may be monosymptomatic (e.g., "seizures"), and the symptoms, particularly chronic pain, may be confined to the neck, head, arm, or low back. The description of symptoms tends to be lengthy and circumstantial, and the patient fails to give details that are necessary for diagnosis. A tangible gain from the illness may be discovered by simple questioning. In civilian life, this is usually in the form of monetary compensation, which, surprisingly, is often less than the patient could earn if he returned to work. Another interesting feature is the frequency with which the patient expresses extreme dissatisfaction with the medical care given him; he is often hostile toward the physicians and nurses. Many of these patients have already been subjected to an excessive number of hospitalizations, and rather dramatic mishaps have allegedly occurred in carrying out diagnostic and therapeutic procedures. The majority of these patients have been suspected and many have been accused of malingering in the past, which may be responsible for the aggressive behavior and resentful attitude of some of them.

Women who suffer injury at work or are involved in auto accidents may exhibit the same symptoms and signs.

ETIOLOGY AND PATHOGENESIS

The theorization of psychoanalysts, that the etiology of both conversion and dissociative symptoms are based on particular psychodynamic mechanisms, is impossible for the authors to affirm or refute. Sociologic and educational factors are probably important for it is generally agreed that hysterical women as a group are less intelligent and less educated than nonhysterical women. A genetic causation must also be considered. Family studies have disclosed that about 20 percent of first degree relatives of female hysterics have the same illness, an incidence ten times that in the general population. This supports the idea that hysteria is a disease (see Goodwin and Guze).

As pointed out by Carothers and by Guze and his colleagues, hysteria and psychopathy (or sociopathy as it is now called) are closely related. Hysteria is the disease of women and sociopathy, mainly of men. This relationship is supported by family studies. First-degree male relatives of hysterical women have an increased incidence of sociopathy and alcoholism; first-degree female relatives of convicted male felons show an increased prevalence of hysteria. Moreover, careful histories of sociopathic girls reveal that many of them develop the full syndrome of hysteria. Women felons often present a mixed picture of hysteria and sociopathy, according to Cloninger and Guze.

DIAGNOSIS

The method of diagnosis subject to the least error is that employed in medicine generally, i.e., obtaining an informative history (from the patient as well as from sources other than the patient) and performing a physical and mental status examination. The characteristic time of onset, the longitudinal history of recurrent multiple complaints, as outlined above, the manner and attitude of the patient, and the absence of symptoms and signs of other medical and surgical disease will permit an accurate diagnosis in the majority of cases.

So-called projective tests (Rorschach and Thematic Apperception Tests), which for a time were popular with dynamic psychiatrists, are not useful in diagnosis and are now used very little. Evidence of extreme suggestibility and the tendency to dramatize symptoms cannot be taken as absolute criteria of the disease, for they appear under certain conditions in individuals who never develop hysteria.

TREATMENT

The treatment of hysteria may be considered from two aspects—the correction of the long-standing basic personality defect, and the removal of the recently acquired physical symptoms. Little or nothing can be done about the former. Psychoanalysts have attempted to modify it by long-term re-education, but their results are unavailable, and there are no control studies for the few reports of therapeutic success. One has the impression that in most cases the underlying illness is so pervasive and so rooted in a personality disorder that nothing can be accomplished except to grant that the patient is inadequate in certain respects and requires medical support. Many psychiatrists, for this reason, are inclined to regard the female hysteric with a lifelong history of ill health as having a severe personality disorder i.e., a psychopathy (see below). In other less-severe cases and especially in those in whom hysterical symptoms have appeared under the pressure of a major crisis, explanatory and supportive psychotherapy appears to be helpful, and the patients have been able thereafter to resume their places in society.

The acute symptoms can usually be controlled by persuasion. Here the best tactic is to treat the patient as though she has had an illness and is now in the process of recovering. The earlier this is done after the development of symptoms, the more likely they are to be relieved. In chronically bedridden patients, strong pressure to get out of bed and resume function must be applied. Compensation and litigation neuroses are quite difficult to treat, and settlement of the patient's claim (''the green poultice'') is usually necessary before the symptoms subside.

The following therapeutic principles should be observed in the classic cases of female hysteria:

1. Hysteria must be treated as a tangible, definite illness. The patient should not be told, ''There is nothing wrong with you,'' or ''It's just your imagination,'' or ''your nerves.'' This at once alienates her, and she almost invariably terminates her relations with the physician. The patient should not be dismissed as a malingerer or a faker of illness.

2. Simple understandable language should be employed in interviews with these patients; abstruse psychologic terms should be avoided. It is unnecessary to employ the term *hysteria* in discussions with these patients or their families, since it has a derogatory connotation which the physician should not imply.

3. The care of the patient should be entrusted to one physician.

4. All indicated examinations and laboratory procedures for the investigation of the chief complaints should be conducted before actual treatment is begun. Once treatment is started, one should avoid, if possible, checking or repeating physical or laboratory examinations.

5. Persuasion and suggestion, both direct and indirect, should be employed. Illustratively, the patient should be repeatedly encouraged, told that she is improving, urged to resume work or household duties and to continue participation in routine activities. Medication should be withheld.

6. There should be several interviews in which the patient is permitted to direct the discussion. She should be assured of the privacy of the interview, of the impersonal, ''morally neutral'' position of the physician, and of the advantages of ''thinking things out more thoroughly.'' Any questions that the patient asks should be answered truthfully, in accordance with the physician's knowledge, in simple, direct terms.

7. Every illness in such patients should be evaluated objectively, so as not to overlook any medical or surgical disease, which may strike a hysterical patient just as it does any other person. Surgical procedures should be used only if strict criteria of surgery-requiring disease are satisfied.

How successful this program will be over a long period of time is not known. The eradication of some recently acquired hysterical symptom is relatively easy. The real test of therapy, however, is whether it enables the patient to adjust satisfactorily to family and society and to perform daily activities effectively, and whether it prevents addiction, unnecessary medical treatments, and operations.

HYPOCHONDRIASIS AND NEUROTIC DEPRESSION

Hypochondriasis (hypochondriacal neurosis) is the morbid preoccupation with bodily functions or physical signs and sensations, leading to the fear or belief of having serious disease. Typically, hypochondriacal symptoms occur in association with other neurotic, psychiatric, and organic syndromes, and many psychiatrists have questioned its status as a nosologic entity. Some psychiatrists still speak of the rigid, obsessive, *hypochondriacal personality,* in which concern for health and relationships with physicians are involved in chronic patterns of maladaptation, and of *hypochondriacal neurosis,* which is a decompensation from a healthier, more mature level of adjustment. Unlike hysterical neurosis and psychophysiologic disorders, in which there also may be morbid preoccupations with physical processes, this neurosis entails no disorder of bodily function. These and other features of hypochondriasis are discussed further on in this chapter.

Also, there is dispute about the existence of *neurotic depression* (depressive neurosis; dysthymic disorder) as a diagnostic entity. That disagreement about this category of illness should exist is not surprising, considering the number of private meanings that are attached to it (see also Chap. 56). A review of some of the writings on this subject discloses that neurotic depression has been distinguished from endogenous depression on the basis of the following criteria: (1) patients with endogenous depressions recover spontaneously, or in response to electroshock or antidepressive drug treatment, in contrast to those with neurotic depressions; (2) patients with endogenous depressions suffer guilt and remorse, whereas the neurotics tend to blame others for their distress; (3) absence of diurnal variation of mood in neurotic depressions, and of insight in endogenous depression; (4) certain differences in heredity, body build, and premorbid personality; and (5) absence of psychotic symptoms (delusions, hallucinations, etc.) in neurotic depression.

Certainly not all psychiatrists agree that a valid distinction exists between the psychotic and neurotic forms of depression. Aubrey Lewis, on the basis of a detailed study of 61 hospitalized depressed patients, denied that any of the foregoing criteria had any differentiating significance.

THE PSYCHOPATHIES AND SEXUAL PERVERSIONS

ANTISOCIAL PERSONALITY (SOCIOPATHY)

Of all the abnormal personality types listed in Table 55-1, the antisocial is the best defined and the one most likely to cause trouble in the family and community. Formerly sociopathy was referred to as psychopathic personality, constitutional psychopathy, and chronic psychopathic inferiority, and was defined as a state in which the individual "is always in trouble, profiting not from experience or punishment, unable to empathize with family or friends or to maintain loyalties to any person, group or code. He is likely to be shallow, callous, and hedonistic, showing marked emotional immaturity with lack of sense of responsibility, lack of judgment, and an ability to rationalize his behavior so that it appears warranted, reasonable and justified." Also included under this heading were certain instances of sexual deviation and of addiction.

Since Prichard first described this condition under the term *moral insanity* in the mid-nineteenth century, there have been many attempts to give it a more precise definition and to avoid using it as a psychiatric wastebasket. At the turn of the century, Koch introduced the term *psychopathic inferiority,* implying that deviations in personality were constitutionally determined. Later the term *psychopathic personality* came into common use. Some authors used this last term indiscriminately to embrace all forms of deviant personalities; others used it in a more restricted sense to define a subgroup of antisocial or aggressive psychopaths. To reduce confusion, the American Psychiatric Association has adopted the term *antisocial personality disorder* to refer to the aggressive or antisocial psychopath. Aubrey Lewis has given a lucid account of the history of the concept of sociopathy.

By far the best modern study of sociopathy is that of L. N. Robins, based on a 30-year follow-up study of 524 cases from a child guidance clinic and 100 controls. Other investigations of note are those of Ehrlich and Keough, who studied 50 patients with sociopathy in a mental hospital, and of Guze et al who studied psychiatric illness in large numbers of felons and their first-degree relatives. The descriptions that follow are taken largely from these writings and those of Reid.

Clinical State This condition, unlike most psychiatric disorders, is manifest by the age of 12 to 15 years, and frequently earlier. It consists essentially of deviant behavior in which individuals seem driven to make trouble in everything they do. Every code imposed by family, school, church, and society is broken. Seemingly the sociopath acts on impulse, but after committing the unsocial act, shows no remorse. The most frequent antisocial activities are theft, incorrigibility, truancy, running away overnight, associating with undesirable characters, staying out late, indiscriminate sexual relations, physical aggression or assault, recklessness and impulsivity, lying without cause, vandalism, abuse of drugs and alcohol and later, inability to work steadily or keep a job. In children or adolescents who exhibited 10 or more of these antisocial symptoms, 43 percent were classed as sociopaths in adulthood. If only 8 or 9 of these traits were present, 29 percent were so classed; if 6 or 7, 25 percent; and 3 to 5, only 15 percent. Conversely, not a single adult sociopath was observed who did not manifest antisocial symptoms in earlier life. Interestingly, a number of other problems of childhood and adolescence, such as enuresis, dirty appearance, sleep walking, irritability, nail biting, oversensitivity, poor eating habits, nervousness, being withdrawn or seclusive, unhappiness, tics, and fears were not predictive of adult sociopathy. None of Robins' patients was mentally defective.

As noted above, more than half the deviant children in Robins' study (even those with 10 or more antisocial manifestations) had lost most of their sociopathic traits by adulthood. This does not mean that they remained psychiatrically normal, however. Of those who did not become adult sociopaths, the large majority developed other adult psychiatric illnesses, particularly addiction to alcohol. Only in the group of children with less than three antisocial symptoms did a reasonable number (one-third) remain well in adult life. Because sociopathic behavior in children may terminate spontaneously or evolve into other disorders, it is advised (in DSM III) that the diagnosis of antisocial personality disorder be reserved for adults; the same behavior pattern in children is designated as *conduct disorder.*

Robins' criteria for making the diagnosis of adult sociopathy were persistent disturbances in at least five of the following so-called life areas—poor work record, marital difficulties, inability to function as a responsible parent, financial irresponsibility and dependency, illegal occupations, multiple arrests, abuse of alcohol, sexual promiscuity, vagrancy, leading a "wild life," social isolation, disciplinary problems in the Armed Forces, lack of guilt, more than nine somatic complaints or a complaint of medical disability, use of aliases, pathologic lying, recklessness, aggressiveness and belligerency, and suicide attempts. These findings in the adult were the same, whether the patients were drawn from the community at large (only 12 percent of Robins' adult sociopaths were in prison at the time of their follow-up examination), from a mental hospital,

or from a group of prisoners (or parolees or probationers). Furthermore, in each of these groups of adult sociopaths, the manifestations of antisocial behavior in childhood were much the same.

Also of interest are Robins' findings that sociopaths show an unusually high incidence of "conversion" symptoms, as well as depressive symptoms and anxiety, and that the neurotic symptoms are in proportion to the sociopathic ones, i.e., the larger the number of antisocial manifestations, the larger the number of neurotic symptoms or the greater the disability from them. These latter symptoms and many other somatic complaints frequently bring the sociopath to the attention of the physician.

The manifestations of sociopathic behavior in children and adults were five to ten times more frequent in the male than the female. Among the latter there was a high incidence of hysterical manifestations, which suggests that female hysteria may be the counterpart of male sociopathy. A search for evidence of encephalitis, often postulated as the basis of sociopathy, was not revealing; Robins could elicit no proof of other brain damage. It has been shown that EEG abnormalities, taking the form of mild to moderate bilateral slowing, are more frequent in criminals and sociopaths than in the normal population. Furthermore the biologic parents of sociopaths also show a higher frequency of such EEG abnormalities than the general population. These and other findings suggest that there may be a genetic predisposition to antisocial personality. More direct evidence of a genetic factor has been provided by Cadoret's studies of adoptees who were separated at birth from antisocial biologic parents; later observations disclosed a higher incidence of antisocial behavior in the adoptees than in controls. Cadoret's study also suggested that childhood hyperactivity and female hysteria (Briquet disease) were phenotypic manifestations of the antisocial personality genotype. The presence of a chromosomal abnormality, e.g., XYY, which has been found in a small number of sex deviants, has not been studied in a controlled manner in sociopaths.

Surveys of the families of sociopaths have also disclosed a high incidence of broken homes, alcoholism, and poverty. Two factors that seem most closely related to the development of sociopathy are a lack of parental discipline and having an antisocial or alcoholic father. However, as Robins' study has shown, if any of these factors are causal, then they must be mediated through the occurrence of deviant behavior in childhood. In the absence of the latter, broken homes, slum neighborhoods, etc., do not lead to adult sociopathy.

Cadoret and his colleagues have presented convincing evidence for gene-environment interaction in the development of adolescent antisocial behavior. They analyzed data from three large adoption studies and found a significant increase in antisocial behaviors when both a genetic factor and an adverse environmental factor were present; the increase with both factors acting together was much greater than the predicted increase from either factor acting alone.

Prognosis This is of interest for several reasons. The relation between deviant behavior in childhood and adolescence and the development of sociopathy and other psychiatric illnesses in adult life has already been discussed. In addition it should be noted that in adult sociopaths, improvement of gross antisocial behavior is possible, occurring in somewhat more than a third of such individuals. Improvement occurs most frequently between the ages of 30 and 40 years (median age 35). This bears out the Gluecks' contention that repetitive criminality diminishes with age. Improvement of sociopathic behavior does not necessarily mean that these individuals have become well-adjusted, but that they have married and are maintaining a home and working. Probably maturation, marriage, assumption of family responsibilities, and fear of imprisonment are the main stabilizing forces; at least these are the ones proffered by sociopaths to explain their improvement.

There is no information as to the best methods of *treatment*. Most psychiatrists have been discouraged by the results of psychotherapy, but whether behavioral therapy, psychoanalysis, or drugs have more to offer cannot be determined from available data.

MALINGERING

This problem arises frequently in connection with both hysteria and sociopathy, and the physician should know how to deal with it. It is not a medical diagnosis, except under the rare circumstances in which a patient is caught in the act of producing a sign of disease or confesses to have done so. The term *malingering* refers to the *conscious and deliberate feigning of illness or disability in order to attain a desired goal*. It does not occur as an isolated phenomenon, and its occurrence must be interpreted as a sign of a serious personality disturbance, often one that prevents effective work or military service, though noteworthy exceptions to this statement can be found.

Certainly there is a close similarity between hysteria and malingering, but the nature of the relationship is nebulous, and there may be great difficulty in establishing a clinical differentiation. As Jones and Llewellyn have observed: "Nothing . . . resembles malingering more than hysteria; nothing, hysteria more than malingering. In both alike we are confronted with the same discrepancy between fact and statement, objective sign and subjective symptom—the outward aspect of health seemingly giving the lie to all the alleged functional disabilities. We may examine the hysterical person and the malingerer, using the same tests, and get precisely the same results in one case as the other."

Most authors cite the following as the main points of difference between the two conditions:

1. The conscious or unconscious quality of the motivation, which always seems more unconscious in the hysteric and more conscious in the malingerer.

2. The influence of persuasion, which is usually effective in hysteria and not in the malingerer.

3. The attitude of the patient. The hysteric appears more genuinely ill and invites examination; the malingerer seems less ill and evades examination.

The tendency of the sociopath to malinger has already been mentioned. Most of the more obvious cases of malingering seen by the authors have been in sociopaths, for which reason comments on the two conditions have been juxtaposed.

In the malingerer one observes pain, hyperesthesia, anesthesia, limping gait, tremor, contracture, paralysis, amaurosis, deafness, stuttering, mutism, amnesia, epileptiform seizures and fugues, unexplained gastrointestinal bleeding, and unexplained skin lesions—in short, the same array of symptoms and signs, singly or in combination, as in the patients with compensation hysteria. A particular form of sociopathy or malingering, which consists essentially of deceiving the medical profession, has been described under the title of *Munchausen's syndrome*—named, not altogether aptly, after a seventeenth century German soldier, Baron von Münchhausen, who invented incredible tales of adventure and daring. Ireland et al, who analyzed 59 well-documented cases (45 men, 14 women), list the following characteristic features, which will be recognized at once by all neurologists with extensive hospital experience: feigned severe illness of a dramatic and emergency nature; factitious evidence of disease, surreptitiously produced by interference with diagnostic procedures or by self-mutilation; a history of many hospitalizations (sometimes more than a hundred), extensive travel, or visits to innumerable physicians; evidence of laparotomy scars and cranial burr holes; pathologic lying; aggressive, unruly, evasive behavior; and, finally, departure from the hospital against medical advice. Unlike the usual forms of compensation hysteria, an ulterior motive is not readily discernible. The psychopathology of this syndrome is quite obscure. It has been regarded as a form of sociopathy, malingering, and compensation hysteria, but the distinctions between them are too ambiguous to be of clinical value. Probably the medical profession has placed too great a reliance on degree of conscious awareness of deception. In such unstable and immature individuals, the terms *conscious, unconscious,* and *deception* are too vague and subjective to serve as useful guides in practical work.

INTERMITTENT EXPLOSIVE DISORDER

From time to time one is confronted by and asked to express a medical opinion about a patient who is uncontrollably aggressive and violent. Some patients have suffered head injuries or other serious brain diseases in the past that have left them handicapped in a number of ways, but their rages and explosive aggressivity make their rehabilitation impossible. Elliott, in a review of what is called the *episodic dyscontrol syndrome,* describes a group of patients who manifest outbursts of verbal and physical violence on a background of seemingly normal personality. However, further study in most instances did reveal some type of "organic brain syndrome." This condition should be set apart from behavioral abnormalities associated with mental retardation, schizophrenia, drug addictions, and alcoholism. Its most characteristic feature is the repetitive, unpredictable episodic violent behavior out of proportion to the provoking situation. Some are subject to seizure disorders, particularly temporal lobe epilepsy, which is not excluded by a normal EEG. These cases aside, the authors believe that most instances of explosive disorder represent a variant of the sociopathy described above. Elliott and Jenkins et al report a beneficial effect of propranolol. Others find lithium, carbamazepine, and phenytoin to be helpful in controlling attacks.

SEXUAL PERVERSIONS

Although sexual perversions are usually included in the section on neurosis or sociopathy in most textbooks of psychiatry, it is a mistake to assume that every sexually perverse individual is neurotic or psychopathic, a position emphasized by Kinsey et al. Some psychiatrists would define any sexual activity that does not lead to reproduction as perverse, but this would place even masturbation and sexual intercourse with contraceptives in this category. Yet all would agree that unusual sexual practices, which become ends in themselves, are deviant in western society.

Much has been written in the psychoanalytic literature about the physiologic development of the sexual instinct from childhood to adult life, and arrests of development are one way of looking at some of the sexual aberrations described below.

Psychosexual Disorders Included under this heading are a variety of psychologically determined sexual deviations, the most common of which are (1) *transsexualism* (the wish to be rid of one's own genitalia and live as a member of the other sex) and (2) *paraphilias* or what were formerly referred to as *sexual deviations.* Included in this latter category are *fetishism* (the use of nonliving objects to achieve sexual excitement); *transvestism* (habitual dressing in the clothes of the opposite sex); zoophilia; pedophilia; exhibitionism; voyeurism; sexual masochism and sadism. These represent special problems rarely encountered by the neurologist, and will not be included here for these reasons. The reader seeking information on these subjects is referred to Kolb's *Modern Clinical Psychiatry* and Meyer's chapter on the paraphilias in the *Comprehensive Textbook of Psychiatry.*

ALCOHOL AND DRUG ADDICTION

These are unquestionably associated with sociopathy, as indicated in the above pages, but they also represent special problems of immense proportions and are therefore discussed in Chaps. 41 and 42.

HOMOSEXUALITY

The homosexual is one who is motivated in adult life by a preferential erotic attraction to members of the same sex. He or she may or may not engage in overt sexual relations with them. Most psychiatrists exclude from the definition of homosexuality those patterns of behavior that are not motivated by specific preferential desire, such as incidental homosexuality of adolescents and the situational homosexuality of prisoners and sailors.

Figures on incidence are difficult to secure. According to the Kinsey reports, approximately 4 percent of American males are exclusively homosexual and up to 10 percent have been "more or less exclusively homosexual for at least three years sometime between the ages of 16 and 65." They report that at least 37 percent of the male population has had overt homosexual experiences sometime between puberty and old age. For females the incidence is lower, perhaps half that for males, and approximately 28 percent have had at some time in their life a homosexual experience. It has been estimated, on the basis of the examination of large numbers of military personnel during World War II, that 1 to 2 percent of male adults are exclusively or predominantly homosexual.

Two main types of male homosexual are recognized. One is exclusively homosexual, functioning in a homosexual ("gay") society and forming strong emotional and social relationships only with other homosexuals. A second type lives in the heterosexual world and may be married and have children; his homosexual activities are intermittent and carried on in secrecy. The first type may be effeminate, with delicate gestures and suggestive gait, special modes of dress, etc., but many in this group do not conform to an effeminate stereotype. The second type may be overtly masculine in his ways and manners; few, if any, are recognizable as homosexuals.

The origins of homosexuality are obscure. We favor the hypothesis that an abnormality of genetic patterning of the immature nervous system (hypothalamus) sets the pattern during early life. A variant of this idea was advanced by Lang—that the constitutional homosexual is an "intersex," by which he meant that the individual was morphologically of one sex but genetically of the other. The intersex could be due to an abnormal balance between genes of the two sexes. A genetic factor is strongly supported by the observations of Kallman that if one of a pair of uniovular twins was homosexual, the other was invariably concordant.

Freudian theory postulates an arrest at or a regression to the earliest ("narcissistic" or "autoerotic") phase in the sexual development of the child. Others postulate that homosexuality is determined by adverse parental attitudes, influence of a dominant aggressive mother on the male homosexual, lack of heterosexual opportunities, and traumatic sexual experiences. All are unsubstantiated. Attempts to show an endocrine basis for homosexuality have also failed.

The most widely held current view is that homosexuality is not a mental or a personality disturbance, though it may at times lead to secondary reactive neurotic or psychotic states (Ross and Talikka). A study by the Kinsey Institute for Sex Research indicates that a homosexual orientation cannot be traced to a single social or psychologic root. Instead, homosexuality seems to arise from a deep-seated predisposition, probably biologic in origin, and as deeply ingrained as heterosexuality.

From the medical point of view it is important to know the types of problems faced by the homosexual. The male homosexual may have few stable relationships, even with other homosexuals, and may spend a great deal of time seeking sexual satisfaction ("cruising"), becoming involved in chance situations which may expose him to robbery, injuries of various sorts, venereal and other diseases (e.g., AIDS, page 612), and blackmail. The female homosexual is less likely to attract notice and tends usually to form a stable relationship with another woman. Female and particularly male homosexuals exhibit a high incidence of neurotic symptoms, especially those of anxiety and depression and benefit from supportive psychotherapy and the medications commonly used to allay these symptoms. Endocrine therapy and psychotropic drugs are not recommended for homosexuality. Other methods of treatment are discouraging, although Bieber et al has claimed a modicum of success, using psychoanalysis.

REFERENCES

BAYER R: *Homosexuality and American Psychiatry. The Politics of Diagnosis.* Basic Books, 1981.

BERG I: School phobia in children of agoraphobic women. *Br J Psychiat* 128:86, 1976.

BIEBER I, DAIN HJ, DINCE PR et al: *Homosexuality: A Psychoanalytic Study.* New York, Basic Books, 1962.

BRIQUET P: *Traité clinique et therapeutique à l'hystérie.* Paris, J-B Ballière et Fils, 1859.

CADORET RJ: Psychopathology in adopted-away offspring of biologic parents with antisocial behavior. *Arch Gen Psychiatry* 35:176, 1978.

CADORET RJ, CAIN C, CROWE RR: Evidence for gene-environment interaction in the development of adolescent antisocial behavior. *Behavior Genetics* 13:301, 1983.

Diagnostic and Statistical Manual of Mental Disorders (DSM III). Washington, American Psychiatric Association, 1980.

CAROTHERS JC: Hysteria, psychopathy and the magic word. *The Mankind Quarterly* 16:93, 1975.

CLONINGER CR, GUZE SB: Psychiatric illness and female criminality: The role of sociopathy and hysteria in antisocial woman. *Am J Psychiatry* 127:303, 1970.

COHEN ME, WHITE PD: Life situations, emotions, and neuro-circulatory asthenia (anxiety neurosis, neurasthenia, effort syndrome). *Proc Assoc Res Nerv Ment Dis* 29:832, 1950.

COHEN ME, WHITE PD, JOHNSON RE: Neurocirculatory asthenia, anxiety neurosis or the effort syndrome. *Arch Intern Med* 81:260, 1948.

EASTON JD, SHERMAN DG: Somatic anxiety attacks and propranolol. *Arch Neurol* 33:689, 1976.

EHRLICH SK, KEOUGH RP: The psychopath in a mental institution. *Arch Neurol Psychiatry* 76:286, 1956.

ELLIOTT FA: Propranolol for the control of belligerent behavior following acute brain damage. *Ann Neurol* 1:489, 1977.

GLUECK S, GLUECK E: *Criminal Careers in Retrospect.* New York, Commonwealth Fund, 1943.

GOODWIN DW, GUZE SB: *Psychiatric Diagnosis,* 3rd ed. New York, Oxford University Press, 1984.

GUZE S: The role of follow-up studies. The contribution to diagnostic classification as applied to hysteria. *Semin Psychiatry* 2:392, 1970.

GUZE SB, GOODWIN DW, CRANE JB: Criminal recidivism and psychiatric illness. *Am J Psychiatry* 127:832, 1970.

INSEL TR (ed): *New Findings in Obsessive-Compulsive Disorders.* Washington, D.C., American Psychiatric Press, 1984.

IRELAND P, SAPIRA JD, TEMPLETON B: Munchausen's Syndrome. *Am J Med* 43:579, 1967.

JENKINS SC, MARUTA T: Therapeutic use of propranolol for intermittent explosive disorders. *Mayo Clin Proc* 62:204, 1987.

JONES AB, LLEWELLYN LJ: *Malingering.* Philadelphia, Lippincott, 1918.

KALLMAN FJ: *Heredity in Health and Mental Disorder.* New York, Norton, 1953.

KINSEY A, POMEROY W, MARTIN C, GEBHARD P: *Sexual Behavior in the Human Female.* Philadelphia, Saunders, 1948.

KINSEY A, POMEROY W, MARTIN C: *Sexual Behavior in the Human Male.* Philadelphia, Saunders, 1948.

KOLB LC: *Modern Clinical Psychiatry,* 9th ed. Philadelphia, Saunders, 1977.

LANG T: Genetic determination of homosexuality. *J Nerv Ment Dis* 92:55, 1948.

LEWIS A: Psychopathic personality: A most elusive category. *Psychol Med* 4:133, 1974.

LEWIS A: Melancholia: A clinical survey of depressive states. *J Ment Sci* 80:277, 1934.

MATUZAS W, GLASS RM: Treatment of agoraphobia and panic attacks. *Arch Gen Psychiatry* 40:220, 1983.

MEYER JK: Paraphilias, in Kaplan HI and Sadock BJ (eds): *Comprehensive Textbook of Psychiatry,* 4th ed. Baltimore, Williams & Wilkins, 1985, chap 23.5, pp 1065–1077.

MODLIN HC: Postaccident anxiety syndrome: Psychosocial aspects. *Am J Psychiatry* 123:1008, 1967.

NEMIAH JC: Neurotic disorders, in Kaplan HI and Sadock BJ (eds): *Comprehensive Textbook of Psychiatry,* 4th ed. Baltimore, Williams & Wilkins, 1985, chap 20, pp 883–957.

PEROUTKA SJ: The selection of anxiolytics in clinical neurology, in Plum F (ed): *Advances in Contemporary Neurology.* Philadelphia, Davis, 1988, chap 4.

PITTS FN, McCLURE JN: Lactate metabolism in anxiety neurosis. *N Engl J Med* 277:1329, 1967.

POLLITT J: Natural history of obsessional states. *Br Med J* 1:194, 1957.

PURTELL JJ, ROBBINS E, COHEN ME: Observations on clinical aspects of hysteria. *JAMA* 146:902, 1951.

REID WH (ed.): *The Psychopath: A Comprehensive Study of Antisocial Disorders and Behaviors.* New York, Brunner-Mazel, 1978.

ROBINS LN: *Deviant Children Grown Up: A Sociological and Psychiatric Study of Sociopathic Personality.* Huntington, NY, Krieger, 1974.

ROBINS E, PURTELL JJ, COHEN ME: Hysteria in men. *N Engl J Med* 246:677, 1952.

ROSENBAUM JF: Current concepts in psychiatry. *N Engl J Med* 36:401, 1982.

ROSS MW, TALIKKA A: Homosexual labelling and cultural control: The role of psychiatry. *Psychiatr Opinion* 16:31, 1979.

SLATER E: A heuristic theory of neurosis. *J Neurol Neurosurg Psychiatry* 7:48, 1944.

SLATER B, SHIELDS J: Genetical aspects of anxiety, in Lader MH (ed): *Studies of Anxiety.* London, Royal Medico-Psychological Association, 1969, pp 62–71.

TYRER P: Classification of anxiety. *Br J Psychiatry* 144:78, 1984.

VAILLANT GE, PERRY JC: Personality disorders, in Kaplan HI and Sadock BJ (eds): *Comprehensive Textbook of Psychiatry,* 4th ed. Baltimore, Williams & Wilkins, 1985, chap 21, pp 958–986.

VON KORFF M, EATON W, KEYL P: The epidemiology of panic attacks and panic disorder. *Am J Epidemiol* 122:970, 1985.

WESTPHAL C: Die Agoraphobie: Eine neuropathische Erscheinung. *Arch Psychiat Nervenkr* 3:138; 219, 1871–1872.

WHEELER EO, WHITE PD, REED EW, COHEN ME: Neurocirculatory asthenia (anxiety neurosis, effort syndrome, neurasthenia): A twenty year follow-up study of one hundred and seventy-three patients. *JAMA* 142:878, 1950.

WINOKUR G, CLAYTON PJ, REICH T: *Manic Depressive Illness.* St. Louis, Mosby, 1969.

WINOKUR G, CROWE RR: Personality disorders, in Freedman AM et al (eds): *Comprehensive Textbook of Psychiatry,* 2nd ed. Baltimore, Williams & Wilkins, 1975, chap 22-1, pp 1279–1297.

WOLPE J: *Psychotherapy by Reciprocal Inhibition.* Stanford, CA, Stanford University Press. 1958.

CHAPTER 56

GRIEF, REACTIVE DEPRESSION, ENDOGENOUS DEPRESSION, MANIC-DEPRESSIVE DISEASE, AND HYPOCHONDRIASIS

In clinical medicine, there are four major categories of psychosis: (1) the confusional-delirious states; (2) the psychoses associated with focal or multifocal cerebral lesions; (3) the affective disorders (manic-depressive and depressive psychoses); and (4) the schizophrenias. The first two categories are discussed in Chaps. 19 and 21. The latter two groups make up the subject matter of this and the following chapter.

Depression is the cause of more human grief and misery than any other single disease to which humankind is subject. This statement is taken from an article by Kline, an authority on the subject, and is shared by everyone in the field of mental health. Although it has been known for over 2000 years (melancholia is described in the writings of Hippocrates), there is still disagreement as to its medical status. Is depression a disease state (kraepelinian concept), or a type of psychologic reaction (meyerian concept)? In other words, is it basically a biologic derangement or a response to stress and conflict with which a person cannot cope?

Before elaborating on this problem, a few words are necessary to explain the grouping of entities listed in the title of this chapter. A depressed or dysphoric mood is the symptom that relates all of them, but the setting in which the depression occurs, differences in certain clinical attributes, and the fact that each requires somewhat different management permit the recognition of a number of distinctive clinical states. Taken together, they are the most frequent of all psychiatric illnesses. At the New England Center Hospital (a tertiary referral center), as indicated on page 1188, they accounted for an estimated 50 percent of psychiatric and 12 percent of all medical admissions. Grief reactions are ubiquitous, but only exceptionally do they require hospitalization.

Depressive states are so often associated with obscure physical symptoms that they are more likely to come to the attention of general physicians and internists than are other psychiatric entities. Moreover, they are frequently misdiagnosed, the symptoms being mistakenly attributed to anemia, low blood pressure, hypothyroidism, migraine, tension headaches, chronic pain syndrome, chronic infection, emotional problems, worry, stress and "nerves." Another reason why physicians should be knowledgeable about depressive illnesses is the danger of suicide, which may be attempted and successfully executed before the depression is recognized. Timely diagnosis may prevent such a tragedy—one that is all the more regrettable since most depressive illnesses can be successfully treated.

NOSOLOGY AND CLASSIFICATION

As remarked in Chap. 24, the term *depression* embraces more than a feeling of sadness and unhappiness. It stands for a complex of disturbed feelings (affect), particularly of hopelessness and loss of self-esteem, associated with decreased energy and libido, abnormalities of thinking and behavior, and prominent physical complaints, the most important of which are insomnia, anorexia, headache, and other types of regional pain. At one extreme are depressive symptoms of psychotic proportions (i.e., these include paranoid or somatic delusions), which create chaos in the life of the patient and anyone close to the patient. At the other extreme are the common feelings of unhappiness, discouragement, and resentment that occur in almost everyone as a reaction to the disappointments of everyday life, such as loss of employment, a failure to gain recognition, or unsuccessful sexual or social adjustment, and which are closely linked in their duration to the persistence of the precipitant factor(s).

Some illnesses in this group, also spoken of as the *affective disorders*, take the form of a relatively pure, uncomplicated depression; others are mixed with anxiety and agitation. Because of an apparent tendency to appear for the first time in middle and late adult life, the latter syndrome has in the past been referred to as *involutional melancholia*. This term takes license with the concept of involution, for such an illness may occur at any time in adult life and have no relationship to the climacteric (Winokur and Cadoret). Some depressions are clearly reactions to real and imaginary life situations. If in proximate relation to the loss of a family member, the condition is called *grief*; if in relation to a life-threatening or disabling medical or neurologic disorder, it is referred to as *induced* or *reactive depression*. As indicated in the preceding chapter, depression may complicate phobic and obsessive-compulsive states and even hysteria; in a sense the depression in these circumstances is also secondary or reactive. Then there are depressions that present as *hypochondriasis*; although the latter psychiatric syndrome may rarely occur as a protracted and obstinate neurosis, the presence of an underlying depression must always be considered when assessing a hypochondriacal patient. *Mania*, which is less frequent than depression, may develop as a relatively pure clinical state, or it may alternate or be intertwined with depression in manic-depressive disease. Lastly, depression may masquerade as a chronic pain, a chronic fatigue state, or some other medical condition; this has been called ''masked depression'' or ''depressive equivalent'' by Pichot and Hassan. In the following pages the *masked depression* as a diagnostic puzzle will be emphasized.

Since *grief* is the most common form of depression that the physician is likely to encounter, it is well to begin our discussion with the contemporary view of this depressive syndrome. Some psychiatrists have suggested that grief is the prototype of all depressive states; others question whether depression and grief are the same process. One school of thought, that of Adolf Meyer and his followers, regards depression as a continuum, with sadness and disappointment at one end and psychotic depressions at the other. The other (kraepelinian) view holds that depression is a disease process, quite independent of social and psychologic forces in the patient's life and that the cause of the illness is ''innate.'' These two disparate concepts are not irreconcilable. An eclectic position is that both are correct—i.e., that there are two basic forms of depression: *exogenous* and *endogenous*. Exogenous (or reactive) depressions have an overt external cause, such as a loss of a loved one, loss of one's fortune or position, or a disabling or life-threatening illness. In this framework, grief would exemplify a reactive or exogenous depression. In contrast, the endogenous

depressions have no apparent external cause; they seem to occur in susceptible individuals as a response to some unknown biologic stimulus. In respect to endogenous depression and manic-depressive psychosis, the genetic data cited further on support the kraepelinian view.

Another semantic problem relates to the differences between grief reaction, reactive depression, and psychoneurotic depression. All three are, in a sense, exogenous or reactive. For reasons to be elaborated, the authors distinguish between these three depressive syndromes; we believe these distinctions to be of therapeutic importance.

There are four main depressive illnesses with which the physician should be acquainted:

1. Grief reaction.

2. Reactive or secondary depression in relation to medical and neurologic diseases.

3. Depression in relation to neurosis.

4. Endogenous or primary depression (with or without agitation and anxiety) and manic-depressive disease.

GRIEF REACTIONS

Grieving is a response to a loss, which may be real (as in the death of a spouse) or, in the opinion of some psychiatrists, symbolized. Psychologic analysis of the typical grief reaction discloses the following characteristics (Lindemann):

1. An intense subjective sensation of mental pain accompanied by a feeling of exhaustion.

2. Preoccupation with the image of the deceased.

3. A sense of guilt concerning the relationship to the deceased.

4. Sometimes an inexplicable and unwarranted hostility toward friends and relatives.

5. A loss of the usual pattern of conduct. Bereaved persons are unable either to initiate or to organize their daily affairs and tend to perform routine tasks in an automatic and uninterested fashion.

The authors cannot vouch for the validity of each of these characteristics, especially 3 and 4, but accept them as a reasonable formulation. There is no doubt, however, that a sense of exhaustion and disorganization of daily activities are invariable accompaniments.

As a rule, the grief reaction lasts for a period of 4 to 12 weeks, by which time it begins to abate, with a gradual resumption of normal activities that come to occupy the mind more and more of the time and expel thoughts of the deceased. Grieving is to be regarded as a natural reaction to personal tragedy, and its absence in circumstances where it should be called forth is believed by psychiatrists to be abnormal. However, the overt expressions of grief are highly individual, depending on personality and cultural and other factors.

Distortions of the normal reaction to personal loss are not infrequent; they are referred to as *pathologic grief.*

1. The most frequent distortion is *prolongation of the reaction,* i.e., there is no sign of resolution by the end of a 3-month period. Mothers who have lost a child tend to suffer for an unduly long period of time, and the elderly who have lost a spouse may never recover completely. Patients with a history of previous depressive episodes may also remain in mourning for longer than usual periods. In general, when a bereaved person has shown no improvement within 3 to 4 months of the loss, one should suspect a pathologic grief reaction and call for psychiatric consultation. Prolonged grief is a not unusual setting for suicide.

2. Another variation of the grief reaction is *delayed* or *postponed grief.* Often, in an attempt to sustain the morale of others or to avoid the unpleasant spectacle of mourning, the patient may show little or no reaction to the loss. This "stiff-upper-lip" attitude is frequently admired and consequently reinforced, especially in Anglo-Saxon and Scandinavian cultures. According to some psychiatrists, the potential danger of this suppressed reaction is that the grief may find expression months or even years later in a delayed depression. (We find this interpretation rather speculative and prefer to believe that the patient later develops an endogenous depression, in which past worries and sources of unhappiness are reinstated.)

3. In an effort to overcome sadness the bereaved person may become hyperactive and even euphoric. The elation is interpreted as a defense against depression. It may give way to a sudden reversal of mood, whereupon the individual is plummeted into a depression. In another variation of unacknowledged grief, bereaved persons embark on a series of social and economic adventures that may end in disaster. They may invest or gamble recklessly, turn away from old friends, or take up high-risk sports such as auto racing or skydiving. Rarely do they recognize the self-punitive nature of their activity or the guilt that is believed to lie behind it. Simply pointing this out sometimes helps such patients.

4. Occasionally patients will acquire the same symptoms as the deceased and may be convinced that they have the same disease. This may be the origin of some of the hypochondriacal ideas that accompany depressive reactions. The identification of this variant of grieving requires only that the examiner, after excluding the presence of disease in the patient for want of clinical evidence, inquire about the illness that took the life of the deceased.

Management of the usual grief reaction consists of maintaining a sympathetic attitude and helping the bereaved person to acknowledge the loss and to face the changes required as a result of it. The sooner the patient comes to a realistic acceptance of the loss and the need to restructure his or her life, the more swiftly the process will reach closure. Stoicism should not be encouraged or reinforced. To express sadness through tears, anguish, and even hostility is helpful for many individuals. The practice of treating grief-stricken patients with antidepressants is seldom effective, for it attempts to suppress what is a natural and necessary human reaction. Early on, undue restlessness, anxiety, and insomnia can be relieved by anxiolytic and sedative medication. Diazepam (Valium), 5 mg tid, or the equivalent dose of chlordiazepoxide (Librium) or oxazepam (Serax) is suitable for daytime sedation and can be used at bedtime for sleep by doubling an individual dose. Each of these drugs has a wide margin of safety, which decreases the danger of its use as a means of committing suicide. The possibility of suicide must be entertained in managing all depressed patients, including mourners, and care must be taken not to supply them with large amounts of hypnotics.

In treating patients with pathologic grief reactions, the help of a psychiatrist should be enlisted, to determine whether the plan of treatment is sound; often these patients require specialized psychiatric help.

REACTIVE DEPRESSION

Depressed patients seldom express feelings of sadness or despair without mentioning physical concomitants, such as easy fatigability, loss of appetite, reduced interest in life and love, and trouble in falling asleep or premature awakening. It follows that whenever these symptoms become manifest in the course of medical disease they should arouse suspicion of a depressive reaction (see Table 56-1).

Chronic pain is a particularly frequent somatic manifestation of depression. The pain may be vague in nature and recalcitrant to straightforward medical and surgical approaches, or, in the beginning, it may have been caused by an arthritic hip, protruded intervertebral disc, or injury. One should question such individuals about recent losses or changes in status, disappointments, or dissatisfactions.

Table 56-1
Depression secondary to neurologic, medical, and surgical diseases and drugs

1. *Neurologic diseases*
   a. Neuronal degenerations—Alzheimer, Huntington, and Parkinson disease
   b. Focal CNS disease—strokes, brain tumors and trauma, multiple sclerosis

2. *Metabolic and endocrine diseases*
   a. Corticosteroids, excess or deficiency
   b. Hypothyroidism, rarely thyrotoxicosis
   c. Cushing syndrome
   d. Addison disease
   e. Hyperparathyroidism
   f. Pernicious anemia
   g. Chronic renal failure/dialysis
   h. B-vitamin deficiencies

3. *Myocardial infarction, open heart surgery, and other operations*

4. *Infectious diseases*
   a. Brucellosis
   b. Viral hepatitis, influenza, pneumonia
   c. Infectious mononucleosis

5. *Cancer, particularly pancreatic*

6. *Parturition*

7. *Medications*
   a. Analgesics and anti-inflammatory agents (other than steroids)—indomethacin, phenacetin, and phenylbutazone
   b. Amphetamines (when withdrawn)
   c. Antibiotics, particularly cycloserine, ethionamide, griseofulvin, isoniazid, nalidixic acid, and sulfonamide
   d. Antihypertensive drugs—clonidine, methyldopa, propranolol, reserpine
   e. Cardiac drugs—digitalis, procainamide
   f. Corticosteroids and ACTH
   g. Disulfiram
   h. L-Dopa
   i. Methysergide
   j. Oral contraceptives

All patients with chronic pain syndromes should be evaluated psychiatrically, as pointed out in Chap. 7.

In a number of major medical illnesses, depressive symptoms occur with such frequency as to constitute important diagnostic and therapeutic problems; contrariwise, in certain chronic, occult diseases, symptoms such as lassitude and fatigue resemble those of a depressive reaction. Hypothyroidism, infectious mononucleosis, infectious hepatitis, carcinoma of the head of the pancreas, metastatic carcinoma of the liver, malnutrition, and frontal lobe tumors may simulate depression for several weeks or months before the diagnosis becomes evident. Drugs such as reserpine, or other *Rauwolfia* derivatives, and the phenothiazines may evoke a depressive reaction; steroids can induce a peculiar psychiatric state in which confusion, insomnia, and depression or elevation of mood are combined. A depressed mood may emerge during the tapering-off period of steroid medication.

Of particular significance is the depression that occurs on learning of a medical or neurologic disease. Often such an emotional reaction, which the physician may tend to ignore, is the dominant manifestation of a devastating disease that threatens the life pattern and independence of the patient. Recognition by the patient that he has suffered a myocardial infarct or stroke, or that he has cancer, multiple sclerosis or Parkinson disease, is almost always followed by some degree of reactive depression.

An example is the depression that follows myocardial infarction (Wishnie). Usually it begins toward the end of the patient's stay in the acute-care ward. Usually, also, it is covert and attracts little attention, the clinical manifestations being at first obscured by bed rest and hypnotic-sedative medication. Discouragement and a gloomy attitude toward the future are the principal indications of the depressive syndrome. The patient may not mention these concerns to the physician, assuming them to be trivial or likely to be misinterpreted as signs of fear or weakness of character. Once the patient is home, the depression becomes much more apparent both to him and his family. Fatigability that approaches exhaustion is the primary complaint and interferes with accustomed activities; it may be described as weakness and falsely attributed to a failing heart. Symptoms of irritability, anxiety, and despondency are next in order of frequency, followed by insomnia and feelings of aimlessness and boredom. When the time comes to return to work, fearful anticipation mounts and often results in long, unwarranted delays in ending the convalescent period. This is more apt to occur when the patient's occupation is physically or mentally stressful.

Although most of these patients ultimately recover without medical assistance (the disorder is, in this sense, self-limited), the toll that depression exacts in terms of mental suffering is enormous. Depression is probably the main cause of extended convalescence and retarded rehabilitation following myocardial infarction. Much of it could be prevented by proper intervention.

The first step in management is recognition of the depressive state. This can be greatly simplified if one assumes that all patients after coronary thrombosis are liable to depression and if a plan to deal with this is started during the acute stage of the illness. Such a program carries no risk for those unusual individuals who may not be depressed, and offers considerable benefit to those who are. One begins by assuring the patient that a sense of sadness and discouragement is normal and to be expected. Next, the patient should be advised that regular activities may not need to be curtailed as much as anticipated. This can be supplemented by giving examples of public figures, such as former Presidents Eisenhower and Johnson, who returned to active life following severe heart attacks. The patient is then given a program of graduated activity consistent with his or her cardiac condition. Physical conditioning is the best antidote for depression in the coronary patient; it raises self-esteem and reinstates a feeling of independence even when bed rest is still required. Once established, this schedule of activity should be carried through convalescence and maintained long after the patient has returned to work.

It is also important, in treating postcoronary depression, to instruct the patient about the disease. Patients have their own ideas about illness, which often do not conform to the facts. Misconceptions must be actively uncovered and corrected. The most prevalent misbeliefs surrounding myocardial infarctions include the following: exertion, even when mild, can kill you; sexual intercourse should never again be attempted; myocardial infarctions tend to recur at orgasm; recurrence is apt to take place on the anniversary of the first infarction; one is likely to die at the same age as did a parent from heart disease; recurrent infarctions are more likely to take place in sleep. After these and other misunderstandings have been corrected, the patient should be told which activities to continue and which to forgo. The spouse and children should be included in the discussions. Warning the patient what to expect reduces the stress of an event and spares much torment. If the physician warns that it is normal to feel weak on returning home from the hospital and that this is not a sign of a failing heart, the patient is less apt to be alarmed when a sense of weakness does occur. The family should not be overprotective.

Sodium amytal, 100 mg tid, in combination with dextroamphetamine, 5.0 mg morning and noon, has been one of the most successful treatments of depression of this type. The tricyclic antidepressants and monoamine oxidase (MAO) inhibitors are generally considered unsafe for use with coronary patients. Electroconvulsive therapy has been successfully and safely employed in postmyocardial infarction patients but should be used only if the depression is severe and persistent enough to warrant it.

An analogous depressive reaction occurs in patients with stroke, and should be managed along the lines indicated

above. It would appear that patients with left anterior lesions, *predominantly* cortical or subcortical (as judged by CT scans), have a greater frequency and severity of depression than patients with lesions in any other location (Starkstein et al). Levine and Finkelstein have reported the occurrence of psychotic depression with hallucinations and delusions in patients with right temporoparietal infarcts.

Other neurologic diseases, such as paralysis agitans (Parkinson disease), are complicated by a depressive reaction in one-quarter to one-half the cases. In this latter disorder, weakness and fatigability, the principal psychologic manifestations, are added to the akinesia, and the resulting therapeutic problem becomes formidable. Another hazard in this disease is the tendency for L-dopa itself to provoke a depression, sometimes with suicidal tendencies and other mental symptoms, such as paranoid ideation and psychotic episodes. The treatment of depression with MAO inhibitors is contraindicated in patients receiving L-dopa. Huntington chorea may cause depression, even before the movement disorder and dementia become conspicuous. In one series, 10 of 101 patients with this disease either committed suicide or attempted it. Also Alzheimer disease is often accompanied by depressive symptoms, in which instance the evaluation of the relative contributions of the affective disorder and the dementia is difficult if not impossible. On several occasions we have had to resort to electroconvulsive therapy to eliminate the depressive factor.

Cancer is another illness that is almost invariably attended by a depressive reaction. An important determinant of the severity of this depressive response is the attitude of the physician. In the nineteenth century, physicians tended to be quite open with their patients and gave an honest diagnosis and a straightforward prognosis. A mid-twentieth century survey of physicians' attitudes toward the truthful disclosure of these vital factors in patients with cancer revealed a disinclination toward candor. There seemed to be a direct relationship between the seriousness of the prognosis and the degree to which truth was hidden. Thus, over 90 percent of dermatologists but less than 20 percent of gynecologists chose to be frank, a disparity that relates to the control each of these specialists can exert over the malignancy. Basal-cell carcinoma can usually be removed entirely and survival ensured; the outlook in carcinoma of the cervix or uterus is far less hopeful. Thus the type of tumor, rather than the physician's attitude, appeared to determine what was said to the patient. It was assumed that the patient, upon hearing that intervention offered uncertain success, would fall into a hopeless depression and that it would therefore be wiser to withhold information that could serve no useful purpose.

In the last few decades there has been a gratifying change in the psychologic management of the cancer patient. It is now generally agreed that the patient should learn the truth in most instances and that withholding or distorting information seriously undermines the doctor-patient relationship. Furthermore, the facts of the illness, if presented with a ray of hope, can be coped with more readily than a tangle of half-truths, hollow reassurances, and furtive falsifications. The notion that patients can be kept blissfully unaware of their jeopardy while their closest relatives are fully informed is not sensible. This approach, which has aptly been called "the conspiracy of silence," not only fails to accomplish its purpose but isolates the patient at a time when all available human support is needed. In being truthful, physicians need not thrust all the harsh realities on each patient the moment the biopsy report returns, but they should make available whatever information is requested and maintain open communications with the patient throughout the course of the illness. Though some individuals cannot bear to hear the truth and ask not to be told, most patients want to know and should be told. The cancer patient often phrases questions indirectly, especially when fearful of the answer. Such a person might talk of buying a new house in an effort to get the doctor's opinion as to whether he or she will survive long enough to justify the purchase. Such questions ought not to pass unnoticed. The physician should ask the patient what he or she means or to rephrase the question to bring out the hidden meaning.

A worry common to patients with cancer, yet seldom mentioned openly, is that the doctor will give up on them. This is particularly so in this era of specialization, when often no one physician is in overall charge. A supportive doctor-patient relationship with mutual trust is the best insurance against the fear of abandonment. Once this has been established, patients are usually able to cope with their depression without specific help from the physician. However, the latter should be ready to supply anxiolytic drugs such as diazepam, 2 to 5 mg qid, if necessary. The dose may be doubled or tripled for use as a hypnotic at bedtime. If depression persists, it is justifiable to try a tricyclic antidepressant or MAO inhibitor.

NEUROTIC DEPRESSION

This term, already introduced in Chap. 55, has little precision. One view is to regard it simply as a depressive syndrome that occurs in an individual who exhibits or who has in the past exhibited the symptoms of anxiety neurosis or one of the other neuroses (hysteria, phobic, or obsessive-compulsive neurosis). Theoretically there is no illogic in assuming that an individual with a neurosis should in addition (one chance in 20) be subject to a hereditary depression. Of course, a depression in response to a serious illness or a grief reaction, i.e., a reactive depression, is as likely to occur in a neurotic individual as in a normal one.

The occurrence of depressive symptoms in response to severe phobias, obsessions and compulsions, i.e., a reactive depression, has also been mentioned in Chap. 55.

The separation of this state from endogenous depression and reactive depression has not received universal acceptance. Some psychiatrists such as Lewis (page 1198) find no basis for separating neurotic from endogenous depression; others stress that there are differences in terms of heredity, prominence of vegetative signs, and delusional thinking, all being more frequent and prominent in endogenous depression. To further confuse the issue, some psychiatrists use the term *depressive neurosis* or *dysthymic disorder* simply to distinguish a relatively mild depression from a more severe or psychotic depression. This is the definition given in DSM III.

ENDOGENOUS DEPRESSION AND MANIC-DEPRESSIVE PSYCHOSIS

DEFINITIONS AND EPIDEMIOLOGY

Manic-depressive disease or psychosis is a disorder of affect (mood), consisting of episodes of depression or mania, or both. Although it has been regarded traditionally as a periodic or cyclic condition in which one major mood swing is followed by an equal but opposite excursion, this is seldom the case. Depression is far more prevalent than mania, and the mixed variety, containing both extremes, is relatively uncommon. Recurrence of episodes of pure mania without interspersed episodes of depression is known, but is exceptional. As a consequence, manic-depressive psychosis has been divided into two subtypes: a *unipolar group,* in which only an endogenous depressive illness occurs, and a *bipolar group,* in which mania occurs, with or without depression (contrary to one's initial impression of the term—that bipolar patients have *both* mania and depression).

Manic-depressive psychosis was given its name by Kraepelin in 1896, and it was with him that our current clinical concept of this disorder originated. He viewed the manic and depressive attacks as opposite poles of the same underlying process, and pointed out that unlike dementia praecox (his name for schizophrenia), manic-depressive psychosis entails no intellectual deterioration with recurrent episodes.

The incidence of manic-depressive disease cannot be stated with precision, mainly because of differing criteria for diagnosis. The apparent increase of the disease in the past 50 years probably reflects a growing awareness of the condition, both among physicians and lay persons. Studies of large groups of patients from isolated areas of Iceland and the Danish islands of Bornholm and Samso, indicate that 5 percent of men and 9 percent of women will develop symptoms of depression or mania, or both, sometime during their lives (Goodwin and Guze). The estimate for an American urban community (New Haven, Connecticut) is higher; the lifetime expectancy for an attack of major depression is 8 to 12 percent in men and twice this number in women (Weissman and Myers). For Western nations in general, if attention is limited to manic-depressive illness, lifetime expectancy is 1 to 2 percent (Klerman).

Manic-depressive psychosis occurs most frequently in middle and later adult years, with a peak age of onset between 55 and 65 for both sexes. However, a significant proportion of patients experience the first attack in childhood, adolescence, or early adult life. Depression is also a significant problem in the elderly; Blazer and Williams, who studied 997 persons over the age of 65 in North Carolina, found symptoms of a major depressive illness in 3.7 percent. The disease is two or three times more frequent among women. There is no known explanation for this difference, but some have speculated that just as many men are depressed, only they deny it or turn to alcohol. It was reported, in the 1930s, to be more common in individuals of Jewish and Irish ethnicity and among those in upper socioeconomic strata, but subsequent studies have not confirmed these findings. The bipolar variety occurs in about 10 percent of patients with affective disorders. Patients in the bipolar group have an earlier age of onset, more frequent and shorter episodes of illness and a greater prevalence of affective disorder among their relatives than do patients with unipolar disease (Winokur).

CLINICAL PRESENTATION

The fully developed endogenous depression may evolve within a few days or it may merge gradually with vague prodromal symptoms that had been present for months. A detailed description of the symptoms and signs of depression was given in Chap. 24. Here it need only be repeated that the patient expresses feelings of sadness, unhappiness, discouragement, hopelessness, and despondency, with loss of self-esteem. Reduced energy for mental and physical activity is universally present, to the point of catatonia in the most severe cases. There is heightened irritability, as well as a lack of interest in all activities that formerly were pleasurable. The mental life of such an individual may narrow to a single-minded concern about his or her physical deterioration, mental decline, or both. In dialogue, the

patient's rejoinders become so stereotyped that the listener can soon predict exactly what is going to be said. There is a poverty of ideation, as well as a notable absence of insight. Consciousness is clear, and though there is usually no evidence of schizophrenic type of thought disorder, delusional ideas and less often hallucinations may be prominent, justifying the term depressive psychosis. The suspicions and delusions are generally congruent with the patient's mood and are not as fixed or bizarre as in schizophrenia. The hallucinations are usually vocal and accusatory; their presence should always raise the possibility of an associated organic disease or drug intoxication.

Frequently, agitation, rather than physical inactivity and mental slowness, is the principal behavioral abnormality. The source of the agitation is an underlying anxiety state. Pacing the floor, particularly in the early morning hours, is characteristic. Such patients tend to be overtalkative and vexed in their manner of expression, so that the examiner is acutely aware of their mental anguish. Attempts at reassurance may meet with initial success, only to be dispelled in the next rush of doubts. These patients remain impervious to reason and logic as these apply to their symptoms, even though they may be able to exercise these functions to a variable degree in other areas of their life.

At its worst the illness takes the form of a depressive stupor; the patient becomes mute, indifferent to nutritional needs, and neglectful even of bowel and bladder functions. The condition at this time resembles catatonia. Such patients must be fed and their other needs attended to until therapy (usually electroconvulsive therapy) brings about improvement.

The most important concern in patients with late life depression is the risk of suicide. Since many of these individuals have reputations for being sound, dependable and stable, and deny being depressed, one's prevailing attitude toward them is to reject the possibility of self-destruction. Because of the high risk of suicide one should seek the advice of a psychiatrist as soon as the diagnosis is suspected.

The *manic phase* is, in most ways, the mirror opposite of the depressed phase, being characterized by a flight of ideas, hyperactivity, and an increased appetite and sex urge. After a minimum of sleep the patient awakes with enthusiasm and expectation. The manic individual appears to possess great drive and confidence, yet lacks the ability to carry out his plans. Headstrong, impulsive, socially intrusive behavior is characteristic. Judgment may be so impaired that the patient may make reckless investments and spend fortunes in gambling and shopping sprees. Setbacks do not perturb the patient but rather act as goads for new activities. Euphoria and expansiveness sometimes bubble over into delusions of power and grandeur, which in turn may make the patient offensively aggressive. Up to a point, the patient's mirth and good spirits may be contagious, and others may join in the laughter; however, if thwarted, the warmth and good humor can suddenly change to anger. Irritability rather than elation may be the prevailing mood. The threshold for paranoid thinking is low, which makes the patient sensitive and suspicious. Personal neglect may reach the point of dishevelment and poor personal hygiene. In its most advanced form, a condition described as *delirious mania,* the patient becomes totally incoherent and altogether disorganized in behavior. At this stage visual and auditory hallucinations and paranoid delusions may be rampant; furthermore, as the term implies, the patient may be disoriented, with clouded sensorium. Fortunately, this extreme is rarely encountered. Rarely also, one observes patients with repeated attacks of mania, without depression at any time.

Hypomania represents a milder degree of the disorder, but this term is also used loosely to depict normal behavior in which the individual is unusually energetic and active. In this latter sense hypomania is a personality trait found in many talented and productive persons, and need not arouse concern unless it is out of character for the individual. This is best determined by questioning the family.

First attacks of either depression or mania last an average of 6 months if untreated although the range of duration of attacks varies greatly. Modern therapy can reduce this by more than half. About 90 percent of manic-depressive patients recover from their first attack. For those who do not recover, there is often some pertinent reason in terms of their family or environment which serves to retard improvement. Attacks tend to be longer in older age groups. About one-half of all depressed patients have one or more recurrences. In a smaller but very significant number (25 percent in Winokur's series), the disease is chronic. In such cases, the patient may become a complete recluse and pass a large segment of his or her life in isolation; and, all treatments have no more than a transitory effect. Variables that are predictive of an unfavorable outcome are high degrees of neuroticism, long duration of illness before treatment, strongly positive family history, and depression secondary to another disorder (Hirschfeld et al).

DIAGNOSIS

According to the third edition of the Diagnostic and Statistical Manual of Mental Disorders (DSM III), the essential diagnostic criteria of endogenous depression consist of a dysphoric mood or loss of interest or pleasure in almost all usual activities in combination with at least four of the following eight symptoms: (1) disturbance of appetite and change in weight; (2) sleep disorder; (3) psychomotor retardation or agitation; (4) decreased sex drive; (5) decreased energy and fatigue; (6) self-reproach, feelings of

worthlessness or guilt; (7) indecisiveness, complaints of memory loss and difficulties in concentrating; (8) thought of death or suicide, or suicide attempts. Each of the four diagnostic symptoms should have been present for at least two weeks.

Adherence to the aforementioned criteria undoubtedly facilitates diagnosis, but not infrequently a single one of these symptoms so dominates the clinical picture as to suggest the diagnosis of another disease state and obscure the presence of an underlying depression.

Complaints of fatigue, weakness, malaise, or widespread aches and pains, for example, suggest a variety of medical diseases such as Addison disease, hypothyroidism, chronic infection, polymyositis, early rheumatoid arthritis, etc. Often the fatigue state is misinterpreted as muscular weakness and this directs a medical search for neuromuscular or other neurologic disease.

Hypochondriacal preoccupation with bowel and digestive functions accounts for repeated visits to the medical clinic. In one study, 21 of 120 hypochondriacal patients were subsequently diagnosed as being depressed (see Woods). Persistent insomnia may be the major complaint of the depressed patient. Early awakening is typical and the morning hours are then the worst period of the day. Other patients have difficulty falling asleep, especially if there is an associated anxiety state. Complaints of loss of memory, and, in males, of impotence and loss of libido are other monosymptomatic presentations; only with a probing inquiry about other disturbances common to depression will the diagnosis become evident.

There are several other clinical situations in which it may prove difficult to recognize an underlying depression. The ones which the authors have found particularly common and troublesome are the following:

1. *Symptoms of depression in patients with chronic pain.* Chronic pain has long been known to have an association with depression. Patients who show this association are far from a homogeneous group. In some patients with chronic pain, the symptoms and signs of depression are quite apparent. If the pain has been present for less than a year and had its onset at the same time as the other depressive symptoms, the response to antidepressant treatment is favorable.

Far more difficult to understand and to manage are patients with persistent pain as the only complaint; the head, face, neck, and lower back are the common loci. An exhaustive search for the source of the pain usually proves unsuccessful, and the conclusion is reached that the pain is "psychogenic." This attribution of pain to some obscure psychologic mechanism is hardly helpful, for usually no amount of exploration will reveal its source. Nevertheless, in a small proportion of such patients, pain will be alleviated by antidepressant drugs, proof, at least in these cases, of the linkage of the pain and depression.

Frequently, in this group of patients, the problem is made even more difficult by repeated surgical operations and dependency on analgesic drugs, which in themselves deplete energy and have other adverse effects. Such patients are to be found among those disabled after multiple operations for prolapsed intervertebral disc or arthritic hips, or those with atypical facial pain, postherpetic neuralgia and so forth. Where the clinical sequence consists of pain as the initial event, followed by chronicity of pain, abuse of drugs, chronic fatigue and depressive symptoms, we tend to view the latter symptoms as reactive, and direct our therapeutic efforts to the relief of both the pain and depression (see page 114).

2. *Depression and alcoholism.* Depression and alcoholism are commonly associated, and it is important to determine which is primary and which is secondary. A depressive syndrome, developing for the first time on a background of alcoholism (secondary depression) is a very common clinical occurrence. In a large series of alcoholics studied by Cadoret and Winokur, a secondary depression occurred in 30 of 61 females and in 41 of 112 males; moreover, once the alcoholism was established, the depression developed much earlier in the women alcoholics than in the men. The opposite occurrence, i.e., the development of alcoholism on the background of a primary depression, is less common. Again, women are disproportionately affected. Moreover, women with primary depression and subsequent alcoholism have a higher incidence of affective disorder in first-degree relatives (Schuckit et al). As mentioned earlier, these differences may be spurious; Winokur's family studies suggest that the same genetic predisposition leads to depression in females and alcoholism and sociopathy in men.

3. *Depression in childhood and adolescents.* We have frequently observed depressive states in children and often they have been misdiagnosed by both internists and psychiatrists. The common manifestations have been chronic headache, refusal to go to school, withdrawal from social activities, anorexia, vomiting and weight loss, and scholastic failure. Nearly all of the cases of so-called male anorexia nervosa have proven to be due to depressive states. Puberty is a time of onset in many cases, but we have seen the disease in late childhood, and it is extremely frequent in high school and college students. It is a tragic mistake not to appreciate this fact and to be treating the nervous disorder by psychotherapy, only to have the patient commit suicide. This has happened to more than a dozen of the children of our colleagues.

4. *Intractable headaches or anorexia.* Either of these may be the most prominent manifestation of depression in a child, adolescent, or young adult (see above).

5. *Anxiety neurosis.* See Chaps. 24 and 55.

6. *Hypochondriasis.* See further on in this chapter.

ETIOLOGY

The following are the main theories that have been proposed to explain the origin of depression.

Genetic Theory The capacity to experience sadness and depression is common to all people. Although there is no question that depression can be provoked by adverse circumstances, some individuals are more liable to depression than others who are subjected to similar degrees of adversity. In general, there seems to be a familial diathesis for most depressive illness, but especially for manic-depressive psychosis and endogenous depression. Much work has been done on the inheritance of depression, most of which has dealt with these two affective disorders. The frequency of these illnesses is increased in the relatives of affected patients (prevalence rate of 14 to 25 percent in first-degree relatives). Furthermore, the type of illness tends to breed true, i.e., the bipolar form is more common among relatives of bipolar patients than among relatives of unipolar patients. Similarly the morbidity risk among first-degree relatives is increased (15 percent, in comparison to 1 to 2 percent risk in the general population). If all twin studies are taken together, there is a concordance rate of 75 percent for monozygotic twins and 20 percent for same-sex dizygotic twins, clearly indicative of a genetic factor. Although the exact pattern of inheritance has not been defined, the authors, from their personal experience, suspect that a dominant mode of heredity is likely. It has been found that depressive disorders in families segregate along with HLA haplotypes, suggesting that a locus on chromosome 6 influences the susceptibility to depressive disorders (Weitkamp et al).

Biochemical Theories The biogenic amines (norepinephrine, serotonin, and dopamine) are the key elements in this theory. Following the observations that antidepressant drugs, such as the tricyclic antidepressants and the MAO inhibitors, exert their effect by increasing one or another of the biogenic amines at the central adrenergic receptor sites (limbic system and hypothalamus) and that drugs that often cause depression (such as reserpine) deplete biogenic amines, the theory followed that naturally occurring depressions might be associated with a deficiency of these latter substances. Indeed measurements of 3-methoxy-4-hydroxyphenylglycol (MHPG), a metabolite of norepinephrine, were found to be subnormal in the CSF of patients with endogenous depression and to be elevated in manic states. Also, 5-hydroxyindoleacetic acid (5-HIAA), a deaminated metabolite of serotonin, was reduced in the CSF of depressed patients (Carroll et al). However, the findings were not consistent. Some investigators interpreted this to mean that all depressions are not the same. At least two subgroups emerged: one with low levels of bioamine metabolites and one with normal levels. Maas, in the study of a small group of depressed patients, reported that those who had low levels of MHPG responded better to imipramine therapy and those with normal levels, to amitriptyline therapy.

Another set of observations, summarized by Schlesser et al, suggests a disorder of the hypothalamic-pituitary-adrenal axis. In a series of cases of endogenous monopolar and bipolar depressions, the parenteral administration of 1 to 2 mg of dexamethasone failed to suppress serum cortisol levels while the patient was ill, but did so after recovery. In a comparable series of reactive depressions there was a normal suppression of serum cortisol levels. Dextroamphetamine restored to some extent the normal response in the patients with endogenous depressions. This test is believed to separate the two large groups of depressed patients and to predict the response to drug therapy, for only the endogenous depressives responded to antidepressant tricyclic and MAO inhibitory drugs. However, subsequent studies (Amsterdam et al, Insel et al) showed that the specificity of this test is less than earlier reports had indicated. In other words, a positive dexamethasone test does not necessarily indicate the presence of endogenous depression. Contrariwise, a normal test does not exclude the diagnosis. Moreover, repeated testing in individual patients may produce variable results, without apparent changes in the clinical state (Charles et al). Another line of laboratory study is the polysomnograph. In approximately one-third of patients with a depression, there is a shortened time between falling asleep and the appearance of the first period of REM sleep, which is characterized by an increase in REM density (number of rapid eye movements) and duration. Although these findings are a consistent biologic marker, they are not specific, occurring also in anorexia nervosa, narcolepsy, and schizophrenia. At the time of writing this edition it must be conceded that there is no reliable biologic test for depression. One must resort to clinical analysis, i.e., the interpretation of symptoms and signs, not only for diagnosis but for the differentiation of special types of depressive reaction.

Research on the amphetamines, cocaine, electroconvulsive shock treatment, and lithium salts has also produced data that agree with the biogenic-amine hypothesis. Although this possibility has received much attention and is generally well accepted, it leaves many questions unanswered. How is a genetic abnormality translated into a disorder of biogenic amines? Why are the therapeutic results so inconsistent with either the tricyclic antidepressants or the MAO inhibitors, both of which should favorably influence the balance of biogenic amines at the proper receptor sites? How can one explain the observation that steroids play a part in the etiology of affective disorders? Further knowledge of the metabolism and physiology of the transmitter function of the biogenic amines is needed before a complete theory can be developed. For readers who seek more information on this subject, the reviews by Willner and by Schildkraut and his colleagues are recommended.

TREATMENT

Enlisting the Help of a Psychiatrist The physician untrained in psychiatry would be rash to attempt the management of these patients without such assistance.

Hospitalization If there is any doubt about the patient's intention of suicide, the patient should be hospitalized. In manic-depressive illness, successive attacks are remarkably similar in the same individual. Thus one can predict the course and intensity of an episode of illness on the basis of the previous one. If a suicide attempt was made in the past, the probability is that it will be made again.

If the depressed patient is psychotic, i.e., suffering from delusions or hallucinations, or is severely agitated, one of the antipsychotic medications (haloperidol, thioridazine, chlorpromazine) should be given initially, before other antidepressant treatment is instituted (see below).

Antidepressant Medication Two categories of antidepressants, the tricyclic compounds and the MAO inhibitors, are the most useful. Imipramine (Tofranil), amitriptyline (Elavil), and doxepin (Sinequan) represent the former; phenelzine (Nardil) and tranylcypromine (Parnate), the latter. In the treatment of depression, most psychiatrists start with imipramine or amitriptyline, because they are the safest. In general, these drugs are equally effective, although an individual patient may have a better response to one than to another. The starting dose is 25 mg/day, which is then raised by 25 mg every 3 to 4 days, as needed. The therapeutic effect of tricyclic medication is often not evident for 2 or 3 weeks after treatment has been initiated. Common side effects are orthostatic hypotension, dry mouth, constipation, tachycardia, urinary hesitancy or retention, tremor, and drowsiness; these compounds should not be given to patients with coronary heart disease. A non-tricyclic antidepressant—trazodone (Desyrel)—has been introduced in the United States. It appears to be as effective as the tricyclic antidepressants in the treatment of depression, without the anticholinergic effects. Trazodone is given initially in a dosage of 150 mg/day, and can be increased by 50 mg every few days until a daily dosage of 400 to 600 mg is reached. Priapism, the mechanism of which is not understood, is the main adverse effect.

If full doses of these drugs, given for 4 to 6 weeks, are ineffective, they should be discontinued and an MAO inhibitor prescribed, after an interval of at least one week. Phenelzine (Nardil) is regarded as the least likely of the MAO inhibitors to produce serious side effects. The usual starting dose is 15 mg tid, which is gradually increased as needed to a maximum of 45 mg tid. The most serious side effect of MAO inhibitors is a hypertensive crisis; therefore, they should be dispensed with extreme caution in patients with hypertension and with cardiovascular or cerebrovascular disease. Patients taking these drugs should avoid foods with a high tyramine content (aged cheese, pickled herring, chicken liver, beer, wines, yeast extract).

Since patients are usually responsive either to the tricyclic drugs or MAO inhibitors but not to both, it is important to find out which of these drugs has been more helpful in the past. This will guide one in current management. Interestingly, it has been found that members of the same family are apt to have a similar response to the same antidepressant.

The authors still find that some depressed patients respond to dextroamphetamine (5 to 10 mg bid, given in the early part of the day), and sodium amytal, 60 to 120 mg tid. These medications, the earliest form of drug therapy for depression, are useful in postmyocardial infarction patients (page 1207) and in patients who are only mildly depressed and still at work, and they have no serious side effects.

Electroconvulsive Therapy (ECT)

Electroconvulsive therapy remains the most effective treatment for severe endogenous depression and can also be used to interrupt manic episodes. The latter often require only two or three treatments. The technique is quite simple. The patient is premedicated with a muscle relaxant [succinylcholine (Anectine)] and then anesthetized by an intravenous injection

of the short-acting barbiturate methohexital (Brevital). An electrode is placed over each temple and an alternating current of about 400 mA and 70 to 120 V is passed between them for 0.1 to 0.5 s. The Anectine prevents strong and injurious muscle spasm. The patient is awake within 5 to 10 min and is up and about in 30 min. The mechanism by which convulsive therapy works is not known. In treating depression, ECT is usually given every other day for 6 to 14 treatments. The only absolute contraindication is the presence of increased intracranial pressure, such as may occur with a neoplasm or hematoma. Its major drawback is a transient impairment of recent memory for the period of treatment and the days that follow, the degree of impairment being related to the number of treatments given. Placing both electrodes on the nondominant side (unilateral ECT) produces less memory disturbance but is thought to be less effective against the depression.

Until the advent of the antidepressant drugs, ECT was the treatment of choice for the agitated depression of middle and late life. Of all the conditions for which ECT is used, it is the one that is most predictably benefited. Close to 90 percent of patients recover within less than 2 months following a course of 6 to 14 treatments. Prior to the use of ECT, this type of depression could be expected to last for 2 to 7 years before remission occurred. Since ECT therapy carries a high risk of confusion and amnesia, most psychiatrists favor the initial use of a neuroleptic agent, such as haloperidol, followed by a trial of a tricyclic compound and MAO inhibitor, before resorting to ECT. These trials, of course, must be conducted in a setting where the chance of suicide is minimized.

Following ECT therapy, maintenance therapy with a tricyclic compound or lithium is necessary to prevent relapse.

Lithium Carbonate

This is the drug of choice in treating the manic phase of manic-depressive disease. Hospitalization is usually required to protect the manic patient from impulsive and often aggressive behavior, which might cause a loss of good standing in the community or jeopardize a career. Chlorpromazine (Thorazine) or haloperidol (Haldol)—or ECT, if these drugs are ineffective—can be used to control the mania until lithium carbonate becomes effective, usually a matter of 4 or 5 days. The usual dosage of lithium is 1 to 3 g daily in divided oral doses, which produces the desired serum level of 1.2 to 1.5 meq/L. The serum level of lithium must be checked frequently, both to ensure that a therapeutic dose is being given and to guard against toxicity (page 903).

Lithium has also proved to be effective in the *milder* degrees of mania, and can be used in such cases without having to hospitalize the patient initially. The continued administration of lithium, given in half the dosage that is used for manic episodes, may prevent further attacks of mania. It is also useful in the prevention of depression in patients with bipolar disease, and in some patients with unipolar disease.

Psychotherapy In all patients with manic-depressive disease, psychotherapy (explanation, reassurance, encouragement) and instruction of the family are of value in helping the patient understand his or her illness and coping with it. The patient and family should be enjoined to seek help at the first hint of relapse.

As a general rule, manic-depressive illness is best managed by a physician who is willing to follow the patient over a long period of time and who is known to the family. Although the prognosis for any individual attack is relatively good, it is wise to arrange for a plan of action that will be set in operation as soon as the first symptoms of a recurrence become manifest. A family physician who has ready access to a psychiatrist best fulfills this need.

SUICIDE

Between 20,000 and 35,000 suicides are recorded annually in the United States, and attempted suicides exceed this number by about 10 times. All psychiatrists agree that these are conservative figures. Suicide is the ninth leading cause of death in America, a figure that emphasizes the importance of recognizing those depressions with a high potential for self-destruction. Every physician should be familiar with the few clues we possess to identify those patients who intend to end their lives.

Manic-depressive psychosis, endogenous depression, depression resulting from a debilitating disease, pathologic grief, and depression in an alcoholic or schizophrenic—all carry the risk of suicide. In manic-depressive disease and endogenous depression, the risk of suicide over the lifetime of the patient is about 15 percent (Guze and Robins). In Robins' series of 134 patients who committed suicide, 47 percent had a depressive illness and 25 percent were alcoholic.

Most suicides are not impulsive but planned. Furthermore, the intention of suicide is more often than not communicated to someone significant in the life of the patient. In Robins' series, 4 out of 5 patients had made medical contact in the year before death. The message may be a direct verbal statement of intent, or indirect, such as giving away a treasured possession or revising a will. It is known that successful suicide is three times more common in men than in women and particularly common among men over 40 years of age. Those with a history of suicide in either mother or father carry a higher risk for self-destruction than those without such a history. A previous

suicide attempt adds to the risk. Most successful suicides give as their motive "a concern about ill health." Chronic illnesses such as alcoholism, cancer, heart disease, and progressive, incurable neurologic conditions all contribute to the risk of suicide. Thus, a portrait of a likely prospect for suicide might be a man in late adult life, in poor health through heavy drinking, who has recently lost his wife, who has attempted suicide before, and whose father committed suicide. However, no single one of these traits stands out as highly significant in terms of predicting suicide. As a consequence, we are left with our clinical judgment and index of suspicion as our main guides. The only rule of thumb is that all suicidal threats are to be taken seriously and all patients who threaten to kill themselves should be evaluated by a psychiatrist. The authors have found that important deterrants of suicide are devotion to Catholicism (suicide is a sin), concern about the suffering it would cause in the family, and fear of death, sincerely expressed by the patient.

Some physicians are reluctant to question depressed patients about the presence of suicidal thoughts on the grounds that this might upset them. More likely it is the physician who is upset by this questioning, for surely the mention of suicide will not alarm persons who are determined to end their lives, nor offend those with no such intention. Rather, a query of this type is apt to be appreciated by the depressed patient because it expresses the physician's concern, and indicates that the patient's behavior is being taken seriously. Should a patient's manner or conversation raise a suspicion of suicidal intent, it should be quickly voiced by the physician. This in itself sometimes brings to awareness unrecognized suicidal urges. If there appears to be an immediate danger of suicide, a bed should be obtained in a general hospital (preferably on the psychiatric ward) and a psychiatrist consulted. The point is to get the patient under cover until a psychiatrist arrives, and since a general hospital is far less threatening than a mental institution the patient is more apt to agree to enter. Once such a person has been admitted to the hospital, precautions against suicide should be initiated, including nurses "around the clock." The psychiatrist can determine the need for more or less security. If the patient refuses hospitalization, the family should be assembled, along with an intimate friend or clergyman, if appropriate, to urge the patient's cooperation. Should all efforts fail, the only recourse is a commitment to a psychiatric ward. Commitment procedures and laws vary from state to state, but all provide for temporary confinement of individuals who are thought to be self-destructive. Although an action of this sort is bound to be stressful for all concerned, prudence and caution are more important than the patient's plea for freedom. Hard feelings engendered by a short period of enforced confinement vanish in time, but those who mourn the loss of a loved one through a preventable suicide are apt to be unforgiving.

Patients who arrive at the hospital having attempted suicide should be under constant surveillance, once consciousness is regained, and a psychiatrist should be consulted. It is unwise to allow the family to keep watch, unless their competence is unquestioned. Among patients who have been hospitalized because of a preoccupation with suicide, a particular danger attends the phase of recovery from depression, when the physician may be lulled into a false sense of security. In either case, the psychiatrist should assume the responsibility for setting up a program of therapy and arrange for transfer to a psychiatric ward, if this is necessary, or for outpatient treatment.

HYPOCHONDRIASIS

A few remarks concerning the status of hypochondriasis as a psychiatric illness are in order. It is a condition that may be defined as the constant preoccupation with matters of health and an exaggerated concern about real or imagined signs and symptoms of illness. A hallmark of hypochondriasis is the failure of reassurance to affect either the symptoms or the patient's conviction of being sick. The most common complaint is pain, often vague and variable, most of which is referable to the head, chest, and lower part of the abdomen. It is a curious fact that over 70 percent of hypochondriacal complaints are related to the left side of the body.

Hypochondriasis is not considered to be a specific psychiatric disorder but is rather the somatic equivalent of depression or anxiety. As such, it is found in a number of psychiatric conditions such as depression (as described earlier in this chapter), schizophrenia, and the neuroses. It is not uncommon to encounter hypochondriacal reactions in otherwise normal individuals during periods of stress. Medical students, for example, traditionally develop symptoms of a variety of diseases during their first exposure to clinical medicine. When adolescents or young adults present hypochondriacal symptoms that are not related to transient episodes of stress, one should suspect a more serious underlying disorder such as depression or schizophrenia.

It is estimated that 85 percent of hypochondriasis is secondary to other mental disorders, chiefly depression, but in about 15 percent of cases there appears to be no associated

illness (*primary hypochondriasis*). In this latter category are the habitués of medical outpatient clinics, who are passed from specialist to specialist, perplexing and angering doctors along the way because their symptoms defy both satisfactory diagnosis and cure. Often referred to as ''crocks,'' these patients seldom benefit from conventional therapy.

The first step in the management of hypochondriasis is to determine whether it is part of another psychiatric syndrome such as depression, neurosis, or schizophrenia. As a rule this question can best be answered by a psychiatrist, and it is advisable to have each case evaluated from this point of view. If depressive symptoms are an important part of the clinical picture, the patient should be given a trial of antidepressant medication as described above. Neurotics and schizophrenics should be treated by a psychiatrist.

The treatment of primary hypochondriasis is difficult, if not impossible, unless the physician keeps in mind the personality of the patient and the therapeutic goals. Hypochondriacs tend to have unalterably rigid and obsessive personalities. For a variety of reasons, these patients need to retain their symptoms, so that the usual concept of ''curing'' is inapplicable. The presence of symptoms provides the context for a relationship with a physician. It is the continuation of this relationship, which is often the only dependable human contact in the patient's life, that motivates some hypochondriacs. Thus it is understandable why the hypochondriac is seldom moved to improve by reassurances that vigor and health will be restored. Physicians are so oriented toward the relief of suffering and the cure of disease that anger and frustration inevitably occur when they meet patients who coexist with their symptoms in an immutable symbiosis. In this situation it is usually the doctor who is the most discomfited. Such patients are best managed by physicians who realize that these are patients who do not necessarily want or expect a cure, who are content with small gains and the avoidance of unnecessary surgery, and who have an interest in the way symptoms persist rather than in any improvement. Since this type of physician is difficult to find, some hospitals have found it economical to utilize staff members who are able to provide such care by establishing special clinics under their leadership; here all hypochondriacs are evaluated and their course is followed. This is probably the most effective method for managing these cases from the standpoint of the physician as well as the patient.

ANOREXIA NERVOSA AND BULIMIA

The special syndrome called *anorexia nervosa* has been difficult to classify. If it has any connection with a psychiatric disease, and this is not established at the present time, it would be with a psychotic depression or an obsessional neurosis.

Anorexia nervosa is a disorder of previously healthy girls and young women, mainly from the upper and middle social classes, who become extremely emaciated as a result of voluntary starvation. It is rare in Orientals and blacks and practically never occurs in males.

As a rule, the syndrome begins shortly after puberty, sometimes later, and rarely it may be delayed until early adult life. Some of the patients have been overweight in childhood and especially in the prepubertal period. Dieting is much talked about and may have been encouraged, especially by the mothers, as a means of becoming more attractive. Sometimes there appears to be a precipitating event, such as leaving home, a disruption of family life, or other stress. Whatever the provocation, food intake is greatly reduced. What is more important, the abnormal eating habits persist even when the patient has become painfully thin, and when counseled to eat normally, she will use every artifice to starve herself. Food is hidden, instead of being eaten, and vomiting may be provoked after a meal or the bowel emptied by laxatives. No amount of persuasion will induce the patient to take adequate amounts of food. The patient shows no concern about her obvious emaciation and remains active. If left alone, these patients waste away and about 5 percent have succumbed to some intercurrent infection.

On physical examination, one is struck with the degree of emaciation; it exceeds that of most of the wasting diseases. Often as much as 30 percent of the body weight will have been lost by the time the patient's family insists on medical consultation. A fine lanugo covers the body and limbs. The skin is thin and dry without its normal elasticity and the nails are brittle. Pubic hair and breast tissue are normal, and in this respect anorexia nervosa is unlike hypopituitary cachexia (Simmonds disease). The extremities are often cold and blue. There are no neurologic signs of nutritional deficiency. The patient is alert and cheerfully indifferent to her condition. Any suggestion that she is unattractively thin or seriously depleted is rejected.

Amenorrhea is practically always present and may precede the extreme weight loss. Luteinizing hormone (LH) concentrations are reduced to pubertal or prepubertal levels. Clomiphene citrate fails to stimulate a rise in LH or follicle-stimulating hormone (FSH) as it does normally. Administration of gonadotropic releasing factor raises the LH and FSH levels, suggesting a hypothalamic disorder. The basal metabolic rate is low; T_3 and T_4 are low, while levels of physiologically inactive 3,3',5'-triiodothyronine (reverse T_3) are normal or increased. Plasma thyrotropin (TSH) and growth hormone levels are normal. Plasma cortisol levels are normal and excretion of 17-hydroxysteroids are slightly reduced. In sum, there is evidence of hypothalamic-pituitary

dysfunction; probably this is not primary but is secondary to starvation. Scheithauer and his colleagues found no definite changes in the pituitary gland in 12 fatal cases. The CT scan shows slight to moderate enlargement of the lateral and third ventricles, which return to normal size as the anorexia subsides.

As to etiology, there are numerous hypotheses. Slater and Roth believe that constitutional factors are important. Earlier signs of hysterical tendencies and of obsessional personality traits are mentioned as being frequent. Neurosis or psychopathy may be found in other members of the family. However, all psychiatrists seem agreed that the patient does not have symptoms that conform to any of the major neuroses or psychoses. In some reported series, depression is a major factor, and it is said that a high percentage of first-degree relatives have manic-depressive disease. Certainly loss of appetite, lack of self-esteem and interest in personal appearance, and self-destructive behavior—common features of anorexia nervosa—are also symptoms of depressive illness, yet the patients do not look despondent or admit to being dejected. Moreover, endogenous depression affects both sexes. The pathologic fear of becoming fat and the obsession with weight might be interpreted as a phobic or obsessional neurosis. A characteristic personality disorder and family constellation are claimed to have been found by psychoanalytically oriented psychiatrists, such as Bruch.

The fact that anorexia nervosa is practically confined to females must figure in any acceptable explanation of the syndrome. Among psychiatric disorders, only hysteria has this sexual predilection. Yet most psychiatrists do not believe anorexia nervosa to be a manifestation of hysteria. The racial-social relationships of the syndrome are also noteworthy. Undoubtedly important also is the fact that anorexia nervosa has its onset in relation to the menarche, at a time when the female exhibits rather large fluctuations in appetite and weight. Obesity before or around puberty is more pronounced in girls than boys. It is as though the appetite-satiety mechanism of the female hypothalamus is unstable.

The most effective *treatment* consists of immediate hospitalization, preferably on a psychiatric ward, winning the patient's confidence, supportive psychotherapy, assignment of one nurse to sit with the patient as each meal is eaten, and a gradual increase of a balanced diet (Anderson). If the patient refuses to eat, tube feeding is the only alternative, and she must understand that it is simply a question of eating voluntarily or being tube-fed. As weight is gained over several weeks the patient becomes more normal in her attitude and will usually continue to recover on this regimen at home. The menses will not return until considerable weight has been gained (to about 10 percent above the weight at the time of the menarche). Our colleagues report an 80 percent success with such a regime, when imipramine 150 mg/day is added. The long-term results are less clear. In several reports there has been a significant relapse rate (up to 50 percent over a period of 3 to 4 years), and many of the survivors are said to lapse into a chronic neurotic state characterized by a persistent preoccupation with food, weight and dieting.

The few adolescent boys that we have seen with this syndrome have recovered on antidepressant medication.

Bulimia This is an eating disorder characterized by massive binge eating, followed by the induction of vomiting and excessive use of laxatives. Insofar as the central psychologic disturbance is the pursuit of thinness at all costs, it is generally conceived as a variant of anorexia nervosa. However, the close relationship with the menarche, emaciation, and endocrinologic disturbances are not as evident in bulimic patients as in those with anorexia nervosa. Pope and his colleagues have reported considerable success in 19 of 20 bulimic patients treated with imipramine and followed for 2 years.

REFERENCES

AMSTERDAM JD, WINOKUR G, CAROFF SN et al: The dexamethasone suppression test in outpatients with primary affective disorder and healthy control subjects. *Am J Psychiatry* 139:287, 1982.

ANDERSON AE: *Practical Comprehensive Treatment of Anorexia Nervosa and Bulimia.* Baltimore, Johns Hopkins University Press, 1985.

BLAZER D, WILLIAMS CD: Epidemiology of dysphoria and depression in an elderly population. *Am J Psychiatry* 137:439, 1980.

BRUCH H: *Eating Disorders: Obesity, Anorexia Nervosa and the Person Within.* New York, Basic Books, 1973.

CADORET R, WINOKUR G: Depression in alcoholism. *Ann NY Acad Sci* 233:34, 1974.

CARROLL BJ, FEINBERG M, GREDEN JF et al: A specific laboratory test for the diagnosis of melancholia. *Arch Gen Psychiatry* 38:15, 1981.

CASSIDY WL, FLANAGAN NB, SPELLMAN M, COHEN ME: Clinical observations in manic-depressive disease. *JAMA* 164:1535, 1957.

CHARLES G, WILMOTTE J, QUENON M et al: Reproducibility of the dexamethasone suppression test in depression. *Biol Psychiat* 17:845, 1982.

Diagnostic a. d Statistical Manual of Mental Disorders, 3rd ed. Washington, D.C., American Psychiatric Association, 1980.

FOSTER DW: Anorexia nervosa and bulimia, in Braunwald E et al (eds): *Harrison's Principles of Internal Medicine,* 11th ed. New York, McGraw-Hill, 1987, pp 397–400.

FREUD S: Mourning and melancholia, in *The Complete Psychological Works of Sigmund Freud.* London, Hogarth, 1957, vol 14, pp 237–258.

GOODWIN DW, GUZE SB: *Psychiatric Diagnosis,* 3rd ed. New York, Oxford University Press, 1984.

GUZE SB, ROBINS E: Suicide and primary affective disorders. *Br J Psychiatry* 117:437, 1970.

HIRSCHFELD RMA, KLERMAN GL, ANDREASEN NC et al: Psychosocial predictors of chronicity in depressed patients. *Br J Psychiatry* 148:648, 1986.

INSEL TR, KALIN NH, GUTTMACHER LB et al: The dexamethasone suppression test in patients with primary obsessive-compulsive disorder. *Psychiatry Res* 6:153, 1982.

KALINOWSKY LB, HIPPUS H: *Pharmacological, Convulsive and Other Somatic Treatments in Psychiatry.* New York, Grune & Stratton, 1969.

KENYON FE: Hypochondriasis: A clinical study. *Br J Psychiatry* 110:478, 1964.

KLERMAN GL: Affective disorders, in Nicholi AM Jr (ed): *The Harvard Guide to Modern Psychiatry.* Cambridge, MA, Harvard, 1978, pp 253–281.

KLINE N: Practical management of depression. *JAMA* 190:732, 1964.

LEVINE DN, FINKELSTEIN S: Delayed psychosis after right temporoparietal stroke or trauma. *Neurology* 32:267, 1982.

LEWIS A: Melancholia: A historical review, in *The State of Psychiatry: Essays and Addresses.* New York, Science House, 1967, pp 71–110.

LEWIS DA, WINOKUR G: Depression. *Medical Grand Rounds* 314:376, 1984.

LINDEMANN E: Symptomatology and management of acute grief. *Am J Psychiatry* 101:141, 1944.

MAAS JW: The clinical and biochemical heterogeneity of the depressive disorders. *Ann Intern Med* 88:556, 1978.

PICHOT P, HASSAN J: Depressions masquées et équivalents dépressifs: problems et de définition et le diagnostic, in Kielholz P (ed): *La Depression Masquée.* Berne, Hans Huber, 1973, pp 62–80.

POPE HG, HUDSON JI, JONES JM et al: Bulimia treated with imipramine. A placebo-controlled double-blind study. *Am J Psychiatry* 140:554, 1983.

ROBINS E: *The Final Months: A Study of the Lives of 134 Persons Who Committed Suicide.* Oxford, England, Oxford University Press, 1981.

SCHEITHAUER BW, KOVACS KT, JARIWALA LK et al: Anorexia nervosa: An immunohistochemical study of the pituitary gland. *Mayo Clin Proc* 63:23, 1988.

SCHILDKRAUT JJ, GREEN AI, MOONEY JJ: Affective disorders: Biochemical aspects, in Kaplan HI, Sadock BJ (eds): *Comprehensive Textbook of Psychiatry,* 4th ed. Baltimore, Williams & Wilkins, 1985, pp 769–778.

SCHLESSER MA, WINOKUR G, SHERMAN BM: Hypothalamic-pituitary-adrenal axis activity in depressive illness. *Arch Gen Psychiatry* 37:737, 1980.

SCHUCKIT M, PITTS FN, REICH T et al: Alcoholism. I. Two types of alcoholism in women. *Arch Gen Psychiatry* 20:301, 1969.

SLATER E, ROTH M: *Mayer-Gross, Slater and Roth Clinical Psychiatry,* 3rd ed. Baltimore, Williams & Wilkins, 1969.

STARKSTEIN SE, ROBINSON RG, PRICE TR: Comparison of cortical and subcortical lesions in the production of poststroke mood disorders. *Brain* 110:1045, 1987.

WEISSMAN NM, MYERS JK: Affective disorders in a U.S. urban community. *Arch Gen Psychiatry* 35:1304, 1978.

WEITKAMP LR, STANCER HC, PERSAD E et al: Depressive disorders and HLA: A gene on chromosome 6 that can affect behavior. *N Engl J Med* 305:1301, 1981.

WILLNER P: Dopamine and depression: A review of recent evidence. *Brain Res Rev* 6:211;225;237, 1983.

WINOKUR G: Mania and depression: Family studies and genetics in relation to treatment, in Lipton MA et al (eds): *Psychopharmacology: A Generation of Progress.* New York, Raven Press, 1978, pp 1213–1221.

WINOKUR G: The types of affective disorder. *J Nerv Ment Dis* 156:82, 1973.

WINOKUR G: CADORET R: The irrelevance of the menopause to depressive disease, in Sachar EJ (ed): *Topics in Psychoendocrinology.* New York, Grune & Stratton, 1975, pp 59–66.

WINOKUR G, CLAYTON PJ, REICH T: *Manic-Depressive Illness.* St. Louis, Mosby, 1969.

WISHNIE HA, HACKETT TP, CASSEM NH: Psychological hazards of convalescence following myocardial infarction. *JAMA* 215:1292, 1971.

WOODS BT: Medical and neurological aspects of depression, in Isselbacher K et al (eds): *Principles of Internal Medicine. Update III.* New York, McGraw-Hill, 1982, pp 167–184.

ZIS AP, GOODWIN FK: The amine hypothesis, in Paykel ES (ed): *Handbook of Affective Disorders.* New York, Guilford, 1982, pp 175–190.

CHAPTER 57

THE SCHIZOPHRENIAS AND PARANOID STATES

SCHIZOPHRENIA

Schizophrenia is the most serious unsolved disease in world society, according to *Medical Research: A Mid-century Survey,* sponsored by the American Foundation (see References). Because of its prevalence (it occurs in about 1 percent of the population) and particularly because of its early onset, chronicity, and associated disability, the same conclusion is probably justified today.

DEFINITIONS

Neurologists and psychiatrists currently accept the idea that schizophrenia comprises a group of closely related disorders characterized by a particular type of disordered thinking, affect, and behavior. The syndromes by which they most commonly manifest themselves differ from those of delirium, confusional states, dementia, and depression in ways that will become clear in the following exposition. Unfortunately diagnosis depends on the recognition of specific psychologic disturbances unsupported by physical findings and laboratory data. This inevitably results in a certain imprecision. In other words, any group of patients classified as schizophrenic will to some extent be ''contaminated'' by patients with diseases that only resemble schizophrenia, whereas variant or incomplete cases of schizophrenia may not have been included. Moreover, there is not full agreement as to whether all the conditions called schizophrenic are the expression of a single disease process. In America, *paranoid schizophrenia* is usually considered to be a type of the common syndrome, whereas in Europe it is generally believed to be a separate disease.

Even the concept of disease with reference to schizophrenia has been criticized. Extreme opinions have claimed that schizophrenia is a product of the imagination of rigid European psychiatrists, or that it is but a social maladjustment, idiosyncratic behavior, or ''creative adaptation to an insane world,'' but these views are seldom taken seriously in medical circles.

HISTORICAL BACKGROUND

Present views of the disease we now call schizophrenia originated with Emil Kraepelin, a Munich neuropsychiatrist, who first clearly separated it from manic-depressive psychosis. He called it *dementia praecox* (adopting the term introduced earlier by Morel) to refer to a deterioration of mental function from a previous level of normalcy, at an early age. At first, Kraepelin believed that ''catatonia'' and ''hebephrenia,'' which had previously been described by Kahlbaum and by Hecker, respectively, as well as the paranoid form of schizophrenia, were separate diseases, but later, by 1898, he had concluded that they were manifestations of a single disease. Onset in adolescence and early adult life and the chronic course, often ending in marked deterioration of the personality, were emphasized as the denominative attributes of all forms of the disease.

Early in the twentieth century, the Swiss psychiatrist, Eugen Bleuler, substituted the term *schizophrenia* for *dementia praecox.* While an improvement, in that the term *dementia* was already being used to specify the clinical effects of another category of disease, it unfortunately implied a ''split personality'' or ''split mind,'' a feature thought by Morton Prince to be typical of a neurosis. Nonetheless schizophrenia became and still is the accepted name for the disease. By the ''splitting'' of psychic functions Bleuler meant the lack of correspondence between ideas and emotions—the inappropriateness of thinking and behavior in relation to the patient's mood and affect (in distinction to manic-depressive disease, in which the patient's morbid thoughts accurately reflect his mood). He also introduced the terms *autism* (''thinking divorced from reality'') and *ambivalence* to describe particular aspects of schizophrenia and called attention to a fourth syndrome, that of *simple schizophrenia.*

Bleuler believed that all the schizophrenic syndromes were composed of primary or basic symptoms, easily remembered as the "four A's" (loose *a*ssociations, flat *a*ffect, *a*mbivalence, and *a*utism), and of secondary or "partial phenomena" such as delusions, hallucinations, negativism, stupor, etc. However interesting this concept proved to be, the psychologic abnormalities are so poorly understood and so difficult to define precisely that this arbitrary division does not seem justified.

Other theories were those of Adolph Meyer and Sigmund Freud. Meyer, who introduced the "psychobiologic approach" to American psychiatry, sought the origins of schizophrenia, as well as other psychiatric syndromes, in the personal and medical history of patients and their habitual reactions to life events. His term for schizophrenia, *parergasia,* never gained wide acceptance. Freud viewed schizophrenia as a manifestation of a "weak ego" and an inability to use the ego defenses to handle anxiety and instinctual forces. As a result, the patient regressed to infantile levels of psychosexual function and a fixation at the narcissistic stage. Berze in 1914 singled out the "insufficiency and lowering of all psychic activity" as being the fundamental defect in schizophrenia and attributed it to organic damage of unknown nature. None of these theories has been corroborated.

In 1937, Langfeldt proposed the concept that schizophrenia consists principally of two different types of psychosis, viz., (1) cases that correspond to the disease considered briefly above, i.e., Kraepelin's dementia praecox and Bleuler's schizophrenia (these cases are characterized, among other things, by a poor prognosis), and (2) cases that occur acutely, on a background of a stable premorbid personality, often with clouding of consciousness and demonstrable precipitating factors. For the latter cases, which could be a manifestation of several diseases, Langfeldt proposed the term *schizophreniform psychoses.* The latter cases tend to have a favorable prognosis.

EPIDEMIOLOGY

Schizophrenia has been found in every racial and social group so far studied. Incidence rates are difficult to evaluate because not all psychiatrists have used the same criteria for diagnosis. Prevalence rates worldwide range from 100 to 500 per 100,000 (probably 150 is nearest the correct value), and expectancy rates are estimated to be as high as 1000 per 100,000, i.e., one chance in 100 that a person will manifest the condition during his or her lifetime. Presumably there are always some undiagnosed cases in every population, which would require the figure to be corrected upward. Most of the statistical data come from North

America, Europe, and Japan, and one cannot be certain that the incidence is the same in other parts of the world, but estimates of a worldwide prevalence of 10 to 20 million and of 4 to 5 million new cases per year seem realistic.

Schizophrenics occupy about half the beds in mental hospitals—more hospital beds than patients with any other single disease. They constitute 20 to 30 percent of all new admissions to psychiatric hospitals (100,000 to 200,000 new cases per year in the United States); at any one time about 300,000 schizophrenics are in hospitals and 1.5 million are living outside. The age of admission to hospital is between 20 and 40, with a peak at 28 to 34 years.

The incidence of schizophrenia has remained more or less the same over the past several decades. Males and females are affected with equal frequency. For unknown reasons the incidence is higher in social classes showing high mobility and disorganization. It has been suggested that deteriorating function caused by the disease results in a "downward drift" to the lowest socioeconomic stratum, where one finds poverty, crowding, limited education, and associated handicaps, but the same data have been used to support the idea that such social factors cause schizophrenia. The fertility of schizophrenics, formerly lowered by institutionalization, is now approaching that of the general population, which will probably result in an increase in their number.

CAUSE AND MECHANISM

Although there is no universal agreement as to the cause of the disease, an increasing weight of evidence favors a genetic factor. Other biologic factors and psychosocial factors are also considered important. The evidence for each will be presented.

Genetic Factors The early studies of Kallmann showed that the expectancy rate for schizophrenia in 5000 siblings of schizophrenic patients was increased from 0.9 percent (the expected rate for the general population) to 11 percent. In 90 sets of fraternal twins, one of whom had schizophrenia, the incidence of disease in the other twin was also 11 percent, the same as in nontwin siblings; in 62 sets of monozygotic twins the incidence in the second twin was 68 percent. In other words, the closer the relatedness of a family member to a schizophrenic, the greater the risk of schizophrenia. Thus, the prospect of a child of one schizophrenic parent having schizophrenia is the same as for the siblings of schizophrenic patients (about 11 percent); if both parents are schizophrenic, the chances are greater than

50 percent that the child will have the disease. Subsequent family studies have repeatedly confirmed these findings (see Goodwin and Guze for a more complete tabulation).

There has been much discussion in the medical literature concerning nature versus nurture, i.e., the relative importance of genetic and environmental factors in the causation of the disease. The available studies lend little support to environmental factors. In the study of Rosenthal, Kety, and their associates, a group of children of schizophrenics were removed at an early age from their natural parents and placed in adoptive homes; these children were compared with a group of adopted children whose natural parents had no known psychiatric disease. Thus the child of the schizophrenic shared the genetic background of his parents but not their environment. Follow-up observations disclosed that the incidence of schizophrenia in the first group of children was about twice that of the second. In two similar studies both Karlsson and Heston showed that children who were separated early in life and reared apart from schizophrenic parents had the same disposition to schizophrenia (11 percent) as children of schizophrenics raised in the homes of their biologic parents. Fischer approached the problem differently. Monozygotic twins, only one of whom was schizophrenic, were identified, and their children were studied; the incidence of schizophrenia in the children of the nonschizophrenic member of the twin pair was the same as in the children of the schizophrenic member.

Rosenthal, Kety, and their associates, in identifying adoptees who developed schizophrenia, included three types of disorder—chronic schizophrenia, latent schizophrenia, and acute schizophrenia. They concluded that the syndrome of schizophrenia was not homogeneous. Among the biologic relatives of the adoptees with chronic schizophrenia there was considerably more schizophrenia and schizophrenia-like illness than among relatives of adoptees with latent and acute schizophrenia. Moreover, typical chronic schizophrenia occurred only in the biologic relatives of adoptees with the same syndrome. There was also an unexpectedly high frequency of chronic, latent, and uncertain forms of schizophrenia in the biologic half siblings of schizophrenic adoptees whose shared parent had one of these diagnoses. The incidence of chronic and latent schizophrenia among the relatives of acute schizophrenia probands was no greater than that in the general population. These findings support the idea of etiologic diversity of schizophrenia, suggested earlier by Matthysse and by Richter.

Although the importance of genetic factors in the etiology of schizophrenia is undeniable, the precise mode of inheritance has not been determined; the findings described above as well as evidence presented by Morton et al and by Böök et al favor a single gene of intermediate (partial or incomplete) dominance.

Other Biologic Factors   Body habitus was singled out long ago by Kretschmer as being linked in some way to schizophrenia. He believed that slender (leptosomic) individuals tended to develop schizophrenia, if they were to become psychotic, and those with a stocky (pyknic) body build became manic-depressive. More modern studies by Sheldon and others have not fully supported this hypothesis.

A great variety of physiologic and endocrine differences between schizophrenic and normal subjects has been claimed. When the observations were controlled, however, the abnormality in question was always found to relate to physical inactivity, neglect, or undernourishment, especially in chronically hospitalized patients, rather than to the disease per se.

There have been many attempts to isolate some metabolic or toxic substance from the blood of schizophrenic patients, which when injected into nonschizophrenic subjects, could reproduce the clinical state. Such positive results as were claimed have been unverified. This is true of the psychotropic copper-containing globulin called *taraxein*, histamine, serotonin or catecholamine metabolites, amino acids, altered macroglobulins, and an erythrocyte-lysing factor. From time to time an aminoaciduria, a folate or vitamin B_{12} deficiency, or some such condition has been discovered in a psychotic patient who is said to have schizophrenia, but isolated findings of this sort, in patients in whom the diagnosis can be questioned, have little meaning.

When certain hallucinogens, such as mescaline and lysergic acid diethylamide (LSD), were first observed to induce hallucinations and abnormalities of thinking, it was hoped that these drugs might provide models of experimental schizophrenia. It was even postulated that in schizophrenia a faulty metabolism of biogenic amines produces such an endogenous psychotogen. This has never been substantiated. When methionine, a potent source of methyl groups, was observed to exacerbate the symptoms of some schizophrenics, it was thought that a primary metabolic fault had been discovered. The presence of increased quantities of dimethoxyphenethylamine and N-methylated indoleamines lent support to this idea. Again, none of these observations has been unequivocally corroborated.

Since the antipsychotic drugs display an affinity for dopamine receptors, it has been widely concluded that these drugs produce their therapeutic effects (and side effects) by receptor blockade. Other hypotheses have proposed a reduction in dopaminergic transmission, implicating neurotransmitters such as norepinephrine, acetylcholine, serotonin, and γ-aminobutyric acid (GABA) which interact or maintain a balance with dopamine (Matthysse and Pope). The original idea of each neurotransmitter regulating a particular function or mental state is probably an oversimplification (for further details see review by Kety).

Since psychoses may complicate corticosteroid administration and certain endocrine disorders (Cushing syndrome, thyrotoxicosis), there have been many attempts to uncover such abnormalities in the schizophrenic patient. All have failed.

Psychosocial Factors Freud's theory of schizophrenia has already been mentioned. He believed that the schizophrenic process represents a fixation at or possibly a regression to the "narcissistic" stage of sexual development. There is no way of affirming or refuting this proposition. The same can be said for the hypothesis that there is a defect in the attention process by which sensations, thoughts, and feelings are "filtered." This results in altered experiences, and the delusions and hallucinations are postulated to be attempts to deal with them.

Intrafamily relationships have been thought by some to be responsible for engendering schizophrenic traits. The picture was painted of the cold, rejecting, but overprotective mother who induces conflicting reaction patterns in her child. The latter is said to be threatened by the intermittent expression of affection, possibility of separation, coercion to conform to family standards, lack of mutual support, etc. Behind all these suggestions is the notion that disturbed interpersonal relations in the family in some way interfere with the normal maturation of personality. Proof is totally lacking that such an environment is unique to the development of schizophrenia. Furthermore, the extent to which these aberrations of family relationship are primary or secondary cannot be ascertained. Unquestionably such explorations have elucidated hitherto unknown aspects of family life, but just how they relate to schizophrenia is anyone's guess.

The observations of Harlow and his associates on the deleterious effects of maternal and peer deprivation in primates suggested the notion that similar deprivations in humans were responsible for the development of schizophrenia. However, such severe degrees of familial deprivation have rarely been documented in humans; and when they were, as in some orphans, the effects were only transitory.

CLINICAL MANIFESTATIONS

Bleuler, adhering to the concept promulgated by Kraepelin, described schizophrenia as

> . . . *a* group of psychoses *whose course is at times chronic, at times marked by intermittent attacks, and*

> *which can stop and retrograde at any stage, but does not permit a full* restitutio ad integrum. *The disease is characterized by a specific type of alteration of thinking, feeling, and relation to the external world which appears no place else in this particular fashion. . . . The fundamental symptoms consist of disturbances of association and affectivity, the predilection for fantasy as against reality, and the inclination to divorce oneself from reality (autism). Furthermore we can add the absence of those very symptoms which play such a great role in certain other diseases as primary disturbances of perception, orientation, memory etc.*

This definition differs only slightly from that of Kraepelin. In his view the fundamental symptoms consisted of "the weakening of judgment, of mental activity and of creative ability, the dulling of emotional interest . . . and the loosening of the inner unity of the psychic life." By this latter phrase he meant "the loss of the inner unity of the activities of intellect, emotion and volition in themselves and among one another"; in particular he stressed the lack of correspondence between emotions and ideas.

Included in the definition, both by Kraepelin and by Bleuler, were a characteristic premorbid personality, an insidious onset in adolescence or early adult life, and a chronic course. Both regarded hallucinations and delusions as secondary or accessory symptoms that could be absent, as in their "dementia praecox simplex" or "simple schizophrenia." Embodied in both their definitions is the concept of disease (rather than a psychopathologic reaction) characterized by chronicity and a unique constellation of symptoms different from delirium, confusion, depression, mania, dementia, and other brain diseases.

Attempts to apply these diagnostic criteria met with difficulty, especially when hallucinations and delusions were absent. In order to overcome this difficulty Schneider proposed that the distinction between primary and accessory manifestations be abandoned. He found that the greatest reliability attached to the occurrence of vocal hallucinations, perceptual delusions (misinterpretation of what the patient sees and hears), and the experience of one's thoughts and actions being broadcasted and being not one's own but influenced by some outside agency (experiences of alienation and influence). This constellation of symptoms, which was precise and easy to recognize, came to be known as Schneider's first-rank symptoms of schizophrenia.

Strict adherence to Schneider's diagnostic criteria,

when applied to a group of patients admitted to the hospital with a diagnosis of schizophrenia, served to identify two groups of patients—those with and those without first-rank symptoms (Taylor). The former responded more poorly to treatment and required a more prolonged period in hospital and higher doses of neuroleptic drugs than the latter. Moreover, the two groups corresponded closely to the two categories of schizophrenic disorders recognized by Robins and Guze on the basis of prognosis. The Schneider-positive, poor-prognosis patients are identifiable with the chronic kraepelinian schizophrenia (also referred to as *nuclear* or *process* schizophrenia); the Schneider-negative patients with good prognosis are probably suffering from some other nonschizophrenic illness or the so-called schizophreniform illness of Langfeldt (see above).

From the neurologic point of view, the central abnormality in schizophrenia appears to be a special disorder of attention and the perception of one's self and the external world. It is unlike the condition that prevails in delirium and other confusional states, dementia and depression. Some patients with chronic schizophrenia, when in remission, show none of the flagrant schneiderian first-rank symptoms and during brief testing of mental status would pass for normal. But on long-term observation they are vague, preoccupied, and unable to think in the abstract, to fully understand figurative statements such as proverbs, and to separate relevant from irrelevant data. There is a circumstantiality and tangentiality about their remarks. They fail to communicate their ideas clearly. Their thinking no longer respects the logical limits of time and space. Parts are confused with the whole, or are clustered together or condensed in an illogical way. Opposites may be considered as identical, and conceptual relationships are distorted. In an analysis of a problem or a situation there is a tendency to be overinclusive rather than underinclusive (as happens in dementia). In conversation and in writing the trend of an argument or thought sequence is often interrupted abruptly, with a resulting disorder of verbal communication.

In more severely affected schizophrenics, thinking is even more disintegrated, and they can do no more than utter a series of meaningless phrases or neologisms; or speech may be reduced to a "word salad." They are unable to attend to the task at hand or to concentrate, and their performance of sequential tasks is interrupted by extraneous ideas, with the result that performance becomes variable and unpredictable, somewhat like that of a confused or delirious patient. At times these patients are talkative and exhibit odd behavior; at other times they are quiet, preoccupied with their own thoughts, and concerned about their

family or others around them or with imagined diseases. Young patients are often quite hypochondriacal, which brings them to the attention of a physician. At the other extreme, they are mute and idle. With remission, they may have only fragmentary memories of events that had occurred during the exacerbation of their illness.

A number of unusual experiences, concerning the relationship of the patients to themselves and to their environment, may be communicated to the examiner, as pointed out by Schneider. They may express the thought that their body is somehow separated from their mind, that they do not feel like themselves, that their body belongs to someone else, or that they are not sure of their own identity or even sex. This is called *depersonalization*. Closely related are the ideas of being under the control of some external agency, of their thoughts being broadcasted, or being made to speak or act in ways that are dictated by others, often through the medium of radar, telepathy, etc. (*passivity feelings*). There are frequently misperceptions and *ideas of reference*—that the remarks or actions of others are subtly directed to themselves. Finally patients may feel that the world about them is changed or unnatural, not in a brief episode like the *jamais vu* of a temporal lobe seizure, but continuously.

Auditory hallucinations are frequent; they consist of voices that are usually accusatory or threatening, or in control of the patient's actions. The voices may or may not be recognized. The voices come from outside the patient or from within and in the latter case cannot be distinguished from the patient's own feelings and thoughts. Visual, olfactory, and other types of hallucinations also occur. The patient believes in the reality of these hallucinations, and they may be part of a delusional system.

The behavior of the individual experiencing these ideas and feelings is correspondingly altered. Early in the course of the illness, normal activities may be interrupted. No longer does the patient function properly in school or at work. Associates and relatives are likely to find the patient's complaints, fears, and bizarre ideas disturbing. The patient may be idle for long periods, preoccupied with inner ruminations, and may withdraw socially. A panic or frenzy of excitement may lead to a visit to an emergency ward (a high degree of anxiety developing for the first time in a young person should always alert one to the possibility of a developing schizophrenia), or the patient may become mute and immobile, i.e., *catatonic*. However, attacks of catatonia are infrequent, and lack of will, drive, assertiveness, etc., are more characteristic of the disease.

Much has been made of the change in affect. Usually the patient's manner is bland or apathetic; he or she may casually express ideas that would be disturbing to a normal person, even smiling or laughing over a morbid idea. To the authors this has not been an impressive feature of the illness. Often one observes agitation and appropriate emotionality in response to a threatening hallucination or delusion, although later there appears increasing indifference and preoccupation, with flat affect, as though the patient had become inured to the abnormal thoughts and feelings.

Other behavioral and delusional features are discussed in relation to the special types of schizophrenia.

SUBTYPES OF SCHIZOPHRENIA

Psychiatrists have traditionally distinguished a number of subtypes of schizophrenia, and this practice will be followed here. These subdivisions should not be considered inviolable, however. Their clinical value has been questioned by Goodwin and Guze who remark on the frequency with which these various types may overlap or change during the course of the illness.

Undifferentiated, or Simple, Schizophrenia In this condition the patient exhibits thought disorder, bland affect, social withdrawal, and impaired work performance, but not hallucinations and delusions. At this stage the diagnosis is uncertain. Any disorder of thinking may be difficult to elicit, but from time to time a peculiar idea emerges in conversation. Terms such as schizoid, latent or borderline schizophrenia, or schizotypal are applied. Eventually, there will be an outbreak of flagrant hallucinations and delusions—an acute schizophrenic episode during which all the aforementioned symptoms worsen. In the acute phase the patient usually needs to be hospitalized and given medication because of a suicidal attempt or some other unexpected action. As a rule, a remission follows, during which the patient is again able to function, but at a level below that which is expected on the basis of his previous abilities and intelligence; and he proves to be lacking in normal drive, initiative, and enterprise. These patients attract notice because they behave in an odd manner, tending to remain by themselves (''loners''), making no effort to adjust to a social group at school, find work, ''have dates,'' or establish or maintain a family unit. If the parents do not provide support and protection, such persons drift from one menial job to another, always shy, withdrawn, and relatively indifferent to their surroundings. Some individuals of this type are found among ''hobos'' and others on the fringes of society.

In this form of schizophrenia, the florid characteristics of catatonia or hebephrenia are not observed and psychotic manifestations are infrequent. Since it may easily be confused with other psychiatric illnesses, the precision of diagnosis is variable (see below, under ''Diagnosis'').

Hebephrenic Schizophrenia (Disorganized Schizophrenia—DSM III) This was believed by Kraepelin to be a particularly malignant form. It tends to occur at an earlier age than the other varieties. The thought disorder is pronounced—there is a striking incoherence of ideas, and the frequent occurrence of hallucinations, delusions, and marked emotional disturbances (periods of excitement alternating with periods of tearfulness and depression) leaves little doubt that the patient is psychotic. The visual and auditory illusions and hallucinations are usually more in the nature of symbolic interpretations than abnormal perceptions. Kraepelin remarked on the changeable, fantastic, and bizarre character of the delusions. Motor symptoms, in the form of stereotyped behavior and mannerisms, are prominent in this form of schizophrenia. Some psychiatrists have been impressed with the fact that hebephrenic patients since their early days are likely to have had a history of tantrums and of being overly pious, shy, fearful, solitary, conscientious, and idealistic—traits that may have marked them as odd or ''queer.'' This latter state is sometimes called *schizoid,* but could just as well represent the early phase of the disease itself (see Chap. 55).

Catatonic Schizophrenia This is the most readily differentiated type. It was originally described by Kahlbaum and considered to be a mental disturbance *sui generis,* until Kraepelin recognized that it was another form of schizophrenia. In 60 percent of cases, the onset is relatively acute. In the other 40 percent, after a long prodrome of slackening interest, apathy, lack of concentration, and dreamy preoccupation, a state of dull stupor supervenes, with mutism, inactivity, refusal of food, and a tendency to maintain one position, ''like a mummy.'' The facial expression is vacant, the lips pursed; the patient lies supine without motion, or sits for hours with hands on knees and head bowed (*catalepsy*). If a limb is lifted by the examiner it will sometimes be held in that position for hours (flexibilitas cerea). Urine and feces are retained, or there is incontinence. The patients must be tube-fed (or will eat mechanically) and have to be dressed and undressed. Pinprick or pinch induces no reaction. Extreme negativism, every command being resisted, characterizes some cases. Echolalia and echopraxia are observed occasionally. Yet these patients may be fully aware of what is said to them or happening around them and will reproduce much of this information during a spontaneous remission or one induced by intravenous sodium amytal. After weeks or months in this state, the patient begins to talk and act more normally, and there is then rapid recovery. In certain phases of catatonia there may be a period of excitement and impulsivity, during which the patient may be suicidal or homicidal.

For reasons that are unclear, this form of schizophrenia is now seen infrequently, and there is increasing recognition of the fact that many of its features are more often manifestations of manic-depressive disease than of schizophrenia.

Acute Schizophrenia This term has been applied to a rapidly evolving florid illness with the main attributes of schizophrenic psychosis. Many psychiatrists are skeptical that such an entity exists, especially when there is no history of familial occurrence or of early schizoid behavior. The majority of such episodes turn out to be manic attacks (Pope and Lipinski); toxic confusional and endocrine psychoses may also simulate acute schizophrenia (the schizophreniform psychosis of Langfeldt). Yet there is no doubt that a small proportion of cases of classic schizophrenia (about 10 percent, according to Kety) will have had an acute episode and long-lasting remission before lapsing into a chronic progressive form of the illness. Unfortunately, these latter patients, at the time of the acute psychosis, cannot be distinguished by competent clinicians from those who have a permanent remission.

Paranoid Schizophrenia This is one of the most frequent subtypes. The mean age of onset is 42 years (Winokur), somewhat later than the preceding types. Multiple, unsystematized, changeable delusions are expressed, some quite fantastic and accompanied by hallucinations. More often than not they are persecutory, but also they may be religious, depressive, and grandiose in nature. Delusional jealousy may be added. Many such patients settle into a chronic hallucinatory psychosis with disorders of thinking, featured by mistrust and suspiciousness. They appear cold, aloof, and indifferent, and many are hypochondriacal.

European psychiatrists, impressed with the lack of schizoid traits in the premorbid period and in the family history, have insisted that paranoid schizophrenia is a separate disease. The studies of Rosenthal and his colleagues in this country tend to bear them out. Also, the clinical and the family studies of Winokur indicate that undifferentiated and hebephrenic schizophrenia are probably different illnesses than paranoid schizophrenia.

There are of course other psychiatric illnesses in which paranoid delusions appear, notably manic-depressive psychosis, dementia, and delirium. Alcoholic auditory hallucinosis stands as a separate illness (see page 878). There is, in addition, a special form of *delusional disorder* (*paranoia*) in which the individual is consumed by a single persecutory, grandiose, or amorous delusional system, without other disorders of thinking. An exotic form is known as *folie à deux,* in which two closely related persons share a delusional system. These several types of paranoia are discussed further in the latter part of the chapter.

Residual Schizophrenia This is an occasionally used designation for the condition in which, after one or several episodes of schizophrenia, patients become nonpsychotic and function reasonably well, though subnormally. In reality they have schizophrenia in remission.

Childhood Schizophrenia This term has been applied to a disorder of children who have a wide variety of developmental and adjustment problems and who at some time become psychotically disturbed; i.e., they become excited, depressed, or hallucinatory and express bizarre ideas. The relation of such illnesses to adult schizophrenia remains unsettled. There is no evidence that such children go on to have schizophrenia later in life. Often organic factors, such as metabolic errors and mental retardation, are demonstrable.

Some psychiatrists speak of infantile autism (page 481) as childhood schizophrenia. The fact that the incidence of schizophrenia is not increased in the families of autistic children supports the idea that they are separate diseases. It is also noteworthy that hardly ever is childhood psychosis recorded in the histories of schizophrenic patients (which is why one should be hesitant to make the diagnosis of schizophrenia during childhood).

OTHER NEUROPSYCHIATRIC ABNORMALITIES

Stevens and others have confirmed the findings of Kraepelin and Bleuler that as many as two-thirds of schizophrenics have some abnormalities on detailed neurologic examination. Studies by Kennard, by Hertzig and Birch, and by Tucker et al found a much higher frequency of "soft signs" in schizophrenics than in a normal population. By soft signs they meant impersistence in assigned tasks, astereognosis and graphesthesia, sensory extinction, hyperreflexia and hyporeflexia, difficulties in coordination, disturbances of balance, abnormal (choreiform) movements, abnormalities of motor activity, adventitial and overflow movements, anisocoria, esotropia, and faults in visual auditory integration. Some of these signs were objectified by the Goldstein-Scherer object sorting test and the Halstead-Reitan tactual performance test. "Soft signs" of this type were noted in 50 percent and correlated with the degree of cognitive disorder. "Hard signs" such as unilateral motor or sensory defects or definite EEG abnormalities were noted in about one-third of all patients. The meaning of these slight abnormalities is conjectural. They are more frequent in the group of schizophrenic patients who are found to have EEG abnormalities and enlarged ventricles (Murray et al).

Sophisticated psychometric testing has disclosed abnormalities not so much in intelligence and memory (which are only slightly reduced in 20 to 30 percent of cases) as in other psychologic functions. Alertness is not impaired, but the maintenance of attention, as evidenced in continuing performance tasks, is reduced (Seidman). Often patients seem oblivious to what happens around them. Except where muteness is a feature, speech is fluent and no measurable alteration of language function or calculation has been reported. In tests of verbal and visual pattern learning, problem solving, and memorizing, Cutting found a surprising degree of impairment in both the acute and chronic schizophrenic (and in patients with retarded depression) not attributable to electroconvulsive therapy, seizures, drugs, or other diseases. Interestingly, in the acute schizophrenic, he found verbal memory more affected than visual pattern memory, in agreement with the findings of Flor-Henry that left-hemispheric functions are more reduced than right. In the chronic schizophrenic there was evidence of bihemispheral derangement.

The high risk of suicide in schizophrenia is often not appreciated. In a 30- to 40-year follow-up study of schizophrenic and manic-depressive patients, Winokur and Tsuang found that in each group the same proportion (about 10 percent) of patients had committed suicide. Suicide occurs most often among young schizophrenics living apart from their families, frightened and discouraged by their symptoms and the difficulties of independent existence. Sometimes the suicide is in response to terrifying and commanding vocal hallucinations. The schizophrenic may also be homicidal, usually in acting upon a delusion that he or she has been wronged by the victim.

Periodically schizophrenic patients are subject to exacerbations of their illness, sometimes at regular intervals, as though determined by a metabolic disorder, e.g., Gjessing's cases, in which attacks of periodic catatonia were associated with shifts in nitrogen balance (see Lehmann). Functional remissions are more frequent and lasting when medication is given and long institutionalization is avoided. Modern therapeutic programs have reduced the number of patients in mental hospitals by 1 to 2 percent per year. However, readmission rates also have risen (revolving-door phenomenon), and the total number of very young and very old patients in hospitals has even increased slightly. The life expectancy of schizophrenics is somewhat reduced, probably because of the malnutrition, neglect, and exposure to infections that occur in public institutions.

NEUROPATHOLOGY

Throughout the modern era of cellular neuropathology, there has been disagreement concerning the status of schizophrenia. Alzheimer and his pupils, who had access to the clinical material of Kraepelin, made a study of 55 cases, including 18 uncomplicated and 6 acute. They noted hypertrophy (ameboid change) of the astrocytes, to which importance was attached because it was not found in cases of manic-depressive psychosis. Further, in the cerebra of deteriorated schizophrenics, an outfall of neurons in the second and third laminae of the frontal cortex was described, along with nuclear swelling, shrinkage of cell bodies, and deposits of lipofuscin. Similar findings were subsequently described by Sioli, Orton, and others.

Dunlap, in 1928, in a highly critical analysis, repudiated all earlier interpretations of these alterations. He pointed out that many changes, such as the dark "sclerotic" nerve cells, were artifacts and that lipofuscin was a nonspecific age change. He asserted also that the neuronal loss described by Alzheimer was based on impression and could not be corroborated by quantitative methods. Similarly, the claim of Oscar Vogt of neuronal loss in the cortex was rejected by his contemporaries, Spielmeyer and Scholz, who were unable to find any consistent cellular abnormality in schizophrenia (see Dunlap for early references).

Unfortunately the matter is not settled even today, for no cases (except those of Vogt) have been rigorously studied by whole-brain serial sections, and no quantitative studies have been made of septal and other central nuclei. Golgi and ultrastructural methods, using reliable techniques, have not been applied. Of course, the absence of a cellular pathologic change does not rule out a disease process, for in delirium tremens, toxic psychosis, and many metabolic diseases of the brain, the lesion is probably subcellular, i.e., molecular. As pointed out by Kety, the disease may ultimately reveal itself by a morphology yet to be explored; in enzymatic, biochemical, or immunologic processes; or in membrane or receptor mechanisms, many of which are now becoming accessible to study.

Of recent interest are observations of sulcal widening and ventricular enlargement in chronic schizophrenics examined by CT scans. Johnstone and associates noted these radiologic abnormalities in 18 cases and associated them with dulling of intellect and affect. Weinberger et al, in 58 chronic schizophrenics under the age of 50 years, found enlargement of the lateral ventricles in 40 percent. Rieder et al, whose patients ranged from 20 to 35 years, found 4 of 17 to have widened sulci.

The exact meaning of these radiologic abnormalities (which have been interpreted as cerebral atrophy) will only become known when the affected regions are subjected to quantitative neuropathologic study. Murray et al, opining that none of the proposed models of hereditary transmission has been convincing, asks whether there are at least two types of schizophrenia—one with ventricular enlargement and a negative family history, and the other (approximately two-thirds of the whole group) with normal ventricles and a positive family history. In the first group of sporadic, "acquired" schizophrenia, environmental factors, such as birth injury and EEG abnormalities (see below), might be more frequent.

A special problem in all morphologic studies relates to the accuracy of the clinical diagnosis. As pointed out by Davison and Bagley, many of the psychologic and behavioral characteristics of schizophrenia occur in Wilson disease, Huntington chorea, chronic alcoholism, metabolic encephalopathies, and temporal lobe epilepsy. Hence one may be observing a clinical syndrome of multiple etiologies, some with an identifiable morphologic substratum. Theoretically, schizophrenia may be affecting the same regions of the brain, but without a presently demonstrable cytopathology.

The EEG has revealed minor abnormalities in 5 to 80 percent of cases, depending on how it is interpreted. Spahn and Patterson report some delta activity in the frontal regions and prominence of postcentral beta activity. And, by depth electrode recording from the septal region, hippocampus, and amygdala, Heath found spike-wave discharges. PET scanning has raised a suspicion of dopamine receptor abnormalities in central ganglionic structures, and Weinberger et al noted a failure of the frontal cortex to increase its blood flow during cognitive activities.

DIAGNOSIS

From a neurologic standpoint, the main distinction to be made is between an acute schizophrenia-like psychosis (schizophreniform reaction; "good-prognosis" schizophrenia) and the chronic disease schizophrenia (nuclear or process schizophrenia). The acute schizophreniform illness takes the form of a delusional-hallucinatory syndrome in which there is little if any disturbance of consciousness. Although such a syndrome is characteristic of schizophrenia, it may occur in the manic phase of manic-depressive disease, alcoholic auditory hallucinosis, temporal lobe epilepsy, chronic amphetamine intoxication, withdrawal from amphetamine after chronic intoxication, and rarely in certain endocrine and metabolic disorders, in which consciousness is not impaired. Whenever this syndrome is recognized, therefore, these several causes need to be differentiated. At the McLean Hospital, less than one out of five of the acute schizophreniform psychoses proves to be due to the disease schizophrenia.

The diagnosis of the disease called schizophrenia involves a different constellation of data. The presence of

the delusional-hallucinatory syndrome always raises the possibility of schizophrenia, but it must be remembered that in chronic schizophrenia or in the remittent form of the disease, the components of this syndrome may be either absent or too subtle to detect during a brief examination. Other data are required for diagnosis. Feighner, Robins, and Guze, who have drawn up a set of diagnostic criteria for research in all the major psychiatric syndromes, state that the diagnosis of schizophrenia is tenable only if there are (1) a chronic illness of at least 6 months' duration and a failure (after an acute episode) to return to the premorbid level of psychosocial adjustment, (2) delusions or hallucinations without significant perplexity or disorientation (i.e., without clouding of consciousness), (3) verbal productions that are so illogical and confusing as to make communication difficult (if the patient is mute, diagnosis should be deferred), and (4) at least three of the following manifestations: (*a*) an adult who is single, (*b*) poor premorbid social adjustment or work history, (*c*) family history of schizophrenia, or (*d*) onset of illness prior to age of 40 years. Important negatives include the absence of a family history of manic-depressive disease, absence of an earlier illness with depressive or manic symptoms, and absence of alcoholism, drug abuse, or other organic disease within a year of onset of the psychosis.

While these criteria are so strict as to exclude certain patients with a schizophrenic illness, those that are included will be found to constitute a fairly homogeneous group. Morrison et al, who used these criteria, noted that after a 10-year period there was practically no change in diagnosis; they had quite reliably separated schizophrenia, the schizophreniform psychoses (in which only the acute delusional-hallucinatory syndrome was present), and manic-depressive psychosis.

In addition to the acute schizophreniform psychosis described above, the authors have encountered the greatest difficulties in the diagnosis of schizophrenia in the following clinical situations:

1. A patient with a normal family and premorbid history, *with an acute illness* having many of the typical features of schizophrenia but *associated with confusion, forgetfulness, and/or clouding of consciousness.* Mood change may be prominent. Thus the illness combines the features of an affective disorder, schizophrenia, and a confusional state. This syndrome is characteristic of corticosteroid psychosis (drug-induced or Cushing disease), thyrotoxic psychosis, puerperal psychosis, PCB intoxication, and the so-called exhaustion psychoses (combat fatigue) of wartime. Usually recovery is complete, and "process schizophrenia" is excluded by the fact that the patient remains well.

2. *Adolescents and young adults whose social relationships are disorganized and who are unusually sensi-*

tive, resentful, rebellious, fearful, discouraged, in trouble with school authorities and the law, using drugs, etc. The latter may have caused seizures, hallucinations, and withdrawal symptoms, or may have resulted in addiction. Such patients are usually classified as having "borderline personality" or "character" disorder that appears to go back to the early years of life; or if they are incorrigible, unable to profit by experience, amoral, and in trouble with social agencies, they are called *sociopaths.* This type of personality disorder and social maladjustment usually turns out not to be schizophrenia, and the most dependable means of determining this fact, at the time the patient is first seen, is the strict application of the criteria of Feighner et al for the diagnosis of schizophrenia (above).

3. There is the opposite type of diagnostic problem, arising in *an individual who has been only marginally competent because of personality problems and many vague neurotic symptoms,* and often requiring prolonged psychotherapy. Many such individuals will be found to have the "pseudoneurotic" or simple form of schizophrenia. Errors in diagnosis usually result from a failure to assess mental status carefully, to search for the typical signs of schizophrenia, and to ascertain the life profile of the disorder.

4. *A chronic delusional-hallucinatory state in an alcoholic patient.* Usually the history will disclose that the illness at first took the form of an acute auditory hallucinosis, characterized by threatening, exteriorized auditory hallucinations to which the patient's emotional reaction was appropriate. Mental clarity was another feature. Only later do a few of these patients drift into a quiet hallucinatory, mildly paranoid state, with rather bland affect. The so-called schizoid personality cannot be detected, and there is usually no family history of schizophrenia. Cases of this type that we have studied had their onset between 45 and 50 years of age, i.e., much later than the age of onset of schizophrenia. For these reasons, this alcoholic, schizophrenia-like illness should be considered different from the "core" or "process" type of schizophrenia.

5. *A patient who is confused or stuporous and seemingly negativistic, refusing or unable to speak, execute commands, or be activated in any way.* By inference one is tempted, if signs of focal cerebral or brainstem disease are absent, to diagnose catatonic schizophrenia, not realizing that catatonia as a phenomenon may be indistinguishable from akinetic mutism and may appear also with widespread disease of the associational cortex, and with severe depression, certain confusional states, and hysteria. The error can be avoided if one makes diagnoses on the basis of positive findings, not on the absence of data. The authors have seen cases of hypoxic and other metabolic encephalopathies, Schilder disease, and Creutzfeldt-Jakob disease mistaken for schizophrenia because of failure to adhere to this principle.

6. *A patient with temporal lobe epilepsy* who, apart from intermittent psychomotor seizures, has long periods (weeks or months) of hallucinations, delusions, bizarre behavior, and disorganization of thinking. Such a mental disturbance often reflects the presence of a persistent temporal-lobe seizure state, which in some cases has been demonstrated by depth electrodes to originate in the amygdaloid area. Other types of psychopathology, such as sexual deviations, may also be associated with temporal lobe epilepsy. In the series reported by Jensen and Larsen, 55 out of 74 patients with temporal-lobe epilepsy exhibited mental disturbances. The nature of the disturbances of emotionality and mentation in such patients is discussed in Chaps. 15 and 25.

7. *Schizophrenics with prominent depressive symptoms who have made repeated suicidal attempts* pose an exceptionally difficult problem in diagnosis. Referred to in the past as schizothymic, to this day it is not certain whether they have schizophrenia or manic-depressive disease or both ("schizoaffective"). When in remission, patients with affective disorders are usually normal, whereas schizophrenic and many schizoaffective psychotics are not.

TREATMENT

It is often possible, once the diagnosis of schizophrenia is established, for an internist or neurologist to assume responsibility for treatment. He soon becomes accustomed to the particular pattern of the patient's behavior and can help support the patient and his or her family during difficult periods. Relapse with psychotic decompensation demands drug therapy, and if there is a hazard of injury or suicide, or difficulty in management at home, hospitalization becomes necessary. Most general hospitals now have facilities for the management of such cases, and many of the state hospitals are able to provide short-term treatment. The aim of hospitalization is to protect the patient, relieve the family of the labor of constant vigilance and supervision, and assure the administration of drugs until the exacerbation spends itself. Later, instead of mere custodial care with restraints, locked doors, and little nursing help, the patient needs a flexible program of planned activities, physiotherapy, vocational and milieu therapy, etc., in a "half-way house," which involves the patient as a contributing member of the clinical unit during the more chronic phases of the disease. The patient can then return to the family and community.

Modern treatment consists essentially of antipsychotic medication. The original drugs were *Rauwolfia* alkaloids and the phenothiazines, particularly chlorpromazine. Several modifications of chlorpromazine have become available, including the piperazine derivatives. The latter [e.g., fluphenazine (Prolixin), trifluoperazine (Stelazine), and perphenazine (Trilafon)] are higher in milligram potency than chlorpromazine. There are also newer molecular types such as the thioxanthenes, e.g., chlorprothixine (Taractan); a butyrophenone, *l*-haloperidol (Haldol); an indole, molindone (Moban); and a tricyclic piperazine, *l*-loxapine (Loxitane). Often these drugs are called *tranquilizers,* with the implication that they reduce anxiety. However, the antipsychotic drugs should not be used for this purpose, since they are less effective and more toxic than the benzodiazepines (Librium, Valium). The antipsychotic drugs not only suppress the psychiatric abnormalities but also have other rather specific ("neuroleptic") effects, probably due to their action as dopamine antagonists in the basal ganglia. Parkinsonian rigidity, motor restlessness (akathisia), dystonia, and several other facial-cervical dyskinesias are common side effects, which once started, may persist long after the drug is discontinued (tardive dyskinesia; see page 901). Many of these extrapyramidal disorders can be controlled by the simultaneous parenteral administration of antihistaminic drugs [e.g., diphenhydramine (Benadryl), 25 mg tid] and the anticholinergic drugs used in the treatment of Parkinson disease [e.g., benztropine mesylate (Cogentin), 0.2 mg tid]. However, the latter drugs must be given cautiously, for they may hamper the antipsychotic action and, if given in large doses, may themselves induce a toxic psychosis. If it becomes necessary to treat the extrapyramidal side effects, it is usually possible to eliminate the anticholinergic drugs after 2 to 3 months without return of symptoms. In chronically medicated patients, in whom tardive dyskinesias are frequent, an increased dose of the antipsychotic drug may suppress the dyskinesia, but only temporarily. Whenever possible, drug therapy should not be prolonged; the use of the lowest possible dose and drug holidays a few times a year are advised. During periods of remission no drug therapy is needed. However, some psychiatrists believe that continuous antipsychotic medication is useful in preventing hospitalization.

The dosages of these antipsychotic drugs need to be individualized. The usual daily dose of chlorpromazine is 300 to 500 mg, but up to 1000 mg or more can be given; the dose of other antipsychotic drugs is equivalent. Since most schizophrenic patients have no insight into their illness and the side effects of the medication are unpleasant, the major difficulty is in getting them to take it, in which case a depot form of fluphenazine can be given once every 1 to 3 weeks. Tolerance and addiction to the antipsychotic drugs do not develop. Turnover rates are low, so that a single dose in 24 h suffices (usually given at bedtime to help with the insomnia).

Electroconvulsive therapy (ECT) is now seldom used except in patients who are stuporous or agitated or who have major affective symptoms, or in exceptional instances where there is no response to medication. Insulin therapy has been abandoned, as has leukotomy. Cingulotomy is still being used in occasional patients who have failed to respond to all other types of therapy.

Massive doses of vitamin C or B (megavitamins) are of no proven value.

Supportive psychotherapy (explanation, reassurance, encouragement) is of course necessary, as in any prolonged illness, and the family needs the same type of help. The physician should be understanding and sympathetic, but also firm and professional. The general purpose of psychotherapy is to assist the patient to obtain a grasp on reality and to strengthen self-esteem and psychologic defenses. Psychoanalytic therapy has been tried with few claims of benefit. Most practicing psychiatrists believe it to have little to offer as a primary mode of treatment.

The two major complications of drug treatment are tardive dyskinesia and the neuroleptic malignant syndrome. The former was described in Chap 42; the latter is described below.

Neuroleptic Malignant Syndrome (NMS)

This complication of neuroleptic treatment of schizophrenia or other psychotic states has become one of the dreaded complications of psychiatric medicine. In 1960 Delay and his colleagues called attention to its occurrence in patients being treated with haloperidal, and since then other of the neuroleptic drugs have been incriminated, particularly the highly potent thioxanthene derivative thiothixine, and the phenothiazines—promazine, chlorpromazine, and thioridazine. Common to all, it is believed, is their dopamine blocking capacity. The incidence of NMS is 0.5 to 1.0 percent of all patients receiving neuroleptics, and the seriousness of the syndrome is reflected in the mortality rate of 15 to 30 percent, if not recognized and treated. It may occur days, weeks, or months after neuroleptic treatment is begun. The syndrome consists of high fever, generalized muscular rigidity, stupor and coma, high CK values (up to 60,000 units) and, in the fatal cases, renal failure presumably due to myoglobinuria. The syndrome bears close resemblance to malignant hyperthermia not only in its clinical aspects but also in its response to dantrolene. If treatment is started early, when consciousness is first altered and the temperature is rising, bromocriptine in oral doses of 5 mg tid (up to 20 mg tid) will terminate the condition in a few hours. Once oral medication can no longer be taken, dantrolene, 0.25 to 3.0 mg/kg intravenously, may be life-saving. Once coma has supervened, circulatory collapse and anuria may prove fatal or leave the patient in a vegative state. The rigor with high fever is the source of muscle damage and myoglobinuria; circulatory collapse may result in hypoxic—ischemic injury. As with malignant hyperthermia, a genetic factor is suspected, provoked possibly by fatigue and dehydration. Meningitis; heat stroke, one of the causes of idiopathic myoglobinuria; lithium intoxication; and acute dystonic reactions figure in the differential diagnosis (Mueller).

PARANOIA AND PARANOID STATES

The term *paranoid* designates patients who show

> . . . *fixed suspicions, persecutory delusions, dominant ideas or grandiose trends logically elaborated and with due regard for reality once the false interpretation or premise has been accepted. Further characteristics are formally correct conduct, adequate emotional reactions, and coherence of the train of thought. (Rosanoff)*

In other words, in pure paranoia there is supposed to be no mental defect other than the delusional system—no dementia, hallucinations, or emotional disturbance. Time was when a large group of the mentally ill were classified as paranoid. But with advancing knowledge of mental illness, fewer and fewer have been left in this category.

The trouble that psychiatrists have taken to couch this definition in negatives implies that paranoia is frequently a feature of other forms of mental illness, notably schizophrenia, manic-depressive, toxic, or alcoholic psychosis, general paresis, etc. This fact about paranoia was known from the beginning, when Heinroth originally described it in 1818 and classified it as a limited disorder of the intellect. Krafft-Ebing, in his monograph on the subject, took pains to distinguish two syndromes: (1) "original paranoia," developing about the time of puberty and attributable to heredity (surely schizophrenia by present-day criteria), and (2) acquired paranoia, developing in late life, particularly in the involutional period (the condition under discussion). Kraepelin remarked that approximately 40 percent of his cases of paranoia developed this symptom early in life and went on to have schizophrenia. The others were true paranoia or a closely related condition which he called *paraphrenia*, a term no longer used.

Figures on the frequency of true paranoia are probably not reliable because they are of necessity based on hospital records. Doubtless there are many individuals with mild forms of the disorder who have never crossed the threshold of a mental hospital. They are relatively harmless, and in their communities are judged to be mildly "cracked," or monomaniacs. Male preponderance is agreed upon (male/female = 2:1), thus differing from schizophrenia, in which males and females are equally affected.

CLINICAL MANIFESTATIONS

It would be inappropriate in a neurology text to give a detailed account of all the many ways in which paranoiacs behave. A simple paradigm will suffice—that of a middle-aged man of uneasy, brooding, asocial, eccentric nature who gradually develops a dominating idea or belief of his own importance, of having in his possession special powers that make him the envy of others who become bent on persecuting him. As the delusion grows he becomes more preoccupied, less efficient, and increasingly suspicious of others, with a tendency to interpret every one of their words, gestures, or actions as having some reference to himself. Only when his behavior becomes noticeably bizarre or when he does something to annoy others does his condition come to medical attention. On examining such a person one is impressed with his capacity for careful reasoning, which betrays good intelligence. Whatever the false belief—delusions of reference, jealousy, and persecution being the most common—the patient's arguments are logical and buttressed cogently by evidence. Also, the views of such patients about other matters are sensible.

As was said, the illness usually does not lead to hospitalization, and if admitted to hospital the patient does not stay long. The querulous paranoiacs are the most annoying. They usually remain in the community, flooding the mails with mimeographed documents accusing people falsely, expressing their worthless opinions about anything and everything.

As the years pass, the patient changes little, though a few such patients may later break down and begin to hallucinate and finally end in a deteriorated state much like schizophrenia. This trend supports Bleuler's opinion, that the illness is often a variant of schizophrenia.

As to causation, there are several interesting ideas. The Freudian school has laid particular emphasis on repressed homosexuality as a major factor. Meyer invoked the long-standing personality disorder, the paranoid constitution. This refers to persons who always have a tendency to biased views, to wonder what others think of them, and to attribute deliberate intentions to indifferent actions. Their behavior seems but an exaggeration of a mild suspiciousness that is part of the personality makeup of most individuals. Finally a break occurs, perhaps preceded by excessive and exhausting work, an emotional upset, an accident or a depressive reaction, after which these individuals can no longer adapt their ideas to the actual facts of their daily lives. All insight is lost. Cameron has presented a detailed discussion of the psychologic mechanisms of paranoia.

The authors' experience with paranoid states in a general hospital has been rather limited. One sees deluded patients, to be sure, but usually their abnormal ideas have referred to health and bodily functions, infidelity of a spouse, theft of possessions, and the like. The abnormal ideas tend to be unsystematized and are usually part of a confusional psychosis, delirium, or dementia. Rarely, a patient comes to the hospital in some other medical context, and it is found that he or she has been living quietly in the community, preoccupied with a bizarre delusional system and appearing neither depressed nor schizophrenic. Of course, paranoid schizophrenics or alcoholics with chronic auditory hallucinosis may also develop some medical problem that brings them to a general hospital. Certainly the neurologist sees delusions most often in depressed patients who decompensate as their depression develops. Among the inmates of a psychiatric hospital for the chronically ill, true paranoia is rare (0.1 percent of admissions, according to Winokur).

MANAGEMENT

The methods and objectives of psychotherapy are discussed fully by Cameron (see References). We have no way of deciding whether psychotherapy has influenced this state. In a general hospital, where nearly all our patients have been depressed or maniacal, we have several times been gratified by the effects of antidepressive medication. In the treatment of patients with pathologic jealousy, Mooney has found phenothiazine drugs to be useful.

From what has been said, the clinical analysis of patients with delusions requires a careful study of mood and intelligence to rule out manic-depressive psychosis and dementia. If either of these two states exists, the treatment proceeds along the lines discussed in Chaps. 56 and 20. A matter of practical importance is for the physician to evaluate carefully the nature of the delusional ideas and try to judge whether the patient is homicidal or suicidal. Occasionally, physicians and others have been killed or maimed by paranoiacs who thought they were being mistreated.

PUERPERAL (POSTPARTUM) PSYCHOSES

The parturitional event, including as it does many biologic factors such as the effects of pain, drugs, eclampsia, hemorrhage, infection, and an abrupt hormonal adjustment, is frequently associated with a disturbance of mood. Obstetricians have repeatedly observed that the woman may feel extraordinarily well immediately postpartum, only to lapse in the next days into a weepy, depressed state in which she is distressed by lack of feeling for her newborn infant. Usually this lasts for only a few days, being quelled by the return home, responsibility for the infant, nursing, etc.

The period after childbirth is one in which there is a strong disposition to psychosis. Opinion varies as to whether there is a special *puerperal psychosis*. Most psychiatrists believe that the psychotic break which may occur at this time is either a confusional-delirious state or a schizophreniform or depressive psychosis, and that these illnesses do not differ from those occurring at other times in life.

As neurologic consultants to the Boston Lying-in Hospital, the authors were impressed with an unusual type of psychosis that they saw on an average of two or three times each year. Usually this psychosis has its onset between 48 and 72 h after a delivery that may have been complicated by excessive bleeding or infection. The patient alternates between periods of noisy hyperactivity and of mutism and inactivity. She is disoriented and incapable of thinking clearly. The baby is rejected as not belonging to her (instances of infanticide are not unknown). Although the illness has some features of delirium, it may merge with a schizophrenic or depressive psychosis that persists for months. We agree with Boyd, who found in a series of cases that about 40 percent were affective, 20 percent schizofreniform, and the remainder, symptomatic psychoses.

Also, in some patients, a depression has followed each of several pregnancies, disabling the patient for months. Some women with manic-depressive disease have had their early depressive attacks only after delivery. In the instances in which we witnessed an acute postpartum schizophrenic episode in patients without family history or prepsychotic schizoid personality, the prognosis for full and lasting recovery seemed better than one usually expects in schizophrenia, i.e., good prognosis schizophrenia. These are only impressions, however.

In the diagnosis of postpartum psychosis, one must also keep in mind the possibility of eclampsia, and the consequences of pituitary infarction (the latter due to circulatory collapse), and hypotensive-hypoxic cerebral injury.

THE ENDOCRINE PSYCHOSES

One of the most provocative observations in contemporary psychiatry is that apparently normal individuals may become psychotic when they develop hyper- or hypothyroidism, the Cushing syndrome, or adrenal insufficiency, or when they receive therapeutic doses of ACTH or cortisone. If these conditions were no more than examples of drug-induced psychosis, they would be interesting enough. The fact is, however, that they differ considerably from the usual toxic deliria or confusional states. The syndrome, reminiscent of puerperal psychosis and some cases of "combat fatigue" seen during World War II, comprises features that are suggestive of manic-depressive psychosis or schizophrenia on the one hand and of the confusional psychoses on the other. These endocrine psychoses have far-reaching medical significance, for they provide experimental models of psychoses that can be created by the manipulation of metabolic factors and by exogenous means.

ACTH AND CORTISONE PSYCHOSIS

These syndromes are now occurring far less frequently than when ACTH and cortisone were first introduced into medicine. Presumably these hormones are now more purified, and there are more reliable data as to safe dosage. The psychosis usually develops over a period of a few days after the patient has received the hormone for one or more weeks. The features are extremely variable. Depression and insomnia are the most frequent symptoms, but some patients become elated, agitated, excited, and talkative, as though under pressure to speak, while others are mute; or the prevailing emotional response may be one of anxiety and panic. Thinking may be confused, illogical, tangential, and incoherent. Hallucinations and sensory misinterpretations may appear. Clouding of the sensorium, disorientation, and confusion, the hallmarks of deliria and the confusional psychoses, have not been prominent in the ACTH and cortisone psychoses. However, the state of awareness is not altogether normal, and at times the patient is frankly bewildered. In the motor sphere there may be incessant activity or immobility, resistiveness, and even negativism verging on catatonia. If the hormone is stopped as soon as the diagnosis is established, the psychosis subsides gradually over several days to weeks, with complete recovery.

In patients with Cushing disease, mental changes are frequent. There is a combination of affective disorder and impairment of cognitive function, easily elicited during mental status testing. The lateral and third ventricles are enlarged. There are glucosteroid receptors in the limbic system, but how they figure in the pathophysiology and morphology of the mental changes is not known.

The mechanism of the acute steroid psychosis is also obscure. From the few available studies it has been learned that the occurrence of the psychosis is not related to the premorbid personality. Although the dosage of ACTH or cortisone has usually been high, there has been no exact correlation between dose level and the occurrence, severity, and duration of the psychosis. Nor does the mental disturbance appear to be related to the rapidity and intensity of the therapeutic response to ACTH and cortisone. Lithium is often effective in controlling the symptoms, allowing continuation of the corticosteroid therapy. The dose is the same as for manic states (page 1214; see also Falk et al).

THYROID PSYCHOSIS

A great deal has been said and written about the pervasive effects of abnormal thyroid function on all organs, including the neuromuscular apparatus and central nervous system. These effects are discussed in Chap. 40, under metabolic diseases of the nervous system (page 866).

The hyperthyroid patient often shows minor changes in emotions and mentation. Restlessness, irritability, apprehension, emotional lability, and at times even agitation and a generalized chorea may occur. Either of two trends may be observed in the relatively rare psychotic thyroid patient. There may be mania with its characteristic increase in psychomotor activity, overtalkativeness, and flight of ideas, or there may be depression with its somber mood, weeping, and anxiety. Visual and auditory hallucinations are present in both groups of cases. The clinical picture is seldom clear. Usually the psychiatrist finds something more than simple mania or agitated depression, i.e., some clouding of the sensorium with perplexity and confusion suggestive of delirium. The condition is said to be related to the premorbid personality, some personality types being more vulnerable, but this point is disputed. The condition is not directly related to the severity of the thyrotoxicosis. Careful studies of cerebral blood flow and metabolism during and after the psychosis have not been done. Treatment of the hyperthyroidism does not result in prompt arrest of the psychic disorder, but usually recovery takes place over a period of months. One must distinguish this illness from other types of recurrent psychosis which happen to be coincidental with or precipitated by hyperthyroidism.

With *myxedema* there is a characteristic slowness and thickness of speech, drowsiness, hypothermia, mental dullness, listlessness and apathy, irritability, and sometimes suspiciousness. The patient may sleep most of the time, having to be awakened for meals. A disturbance of memory, and the lack of genuine symptoms of depression, such as feelings of hopelessness and loss of self-esteem, help to distinguish the mental disorder of myxedema from manic-depressive disease. Nevertheless, unless one thinks of myxedema in all cases of psychomotor retardation, the diagnosis will be missed. Reduced cerebral blood flow and metabolism have been found in myxedema, and with specific therapy these functions are restored to normal.

OTHER ENDOCRINE PSYCHOSES

Mental aberrations much like those in ACTH and cortisone psychoses have been observed in the *Cushing syndrome.* Mental changes in *Addison disease* are frequent but varied. Irritability, confusion, disorientation, and convulsions, with or without hypoglycemia, are the main features. Some of the mental abnormalities may be related to the disturbances of electrolyte balance, but the mechanisms are not well understood.

REFERENCES

AMERICAN FOUNDATION: *Medical Research: A Mid-century Survey.* Boston, Little, Brown, 1956.

BLEULLER E: *Dementia Praecox or the Group of Schizophrenias,* Zinkin J (trans). New York, International Universities Press, 1950.

BÖÖK JA, WETTERBERG L, MODRZEWSKA K: Schizophrenia in a north Swedish geographical isolate 1900–1977. Epidemiology, genetics and biochemistry. *Clin Genet* 14:373, 1978.

BOYD DA: Mental disturbances with childbearing. *Am J Obstet Gynecol* 43:148, 1942.

CAMERON NA: Paranoid conditions and paranoia, in Arieti S, Brody EB (eds): *American Handbook of Psychiatry,* 2nd ed., vol 3. New York, Basic Books, 1974, chap 29, pp 676–693.

CUTTING J: Memory in functional psychoses. *J Neurol Neurosurg Psychiatry* 42:1031, 1979.

DAVISON K, BAGLEY CR: Schizophrenia-like psychoses associated with organic disorders of the nervous system. Review of literature, in *Br J Psychiat. Spec Publ No 4, Current Problems in Neuropsychiatry,* Herrington RN (ed), 1969 pp 113–184.

DELAY J, PICHOT P, LEMPERIERE T: Un neuroleptique majeur nonphenothiazine nonreserpinique. *Ann Med Psychol* 118:145, 1960.

DUNLAP CB: The pathology of the brain in schizophrenia. *Res Publ Assoc Nerv Ment Dis* 5:371, 1928.

FALK WE, MANKE MW, POSKANZER DC: Lithium prophylaxis of corticotropin-induced psychosis. *JAMA* 241:1011, 1979.

FEIGHNER JP, ROBINS E, GUZE SB et al: Diagnostic criteria for use in psychiatric research. *Arch Gen Psychiatry* 26:57, 1972.

FISCHER M: Psychoses in the offspring of schizophrenic twins and their normal co-twins. *Br J Psychiatry* 118:43, 1971.

FLOR-HENRY P: Lateralized temporo-limbic dysfunction and psychopathology. *Ann NY Acad Sci* 280:777, 1976.

GOODWIN DW, GUZE SB: *Psychiatric Diagnosis,* 3rd ed. New York, Oxford University Press, 1984.

HARLOW H: *Learning to Love.* New York, Jason Aronson, 1974.

HEATH RB: Psychosis and epilepsy. Similarities and differences in the anatomico-physiologic substrate, in Koella WP, Trumble MR (eds): *Advances in Biologic Psychiatry,* vol 8. New York, Karger, 1982, pp 166–216.

HERTZIG MA, BIRCH HC: Neurological organization in psychiatrically disturbed patients. *Arch Gen Psychiatry* 19:528, 1968.

HESTON L: Psychiatric disorders in foster home-reared children of schizophrenic mothers. *Br J Psychiatry* 112:819, 1966.

HOLMAN PS, PROCTOR PS, LEVY LR: Eye-tracking dysfunction in schizophrenic patients and their relatives. *Arch Gen Psychiatry* 31:143, 1974.

JENSEN I, LARSEN JK: Mental aspects of temporal lobe epilepsy. *J Neurol Neurosurg Psychiatry* 42:256, 1979.

JOHNSTONE EC, CROW TJ, FRITT CD et al: The dementia of dementia praecox. *Acta Psychiatr Scand* 57:305, 1978.

KALLMANN FJ: The genetic theory of schizophrenia: An analysis of 691 twin index families. *Am J Psychiatry* 103:309, 1946.

KARLSSON JL: *The Biologic Basis of Schizophrenia.* Springfield, IL, Charles C Thomas, 1966.

KARNOSH LJ, HOPE JM: Puerperal psychosis and their sequelae. *Am J Psychiatry* 94:537, 1937.

KENNARD M: Value of equivocal signs in neurological diagnosis. *Neurology* 10:753, 1960.

KETY SS: Genetic and biochemical aspects of schizophrenia, in Nicholi AM Jr (ed): *The Harvard Guide to Modern Psychiatry.* Cambridge, MA, Harvard, 1978, chap 6, pp 93–102.

KETY SS: The syndrome of schizophrenia: Unresolved questions and opportunities for research. *Br J Psychiatry* 136:421, 1980.

KRAEPELIN E: *Dementia Praecox and Paraphrenia,* Barclay RM (trans), Robertson GM (ed). Edinburgh, E & S Livingstone, 1919.

LANGFELDT G: The prognosis in schizophrenia and the factors influencing the course of the disease. *Acta Psychiatr Neurol Scand Suppl* 13, 1937.

LANGFELDT G: The prognosis in schizophrenia. *Acta Psychiatr Neurol Scand Suppl* 110, 1956.

LEHMANN HE: Schizophrenia: Clinical features, in Kaplan HI, Sadock BD (eds): *Comprehensive Textbook of Psychiatry,* 4th ed. Baltimore, Williams & Wilkins, 1985, chap 15.4, pp 680–713.

MATTHYSSE S: Etiologic diversity in the psychoses, in Chung CS, Morton NE (eds): *Genetic Epidemiology.* New York, Academic Press, 1978, pp 311–322.

MATTHYSSE S, POPE A: The approach to schizophrenia through molecular pathology, in Good RA, Day SD, Yunis JJ, (eds): *Molecular Pathology* Springfield, IL, Charles C Thomas, 1975, pp 744–768.

MOONEY H: Pathologic jealousy and psychochemotherapy. *Br J Psychiatry* 111:1023, 1975.

MORRISON J, WINOKUR G, CROWE R, CLANCY J: The Iowa 500: The first follow-up. *Arch Gen Psychiatry* 29:677, 1973.

MORTON LA, KIDD KK, MATTHYSSE SW, RICHARDS RL: Recurrence risks in schizophrenia: Are they model dependent? *Behav Genet* 9:389, 1979.

MUELLER PS: Neuroleptic malignant syndrome. *Psychosomatics* 26:654, 1985.

MURRAY RM, LEWIS SW, REVELEY AM: Towards an etiologic classification of schizophrenia. *Lancet* 1:1023, 1985.

POPE H, LIPINSKI J: Differential diagnosis of schizophrenic and manic-depressive illness. *Arch Gen Psychiatry* 35:811, 1978.

RICHTER D: The impact of biochemistry on the problem of schizophrenia, in Kemali D, Bartholini G, Richter D (eds): *Schizophrenia Today.* Oxford, England, Pergamon Press, 1976, pp 71–86.

RIEDER RO, DONNELLY EF, HERDT JR, WALDMANN IN: Sulcal prominence in young chronic schizophrenic patients: CT scan findings associated with impairment on neuropsychological tests. *Psychiatry Res.* 1:1, 1979.

ROBINS E, GUZE SB: Establishment of diagnostic validity in psychiatric illness: Its application to schizophrenia. *Am J Psychiatry* 126:983, 1970.

ROSANOFF AJ: *Manual of Psychiatry.* New York, Wiley, 1920.

ROSENTHAL D, KETY SS (eds): *The Transmission of Schizophrenia.* New York, Pergamon, 1968.

ROSENTHAL D, WENDER PH, KETY SS et al: Parent-child relationships and psychopathologic disorder in the child. *Arch Gen Psychiatry* 32:466, 1975.

ROSENTHAL D, WENDER PH, KETY SS et al: The adopted-away offspring of schizophrenics. *Am J Psychiatry* 128:307, 1971.

SCHNEIDER K: *Clinical Psychopathology,* Hamilton MW (trans). New York, Grune & Stratton, 1959.

SEIDMAN LJ: Schizophrenia and brain dysfunction. An integration of recent neuro diagnostic findings. *Psychol Bull* 94:195, 1983.

SHELDON WM, STEVENS SS, TUCKER WB: *The Varieties of Human Physique: An Introduction to Constitutional Psychology.* New York, Hafner, 1963.

SPAHN HE, PATTERSON T: Recent studies in psychophysiology of schizophrenia. *Schizophr Bull* 5:481, 1979.

STEVENS JR: An anatomy of schizophrenia? *Arch Gen Psychiatry* 29:177, 1973.

TAYLOR MA: Schneiderian first-rank symptoms and clinical prognostic features in schizophrenia. *Arch Gen Psychiatry* 26:64, 1972.

TUCKER CJ, CAMPION EW, SILBERFARB PM: Sensorimotor functions and cognitive disturbance in psychiatric patients. *Am J Psychiatry* 132:17, 1975.

WEINBERGER DR, BERMAN KF, ZEC RF: Physiologic dysfunction of the dorsolateral prefrontal cortex in schizophrenia. Regional cerebral blood flow evidence. *Arch Gen Psychiatry* 43:114, 1986.

WEINBERGER DR, TORRY EF, NEOPHYTIDES AN, WYATT RJ: Lateral cerebral ventricular enlargement in chronic schizophrenia. *Arch Gen Psychiatry* 36:735, 1979.

WINOKUR G: Delusional disorder (paranoia). *Compr Psychiatry* 18:511, 1977.

WINOKUR G, TSUANG M: The Iowa 500: Suicide in mania, depression and schizophrenia. *Am J Psychiatry* 132:650, 1975.

INDEX

Page references in *italic* indicate tables and illustrations.